The following list gives the common definition of sele[...]cal and nursing terms. An example follows each def[...]

Term	Definition	Term	Definition
laryng(o)-	larynx. *laryng*itis	**-pnea**	breathing. dys*pnea*
lip(o)-	fat. *lip*oma	**pneumo(no)-**	lung. *pneumo*bacillin
lymph(o)-	lymph. *lymph*ocyte	**pod(o)-**	foot. *pod*iatry
mamm(o)-	breast. *mamm*ography	**proct(o)-**	rectum. *proct*itis
mast(o)-	breast. *mast*itis	**pulmo(n)-**	lung. *pulmon*ary
metro-, metra-	uterus. *metro*dynia	**pur-, pyo-**	pus. sup*pur*ation, *pyo*cyte
my(o)-	muscle. *myo*cardium	**pyel(o)-**	pelvis. *pyelo*cystitis
myc(o)-	fungus. *myc*osis	**ren-**	kidney. *ren*iform
myel(o)-	marrow. *myelo*cyte	**rheo-**	flow. *rheo*taxis
myxo-	mucus. *myxo*ma	**rhin(o)-**	nose. *rhin*itis
nephr(o)-	kidney. *nephr*ectomy	**salping(o)-**	fallopian tube. *salpingo*stomy
neur(o)-	nerves. *neuro*blastoma	**sangui-**	blood. *sangui*nolent
nod-	knot. *nod*ule	**sarc(o)-**	flesh. *sarc*oma
nucle(o)-	nucleus. *nucle*otide	**seps-**	decay. *seps*is
oculo-	eye. *oculo*motor	**sial(o)-**	saliva. *sialo*lith
omphal(o)-	navel. *omphalo*cele	**soma(to)-**	body. *somato*genesis
onych(o)-	nail. *onych*olysis	**-spasm**	convulsion. vaso*spasm*
oo-	egg. *oo*blast	**splen(o)-**	spleen. *spleno*megaly
ophthalm(o)-	eye. *ophthalm*ology	**stom(ato)-**	mouth. *stom*atitis
orchi(o)-	testes. *orchio*pathy	**test-**	testicle. *test*osterone
oss-, ost(eo)-	bone. *oss*icle, *osteo*anesthesia	**thel-**	nipple. *thel*itis
ot(o)-	ear. *oto*sclerosis	**-thoracic**	chest. intra*thoracic*
ovo-, ovi-	egg, ova. *ovo*flavin	**thrombo-**	clot. *thrombo*cytopenia
pharyng(o)-	pharynx. *pharyng*itis	**tracheo-**	trachea. *tracheo*tomy
phleb(o)-	vein. *phleb*otomy	**tricho-**	hair. *trich*oid
phren-	diaphragm. *phren*odynia	**vaso-**	vessel. *vaso*dilatation
-plegia	paralysis. para*plegia*	**vesico-**	bladder. *vesico*urethral
pleur(o)-	pleura, rib, side. *pleuro*dynia	**zyg(o)-**	yoke, union. *zyg*ote

THE NURSE'S REFERENCE LIBRARY®

Definitions

Nursing83 Books™
Intermed Communications, Inc.
Springhouse, Pa.

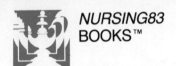

NURSING83 BOOKS™

Intermed Communications Book Division

CHAIRMAN
Eugene W. Jackson

PRESIDENT
Daniel L. Cheney

VICE-PRESIDENT
Timothy B. King

VICE-PRESIDENT, PRODUCTION AND PURCHASING
Bacil Guiley

RESEARCH DIRECTOR
Elizabeth O'Brien

The clinical procedures described and recommended in this publication are based on research and consultation with medical and nursing authorities. To the best of our knowledge, these procedures reflect currently accepted clinical practice; nevertheless, they can't be considered absolute and universal recommendations. For individual application, treatment recommendations must be considered in light of the patient's clinical condition and, before administration of new or infrequently used drugs, in light of latest package-insert information. The publisher disclaims responsibility for any adverse effects resulting directly or indirectly from the suggested procedures, from any undetected errors, or from the reader's misunderstanding of the text.

Library of Congress Cataloging in Publication Data
Main entry under title:

Definitions.

    (The Nurse's reference library)
    "Adapted from Mosby's medical and nursing
dictionary, © 1983"—T.p. verso.
    "Nursing83 books."
    1. Medicine—Dictionaries.   2. Nursing—
Dictionaries.
I. Mosby's medical & nursing dictionary. II. Series.
P121.D39   1983   610'.3'21   83-131
ISBN 0-916730-55-7

NURSE'S REFERENCE LIBRARY® SERIES

Staff for this volume

EDITORIAL DIRECTOR
Helen Klusek Hamilton

CLINICAL DIRECTOR
Minnie Bowen Rose, RN, BSN, MEd

ART DIRECTOR
Sonja Douglas

Editorial Manager: Matthew Cahill
Senior Clinical Editor: Regina Daley Ford, RN, BSN, MA
Clinical Editors: Joanne Patzek DaCunha, RN; Angela D. Lehman, RN; Judith A. Schilling McCann, RN, BSN; Carole Arlene Pyle, RN, BSN, MA, CCRN
Contributing Clinical Editors: Kathleen E. Viall Gallagher, RN, MSN; Mary Chapman Gyetvan, RN, BSEd; Paula Stephens Okun, RN, MSN; Karen Dyer Vance, RN, BSN
Drug Information Editor: Larry N. Gever, RPh, PharmD
Senior Editors: Matthew T. Corso, Peter Johnson
Associate Editors: June F. Gomez, H. Nancy Holmes, William James Kelly, June T. Norris, Patricia Minard Shinehouse
Graphics Coordinator: Lisa Z. Cohen
Assistant Editor: Holly Ann Burdick
Copy Chief: Jill Lasker
Copy Editors: Barbara Hodgson, Jo Lennon, David R. Moreau, Sharyl D. Wolf
Contributing Copy Editors: Andrea F. Barrett; Diane A. Dufresne; Linda A. Johnson; Robert L. Myers, IV; Sandra J. Purrenhage; Evelyn Richardson; Barbara F. Ritter
Production Coordinators: Sally Johnson, Rebecca S. Van Dine
Senior Associate Designer: Kathaleen Motak Singel
Associate Designers: Carol Cameron-Sears, Linda Jovinelly Franklin
Assistant Designers: Jacalyn M. Bove, Christopher Laird
Contributing Designer: Robert Walsh
Illustrators: Len Epstein, Jean Gardner, Robert Jackson, Bob Jones, Dimitri Karentnikov, George Retseck, Dennis Schofield, Joan Walsh
Art Production Manager: Robert Perry
Art Assistants: Diane Fox, Scheryl Franceschini, Don Knauss, Sandra Sanders, Craig T. Simon, Louise Stamper, Ron Yablon
Typography Manager: David C. Kosten
Typography Assistants: Janice Haber, Ethel Halle, Diane Paluba, Nancy Wirs
Production Manager: Wilbur D. Davidson
Quality Control Manager: Robert L. Dean
Editorial Assistants: Maree E. DeRosa, Bernadette M. Glenn, Debra Lee Judy
Researcher: Vonda Heller

Special thanks to Susan M. Glover, RN, BSN, Patricia E. McCulla, Alan M. Rubin, and Anne Moraca-Sawicki, RN, MSN, no longer on the staff, and to Richard Samuel West, who assisted in the preparation of this volume.

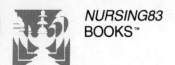

NURSING83
BOOKS™

NURSE'S REFERENCE LIBRARY® SERIES

This volume is part of a series conceived by the publishers of *Nursing83®* magazine and written by hundreds of nursing and medical specialists. This series, the NURSE'S REFERENCE LIBRARY, is the most comprehensive reference set ever created exclusively for the nursing profession. Each volume brings together the most up-to-date clinical information and related nursing practice. Each volume informs, explains, alerts, guides, educates. Taken together, the NURSE'S REFERENCE LIBRARY provides today's nurse with the knowledge and the skills that she needs to be effective in her daily practice and to advance in her career.

Other volumes in the series:

Diseases
Diagnostics
Drugs
Assessment
Procedures

Other publications:

NURSING SKILLBOOK® SERIES

Dealing with Death and Dying
Reading EKGs Correctly
Managing Diabetics Properly
Assessing Vital Functions Accurately
Helping Cancer Patients Effectively
Giving Cardiovascular Drugs Safely

Giving Emergency Care Competently
Monitoring Fluid and Electrolytes Precisely
Documenting Patient Care Responsibly
Combatting Cardiovascular Diseases Skillfully
Coping with Neurologic Problems Proficiently
Nursing Critically Ill Patients Confidently
Using Crisis Intervention Wisely

NURSING PHOTOBOOK™ SERIES

Providing Respiratory Care
Managing I.V. Therapy
Dealing with Emergencies
Giving Medications
Assessing Your Patients
Using Monitors
Providing Early Mobility
Giving Cardiac Care
Performing GI Procedures
Implementing Urologic Procedures

Controlling Infection
Ensuring Intensive Care
Coping with Neurologic Disorders
Caring for Surgical Patients
Working with Orthopedic Patients
Nursing Pediatric Patients
Helping Geriatric Patients
Attending Ob/Gyn Patients
Aiding Ambulatory Patients
Carrying Out Special Procedures

Nursing83 DRUG HANDBOOK™

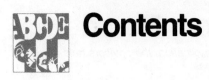 # Contents

Advisory Board

At the time of publication, the advisors held the following positions:

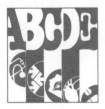

Foreword

Nursing has changed.

Oh, our goal as nurses is still the same. We continue striving to provide our patients with the best nursing care humanly possible. But our path to that goal has become more difficult. Now, more than ever, *humanly* possible also means *technically* and *ethically* possible. Nursing has been made more complicated and more challenging by steady advances in medical knowledge and technology.

Changing Form and Function

Our work has changed in content; it's changed in scope. Recent advances have increased the body of knowledge for which we nurses are responsible, and they've spawned new nursing specialties. New, highly sophisticated equipment has relieved us of many routine aspects of patient care while adding other responsibilities. For example, we've assumed new duties and taken on greater responsibility in such areas as patient assessment, patient teaching, diagnostic testing, and interpretation of increasingly complicated test results. We've moved more and more into positions of administration and management that demand supervisory, planning, and budgeting capabilities as well as advanced nursing skills. And along with this expanding role has come increasing liability for the professional decisions we make and actions we take. To look at just one example, we're now legally liable for recognizing appropriate doses and scheduling of drugs and for identifying any inaccurate orders.

In short, as nurses, we're now expected to know more, to do more, and to accept more legal responsibility for our actions.

Meeting Expectations

To meet these rising expectations, we need ready sources of reliable information—among them, surely, a dictionary that's oriented to the demands of contemporary nursing. DEFINITIONS, the latest volume in the Nurse's Reference Library series, is just such a reference. Prepared and reviewed by professional nurses and other health-care specialists, it contains the latest information and terminology relevant to all phases of modern nursing and to all nurses—student, graduate, the returning nurse, and the seasoned practitioner.

Clearly and precisely worded, the entries in this volume are comprehensive without sacrificing nursing basics. Words are defined in detailed encyclopedic style wherever appropriate. The wide-ranging subject matter emphasizes the newest aspects of nursing practice: contemporary nursing terms and techniques *(nursing process*, including *assessment, planning, implementation*, and *evaluation); new nursing roles (enterostomal therapist, nurse practitioner);* advanced procedures *(cardiac output, phrenic pacemaker, plasmapheresis);* and

Foreword
(continued)

new equipment and the underlying principles that make it work *(fiber-optic duodenoscope, intra-aortic balloon pump, scintillascope)*. DEFINITIONS also includes useful terms from many other disciplines and professions. So, in addition to all the information you'd expect to find about anatomy and physiology, biochemistry, clinical medicine, dentistry, and surgery, you'll also find up-to-date explanations of important terms from . . .

• *administration and management (nursing audit, line position, management by objectives, request for proposal, staff position, union shop).*

• *computer technology,* increasingly important as more and more institutions computerize patient records, interdepartmental medication orders, and supply requests *(byte, echo, edit, menu, software).*

• *law* as related to nursing practice *(deposition, nurse practice act, tort).*

• *pharmacology,* embracing not only generic drug names and classes, but also enzymes, hormones, and vitamins *(propranolol hydrochloride, phenothiazine, chymotrypsin, insulin, ascorbic acid).*

• *psychology and psychiatry,* reflecting the latest theories in mental health and rehabilitation *(behavior therapy, group therapy, interpersonal therapy).*

DEFINITIONS is an appropriate and clinically valuable companion to the previous volumes in the Nurse's Reference Library series. Like the other volumes in this series, it addresses the nurse's special professional needs.

Why a new dictionary? Because the language of nursing has changed. Because *nursing* has changed.

FRANCES J. STORLIE, RN, PhD
Adult Nurse Practitioner
Vancouver, Washington

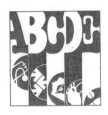

How to Use This Book

In this book, you'll discover tens of thousands of definitions that provide accurate, current, and comprehensive information on nursing practices and concerns. For example, you'll find up-to-date definitions of generic drugs, important drug interactions, in-depth nursing considerations, recommended treatments, and much more. You'll also find more than 700 illustrations and charts that support, clarify, and expand key definitions. And to locate any definition quickly, you'll find a guide word at the upper corner of each page. The guide word on a left-hand page indicates the *first entry* on that page; the guide word on a right-hand page indicates the *last entry* on that page.

Arrangement of Entry Terms
Entry terms—which include single and compound terms, combining forms, standard abbreviations, and acronyms—appear in boldface type for easy reference. These terms appear in *letter-by-letter* alphabetical order, disregarding hyphens and word spaces. For example:

    cricothyrotomy
    cri du chat syndrome
    Crigler-Najjar syndrome

A *compound term*—a noun and one or more modifiers—is alphabetized by its first modifier. So, the definition of I.V.-type traction frame appears under **I.V.-type traction frame**, *not* under **traction frame** or **frame.**

Abbreviations and acronyms appear as entry terms and follow the adopted alphabetical arrangement. Each abbreviation and acronym precedes its spelled-out form and, at times, the cross-reference in which it's defined. For example:

DAT *abbr* Dental Aptitude Test. See **dentist.**

Combining forms (prefixes, suffixes) follow the adopted alphabetical arrangement. The definition of a combining form usually includes examples of usage. For instance:

kinesio- A combining form meaning 'of or pertaining to movement': *kinesiology, kinesioneurosis.*

Entry terms containing *Arabic or Roman numerals* follow terms that are identical except for the numeral. For example, **Beck I operation** precedes **Beck II operation.** Entry terms containing numerals precede those which are identical except for a letter in place of a numeral. For example, T_3 and T_4 precede **Ta.**

Generic drugs derived from the same base and having the same pharmacologic action appear in one entry, which is alphabetized by the generic base. So, to find the definition of **hydrocortisone sodium succinate,** look under **hydrocortisone.** There, you'll find the following entry terms:

hydrocortisone, h. acetate, h. sodium phosphate, h. sodium succinate, h. valerate.

How to Use
This Book
(continued)

Features of Entry Terms
- *Multiple definitions.* When an entry term has more than one meaning, the definitions are numbered according to frequency of use.
- *Plurals.* When the plural of an entry term is irregular, it appears in boldface type after the entry term. Usually, the most common form of a plural appears first. For example:
  carcinoma, *pl.* **carcinomas, carcinomata.**
If the plural form is used more frequently than the singular form, it appears first. For example:
  bacteria, *sing.* **bacterium.**
- *Parts of speech.* When appropriate, alternate parts of speech are listed for the entry term. For instance, if the entry term is an adjective, its verb and noun forms appear in boldface type after the definition. For example:
  agitated . . . —**agitate,** *v.,* **agitation,** *n.*
The abbreviation *adj.* denotes an adjective; *adv.,* an adverb; *n.,* a noun; and *v.,* a verb.

Cross-References
More than 13,000 cross-references, indicated by boldface type, provide rapid access to relevant information. DEFINITIONS uses two basic types of cross-references. The first type directs you to the location of the term's definition. For instance, if you look up **false nucleolus,** the cross-reference specifies the location of the main definition: See **karyosome.** The second type of cross-reference directs you to sources of additional information. For instance, the general entry term **keratitis** refers you to specific types of keratitis: **dendritic keratitis, interstitial keratitis, keratoconjunctivitis sicca,** and **trachoma.** Conversely, the specific entry term **field fever** directs you to the general disease class to which field fever belongs: See also **leptospirosis.**

Other cross-references suggest comparison of related but distinct terms. The entry term **modified radical mastectomy,** for example, contains this cross-reference: Compare **radical mastectomy, simple mastectomy.**

DEFINITIONS: A Valuable Reference
Besides providing encyclopedic definitions of nursing terms, this book contains two valuable appendices. The first appendix, a full-color atlas of human anatomy, provides detailed views of most body systems. The second appendix, a guide to drug interactions, lists the adverse effects of combining classes of prescription drugs, such as digitalis preparations and antihistamines, with other prescription drugs, over-the-counter drugs, foods, and alcoholic beverages. For easy reference, the inside front and back covers contain a summary of the most commonly used medical prefixes and suffixes.

a Symbol for arterial blood.

a- A combining form meaning 'without, not': *abacterial, abaptiston, abasia.*

A Symbol for alveolar gas.

AA *abbr* **1. Alcoholics Anonymous. 2. achievement age.**

AACN *abbr* American Association of Critical-Care Nurses and American Association of Colleges of Nursing.

AAMC *abbr* American Association of Medical Colleges.

AAN *abbr* **American Academy of Nursing.**

AANA *abbr* American Association of Nurse Anesthetists.

AANN *abbr* American Association of Neurological Nurses.

AANNT *abbr* American Association of Nephrology Nurses and Technicians, an organization of nurses and technicians working in the fields of dialysis and renal disease.

AAOHN *abbr* American Association of Occupational Health Nurses.

AAP *abbr* American Association of Pathologists.

AAPA *abbr* American Academy of Physicians' Assistants.

AAPMR *abbr* American Academy of Physical Medicine and Rehabilitation.

AART *abbr* American Association for Respiratory Therapy.

AAUP *abbr* American Association of University Professors.

AAV *abbr* adenoassociated virus.

ab- A combining form meaning 'from, off, away from': *abarthrosis, abarticulation, abaxial.* Also **abs-**.

abalienation **1.** A state of physical deterioration or mental decay. **2.** A state of insanity. —**abalienate**, *v.*, **abalienated**, *adj.*

abandonment of care In law: wrongful cessation of the provision of care to a patient, usually by a physician.

abarthrosis See **synovial joint.**

abarticular **1.** Of or pertaining to a condition that does not affect a joint. **2.** Of or pertaining to a site or structure remote from a joint.

abasia The inability to walk, as in paralytic abasia, which paralyzes the leg muscles. —**abasic, abatic**, *adj.*

abaxial **1.** Of or pertaining to a position outside the axis of a body or structure. **2.** Of or pertaining to a position at the opposite extremity of a structure.

Abbot pump A small portable pump that can be adjusted and finely calibrated to deliver precise amounts of medication in solution through an intravenous infusion set. It is similar to a Harvard pump, but the flow rate may be increased or decreased by smaller increments.

ABC *abbr* **aspiration biopsy cytology.**

abdomen The portion of the body between the thorax and the pelvis. The abdominal cavity contains the lower portion of the esophagus, the stomach, the intestines, the liver, the spleen, and the pancreas. The walls of the abdominal cavity are lined with the parietal layer of the peritoneum, a serous membrane. The covering, or outermost layer of each organ, is formed by the visceral layer of the peritoneum. A small amount of serous fluid in the space between the membranous layers allows the organs to slide freely, as in the normal process of digestion, evacuation, and breathing. Also called belly *(informal).* —**abdominal**, *adj.*

abdominal actinomycosis See **actinomycosis.**

abdominal aorta The portion of the descending aorta that passes from the aortic hiatus of the diaphragm into the abdomen, descending ventral to the vertebral column, and ending at the fourth lumbar vertebra where it divides into the two common iliac arteries. It supplies many different parts of the body, as the testes, ovaries, kidneys, and stomach. Its branches are the celiac, superior mesenteric, inferior mesenteric, middle suprarenals, renals, testicular, ovarian, inferior phrenics, lumbars, middle sacral, and common iliacs.

abdominal aponeurosis The conjoined tendons of the oblique and transverse muscles of the abdomen.

abdominal binder A bandage or elasticized wrap that is applied around the lower part of the torso to support the abdomen. A kind of abdominal binder is a **scultetus binder.**

abdominal fistula An abnormal passage from an abdominal organ to the surface of the body. In a colostomy, a passage from the bowel to an opening on the surface of the abdomen is created surgically.

abdominal hernia A hernia in which a loop of bowel protrudes through the abdominal musculature, often through the site of an old surgical scar. Also called **ventral hernia.** See also **hernia.**

abdominal pregnancy An extrauterine pregnancy in which the conceptus develops in the abdominal cavity after being extruded from the fimbriated end of the Fallopian tube or through a defect in the tube or uterus. The placenta may implant on the abdominal or visceral peritoneum. Abdominal pregnancy may be suspected when the abdomen has enlarged but the uterus has remained small for the length of gestation.

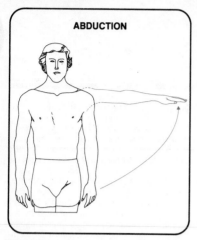

ABDUCTION

Abdominal pregnancies constitute approximately 2% of ectopic pregnancies and approximately 0.01% of all pregnancies. The condition results in perinatal death of the fetus in approximately 90% of cases, maternal death in approximately 6%.

abdominal pulse The pulse of the abdominal aorta.

abdominal reflex A superficial neurological reflex obtained by firmly stroking the skin of the abdomen, normally resulting in a brisk contraction of abdominal muscles in which the umbilicus moves toward the site of the stimulus. This reflex is lost in diseases of the pyramidal tract. See also **superficial reflex.**

abdominal surgery Any operation that involves an incision into the abdomen, usually performed under general anesthesia.

abdomino- A combining form meaning 'pertaining to the abdomen': *abdominocentesis, abdominoscopy, abdominothoracic.*

abdominocentesis See **paracentesis.**

abdominocyesis An abdominal pregnancy.

abdominoscopy A procedure for examining the contents of the peritoneum in which an electrically illuminated tubular device is passed through a trocar into the abdominal cavity. See also **laparoscopy.**

abducens nerve The sixth cranial nerve which originates in the pons in the brainstem. It is a motor nerve controlling the movement of the lateral rectus muscle of the eye.

abducent nerve Either of a pair of cranial nerves essential for lateral eye movements. They branch to the rectus lateralis and pass through a notch below the posterior clinoid process, connecting to two areas in the brain. Also called **nervus abducens, sixth nerve.**

abduction Movement of a limb away from the body. Compare **adduction.**

abduction boots A pair of orthopedic casts for the lower extremities, available in both short-leg and long-leg configurations, with a bar in-

corporated at ankle level to provide hip abduction. Abduction boots are used for postoperative positioning and immobilization after hip adductor releases and to promote proper positioning during healing after surgery to repair structures in the lower extremities.

abductor A structure that draws another part away from the midline of the body, as a muscle that abducts. Compare **adductor.**

Abernethy's sarcoma A malignant neoplasm of fat cells, usually occurring on the trunk.

aberrant 1. Of or pertaining to a wandering from the usual or expected course, as various ducts, nerves, and vessels in the body. 2. In botany and zoology: of or pertaining to an abnormal individual, as certain atypical members of a species.

aberrant ductule A rudimentary structure in the male, situated near the epididymis, that consists of vestigial remains of the caudal part of the embryonic mesonephric tubules. A similar vestigial structure, the paroophoron, is found in the female. See also **appendix epididymis, paradidymis.**

aberrant goiter An enlargement of a supernumerary or ectopic thyroid gland.

abetalipoproteinemia A rare inherited disorder of fat metabolism, characterized by acanthocytosis, low or absent serum betalipoproteins, and hypocholesterolemia. In severe cases steatorrhea, ataxia, nystagmus, motor incoordination, and retinitis pigmentosa occur.

abient Characterized by a tendency to move away from stimuli. Compare **adient.** —**abience,** *n.*

abiogenesis Spontaneous generation; the theory that organic life can originate from inanimate matter. Compare **biogenesis.** —**abiogenetic,** *adj.*

abiosis A nonviable condition or a situation that is incompatible with life. —**abiotic,** *adj.*

abiotrophy A premature depletion of vitality or the deterioration of certain cells and tissues, especially those involved in genetic degenerative diseases. —**abiotrophic,** *adj.*

ablation An amputation, an excision of any part of the body, or a removal of a growth or harmful substance.

ablatio placentae See **abruptio placentae.**

ablepsia The condition of being blind. Also called ablepsy.

abnerval current An electric current that passes from a nerve to and through muscle.

abnormal behavior Maladaptive acts or activities detrimental to the individual and to society. The acts range from the transitory inability to cope with a stressful situation to persistent bizarre or destructive behavior or total disorientation and withdrawal from the realities of everyday life. See also **behavior disorder.**

abnormal psychology In psychology: the study of mental disorders and maladaptive behavior, including neuroses and psychoses, and of normal phenomena like dreams and altered states of consciousness.

ABO blood groups The most important of several systems for classifying human blood based on the antigenic components of the red blood cell. The ABO blood group is identified by the presence or absence of two different antigens, A or B, on the surface of the erythrocyte. The four blood types in this grouping, A, B, AB, and O, are determined by and named for these antigens. Type AB indicates the presence of both antigens; type O the absence of both. Corresponding antibodies, anti-A, and anti-B agglutinins, can be found in the plasma of type O blood. The plasma components of type A and type B blood are, respectively, devoid of anti-A and anti-B agglutinins; both agglutinins are absent from type AB blood plasma. In addition to its significant role in blood banks and transfusion therapy, the ABO blood grouping contributes to forensic medicine, genetics, and, together with the less important blood groups, to anthropology and legal medicine. See also **Rh factor, transfusion.**

aborted systole A contraction of the heart that is usually premature and is not associated with a peripheral pulse.

abortient See **abortifacient.**

abortifacient 1. Producing abortion. 2. An agent that effects abortion.

abortion Spontaneous or induced termination of pregnancy before the fetus has developed enough to be expected to live if born. See also **incomplete abortion, induced abortion, spontaneous abortion, therapeutic abortion.**

abortion-on-demand A concept promoted by pro-choice health advocates that it is the right of a pregnant woman to have an abortion performed at her request. That right may be limited by time of gestation, or it may pertain to any period of gestation.

abortus fever A form of brucellosis, the only one endemic to North America. It is caused by *Brucella abortus*, an organism so named because it causes abortion in cows. Infection in humans results from the ingestion of contaminated milk from cows infected with *B. abortus*, from handling infected meat, or from skin contact with the excreta of living infected animals. Also called **Rio Grande fever.** See also **brucellosis.**

abouchement The junction of a small blood vessel with a large blood vessel.

aboulia See **abulia.**

abrachia The absence of arms. —**abrachial,** *adj.*

abrasion A scraping, or rubbing away of a surface by friction. Abrasion may be the result of trauma, as a skinned knee; of therapy, as in dermabrasion of the skin for removal of scar tissue; or of normal function, as the wearing down of a tooth by mastication. Compare **laceration.** See also **friction burn.** —**abrade,** *v.,* **abrasive,** *adj.*

abreaction An emotional release resulting from mentally reliving or from bringing into consciousness, through the process of catharsis,

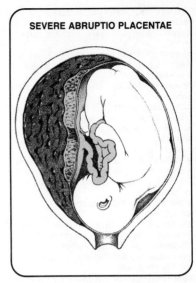

SEVERE ABRUPTIO PLACENTAE

a long-repressed, painful experience. See also **catharsis.**

abrosia The act of fasting or abstaining from food.

abruptio placentae Separation of the placenta implanted in normal position in a pregnancy of 20 weeks or more or during labor prior to delivery of the fetus. It occurs approximately once in 200 births, and, because it often results in severe hemorrhage, it is a significant cause of maternal and fetal mortality. Also called **ablatio placentae, accidental hemorrhage.** Compare **placenta previa.** See also **Couvelaire uterus.**

abscess A cavity containing pus and surrounded by inflamed tissue, formed as a result of suppuration in a localized infection (characteristically, a staphylococcal infection). Healing usually occurs when an abscess drains or is incised. If an abscess is deep in tissue, drainage is effected by means of a sinus tract that connects it to the surface.

absence seizure An epileptic seizure characterized by sudden, momentary loss of consciousness occasionally accompanied by minor myoclonus of the neck or upper extremities, slight symmetrical twitching of the face, or loss of muscle tone. The seizures usually occur many times a day without a warning aura and are most frequent in children and adolescents, especially during puberty. The patient experiencing a typical seizure has a vacant facial expression and ceases all voluntary motor activity; with the rapid return of consciousness, the patient may resume conversation at the point of interruption without realizing what occurred. During and between seizures, the patient's electroencephalogram shows 3-cycle-per-second spike and wave discharges. Anticonvulsant drugs used to prevent absence seizures include clonazepam, ethosuximide, methsuximide, paramethadione, phensuximide, trimethadione, and valproic acid. Formerly called **petit mal** seizure. See also **epilepsy.**

absent without leave (AWOL) In psychiatry: describing a patient who runs away from a psychiatric facility.

absolute alcohol See **dehydrated alcohol.**

absolute growth The total increase in size of an organism or a particular organ or part, as the limbs, head, or trunk.

absorb The act of engorging or taking up various substances.

absorbable gauze A gauzelike material, produced from oxidized cellulose, that can be absorbed. It is applied directly to bleeding tissue for hemostasis.

absorbable gelatin sponge A local hemostatic agent.

absorbed dose In radiotherapy: the energy imparted by ionizing radiation per unit mass of irradiated material at the place of interest. The unit of absorbed dose is the rad, which equals 100 ergs per gram.

absorbent gauze A gauze for absorbing fluids.

absorption 1. The incorporation of matter by other matter through chemical, molecular, or physical action, as the dissolving of a gas in a liquid or the taking up of a liquid by a porous solid. **2.** In physiology: the passage of substances across and into tissues, as the passage of digested food molecules into intestinal cells or the passage of liquids into kidney tubules. 3. In radiology: the absorption of radiant energy by living or nonliving matter with which the radiation reacts.

absorption fever See **puerperal fever.**

abstinence Voluntary avoidance of any substance or the performance of any act for which the person has an appetite.

abstract A condensed scientific article, literary piece, or address.

abstract thinking The final stage in the development of the cognitive thought processes in the child. During this phase thought is characterized by adaptability, flexibility, and the use of abstractions and generalizations. Problem solving is accomplished by drawing logical conclusions from a set of observations, as making hypotheses and testing them. This type of thinking appears from about 12 to 15 years of age, usually after some degree of education.

abulia, aboulia A loss of the ability or a reduced capacity to function voluntarily or to make decisions.

abuse Improper use of equipment, a substance, or a service, as a drug or program, either intentionally or unintentionally. See also **drug abuse.**

abuse of process In law: a civil action for damages in which it is alleged that the legal process has been used in a manner not contemplated by law. This action might be brought by a health practitioner attempting to countersue

a patient or by a psychiatric patient attempting to demonstrate wrongful confinement.

a.c. In prescriptions: *abbr ante cibum,* a Latin phrase meaning 'before meals.'

Ac Symbol for **actinium.**

AC *abbr* **alternating current.**

ac- See **ad-.**

academic ladder The hierarchy of faculty appointments in a university through which a faculty member must advance from instructor, to assistant professor, associate professor, and, finally, to professor.

acampsia A condition in which a joint becomes rigid. See also **ankylosis.**

acantha A spine or a spinous projection. **—acanthoid,** *adj.*

acantho- A combining form meaning 'thorny or spiky': *acanthesthesia, acanthoid, acantholysis.*

acanthocyte An abnormal red blood cell with spurlike projections giving it a thorny appearance. Large numbers are present in abetalipoproteinemia; fewer occur in cirrhosis and in certain malabsorption syndromes. Compare **burr cell.** See also **abetalipoproteinemia, acanthocytosis.**

acanthocytosis The abnormal presence of acanthocytes in the circulating blood system, most commonly associated with abetalipoproteinemia in which as many as 80% of the erythrocytes are acanthocytes. Also called **Bassen-Kornzweig syndrome.** See also **abetalipoproteinemia.**

acanthoma Any benign or malignant tumor arising from the prickle cell layer of the epidermis.

acanthoma adenoides cysticum See **trichoepithelioma.**

acanthoma verrucosa seborrheica See **seborrheic keratosis.**

acanthosis An abnormal thickening of the prickle cell layer of the skin, as in eczema and psoriasis. See also **acanthosis nigricans, epidermis. —acanthotic,** *adj.*

acanthosis nigricans A skin disease characterized by hyperpigmented, warty lesions of the axillae and other body folds. There are benign and malignant forms, the latter associated with cancers of the gastrointestinal tract. See also **acanthosis.**

acardia A rare congenital anomaly in which the heart is absent. It is sometimes seen in a conjoined twin whose survival until birth depended upon the other's circulatory system. **—acardiac,** *adj.*

acardius, acardiacus An acardiac fetus. Also called **fetus acardiacus.**

acardius acephalus An acardiac fetus that lacks a head and most of the upper part of the body.

acardius acormus An acardiac fetus that has a grossly defective trunk.

acardius amorphus An acardiac fetus with a rudimentary body that does not resemble the normal form. Also called acardius anceps.

acariasis Any disease caused by an acarid,

as scrub typhus, which is caused by trombiculid mites.

acarid One of the many mites that are members of the order Acarina, which includes a great number of parasitic and free-living organisms. Most are yet undescribed, but several types are of medical interest because they infect humans. The kinds associated with disease are those acting as intermediate hosts of pathogenic agents, those that directly cause skin or tissue damage, and those that cause loss of blood or tissue fluids. Important as vectors of scrub typhus and other rickettsial agents are the six-legged larvae of trombiculid mites, which are parasitic of humans, many other mammals, and birds.

acaro- A combining form meaning 'pertaining to mites': *acarodermatitis, acaroid, acarophobia.*

accelerated hypertension See **malignant hypertension.**

acceleration An increase in the speed or velocity of an object or reaction. Compare **deceleration.** —**accelerator,** *n.*

acceleration phase In obstetrics: the first period of active labor, characterized by an increased rate of dilatation of the cervical os as charted on a Friedman curve.

acceptable daily intake (ADI) The maximum amount of any substance that can be safely ingested by a human.

acceptance According to Dr. Elisabeth Kübler-Ross, the fifth and final stage of dying. One who reaches this stage comes to terms with impending death and awaits it with quiet expectation. One begins to separate oneself from the news and problems of the world. Communication becomes more nonverbal than verbal. Not all dying patients reach the stage of acceptance. See also **anger, bargaining, denial and isolation,** and **depression.**

acceptor 1. An organism that receives from another person or organism living tissue, as transfused blood or a transplanted organ. **2.** A substance or compound that combines with a part of another substance or compound. Compare **donor.**

accessory 1. A supplement employed chiefly for convenience or for safety, as the electric elevator mechanisms for hospital beds. **2.** In anatomy: a structure that serves one of the main anatomical systems, as the accessory sex organs in men and women or the accessory organs of the skin, as the hair, the nails, and the skin glands.

accessory chromosome An unpaired X or Y sex chromosome. See also **monosome.**

accessory muscle A relatively rare anatomic duplication of a muscle that may appear anywhere in the muscular system.

accessory nerve Either of a pair of cranial nerves essential for speech, swallowing, and certain movements of the head and shoulders. Each nerve has a cranial and a spinal portion, communicates with certain cervical nerves, and connects to the nucleus ambiguus of the brain. Also called **eleventh nerve, nervus accesso-**rius, spinal accessory nerve.

accessory pancreatic duct A small duct opening into the pancreatic duct or duodenum near the mouth of the common bile duct.

accessory phrenic nerve The nerve that joins the phrenic nerve at the root of the neck or in the thorax, forming a loop around the subclavian vein. It may arise from the nerve to the subclavius or from the fifth cervical nerve. Resection of the phrenic nerve to immobilize the diaphragm may be only partially successful if the accessory phrenic nerve is not also resected.

accessory sinus of the nose See **nasal sinus.**

ACCH *abbr* **Association for the Care of Children's Health.**

acclimate, acclimatize The process of adjusting physiologically to a different climate, especially to changes in altitude and in temperature. —**acclimation, acclimatization,** *n.*

accommodation 1. The state or process of adapting or adjusting one thing or set of things to another. **2.** The continuous process or effort of the individual to adapt or adjust to surroundings in order to maintain a state of homeostasis, both physiologically and psychologically. **3.** In sociology: the reciprocal reconciliation of conflicts between individuals or groups concerning habits and customs, usually through a process of compromise, arbitration, or negotiation. Also called **adjustment.** Compare **adaptation.**

accommodation reflex An adjustment of the eyes for near vision, consisting of pupillary constriction, convergence of the eyes, and increased convexity of the lens. Also called **ciliary reflex.** See also **pupillary reflex.**

accomplishment quotient A numerical evaluation of a person's achievement age compared to mental age, expressed as a ratio multiplied by 100. See also **achievement quotient, intelligence quotient.**

accouchement Childbirth; obstetric delivery.

accouchement forcé A dangerous, out-of-date obstetric operation in which the fetus is rapidly delivered through a forcibly dilated cervix.

accountability Responsibility for one's actions.

accreditation A process whereby a professional association or nongovernmental agency grants recognition to a school or institution for demonstrated ability in a special area of practice or training, as the accreditation of hospitals by the Joint Commission of Accreditation for Hospitals or of nursing schools by the National League for Nursing. Compare **certification, licensure.**

accrementition Growth or increase of size by the addition of similar tissue or material, as in cellular division, simple fission, budding, or germination.

accretio cordis An abnormal condition in which there is an adhesion of the pericardium to a structure around the heart.

accretion 1. Growth or increase by the addition of material of the same nature that is

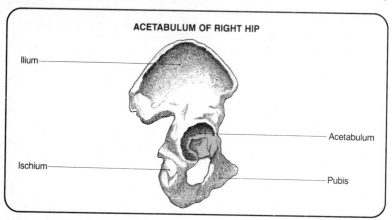

ACETABULUM OF RIGHT HIP

Ilium

Acetabulum

Ischium

Pubis

already present. **2.** The adherence or growing together of parts that are normally separated. **3.** The accumulation of foreign material, especially within a cavity. —**accrete,** *v.,* **accretive,** *adj.*

accretionary growth An increase in size resulting from the accumulation of new tissue through the process of mitosis or the addition of material similar to that which is already present.

acecarbromal A sedative-hypnotic.

acedia A condition of listlessness and a form of melancholy, marked by indifference and sluggish mental processes.

acelius An individual without a body cavity.

acentric **1.** The characteristic of having no center. **2.** In genetics: describing a chromosome fragment that has no centromere.

-aceous A combining form meaning 'pertaining to or of the nature of' something specified: *coriaceous, foliaceous, testaceous.*

acephalo- A combining form meaning 'having no head': *acephalobrachia, acephalus, acephaly.*

acephalobrachia A congenital anomaly in which a fetus lacks both arms and a head.

acephalus A fetus lacking a properly developed head. —**acephalous,** *adj.*

acephaly, acephalia, acephalism A congenital defect in which the head is absent or not properly developed. —**acephalic,** *adj.*

acet- A combining form meaning 'vinegar': *acetify, acetoin, acetyl.*

acetabulum, *pl.* **acetabula** The large, cup-shaped, articular cavity at the juncture of the ilium, the ischium, and the pubis, containing the ball-shaped head of the femur.

acetaminophen A nonnarcotic analgesic and antipyretic agent.

acetate kinase An enzyme that catalyzes the transfer of a phosphate group from adenosine triphosphate to acetate. Also called **acetokinase.**

acetazolamide A diuretic and anticonvulsant agent.

acetazolamide sodium A carbonic anhydrase inhibitor.

Acetest A trademark for a product used to test for the presence of abnormal quantities of acetone in the urine of patients with diabetes mellitus or other metabolic disorders. A large quantity of acetone causes a rapid change in the color of the Acetest tablet. See also **acidosis, ketone bodies.**

acetic acid **1.** A clear, colorless, pungent liquid that is miscible with water, alcohol, glycerin, and ether and that constitutes 3% to 5% of vinegar. Acetic acid is produced commercially by the destructive distillation of wood or from methyl alcohol, or it may be converted from ethyl alcohol by the action of many aerobic bacteria. Various concentrations of acetic acid are used in the manufacture of plastics, dyes, insecticides, cellulose acetate, photographic chemicals, and pharmaceutical preparations, including vaginal jellies and antimicrobial solutions for the treatment of superficial infections of the external auditory canal. **2.** An anti-infective otic agent. Also called ethanoic acid.

acetic acid lotion An astringent.

acetic fermentation The production of acetic acid or vinegar from a weak alcoholic solution.

acetoacetic acid A colorless, oily compound produced in the body by the metabolism of lipids and pyruvates. It is excreted in trace amounts in normal urine and in elevated levels in diabetes mellitus, especially in ketoacidosis. Acetoacetic acid, a ketone body, is also increased during starvation owing to incomplete oxidation of fatty acids. Soluble in water, alcohol, and ether, acetoacetic acid decomposes at temperatures below 100°C (212°F) to acetone and carbon dioxide. Also called **acetone carboxylic acid, acetylacetic acid, diacetic acid.**

acetohexamide An oral sulfonylurea antidiabetic agent.

acetokinase See **acetate kinase.**

acetol kinase An enzyme that catalyzes the transfer of a phosphate group from adenosine triphosphate to hydroxyacetone.

acetone A colorless, aromatic, volatile liquid found in small amounts in normal urine and in larger quantities in the urine of diabetics. Commercially prepared acetone is used to clean the skin before injections and also has many varied industrial uses. Prolonged exposure to the compound can be irritating.

acetone bodies See **ketone bodies.**

acetone carboxylic acid See **acetoacetic acid.**

acetophenazine maleate A phenothiazine antipsychotic agent.

acetophenetidin See **phenacetin.**

acetylacetic acid See **acetoacetic acid.**

acetylcarbromal See **acecarbromal.**

acetylcholine An acetic acid ester of choline, normally present in the body. It has important physiologic functions and is a neurotransmitter at the myoneural junction, in sympathetic and parasympathetic ganglia, and at parasympathetic nerve endings.

acetylcholine chloride A miotic agent.

acetylcoenzyme A (acetyl-CoA) A molecule that is formed in the course of several important metabolic processes. The formation of acetylcoenzyme A is the critical intermediate step between anaerobic glycolysis and the Krebs' citric acid cycle.

acetylcysteine An expectorant.

acetylsalicylic acid See **aspirin.**

ACh *abbr* **acetylcholine.**

achalasia An abnormal condition characterized by the inability of a muscle to relax, particularly the cardiac sphincter of the stomach.

Achard-Thiers syndrome A hormonal disorder seen in postmenopausal women with diabetes, characterized by growth of body hair in a masculine distribution. See also **hirsutism, hypertrichosis.**

ache 1. A pain characterized by persistence, dullness, and, usually, moderate intensity. An ache may be localized, as in a stomach ache, headache, or bone ache, or general, as the myalgia that accompanies a viral infection or a persistent fever. 2. To suffer from a dull, persistent pain of moderate intensity.

achievement age The level of a person's educational development as measured by an achievement test and compared with the normal score for chronological age. Compare **mental age.** See also **developmental age.**

achievement motivation An intrapsychic drive that initiates behavior directed toward the attainment of a particular goal. Compare **physiological motivation, social motivation.**

achievement quotient (AQ) A numerical expression of a person's achievement age, determined by various achievement tests, divided by the chronological age and expressed as a multiple of 100. Compare **intelligence quotient.** See also **accomplishment quotient.**

achievement test A standardized test for the measurement and comparison of an applicant or employee's knowledge or proficiency in various fields of vocational or academic study. Compare **aptitude test, intelligence test, per-**

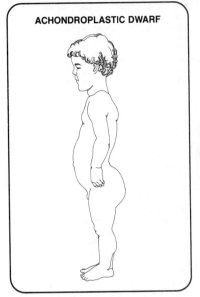

ACHONDROPLASTIC DWARF

sonality test, psychological test.

Achilles tendon See **tendo calcaneus.**

Achilles tendon reflex A deep tendon reflex consisting of plantar flexion of the foot when a sharp tap is given directly to the tendon of the gastrocnemius muscle at the back of the ankle. This reflex is often absent in diabetics and people with peripheral neuropathies. A sluggish return of the flexed foot may be seen in patients with hypothyroidism. A hyperactive reflex may be due to hyperthyroidism or to pyramidal tract disease. Also called **ankle reflex, calcaneal tendon reflex.** See also **deep tendon reflex.**

achlorhydria An abnormal condition characterized by the absence of hydrochloric acid in the gastric juice. See also **pernicious anemia.** —**achlorhydric,** *adj.*

achondroplasia 1. A skeletal condition involving disordered growth of cartilage, often due to nutritional deficiency. See **rickets.** 2. A familial disorder of the growth of cartilage in the epiphyses of the long bones and skull that results in premature ossification, permanent limitation of skeletal development, and dwarfism typified by protruding forehead and by short, thick arms and legs on a normal trunk. Also called **chondrodystrophy.**

achondroplastic dwarf The most common type of dwarf, characterized by disproportionately short limbs, a normal-sized trunk, large head with a depressed nasal bridge and small face, stubby trident hands, and lordosis. The condition results from an inherited defect in bone-forming tissue and is often associated with other defects or abnormalities, although there is usually no involvement of the central nervous system and intelligence is normal. See also **achondroplasia.**

achromatocyte See **achromocyte.**

achromocyte A sickle-shaped, hypochromic erythrocyte, perhaps the result of a ruptured red blood cell that lost hemoglobin. Also called **achromatocyte.**

achylia An absence or severe deficiency of hydrochloric acid and pepsinogen in the stomach. This condition may also occur in the pancreas, when the exocrine portion of that gland fails to produce digestive enzymes. Also called **achylosis.** See also **achlorhydria. —achylous,** *adj.*

achylous 1. Of or pertaining to a lack of gastric juice or other digestive secretions. 2. Of or pertaining to a lack of chyle.

acicular Needle-shaped, as certain leaves and crystals.

acid 1. A compound that yields hydrogenions when dissociated in solution. Acids turn blue litmus red, have a sour taste, and react with bases to form salts. Acids have chemical properties essentially opposite to those of bases. See also **alkali.** 2. *Slang.* Lysergic acid diethylamide. See **lysergide.**

acid- A combining form meaning 'sour, acid': *acidemia, acidophil, aciduric.*

-acid 1. A combining form meaning an 'acid': *diacid, monacid, sulfacid.* 2. A combining form meaning 'pertaining to acid': *subacid, semiacid, superacid.*

acid-base balance A condition existing when the net rate at which the body produces acids or bases equals the net rate at which acids or bases are excreted. The result of acid-base balance is a stable concentration of hydrogen ions in body fluids. See also **acid, base.**

acid-base metabolism The metabolic processes that maintain the balance of acids and bases essential in regulating the composition of body fluids. Acids release hydrogen ions and bases accept them; the number of hydrogen ions present in a solution governs whether it is acid, alkali, or neutral. Hydrogen ions are measured on a pH scale of 1 to 14, with a reading of 7 being neutral. Above 7, the solution is alkaline; below 7, it is acid. Blood is slightly alkaline, ranging from 7.35 to 7.45. Metabolic buffer systems within the body maintain this ratio, and, when it is upset, either acidosis or alkalosis results. See also **acid-base balance, acidosis, alkalosis, pH.**

acid bath A bath taken in water containing a mineral acid to help reduce excessive sweating.

acid burn Damage to tissue caused by exposure to a strong acid. The severity of the burn is determined by the kind of acid and the duration and extent of exposure.

acid dust An accumulation of highly acidic particles of dust. Such substances accumulate in the atmosphere and account for much of the smog hanging over large metropolitan areas. Many respiratory illnesses may be aggravated or caused by such dust.

-acidemia A combining form meaning an 'increased hydrogen-ion concentration in the blood': *lactacidemia, lipacidemia, oxybutyricacidemia.*

acid-fast stain A method of staining used in bacteriology in which a smear on a slide is flooded with carbol-fuchsin stain, decolorized with acid alcohol, and counterstained with methylene blue. Acid-fast organisms resist decolorization and appear red against a blue background when viewed under a microscope. The stain may be performed on any clinical specimen but is most commonly used in examining sputum for *Mycobacterium tuberculosis,* an acid-fast bacillus. A kind of acid-fast stain is the **Ziehl-Neelsen stain.**

acid flush A runoff of precipitation with a high acid content, as may occur during thaws in various parts of the world. Acid flushes may pollute rivers and reservoirs, killing fish and endangering the health of adjacent populations.

acidify 1. To make a substance acid, as through the addition of an acid. 2. To become acid. Compare **alkalinize.**

acid mist Mist containing a high concentration of acid or particles of any toxic chemical, as carbon tetrachloride or silicon tetrachloride. Such chemicals are often used by industry and stored in tanks that may leak their contents into residential areas, becoming especially dangerous if the toxic substance mixes with fog. Inhalation of acid mists may irritate the mucous membranes, the eyes, and the respiratory tract and seriously upset the chemistry of the body.

acidophil 1. A cell or cell constituent with an affinity for acid dyes. 2. An organism that thrives in an acid medium. —**acidophilic,** *adj.*

acidophilic adenoma A tumor of the pituitary gland, characterized by cells that can be stained red with an acid dye. Gigantism and acromegaly are caused by an acidophilic adenoma. Also called **eosinophilic adenoma.**

acidophilus milk Milk inoculated with cultures of *Lactobacillus acidophilus,* used in various enteric disorders to change the bacterial flora of the gastrointestinal tract.

acidosis An abnormal increase in hydrogen ion concentration in the body owing to an accumulation of an acid or the loss of a base. The two main forms of acidosis are named for the cause of the condition. Respiratory acidosis results from respiratory retention of CO_2, and metabolic acidosis results from excessive burning of fats in the absence of usable carbohydrates; anaerobic carbohydrate metabolism; renal acidosis; diarrhea; and intestinal malabsorption. Treatment depends on diagnosis of the underlying pathology and concurrent correction of the acid-base imbalance. Compare **alkalosis.**

acid perfusion test A test to demonstrate sensitivity of the esophagus to acid, a condition suggestive of reflux esophagitis. Normal saline solution and 0.1 normal hydrochloric acid are dripped alternately into the esophagus by means of a nasal-esophageal tube without telling the patient which solution is being infused. A positive response is pain with acid but not with saline. An alternative method is to compare acid barium swallows with neutral barium swallows. If acid sensitivity is present, diffuse spasm of the esophagus may be seen by fluoroscopy when acid barium is infused and no spasm with neutral barium. Also called **Bernstein test.**

acid phosphatase An enzyme that synthesizes phosphate esters of carbohydrates in an acid medium. See also **phosphatase.**

acid poisoning A toxic condition caused by the ingestion of a toxic acid agent, such as hydrochloric, nitric, phosphoric, or sulfuric acids, some of which are ingredients in cleaning compounds. Emergency treatment includes giving copious amounts of water or milk to dilute the acid. Vomiting is not induced, and mild solutions of alkali are not given. Compare **alkali poisoning.**

acid precipitation The precipitation of moisture, as rain or snow, with high acidity caused by release into the atmosphere of pollutants from industry, motor vehicle exhausts, and other sources. Acid precipitation with a pH of 5.6 or less is blamed by various authorities for numerous human health problems, fish kills, and the destruction of timber. Also called acid rain, acid snow.

acid therapy A method for removing warts that employs plaster patches impregnated with acid, as 40% salicylic acid, or with acid drops, as 5% to 16.7% salicylic and lactic acids in flexible collodion. The application is made every 12 to 24 hours for 2 to 4 weeks. Acid therapy is not usually recommended for body areas that perspire heavily or that are likely to become wet or for exposed body parts where the patches would detract from the patient's appearance.

aciduria Acid in the urine.

acinar adenocarcinoma See **acinic cell adenocarcinoma.**

Acinetobacter A genus of nonmotile, aerobic bacteria of the family Neisseriaceae that often occurs in clinical specimens. The *Acinetobacter* contains gram-negative or gram-variable cocci and does not produce spores. This bacterium grows on regular media without serum and is oxidase-negative and catalase-positive.

acinic cell adenocarcinoma An uncommon, low-grade malignant neoplasm that develops in the secreting cells of racemose glands, especially the salivary glands. The tumor consists of cells with clear or slightly granular cytoplasm and small eccentric dark nuclei. Also called **acinar adenocarcinoma, acinous adenocarcinoma.**

acinitis Any inflammation of the tiny, grape-shaped portions of certain glands.

acinous adenocarcinoma See **acinic cell adenocarcinoma.**

acinus, *pl.* **acini** 1. Any small saclike structure in the body. Also called **alveolus.** 2. A subdivision of the lung consisting of the tissue distal to a terminal bronchiole.

ACMC *abbr* **Association of Canadian Medical Colleges.**

acmesthesia A sensation of a pinprick or of a sharp point touching the skin.

acne An inflammatory, papulo-pustular skin eruption, occurring usually on the face, neck, shoulders, and upper back. Its cause is unknown but involves bacterial breakdown of sebum into fatty substances irritating to surrounding subcutaneous tissue. Treatment includes topical and oral antibiotics, topical vitamin A derivatives, benzyl benzoate, and dermabrasion. Kinds of acne include **acne conglobata, acne vulgaris, chloracne, rosacea.** See also **comedo. —acneiform,** *adj.*

acne artificialis An eruption in the skin caused by an external irritant.

acne cachecticorum An eruption or irritation of the skin that may occur in very weak, debilitated patients. It is characterized by soft, mildly infiltrated pustular lesions.

acne conglobata A severe form of acne with abscess, cyst, scar, and keloid formation. Acne conglobata may affect the lower back, buttocks, and thighs as well as the face and chest. Also called **cystic acne.**

acneform Resembling acne.

acneform drug eruption Any one of various skin reactions to a drug, characterized by papules and pustules erupting in acne, with or without comedones.

acnegenic Causing or producing acne.

acne indurata A pathological skin condition characterized by extensive papular lesions that often produce severe scars.

acne keratosa A skin condition characterized by hard conical plugs which usually appear at the corners of the mouth and inflame surrounding tissue.

acne necrotica miliaris A rare, chronic type of folliculitis of the scalp, occurring mostly in adults and characterized by tiny pustules.

acne neonatorum A skin condition of infants caused by sebaceous gland hyperplasia and characterized by the formation of comedones, nodules, and cysts on the nose, cheeks, and forehead.

acne papulosa A common pathological skin condition that develops papular lesions. It is considered a papular form of acne vulgaris.

acne rosacea See **rosacea.**

acne vulgaris A common form of acne seen predominantly in adolescents and young adults. Acne vulgaris is probably an effect of androgenic hormones (which stimulate the production of sebum) and *Corynebacterium acnes* in the piliary canal.

ACNM *abbr* American College of Nurse-Midwives.

ACOG *abbr* American College of Obstetricians and Gynecologists.

acognosia A knowledge of remedies.

aconeus One of seven superficial muscles of the posterior forearm. A small triangular muscle, it originates on the dorsal surface of the lateral condyle and inserts in the olecranon process of the ulna. It is innervated by a branch of the radial nerve, which contains fibers from the seventh and eighth cervical nerves, and it functions to extend the forearm.

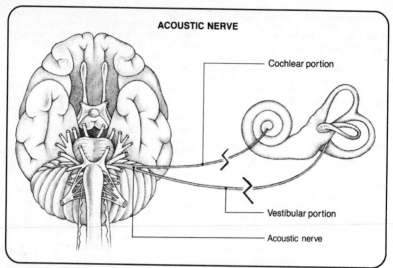

ACOUSTIC NERVE

Cochlear portion

Vestibular portion

Acoustic nerve

acoria A condition characterized by constant hunger, even when the appetite is small.

acorn-tipped catheter A flexible catheter with an acorn-shaped tip, used in various diagnostic procedures, especially in urology.

acou-, acu- A combining form meaning 'pertaining to hearing': *acouesthesia, acoulalion, acouophonia.*

-acousia, -acusia A combining form meaning a '(specified) condition of the hearing': *amblyacousia, bradyacousia, dysacousia.* Also **-acusis, -akusis.**

acousma, *pl.* **acousmas, acousmata** A hallucinatory impression of strange sounds.

acoustic, acoustical Of or pertaining to sound or hearing.

-acoustic 1. A combining form meaning 'pertaining to the hearing organs': *entacoustic, otacoustic.* 2. A combining form meaning 'pertaining to amplified sound waves': *micracoustic, microcoustic, stethacoustic.* Also **-acoustical.**

acoustic microscope A microscope in which the object being viewed is scanned with sound waves and its image reconstructed with light waves. Acoustic microscopes produce excellent resolution of the objects being studied and allow extremely close examination of cells and tissues without risk of marring the specimen.

acoustic nerve Either of a pair of cranial nerves essential to the sense of hearing, having two distinct sets of fibers called the cochlear nerves and the vestibular nerves, and connecting to three areas in the brain. Also called **eighth nerve.**

acoustic neurilemoma See **acoustic neuroma.**

acoustic neurinoma See **acoustic neuroma.**

acoustic neurofibroma See **acoustic neuroma.**

acoustic neuroma A benign tumor that develops from the eighth cranial (acoustic) nerve and grows within the auditory canal. Depending on the location and size of the lesion, tinnitus, increasing deafness, headache, facial numbness, papilledema, dizziness, and an unsteady gait may result. Paresis and difficulty in speaking and swallowing may occur in the later stage. It may be unilateral or bilateral. Also called **acoustic neurilemoma, acoustic neurinoma, acoustic neurofibroma.**

acoustic trauma A gradual loss of hearing caused by exposure to loud noise over an extended period of time or a sudden loss of hearing, partial or complete, caused by an explosion, a severe blow to the head, or other accident. Hearing loss may be temporary or permanent.

acousto-optics A field of physics that studies the generation of light waves by ultrahigh-frequency sound waves.

ACP *abbr* 1. American College of Pathologists. 2. American College of Physicians.

acquired In genetics: of or pertaining to a characteristic, condition, or disease originating after birth and caused, not by hereditary or developmental factors, but by a reaction to environmental influences outside of the organism. Compare **congenital, hereditary.**

acquired immune deficiency syndrome (AIDS) A syndrome that may indicate a defect in cell-mediated immunity. It occurs in patients with no known cause for deficient cellular immunity, in diseases such as Kaposi's sarcoma, *Pneumocystis carinii* pneumonia, and other opportunistic infections. Laboratory tests (histology or culture) generally confirm the diagnosis. A patient with AIDS may have no symptoms or nonspecific symptoms such as fever, weight loss, and generalized, persistent lymphadenopathy. AIDS may be associated with tuberculosis, oral candidiasis, and herpes zoster, as well as malignant neoplasms that may cause or result from immunodeficiency. However, some patients with diseases that are usually associated with AIDS may not be immunodeficient.

acquired immunity   Any form of immunity that is not innate and is obtained during life. It may be natural or artificial and actively or passively induced. **Naturally acquired immunity** is obtained by the development of antibodies resulting from an attack of infectious disease or by the transmission of antibodies from the mother through the placenta to the fetus or to the infant through the colostrum. **Artificially acquired immunity** is obtained by vaccination or by the injection of antiserum. Compare **natural immunity.** See also **active immunity, passive immunity.**

acquired reflex   See **conditioned reflex.**

ACR   *abbr* American College of Radiology.

acrasia   Lack of self control; intemperance.

acrid   Sharp or pungent, bitter and unpleasant to the smell or taste.

acridine   A benzopyridine compound used in the synthesis of dyes and drugs. Its derivatives include fluorescent yellow dyes and the antiseptic agents acriflavine hydrochloride, acriflavine base, and proflavine.

acro-   A combining form meaning 'pertaining to the extremities': *acroagnosis, acroataxia, acrocyanosis.*

acrocentric   Pertaining to a chromosome in which the centromere is located near one of the ends so that the arms of the chromatids are extremely uneven. Compare **metacentric, submetacentric, telocentric.**

acrocephalosyndactylism   See **Apert's syndrome.**

acrocephaly   See **oxycephaly.**

acrochordon   A benign, pedunculated skin tag commonly occurring on the eyelids or neck or in the axillae or groin.

acrocyanosis   A condition characterized by cyanotic discoloration, coldness, and sweating of the extremities, especially the hands, caused by arterial spasm that is usually precipitated by cold or by emotional stress. Warming induces vasodilation, and the blue discoloration becomes mottled with red. Abnormal sympathetic nerve activity or overreaction to certain stimuli may be responsible for the vasospasm that typically occurs in Raynaud's disease and is also seen in rheumatoid arthritis, in scleroderma, and in workers who operate pneumatic air hammers. A kind of acrocyanosis is **peripheral acrocyanosis of the newborn.** Also called **Raynaud's sign.**

acrodermatitis   An eruption of the skin caused by a parasitic mite, which is a member of the order Acarina.

acrodermatitis enteropathica   A rare, chronic disease that afflicts infants characterized by vesicles and bullae of the skin and mucous membranes, alopecia, diarrhea, and failure to thrive. It may be lethal if not treated.

acromegalic eunuchoidism   A rare disorder characterized by genital atrophy and the

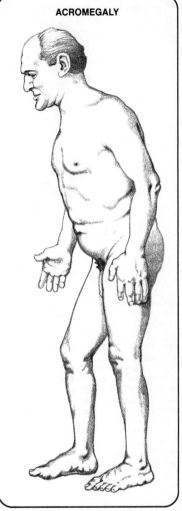

ACROMEGALY

development of female secondary sex characteristics, occurring in men with advanced acromegaly caused by a chromophil adenoma in the anterior pituitary gland. Initially, the gonadal function of the anterior lobe may be stimulated, but with the growth of the tumor, the patient may become impotent, lose facial, axillary, and pubic hair, develop soft skin and a feminine distribution of fat. Also called **retrograde infantilism.**

acromegaly, acromegalia   A chronic metabolic condition characterized by a gradual, marked enlargement and elongation of the bones of the face, jaw, and extremities. The condition, which afflicts middle-aged persons, is caused by the overproduction of growth hormone and is treated by X-ray or surgery, often involving par-

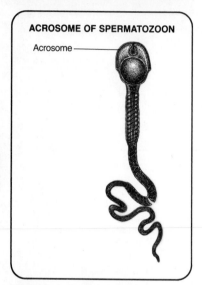

ACROSOME OF SPERMATOZOON

Acrosome

---

tial resection of the pituitary gland. Compare **gigantism**. See also **adenohypophysis, growth hormone**. —**acromegalic**, *adj*.

acromioclavicular articulation The gliding joint between the acromial end of the clavicle and the medial margin of the acromion of the scapula. The joint has six ligaments.

acromion The lateral extension of the spine of the scapula, forming the highest point of the shoulder and connecting with the clavicle at a small oval surface in the middle of the spine. It gives attachment to the deltoideus and trapezius. Also called **acromion process**. Compare **coracoid process**. —**acromial**, *adj*.

acronym A word formed by the initial letters or syllables of other words, as *PEEP*, which is the acronym for *Positive End-Expiratory Pressure*. Most acronyms are composed of the initial capital letters of their full forms and differ from abbreviations in that they are pronounced and treated as words grammatically. —**acronymic**, *adj*.

acroparesthesia 1. An extreme sensitivity at the tips of the extremities of the body, caused by compression of the nerves in the affected area or by polyneuritis. 2. A disease characterized by tingling, numbness, and stiffness in the extremities, especially in the fingers, the hands, and the forearms. It sometimes produces pain, skin pallor, or mild cyanosis. The disease occurs in a simple form, which may produce acrocyanosis, and in an angiospastic form, which may produce gangrene.

acrophobia A pathological fear or dread of high places that results in extreme anxiety. The obsessive phenomenon is most frequently seen in persons who are overconscientious, shy, pedantic, punctilious, or painstakingly addicted to orderliness and symmetry. In many cases, the cause can be traced to some repressed, fear-

producing experience involved with heights, usually occurring in childhood. See also **obsession, phobia**.

acrosomal cap See **acrosome**.

acrosomal head cap See **acrosome**.

acrosomal reaction The pattern of various chemical changes that occur in the anterior of the head of the spermatozoon in response to contact with the ovum and that lead to the penetration by the sperm and fertilization of the ovum.

acrosome The caplike structure surrounding the anterior end of the nucleus of a spermatozoon. It is derived from the Golgi apparatus within the cytoplasm and contains enzymes that function in the penetration of the ovum during fertilization. Also called **acrosomal cap, acrosomal head cap**. See also **acrosomal reaction**. —**acrosomal**, *adj*.

acrotic 1. Of or pertaining to the surface or to the skin glands. 2. Of or pertaining to the absence or the weakness of a pulse.

ACS *abbr* 1. American Cancer Society. 2. American Chemical Society.

ACSM *abbr* American College of Sports Medicine.

act- A combining form meaning 'to do, drive, act': *action, activate, actor*.

ACTH *abbr* **adrenocorticotropic hormone**.

actigraph Any instrument that records changes in the activity of a substance or an organism and produces a graphic record of the process, as an electrocardiograph machine, which produces a record of cardiac activity.

actin A protein found in muscle fibers that acts with myosin to bring about contraction and relaxation. See also **myosin**.

actin- See **actino-**.

acting out The expression of intrapsychic conflict or painful emotion through overt behavior that is usually neurotic, defensive, and unconscious and that may be destructive or dangerous. In controlled situations, like psychodrama, Gestalt therapy, or play therapy, such behavior may be therapeutic in itself and may also serve to reveal to the patient the underlying conflict governing his behavior. See also **transference**.

actinic Of or pertaining to radiation, as sunlight or X-rays.

actinic dermatitis A skin inflammation or rash resulting from exposure to sunlight, X-ray, or atomic particle radiation. Chronic or recurrent actinic dermatitis can predispose to skin cancer. See also **actinic keratosis**.

actinic keratosis A slowly developing, localized thickening of the outer layers of the skin as a result of chronic, excessive exposure to the sun. Treatment of this potentially malignant lesion includes surgical excision, cryotherapy, and topical chemotherapy. Also called **senile keratosis**.

actinin A protein that forms part of the complex of actin and myosin in a muscle fiber. The precise function of actinin is not known, but some researchers believe it may help to maintain the regular architecture of the myofibrils.

actinium (Ac)   A rare, radioactive metallic element. Its atomic number is 89; its atomic weight is 227. It occurs in some ores of uranium.

actino-, actin-   A combining form meaning 'pertaining to a ray or to radiation': *actinocardiogram, actinocutitis, actinogen.*

Actinomyces   A genus of anaerobic, grampositive bacteria. The species that may cause disease in man, *Actinomyces israelii,* is normally present in the mouth and throat. See also **actinomycosis.**

actinomycosis   A chronic, systemic disease characterized by deep, lumpy abscesses that extrude a thin, granular pus through multiple sinuses. The disease occurs worldwide but is seen most frequently in those who live in rural areas. It is not spread from person to person or from animals to humans. The various species of *Actinomyces* are species specific. The causative organism in humans is *A. israelii,* a normal inhabitant of the bowel and mouth. Disease occurs following tissue damage, usually in the presence of another infectious organism. There are three principal forms of actinomycosis. **Abdominal actinomycosis** usually follows an acute inflammatory process in the stomach or intestines, as appendicitis, diverticulum of the large bowel, or a perforation of the stomach. A large mass may be palpated, and sinus tracts may be found in the groin or other area that drains exudate from abscesses deep in the abdomen. Rarely, a pelvic form of abdominal actinomycosis occurs following insertion of an intrauterine contraceptive device. **Cervicofacial actinomycosis** occurs with the spread of the bacterium into the subcutaneous tissues of the mouth, throat, and neck, secondary to dental or tonsillar infection. The process begins with a hard swelling over the angle of the lower jaw and neck. The swelling becomes indurated, and sinus tracts form, draining the pus to the skin. Remarkably little pain accompanies these abscesses, even when they are so deep as to involve the bone of the jaw. **Thoracic actinomycosis** may represent proliferation of the organism from cervicofacial abscesses into the esophagus, or it may result from inhalation of the bacterium into the bronchi. The infection may spread through the lungs, reaching the pleura, or through the esophagus into the mediastinum. Ribs, heart, and the great vessels may then be affected. Fever, cough, draining sinuses, weight loss, night sweats, and, rarely, pleural effusion are characteristic of this form of the disease.

action alternatives   In nursing: any of several possible actions or courses of action chosen by a nurse as part of a goal-oriented nursing care plan and performed to resolve a problem or to modify the effects a particular problem has on a patient.

action current   A current produced in a cell membrane of a nerve or muscle by the electrical activity in the tissue. This current serves to depolarize adjacent membrane areas and thereby initiates a repetition of the action potential along the nerve fiber.

action level   The level of concentration at which an undesirable or toxic component of a food is considered dangerous enough to public health to warrant government prohibition of the sale of that food. The United States Food and Drug Administration tests foods for action levels.

action potential   An electrical impulse consisting of a self-propagating series of polarizations and depolarizations, transmitted across the cell membranes of a nerve fiber during the transmission of a nerve impulse and across the cell membranes of a muscle cell during contraction or other activity of the cell.

activated charcoal   A gastrointestinal absorbent.

activated 7-dehydrocholesterol   See **cholecalciferol.**

activation factor   See **factor XII.**

activator   1. A substance, force, or device that stimulates activity in another substance or structure, especially a substance that activates an enzyme. 2. A substance that stimulates the development of an anatomical structure in the embryo. 3. An internal secretion of the pancreas. 4. An apparatus for making substances radioactive, as a cyclotron or neutron generator.

active algolagnia   See **sadism.**

active assisted exercise   The movement of the body or any of its parts primarily through the individual's own efforts but accompanied by the aid of a therapist or some other device, as an exercise machine. See also **exercise, passive exercise.**

active dental caries   Lesions of the teeth that prolapse toward the pulp.

active euthanasia   The killing of an individual suffering from an incurable illness or an irreparable injury, especially by administering a lethal drug. Also called **mercy killing, positive euthanasia.** Compare **passive euthanasia.**

active exercise   Repetitive movement of a part of the body as a result of voluntary contraction and relaxation of the controlling muscles. Compare **passive exercise.** See also **aerobic exercise, anaerobic exercise.**

active immunity   A form of acquired immunity that results from the production of antibodies in the cells. Antibodies develop naturally after infection or artificially after vaccination.

active movement   Muscular action at a joint owing to voluntary effort without outside help. Compare **passive movement.**

active play   Any activity from which one derives amusement, entertainment, enjoyment, or satisfaction by taking a participatory rather than a passive role. Children of all age groups engage in various forms of active play, from the exploration of objects and toys by the infant and toddler to the formal games, sports, and hobbies of the older child. Compare **passive play.**

active resistance exercise   The movement or exertion of the body or any of its parts

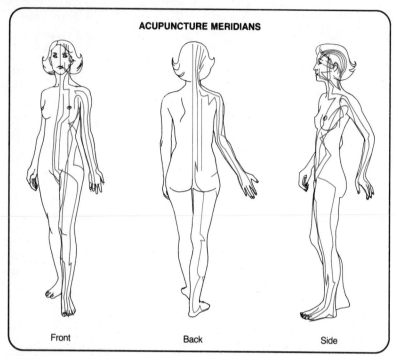

ACUPUNCTURE MERIDIANS

Front   Back   Side

performed totally through the individual's own efforts against a resisting force. See also **progressive resistance exercise.**

active site The place on the surface of an enzyme where its catalytic action occurs.

active transport The movement of materials across the membrane of a cell by means of chemical activity that allows the cell to admit larger molecules than would otherwise be able to enter. Expediting active transport are carrier molecules within the cell that bind themselves to incoming molecules, rotate around them, and disconnect, setting the incoming molecule free inside the cell wall. The entry of large molecules in the process of active transport disturbs the equilibrium of the internal environment of the cell, which compensates for the imbalance by releasing materials through its membrane. Active transport is the means by which the cell absorbs glucose and other substances needed to sustain life and health. Certain enzymes play a role in active transport, providing a chemical "pump" that helps move substances through the cell membrane. Compare **osmosis, passive transport.**

active treatment See **treatment.**

activities of daily living (ADL) The activities usually performed in the course of a normal day in the client's life, as eating, dressing, washing, or brushing the teeth.

ACTP *abbr* adrenocorticotropic polypeptide, a hydrolysate of ACTH (corticotropin).

actual cautery The application of heat, rather than a chemical substance, in the destruction of tissue.

actual charge The amount actually charged or billed by a medical practitioner for a service. The actual charge may not be the same as that paid for the service by an insurance plan.

actual damages See **damages.**

actualize The act of fulfilling a potential, as by a person who may develop capabilities through experience and education.

acu- **1.** A combining form meaning 'pertaining to a needle': *acuclosure, aculeate, acupressure.* **2.** A combining form meaning 'pertaining to hearing': *acuesthesia.* Also **acou-.**

acuminate wart See **condylomatum acuminatum.**

acupressure A therapeutic technique of applying digital pressure in a specified way on designated points on the body to relieve pain, produce anesthesia, or regulate a bodily function.

acupuncture A method of producing analgesia or altering the function of a system of the body by inserting fine, wire-thin needles into the skin at specific sites on the body along a series of lines, or channels, called meridians. The needles are twirled or energized electrically or warmed. Acupuncture originated in the Far East and has gained increasing attention in the West since the early 1970s. Research seeks to determine the usefulness of acupuncture and to understand the mechanisms by which it produces analgesia or alters sensory function. Some studies indicate that the analgesic effect of this technique is reversed by naloxone, suggesting that the release of enkephalin is significantly involved. See also **moxibustion.** **—acupuncturist,** *n.*

acupuncture point One of many discrete points on the skin along the several meridians, or chains of points of the body. Stimulation of any of the various points may induce an increase or decrease in function or sensation in an area or system of the body. The meridians are named and the points numbered to allow specific location of the points to be stimulated in acupuncture, acupressure, or moxibustion.

-acusis See **-acousia.**

acute **1.** Of a disease or disease symptoms: beginning abruptly with marked intensity or sharpness, then subsiding after a relatively short period of time. **2.** Sharp or severe. Compare **chronic.**

acute abdomen An abnormal condition characterized by the acute onset of severe pain within the abdominal cavity. An acute abdomen requires immediate evaluation and diagnosis, as it may indicate a condition that requires surgical intervention. Information about the onset, duration, character, location, and symptoms associated with the pain is critical in making an accurate diagnosis. Also called surgical abdomen.

acute alcoholism Drunkenness or intoxication resulting from excessive consumption of alcoholic beverages. The syndrome is temporary and is characterized by depression of the higher nervous centers, causing impaired motor control, stupor, lack of coordination, and often nausea, dehydration, headache, and other physical symptoms. Compare **chronic alcoholism.**

acute (angle-closure) glaucoma See **glaucoma.**

acute bacterial arthritis See **septic arthritis.**

acute care A pattern of health care in which a patient is treated for an acute episode of illness, for the sequelae of an accident or other trauma, or during recovery from surgery. Acute care is usually given in a hospital by specialized personnel using complex and sophisticated technical equipment and materials, and it may involve intensive care. This pattern of care is often necessary for only a short time, unlike chronic care.

acute childhood leukemia A progressive, malignant disease of the blood-forming tissues that is characterized by the uncontrolled proliferation of immature leukocytes and their precursors, particularly in the bone marrow, spleen, and lymph nodes. It is the most frequent cancer in children, with a peak onset occurring between the ages of 2 and 5 years. NURSING CONSIDERATIONS: Nursing care for the child with acute leukemia involves intensive physical and emotional support during all phases of the disease, its diagnosis, and treatment. Foremost is the preparation of the child and parents for the various diagnostic and therapeutic procedures, including venipuncture, bone marrow aspiration or biopsy, lumbar puncture, and X-ray treatment. Specific medical and nursing management depends on the particular regimen of drug therapy, although most of the chemotherapeutic agents used in treatment cause myelosuppression that may lead to secondary complications of infection, hemorrhage, and anemia. Overwhelming infection is a major problem and one of the most frequent causes of death. Severe neutropenia indicates increased risk of infection. It may occur during immunosuppressive therapy or after prolonged antibiotic therapy. To prevent infection, the nurse isolates the child as much as possible, screens visitors for active infection, institutes strict aseptic procedures, monitors temperature closely, evaluates possible sites of infection (as needle punctures), encourages adequate nutrition, and helps the child to avoid exertion or fatigue, and, at discharge, teaches the child and parents the necessity for avoiding all known sources of infection, primarily the common childhood communicable diseases. Preventive measures to control infection also help to decrease the tendency toward hemorrhage. Special attention is given to skin care, oral hygiene, cleanliness of the perineal area, and restriction of activities that could result in accidental injury. A major nursing consideration is the management of the many side effects resulting from drug toxicity and irradiation, including nausea and vomiting, anorexia, oral and rectal ulceration, alopecia, hemorrhagic cystitis, and peripheral neuropathy, including weakness and numbing of the extremities and severe jaw pain. Although corticosteroid treatment usually increases the appetite and produces a euphoric sense of well-being in the child, it also causes moon face, which is reversed with cessation of the steroid therapy. During maintenance therapy, the nurse continues to provide emotional support and guidance, specifically teaching parents which side effects are normal reactions to drugs and which indicate toxicity and require medical attention. In terminal stages of the disease, relief of discomfort and pain become the primary focus. Effective measures include careful physical handling of the child, frequent position changes, avoidance of pressure on painful areas, and control of annoying environmental factors, as excessive light and noise. Nonsalicylate analgesics are used as needed, depending on the severity of pain.

acute delirium An episode of delirium that is sudden, severe, and transient. See also **delirium.**

acute disease A disease characterized by a relatively short duration of symptoms that are usually severe. An episode of acute disease results in recovery to a state comparable to the patient's state of health and activity prior to the disease, in passage into a chronic phase, or in death. See also **chronic.**

acute epiglottitis, epiglottiditis A severe, rapidly progressing bacterial infection of the upper respiratory tract that occurs in young

ACUTE EPIGLOTTITIS CAUSING AIRWAY OBSTRUCTION

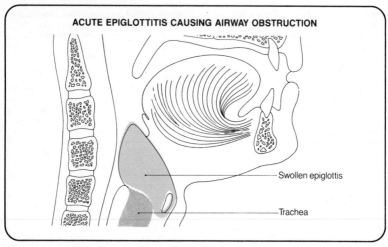

— Swollen epiglottis

— Trachea

children, primarily between the ages of 2 and 7. It is characterized by sore throat, croupy stridor, and an inflamed epiglottis, which may cause sudden respiratory obstruction and be quickly fatal. The infection is generally caused by *Hemophilus influenzae,* type B, although streptococci may occasionally be the causative agent. Transmission occurs by infection with airborne particles or contact with infected secretions. The diagnosis is made by bacteriologic identification of *H. influenzae,* type B, in a specimen taken from the upper respiratory tract or in the blood. An X-ray film of the neck from the side shows an enlarged epiglottis and distention of the hypopharynx, which distinguishes the condition from croup. Direct visualization of the inflamed, cherry-red epiglottis by depression of the tongue or indirect laryngoscopy is also diagnostic but may produce total acute obstruction and is attempted only by trained personnel with equipment to establish an airway or to provide respiratory resuscitation, if necessary.

NURSING CONSIDERATIONS: The nurse may assist intubation or tracheostomy once the diagnosis is confirmed. Intensive nursing care is required for a child with acute epiglottitis. Frequent changing of clothing and bed linen may be necessary to prevent chilling. The most acute phase of the condition passes within 24 to 48 hours and intubation is rarely needed beyond 3 to 4 days. As the child responds to therapy, breathing becomes easier, and there is usually rapid recovery so that bed rest and quiet activity to relieve boredom become primary nursing concerns. The infection may spread, causing such complications as otitis media, pneumonia, and bronchiolitis. Complications of the tracheostomy may also develop, including infection, atelectasis, cannula occlusion, tracheal bleeding, granulation, and stenosis, and delayed healing of the stoma.

acute febrile polyneuritis See **Guillain-Barré syndrome.**

acute glomerulonephritis A noninfectious disease of the glomerulus of the kidney that occurs following a streptococcal infection, most often in childhood. The symptoms are hematuria, proteinuria, decreased production of urine, and edema. Children usually recover completely; adults may develop scar tissue in the glomerulus and consequent decrease of renal function. Treatment may include limitation of dietary protein and sodium, diuretics, antihypertensives, and antibiotics. See also **chronic glomerulonephritis, subacute glomerulonephritis, uremia.**

acute hallucinatory paranoia A form of paranoia in which hallucinations are combined with systematized delusions. Also called **paranoia hallucinatoria.**

acute hallucinosis See **alcoholic hallucinosis.**

acute hemorrhagic leukoencephalitis See **acute necrotizing hemorrhagic encephalopathy.**

acute idiopathic polyneuritis See **Guillain-Barré syndrome.**

acute idiopathic thrombocytopenic purpura See **idiopathic thrombocytopenic purpura.**

acute laryngotracheobronchitis (LTB) See **croup.**

acute lymphoblastic leukemia See **acute lymphocytic leukemia.**

acute lymphocytic leukemia (ALL) A progressive, malignant disease characterized by large numbers of immature cells, closely resembling lymphoblasts, in the bone marrow, the circulating blood, the lymph nodes, the spleen, the liver, and other organs. The number of normal blood cells is reduced. About 80% of the 2,250 cases a year in the United States occur in children, with the greatest number diagnosed between the ages of 2 and 5. The risk of the disease is greatly increased for people with Down's syndrome and for siblings of leukemia patients. The disease has a sudden onset and rapid progression marked by fever, pallor, anorexia, fatigue, anemia, hemorrhage, bone pain, splenomegaly, and recurrent infection. Also called **acute lymphoblastic leukemia.** See also **acute childhood leukemia.**

acute myelocytic leukemia (AML) A malignant neoplasm of blood-forming tissues characterized by the uncontrolled proliferation of immature granular leukocytes that usually have azurophilic Auer rods in their cytoplasm. The typical symptoms, appearing abruptly or, more often, gradually, are spongy bleeding gums, anemia, fatigue, fever, dyspnea, moderate splenomegaly, joint and bone pains, and repeated infections. Chloromas (greenish granulocytic sarcomas) may develop in bone or soft tissue. AML may occur at any age, but it most frequently affects adolescents and young adults. The risk of the disease is increased among people who have been exposed to massive doses of radiation and among individuals with certain blood dyscrasias, as polycythemia vera, primary thrombocytopenia, and refractory anemia. Variants of AML, in which only one cell line proliferates, are erythroid, eosinophilic, basophilic, monocytic, and megakaryocytic leukemias. Also called **acute nonlymphocytic leukemia, granulocytic leukemia, myelogenous leukemia, myeloid leukemia, splenomedullary leukemia, splenomyelogenous leukemia.** See also **acute childhood leukemia.**

acute necrotizing gingivitis A fusospirochetal infection characterized by necrotic, foul-smelling ulcers of the gums and throat, fever, and enlarged lymph nodes in the neck. It is usually associated with poor oral hygiene and is most common in conditions in which there is crowding and malnutrition. Treatment includes peroxide mouth washes, antibiotics, metronidazole, and dental care. Also called **trench mouth, Vincent's angina, Vincent's infection.**

acute necrotizing hemorrhagic encephalopathy A degenerative disease of the brain, characterized by marked edema, numerous minute hemorrhages, necrosis of blood vessel walls, especially those of small veins, demyelination of nerve fibers, and infiltration of the meninges with neutrophils, lymphocytes, and histiocytes. Typical signs are severe headache, fever, and vomiting; convulsions may occur, and the patient may rapidly lose consciousness. Treatment consists of decompression by withdrawing cerebrospinal fluid and administration of large doses of steroids, but the disease is frequently fatal in 1 to 6 days. This kind of encephalopathy is thought to be caused by an immunologic mechanism, but the disease often resembles acute bacterial meningitis or herpes simplex encephalitis. Also called **acute hemorrhagic leukoencephalitis.**

acute nonlymphocytic leukemia See **acute myelocytic leukemia.**

acute pain Severe pain. Compare **chronic pain.** See also **pain intervention.**

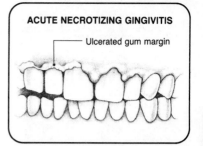

ACUTE NECROTIZING GINGIVITIS

Ulcerated gum margin

acute paranoid disorder A psychopathological condition characterized by a persecutory delusional system of rapid onset, quick development, and short duration, usually lasting less than 6 months. The disorder, which rarely becomes chronic, is most commonly seen in persons who have experienced drastic changes in their environment, such as immigrants, refugees, prisoners, military inductees, and, in a less severe form, those leaving home for the first time.

acute phase The active period in a disease when symptoms are pronounced.

acute promyelocytic leukemia A malignancy of the blood-forming tissues, characterized by severe bleeding, scattered bruises, a low fibrinogen level and platelet count, and the proliferation in bone marrow of promyelocytes and blast cells with distinctive Auer rods.

acute psychosis One of a group of disorders in which the ability to process information is diminished and disordered. The cause of the particular disorder may be a known physiologic abnormality. In other cases, the physiologic abnormality may not be recognized, but the defect in function is clearly present. Delirium and acute brain syndrome are associated with known pathophysiology in the brain and are characterized by disorientation, disturbance of memory, and lapses in consciousness. Acute functional psychosis is associated with unknown pathophysiology and varying signs and symptoms that progress from insomnia and agitation to paranoid or grandiose delusions, mania, emotional lability, and hallucinations.

acute pyogenic arthritis An acute bacterial infection affecting one or more joints, caused by trauma or a penetrating wound and occurring most frequently in children. Typical signs are pain, redness, and swelling in the affected joint, muscular spasms in the area, chills, fever, diaphoresis, and leukocytosis.

acute radial nerve palsy A type of mononeuropathy characterized by damage to the radial nerve and consequent weakening of the muscles of the forearm. It may be caused by excessive compression of the radial nerve against a hard surface in individuals insensitized by the intake of alcohol or sedatives. It may also be caused by the repeated compression of the nerve by weights.

acute radiation exposure Exposure of short duration to intense ionizing radiation,

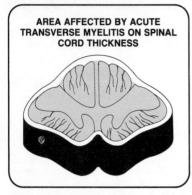

AREA AFFECTED BY ACUTE TRANSVERSE MYELITIS ON SPINAL CORD THICKNESS

usually occurring as the result of an accident in an industrial installation, in a nuclear power plant, or to a vehicle transporting radioactive material or from proximity to a detonated atom bomb. Exposure of the whole body to approximately 10,000 rads causes neurological and cardiovascular breakdown and is fatal within 24 hours. A dose between 500 and 1,200 rads destroys gastrointestinal mucosa, produces bloody diarrhea, and may cause death in several days. Death may occur weeks after exposure to a dose of 200 to 500 rads because of the destructive effect on blood-forming organs, but 600 rads is generally considered the fatal dose.

acute rheumatic arthritis Arthritis that occurs in the acute phase of rheumatic fever.

acute rickets See **infantile scurvy.**

acute schizophrenia A form of schizophrenia that is characterized by the sudden onset of personality disorganization with symptoms that include confusion, emotional turmoil, fear, depression, dreamlike dissociation, and bizarre behavior. Episodes appear suddenly in persons whose previous behavior has been relatively normal and are usually of short duration. Recurrent episodes are common, and, in some instances, a more chronic type of the disorder may develop. Also called **undifferentiated schizophrenia.** See also **schizophrenia, schizophreniform disorder.**

acute transverse myelitis An abnormal condition characterized by inflammation of the entire thickness of the spinal cord, affecting both the sensory and the motor nerves. It is the most destructive form of myelitis and can develop rapidly, accompanied by necrosis and neurologic disorder, which commonly persist after recovery. Patients who develop spastic reflexes soon after the onset of this disease are more likely to recover. This disorder may develop from a variety of causes, as acute multiple sclerosis, measles, pneumonia, and the ingestion of certain toxic agents, as carbon monoxide, lead, and arsenic. Such poisonous substances can destroy the entire circumference of the spinal cord, including the myelin sheaths, the axis cylinders, and the neurons, and can also cause hemorrhage and necrosis. There is no effective treatment and the

prognosis for complete recovery is poor. Any underlying infection is identified and treated accordingly. Some patients with myelitis induced by multiple sclerosis or by various infections have received steroid treatments, but the results of such therapy are inconclusive.

NURSING CONSIDERATIONS: Proper nursing care of the patient with acute transverse myelitis involves frequent assessment of vital signs and constant vigilance for any signs of spinal shock, as hypotension and profuse sweating. Foley catheters must be meticulously maintained to avoid urinary tract infections, and proper skin care is needed to prevent infections and decubitus ulcers. To prevent contractures nurses commonly assist the patient with range-of-motion exercises and assure that the patient is properly aligned. Also important, especially for the patients who develop paraplegia, are physical therapy, bowel and bladder training, and consistent instruction and encouragement throughout the rehabilitation period.

ACVD *abbr* **1.** atherosclerotic cardiovascular disease. **2.** arteriosclerotic cardiovascular disease.

-acy A combining form meaning a 'state or quality of': *anthropocracy, lunacy.*

acyclovir An antiviral agent.

acyesis **1.** The absence of pregnancy. **2.** A condition of sterility in women.

ad- A combining form meaning 'to, toward, addition to, or intensification': *adneural, adoral, adrenal.* Also **ac-, af-, ag-, ap-, as-, at-.**

-ad A combining form meaning 'toward (a specified terminus)': *anteriad, iniad, obeliad.*

A/D *abbr* analog-to-digital.

ADA *abbr* **1.** American Dental Association. **2.** American Diabetes Association. **3.** American Dietetic Association.

adactyly A congenital defect in which one or more digits of the hand or foot are missing.

adamantinoma See **ameloblastoma.**

adamantoblastoma See **ameloblastoma.**

Adam's apple The bulge at the front of the neck produced by the thyroid cartilage of the larynx *(colloquial).* Also called **laryngeal prominence.**

Adams-Stokes syndrome A condition characterized by sudden recurrent episodes of unconsciousness owing to incomplete heart block. Seizures may accompany the episodes. Also called **Stokes-Adams syndrome.**

adaptation A change or response to stress of any kind, as inflammation of the nasal mucosa in infectious rhinitis or an increase in crying in a frightened child. Adaptation may be normal, self-protective, and developmental, as a child learning to talk; it may be all-encompassing, creating further stress, such as polycythemia, naturally occurring at high altitudes, which provides more oxygen-carrying red blood cells but which may also lead to thrombosis, venous congestion, or edema. The degree and nature of adaptation shown by a patient is evaluated regularly by the nurse. It is a measure of the effectiveness of nursing care, the course of the disease, and the ability of the patient to cope with stress. See also **stress.**

adaptation model   In nursing: a conceptual framework that focuses on the patient as an adaptive system, one in which nursing intervention is required when a deficit develops in the patient's ability to cope with the internal and external demands of the environment. These demands are classified in four groups: physiologic needs, the need for a positive self-concept, the need to perform social roles, and the need to balance dependence and independence. The nurse assesses the patient's maladaptive response and identifies the kind of demand that is causing the problem. Nursing care is planned to promote adaptive responses in order to cope successfully with the current stress on the patient's well-being. This model is frequently used as a conceptual framework for programs of nursing education.

adaptation syndrome   See **general adaptation syndrome.**

adaptor RNA   See **transfer RNA.**

addict   A person with a strong physical or psychological dependence on a substance, habit, or practice, especially the use of drugs or alcohol.

addiction   Compulsive, uncontrollable dependence on a substance, habit, or practice to such a degree that cessation causes severe emotional, mental, or physiological reactions. Compare **habituation.**

Addis count   A method for counting red blood cells, white blood cells, epithelial cells, casts, and protein content in a sedimented 12-hour urine sample. Results are expressed as the number of each formed element excreted for each 24-hour period.

Addisonian anemia   See **pernicious anemia.**

Addisonian crisis   See **adrenal crisis.**

Addison's crisis   See **adrenal crisis.**

Addison's disease   A life-threatening condition caused by partial or complete failure of adrenocortical function, often owing to autoimmune processes, infection (especially tubercular or fungal), neoplasm, or hemorrhage in the gland. All three general functions of the adrenal cortex are lost: glucocorticoid, mineralocorticoid, and androgenic. Treatment includes replacement therapy with glucocorticoid and mineralocorticoid drugs, an adequate intake of fluids, control of sodium and potassium balance, and a diet high in carbohydrate and protein. The complications of Addison's disease include high fever, psychotic behavior, and adrenal crisis (Addisonian crisis). Under careful management, the patient's resistance to infection, capacity for work, and general well-being may be maintained. Nurses administer steroid and other drugs, observe the patient for signs of abnormal sodium and potassium levels, monitor body weight and fluid intake and output, and encourage an adequate intake of nutrients. The patient needs protection against stress while in the hospital and instruction in the importance

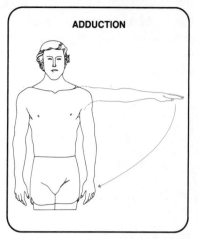

ADDUCTION

of avoiding stress at home. The significance of emotional distress, the value of wearing a medical-alert bracelet or tag, the signs of impending crisis, the use of a prepared kit for emergencies, and the importance of scrupulous attention to drug and diet regimens are emphasized before discharge. Discharge teaching also emphasizes the need to take cortisone after meals or with milk to avoid gastric irritation and the development of ulcers. Also called **Addisonism, Addison's syndrome.** See also **adrenal crisis, hypoadrenalism.**

Addison's keloid   A firm, white or pinkish patch of connective tissue on the skin, sometimes surrounded by a purplish areola. The lesion may involute, leaving a scar. Also called **circumscribed scleroderma, localized scleroderma, morphea.**

Addison's syndrome   See **Addison's disease.**

adduct   To draw any part of the body toward the midline or to draw the digits toward the axial line of the limb.

adduction   Movement of a limb toward the body. Compare **abduction.**

adductor   A muscle that acts to cause adduction. Compare **abductor, tensor.**

adductor brevis   A somewhat triangular muscle in the thigh and one of the five medial femoral muscles. Arising from the inferior ramus of the pubis, between the gracilis and the obturator externus, it passes downward, backward, and to the side to insert into the line leading from the lesser trochanter to the linea aspera of the femur. It is innervated by a branch of the obturator nerve, which contains fibers from the third and fourth lumbar nerves, and it acts to adduct and rotate the thigh medially and to flex the leg. Compare **adductor longus, adductor magnus, gracilis, pectineus.**

adductor canal   The triangular channel found beneath the sartorius muscle and between the adductor longus and vastus medialis through which the femoral vessels and the saphenous

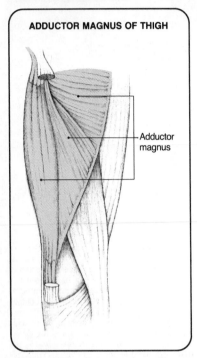

ADDUCTOR MAGNUS OF THIGH

Adductor magnus

nerve pass. Also called **Hunter's canal.**

adductor longus The most superficial of the three adductor muscles of the thigh and one of the five medial femoral muscles. A triangular muscle that arises from the anterior surface of the pubis, it spreads to form a broad fleshy belly, passing downward, backward, and to the side to insert into the linea aspera of the femur, between the vastus medialis and the adductor magnus. It is innervated by a branch of the obturator nerve, which contains fibers from the third and fourth lumbar nerves, and it functions to adduct and flex the thigh. Compare **adductor brevis, adductor magnus, gracilis, pectineus.**

adductor magnus The long, heavy triangular muscle of the medial aspect of the thigh. It arises from the inferior rami of the ischium and pubis and the inferior margin of the ischial tuberosity. The fibers of the muscle insert into the rough surface of the greater trochanter, into the linea aspera via a broad aponeurosis, and into the distal third of the femur via a rounded, thick tendon. The muscle is innervated by the obturator nerve, which contains fibers of the third and fourth lumbar nerves, and by a branch of the sciatic nerve. The adductor magnus acts to adduct the thigh. The proximal portion acts to rotate the thigh medially and to flex it on the hip; the distal portion acts to extend the thigh and rotate it laterally.

aden- See **adeno-.**

adenalgia A condition characterized by pain in any of the glands. Also called **adenodynia.**

adenectomy The surgical removal of any gland.

aden fever See **dengue.**

-adenia A combining form meaning '(condition of the) glands': *anadenia, heteradenia, poradenia.*

adenine arabinoside See **vidarabine.**

adenine-D-ribose See **adenosine.**

adenitis An inflammatory condition of a lymph node or gland. Acute adenitis of the cervical lymph nodes manifests itself as a sore throat and stiff neck, simulating mumps if severe. It is usually a sign of secondary infection related to an oral, pharyngeal, or ear infection. Scarlet fever may cause an acute suppurative cervical adenitis as may infectious mononucleosis. Swelling of the lymph nodes in the back of the neck is often the result of a scalp infection, insect bite, or infestation by head lice. Inflammation of the lymph nodes of the mesenteric portion of the peritoneum often produces pain and other symptoms similar to those of appendicitis. Mesenteric adenitis may be mistaken for appendicitis, but, characteristically, mesenteric adenitis is preceded by a respiratory infection, the pain is less localized and less constant than in appendicitis, and it does not increase in severity. Generalized adenitis is a secondary symptom of syphilis. Therapy requires treatment of the primary infection by the administration of antimicrobial agents, application of warm compresses and, in rare cases, incision and drainage. Compare **acinitis.**

adeno-, aden- A combining form meaning 'pertaining to a gland': *adenocarcinoma, adenocellulitis, adenofibrosis.*

adenoacanthoma A malignant neoplasm derived from glandular tissue with squamous differentiation shown by some of the cells.

adenoameloblastoma, *pl.* **adenoameloblastomas, adenoameloblastomata** A benign tumor of the maxilla composed of ducts lined with columnar or cuboidal epithelial cells. It develops in tissue that normally gives rise to the teeth, and it is most often seen in young people.

adenoassociated virus (AAV) A defective virus that can reproduce only in the presence of adenoviruses. It is not yet known what role, if any, these organisms have in causing disease.

adenocarcinoma, *pl.* **adenocarcinomas, adenocarcinomata** Any one of a large group of malignant, epithelial cell tumors of the glands. Specific tumors are diagnosed and named by cytologic identification of the tissue affected, as an adenocarcinoma of the uterine cervix is characterized by tumor cells resembling the glandular epithelium of the cervix. —**adenocarcinomatous,** *adj.*

adenocarcinoma in situ A localized growth of abnormal glandular tissue that may become malignant. It is most common in the endometrium and in the large intestine.

adenocarcinoma of the kidney See **renal cell carcinoma.**

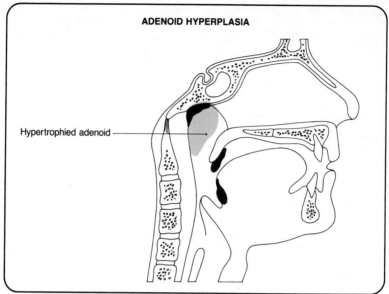

ADENOID HYPERPLASIA

Hypertrophied adenoid

---

adenocele A cystic, glandular tumor.

adenochondroma, *pl.* **adenochondromas, adenochondromata** A neoplasm of cells derived from glandular and cartilaginous tissues, as a mixed tumor of the salivary glands. Also called **chondroadenoma.**

adenocyst, adenocystoma, *pl.* **adenocystomas, adenocystomata** A benign epithelial tumor in which the cells form glandular structures and cysts. A kind of adenocystoma is **papillary adenocystoma lymphomatosum.**

adenocystic carcinoma A malignant neoplasm composed of cords of uniform small epithelial cells arranged in a sievelike pattern around cystic spaces which often contain mucus. The tumor occurs most frequently in the salivary glands, breast, mucous glands of the upper and lower respiratory tract, and, occasionally, in vestibular glands of the vulva. Although it grows slowly, it is malignant and tends to spread along the nerves, causing neurologic damage. Facial paralysis often results from adenocystic carcinoma of the salivary gland. Blood-borne metastases in bones and in the liver have been reported. Also called adenoid cystic carcinoma, **adenomyoepithelioma, cribriform carcinoma, cylindroma, cylindromatous carcinoma.**

adenocyte A mature secretory cell of a gland.

adenodynia See **adenalgia.**

adenoepithelioma, *pl.* **adenoepitheliomas, adenoepitheliomata** A neoplasm consisting of glandular and epithelial components.

adenofibroma, *pl.* **adenofibromas, adenofibromata** A tumor of the connective tissues that contains glandular elements. A kind of adenofibroma is **adenofibroma edematodes.**

adenofibroma edematodes A neoplasm consisting of glandular elements and connective tissue in which there is marked edema, as in a nasal polyp.

adenohypophysis The anterior lobe of the pituitary gland. It secretes growth hormone, thyrotropin, adrenocorticotropic hormone, melanin stimulating hormone, follicle stimulating hormone, luteinizing hormone, prolactin, beta lipotropin, and endorphins. Releasing hormones from the hypothalamus regulate secretion by the anterior pituitary. Adenohypophyseal hormones control activities of the thyroid, gonads, adrenal cortex, breast, and other endocrine glands. Also called **anterior pituitary.**

adenoid See **pharyngeal tonsil.** —**adenoidal,** *adj.*

adenoidal speech An abnormal manner of speaking caused by hypertrophy of the adenoidal tissue that normally exists in the nasopharynx of children. It is often characterized by a muted, nasal quality and may be corrected by a natural reduction of the swollen tissues or by surgical excision of the adenoids.

adenoidectomy Removal of the lymphoid tissue in the nasopharynx. The surgical procedure may be performed because the adenoids are enlarged, causing obstruction, or chronically infected, and normal adenoids may be excised as a prophylactic measure during tonsillectomy. See also **tonsillectomy.**

adenoid hyperplasia A condition in which enlarged adenoid glands cause partial respiratory obstruction, especially in children. Enlarged adenoids, often in association with enlarged tonsils, are a frequent cause of recurrent otitis media, sinusitis, and conduction deafness. Severe nasopharyngeal obstruction can result in alveolar hypoventilation and pulmonary hypertension with congestive heart failure. Treatment is usually surgical removal of the adenoids.

adenoleiomyofibroma, *pl.* **adenoleiomyofibromas, adenoleiomyofibromata** A benign tumor derived from smooth muscle with connective tissue and epithelial elements.

adenolipoma, *pl.* **adenolipomas, adenolipomata** A neoplasm consisting of elements of glandular and fatty tissue.

adenolipomatosis A condition characterized by the growth of numerous adenolipomas in the groin, axilla, and neck.

adenolymphoma, *pl.* **adenolymphomas, adenolymphomata** See **papillary adenocystoma lymphomatosum.**

adenoma, *pl.* **adenomas, adenomata** A benign tumor of glandular epithelium in which the cells of the tumor are arranged in a recognizable glandular structure. An adenoma may cause excess secretion by the affected gland, as acidophilic pituitary adenoma resulting in an excess of growth hormone. Kinds of adenomas include **acidophilic adenoma, basophilic adenoma, fibroadenoma, insulinoma.** —**adenomatous,** *adj.*

-adenoma A combining form meaning a 'tumor composed of glandular tissue or glandlike in structure': *sarcoadenoma, splenadenoma, syringadenoma.*

adenoma sebaceum An abnormal skin condition consisting of multiple, small, yellowish red, waxy papules on the face, composed chiefly of fibrovascular tissue. Adenoma sebaceum is part of the complex known as tuberous sclerosis.

adenomatoid Resembling a glandular tumor.

adenomatosis An abnormal condition in which hyperplasia or tumor development affects two or more endocrine glands, usually the thyroid, adrenals, or pituitary. Also called **multiple endocrine adenomatosis.**

adenomatous goiter An enlargement of the thyroid gland owing to an adenoma or numerous colloid nodules.

adenomyoepithelioma See **adenocystic carcinoma.**

adenomyofibroma, *pl.* **adenomyofibromas, adenomyofibromata** A fibrous tumor that contains glandular and muscular components.

adenomyoma, *pl.* **adenomyomas, adenomyomata** A tumor of the endometrium of the uterus, characterized by a mass of smooth muscle containing endometrial tissue and glands. It usually causes dysmenorrhea.

adenomyomatosis An abnormal condition characterized by the formation of benign nodules resembling adenomyomas, found in the uterus or in parauterine tissue.

adenomyosarcoma, *pl.* **adenomyosarcomas, adenomyosarcomata** A malignant tumor of soft tissue containing glandular elements and striated muscle. A kind of adenomyosarcoma is **Wilms' tumor.**

adenomyosis **1.** A benign neoplastic condition characterized by tumors composed of glandular tissue and smooth muscle cells. **2.** A malignant neoplastic condition characterized by the invasive growth of uterine mucosa in the wall of the uterus or the oviducts.

adenopathy An enlargement of any gland, especially a lymphatic gland. —**adenopathic,** *adj.*

adenosarcoma, *pl.* **adenosarcomas, adenosarcomata** A malignant glandular tumor of the soft tissues of the body.

adenosarcorhabdomyoma, *pl.* **adenosarcorhabdomyomas, adenosarcorhabdomyomata** A tumor composed of glandular elements, embryonal connective tissue, and striated muscle.

adenosine A compound derived from nucleic acid, composed of adenine and a sugar, D-ribose. Adenosine is the major molecular component of the nucleotides adenosine monophosphate, adenosine diphosphate, and adenosine triphosphate and of the nucleic acids deoxyribonucleic acid and ribonucleic acid. Also called **adenine-D-ribose.** See also **adenosine phosphate.**

adenosine 3′:5′-cyclic phosphate See **cyclic adenosine monophosphate.**

adenosine deaminase An enzyme that catalyzes the conversion of adenosine to the nucleoside inosine through the removal of an amino group. See also **adenosine.**

adenosine diphosphate A product of the hydrolysis of adenosine triphosphate.

adenosine hydrolase An enzyme that catalyzes the conversion of adenosine into adenine and pentose.

adenosine kinase An enzyme in the liver and kidney that catalyzes the transfer of a phosphate group from adenosine triphosphate to produce adenosine phosphate.

adenosine monophosphate (AMP) An ester, composed of adenine, D-ribose, and phosphoric acid, that affects energy release in work done by a muscle.

adenosine phosphate **1.** A compound consisting of the nucleotide adenosine attached through its ribose group to one, two, or three phosphoric acid molecules. Kinds of adenosine phosphate, all of which are interconvertible, are **adenosine diphosphate, adenosine monophosphate, adenosine triphosphate. 2.** A therapeutic adjunct for varicose veins and thrombophlebitis.

adenosine triphosphatase (ATPase) An enzyme that catalyzes the hydrolysis of adenosine triphosphate to adenosine diphosphate and inorganic phosphate. Among various enzymes in this group associated with cell membranes and intracellular structures, mitochondrial ATPase is involved in obtaining energy for cellular metabolism and myosin ATPase is involved in muscle contraction.

adenosine triphosphate (ATP) A nu-

MAJOR ADENOVIRAL INFECTIONS

DISEASE	AGE-GROUP	CLINICAL FEATURES
Acute febrile respiratory illness (AFRI)	Children	Nonspecific coldlike symptoms, similar to other viral respiratory illness: fever, pharyngitis, tracheitis, bronchitis, pneumonitis
Acute respiratory disease (ARD)	Adults (usually military recruits)	Malaise, fever, chills, headache, pharyngitis, hoarseness, and dry cough
Viral pneumonia	Children and adults	Sudden onset of high fever, rapid infection of upper and lower respiratory tracts, skin rash, diarrhea, intestinal intussusception
Acute pharyngoconjunctival fever (APC)	Children (particularly after swimming in pools or lakes)	Spiking fever lasting several days, headache, pharyngitis, conjunctivitis, rhinitis, cervical adenitis
Acute follicular conjunctivitis	Adults	Unilateral tearing and mucoid discharge; later, milder symptoms in other eye
Epidemic keratoconjunctivitis (EKC)	Adults	Unilateral or bilateral ocular redness and edema, preorbital swelling, local discomfort, superficial opacity of the cornea without ulceration
Hemorrhagic cystitis	Children (boys)	Adenoviruria, hematuria, dysuria, urinary frequency

cleotide compound present in all cells, where it represents energy storage in the form of high-energy phosphate bonds; free energy is released when **ATP** is hydrolyzed to **ADP** and a phosphate group.

adenosis **1.** A disease in any gland, especially a lymphatic gland. **2.** An abnormal development or enlargement of glandular tissue.

adenovirus Any one of the 31 medium-sized viruses of the Adenoviridae family, pathogenic to man, that cause conjunctivitis, upper respiratory infection, or gastrointestinal infection. After the acute and symptomatic period of illness, the virus may persist in a latent stage in the tonsils, adenoids, and other lymphoid tissue. —**adenoviral,** *adj.*

adenylate To convert a substance to adenylic acid.

adenylate kinase An enzyme in skeletal muscle, the heart, brain, and liver that activates hexokinase to make possible the transfer of phosphate from adenosine diphosphate to fructose or glucose. Also called **myokinase.**

adenylic acid See **adenosine monophosphate.**

adequate and well-controlled studies Clinical and laboratory studies that the sponsors of a new drug are required by law to conduct to demonstrate the truth of the claims made for its safety and effectiveness. See also **control.**

adermia A congenital or acquired skin defect or the absence of skin.

ADH *abbr* **antidiuretic hormone.**

adhere The act of sticking together or becoming fastened, as two surfaces that may be fastened with or as with glue.

adherence **1.** The quality of clinging or being closely attached. **2.** The process in which a person follows rules, guidelines, or standards, especially as a patient follows the prescription and recommendations for a regimen of care.

adhesion A band of scar tissue that binds together two anatomical surfaces which are normally separate from each other. Adhesions are most commonly found in the abdomen where they form following abdominal surgery, inflammation, or injury. A loop of intestine may adhere to unhealed areas and cause an intestinal obstruction if scar tissue develops and constricts the lumen of the bowel, blocking the intestinal flow. The condition is characterized by abdominal pain, nausea and vomiting, distention, and an increase in pulse rate without a rise in temperature. Nasogastric intubation and suction may relieve the blockage. If not, surgery may be necessary to separate adhering surfaces. See also **adhesiotomy, intestinal obstruction.**

adhesiotomy The surgical removal of adhesions, usually performed to relieve an intestinal obstruction. See also **abdominal surgery.**

adhesive absorbent dressing An absorbent dressing on an adhesive backing.

adhesive pericarditis A condition characterized by adhesions between the visceral and the parietal layers of the pericardium or by adhesions between the pericardium and the mediastinum, diaphragm, or chest wall. Adhesions between the pericardial layers may completely obstruct the pericardial cavity. Adhesive pericarditis may seriously impair normal movements of the heart.

adhesive peritonitis An inflammation of the peritoneum, characterized by adhesions between adjacent serous surfaces. This condition may be marked by exudations of serum, fibrin, cells, and pus, accompanied by abdominal pain and tenderness, vomiting, constipation, and fever.

adhesive plaster A strong fabric material covered on one side with an adhesive. Often water-repellent, it may be used to hold bandages and dressings in place, to immobilize a part, or to exert pressure. Also called **adhesive tape.**

adhesive pleurisy Inflammation of the pleura with exudation, causing obliteration of the pleural space through the fusion of the visceral pleural layer covering the lungs and the parietal layer lining the walls of the thoracic cavity.

adhesive skin traction One of two kinds of skin traction in which the therapeutic pull of traction weights is applied with adhesive straps that stick to the skin over the body structure involved, especially a fractured bone. Adhesive skin traction is used only when continuous traction is desired and skin care for the affected area presents no serious problem. The adhesive straps used to secure the traction system to the body area involved spread the pull over a wide area of skin, decreasing the vulnerability of the patient to skin breakdown. Compare **nonadhesive skin traction.**

ADI *abbr* **acceptable daily intake.**

adiathermance The quality of being unaffected by heat waves.

adient Characterized by a tendency to move toward rather than away from stimuli. Compare **abient. —adience,** *n.*

Adie's pupil See **Adie's syndrome.**

Adie's syndrome A pathological condition of the pupil, characterized by abnormal pupillary accommodation. In near vision, the affected pupil contracts and dilates slower than the pupil on the opposite side and does not usually react normally to direct and indirect light. Adie's syndrome is considered a pupillary muscle problem rather than a motor problem and does not indicate any neurological disease. Also called **Adie's pupil.**

adip- See **adipo-.**

adipectomy See **lipectomy.**

adipic Of or pertaining to fatty tissue.

adipo-, adip- A combining form meaning 'pertaining to fat': *adipocele, adipogenesis, adipokinin.*

adipocele A hernia containing fat or fatty tissue. Also called **lipocele.**

adipofibroma, *pl.* **adipofibromas, adipofibromata** A fibrous neoplasm of the connective tissue in which there are fatty components.

adiponecrosis A necrosis of fatty tissue in the body. **—adiponecrotic,** *adj.*

adiponecrosis subcutanea neonatorum An abnormal dermatolgic condition of the newborn characterized by patchy areas of hardened subcutaneous fatty tissue and a bluish-red discoloration of the overlying skin. The lesions, often a result of manipulation during delivery, spontaneously resolve within a period of days to several weeks without scarring. Also called **pseudosclerema, subcutaneous fat necrosis.**

adipose Fatty. Adipose tissue is composed of fat cells arranged in lobules. See also **fat, fatty acid, lipoma.**

adipose tumor See **lipoma.**

adiposogenital dystrophy A disorder occurring in adolescent boys, characterized by genital hypoplasia and feminine secondary sex characteristics, including female distribution of fat. It is caused by hypothalamic malfunction or by a tumor in the anterior pituitary gland. A subnormal body temperature, low blood pressure, and reduced blood sugar are frequently associated with the disorder. Diabetes insipidus often occurs because of hyposecretion of antidiuretic hormone, and involvement of the hypothalamic satiety center may induce overeating and result in pronounced obesity. If a tumor is present, there may be drowsiness and symptoms of increased intracranial pressure. Treatment may include the administration of testosterone and a weight reduction program, excision or radiologic ablation of a tumor, and replacement of hormones, as necessary. Also called **adiposogenital syndrome, Fröhlich's syndrome.**

adiposogenital syndrome See **adiposogenital dystrophy.**

aditus An approach or an entry.

adjunct In health care: an additional substance, treatment, or procedure used for increasing the efficacy or safety of the primary substance, treatment, or procedure or to facilitate its performance. **—adjunctive,** *adj.*

adjunctive psychotherapy A form of psychotherapy that concentrates on improving a person's general mental and physical outlook without trying to resolve basic emotional problems. Some kinds of adjunctive psychotherapy are **music therapy, occupational therapy, physical therapy, recreational therapy.**

adjunct to anesthesia One of a number of drugs of five different classes. Each class of drug has a use in anesthetic procedures, as well as a therapeutic indication in other aspects of health care. Adjuncts to anesthesia are used as premedications, as intravenous supplements to hypnotic or analgesic medications, and as neuromuscular blocking agents, analeptics, and therapeutic gases. Premedications are given to reduce anxiety, sedate the patient, reduce salivation and secretions of the respiratory passages, and prevent bradycardia. Strong analgesics, sedatives and hypnotics, phenothiazenes, anticholinergics, and antianxiety agents are also sometimes prescribed as premedications. Intravenous hypnotic and analgesic supplements, given to augment the effects of nitrous oxide, include morphine, meperidine, diazepam, fentanyl, and droperidol. Neuromuscular blocking agents are given to produce and sustain relaxation of the skeletal muscles during the surgical procedure. These agents are of two kinds: depolarizing or nondepolarizing. Depolarizing agents (including succinylcholine), act by depolarizing the postsynaptic membranes, rendering them refractory to stimulation and producing muscle paralysis. Nondepolarizing agents, including tubocurarine, metocurine, gallamine, and pancuronium, act by competing with acetylcholine for receptor sites on the postjunctional membrane, producing paralysis of the muscles. The use of these agents usually requires assisted or controlled respiration by an anesthetist or anesthesiologist and a careful evaluation of the recovery of neuromuscular transmission in the postoperative period.

adjusted death rate   See **standardized death rate.**

adjustment   See **accommodation.**

adjustment reaction   A temporary disorder of varying severity that occurs as an acute reaction to overwhelming stress in persons of any age who have no apparent underlying mental disorders. Symptoms include anxiety, withdrawal, depression, brooding, temper outbursts, crying spells, attention-getting behavior, enuresis, loss of appetite, aches, pains, and muscle spasms. It can result from such situations as separation of an infant from its mother, the birth of a sibling, loss or change of a job, death of a loved one, or forced retirement. Symptoms usually recede and eventually disappear as stress diminishes. See also **neurotic disorder.**

adjuvant therapy   1. The treatment of a disease with substances that enhance the action of drugs, especially drugs that promote the production of antibodies. 2. In oncology: the use of chemotherapy or radiation therapy in addition to surgery without clinical evidence of metastasis. The goal of therapy is to prevent recurring local or metastatic disease.

ADL   abbr **activities of daily living.**

administration of parenteral fluids   The intravenous infusion of various solutions to maintain adequate hydration, restore blood volume, reestablish lost electrolytes, or provide partial nutrition.

administrator   Overseer of the general effectiveness and efficiency of an agency, who is concerned with organization, planning, development, growth, change, operations, budgets, and evaluation.

adnexa, *sing.* **adnexus**   Tissue or structures in the body that are next to or near another related structure. The ovaries and the fallopian tubes are adnexa of the uterus. —**adnexal,** *adj.*

adolescence   1. The period in development between the onset of puberty and adulthood. It usually begins between the ages of 11 and 13, with the appearance of secondary sex characteristics, and spans the teen years, terminating between 18 and 20 years of age with the ac-

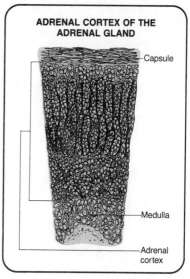

ADRENAL CORTEX OF THE ADRENAL GLAND

Capsule

Medulla

Adrenal cortex

quisition of completely developed adult form. During this period the individual undergoes extensive physical, psychological, emotional, and personality changes. 2. The state or quality of being adolescent or youthful. See also **postpuberty, prepuberty, psychosexual development, psychosocial development, pubarche.**

adolescent   1. Of, pertaining to, or characteristic of adolescence. 2. One in the state or process of adolescence; a teenager.

adolescent vertebral epiphysitis   See **Scheuermann's disease.**

ADP   abbr **adenosine diphosphate.**

adrenal cortex   The greater portion of the adrenal or suprarenal gland, fused with the gland's medulla and producing mineral corticoids, androgens, and glucocorticoids, hormones essential to homeostasis. The outer cortex is normally a deep yellow; the inner part, dark red or brown. It is recognizable in the embryo during the 6th week as a groove in the coelom at the base of the mesentery near the cranial end of the mesonephros.

adrenal cortical carcinoma   A malignant neoplasm of the adrenal cortex that may cause adrenogenital syndrome or Cushing's syndrome. Such tumors vary in size, occur at any age, and are more common in females than in males. Metastases frequently develop in the lungs, liver, and other organs. See also **adrenogenital syndrome, Cushing's syndrome.**

adrenal crisis   An acute, life-threatening state of profound adrenocortical insufficiency in which immediate therapy is required. It is characterized by glucocorticoid deficiency, a drop in extracellular fluid volume, and hyperkalemia. An intravenous isotonic solution of sodium chloride containing a water-soluble glucocorticoid is administered rapidly. Vasopressor agents may be necessary to combat hypotension. If the patient

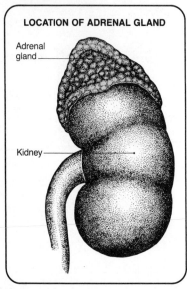

LOCATION OF ADRENAL GLAND

Adrenal gland

Kidney

is vomiting, a nasogastric tube is usually inserted. Total bed rest and the monitoring of blood pressure, temperature, and other vital signs are mandatory. After the first critical hours the patient is followed as for Addison's disease and steroid dosage is tapered to maintenance levels. In all cases the precipitating cause is sought. NURSING CONSIDERATIONS: Nursing care during adrenal crisis includes eliminating all forms of stimuli, especially loud noises or bright lights. The patient is not moved unless absolutely necessary and is not allowed to perform self-care activities. If the condition is identified and treated promptly, the prognosis is good. Discharge instructions include a reminder to the patient to seek medical attention in any stressful situation, whether physiologic or psychologic, in order to prevent a recurrence of the crisis. Also called **Addisonian crisis.** See also **Addison's disease, adrenal cortex.**

adrenalectomy The surgical removal of one or both adrenal glands or the resection of a portion of one or both glands, performed to reduce the excessive secretion of adrenal hormones when an adrenal tumor or a malignancy of the breast or prostate is present. The incision is made under the 12th rib in the rear flank area. Removal of both glands requires steroid replacement therapy. See also **Addison's disease, Cushing's syndrome.**

adrenal gland Either of two secretory organs perched atop the kidneys. Each consists of two parts having independent functions: the cortex and the medulla. The adrenal cortex, in response to adrenocorticotropic hormone secreted by the anterior pituitary, secretes cortisol and androgens. Adrenal androgens serve as precursors that are converted by the liver to testosterone and estrogens. Renin from the kidney controls

adrenal cortical production of aldosterone. The adrenal medulla manufactures the catecholamines epinephrine and norepinephrine.

adrenalize To stimulate or excite.

adrenal virilism The development in a female of male secondary sexual characteristics resulting from excessive production of androgenic hormones or to tumors of the ovary, as arrhenoblastoma, hilus cell tumor, or gynandroblastoma. Also called **virilization.**

adrenarche The intensified activity in the adrenal cortex that occurs at about 8 years of age and increases the elaboration of various hormones, especially androgens.

adrenergic **1.** Of or pertaining to sympathetic nerve fibers of the autonomic nervous system. **2.** Of or pertaining to drugs or hormones that mimic the effects of sympathetic stimulation. **3.** An adrenergic drug. Compare **cholinergic.**

adrenergic blocking agent See **antiadrenergic.**

adrenergic drug See **adrenergic.**

adrenergic fibers Nerve fibers of the autonomic nervous system that release the neurotransmitter norepinephrine. Most postganglionic sympathetic fibers are of this type.

adrenergic receptor A site in a sympathetic effector cell that reacts to adrenergic stimulation. Two types of adrenergic receptors are recognized: alpha-adrenergic receptors and beta-adrenergic receptors. In general, stimulation of alpha receptors is excitatory of the function of the host organ or tissue, and stimulation of the beta-receptors is inhibitory.

-adrenia A combining form meaning '(degree or condition of) adrenal activity': *anadrenia, dysadrenia, hypadrenia.*

adrenocorticotropic, adrenocorticotrophic Of or pertaining to stimulation of the adrenal cortex.

adrenocorticotropic hormone, adrenocorticotrophic hormone (ACTH) A hormone of the anterior pituitary gland that stimulates the growth of the adrenal gland and the secretion of corticosteroids. ACTH secretion, regulated by corticotropin releasing factor (CRF) from the hypothalamus, increases in response to a low level of circulating cortisol and to stress, fever, acute hypoglycemia, and major surgery. Under normal conditions there is a diurnal rhythm in ACTH secretion with an increase beginning after the first few hours of sleep and reaching a peak at the time a person awakens. ACTH stimulates the formation of cyclic adenosine monophosphate (AMP), which is thought to activate the enzyme system that catalyzes the conversion of cholesterol to pregnenolone, the precursor of all steroidal hormones. A purified preparation of ACTH in gelatin is widely used in the treatment of rheumatoid arthritis, acquired hemolytic anemia, intractable allergic states, various dermatologic diseases, and many other disorders. Also called **corticotropin.**

adrenodoxin A protein, produced by the adrenal glands, that participates in the transfer of electrons within animal cells.

adrenogenitalism A condition characterized by hypersecretion of adrenocortical androgens, resulting in somatic masculinization. Excessive production of the hormone may be caused by a virilizing adrenal tumor, congenital adrenal hyperplasia, or an inborn deficiency of enzymes required to transform endogenous androgenic steroids to glucocorticoids. See also **pseudohermaphroditism.**

adrenogenital syndrome An endocrine disorder resulting from abnormal activity of the adrenal cortex. Less than normal amounts of cortisol and more than normal amounts of androgen are produced, causing precocious puberty in boys and masculinization of the external genitalia in girls (pseudohermaphroditism). Most often congenital, the condition may be acquired in adulthood as a result of medication or a tumor that suppresses or stimulates the adrenal glands. Also called **congenital adrenal hyperplasia.** See also **adrenal virilism, pseudohermaphroditism.**

adromia The absence of the conductive capacity of any nerve that normally innervates a muscle.

adult 1. One who is fully developed and matured and who has attained the intellectual capacity and the emotional and psychological stability characteristic of a mature person. **2.** A person who has reached full legal age. Compare **child.**

adult celiac disease See **celiac disease.**

adulteration The debasement or dilution of the purity of any substance, process, or activity by the addition of extraneous material.

adult hemoglobin See **hemoglobin A.**

adult polycystic disease (APD) See **polycystic kidney disease.**

adult respiratory distress syndrome (ARDS) A set of symptoms including decreased compliance of lung tissue, pulmonary edema, and acute hypoxemia. It may be caused by shock, chest trauma, hemorrhage, repeated blood transfusions, disseminated intravascular coagulation, drug overdose, aspiration of gastric contents, or near drowning. The resultant physiologic chain of events leads to pulmonary hypoperfusion, edema, decreased surfactant production, and atelectasis. Treatment may include oxygen therapy by positive end-expiratory pressure (PEEP), mechanical ventilation with PEEP, fluid restriction, diuretics, and corticosteroids. Untreated initially, ARDS may cause death. NURSING CONSIDERATIONS: The symptoms and signs of ARDS include shortness of breath, rapid breathing, flail chest, inadequate oxygenation of the arterial blood, increase in arterial PCO_2 and a decrease in the arterial pH. The changes that occur within the lungs include damage to the membranes of the capillaries, hemorrhage, capillary leaking, interstitial edema, impairment in gas exchange, and ventilation-perfusion abnormalities. These sequelae lead to decreased compliance and increased dyspnea. The patient with ARDS requires constant and meticulous nursing

care, reassurance, and observation for changes in respiratory function and adequacy including signs of hypercapnia, especially comfusion, skin flushing, and behavior changes that include restlessness. Increasing hypoxia may be recognized by tachycardia, elevated blood pressure, and increased peripheral resistance; fulminant respiratory failure is accompanied by falling blood pressure and cyanosis. If PEEP is being used, be alert for sudden disappearance of breath sounds accompanied by signs of respiratory distress—an indication of pneumothorax. Adequate humidification, respiratory therapy, sterile suction techniques, hourly hyperinflation, and position changes are continued as necessary. Weight is taken frequently, X-ray films of the chest are taken and evaluated, and bacteriologic cultures of secretions are performed in the laboratory. Throughout treatment, ventilation is carefully monitored using blood gas studies and spirometry.

adult rickets A disease affecting adults that resembles rickets. See also **osteomalacia, rickets.**

advanced life support (ALS) See **Emergency Medical Technician-Advanced Life Support.**

adventitious Of or pertaining to an accidental condition or an arbitrary action.

adventitious bursa An abnormal bursa that develops as a response to friction or pressure.

adverse drug effect A harmful, unintended reaction to a drug administered at normal dosage.

adynamia Lack of physical and emotional drive owing to psychodynamic weakness. A kind of adynamia is **adynamia episodica hereditaria.** See also **asthenia. —adynamic,** *adj.*

adynamia episodica hereditaria A condition seen in infancy, characterized by muscle weakness and episodes of flaccid paralysis. It is inherited as an autosomal dominant trait. Also called **hyperkalemic periodic paralysis.**

adynamic fever An elevated temperature with a feeble pulse, nervous depression, and a cool, moist skin. Also called **asthenic fever.**

adynamic ileus See **ileus.**

Aedes A genus of mosquito, prevalent in tropical and subtropical regions. Several species are capable of transmitting pathogenic organisms to man, including dengue and yellow fever.

aer- See **aero-.**

aerate The act of charging a substance or a structure with air, carbon dioxide, or oxygen.

aero-, aer- A combining form meaning 'pertaining to air or to gas': *aerobe, aerocystography, aerodontalgia.*

Aerobacter aerogenes See ***Enterobacter cloacae.***

aerobe A microorganism that lives and grows in the presence of free oxygen. Kinds of aerobes are **facultative aerobe, obligate aerobe.** Compare **anaerobe. —aerobic,** *adj.*

aerobic exercise Mild to moderate muscular exertion below the level that produces met-

abolic acidosis. Compare **anaerobic exercise.**
See also **active exercise, passive exercise.**

aerobic glycolysis   See **glycolysis.**

aerobics   See **aerobic exercise.**

aerodontalgia   A painful sensation in the teeth owing to decreased atmospheric pressure, as may occur at high altitudes.

aeroembolism   See **embolism.**

aerophagy, aerophagia   The swallowing of air, usually followed by belching, gastric distress, and flatulence.

aerosinusitis   Inflammation, edema, or hemorrhage of the frontal sinuses, caused by expansion of air within the sinuses when barometric pressure is decreased, as in aircraft at high altitudes. Also called **barosinusitis.**

aerosol   **1.** Nebulized particles suspended in a gas or air. **2.** A pressurized gas containing a finely nebulized medication for inhalation therapy. **3.** A pressurized gas containing a nebulized chemical agent for sterilizing the air of a room.

aerotitis   An inflammation of the ear caused by changes in atmospheric pressure. Also called **barotitis.**

aerotitis media   Inflammation or bleeding in the middle ear owing to a difference between the air pressure in the middle ear and that of the atmosphere, as occurs in sudden changes in altitude, in diving, or in hyperbaric chambers. Symptoms are pain, tinnitus, diminished hearing, and vertigo. Also called **barotitis media.**

-aesthesia, -esthesia   A combining form meaning '(condition of) feeling, perception, or sensation': *allaesthesia, cinaesthesia, hypercryesthesia.*

-aesthetic   See **-esthetic.**

af-   See **ad-.**

afebrile   Without fever.

affect   An outward manifestation of a person's feelings or emotions. —**affective,** *adj.*

affective disorder   See **major affective disorder.**

affective melancholia   The depressive phase of bipolar disorder. See also **depression.**

affect memory   A particular emotional feeling that recurs whenever a significant experience is recalled.

afferent   Proceeding toward a center, as applied to arteries, veins, lymphatics, and nerves. Compare **efferent.**

affidavit   A written statement that is sworn to before a notary public or an officer of the court.

affiliated hospital   A hospital that is associated to some degree with a medical school or health program.

affirmative defense   In law: a denial of guilt or wrongdoing based on new evidence rather than on simple denial of a charge, as a plea of immunity according to a good samaritan law. The defendant bears the burden of proof in an affirmative defense.

afibrinogenemia   A rare, hematologic disorder characterized by a relative lack or absence of fibrinogen in the blood. It may be the result of a primary, congenital blood dyscrasia, or it may be acquired, as in disseminated intravascular coagulation.

African lymphoma   See **Burkitt's lymphoma.**

African sleeping sickness   See **African trypanosomiasis.**

African tick fever   See **relapsing fever.**

African trypanosomiasis   A disease caused by the parasites *Trypanosoma brucei gambiense* or *Trypanosoma brucei rhodesiense,* transmitted to humans by the bite of the tsetse fly. African trypanosomiasis occurs only in the tropical areas of Africa, where tsetse flies are found. The disease progresses through three phases: localized, at the site of invasion of the organism; systemic, marked by fever, chills, headache, anemia, edema of the hands and feet, and enlargement of the lymph glands; and neurologic, marked by symptoms of central nervous system involvement, including lethargy, sleepiness, headache, convulsions, and coma. The disease is fatal unless treated, though it may be years before the patient reaches the neurologic phase. Antimicrobial medication specific for the treatment of trypanosomiasis is available in the United States only from the Centers for Disease Control. Kinds of African trypanosomiasis are **Gambian trypanosomiasis, Rhodesian trypanosomiasis.** Also called **African sleeping sickness, sleeping sickness.** See also **trypanosomiasis, tsetse fly.**

afterbirth   The tissue, fluid, and blood expelled from the uterus after childbirth, including the placenta, the amnion and the chorion, and some amniotic fluid, blood, and blood clots.

afterloading   In radiotherapy: a technique in which an unloaded applicator or needle is placed within the patient at the time of an operative procedure and subsequently loaded with the radioactive source under controlled conditions in which health-care personnel are protected against exposure to radiation. A kind of afterloading is **remote afterloading.**

afterpains   Contractions of the uterus common during the first days postpartum. They tend to be strongest in nursing mothers and multiparas, resolve spontaneously, and rarely require analgesia. The nurse may reassure the mother that afterpains are normal and prove that the uterus is contracting as it should.

Ag   Symbol for **silver.**

ag-   See **ad-.**

AGA   *abbr* **appropriate-for-gestational-age.**

agamete   **1.** Any of the unicellular organisms that reproduce asexually by multiple fission, such as bacteria and protozoa. **2.** Any asexual reproductive cell, as a spore or merozoite, that forms a new organism without fusion with another cell.

agametic, agamous   Asexual; without recognizable sex organs or gametes.

agamic   Reproducing asexually, without the union of gametes; asexual.

agammaglobulinemia   A rare disorder characterized by the absence of the serum immunoglobulin, gamma globulin, associated with an increased susceptibility to infection. The condition may be transient, congenital, or acquired. The transient form is common in infancy before 6 weeks of age when the infant becomes able to synthesize the immunoglobulin. The congenital form is rare, sex-linked, and results in decreased production of antibodies. The acquired form usually occurs in association with a malignant disease, such as leukemia, myeloma, or lymphoma. See also **Bruton's agammaglobulinemia.**

agamocytogeny   See **agamogenesis.** —**agamocytogenic,** *adj.*

agamogenesis   Asexual reproduction, as by budding or simple fission of cells; parthenogenesis. Also called **agamocytogeny, agamogony.** —**agamogenetic, agamogenic,** *adj.*

agamogony   See **agamogenesis.** —**agamogonic,** *adj.*

agamont   See **schizont.**

agamous   See **agametic.**

agar-agar   A dried hydrophilic, colloidal product obtained from certain species of red algae. Because it is unaffected by bacterial enzymes, it is widely used as the basic ingredient in solid culture media in bacteriology. Agaragar is also used as a suspending medium, as an emulsifying agent, and as a bulk laxative. Also called **agar.**

agency   In law: a relationship between two parties in which the first party authorizes the second to act as agent on behalf of the first. It usually implies a contractual arrangement between two parties managed by a third party, the agent.

agenesia corticalis   The failure of the cortical cells of the brain, especially the pyramidal cells, to develop in the embryo, resulting in infantile cerebral paralysis and severe mental retardation.

agenesis, agenesia   **1.** Congenital absence of an organ or part, usually caused by a lack of primordial tissue and failure of development in the embryo. **2.** Impotence or sterility. Compare **dysgenesis.** —**agenic,** *adj.*

agenetic fracture   A spontaneous fracture owing to an imperfect osteogenesis.

ageniocephaly, ageniocephalia   A form of otocephaly in which the brain, cranial vault, and sense organs are intact but the lower jaw is malformed. —**ageniocephalic, ageniocephalous,** *adj.*

agenitalism   A symptom complex owing to the lack of the secretion of the sex hormones, caused by the absence or malfunction of the ovaries or testes.

agenosomia   A congenital malformation characterized by the absence or defective formation of the genitals and protrusion of the intestines through an incompletely developed abdominal wall.

agenosomus   A fetus with agenosomia.

agent   In law: a party authorized to act on behalf of another and to give the other an account of such actions. —**agency,** *n.*

age of majority   The age at which a person is considered to be an adult in the eyes of the law.

agglutination   The aggregation or clumping together of insoluble particles as a result of their interaction with specific antibodies called agglutinins, commonly used in blood typing and in identifying or estimating the strength of immunoglobulins or immune sera. See also **agglutinin, blood typing, precipitin.**

agglutination inhibition test   A serologic technique useful in testing for certain unknown soluble antigens. The unknown antigen is mixed with a known agglutinin. If there is a reaction, the agglutinin can no longer agglutinate the cells or particles that carry its corresponding antigen, and the unknown antigen is thus identified. One type of pregnancy test is based on agglutination inhibition.

agglutinin   A specific kind of antibody whose interaction with antigens is manifested as agglutination. Usually multivalent, agglutinins act on insoluble antigens in stable suspension to form a cross-linking lattice that may clump or precipitate. Compare **precipitin.** See also **agglutination, blood typing, hemagglutination.**

agglutinin absorption   The removal from immune serum of an antibody by treatment with homologous antigen, followed by the centrifugation and separation of the antigen-antibody complex.

agglutinogen   Any antigenic substance that causes agglutination by the production of agglutinin.

aggregate anaphylaxis   An exaggerated reaction of hypersensitivity rapidly induced by the injection of an antigen that forms a soluble antigen-antibody complex.

aggression   A forceful, self-assertive action or attitude that is expressed physically, verbally, or symbolically. It may arise from innate drives or occur as a defense mechanism and is manifested by either constructive or destructive acts directed toward oneself or against others. Kinds of aggression are **constructive aggression, destructive aggression, inward aggression.**

aggressive personality   A personality with behavior patterns characterized by irritability, tantrums, destructiveness, or violence in response to frustration.

aging   The process of growing old, owing in part to a failure of body cells to function normally or to produce new body cells to replace those which are dead or malfunctioning. Normal cell function may be lost through infectious disease, malnutrition, exposure to environmental hazards, or genetic influences. Among body cells that exhibit early signs of aging are those which normally cease dividing after reaching maturity. See also **senile.**

agitated   Describing a condition of psychomotor excitement characterized by purposeless, restless activity. Pacing, crying, and laughing without apparent cause are often exhibited and may serve to release nervous tension associated with anxiety, fear, or other mental stress.

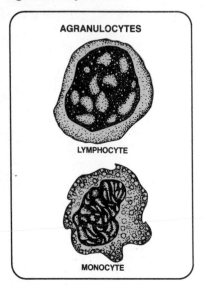

AGRANULOCYTES

LYMPHOCYTE

MONOCYTE

—**agitate,** v., **agitation,** n.
agitated depression A form of depression characterized by severe anxiety accompanied by continuous physical restlessness. See also **depression.**

agitographia A condition characterized by abnormally rapid writing in which words or parts of words are unconsciously omitted. The condition is commonly associated with agitophasia.

agitolalia See **agitophasia.**

agitophasia A condition characterized by abnormally rapid speech in which words, sounds, or syllables are unconsciously omitted, slurred, or distorted. The condition is commonly associated with agitographia. Also called **agitolalia.**

agnathia, agnathy A developmental defect characterized by total or partial absence of the lower jaw. It is usually accompanied by the union or approximation of the ears. Compare **synotia.** See also **otocephaly.** —**agnathous,** adj.

agnathocephalus A fetus with agnathocephaly.

agnathocephaly, agnathocephalia A congenital malformation characterized by the absence of the lower jaw, defective formation of the mouth, and placement of the eyes low on the face with fusion or approximation of the zygomas and the ears. See also **otocephaly.** —**agnathocephalic, agnathocephalous,** adj.

agnathus A fetus with agnathia.

agnogenic myeloid metaplasia See **myeloid metaplasia.**

agnosia Total or partial loss of the ability to recognize familiar objects or persons through sensory stimuli as a result of organic brain damage. The condition may affect any of the senses and is classified accordingly as auditory, visual, olfactory, gustatory, or tactile agnosia. Also called agnosis. See also **autotopagnosia.**

-agnosia A combining form meaning '(condition of the) loss of the faculty to perceive': autotopagnosia, fingeragnosia, paragnosia. Also **-agnosis.**

-agogue, -agog A combining form meaning an 'agent promoting the expulsion of a (specified) substance': lymphagogue, succagogue, uragogue.

agonal thrombus An aggregation of blood platelets, fibrin, clotting factors, and cellular elements that forms in the heart in the process of dying.

agonist **1.** A contracting muscle whose contraction is opposed by another muscle (an antagonist). **2.** A drug or other substance having a specific cellular affinity that produces a predictable response.

agoraphobia An anxiety disorder characterized by a fear of being in an open, crowded, or public place, as a field, tunnel, bridge, congested street, or busy department store, where escape may be difficult or help not available in case of sudden incapacitation. The obsessive phenomenon is observed more often in women than in men and generally can be traced to some sudden loss or separation occurring in childhood. Treatment consists of psychotherapy to uncover the cause of the phobic reaction followed by behavior therapy, specifically the systemic desensitization and flooding techniques for reducing the anxiety and altering the behavioral response. If untreated, fear and avoidance behavior dominate life, and the person refuses to leave home. See also **phobia.**

-agra A combining form meaning a 'pain or painful seizure': cardiagra, podagra, trachelagra.

agranular endoplasmic reticulum See **endoplasmic reticulum.**

agranulocyte Any leukocyte that does not contain cytoplasmic granules, as a monocyte or lymphocyte. Compare **granulocyte.** See also **leukocyte.**

agranulocytosis An abnormal condition of the blood, characterized by a severe reduction in the number of granulocytes (basophils, eosinophils, and neutrophils), resulting in fever, prostration, and bleeding ulcers of the rectum, mouth, and vagina. It is an acute disease and may be an adverse reaction to a medication or the result of radiation therapy.

agraphia An abnormal neurologic condition characterized by loss of the ability to write, resulting from injury to the language center in the cerebral cortex. —**agraphic,** adj.

agrypnia See **insomnia.**

agrypnotic **1.** Insomniac. **2.** A drug or other substance that prevents sleep.

AHA abbr American Hospital Association.

"aha" reaction In psychology: a sudden realization or inspiration, experienced especially during creative thinking. Some psychologists associate great scientific discoveries and artistic inspirations with this reaction, which is not necessarily related to intelligence. The term has apparently replaced aha experience, for-

AIRWAY OBSTRUCTION

FIRST-DEGREE OBSTRUCTION	SECOND-DEGREE OBSTRUCTION	COMPLETE OBSTRUCTION

Foreign body

Inhalation   Expiration

merly used by psychologists, especially those of the Gestalt school, to label experiences in which an individual utters "Aha!" during a moment of revelation.

AHF *abbr* **antihemophilic factor.**

AHH *abbr* **aryl hydrocarbon hydroxylase.**

AI *abbr* **artificial intelligence.**

AID *abbr* **artificial insemination donor.**

AIDS *abbr* **acquired immune deficiency syndrome.**

AIH *abbr* **artificial insemination husband.**

ainhum A pathologic condition of unknown cause that occurs chiefly in the dark-skinned races. Most commonly affecting the fourth or fifth toes, the condition is marked by a fibrous band of tissue that causes a fissured constriction and eventually causes autoamputation of the digit.

air The colorless, odorless gaseous mixture constituting the earth's atmosphere. It consists of 78% nitrogen; 21% oxygen; almost 1% argon; small amounts of carbon dioxide, hydrogen, and ozone; traces of helium, krypton, neon, and xenon; and varying amounts of water vapor.

air bath The exposure of the naked body to warm air for therapeutic purposes. Also called **balneum pneumaticum.**

air cells of the nose See **nasal sinus.**

air conditioner lung See **humidifier lung.**

air embolism The abnormal presence of air in the cardiovascular system, resulting in obstruction of the flow of blood through the vessel. Air may be inadvertently introduced by injection, during intravenous therapy or surgery, or traumatically, as by a puncture wound. See also **decompression sickness, embolus, gas embolism.**

air encephalography See **encephalography.**

airplane splint A splint used for immobilizing a fractured humerus during healing. The splint holds the arm in an abducted position at shoulder level, with the elbow bent. It extends to the waist and may be made of wire or leather, or it may be supported by a plaster body.

air pump A pump that forces air in or out of a cavity or chamber.

air sickness See **motion sickness.**

air thermometer A thermometer using air instead of mercury or alcohol as its expansible medium. See **thermometer.**

airway clearance, ineffective A nursing diagnosis accepted by the Fifth National Conference on the Classification of Nursing Diagnoses. The etiology of the problem is decreased energy or fatigue, infection, obstruction, or secretions of the tracheobronchial tree, perceptual or cognitive impairment, or trauma. The defining characteristics of the condition include abnormal breath sounds, change in the rate or depth of respiration, tachypnea, cough, cyanosis, and dyspnea. See also **nursing diagnosis.**

airway obstruction A mechanical impediment to oxygen delivery or absorption in the lungs, as in bronchospasm, choking, croup, laryngospasm, chronic obstructive lung disease, goiter, tumor, pneumothorax, or the presence of a foreign object.

NURSING CONSIDERATIONS: Acute airway obstruction requires rapid intervention to save the person's life. A bolus of food, a collection of mucus, or a foreign body may be removed manually, by suction, or with the Heimlich maneuver. Obstruction of the airway owing to inflammatory or allergic reaction may be treated with bronchodilating drugs, corticosteroids, intubation, and the administration of oxygen. An emergency tracheotomy may be required if the obstruction cannot be mechanically removed or pharmacologically reduced within a few minutes. See also **aspiration, cardiopulmonary resuscitation, Heimlich maneuver.**

akathisia An abnormal condition characterized by restlessness and agitation, as seen in tardive dyskinesia. —**akathisiac,** *adj.*

akinesia An abnormal state of motor and psychic hypoactivity or muscular paralysis. —**akinetic,** *adj.*

akinetic apraxia The inability to perform a spontaneous movement. See also **apraxia.**

akinetic mutism A state in which a person is unable or refuses to move or to make sounds, resulting from neurological or psychological disturbance.

-akusis See **-acousia.**

Al Symbol for **aluminum.**

-al¹, -ale A combining form meaning 'pertaining to or characterized by': *appendiceal, calyceal, meningeal.*

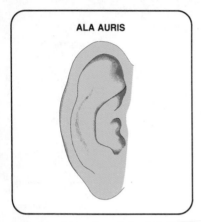

ALA AURIS

-al² A combining form designating a compound containing a member of the aldehyde group: *benzal, chloral, ethanal.*

ala, *pl.* **alae** 1. Any winglike structure. 2. The axilla.

ala auris The auricle of the ear.

ala cerebelli The ala of the central lobule of the cerebellum.

ala cinerea The triangular area on the floor of the fourth ventricle of the brain from which the autonomic fibers of the vagus nerve arise.

ala nasi The outer flaring cartilaginous wall of each nostril.

Al-Anon An international organization that offers guidance and counseling for the relatives, friends, and associates of alcoholics. See also **Alcoholics Anonymous.**

ala of the ethmoid A small projection on each side of the crista galli of the ethmoid bone. Each ala fits into a corresponding depression of the frontal bone.

ala of the ilium The upper flaring portion of the iliac bone.

ala of the sacrum The flat extension of bone on each side of the sacrum.

alar ligament One of a pair of ligaments that connect the axis to the occipital bone and limit rotation of the cranium. Also called **check ligament, odontoid ligament.** Compare **membrana tectoria.**

alarm reaction The first stage of the general adaptation syndrome, characterized by the mobilization of the various defense mechanisms of the body or the mind to cope with a stressful situation of a physical or emotional nature. See also **stress.**

alastrim A mild form of smallpox, thought to be caused by a weak strain of *Poxvirus variolae.* Unlike smallpox, alastrim is rarely fatal. Also called **Cuban itch, milkpox, variola minor.** See also **smallpox.**

Alateen An international organization that offers guidance and counseling for the children of alcoholics. See also **Alcoholics Anonymous.**

ala vomeris An extension of bone on each side of the upper border of the vomer.

alb- A combining form meaning 'white': *albedo, albugo, albumen.*

alba *Latin.* 'White,' as in linea alba.

Albers-Schönberg disease See **osteopetrosis.**

albinism An abnormal congenital condition characterized by partial or total lack of melanin pigment in the body. Total albinos have pale skin that does not tan, white hair, pink eyes, nystagmus, astigmatism, and photophobia. Albinos are prone to severe sunburn, actinic dermatitis, and skin cancer.

Albright's syndrome A disorder characterized by fibrous dysplasia of bone, isolated brown macules on the skin, and endocrine dysfunction. It causes precocious puberty in girls but not in boys. The osseous lesions are reddish-gray, gritty fibromas containing areas of coarse fiber that may be confined to one bone or occur in several, frequently causing deformities. Hyperthyroidism is present in some cases. Treatment may involve osteotomy, curettage, and bone grafts. Also called **Albright-McCune-Sternberg syndrome, osteitis fibrosa disseminata.**

albumin A water-soluble, heat-coagulable protein containing carbon, hydrogen, oxygen, nitrogen, and sulfur. Various albumins are found in practically all animal tissues and in many plant tissues. Determination of the levels and kinds of albumin in urine, blood, and other body tissues is the basis of a number of laboratory diagnostic tests.

albumin A A blood serum constituent that gathers in cancer cells but is deficient in circulation in cancer patients.

albumin (human) A plasma-volume expander.

albuminuria See **proteinuria.**

-albuminuria A combining form meaning a '(specified) condition characterized by excess serum proteins in the urine': *noctalbuminuria, nyctalbuminuria, pseudalbuminuria.*

albuterol A bronchodilator sympathomimetic agent.

Alcock's canal A canal formed by the obturator internus muscle and the obturator fascia through which the pudendal vessels and nerve pass. Also called **pudendal canal.**

alcohol 1. U.S.P.: a preparation containing at least 92.3% and not more than 93.8% by weight of ethyl alcohol, used as a topical antiseptic and solvent. 2. A clear, colorless, volatile liquid that is miscible with water, chloroform, or ether, obtained by the fermentation of carbohydrates with yeast. 3. A compound derived from a hydrocarbon by replacing one or more hydrogen atoms with an equal number of hydroxyl (OH) groups. Depending on the number of hydroxyl radicals, alcohols are classified as monohydric, dihydric, trihydric. Some kinds of alcohol are **rubbing alcohol, sugar alcohol, unsaturated alcohol.**

alcohol bath A procedure for decreasing an elevated body temperature. A tepid solution of 25% to 50% alcohol in water is sponged lightly on each limb, then on the trunk, turning the person only once from supine to prone position and then back again. Some sources recommend the placement of a hot-water bottle at the feet and a cold compress on the head to accelerate heat loss through vasodilation, to promote the comfort of the patient during the procedure, and to reduce the temperature of the circulation to the brain. As the alcohol evaporates quickly, the bed is less likely to get wet, the patient does not need to be dried, and, for an equal result, the solution does not need to be as cold as a plain bath with cold water.

alcoholic cirrhosis See **cirrhosis**.

alcoholic fermentation The conversion of carbohydrates to ethyl alcohol.

alcoholic hallucinosis A form of alcoholic psychosis characterized primarily by auditory hallucinations, abject fear, and delusions of persecution. The condition develops in acute alcoholism shortly after stopping or reducing the intake of alcohol. Also called **acute hallucinosis.** See also **alcoholic psychosis, hallucination.**

alcoholic-nutritional cerebellar degeneration A sudden, severe incoordination in the lower extremity, characteristic of poorly nourished alcoholics. The patient walks, if at all, with an ataxic or wide-based gait. It is important to distinguish between this condition and cerebellar tumors, multiple sclerosis, and other neurologic disorders that have similar motor impairments. Treatment consists of improved nutrition, abstinence from alcohol, and physical therapy. Also called **cerebellar cortical degeneration.** See also **alcoholism.**

alcoholic paranoia Paranoia associated with chronic alcoholism.

alcoholic psychosis Any of a group of severe mental disorders, such as pathological intoxication, delirium tremens, Korsakoff's psychosis, and acute hallucinosis, characterized by brain damage or dysfunction that results from the excessive use of alcohol.

Alcoholics Anonymous (AA) An international nonprofit organization, founded in 1935, consisting of abstinent alcoholics whose purpose is to help alcoholics stop drinking and maintain sobriety through group support, shared experiences, and faith in a power greater than themselves. The AA program, which emphasizes both medical and religious resources for help in overcoming alcoholism, consists of attending meetings and coping with abstinence "one day at a time." Meetings are held at convenient times in factories, schools, churches, hospitals, and many other institutions and community buildings. Similar groups who work with the children, relatives, friends, and associates of alcoholics are Al-Anon and Alateen.

alcoholic trance A state of automatism resulting from intoxication.

alcoholism The extreme dependence on excessive amounts of alcohol, associated with a cumulative pattern of deviant behaviors. Alcoholism is a chronic illness with a slow, insidious

onset, which may occur at any age. The etiology is unknown, but cultural and psychosocial factors are suspect, and families of alcoholics have a higher incidence of alcoholism. Frequent intoxication has cumulative destructive effects on an individual's family and social life, working life, and physical health. The most frequent medical consequences of alcoholism are central nervous system depression and cirrhosis of the liver. The severity of each of these is increased in the absence of food intake. Alcoholic patients also may suffer from alcoholic gastritis, peripheral neuropathies, auditory hallucinations, and cardiac problems. Abrupt withdrawal of alcohol in addiction causes weakness, sweating, and hyperreflexia. The severe form of alcohol withdrawal is called delirium tremens. Extreme caution should be used in administering drugs to the alcoholic patient because of the possibility of additive central nervous system depression. The treatment of alcoholism consists of psychotherapy (especially group therapy, by organizations like Alcoholics Anonymous), electroshock treatments, or drugs that cause an aversion to alcohol. See also **delirium tremens.**

alcohol poisoning Poisoning caused by the ingestion of any of several alcohols, of which ethyl, isopropyl, and methyl are the most common. Ethyl alcohol (grain alcohol) is found in whiskies, brandy, gin, and other beverages. Ordinarily, it is lethal only if large quantities are ingested in a brief period. Isopropyl alcohol is more toxic: ingestion of 236 ml (8 oz) may result in respiratory or circulatory failure. Methyl alcohol (wood alcohol) is extremely poisonous: in addition to nausea, vomiting, and abdominal pain, it may cause blindness, and death may follow the consumption of only 59 ml (2 oz).

aldolase An enzyme found in muscle tissue that catalyzes the step in anaerobic glycolysis involving the breakdown of fructose 1,6-diphosphate to glyceraldehyde 3-phosphate. The enzyme can also catalyze the reverse reaction. See also **glycolysis.**

aldosterone A steroid hormone produced by the adrenal cortex that regulates sodium and potassium balance in the blood.

aldosteronism A condition characterized by hypersecretion of aldosterone, occurring as a primary disease of the adrenal cortex or, more often, as a secondary disorder in response to various extra-adrenal pathologic processes. Primary aldosteronism may be caused by adrenal hyperplasia or by an aldosterone-secreting tumor, as in Conn's syndrome. Secondary aldosteronism is associated with increased plasma renin activity and may be induced by the nephrotic syndrome, hepatic cirrhosis, idiopathic edema, congestive heart failure, trauma, burns, or other kinds of stress. Hypersecretion of aldosterone promotes sodium retention and potassium excretion, leading to increased blood volume and blood pressure, alkalosis, muscular weakness, tetany, paresthesias, nephropathy, ventricular arrhythmias, and other cardiac abnormalities. The electrolyte imbalance in aldosteronism usually causes polydipsia and polyuria. Treatment of primary aldosteronism caused by a tumor may include surgical resection and chemotherapy with the adrenal cytotoxic agent mitotane. Spironolactone, an aldosterone antagonist, is frequently used to treat symptoms of aldosteronism. Also called **hyperaldosteronism.**

aldosteronoma, *pl.* **aldosteronomas, aldosteronomata**   An aldosterone-secreting adenoma of the adrenal cortex that is usually small and occurs more frequently in the left than the right adrenal gland, causing hyperaldosteronism with salt retention, expansion of the extracellular fluid volume, and increased blood pressure.

Aleppo boil   See **oriental sore.**

alert   Highest level of consciousness. Characterized by appropriate responses to auditory, tactile, and visual stimuli and by orientation to time, place, and person.

aleukemic leukemia   A type of leukemia in which the total leukocyte count remains within normal limits and few abnormal forms appear in the peripheral blood. Diagnosis requires tissue examination, usually of the bone marrow. Also called **subleukemic leukemia.** See also **leukemia.**

aleukemic myelosis   See **myeloid metaplasia.**

aleukia   A marked reduction in or the complete absence of white blood cells or blood platelets. Compare **leukopenia, thrombocytopenia.** See also **aplastic anemia.**

aleukocythemic leukemia   See **subleukemic leukemia.**

alexia   An abnormal neurologic condition characterized by an inability to comprehend written words. Compare **dyslexia. —alexic,** *adj.*

alg-   See **algesi-.**

alga, *pl.* **algae**   Any of a large group of nonmotile or motile marine plants containing chlorophyll. Many genera and species of algae are found worldwide; all belong to the phylum Thallophyta. **—algal,** *adj.*

alge-   See **algesi-.**

algesi-, alg-, alge-, algo-   A combining form meaning 'pertaining to pain': *algesia, algesiogenic, algesthenia.*

-algesia   A combining form meaning '(condition of) sensitivity to pain': *asphalgesia, haphalgesia, hyperthermalgesia.*

-algesic   A combining form meaning 'pertaining to sensitivity to pain': *analgesic, hypalgesic, paralgesic.*

-algia   A combining form meaning 'pain, painful condition': *epigastralgia, sacralgia, uteralgia.* Also **-algy.**

-algic   A combining form meaning 'related to pain': *cardialgic, ophthalmalgic, tibialgic.*

algid malaria   A form of malaria caused by the protozoan *Plasmodium falciparum,* characterized by coldness of the skin, profound weakness, and severe diarrhea. See also **falciparum malaria, malaria.**

algo-   See **algesi-.**

algolagnia   A form of sexual perversion characterized by sadism or masochism.

algolagniac   See **sadomasochism.**

algophobia   An anxiety disorder characterized by an abnormal, pervasive fear of experiencing pain or of witnessing pain in others. See also **phobia.**

alienation   **1.** The act or state of being estranged or isolated. **2.** Insanity or mental derangement, now generally restricted to medical jurisprudence or forensic psychiatry. See also **depersonalization.**

alienist   A psychiatrist, especially one who specializes in giving legal evidence concerning the mental competence of persons appearing before a court of law.

alimentary bolus   See **bolus,** definition 1.

alimentary canal   See **digestive tube.**

alimentation   Nourishment. See also **feeding.**

aliphatic acid   An acid of a nonaromatic hydrocarbon characterized by an open carbon chain.

-alis   A combining form meaning 'pertaining to' something specified: *corticalis, rhomboidalis, vesicalis.*

alkali   A compound with the chemical characteristics of a base. Alkalis combine with fatty acids to form soaps, turn red litmus blue, and enter into reactions that form water-soluble carbonates. See also **acid, base. —alkaline,** *adj.*

alkalinity, *n.*

alkali burn   Tissue damage caused by exposure to an alkaline compound like lye. Treatment includes washing the area with copious amounts of water to remove the chemical and applying vinegar or other mildly acidic substance diluted with water to neutralize any remaining acid and to decrease the discomfort. The victim should be immediately taken to a medical facility if the tissue damage is more than slight and superficial. Compare **acid burn.**

-alkaline   A combining form meaning 'of or referring to alkali': *silicoalkaline, subalkaline, vegetoalkaline.*

alkaline ash   Residue in the urine having a pH higher than 7.

alkaline ash–producing foods   Foods that may be ingested in order to produce an alkaline pH in the urine, thereby reducing the incidence of acidic urinary calculi, or that may be avoided in order to reduce the incidence of alkaline calculi. Some of the foods that result in alkaline ash are milk, cream, buttermilk, fruit (except prunes, plums, and cranberries), vegetables (except corn and lentils), almonds, chestnuts, coconuts, and olives.

alkaline bath   A bath taken in water containing sodium bicarbonate, used especially for skin disorders.

alkaline phosphatase   An enzyme, involved in bone mineralization, that hydrolyzes phosphoric esters and functions optimally at 9.3 pH. Most alkaline phosphatase in normal serum is derived from bone, but the enzyme is produced also in the liver, intestinal mucosa, pla-

HOW TO RECOGNIZE ALKALOSIS

CONDITION	SYMPTOMS	SIGNS	BLOOD GAS LEVELS pH	HCO_3^-	$PaCO_2$
Respiratory alkalosis (primary carbon dioxide deficit)	Hyperreflexia, blurred vision, tetany, vertigo, muscle cramps, sighing, diaphoresis	Hyperventilation, latent tetany, positive Chvostek's sign, convulsions	⇑	⇓	⇓
Metabolic alkalosis (primary bicarbonate excess)	Weakness, apathy, leg cramps, paresthesias	Signs of potassium depletion, tetany, respiratory depression, arrhythmia	⇑	⇑	⇑

KEY: ⇓ = decreased ⇑ = increased. Shaded arrows indicate the primary abnormality.

centa, breast, and other tissues. Plasma levels of alkaline phosphatase rise rapidly in the first month of life, fall slowly after the third month, increase again during bone growth in preadolescence; levels decrease in senility, anemia, and malnutrition. Increased concentrations of the enzyme in serum, reflecting increased proliferation or activity of osteoblasts, are found in skeletal disorders, as rickets, osteomalacia, certain malignancies, and Paget's disease; elevated levels occurring in liver disorders, biliary obstruction, or intrahepatic cholestasis reflect impaired hepatic excretory function. Serum alkaline phosphatase is also increased in hyperparathyroidism and in hereditary hyperphosphatasia, characterized by thickness of the calvaria, large areas of increased density at the base of the skull, and deformities of the shafts and epiphyses of long and short bones.

alkalinize, alkalize **1.** To make a substance alkaline, as through the addition of a base. **2.** To become alkaline. Compare **acidify.**

alkali poisoning A toxic condition caused by the ingestion of an alkaline agent like liquid ammonia, lye, and some detergent powders. Emergency treatment includes giving copious amounts of water or milk to dilute the alkali. Vomiting is not induced, and mild acids are not administered. The victim is transported immediately to the hospital for observation of any corrosive damage to the esophagus or of any metabolic abnormality and for mechanical removal of the alkali by gastric intubation and lavage. Compare **acid poisoning.**

alkalosis An abnormal condition of body fluids, characterized by a tendency toward an increased pH, as from an excess of alkaline bicarbonate or a deficiency of acid. Respiratory alkalosis may be caused by hyperventilation, central nervous system disease, congestive heart failure, pulmonary embolism, or early salicylate intoxication. This results in an excess loss of carbon dioxide and a carbonic acid deficit. Metabolic alkalosis may result from loss of acid (such as from prolonged vomiting or nasogastric suction), retention or excess intake of bicarbonate,

or renal mechanisms associated with decreased serum levels of potassium and chloride. Alkalosis is said to be compensated if an adaptive mechanism, as a buffer system, carbon dioxide retention, or bicarbonate excretion, prevents a shift in pH. Treatment of uncompensated alkalosis involves correction of dehydration and various ionic deficits to restore the normal acidbase balance in which the ratio of carbonic acid to bicarbonate is 20:1. Compare **acidosis.**

alkaptonuria A rare inherited disorder resulting from the incomplete metabolism of tyrosine, an amino acid, in which abnormal amounts of homogentisic acid are excreted, staining the urine dark. In this disorder, which is transmitted by an autosomal recessive gene, a key metabolic enzyme is absent from the body. Usually, the condition does not cause symptoms until middle age, at which point ochronosis, a type of arthritis, may develop. —**alkaptonuric,** *adj.*

alkylating agent A substance that promotes alkylation.

ALL *abbr* **acute lymphocytic leukemia.** See also **acute childhood leukemia.**

all- See **allo-.**

allanto- A combining form meaning 'pertaining to a sausage or to the allantois': *allantochorion, allantoid, allantotoxicon.*

allantoidoangiopagus Conjoined twin fetuses of unequal size that are united by the vessels of the umbilical cord. Also called **omphaloangiopagus.** See also **omphalosite.** —**allantoidoangiopagous,** *adj.*

allantois A tubular extension of the yolk sac endoderm that extends with the allantoic vessels into the body stalk of the embryo. In human embryos, allantoic vessels become the umbilical vessels and the chorionic villi. See also **body stalk, umbilical cord.** —**allantoic,** *adj.*

allele **1.** One of two or more alternative forms of a gene that occupy corresponding loci on homologous chromosomes. **2.** Also called **allelomorph.** One of two or more contrasting characteristics transmitted by alternative genes.

allelo- A combining form meaning 'pertain-

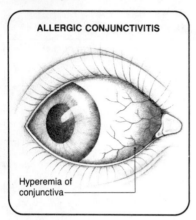

ALLERGIC CONJUNCTIVITIS

Hyperemia of
conjunctiva

ing to another': *allelocatalysis, allelomorph, allelotaxis.*

allelomorph   See **allele.**

allergen   A substance that can produce a hypersensitive reaction in the body but is not necessarily intrinsically harmful. Such a substance may be a protein or a nonprotein. Some common allergens are pollen, animal dander, house dust, feathers, and various foods. Some studies indicate that one of every six Americans is hypersensitive to one or more allergens. The bodies of normal individuals develop a natural or acquired immunity to allergens, but in less fortunate individuals the immune system may be overly sensitive to foreign substances and to others produced naturally by the body. The body normally protects itself against allergens or antigens by the complex chemical reactions of the humoral immune and the cell-mediated immune systems. Methods to identify specific allergens affecting individuals continue to improve. The most common method involves a skin test in which several allergens can be examined simultaneously. —**allergenic,** *adj.*

allergenic   Of or pertaining to a substance that tends to cause hypersensitivity reactions in certain individuals.

allergic   **1.** Of or pertaining to allergy. **2.** Having an allergy.

allergic alveolitis   See **hypersensitivity pneumonitis.**

allergic asthma   A form of asthma caused by the exposure of the bronchial mucosa to an inhaled airborne antigen. This allergen causes the production of antibodies that bind to mast cells in the bronchial tree. The mast cells then release histamine, which stimulates contraction of bronchial smooth muscle and causes mucosal edema. Psychological factors may provoke asthma attacks in bronchi already sensitized by allergens. Hyposensitization treatments are more effective for pollen sensitivity than for house dust, animal hair, molds, and insects. Often, a diurnal pattern of histamine release is seen, causing variable degrees of bronchospasm at different times of the day. Also called **extrinsic asthma.**

Compare **intrinsic asthma.** See also **asthma, status asthmaticus.**

allergic bronchopulmonary aspergillosis   A form of aspergillosis that occurs in asthmatics when the fungus *Aspergillus fumigatus,* growing within the bronchial lumen, causes a Type I or Type III hypersensitivity reaction. The characteristics of the condition are similar to those of asthma, including dyspnea and wheezing. Chest examination and pulmonary function tests may reveal airway obstruction. Serologic tests usually reveal precipitating antibodies to *A. fumigatus.* Bacteriologic and microscopic examination of sputum may reveal *A. fumigatus* in addition to Charcot-Leyden crystals. Eosinophilia is usually also present. Compare **aspergillosis.**

allergic conjunctivitis   An abnormal condition characterized by hyperemia of the conjunctiva owing to an allergy. Common allergens that cause this condition are pollen, grass, topical medications, air pollutants, occupational irritants, and smoke. The condition is bilateral, usually starts before puberty, and commonly recurs in a seasonal pattern.

allergic coryza   Acute rhinitis caused by exposure to any allergen to which the person is hypersensitive.

allergic cutaneous angiitis   See **allergic vasculitis.**

allergic interstitial pneumonitis   See **hypersensitivity pneumonitis.**

allergic reaction   A hypersensitive response to an allergen to which an organism has previously been exposed and to which the organism has developed antibodies. Subsequent exposure causes the release of histamine and a variety of symptoms, including urticaria, eczema, dyspnea, bronchospasm, diarrhea, rhinitis, sinusitis, laryngospasm, and anaphylaxis. Eosinophilia is usually present, revealed in a differential white blood cell count.

allergic rhinitis   Inflammation of the nasal passages, usually associated with watery nasal discharge and itching of the nose and eyes, owing to a localized sensitivity reaction to house dust, animal dander, or an antigen, commonly pollen. The condition may be seasonal, as in hay fever, or perennial, as in allergy to dust.

allergic vasculitis   An inflammatory condition of the blood vessels that is induced by an allergen. Disseminated intravascular inflammation sometimes occurs in patients treated with iodides, penicillin, sulfonamides, and thioureas. Allergic cutaneous vasculitis is characterized by itching, malaise, a slight fever, and the presence of papules, vesicles, urticarial wheals, or small ulcers on the skin.

allergy   A hypersensitive reaction to intrinsically harmless antigens, most of which are environmental. Studies show that one of every six Americans has a severe allergy and that more than 20 million Americans have allergic reactions to airborne or inhaled allergens, as cigarette smoke, house dust, and pollens. Allergic rhinitis, which is associated with airborne allergens, affects predominantly young children and adolescents but occurs in all age-groups. Allergies are classified according to Types I, II, III, and IV hypersensitivity. Types I, II, and III involve different immunoglobulin antibodies and their interaction with different antigens. Type IV allergy is associated with contact dermatitis and T cells that react directly with the antigen and cause local inflammation. Allergies are divided into those that produce immediate or antibody-mediated reactions and those that produce delayed or cell-mediated reactions. Immediate allergic reactions involve Types I, II, and III hypersensitivity and antigen-antibody reactions that activate certain enzymes, creating an imbalance between these enzymes and their inhibitors. Immediate allergic reactions also release certain substances into the circulation, as histamine, bradykinin, acetylcholine, gamma globulin G, and leukotaxine. Delayed allergic reactions are caused by antigens but do not seem to depend on antibodies. Depending on the type of hypersensitivity involved, some common symptoms of allergy are bronchial congestion, conjunctivitis, edema, fever, urticaria, and vomiting. Severe allergic reactions, as anaphylaxis, can cause systemic shock and death. Symptoms of limited duration, as those associated with hay fever, serum sickness, bee stings, and urticaria, can be suppressed by glucocorticoids administered as supplements to primary therapy. The effect of such steroids may be considerably delayed. Severe allergic reactions, as anaphylaxis and angioneurotic edema of the glottis, commonly require immediate therapy with epinephrine administered subcutaneously. When allergic reactions are life-threatening, steroids, as dexamethasone sodium phosphate, may be administered intravenously. For milder diseases, as serum sickness and hay fever, antihistamines are usually administered. See also **allergy testing.**

allergy testing   Any one of the various procedures used in identifying the specific allergens that afflict the patients involved. Such tests are helpful in prescribing treatment to prevent allergic reactions or to reduce their severity. Skin testing is the most common kind of procedure for allergy testing and commonly exposes the patient to small quantities of the suspected allergens. Positive reactions usually occur within 20 minutes and are commonly manifested as varying degrees of erythema. Factors considered in performing allergy tests include the medical history of the patient, the allergy history, the environment, and the diet. Individuals to be tested are usually instructed to discontinue the use of any antihistamines at least 24 hours before the test, as these drugs can interfere with normal test responses. The most common kinds of allergy testing include the intradermal, scratch, patch, conjunctival, and use tests.

allied health personnel   See **paramedical personnel.**

alligator forceps   1. A forceps with heavy teeth and a double clamp, employed in orthopedic surgery. **2.** A forceps with long, thin, angular handles and interlocking teeth.

allo-, all-   A combining form meaning 'differing from the normal, reversal, or referring to another': *allobiosis, allochezia, allopathy.*

allodiploid, allodiploidic   1. Of or pertaining to an individual, organism, strain, or cell that has two genetically distinct sets of chromosomes derived from different ancestral species, as occurs in hybridization. **2.** Such an individual, organism, strain, or cell.

allodiploidy   The state or condition of having two genetically distinct sets of chromosomes derived from different ancestral species.

alloeroticism, alloerotism   See **heteroeroticism.**

allogamy   See **cross-fertilization. —allogamous,** *adj.*

allohexaploid, allohexaploidic   See **allopolyploid.**

allometric growth   The increase in size of different organs or parts of an organism at various rates. Also called **heterauxesis.** Compare **isometric growth.** See also **allometry.**

allometron   A quantitative change in the proportional relationship of the parts of an organism as a result of the evolutionary process.

allometry   The measurement and study of the changes in proportions of the various parts of an organism in relation to the growth of the whole or within a series of related organisms. **—allometric,** *adj.*

allopathic physician   A physician who treats disease and injury with active interventions, as medical and surgical treatment, intended to bring about effects opposite from those produced by the disease or injury. Almost all practicing physicians in the United States are allopathic. Compare **chiropractic, homeopathy.**

allopathy   A system of medical therapy in which a disease or an abnormal condition is treated by creating an environment that is antagonistic to the disease or condition, as an antibiotic toxic to a pathogenic organism is given in an infection or an iron supplement may be given to increase the synthesis of hemoglobin in iron deficiency anemia.

allopentaploid, allopentaploidic   See **allopolyploid.**

alloplastic maneuver   In psychology: a process that is part of adaptation, involving an adjustment or change in the external environment. Compare **autoplastic maneuver.**

alloploid, alloploidic   See **allodiploid, alloploidy.**

alloploidy   See **allodiploidy, allopolyploidy.**

allopolyploid, allopolyploidic   1. Of or pertaining to an individual, organism, strain, or cell that has more than two genetically distinct sets of chromosomes derived from two or more different ancestral species, as occurs in hybridization. They are referred to as allotriploid, allotetraploid, allopentraploid, allohexaploid, and so on, depending on the number of

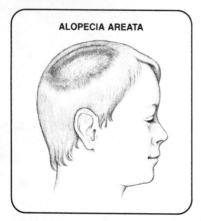

ALOPECIA AREATA

multiples of haploid sets of chromosomes they contain. **2.** Such an individual, organism, strain, or cell. Compare **autopolyploid.**

allopolyploidy The state or condition of having more than two genetically distinct sets of chromosomes from two or more ancestral species. Compare **autopolyploidy.**

allopurinol A drug used to treat hyperuricemia and gout.

all or none law The principle that the heart muscle, under any stimulus above the threshold level, regardless of the intensity, will either contract to the maximum extent or not at all. The principle also applies to single strands of muscle and nerve fibers, although the degree of response when an entire muscle or nerve trunk is stimulated depends on the number of fibers stimulated. Also called **Bowditch's law.**

allotetraploid, allotetraploidic See **allopolyploid.**

allotrio- A combining form meaning 'strange or foreign': *allotriodontia, allotriogeustia, allotriophagy.*

allotriploid, allotriploidic See **allopolyploid.**

allowable charge The maximum amount that a third party, usually an insurance company, will pay to reimburse a provider for a specific service.

allowable costs Components of an institution's costs that are reimbursable as determined by a payment formula. In general, costs of services not considered to be reasonable or necessary to the proper delivery of health services are excluded from allowable costs.

alloy A mixture of two or more metals or of substances with metallic properties. Most alloys are formed by mixing molten metals that dissolve in each other. A number of alloys have medical applications, as those used for prostheses and in dental amalgams. See also **amalgam.**

aloe The inspissated juice of various species of *Aloe* trees, formerly used as a cathartic but generally discontinued because it often causes severe intestinal cramps.

alopecia Partial or complete lack of hair re-sulting from normal aging, endocrine disorder, drug reaction, anticancer medication, or skin disease. Also called **baldness.** Kinds of alopecia include **alopecia areata, alopecia totalis, alopecia universalis.**

alopecia areata A disease of unknown cause in which there are well-defined bald patches on the head and other hairy parts of the body. The condition is usually self-limited and clears completely within 6 to 12 months without treatment. Recurrences are common.

alopecia totalis An uncommon condition characterized by the loss of all the hair on the scalp. The cause in unknown, and the baldness is usually permanent. No treatment is known. Compare **alopecia areata, alopecia universalis.**

alopecia universalis A lack of hair on all parts of the body, occasionally an extension of alopecia areata. Compare **alopecia totalis.**

alpha The first letter of the Greek alphabet, often used in chemical nomenclature to distinguish one variation in a chemical compound from others.

alpha-adrenergic blocking agent See **antiadrenergic.**

alpha-adrenergic receptor See **alpha receptor.**

alpha-aminoisovalerianic acid See **valine.**

alpha-chymotrypsin A proteolytic enzyme that aids in cataract extraction.

alpha fetoprotein (AFP) A protein normally synthesized by the liver, yolk sac, and gastrointestinal tract of a human fetus, but which may be found elevated in the sera of adults having certain malignancies. AFP measurements in amniotic fluid are used for early diagnosis of fetal neural defects, as spina bifida and anencephaly. Elevated serum levels may be present in ataxia telangiectasia, hereditary tyrosinemia, cirrhosis, alcoholic hepatitis, and viral hepatitis. Although not a specific marker for malignancies, AFP may be used to monitor effectiveness of surgical and chemotherapeutic management of hepatomas and germ cell neoplasms.

alpha-galactosidase A form of the enzyme that catalyzes the conversion of alpha-D-galactoside to D-galactose.

alpha hemolysis The development of a greenish zone around a bacterial colony growing on blood-agar medium, characteristic of pneumococci and certain streptococci and caused by the partial decomposition of hemoglobin. Compare **beta hemolysis.**

alpha-hydroxypropionic acid See **lactic acid.**

alpha-methyldopa See **methyldopa.**

alphaprodine hydrochloride A narcotic and opioid analgesic agent.

alpha receptor Any one of the postulated adrenergic components of receptor tissues that responds to norepinephrine and to various blocking agents. The activation of the alpha receptors causes such physiological responses as increased peripheral vascular resistance, dilation of the pupils, and contraction of pilomotor muscles. Also called **alpha-adrenergic receptor.** Compare **beta receptor.**

alpha rhythm See **alpha wave.**

alpha state A condition of relaxed, peaceful wakefulness devoid of concentration and sensory stimulation. It is characterized by the alpha rhythm of brain wave activity, as recorded by an electroencephalograph, and is accompanied by feelings of tranquillity and a lack of tension and anxiety. Biofeedback training and meditation techniques are used as means of achieving the state.

Alpha Tau Delta A national fraternity for professional nurses.

alpha tocopheryl See **vitamin E.**

alpha wave One of the four types of brain waves, characterized by a relatively high voltage or amplitude and a frequency of 8 to 13 Hz. Alpha waves are the 'relaxed' waves of the brain and constitute the majority of waves recorded by electroencephalograms registering the activity of the parietal and the occipital lobes and the posterior parts of the temporal lobes when the individual is awake but nonattentive and relaxed, with the eyes closed. Opening and closing the eyes affect the patterns of both the alpha waves and the beta waves. Also called **alpha rhythm.** Compare **beta wave, delta wave, theta wave.**

alprazolam A benzodiazepine antianxiety agent.

alprostadil Palliative therapy for temporary maintenance of patency of ductus arteriosus.

ALS *abbr* **1. antilymphocyte serum. 2. advanced life support.** See **Emergency Medical Technician-Advanced Life Support. 3. amyotrophic lateral sclerosis.**

alseroxylon A sympathetic antihypertensive agent that acts peripherally.

altered state of consciousness (ASC) Any state of awareness that differs from the normal awareness of a conscious person. Altered states of consciousness have been achieved, especially in Eastern cultures, by many individuals using various techniques, as long fasting, deep breathing, whirling, and chanting. Researchers now recognize that such practices can affect the chemistry of the body and help to induce the desired state. Experiments suggest that telepathy, mystical experiences, clairvoyance, and other altered states of consciousness may be subconscious capabilities in most individuals and can be used to improve health and help fight disease.

alternate generation, alternations of generations A type of reproduction in which a sexual generation alternates with one or more asexual generations, as in many plants and lower animals.

alternating current (AC) An electrical current that reverses direction and changes in magnitude, according to a consistent sinusoidal pattern.

alternating pulse A regular, steady pulse

in which a strong beat is followed by a weak one. It is characteristic of left-ventricular failure. Also called **pulsus alternans.**

alternative inheritance The acquisition of all genetic traits and conditions from one parent, as in self-pollinating plants and self-fertilizing animals.

altitude sickness A syndrome associated with the relatively low concentrations of oxygen in the atmosphere at altitudes encountered during mountain climbing or travel in unpressurized aircraft. The acute symptoms may include dizziness, headache, irritability, breathlessness, and euphoria. Older people and those affected by pulmonary or cardiac disorders may suffer pulmonary edema, heart failure, or prostration, requiring emergency treatment and removal to lower altitudes. A chronic form of altitude sickness is characterized by an increased production of red blood cells, resulting in blood that is thick and difficult to move through the circulatory system. See also **polycythemia.**

alum A topical astringent, used primarily in lotions and douches. Alum is applied topically as a 0.5% to 5% solution. It is not to be confused with caustic pencils made from silver nitrate.

alum bath A bath taken in water containing alum, used primarily for skin disorders.

aluminum (Al) A widely used metallic element and the third most abundant of all the elements. Its atomic number is 13; its atomic weight is 26.97. It occurs in the ores feldspar, mica, and kaolin but most abundantly in bauxite. Aluminum is commonly obtained by purifying bauxite to produce alumina, which is reduced to aluminum. It is light and durable and used extensively in the manufacture of aircraft components, prosthetic devices, and dental appliances. It is also a component of many antacids, antiseptics, astringents, and styptics. Aluminum salts, as aluminum hydroxychloride, can cause allergic reactions in susceptible individuals. Aluminum hydroxychloride is the most commonly used agent in antiperspirants and is also effective as a deodorant.

aluminum acetate An astringent.

aluminum carbonate, a. hydroxide, a. phosphate Used as antacids.

aluminum paste An emollient and protectant.

aluminum sulfate An astringent.

alve- A combining form meaning 'trough, channel, cavity': *alvei, alveolate, alveolus.*

alveolar adenocarcinoma A neoplasm in which the tumor cells form alveoli.

alveolar canal Any of the canals of the maxilla through which the posterior superior alveolar blood vessels and the nerves to the upper teeth pass. Also called **dental canal.**

alveolar cell carcinoma A malignant pulmonary neoplasm that arises in a bronchiole and spreads along alveolar surfaces. The tumor consists of cuboidal or nonciliated columnar epithelial cells with abundant eosinophilic cytoplasm that may contain droplets of mucus. This form of lung cancer, which occurs less fre-

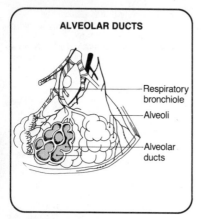

ALVEOLAR DUCTS

Respiratory bronchiole

Alveoli

Alveolar ducts

quently than bronchogenic squamous cell carcinoma or oat cell carcinoma, is characterized clinically by a severe cough and copious sputum. Also called **bronchiolar carcinoma.**

alveolar duct The terminal segment of a respiratory bronchiole in the lung.

alveolar fistula See **dental fistula.**

alveolar soft part sarcoma A tumor in subcutaneous or fibromuscular tissue, consisting of numerous large round or polygonal cells in a netlike matrix of connective tissue.

alveolitis See **hypersensitivity pneumonitis.**

alveolo- A combining form meaning 'pertaining to an alveolus': *alveoloclasia, alveolodontal, alveoloplasty.*

alveolus A small saclike structure. See also **dental alveolus, pulmonary alveolus.** —**alveolar,** *adj.*

alymphocytosis An abnormal reduction in the total number of lymphocytes circulating in the blood. It is similar to lymphocytopenia but usually implies a more severe reduction. Compare **aplastic anemia, lymphocytopenia.** See also **leukocyte, lymphocyte.**

Alzheimer's disease Presenile dementia, characterized by confusion, restlessness, agnosia, speech disturbances, inability to carry out purposeful movements, and hallucinosis. The patient may become hypomanic, refuse food, and lose sphincter control without local impairment. The disease usually begins in later middle life with slight defects in memory and behavior and occurs with equal frequency in men and women. Typical pathologic features are miliary plaques in the cortex and fibrillary degeneration within pyramidal ganglion cells. Treatment can only be palliative, but maintaining proper nutrition may delay the progression of the disease.

Am Symbol for **americium.**

AMA *abbr* **American Medical Association.**

amalgam 1. A mixture or combination. 2. An alloy of mercury and another metal or metals.

Amanita A genus of mushrooms. Some species, as *Amanita phalloides,* are poisonous,

causing hallucinations, gastrointestinal upset, and pain that may be followed by liver, kidney, and central nervous system damage.

amantadine hydrochloride An antiviral antibiotic.

amasesis The inability to chew food, caused by paralysis of the muscles of mastication, impaired teeth, poorly fitted dentures, or a psychiatric problem.

amastia Absence of the breasts in women caused by a congenital defect, an endocrine disorder resulting in faulty development, lack of development of secondary sex characteristics, or a bilateral mastectomy. Also called **amazia.**

amaurosis Blindness, especially lack of vision resulting from an extraocular cause, as disease of the optic nerve or brain, diabetes, renal disease, or systemic poisoning produced by excessive use of alcohol or tobacco. Unilateral or, more rarely, bilateral amaurosis may follow an emotional shock and may continue for days or months. Amaurosis may accompany an attack of acute gastritis. One kind of congenital amaurosis is transmitted as an autosomal recessive trait. —**amaurotic,** *adj.*

amaurosis congenita of Leber See **Leber's congenital amaurosis.**

amaurosis fugax Transient episodic blindness. Compare **amaurosis.**

amaurosis partialis fugax Transitory partial blindness, usually caused by vascular insufficiency of the retina or optic nerve as a result of carotid artery disease.

amaurotic familial idiocy See **Tay-Sachs disease.**

amazia See **amastia.**

amb- See **ambo-.**

ambenonium chloride A cholinergic (parasympathomimetic) agent.

amber mutation In molecular genetics: a genetic alteration in which a polypeptide chain terminates prematurely, because the triplet of nucleotides that normally code for the next amino acid in the chain becomes UAG, the uracil-adenine-guanine sequence that signals the end of the chain. Also called **nonsense mutation, ochre mutation.**

ambi- A combining form meaning 'on both sides': *ambidexterity, ambilateral, ambiversion.*

ambient air standard The maximum tolerable concentration of any air pollutant, as lead, nitrogen dioxide, sodium hydroxide, or sulfuric dioxide. Federal authorities in the United States have indicated that only Los Angeles, Chicago, Salt Lake City, and metropolitan New York may not meet the ambient air standard for nitrogen dioxide and that those cities and many others throughout the world have an atmosphere polluted by various toxic chemicals that are dangerous to breathe. Research and medical evidence show the strong correlation between many diseases and toxic chemicals, but little is known about the precise effects and movement of airborne pollutants.

ambiguous genitalia External genitalia

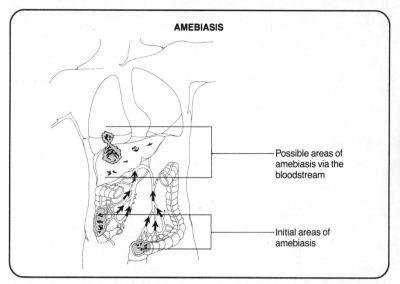

AMEBIASIS

Possible areas of amebiasis via the bloodstream

Initial areas of amebiasis

that are not normal and morphologically typical of either sex, as occurs in pseudohermaphroditism.

ambivalence 1. A state in which a person experiences conflicting feelings, attitudes, drives, desires, or emotions, as love and hate, tenderness and cruelty, pleasure and pain. To some degree, ambivalence is normal. Treatment in severe, debilitating cases consists of psychotherapy appropriate to the underlying cause. 2. Uncertainty and fluctuation owing to an inability to make a choice between opposites. 3. A continuous oscillation or fluctuation. —**ambivalent,** *adj.*

ambivert A person who possesses some of the characteristics of both introversion and extroversion.

amblyopia Reduced vision in an eye that appears to be structurally normal when examined with an ophthalmoscope. Kinds of amblyopia are **suppression amblyopia, toxic amblyopia.**

ambo-, amb- A combining form meaning 'both or on both sides': *ambomaleal.*

ambulatory Able to walk, hence describing a patient who is not confined to bed; or designating a health service for people who are not hospitalized.

ambulatory automatism Aimless wandering or moving about or performance of mechanical acts without conscious awareness of the behavior. See also **fugue, poriomania.**

ambulatory care All health services provided on an outpatient basis to those who visit a hospital or other health-care facility and depart after treatment on the same day.

amcinonide A topical anti-inflammatory agent.

ameba, amoeba A microscopic, single-celled, parasitic organism. Several species may infect man, including *Entamoeba histolytica* and *Escherichia coli.* See also **amebiasis.** —**amebic,** *adj.*

-ameba, -amoeba A combining form meaning a '(specified) protozoan': *caudameba, Dientameba, Entameba.*

amebiasis, amoebiasis An infection of the intestine or liver by species of pathogenic amebae, particularly *Entamoeba histolytica,* acquired by ingesting food or water contaminated with infected feces. Mild amebiasis may be asymptomatic; severe infection may cause profuse diarrhea, acute abdominal pain, jaundice, anorexia, and weight loss. It is most serious in infants, the elderly, and debilitated people. Metronidazole is usually effective in curing the infection. See also **ameba, amebic abscess, amebic dysentery, hepatic amebiasis.**

amebic abscess A collection of pus formed by disintegrated tissue in a cavity, usually in the liver, caused by the protozoan parasite *Entamoeba histolytica.* Cysts of the organism, ingested in fecally contaminated food or water, pass through the digestive tract into the intestine, where active trophozoites of the parasite are released. The trophozoites enter the intestinal mucosa, causing ulceration, nausea, vomiting, abdominal pain, and severe diarrhea, and they may invade the liver and produce an abscess.

amebic dysentery An inflammation of the intestine caused by infestation with *Entamoeba histolytica* and characterized by frequent, loose stools flecked with blood and mucus. Intestinal amebiasis is often accompanied by symptoms of liver involvement. Also called **intestinal amebiasis.** See also **amebiasis,** *Entamoeba histolytica,* **hepatic amebiasis.**

amelanotic Of or pertaining to tissue that is unpigmented because it lacks melanin.

amelia 1. A birth defect, marked by the absence of one or more limbs. The term may be modified to indicate the number of legs or arms missing at birth, as **tetramelia.** 2. A psychological trait of apathy or indifference associated with certain forms of psychosis.

amelification The differentiation of ameloblasts, or enamel cells, into the enamel of the teeth.

ameloblast An epithelial cell from which the enamel of the teeth is formed. —**ameloblastic,** *adj.*

ameloblastic fibroma An odontogenic neoplasm in which there is a simultaneous proliferation of mesenchymal and epithelial tissues but no development of dentin or enamel.

ameloblastic hemangioma A highly vascular tumor of cells covering the dental papilla. See also **hemangioma.**

ameloblastic sarcoma A malignant odontogenic tumor, characterized by the proliferation of epithelial and mesenchymal tissue without the formation of dentin or enamel.

ameloblastoma A highly destructive, malignant, rapid growing tumor of the jaw.

amelodentinal Pertaining to both the enamel and dentin of the teeth.

amelogenesis The formation of the enamel of the teeth. —**amelogenic,** *adj.*

amelogenesis imperfecta A hereditary dental defect characterized by a brown coloration of the teeth and resulting from either severe hypocalcification or hypoplasia of the enamel. The condition, which is inherited as an autosomal dominant trait, is classified according to severity as agenesis, in which there is complete lack of enamel; enamel hypoplasia, in which defective matrix formation causes the enamel to be normal in quality of hardness but deficient in quantity; or enamel hypocalcification, in which defective maturation of the ameloblasts results in the normal quantity of enamel, though it is soft and undercalcified in context. Also called **hereditary brown enamel, hereditary enamel hypoplasia.** Compare **dentinogenesis imperfecta.** See also **enamel hypocalcification, enamel hypoplasia.**

amenorrhea The absence of menstruation. Amenorrhea is normal prior to sexual maturity, during pregnancy, after menopause, and during the intermenstrual phase of the monthly hormonal cycle but is otherwise caused by dysfunction of the hypothalamus, pituitary gland, ovary, or uterus, by the congenital absence or surgical removal of both ovaries or the uterus, or by medication. Primary amenorrhea is the failure of menstrual cycles to begin. Secondary amenorrhea is the cessation of menstrual cycles once established. See also **hypothalamic amenorrhea, post-pill amenorrhea.** —**amenorrheic.** *adj.*

amentia 1. See **mental retardation.** 2. A state of mind that is characterized by apathy and disorientation, bordering on stupor, as in Stearns' alcoholic amentia. Also called **confusional insanity.**

American Academy of Nursing (AAN) The honorary organization of the American Nurses' Association, created to recognize superior achievement in nursing in order to promote advances and excellence in nursing practice and education. A person who is elected to membership is given the title of Fellow of the American Academy of Nursing and may use the abbreviation FAAN as an honorific.

American Journal of Nursing The professional journal of the American Nurses' Association (ANA). The journal contains articles and papers of general and specialized clinical interest to nurses and is the principal resource regarding the profession and employment in the profession in the United States. It is one of five magazines published by the American Journal of Nursing Company of which ANA is the sole owner.

American leishmaniasis A group of mucocutaneous infections caused by various species of *Leishmania,* characterized by disfiguring ulcerative lesions of the nose, mouth, and throat. These infections are most prevalent in southern Mexico and in Central and South America. Illness may be prolonged, rendering patients susceptible to serious secondary infections. Kinds of American leishmaniasis are **chiclero's ulcer, espundia, forest yaws, uta.** Also called **mucocutaneous leishmaniasis, New World leishmaniasis.** See also **leishmaniasis.**

American Medical Association (AMA) A professional association whose membership is made up of approximately half of the total licensed physicians in the United States, including practitioners in all recognized medical specialties as well as general primary care physicians. The AMA is governed by a Board of Trustees and House of Delegates who represent various state and local medical associations as well as such government agencies as the Public Health Service and medical departments of the Army, Navy, and Air Force. The AMA maintains directories of all qualified physicians (including nonmembers) in the United States, including graduates of foreign medical colleges, evaluates prescription and nonprescription drugs, advises congressional and state legislators regarding proposed health-care laws, and publishes a variety of journals that report on scientific and socioeconomic developments in the field of medicine. See also **British Medical Association.**

American mountain fever See **Colorado tick fever.**

American Nurses' Association (ANA) The national professional association of registered nurses in the United States. It was founded in 1896 to improve standards of health and the availability of health care given in order to foster high standards for nursing, to promote the professional development of nurses, and to advance the economic and general welfare of nurses. The ANA is made up of 53 constituent associations from 50 states, the District of Columbia, Guam, and the Virgin Islands, representing more than 900 district associations. National conventions are held biennially in even-numbered years. Members may join one or more of the five Divisions on Nursing Practice: Community Health; Gerontological; Maternal and Child Health; Medical-Surgical; and Psychiatric and Mental Health Nursing. These Divisions are coordinated by the Congress for Nursing Practice. The Congress evaluates changes in the scope of practice, monitors scientific and educational developments, encourages research, and develops statements that describe ANA policies regarding legislation affecting nursing practice. Other commissions within the Association include the Commission on Nursing Education, the Commission on Nursing Services, the Commission on Nursing Research, and the Economic and General Welfare Commission (E and GW), which functions at the local, state, and national level. The programs of the E and GW Commission are intended to ensure fair compensation for nurses, working conditions that are conducive to high quality nursing care, and a pool of qualified nurses adequate for the health-care needs of the country. In addition, the ANA is politically active on the federal level in all issues relevant to nursing. Statistical services enable the Association to fulfill its role as the most authoritative source of data on nursing in the United States. The publications of the ANA include the *American Nurse*, a newspaper, the *Publications List*, and *The American Journal of Nursing*, the professional journal of the Association.

American Red Cross One of more than 120 national organizations that seek to reduce human suffering through various health, safety, and disaster relief programs in affiliation with the International Committee of the Red Cross. The Committee and all Red Cross organizations evolved from the Geneva Convention of 1864, following the example and urging of Swiss humanitarian Jean Henri Dunant, who aided wounded French and Austrian soldiers at the Battle of Solferino in 1859. The American Red Cross has more than 130 million members in about 3,100 chapters throughout the United States. Volunteers comprise the entire staffs of about 1,700 chapters. Other chapters maintain small paid staffs and some professionals but depend largely on volunteers. The American Red Cross blood program collects and distributes more blood than any other single agency in the United States and coordinates distribution of blood and blood products to the U.S. Defense Department on request or during national emergencies. The organization annually collects about 4 million blood donations and gives blood to more than 4,000 hospitals. American Red Cross nursing and health programs include courses in the home on parenthood, prenatal and postnatal care, hygiene, and venereal disease. Nursing students are enrolled for service in American Red Cross community programs and during disasters. Four area offices at Alexandria, Virginia; Atlanta; St. Louis; and San Francisco supervise and assist 70 divisions of the American Red Cross and direct field staff members assigned to military installations. National headquarters of the organization is at 17th and D Streets, NW, Washington, D.C. 20006. The President of the United States is honorary chairman of the organization, for which a 50-member board of governors, all volunteers, develops policy. The symbol of the American Red Cross, like that of most other Red Cross societies throughout the world, is a red cross on a field of white; in Switzerland it is a white cross on a red field; in Muslim countries, a red crescent; in Israel, a red star of David; and, in Iran, a red lion and sun.

American trypanosomiasis See **Chagas' disease.**

American Type Culture Collection (ATCC) A nonprofit, nongovernmental organization that is concerned with the preservation of specimens of cellular and microbiological cultures and with the distribution of the cultures to research centers and laboratories in the academic, scientific, and medical communities.

americium (Am) A manmade radioactive element of the actinide group. Its atomic number is 95; its atomic weight is 243.

Ameslan Acronym for American Sign Language, a method of communication with the deaf that relies primarily on the position, shape, and motion of the hands and fingers for the transmission of concepts and messages.

amethopterin See **methotrexate.**

ametropia A condition characterized by an optical defect involving an error of refraction, as astigmatism, hyperopia, myopia. —**ametropic,** *adj.*

amide-compound local anesthetic Any of more than two dozen compounds that are safe, versatile, and effective local anesthetics. If hypersensitivity to a drug in this group precludes its use, one of the ester-compound local anesthetics may provide analgesia without adverse effect. Some kinds of amide-compound local anesthetics are **bupivacaine, dibucaine, etiodocaine, lidocaine, mepivacaine, prilocaine.**

amido- A combining form meaning 'the presence of the radical NH_2 along with the radical CO': *amido-acetal, amidobenzene, amidopyrine.*

amidobenzene See **aniline.**

amikacin sulfate An aminoglycoside antibiotic.

amiloride A potassium-sparing diuretic.

amine In chemistry: any organic compound that contains nitrogen.

amine pump *Informal.* An active transport system in the presynaptic nerve endings that takes up released amine neurotransmitters. Adverse reactions to some drugs, notably tricyclic antidepressants, block this function, resulting in a high concentration of norepinephrine in cardiac tissue and resultant tachycardia and arrhythmia. See also **monoamine oxidase inhibitor.**

aminoacetic acid A nonessential amino acid occurring as a natural ingredient of many

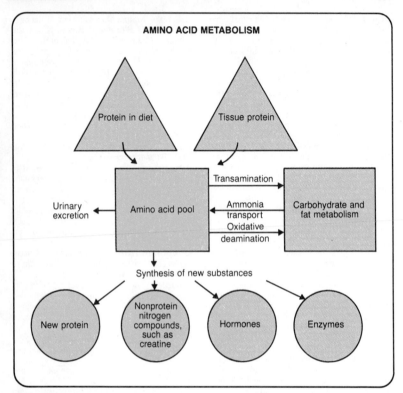

AMINO ACID METABOLISM

proteins; as a synthetic compound, it is used as a dietary supplement and a gastric antacid. Also called **glycine, glycocoll.**

amino acid　An organic chemical compound composed of one or more basic amino groups and one or more acidic carboxyl groups. Of the more than 100 amino acids that occur in nature, 20 are the building blocks of peptides, polypeptides, and proteins. See also **essential amino acid.**

amino acid solution　A supplement for protein-depleted patients.

aminoaciduria　The abnormal presence of amino acids in the urine that usually indicates an inborn metabolic defect, as in cystinuria.

aminobenzene　See **aniline.**

aminobenzoic acid　A metabolic product of the catabolism of the amino acid tryptophan. Also called **anthralinic acid.**

aminocaproic acid　A systemic hemostatic agent.

aminoglutethimide　An antineoplastic that alters hormone balance.

aminoglycoside antibiotic　See **antibiotic.**

amino oxidase　See **monoamine oxidase.**

aminophylline　A respiratory tract spasmolytic agent. Also called **theophylline ethylenediamine.**

aminosalicylic acid　A second-line tuberculostatic antibacterial.

aminosuccinic acid　See **aspartic acid.**

aminotransferase　See **transaminase.**

amitosis　Direct cell division in which there is simple fission of the nucleus and cytoplasm. It does not involve the complex stages of chromatin separation of the chromosomes that occur in mitosis. —**amitotic,** *adj.*

amitriptyline hydrochloride　A tricyclic antidepressant.

AML　*abbr* **acute myelocytic leukemia.**

ammoni-　A combining form meaning 'pertaining to ammonium': *ammoniemia, ammonirrhea, ammoniuria.*

ammonia　1. A colorless aromatic gas consisting of nitrogen and hydrogen, produced by the decomposition of nitrogenous organic matter. Some of its many uses are as a detergent and an emulsifier. 2. (**aromatic spirits**) A respiratory stimulant.

ammoniacal fermentation　The production of ammonia and carbon dioxide from urea by the enzyme urease.

ammoniated mercury　A dermatomucosal agent used to treat psoriasis and other skin conditions.

ammonium chloride　An expectorant and systemic acidifier.

amnesia　A loss of memory owing to brain damage or to severe emotional trauma. Kinds of amnesia are **anterograde amnesia,** hysterical amnesia, posttraumatic amnesia, **retrograde amnesia.**

amnestic apraxia The inability to carry out a movement in response to a request owing to a lack of ability to remember the request rather than to a loss of motor function. See also **apraxia.**

amnio- A combining form meaning 'pertaining to the amnion': *amniogenesis, amnioma, amniorrhexis.*

amniocentesis The needle aspiration of a small amount of amniotic fluid for laboratory analysis. This obstetric procedure is usually performed between the 16th and 20th weeks of gestation to diagnose various genetic defects, including chromosomal abnormalities, neural tube defects, and Tay-Sachs disease. It is also performed to discover the sex of the fetus if certain sex-linked genetic defects are suspected. Later in pregnancy amniocentesis may be performed to assess fetal maturity by testing the lecithin-sphingomyelin (L/S) ratio in the laboratory prior to therapeutic termination of pregnancy. The fluid may be tested for the concentration of creatinine, another indicator of fetal maturity. When postmaturity is suspected, amniocentesis is performed to examine the amniotic fluid for meconium. Maternal and fetal infection with attendant morbidity or mortality may occur, but it is rare. Premature rupture of the membranes, premature labor, or trauma to the fetus or umbilical cord may occur. The procedure is not usually performed for genetic diagnosis unless the mother plans to terminate the pregnancy if the procedure indicates the presence of a genetic disease or abnormality.

amnion A membrane, continuous with and covering the fetal side of the placenta, that forms the outer surface of the umbilical cord and becomes the outermost layer of the skin of the developing fetus. Compare **chorion.**

amniotic fluid A liquid produced by the fetal membranes and the fetus. It surrounds the fetus throughout pregnancy, usually totaling about 1,000 ml at term. In addition to providing the fetus with physical protection, the amniotic fluid is a medium of active chemical exchange. It is secreted and resorbed by cells lining the amniotic sac at a rate of 500 ml/hour at term, and is swallowed, metabolized, and excreted as fetal urine at a rate of 50 ml/hour. Its chemical constituents are those of maternal and fetal plasma in different concentrations. Its pH is close to neutral. Amniotic fluid itself is clear, though desquamated fetal cells and lipids give it a cloudy appearance.

amniotic sac A thin-walled bag that contains the fetus and amniotic fluid during pregnancy, having a capacity of 4 to 5 liters at term. The wall of the sac extends from the margin of the placenta. The amnion, chorion, and decidua that make up the wall are each a few cell layers thick. They are closely applied though not fused to each other and to the wall of the uterus. The intact sac and its fluid provide for the equilibration of hydrostatic pressure within the uterus,

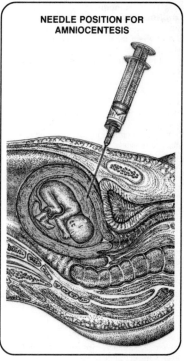

NEEDLE POSITION FOR AMNIOCENTESIS

and, during labor, effect the uniform transmission of the force of uterine contractions to the cervix for dilatation. See also **amnion, chorion, decidua.**

amobarbital, a. sodium A barbiturate sedative-hypnotic agent.

amoeba See ameba.

-amoeba See -ameba.

amoebiasis See amebiasis.

amoebic dysentery See amebic dysentery.

amorph An inactive gene; a mutant allele that has little or no effect on the expression of a trait. Compare **antimorph, hypermorph, hypomorph.**

amorphic In genetics: of or pertaining to a gene that is inactive or nearly inactive so that it has no determinable effect.

amoxapine A tricyclic antidepressant.

amoxicillin trihydrate A penicillin antibiotic.

AMP *abbr* adenosine monophosphate.

ampere A unit of measurement of the amount of electrical current. An ampere, according to the meter-kilogram-second (MKS) system, is the amount of current passed through a resistance of 1 ohm by an electrical potential of 1 volt. The standard international ampere is the amount of current that deposits 0.001118 g of silver per second when passed, according to certain specifications, through a silver nitrate solution. See also **ohm, volt.**

amph- See **amphi-**.

amphetamine A central nervous system stimulant used in treating narcolepsy, as part of a program for the management of children with attention deficit disorder, and as an adjunct to diet in treating exogenous obesity. Amphetamine increases systolic and diastolic blood pressures and acts as a weak bronchodilator and respiratory stimulant; it has a high potential for abuse, resulting in tolerance, psychological dependence, and severe social disability. Overdosage of the drug may cause nausea, vomiting, diarrhea, abdominal cramps, cardiac arrhythmias, restlessness, tremor, hyperreflexia, tachypnea, confusion, assaultiveness, hallucinations, and panic states. Also called **speed** (slang).

amphetamine hydrochloride, a. phosphate, a. sulfate Amphetamine central nervous system stimulants.

amphi-, amph- A combining form meaning 'on both sides': amphiarthrosis, amphiaster, amphibious.

amphiarthrosis See **cartilaginous joint**.

amphigenesis See **amphigony**.

amphigenetic 1. Produced by the union of gametes from both sexes. 2. Bisexual; having both testicular and ovarian tissue.

amphigonadism True hermaphroditism; having both testicular and ovarian tissue. —**amphigonadic**, adj.

amphigonous inheritance The acquisition of genetic traits and conditions from both parents. Also called **biparental inheritance, duplex inheritance**.

amphigony Sexual reproduction. Also called **amphigenesis**. —**amphigonic**, adj.

amphikaryon A nucleus containing the diploid number of chromosomes. —**amphikaryotic**, adj.

amphimixis 1. The union of germ cells in reproduction so that both maternal and paternal hereditary characteristics are derived; interbreeding. 2. In psychoanalysis: the union and integration of oral, anal, and genital libidinal impulses in the development of sexuality.

ampho- A combining form meaning 'both': amphochromophil, amphodiplopia, amphogenic.

amphoric breath sound An abnormal, hollow blowing sound heard with a stethoscope. It indicates a cavity opening into the bronchus, or a pneumothorax.

amphotericin B An antifungal agent.

ampicillin, a. sodium Penicillin antibiotic agents.

amplification In molecular genetics: 1. A process in which the amount of plasmid DNA is increased in proportion to the amount of bacterial DNA by treatment with certain substances, including chloramphenicol. 2. The replication in bulk of an entire gene library. —**amplify**, v.

amplitude Width or breadth of range or extent, as amplitude of accommodation or amplitude of convergence.

amplitude of accommodation The total accommodative power of the eye, determined by the difference between the refractive power for farthest vision and that for nearest vision.

amplitude of convergence The difference in the power needed to turn the eyes from their far point to their near point of convergence.

ampule, ampoule, ampul A small, sterile glass or plastic container that usually contains a single dose of a solution to be administered parenterally.

ampulla, pl. **ampullae** A dilated segment of a canal or duct; **a. ductus deferens,** dilatation of the vas deferens just before it joins the duct of the seminal vesicle; **a. of lacrimal duct,** dilatation of the lacrimal duct just before it opens into the lacrimal sac; **a. of rectum,** dilatation proximal to the anal canal; **a. of semicircular canal,** dilatation at the end of this canal that contains an ampulla of a semicircular duct; **a. of semicircular ducts,** dilatation near their joining with the utricle; **a. of uterine tube,** dilatation of the distal end of a uterine tube ending in an infundibulum; **a. of vas deferens,** dilatation of the ductus deferens at the base of the bladder; **a. of Vater,** dilatation of the duodenal end of the drainage systems of the pancreatic and common bile ducts.

ampullary tubal pregnancy A kind of tubal pregnancy in which implantation occurs in the ampulla of one of the Fallopian tubes. See also **tubal pregnancy**.

amputation The surgical removal of a part of the body or a limb or part of a limb, performed to treat recurrent infections or gangrene in peripheral vascular disease, to remove malignant tumors, and in severe trauma. Kinds of amputation include **closed amputation, open amputation, primary amputation, secondary amputation**.

amputation neuroma A form of traumatic neuroma that may develop near the stump after the amputation of an extremity.

amputee A person who has had one or more extremities traumatically, congenitally, or surgically removed. See also **congenital amputation**.

amsler grid A checkerboard grid of intersecting dark horizontal and vertical lines with one dark spot in the middle. To discover a visual field defect, the person simply covers or closes one eye, and looks at the spot with the other. A visual field defect is perceived as a defect, distortion, blank, or other fault in the grid. The person may record the defects directly on a paper copy of the grid that may be kept as a permanent record.

Amsterdam dwarf A person affected with de Lange's syndrome, in which short stature and severe mental retardation are associated with many other abnormalities.

amyelinic Without myelin; having no medullary sheath.

amyelinic neuroma A tumor that contains only nonmyelinated nerve fibers.

amyl- See **amylo-**.

amyl alcohol A colorless, oily liquid that is

only slightly soluble in water but can be mixed with ethyl alcohol, chloroform, or ether.

amyl alcohol tertiary See **amylene hydrate.**

amylase An enzyme that catalyzes the hydrolysis of starch into smaller carbohydrate molecules. Alpha-amylase, found in saliva, pancreatic juice, malt, certain bacteria, and molds, catalyzes the hydrolysis of starches to dextrins, maltose, and maltotriose. Beta-amylase, found in grains, vegetables, and malt, is involved in the hydrolysis of starch to maltose. See also **enzyme.**

amylasuria Excessive amylase in the urine.

amylene hydrate A clear, colorless liquid with a camphorlike odor, miscible with alcohol, chloroform, ether, or glycerin and used as a solvent and a hypnotic.

amylic fermentation The formation of amyl alcohol from sugar.

amyl nitrite A coronary vasodilator.

amylo-, amyl- A combining form meaning 'pertaining to starch': *amyloclast, amylodextrin, amyloid.*

amyloidosis A disease in which a waxy, starchlike, glycoprotein (amyloid) accumulates in tissues and organs, impairing their function. There are two major forms of the condition. Primary amyloidosis usually occurs with multiple myeloma. Patients with secondary amyloidosis usually suffer from another chronic infectious or inflammatory disease, as tuberculosis, osteomyelitis, rheumatoid arthritis, or Crohn's disease. The cause of both types of amyloidosis is unknown. Almost all organs are affected, most often the heart, lungs, tongue, and intestines in primary amyloidosis, and the kidneys, liver, and spleen in the secondary type. Diagnosis is made through biopsy of the suspected organ. There is no known cure for amyloidosis, and treatment in the secondary type is aimed at alleviating the underlying chronic disease. Patients with renal amyloidosis are frequently candidates for kidney dialysis and transplantation.

amylopectinosis See **Andersen's disease.**

amyotonia An abnormal condition of skeletal muscle, characterized by a lack of tone, weakness, and wasting, usually the result of motor neuron disease. —**amyotonic,** *adj.*

amyotonia congenita See **Oppenheim's disease.**

amyotrophic lateral sclerosis (ALS) A degenerative disease of the motor neurons, characterized by atrophy of the muscles of the hands, forearms, and legs, spreading to involve most of the body. It results from degeneration of the motor neurons of the anterior horns and cortico spinal tracts, beginning in middle age and progressing rapidly, causing death within 2 to 5 years. There is no known treatment.Also called **Lou Gehrig's disease.** See also **Aran-Duchenne muscular atrophy.**

an- **1.** A combining form meaning 'upward, backward, excessive,' or 'again': *anelectrotonic, anion, anode.* **2.** A combining form meaning 'not': *anaerogenic, anaphia.* Also **ana-.**

-an, -ian A combining form meaning 'belonging to, characteristic of, similar to': *amphibian, protozoan salpingian.*

ANA *abbr* **American Nurses' Association.**

ana- See **an¹.**

anabolic steroid Any one of several compounds derived from testosterone or prepared synthetically to promote general body growth, to oppose the effects of endogenous estrogen, or to promote masculinizing effects. All such compounds cause a mixed androgenic-anabolic effect. Anabolic steroids are prescribed in the treatment of aplastic anemia, red-cell aplasia, and hemolytic anemia and in anemias associated with renal failure, myeloid metaplasia, and leukemia. Some common compounds used in such therapies are calusterone, methandriol, and nandrolone. Anabolic steroids used in the palliation of carcinoma of the breast in women carry the risk of causing masculinization. The earliest symptoms of such undesirable effects are acne, growth of facial hair, and hoarsening or deepening of the voice. Continued use of these compounds in women may also produce prominent musculature, excessive body hair, and hypertrophy of the clitoris.

anabolism Constructive metabolism characterized by the conversion of simple substances into the more complex compounds of living matter. Compare **catabolism.** —**anabolic,** *adj.*

anaclisis **1.** A condition, normal in childhood but pathologic in adulthood, in which a person is emotionally dependent on other people. **2.** A condition in which a person consciously or unconsciously chooses a love object because of a resemblance to the mother, father, or other person who was an important source of comfort and protection in infancy. —**anaclitic,** *adj.*

anaclitic depression A syndrome occurring in infants, usually following sudden separation from the mothering person. Symptoms include apprehension, withdrawal, incessant crying, refusal to eat, sleep disturbances, and, eventually, stupor leading to severe impairment of the infant's physical, social, and intellectual development. If the mothering figure or a substitute is made available within 1 to 3 months, the infant recovers quickly with no long-term effects. See also **hospitalism.**

anacrotic pulse On a sphygmographic tracing: a pulse characterized by one transient drop in amplitude on the curve of the primary elevation. It is seen in valvular aortic stenosis.

anadicrotic pulse On a sphygmographic tracing: a pulse characterized by two transient drops in amplitude on the curve of primary elevation.

anadidymus Conjoined twins that are united in the upper portion of the body but are separated in the lower half.

anadipsia Extreme thirst, often occurring in the manic phase of manic-depressive psychosis. The condition is the result of dehydration owing to the excessive perspiration, continuous urination, and relentless physical activity pro-

ANAL CANAL

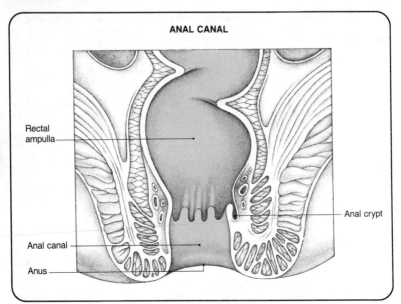

Rectal ampulla

Anal crypt

Anal canal

Anus

duced by the intense excitement characteristic of the manic phase.

anaerobe A microorganism that grows and lives in the complete or almost complete absence of oxygen. Anaerobes are widely distributed in nature and in the body. Some kinds of anaerobes are **facultative anaerobe, obligate anaerobe.** Compare **aerobe.** See also **anaerobic infection.** —**anaerobic,** *adj.*

anaerobic **1.** Pertaining to the absence of air or oxygen. **2.** Able to grow and function without air or oxygen.

anaerobic exercise Muscular exertion sufficient to result in metabolic acidosis owing to accumulation of lactic acid as a product of muscle metabolism. Compare **aerobic exercise.** See also **active exercise, passive exercise.**

anaerobic glycolysis See **glycolysis.**

anaerobic infection An infection caused by an anaerobic organism, usually occurring in deep puncture wounds that exclude air or in tissue that has diminished oxygen-reduction potential as a result of trauma, necrosis, or overgrowth of bacteria. Kinds of anaerobic infection are **gangrene, tetanus.** See also *Clostridium.*

anaerobic myositis See **gas gangrene.**

anakatadidymus Conjoined twins that are united in the middle but separated at the upper and lower parts of the body.

anal Of or pertaining to the anus.

anal agenesis See **imperforate anus.**

anal canal The final portion of the alimentary tract, about 4 cm (1½ inches) long, between the rectal ampulla and the anus.

anal character In psychoanalysis: a kind of personality exhibiting patterns of behavior originating in the anal phase of infancy, char-

acterized by extreme orderliness, obstinacy, perfectionism, cleanliness, punctuality, and miserliness, or their extreme opposites. See also **anal stage, psychosexual development.**

anal crypt The depression between rectal columns that encloses networks of veins that, when inflamed and swollen, are called hemorrhoids.

analeptic A substance that quickens central nervous system (CNS) activity by increasing the rate of neuronal discharge or by blocking an inhibitory neurotransmitter. Many natural and synthetic compounds stimulate the CNS, but only a few are used therapeutically. Caffeine, a potent CNS stimulant, helps restore mental alertness and overcome respiratory depression but may cause nausea, nervousness, tinnitus, tremor, tachycardia, extra systoles, diuresis, and scintillating scotoma. Amphetamines, sympathomimetic amines with CNS-stimulating activity, help treat narcolepsy and obesity but have a high potential for abuse and may cause dizziness, restlessness, tachycardia, increased blood pressure, headache, mouth dryness, an unpleasant taste, gastrointestinal symptoms, and urticaria. Doxapram, ethamivan, and nikethamide stimulate the respiratory center and restore consciousness after anesthesia or acute sedative-hypnotic intoxication.

anal eroticism, anal erotism In psychoanalysis: libidinal fixation at or regression to the anal stage of psychosexual development, often reflected in such personality traits as miserliness, stubbornness, and overscrupulousness. Compare **oral eroticism.** See also **anal character.**

anal fissure A linear ulceration or laceration of the skin of the anus.

anal fistula An abnormal opening on the cutaneous surface near the anus, usually resulting from a local crypt abscess and also common in Crohn's disease. A perianal fistula may or may not communicate with the rectum. Also called **fistula in ano.**

analgesia A lack of pain without loss of consciousness.

analgesia algera See **anesthesia dolorosa.**

analgesic 1. Relieving pain. 2. A drug that relieves pain.

analgesic cocktail *Informal.* An individualized mixture of drugs used for pain relief in specific syndromes. See also **lytic cocktail.**

anal membrane See **cloacal membrane.**

anal membrane atresia See **imperforate anus.**

analog, analogue 1. A substance, tissue, or organ that is similar in appearance or function to another but differing in origin or development, as the eye of a fly and the eye of a human. 2. A drug or other chemical compound that resembles another in structure or constituents but has different effects. Compare **homolog.**

anal reflex A superficial neurological reflex obtained by stroking the skin or mucosa of the region around the anus, which normally results in a contraction of the external anal sphincter. This reflex may be lost in disease of the pyramidal tract above the upper lumbar spine level. See also **superficial reflex.**

anal sadism In psychoanalysis: a sadistic form of anal eroticism, manifested by such behavior as aggressiveness and selfishness. Compare **oral sadism.**

anal stage In psychoanalysis: the pregenital period in psychosexual development, occurring between the ages of 1 and 3 years, when preoccupation with the function of the bowel and the sensations associated with the anus are the predominant source of pleasurable stimulation. It is regarded as an important determinant of ultimate personality type. Adult patterns of behavior associated with fixation on this stage include either extreme neatness, orderliness, cleanliness, perfectionism, and punctuality, or their extreme opposites. See also **anal character, psychosexual development.**

anal stenosis See **imperforate anus.**

analysand A person undergoing psychoanalysis.

analysis 1. The separation of substances into their constituent parts and the determination of the nature, properties, and composition of compounds. 2. In chemistry: qualitative analysis is the determination of the elements present in a substance; quantitative analysis is the determination of how much of each element is present in a substance. 3. *Informal.* Psychoanalysis. —**analytic,** *adj.* **analyze,** *v.*

analysis of variance (ANOVA) A series of statistical procedures for determining the differences, attributable to chance alone, among two or more groups of scores.

analyst 1. A psychoanalyst. 2. A person who

analyzes the chemical, physical, or other properties of a substance or product.

analytic psychology 1. The system in which phenomena, such as sensations and feelings, are analyzed and classified by introspective rather than by experimental methods. Compare **experimental psychology.** 2. A system of analyzing the psyche according to the concepts developed by Carl Gustav Jung. It differs from the psychoanalysis of Sigmund Freud in stressing a racial or collective unconscious and a mystical, religious factor in the development of the personal unconscious and in minimizing the importance of sexual influence on early emotional and psychological development. Also called **Jungian psychology.**

analyzing In five-step nursing process: a category of nursing behavior in which the healthcare needs of the client are identified and the goals of care are selected. The nurse interprets data, identifies problems involving the client, the client's family, and significant others, establishes priorities among goals, integrates the information, and projects the expected outcomes of nursing activities. Although analyzing follows assessing and precedes planning in the five steps of the nursing process, in practice, analyzing is integral to effective nursing practice at all steps of the process. See also **evaluating, implementation.**

anamnesis 1. Remembrance of the past. 2. The accumulated data concerning a medical or psychiatric patient and the patient's background, including family, previous environment, experiences, and particularly, recollections, for use in analyzing his condition. Compare **catamnesis.**

anaphase The third of four stages of nuclear division in mitosis and in each of the two divisions of meiosis. In mitosis and the second meiotic division, the centromeres divide and the two chromatids, which are arranged along the equatorial plane of the spindle, separate and move to the opposite poles of the cell, forming daughter chromosomes. In the first meiotic division, the pairs of homologous chromosomes separate from each other and move intact to the opposite poles of the spindle. See also **interphase, meiosis, metaphase, mitosis, prophase, telophase.**

anaphylactic hypersensitivity An IgE or IgG dependent, immediate-acting humoral hypersensitivity response to an exogenous antigen. An intradermal skin test produces a wheal-and-flare reaction and edema within 30 minutes. Histamine, kinins, and other substances are released from mast cells, causing vasodilation and muscle contraction. Systemic anaphylaxis, atopic allergies, hayfever, and insect-sting reactions are all anaphylactic hypersensitivity reactions. Also called **type I hypersensitivity.** Compare **cell-mediated immune response, cytotoxic hypersensitivity, immune complex hypersensitivity.** See also **anaphylactic shock.**

anaphylactic shock A severe and some-

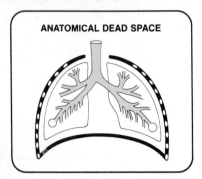

ANATOMICAL DEAD SPACE

times fatal systemic hypersensitivity reaction to a sensitizing substance, as a drug, vaccine, food, serum, allergen extract, insect venom, or chemical. This condition may occur within seconds from the time of exposure to the sensitizing factor and is commonly marked by respiratory distress and vascular collapse. The more quickly any systemic atopic reaction occurs in the individual after exposure, the more severe the associated shock is likely to be. The involved allergen enters the systemic circulation and triggers an incomplete humoral response that allows the allergen to combine with IgE and cause the release of histamine. Also entering into the reaction are IgG and IgM, which cause the release of complement fractions, further stimulating histamine action. If the patient is conscious and normotensive, treatment requires the immediate injection of epinephrine intramuscularly or subcutaneously with vigorous massage of the injection site to assure faster distribution of the drug. If the patient is unconscious, epinephrine is administered intravenously. The airway is maintained and the patient is carefully monitored for signs of laryngeal edema, which may require the insertion of an endotracheal tube or a tracheotomy and oxygen therapy.
NURSING CONSIDERATIONS: Nursing care of patients experiencing anaphylactic shock requires the performance of appropriate emergency treatment and the close monitoring of the patient for hypotension and decreased circulatory volume; volume expanders, as plasma, saline, and albumin, are often ordered. After the emergency, other medications, as subcutaneous epinephrine, corticosteroids, and diphenhydramine I.V. are administered as prescribed; blood pressure, central venous pressure, and urinary output are monitored. Patients with allergies that produce anaphylactic shock are instructed to avoid offending allergens; patients with insect sting allergies are instructed to carry emergency anaphylactic kits when outdoors. Such kits contain epinephrine, antihistamine, and tourniquets.
anaphylactoid purpura See **Henoch-Schönlein purpura.**
anaphylaxis An exaggerated hypersensitivity reaction to a previously encountered antigen. The response, which is mediated by antibodies of the IgE class of immunoglobulins, causes the

release of histamine, kinin, and substances that affect smooth muscle. The reaction may be a localized wheal and flare of generalized itching, hyperemia, angioedema, and, in severe cases, vascular collapse, bronchospasm, and shock. The severity of symptoms depends on the original sensitizing dose of the antigen, the amount and distribution of antibodies, and the route of entry and size of the dose of antigen producing anaphylaxis. Insect stings, contrast media containing iodide, aspirin, antitoxins prepared with animal serum, and allergens used in testing and desensitizing patients who are hypersensitive produce anaphylaxis in some individuals. Kinds of anaphylaxis are **aggregate anaphylaxis, antiserum anaphylaxis, cutaneous anaphylaxis, cytotoxic anaphylaxis, indirect anaphylaxis, inverse anaphylaxis.** —**anaphylactic, anaphylactoid,** adj.
anaplasia A change in the structure of cells and in their orientation to each other characterized by a loss of differentiation and reversion to a more primitive form. Anaplasia is characteristic of malignancy. Compare **metastasis.** —**anaplastic,** adj.
anaplastic astrocytoma See **glioblastoma multiforme.**
anasarca Generalized, massive edema. Anasarca is often observed in edema associated with renal disease when fluid retention continues for an extended period of time. See also **edema.** —**anasarcous,** adj.
anastomosis, pl. **anastomoses** A surgical joining of two ducts or blood vessels to allow flow from one to the other. It may be performed to bypass an aneurysm or a vascular or arterial occlusion. Kinds of anastomoses are end-to-end anastomosis, side-to-side anastomosis. See also **aneurysm, bypass.**
anastomosis at elbow joint A convergence of blood vessels at the elbow joint, consisting of various veins and portions of the brachial and deep brachial arteries and their branches.
anatomical dead space An area in the trachea, bronchi, and air passages containing air that does not reach the alveoli during respiration. As a general rule, the volume of air in the anatomical dead space in milliliters is approximately equal to the weight in pounds of the involved individual. Certain lung disorders, as emphysema, increase the amount of anatomical dead space. Compare **physiological dead space.**
anatomical position A position of the body in which a person stands erect, facing directly forward, feet pointed forward slightly apart, arms hanging down at the sides with palms facing forward. This is the standard neutral position of reference used to describe sites or motions of various parts of the body. See also **body position.**
anatomical snuffbox A small, cuplike depression on the back of the hand near the wrist, formed by the tendons reaching toward the thumb and index finger as the thumb is

abducted, the wrist flexed, and the digits extended.

anatomic curve The curvature of the different segments of the vertebral column. In the lateral contour of the back, the cervical curve appears concave, the thoracic curve appears convex, and the lumbar curve appears concave.

anatomy **1.** The study, classification, and description of structures and organs of the body. Kinds of anatomy are **applied anatomy, comparative anatomy, descriptive anatomy, gross anatomy, microscopic anatomy, pathological anatomy, surface anatomy. 2.** The structure of an organism. **3.** A text on anatomy. **4.** Dissection of a body.

-ance See **-ency.**

ancrod The venom of the Malayan pit viper, used to remove fibrinogen from the circulation, thus preventing clotting of the blood.

-ancy See **-ency.**

ancylo-, anchylo-, ankylo- A combining form meaning 'bent or in the form of a loop': *ancylostomatic, ancylostomiasis, ancylostomoanemia.*

Ancylostoma A genus of nematode that includes *Necator americanus,* the most common North American hookworm.

ancylostomiasis Hookworm disease, more specifically that caused by *Ancylostoma duodenale, A. braziliensis,* or *A. canium.* Infection by *A. duodenale* is generally more harmful and less responsive to treatment than that by *Necator americanus,* which is the hookworm most often found in the southern United States. Clinical manifestations and treatment are similar for all types of hookworms. See also **hookworm.**

Andersen's disease A rare glycogen-storage disease characterized by a genetic deficiency of branching enzyme (amylo-1:4, 1:6 transglucosisase), causing the deposition in tissues of abnormal glycogen with long inner and outer chains. Infants with the disease are normal at birth but fail to thrive and soon show hepatomegaly, splenomegaly, and hypotonic muscles, associated with the progressive development of liver cirrhosis or heart failure of unknown mechanisms. Diagnosis is by enzyme assays of white blood cells and fibroblasts. There is no specific therapy for the disease, which is usually fatal in the first few years of life. Also called **amylopectinosis, Cori's disease, glycogen storage disease, type IV.**

andr- See **andro-.**

andreioma See **arrhenoblastoma.**

andreoblastoma See **arrhenoblastoma.**

andro-, andr- A combining form meaning 'pertaining to man or to the male': *androcyte, androgen, androgone.*

androgamone A gamone secreted by the male gamete.

androgen A class of hormones that increases male characteristics. Natural hormones, as testosterone and its esters and analogs, are primarily used as substitutional therapy during the male climacteric. See also **anabolism. —androgenic,** *adj.*

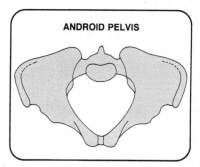

ANDROID PELVIS

androgynous **1.** Of a man or woman: having some characteristics of both sexes. Social role, behavior, personality, and appearance are reflections of individuality and are not determined by gender. **2.** Hermaphroditic. Compare **gynandrous. —androgyny,** *n.*

android pelvis A type of pelvis in which the structure is characteristic of the male. It is not uncommon in women. The bones are thick and heavy and the inlet is heart-shaped. The sacrum inclines anteriorly, the side walls are convergent, and the pubic arch is small. The diameters of the midplane and the outlet are smaller than in the normal gynecoid pelvis, and vaginal delivery is likely to be difficult unless the overall pelvis is large and the fetus small.

androma See **arrhenoblastoma.**

androsterone Originally believed to be the principal male sex hormone, it is used less frequently since the discovery of testosterone. The greater potency of several other male sex hormones has relegated androsterone largely to historical biochemical interest. See also **testosterone.**

-ane A combining form designating hydrocarbons of the paraffin series: *butane, lindane, xylane.*

anemia A disorder characterized by a decrease in hemoglobin in the blood to levels below the normal range. According to the pathophysiological classification, anemia is a reflection of any one (or more) of three basic processes: decreased hemoglobin or red cell production, increased red cell destruction, or blood loss. A separate and distinct morphological classification system describes anemia by the hemoglobin content of the red cells (normochromic or hypochromic) and by differences in red cell size (macrocytic, normocytic, or microcytic). Depending on its severity, anemia may be accompanied by some or all of a number of clinical findings that stem directly from the diminished oxygen-carrying capacity of the blood. These include fatigue, exertional dyspnea, dizziness, headache, insomnia, and pallor, especially of the mucous membranes. Anorexia and dyspepsia, palpitations, tachycardia, cardiac dilatation and systolic murmurs also occur. The therapeutic response to anemia is highly variable and depends on the specific causative factors involved. Moderate to severe anemia, with hemoglobin levels that are below 7 to 8 g/dl, may call for transfusion of one or more units of blood, especially if the condition is acute and accompanied by specific clinical signs. Depending on the kind of anemia, treatment aims at providing supplements of the deficient component, eliminating the cause of the blood loss, or alleviating the hemolytic component. The latter may involve the administration of adrenal corticosteroids or, possibly, splenectomy.

NURSING CONSIDERATIONS: The nurse emphasizes to the patient the importance of adequate diet to supply blood building components. The patient's need for rest is stressed, especially in the face of cardiac and respiratory symptoms. The time needed for recovery and the need for repeated blood tests to evaluate the progress of therapy are outlined. The patient is also cautioned, where applicable, to be alert for signs of increasing anemia or resumption of blood loss. When transfusions are given, the nurse is alert for indications of a transfusion reaction. —**anemic,** *adj.*

-anemia, -anaemia   A combining form meaning '(condition of) red blood cell deficiency or its remedy': *achylanemia, melanemia, sulfanemia.* Also **-nemia.**

anemia of pregnancy   A condition of pregnancy characterized by a reduction in the concentration of hemoglobin in the blood. It may be physiologic or pathologic. In physiologic anemia of pregnancy, the reduction in concentration results from dilution because the plasma volume expands more than the red blood cell volume. The hematocrit in pregnancy normally drops several points below the level it was before pregnancy. In pathologic anemia of pregnancy, the oxygen-carrying capacity of the blood is deficient owing to disordered erythrocyte production or excessive loss of erythrocytes through destruction or bleeding. Pathologic anemia is a common complication of pregnancy occurring in approximately one half of all pregnancies. Disordered production of erythrocytes may result from nutritional deficiency of iron, folic acid, or vitamin B_{12} or from chronic disease, malignancy, chronic malnutrition, or exposure to toxins. Destruction of erythrocytes may result from inflammation, chronic infection, sepsis, autoimmune disorders, microangiopath, or a hematologic disease in which the red cells are abnormal.

anemic anoxia   A condition characterized by a deficiency of oxygen in body tissues, resulting from a decrease in the number of erythrocytes in the blood or in the amount of hemoglobin.

anemo-   A combining form meaning 'pertaining to the wind': *anemopathy, anemophobia, anemotropism.*

anencephaly   Congenital absence of the brain and spinal cord in which the cranium does not close and the vertebral canal remains a groove. Transmitted genetically, anencephaly is not compatible with life. It can be detected early in gestation by amniotic fluid tap and analysis or by ultrasonography. See also **neural tube defect.**

anergic stupor   A kind of dementia characterized by quietness, listlessness, and nonresistance.

anergy   **1.** Lack of activity. **2.** An immunodeficient condition characterized by a lack of or diminished reaction to an antigen or group of antigens. This state may be seen in advanced tuberculosis and other serious infections and in some malignancies. —**anergic,** *adj.*

aneroid   Not containing a liquid; used especially to describe a device that does not contain liquid (such as an aneroid sphygmomanometer, which does not contain a column of liquid mercury), in contrast to a device performing a similar function that does contain liquid.

anesthesia   The absence of normal sensation, especially sensitivity to pain, as induced by an anesthetic substance or by hypnosis or as occurs with traumatic or pathophysiologic damage to nerve tissue. Anesthesia induced for medical or surgical purposes may be topical, local, regional, or general and is named for the anesthetic agent used, the method or procedure followed, the area or organ anesthetized, or the age or class of patient served. See also specific anesthetic agents and forms of anesthesia.

anesthesia dolorosa   A severe, spontaneous, paradoxical pain in an anesthetized area. Also called **analgesia algera.**

anesthesia machine   An apparatus for administering inhalant anesthetic agents. Although there are many different models, all have the following features: an accommodation for a source of gas; a meter to measure the flow of gas; vessels for volatilizing and mixing the anesthetic agents and the carrier gases; and a system for delivery of the gas to the patient.

anesthesia patients, classification of   The system by which the American Society of Anesthesiologists classifies anesthesia patients in five categories by anesthetic risk factors. Class I includes patients who are generally healthy, without serious organic, physiologic, biochemical, or psychiatric problems, and for whom anesthesia is required only for a local condition, as an inguinal hernia or fibroid uterus. Class II includes patients who have mild to moderate systemic problems, whether involving or extraneous to the condition requiring anesthesia, as anemia, mild diabetes, essential hypertension, extreme obesity, or chronic bronchitis. Class III includes patients who have severe systemic disturbances or disease, whether or not related to the procedure requiring surgical anesthesia. Class IV includes patients who are suffering from a life-threatening, but not necessarily terminal, condition that may or may not be related to the intended surgical procedure. Class V includes the moribund patient who has little chance of survival, as a person in shock with a burst abdominal aneurysm or a massive pulmonary embolus. The letter E is added to the roman numeral to indicate an emergency procedure, as a

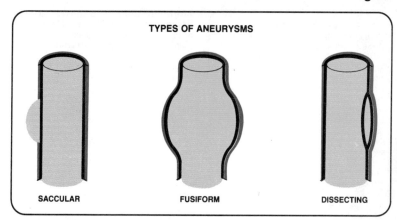

TYPES OF ANEURYSMS

SACCULAR   FUSIFORM   DISSECTING

patient scheduled for an elective herniorrhaphy who becomes an emergency case when the hernia becomes an obstruction.

anesthesia screen A metal, inverted U-shaped frame that attaches to the sides of an operating table, 30 to 45 cm (12 to 18 inches) above a patient's upper chest. It is covered with a sheet to prevent contamination of an operative site on the chest or abdomen by airborne infection from the patient or the anesthetist and to provide a wide sterile field for the surgeon.

anesthesiologist A physician trained in the administration of anesthetics and in the provision of respiratory and cardiovascular support during anesthetic procedures. Compare **nurse anesthetist.**

anesthesiology The branch of medicine that is concerned with the relief of pain and with the administration of medication to relieve pain during surgery. It is a specialty requiring competency in general medicine, a broad understanding of surgical procedures, a wide knowledge of clinical pharmacology, biochemistry, cardiology, and respiratory physiology. See also **anesthesiologist, nurse anesthetist.**

anesthetist **1.** A person who administers anesthesia. **2.** An anesthesiologist. See also **nurse anesthetist.**

anetoderma An idiopathic, patchy atrophy and looseness of skin for which there is no known effective treatment.

aneuploid, aneuploidic **1.** Of or pertaining to an individual, organism, strain, or cell that has a chromosome number that is not an exact multiple of the normal, basic haploid number characteristic of the species. Variation occurs through individual chromosomes rather than an entire set so that there are more or less than the normal diploid number found in the somatic cell. **2.** Such an individual, organism, strain, or cell. Compare **euploid.** See also **monosomy, trisomy.**

aneuploidy Any variation in chromosome number that involves individual chromosomes rather than entire sets. There may be fewer chromosomes, as in Turner's syndrome, or more

chromosomes, as in Down's syndrome. Such individuals have various abnormal physiological and morphological traits. Compare **euploidy.** See also **monosomy, trisomy.**

aneurysm A localized dilatation of the wall of a blood vessel, usually caused by atherosclerosis and hypertension, or, less frequently, by trauma, infection, or a congenital weakness in the vessel wall. Aneurysms are most prominent and significant in the aorta but also occur in peripheral vessels and are fairly common in the lower extremities of older people, especially in the popliteal arteries. An arterial aneurysm may be a saccular distention affecting only part of the circumference of the vessel; it may be a fusiform or cylindroid dilatation of a section of the vessel; or it may be a longitudinal dissection between layers of the vascular wall. A sign of an arterial aneurysm is a pulsating swelling that produces a blowing murmur on auscultation with a stethoscope. An aneurysm may rupture, causing hemorrhage, or thrombi may form in the dilated pouch and give rise to emboli that may obstruct smaller vessels. Kinds of aneurysms include **aortic aneurysm, berry aneurysm, cerebral aneurysm, compound aneurysm, dissecting aneurysm, mycotic aneurysm, racemose aneurysm, Rasmussen's aneurysm, ventricular aneurysm.** —aneurysmal, *adj.*

aneurysm needle A needle equipped with a handle, used to ligate aneurysms.

ANF *abbr* **1. American Nurses' Foundation. 2. antinuclear factor.**

anger According to Elisabeth Kübler-Ross, the second stage of dying. The person in this stage feels anger, envy, rage, and resentment. He often projects this anger randomly onto his environment: his doctors, nurses, and family. See also **acceptance, bargaining, denial and isolation, depression.**

angi- See **angio-.**

angiitis An inflammatory condition of a vessel, chiefly a blood or lymph vessel. A kind of angiitis is **consecutive angiitis.** See also **vasculitis.**

ANGIOCATHER
(OVER-THE-NEEDLE CATHETER)

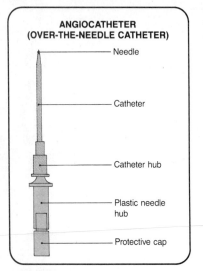

- Needle
- Catheter
- Catheter hub
- Plastic needle hub
- Protective cap

angina 1. A spasmodic, cramplike choking feeling. 2. A term now used primarily to denote the paroxysmal thoracic pain and choking feeling caused by anoxia of the myocardium (angina pectoris). 3. A descriptive feature of various diseases characterized by a feeling of choking, suffocation, or crushing pressure and pain. Kinds of angina are **intestinal angina, Ludwig's angina, Prinzmetal's angina.** —**anginal,** *adj.*

-angina A combining form meaning 'severe ulceration, usually of the mouth or throat': *herpangina, juxtangina, monocytangina.*

angina decubitus A condition characterized by periodic attacks of angina pectoris that occur when the person is lying down.

angina dyspeptica A painful condition caused by gaseous distention of the stomach that mimics angina pectoris.

angina epiglottidea A painful condition caused by inflammation of the epiglottis.

angina pectoris A paroxysmal thoracic pain caused most often by myocardial anoxia owing to atherosclerosis of the coronary arteries. The pain radiates down the inner aspect of the left arm and is frequently accompanied by a feeling of suffocation and impending death. Attacks of angina pectoris are often related to exertion, emotional stress, and exposure to intense cold. The pain may be relieved by rest and vasodilation of the coronary arteries by medication, as with nitroglycerin.

angina sine dolore A painless episode of coronary insufficiency.

angina trachealis See **croup.**

angio-, angei-, angi- A combining form meaning 'pertaining to a vessel, usually a blood vessel': *angioblastic, angiochondroma, angioglioma.*

angioblastic meningioma A tumor of the blood vessels of the meninges covering the spinal cord or the brain.

angioblastoma, *pl.* **angioblastomas, angioblastomata** A tumor of blood vessels in the brain. Kinds of angioblastomas are **angioblastic meningioma, cerebellar angioblastoma.**

angiocardiogram A radiograph of the heart and the vessels of the heart. A radiopaque substance is injected forcibly into a vein in the antecubital space and X-rays are taken as the radiopaque contrast medium passes through the heart and its vessels. Nausea and vomiting are common untoward reactions; urticaria, shortness of breath, or anaphylaxis may also occur.

angiocatheter A small hollow, flexible tube used to provide venous access for delivery of drugs or fluids. A needle fits inside a catheter. Once inserted, the needle is removed, leaving only the catheter in place. Also called angiocath, over-the-needle catheter (ONC).

angiochondroma, *pl.* **angiochondromas, angiochondromata** A cartilaginous tumor characterized by an excessive formation of blood vessels.

angioedema See **angioneurotic edema.**

angioendothelioma See **hemangioendothelioma.**

angiofibroma, *pl.* **angiofibromas, angiofibromata** An angioma containing fibrous tissue. Also called **fibroangioma.**

angioglioma, *pl.* **angiogliomas, angiogliomatas** A highly vascular tumor composed of neuroglia.

angiography The X-ray visualization of the internal anatomy of the heart and blood vessels following the intravascular introduction of radiopaque contrast medium. The procedure is used as a diagnostic aid in myocardial infarction, vascular occlusion, calcified atherosclerotic plaques, cerebrovascular accident, portal hypertension, renal neoplasms, renal artery stenosis as a causative factor in hypertension, pulmonary emboli, and congenital and acquired lesions of pulmonary vessels. The contrast medium may be injected into an artery or vein or introduced into a catheter inserted in a peripheral artery and threaded through the vessel to a visceral site. Since the iodine in the contrast medium may cause a marked allergic reaction in some patients, testing for hypersensitivity is indicated before the radiopaque substance is used. After the procedure, the patient is monitored for signs of bleeding, and bed rest for a number of hours is indicated. —**angiographic,** *adj.*

angiohemophilia See **Von Willebrand's disease.**

angiokeratoma, *pl.* **angiokeratomas, angiokeratomata** A vascular, horny neoplasm on the skin, characterized by clumps of dilated blood vessels, clusters of warts, and thickening of the epidermis, especially the scrotum and the dorsal aspect of the fingers and toes.

angiokeratoma circumscriptum A rare skin disorder characterized by discrete papules and nodules in small patches on the legs or on the trunk.

angiokeratoma corporis diffusum An uncommon familial disease in which phospholipids are stored in many parts of the body, especially the blood vessels, causing vasomotor, urinary, and cutaneous disorders, and, in some cases, muscular abnormalities. Characteristic signs of the disease are edema, hypertension, and cardiomegaly, especially enlargement of the left ventricle; diffuse nodularity of the skin; albumin, erythrocytes, leukocytes, and casts in the urine; and vacuoles in muscle bundles. Also called **Fabry's disease, Fabry's syndrome.**

angiolipoma, *pl.* **angiolipomas, angiolipomata** A benign neoplasm containing blood vessels and tissue. Also called **lipoma cavernosum, telangiectatic lipoma.**

angioma, *pl.* **angiomas, angiomata** Any benign tumor made up primarily of blood vessels (hemangioma) or lymph vessels (lymphangioma). Most angiomas are congenital; some, like cavernous hemangiomas, disappear spontaneously.

-angioma A combining form meaning a 'tumor composed chiefly of blood and lymph vessels': *fibroangioma, glomangioma, telangioma.*

angioma arteriale racemosum A vascular neoplasm characterized initially by the intertwining of many small, newly formed, dilated blood vessels. Subsequently, normal blood vessels become affected.

angioma cavernosum See **cavernous hemangioma.**

angioma cutis A nevus composed of a network of dilated blood vessels.

angioma lymphaticum See **lymphangioma.**

angioma serpiginosum A cutaneous disease characterized by rings of tiny vascular points resembling grains of pepper. Also called **Hutchinson's disease.**

angiomatosis A condition characterized by the presence of numerous vascular tumors. A kind of angiomatosis is **Osler-Weber-Rendu syndrome.**

angiomyoma, *pl.* **angiomyomas, angiomyomata** A tumor composed of vascular and muscular tissue elements.

angiomyoneuroma, *pl.* **angiomyoneuromas, angiomyoneuromata** See **glomangioma.**

angiomyosarcoma, *pl.* **angiomyosarcomas, angiomyosarcomata** A tumor containing vascular, muscular, and connective tissue elements.

angioneuroma, *pl.* **angioneuromas, angioneuromata** See **glomangioma.**

angioneurotic anuria An abnormal condition characterized by an almost complete absence of urination caused by destruction of tissue in the renal cortex. See also **anuria.**

angioneurotic edema An acute, painless, dermal, subcutaneous, or submucosal swelling of short duration involving the face, neck, lips, larynx, hands, feet, genitalia, or viscera. It may result from food or drug allergy, infection, or emotional stress, or it may be hereditary. Treat-

ment depends upon the cause. For severe forms, intubation, tracheotomy, or subcutaneous injections of epinephrine may be necessary to prevent respiratory obstruction. Prevention depends on the identification and avoidance of etiologic factors. Also called **angioedema.** See also **anaphylaxis, hives, serum sickness, urticaria.**

angiosarcoma A rare, malignant tumor consisting of endothelial and fibroblastic tissue. Also called **hemangiosarcoma.** Compare **angioma.**

angiotensin A polypeptide occurring in the blood causing vasoconstriction, increased blood pressure, and the release of aldosterone from the adrenal cortex. Angiotensin is formed by the action of renin on angiotensinogen, an alpha-2-globulin that is produced in the liver and constantly circulates in the blood. Renin, elaborated by juxtaglomerular cells in the kidney in response to decreased blood volume and serum sodium, acts as an enzyme in the conversion of angiotensinogen to angiotensin I, which is rapidly hydrolyzed to form the active compound angiotensin II. The vasoconstrictive action of angiotensin II decreases the glomerular filtration rate and the concomitant action of aldosterone promotes sodium retention, with the result that blood volume and sodium reabsorption increase. Plasma angiotensin increases during the luteal phase of the menstrual cycle and is probably responsible for an elevated level of aldosterone during that period. Angiotensin is inactivated by peptidases, called angiotensinases, in plasma and tissues.

angle 1. The space or the shape formed at the intersection of two lines, planes, or borders. The divergence of the lines, planes, or borders may be measured in degrees of a circle. 2. In anatomy and physiology: the geometric relationships between the surfaces of body structures and the positions affected by movement.

angstrom, angstrom unit A unit of measure of length equal to 0.1 millimicron (one ten-billionth of a meter).

angular movement One of the four basic kinds of movement allowed by the various joints of the skeleton in which the angle between two adjoining bones is decreased, as in flexion, or increased, as in extension. Compare **circumduction, gliding, rotation.**

angular vein One of a pair of veins of the face, formed by the junction of the frontal and the supraorbital veins. At the root of the nose, each angular vein receives the flow of venous blood from the infraorbital, the superior palpebral, the inferior palpebral, and the external nasal veins, becoming the first part of one of the two facial veins.

angulated fracture A fracture in which the fragments of bone are angulated.

anhedonia The inability to feel pleasure from ordinarily pleasurable experiences. Compare **analgesia. —anhedonic,** *adj.*

anhidrosis An abnormal condition characterized by inadequate perspiration. —**anhidrotic,** *adj.*

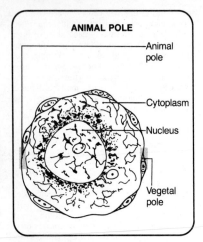

ANIMAL POLE

Animal pole

Cytoplasm

Nucleus

Vegetal pole

anhidrotic 1. Of or pertaining to anhidrosis. 2. An agent that reduces or suppresses sweating.

anicteric hepatitis A mild form of hepatitis in which there is no jaundice (icterus), usually seen in infants and young children. Symptoms include anorexia, gastrointestinal disturbances, and slight fever. SGOT and SGPT are elevated. The infection may be mistaken for flu or go unnoticed. Compare **hepatitis.** See also **icterus, jaundice.**

anidean, anidian, anidous Formless; shapeless; denoting an undifferentiated mass, as an anideus.

anideus An anomalous, rudimentary conceptus consisting of a simple rounded mass with little indication of the body parts. A kind of anideus is **embryonic anideus.** Also called **fetus anideus.**

aniline An oily, colorless poisonous liquid with a strong odor and burning taste, formerly extracted from the indigo plant and now made synthetically using nitrobenzene in the manufacture of aniline dyes. Industrial workers exposed to aniline are at risk of developing methemoglobinemia and bone marrow depression. Also called **amidobenzene, aminobenzene.**

anilinparasulfonic acid See **sulfanilic acid.**

anima 1. The soul or life. 2. The active ingredient in a drug. 3. In Jungian psychology: a person's true, inner, unconscious being or personality, as distinguished from overt personality, or persona. 4. In analytic psychology: the female component of the male personality. Compare **animus.**

animal pole The active, formative part of the ovum protoplasm that contains the nucleus and bulk of the cytoplasm and where the polar bodies form. In mammals it is also the site where the inner cell mass gives rise to the ectoderm. Also called **germinal pole.** Compare **vegetal pole.**

animal starch See **glycogen.**

animus 1. The active or rational soul; the animating principle of life. 2. The male component of the female personality. 3. In psychiatry: a deep-seated antagonism that is usually controlled but may erupt with virulence under stress. Compare **anima.**

anion 1. A negatively charged ion which is attracted to the positive electrode (anode) in electrolysis. 2. A negatively charged atom, molecule, or radical. Compare **cation.**

anion-exchange resin Any one of the simple organic polymers with high molecular weights that exchange anions with other ions in solution. Anion-exchange resins are used as antacids in treating ulcers. Compare **cation-exchange resin.**

anion gap The difference between the concentrations of serum cations and anions, determined by measuring the concentrations of sodium cations and chloride and bicarbonate anions. It is helpful in the diagnosis and treatment of acidosis, and it is estimated by subtracting the sum of sodium and bicarbonate concentrations in the plasma from that of sodium. It is normally about 8 to 14 mEq/liter and represents the negative charges contributed to plasma by unmeasured ions or ions other than those of chloride and bicarbonate, mainly phosphate, sulfate, organic acids, and plasma proteins. Anions other than chloride and bicarbonate normally constitute about 12 mEq/liter of the total anion concentration in plasma. Acidosis can develop with or without an associated anion increase. An increase in the anion gap often suggests diabetic ketoacidosis, drug poisoning, renal failure, or lactic acidosis and usually warrants further laboratory tests.

anise The fruit of the *Pimpinella anisum* plant. Extract of anise is used in the preparation of carminatives and expectorants.

aniseikonia An abnormal ocular condition in which each eye perceives the same image as being of a different size.

anisindione An oral anticoagulant of the indandione type.

aniso- A combining form meaning 'unequal or dissimilar': *anisochromia, anisodont, anisognathous.*

anisocytosis An abnormal condition of the blood characterized by red blood cells of variable and abnormal size. Compare **poikilocytosis.** See also **macrocytosis, microcytosis.**

anisogamete A gamete that differs considerably in size and structure from the one with which it unites, as the macrogamete and microgamete of certain sporozoa. Compare **heterogamete, isogamete.** —**anisogametic,** *adj.*

anisogamy Sexual conjugation of gametes that are of unequal size and structure, such as in certain thallophytes and sporozoa. Compare **heterogamy, isogamy.** —**anisogamous,** *adj.*

anisokaryosis Significant variation in the size of the nucleus of cells of the same general type. —**anisokaryotic,** *adj.*

anisometropia An abnormal ocular condition characterized by a difference in the refractive powers of the eyes.

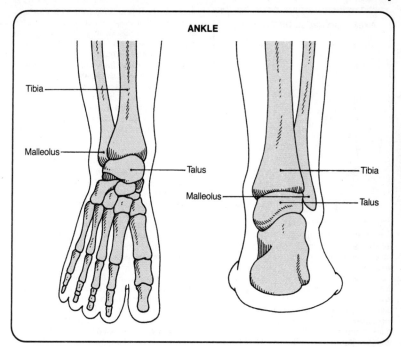

ANKLE

Tibia

Malleolus

Talus

Malleolus

Tibia

Talus

anisopoikilocytosis An abnormal condition of the blood characterized by red blood cells of variable and abnormal size and shape. See also **anisocytosis, erythrocyte, morphology, poikilocytosis.**

anisotropine methylbromide A gastrointestinal anticholinergic agent.

ankle **1.** The joint of the tibia, the talus, and the malleolus. **2.** The part of the leg where this joint is located.

ankle reflex See **Achilles tendon reflex.**

ankylo- See **ancylo-.**

ankylosing spondylitis A chronic inflammatory disease of unknown etiology, first affecting the spine and adjacent structures and commonly progressing to eventual fusion (ankylosis) of the involved joints. In extreme cases, the patient develops a forward flexion of the spine, called a 'poker spine' or 'bamboo spine.' The disease primarily affects males under the age of 30, and generally burns itself out after a course of 20 years. There is a strong hereditary tendency. In addition to the spine, the joints of the hip, shoulder, neck, ribs, and jaw are often involved. When the costovertebral joints are involved, the patient may have difficulty in expanding the rib cage while breathing. Ankylosing spondylitis is a systemic disease, often affecting the eyes and the heart. Many patients with the disease also have inflammatory bowel disease. The aim of treatment is to reduce pain and inflammation in the involved joints, usually with nonsteroidal anti-inflammatory drugs. Physical therapy aids in keeping the spine as erect as possible to prevent flexion contractures. In advanced cases, surgery may be performed to straighten a badly deformed spine. Also called Marie-Strumpell disease. Compare **rheumatoid arthritis.** See also **ankylosis.**

ankylosis **1.** Fixation of a joint, often in an abnormal position, usually resulting from destruction of articular cartilage and subchondral bone, as occurs in rheumatoid arthritis. **2.** Surgically induced fixation of a joint to relieve pain or provide support. Also called **arthrodesis, fusion.**

anlage In embryology: the undifferentiated layer of cells from which a particular organ, tissue, or structure develops; primordium rudiment. See also **blastema.**

ANLL *abbr* acute nonlymphocytic leukemia. See **acute myelocytic leukemia.**

annular Describing a ring-shaped lesion surrounding a clear, normal, unaffected disk of skin.

annular ligament A ligament that encircles the head of the radius and holds it in the radial notch of the ulna. Distal to the notch, the annular ligament forms a complete fibrous ring.

anodmia See **anosmia.** —**anodmatic, anodmic,** *adj.*

anodontia A congenital defect in which some or all of the teeth are missing.

anodyne A drug that relieves or lessens pain. Compare **analgesic.**

anomalo- A combining form meaning 'uneven or irregular': *anomalopia, anomaloscope, anomalotrophy.*

anomaly **1.** Deviation from what is regarded

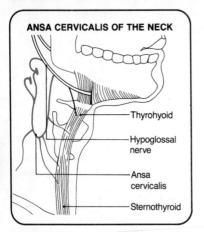

ANSA CERVICALIS OF THE NECK

— Thyrohyoid

— Hypoglossal nerve

— Ansa cervicalis

— Sternothyroid

as normal. **2.** Congenital malformation, as the absence of a limb or the presence of an extra finger. —**anomalous,** *adj.*

anomia A form of aphasia characterized by the inability to name objects, caused by a lesion in the temporal lobe of the brain.

anomie, anomy A state of apathy, alienation, anxiety, personal disorientation, and distress, resulting from the loss of social norms and goals previously valued.

anoopsia A strabismus in which one or both eyes are deviated upward.

Anopheles A genus of mosquito, many species of which transmit malaria-causing parasites to man. These mosquitoes are characterized by long thin palps. See also **malaria.**

anopia Blindness resulting from a defect in or the absence of one or both eyes.

-anopia, -anopsia 1. A combining form meaning '(condition involving) nonuse or arrested development of the eye': *hemianopia, hesperanopia, duadrantopia.* **2.** A combining form meaning '(condition of) defective color vision': *cyanopia, deuteranopia, tritanopia.*

anorchia, anorchism Congenital absence of one or both testes.

anorectal Of or pertaining to the anal and rectal portions of the large intestine.

anorectic 1. Of or pertaining to anorexia. **2.** Lacking appetite. **3.** Causing a loss of appetite, as an anorexiant drug. —**anorectous, anorexiant,** *adj.*

anorexia Lack or loss of appetite, resulting in the inability to eat. The condition may result from poorly prepared food or unattractive surroundings, unfavorable company, or psychological causes. Compare **pseudoanorexia.** See also **anorexia nervosa.** —**anorexic,** *adj.*

anorexia nervosa A psychoneurotic disorder characterized by prolonged refusal to eat, resulting in emaciation, amenorrhea, emotional disturbance concerning body image, and abnormal fear of becoming obese. The condition is seen primarily in adolescents, predominantly girls, and is usually associated with emotional

stress or conflict, as anxiety, irritation, anger, and fear, which may accompany a major change in the person's life. Goals of treatment are to improve nourishment and to overcome the underlying emotional conflicts.

anosmia Loss or impairment of the sense of smell, commonly occurring as a temporary condition resulting from a head cold or respiratory infection or when intranasal swelling or other obstruction prevents odors from reaching the olfactory region. It becomes a permanent condition when the olfactory neuroepithelium or any part of the olfactory nerve is destroyed as a result of intracranial trauma, neoplasms, or disease, as atrophic rhinitis or the chronic rhinitis associated with the granulomatous diseases. In some instances, the condition may be caused by psychological factors, as a phobia or fear associated with a particular smell. Kinds of anosmia are **anosmia gustatoria, preferential anosmia.** Also called **anodmia, anosphrasia, olfactory anesthesia.** —**anosmatic, anosmic,** *adj.*

anosmia gustatoria The inability to smell foods.

anosognosia An abnormal condition characterized by a real or feigned inability to perceive a defect, especially paralysis, on one side of the body, possibly attributable to a lesion in the right parietal lobe of the brain.

anosphrasia, anosphresia See **anosmia.**

ANOVA *abbr* **analysis of variance.**

anovulation Failure of the ovaries to produce, mature, or release eggs, owing to ovarian immaturity or postmaturity; to altered ovarian function, as in pregnancy and lactation; to primary ovarian dysfunction, as in ovarian dysgenesis; or to disturbance of the interaction of the hypothalamus, pituitary gland, and ovary, caused by stress or disease. Hormonal contraceptives prevent conception by suppressing ovulation. Anovulation may be an adverse side effect of other medications prescribed in the treatment of other disorders. —**anovulatory,** *adj.*

anoxia An abnormal condition characterized by a relative or a total lack of oxygen. Anoxia may be local or systemic and may be the result of an inadequate supply of oxygen to the respiratory system or of an inability of the blood to carry oxygen to the tissues or of the tissues to absorb the oxygen from the circulation. Kinds of anoxia include cerebral anoxia, stagnant anoxia. —**anoxic,** *adj.*

-ans A combining form meaning '-ing': *aberrans, penetrans, proliferans.*

ansa, *pl.* **ansae** In anatomy: a looplike structure resembling a curved handle of a vase.

ansa cervicalis One of three loops of nerves in the cervical plexus, branches of which innervate the infrahyoid muscles. It has a superior root, which connects with the hypoglossal nerve and contains fibers of the first and the second cervical nerves, and an inferior root, which connects with the second and the third cervical nerves. Also called **ansa hypoglossi.**

ansa hypoglossi See **ansa cervicalis.**
answer In law: the response of a defendant to the complaint of a plaintiff. The answer contains a denial of the plaintiff's allegations and may also contain an affirmative defense or a counterclaim. It is the principal pleading on the part of the defense and is prepared in writing, usually by the defense attorney, and submitted to the court.
ant- See **anti-.**
antacid **1.** Opposing acidity. **2.** A drug or dietary substance that buffers, neutralizes, or absorbs hydrochloric acid in the stomach. Most antacids are not absorbed systemically. Antacids containing aluminum and calcium are constipating; those containing magnesium have a laxative effect.
antagonist **1.** One who contends with or is opposed to another. **2.** In physiology: any agent, such as a drug or muscle, that exerts an opposite action to that of another. Kinds of antagonists include antimetabolite, associated antagonist, direct antagonist. Compare **agonist. 3.** In dentistry: a tooth in the upper jaw that articulates during mastication or occlusion with a tooth in the lower jaw. —**antagonistic,** *adj.,* **antagonize,** *v.*
antagonist drug A drug that opposes the action of another drug by neutralization, by receptor-site blockade, or by other means. See also **narcotic antagonist.**
ante- A combining form meaning 'before in time or in place': *anteflexion, antenatal, antepartal.*
anteflexion An abnormal position of an organ in which the organ is tilted acutely forward, folded over on itself.
antenatal See **prenatal.**
antenatal diagnosis See **prenatal diagnosis.**
antepartal care Care of a pregnant woman during the time in the maternity cycle that begins with conception and ends with the onset of labor. A medical, surgical, gynecologic, obstetric, social, and family history is taken with particular emphasis on the discovery of familial or transmissable diseases. A physical examination is performed, including a pelvic examination, a pap smear, and tests for *Neisseria gonorrhea, Candida albicans,* and *Trichomonas vaginalis.* Blood pressure, weight, urinalysis for sugar and protein, measurement of the height of the fundus, and auscultation of the fetal heart are routinely performed at monthly intervals or even more frequently. Laboratory tests are performed to determine blood type and Rh factor, hematocrit, and hemoglobin. A serologic test for syphilis is performed and various diagnostic studies may be done. Amniocentesis may be performed if certain fetal abnormalities are suspected.
NURSING CONSIDERATIONS: The parents are encouraged to discuss their concerns about the pregnancy, to understand the physiological processes, to report decreased fetal activity, to take a preparation-for-labor class, and to plan for the infant's needs. The basic goal of prenatal care is a healthy mother, who is ready emotionally and physically to give birth to a healthy baby. Increasingly, that goal has come to include the mother's and father's satisfaction with the birth itself and a minimal use of obstetric intervention. Information, emotional support, good nutrition, and careful observation help most mothers to achieve healthy, happy intrapartal and postpartal periods of the maternity cycle. See also **intrapartal care, postpartal care.**
anterior **1.** The front of a structure. **2.** Of or pertaining to a surface or part situated toward the front or facing forward. Also called **ventral.** Compare **posterior.**
anterior asynclitism See **asynclitism.**
anterior atlantoaxial ligament One of five ligaments connecting the atlas to the axis. It is fixed to the inferior border of the anterior arch of the atlas and to the ventral surface of the body of the axis. Compare **posterior atlantoaxial ligament.**
anterior atlanto-occipital membrane One of two broad, densely woven fibrous sheets that form part of the atlanto-occipital joint between the atlas and the occipital bone. It is continuous with two articular capsules and strengthened ventrally by a strong, rounded cord connecting the base of the occipital bone to the anterior arch of the atlas. Also called anterior atlanto-occipital ligament. Compare **posterior atlanto-occipital membrane.**
anterior cardiac vein One of several small vessels that return deoxygenated blood from the ventral portion of the myocardium of the right ventricle to the right atrium. In some individuals, the right marginal vein opens into the right atrium, and, in those instances, is regarded as one of the anterior cardiac veins. See also **coronary sinus.**
anterior common ligament See **anterior longitudinal ligament.**
anterior crural nerve See **femoral nerve.**
anterior cutaneous nerve One of a pair of cutaneous branches of the cervical plexus. It arises from the second and the third cervical nerves, bends around the middle of the sternocleidomastoideus, crosses the muscle obliquely, passes beneath the platysma, and divides into the ascending and the descending branches. The ascending branches pass upward, pierce the platysma, and are distributed to the cranial, the ventral, and the lateral parts of the neck. The descending branches are distributed to the skin of the ventral and the lateral parts of the neck as far down as the sternum.
anterior fontanel See **fontanel.**
anterior longitudinal ligament The broad, strong ligament attached to the ventral surfaces of the vertebral bodies. It extends from the occipital bone and the anterior tubercle of the atlas to the sacrum. Also called **anterior common ligament.** Compare **posterior longitudinal ligament.**
anterior mediastinal node A node in one of the three groups of thoracic visceral nodes of

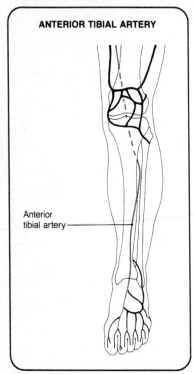

ANTERIOR TIBIAL ARTERY

Anterior
tibial artery

the lymphatic system that drain lymph from the nodes of the thymus, pericardium, and sternum. They are located ventral to the brachiocephalic veins and to the arterial trunks from the aortic arch. The efferents of the nodes form the right and the left bronchomediastinal trunks. Compare **posterior mediastinal node.** See also **lymph, lymphatic system, lymph node.**

anterior mediastinum A caudal portion of the mediastinum in the middle of the thorax, bounded ventrally by the body of the sternum and parts of the fourth through the seventh ribs and dorsally by the parietal pericardium, extending downward as far as the diaphragm. It contains a few lymph nodes, a few vessels, and a thin layer of subserous fascia, which is separated from the endothoracic fascia by a fascial cleft. Compare **middle mediastinum, posterior mediastinum, superior mediastinum.**

anterior nares The ends of the nostrils that open anteriorly into the nasal cavity and allow the inhalation and the exhalation of air. Each is an oval opening that measures about 1.5 cm (⅝ inch) anterioposteriorly and about 1 cm (½ inch) in diameter. The anterior nares connect with the nasal fossae. Also called **nostrils.** Compare **posterior nares.**

anterior neuropore The opening of the embryonic neural tube in the anterior portion of the forebrain. It closes at the 20-somite stage, which indicates the end of horizon XI in the numerical anatomical charting of human embryonic development. Compare **posterior neuropore.** See also **horizon.**

anterior pituitary See **adenohypophysis.**

anterior tibial artery One of the two divisions of the popliteal artery, arising in back of the knee, dividing into six branches, and supplying various muscles of the leg and foot. Its six branches are the posterior tibial recurrent, fibular, anterior tibial recurrent, muscular, anterior medial malleolar, and anterior lateral malleolar. Compare **posterior tibial artery.**

anterior tibial node One of the small lymph glands of the lower limb, lying on the interosseous membrane near the proximal portion of the anterior tibial vessels. Compare **inguinal node, popliteal node.**

anterograde amnesia The inability to recall events of long ago with normal recall of recent events. Compare **anterograde memory.**

anterograde memory The ability to recall events of long ago but not those of recent occurrence. Compare **anterograde amnesia.** Also called **senile memory.**

anteroposterior From the front to the back of the body, commonly associated with the direction of the roentgenographic beam.

anteversion An abnormal position of an organ in which the organ is tilted forward on its axis, away from the midline.

anthelmintic 1. Of or pertaining to a substance that destroys or prevents the development of parasitic worms, as filariae, flukes, hookworms, pinworms, roundworms, schistosomes, tapeworms, trichinae, and whipworms. 2. An anthelmintic drug. An anthelmintic may interfere with the parasites' carbohydrate metabolism, inhibit their respiratory enzymes, block their neuromuscular action, or render them susceptible to destruction by the host's macrophages. Among a number of drugs used in treating specific helmintic infections are piperazine, pyrantel pamoate, pyrvinium pamoate, mebandazole, niclosamide, diethylcarbamazine, and theabendazole.

-anthema A combining form meaning a '(specified) type of eruption, rash': *eisanthema, enanthema, exanthema.*

anthraco- A combining form meaning 'pertaining to a carbuncle or to carbon dioxide': *anthracoid, anthraconecrosis, anthracosis.*

anthracosis A chronic lung disease occurring in coal miners, characterized by the deposit of coal dust in the lungs and the formation of black nodules on the bronchioles and resulting in focal emphysema. The condition is aggravated by cigarette smoking. There is no specific treatment; most cases are asymptomatic and the progress of the condition may be halted by the prevention of further exposure to coal dust. Also called **black lung, coalworker's pneumoconiosis, miner's pneumoconiosis.** See also **inorganic dust.**

anthracosis linguae See **parasitic glossitis.**

anthralin A dermatomucosal agent used to

treat psoriasis and other skin conditions.

anthralinic acid See **aminobenzoic acid.**

anthrax A disease affecting primarily farm animals (cattle, goats, pigs, sheep, and horses), caused by the bacterium *Bacillus anthracis.* Anthrax in animals is usually fatal. Humans most often acquire it when a break in the skin comes into direct contact with infected animals and their hides, but they may also contract a pulmonary form of anthrax by inhaling the spores of the bacterium. The cutaneous form begins with a reddish-brown lesion that ulcerates and then forms a dark scab. The signs and symptoms that follow include internal hemorrhage, muscle pain, headache, fever, nausea, and vomiting. The pulmonary form, called woolsorter's disease, is often fatal unless treated early. Treatment for both forms is penicillin G or tetracycline. A vaccine is available for veterinarians and for others for whom anthrax is an occupational hazard. Also called **malignant pustule.**

anthropo- A combining form meaning 'pertaining to a human being': *anthropocentric, anthropocracy, anthropoid.*

anthropoid pelvis A type of pelvis in which the inlet is oval; the anteroposterior diameter is much greater than the transverse and, owing to the posterior inclination of the sacrum, the posterior portion of the space in the true pelvis is much greater than the anterior portion. The side walls are somewhat convergent and the ischial spines are prominent. If the pelvis is large, vaginal delivery is not compromised, but the occiput posterior position of the fetus is favored. This type of pelvis is present in 40% of nonwhite women and in more than 25% of white women.

anti-, ant- A combining form meaning 'against or over against': *antialexin, antibiosis, antichlorotic.*

antiadrenergic 1. Of or pertaining to the blocking of the effects of impulses transmitted by the adrenergic postganglionic fibers of the sympathetic nervous system. 2. An antiadrenergic agent. Drugs that block the response to norepinephrine by alpha-adrenergic receptors reduce the tone of smooth muscle in peripheral blood vessels, causing increased peripheral circulation and decreased blood pressure. Alphablocking agents include ergotamine derivatives, used in treating migraine; phenoxybenzamine and phentolamine, administered for Raynaud's disease, pheochromocytoma, and diabetic gangrene; and tolazoline hydrochloride, administered to patients with spastic vascular disease. Agents that block beta-adrenergic receptors decrease the rate and force of heart contractions among other effects. Propranolol and its congeners are beta-blocking agents. Also called **sympatholytic.** Compare **adrenergic.**

antiadrenergic drug See **antiadrenergic.**

antianemic 1. Of or pertaining to a substance or procedure that counteracts or prevents a deficiency of erythrocytes. 2. An agent used to treat or to prevent anemia. Whole blood is transfused in the treatment of anemia resulting from

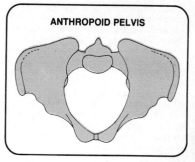

ANTHROPOID PELVIS

acute blood loss, and packed red cells are usually administered when the deficiency is caused by chronic blood loss. Transfusions of blood components are used in the treatment of aplastic anemia. Iron-deficiency anemia, the most common form of anemia, is usually treated with oral preparations of ferrous sulfate, fumarate, or gluconate, but a parenteral preparation is indicated for people who are unable to absorb iron from the gastrointestinal tract or for those who develop nausea and diarrhea when taking iron orally. Cyanocobalamin is administered parenterally in the treatment of pernicious anemia. Folic acid is prescribed to correct a deficiency of that vitamin in the anemias accompanying general malnutrition or alcoholic cirrhosis and to treat the common anemia of infants who are on a milk diet exclusively. A combination of folic acid and vitamin B_{12} is prescribed for people who are anemic owing to an inadequate dietary intake of both vitamins.

antiantibody An immunoglobulin formed as the result of the administration of an antibody that acts as an immunogen. The antiantibody then interacts with the antibody. See also **antibody, immune gamma globulin.**

antianxiety agent See **sedative-hypnotic.**

antiarrhythmic 1. Of or pertaining to a procedure or substance that prevents, alleviates, or corrects an abnormal cardiac rhythm. 2. An agent used to treat a cardiac arrhythmia. A defibrillator that delivers a precordial electric shock is often used to restore a normal rhythm to rapid, irregular atrial or ventricular contractions. A pacemaker may be implanted in a patient with an extremely slow heart rate or other arrhythmia. The electrode catheter of an external pacemaker may be threaded through a vein to the heart in cases of ventricular standstill or complete heart block. Two of the major antiarrhythmic drugs are lidocaine, which increases the threshhold of electrical stimulation in the ventricles during diastole, and a combination of disopyramide, procainamide, and quinidine, which decrease the excitability of the myocardium and prolong the refractory period. The beta-adrenergic blocking agent propranolol may be used in treating arrhythmias. Isoproterenol is indicated for complete heart block and ventricular arrhythmias requiring an increased force of cardiac contractions to establish a normal rhythm. Atropine may be used in the treatment of bradycardia, a sedative in the treatment of tachycardia, and digitalis in the treatment of atrial fibrillation. See also **arrhythmia**.

antibacterial 1. Of or pertaining to a substance that kills bacteria or inhibits their growth or replication. 2. An antibacterial agent. Antibiotics synthesized chemically or derived from various microorganisms exert their bactericidal or bacteriostatic effect by interfering with the production of the bacterial cell wall, by interfering with protein synthesis, nucleic acid synthesis, or cell membrane integrity, or by inhibiting critical biosynthetic pathways in the bacteria.

antiberiberi factor See **thiamine**.

antibiotic 1. Of or pertaining to the ability to destroy or interfere with the development of a living organism. 2. An antimicrobial agent, derived from cultures of a microorganism or produced semisynthetically, used to treat infections. The penicillins, derived from species of the fungus *Penicillium* or manufactured semisynthetically, consist of a thiazolidine ring fused to a beta-lactam ring connected to side chains; these agents exert their action by inhibiting mucopeptide synthesis in bacterial cell walls during multiplication of the organisms. Penicillin G and V are widely used in treating many gram-positive coccal infections but are inactivated by the enzyme penicillinase produced by strains of staphylococci; cloxacillin, dicloxacillin, methicillin, nafcillin, and oxacillin are penicillinase-resistant penicillins. Broad-spectrum penicillins effective against gram-negative organisms are ampicillin, carbenicillin, and amoxicillin. Hypersensitivity reactions, as rash, fever, bronchospasm, vasculitis, and anaphylaxis, are relatively common side effects of penicillin therapy. Aminoglycoside antibiotics, composed of amino sugars in glycoside linkage, interfere with the synthesis of bacterial proteins and are used primarily for the treatment of infections caused by gram-negative organisms. The aminoglycosides include gentamicin derived from *Micromonospora*, semisynthetic amikacin, kanamycin, neomycin, streptomycin, and tobramycin. These agents commonly cause nephrotoxic and ototoxic reactions as well as gastrointestinal disturbances. Macrolide antibiotics, consisting of a large lactone ring and deoxamino sugar, interfere in protein synthesis of susceptible bacteria during multiplication without affecting nucleic acid synthesis. Oleandomycin, which is added to feed to improve the growth of poultry and swine, and broad-spectrum erythromycin, used to treat various gram-positive and gram-negative infections and intestinal amebiasis, are macrolides derived from species of *Streptomyces*. Erythromycin may cause mild allergic reactions and gastrointestinal discomfort, but nausea, vomiting, and diarrhea occur infrequently with the usual oral dose. Polypeptide antibiotics derived from species of *Streptomyces* or certain soil bacilli vary in their spectra; most of these agents are nephrotoxic and ototoxic.

Bacitracin and vancomycin are polypeptides used to treat severe staphylococcal infections; capreomycin is an antituberculosis agent; and gramicidin is included in ointments for topical infections. Antifungals, including amphotericin B and nystatin, apparently bind to sterols in fungus cell membranes and change their permeability; griseofulvin grossly distorts terminal hyphae of fungi. Amphotericin B is effective against many kinds of fungi; it may cause fever, vomiting, diarrhea, generalized pains, anemia, renal dysfunction, and other adverse effects when administered intravenously. Oral griseofulvin is used to treat various fungal infections of the skin and nails and may cause hypersensitivity reactions, gastrointestinal disturbances, fatigue, and insomnia. Nystatin is applied locally for the treatment of oral and vaginal candidiasis; candicidin is also used for vaginal candidiasis. The tetracyclines, including the prototype derived from *Streptomyces*, demeclocycline, doxycycline, minocycline, and oxytetracycline, are active against a wide range of gram-positive and gram-negative organisms and some rickettsiae. Antibiotics in this group are primarily bacteriostatic and are thought to exert their effect by inhibiting protein synthesis in the organisms. Tetracycline therapy may cause gastrointestinal irritation, photosensitivity, renal toxicity, and hepatic toxicity, and administration of a drug of this group during the last half of pregnancy, during infancy, or before the age of eight may result in permanent discoloration of the teeth. The cephalosporins, derived from the soil fungus *Cephalosporium* or produced semisynthetically, inhibit bacterial cell wall synthesis, resist the action of penicillinase, and are used in treating infections of the respiratory tract, urinary tract, middle ear, and bones, as well as septicemia caused by a wide range of gram-positive and gram-negative organisms. The group includes cefadroxil, cefamandole, cefazolin, cephalexin, cephaloglycin, cephalothin, cephapirin, and cephradine. Treatment with a cephalosporin may cause nausea, vomiting, diarrhea, enterocolitis, or an allergic reaction, as rash, angioedema, or exfoliative dermatitis; use of antibiotics in this group is contraindicated in patients who have shown hypersensitivity to a penicillin. Chloramphenicol, a broad-spectrum antibiotic initially derived from *Streptomyces venezuelae*, inhibits protein synthesis in bacteria by interfering with the transfer of activated amino acids from soluble RNA to ribosomes. Since the drug may cause life-threatening blood dyscrasias, its use is reserved for the treatment of acute typhoid fever, serious gram-negative infections (including *Hemophilus influenzae* meningitis), meningitis, and rickettsial diseases.

antibiotic sensitivity tests A laboratory method for determining the susceptibility of bacterial infections to therapy with antibiotics. After the infecting organism has been recovered from a clinical specimen, it is cultured and tested against several antibiotic drugs, often in two groups, gram-positive and gram-negative. If the

WHAT ANTICHOLINERGICS DO

INNERVATED ORGAN	When body naturally releases neurohormone acetylcholine:	When cholinergic blockers are given:
Heart	▼	▲
Bronchioles	▲	▼
GI tract	▲	▼
Bladder	▲	▼
Bladder sphincter	▼	
Blood vessels	▼	▲
Sweat and salivary glands	▲	▼

KEY: ▼ = relaxes or dilates   ▲ = constricts or stimulates

growth of the organism is inhibited by the action of the drug, it is reported as sensitive to that antibiotic. If the organism is not susceptible to the antibiotic in question, it is reported as resistant to that drug. See also **Gram's stain.**

antibody An immunoglobulin, essential to the immune system, produced by lymphoid tissue in response to bacteria, viruses, or other antigenic substances. An antibody is specific to an antigen. Each class of antibody is named for its action. Among the many antibodies are agglutinins, bacteriolysins, opsonins, precipitin. See also **epitope, plasma protein, T cell.**

antibody instructive theory A theory that each antigenic contact in the life of an individual develops a new antibody, as when an immunoglobulin-covered B cell comes in contact with an antigen and subsequently produces plasma cells and memory cells. The theory maintains that the random contact of B cells with antigens induces the reticuloendothelial system to instruct memory cells to produce antibodies against antigens at any time. Compare **antibody specific theory.**

antibody specific theory A theory maintaining that the body develops antibody patterns before or shortly after birth and can recognize any antigen and increase antibodies specific to that antigen at any time. The theory holds that the body contains an enormous number of diverse clones of cells, each genetically programmed to synthesize a different antibody. This theory further maintains that any antigen entering the body selects the specific clone programmed to synthesize the antibody for that antigen and stimulates the cells of the clone to proliferate and produce more of the same antibody. Also called **clonal selection theory.** Compare **antibody instructive theory.**

antibromic See **deodorant.**

anticholinergic **1.** Of or pertaining to a blockade of acetylcholine receptors, which results in the inhibition of the transmission of parasympathetic nerve impulses. **2.** An anticholinergic agent that functions by competing with the neurotransmitter acetylcholine for its receptor sites at synaptic junctions. Anticholinergic drugs reduce spasms of smooth muscle in the bladder, bronchi, and intestine; relax the iris sphincter; decrease gastric, bronchial, and salivary secretions; decrease perspiration; and accelerate impulse conduction through the myocardium by blocking vagal impulses. Many anticholinergic agents reduce parkinsonian symptoms; atropine in large doses stimulates the central nervous system and in small doses acts as a depressant. Among numerous cholinergic blocking agents are anisotropine methylbromide, belladonna, glycopyrrolate, hyoscyamine sulfate, methixene hydrochloride, and scopolamine. Various members of the group are used to treat spastic disorders of the gastrointestinal tract, to

USE OF ANTICONVULSANTS IN EPILEPTIC-TYPE SEIZURES

DRUG CATEGORY	GRAND MAL	PETIT MAL	MYOCLONIC	MIXED	PSYCHO-MOTOR	STATUS EPILEPTICUS
Barbiturate derivatives	✔	✔	✔	✔	✔	
Benzodiazepine derivatives		✔	✔			✔
Hydantoin derivatives	✔			✔	✔	✔
Oxazolidone derivatives		✔				
Succinimide derivatives		✔				
Miscellaneous						
Acetazolamide		✔				
Bromides*	✔	✔	✔	✔	✔	
Carbamazepine	✔			✔	✔	
Valproic acid		✔				

*Rarely used as drug of first or second choice

reduce salivary and bronchial secretions pre-operatively, or to dilate the pupil. Also called **parasympatholytic.** Compare **cholinergic.**

anticholinergic agent See **anticholinergic.**

anticholinesterase A drug that inhibits or inactivates the action of acetylcholinesterase. Drugs of this class cause acetylcholine to accumulate at the junctions of various cholinergic nerve fibers and their effector sites or organs, allowing potentially continuous stimulation of cholinergic fibers throughout the central and peripheral nervous systems. Anticholinesterase drugs include neostigmine, edrophonium, and pyridostigmine. Neostigmine and pyridostigmine are prescribed in the treatment of myasthenia gravis; edrophonium in the diagnosis of myasthenia gravis and the treatment of overdosage of curariform drugs. Many agricultural insecticides have been developed from anticholinesterases; these are the highly toxic chemicals called organophosphates. Nerve gases developed as potential chemical-warfare agents contain potent, irreversible forms of anticholinesterase.

anticipatory guidance The psychological preparation of a patient to help relieve fear and anxiety of an event expected to be stressful, as the preparation of a child for surgery by explaining what will happen and what it will feel like and the showing of equipment or the part of the hospital where the child will be.

anticoagulant 1. Of or pertaining to a substance that prevents or delays coagulation of the blood. 2. An anticoagulant drug. Heparin, obtained from the liver and lungs of domestic animals, is a potent anticoagulant that interferes with the formation of thromboplastin, with the conversion of prothrombin to thrombin, and with the formation of fibrin from fibrinogen. Synthetic coumarin and phenindione derivatives administered orally are vitamin K antagonists that prevent coagulation by inhibiting the formation of certain clotting factors.

anticodon In genetics: a sequence of three nucleotides in transfer RNA that pairs complementarily with a specific codon of messenger RNA during protein synthesis to specify a particular amino acid in the polypeptide chain. See also **genetic code, transcription, translation.**

anticonvulsant 1. Of or pertaining to a substance or procedure that prevents or reduces the severity of epileptic or other convulsive seizures. 2. An anticonvulsant drug. Hydantoin derivatives, especially sodium diphenylhydantoin, apparently exert their anticonvulsant effect by stabilizing the cell membrane and decreasing intracellular sodium, with the result that the excitability of the epileptogenic focus is reduced. Phenytoin prevents the spread of excessive discharges in cerebral motor areas and suppresses dysrhythmias originating in the thalamus, frontal lobes, and other brain areas. Phenacemide and primidone are also used in treating grand mal epilepsy.

antidepressant 1. Of or pertaining to a substance or a measure that prevents or relieves depression. **2.** An antidepressant agent. Tricyclic antidepressant agents, as amitryptyline and imipramine, block re-uptake of amine neurotransmitters, but the exact mechanism of the antidepressant action of these drugs is unknown. Monoamine oxidase (MAO) inhibitors, as isocarboxazid, pargyline, phenelzine, and tranylcypromine, increase the concentration of epinephrine, norepinephrine, and serotonin in storage sites in the nervous system, and it is theorized that this increased level of monoamines in the brain stem is responsible for the drugs' antidepressant effect. Some MAO inhibitors also have antihypertensive action.

antidiuretic 1. Of or pertaining to the suppression of urine formation. **2.** An antidiuretic agent, such as antidiuretic hormone (vasopressin). —**antidiuresis,** *n.*

antidiuretic hormone (ADH) A hormone that decreases the production of urine by increasing the reabsorption of water by the renal tubules. ADH is secreted by cells of the hypothalamus and stored in the posterior lobe of the pituitary gland. It is released in response to a decrease in blood volume, an increased concentration of sodium or other substances in plasma, or by pain, stress, or the action of certain drugs. ADH can cause contraction of smooth muscle in the gastrointestinal tract and blood vessels, especially capillaries, arterioles, and venules. Acetylcholine, methacoline, nicotine, large doses of barbiturates, anesthetics, epinephrine, and norepinephrine stimulate ADH release; ethanol and phenytoin inhibit production of the hormone. Synthetic ADH is used in the treatment of diabetes insipidus. Also called **vasopressin.**

antidote A drug or other substance that opposes or antagonizes the action of a poison. An antidote may be mechanical, acting to coat the stomach and prevent absorption of the poison; chemical, acting to make the toxin inert; or physiologic, acting to oppose the action of the poison, as a sedative given to a person who has ingested a large amount of a stimulant.

antidromic conduction The conduction of a neural impulse backward from a receptor in the midportion of an axon. As synaptic junctions allow conduction in one direction only, any backward, antidromic impulses that occur fail to pass the synapse, dying at that point. Compare **orthodromic conduction.**

antiembolism hose Elasticized stockings worn to prevent the formation of emboli and thrombi, especially in patients after surgery or those restricted to bed. Return flow of the venous circulation is promoted, preventing venous stasis and dilation of the veins, conditions that predispose to thromboembolic disorders.

antiemetic 1. Of or pertaining to a substance or procedure that prevents or alleviates nausea and vomiting. **2.** An antiemetic drug or

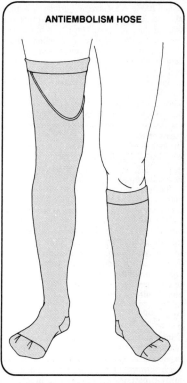

ANTIEMBOLISM HOSE

agent. Belladonna derivatives, bromides, barbiturates and other sedatives, and substances that protect the stomach lining, as lime water or mild gastric astringents, have weak antiemetic properties. Chlorpromazine and other phenothiazines are the most effective antiemetic agents. In motion sickness scopolamine and antihistamines provide relief. Marijuana may alleviate the nausea induced by certain antineoplastic drugs in cancer patients.

antiepileptic See **anticonvulsant.**

antifebrile See **antipyretic.**

antifungal 1. Of or pertaining to a substance that kills fungi or inhibits their growth or reproduction. **2.** An antifungal, antibiotic drug. Amphotericin B, effective against a broad spectrum of fungi, probably acts by binding to sterols in the fungal cell membrane and changing the membrane's permeability. Griseofulvin, another broad-spectrum antifungal agent, binds to the host's new keratin and renders it resistant to further fungal invasion. Miconazole inhibits the growth of common dermatophytes, including yeastlike *Candida albicans,* and nystatin is effective against yeast and yeastlike fungi.

antigen A substance, usually a protein, that causes the formation of an antibody and reacts specifically with that antibody.

antigen-antibody reaction A process of the immune system in which immunoglobulin-coated B cells recognize an intruder or antigen and stimulate antibody production to protect the body against infection. The T cells of the body assist in the antigen-antibody reaction, but the B cells play the key role. Antigen-antibody reactions activate the complement system of the body, amplifying the humoral immunity response of the B cells and causing lysis of the antigenic cells. Antigen-antibody reactions involve the binding of antigens to antibodies to form antigen-antibody complexes that may render the toxic antigen harmless, agglutinize antigens on the surface of microorganisms, or activate the complement system by exposing the complement-binding sites on the antibody molecule. Complement protein immediately binds to these sites and triggers the activity of the other complement proteins to produce cytolysis of the antigen cells. The antigen-antibody reaction may start immediately with antigen contact, or it may start 48 hours later. Antigen-antibody reactions are essential to the immune response of the body and are precipitated by contact of antigenic protein molecules with antibody protein molecules. The antigen-antibody reactions occur and antigen-antibody complexes are formed when unique areas on the surfaces of antigen molecules fit precisely into appropriate concave combining sites on the surfaces of antibody molecules. Various amounts of IgM, IgG, IgA, IgE, and IgD are normally present during any antigenic challenge. Antigenic-antibody reactions normally produce immunity, but they can also produce allergy, autoimmunity, and fetomaternal hematologic incompatibility. In immediate allergic reactions, antigens provoke the production of specific antibodies that may circulate freely in the serum or may become attached to specific cells. Antigen-antibody reaction in the immediate allergic response activates certain enzymes and causes an imbalance between these enzymes and their inhibitors. Simultaneously released into the circulation are certain pharmacologically active substances, as acetylcholine, bradykinin, histamine, gamma globulin G, and leukotaxine. Autoimmunity makes it impossible for the immune system to distinguish between self and a foreign substance.

antigen determinant A small area on the surface of an antigen molecule that fits a combining site of an antibody molecule and binds the antigen in the formation of an antigen-antibody complex. Antigen determinants commonly consist of a sequence of amino acids that decrees the shape of these reactive areas. Also called **epitope.**

antigenicity The quality of causing the production of antibodies. The degree of antigenicity depends on the kind and amount of the particular substance, the condition of the host, and the degree to which the host is sensitive to the antigen and able to produce antibodies.

antigerminal pole See **vegetal pole.**

antiglobulin An antibody against human globulin, occurring naturally or prepared in laboratory animals. Specific antiglobulins are used in the detection of specific antibodies, as in blood typing. See also **antiglobulin test, Coomb's test, precipitin.**

antiglobulin test A test for the presence of antibodies that coat and damage red blood cells as a result of any of several diseases or conditions. The test can detect Rh antibodies in maternal blood and is used to anticipate hemolytic disease of the newborn. It is also used to diagnose and screen for autoimmune hemolytic anemias and to determine the compatibility of blood types. When exposed to a sample of the patient's serum, the antiglobulin serum will cause agglutination if human globulin antibody or its complement is present. Also called **Coombs' test.** See also **autoimmune disease, erythroblastosis fetalis.**

antihemophilic C factor See **plasma thromboplastin antecedent.**

antihemophilic factor (AHF) A systemic hemostatic agent used to treat factor VIII deficiency.

antihistamine Any substance capable of reducing the physiological and pharmacological effects of histamine, including a wide variety of drugs that block histamine receptors. Many such drugs are readily available as nonprescription medicines for the management of allergies. Toxicity resulting from the overuse of antihistamines and their accidental ingestion by children is common and sometimes fatal. These substances do not stop the release of histamine, and the ways in which they act on the central nervous system (CNS) are not completely understood. The antihistamines are divided into H_1 and H_2 blockers depending on the responses to histamine they prevent. The H_1 blocking drugs, as the alkylamines, ethanolamines, ethylenediamines, and piperazines, are effective in the symptomatic treatment of acute exudative allergies, as pollinosis and urticaria. The H_2 blocking drugs, as cimetidine, are effective in the control of gastric secretions and are often used in the treatment of duodenal ulcers. Antihistamines can both stimulate and depress the CNS. The side effects of H_1 blockers may include sedation, nausea, constipation, and dryness of the throat and respiratory tract. About 25% of the individuals who use antihistamines experience some bothersome reaction. —**antihistaminic,** adj.

antihypertensive 1. Of or pertaining to a substance or procedure that reduces high blood pressure. 2. An antihypertensive agent. Various drugs achieve their antihypertensive effect by depleting tissue stores of catecholamines in peripheral sites, by stimulating pressor receptors in the carotid sinus and heart, by blocking autonomic nerve impulses that constrict blood vessels, by stimulating central inhibitory alpha-adrenergic receptors, or by direct vasodilation. Thiazides and other diuretic agents reduce blood pressure by decreasing blood volume. Among the numerous drugs used to treat hypertension are rauwolfia and veratrum alkaloids, diazoxide, guanethidine, methyldopa, pargyline hydrochloride, and trimethaphan camsylate.

anti-inflammatory **1.** Of or pertaining to a substance or procedure that counteracts or reduces inflammation. **2.** An anti-inflammatory drug or agent. Betamethasone, prednisolone, prednisone, and other synthetic glucocorticoids are used extensively in treating inflammation. The basis of the anti-inflammatory effect of salicylates and nonsteroidal anti-inflammatory agents, as phenylsutazone and indomethacin, appears to involve inhibition of prostaglandin biosynthesis.

antilipidemic **1.** Of or pertaining to a regimen, diet, or agent that reduces the amount of lipids in the serum. **2.** A drug used to reduce the amount of lipids in the serum. Antilipidemic diets and drugs are prescribed to reduce the risk of atherosclerotic cardiovascular disease (ACVD) based on two facts: atheromatous plaques contain free cholesterol, and lower serum cholesterol levels and less coronary heart disease are found in populations consuming a low-fat diet than in those on a high-fat diet. Although it has not been proven that food intake affects the development of ACVD, a prudent low-fat diet with polyunsaturates replacing saturated fats is considered a valuable preventive measure by many cardiologists. A number of pharmacologic agents are used to reduce serum lipids, but it is not established whether drug-induced lowering of serum cholesterol or triglyceride levels has a beneficial effect, no effect, or a detrimental effect on ACVD morbidity or mortality. Clofibrate reduces very low density lipoproteins in serum; the drug may reduce the risk of a second, non-fatal myocardial infarction but it increases the risk of cholelithiasis, cardiac arrhythmias, intermittent claudication, and thromboembolism. Cholestyramine exerts its antilipidemic action by combining with bile acids in the intestine to form an insoluble complex that is excreted in the feces; it may reduce serum cholesterol markedly, but it prevents the absorption of essential fat-soluble vitamins and may be associated with several serious side effects. Colestipol also binds and removes bile acids from the intestine; sitosterol may interfere with intestinal absorption of cholesterol, but the exact mechanism of its action and that of antilipidemic probucol are unknown. Dextrothyroxine lowers serum lipid levels by stimulating hepatic catabolism and excretion of cholesterol and its metabolites. See also **hyperlipidemia.**

antilymphocyte serum (ALS) A serum prescribed as an immunosuppressive agent for the reduction of rejection reactions in organ transplant and as an adjunct in chemotherapy for malignant neoplasms. Its effects have been promising in some cases of leukemia and in kidney transplant. It is associated with some adverse effects, as serious serum sickness, generalized infection, anaphylaxis, and antigen-antibody–induced glomerulonephritis.

antimalarial **1.** Of or pertaining to a substance that destroys or suppresses the development of malaria plasmodia or to a procedure that exterminates the mosquito vectors of the disease, as spraying insecticides or draining swamps. **2.** An antimalarial drug that destroys or prevents the development of plasmodia in human hosts. Chloroquine hydrochloride and hydroxychloroquine sulfate are effective against *Plasmodium vivax*, *P. malariae*, and certain strains of *P. falciparum*.

antimetabolite A drug or other substance that resembles a normal human metabolite and interferes with its function in the body, usually by competing for the metabolite's receptors or enzymes. Among the antimetabolites used as antineoplastic agents are the folic acid analog methotrexate and the pyrimidine analogs fluorouracil and floxuridine. Antineoplastic mercaptopurine, an analog of the nucleotide adenine and the purine base hypoxanthine, is a metabolic anatagonist of both compounds. Thioguanine, another member of a large series of purine analogs, interferes with nucleic acid synthesis. Cytarabine, used in the treatment of acute myelocytic leukemia, is a synthetic nucleoside that resembles cytidine and kills cells actively synthesizing DNA, apparently by inhibiting the enzyme DNA polymerase.

antimicrobial See **antibacterial.**

antimitochondrial antibody An antibody that acts specifically against mitochondria. These antibodies are not normally present in the blood of healthy people. A laboratory test for the presence of the antibodies in the blood is a valuable diagnostic aid in liver disease, as a biopsy of the liver may not yield affected tissue. Low titers may occur in chronic hepatitis, drug-induced hepatotoxicity, and various other diseases. High titers are virtually diagnostic of primary biliary cirrhosis.

antimony A bluish, crystalline metallic element occurring in nature, both free and as salts. Various antimony compounds are used in the treatment of filariasis, leishmaniasis, lymphogranuloma, schistosomiasis, and trypanosomiasis and as an emetic. See also **antimony potassium tartrate.**

antimony poisoning Poisoning caused by the ingestion or inhalation of antimony or antimony compounds, characterized by vomiting, sweating, diarrhea, and a metallic taste in the mouth. Irritation of the skin or mucous membrane may result from external exposure. Severe poisoning resembles arsenic poisoning. British antilewisite is used for chelation. Antimony and antimony compounds are common ingredients of many substances used in medicine and industry.

antimony potassium tartrate An antischistosomal.

antimorph A mutant gene that inhibits or antagonizes the normal influence of its allele in the expression of a trait. Compare **amorph, hypermorph, hypomorph.**

antimuscarinic Inhibiting the stimulation of the postganglionic parasympathetic receptor.

antimutagen **1.** Any substance that reduces the rate of spontaneous mutations or counteracts or reverses the action of a mutagen. **2.** Any tech-

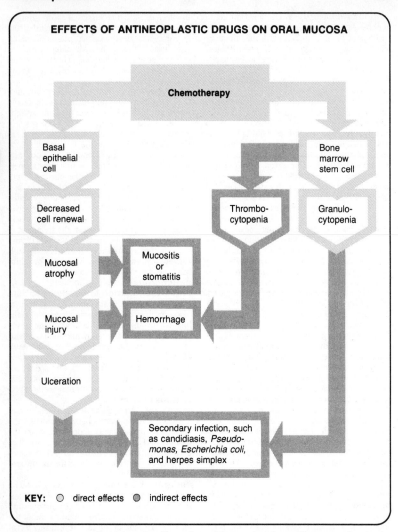

EFFECTS OF ANTINEOPLASTIC DRUGS ON ORAL MUCOSA

Chemotherapy

Basal epithelial cell — Bone marrow stem cell

Decreased cell renewal — Thrombo-cytopenia — Granulo-cytopenia

Mucosal atrophy — Mucositis or stomatitis

Mucosal injury — Hemorrhage

Ulceration

Secondary infection, such as candidiasis, *Pseudomonas, Escherichia coli,* and herpes simplex

KEY: ○ direct effects ◉ indirect effects

nique that protects cells against the effects of mutagenic agents. **—antimutagenic,** *adj.*
antineoplastic **1.** Of or pertaining to a substance, procedure, or measure that prevents the proliferation of malignant cells. **2.** A chemotherapeutic agent that controls or kills cancer cells. Drugs used in the treatment of cancer are cytotoxic but are generally more damaging to dividing cells than to resting cells. Cycle-specific antineoplastic agents are more effective in killing proliferating cells than in killing resting cells, and phase-specific agents are most active during a specific phase of the cell cycle. Most anticancer drugs prevent the proliferation of cells by inhibiting the synthesis of DNA by various mechanisms. Alkylating agents, as nitrogen mustard derivatives, ethylenimine derivatives, and alkyl sulfonates, interfere with DNA replication by causing cross-linking of DNA strands and abnormal pairing of nucleotides. Antimetabolites exert their action by interfering with the formation of compounds required for cell division. Methotrexate, a folic acid analog, and 5-fluorouracil, a pyrimidine analog, inhibit enzymes required for the formation of the essential DNA constituent thymidine. Hypoxanthine analog 6-mercaptopurine and 6-thioguanine, an analog of guanine, interfere with the biosynthesis of purine. Vinblastine and vincristine, alkaloids derived from the periwinkle plant, disrupt cell division by interfering with the formation of the mitotic spindle. Antineoplastic antibiotics, as doxorubicin, daunomycin, and mitomycin, block or inhibit DNA synthesis, while actinomycin-D

COMPARATIVE INCIDENCE OF ANTINUCLEAR ANTIBODIES (ANA)

DISEASE	INCIDENCE OF POSITIVE ANA
Systemic lupus erythematosus (SLE)	95% to 100%
Lupoid hepatitis	95% to 100%
Felty's syndrome	95% to 100%
Progressive systemic sclerosis (scleroderma)	75% to 80%
Drug-associated SLE-like syndrome: (hydralazine, procainamide, isoniazid)	~50%
Sjögren's syndrome	40% to 75%
Normal old age	~40%
Rheumatoid arthritis	25% to 60%
Healthy family member of SLE patient	~25%
Chronic discoid lupus erythematosus	15% to 50%
Juvenile arthritis	15% to 30%
Polyarteritis nodosa	15% to 25%
Miscellaneous diseases	10% to 50%
Dermatomyositis, polymyositis	10% to 30%
Rheumatic fever	~5%
Normal persons (general population)	~5%

and mithramycin interfere with RNA synthesis. Cytotoxic chemotherapeutic agents may be administered orally, intravenously, topically, intrathecally, or into a body cavity. All have untoward and unpleasant side effects and are potentially immunosuppresive and dangerous. Estrogens, corticosteroids, and androgens, although not considered antineoplastic agents, frequently cause tumor regression when administered in high doses to patients with hormone-dependent cancers. See also **alkylating agent, antimetabolite.**

antineoplastic antibiotic A chemical substance derived from a microorganism or a synthetic analog of the substance, used in cancer chemotherapy. Actinomycin-D, employed in the treatment of Wilms' tumor, testicular carcinoma, choriocarcinoma, rhabdomyosarcoma, and some other sarcomas, exerts its antineoplastic effect by interfering with RNA synthesis. Mithramycin, with a similar mechanism of action, is also administered for testicular cancer and for trophoblastic neoplasms. Doxorubicin, a broad spectrum agent that is especially useful in treating breast carcinoma, lymphomas, sarcomas, and acute leukemia—and closely related daunomycin, which is also effective in acute leukemias—block the biosynthesis of RNA. Mitomycin-C, prescribed for gastric, breast, cervical, and head and neck carcinomas, cross-links strands of DNA. Bleomycin, used in the treatment of squamous cell carcinomas of the head and neck, testicular carcinoma, and lymphomas, damages DNA and prevents its repair. Antineoplastic antibiotics depress bone marrow and usually cause nausea and vomiting; several cause alopecia. Doxorubicin and daunomycin may be cardiotoxic, and mitomycin and bleomycin may produce pulmonary changes.

antineoplastic hormone A chemical substance produced by an endocrine gland or a synthetic analog of the naturally occurring compound, used to control certain disseminated cancers. Hormonal therapy is designed to counteract the effect of an endogenous hormone required for the growth of the tumor. The estrogens diethylstilbestrol (DES) and ethinyl estradiol are employed in palliative treatment of a prostatic carcinoma that is nonresectable or unresponsive to radiotherapy. An androgen, as testosterone propionate, testolactone, or fluoxymesterone, may be administered postoperatively to control disseminated breast cancer in women whose tumors are estrogen dependent. The antiestrogen tamoxifen produces responses in many patients with advanced estrogen-dependent breast cancer. Parodoxically, large doses of estrogen, frequently used to control disseminated breast cancer in postmenopausal women, apparently check the growth of tumors by inhibiting the secretion of estrogen by the adrenal gland. Some progestins produce a favorable response in women with disseminated endometrial carcinoma and, occasionally, in patients with prostatic or renal cancers. These progestins include megestrol acetate, medroxyprogesterone acetate, and hydroxyprogesterone caproate.

antinuclear antibody An antibody directed at components of cellular nuclei, as DNA, found in patients with various diseases, as systemic lupus erythematosus.

antiparallel In molecular genetics: the condition in which molecules, as strands of DNA, are parallel but point in opposite directions.

antiparasitic **1.** Of or pertaining to a substance or procedure that kills parasites or inhibits their growth or reproduction. **2.** An an-

EXTRAPYRAMIDAL SYMPTOMS (EPS) CAUSED BY ANTIPSYCHOTIC DRUGS

SYMPTOMS	DEFINITIONS
Akathisia	Discomforting feeling of insomnia, restlessness, and compulsion to walk about, with marked inability to sit still. Symptoms are first seen in 2 to 4 weeks, with a peak in 6 to 10 weeks. They decline in 12 to 16 weeks.
Akinesia	Diminished muscular movements, weakness, unusual numbness or tingling sensations. Symptoms are first seen during the first 2 weeks, with a peak in 1 week. They decline in 3 to 4 weeks.
Dystonia	Uncoordinated jerking or spastic movements of neck, face, eyes, tongue, torso, arm or leg muscles; backward rolling of the eyes in their sockets (oculogyric crisis); sideways twisting of the neck (torticollis); protrusion of the tongue ("thick" tongue); drooling; spasms of back muscles (opisthotonos). Symptoms are seen in the first few days, with a peak in 1 week. They decline in 2 weeks.
Rigidity	Abnormally high muscle tone or tension, "cogwheel" resistance to movement, unchanging blank facial expression (masked facies), stiff mechanical gait. Symptoms are first seen in ½ to 2 weeks, with a peak in 2 to 4 weeks. They decline in 5 to 10 weeks.
Tremor	Fine quivering motions due to alternating rapid contractions, especially of the arm muscles. Symptoms are first seen in ½ to 2 weeks, with a peak in 2 to 6 weeks. They decline in 8 to 16 weeks.

tiparasitic drug including amebicides, anthelmintics, antimalarials, schistosomicides, trichomonacides, and trypanosomicides.

antiparkinsonian Of or pertaining to a substance or procedure used to treat parkinsonism. Drugs for this neurological disorder are of two kinds: those that compensate for the lack of dopamine in the corpus striatum of parkinsonism patients, and anticholinergic agents that counteract the activity of the abundant acetylcholine in the striatum. Synthetic levodopa, a dopamine precursor that crosses the blood-brain barrier, is administered to patients to reduce the rigidity, sluggishness, dysphagia, drooling, and instability characteristic of the disease, but the drug does not alter the relentless course of the disorder. Centrally active cholinergic blockers, notably benztropine, biperiden, procyclidine, and trihexyphenidyl, may relieve tremors and rigidity and improve mobility. The antiviral agent amantadine is often effective in the treatment of parkinsonism; the mechanism of its action is not established, but it apparently causes an increased release of dopamine in the brain. Extrapyramidal symptoms similar to idiopathic parkinsonism are frequently induced by antipsychotic drugs. See also **tardive dyskinesia.**

antiperistaltic 1. Of or pertaining to a substance that inhibits or diminishes peristalsis. 2. An antiperistaltic agent. Narcotics, as paregoric, diphenoxylate, and loperamide hydrochloride, are antiperistaltic agents used to provide symptomatic relief in diarrhea. Anticholinergic (parasympatholytic) drugs reduce spasms of intestinal smooth muscle and are frequently prescribed to decrease excessive gastrointestinal motility.

antipernicious anemia factor See **cyanocobalamin.**

antipruritic 1. Of or pertaining to a substance or procedure that tends to relieve or prevent itching. 2. An antipruritic drug. Topical anesthetics, corticosteroids, and antihistamines are used as antipruritic agents.

antipsychotic 1. Of or pertaining to a substance or procedure that counteracts or diminishes symptoms of a psychosis. 2. An antipsychotic drug. Phenothiazine derivatives are the most frequently prescribed antipsychotics for use in the treatment of schizophrenia and other major affective disorders. They apparently act by enhancing the filtering mechanisms of the reticular formation in the brain stem. Common side effects of phenothiazines are a dry mouth, blurred vision, and extrapyramidal reactions requiring treatment with antiparkinsonian agents. See also **antidepressant, neuroleptic, tranquilizer.**

antipyretic 1. Of or pertaining to a substance or procedure that reduces fever. 2. An antipyretic agent. Such drugs usually lower the thermodetection set point of the hypothalamic heat regulatory center, with resulting vasodilation and sweating. Widely used antipyretic agents are acetaminophen, administered orally or through rectal suppositories, aspirin, and other salicylates. Also called **antifebrile, antithermic, febrifuge.**

antipyretic bath A procedure in which the patient's body temperature is reduced by use of tepid water.

antiscorbutic vitamin See **ascorbic acid.**
antisense In molecular genetics: a strand of DNA containing the same sequence of nucleotides as messenger RNA (mRNA).
antisepsis Destruction of microorganisms to prevent infection. —**antiseptic,** *adj.*
antiseptic **1.** Tending to inhibit the growth and reproduction of microorganisms. **2.** A substance that tends to inhibit the growth and reproduction of microorganisms.
antiseptic dressing A dressing treated with an antiseptic, germicide, or bacteriostat, applied to a wound or an incision to prevent or treat infection.
antiseptic gauze Gauze permeated with an antiseptic solution, sometimes packaged in individual, sealed packets.
antiserum, *pl.* **antisera, antiserums** Serum of an animal or human containing antibodies against a specific disease, used to confer passive immunity to that disease. Antisera do not provoke the production of antibodies. There are two types of antiserum. Antitoxin is an antiserum that neutralizes the toxin produced by specific bacteria, but it does not kill the bacteria. Antimicrobial serum acts to destroy bacteria by making them more susceptible to the leukocytic action. Polyvalent antiserum acts on more than one strain of bacteria; univalent antiserum acts on only one strain. Antibiotic drugs have largely replaced antimicrobial antisera. Caution is always to be used in giving antiserum of any kind, as hepatitis or hypersensitivity reactions can occur. Also called **immune serum.** Compare **vaccine.**
antiserum anaphylaxis An exaggerated reaction of hypersensitivity in a normal person caused by the injection of serum from a sensitized individual. Also called **passive anaphylaxis.**
antisocial personality A person who exhibits attitudes and overt behavior contrary to the customs, standards, and moral principles accepted by society. Also called **psychopathic personality, sociopathic personality.** See also **antisocial personality disorder.**
antisocial personality disorder A condition characterized by repetitive behavioral patterns that lack moral and ethical standards and bring a person into continuous conflict with society. Symptoms include aggressiveness, callousness, impulsiveness, irresponsibility, hostility, a low frustration level, a marked emotional immaturity, and poor judgment. A person who has this disorder neglects the rights of others, is incapable of loyalty to others or to social values, is unable to feel guilt or to learn from experience, is impervious to punishment, and tends to rationalize his behavior or to blame it on others. The disorder is usually recognized before adulthood and often persists throughout life. Adverse environmental influences, biological deficiencies, and unconscious conflicts resulting from aberrant family relationships may contribute to the development of the disorder. Most individuals with this condition manage to

function in society despite frequent bouts with authorities, but many are referred by courts to prisons. Also called **antisocial reaction.** See also **psychopath.**
antisocial reaction See **antisocial personality disorder.**
antistreptolysin-O test (ASOT, ASLT) A streptococcal antibody test for finding and measuring serum antibodies to streptolysin-O, an exotoxin produced by most group A and some group C and G streptococci. The test is often used as an aid in the diagnosis of rheumatic fever. A low titer of antistreptolysin-O antibody is present in most people, since streptococcal infection is common. Elevated or increasing titers indicate a recent infection. See also **Lancefield's classification.**
antithermic See **antipyretic.**
antithyroid drug Any one of several preparations that can inhibit the synthesis of thyroid hormones and are commonly used in the treatment of hyperthyroidism. The major antithyroid drugs are thioamides, as propylthiouracil, methimazole, and carbimazole. In the body, such substances interfere with the incorporation of iodine into the tyrosyl residues of thyroglobulin required for the production of the hormones thyroxine and triiodothyronine. These drugs are often used to control hyperthyroidism during an anticipated remission and before a thyroidectomy. Such substances cross the placenta, can cause fetal hypothyroidism and goiter, and are contraindicated for mothers who breast-feed their children.
antitoxin A subgroup of antisera usually prepared from the serum of horses immunized against a particular toxin-producing organism, as botulism antitoxin given therapeutically in botulism and tetanus and diptheria antitoxins given prophylactically to prevent those infections.
antitrust In law: against the operation, establishment, or maintenance of a monopoly in the manufacture, production, or sale of a commodity, providing of a service, or practice of a profession.
antitussive **1.** Against a cough. **2.** Any of a large group of narcotic and nonnarcotic drugs that act on the central and peripheral nervous systems to suppress the cough reflex. Because the cough reflex is necessary for clearing the upper respiratory tract of obstructive secretions, antitussives should not be used with a productive cough. Codeine and hydrocodone are potent narcotic antitussives. Dextromethorphan is an equally effective antitussive with no dependence liability. Antitussives are administered orally, usually in a syrup with a mucolytic or expectorant and alcohol, or, sometimes, in a capsule with an antihistaminic and a mild analgesic.
antivenin A suspension of venom-neutralizing antibodies prepared from the serum of immunized horses. Antivenin confers passive immunity and is given as a part of emergency first aid treatment for various snake and insect bites.

SIGNS OF ANXIETY

Appearance
↑ Muscle tension (rigidity)
Skin blanches, pales
↑ Perspiration, clammy skin
Fatigue
↑ Small motor activity (restlessness, tremor)

Behavior
↓ Attention span
↓ Ability to follow directions
↑ Acting out
↑ Somatizing
↑ Immobility

Conversation
↑ Number of questions
Constant seeking of reassurance
Frequent shifting of topics of conversation
Describes fears with sense of helplessness
Avoids focusing on feelings
Focuses on equipment or procedures

Physiological signs mediated through autonomic nervous system
↑ Heart rate
↑ Rate or depth of respirations
Rapid, extreme shifts in body temperature, blood pressure, and menstrual flow
Diarrhea
Urinary urgency
Dryness of mouth
↓ Appetite
↑ Perspiration
Dilation of pupils

antiviral Destructive to viruses.

antivitamin A substance that inactivates a vitamin.

antixerophthalmic vitamin See **vitamin A**.

antr- See **antro-**.

antral gastritis An abnormal narrowing of the antrum, or distal portion of the stomach. The narrowing is not a true gastritis, but a radiographic finding which may represent gastric ulcer or tumor. Compare **gastritis.**

antro-, antr A combining form meaning 'pertaining to an antrum or sinus': *antrocele, antrodynia, antrophore.*

antrum cardiacum A constricted passage from the esophagus to the stomach, lying just inside the opening formed by the cardiac sphincter.

anuresis See **anuria. —anuretic,** *adj.*

anuria The inability to urinate, the cessation of urine production, or a urinary output of less than 100 to 250 ml (3.4 to 8.4 oz) per day. Anuria may be caused by kidney failure or dysfunction, a decline in blood pressure below that required to maintain filtration pressure in the kidney, or an obstruction in the urinary passages. A rapid decline in urinary output, leading ultimately to anuria and uremia, occurs in acute renal failure. Kinds of anuria include **angioneurotic anuria** and **obstructive anuria.** Also called **anuresis. —anuric,** *adj.*

anus The opening at the end of the anal canal.

anxietas A state of anxiety, nervous restlessness, or apprehension, often accompanied by a feeling of oppression in the epigastrium. Kinds of anxietas are **anxietas presenilis, restless legs syndrome.**

anxietas presenilis A state of extreme anxiety caused by approaching senility.

anxietas tibiarum See **restless legs syndrome.**

anxiety A state or feeling of uneasiness, agitation, uncertainty, and fear resulting from the anticipation of some threat or danger, usually of intrapsychic rather than external origin, whose source is generally unknown or unrecognized. The condition may result as a rational response to a tension-producing situation, like applying for a job, or from a general concern about life's uncertainties. It is a pathologic condition if it is not based in reality and if it is so severe that it results in the inability to function. Kinds of anxiety include **castration anxiety, free-floating anxiety, separation anxiety, situational anxiety.**

anxiety attack An acute, psychobiological reaction manifested by intense anxiety and panic. Symptoms vary according to the intensity of the attack but typically include palpitations, shortness of breath, dizziness, faintness, profuse sweating, pallor of the face and extremities, gastrointestinal discomfort, and a vague feeling of imminent death. Attacks usually occur suddenly, last from a few seconds to an hour or longer, and vary in frequency from several times a day to once a month. Treatment consists of reassurance, administration of a sedative, if necessary, and appropriate psychotherapy to identify the stresses perceived as threatening. See also **anxiety, anxiety neurosis.**

anxiety neurosis A neurotic disorder characterized by persistent anxiety. The symptoms range from mild, chronic tenseness, with feelings of timidity, fatigue, apprehension, and indecisiveness, to more intense states of restlessness and irritability that may lead to aggressive acts or indecisiveness. In extreme cases, the overwhelming emotional discomfort is accompanied by physical reactions, including tremor, sustained muscle tension, tachycardia, dyspnea, hypertension, increased respiration, and profuse perspiration. Other physical signs include changes in skin color, nausea, vomiting, diarrhea, restlessness, immobilization, insomnia, and changes in appetite, all occurring without underlying organic cause. The symptoms of anxiety may be controlled with medication, such as tranquilizers, but psychotherapy is the preferred treatment and sometimes cures the neurosis. Also called **anxiety reaction,** anxiety state. See also **anxiety, anxiety attack.**

anxiety reaction   See **anxiety neurosis.**

AORN   *abbr* **Association of Operating Room Nurses.**

aorta   The main trunk of the systemic arterial circulation, comprised of four parts: the ascending aorta, the arch of the aorta, the thoracic portion of the descending aorta, and the abdominal portion of the descending aorta. It starts at the aortic opening of the left ventricle, where it has a diameter of about 3 cm (1⅛ inches), rises a short distance toward the neck, bends to the left and dorsally over the root of the left lung, descends within the thorax on the left side of the vertebral column, and passes through the aortic hiatus of the diaphragm into the abdominal cavity. Opposite the caudal border of the fourth lumbar vertebra, it narrows to about 1.75 cm (¾ inch) in diameter and branches into the two common iliac arteries.

aortic aneurysm   A localized dilatation of the wall of the aorta caused by atherosclerosis, hypertension, or, less frequently, by syphilis. The lesion may be a saccular distention, a fusiform or cylindroid swelling of a length of the vessel, or a longitudinal dissection between the outer and middle layers of the vessel wall. Syphilitic aneurysms almost always occur in the thoracic aorta and usually involve the aortic arch, while more common atherosclerotic aneurysms are usually in the abdominal section of the great vessel below the renal arteries and above the bifurcation of the aorta. These lesions often contain atheromatous ulcers covered by thrombi that may discharge emboli, causing obstruction of smaller vessels. A bulging abdominal aortic aneurysm may impinge on a ureter, vertebra, or other adjacent structure, causing pain. A pulsatile mass may be detected in a routine examination, but in many cases the first sign is life-threatening hemorrhage, resulting from rupture of the lesion. A diagnosis of an unruptured aneurysm may be made using X-rays of the abdomen, which show a ring of calcification around the dilatation, or with an angiogram. Treatment of small chronic aneurysms includes the use of antihypertensive drugs to reduce pressure on the weak area of the vessel, analgesics to relieve pain, and agents to reduce the force of cardiac contraction. Acute or large aneurysms are resected, and the segment of the aorta is replaced with synthetic prostheses. Cardiopulmonary bypass is required during surgical repair of an aneurysm of the ascending, trans-

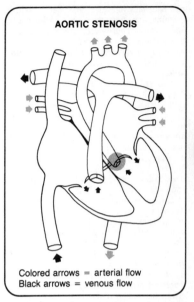

AORTIC STENOSIS

Colored arrows = arterial flow
Black arrows = venous flow

verse, or descending aorta but not for an abdominal aneurysm. Common postoperative complications are renal failure and ileus. See also **dissecting aneurysm.**

aortic arch   See **arch of the aorta.**

aortic arch syndrome   Any of a group of occlusive conditions of the aortic arch producing a variety of symptoms related to obstruction of the large branch arteries, including the innominate, left common carotid, or left subclavian. Such conditions as atherosclerosis, Takayasu's disease, and syphilis may cause aortic arch syndrome. The symptoms include syncope, temporary blindness, hemiplegia, aphasia, and memory loss.

aortic body reflex   A normal chemical reflex initiated by a decrease in oxygen concentration in the blood and, to a lesser degree, by increased carbon dioxide and hydrogen ion concentrations that act on chemoreceptors in the wall of the arch of the aorta and result in nerve impulses that cause the respiratory center in the medulla to increase respiratory activity. See also **carotid body reflex.**

aortic regurgitation   See **regurgitation,** definition 2.

aortic stenosis   A cardiac anomaly characterized by a narrowing or stricture of the aortic valve owing to congenital malformation or to fusion of the cusps, as may result from rheumatic fever. Aortic stenosis obstructs the flow of blood from the left ventricle into the aorta, causing decreased cardiac output and pulmonary vascular congestion. Clinical manifestations include faint peripheral pulses, exercise intolerance, anginal pain, and a systolic murmur. Diagnosis is confirmed by cardiac catheterization and echocardiography. Surgical repair is usually indicated, followed by frequent examinations, since recurrence of the stenosis and bacterial endocarditis are relatively common sequelae. Children with aortic stenosis are usually restricted from strenuous, competitive sports activities. See also **congenital cardiac anomaly.**

aortic valve A tricuspid valve in the heart between the left ventricle and the aorta. It is composed of three semilunar cusps that close in diastole to prevent blood from flowing back into the left ventricle from the aorta. The three cusps are separated by sinuses which resemble tiny buckets when they are filled with blood. These cup-shaped flaps grow from the lining of the aorta and, in systole, open to allow oxygenated blood to flow from the left ventricle into the aorta and on to the peripheral circulation. Compare **mitral valve, pulmonary valve.**

aortitis An inflammatory condition of the aorta, occurring most frequently in tertiary syphilis and occasionally in rheumatic fever.

aortography A radiographic process in which the aorta and its branches are injected with any of various contrast media for visualization. —**aortographic,** *adj.*

aortopulmonary fenestration A congenital anomaly characterized by an abnormal fenestration in the ascending aorta and the pulmonary artery cephalad to the semilunar valve, allowing oxygenated and unoxygenated blood to mix, resulting in a decrease in the oxygen available in the peripheral circulation.

aosmic Anosmic.

ap- **1.** See **apo-.** **2.** See **ad-.**

APA *abbr* American Podiatric Association, American Psychiatric Association, American Psychoanalytic Association, American Psychological Association, and American Psychopathological Association.

apathy An absence or suppression of emotion, feeling, concern, or passion; an indifference to things generally found to be exciting or moving. The condition is commonly seen in patients with neurasthenic neurosis and schizophrenia. —**apathetic,** *adj.*

APC *abbr* aspirin, phenacetin, caffeine.

APD *abbr* adult polycystic disease. See **polycystic kidney disease.**

apepsia nervosa See **anorexia nervosa.**

aperient See **aperitive.**

aperitive **1.** A mild laxative. **2.** Acting as a mild laxative. Also called **aperient.**

Apert's syndrome A rare condition characterized by an abnormal craniofacial appearance in combination with partial or complete syndactyly of the hands and the feet. The specific cause of Apert's syndrome is not known, but the condition appears to be the result of a primary germplasm defect. Characteristic features of this condition include premature synostosis of the cranial bones, with resultant growth disturbances. Some signs of Apert's syndrome are a peaked and vertically elongated head, widespread and bulging eyes, and a high, arched posterior palate with bony defects of the maxilla and the mandible. The degree of syndactyly varies greatly and may be complete, with the apparent fusion of all the digits externally. The treatment of Apert's syndrome usually includes an osteotomy of the cranial bones to prevent increased intracranial pressure. The syndactyly may be surgically corrected, the specific procedure depending on the severity of the deformity. Also called **acrocephalosyndactylism.**

aperture An opening or hole in an object or anatomical structure. See specific apertures.

aperture of frontal sinus An external opening of the frontal sinus into the nasal cavity.

aperture of glottis An opening between the true vocal cords and the arytenoid cartilages.

aperture of larynx An opening between the pharynx and larynx.

aperture of sphenoid sinus A round opening between the sphenoid sinus and nasal cavity, situated just above the superior nasal concha.

apex, *pl.* **apices** The top, the end, or the tip of a structure, as the apex of the heart, the apices of the teeth.

apex beat A pulsation of the left ventricle of the heart, palpable and sometimes visible at the fifth intercostal space, approximately 9 cm (3½ inches) to the left of the midline.

apexcardiogram A graphic representation of the pulsations of the precordium in the region of the cardiac apex.

apex cordis The pointed lower border of the heart. It is directed downward, forward, and to the left, and is usually located at the level of the fifth intercostal space.

apex pulmonis The rounded upper border of each lung, projecting above the clavicle into the root of the neck.

Apgar score The evaluation of an infant's physical condition, usually performed 1 minute and 5 minutes after birth, based on a rating of five factors that reflect the infant's ability to adjust to extrauterine life. A pediatrician, Virginia Apgar, M.D., developed the system for the rapid identification of infants requiring immediate intervention or transfer to an intensive-care nursery. The infant's heart rate, respiratory effort, muscle tone, reflex irritability, and color are scored from a low value of zero to a normal value of two. The five scores are combined, and the totals at 1 minute and 5 minutes are noted; for example, Apgar 9/10 is a score of 9 at 1 minute and 10 at 5 minutes. A score of 0 to 3 represents severe distress, a score of 4 to 7 indicates moderate distress, and a score of 7 to 10 indicates an absence of difficulty in adjusting to extrauterine life.

NURSING CONSIDERATIONS: A low 1-minute score requires immediate intervention, including giving oxygen, clearing the nasopharynx, and usually transfer to an intensive care nursery. An infant with a low score that persists at 5 minutes requires expert care, which may include assisted ventilation, umbilical catheterization, cardiac massage, blood gas evaluation, medication to correct acid-base deficit, or medication to reverse the effects of maternal medication.

APHA *abbr* American Protestant Health Association and American Public Health Association.

aphagia A condition characterized by the loss of the ability to swallow owing either to organic or to psychological causes. See also **dysphagia.**

aphagia algera A condition characterized by the refusal to eat or swallow because doing so causes pain.

aphakia, aphacia In ophthalmology: a condition in which part or all of the crystalline lens of the eye is absent. —**aphakic, aphacic,** *adj.*

aphasia An abnormal neurologic condition in which language function is defective or absent owing to an injury to certain areas of the cerebral cortex. The deficiency may be sensory or receptive, in which language is not understood, or expressive or motor, in which words cannot be formed or expressed. Sensory aphasia may be complete or partial, affecting specific language functions, as in dyslexia or alexia. Expressive aphasia may be complete, as in dysphasia, in which speech is impaired or as in agraphia, in which writing is affected; or it may be partial, diminishing either or both functions. Most commonly, the condition is a mixture of incomplete expressive and receptive aphasia. See also **Broca's area.**

-aphia A combining form meaning a 'condition of the sense of touch': *araphia, hyperaphia, paraphia.* Also **-haphia.**

aphonia A condition characterized by loss of the ability to produce normal speech sounds owing to overuse of the vocal cords, organic disease, or psychological causes, such as hysteria. See also **speech dysfunction.** —**aphonic, aphonous,** *adj.*

aphonia clericorum A condition characterized by a loss of the voice from overuse.

aphonia paralytica A condition characterized by a loss of the voice owing to paralysis or disease of the laryngeal nerves.

aphonia paranoica An inability to speak that lacks an organic basis and that is characteristic of some forms of mental illness.

aphonic speech Abnormal speech in which vocalizations are whispered.

-aphrodisia A combining form meaning a '(specified) condition of sexual arousal': *anaphrodisia, hypaphrodisia.*

aphronia In psychiatry: a condition characterized by an impaired ability to make common-sense decisions. —**aphronic,** *n., adj.*

aphthous fever An acute, extremely contagious, rhinovirus infection of cloven-hooved animals. It is characterized by the development of ulcers on the skin around the mouth, on the mucous membrane in the mouth, and on the udders. Horses are immune. Uncommonly, the virus is transmitted to man by direct contact with infected animals or their secretions or with contaminated milk. Also called **foot-and-mouth disease.**

aphthous stomatitis A recurring condi-

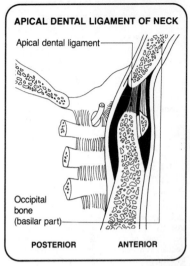

APICAL DENTAL LIGAMENT OF NECK

Apical dental ligament

Occipital bone (basilar part)

POSTERIOR   ANTERIOR

tion characterized by the eruption of painful ulcers (commonly called canker sores) on the mucous membranes of the mouth. The cause is unknown, but there is evidence to suggest that aphthous stomatitis is an immune reaction. See also **canker sore.**

APIC *abbr* American Association for Practitioners of Infection Control.

apical dental ligament A ligament connecting the axis to the occipital bone. It extends from the process of the axis to the anterior margin of the foramen magnum and lies between the two alar ligaments, blending with the anterior atlanto-occipital membrane. It is considered a rudimentary intervertebral disc and contains traces of the embryonic notochord.

aplasia 1. A developmental failure resulting in the absence of an organ or tissue. 2. In hematology: a failure of the normal process of cell generation and development. See also **aplastic anemia, hyperplasia.** —**aplastic,** *adj.*

aplasia cutis congenita The congenital absence of a localized area of skin. The defect occurs predominantly on the scalp, less frequently on the limbs and trunk, and is usually covered by a thin, translucent membrane or scar tissue, or it may be raw and ulcerated. The conditon is genetically transmitted, although the mode of inheritance is not known.

aplastic 1. Pertaining to the absence or defective development of a tissue or organ. 2. Failure of a tissue to produce normal daughter cells by mitosis. See also **aplastic anemia.** —**aplasia,** *n.*

aplastic anemia A deficiency of all of the formed elements of the blood, representing a failure of the cell-generating capacity of the bone marrow. It may be caused by neoplastic disease of the bone marrow, or, more commonly, by destruction of the bone marrow by exposure to toxic chemicals, ionizing radiation, or some an-

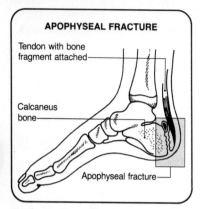

APOPHYSEAL FRACTURE

Tendon with bone fragment attached

Calcaneus bone

Apophyseal fracture

tibiotics or other medications. Rarely, an idiopathic form of the disease occurs.

apnea An absence of spontaneous respiration. Kinds of apnea include **cardiac apnea, deglutition apnea, periodic apnea of the newborn, primary apnea, reflex apnea, secondary apnea.** —**apneic,** *adj.*

apo-, ap- A combining form meaning 'separation or derivation from': *apobiosis, apocarteresis, aponeurosis.*

apocrine gland One of the large, deep exocrine glands located in the axillary, anal, genital, and mammary areas of the body. The apocrine glands secrete sweat that has a strong, characteristic odor. Compare **eccrine gland.** See also **exocrine gland.**

apodial symmelia See **sirenomelia.**

apomorphine hydrochloride An emetic.

aponeurosis, *pl.* **aponeuroses** A strong sheet of fibrous connective tissue that serves as a tendon to attach muscles to bone or as fascia to bind muscles together.

aponeurosis of the obliquus externus abdominis The strong membrane that covers the entire ventral surface of the abdomen and lies superficial to the rectus abdominis. Fibers from both sides of the aponeurosis interlace in the midline to form the linea alba. The upper part of the aponeurosis serves as the inferior origin of the pectoralis major; the lower part ends in the inguinal ligament.

apophyseal fracture A fracture that separates an apophysis of a bone from the main osseous tissue at a point of strong tendinous attachment.

apophysis A protuberance or swelling, especially a bony outgrowth that is not separated from the bone.

apophysitis A condition characterized by the inflammation of an apophysis. Apophysitis occurs most frequently as a disorder of the foot caused by disease of the epiphysis of the quadrangular bone at the back of the tarsus.

apoplexy 1. A cerebrovascular accident, resulting in paralysis. 2. A hemorrhage within an organ. —**apoplectic,** *adj.*

apothecaries' measure A system of grad-

uated liquid volumes originally based on the minim, formerly equal to one drop of water but now standardized to 0.06 ml. In this system 60 minims equal 1 fluid dram, 8 fluid drams equal 1 fluid ounce, 16 fluid ounces equal 1 pint, 2 pints equal 1 quart, 4 quarts equal 1 gallon. See also **apothecaries' weight, metric system.**

apothecaries' weight A system of graduated amounts arranged in order of heaviness and based upon the grain, formerly equal to the weight of a plump grain of wheat but now standardized to 65 mg. In this system 20 grains equal 1 scruple, 3 scruples equal 1 dram, 8 drams equal 1 ounce, 12 ounces equal 1 pound. Compare **avoirdupois weight.** See also **apothecaries' measure, metric system.**

appellant In law: a party that brings an appeal to an appellate court. Having lost the case in a lower court, the appellant requests the court to reconsider the case.

appellate court A court of law that has the power to review the decision of a lower court. It does not make a new determination of the facts of the case; it reviews only the way in which the law was applied in the case.

appellee In law: a party in an appeal that won the case in a lower court. The appellee argues that the decision of the lower court should not be modified by the appellate court.

appendage An accessory structure attached to another part or organ. Also called **appendix.**

appendectomy The surgical removal of the vermiform appendix through an incision in the right lower quadrant of the abdomen. See also **abdominal surgery, peritonitis.**

appendiceal, appendicial, appendical Of or pertaining to the vermiform appendix.

appendicitis Inflammation of the vermiform appendix, usually acute, which if undiagnosed leads rapidly to perforation and peritonitis. The most common symptom is constant pain in the right lower quadrant of the abdomen around McBurney's point, which the patient describes as having begun as intermittent pain in midabdomen. To decrease the pain, the patient keeps his knees bent to avoid tension of abdominal muscles. Appendicitis is characterized by vomiting, a low-grade fever of 37.2° to 38.9°C (99° to 102°F), an elevated white blood count, rebound tenderness, a rigid abdomen, and decreased or absent bowel sounds. The inflammation is caused by an obstruction, as a hard mass of feces or a foreign body, in the lumen of the appendix, fibrous disease of the bowel wall, an adhesion, or a parasitic infestation. Treatment is appendectomy, within 24 to 48 hours of the first symptoms, because delay usually results in rupture and peritonitis as fecal matter is released into the peritoneal cavity. Appendicitis is most apt to occur in teenagers and young adults and is more frequent in males. See also **appendectomy, appendix, McBurney's point, perforate, peritonitis.**

appendix, *pl.* **appendixes, appendices** 1. Accessory part of main structure. Also called **appendage.** 2. See **vermiform appendix.**

appendix dyspepsia　An abnormal condition characterized by the impairment of the digestive function associated with chronic appendicitis. See also **dyspepsia.**

appendix epididymidis　A cystic structure sometimes found on the head of the epididymis. It represents a remnant of the mesonephros.

appendix epiploica, *pl.* **appendices epiploicae**　One of the fat pads, 2 to 10 cm (¾ to 4 inches) long, scattered through the peritoneum along the colon and the upper part of the rectum, especially along the transverse and the sigmoid parts of the colon.

appendix vermiformis　See **vermiform appendix.**

apperception　**1.** Mental perception or recognition. **2.** In psychology: a conscious process of understanding or perceiving in terms of a person's previous knowledge, experiences, emotions, and memories. —**apperceptive,** *adj.*

applied anatomy　The study of the structure and morphology of the organs of the body as it relates to the diagnosis and treatment of disease. Also called practical anatomy. Kinds of applied anatomy are **pathological anatomy** and **surgical anatomy.**

applied chemistry　The application of the study of chemical elements and compounds to industry and the arts.

applied psychology　**1.** The interpretation of historical, literary, medical or other data according to psychological principles. **2.** Any branch of psychology that emphasizes practical rather than theoretical approaches and objectives, as clinical psychology, child psychology, industrial psychology, educational psychology.

applied science　See **science.**

appositional growth　An increase in size by the addition of new tissue or similar material at the periphery of a particular part or structure, as in the addition of new layers in bone and tooth formation. Compare **interstitial growth.**

approach-approach conflict　A conflict resulting from the simultaneous presence of two or more incompatible impulses, desires, or goals, each of which is desirable. Also called **double-approach conflict.** See also **conflict.**

approach-avoidance conflict　A conflict resulting from the presence of a single goal or desire that is both desirable and undesirable. See also **conflict.**

appropriate-for-gestational-age (AGA) infant　A newborn infant whose size, growth, and maturation is normal for gestational age, whether delivered prematurely, at term, or later than term. Such infants, if born at term, fall within the average range of size and weight on intrauterine growth curves, measuring from 48 to 53 cm (18⅞ to 20⅞ inches) in length and weighing between 2,700 and 4,000 g (6 and 8¾ lb).

apractognosia　See **constructional apraxia.**

apraxia　An impairment in the ability to perform purposeful acts or to manipulate objects.

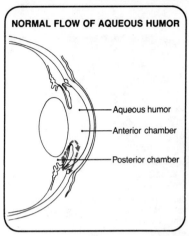

NORMAL FLOW OF AQUEOUS HUMOR

— Aqueous humor

— Anterior chamber

— Posterior chamber

The condition is primarily neurologic but occurs in several forms. **Sensory apraxia** is characterized by impairment caused by a loss of the perception of the use of an object. **Motor apraxia** is characterized by an inability to use an object or perform a task without any loss of perception of the use of the object or the goal of the task. **Amnestic apraxia** is characterized by an inability to perform the function owing to an inability to remember the command to perform it. —**apraxic,** *adj.*

aprobarbital　A barbiturate sedative-hypnotic agent.

APTA　*abbr* American Physical Therapy Association.

aptitude　A natural ability, tendency, talent, or capability to learn, understand, or acquire a particular skill; mental alertness.

aptitude test　Any of a variety of standardized tests for measuring an individual's ability to learn certain skills. Compare **achievement test, intelligence test, personality test, psychological test.**

AQ　*abbr* achievement quotient.

aqua amnii　See **amniotic fluid.**

aqua pad　A hollow pad with circulating fluid that produces heat or cold. Depending on its size, the pad provides a local or systemic effect.

aqueduct of Sylvius　See **cerebral aqueduct.**

aqueous　**1.** Watery or waterlike. **2.** A medication prepared with water. See also **aqueous humor.**

aqueous humor　The clear, watery fluid circulating in the anterior and posterior chambers of the eye. It is produced by the ciliary processes and is reabsorbed into the venous system at the iridocorneal angle by means of the sinus venosus, or canal of Schlemm.

AR　*abbr* assisted respiration.

Ar　Symbol for argon.

arabinosylcytosine　See **cytarabine.**

arachidonic acid　An essential fatty acid

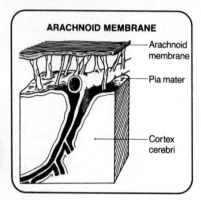

ARACHNOID MEMBRANE

Arachnoid membrane

Pia mater

Cortex cerebri

that is a component of lecithin and a basic material for the biosynthesis of some prostaglandins.

arachn- See arachno-.

arachno-, arachn- A combining form meaning 'pertaining to the arachnoid membrane or to a spider': *arachnoidal, arachnoidea, arachnolysin.*

arachnodactyly A congenital condition of having long, thin, spiderlike fingers and toes. See **Marfan's syndrome.**

arachnoid A delicate, fibrous structure resembling a cobweb or spiderweb, as the arachnoid membrane that forms the middle of three protective layers of meninges surrounding the brain and spinal cord. —**arachnoidal,** *adj.*

arachnoidea encephali The part of the arachnoid membrane enclosing the brain.

arachnoidea spinalis The part of the arachnoid membrane enclosing the spinal cord. See **arachnoid membrane.**

arachnoid membrane A thin, delicate membrane enclosing the brain and the spinal cord, interposed between the pia mater and the dura mater. The subarachnoid space lies between the arachnoid membrane and the pia, and the subdural space lies between the arachnoid membrane and the dura. Also called **arachnoid.**

Aran-Duchenne muscular atrophy A form of amyotrophic lateral sclerosis affecting the hands, arms, shoulders, and legs at the onset before becoming more generalized.

arbitration The hearing and resolution of controversy by a neutral person chosen by the opposing parties or appointed under statutory authority.

arbitrator An impartial person appointed to resolve a dispute between parties. The arbitrator listens to the evidence as presented by the parties in an informal hearing and attempts to arrive at a resolution acceptable to both parties. —**arbitration,** *n.*

arbovirus Any one of more than 300 arthropod-borne viruses that cause infections characterized by a combination of two or more of the following: fever, rash, encephalitis, and bleeding into the viscera or skin. Dengue, yellow fever, and equine encephalitis are three common arboviral infections. Treatment is symptomatic for all arbovirus infections. Vaccines have been developed to prevent infection from some arboviruses.

arch- See archi-.

arche- See archi-.

archenteric canal See neurenteric canal.

archenteron, *pl.* **archentera** The primitive digestive cavity formed by the invagination of the blastula in the embryonic development of many animals. It corresponds to the tubular cavity in the vertebrates that connects the amniotic cavity with the yolk sac. Also called **archigaster, coelenteron, gastrocoele, primitive gut.** See also **gastrula.** —**archenteric,** *adj.*

archetype 1. An original model or pattern from which a thing or group of things is made or evolves. 2. In analytic psychology: an inherited primordial idea or mode of thought derived from the experiences of the human race and present in the unconscious of the individual in the form of drives, moods, and concepts. See also **anima.** —**archetypal, archetypic, archetypical,** *adj.*

archi- arch-, arche- A combining form meaning 'first, beginning, or original': *archenteron, archiblastoma, archicyte.*

archiblastoma, *pl.* **archiblastomas, archiblastomata** A tumor composed of cells derived from the layer of tissue surrounding the germinal vesicle.

archigaster See archenteron.

archinephric canal See pronephric duct.

archinephric duct See pronephric duct.

archinephron, *pl.* **archinephra** See pronephros. —**archinephric,** *adj.*

archistome See blastopore.

archo- A combining form meaning 'pertaining to the rectum or anus': *archocele, archoptoma, archostenosis.*

arch of the aorta One of the four portions of the aorta, giving rise to three arterial branches called the brachiocephalic, left common carotid, and the left subclavian arteries. The arch rises at the level of the cranial border of the second sternocostal articulation of the right side, passes to the left in front of the trachea, bends dorsally, and becomes part of the descending aorta. Also called **aortic arch.**

arcing spring contraceptive diaphragm A kind of contraceptive diaphragm in which the flexible metal spring that forms the rim is a combination of a flexible coil spring and a flat, band spring made of stainless steel. The rubber dome is approximately 3.8 cm (1½ inches) deep, and the diameter of the rubber-covered rim is between 5.5 and 10 cm (2⅛ and 4 inches). Ten sizes, in increments of 0.5 cm (⅕ inch), allow the clinician to fit the diaphragm to each individual woman. The kind of spring and the size of the rim in millimeters are stamped on the rim, as, for example, 75 mm arcing spring. This kind of diaphragm is prescribed for a woman whose vaginal musculature is relaxed and does not afford strong support, as in first degree cystocele, rectocele, or uterine prolapse; if the uterus is in an abnormal position, the arcing spring may offer better protection than the coil or flat spring, being stronger and better able to prevent the diaphragm from slipping out of the fornices of the vagina, thereby leaving the cervix exposed. Many women who have had a vaginal delivery are fitted with an arcing spring diaphragm, as some loss of vaginal muscle tone commonly occurs. An unusually long or short vagina or a vagina of unusual contour may often be well fitted with an arcing spring diaphragm. It is the most commonly prescribed kind of diaphragm, and, while heavier than the other kinds, is usually found to be comfortable to use. Compare **coil spring contraceptive diaphragm, flat spring contraceptive diaphragm.** See also **contraceptive diaphragm fitting.**

ARDS *abbr* **adult respiratory distress syndrome.**

area In anatomy: a limited anatomical space that contains a specific structure of the body or within which certain physiologic functions predominate, as the aortic area and the association areas of the cerebral cortex.

arenavirus Any one of a group of viruses usually transmitted to man by oral or cutaneous contact with the excreta of wild rodents. Individual arenaviruses are identified with specific geographical areas, as **Bolivian hemorrhagic fever,** in one river valley in Bolivia; **Lassa fever,** in Nigeria, Liberia, and Sierra Leone; and **Argentine hemorrhagic fever,** in two agricultural provinces in Argentina.

areola, *pl.* **areolae** **1.** A small space or a cavity within a tissue. **2.** A circular area of a different color surrounding a central feature, as the discoloration about a pustule or vesicle. **3.** The part of the iris around the pupil.

areola mammae The pigmented, circular area surrounding the nipple of each breast. Also called **areola papillaris.**

areola papillaris See **areola mammae.**

areolar gland One of the large sebaceous glands in the areolae encircling the nipples on the breasts of women. The areolar glands secrete a lipoid fluid that lubricates and protects the nipple during nursing, and contain smooth muscle bundles that cause the nipples to become erect when stimulated. Also called **gland of Montgomery.**

areolar tissue A kind of connective tissue having little tensile strength and consisting of loosely woven fibers and areolae. Also called **fibroareolar tissue.** Compare **fibrous tissue.**

argentaffin cell A cell containing serotonin-secreting granules that stain readily with silver and chromium parts. Such cells occur in most regions of the gastrointestinal tract and are especially abundant in the crypts of Lieberkühn. Also called **enterochromaffin cell, Kulchitsky's cell.** See also **carcinoid, carcinoid syndrome.**

argentaffinoma, *pl.* **argentaffinomas, argentaffinomata** A carcinoid tumor arising most often from argentaffin cells (Kultschitz-

ky's cells) in epithelium of the crypts of Lieberkühn in the gastrointestinal tract. The neoplasm, which occurs chiefly in middle-aged or elderly persons, may be a nodule or plaque in the early stage and a growth encircling the bowel in the later stage. Highly vascular tumors formed of silver-staining argentaffin cells may also develop in the bronchi.

argentaffinoma syndrome See **carcinoid syndrome.**

Argentine hemorrhagic fever See **arenavirus.**

arginine A crystalline basic amino acid produced by the decomposition of vegetable tissues, protamines, and proteins. Also prepared synthetically.

argininemia An autosomal recessive disorder characterized by an increased amount of arginine in the blood caused by a deficiency of arginase. Without arginase, ammonia cannot be metabolized into urea. Partial deficiency may result in hyperammonemia, metabolic alkalosis, convulsions, hepatomegaly, mental retardation, and growth failure; total deficiency is fatal. See also **ammonia, urea.**

argon (Ar) A colorless, odorless, chemically inactive gas and one of the six rare gases in the atmosphere. Its atomic number is 18; its atomic weight is 39.9.

Argyll Robertson pupil A pupil that constricts on accommodation but not in response to light. It is most often seen in advanced neurosyphilis.

ariboflavinosis A condition caused by deficiency of vitamin B_2 in the diet and characterized by lesions at the corners of the mouth, on the lips, and around the nose and eyes, by seborrheic dermatitis, and by various visual disorders. See also **riboflavin.**

arithmetic mean See **mean,** definition 2.

arm cylinder cast An orthopedic device of plaster of paris or fiberglass used for immobilizing the upper limb from the wrist to the upper arm. It is most often applied to aid the healing of a dislocated elbow, for postoperative immobilization or positioning of the elbow, or in the correction or the maintenance of a correction of a deformity of the elbow.

Arnold-Chiari malformation A congenital herniation of the brain stem and lower cerebellum through the foramen magnum into the cervical vertebral canal, often associated with hydrocephalus and spina bifida. See also **neural tube defect.**

aromatic alcohol A fatty alcohol in which part of the hydrogen of the alcohol radical is replaced by a phenyl hydrocarbon.

aromatic bath A medicated bath in which aromatic substances or essential oils are added to the water.

arrest To inhibit, restrain, or stop, as to arrest the course of a disease. See also **cardiac arrest.**

arrested dental caries Dental caries in which the area of decay has stopped progressing and infection is not present but in which the demineralized area remains a cavity.

HOW ARRHYTHMIAS AFFECT THE CARDIOVASCULAR SYSTEM	
ARRHYTHMIA	**EFFECTS**
Paroxysmal tachycardia	• Reduced cardiac output, with associated symptoms • Increased oxygen demands on myocardium • Decreased coronary blood supply • Possible progression to atrial fibrillation, ventricular tachycardia, and ventricular fibrillation
Atrial fibrillation with rapid ventricular response	• Compromised cardiac output • Decreased coronary blood supply • Increased oxygen consumption • Loss of "atrial kick"
Ventricular tachycardia	• Decreased ventricular filling • Rapid fall in cardiac output • Development of dyspnea, angina, hypotension, oliguria, syncope • Possible progression to ventricular fibrillation
Ventricular fibrillation	• Failure of normal cardiac contraction sequence • Loss of consciousness, seizures, apnea, death

arrested development The cessation of one or more phases of the developmental process in utero before normal completion, resulting in congenital anomalies. Also called **developmental arrest.**

arrheno- A combining form meaning 'male': *arrhenoblastoma, arrhenogenic, arrhenoplasm.*

arrhenoblastoma An ovarian neoplasm whose cells mimic those in testicular tubules and secrete male sex hormone, causing virilization in females. Also called **andreioma, andreoblastoma, androma, Sertoli-Leydig cell tumor.**

arrhenoma See **arrhenoblastoma.**

arrhythmia, arrythmia Any deviation from the normal pattern of the heartbeat. Kinds of arrhythmias include **asystole, atrial fibrillation, atrioventricular block, premature ventricular contraction, sinoatrial block. —arrhythmic, arrhythmical,** *adj.*

arsenic (As) An element that occurs throughout the earth's crust in metal arsenides, arsenious sulfides, and arsenious oxides. Its atomic number is 33; its atomic weight is 74.9. The arsenic atom occurs in the elemental form and in trivalent and pentavalent oxidation states. This element has been used for centuries as a therapeutic agent and as a poison and continues to have limited use in some trypanocidal drugs, as melarsoprol and tryparsamide. The pentavalent forms of arsenicals are rapidly excreted and cause much less toxicity than the trivalent forms. Chronic exposure to inorganic arsenicals, especially the trivalent compounds, may cause severe damage to the gastrointestinal lining, kidneys, central nervous system, bone marrow, liver, and blood system. Small doses of inorganic arsenic cause mild vasodilation; larger doses induce capillary dilation, cardiac disorders, and diminished blood volume. Various studies show a strong connection between the intensity and duration of exposure to arsenic and lung cancer in metal workers. Federal restrictions on arsenic levels in food and occupational environments have greatly reduced the incidence of both acute and chronic arsenic poisoning.

arsenic poisoning Poisoning caused by the ingestion or inhalation of arsenic or a substance containing arsenic, an ingredient in some pesticides, herbicides, dyes, and medicinal solutions. Small amounts absorbed over a period of time may result in chronic poisoning, producing nausea, headache, coloration and scaling of the skin, hyperkeratoses, anorexia, and white lines across the fingernails. Ingestion of large amounts of arsenic results in severe gastrointestinal pain, diarrhea, vomiting, and swelling of the extremities. Renal failure and shock may occur, and death may result.

arteri- See **arterio-.**

arteria alveolaris inferior See **inferior alveolar artery.**

arterial Of or pertaining to an artery.

arterial blood gas The oxygen and carbon dioxide in arterial blood, measured by various methods to assess the adequacy of ventilation and oxygenation, and the acid-base status. The oxygen content of arterial blood, normally 15 to 23 volumes %, is decreased in chronic obstructive lung disease, flail chest, kyphoscoliosis, neuromuscular impairment, obesity, hypoventilation, and postoperative respiratory complications. Oxygen saturation of hemoglobin is normally 94% or higher. The partial pressure of oxygen (PaO_2), normally 75 to 100 mmHg, is increased in polycythemia and hyperventilation and decreased in anemias, cardiac decompensation, chronic obstructive pulmonary disease, and certain neuromuscular disorders. The carbon dioxide content, normally 46%, is increased in emphysema and aldosteronism and by severe vomiting; it is decreased in starvation, acute renal failure, diabetic acidosis, and severe diarrhea. The HCO_3^- level is normally 22 to 26 mEq/L. Partial pressure of carbon dioxide, normally 35 to 45 mmHg, may be higher in emphysema, obstructive lung disease, and reduced function of the respiratory center and lower in pregnancy and in the presence of pulmonary emboli and anxiety. The normal pH of arterial blood is 7.35 to 7.42.

arterial circle of Willis The anastomosis at the base of the brain, formed by the anterior and the posterior cerebral arteries and branches of the internal carotid and the basilar arteries. The three arterial trunks that supply each cerebral hemisphere arise from the arterial circle of Willis. The trunks are the anterior, giving rise to the two anterior cerebral arteries, the anterolateral, giving rise to the two middle cerebral arteries, and the posterior, giving rise to the two posterior cerebral arteries.

arterial insufficiency Inadequate blood flow in arteries caused by occlusive atherosclerotic plaques or emboli, damaged, diseased, or intrinsically weak vessels, arteriovenous fistulas, aneurysms, hypercoagulability states, or heavy use of tobacco. Signs of arterial inadequacy include pale, cyanotic, or mottled skin over the affected area, absent or decreased sensations, tingling, diminished sense of temperature, muscle pains, as intermittent claudication in the calf following continuous exercise, reduced or absent peripheral pulses, and, in advanced disease, atrophy of muscles of the involved extremity. Arterial insufficiency may be diagnosed by checking and comparing peripheral pulses in contralateral extremities, by angiography, by ultrasound using a Doppler device, and by skin temperature tests.

arterial insufficiency of lower extremities A condition characterized by hardening, thickening, and loss of elasticity of the walls of peripheral arteries causing decreased circulation, sensation, and function. Symptoms include sharp, cramping pain during exercise or rest at night, numbness, skin changes ranging from pallor to ulceration, and loss of hair on the legs. Pedal and popliteal pulses may be diminished or absent. Laboratory studies usually show elevated plasma lipids.

arterial pressure The stress exerted by the circulating blood on the walls of the arteries. The amount of arterial pressure in an individual is the product of the cardiac output and the systemic vascular resistance. A number of extrinsic and intrinsic factors serve to regulate and to maintain a reasonably constant arterial pressure. Extrinsic factors include neurological stimulation, catecholamines, prostaglandins, and other hormones. Intrinsic factors include chemoreceptors and pressure-sensitive receptors in the arterial walls that act to cause vasoconstriction or vasodilation. Arterial blood pressure is commonly measured with a sphygmomanometer and stethoscope. Stress, hypervolemia, hypovolemia, and various drugs may alter the arterial pressure. See also **blood pressure.**

arterial wall The fibrous enclosure of the many vessels that carry oxygenated blood from the heart to structures throughout the body, and of the pulmonary arteries that carry venous blood from the heart to the lungs. The arteries, like the veins, are cylindrical tubes enclosed by layers of different kinds of tissue. The inner layer is composed of a membrane of endothelium, a subendothelial layer of delicate connective tissue, and an internal elastic membrane. The endothelium of the inner layer is composed of a single layer of simple squamous cells and is continuous with the endothelium of the capillaries and the endocardium of the heart. The middle layer of tissue around each artery comprises most of the arterial wall and is composed of circular sheets of smooth muscle cells and elastic tissue. The outer layer consists of areolar connective tissue with a fine network of collagenous and elastic fibers. Most of the arteries in the body are of medium size, with a diameter of about 4 mm.

arterio-, arteri- A combining form meaning 'pertaining to an artery': *arteriosclerosis, arteriovenous, arteritis.*

arteriogram An X-ray of an artery injected with a radiopaque medium. See also **arteriography.**

arteriography A method of radiologic visualization of arteries performed after radiopaque contrast medium is introduced into the bloodstream or into a specific vessel by injection or through a catheter. See also **angiography.** —**arteriographic,** *adj.*

arteriola See arteriole.

arteriole One of the blood vessels of the smallest branch of the arterial circulation. Blood flowing from the heart is pumped through the arteries to the arterioles to the capillaries into the veins and returned to the heart. The muscular wall of the arterioles constricts and dilates in response to neurochemical stimuli; thus, arterioles play a significant role in peripheral vascular resistance and in regulation of blood pressure.

arteriosclerosis A common arterial disorder characterized by thickening, loss of elasticity, and calcification of arterial walls, resulting in a decreased blood supply, especially to the cerebrum and lower extremities. The condition often develops with aging, and in hypertension, nephrosclerosis, scleroderma, diabetes, and hyperlipidemia. Typical signs include intermittent claudication, changes in skin temperature and color, altered peripheral pulses, bruits over an involved artery, headache, dizziness, and memory defects. The use of vasodilators and exercise to stimulate collateral circulation may relieve symptoms of arteriosclerosis, but there is specific treatment for the disorder.

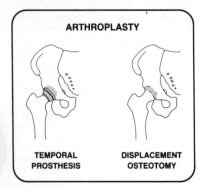

ARTHROPLASTY

TEMPORAL
PROSTHESIS

DISPLACEMENT
OSTEOTOMY

Preventive measures include therapy of predisposing diseases, continued activity in later life, adequate rest, and avoidance of stress. Kinds of arteriosclerosis are **atherosclerosis, Mönckeberg's arteriosclerosis.**
arteriovenous   Of or pertaining to arteries and veins.
arteriovenous angioma of the brain   A congenital tumor consisting of a tangle of coiled, usually dilated arteries and veins, islets of sclerosed brain tissue, and, occasionally, cartilaginous cells. The lesion, which may be distinguished by an intracranial bruit, generally arises in the vascular system of the pia mater and may grow to project deeply into the brain, causing seizures and progressive hemiparesis.
arteriovenous fistula   An abnormal communication between an artery and vein occurring congenitally or resulting from trauma, infection, arterial aneurysm, or a malignancy. A continuous murmur and palpable thrill may be detected over the fistula and may be obliterated by compressing the feeding artery; this maneuver may slow the heart beat (Branham's sign). Chronic arteriovenous fistulas may give rise to varicosities, cutaneous ulcers, and cardiac enlargement. A congenital fistula may result in a cavernous hemangioma. If an arteriovenous fistula is limited in size and is in an accessible location, it can be treated by surgical excision. An arteriovenous fistula is often created surgically to provide access to the bloodstream of patients receiving hemodialysis.
arteritis   An inflammatory condition of the inner layers or the outer coat of one or more arteries, occurring as a clinical entity or accompanying another disorder, as rheumatoid arthritis, rheumatic fever, polymyositis, or systemic lupus erythematosus. Kinds of arteritis include **infantile arteritis, rheumatic arteritis, Takayasu's arteritis, temporal arteritis.** See also **endarteritis, periarteritis.**
arteritis umbilicalis   A septic inflammation of the umbilical artery in newborn infants, usually by the bacteria of the species *Clostridium tetani.*
artery   One of the large blood vessels of arterial circulation carrying blood from the heart to the arterioles. The wall of an artery has three layers: the **tunica adventitia,** the outer coat; the **tunica media,** the middle coat; and the **tunica intima,** the inner coat. See also **arteriole.**
artery forceps   Any forceps used for grasping, compressing, and holding the end of an artery during ligation. Generally self-locking, its handles are scissorlike. Also called **hemostatic forceps.**
arthr-, arthro-   A combining form meaning 'pertaining to a joint': *arthralgia, arthrocentesis.*
arthralgia   Any pain that affects a joint. —**arthralgic,** *adj.*
-arthria   A combining form meaning a '(specified) condition involving the ability to articulate': *anarthria, dysarthria, pararthria.*
-arthritic   A combining form meaning 'pertaining to an arthritic condition': *antarthritic, antiarthritic, postarthritic.* Also -**arthrical.**
arthritis   Any inflammatory condition of the joints, characterized by pain and swelling. See also **osteoarthritis, rheumatoid arthritis.**
arthritis deformans   See **rheumatoid arthritis.**
arthrocentesis   The puncture of a joint with a needle and the withdrawal of fluid, performed to obtain samples of synovial fluid for diagnostic purposes.
arthrodesis   See **ankylosis,** definition 2.
arthrodia   See **gliding joint.**
arthrogryposis multiplex congenita   Fibrous stiffness of one or more joints, present at birth, often associated with incomplete development of the muscles that move the involved joints and degenerative changes of the motor neurons that innervate those muscles. The cause of this rare condition is unknown.
arthropathy   Any disease or abnormal condition affecting a joint. —**arthropathic,** *adj.*
arthroplasty   The surgical reconstruction or replacement of a painful, degenerated joint to restore mobility to a joint in osteoarthritis, rheumatoid arthritis, or to correct a congenital deformity. One of two procedures is used: either the bones of the joint are reshaped and soft tissue or a metal disc is placed between the reshaped ends (displacement osteotomy), or all or part of the joint is replaced with a metal or plastic prosthesis (temporal prosthesis). Preoperative care includes the typing and cross-matching of blood. Postoperatively, the patient is immediately placed in traction to immobilize the affected limb. Exercise to increase muscle strength and range of motion is allowed in a slow, progressive schedule. Frequent checks of distal circulation are necessary if a cast is in place. The nurse watches for signs of surgical shock, thrombophlebitis, pulmonary embolism, or fat embolism. Antibiotics are usually given to prevent infection, which is the most common cause of failure of the surgery. See also **osteoarthritis.**
arthropod   A member of the Arthropoda, a large phylum of animal life which includes crabs and lobsters as well as mites, ticks, spiders, and insects. Arthropods generally are distinguished

by a jointed exoskeleton (shell) and paired, jointed legs; they bite, sting, cause allergic reactions, and carry viruses and other disease agents.

arthroscopy   The examination of the interior of a joint, performed by inserting a specially designed endoscope through a small incision. The procedure, used chiefly in knee problems, permits biopsy of cartilage or synovium, the diagnosis of a torn meniscus, and, in some instances, the removal of loose bodies in the joint space. —**arthroscopic,** *adj.*

Arthus reaction   A rare, severe, immediate hypersensitivity reaction to a foreign substance, which is usually not irritating but, in certain individuals is antigenic. An acute local inflammatory reaction occurs at the site of injection. A sterile abscess may form that is slow to heal and that may become necrotic and secondarily infected. Also called Arthus phenomenon.

articul-   A combining form meaning 'pertaining to a joint': *articular, articulatio.*

articular capsule   An envelope of tissue that surrounds a freely moving joint, composed of an external layer of white fibrous tissue and an internal synovial membrane. See also **fibrous capsule.**

articular cartilage   See **cartilage.**

articular disc   The platelike end of certain bones in movable joints, developed from unabsorbed mesoderm and sometimes closely associated with surrounding muscles or with cartilage.

articular fracture   A fracture involving the articular surfaces of a joint.

articulatio cubiti   See **elbow joint.**

articulatio ellipsoidea   See **condyloid joint.**

articulatio genus   See **knee joint.**

articulation   See **joint.**

articulation of the pelvis   Any one of the connections between the bones of the pelvis, involving four groups of ligaments. The first group connects the sacrum and the ilium; the second, the sacrum and the ischium; the third, the sacrum and the coccyx; and the fourth, the two pubic bones.

articulatio plana   See **gliding joint.**

articulatio sellaris   See **saddle joint.**

artifact   Anything extraneous or irrelevant, as a substance, structure, piece of information, etc.

artificial fever   An elevated body temperature produced by artificial means, as the injection of malarial parasites or of a vaccine known to produce fever symptoms, or by applying heat to the body. An artificial fever may be prescribed for a patient to arrest a disease that is sensitive to elevated body temperatures. Also called **fever therapy.**

artificial insemination   The introduction of semen into the vagina or uterus by mechanical or instrumental means rather than by sexual intercourse. The procedure is planned to coincide with the expected time of ovulation so that fertilization can occur. Kinds of artificial insemination are **artificial insemination donor,**

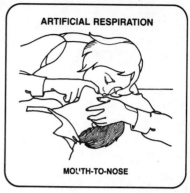

ARTIFICIAL RESPIRATION

MOUTH-TO-NOSE

artificial insemination husband. Also called artificial impregnation.

artificial insemination donor (AID)   Artificial insemination in which the semen specimen is provided by an anonymous donor. The procedure is used primarily in cases where the husband is sterile. Also called **heterologous insemination.** Compare **artificial insemination husband.**

artificial insemination husband (AIH)   Artificial insemination in which the semen specimen is provided by the husband. The procedure is used primarily in cases of impotency or when the husband is incapable of sexual intercourse because of some physical disability. Also called **homologous insemination.** Compare **artificial insemination donor.**

artificial intelligence (AI)   The capability of a device, as an industrial robot, to perform functions previously thought to require human intelligence. Computer technology produces many instruments and systems that mimic and surpass some human capabilities, as speed of counting, correlating, sensing, and deducing.

artificial kidney   See **hemodialysis, peritoneal dialysis.**

artificial limb   See **prosthesis.**

artificial lung   See **Drinker respirator.**

artificially acquired immunity   See **acquired immunity.**

artificial pacemaker   See **cardiac pacemaker.**

artificial respiration   The process of maintaining respiration by manual or mechanical means when normal breathing has stopped. Effective ventilation of the lungs may fail because of bronchial obstruction by swelling, a foreign body, increased secretions, neuromuscular weakness, status asthmaticus, exhaustion, pharmacologic depression, or trauma to the chest wall. Before attempting to administer artificial respiration, the airway is tested and any obstruction removed; the pulse is palpated and the need for cardiopulmonary resuscitation is evaluated. See also **cardiopulmonary resuscitation, resuscitation, ventilator.**

artificial selection   The process by which the genotypes of successive plant and animal

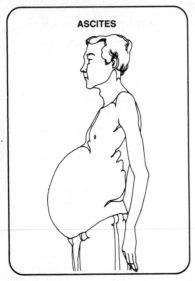

ASCITES

generations are determined through controlled breeding. Compare **natural selection.**

artificial tears   Solution used to stimulate natural tears; used to reduce eye irritation.

aryl hydrocarbon hydroxylase (AHH) An enzyme that converts carcinogenic chemicals in tobacco smoke and in polluted air into active carcinogens within the lungs. Aryl hydrocarbon hydroxylase is the subject of numerous studies to determine why some smokers develop cancer and others do not. Experimental blood tests indicate that the level of aryl hydrocarbon hydroxylase may be a factor in hereditary predisposition of a cigarette smoker to cancer.

As   Symbol for **arsenic.**

as-   See **ad-.**

ASA   *abbr* **American Society of Anesthesiologists.**

asbestosis   A chronic lung disease caused by the inhalation of asbestos fibers that results in the development of alveolar, interstitial, and pleural fibrosis. Asbestos miners and workers are most frequently affected, but the disease sometimes occurs in other people who have been exposed to asbestos building materials. Chest X-ray films show the characteristic small linear opacities distributed throughout the lungs. The disease is progressive: shortness of breath develops, eventually, in respiratory failure. Cigarette smoking and continuous exposure to asbestos aggravate the condition. Fatal mesothelial tumors sometimes occur. There is no treatment. See also **chronic obstructive lung disease, inorganic dust.**

ASC   *abbr* **altered state of consciousness.**

ascariasis   An infection caused by a parasitic worm, *Ascaris lumbricoides,* that migrates through the lungs in its larval stage. The eggs are passed in human feces, contaminating the soil and allowing transmission to the mouths of others through hands, water, or food. After hatching in the small intestine, the larvae travel through the wall of the intestine, whence they are carried by the lymphatics and blood to the lungs. Early respiratory symptoms of coughing, wheezing, and fever are caused by the passage through the respiratory tract. The larvae are swallowed, they mature in the jejunum, where they release eggs, and the cycle is repeated. Intestinal infection may result in abdominal cramps and obstruction. In children, migration of the adult worms into the liver, gall bladder, or peritoneal cavity may cause death. The infective eggs are readily identified in the feces. The disease can be prevented by educating people, especially children, about good sanitation habits and handwashing.

Ascaris   A genus of large parasitic intestinal roundworms, as *Ascaris lumbricoides,* a cause of ascariasis, found throughout temperate and tropical regions.

ascending aorta   One of the four main sections of the aorta, branching into the right and left coronary arteries, rising from the semilunar valve of the heart, curving to the right near the cranial border of the second right costal cartilage, and lying about 6 cm (2½ inches) deep to the dorsal surface of the sternum. It is about 5 cm (2 inches) long and has three small aortic sinuses at its origin, opposite the aortic valve.

ascending colon   The segment of the colon that extends from the cecum in the lower right side of the abdomen to the transverse colon at the hepatic flexure on the right side, usually at the level of the umbilicus.

ascending current   See **centripetal current.**

ascending oblique muscle   See **obliquus internus abdominis.**

ascending pharyngeal artery   One of the smallest arteries that branch from the external carotid artery, deep in the neck, supplying various organs and muscles of the head, as the tympanic cavity, the longi capitis, and the colli. It divides into five branches, the pharyngeal, palatine, prevertebral, inferior tympanic, and posterior meningeal.

ascending urography   See **urography.**

Ascheim-Zondek (AZ) test   An obsolete biologic test for pregnancy.

ascites   An abnormal intraperitoneal accumulation of a fluid containing large amounts of protein and electrolytes. Ascites may be detectable when more than 500 ml (17 oz) of fluid has accumulated. The condition may be accompanied by general abdominal swelling, hemodilution, edema, or a decrease in urinary output. Identification of ascites is made through auscultation, percussion, and palpation. Ascites is a complication of cirrhosis, congestive heart failure, nephrosis, malignant neoplastic disease, peritonitis, or various fungal and parasitic diseases. See also **paracentesis.** —**ascitic,** *adj.*

ascites adiposus   See **chylous ascites.**

ascites precox   An abnormal accumulation of fluid within the peritoneal cavity preceding

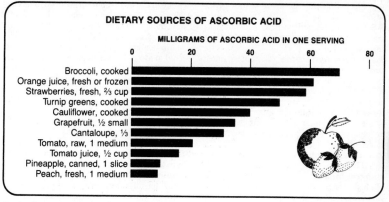

DIETARY SOURCES OF ASCORBIC ACID

MILLIGRAMS OF ASCORBIC ACID IN ONE SERVING

	0	20	40	60	80

Broccoli, cooked
Orange juice, fresh or frozen
Strawberries, fresh, ⅔ cup
Turnip greens, cooked
Cauliflower, cooked
Grapefruit, ½ small
Cantaloupe, ⅓
Tomato, raw, 1 medium
Tomato juice, ½ cup
Pineapple, canned, 1 slice
Peach, fresh, 1 medium

the development of generalized edema associated with pericarditis. See also **ascites**.

ascorbemia The presence of ascorbic acid in the blood in amounts greater than normal, usually reflecting only an excess of ascorbic acid in the diet.

ascorbic acid A water soluble, white crystalline vitamin present in citrus fruits, tomatoes, berries, potatoes, and fresh, green, leafy vegetables, such as broccoli, brussels sprouts, collards, turnip greens, parsley, sweet peppers, and cabbage. It is essential for the formation of collagen and fibrous tissue for normal intercellular matrices in teeth, bone, cartilage, connective tissue, and skin, and for the structural integrity of capillary walls. It also aids in fighting bacterial infections and interacts with other nutrients. Signs of deficiency are bleeding gums, tendency to bruising, swollen or painful joints, nosebleeds, anemia, lowered resistance to infections, and slow healing of wounds and fractures. Severe deficiency results in scurvy. An excess of ascorbic acid may cause a burning sensation during urination, diarrhea, skin rash, and nausea, and may disturb the absorption and metabolism of vitamin B_{12}. Tests for glycosuria, uric acid, and iron may be inaccurate when large amounts of the vitamin are being administered. Also called **antiscorbutic vitamin, cevitamic acid, vitamin C.** See also **ascorbemia, bioflavonoid, scurvy.**

ascorburia The presence of ascorbic acid in the urine in amounts greater than normal, usually reflecting only an excess of ascorbic acid in the diet.

ASD *abbr* **atrial septal defect.**

-ase A combining form used in naming enzymes: *lipoidase, oxidase, protease.*

asepsis 1. The absence of germs. 2. Medical asepsis, the removal or destruction of disease organisms or infected material. 3. Surgical asepsis, protection against infection before, during, or following surgery by the use of sterile technique. —**aseptic**, *adj*.

aseptic fever A fever not associated with infection. Mechanical trauma, as in a crushing injury, can cause fever even when no pathogenic

microorganism is present. Although the exact mechanism is not understood, fever in such cases is believed to result from the breakdown of leukocytes or from the absorption of avascular tissue.

aseptic gauze 1. Sterile gauze prepared and packed for surgical use. 2. Any gauze that is free of microorganisms.

aseptic meningitis An inflammation of the meninges that is caused by one of a number of viruses, including coxsackieviruses, nonparalytic polio viruses, echoviruses, and mumps. The disease is especially common in children during the late summer and early fall. In about one third of the cases no pathogen can be demonstrated, but analysis of cerebrospinal fluid reveals increased numbers of white blood cells, normal glucose concentration, and no bacteria. Symptoms vary depending upon the causative agent and may include fever, headache, stiff neck and back, nausea, and skin rash. No specific treatment is available. Supportive therapy is directed toward maintaining hydration and controlling the fever. Complete recovery, without complication or residual effect, is usual.

Asepto syringe A trade name for a bulb-fitted, blunt-tipped syringe used primarily for irrigation of wounds.

asexual 1. Not sexual. 2. Of or pertaining to an organism that has no sexual organs. 3. Of or pertaining to a process that is not sexual. —**asexuality**, *n*.

asexual dwarf An adult dwarf whose genital organs are underdeveloped.

asexual generation Any type of reproduction that occurs without the union of male and female gametes, as fission, budding, sporulation, or parthenogenesis. Also called **direct generation, nonsexual generation.**

asexualization The process of making one incapable of reproduction; sterilization of an individual or animal by castration, vasectomy, removal of the ovaries, or other means.

asexual reproduction A type of reproduction found in plants and lower animals in which new organisms are formed without the union of gametes, as occurs in budding, fission, and spore formation. Compare **sexual generation.**

ASHA *abbr* American School Health Association and American Speech-Language-Hearing Association.

Asherman syndrome Secondary amenorrhea in a hormonally normal woman, caused by obliteration of the endometrial cavity by adhesions that form as a result of curettage or infection.

Asian flu See **influenza.**

-asis A combining form meaning an 'action, process, or result of': *basis, metabasis, oxydasis.*

ASLT *abbr* **antistreptolysin-O test.**

ASOT *abbr* **antistreptolysin-O test.**

asparaginase **1.** An enzyme that catalyzes the hydrolysis of asparagine to asparaginic acid and ammonia. **2.** An antineoplastic agent derived from *Escherichia coli.*

aspartate kinase An enzyme that catalyzes the transfer of a phosphate group from adenosine triphosphate to aspartate to produce phosphoaspartate.

aspartate transaminase An enzyme that catalyzes the breakdown of the amino acid aspartic acid to fumaric acid and ammonia by transferring an amino group from the aspartic acid molecule to another molecule.

aspartic acid A nonessential amino acid present in sugar cane, beet molasses, and the breakdown products of many proteins. Pure aspartic acid is a water-soluble, colorless crystalline substance. In the Krebs' citric acid cycle, aspartic acid and oxaloacetic acid are interconvertible. Aspartic acid is used in culture media, dietary supplements, detergents, fungicides, and germicides. Also called **aminosuccinic acid.**

aspergillic acid An antibiotic substance derived from *Aspergillus flavus,* an aflatoxin-producing mold found on corn, grain, and peanuts.

aspergillosis An infection caused by a fungus of the genus *Aspergillus,* most commonly affecting the ear but capable of causing inflammatory, granulomatous lesions on or in any organ. The infection is relatively uncommon and typically occurs in a person already weakened by some other disorder. Topical fungicides can be used on the skin; amphotericin B is used to treat systemic aspergillosis, especially if it has spread to the lungs. The prognosis, as for most systemic fungal infections, is poor.

Aspergillus A genus of fungi that is a common contaminant in the laboratory and a cause of nosocomial infection. The fungus has hyphae and spores, lives in the soil, is ubiquitous, and proliferates rapidly. Inhalation of the spores of the two pathogenic species, *Aspergillus fumigatus* and *A. flavus,* is common, but infection is rare.

aspermia Lack of formation or ejaculation of semen.

asphyxia Severe hypoxia leading to hypoxemia and hypercapnea, loss of consciousness, and, if not corrected, death. Some of the more common causes of asphyxia are drowning, electric shock, aspiration of vomitus, lodging of a foreign body in the respiratory tract, inhalation of toxic gas or smoke, and poisoning. Artificial ventilation and oxygen are promptly administered to avoid damage to the brain. The underlying cause is then treated. See **artificial respiration.** —**asphyxiate,** *v.,* **asphyxiated,** *adj.*

aspirating needle A long hollow needle used to remove fluid from a cavity, vessel, or structure of the body.

aspiration **1.** The act of taking a breath, inhaling. **2.** The act of withdrawing a fluid, as mucus or serum, from the body by a suction device. See also **aspiration pneumonia.** —**aspirate,** *n.*

aspiration biopsy The removal of living tissue for microscopic examination by suction through a fine needle attached to a syringe. The procedure is used primarily to obtain cells from a lesion containing fluid or when fluid is formed in a serous cavity. See also **cytology, needle biopsy.**

aspiration biopsy cytology (ABC) A microscopic examination of cells obtained directly from living body tissue by aspiration through a fine needle. It is used primarily as a diagnostic procedure, generally as a technique for detecting nuclear and cytoplasmic changes in cancerous tissue. Compare **exfoliative cytology.**

aspiration of vomitus The inhalation of regurgitated gastric contents into the pulmonary system. See also **aspiration, aspiration pneumonia.**

aspiration pneumonia An inflammatory condition of the lungs and bronchi caused by the inhalation of vomitus containing acid gastric contents. Aspiration pneumonia most often occurs during anesthesia or recovery from anesthesia or during a seizure of acute alcoholic intoxication or other condition characterized by vomiting and a decreased level of consciousness. Treatment requires prompt suctioning of the bronchi and the administration, under pressure, of 100% oxygen. Continued artificial ventilation may be required. Corticosteroids are usually given to diminish inflammation. The sputum is cultured regularly, and any bacterial infection thus diagnosed is treated with an appropriate antibiotic. As long as oxygen is required, frequent analyses of the levels of gases in the blood are performed.

NURSING CONSIDERATIONS: The pulse rate and quality of respirations, level of consciousness, and the color of the skin are carefully monitored. Infection and respiratory failure are frequent complications. Aspiration pneumonia may be avoided by correctly positioning unconscious patients with the head low and turned to the side and by paying careful attention to the maintenance of an adequate airway. An oral airway is left in place until the patient can take it out, and secretions are removed by suction as necessary. See also **pneumonia.**

aspirator Any instrument that removes a

substance from body cavities by suction, as a bulb syringe, piston pump, or hypodermic syringe.

aspirin A salicylate nonnarcotic analgesic and antipyretic agent to treat mild to moderate pain and arthritis.

aspirin poisoning See **salicylate poisoning.**

ASRT *abbr* **American Society of Radiologic Technologists.**

Assam fever See **kala-azar.**

assault **1.** An unlawful act that places another person, without that person's consent, in fear of immediate bodily harm or battery. The act must be presently possible, thus causing well-founded apprehension in the victim of the assault. **2.** The act of committing an assault. **3.** To threaten a person with bodily harm or injury.

assertion training See **assertive training.**

assertive training A technique used in behavior therapy to help individuals become more self-assertive and self-confident in interpersonal relationships. It focuses on the direct, honest statement of feelings and beliefs, both positive and negative. The technique is learned by role playing in a therapeutic setting, usually in a group, followed by practice in actual situations. Also called **assertion training.**

assessing In five-step nursing process: a category of nursing behavior that includes gathering, verifying, and communicating information relative to the client. The nurse collects information from verbal interactions with the client, the client's family, and significant others; examines standard data sources for information; systematically checks for symptoms and signs; determines the client's ability to perform self-care activities; assesses the client's environment; and identifies reactions of the staff (including the nurse who is performing the assessment) to the client and to the client's family and significant others. To verify the data the nurse confirms the observations and perceptions by gathering additional information; discusses the orders and decisions made by other members of the staff with them, when indicated; and personally evaluates and checks the patient's condition. The nurse reports the information that has been gathered and verified. Although assessing is the first of the five steps of the nursing process, preceding analyzing, in practice assessing is integral to effective nursing practice at all steps of the process. See also **evaluating, implementation, planning.**

assessment In medicine and nursing: **1.** An evaluation or appraisal of a patient's condition. **2.** The process of gathering data needed to formulate a nursing diagnosis. **3.** In a problem-oriented medical record: an examiner's evaluation of the disease or condition based on the patient's subjective report of the symptoms and course of the illness or condition and the examiner's objective findings, including data obtained through laboratory tests, physical examination, and medical history. See also **nursing**

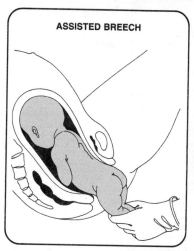

ASSISTED BREECH

assessment, problem-oriented medical record. —**assess,** *v.*

assimilation **1.** The process of incorporating nutritive material into living tissue; the end stage of the nutrition process, following digestion and absorption or occurring simultaneously with absorption. **2.** In psychology: the incorporation of new experiences into a person's pattern of consciousness. Compare **apperception.** **3.** In sociology: the process in which a person or a group of people of different ethnic backgrounds become absorbed into a new culture. —**assimilate,** *v.*

assisted breech An obstetrical operation in which a baby being born feet or buttocks first is permitted to deliver spontaneously as far as its umbilicus and is then extracted. Also called **partial breech extraction.** Compare **breech extraction.**

assisted ventilation See **IPPB.**

associate degree in nursing An academic degree after satisfactory completion of a 2-year course of study, usually at a community or junior college. The recipient is eligible to take the national licensing examination to become a registered nurse. An associate degree in nursing is not available in Canada.

associate nurse *U.S.* **1.** In primary nursing: a nurse who is responsible for implementing a primary nurse's care plans. **2.** In some states, a registered nurse who holds a diploma from a hospital school of nursing or an associate degree from a 2-year academic school of nursing.

association **1.** A connection, union, joining, or combination of things. **2.** In psychology: the connection of remembered feelings, emotions, sensations, thoughts, or perceptions with particular persons, things, or ideas. Kinds of association are **association of ideas, clang association, controlled association, dream association, free association.**

association area Any part of the cerebral cortex involved in the integration of sensory in-

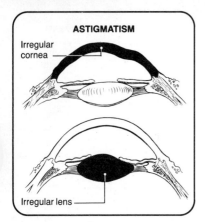

ASTIGMATISM

Irregular cornea

Irregular lens

formation. Also called **association cortex.**

association cortex See **association area.**

association of ideas A mental connection established between similar or simultaneously occurring ideas, feelings, or perceptions.

association test A technique used in psychiatric diagnosis and in educational and psychological evaluation in which a person is asked to respond to a stimulus word with the first word that comes to mind. The time taken to respond and the associations offered are compared with pretested responses and are classified and enumerated for diagnostic significance. Also called **word association test.**

associative play A form of play in which a group of children participate in similar or identical activities without formal organization, group direction, group interaction, or a definite goal. The children may borrow or lend toys or pieces of play equipment and they may imitate others in the group, but each child acts independently, as on a playground or among a group riding tricycles or bicycles. Compare **cooperative play.** See also **parallel play, solitary play.**

astatine (At) A very unstable, radioactive element that occurs naturally in very small amounts. Its atomic number is 85; its atomic weight is 210.

-aster A combining form meaning 'star-shaped': *cytaster, diaster, oleaster.*

astereognosis A neurologic disorder characterized by an inability to identify objects by touch.

asterixis A hand-flapping tremor, often accompanying metabolic disorders. The tremor is usually induced by extending the arm and dorsiflexing the wrist. Asterixis is seen frequently in hepatic coma. Also called **flapping tremor, liver flap.**

asteroid body An irregular star-shaped structure that develops in the giant cells in certain diseases, including sarcoidosis, actinomycosis, and nocardiosis.

asthenia **1.** The lack or loss of strength or energy; weakness; debility. **2.** In psychiatry: lack of dynamic force in the personality. Kinds of

asthenia include asthenia gravis hypophyseogenea, myalgic asthenia, neurocirculatory asthenia, tropical anhidrotic asthenia. See also **adynamia.** —**asthenic,** *adj.*

-asthenia A combining form meaning '(condition of) depleted vitality': *gangliasthenia, neurasthenia, phlebasthenia.*

asthenic fever An abnormal rise in body temperature associated with mental depression and characterized by a weak pulse and cool, moist skin.

asthenic habitus A body structure characterized by a slender build with long limbs, an angular profile, and prominent muscles or bones.

asthenic personality A personality characterized by low energy, lack of enthusiasm, and oversensitivity to physical and emotional strain. A person who has this kind of personality may be easily fatigued and self-pitying, and he may place the burden of his physical and emotional difficulties on others.

asthma A respiratory disorder characterized by recurring episodes of paroxysmal dyspnea, wheezing on expiration, coughing, and viscous mucoid bronchial secretions. The episodes may be precipitated by inhalation of allergens or pollutants, infection, vigorous exercise, or emotional stress. Treatment includes elimination of the causative agent, hyposensitization, aerosol or oral bronchodilators, and short-term use of corticosteroids. Beta-adrenergic drugs, barbiturates, and narcotics are contraindicated. Repeated attacks often result in emphysema and permanent obstructive lung disease. See also **allergic asthma, intrinsic asthma, status asthmaticus.**

-asthma A combining form meaning '(condition of) labored breathing': *acetonasthma, cardiasthma, corasthma.*

asthma crystal See **Charcot-Leyden crystal.**

-asthmatic A combining form meaning 'pertaining to asthma, its symptoms, or its treatment': *antiasthmatic, nonasthmatic, postasthmatic.*

asthmatic eosinophilia A form of eosinophilic pneumonia, characterized by allergic bronchospasm, by expectoration of bronchial casts containing eosinophils and mycelium, and by cough and fever. The condition usually occurs in the fourth or fifth decade of life, and is twice as common in women as in men. It is a result of hypersensitivity to *Aspergillus fumigatus* or *Candida albicans.* Untreated, the condition may result in pleural effusion, pericarditis, ascites, encephalitis, hepatomegaly, and respiratory failure. Treatment is similar to that for asthma and includes administration of corticosteroids and antibiotics. Desensitization to the allergen is not usually effective. See also **allergic asthma, eosinophilic pneumonia.**

astigmatism An abnormal condition of the eye in which the light rays cannot be focused clearly in a point on the retina because the spherical curve of the cornea or lens is not equal in all meridians. Vision is blurred and eye use causes discomfort. The person cannot accommodate to correct the problem. The condition usually may be corrected with contact lenses or with eyeglasses ground to neutralize the defect.

astragalus, *pl.* **astragali** See **talus.**

astringent 1. A substance that causes contraction of tissues upon application, usually used locally. **2.** Having the quality of an astringent. **—astringency,** *n.*

astringent bath A bath in which alum, tannic acid, or another astringent is added to the water.

astro- A combining form meaning 'pertaining to a star, or star-shaped': *astroblastoma, astrocytoma, astrophorous.*

astroblastoma, *pl.* **astroblastomas, astroblastomata** A malignant neoplasm of the brain and spinal cord. Cells of an astroblastoma lie around blood vessels or, in some cases, cluster around connective tissue septa.

astrocytic glioma See **astrocytoma.**

astrocytoma, *pl.* **astrocytomas, astrocytomata** A primary tumor of the brain composed of astrocytes and characterized by slow growth, cyst formation, invasion of surrounding structures, and, often, the development of a highly malignant glioblastoma within the tumor mass. Complete surgical resection of an astrocytoma may be possible early in the development of the tumor.

astrocytosis An increase in the number of neuroglial cells with fibrous or protoplasmic processes frequently observed in an irregular area adjacent to degenerative lesions, as abscesses, certain brain neoplasms, and encephalomalacia. Astrocytosis represents a reparative process, and in some cases it may be diffuse in a fairly large region.

asymmetrical, asymmetric Of the body or parts of the body: unequal in size or shape; different in placement or arrangement about an axis. Compare **symmetrical. —asymmetry,** *n.*

asymmetric tonic neck reflex See **tonic neck reflex.**

asynclitism Presentation of a parietal aspect of the fetal head to the maternal pelvic inlet in labor, the sagittal suture being parallel to the transverse diameter of the pelvis but anterior or posterior to it. In normal labor, the fetal head usually engages with some degree of asynclitism. Anterior asynclitism, in which the anterior parietes present, is called Nägele's obliquity. Posterior asynclitism is called Litzmann's obliquity. See also **engagement, cardinal movements of labor.**

asynergy 1. A condition characterized by faulty coordination among groups of organs or muscles that normally function harmoniously. **2.** The state of muscle antagonism found in cerebellar disease. See also **ataxia, cerebellum.**

asyntaxia Any interference with the orderly sequence of growth and differentiation of the fetus during embryonic development, resulting in one or more congenital anomalies. A kind of asyntaxia is **asyntaxia dorsalis.** See also **developmental anomaly.**

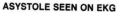

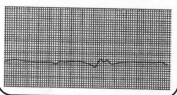

ASYSTOLE SEEN ON EKG

asyntaxia dorsalis Failure of the neural tube to close during embryonic development. See also **neural tube defect.**

asystole The absence of a heartbeat, as distinguished from fibrillation in which electrical activity persists but contraction ceases. Cardiotoxic asystole is characterized by a brief period of cardiac arrest caused by an acceleration in the heart rate. Asystole requires immediate cardiopulmonary resuscitation with cardiac massage and adequate ventilation. If these measures fail to initiate heart contractions, a discharge with a defibrillator may be administered and, if that is ineffective, an intracardiac injection of epinephrine may be given (taking care to avoid direct myocardial injection), or 5 to 10 ml of 1.0% calcium chloride may be injected into the ventricular cavity. Also called **cardiac arrest, cardiac standstill, ventricular standstill. —asystolic,** *adj.*

at- See **ad-.**

At Symbol for **astatine.**

atavism The appearance in an individual of traits or characteristics more like those of a grandparent or earlier ancestor than of the parents. Atavistic data may offer clues to an examining physician of genetic or familial health factors. **—atavistic,** *adj.*

ataxia An abnormal condition characterized by impaired ability to coordinate movement. A staggering gait and postural imbalance are caused by a lesion in the spinal cord or cerebellum, which might be the sequela of birth trauma, congenital disorder, infection, degenerative disorder, neoplasm, toxic substance, or head injury. See also **hereditary ataxia.**

ataxic aphasia See **motor aphasia.**

ataxic speech Abnormal speech characterized by faulty formation of the sounds owing to neuromuscular dysfunction.

ATCC *abbr* **American Type Culture Collection.**

-ate[1] 1. A combining form meaning 'acted upon or being in a (specified) state': *degenerate, disparate, enucleate.* **2.** A combining form meaning 'possessing': *caudate, cuspidate, longipedate.*

-ate[2] 1. A combining form meaning a 'chemical compound derived from a (specified) source': *opiate, silicate, sulfate.* **2.** A combining form meaning an 'acid compound': *acetate, oxalate, phosphate.*

atelectasis An abnormal condition characterized by the collapse of lung tissue, pre-

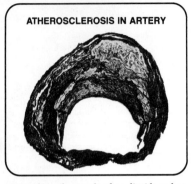

ATHEROSCLEROSIS IN ARTERY

venting the exchange of carbon dioxide and oxygen during respiration. Symptoms include diminished breath sounds, a mediastinal shift toward the side of the collapse, fever, and increasing dyspnea. The condition may be caused by obstruction of the major airways and bronchioles, by pressure on the lung from fluid or air in the pleural space, or by pressure from a tumor outside the lung. As the remaining portions of the lung eventually hyperinflate, oxygen saturation of the blood is often nearly normal. Loss of functional lung tissue may secondarily cause increased heart rate, blood pressure, and respiratory rate. The retained secretions are rich in nutrients for the growth of bacteria, a condition often leading to stasis pneumonia in critically ill patients. See also **postoperative atelectasis, primary atelectasis.**

atelectatic rale An abnormal intermittent crackling sound heard during auscultation of the chest. It usually disappears after the individual being examined coughs or breathes deeply several times.

ateliotic dwarf A dwarf whose skeleton is incompletely formed, resulting from the nonunion of the epiphyses and diaphyses during bone development.

atelo- A combining form meaning 'imperfect or incomplete': *atelocardia, ateloglossia, atelopodia.*

atenolol A sympatholytic antihypertensive used as a beta-adrenergic blocker.

atheroma, *pl.* **atheromas, atheromata** An abnormal mass of fat or lipids, as in a sebaceous cyst or in deposits in an arterial wall. —**atheromatous,** *adj.*

atheromatosis The development of many atheromas.

atherosclerosis A common arterial disorder characterized by yellowish plaques of cholesterol, lipids, and cellular debris in the inner layers of the walls of large- and medium-sized arteries. With the formation of the plaques, the vessel walls become thick, fibrotic, and calcified, and the lumen narrows, resulting in reduced circulation in organs and areas normally supplied by the artery. Atheromatous lesions are major causes of coronary heart disease, angina pectoris, myocardial infarction, and other car-

diac disorders. The pathogenesis of atherosclerosis is not clear; it may be induced by injury to arterial endothelium, the proliferation of smooth muscle in vessel walls, or the accumulation of lipids in hyperlipidemia caused by dietary excesses, faulty carbohydrate metabolism, or a genetic defect, as in hyperlipidemia Type II. Atherosclerosis usually occurs with aging and is often associated with obesity, hypertension, and diabetes. Segments of arteries obstructed or severely damaged by atheromatous lesions may be replaced by patch grafts or bypassed, as in coronary bypass surgery, or the lesion may be removed from the vessel in an endarterectomy. Antilipidemic agents do not reverse atherosclerosis, but a diet low in cholesterol, calories, and saturated fats, adequate exercise, and the avoidance of smoking and stress may help to prevent the disorder. See also **arteriosclerosis.**

athetosis A neuromuscular condition characterized by slow, writhing, continuous, and involuntary movement of the extremities, as seen in some forms of cerebral palsy and in motor disorders resulting from lesions in the basal ganglia.

athiaminosis A condition resulting from lack of thiamine in the diet. See also **beriberi, thiamine.**

athlete's foot See tinea.

athlete's heart The typical, enlarged heart of an athlete trained for endurance, characterized by a slow rate of contractions, an increased pumping capacity, and greater than average ability to deliver oxygen to skeletal muscles.

athletic habitus A physique characterized by a well-proportioned, muscular body with broad shoulders, thick neck, deep chest, and flat abdomen. Compare **asthenic habitus.** See also **mesomorph.**

atlanto-occipital joint One of a pair of condyloid joints formed by the articulation of the atlas of the vertebral column with the occipital bone of the skull. It includes two articular capsules, two membranes, and two lateral ligaments. The atlanto-occipital joint permits nodding and lateral movements of the head.

atlas The first cervical vertebra, articulating with the occipital bone and the axis.

atmo- A combining form meaning 'pertaining to steam or vapor': *atmocausis, atmolysis, atmotherapy.*

atmosphere **1.** The natural body of air, composed of approximately 20% oxygen, 78% nitrogen, and 2% carbon dioxide and other gases, that covers the surface of the earth. **2.** An envelope of gas, which may or may not duplicate the natural atmosphere in chemical components. **3.** A unit of gas pressure that is usually defined as being equivalent to the average pressure of the earth's atmosphere at sea level, or about 14.7 psi. —**atmospheric,** *adj.*

atmospheric pressure The pressure exerted by the weight of the atmosphere. The atmospheric pressure at sea level is approximately 15 psi. With increasing altitude the pressure decreases: at 9,144 m (30,000 feet), approximately the height of Mt. Everest, the air pressure is 4.3 psi. Also called **barometric pressure.**

atom   **1.** In physics: the smallest division of an element that exhibits all the properties and characteristics of the element. It is comprised of neutrons, electrons, and protons. The number of protons in the nucleus of every atom of any given element is the same and is called its atomic number. **2.** *Nontechnical.* The amount of any substance that is so small further division is not possible. **3.** *Informal.* A minute amount of any substance. —**atomic,** *adj.*

atomic number   The number of protons in the nucleus of every atom of a particular element. The atomic number equals the number of electrons, and their number and arrangement determine the chemical characteristics of the atom, with the exception of its atomic weight and radioactivity. See also **atom, electron, proton.**

atomic weight   The relative mass of an atom based on the weight of an atom of carbon 12.

atomize   See **nebulize.**

atomizer   A device for reducing a liquid and ejecting it as a fine spray or vapor.

atonia   An abnormal lack of muscle tone. —**atonic,** *adj.*

atonia constipation   Constipation caused by the failure of the colon to respond to the normal stimuli for evacuation. It may occur in elderly or bedridden patients or after prolonged dependence on laxatives. To prevent impaction of fecal material in the colon and rectum, a moderately irritant oral laxative or a mild suppository may be recommended. Patients are encouraged to develop regular, unhurried bowel habits and may be given a diet rich in fruits and vegetables. If fecal impaction develops, it may be removed by means of a mild enema or manual disimpaction, with the use of anesthetic agents. Also called **lazy colon.** See also **fecalith, inactive colon.**

atonic   **1.** Weak. **2.** Lacking normal tone, as in the case of a muscle that is flaccid. **3.** Lacking vigor, as an atonic ulcer, which heals slowly. —**atony,** *n.*

atonic bladder   See **flaccid bladder.**

atonic impotence   See **impotence.**

atopic   Of or pertaining to a hereditary tendency to develop immediate allergic reactions, as asthma, atopic dermatitis, or vasomotor rhinitis, owing to the presence of an antibody (atopic reagin) in the skin and sometimes the bloodstream. —**atopy,** *n.*

atopic asthma   See **extrinsic asthma.**

atopic dermatitis   An intensely pruritic, often excoriated, maculo-papular inflammation commonly found on the face and antecubital and popliteal areas of allergy-prone individuals. Although it may occur at any age, it is most common in infants and clears completely in half the cases by 18 months of age. Treatment includes discovery and avoidance of allergens, and application of topical and parenteral corticosteroids, tar ointments, antihistamines, and wet compresses of Burow's solution. Also called **atopic eczema, infantile eczema.** Compare

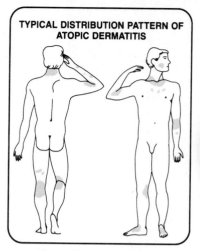

TYPICAL DISTRIBUTION PATTERN OF ATOPIC DERMATITIS

contact dermatitis. See also **atopic.**

atopic eczema   See **atopic dermatitis.**

atopic reagin   See **reagin.**

atoxic   See **nontoxic.**

ATP   *abbr* **adenosine triphosphate.**

ATPase   *abbr* **adenosine triphosphatase.**

ATPD   *abbr* Ambient temperature, ambient pressure, dry.

ATPS   *abbr* Ambient temperature, ambient pressure, saturated (with water vapor).

atresia   The absence of a normal body opening, duct, or canal, as the anus, vagina, or external ear canal. —**atresic, atretic,** *adj.*

-atresia   A combining form meaning a 'condition of occlusion': *gynatresia, hedratresia, urethratresia.*

atresic teratism   A congenital anomaly in which any of the normal openings of the body, as the mouth, nares, anus, or vagina, fail to form.

atreto-   A combining form meaning 'closed, or imperforate': *atretoblepharia, atretolemia, atretorrhinia.*

atrial appendix   See **auricle.**

atrial failure   An abnormal condition characterized by the failure of the atrium to fill adequately and distend the associated ventricle. The atria provide a pumping function and a reservoir function for the heart, and normally contribute 15% to 20% of ventricular filling. Tachycardia commonly increases this proportion. In normal individuals or in patients with mild heart disease, loss of the atrial pumping function may not change cardiac output at rest, but may decrease the output during exercise. Heart failure caused by atrial failure may occur with the onset of atrial fibrillation in patients who have compensated heart disease. Such individuals may develop congestive heart failure even when under treatment with digitalis to control the ventricular response rate. Atrial fibrillation very rarely produces heart failure in people with otherwise normal hearts.

atrial fibrillation   A condition characterized

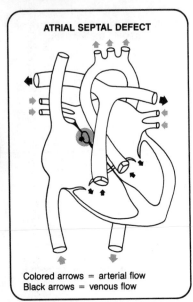

ATRIAL SEPTAL DEFECT

Colored arrows = arterial flow
Black arrows = venous flow

by rapid, random contractions of the atria, causing irregular ventricular beats at the rate of 130 to 150/minute. The atria may discharge more than 350 impulses/minute, but some do not pass the atrioventricular junction. The ventricles cannot contract in response to all the stimuli that are received, and ventricular contractions become disordered. The arrhythmia occurs most frequently in rheumatic heart disease, mitral stenosis, and atrial infarction. The rapid pulsations result in a decreased cardiac output, and the disorganized contractions of the atria promote thrombus formation in the upper chambers. Treatment consists of the administration of digitalis or of quinidine or the use of electric shock to restore a normal sinus rhythm.

atrial gallop An abnormal cardiac rhythm in which a low-pitched, extra sound is heard late in diastole on auscultation of the heart. It indicates increased resistance to ventricular filling and is frequently heard in hypertensive cardiovascular disease, coronary artery disease, and aortic stenosis. Also called S_4. See also **gallop, heart sound.**

atrial myxoma A benign, pedunculated gelatinous tumor that originates in the interatrial septum of the heart. It may cause palpitations, disseminated neuritis, nausea, weight loss, fatigue, dyspnea, fever, and, occasionally, sudden loss of consciousness owing to obstruction of the flow of blood through the heart.

atrial septal defect (ASD) A congenital cardiac anomaly characterized by an abnormal opening between the two atria. The severity of the condition depends on the size and location of the defect, which is dependent on the stage at which embryonic development was arrested. The defects are classified as ostium secundum de-

fect, in which the aperture in the septum secundum of the fetal heart fails to close; ostium primum defect, in which there is inadequate development of the endocardial cushions; and sinus venosus defect, in which the superior portion of the atrium fails to develop. Atrial septal defects cause an increased flow of oxygenated blood into the right side of the heart, which is usually well tolerated, because it is delivered under much lower pressure than in ventricular septal defect. Clinical manifestations include right atrial and ventricular enlargement, a characteristic harsh, scratchy systolic murmur, and a fixed splitting of the second heart sound, which does not vary with respiration. X-rays and electrocardiograms generally show right atrial and ventricular enlargement, although definitive diagnosis is made by cardiac catheterization. Surgical closure is indicated in most cases but, unless the defect is severe, is usually postponed until later childhood to prevent complications during early adulthood, as atrial arrhythmias, bacterial endocarditis, and congestive heart failure. Also called **atrioseptal defect.** See also **congenital cardiac anomaly.**

atrio- A combining form meaning 'pertaining to the atrium of the heart': *atriocommisuropexy, atrionector, atrioseptopexy.*

atrioseptal defect See **atrial septal defect.**

atrioventricular (AV) block The slowed conduction or stoppage of the cardiac excitatory impulse, occurring at the atrioventricular node, bundle of His, or its branches. Kinds of AV block include first-degree block, with prolonged AV conduction, second-degree block, with partial AV block (can be either Mobitz Type I or Mobitz Type II), and third-degree block, with complete atrioventricular block. An overdose of digitalis, degenerative or inflammatory cardiac disease, or acute myocardial infarction may precipitate the condition. AV block is a common indication for the insertion of a cardiac pacemaker.

atrioventricular bundle See **bundle of His.**

atrioventricular (AV) node An area of specialized cardiac muscle that receives the cardiac impulse from the sinoatrial (SA) node and conducts it to the atrioventricular bundle of His and thence to the walls of the ventricles. The AV node is located in the septal wall of the right atrium.

atrioventricular septum A small portion of membranous septum that separates the atria from the ventricles.

atrioventricular valve A valve in the heart through which blood flows from the atria to the ventricles. The valve between the left atrium and left ventricle is the mitral valve; the right atrioventricular valve is the tricuspid valve.

at risk The state of an individual or population being vulnerable to a particular disease or injury. The factors determining risk may be environmental or physiological. An example of an environmental factor is exposure to harmful substances or organisms. An example of a physiological factor is genetic predisposition to a disease.

atrium, *pl.* **atria** A chamber or cavity, especially the right and left atria of the heart.

atrium of the heart One of the two upper chambers of the heart. The right atrium receives deoxygenated blood from the superior vena cava, the interior vena cava, and the coronary sinus. The left atrium receives oxygenated blood from the pulmonary veins. Blood is emptied into the ventricles from the atria during diastole.

-atrophia 1. A combining form meaning a 'condition of malnutrition': *metatrophia, metratrophia, pantatrophia.* **2.** A combining form meaning a 'progressive decline of a body part': *dermatrophia, neuratrophia, splenatrophia.* Also **-trophy.**

atrophic arthritis See **rheumatoid arthritis.**

atrophic catarrh An abnormal condition characterized by inflammation and discharge from the mucous membranes of the nose, accompanied by the loss of mucosal and submucosal tissue. Compare **hypertrophic catarrh.** See also **catarrh.**

atrophic fracture A spontaneous fracture caused by atrophy, as in the bones of an elderly person.

atrophic gastritis A chronic inflammation of the stomach, associated with degeneration of the gastric mucosa. Seen in elderly patients and in persons with pernicious anemia, atrophic gastritis may cause epigastric pain. Even though less acid is being produced by the stomach, antacids are helpful in relieving discomfort. See also **gastritis, pernicious anemia.**

atrophy A wasting or diminution of size or physiological activity of a part of the body owing to disease or other influences. A skeletal muscle may undergo atrophy because of lack of physical exercise or as a result of neurologic or musculoskeletal disease. Cells of the brain and central nervous system may atrophy in old age because of restricted blood flow to those areas. See also **aging. —atrophic,** *adj.*

atropine sulfate 1. An antiarrhythmic agent. **2.** A cholinergic blocking (parasympatholytic) agent. **3.** A gastrointestinal anticholinergic agent. **4.** A mydriatic agent.

attachment 1. The state or quality of being affixed or attached. **2.** In psychiatry: a mode of behavior in which one individual relates in an affiliative or dependent manner to another; a feeling of affection or loyalty that binds one person to another. Such relationships develop at critical periods during life and any failure to form these attachments, because of lack of opportunity or the inability to relate, can lead to personality deviation disorders or maladaptive behavior. See **bonding. 3.** In dentistry: any device, as a retainer or artificial crown, used to secure a partial denture to a natural tooth in the mouth.

attending physician The physician who is responsible for a particular, usually private, patient. In a university setting, an attending phy-

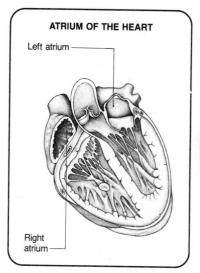

ATRIUM OF THE HEART

Left atrium

Right atrium

sician often also has teaching responsibilities and holds a faculty appointment. Also called **attending** *(informal).*

attention deficit disorder A syndrome affecting children, adolescents, and, rarely, adults characterized by learning and behavior disabilities. The symptoms may be mild or severe and are associated with functional deviations of the central nervous system without signs of major neurologic or psychiatric disturbance. The people affected are usually of normal or above average intelligence. Symptoms include impairment in perception, conceptualization, language, memory, and motor skills, decreased attention span, increased impulsivity and emotional lability, and usually, but not always, hyperactivity. The condition is ten times more prevalent in boys than in girls and may result from genetic factors, biochemical irregularities, or perinatal injury or disease. There is no known cure, and symptoms often subside or disappear with time. Medication with methylphenidate, permoline, or the dextroamphetamines is frequently prescribed for children with hyperactive symptoms, and some form of psychotherapeutic counseling is often recommended. Some treatments include abstinence from certain foods and food additives. Also called **hyperactivity, hyperkinesis, minimal brain dysfunction.** See also **learning disability.**

attic, the See **epitympanic recess.**

attitudinal reflex Any reflex initiated by a change in position of the head or by a change in position of the head with respect to the position of the body. Kinds of attitudinal reflexes include **tonic labyrinthine reflex, tonic neck reflex.** Also called **statotonic reflex.**

attrition The process of wearing away or wearing down by friction.

-ature A noun-forming combining form: *armature, ligature, tubulature.*

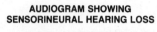

**AUDIOGRAM SHOWING
SENSORINEURAL HEARING LOSS**

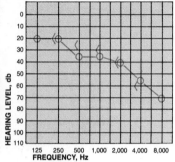

< = Air-conduction threshold
O = Bone-conduction threshold

Au Symbol for **gold.**

audioanalgesia The use of music to enhance relaxation and to distract a patient's mind from pain, as during dentistry. The procedure has also been tried experimentally during labor.

audiogram A chart showing the acuteness of hearing of an individual as indicated by the ability to hear sounds and to distinguish different speech sounds. See also **audiometry.**

audiology A field of research devoted to the study of hearing, especially impaired hearing that cannot be corrected by medical means. —**audiologic,** *adj.*

audiometer An electrical device for testing the hearing and for measuring bone and air conduction.

audiometry The testing of the acuity of the sense of hearing. Various audiometric tests determine the lowest intensity of sound at which an individual can perceive an auditory stimulus (hearing threshold), hear different frequencies, and distinguish different speech sounds. Pure tone audiometry assesses the person's ability to hear frequencies, usually ranging from 125 to 8,000 hertz (Hz) and can indicate if a hearing loss is caused by a middle-ear problem or by one in the inner ear or the auditory nerve. Speech audiometry tests the ability to repeat selected words. Impedance audiometry is an objective method of assessing the conductive mechanism of the middle ear by measuring muscle responses to sound with a probe inserted in the ear canal. Cortical audiometry indicates auditory acuity by measuring and averaging electrical potentials evoked from the cortex of the brain by pure tones. Localization audiometry is a method for measuring the individual's ability to locate the source of a pure tone received binaurally in a sound field. —**audiometric,** *adj.*

audit A methodical examination; to examine with intent to verify. Nursing audits examine standards of nursing care.

auditory ossicles The incus, the malleus,

and the stapes, small bones in the middle ear that articulate with each other and the tympanic membrane. Sound waves are transmitted through them as the tympanic membrane vibrates.

auditory tube See **eustachian tube.**

Auer body See **Auer rod.**

Auer rod An abnormal, needle-shaped or round, pink-staining inclusion in the cytoplasm of myeloblasts and promyelocytes in acute myelogenous or myelomonocytic leukemia. These inclusions contain enzymes such as acid phosphatase, peroxidase, and esterase, and may represent abnormal derivatives of cytoplasmic granules. The finding of Auer rods in stained smears of blood may help to differentiate acute myelogenous leukemia from acute lymphoblastic leukemia. Also called **Auer body.**

aur- A combining form meaning 'pertaining to the ear': *auralgan, auricle, auricular.*

aura, *pl.* **aurae, auras** **1.** A sensation, as of light or warmth, that may precede an attack of migraine or an epileptic seizure. **2.** An emanation of light or color surrounding a person as seen in Kirlian photography and studied in current nursing research in healing techniques.

aural **1.** Of or pertaining to the ear or hearing. **2.** Of or pertaining to an aura. —**aurally,** *adv.*

aural forceps A dressing forceps with fine, bent tips, used in aural surgery.

auricle **1.** The external ear. Also called **pinna. 2.** The left or right cardiac atrium, so named because of its earlike shape.

auricular **1.** Of or pertaining to the auricle of the ear. **2.** Otic.

auricularis anterior One of three extrinsic muscles of the ear. Arising from the anterior portion of the fascia in the temporal area and inserting into a projection in front of the helix, it is innervated by the temporal branch of the facial nerve and functions to move the auricula forward and upward. Some people can voluntarily contract the auricularis anterior to move the ears. Compare **auricularis posterior, auricularis superior.**

auricularis posterior One of three extrinsic muscles of the ear. Arising from the mastoid area of the temporal bone by short aponeurotic fibers and inserting into the lower part of the cranial surface of the concha, it is innervated by the posterior auricular branch of the facial nerve and serves to draw the auricula backward. Compare **auricularis anterior, auricularis superior.**

auricularis superior A thin, fan-shaped muscle that is one of three extrinsic muscles of the ear. It arises in the fascia of the temporal area and converges to insert into the cranial surface of the auricula with a thin, flattened tendon. It is innervated by a temporal branch of the facial nerve and acts to draw the auricula upward. Compare **auricularis anterior, auricularis posterior.**

auriculoventriculostomy A surgical procedure that directs cerebrospinal fluid into the general circulation in the treatment of hydrocephalus, usually in the newborn. In this procedure, a polyethylene tube is passed from the lateral ventricle through a burr hole in the parietal skull area under the scalp and into the jugular vein for the discharge of cerebrospinal fluid into the superior vena cava or the right atrium. The insertion of the tube into these structures, which have one-way valves, avoids reflux of the blood into the ventricles and continues the drain of excess cerebrospinal fluid when ventricular pressure increases. This procedure is performed to correct the communicating and the obstructive forms of hydrocephalus.

auriosis See **chrysiasis.**

aurothioglucose A gold salt used to treat rheumatoid arthritis.

auscultation The act of listening for sounds within the body to evaluate the condition of the heart, lungs, pleura, intestines, or other organs or to detect the fetal heart sound. Auscultation may be performed directly but most commonly a stethoscope is used to determine the frequency, intensity, duration, and quality of the sounds. —**auscultate,** v.

auscultatory percussion See **auscultation, percussion.**

Australia antigen Hepatitis B surface antigen (HBsAG), found in the serum of a person who has acute or chronic serum hepatitis or who is a carrier for that virus. Extremely dilute concentrations of the antigen can cause the disease. Medical personnel must take adequate precautions to avoid autoinoculation, especially in dialysis units, blood banks, and laboratories. Blood banks routinely screen for Australia antigen to avoid causing active hepatitis infection in a transfusion recipient. See also **hepatitis.**

Australian Q fever See **Q fever.**

autacoid Any of a group of substances, as hormones, that are produced in one organ and are transported via blood or lymph as a means to control a physiologic process in another part of the body.

autism A mental disorder characterized by extreme withdrawal and an abnormal absorption in fantasy, accompanied by delusion, hallucination, and an inability to communicate verbally or to otherwise relate to people. Schizophrenic children are often autistic. See also **infantile autism.** —**autistic,** adj.

auto- A combining form meaning 'pertaining to self': autoblast, autocatharsis, autoclasis.

autoantibody An immunoglobulin that reacts against a normal constituent in a person's body, as nuclear material in the patient with systemic lupus erythematosus. There are several mechanisms that may trigger the production of autoantibodies. An antigen formed during fetal development and then sequestered may be released as a result of infection or trauma and elicit the synthesis of autoantibodies, as occurs in autoimmune thyroiditis, sympathetic uveitis, and aspermia. Antibodies produced against certain streptococcal antigens during infection may cross-react with myocardial tissue, causing rheumatic heart disease, or with glomerular

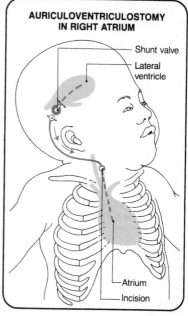

AURICULOVENTRICULOSTOMY IN RIGHT ATRIUM

Shunt valve
Lateral ventricle
Atrium
Incision

basement membrane, causing glomerulonephritis. Normal body proteins may be converted to autoantigens by chemicals, infectious organisms, or therapeutic drugs. Autoantibodies are found against gastric parietal cells in pernicious anemia, against platelets in autoimmune thrombocytopenia, and against antigens on the surface of erythrocytes in autoimmune hemolytic anemia.

autoantigen An endogenous body constituent that stimulates the production of autoantibody and a resulting autoimmune reaction against one or more tissues of the person in whom the abnormal reaction occurs. See also **autoantibody.**

autochthonous idea An idea that originates in the unconscious and arises spontaneously in the mind, independent of the conscious train of thought.

autodiploid, autodiploidic 1. Of or pertaining to an individual, organism, strain, or cell containing two genetically identical or nearly identical chromosome sets that are derived from the same ancestral species and result from the duplication of the haploid set. 2. Such an individual, organism, strain, or cell. Compare **allodiploid.** See also **autopolyploid.**

autodiploidy The state or condition of having two genetically identical or nearly identical chromosome sets from the same ancestral species. Such a state enables cell division to occur in a normal manner. Compare **allodiploidy.**

autoeroticism 1. Sensual, usually sexual, gratification of the self, usually obtained through the stimulus of one's own body without the participation of another person and derived from such acts as stroking, masturbation, fantasy, or from other oral, anal, or visual sources of stimulation. **2.** Sexual feeling or desire occurring without any external stimulus. **3.** In Freudian psychoanalytic theory: an early phase of psychosexual development, occurring in the oral and the anal stages. Also called **autoerotism.** Compare **heteroeroticism.** —**autoerotic,** *adj.*

autoerotism See **autoeroticism.**

autoerythrocyte sensitization An unusual disorder characterized by the spontaneous appearance of painful, hemorrhagic spots on the anterior aspects of the arms and legs, resulting from hypersensitivity to the patient's own red blood cells. Autoimmune hemolytic anemia, an extreme example of hypersensitivity to antigens on the surface of the patient's erythrocytes, may cause fulminant hemolysis, fever, abdominal pain, hyperbilirubinemia, thrombosis, and shock.

autoerythrocyte sensitization syndrome See **Gardener-Diamond syndrome.**

autogenesis 1. Abiogenesis. **2.** Self-produced; originating from within the organism. Also called **autogeny.** Compare **heterogenesis, homogenesis.** —**autogenetic,** *adj.*

autogenous 1. Self-generating. **2.** Originating from within the organism, as a toxin or vaccine.

autogeny See **autogenesis.** —**autogenic,** *adj.*

autograft Surgical transplantation of any tissue from one part of the body to another location in the same individual. Autografts are commonly used to replace skin lost in severe burns.

autographism See **dermatographia.**

autohexaploid, autohexaploidic See **autopolyploid.**

autoimmune disease One of a large group of diseases characterized by the subversion or alteration of the function of the immune system of the body. Antigens normally present in the internal cells stimulate the development of antibodies, and the antibodies, unable to distinguish antigens of the internal cells from external antigens, act against the internal cell to cause localized and systemic reactions. These reactions affect the epithelial and the connective tissues of the body, causing a variety of diseases that can be divided into two general categories: the collagen diseases (including systemic lupus erythematosus, dermatomyositis, periarteritis nodosa, scleroderma, and rheumatoid arthritis) and the autoimmune hemolytic disorders (including idiopathic thrombocytopenic purpura, acquired hemolytic anemia, and autoimmune leukopenia). The precise pathophysiologic processes and the etiology of these diseases are unknown and remain under study. Therapy includes corticosteroid, anti-inflammatory, and immunosuppressive drugs. The symptoms are treated specifically, as a transfusion for hemorrhage, analgesics for pain, and physical therapy for the prevention of contracture. Diet may be regulated for specific needs. Surgical treatment may be corrective or preventive, as a hip replacement in rheumatoid arthritis or a splenectomy in thrombocytopenic purpura.

NURSING CONSIDERATIONS: Many of these diseases are characterized by periods of crisis and periods of remission. During a crisis, the patient may be hospitalized and require extensive nursing care, with relief from pain, applications of heat or cold, range of motion exercises, or assistance in movement and ambulation. The nurse observes for signs of hemorrhage, puts side rails or a trapeze in place, if necessary, protects the person from infection, and prevents chilling or overheating. As the patient is in particular need of emotional support, the nurse helps the person to verbalize feelings of anger and frustration, to recognize limitations, to focus on strengths, to set realistic goals, and to understand the disease process. It is important also to teach the patient and the family the side effects of the drugs being prescribed as well as how the drugs are to be taken.

autoimmunity An abnormal characteristic or condition in which the body reacts against constituents of its own tissues. Some authorities believe autoimmunity indicates an inability of the immune system in the body to distinguish between autoantigens and foreign substances because of some change in the function of the cellular components of the immune system. Autoimmunity may result in hypersensitivity and autoimmune disease. It is not yet fully understood, but there are several common theories to explain autoimmunity, as the forbidden clone theory, the sequestered antigens theory, and the immune complex activity theory.

automatic behavior See **automatism.**

automatic bladder See **spastic bladder.**

automatic infiltration detector A temperature-sensitive device that activates an alarm and automatically stops an intravenous infusion when infiltration of the intravenous fluid occurs. The device detects any cooling of the skin at the intravenous site, a common sign of infiltration. The detector is usually secured to the skin with tape and attaches by a small cable to the fluid monitoring circuit of an intravenous pump.

automatism 1. In physiology: involuntary function of an organ system independent of apparent external stimuli, as the beating of the heart, or dependent upon external stimuli but not consciously controlled, as the dilation of the pupil of the eye. **2.** In philosophy: the theory that the body acts as a machine and that the mind, the processes of which are solely dependent on brain activity, is a noncontrolling adjunct of the body. **3.** In psychology: mechanical, repetitive, and undirected behavior that is not consciously controlled, as seen in psychomotor epilepsy, hysterical states, and such acts as sleepwalking. Kinds of automatism include **ambulatory automatism, command automatism, posttraumatic automatism.** Also called **automatic behavior.**

autonomic Of or pertaining to the autonomic nervous system.

autonomic drug Any of a large group of

drugs that mimic or modify the function of the autonomic nervous system.

autonomic dysreflexia   A dysreflexia that is the result of impaired function of the autonomic nervous system.

autonomic nervous system   The part of the nervous system that regulates involuntary vital function, including the activity of the cardiac muscle, the smooth muscle, and the glands. It has two divisions: the sympathetic nervous system accelerates heart rate, constricts blood vessels, and raises blood pressure; the parasympathetic nervous system slows heart rate, increases intestinal peristalsis and gland activity, and relaxes sphincters.

autonomic reflex   Any of a large number of normal reflexes governing and regulating the functions of the viscera. Autonomic reflexes control such activities of the body as blood pressure, heart rate, peristalsis, sweating, and urination.

autonomous bladder   See **flaccid bladder.**

autonomy   The quality of having the ability or tendency to function independently. —**autonomous,** *adj.*

autopentaploid, autopentaploidic   See **autopolyploid.**

autoplastic maneuver   In psychology: a process that is part of adaptation, involving an adjustment within the self. Compare **alloplastic maneuver.**

autopolyploid, autopolyploidic   1. Of or pertaining to an individual, organism, strain, or cell that has more than two genetically identical or nearly identical sets of chromosomes that are derived from the same ancestral species. They result from the duplication of the haploid chromosome set and are referred to as autotriploid, autotetraploid, autopentaploid, autohexaploid, and so on, depending on the number of multiples of the haploid chromosomes they contain. 2. Such an individual, organism, strain, or cell. Compare **allopolyploid.** See also **allodiploid.**

autopolyploidy   The state or condition of having more than two identical or nearly identical sets of chromosomes. Compare **allopolyploid.**

autopsy   A postmortem examination performed to confirm or determine the cause of death. Also called **necropsy, thanotopsy.** —**autopsic, autopsical,** *adj.,* **autopsist,** *n.*

autopsy pathology   The study of disease by the examination of the body after death by a pathologist. The organs and tissues are first described by their appearance at the time of dissection, then by their appearance in the microscopic examination of small representative samples of tissue taken for their diagnostic value.

autoserous treatment   Therapy of an infectious disease by inoculating the patient with the patient's own serum.

autosite   The larger, more normally formed member of unequal or asymmetrical, conjoined twins upon whom the other smaller fetus is dependent for various physiologic functions and

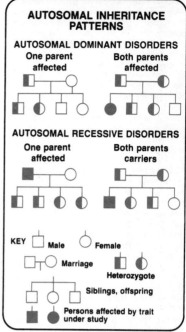

AUTOSOMAL INHERITANCE PATTERNS

AUTOSOMAL DOMINANT DISORDERS

One parent affected   Both parents affected

AUTOSOMAL RECESSIVE DISORDERS

One parent affected   Both parents carriers

KEY   □ Male   ○ Female

□─○ Marriage

▌ ◖ Heterozygote

Siblings, offspring

Persons affected by trait under study

for nutrition and growth. Compare **parasitic fetus.** —**autositic,** *adj.*

autosomal   1. Pertaining to or characteristic of an autosome. 2. Pertaining to any condition transmitted by an autosome.

autosomal-dominant inheritance   A pattern of inheritance in which the transmission of a dominant gene on an autosome causes a characteristic to be manifested. Males and females are affected with equal frequency. Affected individuals have an affected parent (unless the condition is the result of a fresh mutation). Half of the children of a heterozygous affected parent are affected. All of the children of a homozygous affected parent are affected. Normal children of an affected parent do not carry the trait. Traits can be traced vertically through previous generations. A family history may be illustrated by drawing a pedigree. The first case, the propositus, appears suddenly in the pedigree, usually as a mutation. Achondroplasia, osteogenesis imperfecta, polydactyly, and Marfan's syndrome are autosomal-dominant disorders. Compare **autosomal-recessive inheritance.**

autosomal inheritance   A pattern of inheritance in which the transmission of traits depends on the presence or absence of certain genes on the autosomes. The pattern may be dominant or recessive, and males and females are affected with equal frequency. The majority of hereditary disorders are the result of a defective gene on an autosome. See also **autosomal-dominant inheritance, autosomal-recessive inheritance.**

autosomal-recessive inheritance A pattern of inheritance in which the transmission of a recessive gene on an autosome results in a carrier state if the person is heterozygous for the trait and in the affected state if the person is homozygous for the trait. Males and females are affected with equal frequency. Affected individuals have unaffected parents who are heterozygous for the trait. One fourth of the children of two unaffected heterozygous parents are affected. All of the children of two homozygous affected parents are affected. The children of a couple in which one parent has the trait and the other does not are all carriers who show no effect of the trait. There is usually no family history of the trait; it becomes manifest when two unaffected parents who are heterozygous for a particular recessive gene have a child who is homozygous for the trait. Cystic fibrosis, phenylketonuria, and galactosemia are examples of autosomal-recessive inheritance.

autosome Any chromosome that is not a sex chromosome and that appears as a homologous pair in the somatic cell. Humans have 22 pairs of autosomes, which are involved in transmitting all genetic traits and conditions other than those that are sex-linked. Also called **euchromosome.**

autosplenectomy A progressive shrinking of the spleen, which may occur in sickle-cell anemia. The spleen is replaced by fibrous tissue and becomes nonfunctional.

autosuggestion An idea, thought, attitude, or belief suggested to oneself, often as a formula or incantation, as a means of controlling one's behavior. Compare **suggestion.**

autotetraploid, autotetraploidic See **autopolyploid.**

autotopagnosia The inability to recognize or localize the various parts of the body owing to organic brain damage. Also called **body-image agnosia.** See also **proprioception.**

autotriploid, autotriploidic See **autopolyploid.**

autumn fever See **leptospirosis.**

auxanology The scientific study of growth and development. —**auxanologic, auxanological,** adj.

auxesis, pl. **auxeses** An increase in size or volume owing to cell expansion rather than to an increase in the number of cells or tissue elements; hypertrophy. Also called **auxetic growth.** Compare **merisis.** —**auxetic,** adj., n.

auxo- A combining form meaning 'pertaining to growth, to acceleration, or to stimulation': auxochrome, auxocyte, auxotonic.

AV abbr atrioventricular, arteriovenous.

avantin See **isopropyl alcohol.**

avascular **1.** Of a tissue area: not receiving a sufficient supply of blood. The reduced flow may be the result of blockage by a blood clot, the deliberate stoppage of flow during surgery, or of measures taken to control a hemorrhage. **2.** Of a kind of tissue: not having blood vessels.

aversion conditioning See **aversion therapy.**

aversion therapy A form of behavior therapy in which punishment or unpleasant or painful stimuli, like electric shock or drugs that induce nausea, are used in the suppression of undesirable behavior. The procedure is used in treating such conditions as drug abuse, alcoholism, gambling, overeating, smoking, and various sexual deviations. Also called **aversive conditioning.** See also **behavior therapy.**

aversive stimulus A stimulus, as electric shock, that causes psychic or physical pain. See also **aversion therapy.**

avitaminosis A condition resulting from a deficiency of or the lack of absorption or utilization of one or more essential vitamins in the diet. Also called **hypovitaminosis.** Compare **hypervitaminosis.** See also specific vitamins.

AV nicking A vascular abnormality on the retina of the eye, visible on ophthalmologic examination, in which a vein is compressed by an arteriovenous crossing. The vein appears 'nicked,' owing to constriction or spasm. It is a sign of hypertension, arteriosclerosis, and other vascular conditions.

Avogadro's law A law in physics stating that equal volumes of all gases at a given temperature and pressure contain the identical number of molecules.

avoidance In psychiatry: a conscious or unconscious defense mechanism, physical or psychological in nature, by which an individual tries to avoid or escape from unpleasant stimuli, conflicts, or feelings, as anxiety, fear, pain, or danger.

avoidance-avoidance conflict A conflict resulting from the confrontation of two or more alternative goals or desires that are equally aversive and undesirable. Also called **double-avoidant conflict.** See also **conflict.**

avoidance conditioning The establishment of certain patterns of behavior in order to avoid unpleasant or painful stimuli.

avoirdupois weight The English system of weights in which there are 7,000 grains, 256 drams, or 16 ounces to one pound. One ounce in this system equals 28.35 grams and one pound equals 453.5 grams. Compare **apothecaries' weight.** See also **metric system.**

avulsed teeth Teeth that have been forcibly displaced from their normal position. In some cases they can be surgically reimplanted, but this procedure is not often successful. See also **avulsion.**

avulsion The separation, by tearing, of any part of the body from the whole, as an umbilical cord torn in the process of delivering the placenta. —**avulse,** v.

avulsion fracture A fracture caused by the tearing away of a fragment of bone where a strong ligamentous or tendinous attachment forcibly pulls the fragment away from osseous tissue.

ax- A combining form meaning 'pertaining to an axis': axial, axofugal. Also **axio-, axon-.**

axial current The central part of the blood current.

axial gradient **1.** The variation in metabolic rate in different parts of the body. **2.** The development toward the body axis or its parts in relation to the metabolic rate in the various parts.

axial illumination See **illumination.**

axial neuritis See **parenchymatous neuritis.**

axilla, *pl.* **axillae** A pyramid-shaped space forming the underside of the shoulder between the upper part of the arm and the side of the chest. Also called armpit.

axillary anesthesia See **brachial plexus anesthesia.**

axillary artery One of a pair of continuations of the subclavian arteries that start at the outer border of the first rib and ends at the distal border of the teres major, where it becomes the brachial artery. It has three parts and six branches, supplying various chest and arm muscles, as the pectorals, deltoid, and subclavius. The six branches are the highest thoracic, thoracoacromial, lateral thoracic, subscapular, posterior humeral circumflex, and the anterior humeral circumflex.

axillary nerve One of the last two branches of the posterior cord of the brachial plexus before the posterior cord becomes the radial nerve. The axillary nerve passes over the insertion of the subscapularis, crosses the teres minor, and leaves the axilla, accompanied by the posterior humeral circumflex artery. It passes through the quadrilateral space bounded by the neck of the humerus, the two teres muscles, and the long head of the triceps and divides into a posterior branch and an anterior branch. The posterior branch innervates the teres minor, part of the deltoideus, and part of the skin overlying the deltoideus; the anterior branch winds around the neck of the humerus and innervates the deltoideus. Some fibers of the nerve also supply the capsule of the shoulder joint.

axillary node One of the lymph glands of the axilla that help to fight infections in the chest, armpit, neck, and arm and to drain lymph from those areas. The 20 to 30 axillary nodes are divided into the lateral group, the anterior group, the subscapular or posterior group, the central group, and the medial or infraclavicular group. The lateral group is associated with lymphatic vessels that drain the whole arm; the anterior group with vessels that drain the thoracic muscles; the posterior group with vessels that drain the dorsal muscles of the neck and the muscles of the thoracic wall; the central group with vessels that drain the lymph from the nodes of the three preceding groups; the infraclavicular group with afferent vessels that drain lymph from the breast and efferent vessels that form the subclavian lymphatic trunk. See also **lymphatic system, lymph node.**

axillary vein One of a pair of veins of the upper limb that begins at the junction of the basilic and the brachial veins near the distal border of the teres major and becomes the subclavian vein at the outer border of the first rib. It receives deoxygenated blood from the venous

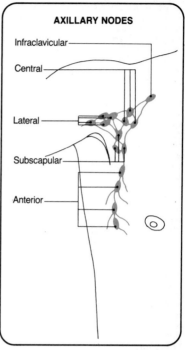

AXILLARY NODES

Infraclavicular
Central
Lateral
Subscapular
Anterior

tributaries that correspond to the branches of the axillary artery and, near its termination, from the cephalic vein. It contains a pair of valves at the distal border of the subscapularis. Compare **subclavian vein.**

axio- See **ax-.**

axis, *pl.* **axes** **1.** In anatomy: a line that passes through the center of the body, or a part of the body, as the frontal axis, binauricular axis, basifacial axis. **2.** The second cervical vertebra about which the atlas rotates, allowing the head to be turned, extended, and flexed. Also called **epistropheus, odontoid vertebra.**

axis traction **1.** The process of pulling a baby's head with obstetric forceps in a direction in line with the path of least resistance, following the curve of Carus through the mother's birth canal. **2.** *Informal.* Any mechanical device attached to obstetric forceps to facilitate pulling in the proper direction.

axoaxonic synapse A type of synapse in which the axon of one neuron comes in contact with the axon of another neuron.

axodendritic synapse A type of synapse in which the axon of one neuron comes in contact with the dendrites of another neuron.

axodendrosomatic synapse A type of synapse in which the axon of one neuron comes in contact with both the dendrites and the cell body of another neuron.

axon The cylindrical extension of a nerve cell that conducts impulses away from the neuron cell body. Axons may be bare or sheathed in myelin. Also called axis cylinder. Compare **dendrite.**

axon- See **ax-.**

axon flare Vasodilation, reddening, and increased sensitivity of skin surrounding an injured area, caused by an axon reflex. Axon flare or reflex is considered part of a triple response in which injury or stroking of the skin results in local reddening, the release of histamine or a histaminelike substance, a surrounding flare, and wheal formation. A pin prick in the involved area causes more intense pain than a similar stimulus prior to injury.

axoplasmic flow The continuous pulsing, undulating movement of the cytoplasm between the cell body of a neuron, where protein synthesis occurs, and the axon fiber in order to supply the substances vital to the axon for the maintenance of activity and for repair. The nerve fiber is totally dependent on the cell body for metabolites and any interruption in the axoplasmic flow caused by disease or trauma results in the degeneration of the unsupplied areas of the axon.

axosomatic synapse A type of synapse in which the axon of one neuron comes in contact with the cell body of another neuron.

azatadine maleate An antihistamine.

azathioprine An antimetabolite chemotherapy drug.

azo- A combining form meaning 'containing nitrogen': *azocarmine, azoimide, azorubin.*

azoospermia Lack of spermatozoa in the semen. It may be caused by testicular dysfunction or by blockage of the tubules of the epididymis, or it may be induced by vasectomy. Infertility but not impotence is associated with azoospermia. Compare **oligospermia.**

azotemia The retention in the blood of excessive amounts of nitrogenous compounds. This toxic condition is caused by failure of the kidneys to remove urea from the blood and is characteristic of uremia. See also **uremia. —azotemic,** *adj.*

AZ test See **Ascheim-Zondek test.**

azul, azula See **pinta.**

azygosperm See **azygospore.**

azygospore A spore that is produced directly from a gamete that does not undergo conjugation, as in certain algae and fungi. Also called **azygosperm.**

azygous, azygos Occurring as a single entity or part, as any unpaired anatomical structure; not part of a pair. **—azygos,** *n.*

azygous vein One of the seven veins of the thorax. Beginning opposite the first or second lumbar vertebra, it rises through the aortic hiatus in the diaphragm and passes to the right of the vertebral column to the fourth thoracic vertebra, then arches ventrally over the root of the right lung, and ends in the superior vena cava. It receives numerous veins, as the hemiazygous veins, several esophageal veins, and the right bronchial vein. Compare **internal thoracic vein, left brachiocephalic vein, right brachiocephalic vein.**

B

B Symbol for **boron.**

Ba Symbol for **barium.**

BA *abbr* Bachelor of Arts.

Babcock's operation The extirpation of a varicosed saphenous vein by inserting an acorn-tipped sound, tying the vein to the sound, and drawing it out.

babesiosis An infection caused by protozoa of the genus *Babesia.* The infective organism is introduced into the host through the bite of ticks of the species *Ixodes dammini.* Symptoms include headache, fever, nausea and vomiting, myalgia, and hemolysis. Also called babesiasis.

Babinski's reflex Dorsiflexion of the big toe with extension and fanning of the other toes elicited by firmly stroking the lateral aspect of the sole of the foot. The reflex is normal in newborn infants and abnormal in children and adults in whom it may indicate a lesion in the pyramidal tract. Also called Babinski's sign.

bacampicillin A penicillin antibiotic.

bachelor of science in nursing (BSN) An academic degree awarded upon satisfactory completion of a four-year course of study in an institution of higher learning. The recipient is eligible to take the national certifying examination to become a registered nurse. A BSN degree is prerequisite to advancement in most systems and institutions that employ nurses. Compare **associate degree in nursing, diploma program in nursing.**

bacill- A combining form meaning 'pertaining to any rod-shaped bacterium': *bacillemia, bacillicidal, bacillosis.*

Bacillaceae A family of Schizomycetes of the order Eubacteriales, consisting of gram-positive, rod-shaped cells that can produce cylindrical, ellipsoid, or spherical endospores situated terminally, subterminally, or centrally. These cells are chemoheterotropic and mostly saprophytic, commonly appearing in soil. Some are parasitic on insects and animals and are pathogenic. The family includes the genus *Bacillus,* which is aerobic, and the genus *Clostridium,* which is facultatively anaerobic.

bacillary dysentery See **shigellosis.**

bacille Calmette-Guérin (BCG) An attenuated strain of tubercle bacilli, used in many countries as a vaccine against tuberculosis, most often administered intradermally, using a multiple-puncture disk. It appears to prevent the more serious forms of tuberculosis and to give some protection to persons living in areas where tuberculosis is prevalent. BCG is also administered to stimulate the immune response in people who have certain kinds of malignancy. It induces a positive tuberculin reaction and may

mask early, active infection by removing the diagnostic sign of conversion from the negative to the positive skin reaction. See also **tuberculin test, tuberculosis.**

bacilliform Rod-shaped in form, like a bacillus.

bacilluria The presence of bacilli in the urine.

Bacillus A genus of aerobic, gram-positive, spore-producing bacteria in the family Bacillaceae, order Eubacteriales, including 33 species, 3 of which are pathogenic and the rest saprophytic soil forms. Many microorganisms formerly classified as *Bacillus* are now classified in other genera. See also **Bacillaceae.**

Bacillus anthracis A species of gram-positive, facultative anaerobe that causes anthrax. The spores of this organism, if inhaled, can cause a pulmonary form of anthrax; spores can live for many years in animal products, as hides and wool, and in soil. See also **anthrax, woolsorter's disease.**

bacillus Calmette-Guérin vaccine See **BCG vaccine.**

bacitracin An antibiotic local and ophthalmic anti-infective agent.

backache Pain in the lumbar, lumbosacral, or cervical regions of the back, varying in sharpness and intensity. Causes may include muscle strain or other muscular disorders or pressure on the root of a nerve, as the sciatic nerve, owing in turn to a variety of factors, including a ruptured vertebral disk. Treatment may include heat, ultrasound, and devices to provide support for the affected area while in bed or while standing or sitting, bed rest, surgical intervention, and medications to relieve pain and relax spasm of the muscle of the affected area.

backcross In genetics: **1.** The cross of a first filial-generation hybrid with one of the parents or with a genotype that is identical to the parental strain. **2.** The organism or strain produced by such a cross.

background radiation Naturally occurring radiation emitted by materials in the soil, ground waters, and building material, radioactive substances in the body [especially potassium 40 (^{40}K)], and cosmic rays from outer space. The average person is exposed each year to 44 milliradians (mrads) of cosmic radiation, 44 mrads external terrestrial radiation, and 18 mrads naturally occurring internal radioactive sources.

back pressure Pressure that builds in a vessel or a cavity as fluid is accumulated. The pressure increases and extends backward if the normal mechanism for egress or passage of the fluid is not restored. See also **backward failure.**

backward failure Cardiac failure marked

by elevated venous pressure and diminished arterial pressure, most commonly beginning as left ventricular failure that results in decreased output. Backward failure develops when the ventricle cannot empty and the blood backs up in the pulmonary veins and the lungs, causing pulmonary edema.

baclofen A skeletal muscle relaxant.

bacter- See **bacterio-**.

bacteremia The presence of bacteria in the blood. Undocumented bacteremias occur frequently and usually abate spontaneously. Bacteremia is demonstrated by blood culture. Antibiotic treatment, if given, is specific for the organism found and appropriate to the locus of infection. Compare **septicemia**. See also **septic shock**. —**bacteremic**, adj.

bacteremic shock See **septic shock**.

-bacteria A combining form meaning 'genus of microscopic plants forming the class Schizomycetes': lysobacteria, nitrobacteria, streptobacteria.

bacteria, sing. **bacterium** Any of the small unicellular microorganisms of the class Schizomycetes. The genera vary morphologically, being spherical (cocci), rod-shaped (bacilli), spiral (spirochetes), or comma-shaped (vibrios). The nature, severity, and outcome of any infection caused by a bacterium are characteristic of that species.

bacterial aneurysm See **mycotic aneurysm**.

bacterial endocarditis An acute or subacute bacterial infection of the endocardium, or the heart valves, or both. The condition is characterized by heart murmur, prolonged fever, bacteremia, splenomegaly, and embolism. The acute variety progresses rapidly and is usually caused by staphylococci or pneumococci. The subacute variety is usually caused by lodging of streptococcus viridans in valves of the heart damaged by rheumatic fever. Prompt treatment of both types with antibiotics, as penicillin, cephalosporin, or gentamicin given intravenously, is essential to prevent destruction of the valves and cardiac failure. See also **endocarditis, subacute bacterial endocarditis**.

bacterial food poisoning A toxic condition resulting from the ingestion of food contaminated by certain bacteria. Acute infectious gastroenteritis caused by various species of salmonella is characterized by fever, chills, nausea, vomiting, diarrhea, and general discomfort beginning 8 to 48 hours after ingestion and continuing for several days. Similar symptoms caused by staphylococcus, usually S. aureus, appear much sooner and rarely last more than a few hours. Food poisoning caused by the neurotoxin of Clostridium botulinum is characterized by gastrointestinal symptoms, disturbances of vision, weakness or paralysis of muscles, and, in severe cases, respiratory failure. See also **botulism**.

bacterial kinase 1. A kinase of bacterial origin. 2. A bacterial enzyme that activates plasminogen, the precursor of plasmin.

bacterial plaque A film comprised of microorganisms that attaches to the teeth and often causes caries and infections of the gums. Mucin secreted by the salivary glands is also a component of plaque; it varies in thickness and consistency depending on individual metabolism, dental hygiene, diet, and environmental factors. Also called **dental plaque**.

bacterial protein Any protein produced by a bacterium.

bactericidal Destructive to bacteria. Compare **bacteriostatic**.

bactericidin An antibody that kills bacteria in the presence of complement.

bacterio-, bacter- A combining form meaning 'pertaining to any bacterial microorganism': bacteriogenic, bacteriophytoma, bacteriosis.

bacteriocidal Capable of acting to kill bacteria. Compare **bacteriostatic**.

bacteriologist A specialist in bacteriology.

bacteriology The scientific study of bacteria. —**bacteriologic, bacteriological**, adj.

bacteriolysin An antibody that causes the breakdown of a particular species of bacterial cell. Complement is usually also necessary for this reaction. See also **bacteriolysis**.

bacteriolysis The breakdown of bacteria intracellularly or extracellularly. See also **bacteriolysin**. —**bacteriolytic**, adj.

bacteriophage Any virus that causes lysis of host bacteria, including the blue-green 'algae.' Bacteriophages resemble other viruses in that each is composed of either ribonucleic acid or deoxyribonucleic acid. They vary in structure from simple fibrous bodies to complex forms with contractile 'tails.' Bacteriophages associated with temperate bacteria may be genetically intimate with the host and are named after the bacterial strain for which they are specific, as coliphage and corynebacteriophage. —**bacteriophagic**, adj., **bacteriophagy**, n.

bacteriostatic Tending to restrain the development or the reproduction of bacteria. Compare **bacteriocidal**.

bacteriuria The presence of bacteria in the urine. The presence of more than 100,000 pathogenic bacteria/ml of urine is usually considered significant and diagnostic of urinary tract infection. See also **urinary tract infection**.

bacteroid, bacterioid 1. Of, pertaining to, or resembling bacteria. 2. A structure that resembles a bacterium. —**bacteroidal, bacterioidal**, adj.

Bacteroides A genus of obligate anaerobic bacilli normally found in the colon, mouth, genital tract, and upper respiratory system. Severe infection may result from the invasion of the bacillus through a break in the mucous membrane into the venous circulation, where thrombosis and bacteremia may occur. Foul-smelling abcesses, gas, and putrefaction are characteristic of infection. Of the 30 species, Bacteroides fragilis is the most common and virulent.

BAEP abbr **brain stem auditory evoked potential**.

bag **1.** A flexible or dilatable sac or pouch designed to contain gas, fluid, or semisolid material such as crushed ice. An Ambu bag (also called a manual resuscitation bag) is used to control the flow of respiratory gases entering the lungs of a patient. Several types of bags are used in medical or surgical procedures to dilate the anus, vagina, or other body openings. **2. Bag of waters,** the membranous sac of amniotic fluid surrounding the fetus in the uterus of a pregnant woman. Also called **amnion.**

bagasse The crushed fibers or the residue of sugar cane.

bagassosis A self-limiting lung disease caused by an allergic response to bagasse, the fungi-laden, dusty debris remaining after the syrup has been extracted from sugar cane. It is characterized by fever, dyspnea, and malaise. Treatment may include oral administration of corticosteroid drugs. To prevent the recurrence of this disease, the antigen should be avoided. See also **hypersensitivity pneumonitis, organic dust.**

bagging *Informal.* The artificial respiration performed with a ventilator or respirator bag, as an Ambu bag or Hope resuscitator.

bag of waters See **bag.**

Bain Breathing Circuit A continuous-flow anesthetic system that does not require a soda-lime absorber.

Bainbridge reflex A cardiac reflex consisting of an increased pulse rate, resulting from stimulation of stretch receptors in the wall of the left atrium. It may be produced by the infusion of large amounts of intravenous fluids.

BAL *abbr* **British antilewisite.**

balance **1.** A weighing instrument. **2.** A normal state of physiologic equilibrium. **3.** A state of mental or emotional equilibrium. **4.** To bring into equilibrium. —**balanced,** *adj.*

balanced anesthesia *Informal.* One of a number of variable techniques of general anesthesia in which no single anesthetic agent or preset proportion of the combination of agents is used; rather, an individualized mixture of anesthetics is prescribed according to the needs of a particular patient for a particular operation. One type of balanced anesthesia may combine a local or regional anesthetic with general anesthetic agents; another may combine a muscle relaxant, an analgesic, oxygen, an anesthetic gas, and a sedative.

balanced diet A diet containing all of the essential nutrients that cannot be synthesized in adequate quantities by the body, in amounts adequate for growth, energy needs, nitrogen equilibrium, repair of wear, and maintenance of normal health.

balanced polymorphism The recurrence in a population of an equalized mixture of homozygotes and heterozygotes for specific genetic traits, which are maintained from generation to generation by the forces of natural selection. Compare **genetic polymorphism.**

balanced suspension A system of splints, ropes, slings, pulleys, and weights for suspend-

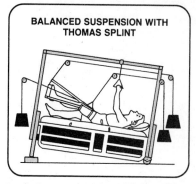

BALANCED SUSPENSION WITH THOMAS SPLINT

ing the lower extremities of the body, used as an aid to healing and recuperation from fractures or from surgical procedures.

balanced traction A system of balanced suspension that supplements traction in the treatment of fractures of the lower extremities or following various operations affecting the lower parts of the body.

balanced translocation The transfer of segments between nonhomologous chromosomes in such a way that there are changes in the configuration but not in the total number of chromosomes, so that each cell or gamete contains no more or no less than the normal amount of diploid or haploid genetic material. See also **translocation.**

balanic Of or pertaining to the glans penis or the glans clitoridis.

balanitis Inflammation of the glans penis.

balanitis xerotica obliterans A chronic skin disease of the penis, characterized by a white, indurated area surrounding the meatus.

balano- A combining form meaning 'pertaining to the glans penis': *balanocele, balanoplasty, balanoposthitis.*

balanoplasty An operation involving plastic surgery of the glans penis.

balanoposthitis A generalized inflammation of the glans penis and prepuce, characterized by soreness, irritation, and discharge, occurring as a complication of bacterial or fungal infection. Smear and culture can determine the causative agent, often a common venereal disease, whereupon specific antimicrobial therapy can be instituted. Circumcision may be considered in severe cases. To relieve discomfort, the inflamed area can be irrigated with a warm saline solution several times a day.

balanopreputial Of or pertaining to the glans penis and the prepuce.

balanorrhagia Balanitis in which pus is discharged copiously from the penis.

balantidiasis An infection caused by ingestion of cysts of the protozoan *Balantidium coli.* In some cases the organism is a harmless inhabitant of the large intestine, but infection with *B. coli* usually causes diarrhea. The diagnosis requires identification of cysts and trophozoites in the stool or in the exudate from intestinal

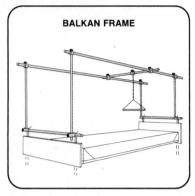

BALKAN FRAME

ulcers. Metronidazole is usually prescribed to treat the infection.

Balantidium coli The largest and the only ciliated protozoan species that is pathogenic to man, causing balantidiasis. The organism is seen in two life stages: the motile trophozoite and the encysted cercaria. It is a normal inhabitant of the domestic hog and is transmitted to man by the ingestion of cysts excreted by the hog.

baldness Absence of hair, especially from the scalp. See also **alopecia.**

Balkan frame An overhead, rectangular frame, attached to the bed of a patient undergoing orthopedic treatment, for use in attaching splints, suspending or changing the position of immobilized limbs, and for continuous traction involving weights and pulleys.

ball A relatively spherical mass, as one of the chondrin balls imbedded in hyaline cartilage.

ball-and-socket joint A synovial joint in which the globular head of an articulating bone is received into a cuplike cavity, allowing the distal bone to move around an indefinite number of axes with a common center, as in hip and shoulder joints. Also called **enarthrosis, spheroidea.** Compare **condyloid joint, pivot joint, saddle joint.**

ballism See **ballismus.**

ballismus An abnormal condition characterized by violent flailing motions of the arms and, occasionally, the head, resulting from injury to the subthalamic nucleus. Hemiballismus is a unilateral form of the condition. Also called **ballism.**

ballistocardiogram A record of the movement of the body toward the head and toward the feet caused by the thrust of the heart during systolic ejection of the blood into the aorta and the pulmonary arteries. The ballistocardiogram is a sensitive tool that is useful in measuring cardiac output and the force of contraction of the heart.

balloon septostomy See **Rashkind procedure.**

balloon-tip catheter A catheter bearing a nonporous inflatable sac around its distal end. After insertion of the catheter the sac can be inflated with air or sterile water, introduced via injection into a special port at the proximal end of the catheter. The inflated sac serves to secure the catheter in the correct position. Kinds of balloon-tip catheters include **Foley catheter, Swan-Ganz catheter.**

ballottable head A fetal head that has not descended and become fixed in the maternal bony pelvis.

ballottement A technique of palpating a floating structure by bouncing it gently and feeling it rebound. Ballottement of a fetus within a uterus is an objective sign of pregnancy. In late pregnancy, a fetal head that can be ballotted is said to be floating or unengaged, as differentiated from a fixed or an engaged head which cannot be easily dislodged from the pelvis.

ball thrombus A relatively round, coagulated mass of blood containing platelets, fibrin, and cellular fragments, which may obstruct a blood vessel or an orifice, usually the mitral valve of the heart.

ball-valve action The intermittent opening and closing of an orifice by a buoyant, ball-shaped mass that acts as a valve. Some kinds of objects that may act in this manner are kidney stones, gallstones, and blood clots.

balm **1.** A healing or a soothing substance, as any of various medicinal ointments. **2.** An aromatic plant of the genus *Melissa* that relieves pain.

balneology A field of medicine that deals with the chemical compositions of various mineral waters and their healing characteristics, especially in baths. —**balneologic,** *adj.*

balneotherapy A use of baths in the treatment of many diseases and conditions.

balneum pneumaticum See **air bath.**

balsam Any of a variety of resinous saps, generally from evergreens, usually containing benzoic or cinnamic acid. Balsam is sometimes used in rectal suppositories and dermatologic agents as a counterirritant.

bamboo spine The characteristically rigid spine of advanced ankylosing spondylitis. Also called **poker spine.** See also **ankylosing spondylitis.**

band **1.** In anatomy: a bundle of fibers, as seen in striated muscle, that encircles a structure or binds one part of the body to another. **2.** In dentistry: a strip of metal that fits around a tooth and serves as an attachment for orthodontic components. **3.** *Informal.* The immature form of a segmented granulocyte characterized by a sausage-shaped nucleus. It is the only immature leukocyte normally found in the peripheral circulation. Bands represent 3% to 5% of the total white cell volume. An increase in the relative number of bands indicates bacterial infection or acute stress to the bone marrow. Also called **stab form.**

bandage **1.** A strip or roll of cloth or other material that may be wound around a part of the body in a variety of ways to secure a dressing, maintain pressure over a compress, or immobilize a limb or other part of the body. **2.** To apply a bandage.

bandage shears A sturdy pair of scissors used to cut through bandages. The blades of most bandage shears are angled to the shaft of the instrument, and the lower blade has a rounded blunt protuberance to facilitate insertion under the bandage without harming the patient's skin.

band cell Any one of the developing granular leukocytes in circulating blood, characterized by a curved or indented nucleus. Band cells are intermediate leukocytic forms between metamyelocytes and adult leukocytes with segmented nuclei.

banding In genetics: any of several techniques of staining chromosomes with fluorescent stains or chemical dyes that produce a series of lateral light and dark areas whose intensity and position are characteristic for each chromosome. Banding patterns are identified according to the staining technique used, as C-banding, G-banding, Q-banding, and R-banding. Also called chromosome banding.

Bandl's ring See **pathologic retraction ring.**

Bangkok hemorrhagic fever See **dengue.**

bank blood Anticoagulated, preserved blood collected from doners in units of 500 ml and stored under refrigeration for future use. Dated and identified as to blood type, it is stored for a usual maximum period of 21 days. Bank blood may be used directly after cross-matching against the recipient's blood or for the extraction and preparation of any of its components. See also **packed cells, pooled plasma, whole blood.**

Banting treatment A therapeutic regimen for the treatment of obesity, consisting of a low-carbohydrate, high-protein diet. Also called Banting diet.

Banti's syndrome A serious, progressive disorder involving several organ systems, characterized by portal hypertension, splenomegaly, anemia, leukopenia, gastrointestinal tract bleeding, and cirrhosis of the liver. Obstruction of the blood vessels that lie between the intestines and the liver leads to venous congestion, an enlarged spleen, and abnormal destruction of red and white blood cells. Early symptoms are weakness, fatigue, and anemia. Surgical removal of the spleen and creation of a portacaval shunt to improve portal circulation are sometimes necessary. Since the syndrome is often a complication of alcoholic cirrhosis of the liver, medical treatment includes prescribing improved nutrition, vitamins, abstinence from alcohol, and rest. Also called **Banti's disease.** See also **cirrhosis, portacaval shunt, portal hypertension.**

bar- See **baro-.**

baralyme (BL) A chemical compound used to absorb exhaled carbon dioxide in an anesthesia rebreathing system.

Bárány's symptom See **caloric test.**

barber's itch See **sycosis barbae.**

barbital A barbiturate sedative-hypnotic agent.

barbiturate A derivative of barbituric acid that acts as a sedative or hypnotic.

-barbituric A combining form meaning an 'acid used medicinally for its soporific effects': *dibromobarbituric, isobarbituric, phenylethylbarbituric.*

barbiturism 1. Acute or chronic poisoning by any of the derivatives of barbituric acid. Ingestion of such preparations in excess of therapeutic quantities may be fatal or may produce physiologic, pathologic, and psychologic changes, as depressed respiration, cyanosis, disorientation, and coma. 2. Addiction to a barbiturate.

Bard-Pic syndrome A condition characterized by progressive jaundice and cachexia, associated with advanced pancreatic cancer.

Bard's sign The increased oscillations of the eyeball in organic nystagmus when the patient tries to visually follow a target moved from side to side across the line of sight. Such oscillations usually cease during the same test if the patient has congenital nystagmus.

bargaining According to Dr. Elisabeth Kübler-Ross, the third stage of dying. The dying person tries to make an agreement, usually with God, in hope of postponing the inevitable. See **acceptance, anger, denial and isolation,** and **depression.**

bar graph A graph in which frequencies are represented by bars extending from the ordinate or the abscissa, allowing the distribution of the entire sample to be seen at once.

bariatrics The field of medicine that focuses on the treatment and the control of obesity and diseases associated with obesity.

barium (Ba) A pale yellow, metallic element classified with the alkaline earths. Its atomic number is 56; its atomic weight is 137.36. The acid-soluble salts of barium are poisonous. Barium carbonate, formerly used in medicine, is now used to prepare the cardiac stimulant, barium chloride; fine, milky barium sulfate is used as a contrast medium in radiography of the digestive tract.

barium enema A rectal infusion of barium sulfate, a radiopaque contrast medium, which is retained in the lower intestinal tract during radiographic studies for diagnosing obstruction, tumors, or other abnormalities, such as ulcerative colitis. Also called **contrast enema.**

barium meal The ingestion of barium sulfate, a radiopaque contrast medium, for the radiographic examination of the esophagus, stomach, and intestinal tract in the diagnosis of such conditions as dysphagia, peptic ulcer, and fistulas. The movement of the barium through the gastrointestinal tract is followed by fluoroscopy, X-rays, or both. Also called **barium swallow.**

barium sulfate A radiopaque medium used as a diagnostic aid in radiography.

barium swallow See **barium meal.**

barley-malt extract A bulk-forming laxative.

Barlow's disease See **infantile scurvy.**

Barlow's syndrome An abnormal cardiac condition characterized by an apical systolic murmur, a systolic click, and an electrocardiogram indicating inferior ischemia. These signs

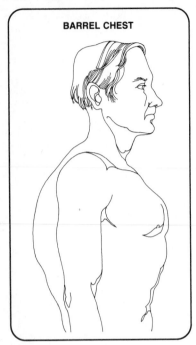

BARREL CHEST

are associated with mitral regurgitation caused by prolapse of the mitral valve. Also called **electrocardiographic-auscultatory syndrome.**

baro-, bar- A combining form meaning 'pertaining to pressure': *baresthesia, barognosis, barospirator.*

barognosis, *pl.* **barognoses** The ability to estimate weight.

baroreceptor One of the pressure-sensitive nerve endings in the walls of the atria of the heart, the vena cava, the aortic arch, and the carotid sinus. Baroreceptors stimulate central reflex mechanisms that allow physiologic adjustment and adaptation to changes in blood pressure via vasodilatation or vasoconstriction. Baroreceptors are essential for homeostasis.

barosinusitis See **aerosinusitis.**

barotitis See **aerotitis.**

barotitis media See **aerotitis media.**

barotrauma Physical injury sustained as a result of exposure to increased environmental pressure, as barotitis media, or rupture of the lungs or paranasal sinuses, as may occur among deep-sea divers or caisson workers.

Barr body See **sex chromatin.**

barrel chest A large, rounded thorax, considered normal in some stocky individuals and certain others who live in high-altitude areas and consequently develop increased vital capacities. Barrel chest, however, may also be a sign of pulmonary emphysema.

Barr-Epstein virus See **Epstein-Barr virus.**

Barré's sign The inability of a hemiplegic

to maintain a flexed position on the side of the lesion; when placed in a prone attitude with the lower limbs flexed at the knees, the leg on the side of the lesion extends.

Barrett's esophagus See **Barrett's syndrome.**

Barrett's syndrome A disorder of the lower esophagus marked by a benign ulcerlike lesion in columnar epithelium, resulting most often from chronic irritation of the esophagus by gastric reflux of acidic digestive juices. Major symptoms include dysphagia and heartburn. Symptoms may be relieved by eating frequent small meals, avoiding foods that produce gas, taking antacid medication, and elevating the head of the bed to prevent passive reflux when lying down.

barrier A wall or other obstacle that can restrain or block the passage of substances. Barrier methods of contraception, as the condom or cervical diaphragm, prevent the passage of spermatazoa into the uterus. Membranes and cell walls of body tissues function as screenlike barriers to permit the movement of water or certain other molecules from one side to the other while preventing the passage of other substances. Barriers in kidney tissues adjust automatically to regulate the retention or excretion of water and other substances according to the needs of organ systems elsewhere in the body.

barrier nursing Nursing care of a patient in isolation, performed to prevent the spread of infection by creating an aseptic barrier around the patient. Gown, mask, and gloves are worn by staff or visitors entering the room; the number of staff entering the room is kept to a minimum, and visitors are limited. Contaminated substances are handled according to strict protocols. Specific techniques vary with the indication for isolation.

bartholinitis An inflammatory condition of one or both Bartholin's glands, caused by bacterial infection. Usually, the causative microorganism is a species of *Streptococcus* or *Staphylococcus* or a strain of gonococci. The condition is characterized by swelling of one or both glands, pain, and the development of an abscess in the infected gland. A fistula may develop from the gland to the vagina, anus, or perineum. Treatment includes local application of heat, often by soaking in hot water, antibiotics, or, if necessary, incision of the gland and drainage of the purulent material or excision of the entire gland and its duct.

Bartholin's cyst A cyst that arises from one of the vestibular glands or from its ducts, filling with a clear fluid, which replaces the suppurative exudate characteristic of chronic inflammation.

Bartholin's duct The major duct of the sublingual gland.

Bartholin's gland One of two small, mucus-secreting glands located on the posterior and lateral aspect of the vestibule of the vagina. Also called **greater vestibular gland.**

Bartonella A genus of small, gram-negative flagellated pleomorphic coccobacilli. Members of the genus are intracellular parasites that infect red blood cells and the epithelial cells of the lymph nodes, liver, and spleen. They are transmitted at night by the bite of a sandfly of the genus *Phlebotomus*. The only known species of *Bartonella* is *B. bacilliformis*, the organism that causes bartonellosis. Owing to its distinctive appearance, it is easily identified on microscopic examination of a smear of blood stained with Wright's stain.

bartonellosis An acute infection caused by *Bartonella bacilliformis*, transmitted by the bite of a sandfly. It is characterized by fever, severe anemia, bone pain, and, several weeks after the first symptoms are observed, by multiple nodular or verrucose skin lesions. The disease is endemic in the valleys of the Andes in Peru, Colombia, and Ecuador. The treatment usually includes chloramphenicol, penicillin, streptomycin, or tetracycline. Untreated, the infection is often fatal. Also called **Carrión's disease, Oroya fever, verruga peruana.**

Barton forceps See **obstetric forceps.**

Barton's fracture A fracture of the distal articular surface of the radius, which may be accompanied by the dorsal dislocation of the carpus on the radius.

Bartter's syndrome A rare hereditary disorder, characterized by hyperplasia of the juxtaglomerular apparatus and secondary hyperaldosteronism. Renin and angiotensin levels may be elevated, but blood pressure usually remains normal. Early signs in childhood are abnormal physical growth and mental retardation, often accompanied by chronic hypokalemia and alkalosis.

bary- A combining form meaning 'heavy or difficult': *baryecoia, baryencephalia, baryphonia.*

basal Pertaining to or situated near the base.

basal anesthesia 1. A state of unconsciousness just short of complete surgical anesthesia in depth, in which the patient does not respond to words but still reacts to a pinprick or other noxious stimuli. 2. Narcosis produced by injection or infusion of potent sedatives alone, without added narcotics or anesthetic agents. 3. Any form of anesthesia in which the patient is completely unconscious, in contrast to awake anesthesia. Also called **narcoanesthesia.**

basal body temperature The temperature of the body taken in the morning, orally or rectally, after at least 5 hours of sleep and before doing anything else, including getting out of bed, smoking a cigarette, moving around, talking, eating, or drinking.

basal body temperature method of family planning A natural method of family planning that relies on the identification of the fertile period of the menstrual cycle by noting the progesterone mediated rise in basal body temperature of 0.3°C to 0.5°C (0.5°F to 1.0°F) that occurs with ovulation. The rate and pattern of the increase varies greatly from woman to woman, and somewhat from cycle to cycle in any one woman. Several cycles are observed and

careful records are kept in which the woman takes her oral or rectal temperature at the same time every morning, before doing anything else. Talking, smoking, eating, or even posture changes may alter the temperature. Other factors, including infection, stress, a bad night's sleep, medication, or environmental temperature, may also alter it. If any of these are present the woman notes them on her record. The fertile period is considered to continue until the temperature is above the baseline for 5 days; the rise occurs slowly during all 5 days or increases rapidly, reaching a plateau at which it remains for 3 or 4 days. The days following that period are considered 'safe,' unfertile days. Abstinence is required from 6 days before the earliest day on which ovulation was noted to occur during the preceding 6 months until the 5th day after the rise in temperature in the current cycle. Another way of calculating the possible beginning of the fertile days is to subtract 19 days from the shortest complete menstrual cycle of the preceding 6 months. The basal body temperature method is more effective when used with the ovulation method than is either method used alone. The combination of these methods is called the symptothermal method of family planning. Compare **calendar method of family planning, ovulation method of family planning.**

basal bone 1. In prosthodontics: the osseous tissue of the mandible and the maxillae, except for the rami and the processes, that provides support for artificial dentures. 2. In orthodontics: the fixed osseous structure that limits the movement of teeth in the creation of a stable occlusion.

basal cell Any one of the cells in the base layer of stratified epithelium.

basal cell acanthoma See **basal cell papilloma.**

basal cell carcinoma A malignant, epithelial cell tumor that begins as a papule and enlarges peripherally, developing a central crater that erodes, crusts, and bleeds. Metastasis is rare, but local invasion destroys underlying and adjacent tissue. In 90% of cases, the lesion is seen between the hairline and the upper lip. The primary cause of the cancer is excessive exposure to the sun or to X-rays. Treatment is eradication of the lesion, often by electrodesiccation or cryotherapy. Also called **basal cell epithelioma, basaloma, carcinoma basocellulare, hair matrix carcinoma.** See also **rodent ulcer.**

basal cell epithelioma See **basal cell carcinoma.**

basal cell papilloma A benign, epidermal neoplasm characterized by multiple yellow or brown raised oval lesions that usually develop in middle age. Also called **basal cell acanthoma, seborrheic keratosis.**

basal ganglia The islands of gray matter within each cerebral hemisphere, the most important being the caudate nucleus, the putamen, and the pallidium. The basal ganglia are surrounded by the rings of the limbic system and lie between the thalamus of the diencephalon and the white matter of the hemisphere.

basal lamina A thin, noncellular layer of ground substance lying just under epithelial surfaces. Constituting the uppermost layer of the basement membrane, it can be examined with an electron microscope. Also called **basement lamina.**

basal layer See **stratum basale.**

basal membrane A sheet of tissue that forms the outer layer of the choroid and lies just under the pigmented layer of the retina. It is composed of elastic fibers and a thin homogenous layer.

basal metabolic rate (BMR) The amount of energy used in a unit of time by a fasting, resting subject to maintain vital functions. The rate, determined by the amount of oxygen utilized, is expressed in calories consumed per hour per square meter of body surface area or per kilogram of body weight.

basal metabolism The amount of energy needed to maintain essential basic body functions, as respiration, circulation, temperature, peristalsis, and muscle tone, measured when the subject is awake and at complete rest, has not eaten for 14 to 18 hours, and is in a comfortable, warm environment. It is expressed as a basal metabolic rate, according to large calories/hour/ square meter of body surface.

basaloid carcinoma A rare, malignant neoplasm of the anal canal containing areas which resemble basal cell carcinoma of the skin, though a basaloid carcinoma is the more rapidly invasive and malignant of the two. The tumor may spread to the skin of the perineum.

basaloma See **basal cell carcinoma.**

basal temperature The temperature of a healthy individual immediately following at least 8 hours of relaxed sleep and a fast of 14 to 18 hours.

base 1. A chemical compound that combines with an acid to form a salt. Compare **alkali.** 2. A molecule or radical that takes up or accepts protons. 3. The major ingredient of a compounded material, particularly one that is used as a medication. Petroleum jelly is frequently used as a base for ointments.

base analogue An analogue of one of the purine or the pyrimidine bases normally found in ribonucleic acid or deoxyribonucleic acid.

Basedow's goiter An enlargement of the thyroid gland, characterized by the hypersecretion of thyroid hormone following iodine therapy.

basement lamina See **basal lamina.**

basement membrane The fragile, noncellular layer of tissue that secures the overlying layers of stratified epithelium. It is the deepest layer, may contain reticular fibers, and can be selectively stained with silver stains.

base of the heart The portion of the heart opposite the apex, directed to the right side of the body. It forms the upper border of the heart, lies just below the second rib, and involves primarily the left atrium, part of the right atrium, and the proximal portions of the great vessels.

Passing between the base of the heart and the bodies of the fifth to the eighth thoracic vertebrae are the descending aorta, the esophagus, and the thoracic duct.

base of the skull The floor of the skull, containing the anterior, middle, and posterior cranial fossae and numerous foramina, as the optic foramen, foramen ovale, foramen lacerum, and foramen magnum.

base pair A pair of nucleotides in a nucleic acid. One of the pair must be a purine, the other a pyrimidine. Base pairing finds guanine paired with cytosine and adenine paired with thymine.

base pairing In molecular genetics: the association in nucleic acids of the purine bases adenine and guanine with the pyrimidine bases cytosine, thymine, and uracil. In DNA, adenine always pairs with thymine, and guanine always pairs with cytosine. In RNA, adenine invariably pairs with uracil, and guanine invariably pairs with cytosine.

base ratio The ratio of molar quantities of the bases in ribonucleic and deoxyribonucleic acids.

bas-fond The bottom or fundus of any structure, especially the fundus of the urinary bladder.

basi-, basio- A combining form meaning 'pertaining to a foundation or a base': *basicranial, basilaris, basiotribe.*

-basia A combining form meaning 'ability to walk': *abasia, brachybasia, dysbasia.*

BASIC *abbr* Beginners' All-purpose Symbolic Instruction Code, a programming language widely used on personal computers and small business systems.

-basic A combining form meaning 'relating to or containing alkaline compounds': *ammonobasic, polybasic, tribasic.*

basic amino acid An amino acid that has a positive electric charge in solution. The basic amino acids are arginine, histidine, and lysine.

basic health services The minimum degree of health care considered to be necessary to maintain adequate health and protection from disease.

basilar Of or pertaining to a base or a basal area.

basilar artery The single arterial trunk formed by the junction of the two vertebral arteries at the base of the skull, extending from the inferior to the superior border of the pons, dividing into the left and right cerebral arteries, and supplying the internal ear and parts of the brain through the five branches of each artery. The branches are the pontine, labyrinthine, anterior inferior cerebellar, superior cerebellar, and posterior cerebral.

basilar artery insufficiency syndrome The composite of clinical indicators associated with insufficient blood flow through the basilar artery, a condition that may be caused by arterial occlusion. Some of the common signs of this syndrome are dizziness, blindness, numbness, depression, dysarthria, dysphagia, and weakness on one side of the body.

basilar membrane The cellular structure that forms the floor of the cochlear duct and is supported by bony and fibrous projections from the cochlear wall. It provides a fibrous base for the spiral organ of Corti.

basilar plexus The venous network interlaced between the layers of the dura mater over the basilar portion of the occipital bone. It connects the two petrosal sinuses and communicates with the anterior vertebral venous plexus.

basilar sulcus The sulcus that cradles the basilar artery, in the midline of the pons.

basilic vein One of the four superficial veins of the arm, beginning in the ulnar part of the dorsal venous network and running proximally on the posterior surface of the ulnar side of the forearm. It veers toward the anterior surface of the forearm distal to the elbow and is joined by the median cubital vein; then ascends obliquely between the biceps brachii and the pronator teres and crosses the brachial artery. It then runs proximally along the medial border of the biceps brachii, pierces the deep fascia, and ascends to join the brachial vein to form the axillary vein. Compare **dorsal digital vein, median antebrachial vein.**

basiloma, *pl.* **basilomas, basilomata** A carcinoma composed of basal cells. A kind of basiloma is **basiloma terebrans.** Also called basaloma. See also **basal cell carcinoma.**

basiloma terebrans A basal cell epithelioma that is invasive.

basio- See **basi-.**

basioccipital Of or pertaining to the basilar process of the occipital bone.

basion The midpoint on the anterior margin of the foramen magnum of the occipital bone, opposite the opisthion in the middle of the posterior margin.

basis pedunculi cerebri See **crus cerebri.**

basophil A granulocytic white blood cell characterized by a segmented nucleus that contains granules that stain blue when exposed to a basic dye. Basophils represent 1% or less of the total white blood cell count. The relative number of basophils increases in myeloproliferative diseases and decreases in severe allergic reactions. Compare **eosinophil, neutrophil.** See also **agranulocyte, differential white blood cell count, granulocyte, leukocyte, polymorphonuclear leukocyte.**

basophilic adenoma A tumor of the pituitary gland composed of cells that can be stained with basic dyes. Cushing's syndrome is often caused by a basophilic adenoma. Compare **acidophilic adenoma, chromophobic adenoma.**

basophilic leukemia An acute or chronic malignant neoplasm of blood-forming tissues, characterized by large numbers of immature basophilic granulocytes in peripheral circulation and in tissues. See also **acute myelocytic leukemia.**

basophilic stippling The abnormal presence of punctate, basophilic granules in the red blood cells, observed under the microscope on

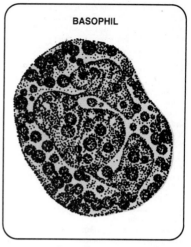

BASOPHIL

a gram-stained smear of the blood. Stippling is characteristic of lead poisoning. See also **basophil, lead poisoning.**

basosquamous cell carcinoma A malignant epidermal tumor composed of basal and squamous cells.

Bassen-Kornzweig syndrome See **abetalipoproteinemia.**

bath In the hospital: a cleansing procedure performed daily by or for almost all patients to help prevent infection, preserve the unbroken condition of the skin, stimulate circulation, promote oxygen intake, maintain muscle tone and joint mobility, and provide comfort.

bathesthesia, bathyesthesia A deep sensibility, as that associated with organs or structures beneath the surface of the body, as muscles and joints.

bathmic evolution See **orthogenic evolution.**

batho- See **bathy-.**

bathy-, batho- A combining form meaning 'pertaining to depth, deep': *bathycentesis, bathypnea, bathomorphic.*

bathycardia An abnormal but nonpathological condition characterized by an unusually low position of the heart.

battered woman syndrome (BWS) Repeated episodes of physical assault on a woman by the man with whom she lives, often resulting in serious physical and psychological damage to the woman. Such violence tends to follow a predictable pattern. The first phase is characterized by the man acting increasingly irritable, edgy, and tense. Verbal abuse, insults, and criticism increase, and shoves or slaps begin. The second phase is the time of the acute, violent activity. As the tension mounts, the woman becomes unable to placate the man, and she may argue or defend herself. The man uses this as the justification for his anger and assaults her, often saying that he is "teaching her a lesson." The third stage is characterized by apology and remorse on the part of the man, with promises of change. The calm continues until tension builds again. The battered woman syndrome occurs at all socioeconomic levels, and one half to three quarters of female assault victims are the victims of an attack by a lover or husband. It is estimated that between one and two million women a year are beaten by their husbands. Men who grew up in homes in which the father abused the mother are more likely to beat their wives than are men who lived in nonviolent homes. Personal and cultural attitudes also affect the incidence of wife-battering. Aggressive behavior is a normal part of male socialization in most cultures; physical aggression may be condoned as a means of resolving a conflict. A personality profile obtained by psychological testing reveals the typical battered woman to be reserved, withdrawn, depressed, and anxious, with low self-esteem, a poorly integrated self-image, and a general inability to cope with life's demands. The parents of such women encouraged compliance, were not physically affectionate, and socially restricted their daughters' independence, preventing the widening of social contact that normally occurs in adolescence. Victims of the battered woman syndrome are often afraid to leave the man and the situation; change, loneliness, and the unknown are perceived as more painful than the beatings. Nurses are in an excellent position to offer assistance to battered women in several ways, as encouraging a woman to talk about the battering and the injuries may help her to admit what she may have been too embarrassed to reveal even to her parents. A realistic appraisal of the situation is then possible; the woman wants to hear that the nurse thinks the battering will not recur but the nurse can tell her only that the usual pattern is for the abuse to continue and to become more severe. The woman may be referred to the social service department or given directions for contacting special community agencies, as a battered women's shelter or a hotline to a counseling service. Caring for and counseling a battered woman often require great patience, because she is usually ambivalent about her situation and may be confused to the point of believing that she deserves the assaults she has suffered. Records are maintained to document the extent of the problem, including the form of abuse reported, the injuries sustained, and a summary of similar incidents and previous admissions.

battery 1. A complex of two or more electrolytic cells connected together to form a single source providing direct current or voltage. 2. A series or a combination of tests to determine the cause of a particular illness or the degree of proficiency in a particular skill or discipline. 3. In law: physical contact with another person without that person's consent, such as administration of unwanted medical or nursing care. See **assault.**

Battey bacillus Any of a group of atypical mycobacteria, including *Mycobacteria avium* and *M. intracellulare*, that cause a chronic pulmo-

nary disease resembling tuberculosis. These organisms are resistant to most of the common bacteriostatic and antibiotic medications. Surgical resection of involved lung tissue may be necessary and may improve the outcome in serious cases. Rest, good nutrition, and general supportive care are usually recommended. Compare **tuberculosis.**

battledore placenta A placenta to which the umbilical cord is attached at the periphery.

Battle's sign A small hemorrhagic spot behind the ear that appears in a fracture of a bone of the lower skull.

Baudelocque's diameter See **external conjugate.**

Baudelocque's method In obstetrics: a maneuver used to convert a face presentation to a vertex presentation. The operator flexes the fetal head vaginally and applies counterpressure to the back of the head abdominally while an assistant rotates the fetus in the direction of flexion until the vertex is fixed in the pelvis.

Baynton's bandage A spiral adhesive wrap applied to the leg over a dressing, used in the treatment of indolent ulcers of the leg.

BBB *abbr* **blood-brain barrier.**

B cell A type of lymphocyte that originates in the bone marrow. A precursor of the plasma cell, which upon suitable antigenic stimulation is one of the two lymphocytes that play a major role in the body's immunologic response. See also **plasma cell, T cell.**

BCG *abbr* **bacillus Calmette-Guérin.**

BCG vaccine An active immunizing agent prepared from bacillus Calmette-Guérin.

B complex vitamins A large group of water soluble substances that includes **biotin, choline, cyanocobalamin** (vitamin B_{12}), **folic acid, inositol, niacin** (vitamin B_3), **para-aminobenzoic acid, pyridoxine** (vitamin B_6), **riboflavin** (vitamin B_2), and **thiamine** (vitamin B_1). The B complex vitamins are essential in converting carbohydrates into glucose to provide energy, for metabolism of fats and proteins, for normal functioning of the nervous system, for maintenance of muscle tone in the gastrointestinal tract, and for the health of skin, hair, eyes, mouth, and liver. They are found in brewer's yeast, liver, whole-grain cereals, nuts, eggs, meats, fish, and vegetables and are produced by the intestinal bacteria. See also specific vitamins.

b.d See **b.i.d.**

Be Symbol for **beryllium.**

beaded 1. Of or having a resemblance to a row of beads. 2. Of or pertaining to bacterial colonies that develop along the inoculation line in various stab cultures. 3. Of or pertaining to stained bacteria that develop more deeply stained beadlike granules.

beaker cell See **goblet cell.**

BEAM *abbr* **brain electrical activity map.**

bean The pod-enclosed flattened seed of numerous leguminous plants. Beans used in pharmocological preparations are alphabetized by specific name.

Becker's muscular dystrophy A chronic

degenerative disease of the muscles, characterized by progressive weakness and onset between
8 and 20 years of age. It occurs less frequently,
progresses more slowly, and has a better prognosis than the more common pseudohypertrophic form of muscular dystrophy. The pathophysiology of the disease is not understood; it is
transmitted genetically as an autosomal recessive trait. Also called **benign pseudohypertrophic muscular dystrophy.**

Beck I operation   A surgical procedure to
provide collateral circulation to the heart. The
operation roughens the surface of the epicardium and the parietal lining of the pericardium,
applies an irritant to these surfaces and partially
closes the coronary sinus at its entrance to the
right atrium. The surgeon then grafts the parietal pericardium and the mediastinal fat to the
myocardium.

Beck II operation   An operation in two stages
that provides collateral circulation to the heart.
In the first stage, a venous graft is placed between the aorta and the coronary sinus to shunt
arterial blood. In the second stage of the procedure, executed 2 to 3 weeks after the first stage,
the coronary sinus is partially closed to raise
pressure within the sinus and force oxygenated
blood from the aorta to flow into the coronary
vessels.

Beck's triad   A combination of three symptoms that characterize cardiac compression: high
venous pressure, low arterial pressure, and a
small, quiet heart.

Beckwith's syndrome   A hereditary disorder of unknown etiology associated with neonatal hypoglycemia and hyperinsulinism. Clinical manifestations include gigantism,
macroglossia, omphalocele or umbilical hernia,
visceromegaly, hyperplasia of the kidney and
pancreas, extreme enlargement of the cells of
the adrenal cortex, and often various other abnormalities. Treatment consists of adequate glucose, diazoxide, and glucocorticoid therapy.
Subtotal pancreatectomy is often necessary in
cases of beta-cell hyperplasia, nesidioblastosis,
or beta-cell tumor of the pancreas.

Beckwith-Wiedemann syndrome   See
EMG syndrome.

beclomethasone dipropionate   A corticosteroid administered by nasal inhalation.

bed   In anatomy: a supporting matrix of tissue, as the nail beds of modified epidermis over
which the fingernails and the toenails move as
they grow.

bedbug   A blood-sucking arthropod of the
species *Cimex lectularius* that feeds on humans
and other animals. The bedbug can be removed
after covering it with petrolatum. The bite, which
causes itching, pain, and redness, can be treated
with a lotion or cream containing a corticosteroid or other topical anti-inflammatory or analgesic preparation.

Bednar's aphthae   The small, yellowish,
slightly elevated ulcerated patches that normally
occur on the posterior portion of the hard palate
of newborn babies. Compare *Candida albi-*
cans, **Epstein's pearls.**

bedside manner   **1.** The behavior of a nurse
or doctor as perceived by a patient. **2.** An agree-
able and satisfying professional demeanor in the
eyes of a patient.

bedsore   See **decubitus ulcer.**

Bee-cell pessary   See **pessary.**

beef tapeworm   See *Taenia saginata.*

beef tapeworm infection   An infection
caused by the tapeworm *Taenia saginata*, transmitted to humans when they eat contaminated
beef. The adult worm can live for years in the
intestine of humans without causing any symptoms. The infection is rarely found in the U.S.
because beef is carefully inspected before being
made available, but it is commonly found in
other parts of the world. See **tapeworm infection.**

bee sting   An injury that is caused by the
venom of bees, usually accompanied by pain and
swelling. The stinger of the honeybee usually
remains implanted in the victim and should be
removed. Pain may be alleviated by the application of an ice pack or a paste of sodium bicarbonate and water. Serious reactions may result from multiple stings, stings occurring on
some areas of the head, or the injection of venom
directly into the circulatory system. In a hypersensitive person, a single bee sting may result
in death owing to anaphylactic shock and bronchospasm. Hypersensitive individuals are encouraged to carry emergency treatment supplies
with them when the possibility of bee sting exists. Compare **wasp.**

behavior   **1.** The manner in which a person
acts or performs. **2.** Any or all of the activities
of a person, including physical actions, which
are observed directly, and mental activity, which
is inferred and interpreted. Kinds of behavior
include **abnormal behavior, automatic behavior, invariable behavior, variable behavior.**

behavioral objective   A goal in therapy or
research that concerns an act or a specific behavior or pattern of behaviors.

behavioral reflex   See **conditioned response.**

behavioral science   Any of the various interrelated disciplines, as psychiatry, psychology,
sociology, and anthropology, that observe and
study human activity, including psychological
and emotional development, interpersonal relationships, values, and mores.

behavior disorder   Any of a group of antisocial behavior patterns occurring primarily
in children and adolescents, as overaggressive-
ness, overactivity, destructiveness, cruelty,
truancy, lying, disobedience, perverse sexual
activity, criminality, alcoholism, and drug addiction. The most common motivating force for
such reactions is hostility, which is manifested
either overtly or covertly and is precipitated by
a disturbed relationship between the child and
his parents, an unstable home situation, and, in
some cases, by organic brain dysfunction. Behavior disorders may be symptomatic of other

neuroses or psychoses, as childhood schizophrenia. Treatment may include psychotherapy, milieu therapy, medication, and family counseling. See also **antisocial personality disorder.**

behaviorism A school of psychology founded by John B. Watson that studies and interprets behavior by observing measurable responses to stimuli without reference to consciousness, mental states, or subjective phenomena, as ideas and emotions. See also **neobehaviorism.**

behaviorist A disciple of the school of behaviorism.

behavioristic psychology See **behaviorism.**

behavior modification See **behavior therapy.**

behavior systems model A conceptual framework describing factors that may affect the stability of a person's behavior. The model examines systems of behavior, not the behavior of an individual at any particular time. In this model, behavior is defined as an integrated response to stimuli. Several subsystems of behavior form man's eight microsystems, which are: ingestion, elimination, dependency, sex, achievement, affiliation, aggression, and restoration. Each subsystem comprises several structural components called imperatives, which are goal, set, choice, action, and support. The goal of nursing care is to attain, maintain, or restore balance of the subsystems of behavior for the stability of the patient.

behavior therapy A kind of psychotherapy that attempts to modify observable, maladjusted patterns of behavior by the substitution of a new response or set of responses to a given stimulus. The treatment techniques involve the methods, concepts, and procedures derived from experimental psychology and include assertiveness training, aversion therapy, contingency management, flooding, modeling, operant conditioning, and systemic desensitization. Also called **behavior modification.** See also **biofeedback.**

Behçet's disease A rare and severe illness of unknown cause, mostly affecting young males and characterized by severe uveitis and retinal vasculitis. Some other signs are optic atrophy and aphthalike lesions of the mouth and the genitals, indicating diffuse vasculitis. Also called **Behçet's syndrome.**

Behla's bodies See **Plimmer's bodies.**

BEI *abbr* **butanol extractable iodine.**

bejel A nonvenereal form of syphilis prevalent among children in the Middle East and North Africa, caused by the spirochete *Treponema pallidum II.* It is transmitted by person-to-person contact and by the sharing of drinking and eating utensils. The primary lesion is usually on or near the mouth, appearing as a mucous patch, followed by the development of pimplelike sores on the trunk, arms, and legs. Chronic ulceration of the nose and soft palate occurs in the advanced stages of the infection. Destructive changes in the tissues of the heart, central nervous system, and mouth, often associated with the ve-

nereal form of syphilis, rarely develop. Intramuscular injection of penicillin is effective in curing the infection, but if extensive tissue destruction has occurred, scar tissue forms and may be permanently disfiguring.

Békésy audiometry A method of testing hearing in which the subject presses a signal button while listening to a pure tone that is progressively diminished in intensity and releases the button when the sound no longer is heard.

bel A unit that expresses intensity of sound. It is the logarithm (to the base 10) of the ratio of the power of any specific sound to the power of a reference sound. The most common reference sound has a power of 10^{-16} watts per square cm, or the approximate minimum intensity of sound at 1,000 cycles per second that is perceptible to the human ear. An increase of 1 bel approximately doubles the intensity or loudness of most sounds.

belching See **eructation.**

belladonna **1.** The dried leaf and flowering or fruiting tops of *Atropa belladonna*, a common perennial called deadly nightshade, containing the alkaloids hyoscyamine and atropine. **2.** A gastrointestinal anticholinergic agent.

bellows murmur A blowing sound, as air moving in and out of a bellows.

Bell's law An axiom stating that the ventral spinal roots are motor and the dorsal spinal roots are sensory. Also called **Bell-Magendie law, Magendie's law.**

Bell's mania A mood disorder characterized by acute delirium. See also **delirium, mania.**

Bell's palsy A paralysis of the facial nerve, resulting from trauma to the nerve, compression of the nerve by a tumor, or, most often, from an unknown cause. Any or all branches of the nerve may be affected. The person may not be able to open an eye or close the mouth. The condition may be unilateral or bilateral, transient or permanent. Plastic surgery may reduce the deformity.

Bell's phenomenon A sign of peripheral facial paralysis, manifested by the upward and outward rolling of the eyeball when the affected individual tries to close the eye.

belonephobia A morbid fear of sharp-pointed objects, especially needles and pins.

Bence Jones protein A protein found almost exclusively in the urine of patients with multiple myeloma. The protein constitutes the light chain component of myeloma globulin. See also **multiple myeloma, protein.**

bench research *Informal.* In medicine: any research done in a controlled laboratory setting using other than human subjects.

bending fracture A fracture indirectly caused by the bending of an extremity, as of the foot or of the big toe.

bendroflumethiazide A thiazide diuretic.

bends, the See **decompression sickness.**

Benedict's qualitative test A test for sugar in the urine based on the reduction by glucose of cupric ions to a colored cuprous oxide pre-

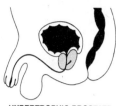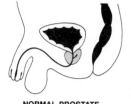

BENIGN PROSTATIC HYPERTROPHY

HYPERTROPHIC PROSTATE   NORMAL PROSTATE

cipitate when it is placed in an alkaline solution.
benign Of a tumor: noncancerous and therefore not an immediate threat, even though treatment eventually may be required for health or cosmetic reasons. Compare **malignant.**
benign hypertension A misnomer implying an innocent elevation of blood pressure. Since any sustained elevation of blood pressure may adversely affect health, it is incorrect to refer to the condition as 'benign.' Compare **malignant hypertension.** See also **essential hypertension.**
benign intracranial hypertension See **pseudotumor cerebri.**
benign juvenile melanoma A benign, pink or fuchsia raised papule with a scaly surface, usually on a cheek and occurring most commonly in children between the ages of 9 and 13 years. It may be mistaken for a malignant melanoma. Also called **compound melanocytoma, spindle cell nevus, Spitz nevus.**
benign mesenchymoma A benign neoplasm that has two or more definitely recognizable mesenchymal elements in addition to fibrous tissue.
benign neoplasm A tumor, characteristically localized, that has a fibrous capsule, limited potential for growth, a regular shape, and cells that are well differentiated. A benign neoplasm does not invade surrounding tissue or metastasize to distant sites. It causes harm only by pressure and does not usually recur after surgical excision. Some kinds of benign neoplasms are **adenoma, fibroma, hemangioma, lipoma.** See also **malignant neoplasm.**
benign prostatic hypertrophy Enlargement of the prostate gland, common among men by the age of 50. The condition is not malignant or inflammatory but is usually progressive and may lead to obstruction of the urethra and to interference with the flow of urine, possibly causing frequency of urination, the need to urinate during the night, pain, and urinary tract infections. Treatment consists of conservative measures: regular sexual release, hot baths, prostatic massage, avoidance of alcohol or excessive fluid intake, and voiding upon the urge to do so. Surgical resection of the enlarged prostate is sometimes necessary. Compare **prostatitis.** See also **prostatectomy.**
benign pseudohypertrophic muscular

dystrophy See **Becker's muscular dystrophy.**
benign stupor A state of apathy or lethargy, as occurs in severe depression.
benign tumor A neoplasm that does not invade other tissues or metastasize in other sites. A benign tumor is usually well encapsulated, and its cells exhibit less anaplasia than those of a malignant growth.
Bennet's small corpuscle See **Drysdale's corpuscle.**
Bennett's fracture A fracture that runs obliquely through the base of the first metacarpal bone and into the carpometacarpal joint, detaching the greater part of the articular facet. Bennett's fracture may be associated with dorsal subluxation or with dislocation of the first metacarpal.
bent fracture An incomplete greenstick fracture.
bentonite Colloidal, hydrated aluminum silicate, which, when added to water, swells to approximately 12 times its dry size. It is used as a bulk laxative and as a base for skin care preparations.
benzalkonium chloride A disinfectant; also used as an ophthalmic anti-infective.
benzathine penicillin G See **penicillin G benzathine.**
benzene poisoning A toxic condition caused by ingestion of benzene, the inhalation of benzene fumes, or exposure to such benzene-related products as toluene or xylene, characterized by nausea, headache, dizziness, and incoordination. In acute cases, respiratory failure or ventricular fibrillation may cause death. Chronic exposure may result in aplastic anemia or a form of leukemia. Benzene poisoning by inhalation is treated with ventilatory assistance and oxygen; poisoning by ingestion is treated with gastric intubation, removal of the poison, and lavage. See also **nitrobenzene poisoning.**
benzocaine An antipruritic and topical anesthetic for application to oral mucous membranes; also a local anesthetic for otic use.
benzodiazepine derivative One of a group of psychotropic agents, including the tranquilizers chlordiazepoxide, diazepam, oxazepam, and chlorazepate, prescribed to alleviate anxiety; and the hypnotics flurazepam and temazepam, prescribed in the treatment of insomnia.

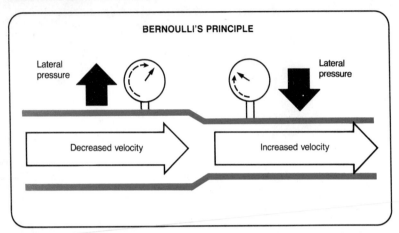

BERNOULLI'S PRINCIPLE

Lateral pressure

Lateral pressure

Decreased velocity

Increased velocity

benzoic acid A keratolytic agent, usually used with salicylic acid as an ointment in the treatment of athlete's foot and ringworm of the scalp.

benzonatate A nonnarcotic antitussive agent.

benzotropine mesylate A cholinergic-blocking (parasympatholytic) agent.

benzoyl peroxide A dermatomucosal agent used to treat acne vulgaris.

benzphetamine hydrochloride An amphetaminelike central nervous system stimulant.

benzquinamide hydrochloride An antiemetic agent.

benzthiazide A thiazide diuretic agent.

benzyl alcohol A clear, colorless, oily liquid, derived from certain balsams, used as a topical anesthetic and as a bacteriostatic agent in solutions for injection. Also called **phenyl carbinol, phenyl methanol.**

benzyl benzoate lotion A scabicide and pediculicide.

benzyl carbonol See **phenylethyl alcohol.**

Berger rhythm See **alpha wave.** Also called **Berger wave.**

Berger wave See **alpha wave.**

Bergonié-Tréboneau law In radiotherapy: a rule stating that the radiosensitivity of tissue depends on the number of undifferentiated cells, their mitotic activity, and the length of time they are actively proliferating.

beriberi A disease of the peripheral nerves owing to a deficiency of or an inability to assimilate thiamine. It is frequently caused by a diet limited to polished white rice, and it occurs in endemic form in eastern and southern Asia. Rare cases in the United States are associated with stressful conditions, as hypothyroidism, infections, pregnancy, lactation, and chronic alcoholism. Symptoms are fatigue, diarrhea, appetite and weight loss, disturbed nerve function causing paralysis and wasting of limbs, edema, and heart failure. Appropriate dietary adjustments and supplementary vitamin B can prevent or correct this disease. Also called **athiaminosis, kakke disease.** See also **thiamine.**

berkelium (Bk) An artificial radioactive transuranic element. Its atomic number is 97; its atomic weight is 247.

Berlock dermatitis An abnormal skin condition, characterized by hyperpigmentation and skin lesions, caused by a unique reaction to psoralen-type photosynthesizers commonly used in perfumes, colognes, and pomades, as oil of bergamot. This condition affects mostly women and children and may result from the use of products containing psoralens and from exposure to ultraviolet light. Although only about 5% of the radiation of the sun is ultraviolet light and much of that is absorbed by oxygen and ozone, the level of ultraviolet radiation reaching the earth, especially on a sunny day, is sufficient to cause the lesion to appear.

NURSING CONSIDERATIONS: Patients with Berlock dermatitis benefit from advice about the complications of prolonged exposure to sunlight and ultraviolet light. They also appreciate the justifiable reassurance that the lesions will vanish within a few months.

Bernard-Soulier syndrome A coagulation disorder characterized by an absence of or a deficiency in the ability of the platelets to aggregate owing to the relative lack of an essential glycoprotein in the membranes of the platelets. On microscopic examination, the platelets appear large and dispersed. The use of aspirin may provoke hemorrhage in people who have this condition. Following trauma and surgery, loss of blood may be greater than normal and transfusion may be required.

Bernoulli's law A law of chemistry stating that the velocity of a gas or a fluid flowing through a tube is inversely proportional to the pressure it exerts against the side of the tube: the greater the velocity, the lower the pressure.

Bernoulli's principle In physics: a principle stating that the sum of the velocity and the kinetic energy of a fluid flowing through a tube is constant. The greater the velocity, the less the lateral pressure on the wall of the tube. Thus, if an artery is narrowed by an atherosclerotic

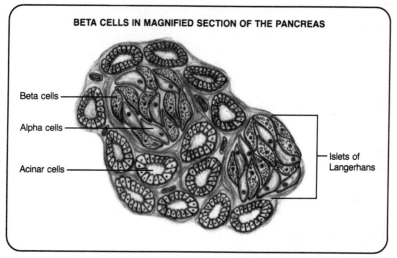

BETA CELLS IN MAGNIFIED SECTION OF THE PANCREAS

Beta cells

Alpha cells

Acinar cells

Islets of Langerhans

plaque, the flow of blood through the constriction increases in velocity and decreases in lateral pressure.

Bernstein test   See **acid perfusion test.**

berry aneurysm   A small, saccular dilatation of the wall of a cerebral artery, occurring most frequently at the junctures of vessels in the circle of Willis. A berry aneurysm may be the result of a congenital developmental defect and may rupture without warning, causing intracranial hemorrhage.

berylliosis   Poisoning that results from the inhalation of fine dusts, mists, or vapors containing beryllium or beryllium compounds. Berylliosis is characterized by granulomas throughout the body and by diffuse pulmonary fibrosis, resulting in a dry cough, shortness of breath, and chest pain. Symptoms may not appear for several years following exposure. See also **inorganic dust.**

beryllium (Be)   A steel-gray, light-weight metallic element. Its atomic number is 4; its atomic weight is 9.012. Beryllium occurs naturally as beryl and is used in metallic alloys and in fluorescent powders. Inhalation of beryllium fumes or particles may cause the formation of granulomas in the lungs, skin, and subcutaneous tissues. See also **berylliosis.**

bestiality   1. A brutal or animal-like character or nature. 2. Conduct or behavior that is characterized by beastlike appetites or instincts. 3. Sexual relations between a human being and an animal. 4. Sodomy. Also called **zooerastia.** See also **zoophilia.**

beta (β)   The second letter of the Greek alphabet, employed as a combining form with chemical names to distinguish one of two or more isomers or to indicate the position of substituted atoms in certain compounds. Compare **alpha.**

beta-adrenergic blocking agent   See **antiadrenergic.**

beta-adrenergic receptor   See **beta receptor.**

beta-adrenergic stimulating agent   See **adrenergic.**

beta-carotene   An ultraviolet screen.

beta cells   1. Insulin-producing cells situated in the islets of Langerhans. They contain granules that are soluble in alcohol and tend to be concentrated in the central portion of each islet. The insulin-producing function of the beta cells tends to accelerate the movement of glucose, amino acids, and fatty acids out of the blood and into the cellular cytoplasm, countering glucagon function of alpha cells. 2. The basophilic cells of the anterior lobe of the pituitary gland.

beta fetoprotein   A protein found in fetal liver and in some adults with liver disease. It is identical to normal liver ferritin. See also **alpha fetoprotein, ferritin, fetoprotein.**

beta-galactosidase   See **lactase.**

beta hemolysis   The development of a clear zone around a bacterial colony growing on blood-agar medium, characteristic of certain pathogenic bacteria. Compare **alpha hemolysis.**

beta-hemolytic streptococci   The pyogenic streptococci of groups A, B, C, E, F, G, H, K, L, M, and O that cause hemolysis of red blood cells in blood agar in the laboratory. These organisms cause most of the acute streptococcal infections seen in humans, including rheumatic fever, scarlet fever, many cases of pneumonia and septicemia, and streptococcal sore throat. Penicillin is usually prescribed to treat these infections when they are suspected, even before the results of the bacteriologic culture are available, because it is known that these organisms as a group are sensitive to the effects of penicillin and because the sequelae of untreated streptococcal infection may include glomerulonephritis and rheumatic fever.

beta-ketobutyric acid   See **acetoacetic acid.**

betamethasone, b. acetate, b. benzoate, b. diproprionate, b. disodium phosphate, b. sodium phosphate, b. valerate Topical anti-inflammatory agents.

beta particle An electron or positron emitted from the nucleus of an atom during radioactive decay of the atom.

beta receptor Any one of the postulated adrenergic components of receptor tissues that responds to epinephrine and such blocking agents as propranolol. Activation of beta receptors causes various physiological reactions, as relaxation of the bronchial muscles, increased cardiac rate, and the force of cardiac contraction. Also called **beta-adrenergic receptor.** Compare **alpha receptor.**

beta rhythm See **beta wave.**

betatron A cyclic accelerator that produces high-energy electrons by magnetic induction. The magnetic field of the betatron deflects electrons into a circular orbit, and an increasing magnetic orbital flux produces an induced circumferential electric field which accelerates the electrons.

beta wave One of the four types of brain waves, characterized by relatively low voltage and a frequency of more than 13 Hz. Beta waves are the 'busy waves' of the brain, recorded by electroencephalograph from the frontal and the central areas of the cerebrum when the patient is awake and alert with eyes open. Also called **beta rhythm.** Compare **alpha wave, delta wave, theta wave.**

bethanechol chloride A cholinergic (parasympathomimetic) agent.

bezoar A hard ball of hair and vegetable fiber that may develop within the intestines of humans but more often is found in the stomachs of ruminants.

B-galactosidase See **lactase.**

bhang, bang An Asian Indian hallucinogenic, composed of dried leaves and the young stems of uncultivated *Cannabis sativa.* It is usually ingested as a boiled mixture with milk, sugar, or water; it produces euphoria. It also may be smoked or chewed. See also **cannabis.**

bi- 1. See **bio-.** 2. A combining form meaning 'twice, two': *biarticular, bicapsular, bicaudal.* Also **bis-.**

Bi Symbol for **bismuth.**

-bia A combining form meaning 'creature possessing a mode of life': *aerobia, coenobia, Euphorbia.*

bias 1. An oblique or a diagonal line. 2. A prejudiced or subjective attitude. 3. In statistics: the systematic distortion of a statistic caused by a particular sampling process. 4. In electronics: a voltage applied to an electronic device, as a vacuum tube or a transistor, to control operating limits.

bicarbonate of soda See **sodium bicarbonate.**

biceps See **biceps brachii.**

biceps brachii The long fusiform muscle of the upper arm on the anterior surface of the humerus, arising in two heads from the scapula. The short head arises in a thick flat tendon from the corocoid process; the long head arises in the glenoid cavity. Both parts of the muscle converge in a flattened tendon that inserts into the radius of the forearm. The biceps brachii is innervated by branches of the musculocutaneous nerve, containing fibers from the fifth and the sixth cervical nerves. It flexes the arm and the forearm and supinates the hand. The long head draws the humerus toward the glenoid fossa, strengthening the shoulder joint. Also called **biceps, biceps flexor cubiti.** Compare **brachialis, triceps brachii.**

biceps femoris One of the posterior femoral muscles. It has two heads at its origin. The long head arises from the tuberosity of the ischium and from the inferior part of the sacrotuberous ligament; the short head arises from the linea aspera and from the lateral intermuscular septum. The fibers passing from both heads join in a tendon that inserts into the lateral side of the fibula and, by a few fibers, into the lateral condyle of the tibia. The tendon of insertion forms the lateral hamstring. The long head of the muscle is innervated by branches of the sciatic nerve containing fibers from the first three sacral nerves. The short head is innervated by a branch of the peroneal nerve containing fibers from the fifth lumbar and first two sacral nerves. The biceps femoris flexes the leg and rotates it laterally and extends the thigh and tends to rotate it laterally. Also called **hamstring muscle.**

biceps flexor cubiti See **biceps brachii.**

biceps reflex A contraction of a biceps muscle produced when the tendon is tapped with a percussor in testing deep tendon reflexes.

biconcave Concave on both sides, especially as applied to a lens. —**biconcavity,** *n.*

biconvex Convex on both sides, especially as applied to a lens. —**biconvexity,** *n.*

bicornate Having two horns or processes.

bicuspid 1. Having or ending in two cusps or points. 2. One of the two teeth between the molars and canines of the upper and lower jaw. Also called **premolar tooth.**

bicuspid valve See **mitral valve.**

b.i.d. In prescriptions: *abbr bis in die,* a Latin phrase meaning 'twice a day.'

bidactyly An abnormal condition in which the second, third, and fourth digits on the same hand are missing and only the first and fifth are represented. Also called **lobster-claw deformity.** —**bidactylous,** *adj.*

bidermoma, *pl.* **bidermomas, bidermomata** A teratoid neoplasm composed of cells and tissues originating in two germ layers.

biduotertian fever A form of malaria characterized by overlapping paroxysms of chills, fever, and other symptoms, caused by infection with two strains of *Plasmodium,* each having its own cycle of symptoms, as in quartan and tertian malaria. See also **malaria.**

bifid Split into two parts.

bifocal 1. Of or pertaining to the characteristic of having two foci. 2. Of a lens: having two areas of different focal lengths.

bifurcation A splitting into two branches,

as the trachea, which branches into the two bronchi at about the level of the fifth thoracic vertebra.

Bigelow's lithotrite   A long-jawed lithotrite, passed through the urethra, for crushing a calculus in the bladder.

bigeminal pulse   An abnormal pulse in which two beats in close succession are followed by a pause during which no pulse is felt. See also **trigeminal pulse, trigeminy.**

bigeminy   1. An association in pairs. 2. A cardiac arrhythmia characterized by two beats in rapid succession followed by a longer interval. The arrhythmia is usually related to premature ventricular beats. **—bigeminal,** *adj.*

bilabe   A narrow forceps used to remove small calculi from the bladder.

bilaminar   Of or pertaining to the characteristic of having two layers, as the basal lamina and the reticular lamina that constitute the basement membrane of the epithelium.

bilaminar blastoderm   The stage of embryonic development prior to mesoderm formation, in which only the ectoderm and entoderm primary germ layers have formed. Compare **trilaminar blastoderm.**

bilateral   1. Having two sides. 2. Occurring or appearing on two sides. A patient with bilateral hearing loss may have partial or total deafness in both ears. 3. Having two layers.

bilateral long leg spica cast   An orthopedic device of plaster of paris, fiberglass, or other casting material that encases and immobilizes the trunk cranially as far as the nipple line and both legs caudally as far as the toes. A horizontal crossbar to improve immobilization connects the parts of the cast encasing both legs at ankle level. The bilateral long leg spica cast is used to aid the healing of fractures of the hip, the femur, the acetabulum, or the pelvis and for the correction or maintenance of the correction of a hip deformity. Compare **one-and-a-half spica cast, unilateral long leg spica cast.**

bile   A bitter, yellow-green secretion of the liver. Stored in the gallbladder, bile receives its color from the presence of bile pigments, as bilirubin. Bile passes from the gallbladder through the common bile duct in response to the presence of a fatty meal in the duodenum. Bile emulsifies these fats, preparing them for further digestion and absorption in the small intestine. Any interference in the flow of bile will result in the presence of unabsorbed fat in the feces and in jaundice. Also called **gall.** See also **biliary obstruction, jaundice. —biliary,** *adj.*

bile acid   A steroid acid of the bile, produced during the metabolism of cholesterol. On hydrolysis, bile acid yields glycine and cholic acid.

bile salts   A digestant used to treat uncomplicated constipation.

bile solubility test   A bacteriologic test used in the differential diagnosis of pneumococcal and streptococcal infection. A broth culture of each organism is placed into two tubes. Ox bile is added to one and salt to the other. Pneumococci dissolve in ox bile, resulting in a clear solution; streptococci do not dissolve, resulting in a cloudy solution. The tube with salt is used for comparative purposes.

Bilharzia   See *Schistosoma.*

bilharziasis   See **schistosomiasis.**

bili-   A combining form meaning 'pertaining to the bile': *biliary, bilidigestive, bilifuscin.*

biliary   Referring to bile or to the gallbladder and its ducts, which transport bile. These are often called the biliary tract or the biliary system. See also **bile, biliary calculus.**

biliary atresia   Congenital absence or underdevelopment of one or more of the biliary structures, causing jaundice and early liver damage. As the condition worsens, the child may show retarded growth and develop portal hypertension. Surgery can correct the defective ducts in only a small percentage of cases. Most infants die in early childhood from biliary cirrhosis. It is essential for the physician to distinguish between this condition and neonatal hepatitis, which is treatable. See also **biliary cirrhosis.**

biliary calculus   A stone formed in the biliary tract, consisting of bile pigments and calcium salts. Biliary calculi may cause jaundice, right upper quadrant pain, obstruction, and inflammation of the gallbladder. If stones cannot pass spontaneously into the duodenum, intravenous cholangiography will reveal their location, and they can be surgically removed. Also called **choledocholithiasis, gallstones.** See also **cholangitis, cholecystitis, cholelithiasis.**

biliary cirrhosis   An inflammatory condition in which the flow of bile through the ductules of the liver is obstructed. Biliary cirrhosis most commonly affects women in their middle years, and its cause is unknown. It is characterized by abdominal pain, jaundice, steatorrhea, and enlargement of the liver and spleen. The disease is a slowly progressive one and in its end stages closely resembles cirrhosis of the liver. There is no specific medical or surgical treatment. Care must be taken to rule out obstruction of the biliary structures outside the liver, because the latter condition can be treated successfully. Compare **biliary calculus, biliary obstruction.**

biliary colic   A type of smooth-muscle or visceral pain specifically associated with the passing of stones through the bile ducts. Also called cholecystalgia. See also **biliary calculus.**

biliary duct   A duct through which bile passes from the liver to the duodenum.

biliary fistula   An abnormal passage from the gallbladder, a bile duct, or the liver to an internal organ or the surface of the body. Biliary fistulae opening into the colon, duodenum, hepatic duct, peritoneal cavity, pleural space, or skin are complications in cholelithiasis; a gallstone entering the duodenum may become impacted, usually in the ileocecal valve, and cause intestinal obstruction.

biliary obstruction   Blockage of the common or cystic bile duct, usually caused by one or more gallstones. It impedes bile drainage and

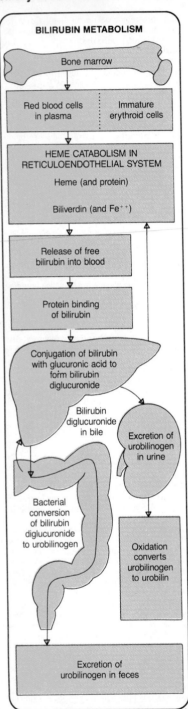

BILIRUBIN METABOLISM

Bone marrow

Red blood cells in plasma | Immature erythroid cells

HEME CATABOLISM IN RETICULOENDOTHELIAL SYSTEM

Heme (and protein)

Biliverdin (and Fe^{++})

Release of free bilirubin into blood

Protein binding of bilirubin

Conjugation of bilirubin with glucuronic acid to form bilirubin diglucuronide

Bilirubin diglucuronide in bile

Excretion of urobilinogen in urine

Bacterial conversion of bilirubin diglucuronide to urobilinogen

Oxidation converts urobilinogen to urobilin

Excretion of urobilinogen in feces

produces an inflammatory reaction. Uncommon causes of biliary obstruction include choledochal cysts, pancreatic and duodenal tumors, Crohn's disease, pancreatitis, echinococcosis, ascariasis, and sclerosing cholangitis. Stones, consisting chiefly of cholesterol, bile pigment, and calcium, may form in the gallbladder and in the hepatic duct in persons of either sex at any age but are more common in middle-aged women. Increased amounts of serum cholesterol in the blood, as occurs in obesity, diabetes, hypothyroidism, biliary stasis, and inflammation of the biliary system, promote the formation of gallstones. Cholelithiasis may be asymptomatic until a stone lodges in a biliary duct, but the patient usually has a prior history of indigestion and discomfort after eating fatty foods. Cholecystectomy is usually the definitive treatment, but in most cases surgery is delayed until the patient's condition is stabilized and any prothrombin deficiency (owing to vitamin K malabsorption) is corrected.

NURSING CONSIDERATIONS: The patient may experience intense pain as obstruction causes biliary colic. Instruction is given on the importance of adhering to a low-fat diet and reporting recurrence of symptoms if discharge occurs prior to surgery. Cholecystectomy usually requires several days of intensive nursing care and support. See **cholecystectomy.**

biliary tract cancer A relatively rare malignancy in an extrahepatic bile duct, occurring slightly more often in men than in women, characterized by progressive jaundice, pruritus, weight loss, and, in the later stages, by severe pain. Transhepatic cholangiography and X-rays following the introduction of a contrast medium into the common bile duct and pancreatic duct are used to identify and determine the site of the lesion. Results of laboratory studies indicative of extrahepatic biliary obstruction include greater than normal levels of serum alkaline phosphatase and bilirubin in the blood. If the tumor is in the ampulla of Vater, occult blood may be found in the stool. The tumor is an adenocarcinoma; it may be papillary or flat and ulcerated. It is generally inoperable if it is located in the hepatic or common bile duct, but periampullary lesions may be treated by pancreatoduodenectomy. In cases of an inoperable tumor, various surgical procedures may be performed palliatively to improve the flow of bile. Preoperative, postoperative, and palliative irradiation are also used. With the exception of a rare remission induced by 5-fluorouracil, chemotherapy is not effective in treating these lesions.

biligulate Having two tongues or two tongue-like structures.

bilious 1. Of or pertaining to bile. 2. Characterized by an excessive secretion of bile. 3. Characterized by a disorder affecting bile.

bilirubin The orange yellow pigment of bile, formed principally by the breakdown of hemoglobin in red blood cells after termination of their normal lifespan. Water-insoluble, unconjugated bilirubin normally travels in the blood-

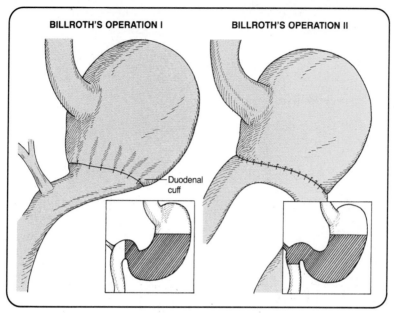

BILLROTH'S OPERATION I   BILLROTH'S OPERATION II

Duodenal
cuff

stream to the liver, where it is converted to a water-soluble, conjugated form and excreted into the bile. In a healthy person, about 250 mg of bilirubin are produced daily, and the majority of that is eventually excreted from the body in the stool. The characteristic yellow pallor of jaundice is caused by the accumulation of bilirubin in the blood and in the tissues of the skin. Testing for bilirubin in the blood provides valuable information for diagnosing and evaluating liver disease, biliary obstruction, and hemolytic anemia. See also **jaundice, van den Bergh test.**

biliuria   The presence of bile in the urine.

biliverdin   A greenish bile pigment formed in the breakdown of hemoglobin and converted to bilirubin. See also **bile, bilirubin.**

Billroth's operation I   The surgical removal of the pylorus in the treatment of gastric cancer. The proximal end of the duodenum is anastomosed to the stomach.

Billroth's operation II   The surgical removal of the pylorus and duodenum. The cut end of the stomach is anastomosed to the jejunum through the transverse mesocolon.

bilobulate, bilobular   Having two lobes.

bilocular, biloculate   In biology: **1.** Divided into two cells. **2.** Containing two cells.

bimanual   Of or pertaining to the functioning of both hands.

binary fission   Direct division of a cell or nucleus into two equal parts. It is the common form of asexual reproduction of bacteria, protozoa, and other lower forms of life. Also called **simple fission.** Compare **multiple fission.**

binaural stethoscope   A stethoscope having two earpieces.

bind   **1.** To bandage or wrap in a band. **2.** To join together with a band or with a ligature. **3.** In chemistry: to combine or unite molecules by employing reactive groups within the molecules or by using a binding chemical. Binding is especially associated with chemical bonds that are fairly easily broken, as in the bonds between toxins and antitoxins.

binder   A broad bandage that most commonly surrounds and supports the chest or abdomen. See **abdominal binder, chest binder.**

Binet age   The mental age of an individual, especially a child, as determined by the Binet-Simon tests, which are evaluated on the basis of tested intelligence of the normal individual at any given age. The Binet age corresponding to 'profoundly retarded' is 1 to 2 years; to 'severely retarded,' 3 to 7 years; and to 'mildly retarded,' 8 to 12 years.

binocular   **1.** Pertaining to both eyes, especially regarding vision. **2.** A microscope, telescope, or field glass that can accommodate viewing by both eyes.

binocular fixation   The process of having both eyes directed at the same object at the same time. This is essential to having good depth perception.

binocular ophthalmoscope   An ophthalmoscope having two eyepieces for stereoscopic examination of the eye.

binocular parallax   The difference in the angles formed by the sight lines to two objects situated at different distances from the eyes. Binocular parallax is a major factor in depth perception. Also called **stereoscopic parallax.**

binocular perception   The visual ability to judge depth or distance by virtue of having two eyes.

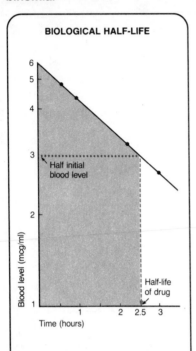

BIOLOGICAL HALF-LIFE

Half initial blood level

Half-life of drug

Blood level (mcg/ml)

Time (hours)

This diagram shows the time required (2½ hours) for the blood level of gentamicin to fall to 3 mcg/ml, one half its peak level of 6 mcg/ml.

binomial Containing two names or terms.

binovular Developing from two distinct ova, as in dizygotic twins. Also called **diovular.** Compare **uniovular.**

binovular twins See **dizygotic twins.**

bio- A combining form meaning 'pertaining to life': *bioassay, biogenesis, biolysis, biosynthesis.* Also **bi-.**

bioassay The laboratory determination of the concentration of a drug or other substance in a specimen by comparing its effect on an organism, an animal, or an isolated tissue with that of a standard preparation. Also called **biological assay.**

bioavailability The degree of activity or amount of an administered drug or other substance that becomes available for activity in the target tissue.

biochemical genetics See **molecular genetics.**

biochemistry The chemistry of living organisms and life processes. Also called **biological chemistry, physiological chemistry.**

bioequivalent In pharmacology: **1.** Of or pertaining to a drug that has the same effect on the body as another drug, usually one nearly

identical in its chemical formulation. **2.** A bioequivalent drug. —**bioequivalence,** *n.*

biofeedback A process providing a person with visual or auditory information about the autonomic physiologic functions of the body, as blood pressure, muscle tension, and brain wave activity, usually through use of instrumentation. By trial and error, the person learns to consciously control these processes, which were previously regarded as involuntary. Biofeedback may be used clinically to treat many conditions, as hypertension, insomnia, and migraine headache.

bioflavonoid A generic term for any of a group of colored flavones found in many fruits and essential for the absorption and metabolism of ascorbic acid. The bioflavonoids are needed for the maintenance of collagen and of the capillary walls and may aid in protection against infection. The components are citrin, hesperidin, rutin, flavones, and flavonoids. Rich sources include lemons, grapes, plums, grapefruit, black currants, apricots, buckwheat, cherries, blackberries, and rose hips. Deficiency can result in a tendency to bleed or bruise easily. The bioflavonoids are completely nontoxic. Also called **vitamin P.** See also **ascorbic acid.**

biogenesis, biogeny **1.** The doctrine that living material can originate only from preexisting life and not from inanimate matter. **2.** The origin of life and living organisms; ontogeny and phylogeny. —**biogenetic,** *adj.*

biogenetic law See **recapitulation theory.**

biogenic **1.** Produced by the action of a living organism, as fermentation. **2.** Essential to life and the maintenance of health, as food, water, and proper rest.

biogenic amine One of a large group of naturally occurring biologically active compounds, most of which act as neurotransmitters. The most dominant, norepinephrine, is involved in such physiologic functions as emotional reactions, memory, sleep, and arousal from sleep. Other biochemicals of the group include three catecholamines: histamine, serotonin, and dopamine. These substances are active in regulating blood pressure, elimination, body temperature, and many other centrally mediated bodily functions.

biogenous **1.** Biogenetic. **2.** Biogenic.

biogeny See **biogenesis.**

biological, biologic Any medicinal preparation made from living organisms or the products of living organisms. Kinds of biologicals are **antigens, antitoxins, serums, vaccines.**

biological assay See **bioassay.**

biological chemistry See **biochemistry.**

biological half-life The time required for the body to eliminate one half of an administered dosage of any substance by regular physiological processes. The time required is approximately the same for both the stable and radioactive isotopes of a specific element. See also **effective half-life, half-life.**

biological vector See **vector.**

biologic psychiatry A school of psychiatric thought that stresses the physical, chemical, and neurological causes of and treatments for mental and emotional disorders.

biology The scientific study of plants and animals. Some branches of biology are biometry, ecology, molecular biology, and paleontology.

biome The total group of biological communities existing in and characteristic of a given geographic region, as a desert, woodland, or marsh. A biome includes all plants, animals, and microorganisms of a particular region.

biomechanics The study of mechanical laws and their application to living organisms, especially the human body and its locomotor system. —**biomechanical,** adj.

biomedical engineering A system of techniques in which knowledge of biological processes is applied to solve practical medical problems and to answer questions in biomedical research.

bionics The science of applying electronic principles and devices, as computers and solid-state miniaturized circuitry, to medical problems, as artificial pacemakers used to correct abnormal heart rhythms. —**bionic,** adj.

biophore According to Weismannism, the basic hereditary unit contained in the germ plasm from which all living cells develop and all inherited characteristics are transmitted. Compare **gemmule.**

biopsy 1. The removal of a small piece of living tissue from an organ or other part of the body for microscopic examination to confirm or establish a diagnosis, estimate prognosis, or follow the course of a disease. 2. The tissue excised for examination. 3. *Informal.* To excise tissue for examination. Kinds of biopsy include **aspiration biopsy, needle biopsy, punch biopsy, surface biopsy.** —**bioptic,** adj.

biopsychic Of or pertaining to psychic factors as they relate to living organisms.

biopsychology See **psychobiology.**

biopsychosocial Of or pertaining to the complex of biological, psychological, and social aspects of life.

biorhythm Any cyclic, biological event or phenomenon, as the sleep cycle, the menstrual cycle, or the respiratory cycle. —**biorhythmic,** adj.

-biosis A combining form meaning 'life': *macrobiosis, necrobiosis, otobiosis.*

biostatistics Numerical data on births, deaths, diseases, injuries, and other factors affecting the general health and condition of human populations. Also called **vital statistics.**

biosynthesis Any one of thousands of chemical reactions continually occurring throughout the body in which simple molecules form complex biomolecules, especially the carbohydrates, the lipids, the proteins, the nucleotides, and the nucleic acids. Biosynthetic reactions constitute the anabolism of the body. —**biosynthetic,** adj.

biotaxis The ability of living cells to develop into certain forms and arrangements. See also **cytoclesis.** —**biotactic,** adj.

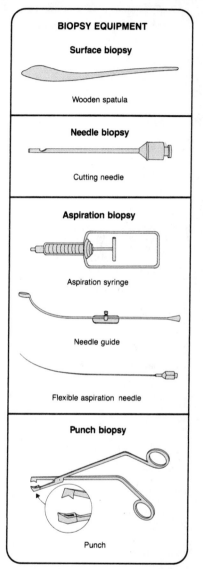

BIOPSY EQUIPMENT

Surface biopsy

Wooden spatula

Needle biopsy

Cutting needle

Aspiration biopsy

Aspiration syringe

Needle guide

Flexible aspiration needle

Punch biopsy

Punch

biotaxy 1. Biotaxis. 2. The systematic classification of living organisms according to their anatomical characteristics; taxonomy.

biotechnology The study of the relationships between humans or other living organisms and machinery, as the health effects of word processor equipment on office workers or the ability of airplane pilots to perform tasks when traveling at supersonic speeds.

-biotic A combining form meaning: 1. 'Pertaining to life': *anabiotic, microbiotic.* 2. 'Possessing a (specified) mode of life': *endobiotic, photobiotic, symbiotic.*

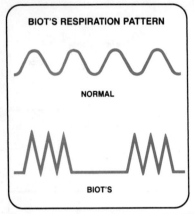

BIOT'S RESPIRATION PATTERN

NORMAL

BIOT'S

biotin A colorless, crystalline, water-soluble B complex vitamin that acts as a coenzyme in fatty acid production and in the oxidation of fatty acids and carbohydrates. It also aids in the utilization of protein, folic acid, pantothenic acid, and vitamin B_{12}. Rich sources are egg yolk, beef liver, kidney, unpolished rice, brewer's yeast, peanuts, cauliflower, and mushrooms. Since biotin is synthesized by intestinal bacteria, naturally occurring deficiency disease is unknown, although it can be induced by large quantities of raw egg whites in the diet. Also called **vitamin H.**

biotin deficiency syndrome An abnormal condition caused by a deficiency of biotin, characterized by dermatitis, hyperesthesia, muscle pain, anorexia, slight anemia, and changes in electrocardiographic activity of the heart. The average daily requirement of biotin for an adult is 100 to 200 μg; the average American diet provides 100 to 300 μg of the vitamin.

biotope A specific biological habitat or site.

biotransformation The chemical changes a substance undergoes in the body, as by the action of enzymes. See also **metabolic.**

Biot's respiration An abnormal respiratory pattern, characterized by irregular periods of apnea alternating with periods of breathing in which each breath has the same depth and is faster and deeper than normal. Biot's respiration is symptomatic of meningitis or increased intracranial pressure.

biparental inheritance See **amphigonous inheritance.**

biparietal Of or pertaining to the two parietal bones of the head, as the biparietal diameter.

biparietal diameter The distance between the protuberances of the two parietal bones of the skull.

bipartite Having two parts.

biped **1.** Having two feet. **2.** Any animal with only two feet.

bipedal Capable of locomotion on two feet.

bipenniform Of bodily structure: having the bilateral symmetry of a feather, as the pattern formed by the fasciculi that converge on both sides of a muscle tendon in the rectus femoris. Compare **multipenniform, penniform, radiate.**

biperiden hydrochloride, b. lactate Cholinergic-blocking (parasympatholytic) agents.

biphasic Having two phases, parts, aspects, or stages.

bipolar **1.** Having two poles, as in certain electrotherapeutic treatments using two poles or in certain methods of bacterial staining that affect only the two poles of the microorganism under study. **2.** Of a nerve cell: having an afferent and an efferent process.

bipolar disorder A major affective disorder characterized by episodes of mania and depression. One or the other phase may be predominant at any given time, one phase may appear alternately with the other, or elements of both phases may be present simultaneously. Characteristics of the manic phase are excessive emotional displays, excitement, euphoria, hyperactivity accompanied by elation, boisterousness, impaired ability to concentrate, decreased need for sleep, and seemingly unbounded energy, often accompanied by delusions of grandeur. In the depressive phase, marked apathy and underactivity are accompanied by feelings of profound sadness, loneliness, guilt, and lowered self-esteem. Causes of the disorder are multiple and complex, often involving biological, psychological, interpersonal, and social and cultural factors. Treatment includes antidepressants, tranquilizers and antianxiety drugs, or the use of electroconvulsive therapy for persons who present an immediate and serious risk of suicide, followed by long-term psychotherapy. Careful nursing observation is important during depression, particularly during the recovery from depression, because of the possibility of suicide.

bipolar lead **1.** An electrocardiographic conductor having two electrodes placed on different body regions, with each electrode contributing significantly to the record. **2.** *Informal.* A tracing produced by such a lead on an electrocardiograph.

bipotentiality The characteristic of acting or reacting according to either of two potentials.

bird breeder's lung See **pigeon breeder's lung.**

bird-headed dwarf A person affected with Seckel's syndrome, a congenital disorder characterized by a proportionate shortness of stature; a proportionately small head with hypoplasia of the jaws, large eyes, and a beaklike protrusion of the nose; mental retardation; and various other skeletal, cutaneous, and genital defects. Also called **nanocephalic dwarf.**

birth The act or process of being born.

birth canal *Informal.* The passage that extends from the inlet of the true pelvis to the vaginal orifice through which an infant passes during vaginal birth.

birth control Use of a drug, device, or practice to prevent or to delay pregnancy. See also **contraception.**

birth defect   See **congenital anomaly.**

birthing chair   A chair used in labor and delivery to promote the comfort of the mother and the efficiency of parturition. The chair may be specially designed, having many technical features, or it may be a simple three-legged stool with a high, slanted back and a circular seat with a large central hole in it. The newer birthing chairs allow the woman to sit straight up or to recline. The chair has a lower section that may be removed or folded out of the way. The upright position appears to shorten the time in labor, particularly the second or expulsive stage of labor, probably owing to gravity and increased participation of the mother. The chair is not suitable for use with anesthesia.

birthmark   Any localized skin discoloration or blemish, flat or raised, present at birth or appearing shortly thereafter. Kinds of birthmarks include **mole, nevus.**

birthrate   The proportion of the number of births in a specific area during a given period to the total population of that area, usually expressed as the number of births per 1,000 of population. Compare **crude birthrate, refined birthrate, true birthrate.**

birth trauma   **1.** Any physical injury suffered by an infant during the process of delivery. **2.** The supposed psychic shock, according to some psychiatric theories, that an infant suffers during delivery.

birth weight   The measured weight of an infant at birth, usually about 3,500 g (7.5 lb) in the United States. Of newborns, 97% weigh between 2,500 g (5.5 lb) and 4,500 g (10 lb). Infants weighing less than 2,500 g at term are considered **small for gestational age.** Infants weighing more than 4,500 g are considered **large for gestational age** and are often the offspring of diabetic mothers.

bis-   A combining form meaning 'twice, two': *bisacromial, bisaxillary, bisferious, bisiliac.* Also **bi-.**

bisacodyl   A stimulant laxative.

bisect   To divide into two equal lengths or parts.

bisexual   **1.** Hermaphroditic; having gonads of both sexes. **2.** Possessing physical or psychological characteristics of both sexes. **3.** Engaging in both heterosexual and homosexual activity. **4.** Desiring sexual contact with persons of both sexes.

bisexual libido   In psychoanalysis: the tendency in a person to seek sexual gratification with people of either sex.

bishydroxycoumarin   See **dicumarol.**

bismuth (Bi)   A reddish, crystalline, trivalent metallic element. Its atomic number is 83; its atomic weight is 209. It is combined with various other elements, as oxygen, to produce numerous salts used in the manufacture of many pharmaceutical substances.

bismuth subcarbonate, b. subgallate, b. subsalicylate   Antidiarrheal agents.

bit   In data processing: the smallest unit of information for data storage. Compare **byte.**

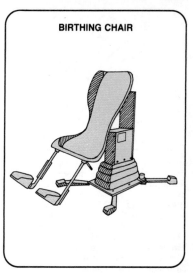

BIRTHING CHAIR

bite block   See **occlusion rim.**

bitegage   A prosthetic dental device that helps attain proper occlusion of the teeth rooted in the maxilla and the mandible.

bitelock   A dental device for retaining the occlusion rims in the same relation outside the mouth as inside the mouth.

bitemporal   Of or pertaining to both temples or both temporal bones.

biteplate   A device used in dentistry as a diagnostic or a therapeutic aid for prosthodontics or for orthodontics. It is fabricated of wire and plastic, worn in the palate, and may also be used to correct temperomandibular joint problems or as a splint in restoring the full mouth.

bithionol (TBP)   A pale gray powder, soluble in acetone, alcohol, or ether, used as a local antiseptic and administered orally in the treatment of infestations of the giant liver fluke *(Fasciola gigantica)* and of the lung fluke *(Paragonimus westermani)* that cause parasitic hemoptysis in Asiatic countries.

Bithynia   A genus of snails, species of which act as intermediate hosts to *Opisthorchis.*

biting in childhood   A natural behavior trait and reflex action in infants, acquired at about 5 to 6 months of age in response to the introduction of solid foods in the diet and the beginning of the teething process. In the psychosocial development of the infant, biting is the first learned aggressive action, and through it the infant learns to control the environment. The behavior also confronts the infant with one of the first inner conflicts, because biting can produce both pain and pleasure. Biting during breastfeeding causes withdrawal of the nipple and anxiety in the mother, yet it also serves as a means of soothing teething discomfort. Toddlers and older children often use biting for expressing aggression toward their parents and other children. Most children normally outgrow the

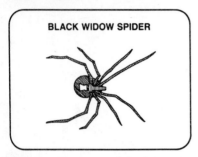

BLACK WIDOW SPIDER

tendency unless severe maladaptive or emotional problems are present. See also **psychosexual development, psychosocial development.**

Bitot's spots   White or gray triangular deposits on the bulbar conjunctiva adjacent to the lateral margin of the cornea, a clinical sign of vitamin A deficiency.

bitrochanteric lipodystrophy   An abnormal and excessive deposition of fat on the buttocks and the outer aspect of the upper thighs, occurring most commonly in women. See also **lipodystrophy.**

bitterling test   A test for pregnancy in which the small, carplike bitterling fish of Japan is immersed in a quart of fresh water containing two teaspoonsful of the urine of the woman being tested. If she is pregnant, the long oviduct of the bitterling grows from its belly.

biuret test   A method for detecting urea and other soluble proteins in serum.

bivalent   **1.** In genetics: a pair of synapsed homologous chromosomes that are attached to each other by chiasmata during the early first meiotic prophase of gametogenesis. The structure serves as the basis for the tetrads from which gametes are produced during the two meiotic divisions. Also called **divalent. 2.** In chemistry: See **valence,** definition 1. —**bivalence,** *n.*

bivalent chromosome   A pair of synapsed homologous chromosomes during the early stages of gametogenesis. See also **bivalent.**

bivalve cast   An orthopedic cast used for immobilizing a section of the body for the healing of one or more broken bones or for correction or the maintenance of correction of an orthopedic deformity. The bivalve cast is cut in half to monitor and detect pressure under the cast, especially with a patient who has decreased sensation or who has no sensation in the portion of the body surrounded by the cast. An area of the skin that is subjected to prolonged pressure from a cast may become infected, and early signs of pressure are almost impossible to detect. The bivalve cast is cut into anterior and posterior portions to facilitate inspection of the patient's skin. If dangerous pressure areas are detected, "windows" are then cut out of the cast over the pressure areas to relieve the problem.

bizarre leiomyoma   See **epithelioid leiomyoma.**

Bk   Symbol for **berkelium.**

Black Death   *Informal.* Bubonic plague, especially the epidemic in the 14th century that killed over 25,000,000 people in Europe. See also **bubonic plague, plague, Yersinia pestis.**

Blackfan-Diamond syndrome   A rare congenital disorder evident in the first 3 months of life, characterized by severe anemia and very low reticulocyte count, but normal numbers of platelets and white cells. Also called congenital hypoplastic anemia. See also **anemia.**

black fever   See **kala-azar.**

black hairy tongue   See **parasitic glossitis.**

blackhead   See **comedo.**

black light   See **Wood's light.**

black lung   See **anthracosis.**

black lung disease   See **pneumoconiosis.**

blackout   *Informal.* A temporary loss of vision or consciousness resulting from cerebral ischemia.

black plague   See **bubonic plague.**

black tongue   See **parasitic glossitis.**

blackwater fever   A serious complication of chronic falciparum malaria, characterized by jaundice, hemoglobinuria, acute renal failure, and the passage of bloody dark red or black urine owing to massive intravascular hemolysis. Death occurs in 20% to 30% of all cases; mortality is particularly high among Europeans. See also **falciparum malaria, malaria.**

black widow spider   A poisonous arachnid found in many parts of the world. The venom injected with its bite causes perspiration, abdominal cramps, nausea, headaches, and dizziness of various levels of intensity. Small children, old people, and those with heart conditions are most severely affected and may require hospitalization and the administration of an antivenin.

black widow spider antivenin   A passive immunizing agent.

bladder   **1.** A membranous sac serving as a receptacle for secretions. **2.** The urinary bladder.

bladder cancer   The most common malignancy of the urinary tract. It is characterized by a tumor or by multiple growths that tend to recur in a more aggressive form. Malignant neoplasia of the bladder occurs 2.3 times more often in men than in women and is more prevalent in urban than in rural areas. The risk for developing bladder cancer is increased with cigarette smoking; exposure to carcinogens, as aniline dyes; and the use of beta-naphthylamine, mixtures of aromatic hydrocarbons, or benzidine and its salts, used in chemical, paint, plastics, rubber, textile, petroleum, and wood industries and in medical laboratories. Other predisposing factors are chronic urinary tract infections, calculous disease, and schistosomiasis; in Egypt, where *Schistosoma haematobium* infestations are extremely common, the bladder is the most frequent site of cancer. Early symptoms of a bladder cancer include hematuria, frequent urination, dysuria, and cystitis. Urinalysis, excretory urography, cystoscopy, or transurethral biopsy are performed for diagnosis. The majority of bladder malignancies are transitional cell carcinomas; a small percentage are squamous cell carcinomas or adenocarcinomas. Superficial or multiple lesions may be treated by fulguration or open loop resection. A segmental resection is usually performed if the tumor is at the dome or in a lateral wall of the bladder, but total cystectomy may be performed for an invasive lesion of the trigone. In patients requiring cystectomy, a conduit is constructed to divert urine to the colon, to a rectal bladder, or to an abdominal stoma. External radiation may be administered preoperatively or as palliation for inoperable lesions. Internal radiation, the introduction of radioisotopes by means of a balloon of a catheter, or the implantation of radon seeds may be used in treating small localized tumors on the bladder wall. Medications that are often used as palliatives are 5-fluorouracil and adriamycin. See also **cystectomy.**

bladder flap *Informal.* The vesicouterine fold of peritoneum that is incised during low cervical cesarean section so that the bladder can be separated from the uterus to expose the lower uterine segment for incision. The flap is reapproximated with sutures during closure to cover the uterine incision. See also **cesarean section.**

Blalock-Taussig procedure Surgical construction of a shunt as a temporary measure to overcome congenital pulmonary stenosis, as in an infant born with tetralogy of Fallot. Preoperatively, a cardiac catheterization is done to identify the defect or defects, and the levels of arterial blood gases are analyzed. Hypothermia anesthesia and a cardiac bypass machine are utilized. The subclavian artery is joined end-to-end with the pulmonary artery, directing blood from the systemic circulation to the lungs. See also **heart surgery.**

blanch **1.** Causing to become pale. **2.** Whitening or bleaching a surface or substance. **3.** Becoming white or pale, as from vasoconstriction accompanying fear or anger.

bland Mild or having a soothing effect.

bland diet A diet that is mechanically, chemically, physiologically, and, sometimes, thermally nonirritating. It is often prescribed in the treatment of peptic ulcer, ulcerative colitis, gallbladder disease, diverticulosis and diverticulitis, gastritis, idiopathic spastic constipation, and mucous colitis, and after abdominal surgery. The diet may include eggs, meat, poultry, fish, and enriched fine cereals; milk is usually an important ingredient. See also **sippy diet.**

blanket bath The procedure of wrapping the patient in a wet pack and then in blankets.

-blast A combining form meaning an 'embryonic state of development': *leucoblast, megaloblast, osteoblast.*

blast cell Any immature cell, as an erythroblast, a lymphoblast, or a neuroblast.

blastema, *pl.* **blastemas, blastemata** **1.** Any mass of living protoplasm capable of growth and differentiation, specifically the primordial undifferentiated cellular material from

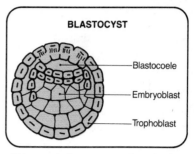

BLASTOCYST

— Blastocoele
— Embryoblast
— Trophoblast

which a particular organ or a tissue develops. **2.** In certain animals, a group of cells capable of regenerating a lost or damaged part or of giving rise to a complete organism in asexual reproduction. **3.** The budding or sprouting area of a plant. —**blastemal, blastematic, blastemic,** *adj.*

-blastema A combining form meaning a 'mass of living substance': *epiblastema, scleroblastema, scytoblastema.*

blastid, blastide The site in the fertilized ovum where the pronuclei fuse and the nucleus forms.

blastin Any substance that provides nourishment for or stimulates the growth or proliferation of cells, as allantoin.

blasto- A combining form meaning 'pertaining to an early embryonic or developing stage': *blastocele, blastocytoma, blastomatosis.*

blastocoele, blastocoel, blastocele The fluid-filled cavity of the blastocyst in mammals and the blastula or discoblastula of lower animals. The cavity increases the surface area of the developing embryo for better absorption of nutrients and oxygen. Also called **cleavage cavity, segmentation cavity, subgerminal cavity.**

blastocyst The embryonic form that follows the morula in human development. It is a spherical mass of cells having a central, fluid-filled cavity (blastocoele) surrounded by two layers of cells. The outer layer (trophoblast) later forms the placenta; the inner layer (embryoblast) later forms the embryo. Implantation in the wall of the uterus usually occurs at this stage, on approximately the 8th day after fertilization. Also called **blastula.**

blastocyte An undifferentiated embryonic cell prior to germ layer formation. —**blastocytic,** *adj.*

blastocytoma See **blastoma.**

blastoderm The layer of cells forming the wall of the blastocyst in mammals and the blastula in lower animals during the early stages of embryonic development. It is produced by the cleavage of the fertilized ovum and gives rise to the primary germ layers (the ectoderm, mesoderm, and endoderm) from which the embryo and all of its membranes are derived. In animals in which the ovum contains a large amount of yolk and undergoes partial cleavage, the cells form a small caplike structure, or cellular disk,

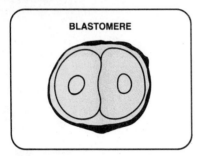

BLASTOMERE

above the yolk mass. Kinds of blastoderm are **bilaminar blastoderm, embryonic blastoderm, extraembryonic blastoderm, trilaminar blastoderm.** Also called **germinal membrane.** —**blastodermal, blastodermic,** *adj.*

blastodisc, blastodisk The disklike nonyolk area of the protoplasm surrounding the animal pole where cleavage occurs in a fertilized ovum containing a large amount of yolk, as in birds and reptiles. As cleavage continues the blastomeres form a convex structure, the blastula, which eventually develops into the embryo.

blastogenesis 1. Asexual reproduction by budding. 2. The theory of the transmission of hereditary characteristics by the germ plasm, as opposed to the theory of pangenesis. 3. The early development of the embryo during cleavage and formation of the germ layers. 4. The process of transforming small lymphocytes in tissue culture into large blastlike cells by exposure to phytohemagglutin or other substances, often for the purpose of inducing mitosis. —**blastogenetic,** *adj.*

blastogenic 1. Originating in the germ plasm. 2. Initiating tissue proliferation. 3. Relating to or characterized by blastogenesis.

blastogeny The early stages in ontogeny; the germ plasm history of an organism or species, which traces the history of the inherited characteristics.

blastokinin A globulin, secreted by the uterus in many mammals, that may stimulate and regulate the implantation process of the blastocyst in the uterine wall. Also called **uteroglobulin.**

blastolysis Destruction of a germ cell or blastoderm. —**blastolytic,** *adj.*

blastoma, *pl.* **blastomas, blastomata** A neoplasm of embryonic tissue developing from the blastema of an organ or tissue. A blastoma derived from a number of scattered cells is pluricentric and one arising from a single cell or group of cells is unicentric. Also called **blastocytoma.** —**blastomatous,** *adj.*

blastomatosis The development of many tumors derived from embryonic tissue.

blastomere One of a pair of cells that develops in the first mitotic division of the segmentation nucleus of a fertilized ovum. The two blastomeres divide and subdivide to form the morula in the first several days of pregnancy. —**blastomeric,** *adj.*

blastomerotomy The destruction or the

separation of blastomeres, either caused naturally or induced artificially. Also called **blastotomy.** —**blastomerotomic,** *adj.*

Blastomyces A genus of yeastlike fungus, usually including the species *B. dermatitidis,* which causes North American blastomycosis, and *Paracoccidioides brasiliensis,* which causes South American blastomycosis.

blastomycosis An infectious disease caused by a yeastlike fungus, *Blastomyces dermatitidis,* that usually affects only the skin but may invade the lungs, kidneys, central nervous system, and bones. The disease is most common in young men living in North America, particularly the southeastern United States, but outbreaks have occurred in Africa and Latin America. Skin infections often begin as small papules on the hand, face, neck, or other exposed areas where there has been a cut, bruise, or other injury and spread gradually and irregularly into surrounding areas. When the lungs are involved, X-ray films of the chest show tumors resembling cancer. The person usually has a cough, dyspnea, chest pain, chills, and a fever with heavy sweating. Diagnosis is made by identification of the disease organism in a culture of specimens from lesions. Treatment usually involves the administration of a fungicidal antibiotic, amphotericin B. Recovery usually begins within the first week of treatment. Also called **Gilchrist's disease.** See also **fungus, mycosis.**

blastopore In embryology: the invagination into a blastula that occurs in the process of the blastula becoming a gastrula.

blastoporic canal See **neurenteric canal.**

blastosphere See **blastocyst.** —**blastospheric,** *adj.*

blastotomy See **blastomerotomy.** —**blastotomic,** *adj.*

blastula See **blastocyst.**

-blastula A combining form meaning an 'early embryonic stage in the development of a fertilized egg': *coeloblastula, diblastula, steroblastula.*

blastulation The transformation of the morula into a blastocyst or blastula by the development of a central cavity, the blastocoele.

BLB mask *abbr* **Boothby-Lovelace-Bulbulian mask.**

bleb An accumulation of fluid under the skin, usually associated with lesions that are smaller than normal blisters. —**blebby,** *adj.*

bleed 1. To lose blood from the blood vessels of the body. The blood may flow externally, through an orifice or a break in the skin, or it may flow internally, into a cavity, an organ, or the spaces between the tissues. The color, quantity, and source of the blood are noted. 2. To cause blood to flow from a vein or an artery.

bleeder *Informal.* 1. A person who has hemophilia or any other vascular or hematologic condition associated with a tendency to hemorrhage. 2. A bleeding blood vessel, especially one cut during a surgical procedure.

bleeding The release of blood from the vascular system as a result of damage to or inadequacy of one or more blood vessels. See also **blood clotting.**

bleeding time The time required for blood to stop flowing from a tiny wound. Bleeding time may be measured by Duke, Ivy, or Template methods; the Template method is the most accurate and widely used. Normal bleeding time is 1 to 3 minutes for the Duke method, 1 to 7 minutes for the Ivy, and 2 to 8 minutes for the Template. Prolonged bleeding times most often result from uremia, a platelet function disorder, or ingestion of aspirin or other antiinflammatory medications. See also **hemostasis.**

blending inheritance The apparent fusion in the offspring of distinct, dissimilar characteristics of the parents, usually of a quantitative nature, as height, with segregation of the specific traits failing to appear in successive generations. This pre-Mendelian concept of inheritance is now explained in terms of multiple pairs of genes that have a cumulative effect. See also **polygene.**

blenn- See **blenno-.**

blenno-, blenn- A combining form meaning 'pertaining to mucus': *blennemesis, blennostasis, blennothorax.*

blennorrhea 1. Excessive discharge of mucus. See also **pharyngoconjunctival fever. 2.** Gonorrhea. Also called **blennorrhagia.**

bleomycin sulfate An antibiotic used in cancer chemotherapy.

blephar- See **blepharo-.**

blepharal Of or pertaining to the eyelids.

-blepharia A combining form meaning '(condition of the) eyelid': *ablepharia, atretoblepharia, macroblepharia.*

blepharitis An inflammatory condition of the lash follicles and Meibomian glands of the eyelids, characterized by swelling, redness, and crusts of dried mucus on the eyelids. **Ulcerative blepharitis** is caused by bacterial infection. **Nonulcerative blepharitis** may be caused by psoriasis, seborrhea, or an allergic response.

blepharo-, blephar- A combining form meaning 'pertaining to the eyelid or eyelash': *blepharochalasis, blepharal, blepharelosis.*

blepharoadenoma, *pl.* **blepharoadenomas, blepharoadenomata** A glandular epithelial tumor of the eyelid.

blepharoatheroma, *pl.* **blepharoatheromas, blepharoatheromata** A tumor of the eyelid.

blepharoncus A neoplasm of the eyelid.

blepharoplegia Paralysis of the eyelid.

-blepsia A combining form meaning '(condition of) sight': *acyanoblepsia, chionablepsia, hemiablepsia.* Also **-blepsy.**

-blepsy See **-blepsia.**

blight Any disease of plants caused by fungus.

blighted ovum A fertilized ovum that fails to develop. On X-ray or ultrasonic visualization it appears to be a fluid-filled cyst attached to the wall of the uterus. It may be empty, or it may contain amorphous parts. Many first trimester spontaneous abortions represent the expulsion of a blighted ovum.

blind fistula An abnormal passage with only one open end; the opening may be on the body surface or on or within an internal organ or structure. Also called **incomplete fistula.**

blind loop A redundant segment of intestine. Bacterial overgrowth occurs and may lead to malabsorption, obstruction, and necrosis. Blind loops may be inadvertently created by surgical procedures, as side-to-side ileotransverse colostomy.

blindness The inability to see.

blind spot 1. A normal gap in the visual field occurring when an image is focused on the space in the retina occupied by the optic disk. **2.** An abnormal gap in the visual field owing to a lesion on the retina or in the optic pathways or to hemorrhage or choroiditis, often perceived as light spots or flashes.

blister A vesicle or bulla.

bloat A swelling or filling with gas, as the distention of the abdomen from swallowing air or from intestinal gas.

block anesthesia See **conduction anesthesia.**

blocking 1. Preventing the transmission of a nerve impulse by the injection of an anesthetic. **2.** Interrupting an intracellular biosynthetic process, as by the injection of actinomycin D. **3.** Being unable to remember or involuntarily interrupting a train of thought or speech, usually owing to emotional or mental conflict. **4.** Repressing an idea or emotion to keep it from obtruding into the consciousness.

blocking antibody An antibody that fails to cross-link and cause agglutination. When such antibodies are present in high concentration, they tend to interfere with the action of other antibodies by occupying all of the antigenic sites. See also **antigen-antibody reaction, hapten.**

blood The liquid pumped by the heart through all of the arteries, veins, and capillaries. It consists of a clear yellow fluid, called plasma, and the formed elements, a series of different cell types, all with varying functions. The major function of the blood is to transport oxygen and nutrients to the cells and to remove from the cells carbon dioxide and other waste products for detoxification and elimination. The normal adult has a total blood volume of 7% to 8% of body weight. This is approximately equivalent to 70 ml/kg of body weight for men and about 65 ml/kg for women. It moves at a speed of about 30 cm/second, with a complete circulation time of 20 seconds. Compare **lymph.** See also **blood cell, erythrocyte, leukocyte, plasma, platelet.**

blood agar A culture medium consisting of blood and nutrient agar, used in bacteriology to cultivate certain microorganisms, including *Staphylococcus epidermidis, Diplococcus pneumoniae,* and *Clostridium perfringens.*

blood bank An organizational unit responsible for collecting, processing, and storing blood to be used for transfusion and other purposes.

BLOOD CLOT FORMATION

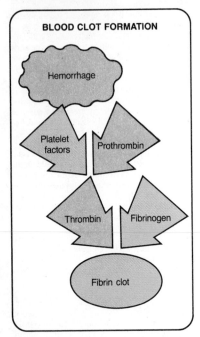

Hemorrhage

Platelet factors

Prothrombin

Thrombin

Fibrinogen

Fibrin clot

It is usually a subdivision of a laboratory in a hospital and is often charged with the responsibility for all serological testing. See also **bank blood, component therapy, transfusion.**

blood-brain barrier (BBB) An anatomical-physiological feature of the brain thought to consist of walls of capillaries in the central nervous system and surrounding glial membranes. The barrier separates the parenchyma of the central nervous system from blood. The blood-brain barrier functions in preventing or slowing the passage of various chemical compounds, radioactive ions, and disease-causing organisms, as viruses, from the blood into the central nervous system.

blood buffers A system of buffers, composed primarily of dissolved carbon dioxide and bicarbonate ions, that functions in maintaining the proper pH of the blood. See also **buffer, pH.**

blood cell Any one of the formed elements of the blood, including red cells (erythrocytes), white cells (leukocytes), and platelets (thrombocytes). Together they normally constitute about 50% of the total volume of the blood. See also **erythrocyte, leukocyte, platelet.**

blood clot A semisolid, gelatinous mass, the end result of the clotting process in blood. It ordinarily consists of red cells, white cells, and platelets enmeshed in an insoluble fibrin network. Compare **embolus, thrombus.** See also **blood clotting, fibrinogen.**

blood clotting The conversion of blood from a free-flowing liquid to a semisolid gel. Although it can occur within the intact blood vessel, the process usually starts with tissue dam-

age and exposure of the blood to air. Within seconds of injury to the vessel wall, platelets clump at the site. If normal amounts of calcium, platelets, and tissue factors are present, prothrombin will be converted to thrombin. Thrombin then acts as a catalyst for the conversion of fibrinogen to a mesh of insoluble fibrin, in which all of the formed elements are immobilized. Also called **blood coagulation.** Compare **hemostasis.** See also **anticoagulant.**

blood coagulation See **blood clotting.**

blood count *Nontechnical.* A computation of the number of cells per cubic millimeter of blood performed for a variety of diagnostic purposes. Approximately 4.5 and 5.0 million red cells per cubic millimeter are considered normal for women and men, respectively. Normally, leukocytes range between 5,000 and 10,000 cells per cubic millimeter. The relative number of the types of white cells is also important for diagnostic purposes and is reported as a percentage of the total white count. See also **anemia, differential white blood cell count, platelet.**

blood culture medium A liquid enrichment medium for the growth of bacteria in the diagnosis of blood infections. It contains a suspension of brain tissue in meat broth with dextrose, peptone, and citrate and has a pH of 7.4.

blood donor Anyone who donates blood to a blood bank or directly to another person. See also **blood bank, transfusion.**

blood dyscrasia A pathologic condition in which any of the constituents of the blood are abnormal or are present in abnormal quantity, as in leukemia or hemophilia.

blood fluke A parasitic flatworm of the class Trematoda, genus *Schistosoma,* including the species *S. haematobium, S. japonicum,* and *S. mansoni.* See also *Schistosoma,* **schistosomiasis.**

blood gas Gas dissolved in the liquid part of the blood. Blood gases include oxygen, carbon dioxide, and nitrogen.

blood gas determination An analysis of the pH of the blood and the concentration and pressure of oxygen, carbon dioxide, and hydrogen ion in the blood. It can be performed rapidly as an emergency procedure to assess acid-base balance and ventilatory status. See also **acid-base balance, acidosis, alkalosis, oxygenation, pH.**

blood glucose See **blood sugar.**

blood group The classification of blood based on the presence or absence of genetically determined antigens on the surface of the red cell. More than 14 different grouping systems have been described; their relative importance depends on their clinical significance in transfusion therapy. See also **ABO blood groups.**

blood island One of the clusters of mesodermal cells that proliferate on the outer surface of the embryonic yolk sac and give it a lumpy appearance. The outermost cells flatten into primitive endothelium; the inner cells develop primitive blood plasma and elaborate hemoglobin within their cytoplasm.

blood lavage The removal of toxic elements from the blood by the injection of serum into the veins.

blood patch See **epidural blood patch.**

blood plasma The liquid portion of the blood, free of its formed elements and particles. Plasma represents approximately 50% of the total volume of blood and contains glucose, proteins, amino acids, and other nutritive materials, urea and other excretory products, as well as hormones, enzymes, vitamins, and minerals. Compare **serum.** See also **blood, plasma protein, pooled plasma.**

blood poisoning See **septicemia.**

blood pressure (BP) The pressure exerted by the circulating volume of blood on the walls of the arteries, the veins, and the chambers of the heart. Overall blood pressure is maintained by the complex interaction of the homeostatic mechanisms of the body, moderated by the volume of the blood, the lumen of the arteries and arterioles, and the force of the cardiac contraction. Although varying with age and physical condition, normal blood pressure in the aorta and the large arteries of a healthy young adult is approximately 120 mmHg during systole and 80 mmHg in diastole. The pulse pressure is approximately 50 mmHg.

blood pump 1. A pump for regulating the flow of blood into a blood vessel during transfusion. 2. A component of a heart-lung machine that pumps the blood through the machine for oxygenation and then through the peripheral circulatory system of the body. See also **oxygenation.**

blood serum See **serum.**

blood substitute A substance used as a replacement for circulating blood or for extending its volume. Plasma, human serum albumin, packed red cells, platelets, leukocytes, and concentrates of clotting factors are often administered in place of whole blood transfusions in the treatment of various disorders. Substances that are sometimes used in solution to expand blood volume include dextran, hetastarch, albumin solutions, or plasma protein fraction. Perfluorocarbon emulsions that are being tested as blood substitutes are able to carry oxygen to tissues, have a long shelf-life without refrigeration, and do not induce antigen-antibody reactions.

blood sugar 1. One of a group of closely related substances, as glucose, fructose, and galactose, that are normal constituents of the blood and are essential for cellular metabolism. 2. *Nontechnical.* The concentration of glucose in the blood. It is represented in milligrams of glucose per deciliter of blood. See also **hyperglycemia, hypoglycemia.** Also called **blood glucose.**

blood test 1. Any test that determines something about the characteristics or properties of the blood.

blood transfusion The administration of whole blood or a component, such as packed red cells, to replace blood lost through trauma, surgery, or disease.

NORMAL BLOOD PRESSURE	
AGE	**AVERAGE READING**
Under 1 year	63 mean (using flush technique)
2 years	96/30
4 years	98/60
6 years	105/60
10 years	112/64
Adolescent	120/75
Adult	120/80

blood typing Identification of genetically determined antigens on the surface of the red blood cell, used to determine a person's blood group. Usually a blood bank procedure, it is the first step in testing donor's and recipient's blood to be used in transfusion and is followed by cross matching. See also **ABO blood groups, blood group, Rh factor, transfusion reaction.**

blood urea nitrogen (BUN) The amount of nitrogenous substance present in the blood as urea. BUN is a rough indicator of kidney function. It is elevated in kidney failure, shock, gastrointestinal bleeding, diabetes mellitus, and some tumors. BUN levels are decreased in liver disease, malnutrition, and normal pregnancy. See also **azotemia.**

blood vessel Any one of the network of tubes that carries blood. Kinds of blood vessels are **arteries, arterioles, capillaries, veins, venules.**

blood-warming coil A device constructed of coiled plastic tubing, used for warming reserve blood before massive transfusions, as those often required for patients who develop extensive gastrointestinal bleeding. Administration of cold blood in such transfusions may cause the patient to go into shock. The blood-warming coil is a prepackaged, sterile, single-use device. Compare **electric blood warmer.**

bloody show See **vaginal bleeding.**

blow-out fracture A fracture of the floor of the orbit caused by a blow that suddenly increases the intraocular pressure.

blue baby An infant born with cyanosis caused either by a congenital heart lesion, such as transposition of the great vessels or tetralogy of Fallot, or by incomplete expansion of the lungs (congenital atelectasis). Tetralogy of Fallot is the most common congenital cyanotic cardiac lesion. Congenital cyanotic heart lesions are diagnosed by cardiac catheterization, angiography, or echocardiography and are corrected surgically, preferably in early childhood. See also **congenital cardiac anomaly, tetralogy of Fallot.**

blue bloater See **chronic bronchitis.**

blue fever *Informal.* Rocky Mountain spotted fever, so named for the dark cyanotic discoloration of the skin following the initial rickettsial infection. See also **rickettsiosis, Rocky Mountain spotted fever, typhus.**

blue nevus A sharply circumscribed, usually benign, steel-blue skin nodule with a diameter between 2 and 7 mm. It is found on the face or upper extremities, grows very slowly, and persists throughout life. Nodular blue nevi found on the buttocks or in the sacrococcygeal region occasionally become malignant. Any sudden change in the size of such a lesion demands surgical attention and biopsy. The dark color is caused by large, densely packed melanocytes deep in the dermis of the nevus. Compare **melanoma.**

blue phlebitis See **phlegmasia cerulea dolens.**

blue spot **1.** One of a number of small greyish-blue spots that may appear near the armpits or around the groins of individuals infested with lice, as in pediculosis corporis and pediculosis pubis. These spots are usually less than 1 cm (½ inch) in diameter and are caused by a substance in the saliva of lice that converts bilirubin to biliverdin. Also called **macula cerulea.** **2.** One of a number of dark blue or mulberry-hued round or oval spots that may appear congenitally in the sacral regions of certain children under 5 years of age. They usually disappear spontaneously as the affected individual matures. Also called **Mongolian spot.**

blunt dissection A dissection performed by separating tissues along natural lines of cleavage, without cutting.

blunthook **1.** A sturdy hook-shaped bar used in obstetrics for traction between the abdomen and the thigh in cases of difficult breech deliveries. **2.** A hook-shaped device with a blunt end used in embryotomy.

blush A brief, diffuse erythema of the face and neck, commonly the result of dilatation of superficial small blood vessels in response to heat or sudden emotion.

B/M Symbol for black male, often used in the initial identifying statement in a patient record.

BM *abbr* **bowel movement.**

BMA *abbr* **British Medical Association.**

BMR *abbr* **basal metabolic rate.**

BOA *abbr* **born out of asepsis.**

board certification In medicine: a process in which an individual is tested in a medical specialty or subspecialty. Physicians are approved to practice after successfully completing requirements of specialty or subspecialty Boards. The various medical professional organizations provide board certification examinations. Successful candidates are called Fellows, such as Fellow of the American College of Surgeons (FACS). Board certification is required for professional practice in a hospital, including the admission of patients, the use of hospital resources, or the performance of certain diagnostic tests or surgery.

board certified In medicine: denoting a physician who has passed the certification examination administered by a medical specialty board and has been certified as a specialist in a particular field of medicine.

board eligible In medicine: denoting a physician who has completed the educational requirements necessary for eligibility to take the specialty board examinations.

board of health An administrative body acting on a municipal, county, state, provincial, or national level. The functions, powers, and responsibilities of boards of health vary with the locales. Each board is generally concerned with the recognition of the health needs of the people and the coordination of projects and resources to meet and identify these needs. Among the tasks of most boards of health are prevention of disease, health education, and implementation of laws pertaining to health.

Boas' test **1.** A test for hydrochloric acid in the contents of the stomach. **2.** A test for gastric motility in which a fasting patient drinks water which has been tinted green with chlorophyll solution. After 30 minutes, the contents of the stomach are aspirated and the amount of tinted water that has passed through the stomach is determined.

body **1.** The whole structure of an individual with all the organs. **2.** A cadaver or a corpse. **3.** The largest or the main part of any organ, as the body of the tibia or the body of the vastus lateralis. Also called **corpus, soma.**

body fluid A fluid contained in the three fluid compartments of the body, the blood plasma of the circulating blood, the interstitial fluid between the cells, and the cell fluid within the cells. Blood plasma and interstitial fluid make up the extracellular fluid; the cell fluid is the intracellular fluid. The chemical constituents of the fluids vary greatly; for example, sodium is present in large amounts in both compartments of the extracellular fluid but is nearly absent in the intracellular fluid; protein is present in the blood plasma and cell fluid, but not in the interstitial fluid.

body image A person's subjective concept of his physical appearance. The mental representation, which may be realistic or unrealistic, is constructed from self-observation, the reactions of others, and a complex interaction of attitudes, emotions, memories, fantasies, and experiences, both conscious and unconscious. A marked inability to conceptualize one's personal body characteristics may be caused by organic brain damage, as in autotopagnosia; by a physical disability, as the loss of a limb; or by psychological and emotional disturbances, as in anorexia nervosa.

body-image agnosia See **autotopagnosia.**

body jacket An orthopedic cast that encases the trunk of the body but does not extend over the cervical area; it may be equipped with shoulder straps. It is used to help immobilize the trunk for the healing of spinal injuries and scoliosis and for postoperative positioning and immobilization after spinal surgery.

body language A set of nonverbal signals, including body movements, postures, gestures, spatial positions, facial expressions, and bodily adornment, that give expression to various physical, mental, and emotional states.

body mechanics The field of physiology that studies muscular actions and the function of muscles in maintaining the posture of the body.

body movement Motion of all or part of the body, especially at a joint or joints. Some kinds of body movements are **abduction, adduction, extension, flexion, rotation.**

body odor A fetid smell associated with stale perspiration. Freshly secreted perspiration is odorless, but after exposure to the atmosphere and bacterial activity at the surface of the skin, chemical changes occur to produce the odor. Body odors also can be the result of discharges from a variety of skin conditions, including cancer, fungus, hemorrhoids, leukemia, and ulcers. See also **bromhidrosis.**

body of Retzius Any one of the masses of protoplasm containing pigment granules at the lower end of a hair cell of the organ of Corti in the internal ear.

body position Attitude or posture of the body. Some kinds of body position are **anatomical, decubitus, Fowler's position, prone, supine, Trendelenburg's position.**

body-righting reflex Any one of the neuromuscular responses to restore the body to its normal upright position when it has been displaced. The righting reflexes involve complicated mechanisms and processes associated with the structures of the internal ear, as the utricle, the saccule, the macula, and the semicircular canals. Also involved in the righting mechanism are receptors for the vestibular branch of the eighth cranial nerve. Any change in the position of the head produces a change in the pressure on the gelatinous membrane of the macula and causes tiny otoliths within the membrane to pull on hair cells, stimulating adjacent receptors of the vestibular nerve. The fibers of the nerve transmit impulses to the brain, producing a sense of position of the head by a sensation of change in the gravitational pull, activating muscles that tend to restore the body to its optimum position. Also activating righting reflexes are proprioceptors in muscles and tendons and visual nerve impulses. Interruption of the impulses associated with body-righting reflexes may disturb equilibrium and cause nausea and vomiting.

body stalk The elongated part of the embryo that is connected to the chorion. The stalk first extends from the posterior end of the embryo to the chorion but later moves to the midventral region and forms the lengthening umbilical cord. As the embryo develops and the amnion expands, the umbilical cord comes to enclose the body stalk and the yolk sac.

body surface area (BSA) See **surface area.**

body systems model In nursing education: a conceptual framework in which illness is studied in relation to the functional systems of the body, as the circulatory, nervous, gastrointestinal, and reproductive. In this model, nursing care is directed toward manipulating the patient's environment in such a way that the signs and symptoms of the health problem are alleviated. As the body systems model focuses on the disease rather than the patient, current educational programs tend to integrate it with other concepts that allow the nurse to approach the patient in a more holistic framework, recognizing the complexity of the external and internal agents that contribute to illness and to health.

body temperature The level of heat produced and sustained by the body processes. Variations and changes in body temperature are major indicators of disease and other abnormalities. Heat is generated within the body through metabolism of food and lost from the body surface through radiation, convection, and evaporation of perspiration. Heat production and loss are regulated and controlled in the hypothalamus and brain stem. Fever is usually a function of an increase in the generation of heat, but some abnormal conditions, as congestive heart failure, produce slight elevations of body temperature through impairment of the heat-loss function. Contributing to the failure to dissipate heat are reduced activity of the heart, lower rate of blood flow to the skin, and the insulating effect of edema. Diseases of the hypothalamus or interference with the other regulatory centers may produce abnormally low body temperatures. Normal adult body temperature, as measured orally, is 37°C (98.6°F). Oral temperatures ranging from 35.8°C (96.5°F) to 37.2°C (99°F) are consistent with good health, depending on the physical activity of the person, the ambient temperature, and the particular, normal body temperature for that person. Axillary temperature is usually 1°F lower than the oral temperature. Rectal temperatures may be 0.5° to 1°F higher than oral readings. Body temperature appears to vary 1° to 2°F throughout the day, with lows recorded early in the morning and peaks between 6 P.M. and 10 P.M. This diurnal variation may increase in range during a fever. While adult body temperature, normal and abnormal, tends to vary within a relatively narrow range, the temperatures of children respond more dramatically and rapidly to disease, changes in ambient temperature, and levels of physical activity.

Boeck's sarcoid See **sarcoidosis.**

boil A skin abscess. See **furuncle.**

boiling point The temperature at which a substance passes from the liquid to the gaseous state at a particular atmospheric pressure. See also **evaporation.**

bole Any of a variety of soft, friable clays of various colors, although usually red from iron oxide. They consist of hydrous silicate of aluminum, are used as pigments, and were once commonly used as absorbents and astringents. See also **kaolin.**

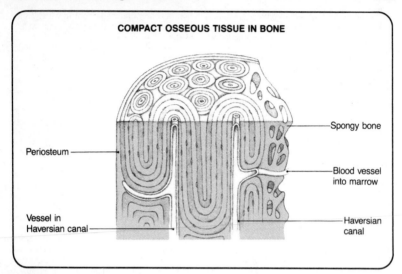

COMPACT OSSEOUS TISSUE IN BONE

Spongy bone

Periosteum

Blood vessel
into marrow

Vessel in
Haversian canal

Haversian
canal

Bolivian hemorrhagic fever An infectious disease caused by an arenavirus, generally transmitted from infected rodents to humans through contamination of food by rodent urine, though direct transmission between people has also been observed. After an incubation period of from 1 to 2 weeks, the patient experiences chills, fever, headache, muscle ache, anorexia, nausea, and vomiting. As the disease progresses, hypotension, dehydration, bradycardia, pulmonary edema, and internal hemorrhages may occur. The mortality may reach 30%; pulmonary edema is the most common cause of death. There is no specific therapy. Peritoneal dialysis is sometimes performed. Also called **Machupo.** See also **Argentine hemorrhagic fever, Lassa fever.**

bolus **1.** A dose of a medication or a contrast material, radioactive isotope, or other pharmaceutical preparation injected all at once intravenously. **2.** A large round preparation of medicinal material for oral ingestion, usually soft and not prepackaged. **3.** A round mass, specifically a masticated lump of food ready to be swallowed. Also called **alimentary bolus. 4.** See **bole.**

Bombay phenotype A rare genetic trait involving the phenotypic expression of the ABO blood groups. The gene for the H antigen, which in the usual dominant form of HH or Hh is responsible for the precursor necessary for the production of the A and B antigens, is homozygous recessive in individuals with this trait so that the expression of the A, B, and H antigens is suppressed. Cells of such individuals are phenotypically of blood type O even though they are genotype AB, and the serum contains anti-A, anti-B, and anti-H antigens. In such cases the offspring from two phenotypic O blood type parents may be blood type AB. The phenomenon is an example of the intricate interaction of linked genes in which one gene on a chromosome controls the expression or suppression of another gene that is not its allele. The trait is named for the city in which it was first reported. See also **ABO blood groups.**

bonding The attachment process that occurs between an infant and the parents, especially the mother, and is significant in the formation of affectionate ties that later influence both the physical and psychological development of the child. The process is reciprocal and is usually initiated immediately following birth by placing the nude infant on the mother's abdomen so that both the parents and child can see and touch one another and begin to interact. The newborn is in an alert, reactive state for about 30 minutes to 1 hour after birth and displays such behavior as crying, sucking, clinging, grasping, and following with the eyes, which in turn stimulates the expression of the parenting instincts. Especially important in initiating bonding is eye-to-eye contact, fondling of the infant, soothing talk, and other affectionate behavior that begins to create positive emotional ties. Another essential element is the amount of contact that occurs between parents and the newborn, especially crucial with premature and high-risk infants. New concepts in normal delivery procedures, especially the trend toward more natural childbirth, allowing the father to participate and even to assist in the delivery, and the parental involvement in the care of premature and ill newborns help to facilitate stronger parent-infant relationships. Also called **maternal-child attachment.** See also **maternal deprivation syndrome, maternal-infant bonding.**

bone **1.** The dense, hard, and slightly elastic connective tissue, comprising the 206 bones of the human skeleton. It is composed of compact osseous tissue surrounding spongy cancellous tissue permeated by many blood vessels and nerves and enclosed in membranous periosteum. Long bones contain yellow marrow in longitudinal cavities and red marrow in their articular ends. Red marrow also fills the cavities of the flat and the short bones, the bodies of the vertebrae, the cranial diploe, the sternum, and the ribs. Blood cells are produced in active red marrow. Osteocytes form bone tissue in concentric rings around an intricate Haversian system of interconnecting canals that accommodates blood vessels, lymphatic vessels, and nerve fibers. **2.** Any single element of the skeleton, as a rib, the sternum, or the femur. See also **connective tissue.**

bone cancer A skeletal malignancy occurring as a primary sarcomatous tumor in an area of rapid growth or, more frequently, as a metastasis from cancer elsewhere in the body. Primary bone tumors are comparatively rare, but the incidence peaks during adolescence, then decreases, and rises slowly after the age of 35. In adults bone cancer is strongly linked to exposure to ionizing radiation, especially in applying paints containing radium to watch dials. Paget's disease, hyperparathyroidism, chronic osteomyelitis, old bone infarcts, and fracture callosities increase the risk of bone tumors, but most osseous malignancies are metastatic lesions found most often in the spine or pelvis and less often in sites away from the trunk. Bone cancers progress rapidly but are often difficult to detect; pain that increases at night may be the only symptom. X-rays, radioisotopic scans, arteriography, and biopsies are diagnostic; alkaline phosphatase levels are elevated in osteoblastic tumors, and serum calcium and urinary calcium are increased in highly destructive lesions; but in other bone lesions, blood studies are often equivocal. The most common osseous malignancies are osteosarcomas, followed by chrondrosarcomas, fibrosarcomas, and Ewing's sarcoma. Surgical treatment consists of local resection of slow-growing tumors or amputation, including the joint above the tumor, if the lesion is particularly virulent and fast-growing. Radiotherapy may be administered preoperatively or as the primary form of treatment of radiosensitive tumors, as Ewing's sarcoma, reticulum cell sarcoma, and multiple myeloma. Chemotherapy is often effective in curing Ewing's tumors. The use of interferon and other forms of immunotherapy is experimental.

bone-cutting forceps A kind of forceps that has long handles, single or double joints, and heavy blades.

bone marrow Specialized, soft tissue filling the spaces in cancellous bone of the epiphyses. Fatty, **yellow marrow** is found in the compact bone of most adult epiphyses. **Red marrow** is found in many bones of infants and children and in the spongy bone of the proximal epiphyses of the humerus and femur and in the sternum, ribs, and vertical bodies of adults. It is composed of myeloid tissue and is essential in the manufacture and maturation of both red and white blood cells.

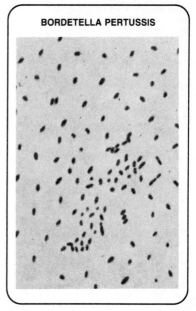

BORDETELLA PERTUSSIS

Bonnevie-Ullrich syndrome See **Turner's syndrome.**

booster injection The administration of an antigen, as a vaccine or toxoid, usually in a smaller amount than the original immunization, given to maintain the immune response at an appropriate level.

Boothby-Lovelace-Bulbulian (BLB) mask An apparatus for administering oxygen, consisting of a mask fitted with an inspiratory-expiratory valve and a rebreathing bag.

boracic acid See **boric acid.**

borax bath A medicated bath in which borax and glycerin are added to the water.

borborygmus, *pl.* **borborygmi** An audible abdominal sound produced by hyperactive intestinal peristalsis. Borborygmi are rumbling, gurgling, and tinkling noises heard in auscultation. Although increased intestinal activity may be noted in cases of gastroenteritis and diarrhea, true borborygmi are more intense and episodic. Borborygmi accompanied by vomiting, distension, and intestinal cramps suggest a mechanical obstruction of the small intestine.

borderline schizophrenia See **latent schizophrenia.**

Bordetella A genus of gram-negative coccobacilli, some species of which are pathogens of the respiratory tract of man, including *Bordetella bronchiseptica, B. parapertussis,* and *B. pertussis.* See also **parapertussis, pertussis.**

boric acid An ophthalmic and otic anti-infective agent. Also called **boracic acid, orthoboric acid.**

Bornholm disease A viral disease of epidemic potential that appears as a sudden pain in the area of the diaphragm, accompanied by malaise, nausea, headache, and intermittent fever. Also called **epidemic pleurodynia.**

born out of asepsis (BOA) In a hospital: a newborn infant that was not delivered in the usual place in an obstetric unit. Depending on the policy of the institution, a BOA-designated infant may have been born on the way to the hospital, in the hospital, on the way to the delivery suite, or in a labor room.

boron (B) A nonmetallic element, similar to aluminum. Its atomic number is 5; its atomic weight is 10.8. Elemental boron occurs in the form of dark crystals and as a greenish-yellow amorphous mass. Certain concentrations of this element are toxic to plant and animal life, but some plants need traces of boron for their normal growth. It is the characteristic element of boric acid, which is used chiefly as a dusting powder and ointment for minor skin disorders. Boric acid in solution was formerly extensively employed as an anti-infective and eyewash, but the high incidence of toxic reactions and fatalities associated with these preparations has greatly reduced their use.

Borrelia A genus of coarse, unevenly coiled, helical spirochetes, several species of which cause tickborne and louseborne relapsing fever. The organism is spread to offspring from generation to generation. This does not occur in lice. Many animals serve as reservoirs and hosts for *Borrelia.* The spirochete may be identified by microscopic examination of a smear of blood stained with Wright's stain; it is also easily inoculated onto culture media for bacterial culture and identification.

Bostock's catarrh See **hay fever.**

Boston exanthem An epidemic disease characterized by scattered, pale red maculopapules on the face, chest, and back, occasionally accompanied by small ulcerations on the tonsils and soft palate. There is little or no adenopathy, and the rash disappears spontaneously in 2 or 3 weeks. It is caused by echovirus 16 and requires no treatment. Compare **herpangina.**

bottle-feeding Feeding an infant or young child from a bottle with a rubber nipple on the end, sometimes called artificial feeding because it is done as a substitute for or supplement to breast-feeding.

bottle-mouth syndrome See **nursing-bottle caries.**

botulism An often fatal form of food poisoning caused by an endotoxin produced by the bacillus *Clostridium botulinum.* The toxin is ingested in food contaminated by *C. botulinum,* although it is not necessary for the live bacillus to be present if the toxin has been produced. In rare instances, the toxin may be introduced into the human body through a wound contaminated by the organism. Botulism differs from most other types of food poisoning in that it develops without gastric distress and may not occur for from 18 hours to 1 week after the contaminated food has been ingested. Botulism is characterized by a period of lassitude and fatigue followed by visual disturbances, as double vision, difficulty in focusing the eyes, and loss of ability of the pupil to accommodate to light. Muscles may become weak, and the patient often develops dysphagia. Nausea and vomiting occur in less than half the cases. Hospitalization is required and antitoxins are administered. Sedatives are given, mainly to relieve anxiety. Approximately two thirds of the cases of botulism are fatal, usually as a result of respiratory complications. For those who survive, recovery is slow. Most botulism occurs after eating improperly canned or cooked foods. See also *Clostridium.*

bouba See **yaws.**

Bouchard's node An abnormal cartilaginous or bony enlargement of a proximal interphalangeal joint of a finger, usually occurring in degenerative diseases of the joints. Compare **Heberden node.**

bougie A thin, cylindrical instrument made of rubber, waxed silk, or other flexible material for insertion into canals of the body in order to dilate, examine, or measure them.

-boulia See **-bulia.**

boulimia See **bulimia.**

bounding pulse A pulse that, on palpation, feels full and springlike owing to an increased thrust of cardiac contraction or an increased volume of circulating blood within the elastic structures of the vascular system.

bouquet fever See **dengue.**

Bourneville's disease See **tuberous sclerosis.**

boutonneuse fever An infectious disease caused by *Rickettsia conorii,* transmitted to humans through the bite of a tick. The onset of the disease is characterized by a lesion called a tache noire, or black spot, at the site of the infection, fever lasting from a few days to 2 weeks, and a papular erythematous rash that spreads over the body to include the skin of the palms and soles. Treatment usually involves administration of antibiotics. There is no prophylactic medication available, and prevention depends primarily upon avoiding ticks. The disease is similar to Rocky Mountain spotted fever and to other rickettsial diseases. It is prevalent in parts of Europe, Asia, Africa, and the Middle East. See also **rickettsiosis, Rocky Mountain spotted fever.**

Bowditch's law See **all or none law.**

bowel See **intestine.**

bowel elimination, alteration in: constipation. A nursing diagnosis accepted by the Fifth National Conference on the Classification of Nursing Diagnoses. The etiology of the condition is to be developed at a later conference. The defining characteristics include decreased activity level; decreased frequency of elimination; a hard, formed stool; a palpable rectal mass; a reported feeling of pressure or fullness in the rectum, and straining at stool. Abdominal pain, appetite impairment, back pain, headache, and interference with daily living may also be present. See also **nursing diagnosis.**

bowel elimination, alteration in: diar-

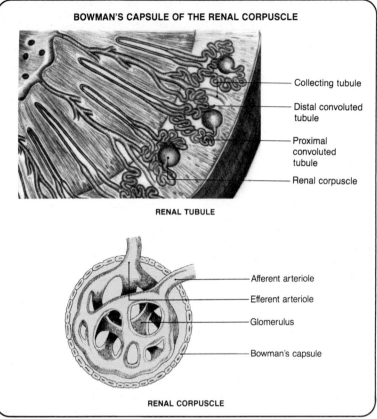

BOWMAN'S CAPSULE OF THE RENAL CORPUSCLE

— Collecting tubule

— Distal convoluted tubule

— Proximal convoluted tubule

— Renal corpuscle

RENAL TUBULE

— Afferent arteriole

— Efferent arteriole

— Glomerulus

— Bowman's capsule

RENAL CORPUSCLE

rhea A nursing diagnosis accepted by the Fifth National Conference on the Classification of Nursing Diagnoses. The etiology of the condition is to be developed at a later conference. The defining characteristics include abdominal pain, cramping, increased frequency of elimination, increased frequency of bowel sounds, loose or liquid stools, and urgency of defecation. A change in the color of the feces may also be noted. See also **nursing diagnosis.**

bowel elimination, alteration in: incontinence A nursing diagnosis accepted by the Fifth National Conference on the Classification of Nursing Diagnoses. The etiology of the condition is to be developed at a later conference. The defining characteristic of the problem is the involuntary passage of stool. See also **nursing diagnosis.**

bowel training A method of establishing regular evacuation by reflex conditioning, used in the treatment of fecal incontinence, impaction, chronic diarrhea, and autonomic hyperreflexia. In patients with autonomic hyperreflexia, distention of the rectum and bladder causes paroxysmal hypertension, restlessness, chills, diaphoresis, headache, elevated temperature, and

bradycardia.

Bowen's disease See **intraepidermal carcinoma.**

Bowen's precancerous dermatosis See **intraepidermal carcinoma.**

bowleg See **genu varum.**

Bowman's capsule The cup-shaped end of a renal tubule containing a glomerulus. Also called **glomerular capsule.**

box bath See **cabinet bath.**

boxer's fracture A fracture of one or more metacarpal bones, usually the fourth or the fifth, caused by punching a hard object. Such a fracture is often distal, angulated, and impacted.

Boyle's law In physics: a law stating that the product of the volume and pressure of a gas compressed at a constant temperature remains constant.

BP *abbr* **blood pressure.**

Br Symbol for **bromine.**

brace An orthopedic device, sometimes jointed, to support and hold any movable part of the body in the correct position to allow function, as a leg brace permits walking and standing. Compare **splint.**

brachi- A combining form meaning 'pertaining to the arm': *brachialgia, brachiation, brachiocyllosis.*

-brachia A combining form meaning an 'anatomical condition involving an arm': *acephalobrachia, diantebrachia, monobrachia.*

brachial Of or pertaining to the arm.

brachial artery The principal artery of the upper arm that is the continuation of the axillary artery. It has three branches and terminates at the bifurcation of its main trunk into the radial artery and the ulnar artery.

brachialis A muscle of the upper arm, covering the anterior part of the elbow joint and the distal half of the humerus. It arises from the anterior surface of the humerus and inserts, by a thick tendon, into the tuberosity of the coronoid process of the ulna. It is innervated by a branch of the musculocutaneous nerve, containing fibers from the fifth and the sixth cervical nerves, and functions to flex the forearm. Compare **biceps brachii, triceps brachii.**

brachial plexus A network of nerves in the neck, passing under the clavicle and into the axilla, originating in the fifth, sixth, seventh, and eighth cervical and first thoracic spinal nerves and innervating the muscles and skin of the chest, shoulders, and arms.

brachial plexus anesthesia An anesthetic block of the region innervated by the anterior divisions of the last four cervical and first thoracic nerves. The plexus extends from the transverse processes to the apex of the axilla, where the terminal nerves are formed. Because of the anatomy of the area, many approaches are possible, the axillary being most common; supraclavicular and interscalene are also used. Perivascular axillary block has the least incidence of complications, it being limited to minimal extravasation of blood. Other approaches may result in Horner's syndrome, phrenic nerve palsy, pneumothorax, recurrent laryngeal paralysis, sensory deficits, paresthesias, or hematomas. See also **regional anesthesia.**

brachial plexus paralysis See **Erb's palsy.**

brachial pulse The pulse of the brachial artery, palpated in the antecubital space.

brachiocephalic arteritis See **Takayasu's arteritis.**

brachiocephalic artery One of the three arteries that branch from the arch of the aorta, running about 5 cm (2 inches) from the level of the cranial border of the second right costal cartilage, ascending cranially, dorsally, and obliquely to the right, and dividing into the right common carotid and the right subclavian arteries.

brachiocephalic trunk See **brachiocephalic artery.**

brachioradialis The most superficial muscle on the radial side of the forearm. It arises from the lateral supracondylar ridge of the humerus and from the lateral intermuscular septum and inserts, by a flat tendon, into the styloid process of the radius. It is innervated by a branch of the radial nerve, which contains fibers from the fifth and the sixth cervical nerves, and it functions to flex the forearm.

brachioradialis reflex A deep tendon reflex, elicited by striking the lateral surface of the forearm proximal to the distal head of the radius, characterized by normal slight elbow flexion and forearm supination. It is accentuated by disease of the pyramidal tract above the level of the fifth cervical vertebra. See also **deep tendon reflex.**

-brachium A combining form meaning 'arm or armlike growth': *antibrachium, prebrachium, pontibrachium.*

brachy- A combining form meaning 'short': *brachycheilia, brachygnathia, brachyskelous.*

brachycephaly, brachycephalia, brachycephalism A congenital malformation of the skull in which premature closure of the coronal suture results in excessive lateral growth of the head, giving it a short, broad appearance with a cephalic index of between 81 and 85. See also **craniostenosis.** —**brachycephalic, brachycephalous,** *adj.*

Bradford frame A rectangular orthopedic frame made of pipes to which heavy movable straps of canvas are attached, running from side to side to support a patient in a prone or supine position. The straps can be removed to permit the patient to urinate or defecate while remaining immobile.

Bradford solid frame A rectangular orthopedic device of metal covered with canvas to aid in immobilization, especially of children in traction. The Bradford solid frame provides support for the entire body and is especially appropriate for patients who are under 5 years of age, hyperactive, or mentally retarded. The main purpose of the device is to assist in maintaining proper immobilization, positioning, and alignment by controlling movement. The Bradford solid frame is not placed directly on a bed but elevated at both ends by plywood blocks or by other suitable devices. It is most often used with Bryant traction but never with balanced suspension traction, cervical traction, cervical tongs, or certain other kinds of traction.

Bradford split frame A rectangular orthopedic device of metal covered with two separate pieces of canvas fastened at both ends of the frame. Used especially in pediatrics to aid in the immobilization of children in traction, it is divided in the middle by a large opening designed to accommodate the excretory functions of an incontinent patient in a hip spica cast. The division also allows for the upper and lower extremities of the patient to be elevated separately and for the maintenance of a clean and dry cast.

Bradley method A method of psychophysical preparation for childbirth developed by Robert Bradley, MD, comprising education about the physiology of childbirth, exercise and nutrition during pregnancy, and techniques of breathing and relaxation for control and comfort during labor and delivery. The father is extensively involved in the classes and acts as the mother's coach during labor. The first stage of labor is divided into two parts. During the latent

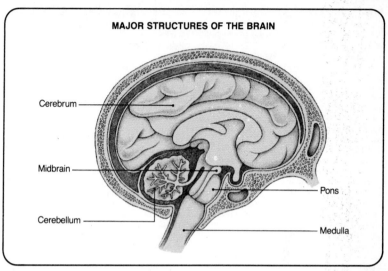

MAJOR STRUCTURES OF THE BRAIN

Cerebrum

Midbrain

Cerebellum

Pons

Medulla

phase, the woman is encouraged to carry on her normal activities until she feels the need to concentrate on the contractions. During the active phase, the uterine cervix dilates from about 5 cm (2 inches) to 10 cm (4 inches), the contractions occur every 1½ to 3 minutes and last from 40 to 90 seconds, the interval between contractions tends to decrease, and the length and intensity of the contractions tend to increase. The father helps the mother to relax by repeating reminders to relax the various parts of her body, by massaging and touching her as he has learned she finds relaxing, and by arranging and rearranging pillows to support her in a lounge chair position. During contractions, she breathes deeply and slowly in through the nose and out through the mouth. Her abdominal wall lifts with each inhalation and falls with each exhalation. She may close her eyes and try to visualize the baby's head pressing against the cervix, causing it to dilate. She is encouraged by the close support of the father, the midwife or obstetrician, and the nurse. During the second stage of labor, the uterine cervix is fully dilated, the contractions are strong and expulsive, occurring every 1½ to 2 minutes and lasting 60 to 90 seconds. The mother, feeling the urge to bear down and push, allows her knees to fall away from each other without forcibly drawing her thighs against her abdomen as in other methods. She breathes in and out deeply once or twice, waiting for the contraction to build in strength, then she bears down while holding her breath. She pushes as hard as necessary to relieve the pressure or urgency of the contraction. The father may count seconds for her so that she can push for 10 or for 15 seconds, as necessary. He also checks to see that her legs and buttocks are relaxed, and he reminds her to keep her perineum relaxed, to concentrate, and to let the baby out. As the baby is born, with the mother still in a semisitting po-

sition, the infant is placed on her abdomen and then nursed. The mother is given a glass of orange juice and often walks back to her room with the father and the baby. Among the advantages of the method are its simplicity, the involvement of the father, and the realistic approach to the efforts and discomfort of labor. Also called **husband-coached childbirth.** Compare **Lamaze method, Read method.**

brady- A combining form meaning 'slow, dull': *bradyacusia, bradydiastalsis, bradyphagia.*

bradycardia An abnormal circulatory condition in which the myocardium contracts steadily but at a rate of less than 60 contractions a minute. The heart normally slows during sleep, and, in some physically fit people, the pulse may be quite slow. Pathologic bradycardia may be symptomatic of a brain tumor, digitalis toxicity, or vagotonus. Cardiac output is decreased, causing faintness, dizziness, chest pain, and, eventually, syncope and circulatory collapse. Treatment may include administration of atropine, implantation of a pacemaker, or reduction of digitalis dosage.

bradykinesia An abnormal condition characterized by slowness of all voluntary movement and speech, as caused by parkinsonism, other extrapyramidal disorders, and certain tranquilizers.

bradypnea Abnormally slow but regular respiration. Also called oligopnea. See also **respiratory rate hypopnea.**

Braille A system of printing for the blind consisting of raised dots or points that can be read by touch.

brain The portion of the central nervous system contained within the cranium. It consists of the cerebrum, cerebellum, pons, medulla, and midbrain. Specialized cells in its mass of convoluted gray or white tissue coordinate and regulate the functions of the central nervous system.

brain concussion   A violent jarring, shaking, or other blunt, nonpenetrating injury to the brain caused by a sudden change in momentum of the head. Characteristically, after a mild concussion there may be a transient loss of consciousness followed, on awakening, by a headache. Severe concussion may cause prolonged unconsciousness and disruption of certain vital functions of the brain stem, as respiration and vasomotor stability. Treatment after concussion consists principally of obtaining history of trauma and observing for signs of intracranial bleeding. Also called **concussion.**

brain death   An irreversible form of unconsciousness characterized by a complete loss of brain function while the heart continues to beat. The legal definition of this condition varies from state to state. The usual clinical criteria for brain death include the absence of reflex activity, movements, and respiration. The pupils are dilated and fixed. As hypothermia, anesthesia, poisoning, or drug intoxication may cause deep physiologic depression that resembles brain death, a diagnosis of brain death requires that the electrical activity of the brain be evaluated and shown to be absent on two electroencephalograms performed 12 to 24 hours apart. Also called **irreversible coma.** Compare **coma, sleep, stupor.**

brain electrical activity map (BEAM)   A topographic map of the brain created by a computer that is able to respond to the electrical potentials evoked in the brain by a flash of light. Potentials recorded at 4-millisecond intervals are converted into a many-colored map of the brain showing them to be positive or negative. The waves may be observed traveling through the brain. If the wave is disordered, blocked, too small, or too large, there may be a tumor or other lesion causing the abnormal pattern.

brain fever   *Informal.* Any inflammation of the brain tissues or meninges. See also **encephalitis.**

brain scan   A diagnostic procedure employing radioisotope imaging techniques to localize and identify intracranial masses, lesions, tumors, or infarcts. Radioisotopes are injected intravenously to circulate to the brain where they accumulate in abnormal tissue. The radioisotopes are traced and photographed by a scintillator, or scanner, and the size and location of the abnormality are determined. The nature and rate of accumulation of radioisotopes in pathologic tissue in some cases are diagnostic of a particular lesion. Compare **computerized axial tomography.** See also **isotope, radioisotope.**

brain stem   The portion of the brain comprising the medulla oblongata, the pons, and the mesencephalon. It performs motor, sensory, and reflex functions and contains the corticospinal and the reticulospinal tracts. The 12 pairs of cranial nerves from the brain arise mostly from the brain stem. Compare **medulla oblongata, mesencephalon, pons.**

brain stem auditory evoked potential (BAEP)   The most reliable evoked potential for predicting nerve damage during surgery in the auditory nerve region. A clicking sound is made and the EEG waves from the auditory area of the patient's brain are observed. Cessation or absence of electrical activity may indicate damage or destruction.

brain tumor   A neoplasm of the intracranial portion of the central nervous system that is usually invasive but does not spread beyond the cerebrospinal axis. Brain tumors, which are not rare, cause significant morbidity and mortality, but increasing numbers are successfully treated. Intracranial tumors in children are usually the result of a developmental defect. In adults 20% to 40% of malignancies in the brain are metastatic lesions from cancers in the breast, lung, gastrointestinal tract, kidney, or any site of a malignant melanoma. The etiology of primary brain tumors is not known. Symptoms of a brain tumor are often those of increased intracranial pressure, as headache, nausea, vomiting, papilledema, lethargy, and disorientation. Various localizing signs also occur, as loss of vision in the eye on the side of an occipital neoplasm. Diagnostic measures include visual field and funduscopic examinations, skull X-rays, electroencephalography, cerebral angiography, brain scanning, computerized axial tomography, and spinal fluid studies. Lumbar puncture may not be performed if increased intracranial pressure is obvious. A broad spectrum of tumors may be found in the brain, but gliomas, chiefly astrocytomas, are the most common malignancies. Rapidly growing medulloblastomas often occur in children. Benign meningiomas are the only intracranial neoplasms more common in women than in men. Craniopharyngiomas, generally found in children and young adults, are benign but impinge on critical structures and are difficult to remove. Schwannomas most often arise from the eighth cranial nerve and cause deafness; but they are generally benign. Surgery is the initial treatment for most primary tumors of the brain. Radiotherapy is indicated for inoperable lesions, medulloblastomas, tumors with multiple foci, and as postoperative treatment of residual tumor tissue. Beams of neutrons and high energy pi-mesons currently show promise in the treatment of highly malignant brain lesions. The blood-brain barrier impedes the effect of some antineoplastic agents but responses are obtained in some cases treated with procarbazine and various nitrosoureas administered alone or with vincristine. Compare **spinal cord tumor.**

bran bath   A bath in which bran has been boiled in the water, used for the relief of skin irritation.

branched chain ketoaciduria   See **maple syrup urine disease.**

branched tubular gland   One of the many multicellular glands with one excretory duct from two or more tube-shaped secretory branches, as some of the gastric glands.

branchial fistula   A congenital, abnormal passage from the pharynx to the external surface

ANATOMY OF THE BREAST

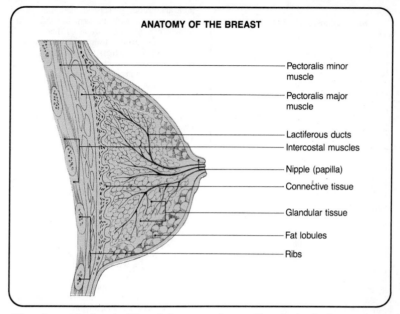

- Pectoralis minor muscle
- Pectoralis major muscle
- Lactiferous ducts
- Intercostal muscles
- Nipple (papilla)
- Connective tissue
- Glandular tissue
- Fat lobules
- Ribs

of the neck, resulting from the failure of a branchial cleft to close during fetal development. Introduction of a sound into a branchial fistula may cause pallor and arrhythmic pounding of the heart. Also called **cervical fistula.**

brand name See **trade name.**

brassfounder's ague See **metal fume fever.**

brassy eye See **chalkitis.**

Braun's canal See **neurenteric canal.**

Braxton-Hicks contraction Irregular tightening of the pregnant uterus that begins in the first trimester and increases in frequency, duration, and intensity as pregnancy progresses. Contractility of uterine muscle increases in pregnancy. Near term, strong Braxton-Hicks contractions are often difficult to distinguish from the contractions of true labor. Also called false labor.

Brazilian trypanosomiasis See **Chagas' disease.**

breach of contract The failure to perform as promised or agreed in a contract. The breach may be complete or partial and may occur by repudiation, by failure to recognize the contract, or by prevention or hindrance of performance.

breach of duty 1. The failure to perform an act required by law. 2. The performance of an act in an unlawful way.

breakbone fever See **dengue.**

breast 1. The anterior aspect of the chest. 2. A mammary gland.

breast cancer A malignant neoplastic disease of breast tissue, the most common malignancy in women in the United States. The incidence increases exponentially with age from the third to the fifth decade and reaches a second peak at age 65, suggesting that breast cancer in premenopausal women may be related to ovarian hormonal function and in postmenopausal patients to adrenal function. Based on the great prevalence of breast cancer in affluent countries, especially in high socioeconomic groups, it is thought that a high fat diet may be a causative factor, but the relationship is unproven and the etiology is unknown. Risk factors include a family history of breast cancer, nulliparity, exposure to ionizing radiation, early menarche, late menopause, obesity, diabetes, hypertension, chronic cystic disease of the breast, and, possibly, postmenopausal estrogen therapy. Women who are over 40 when they bear their first child and patients with malignancies in other body sites also have an increased risk of developing breast cancer. Initial symptoms, detected in most cases by self-examination, include a small painless lump, thick or dimpled skin, or nipple retraction. The diagnosis may be established by a careful physical examination, mammography, and cytologic examination of tumor cells obtained by biopsy. Tumors are more common in the left than in the right breast and in the upper and outer quadrant than in the other quadrants. Metastasis through the lymphatic system to axillary lymph nodes and to bone, lung, brain, and liver is common, but there is evidence that primary carcinomas of the breast may exist in multiple sites and that tumor cells may enter the blood stream directly without passing through lymph nodes. Surgical treatment, depending on the assessment of the tumor, may be a radical, modified radical, or simple mastectomy, with dissection of axillary nodes, or a lumpectomy. Postoperative radiotherapy, chemotherapy, or

BREAST-FEEDING POSITIONS

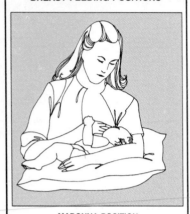

MADONNA POSITION

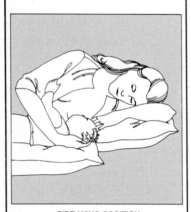

SIDE-LYING POSITION

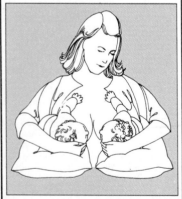

FOOTBALL POSITION

both are usually prescribed. Less than 1% of breast cancers occur in men, but those with Klinefelter's syndrome are at 60 times greater risk. See also **lumpectomy, mastectomy.**

breast examination A process in which the breasts and their accessory structures are observed and palpated in assessing the presence of changes or abnormalities that could indicate malignant disease. The breasts are observed with the patient sitting with her arms at her sides; sitting with her arms over her head, back straight; leaning forward; and, finally, sitting upright, as she contracts the pectoral muscles. The breasts are observed for symmetry of shape and size and for surface characteristics, including moles or nevi, hyperpigmentation, retraction or dimpling, edema, abnormal distribution of hair, focal vascularity, or lesions. With the patient still sitting, the axillary nodes and the supraclavicular and subclavicular areas are palpated. With the patient lying down on her back, each breast is shifted medially, and the glandular area in each is palpated with the flat of the fingers of a hand in concentric circles or in a pattern like the spokes of a wheel, from the periphery inward. The areolar areas, the nipples, and the tail of Spence in the upper outer quadrant extending toward the axilla are then palpated. See also **self-breast examination.**

breast-feeding Suckling or nursing. **1.** Giving an infant milk from the breast. **2.** Taking milk from the breast. See **breast milk, lactation.**

breast milk Human milk, the ideal food for most infants. It is easily digested, clean, and warm. It confers some immunities (bronchiolitis and gastroenteritis are rare in breast-fed children) and promotes emotional bonding between mother and child. Infants fed breast milk are less likely to become obese or to develop dental malocclusions. Breast-feeding encourages postpartum uterine involution and slows the natural return of the menses, providing a measure of contraception.

breast milk jaundice Jaundice and hyperbilirubinemia in breast-fed infants that occur in the first weeks of life as a result of a metabolite in the mother's milk that inhibits the infant's ability to conjugate bilirubin to protein for excretion. Breast milk jaundice usually occurs after the 5th day of life and peaks toward the end of the 2nd or 3rd week. Serum bilirubin levels usually exceed 5 mg/100 ml but rarely reach dangerous levels of 20 mg/100 ml, at which kernicterus may develop. The infant seems normal and healthy but skin and sclera are jaundiced. Also called neonatal jaundice.

breast pump A device for withdrawing milk from the breast.

breast self-examination (BSE) See **self-breast examination.**

breathing See **respiration.**

breathing pattern: ineffective A nursing diagnosis accepted by the Fifth National Conference on the Classification of Nursing Diagnoses. The etiology of the condition includes

ABNORMAL BREATH SOUNDS

TYPE	LOCATION	CAUSE	DESCRIPTION
Rales	All lung fields. Heard in lung bases first with pulmonary edema, usually during inspiratory phase	Air passing through moisture, especially in the small airways and alveoli	Light crackling, popping, nonmusical; can be further classified by pitch: high, medium, or low
Rhonchi	In larger airways, usually during expiratory phase	Fluid or secretions in the large airways or narrowing of large airways	Coarse rattling, usually louder and lower pitched than rales; can be described as sonorous, bubbling, moaning, musical, sibilant, and rumbly
Wheezes	All lung fields	Narrowed airways	Creaking, groaning; always high-pitched, musical squeaks
Pleural friction rub	Anterolateral lung field, on both inspiration and expiration (with the patient in an upright position)	Inflamed parietal and visceral pleural linings rubbing together	Superficial squeaking or grating

neuromuscular impairment, pain, musculoskeletal impairment, impairment of perception or cognition, anxiety, decreased energy, and fatigue. The defining characteristics of the problem include dyspnea, shortness of breath, tachypnea, fremitus, abnormal concentrations of arterial blood gases, cyanosis, cough, nasal flaring, change in depth of respiration, pursed-lip breathing or prolonged expiratory phase, increased anteroposterior diameter of the chest, use of accessory muscles of breathing, and altered excursion of the chest wall with respiration. See also **nursing diagnosis.**

breathing tube A device inserted into the trachea through the mouth or nose to assure a patent airway for adequate respiration during artificial or assisted ventilation. See also **extubation, intubation.**

breathlessness See **dyspnea.**

breath sound The sound of air and carbon dioxide passing in and out of the respiratory system as heard with a stethoscope. Vesicular and tracheal breath sounds are normal. Decreased breath sounds may indicate an obstruction of an airway, collapse of a portion or all of a lung, thickening of the pleurae of the lungs, emphysema, or other chronic obstructive lung disease.

breech birth Parturition in which the feet, knees, or buttocks emerge first. Breech birth is often hazardous: the body may deliver easily but the head may become trapped by an incompletely dilated cervix because a neonate's head is usually larger than the body. See also **assisted breech, version and extraction.**

breech extraction An obstetrical operation in which a neonate being born feet or buttocks first is grasped before any part of the trunk is born and delivered by traction. Compare **assisted breech.**

breech presentation Intrauterine position of the fetus in which the buttocks or feet present, occurring in approximately 3% of labors. Kinds of breech presentation are **complete breech, footling breech, frank breech.** Compare **vertex presentation.** See also **breech birth.**

bregma The junction of the coronal and sagittal sutures on the top of the skull. —**bregmatic,** *adj.*

Brenner tumor An uncommon, benign ovarian neoplasm consisting of nests or cords of epithelial cells containing glycogen that are enclosed in fibrous connective tissue. The tumor may be solid or cystic and is sometimes difficult to distinguish from certain granulosa-theca cell neoplasms.

brepho- A combining form meaning 'pertaining to an embryo, fetus, or newborn infant': *brephoplastic, brephopolysarcia, brephotrophic.*

bretylium tosylate An antiarrhythmic agent.

brevi- A combining form meaning 'short': *brevicollis, breviflexor, breviradiate.*

brewer's yeast A preparation containing the dried pulverized cells of a yeast, as *Saccharomyces cerevisiae*, that is used as a leavening agent and as a dietary supplement. It is one of the best sources of the B complex vitamins and of many minerals and is also a high grade of protein. Brewer's yeast may protect against toxicity of large doses of vitamin D, is used to prevent constipation, and is a good source of enzyme-producing agent.

bridge of Varolius See **pons.**

bridging **1.** A nursing technique of positioning a patient so that bony prominences are free of pressure on the mattress by using pads, bolsters of foam rubber, or pillows to distribute body weight over a larger surface. **2.** A nursing technique for supporting a part of the body, as the testicles in treating orchitis using a Bellevue bridge made of a towel or other material.

brief psychotherapy In psychiatry: treatment directed toward the active resolution of personality or behavioral problems rather than toward the speculative analysis of the unconscious. It usually concentrates on a specific problem or symptom and is limited to a specified number of sessions with the therapist.

Bright's disease A kidney disease, especially glomerulonephritis.

Brill-Symmer's disease See **giant follicular lymphoma.**

Brill-Zinsser disease A mild form of typhus that recurs in a person who appears to have completely recovered from a severe case of the disease. Some rickettsiae remain in the body after the symptoms of the disease abate, causing the recurrence of symptoms, especially when stress, illness, or malnutrition weaken the person. Treatment with antibiotics may eradicate the organism. See also **endemic typhus, epidemic typhus, rickettsiosis, typhus.**

Briquet's syndrome See **somatization disorder.**

Brissaud's dwarf A person affected with infantile myxedema in which short stature is associated with hypothyroidism.

British antilewisite (BAL) A heavy metal antagonist. Also called **dimercaprol.**

British Medical Association (BMA) A national professional organization of physicians in the United Kingdom.

British Pharmacopoeia The official British reference work setting forth standards of strength and purity of medications and containing directions for their preparation in order to ensure that the same prescription written by different doctors and filled by different pharmacists will contain exactly the same ingredients in the same proportions.

brittle diabetes A chronic, difficult to control disease of carbohydrate metabolism, characterized by inexplicable oscillations between hypoglycemia and ketoacidosis. See also **diabetes mellitus.**

broad beta disease A familial type of hyperlipoproteinemia in which a lipoprotein, high in cholesterol and triglycerides, accumulates in the blood. The condition, which affects males in their 20s and females in their 30s and 40s, is characterized by yellowish nodules (xanthomas) on the elbows and knees, peripheral vascular disease, and elevated serum cholesterol levels. People with this disease are at risk of developing early coronary disease. Therapy includes dietary measures to reduce weight and serum lipids. See also **hyperlipoproteinemia.**

broad ligament A folded sheet of peritoneum draped over the uterine tubes, the uterus, and the ovaries. It extends from the sides of uterus to the sidewalls of the pelvis, dividing the pelvis from side to side and creating the vesicouterine fossa and pouch in front of the uterus and the rectouterine fossa and pouch behind it. Also called **ligamentum latum uteri.**

Broca's area An area involved in speech production, situated on the inferior frontal gyrus of the brain.

Brodie's abscess A form of osteomyelitis consisting of an indolent staphylococcal infection of bone, usually in the metaphysis of a long bone of a child, characterized by a necrotic cavity surrounded by dense granulation tissue. See also **osteomyelitis.**

Brodmann's areas The 47 different areas of the cerebral cortex that are associated with specific neurologic functions and distinguished by different cellular components. Compare **motor area.** See also **cerebral cortex.**

brom-, bromo- A combining form meaning 'odor, stench': *bromacetone, bromhidrosis.*

bromelains An orally administered enzyme used to treat internal traumatic injuries.

bromhidrosis An abnormal condition in which the apocrine sweat has an unpleasant odor. The odor is usually caused by bacterial decomposition of perspiration on the skin. Treatment includes frequent bathing, changing of socks and underclothes, and the use of deodorants, antibacterial soaps, and dusting powders. Also called **body odor.**

bromide **1.** A compound in which the negative element is bromine. **2.** A bromine salt used to treat major motor and myoclonic seizures.

bromine (Br) A toxic, red-brown, liquid element of the halogen group. Its atomic number is 35; its atomic weight is 79.909. Bromine is used in industry, in photography, in the manufacture of organic chemicals and fuels, and in medications. Bromine gives off a red vapor that is extremely irritating to the eyes and the respiratory tract. Liquid bromine is irritating to the skin; bromates used as neutralizers in cold wave products are toxic if ingested. Bromides are binary compounds of bromine. See also **bromide.**

bromo- See **brom-.**

bromocriptine mesylate A drug used to treat hyperprolactinemia.

bromoderma An acneiform, bullous, or nodular skin rash, occurring as a hypersensitivity reaction to ingested bromides.

brompheniramine maleate An alkylamine antihistamine.

Brompton's cocktail An analgesic solution containing alcohol, morphine, methadone or heroin, cocaine, and, in some cases, a phenethiazine. The cocktail is administered in the control of pain in the terminally ill patient. Given frequently in small doses, it may relieve pain for many months. It was developed at the Brompton Hospital in England. Also called Brompton's mixture.

Bromsulphalein (BSP) test A trade name for sulfobromophthalein, a dye prepared for use in a highly sensitive, nonspecific test that measures the ability of liver cells to remove the sulfobromophthalein from the blood. The test is rarely indicated because it may cause severe allergic reactions and cannot indicate specific liver dysfunction. See also **sulfobromophthalein.**

bronch- A combining form meaning 'pertaining to the bronchus': *bronchiectasis, bronchiotetany, bronchodilation.*

bronchial breath sound An abnormal sound heard with a stethoscope over the lungs, indicating consolidation owing to pneumonia or compression. Expiration and inspiration produce loud, high-pitched sounds of equal duration.

bronchial fremitus A vibration that can be palpated or auscultated on the chest wall over a bronchus congested by secretions that rattle as the air passes during respiration.

bronchial hyperreactivity An abnormal respiratory condition characterized by reflex bronchospasm in response to histamine or a cholinergic drug. It is a universal feature of asthma and is used in the differential diagnosis of asthma and heart disease. An asthmatic person experiences episodes of bronchospasm in response to the cholinergic effect of endogenous histamine and to exposure via inhalation of histamine or a cholinergic drug like methacholine in testing for asthma.

bronchial tree An anatomical complex of the bronchi and the bronchial tubes. The bronchi branch from the trachea and the bronchial tubes branch from the bronchi. The right bronchus is wider and shorter than the left bronchus, and it diverges less abruptly from the trachea. The right bronchus branches into three subsidiary bronchi, one passing to each of the three lobes that comprise the right lung. The left bronchus is smaller in diameter but about twice as long as the right bronchus and passes inferior to the pulmonary artery before branching into the bronchi for the inferior and the superior lobes of the left lung.

bronchiectasis An abnormal condition of the bronchial tree, characterized by irreversible dilatation and destruction of the bronchial walls. The condition is sometimes congenital, but is more often a result of bronchial infection or of obstruction by a tumor or an aspirated foreign body. Symptoms of bronchiectasis include a constant cough productive of copious purulent sputum, hemoptysis, chronic sinusitis, clubbing of fingers, and persistent moist, coarse rales. Some of the complications of bronchiectasis are pneumonia, lung abscess, empyema, brain abscess, and amyloidosis. Treatment includes frequent postural drainage, antibiotics, and, rarely, surgical resection of the affected part of the lungs.

bronchiolar carcinoma See **alveolar cell carcinoma.**

bronchiole A small airway of the respiratory system extending from the bronchi into the lobes of the lung. There are two divisions of bronchioles: the terminal bronchioles pass inspired air from the bronchi to the respiratory bronchioles and expired waste gases from the respiratory bronchioles to the bronchi. The respiratory bronchioles function similarly, allowing the exchange of air and waste gases between the alveolar ducts and the terminal bronchioles. —**bronchiolar,** *adj.*

bronchiolitis An acute viral infection of the lower respiratory tract that occurs primarily in infants aged 2 to 12 months, characterized by expiratory wheezing, respiratory distress, and obstruction at the level of the bronchioles. The most common causative agents are the respiratory syncytial viruses (RSV) and the parainfluenza viruses. *Mycoplasma pneumoniae,* the rhinoviruses, the enteroviruses, and measles virus are less common etiologic agents. Transmission occurs by infection with airborne particles or by contact with infected secretions. The focus of care is to promote rest and to conserve the child's energy by reducing anxiety and apprehension; to increase the ease of breathing with humidity and oxygen as needed; to aid in changing position for comfort; and to induce drainage of secretions or to suction when necessary. Fever is usually controlled by the cool atmosphere of the mist tent and by administering antipyretics as needed. Frequent changing of clothing and bed linen is often necessary in a mist environment to reduce chilling. Vital signs and breath sounds are continuously monitored to detect early signs of respiratory distress. Children with bacterial infections are isolated to prevent cross-contamination.

bronchitis An acute or chronic inflammation of the mucous membranes of the tracheobronchial tree. Acute bronchitis is characterized by a productive cough, fever, hypertrophy of mucus-secreting structures, and back pain. Caused by the spread of upper respiratory viral infections to the bronchi, it is often observed with or following childhood infections, such as measles, whooping cough, diphtheria, and typhoid fever. Treatment includes bedrest, aspirin, expectorants, and appropriate antibiotic therapy. Chronic bronchitis is distinguished by an excessive secretion of mucus in the bronchi with a productive cough for at least 3 consecutive months in at least 2 successive years. Additional symptoms are frequent chest infections, cyanosis, hypoxemia, hypercapnia, and a marked tendency for the development of cor pulmonale and respiratory failure. Causes of chronic bronchitis include cigarette smoking, air pollution, chronic infections, and abnormal physical development of the bronchi that distorts the structures sufficiently to interfere with bronchial drainage. Most common in adults, it is often a complication of cystic fibrosis in children. Treatment includes the cessation of cigarette smoking, avoidance of other potentially toxic airway irritants, the use of expectorants, and postural drainage. Currently, prophylactic antibiotics, steroids, and desensitization therapy are not recommended.

bronchodilator A substance, especially a drug, that relaxes the smooth muscle of the bronchioles to improve ventilation to the lungs. Pharmacologic bronchodilators are prescribed to improve aeration in asthma, bronchiectasis, bronchitis, and emphysema. Commonly used bronchodilators include ephedrine, isoproterenol, theophyllin, and the various derivatives and combinations of these drugs. Beclomethasone and triamcinolone are available in aerosol form. The adverse effects of bronchodilators vary, depending on the particular class of the bronchodilating drug. In general, bronchodilators are given with caution to people who have impaired cardiac function. Nervousness, irritability, gastritis, or palpitations of the heart may occur.

bronchofibroscopy See fiberoptic bronchoscopy.

bronchogenic carcinoma One of the more than 90% of malignant lung tumors that originate in bronchi. Lesions, usually the result of cigarette smoking, may cause coughing and wheezing, fatigue, chest tightness, aching joints, and, in the late stages, bloody sputum, clubbing of the fingers, weight loss, and pleural effusion. Diagnosis is made by bronchoscopy, sputum cytology, lymph node biopsy, and radioisotope scanning procedures, but exploratory surgery may be required. About 45% of the tumors are squamous cell or epidermoid carcinomas, 33% are oat cell carcinomas, and 15% to 20% are adenocarcinomas. Surgery is the most effective treatment, but approximately 50% of cases are advanced and inoperable when first seen. Palliative treatment includes radiotherapy and chemotherapy.

bronchopneumonia An acute inflammation of the lungs and bronchioles, characterized by chills, fever, high pulse and respiratory rates, bronchial breathing, cough with purulent bloody sputum, severe chest pain, and abdominal distension. The disease is usually a result of a spread of bacterial infection from the upper respiratory tract to the lower respiratory tract, caused by *Mycoplasma pneumoniae, Staphylococcus pyogenes,* or *Streptococcus pneumoniae.* Atypical forms of bronchopneumonia may occur in viral and rickettsial infections. The most common cause in infancy is the respiratory syncytial virus. The condition results in pleural effusion, empyema, lung abscess, peripheral thrombophlebitis, respiratory failure, congestive heart failure, and jaundice. Treatment includes an antibiotic, often penicillin or ampicillin, oxygen therapy, supportive measures to keep the bronchi clear of secretions, and relief of pleural pain. Compare **aspiration pneu-**

monia, eosinophilic pneumonia, interstitial pneumonia.

bronchopulmonary Of or pertaining to the bronchi and the lungs.

bronchoscope A rigid or flexible tube for visual examination of the bronchi. The fiberoptic bronchoscope contains fibers that carry light down the tube and project an enlarged image up the tube to the viewer. The bronchoscope is used to examine the bronchi, to secure a specimen for biopsy or culture, or to aspirate a foreign body from the respiratory tract. See also **fiberoptic bronchoscopy. —bronchoscopic,** *adj.*

bronchoscopy The visual examination of the tracheobronchial tree, using the standard rigid, tubular metal bronchoscope or the narrower, flexible fiberoptic bronchoscope, which has greatly expanded the diagnostic and therapeutic applications of the procedure. In addition to visualization, the procedure can be used for suctioning, for obtaining a biopsy and fluid or sputum for examination, for removal of foreign bodies, and for diagnosing such conditions as localized atelectasis, bronchial obstruction, lung abscess, and tracheal extubation. See also **bronchoscope. —bronchoscopic,** *adj.*

bronchospasm An abnormal contraction of the smooth muscle of the bronchi, resulting in an acute narrowing and obstruction of the respiratory airway. A cough with generalized wheezing usually indicates this condition. Bronchospasm is a chief characteristic of asthma and bronchitis. Treatment includes the use of active bronchodilators, catecholamines, corticosteroids, or methylxanthines, and of preventive drugs, as cromolyn sodium. See also **asthma, bronchitis.**

bronchus, *pl.* **bronchi** Any one of several large air passages in the lungs through which pass inspired air and exhaled waste gases. Each bronchus has a wall consisting of three layers. The outermost layer is made of dense fibrous tissue, reinforced with cartilage. The middle layer is a network of smooth muscle. The innermost layer consists of ciliated mucous membrane. Kinds of bronchi are **lobar bronchus, primary bronchus, secondary bronchus, segmental bronchus.** See also **arteriole, bronchiole. —bronchial,** *adj.*

Brooke formula A formula developed at the Brooke Army Medical Center for calculating fluid and electrolyte replacement in burns. Some others include the **Evans formula,** the **MGM formula,** and the **Parkland** or **Baxter formula.**

Brown-Séquard's treatment See **organotherapy.**

Brown-Séquard syndrome A traumatic neurologic disorder resulting from compression of one side of the spinal cord, above the 10th thoracic vertebrae, characterized by spastic paralysis on the injured side of the body, loss of postural sense, and loss of the senses of pain and heat on the uninjured side of the body.

brown spider A poisonous arachnid, also

known as the brown recluse or violin spider, found in both North and South America. The venom from its bite usually creates a blister surrounded by concentric white and red circles. This so-called bull's-eye appearance is helpful in distinguishing it from other spider bites. The wound ordinarily ulcerates and sometimes becomes infected. Pain, nausea, fever, and chills are common, but the reaction is usually self-limiting.

Brucella abortus See abortus fever.

brucellosis A disease caused by any of several species of the gram-negative coccobacillus *Brucella*. Brucellosis is most prevalent in rural areas among farmers, veterinarians, meat packers, slaughterhouse workers, and livestock producers. Primarily a disease of animals (including cattle, pigs, and goats), humans usually acquire it by ingesting contaminated milk or milk products or through a break in the skin. It is characterized by fever, chills, sweating, malaise, and weakness. The fever often comes in waves, rising in the evening and subsiding during the day, occurring at intervals separated by periods of remission. Other signs and symptoms may include anorexia and weight loss, headache, muscle and joint pain, and an enlarged spleen. In some patients, the disease is acute; more often, it is chronic, recurring over a period of months or years. Although brucellosis itself is rarely fatal, treatment is important because such serious complications as pneumonia, meningitis, and encephalitis can develop. Tetracycline plus streptomycin is the treatment of choice; bed rest is also important. Also called **Cyprus fever, Malta fever, Mediterranean fever, rock fever, undulant fever.** See also abortus fever.

Bruch's disease See Marseilles fever.

Brudzinski's sign An involuntary flexion of the knee when the neck is passively flexed, seen in patients with meningitis.

bruise See ecchymosis.

bruit An abnormal sound or murmur heard while auscultating an organ or gland, as the liver or thyroid. The specific character of the bruit, its location, and when it occurs in a cycle of other sounds are all of diagnostic importance.

Brushfield's spots Pinpoint, white or light yellow spots on the iris of a child with Down's syndrome. Occasionally they are seen in normal infants, but their absence may help to rule out Down's syndrome.

Bruton's agammaglobulinemia A sex-linked, inherited condition characterized by the absence of gamma globulin in the blood. Patients with this syndrome are deficient in antibodies and susceptible to repeated infections. Compare **agammaglobulinemia.**

bruxism The compulsive, unconscious grinding of the teeth, especially during sleep or as a mechanism for the release of tension during periods of extreme stress in the waking hours. Also called **bruxomania.**

bruxomania See bruxism.

bry- A combining form meaning 'full of life': *bryocyte, bryocytole, bryocytic.*

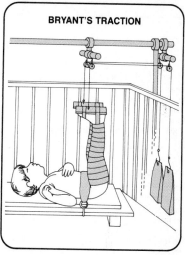

BRYANT'S TRACTION

Bryant's traction An orthopedic mechanism used only with infants to immobilize both lower extremities in the treatment of a fractured femur or in the correction of the congenital dislocation of the hip. This mechanism consists of a traction frame supporting weights, connected by ropes that run through pulleys to traction foot plates worn by the infant involved. The traction pull elevates the lower extremities to a vertical position with the patient supine, the trunk and the lower extremities forming a right angle. The weight applied to the traction mechanism is usually less than 15.9 kg (35 lb) Compare **Buck's traction.**

BSA *abbr* **body surface area.** See surface area.

BSE *abbr* **breast self-examination.** See self-breast examination.

BSN *abbr* **bachelor of science in nursing.**

BSP *abbr* **Bromsulphalein (test).**

BTPD *abbr* body temperature, ambient pressure, dry.

BTPS *abbr* body temperature, ambient pressure, saturated (with water vapor).

buba See yaws.

bubbling rale An abnormal chest sound characteristic of moisture moving in the lungs. Compare **amphoric breath sound, atelectatic rale, dry rale.**

bubo *pl.* **buboes** A greatly enlarged, inflamed lymph node usually in the axilla or groin, associated with such diseases as chancroid, lymphogranuloma venereum, and plague. Treatment includes specific antibiotic therapy, application of moist heat, and sometimes, incision and drainage.

bubonic plague The most common form of plague, characterized by painful buboes in the axilla, groin, or neck; fever often rising to 41°C (106°F), prostration with a rapid, thready pulse; hypotension; delirium; and bleeding into the skin from the superficial blood vessels. The

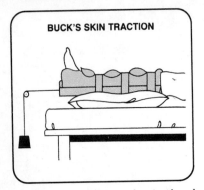

BUCK'S SKIN TRACTION

symptoms are caused by an endotoxin released by a bacillus, *Yersinia pestis*, introduced into the body by the bite of a rat flea that has bitten an infected rat. Inoculation with plague vaccine confers partial immunity; infection provides lifetime immunity. Treatment includes antibiotics, supportive nursing care, surgical drainage of buboes, isolation, and stringent precautions against spread of the disease. Conditions favor a plague epidemic when a large infected rat population lives with a large nonimmune human population in a damp, warm climate. Improved sanitary conditions and the eradication of rats and rat fleas may prevent outbreaks of the disease. Killing the rats and not the fleas promotes human infection. Also called **Black Death, black plague**. Compare **pneumonic plague, septicemic plague**. See also **bubo**.

bucca-　See **bucco-**.

buccal　Of or pertaining to the inside of the cheek, the surface of a tooth, or the gum next to the cheek.

buccal administration of medication Oral administration of a drug, usually in the form of a tablet, by placing it between the cheek and the teeth or gum until it dissolves.

buccal fat pad　A fat pad in the cheek under the subcutaneous layer of the skin, over the buccinator. It is particularly prominent in infants and is often called a sucking pad.

bucci-　See **bucco-**.

buccinator　The main muscle of the cheek, one of the 12 muscles of the mouth. It arises from the maxilla above and the mandible below, inserting in the lips; its superficial surface is covered by the buccopharyngeal fascia and the buccal fat pad. Its deep part is pierced by the duct of the parotid gland opposite the second molar tooth. The buccinator, innervated by buccal branches of the facial nerve, compresses the cheek, acting as an important accessory muscle of mastication by holding food under the teeth.

bucco-, bucca-, bucci-　A combining form meaning 'pertaining to the cheek': *buccocervical, buccodistal, buccogingival*.

buccopharyngeal　Of or pertaining to the cheek and the pharynx or to the mouth and the pharynx.

bucket-handle fracture　A fracture that produces a tear in a semilunar cartilage along the medial side.

bucking　*Informal.* **1.** Gagging on an endotracheal tube. **2.** Involuntarily resisting insufflation by a positive pressure respirator.

Buck's skin traction　An orthopedic procedure that applies traction to the lower extremity, with the hips and the knees extended. It is used to help in the treatment of hip and knee contractures, in postoperative positioning and immobilization, and in disease processes of the hip and the knee. This type of traction may be unilateral, involving one leg, or bilateral, involving both legs.

Buck's traction　One of the most common orthopedic mechanisms by which pull is exerted on the lower extremity with a system of ropes, weights, and pulleys. Buck's traction, which may be unilateral or bilateral, is used to immobilize, position, and align the lower extremity in the treatment of contractures and diseases of the hip and knee. The mechanism commonly consists of a metal bar extending from a frame at the foot of the patient's bed, supporting traction weights connected by a rope passing through a pulley to a cast or a splint around the affected body structure. Compare **Bryant's traction**.

buclizine hydrochloride　An antiemetic agent.

Budd-Chiari syndrome　A disorder of hepatic circulation, marked by venous obstruction, which leads to liver enlargement, ascites, extensive development of collateral vessels, and severe portal hypertension. Also called **Chiari's syndrome, Rokitansky's disease**.

budding　A type of asexual reproduction in which the cell produces a budlike projection containing chromatin that eventually separates from the parent and develops into an independent organism. It is a common form of reproduction in the lower animals and plants, as sponges, yeasts, and molds.

Buerger's disease　See **thromboangiitis obliterans**.

buffer　A substance or group of substances that absorbs hydrogen ions when a base is added to the system and that releases hydrogen ions upon the addition of an acid. Buffers minimize changes of pH in a chemical system. Among the functions carried out by buffer systems in the body are maintenance of the acid-base balance of the blood and maintenance of the proper pH in kidney tubules. See also **blood buffers, pH**.

buffy coat transfusion　See **granulocyte transfusion**.

bulbar conjunctiva　See **conjunctiva**.

bulbar paralysis　A degenerative neurologic condition characterized by progressive paralysis of the lips, tongue, mouth, pharynx, and larynx. The condition occurs most commonly in people over 50 years of age, in multiple sclerosis, and in amyotrophic lateral sclerosis.

bulbourethral gland　One of two small glands located on each side of the prostate, draining to the urethra. Bulbourethral glands secrete a fluid component of the seminal fluid.

BUNDLE OF HIS IN THE HEART'S CONDUCTION SYSTEM

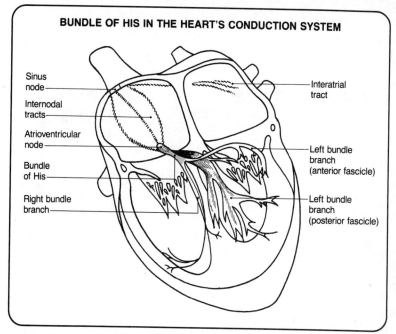

Sinus node
Internodal tracts
Atrioventricular node
Bundle of His
Right bundle branch

Interatrial tract
Left bundle branch (anterior fascicle)
Left bundle branch (posterior fascicle)

bulb syringe A blunt-tipped, flexible syringe usually made of rubber or plastic. Bulb syringes are used primarily for irrigating external orifices, as the auditory canal.

bulbus oculi See **eye**.

-bulia A combining form meaning '(condition of the) will': *abulia, parabulia, hyperbulia.* Also **-boulia.**

bulimia, boulimia An insatiable craving for food, often resulting in episodes of continous eating followed by periods of depression and self-deprivation. —**bulemic,** *n., adj.*

bulk See **dietary fiber.**

bulk cathartic A cathartic that acts by softening and increasing the mass of fecal material in the bowel. Bulk cathartics contain a hydrophilic agent like methylcellulose or psyllium seed.

bulla, *pl.* **bullae** A thin-walled blister of the skin or mucous membranes greater than 1 cm (½ inch) in diameter containing clear, serous fluid. Compare **vesicle.** —**bullous,** *adj.*

bulldog forceps Short, spring forceps for clamping an artery or vein for hemostasis. The jaws may be padded to avoid injury to vascular tissue.

bullet forceps A kind of forceps that has thin, curved, serrated blades designed for extracting a foreign object, as a bullet, from the base of a puncture wound.

bullous myringitis An inflammatory condition of the ear, characterized by fluid-filled vesicles on the tympanic membrane and the sudden onset of severe pain in the ear. The condition often occurs with bacterial otitis media. Treatment includes the administration of antibiotics,

analgesics, and surgical draining of the vesicles. See also **otitis media.**

BUN *abbr* **blood urea nitrogen.**

-bund A combining form meaning 'prone to' something specified: *furibund, moribund.*

bundle branch block An abnormality in the conduction of the cardiac impulse through the fibers of the bundle of His. If many fibers are affected, the heart rate is reduced; the pacemaker function is relegated to the ventricles and peripheral perfusion is impaired. The condition may occur following myocardial infarction, in ischemic heart disease, or in certain degenerative neurological diseases. An artificial pacemaker may be used to maintain adequate cardiac function.

bundle of His A band of fibers in the myocardium through which the cardiac impulse is transmitted from the atrioventricular (AV) node to the ventricles. The bundle of His begins at the AV node, follows the membranous septum of the heart and divides to form the left bundle branch and the right bundle branch. The right bundle branch continues toward the apex and spreads throughout the right ventricle. The left bundle branch penetrates the fibrous septum and spreads throughout the left ventricle. The ends of both bundle branches within the ventricles are composed of Purkinje fibers. Also called **atrioventricular bundle, His bundle.**

bunion An abnormal enlargement of the joint at the base of the great toe. It is caused by inflammation of the bursa, usually as a result of chronic irritation and pressure from poorly fitted shoes. It is characterized by soreness, swell-

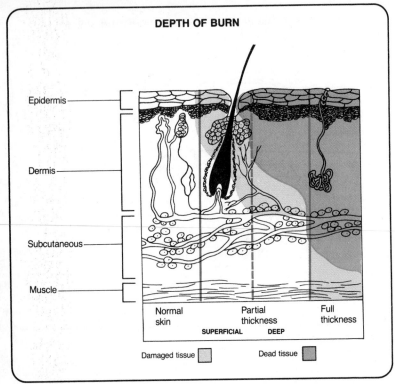

DEPTH OF BURN

Epidermis

Dermis

Subcutaneous

Muscle

| Normal skin | Partial thickness | Full thickness |

SUPERFICIAL   DEEP

Damaged tissue ☐   Dead tissue ☐

ing, thickening of the skin, and lateral displacement of the great toe.

Bunyamwera arbovirus One of a group of arthropod-borne viruses that infect man, carried by mosquitoes from rodent hosts causing a mild disease characterized by headache, weakness, low-grade fever, myalgia, and a rash. Convalescence is prolonged. Outbreaks have occurred in North America, South America, Africa, and Europe.

buphthalmos See **congenital glaucoma.**

bupivacaine hydrochloride An amide local anesthetic agent.

Burkitt's lymphoma A malignant neoplasm composed of undifferentiated lymphoreticular cells that form a large osteolytic lesion in the jaw or, in children, an abdominal mass. The tumor, which is seen chiefly in Central Africa, is characteristically a gray-white mass with a brainlike consistency, sometimes containing areas of hemorrhage and necrosis. Central nervous system involvement often occurs, and other organs may be affected. The Epstein-Barr virus (EBV), a herpesvirus, may be the cause of this lymphoma. Chemotherapy usually results in rapid shrinking of the osteolytic lesion and complete cure of the disease. Also called **African lymphoma, Burkitt's tumor.**

Burkitt's tumor See **Burkitt's lymphoma.**

burn Any injury to tissues of the body caused by heat, electricity, chemicals, or gases in which the extent of the injury is determined by the amount of exposure of the cell to the agent and to the nature of the agent. The treatment of burns includes pain relief, careful asepsis, prevention of infection, maintenance of the balance in the body of fluids and electrolytes, and good nutrition. Severe burns of any etiology may cause shock, which is treated before the wound. See also **chemical burn, electrocution, thermal burn.**

burn center A health-care facility that is designed to care for patients who have been severely burned. A network of burn centers has been established throughout the United States and Canada that provide sophisticated advanced techniques of care for burn victims.

burnout The condition of having no energy left to care, resulting from chronic, unrelieved job-related stress and characterized by physical and emotional exhaustion and, sometimes, by physical illness. The professional loses concern for the clients; no longer has positive feelings, sympathy, or respect for patients; and often develops cynical, dehumanized perceptions of people, labeling them in a derogatory manner. Causes of burnout peculiar to the nursing profession often include stressful, even dangerous, work environments; lack of support; lack of respectful relationships within the health-care team; low pay scales, with a broadening gulf between nurse's and physician's salaries; shift changes and long work hours with overtime causing shifts to last from 12 to 16 hours; general understaffing of hospitals; pressure from the responsibility of providing continuous high-level care over long periods of time; frustration and disillusionment resulting from the difference between job realities and job expectations; and sexism.

burn therapy The management of a patient burned by flames, a hot liquid, explosives, chemicals, or electric current. Burn therapy aims to prevent infection and further destruction of soft tissue, cartilage, or bone; to promote cosmetic healing; and to retain body function. Therapy depends on the type and extent of burns and ranges from simple cool-water immersion or soaks for minor burns to hydrotherapy, debridement, and skin grafts for severe burns.

Burow's solution A liquid preparation containing aluminum sulfate, acetic acid, precipitated calcium carbonate, and water, used as a topical astringent, antiseptic, and antipyretic for a wide variety of skin disorders. Also called **aluminum acetate solution.**

burr cell One of a variety of cells or cell fragments that have spicules, or tiny projections on the surface. Compare **acanthocyte.** Also called echinocyte

burrowing flea See *Tunga penetrans.*

bursa, *pl.* **bursae** **1.** A fibrous sac between certain tendons and the bones beneath them. Lined with a synovial membrane that secretes synovial fluid, the bursa acts as a small cushion that allows the tendon as it contracts and relaxes to move over the bone. See also **adventitious bursa, bursa of Achilles, olecranon bursa, prepatellar bursa. 2.** A sac or closed cavity. See also **omental bursa, pharyngeal bursa.**

bursa of Achilles Bursa separating the tendon of Achilles and the calcaneus.

bursitis An inflammation of the bursa, the connective tissue structure surrounding a joint. Bursitis may be precipitated by arthritis, infection, injury, or excessive or traumatic exercise or effort. The chief symptom is severe pain of the affected joint, particularly on movement. The goals of treatment for bursitis include the control of pain and the maintenance of joint motion. A frequent measure used for the relief of acute pain is an intrabursal injection of an adrenocorticosteroid, followed by procaine infusion. Other commonly used treatments are analgesics, antiinflammatory agents, cold, and immobilization of the inflamed site. After the inflammatory process has subsided, heat may be helpful. In chronic cases surgery may be required to remove calcium deposits. Some kinds of bursitis are **housemaid's knee, miner's elbow, weaver's bottom.** See also **rheumatism.**

bursting fracture Any fracture that disperses multiple bone fragments, usually at or near the end of a bone.

Buschke's disease See **cryptococcosis.**

busulfan An alkylating agent used in cancer chemotherapy.

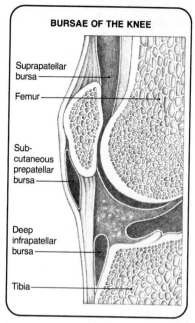

BURSAE OF THE KNEE

Suprapatellar bursa

Femur

Subcutaneous prepatellar bursa

Deep infrapatellar bursa

Tibia

butabarbital, b. sodium Barbiturate sedative-hypnotic agents.

butanoic acid See **butyric acid.**

butanol extractable iodine (BEI) Iodine in the blood that can be separated from plasma proteins by extraction with the organic solvent butanol. Measurement of BEI indicates the level of thyroid hormone in the blood.

butaperazine maleate An antipsychotic.

butorphanol tartrate A narcotic analgesic with narcotic antagonist activity.

butterfly bandage A narrow adhesive strip with broader winglike ends used to approximate the edges of a superficial wound and to hold the sides together as they heal. It is used in place of a suture in certain cases. Also called **butterfly.**

butterfly fracture A bone break in which the center fragment contained by two cracks forms a triangle.

butterfly rash An erythematous, scaling eruption of both cheeks joined by a narrow band of rash across the nose. It is seen in lupus erythematosus, rosacea, and seborrheic dermatitis.

buttermilk **1.** The slightly sour-tasting liquid residue remaining after the solids in cream have been churned into butter. It is nearly fat free and, except for a relatively low content of vitamin A, is nutritionally comparable with whole milk. **2.** Cultured milk made by the addition of certain organisms to fat-free milk.

buttock See **nates.**

buttonhole A small slitlike hole in the wall of a structure or a cavity of the body.

buttonhole fracture Any fracture caused by the perforation of a bone by a bullet.

button suture A technique in suturing in

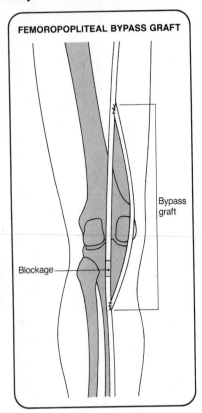

FEMOROPOPLITEAL BYPASS GRAFT

Bypass graft

Blockage

which the ends of the suture material are passed through buttons on the surface of the skin and tied. It is used to prevent the suture from cutting through the skin.

butyl A hydrocarbon radical, the compounds of which are obtained from petroleum. Butyl compounds, some of which are toxic and irritating, are used in a variety of industrial and medical applications, including anesthesia.

butyl alcohol A clear liquid derived from beet molasses.

butyr- A combining form meaning 'pertaining to butter': *butyraceous, butyric, butyrinase.*

butyric acid A fatty acid occurring in rancid butter, feces, urine, perspiration, and, in trace amounts, in the spleen and blood. Butyric acid is used in the preparation of flavorings, emulsifying agents, and pharmaceuticals. Also called **butanoic acid, propylformic acid.**

butyric fermentation The conversion to butyric acid of carbohydrates.

butyrophenone One of a small group of major tranquilizers used in treating psychosis, to decrease the choreic symptoms of Huntington's chorea and the tics and coprolalia of Gilles de la Tourette's syndrome, and as an adjunct in neuroleptic anesthesia. The two principal butyrophenones are haloperidol and droperidol. Butyrophenones are pharmacologically and clinically similar to the phenothiazines.

BWS *abbr* **battered woman syndrome.**

bypass Any one of various surgical procedures to divert the flow of blood or other natural fluids from normal anatomical courses. A bypass may be either temporary or permanent. Bypass surgery is commonly performed in the treatment of cardiac and gastrointestinal disorders.

byssinosis An occupational respiratory disease characterized by shortness of breath, coughing, and wheezing. The condition is an allergic reaction to dust or fungi in cotton, flax, and hemp fibers. The symptoms are typically more pronounced on Mondays when the workers return after a weekend break and are reversible in the early stages. Prolonged exposure of many years results in chronic airway obstruction, bronchitis, and emphysema with fibrosis, leading to respiratory failure, pulmonary hypertension, and cor pulmonale. Treatment is symptomatic for the irreversible changes of emphysema and chronic bronchitis. Compare **pneumoconiosis.**

byte In data processing: series of adjacent binary digits that a computer processes as a unit. Compare **bit.**

c Symbol for capillary blood.

c *abbr* **curie.**

C Symbol for concentration of gas in the blood.

Ca Symbol for **calcium.**

cabinet bath A bath in which the patient is enclosed in a cabinet, except for the head, and heated by hot air or radiant heat. Also called **box bath.**

Cabot's splint A metal splint worn behind the thigh and leg for support.

cac- See **caco-.**

cacao **1.** Cocoa. **2.** The substance *Theobroma cacao.* **3.** The seeds of *Theobroma cacao.*

cacesthesia Any morbid feeling or disordered sensibility. —**cacesthetic,** *adj.*

cachet Any lenticular edible capsule that encloses a dose of medicine.

cachexia General ill health and malnutrition, marked by weakness and emaciation, usually associated with serious disease, as tuberculosis or cancer. Also called cachexy. —**cachectic,** *adj.*

cachinnation An excessive laughter for no apparent reason, often part of the behavioral pattern in schizophrenia. —**cachinnate,** *v.*

caco-, cac- A combining form meaning 'ill, bad': *cacodontia, cacogeusia, cacosmia.*

cacodemonomania An abnormal mental condition in which the patient claims to be possessed by an evil spirit.

cacophony, *pl.* **cacophonies** A harsh or discordant sound or a mixture of confused, different sounds. —**cacophonic, cacophonous,** *adj.*

cadaver A dead body used for dissection and study.

cadmium (Cd) A metallic, bluish-white element that resembles tin. Its atomic number is 48; its atomic weight is 112.40. Cadmium has many uses in industry and was formerly used in medications. Such medications have been replaced by less toxic drugs. Cadmium bromide, used in engraving, lithography, and photography, can cause severe gastrointestinal symptoms if swallowed. Cadmium may also cause poisoning by inhalation of fumes from metal-plating processes or by the ingestion of acidic foods prepared and stored in cadmium-lined containers, as lemonade in certain metal cans.

cadmium poisoning Poisoning resulting from the inhalation of cadmium in fumes created by welding, smelting, or other industrial processes involving solder. The effects may include vomiting, dyspnea, headache, prostration, pulmonary edema, and, possibly, years later, cancer. Treatment for acute poisoning includes intravenous fluids and hyperbaric oxygen.

caduceus The wand of the god Hermes or Mercury, used as the symbol for the U.S. Army Medical Corps. It is represented as a staff with two serpents coiled around it and is often confused with the staff of Æsculapius.

caenogenesis See **cenogenesis.**

café-au-lait spot A pale tan macule the color of coffee with milk. Several café-au-lait spots developing simultaneously are associated with neurofibromatosis, but occasional café-au-lait spots occur normally. See also **neurofibromatosis.**

caffeine, c. citrate, c. sodium benzoate injection Mild central nervous system stimulants.

-caine A combining form naming synthetic alkaloid anesthetics: *isocaine, metycaine, neurocaine.*

caisson disease See **decompression sickness.**

calabar swelling An abnormal condition characterized by fugitive, swollen lumps of subcutaneous tissue caused by a parasitic, filarial worm endemic to central and west Africa. The swollen areas migrate with the worm through the body at a speed of about 1 cm/minute and may become as large as a small egg. At times the worm may move under the conjunctiva of the eye and may live in the anterior chamber of the eye. Treatment includes the oral administration of diethylcarbamazine, which destroys the adult worms and their offspring. Antihistamines and other medications may be given. See also *Loa loa*, **loiasis.**

calamine A topical astringent and protectant.

calc- A combining form meaning: **1.** 'Pertaining to lime or limestone': *calcarea, calcariuria, calciosis.* **2.** 'Pertaining to the heel': *calcaneocavus, calcaneum, calcanodynia.*

calcaneal Of or pertaining to the calcaneus at the back of the tarsus.

calcaneal spurs Abnormal, often painful, bony outgrowths on the lower surface of the calcaneus, resulting from chronic traumatic pressure on the heel.

calcaneal tendon See **tendo calcaneus.**

calcaneal tendon reflex See **Achilles tendon reflex.**

calcaneal tuberosity A transverse elevation on the plantar surface of the calcaneus to which are attached the abductor digiti minimi, the long plantar ligament, and various other muscles, including the abductor hallucis and the flexor digitorum brevis.

calcaneodynia A painful condition of the heel.

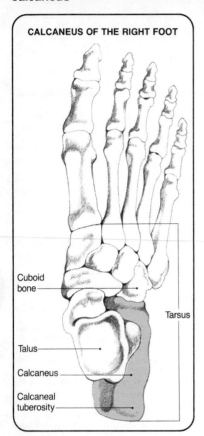

CALCANEUS OF THE RIGHT FOOT

Cuboid bone

Tarsus

Talus

Calcaneus

Calcaneal tuberosity

calcaneus The heel bone. The largest of the tarsal bones, it articulates proximally with the talus and distally with the cuboid. —**calcaneal, calcanean,** *adj.*

calcar, *pl.* **calcaria** A spur or a structure that resembles a spur.

calcareous Of or pertaining to calcium or lime.

calcarine **1.** Having the shape of a spur. **2.** Of or pertaining to the calcar.

calcarine fissure A fissure between the cuneus and the lingual gyrus on the medial surface of the occipital lobe of the brain. Also called calcarine sulcus.

calcifediol A parathyroid-like agent.

calciferol The general term for the fat-soluble vitamins chemically related to the steroids and essential for the normal formation of bones and teeth and for the absorption of calcium and phosphorus from the gastrointestinal tract. The two types of vitamin D are **ergocalciferol** (vitamin D_2) and **cholecalciferol** (vitamin D_3). The vitamin is present in natural foods in small amounts, and requirements are usually met by artificial enrichment of various foods, especially milk and dairy products, and exposure to sun-

light. Ultraviolet rays activate a form of cholesterol in the oil of the skin and convert it to a form of the vitamin, which is then absorbed. The natural foods containing vitamin D are of animal origin and include saltwater fish, especially salmon, sardines, and herring; organ meats; fish-live oils; and egg yolk. Deficiency of the vitamin results in rickets in children, osteomalacia, osteoporosis, and osteodystrophy. Hypervitaminosis D produces a toxicity syndrome characterized by anorexia, vomiting, headache, drowsiness, diarrhea, and calcification of the soft tissues of the heart, blood vessels, renal tubules, and lungs. Treatment consists of discontinuing the vitamin dosage and initiating a low-calcium diet until symptoms resolve.

calcific aortic disease An abnormal condition characterized by small deposits of calcium in the aorta.

calcification The accumulation of calcium salts in tissues. Normally, about 99% of all the calcium entering the human body is deposited in the bones and teeth; the remaining 1% is dissolved in body fluids, as the blood. Disorders affecting the delicate balance between calcium and other minerals, parathyroid hormone, and vitamin D can result in calcium deposits in arteries, kidneys, lung alveoli, and other tissues, interfering with usual organ functions. See also **calcitonin, calcium, calculus.**

calcified fetus See **lithopedion.**

calcinosis A condition marked by the deposition of calcium salts in various tissues of the body.

calcitonin A hormone produced in parafollicular cells of the thyroid that participates in regulating the blood level of calcium and stimulates bone mineralization. A synthetic preparation of the hormone is used in the treatment of certain bone disorders. Calcitonin acts to reduce the blood level of calcium and to inhibit bone resorption, while parathyroid hormone acts to increase blood calcium and bone resorption. Calcitonin has a short-term effect in enhancing bone formation and causes transient decreases in the volume and acidity of gastric juice and in the volume of amylase and trypsin in pancreatic juice. The hormone also promotes the excretion of phosphate, sodium, and calcium by decreasing their reabsorption in kidney tubules. The secretion of calcitonin is regulated by the amount of calcium in plasma, and an infusion of calcium may increase the concentration of the circulating hormone two- to threefold. Men usually have a higher level of plasma calcitonin than women.

calcitonin (Salmon) A parathyroid-like agent.

calcitriol A parathyroid-like agent.

calcium (Ca) An alkaline earth metal element. Its atomic number is 20; its atomic weight is 40. Its metallic form is a white, flammable solid, somewhat harder than lead. Calcium is commonly produced by the electrolysis or by the thermal dissociation of calcium chloride. Calcium is the fifth most abundant element in the

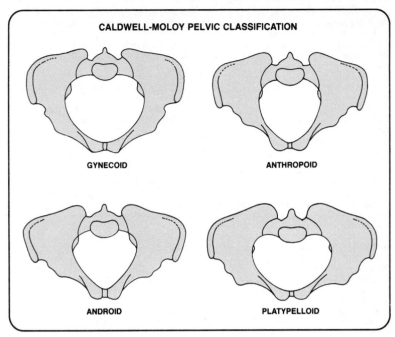

CALDWELL-MOLOY PELVIC CLASSIFICATION

GYNECOID

ANTHROPOID

ANDROID

PLATYPELLOID

human body and occurs mainly in the bone. The body requires calcium ions for the transmission of nerve impulses, muscle contraction, blood coagulation, cardiac functions, and other processes. It is a component of extracellular fluid and of the cells of soft tissue. The average daily human intake of calcium varies from 200 to 2,500 mg. In the United States dairy products are the major dietary sources of this element. More than 90% of the calcium in the body is stored in the skeleton, which constantly exchanges its supplies with the calcium of the interstitial fluids. The endocrine system controls the concentration of ionized calcium in the plasma. Only a fraction of this amount is ionized and diffusable; the rest is bound to proteins, especially albumin. It is the ionized, diffusable portion of calcium that figures in the physiological changes associated with hypocalcemia. About one third of the calcium ingested by humans is absorbed, primarily in the small bowel. Vitamin D, calcitonin, and parathyroid hormone are essential in the metabolism of calcium. The degree of cell permeability varies inversely with calcium ion concentration. Abnormally high levels of ionized calcium in the extracellular fluid can produce muscle weakness, lethargy, and coma. A relatively small decrease from the normal level of this element can produce tetanic seizures.

calcium carbonate An antacid.

calcium chloride, c. gluceptate, c. gluconate, c. lactate Sources of calcium ions for electrolyte therapy.

calcium polycarbophil A bulk-forming laxative and antidiarrheal.

calcium pump A theoretical, energy-requiring mechanism for transmitting calcium ions across a cell membrane from a region of low calcium ion concentration to one of higher concentration. Compare **sodium pump.**

calculus, *pl.* **calculi** A pathological stone formed of mineral salts. Calculi are usually found within hollow organs or ducts and can cause obstruction and inflammation. Kinds of calculi include **biliary calculus,** renal calculus. Also called **stone.**

Caldwell-Moloy pelvic classification A system for classifying the structure of the bony pelvis of the female. The types in this system are android, anthropoid, gynecoid, and platypelloid. The sacrum, sidewalls, sacrosciatic notch, ischial spines, pubic arch, and ischial tuberosities are the anatomic points of reference used to determine pelvic type. The classification system requires that a mixed pelvis be named for the character of its posterior section with the name of the type characterized by the anterior portion following a hyphen, as in a gynecoid-android pelvis. See also **pelvic classification.**

calefacient **1.** Making or tending to make anything warm or hot. **2.** An agent that imparts a sense of warmth when applied, as a hot-water bottle or a hot compress.

calendar method of family planning A natural method of family planning in which the fertile period of a woman's menstrual cycle is identified by an examination of at least six menstrual cycles recorded on a calendar. If the length of the cycle varies, 12 cycles are recorded. It is assumed that ovulation occurs 14 days before the onset of menstruation and that during the 4 days before the expected or usual day of ovulation, the day of ovulation, and the 3 days after ovulation, fertilization may occur. Abstinence is required during the fertile period. In a woman with a regular cycle this period is from the 18th to the 11th days prior to the first day of the next menstrual period. However, if the cycle varies in length, the number of variance days between the shortest and longest cycles is added to the period of abstinence, allowing for the earliest and latest day of ovulation and the surrounding 'unsafe days.' Thus, if menstruation occurs every 24 to 30 days, abstinence would be required from the 6th to the 19th days of the cycle. The calendar method is more effective as an adjunct to the symptothermal method of family planning than if used alone. Also called **natural family-planning method.** Compare **basal body temperature method of family planning, ovulation method of family planning, symptothermal method of family planning.**

calf, *pl.* **calves** The fleshy mass at the back of the leg below the knee, composed chiefly of the gastrocnemius muscle.

caliber, calibre The diameter of a tube or a canal, as any of the blood vessels.

California encephalitis A common, acute viral infection that affects the central nervous system. Epidemics occur mainly in the Midwest, on the Eastern Seaboard, and in Texas and Louisiana. The virus was first isolated in California. The infection generally follows one of two clinical courses. The mild form is characterized by headache, malaise, gastrointestinal symptoms, and a fever that may reach 40°C (104°F). The more severe form may be marked by a sudden onset of fever, vomiting, headaches, lethargy, and signs of neurologic involvement, as loss of reflexes, disorientation, seizure, loss of consciousness, and flaccid paralysis. Recovery usually begins in a week. Mortality is very low, but a significant number of patients have neurologic sequelae for a year or more. Treatment usually involves administration of anticonvulsant and sedative medications. See also **arbovirus, encephalitis.**

californium (Cf) An artificial element in the actinide group. Its atomic number is 98. Californium isotopes discovered so far have atomic weights ranging from 244 to 245.

calipers An instrument with two hinged, adjustable, curved legs, used to measure the thickness or the diameter of a convex body or solid.

caliper splint A splint for the leg consisting of two metal rods running from the back of a band around the thigh or from a cushioned ring around the lower portion of the pelvis. The rods are attached to a metal plate under the shoe below the arch of the foot.

Calliphoridae A family of flies that belongs to the order Diptera, serves as pathogenic vectors, and may cause myiasis in humans. These flies include the genera *Auchmeromyia, Calliphora, Chrysomyia, Cochliomyia, Cordylobia, Lucilia, Phaenicia,* and *Phormia.*

callomania An abnormal psychological condition characterized by delusions of personal beauty.

callosal fissure A groove following the convex aspect of the corpus callosum.

callosity See **callus.**

callosomarginal fissure A long, irregular groove on the medial surface of a cerebral hemisphere. It divides the cingulate gyrus from the medial frontal gyrus and from the paracentral lobule. Also called **cingulate sulcus.**

callus **1.** A common, usually painless thickening of the epidermis at locations of external pressure or friction. Also called **callosity.** Compare **corn.** **2.** Bony deposit formed between and around the broken ends of a fractured bone during healing. —**callous,** *adj.*

calmodulin A polypeptide protein that mediates a variety of biochemical and physiological processes, including the contraction of muscles and the release of norepinephrine. Depending on its form and function, calmodulin may act independently of, in concert with, or antagonistically to reactions involving cyclic adenosinemonophosphate.

calor Heat, as that generated by inflammation of tissues or that from the normal metabolic processes of the body.

calor- A combining form meaning 'pertaining to heat': *calorie, calorifacient, calorization.*

caloric Of or pertaining to heat or calories.

caloric test A procedure for determining if the ear is diseased or normal. The test alternately irrigates the ear with hot water and cold water. If the ear is normal the hot water irrigation produces a rotatory nystagmus toward the irrigated side. Cold water irrigation produces a rotatory nystagmus away from the irrigated side. If the ear is diseased, irrigation produces no nystagmus. Also called **Bárány's symptom.**

calorie **1.** The amount of heat required to raise 1 g of water 1°C at atmospheric pressure. Also called **gram calorie,** small calorie. **2.** A quantity of heat equal to 1,000 small calories. Also called **great calorie, kilogram calorie, large calorie.** **3.** A unit, equal to the large calorie, used to denote the heat expenditure of an organism and the fuel or energy value of food. —**caloric,** *adj.*

calorific Pertaining to the production of heat.

calorigenic Of or pertaining to a substance or process that produces or increases production of heat or energy or that increases the consumption of oxygen.

calorimeter A device used for measuring quantities of heat generated by friction, by chemical reaction, or by the human body. —**calorimetric,** *adj.*

calorimetry The measurement of the amounts of heat radiated and the amounts of heat absorbed. Compare **direct calorimetry, indirect calorimetry.** —**calorimetric,** *adj.*

calvaria The skull cap or superior portion of the skull, which varies greatly in shape from individual to individual. In some persons, the calvaria is relatively oval; in others it is more circular. It is traversed by the coronal suture between the frontal and the parietal bones, by the sagittal suture in the midline between the two parietal bones, and by the upper part of the lambdoid suture between the parietal bones and the occipital bone. The inner surface of the calvaria is indented to accept the convolutions of the cerebrum and furrowed for the branches of the meningeal vessels. It also contains the superior sagittal sinus, affords attachment at its margins for the falx cerebri, and posteriorly, in some individuals it accommodates the openings of the parietal foramina. The soft spots in the skull of an infant are situated on the surface of the calvaria at the junction of the sagittal and the coronal sutures and at the junction of the sagittal and lambdoid sutures. See also **bregma.**

calvities   The condition of baldness. **—calvous,** *adj.*

calyx, *pl.* **calyces, calyxes**   **1.** A cup-shaped organ. **2.** A renal calyx. **3.** The wall of an ovarian follicle after expulsion of the ovum at ovulation.

cambium layer   **1.** The loose, inner cellular layer of the periosteum that develops during ossification.

camera   In anatomy: any cavity or chamber, as those of the eye or the heart.

camphor   An antipruritic and counterirritant. Also called **camphora, gum camphor.**

camphora   See **camphor.**

camphor bath   An air bath in which the air is filled with camphor vapor.

camphor salicylate   A crystalline substance formed by the fusion of camphor and salicylic acid, used in skin ointments and administered internally for diarrhea.

camptodactyly   The permanent flexion of one or more fingers. **—camptodactylic,** *adj.*

camptomelia   A congenital anomaly characterized by bending of one or more limbs causing permanent bowing or curving of the affected area. **—camptomelic,** *adj.*

Canadian Association of University Schools of Nursing (CAUSN)   A national Canadian organization of nursing schools affiliated with institutions of higher learning.

Canadian Association of University Teachers (CAUT)   A national Canadian organization representing the interests of all who teach in the universities of the provinces and territories of Canada. The official languages of the CAUT are French and English.

Canadian crutch   A wooden or metal device that helps a disabled patient stand or walk. It consists of two uprights with a crosspiece to accommodate the hand and a concave crosspiece that fits the armpit for support.

***Canadian Journal of Public Health* (CJPH)**   The official publication of the Canadian Public Health Association.

***Canadian Medical Association Journal* (CMAJ)**   The official publication of the Canadian Medical Association.

Canadian Nurses' Association (CNA)   The official national organization for the professional registered nurses of Canada who are members of one of the 10 provincial nurses' associations and the Northwest Territory's association. The CNA, a federation of these 11 associations, is supported by contributions of the 140,000 members of the regional associations. The chief objective of the CNA is to promote conditions conducive to the good health of the people and to good patient care. It is concerned with the quality and quantity of nurses available, the standards of preparation for nurses, the social and economic welfare of nurses, the advancement of competence and expertise within the profession, the promotion of unity and understanding among the members, and the representation of the organized profession of nurses nationally and internationally. A board of 23 elected volunteers and a permanent staff working at CNA House in Ottawa manage the affairs of the organization. Among the services provided are a research and advisory unit that studies trends in nursing and health and prepares briefs, when necessary; a library containing reference works, the archives of the CNA, and up-to-date lists of educational programs in nursing; an information service that collects and disseminates information about nursing and publishes *The Canadian Nurse* and *L'Infirmière Canadienne;* a labor relations service; a testing service; a governmental liaison service; and an international service that facilitates a working relationship with various organizations, as the World Health Organization and the Pan American Health Organization. All services are provided in the two official languages, English and French.

Canadian Nurses' Association Testing Service (CNATS)   The organizational affiliate of the Canadian Nurses' Association that is concerned with testing the graduates of approved schools of nursing to qualify as registered nurses.

Canadian Nurses' Foundation (CNF)   A national Canadian foundation organized to support scholarship in nursing. The CNF awards financial support to nurses undertaking graduate studies in nursing and to nurses planning research in nursing.

Canadian Nurses' Respiratory Society (CNRS)   An organization of nurses working with, or interested in alleviating the problems of, respiratory disease. The CNRS, an affiliate of the Canadian Nurses' Association, is a section of the Canadian Lung Association.

Canadian Orthopedic Nurses' Association (CONA)   A national Canadian organization concerned with the nursing care of orthopedic patients and the continuing education of nurses working in orthopedics. Membership includes orthopedic nurses and other professionals concerned with orthopedics.

Canadian Public Health Association (CPHA)   A national Canadian organization concerned with issues in public health and epidemiology. Membership is open to professionals and to others interested in these issues.

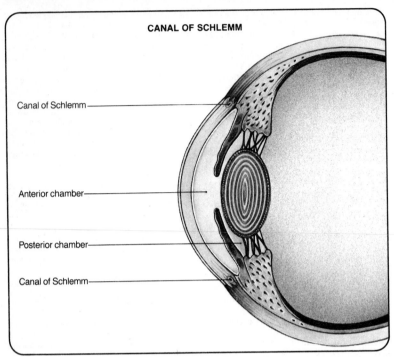

CANAL OF SCHLEMM

Canal of Schlemm

Anterior chamber

Posterior chamber

Canal of Schlemm

canal In anatomy: a narrow tube or channel. Some kinds of canals are **adductor canal, Alcock's canal, alveolar canal.**

canaliculus, *pl.* **canaliculi** A very small tube or channel, like the tiny Haversian canaliculi throughout bone tissue.

canalization The formation of canals or of passages through any tissue.

canal of Schlemm A tiny vein at the angle of the anterior chamber of the eye that connects with the pectinate villi, draining the aqueous humor and funneling it into the bloodstream. Also called **Schlemm's canal.**

cancellous Of tissue: latticelike, porous, spongy. Cancellous tissue is normally present in the interior of many bones, where the spaces are usually filled with marrow.

cancer **1.** A neoplasm characterized by the uncontrolled growth of anaplastic cells that tend to invade surrounding tissue and metastasize to distant body sites. **2.** Any of a large group of malignant neoplastic diseases characterized by the presence of malignant cells. Each cancer is distinguished by the nature, site, or clinical course of the lesion. The basic etiology of cancer is undetermined, but many potential causes are recognized. More than 80% of cancer cases are attributed to cigarette smoking, exposure to carcinogenic chemicals, ionizing radiation, and ultraviolet rays; overexposure to the sun is the major cause of skin cancer. Many viruses induce malignant tumors in animals, and viral particles are detected in some human tumors; but there is no clear evidence that any microorganism causes human cancer. The high incidence of various kinds of cancer in certain families suggests that genetic susceptibility is an important factor. An excess rate of malignant tumors in organ transplant recipients following immunosuppressive therapy indicates that the immune system plays a major role in controlling the proliferation of anaplastic cells. The basic defect may be a biochemical anomaly that triggers abnormal cell growth and glucose metabolism and in which certain vital proteins and respiratory enzymes are reduced. The incidence of different kinds of cancer varies markedly with sex, age, ethnic group, and geographic location. In the United States, cancer is second only to heart disease as a cause of mortality and is the leading cause of death of children between the ages of 3 and 14. The most common sites for the development of malignant tumors are the lung, breast, colon, uterus, oral cavity, and bone marrow. Surgery remains the major form of treatment, but irradiation is widely used as preoperative, postoperative, or primary therapy; chemotherapy, with single or multiple antineoplastic agents, is often highly effective. Many malignant lesions are curable if detected in the early stages. Depending on the site, the warning signal may be a change in bowel or bladder habits, a nonhealing sore, unusual bleeding or discharge, a thickening or lump in the breast or elsewhere, indigestion or dysphagia, an obvious change in a wart or mole, or a nagging cough or persistent hoarseness.

cancer bodies   See **Russell's bodies.**

cancericidal   Of or pertaining to a substance or procedure capable of destroying cancer cells.

cancer in situ   See **carcinoma in situ.**

cancer of the small intestine   A neoplastic disease of the duodenum, jejunum, or ileum. Its characteristics vary, depending on the kind of tumor and the site, but may include abdominal pain, vomiting, weight loss, diarrhea, intermittent bowel obstruction, gastrointestinal bleeding, or a mass deep in the right abdomen. Diagnosis is made with barium X-ray examination, but such studies may be inconclusive until lesions are large. Adenocarcinomas, the most common tumors, occur more frequently in the duodenum or upper jejunum and form polypoid or constricting napkin-ring growths. Lymphomas, found most often in the lower small intestine, may impair bowel motility by invading nerves and, in some cases, are associated with a malabsorption syndrome. Less common tumors of the small intestine are carcinoids, usually found in the ileum, and sarcomas, usually seen in the jejunum and ileum. A leiomyosarcoma may sometimes form a large extraluminal mass but does not metastasize, unlike other cancers of the small intestine. Surgery, including a wide resection of mesenteric lymph nodes, is indicated for adenocarcinomas. Irradiation is not effective in ablation of these tumors but is recommended postoperatively for lymphomas to treat metastatic lesions in mesenteric lymph nodes, the liver, and spleen. Resection of carcinoids is advised to prevent bowel obstruction even if metastatic disease is present, and some patients with these lesions may respond to chemotherapeutic agents, as cyclophosphamide, 5-fluorouracil, methotrexate, and streptozotocin. Cancer of the small intestine, which is uncommon considering the great length and surface area of that organ, occurs slightly more often in men than in women.

cancer staging   A system for describing the extent of a malignant tumor and its metastases, used to plan appropriate treatment and predict prognosis. Staging involves a careful physical examination, diagnostic procedures, and, ultimately, surgical exploration. The standardized system developed by the American Joint Committee for Cancer Staging and End Results Reporting uses the letter T to represent the tumor, N for the regional lymph node involvement, M for distant metastases, and numerical subscripts in each category to indicate the degree of dissemination. According to this system $T_1N_0M_0$ designates a small, localized tumor; $T_2N_1M_0$ is a larger primary tumor that has extended to regional nodes; and $T_4N_3M_3$ is a very large lesion involving regional nodes and distant sites. The Ann Arbor System classifies Hodgkin's disease as Stages I to IV according to the number and location of involved lymph nodes in relation to the diaphragm and the involvement of extralymphatic organs or tissues, based on numerous diagnostic procedures and by a staging lapa-

rotomy. Other systems may be used for staging breast carcinoma, colorectal cancer, and cutaneous melanoma.

cancer-ulcer   A carcinomatous ulceration.

cancr-, chancr-   A combining form meaning 'pertaining to cancer': *cancriform, cancroid, cancrology.*

cancriform   Of or pertaining to a lesion resembling a cancer.

cancroid   **1.** Of or pertaining to a lesion resembling a cancer. **2.** A moderately malignant skin cancer.

candicidin   An antifungal agent.

Candida   A genus of yeastlike fungi including the common pathogen, *Candida albicans.*

Candida albicans   A common, budding, yeastlike, microscopic fungal organism normally present in the mucous membranes of the mouth, intestinal tract, vagina, and on the skin of healthy people. Under certain circumstances, it may cause superficial infections of the mouth or vagina and, less commonly, serious invasive systemic infection and toxic reaction. See also **candidiasis.**

candidiasis   Any infection caused by a species of *Candida,* usually *Candida albicans,* characterized by pruritus, a white exudate, peeling, and easy bleeding. Diaper rash, intertrigo, vaginitis, and thrush are common topical manifestations of candidiasis. Endocarditis, other inflammatory conditions of the heart and liver, and infection of the kidney, spleen, and lungs sometimes occur in debilitated patients. Treatment includes the oral and topical administration of antifungal drugs, as nystatin, clotrimazole, and, rarely, amphotericin-B. Gentian violet, painted on the inflamed mucosa of the mouth or vagina or, in intertrigo or diaper rash, on the skin, is messy but effective.

Candiru fever   An arbovirus infection transmitted to humans by the bite of a sandfly, characterized by an acute fever, headache, and muscle aches. Recovery occurs, without treatment, within a few days. Candiru fever occurs mainly in the forests of Brazil. See also **arbovirus, phlebotomus fever.**

candy-striper   *Informal.* A hospital volunteer, named for the striped pink-and-white uniforms traditionally worn by the young people who perform this service.

cane-cutter's cramp   See **heat cramp.**

canefield fever   See **field fever.**

canine tooth   Any one of the four teeth, two in each jaw, situated immediately lateral to the incisor teeth in the human dental arches. The canine teeth are larger and stronger than the incisors, and they project beyond the level of the other teeth in both arches. Their roots sink deeply into the bones, causing marked prominences on the alveolar arch. The canines erupt as deciduous teeth about 16 to 20 months after birth. The eruption of the permanent canines occurs during the 11th or the 12th year of life.

canker   An ulcer or sore, especially in the mouth. Also called **aphthous stomatitis.**

canker sore   An ulcerous lesion of the mouth,

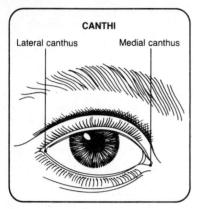

CANTHI

Lateral canthus   Medial canthus

characteristic of aphthous stomatitis. See also **aphthous stomatitis.**

cannabis   A psychoactive drug derived from the flowering tops of hemp plants. It is employed effectively as an antiemetic in some cancer patients to counter the nausea and vomiting associated with chemotherapy. Cannabis is controlled under Schedule I of the Comprehensive Drug Abuse Prevention and Control Act of 1970 and may be legally obtained by approved cancer centers for research and other special medical applications authorized by the Drug Enforcement Administration of the U.S. Department of Justice. The common hemp from which cannabis is obtained is a herbaceous annual of which *Cannabis sativa* is the sole species. The two subspecies are *indica* and *americana.* All parts of the plant contain psychoactive substances or cannabinoids, the highest concentrations of which are in the flowering tops of the plant. The cannabinoids synthesized by the hemp plant include cannabinol, cannabidiol, cannabinolic acid, cannabigerol, cannabicyclol, and several isomers of tetrahydrocannabinol (THC). THC is believed to cause the most characteristic psychological effects, which include alterations of mood, memory, motor coordination, cognitive ability, and self-perception. Most users of cannabis smoke marijuana cigarettes containing dried and chopped leaves of the hemp plant. Other users ingest the drug. Low doses of cannabis seldom impair the ability to perform simple motor tasks but commonly hinder more complex actions, as driving and flying, which involve complex sensory perception, concentration, and information processing. Cannabis may also enhance the nondominant senses of touch, taste, and smell. Higher doses in some persons can produce delusions, paranoid feelings, anxiety, and panic. This drug also increases the heart rate and systolic blood pressure. Pharmacological effects of smoking marijuana occur within minutes after smoking begins and produce peak plasma concentrations of THC within 10 to 30 minutes. The effects of one cigarette rarely last more than 2 or 3 hours. Marijuana is about three times more powerful when smoked than when taken orally. The smoking of marijuana has increased throughout the world since the 1960s, and, in 1977, approximately 60% of young adults polled in the United States reported some experience with the drug. Research indicates that some cannabinoids may be therapeutic as anticonvulsants and helpful in reducing intraocular pressure associated with glaucoma. Also called **bhang, ganja, grass, hashish, marijuana, pot, reefer.**

cannabism   A condition associated with overuse of cannabis, characterized by increased heart rate, hallucinations, delusions, and a confused anxiety state. In its acute stage, cannabism usually responds to simple reassurance. Effects of frequent and prolonged cannabis use are still being investigated. See **tetrahydrocannabinol.**

cannon wave   A radical 'a' wave in the jugular pulse, characteristic of a complete heart block and of premature ventricular beats of the heart. Cannon waves are caused by the contraction of the right atrium of the heart after contraction of the right ventricle has closed the tricuspid valve.

cannula, *pl.* **cannulas, cannulae**   A flexible tube containing a stiff, pointed trocar that may be inserted into the body, guided by the trocar. As the trocar is removed, a body fluid may be passed through the cannula to the outside. —**cannular, cannulate,** *adj.*

cannulation, cannulization   The insertion of a cannula into a body duct or cavity, as into the trachea, bladder, or a blood vessel. —**cannulate, cannulize,** *v.*

cantharidin   A topical keratolytic agent.

cantharis, *pl.* **cantharides**   The dried insects *Cantharis vesicatoria* containing cantharidin, formerly used as a topical vesicant. Also called **Spanish fly.**

cantho-   A combining form meaning 'pertaining to the canthus': *cantholysis, canthorraphy, canthotomy.*

canthus, *pl.* **canthi**   The angle at the medial and the lateral margins of the eyelids. The medial canthus opens into a small space containing the opening to a lacrimal duct. Also called **palpebral commissure. —canthic,** *adj.*

Cap   *abbr* Latin *capiat* 'let him or her take,' used in medicinal prescriptions.

CAP   In molecular genetics: an abbreviation for **catabolic activator protein.** CAP participates in initiating the transcription of RNA in organisms without a true nucleus, as bacteria.

capeline bandage   A caplike covering used for protecting the head, shoulder, or a stump. Also called Hippocrates' bandage.

capillaritis   An abnormal condition characterized by a progressive pigmentary disorder of the skin without inflammation but with dilatation. It does not involve any systemic problems and runs a benign self-limiting course.

capillarity   See **capillary action.**

capillary   One of the tiny blood vessels (about 0.008 mm in diameter) joining arterioles and venules. Through their walls, which consist of a single layer of endothelial cells, blood and tissue cells exchange various substances.

capillary action   The action involving molecular adhesion by which the surface of a liquid in a tube is either elevated or depressed, depending on the cohesiveness of the liquid molecules. The more cohesive the molecules, the more elevated will be the surface of the liquid. Less cohesive liquid molecules will adhere to the surfaces of the tube in which they are contained and depress the surface of the liquid. Also called **capillarity.**

capillary angioma   See **cherry angioma.**

capillary bed   A capillary network.

capillary flames   See **telangiectatic nevus.**

capillary fracture   Any thin hairlike fracture.

capillary hemangioma   A blood-filled birthmark or benign tumor consisting of closely packed, small blood vessels. Commonly found in infants, a capillary hemangioma first grows, then spontaneously disappears in early childhood without treatment. Surgical removal will not usually be attempted unless frequent trauma and bleeding are present. Also called **hemangioma simplex, strawberry hemangioma, strawberry mark.** Compare **cavernous hemangioma, nevus flammeus.**

capillovenous   Of or pertaining to the venous capillaries.

capillus, *pl.* **capilli**   One of the hairs of the body, especially one of the hairs of the scalp.

capit-   A combining form meaning 'pertaining to the head': *capitate, capitopedal, capitular.*

capitate   Having the shape of a head.

capitate bone   One of the largest carpal bones, located at the center of the wrist and presenting a rounded head that fits the concavity of the scaphoid and the lunate bones. Various ligaments are attached to the rough dorsal and palmar surfaces. The capitate articulates with the scaphoid and lunate proximally; the second, third, and fourth metacarpals distally; the trapezoid on the radial side; and the hamate on the ulnar side. Also called **os capitatum, os magnum.**

capitulum, *pl.* **capitula**   A small, rounded prominence on a bone where it articulates with another bone.

capitulum humeri   A rounded eminence at the distal end of the humerus. It articulates with the radius.

-capnia   A combining form meaning '(condition of) carbon dioxide content in the blood': *acapnia, eucapnia, hypocapnia.*

capnograph   An instrument used in anesthesia, respiratory physiology, and respiratory therapy to produce a tracing, or capnogram, which shows the proportion of carbon dioxide in expired air.

capreomycin sulfate   An antitubercular agent.

capric acid   A white, crystalline substance with a rancid odor, occurring as a glyceride in natural oils. Capric acid is used in the produc-

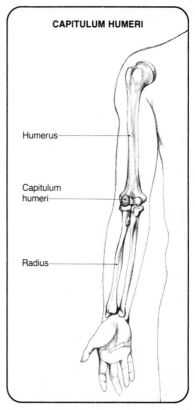

CAPITULUM HUMERI

Humerus

Capitulum humeri

Radius

tion of perfumes, flavors, wetting agents, and food additives. Also called **decanoic acid, decoic acid.**

caps-, kaps-   A combining form meaning 'capsule or container': *capsitis, capsulation, capsuloplasty.*

capsid   The layer of protein enveloping a virion. A capsid is composed of structural units, called capsomeres, and its symmetry may be cubic or helical.

capsula, *pl.* **capsuli**   See **capsule.**

capsular swelling test   See **quellung reaction.**

capsule   1. A small, soluble container, usually made of gelatin, used for enclosing a dose of medication for swallowing. Compare **tablet.** 2. A membranous shell surrounding certain microorganisms, as the pneumococcus bacterium. 3. A well-defined anatomical structure that encloses an organ or part, as the capsule of the adrenal gland.

capsulectomy   The surgical excision of a capsule, usually the capsule of a joint or the capsule of the lens of the eye.

capsule of Tenon   See **fascia bulbi.**

capsule of the kidney   The fatty enclosure of the kidney, consisting of adipose tissue continuous at the hilus with the fat of the renal sinus. This investment of perirenal fat covers the fibrous capsule and helps to protect the organ from bumps and shocks. Compare **Bowman's capsule.**

capsuloma, *pl.* **capsulomas, capsulomata** A neoplasm of the renal capsule or the subcapsular area.

capsulotomy An incision into the capsule of the eye, as in an operation to remove a cataract.

captain-of-the-ship doctrine The medicolegal principle that the physician is ultimately responsible for all patient-care activities and thus may be held accountable and may be sued for negligence or malpractice when the act at issue is performed by an employee or other person under the physician's control, even if not ordered by the physician.

captopril An antihypertensive enzyme inhibitor.

caput, *pl.* **capita 1.** The head. **2.** The enlarged or prominent extremity of an organ or part. Some kinds of capita include **caput costae, caput epididymidis, caput femoris, caput fibulae, caput humeri, caput mallei, caput mandibulae, caput ossis metacarpalis, caput phalangis, caput radii, caput stapedis, caput succedaneum.**

caput costae The head of a rib; it articulates with a vertebral body.

caput epididymidis The head of the epididymis.

caput femoris The head of the femur; it fits into the acetabulum.

caput fibulae The head of the fibula; it articulates with the lateral condyle of the tibia.

caput humeri The head of the humerus; it fits into the glenoid cavity of the scapula.

caput mallei The head of the malleus.

caput mandibulae The articular process of the ramus of the mandible.

caput ossis metacarpalis The metacarpal head; it articulates with the proximal phalanx of the same digit.

caput phalangis The articular head at the distal end of the proximal and middle phalanges.

caput radii The head of the radius; it articulates with the capitulum of the humerus.

caput stapedis The head of the stapes.

caput succedaneum A localized pitting edema in the scalp of a fetus that may overlie sutures of the skull. It is usually formed during labor as a result of the circular pressure of the cervix on the fetal occiput. On vaginal examination the swelling may be mistaken for unruptured membranes. If the caput enlarges appreciably during labor, it may give an erroneous impression of fetal descent on successive examinations. At birth the baby's head may appear markedly deformed, but the swelling begins to resolve immediately and is usually gone in a few days. Compare **cephalhematoma, molding.**

carate See **pinta.**

carbachol A miotic agent.

carbamate kinase A liver enzyme that cat-

alyzes the transfer of a phosphate group from adenosine triphosphate, associated with ammonia and carbon dioxide, to form adenosine diphosphate and carbamoylphosphate.

carbamazepine An anticonvulsant agent.

carbamide peroxide A topical anti-infective and ceruminolytic agent.

carbarsone An amebicide.

carbazochrome salicylate A local hemostatic agent.

carbenicillin disodium, c. indanyl sodium Penicillin antibiotics.

carbidopa A DOPA decarboxylase inhibitor often combined with levodopa.

carbinoxamine maleate An ethanolamine antihistamine.

carbo-, carbon- A combining form meaning 'carbon, charcoal': *carbonate, carboneol, carbonometry.*

carbocyclic See **closed-chain.**

carbohydrate Any of a group of organic compounds, the most important being sugar, starch, cellulose, and gum. They are classified according to molecular structure as mono-, di-, tri-, poly-, and heterosaccharides. Carbohydrates constitute the main source of energy for all body functions and are necessary for the metabolism of other nutrients. They are synthesized by all green plants and, in the body, are either absorbed immediately or stored in the form of glycogen. Cereals, vegetables, fruits, rice, potatoes, legumes, and flour products are the major sources of carbohydrates. They can also be manufactured in the body from some amino acids and the glycerol component of fats. Symptoms of deficiency include fatigue, depression, breakdown of essential body protein, and electrolyte imbalance. Excessive consumption of carbohydrates may result in tooth decay, obesity, diabetes mellitus, hypertension, cardiovascular disease, anemia, cancer, and kidney dysfunction.

carbohydrate metabolism The sum of the anabolic and catabolic processes of the body involved in the synthesis and breakdown of carbohydrates, principally galactose, fructose, and glucose. Some of the processes are glycogenesis, glyconeogenesis, and glycolysis. Energy-rich phosphate bonds are produced in many metabolic reactions requiring carbohydrates.

carbolated camphor A mixture of 1.5 parts camphor with 1.0 parts each of alcohol and phenol, used as an antiseptic dressing for wounds.

carbol-fuchsin solution A local anti-infective agent. Also called **Castellani's paint.**

carbolic acid A poisonous, colorless-to-pale-pink crystalline compound obtained from coal tar distillation and converted to a clear liquid with a strong odor and burning taste by the addition of 10% water. Low concentrations of carbolic acid are used in antiseptic preparations. Also called **hydroxybenzene, oxybenzene, phenic acid, phenol, phenylic acid, phenylic alcohol.**

carbolic acid poisoning See **phenol poisoning.**

carbon (C) A nonmetallic, chiefly tetravalent element. Its atomic number is 6; its atomic weight is 12.011. Carbon occurs in pure form in diamond and graphite and is a component of all living tissue. Most of the study of organic chemistry focuses on the vast number of carbon compounds. Carbon occurs in impure form in charcoal, coke, and soot, and in the atmosphere as carbon dioxide. Carbon is essential to the chemistry of the body, participating in many metabolic processes and acting as a component of carbohydrates, amino acids, triglycerides, deoxyribonucleic and ribonucleic acids, and many other compounds. Carbon dioxide produced in glycolysis is important in the acid-base balance of the body and in controlling respiration. Carbon is a component of carbon monoxide, which can be lethal if inhaled, and of many hydrocarbons, the fumes of which can cause death from respiratory failure. Brief incidental exposures to low concentrations of solvent vapors that contain carbon, as gasoline, lighter fluids, aerosol sprays, and spot removers, may be relatively harmless, but exposures to concentrations of hydrocarbon vapors often found in the home and in manufacturing environments may be dangerous. Many occupational pulmonary diseases, as coal worker's pneumoconiosis, black lung disease, aluminosis (bauxite lung), baritosis, berylliosis, and byssinosis, are caused by chronic inhalation of dusts containing carbon compounds. See also **carbon 11, carbon 14.**

carbon- See **carbo-.**

carbon 11 A radioisotope of carbon with a half-life of 20 minutes. It is produced by a cyclotron and emits positrons. Compare **carbon 14.**

carbon 14 A beta-emitter with a half-life of 5,600 years. It occurs naturally, arising from cosmic rays, and is used as a tracer in studying various aspects of metabolism and in dating relics which contain natural carbonaceous materials. Compare **carbon 11.**

carbon arc lamp An electric lamp producing a strong white light of adjustable intensity from an arc of current between carbon electrodes.

carbon cycle The steps by which carbon in the form of carbon dioxide is extracted from and returned to the atmosphere by living organisms, especially human beings. The process starts with the photosynthetic production of carbohydrates by plants, progresses through the consumption of carbohydrates by animals and human beings, and ends with the exhalation of carbon dioxide by those same animals and human beings, and also with the release of carbon dioxide during the decomposition of dead plants and animals. Various chemical processes intervene between the ingestion of carbohydrates and the release of carbon dioxide. Carbohydrate metabolism starts with the movement of glucose through cell membranes and subsequently involves glycolysis, the processes of the citric acid cycle, electron transport, and oxidative phosphorylation. See also **Krebs' citric acid cycle.**

carbon dioxide (CO₂) A colorless, odorless gas produced by the oxidation of carbon. Carbon dioxide, as a product of cell respiration, is carried by the blood to the lungs and is exhaled. The acid-base balance of body fluids and tissues is affected by the level of carbon dioxide and its carbonate compounds. Solid carbon dioxide (dry ice) is used in the treatment of some skin conditions.

carbon dioxide bath A bath taken in water that is saturated with carbon dioxide. See also **Nauheim bath.**

carbon dioxide tension The partial pressure of carbon dioxide gas, expressed as $PaCO_2$, which is proportional to its percentage in the blood or lungs. It is expressed quantitatively in mmHg. Alveolar $PaCO_2$ directly reflects adequate pulmonary gas exchange in relation to blood flow. A high rate of ventilation causes a lower alveolar $PaCO_2$; a lower rate of breathing leads to higher amounts of alveolar and blood carbon dioxide. The $PaCO_2$ is measured by glass electrodes in samples of arterial blood. Normal values for arterial and alveolar carbon dioxide tension are between 35 and 45 mmHg. Higher levels occur in conditions of slow blood flow or increased metabolic rate. Below-normal values are caused by hyperventilation, respiratory alkalosis, or rapid rates of blood flow. See also **carbon dioxide, hypercapnia, hyperventilation, hypoventilation.**

carbon monoxide A colorless, odorless, poisonous gas produced by the combustion of carbon or organic fuels in a limited oxygen supply, as in the cylinders of an internal combustion engine. Carbon monoxide combines irreversibly with hemoglobin, preventing the formation of oxyhemoglobin and reducing the oxygen supply to the tissues. Prolonged exposure to high levels of carbon monoxide results in asphyxiation.

carbon monoxide poisoning A toxic condition in which carbon monoxide gas has been inhaled and absorbed in the lungs, displacing oxygen from the red blood cells and decreasing the capacity of the blood to carry oxygen to the cells of the body. Characteristically, headache, dyspnea, drowsiness, confusion, cherry-pink skin, unconsciousness, and apnea occur in sequence as the level of carbon monoxide in the blood increases. The most common source of carbon monoxide in cases of poisoning is exhaust fumes from an automobile. Treatment includes removal of the victim from the toxic environment, resuscitation, and administration of oxygen.

carbon tetrachloride A colorless, volatile, toxic liquid used as a solvent and in fire extinguishers. Ingestion of the liquid or inhalation of the fumes usually results in weakness, mental confusion, nausea, depression, abdominal pain, and convulsions. In poisoning by inhalation, ventilatory assistance and oxygen may be necessary. In poisoning by ingestion, removal of the poison and gastric lavage with saline solution are the usual treatments. Carbon tetrachloride is particularly toxic to the kidneys

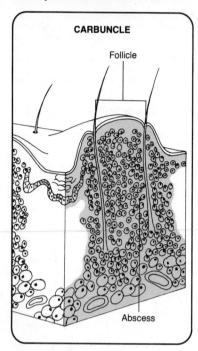

CARBUNCLE

Follicle

Abscess

and liver: permanent damage to these organs may result.

carboprost tromethamine An oxytocic agent.

carboxyhemoglobin A compound produced by the exposure of hemoglobin to carbon monoxide. Carbon monoxide from the environment is inhaled into the lungs, absorbed through the alveoli, and bound to hemoglobin in the blood, blocking the sites for oxygen transport. Oxygen levels decrease and, when the decrease is excessive, hypoxia and anoxia result. See also **carbon monoxide poisoning, oxyhemoglobin.**

carboxyl A monovalent radical COOH characteristic of organic acids. The hydrogen of the radical can be replaced by metals to form salts.

carbuncle A cluster of staphylococcal abscesses or boils containing purulent matter in deep, interconnecting, subcutaneous pockets. Eventually, pus discharges to the skin surface through numerous openings. Common sites for carbuncles are the back of the neck and the buttocks. Diabetes mellitus and hypogammaglobulinemia may be associated diseases. Treatment may include the use of antibiotics, hot compresses, and surgical drainage.

carbunculosis An abnormal condition, characterized by the bacterial infection of the hair follicle resulting in the formation of deep, painful abscesses that drain through multiple openings onto the skin surface, usually around hair follicles. Carbunculosis is a form of folliculitis, most commonly caused by the coagulase-positive *Staphylococcus aureus.* The lesions caused by this condition may result in fever and malaise.

carcin- A combining form meaning 'pertaining to cancer': *carcinelcosis, carcinogen.*

carcinectomy The excision of a cancer.

carcinoembryonic antigen (CEA) An antigen present in very small quantities in adult tissue. A greater than normal amount is suggestive of cancer. Tests for its presence aid in screening, in evaluating recurrent or disseminated disease, and in gauging the success of surgical ablation of malignant tumors.

carcinogen A substance that causes the development of a cancer.

carcinogenic Of or pertaining to the ability to cause the development of a cancer. Also called **cancerigenic, cancerogenic.**

carcinogenicity Of or pertaining to the ability to cause the development of a cancer.

carcinoid A small yellow tumor derived from argentaffin cells in the gastrointestinal mucosa that secrete serotonin, other catecholamines, and similar compounds. Carcinoid tumors spread slowly locally but may later metastasize widely. Their secretions often cause systemic symptoms. Also called **argentaffinoma, Kulchitsky-cell carcinoma.** See also **argentaffin cell, carcinoid syndrome.**

carcinoid syndrome The systemic effects of serotonin-secreting carcinoid tumors manifested by flushing, diarrhea, cramps, skin lesions resembling pellagra, labored breathing, palpitations, and valvular heart disease, especially of the pulmonary valve. Also called **argentaffinoma syndrome.** See also **carcinoid.**

carcinolysis The destruction of cancer cells, as by the action of an antineoplastic drug. —**carcinolytic,** *adj.*

carcinoma, *pl.* **carcinomas, carcinomata** A malignant epithelial neoplasm that tends to invade surrounding tissue and to metastasize to distant regions of the body. It develops most frequently in the skin, large intestine, lungs, stomach, prostate gland, cervix, or breast. The tumor is characteristically firm, irregular and nodular, with a well-defined border in some places; as a result, it usually cannot be clearly dissected and excised without removing normal surrounding tissue. Macroscopically, it is whitish with diffuse, dark hemorrhagic patches, and it has yellow areas of necrosis in the center. Microscopically, the tumor cells are characterized by anaplasia, abnormal size and shape, disproportionately large nuclei, and clumps of nuclear chromatin. —**carcinomatous,** *adj.*

-carcinoma A combining form meaning 'a malignant tumor composed of epithelial cells, with a tendency to metastasize': *ophthalmocarcinoma, osteocarcinoma, phlebocarcinoma.*

carcinoma basocellulare See **basal cell carcinoma.**

carcinoma cutaneum 1. See **basal cell carcinoma.** 2. See **squamous cell carcinoma.**

carcinoma en cuirasse A rare neoplasm accompanying advanced breast cancer and characterized by progressive fibrosis and rigidity of the skin of the chest, neck, back, and, occasionally, the abdomen. Another type, an extraperitoneal extension of gelatinous carcinoma of the rectum, encases the abdominal cavity in a rigid shell.

carcinoma fibrosum See **scirrhous carcinoma.**

carcinoma gigantocellulare See **giant cell carcinoma.**

carcinoma in situ A malignant neoplasm that has not invaded the basement membrane but shows cytologic characteristics of invasive cancer. Such neoplastic changes in stratified squamous or glandular epithelium are frequently seen on the uterine cervix and also occur in the anus, bronchi, buccal mucosa, esophagus, eye, lip, penis, uterine endometrium, vagina, and in the lesions of senile keratosis. Cervical carcinoma in situ is treated successfully by various methods, including cryosurgery, electrocautery, and simple hysterectomy. Lesions of this kind in pregnant women sometimes regress in the months after delivery. Also called **cancer in situ, intraepithelial carcinoma, preinvasive carcinoma.** See also **erythroplasia of Queyrat.**

carcinoma lenticulare A form of carcinoma tuberosum or scirrhous skin cancer characterized by the development of many small, relatively flat nodules that often coalesce to form larger areas resembling a fungous infection.

carcinoma medullare See **medullary carcinoma.**

carcinoma molle See **medullary carcinoma.**

carcinoma mucocellulare See **Krukenberg's tumor.**

carcinoma scroti An epithelial cell carcinoma of the scrotum.

carcinoma simplex An undifferentiated epithelial tumor in which the stroma and neoplastic epithelial cells do not have a definite microscopic pattern.

carcinoma spongiosum A carcinoma that is soft and spongy with small and large cavities in it. See also **medullary carcinoma.**

carcinoma telangiectaticum A neoplasm of the capillaries of the skin causing dilatation of the vessels and red spots on the skin that blanch with pressure.

carcinomatoid Resembling a carcinoma.

carcinomatosis An abnormal condition characterized by the extensive spread of carcinoma throughout the body.

carcinoma tuberosum See **tuberous carcinoma.**

carcinoma villosum See **villous carcinoma.**

carcinomectomy See **carcinectomy.**

carcinophilia The property in which there is an affinity for carcinomatous tissue. —**carcinophilic,** *adj.*

carcinosarcoma, *pl.* **carcinosarcomas, carcinosarcomata** A malignant neoplasm composed of carcinomatous and sarcomatous cells. Tumors of this type may occur in the esophagus, thyroid gland, and uterus.

carcinosis, *pl.* **carcinoses** A condition characterized by the development of many carcinomas throughout the body. Kinds of carcinoses are **carcinosis pleurae, miliary carcinosis. Also called carcinomatosis.**

carcinosis pleurae A secondary malignancy of the pleura in which nodules develop throughout the membranes.

carcinostatic Of or pertaining to the tendency to slow or halt the growth of a carcinoma.

carcinous Carcinomatous.

card-, cardio- A combining form meaning 'heart': *cardioclasis, cardiography, cardiomegaly.*

cardia 1. The opening between the esophagus and the cardiac portion of the stomach. 2. The portion of the stomach surrounding the esophagogastric connection, characterized by the absence of acid cells. 3. An obsolete term formerly and vaguely used to describe the heart and the region around the heart. —**cardiac,** *adj.*

cardia- See **cardio-.**

-cardia A combining form meaning 'a type of heart action or location': *araiocardia, brachycardia, miocardia.*

cardiac 1. Of or pertaining to the heart. 2. Pertaining to a person with heart disease. 3. Of or pertaining to the proximal part of the stomach.

-cardiac 1. A combining form meaning 'to characterize types and locations of heart ailments': *gravidocardiac, intracardiac, precardiac.* 2. A combining form meaning 'to identify heart ailment patients': *diplocardiac, hemicardiac, phrenopericardiac.*

cardiac aneurysm See **ventricular aneurysm.**

cardiac apnea Abnormal, temporary absence of respiration, as in Cheynes-Stokes respiration.

cardiac arrest See **cardiac standstill.**

cardiac arrhythmia An abnormal rate or rhythm of atrial or ventricular myocardial contraction. The condition may be caused by a defect in the ability of the sinoatrial node to maintain its pacemaker function, or by a failure of the bundle of His, the bundle branches, or the Purkinje network to conduct the contractile impulse. Increased metabolic demand, as in exercise or fever, or altered metabolic function, as in acidosis, alkalosis, hypokalemia, or hypocalcemia, results in an arrhythmia if the capacity of the heart to adjust to the particular stress is exceeded. Kinds of arrhythmia include **atrioventricular block, bradycardia, extrasystole, premature atrial contraction, premature ventricular contraction, tachycardia.**

cardiac asthma An attack of asthma associated with heart disease, as ventricular failure, and characterized by predominant pulmonary congestion with some bronchoconstriction.

cardiac catheter A long, fine catheter designed to be passed into the heart through a

CARDIAC CATHETERIZATION

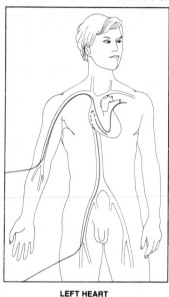

LEFT HEART

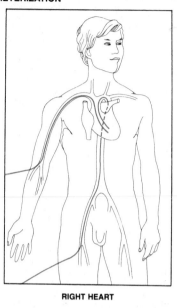

RIGHT HEART

blood vessel. Used for diagnosis, it allows determination of blood pressure and flow rate in the vessels and chambers of the heart and identification of abnormal anatomy. Medication may be instilled directly into a coronary vessel, often with visualization by tomography.

cardiac catheterization A diagnostic procedure in which a catheter is introduced into a large vein, usually of an arm or a leg, and threaded through the venous system to the heart. A sterile radiopaque catheter 100 to 125 cm (40 to 50 inches) in length is passed through an incision into the vein, through the vein to the superior vena cava, and into the right atrium and other structures to be studied. The course of the catheter is followed with fluoroscopy, and radiographs may be taken. An electrocardiogram is monitored on an oscilloscope. As the catheter tip passes through the chambers and vessels of the heart, the pressure of the flow of blood is monitored, and samples of the blood are taken to study the oxygen content. Formerly, only the right side of the heart could be catheterized; now, the left side may also be studied, but it requires passage through the arterial circulation into the left ventricle. Many conditions may be accurately identified and assessed using cardiac catheterization, including congenital heart disease, tricuspid stenosis, and valvular incompetence. Among the risks of the procedure are local infection, cardiac arrhythmia and thrombophlebitis.

NURSING CONSIDERATIONS: Cardiac catheterization takes from 1 to 3 hours and the patient has to lie still during the entire procedure. It is not painful, but, because anxiety producing, the patient needs explanation and emotional support. A young child may need anesthesia in order to lie still. An antibiotic is often given the day before. The pulse on the operative side and the blood pressure on the other side of the body are monitored frequently after the procedure. The temperature may be elevated for several hours, and there may be pain at the site of the incision. The nurse observes for signs of infection, thrombophlebitis, and cardiac arrhythmia. Cardiac catheterization is often performed by a special team in a special laboratory.

cardiac compression See **cardiac tamponade.**

cardiac conduction defect Any impairment of the electrical pathways and the specialized muscular fibers that conduct action impulses to contract the atria and the ventricles. Conduction defects may develop in the sinus node, the atrioventricular node, the bundle of His, the left or the right fiber bundles, or the Purkinje fibers. Defective transmission of cardiac impulses along the conduction routes may be caused by ischemic coronary disease or by an occlusion, a lesion, or other pathological factor.

cardiac cycle The cycle of events during which an electrical impulse is conducted through special fibers over the muscle of the myocardium, from the sinoatrial node of the atrioventricular node, to the bundle of His and the bundle branches, and to the Purkinje fibers, causing contraction of the atria followed by contraction of the ventricles. Contraction occurs with depolarization of the muscle fibers; recovery requires repolarization. Deoxygenated blood enters the right atrium of the heart from the superior vena cava and is pumped through the tricuspid valve into the right ventricle. With ventricular contraction, the blood is pumped through the semilunar valve into the pulmonary artery and the lungs for oxygenation. Oxygen-rich blood is returned to the heart through the branches of the pulmonary veins to the left atrium and is then passed through the mitral valve into the left ventricle. With ventricular contraction, the blood is pumped through the aortic semilunar valve into the aorta for peripheral circulation. The contractions of the left and the right atria are nearly simultaneous; they precede the nearly simultaneous contractions of the ventricles. The atria begin to repolarize during ventricular depolarization. On electrocardiogram, the cycle is shown as a series of waves, called P, Q, R, S, and T waves, that includes the QRS complex and, as two segments that connect the waves, the PR segment and the ST segment. Structural, chemical, or electrical abnormalities may cause a large variety of abnormalities in electrical conduction, muscular contraction, and blood flow in the heart. The EKG may reflect these abnormalities by changes in the shape and duration of the waves and segments of the EKG that represent phases of the cardiac cycle. See also specific waves and specific segments.

cardiac impulse   The movement of the thorax, caused by the beating of the heart. It is readily palpable and easily recorded.

cardiac massage   Repeated, rhythmic compression of the heart applied directly, during surgery, or through the intact chest wall in an effort to maintain circulation after cardiac arrest or ventricular fibrillation. See also **cardiopulmonary resuscitation.**

cardiac monitor   A device for the continuous observation of cardiac function. It may include electrocardiograph and oscilloscope readings, recording devices, and a visual or audible record of heart function and rhythm. An alarm system may be set to alert staff of variation from a certain rate.

cardiac monitoring   A continuous check on the functioning of the heart with an electronic instrument that provides an electrocardiographic reading on an oscilloscope. Each ventricular contraction of the heart is indicated by either a flashing light or an audible sound. The indicator is often integrated with an alarm system that is triggered by a pulse rate above or below predetermined limits. The procedure is performed most often in an intensive care unit, although devices are available for patients who are ambulatory.

cardiac murmur   An abnormal sound associated with the flow of blood through the heart, which may indicate incomplete closing of one or more heart valves or may be a sign of valvular stenosis. Murmurs are classified as systolic or diastolic. Depending on various characteristics,

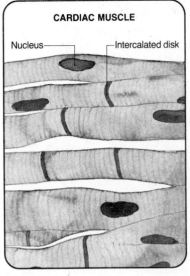

CARDIAC MUSCLE

Nucleus — Intercalated disk

as intensity, frequency, and duration, a cardiac murmur may be a benign or a pathogenic sign. Also called **heart murmur.**

cardiac muscle   A special striated muscle of the myocardium, containing dark intercalated discs at the junctions of abutting fibers. Cardiac muscle is an exception among involuntary muscles, which are characteristically smooth. Its contractile fibrillae resemble those of skeletal muscle but are only one-third as large in diameter, are richer in sarcoplasm, and contain centrally located instead of peripheral nuclei. Studies with the electron microscope indicate that the intercalated discs in cardiac muscle represent cell boundaries. The connective tissue of cardiac muscle is sparser than that of skeletal muscle.

cardiac output   The volume of blood expelled by the ventricles of the heart, equal to the amount of blood ejected at each beat (the stroke output) multiplied by the number of beats in the period of time used in the computation. Cardiac output is commonly measured by the thermodilution technique in which a catheter with a thermistor electrode at the tip is inserted in the pulmonary artery, and a certain amount of a cold solution is injected through the lumen of the catheter into the right atrium. The thermistor determines the temperature of the solution when it reaches the pulmonary artery, and the output is calculated on the basis of the temperature change; the increase in the temperature of the solution is inversely related to the functioning of the heart. A normal heart in a resting adult ejects from 2.5 to 3.6 liters (2¾ to 3¾ qt) of blood per minute. A decreased output at rest is usually indicative of a late stage in abnormal cardiac performance; its failure to increase during exercise occurs much earlier in a malfunctioning heart.

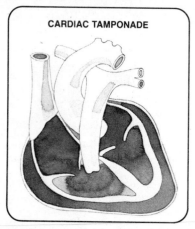

CARDIAC TAMPONADE

lanoside, lanatoside, and ouabain, increase the force of myocardial contractions and decrease the heart rate and conduction velocity, allowing more time for the ventricles to relax and become filled with blood. These glycosides, which are composed of a steroid nucleus, lactone ring, and a sugar, are used in the treatment of congestive heart failure, atrial flutter and fibrillation, paroxysmal atrial tachycardia, and cardiogenic shock. Epinephrine, a potent vasopressor and cardiac stimulant, is sometimes used to restore heart rhythm in cardiac arrest but is not employed in treating heart failure or cardiogenic shock. Isoproterenol hydrochloride, which is related to epinephrine, may be used in treating heart block. Dobutamine hydrochloride and dopamine are employed in the short-term treatment of cardiac decompensation owing to depressed contractility.

cardiac tamponade　　Compression of the heart produced by the accumulation in the pericardial sac of fluid or of blood resulting from the rupture of a blood vessel of the myocardium, as by a penetrating wound. Signs of cardiac tamponade may include distended neck veins, hypotension, decreased heart sounds, tachypnea, peripheral pulses that are weak or absent or that fall sharply during inspiration (pulsus paradoxus), elevated cerebrovascular pressure, reduced left atrial pressure, and a pericardial friction rub. The patient, who is usually anxious and restless, may sit upright or lean forward, and the skin may be pale, dusky, or cyanotic. The electrocardiogram generally shows decreased cardiac voltage and the chest X-ray may reveal an enlarged heart shadow ("water bottle" heart). Cardiotonic and antiarrhythmic drugs and measures for controlling pain are administered as ordered. Aspiration of the fluid or blood in the pericardial sac (pericardiocentesis) is performed for diagnosis and for therapy. If surgery is indicated, the patient is prepared for the procedure, and the bleeding vessel or vessels are ligated.

NURSING CONSIDERATIONS: The patient with life-threatening cardiac tamponade is usually cared for in an intensive care unit. A drain may be put in place in the pericardial sac. Coughing and deep breathing are painful, and recovery may be lengthy and difficult. The patient requires extensive physical and emotional care.

cardiac output, alteration in: decreased　A nursing diagnosis accepted by the Fifth National Conference on the Classification of Nursing Diagnoses. The etiology of the condition is to be developed at a later conference. The defining characteristics include variations in blood pressure, arrhythmias, fatigue, jugular vein distention, color changes of the skin and mucous membranes, oliguria, decreased peripheral pulses, cold and clammy skin, rales, dyspnea, orthopnea, and restlessness. Other characteristics that often occur are mental status change, shortness of breath, syncope, vertigo, edema, cough, frothy sputum, cardiac gallop, and weakness. See also **nursing diagnosis.**

cardiac plexus　One of several nerve complexes situated close to the arch of the aorta. The cardiac plexuses contain sympathetic and parasympathetic nerve fibers, which leave the plexuses, accompany the right and the left coronary arteries, and enter the heart. Some of the fibers from the plexuses terminate in the sinoatrial node; others terminate in the atrioventricular node and in the atrial myocardium.

cardiac reserve　The potential capacity of the heart to function well beyond its basal level, responding to the demands of various physiological and psychological changes.

cardiac sphincter　A ring of muscle fibers at the juncture of the esophagus and stomach.

cardiac standstill　The complete cessation of contractions of the heart, resulting in circulatory failure, unconsciousness, respiratory arrest, and death. Cardiac standstill requires immediate cardiopulmonary resuscitation, open cardiac massage, or stimulation of the heart with an electric current. It may be caused by myocardial infarction, chronic disorder of the conduction system of the myocardium, systemic diseases, or metabolic disturbance. Also called cardiac arrest, cardioplegia, cardiopulmonary arrest.

cardiac stimulant　A pharmacologic agent which increases the action of the heart. Cardiac glycosides, as digitalis, digitoxin, digoxin, de-

cardiac valve　See **heart valve.**

cardinal frontal plane　The plane that divides the body into front and back portions. Also called **vertical plane.**

cardinal horizontal plane　The plane that divides the body into upper and lower portions. Also called **transverse plane.**

cardinal ligament　A sheet of subserous fascia extending across the pelvic floor as a continuation of the broad ligament. It is embedded in the adipose tissue on each side of the vagina and is formed by the fasciae of the vagina and the cervix converging at the lateral borders of these organs. The ligament forms ventral and dorsal extensions at the lateral portion of the pelvic diaphragm. The ventral extension joins the tissue supporting the bladder. The dorsal extension blends with the uterosacral ligaments. The vaginal arteries course across the pelvis in close association with the cardinal ligament. See also **broad ligament.**

cardinal movements of labor　The typical sequence of positions assumed by the fetus as it descends through the pelvis during labor and delivery, usually designated as engagement, flexion, descent, internal rotation, extension, and external rotation or restitution. The birth canal is a curved cylinder; the head must enter it in a downward, transverse direction but exit it in a more forward, anteroposterior direction. In a vertex presentation, engagement of the head in the pelvic inlet requires flexion of the head with chin on chest. Following descent, the head must undergo extension to turn forward and be born under the symphysis. The pelvic inlet is somewhat heart-shaped and the fetal head enters it facing obliquely; but the pelvic outlet is somewhat diamond-shaped and the head usually exits it facing posteriorly and must undergo internal rotation to do so. Following delivery of the head, the shoulders remain for a time in the oblique plane and the head undergoes external rotation or restitution to allow the widest diameter of the shoulders to be delivered from the longer anteroposterior diameter of the pelvic outlet.

cardinal position of gaze　In ophthalmology: one of six positions to which the normal eye may be turned. Each position requires the function of a specific ocular muscle and a cranial nerve. The positions and the corresponding muscles and nerves are as follows:
　Straight nasal: medial rectus and the third cranial nerve.
　Up nasal: inferior oblique and the third cranial nerve.
　Down nasal: superior oblique and the fourth cranial nerve.
　Straight temporal: lateral rectus and the sixth cranial nerve.
　Up temporal: superior rectus and the third cranial nerve.
　Down temporal: inferior rectus and the third cranial nerve.

cardinal sagittal plane　The plane that divides the body into left and right portions. Also called **midsagittal plane.**

cardinal symptom　See **symptom.**

cardio-, cardia-　A combining form meaning 'pertaining to the heart': *cardiocele, cardiocirrhosis, cardiodynia.*

cardioactive　Affecting the heart.

cardiocirculatory　Of or pertaining to the heart and the circulation.

cardiogenic shock　An abnormal condition often characterized by low cardiac output in association with acute myocardial infarction and congestive heart failure. This condition is difficult to diagnose because of complex hemodynamic variations in affected individuals. Although low cardiac output is a common sign

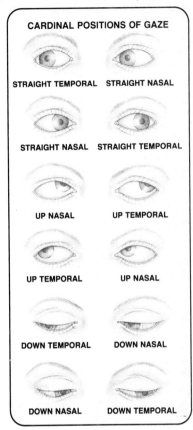

CARDINAL POSITIONS OF GAZE

STRAIGHT TEMPORAL　　STRAIGHT NASAL

STRAIGHT NASAL　　STRAIGHT TEMPORAL

UP NASAL　　UP TEMPORAL

UP TEMPORAL　　UP NASAL

DOWN TEMPORAL　　DOWN NASAL

DOWN NASAL　　DOWN TEMPORAL

of this disorder, cardiogenic shock may also occur in association with normal or higher-than-normal output. Fast determination of blood volume is important to proper therapy. Cardiogenic shock is fatal in about 80% of cases, and immediate therapy is necessary to save affected individuals. Depending on the signs, therapy may include the administration of fluids, diuretics, or vasoactive drugs and the application of various devices, as pacing catheters. A variety of surgical procedures may be part of the therapy but are not usually employed.

cardiogram　An electronically recorded tracing of cardiac activity.

cardiography　The technique of graphically recording the movements of the heart by means of a cardiograph.

cardioinhibitor　A substance, as a drug, that inhibits heart action.

cardiologist　A physician specializing in the diagnosis and treatment of disorders of the heart.

cardiology　The study of the anatomy, normal functions, and disorders of the heart.

cardiolysis　An operation that separates the heart and the pericardium from the sternal periosteum in a procedure to correct adhesive mediastinopericarditis. The operation resects the ribs and the sternum over the pericardium.

cardiomegaly Hypertrophy of the heart, caused most frequently by hypertension and also occurring in arteriovenous fistula, congenital aortic stenosis, ventricular septal defect, patent ductus arteriosus, and Paget's disease. In athletes, an enlarged, well-functioning heart is a normal finding.

cardiomyopathy Any disease that affects the myocardium. Three types of cardiomyopathy are congestive, restrictive, and hypertrophic.

cardioplegia See **cardiac standstill.**

cardiopulmonary Of or pertaining to the heart and the lungs.

cardiopulmonary arrest See **cardiac standstill.**

cardiopulmonary bypass A procedure used in heart surgery in which the blood is diverted from the heart and lungs by means of a pump oxygenator and returned directly to the aorta.

cardiopulmonary resuscitation (CPR) A basic emergency procedure for life support, consisting of artificial respiration and manual external cardiac massage. It is used in cases of cardiac arrest to establish effective circulation and ventilation in order to prevent irreversible cerebral damage owing to anoxia. External cardiac massage compresses the heart between the lower sternum and the thoracic vertebral column. During compressions, blood is forced into systemic and pulmonary circulation, and venous blood refills the heart when the compression is released. Mouth-to-mouth breathing or a mechanical form of ventilation is used concomitantly with CPR in order to oxygenate the blood being pumped through the circulatory system.

cardiorrhaphy An operation in which the heart muscle is sutured.

cardioscope An obsolete device for inspecting and manipulating the internal structures of the heart.

cardiospasm A form of achalasia characterized by a failure of the cardia at the distal end of the esophagus to relax, causing dysphagia and regurgitation and sometimes requiring surgical division of the muscle.

cardiotachometer An instrument that continuously monitors and records the heartbeat.

cardiotomy **1.** An operation in which the heart is incised. **2.** An operation in which the cardiac end of the stomach or cardiac orifice is incised.

cardiotonic **1.** Of or pertaining to a substance that tends to increase the efficiency of contractions of the heart muscle. **2.** A pharmacologic agent that increases the force of myocardial contractions. Cardiac glycosides, derived from certain plant alkaloids, exert a tonic effect by altering the transport of electrolytes across the myocardial membrane, causing an increased influx of sodium and calcium and an increased efflux of potassium. Digitalis, digitoxin, and digoxin, widely used cardiac glycosides obtained from leaves of a species of foxglove, increase the force of myocardial contractions, extend the refractory period of the atrioventricular node, and, to a lesser degree, affect the sinoatrial node and the heart's conduction system. Other cardiac glycosides are ouabain and strophanthin, obtained from species of *Strophanthus;* scillaridin, derived from squill; and bufotalin, obtained from the skin and saliva of a European toad.

cardiotoxic Having a toxic or injurious effect on the heart.

cardiovascular Of or pertaining to the heart and blood vessels.

cardiovascular assessment An evaluation of the condition, function, and abnormalities of the heart and circulatory system.

cardiovascular disease Any one of numerous abnormal conditions characterized by dysfunction of the heart and blood vessels. Some common kinds of cardiovascular disease are **atherosclerosis, cor pulmonale, hypertension,** and **rheumatic heart disease.** In the United States cardiovascular disease is second to cancer as the leading cause of death, accounting for about 50% of all deaths from disease annually. More than a quarter of a million persons under age 65 die each year from this disorder; about half of such deaths are attributed to atherosclerosis. The prevalent kinds of cardiovascular disease are the rheumatic, the syphilitic, and the traumatic varieties.

cardiovascular system The network of structures, including the heart and the blood vessels, that pump and convey the blood throughout the body. The system includes thousands of miles of vessels, capillaries, and venules and is vital to maintaining homeostasis. Numerous control mechanisms of the system assure that the blood is delivered to the structures where it is most needed and at the proper rate. The system delivers nutrients and other essential materials to the fluids surrounding the cells and removes waste products, which are conveyed to excretory organs, as the kidneys and the intestine. The cardiovascular system functions in close association with the respiratory system, transporting oxygen inhaled into the lungs and conveying carbon dioxide to the lungs for expiration. Sympathetic and parasympathetic impulses from the medulla and cardiac baroreceptors sensitive to changes in pressure control the function of the heart, which pumps the oxygenated blood carried by the arteries and receives deoxygenated blood from the veins. Cardiovascular diseases affect a large number of individuals throughout the world, and half a million Americans die each year from coronary diseases. A variety of factors, as diet, exercise, and stress, affect the cardiovascular system.

cardioversion The restoration of the heart's sinus rhythm by delivery of a synchronized electrical shock through two metal paddles placed on the patient's chest. Cardioversion is used in the treatment of atrial fibrillation and in ventricular, nodal, and atrial arrhythmias.

carditis An inflammatory condition of the muscles of the heart, usually resulting from infection. In most cases more than one layer of muscles is involved. Chest pain, cardiac arrhythmia, circulatory failure, and damage to the structures of the heart may occur. Kinds of carditis are **endocarditis, myocarditis, pericarditis.**

career ladder In nursing education: a pathway for upward mobility that begins with a course of study in practical nursing or a program that grants an associate degree in nursing. On completion of this basic level, the candidate may continue up the ladder, taking a baccalaureate program in nursing. After this, the person may continue on to a masters and a doctoral program.

care of the sick In public health nursing: the care of sick patients in their homes, as distinguished from health supervision. Public health nursing agencies are reimbursed for the nursing services rendered by the nurses according to the kind of service rendered, as a sick visit or a health supervision visit. Compare **health supervision.**

caries An abnormal condition of a tooth or a bone characterized by decay, disintegration, and destruction of the structure. Kinds of caries include **dental caries, radiation caries, spinal caries.**

carina, *pl.* **carinae** Any structure shaped like a ridge or keel, as the carina of the trachea, which projects from the lowest tracheal cartilage.

cariogenic Tending to produce caries.

carisoprodol A skeletal muscle relaxant.

carminative 1. Of or pertaining to a substance that relieves flatulence and abdominal distention. 2. A carminative agent that relieves gaseous distention and painful spasms, especially after meals. Volatile oils of anise, bitter almond, cinnamon, fennel, peppermint, spearmint, and wintergreen, which have a soothing effect passing through the stomach, were formerly used as carminatives, but they are rarely used in modern medicine except as flavoring agents.

carmine dye A red coloring substance, produced by the addition of alum to an extract of cochineal, used for staining specimens in histology.

carmustine (BCNU) An alkylating agent used as in chemotherapy.

carneous Having the quality of flesh.

carnitine A naturally-occuring amino acid found in skeletal muscle, essential for long-chain fatty acid oxidation.

carnivore An animal belonging to the order *Carnivora*, classified as a flesheater, with appropriate teeth and a characteristically simple stomach and a short intestine for such a diet. **—carnivorous,** *adj.*

carotene, carotin, carrotene, carrotine A red or orange hydrocarbon found in carrots, sweet potatoes, milk fat, egg yolk, and leafy vegetables, as beet greens, spinach, and broccoli.

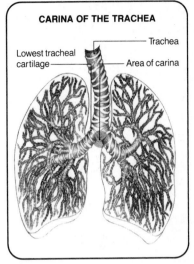

CARINA OF THE TRACHEA

Lowest tracheal cartilage — Trachea — Area of carina

Carotene is a provitamin and in the body is converted into vitamin A. An inability to utilize carotene results in vitamin A deficiency. See also **vitamin A.**

carotenemia The presence of carotene in the blood resulting in an abnormal yellow appearance of the plasma and skin. The conjunctivae are not discolored. Also called **pseudojaundice.** Compare **hyperbilirubinemia.** See also **icterus, jaundice.**

carotenoid, carotinoid Any of a group of red, yellow, or orange highly unsaturated pigments that are found in some animal tissue and in foods, as carrots, sweet potatoes, and leafy green vegetables. Many of these substances, as carotene, are necessary for the formation of vitamin A in the body, while others, including lycopene and xanthophyll, show no vitamin A activity.

carotenosis See **carotenemia.**

carotid Of or pertaining to the carotid artery. See also **carotid body, carotid sinus.**

carotid body A small structure containing neural tissue at the bifurcation of the carotid arteries. It monitors the oxygen content of the blood and assists in regulating respiration.

carotid body reflex A normal chemical reflex initiated by a decrease in oxygen concentration in the blood and, to a lesser degree, by increased carbon dioxide and hydrogen ion concentrations that act on chemoreceptors at the bifurcation of the common carotid arteries and result in nerve impulses that cause the respiratory center in the medulla to increase respiratory activity. See also **aortic body reflex.**

carotid body tumor A benign, round, firm growth that develops at the bifurcation of the common carotid artery. The tumor usually has no effect but it sometimes may cause dizziness, nausea, and vomiting, especially if it impedes the flow of blood as pressure is increased in the

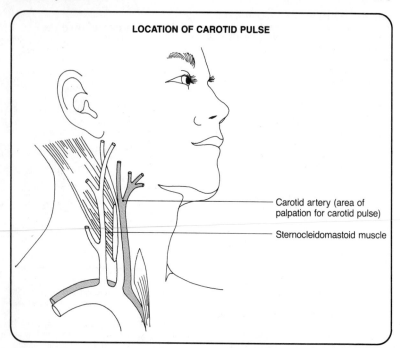

LOCATION OF CAROTID PULSE

Carotid artery (area of palpation for carotid pulse)

Sternocleidomastoid muscle

vascular system. It may be surgically excised in some cases.

carotid plexus Any one of three nerve plexuses associated with the carotid arteries. Compare **common carotid plexus, external carotid plexus, internal carotid plexus.**

carotid pulse The pulse of the carotid artery, palpated by gently pressing a finger in the groove between the larynx and the sternocleidomastoid muscle in the neck.

carotid sinus A dilatation of the arterial wall at the bifurcation of the common carotid artery. It contains sensory nerve endings from the vagus nerve that respond to changes in blood pressure.

carotid sinus reflex The decrease in the heart rate as a reflex reaction from pressure on or within the carotid artery at the level of its bifurcation. This reflex starts in the sinus of the internal carotid artery. See also **carotid sinus syndrome.**

carotid sinus syndrome A temporary loss of consciousness that sometimes accompanies convulsive seizures because of the intensity of the carotid sinus reflex when pressure builds in one or both carotid sinuses.

carotodynia A tenderness along the length of the common carotid artery.

-carp A combining form meaning 'fruit': *archicarp, ascocarp, pericarp.*

carpal Of or pertaining to the carpus, or wrist.

-carpal A combining form referring to the wrist: *extracarpal, radiocarpal, trapeziometacarpal.*

carpal tunnel A conduit for the median nerve and the flexor tendons, formed by the carpal bones and the flexor retinaculum.

carpal tunnel syndrome A common painful disorder of the wrist and hand, induced by compression on the median nerve between the inelastic carpal ligament and other structures within the carpal tunnel. The syndrome is seen more often in women, especially in pregnant and in menopausal women. Symptoms may result from trauma, synovitis, or tumor, or may develop with rheumatoid arthritis, amyloidosis, agromegaly, or diabetes. The median nerve innervates the palm and the radial side of the hand; compression of the nerve causes weakness, pain with opposition of the thumb, and burning, tingling, or aching, sometimes radiating to the forearm and to the shoulder joint. Weakness and atrophy of muscles may increase from lack of use, impairing thumb and finger dexterity. Pain may be intermittent or constant and is often most intense at night. Symptomatic treatment usually relieves mild symptoms of recent onset, but if the pain becomes disabling, the injection of corticosteroids often brings dramatic relief. Surgical division of the volar carpal ligament to relieve nerve pressure is usually curative. Nursing treatment includes emotional support, nocturnal splinting of the hand and forearm, elevation of the arm to relieve the swelling of soft tissue, and encouragement of mild wrist and finger movements to prevent atrophy of muscles.

carphenazine maleate A phenothiazine

used as an antipsychotic agent.

carpopedal spasm   A spasm of the hand, thumbs, foot, or toes that sometimes accompanies tetany.

carpus   The wrist, made up of eight bones arranged in two rows. The proximal row consists of the scaphoid, lunate, triangular, and pisiform. The distal row consists of the trapezium, trapezoid, capitate, and hamate.

Carrel-Lindbergh pump   See **Lindbergh pump.**

carrier   **1.** A person or animal who harbors and spreads an organism causing disease in others but who does not become ill. **2.** One whose chromosomes carry a recessive gene.

Carrión's disease   See **bartonellosis.**

cartilage   A nonvascular supporting connective tissue composed of various cells and fibers, found chiefly in the joints, the thorax, and various rigid tubes, as the larynx, trachea, nose, and ear. Temporary cartilage, as that comprising most of the fetal skeleton at an early stage, is later replaced by bone. Permanent cartilage remains unossified, except in certain diseases and, sometimes, in advanced age. Kinds of permanent cartilage are **hyaline cartilage, white fibrocartilage, yellow cartilage. —cartilaginous,** *adj.*

cartilage-hair hypoplasia   A genetic disorder, inherited as an autosomal recessive trait, characterized by dwarfism caused by hypoplasia of the cartilage, multiple skeletal abnormalities, and excessively sparse, short, fine, brittle hair that is usually light colored. The condition is found primarily among Amish people in the United States and Canada.

cartilaginous joint   A slightly movable joint in which cartilage unites bony surfaces. Two types of articulation involving cartilaginous joints are synchondrosis and symphysis. Also called **amphiarthrosis, junctura cartilaginea.** Compare **fibrous joint, synovial joint.**

CARTOS   Acronym for *c*omputer-*a*ided *r*econstruction by *t*racing *o*f *s*erial sections, a technique in which serial, hand-drawn copies of electron micrographs are programmed on a computer for display on a television screen. The image can be manipulated for study of all dimensions of the structure.

caruncle, caruncula   A small, fleshy projection, as one of the lacrimal caruncles at the inner canthus of the eye or the hymenal caruncles that are the hymenal remnants.

carunculae hymenales   Remnants of a ruptured hymen that appear as irregular projections of normal skin around the introitus to the vagina. Also called hymeneal tags.

caryo-, karyo-   A combining form meaning 'pertaining to a nucleus': *caryokinesis, caryophyllus.*

cascade   Any process that develops in stages, with each stage dependent on the preceding one, often producing a cumulative effect.

cascara sagrada   A stimulant laxative.

caseation   A form of tissue necrosis in which there is loss of cellular outline and the appearance is that of crumbly cheese. It is typical of tuberculosis. **—caseate,** *v.* **caseous,** *adj.*

caseation necrosis   Necrosis that transforms tissue into a dry cheeselike mass.

case fatality rate   The number of deaths caused by any specific disease, expressed as a percentage of the total number of cases of the disease.

caseous   Cheeselike, describing the mixture of fat and protein that appear in some body tissues undergoing necrosis.

caseous fermentation   The coagulation of soluble casein through the action of rennin.

cast   **1.** A stiff, solid dressing formed with plaster of Paris or other material, such as fiberglass, around a limb or other body part to immobilize it during healing. **2.** A mold of a part or all of a patient's teeth and internal jaw area for fitting prostheses or dentures. **3.** A tiny structure formed by deposits of mineral or other substances on the walls of renal tubules, bronchioles, or other organs. Casts often appear in samples of urine or blood collected for laboratory examination. **4.** The deviation of an eye from the normal parallel lines of vision, as in strabismus.

Castellani's paint   A liquid applied topically to large areas of the skin, as a disinfectant for treatment of fungal infection. Castellani's paint consists of phenol, resorcinal, boric acid, acetone, and basic fuchsin. See also **paint.**

castor oil   A stimulant laxative.

castration   The surgical excision of one or both testicles or ovaries, performed most frequently to reduce the production and secretion of certain hormones that may stimulate the proliferation of malignant cells in women with breast cancer and in men with cancer of the prostate. The patient must be informed that bilateral excision of the gonads causes sterility. See also **oophorectomy, orchidectomy.**

castration anxiety   **1.** The fantasized fear of injury or loss of the genital organs, often as the reaction to a repressed feeling of punishment for forbidden sexual desires. It may also be caused by some apparently threatening everyday occurrence, such as a humiliating experience, loss of a job, or loss of authority. **2.** A general threat to the masculinity or femininity of a person or an unrealistic fear of bodily injury or loss of power. Also called anxiety complex. See also **anxiety neurosis.**

castration complex   See **castration anxiety.**

casuistics   The recording and the study of the cases of any disease.

CAT   Acronym for **computerized axial tomography.**

cata-, cat-   A combining form meaning 'down, under, against, with': *catabasis, catabolic, catacausis.*

catabasis, *pl.* **catabases**   The phase in which a disease declines. **—catabatic,** *adj.*

catabiosis   The normal aging of cells. **—catabiotic,** *adj.*

catabolic activator protein   See **CAP.**

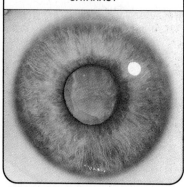

CATARACT

catabolism A complex, metabolic process in which energy is liberated for use in work, energy storage, or heat production by the oxidation of carbohydrates, fats, and proteins. Carbon dioxide and water are produced as well as energy. Compare **anabolism.** —**catabolic,** *adj.*

catacrotism An anomaly of the pulse, characterized by a small additional wave in the descending limb of the pulse tracing. —**catacrotic,** *adj.*

catalepsy An abnormal state characterized by a trancelike level of consciousness and postural rigidity. It occurs in hypnosis and in certain organic and psychological disorders, as schizophrenia, epilepsy, and hysteria.

catalysis An increase in the rate of any chemical reaction, caused by a chemical material that is neither part of the process itself nor consumed or affected by the reaction. Compare **negative catalysis.** See also **catalyst.** —**catalytic,** *adj.*

catalyst A substance that influences the rate of a chemical reaction without being permanently altered by the process. Most catalysts, including enzymes in living organisms, accelerate chemical reactions; negative catalysts retard such reactions. See also **enzyme.**

-catalytic A combining form meaning 'pertaining to a chemical reaction caused by an agent unchanged by the reaction': *allelocatalytic, autocatalytic, photocatalytic.* Also **-catalytical.**

catamnesis The medical history of a patient from the onset of an illness.

cataphylaxis **1.** The migration of leukocytes and antibodies to the site of an infection. **2.** The deterioration of the natural defense system of the body. —**cataphylactic,** *adj.*

cataplexy A condition characterized by sudden muscular weakness and hypotonia, caused by emotions, as anger, fear or surprise, often associated with narcolepsy. —**cataplectic,** *adj.*

cataract An abnormal progressive condition of the lens of the eye, characterized by loss of transparency. A gray-white opacity that forms within the lens, behind the pupil. Most cataracts are caused by degenerative changes, occurring most often after 50 years of age. The tendency to develop cataracts is inherited. Trauma, as a puncture wound, may result in cataract formation; less often, exposure to such poisons as dinitrophenol or naphthalene causes them. Congenital cataracts are usually hereditary but may be caused by viral infection during the first trimester of gestation. If cataracts are untreated, sight is eventually lost. At first vision is blurred; then, bright lights glare diffusely, and distortion and double vision may develop. Uncomplicated cataracts of old age (**senile cataracts**) are usually treated with excision of the lens and prescription of special contact lens or glasses. The soft cataracts of children and young adults may either be incised and drained or fragmented by ultrasound, followed by irrigation and aspiration of the fragments through a minute incision.

catarrh Inflammation of the mucous membranes with discharge, especially inflammation of the air passages of the nose and the trachea. —**catarrhal, catarrhous,** *adj.*

catarrhal dysentery See **sprue.**

catastrophic care A pattern of medical and nursing care that involves intensive, highly technical life-support care of an acutely ill or severely traumatized patient.

catastrophic health insurance Health insurance that awards benefits to pay for the cost of severe or lengthy disability or illness. Benefits on some policies are not paid until a specified minimum amount, paid by the insured, is exceeded. Most policies have a limit in total benefits paid, and payment for certain kinds of services may either be precluded or limited to a maximum indemnity.

catastrophic reaction The uncoordinated response to a drastic shock or a sudden threatening condition, as often occurs in the victims of car crashes and disasters.

catatonia A state or condition characterized by conspicuous motor disturbance, manifested usually as immobility with extreme muscular rigidity, or, less commonly, as excessive, impulsive activity. See also **catatonic schizophrenia.** —**catatonic,** *adj.*

catatonic schizophrenia A form of schizophrenia characterized by alternating periods of extreme withdrawal and extreme excitement. During the withdrawal stage stupor, muscular rigidity, mutism, blocking, negativism, catalepsy, and cerea flexibilitas may be seen; during the period of excitement, purposeless and impulsive activity may range from mild agitation to violence. Either phase may last for a period of hours, days, or weeks, and the change to the alternate phase is usually abrupt and rapid. Treatment may include tranquilizers, an antidepressant or antianxiety drug, followed by long-term psychotherapy. See also **catatonia.**

cat-bite fever See **cat-scratch fever.**

catchment area The specific geographical area for which a particular institution, especially a mental health center, is responsible.

catch-up growth An acceleration of the growth rate following a period of growth retardation owing to a secondary deficiency, as acute malnutrition or severe illness. The phenomenon, which is routinely seen in premature infants, involves rapid increase in weight, length, and head circumference and continues until the normal individual growth pattern is resumed. The severity, duration, and the developmental timing at which the deficiency occurs may result in some growth inadequacy or permanent deficit, especially in such tissue as the brain.

cat-cry syndrome A rare, congenital disorder recognized at birth by a kittenlike cry which may prevail for weeks, then disappear. Other characteristics include low birth weight, microcephaly, "moon face," wide-set eyes, strabismus, and low-set misshaped ears. Infants are hypotonic; heart defects and mental and physical retardation are common. Also called **cri du chat syndrome.**

catecholamine Any one of a group of sympathomimetic compounds composed of a catechol molecule and the aliphatic portion of an amine. Some catecholamines are produced naturally by the body and function as key neurological chemicals. Catecholamines are also synthesized as drugs used in the treatment of various disorders, as anaphylaxis, asthma, cardiac failure, and shock. Some important endogenous catecholamines are dopamine, epinephrine, and norepinephrine. Norepinephrine mediates a host of physiologic and metabolic responses that follow the stimulation of the sympathetic nerves. In response to stress, the adrenal medulla is stimulated, causing the elevation of epinephrine and norepinephrine concentrations in the circulation. Epinephrine dilates blood vessels to the skeletal muscles. Norepinephrine slightly constricts these blood vessels. Both compounds stimulate the myocardium. Dopamine is found primarily in the basal ganglia of the central nervous system (CNS), but dopaminergic nerve endings and specific receptors for this compound have been found in other CNS areas. The major functions of catecholamines and drugs that mimic their actions include the peripheral excitation of certain muscles, peripheral inhibition of certain muscles, cardiac excitation, metabolic actions, endocrine actions and CNS actions. Differences in the actions of the catecholamines depend on alpha and beta receptors in nerve terminals throughout the body. The brain contains separate neuronal systems that use dopamine, epinephrine, and norepinephrine. More than half of the catecholamine content of the CNS is dopamine, large quantities of which are found in the basal ganglia, the central nucleus of the amygdala, the median eminence, the olfactory tubercle and the restricted fields of the frontal cortex. The hypothalamus and certain zones of the limbic system contain relatively large amounts of norepinephrine, which is also found in lesser amounts in other brain areas. Neurons in the CNS that contain epinephrine are situated primarily in the medullary reticular formation. Catecholamines act directly on sympathetic effector cells by binding to receptors in cellular plasma membranes. Sympathomimetic drugs influence biochemical reactions and functional responses in all the tissues they effect.

cat-eye syndrome A rare, congenital autosomal anomaly, marked by the presence of an extra, small chromosome 22 and pupils that resemble the vertical pupils of a cat. Anal atresia, heart abnormalities, and severe mental retardation are common.

categorical data In research: any data that are classified by name rather than by number, as race, religion, ethnicity, or marital status.

catgut A nonabsorbable suture material, prepared from the intestines of sheep, used to close surgical wounds. Compare **chromic.**

catharsis 1. A cleansing or purging. —**cathartic,** *n.* 2. The therapeutic release of pent-up feelings and emotions by open discussion of ideas and thoughts. 3. In psychoanalysis: the process of bringing repressed ideas and feelings into the consciousness by the technique of free association, often in conjunction with hypnosis and the use of hypnotic drugs. Also called **psychocatharsis.** See also **abreaction.** —**cathartic,** *adj.*

cathartic 1. Of or pertaining to a substance that causes evacuation of the bowel. 2. A cathartic agent that promotes bowel evacuation by stimulating peristalsis, increasing the fluidity or bulk of intestinal contents, softening the feces, or lubricating the intestinal wall. The term *cathartic* implies a fluid evacuation; this is in contrast to *laxative,* which implies the elimination of a soft, formed stool. Cathartics that increase peristalsis, usually by irritating intestinal mucosa, include certain plant substances, as aloe, colocynth, croton oil, podophyllum senna, phenolphthalein, bisacodyl, and dehydrocholic acid. Saline cathartics, as sodium sulfate, magnesium sulfate, and magnesium hydroxide, dilute the intestinal contents by retaining water through osmotic forces. Suppositories containing sodium biphosphate, sodium acid pyrophosphate, and sodium bicarbonate induce defecation when the salts react to form carbon dioxide and the expanding gas stimulates peristalsis. Also called **coprogogue.** See also **laxative.** —**catharsis,** *n.*

-cathartic A combining form meaning 'pertaining to cleaning': *cephalocathartic, emetocathartic, hematocathartic.*

catheter A hollow, flexible tube that can be inserted into a vessel or cavity of the body to withdraw or to instill fluids. Most catheters are made of soft plastic or rubber and may be used for treatment or diagnosis. Kinds of catheters include **acorn-tipped catheter, Foley catheter.**

catheterization The introduction of a catheter into a body cavity or organ to inject or remove a fluid. The most common procedure is the insertion of a catheter into the bladder through the urethra for the relief of urinary retention and for emptying the bladder completely before surgery. It is also used when a urine specimen may otherwise be contaminated, as when a woman is menstruating. Self-catheterization is taught to those patients with neurogenic bladder. Sterile, aseptic techniques are necessary to prevent infection; trauma is also to be avoided, particularly to the male urethra and when the procedure is performed on children, who are frightened by the technique and cannot cooperate. For indwelling catheters, attention is given to maintaining continuous free drainage and to routine care measures to prevent infection. Kinds of catheterization are **cardiac catheterization, hepatic vein catheterization, laryngeal catheterization.** See also **Foley catheter.** —**catheterize,** *v.*

cathexis The conscious or unconscious attachment of emotional feeling and importance to a specific idea, person, or object. —**cathectic,** *adj.*

cathode ray A stream of electrons emitted by the negative electrode of a gaseous discharge device when the cathode is bombarded by positive ions, as in a cathode ray tube, an oscilloscope, and a television picture tube. The ray itself is usually focused by a series of electromagnets that control its direction and position on a screen coated with a phosphor in order to create a visible pattern.

cathode ray oscilloscope An instrument that produces a visual representation of electrical variations by means of the fluorescent screen of a cathode-ray tube. Oscilloscopes have many applications in medicine and in nursing, as the displaying of patients' brain waves and heart beats for monitoring and diagnostic purposes.

cation A positively charged ion that in solution is attracted to the negative electrode.

cation-exchange resin Any one of various insoluble organic polymers with high molecular weights that exchange their cations for other ions in solution. Cation-exchange resins are used especially to restrict intestinal sodium absorption in patients with edema. Compare **anion-exchange resin.**

catling, catlin A long, sharp, double-edged knife used in amputation.

catoptric Of or pertaining to a reflected image.

CAT scan See **computerized axial tomography.**

cat-scratch fever A disease that results from the scratch or bite of a healthy cat. Inflammation and pustules are found on the scratched skin, and lymph nodes in the neck, head, groin, or axilla swell 2 weeks later. Although patients are rarely ill, fever and malaise may occur. No treatment is required. The cat-scratch skin test is available to help in the diagnosis. Also called **cat-scratch disease.**

cat's eye amaurosis A monocular blindness, with a bright reflection from the pupil caused by a white mass in the vitreous humor resulting from inflammation or a malignant lesion.

caud- A combining form meaning 'pertaining to a tail': *caudal, caudalward, caudocephalad.*

caudad Toward the tail or end of the body, away from the head. Compare **cephalad.**

cauda equina The lower end of the spinal cord at the first lumbar vertebrae and the bundle of lumbar, sacral, and coccygeal nerve roots that emerge from the spinal cord and descend through the spinal canal of the sacrum and coccyx before reaching the intervertebral foramina of their particular vertebrae. The cauda equina looks like a horse's tail.

caudal Signifying a position toward the distal end of the spine.

caudal anesthesia The injection of a local anesthetic agent into the caudal portion of the spinal canal through the sacrum. Caudal anesthesia has largely been replaced by epidural anesthesia because of the difficulty of controlling the level of anesthesia, the need for large volumes (10 to 15 ml) of anesthetic solution, a high (5% to 10%) rate of failure, frequent neurologic complications, arterial hypotension, and, in obstetrics, reduced force of labor. Other complications of caudal anesthesia include maternal infection and inadvertent injection into the fetus. See also **regional anesthesia.**

caudate Having a tail.

caudate process A small elevation of tissue that extends obliquely from the lower extremity of the caudate lobe of the liver to the visceral surface of the right lobe. It separates the fossa for the gallbladder from the beginning of the fossa for the inferior vena cava.

caul The intact amniotic sac surrounding the fetus at birth. The sac usually ruptures or is ruptured during the course of labor or delivery; when it remains intact it must be torn or cut to allow the baby to breathe.

cauliflower ear A thickened, deformed ear caused by repeated trauma, as suffered by boxers. Plastic surgery may be a means of restoring the normal appearance of the ear.

caumesthesia An abnormal condition in which a patient has a low temperature but experiences a sense of intense heat. —**caumesthetic,** *adj.*

causalgia A severe sensation of burning pain, often in an extremity, sometimes with local erythema of the skin. It is the result of injury to a peripheral sensory nerve.

causal hypothesis In research: a hypothesis that predicts a cause and effect relationship among the variables to be studied.

causal hypothesis testing study In nursing research: an experimental design used in testing a hypothesis that predicts a cause and effect relationship within the data to be studied.

causality In research: a relationship between one phenomenon or event (A) and another (B) in which A precedes and causes B and the direction of influence and the nature of the effect are predictable and reproducible and may be empirically observed. Causality is difficult to prove; some social scientists state that it is impossible to prove a causal relationship.

causation In law: the existence of a reasonable connection between the misfeasance, malfeasance, or nonfeasance of the defendant and the injury or damage suffered by the plaintiff. In a lawsuit in which negligence is alleged, the harm suffered by the plaintiff must be proven to result directly from the negligence of the defendant; causation must be demonstrated.

cause Any process, substance, or organism that produces an effect or condition.

CAUSN *abbr* **Canadian Association of University Schools of Nursing.**

CAUT *abbr* **Canadian Association of University Teachers.**

cautery **1.** A device or agent that scars and burns the skin, as in the coagulation of tissue by heat or caustic substances. **2.** A destructive effect produced by a cauterizing agent.

cautery knife A surgical knife that cuts tissue and cauterizes it to prevent bleeding. The knife is connected to an electrical source which generates the heat necessary for cauterization.

cav- A combining form meaning 'hollow': *cavascope, cavernome, cavity.*

cavalry bone See **rider's bone.**

cavernoma, *pl.* **cavernomas, cavernomata** See **cavernous hemangioma.**

cavernous Containing cavities or hollow spaces. See also **cavernous hemangioma.**

cavernous angioma See **cavernous hemangioma.**

cavernous body of the clitoris See **corpus cavernosum clitoridis.**

cavernous body of the penis See **corpus cavernosum penis.**

cavernous hemangioma A benign, congenital tumor consisting of large, blood-filled, cystic spaces. The scalp, face, and neck are the most common sites, but these tumors have been found in the liver and other organs. Superficial cavernous hemangiomas are friable and easily infected if the skin is broken. Treatment includes observation, irradiation, sclerosing solutions, and surgery. Compare **capillary hemangioma, nevus flammeus.**

cavernous lymphangioma See **lymphangioma cavernosum.**

cavernous rale An abnormal hollow, metallic sound heard during auscultation of the thorax. It is caused by contraction and expansion of a pulmonary cavity during respiration and indicates a pathological condition.

cavernous sinus One of a pair of irregularly shaped, bilateral venous channels between the sphenoid bone of the skull and the dura mater. It is one of the five anterior inferior venous sinuses that drain the blood from the dura mater into the internal jugular vein. Like the other anterior inferior sinuses, the cavernous sinus has no valves. Coursing through the sinus are the oculomotor nerve, the trochlear nerve, the abducent nerve, the ophthalmic and the maxillary divisions of the trigeminal nerve, and the internal carotid artery. The cavernous sinus receives the superior and the inferior ophthalmic veins, some of the cerebral veins, and the sphenoparietal sinus, and joins the cavernous sinus from the opposite side through the intercavernous sinuses. The cavernous sinus drains into the inferior petrosal sinus, thence into the internal jugular vein.

cavernous sinus syndrome An abnormal condition characterized by edema of the conjunctiva, the upper eyelid, and the root of the nose, and by paralysis of the third, the fourth, and the sixth nerves. It is caused by a thrombosis of the cavernous sinus.

cavernous sinus thrombosis A syndrome, usually secondary to infections near the eye or nose, characterized by orbital edema, venous congestion of the eye, and palsy of the nerves supplying the extraocular muscles. The infection may spread to involve the cerebrospinal fluid and meninges. Treatment is with antibiotics and, sometimes, with anticoagulants. Prevention includes avoidance of squeezing pimples and other skin lesions in the area of the nose and central face.

cavitary **1.** Denoting the presence of one or more cavities. **2.** Any entozoon having a body cavity or an alimentary canal.

cavitate The act of rapidly forming and collapsing vapor pockets in a flowing fluid with low pressure areas, often causing damage to surrounding structures.

cavitation **1.** The formation of cavities within the body, as those formed in the lung by tuberculosis. **2.** Any cavity within the body, as the pleural cavities.

cavity **1.** A hollow space within a larger structure, as the peritoneal cavity or the oral cavity. **2.** *Nontechnical.* A space in a tooth formed by dental caries.

cavogram An angiogram of the inferior or superior vena cava.

cavum, *pl.* **cava 1.** Any hollow or cavity. **2.** The inferior or superior vena cava.

CBC *abbr* **complete blood count.**

CBF *abbr* **cerebral blood flow.**

CBS *abbr* **chronic brain syndrome.**

CCRN *abbr* Certified Critical-Care Registered Nurse.

CCU *abbr* **coronary care unit.**

Cd Symbol for **cadmium.**

CDC *abbr* **Centers for Disease Control.**

Ce Symbol for **cerium.**

CEA *abbr* **carcinoembryonic antigen.**

ceasmic Pertaining to or characterized by a fissure or abnormal cleavage of parts.

ceasmic teratism A congenital anomaly, caused by developmental arrest, in which parts of the body that should be fused remain in their fissured embryonic state, as in cleft palate.

cec- A combining form meaning 'pertaining to a cecum': *cecitis, cecectomy, cecoplication.*

cecal, caecal **1.** Of or pertaining to the cecum. **2.** Of or pertaining to the optic disk or the blind spot in the retina.

cecal appendix See **vermiform appendix.**

cecocolostomy **1.** A surgical operation that creates an anastomosis between the cecum and the colon. **2.** The anastomosis produced by this operation.

cecofixation See **cecopexy.**

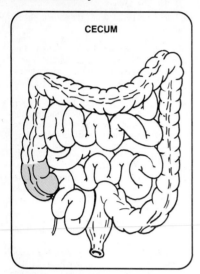

CECUM

cecoileostomy A surgical operation that connects the ileum with the cecum. Also called **ileocecostomy.**

cecopexy A surgical operation that fixes or suspends the cecum to correct its excessive mobility. Also called **cecofixation.**

cecostomy The surgical construction of an opening into the cecum, performed as a temporary measure to relieve intestinal obstruction in a patient who cannot tolerate major surgery. Twenty-four hours before surgery, if time permits, a low residue diet is given with only clear liquids allowed. Cleansing enemas and antibiotics are prescribed to reduce the number of bacteria in the bowel. I.V. fluids and electrolytes are given, and a nasointestinal tube is inserted. With the patient under local anesthesia, a tube is inserted into the cecum to allow drainage of feces. The procedure may also be done to decompress the large bowel and prevent distention until peristalsis is restored after intestinal surgery. Postoperatively, the tube is connected to a drainage bottle. The nurse irrigates the cecostomy tube with saline solution as necessary, allowing the solution to flow in and out by gravity, if possible. Frequent changes of dressings are needed to keep the skin clean and dry. An ileostomy bag may be used. When edema and inflammation have subsided, the obstruction is resected, the healthy sections of bowel reconnected, and the cecostomy closed. See also **abdominal surgery, intestinal obstruction.**

cecum A cul-de-sac constituting the first part of the large intestine.

cefaclor A cephalosporin antibiotic.

cefadroxil monohydrate A cephalosporin antibiotic.

cefamandole naftate A cephalosporin antibiotic.

cefazolin sodium A cephalosporin antibiotic.

cefotaxime A cephalosporin antibiotic.

cefoxitin sodium A cephalosporin antibiotic.

cel-, coel A combining form meaning: **1.** 'A cavity of the body': *celarium, celoschisis, celozoic.* **2.** 'A swelling or tumor, hernia': *celectome, celology, celosomia.*

-cele A combining form meaning: **1.** A 'tumor or swelling': *hematoscheocele, oodeocele, tracheocele.* **2.** A 'cavity': *paracele, orchidocele, syringocele.* Also **-coel, -coele.**

celiac artery A thick visceral branch of the abdominal aorta, arising caudal to the diaphragm, usually dividing into the left gastric, the common hepatic, and the splenic arteries.

celiac disease A chronic inability to tolerate foods containing gluten or wheat protein. The disease affects adults and young children, who suffer from abdominal distention, vomiting, diarrhea, muscle wasting, and extreme lethargy. A characteristic sign is a pale, foulsmelling stool that floats on water owing to its high fat content. There may be a secondary lactose intolerance, and it may become necessary to eliminate all milk and dairy products from the diet. Most patients respond well to a highprotein, high-calorie, gluten-free diet. Rice and corn are good substitutes for wheat, and any vitamin or mineral deficiencies can be corrected with oral preparations. Prognosis for full recovery is excellent. Failure to respond generally indicates misdiagnosis. Also called **celiac sprue, nontropical sprue.** Compare **malabsorption syndrome.**

celiac plexus See **solar plexus.**

celiac rickets Arrested growth and osseous deformities resulting from malabsorption of fat and calcium. See **celiac disease, rickets.**

celio- A combining form meaning 'pertaining to the abdomen': *celioma, celiopathy, celiorrhaphy.*

celiocolpotomy An incision into the abdomen through the vagina.

celioma, *pl.* **celiomas, celiomata** An abdominal neoplasm, especially a mesothelial tumor of the peritoneum.

celioscope See **laparoscope.**

celiothelioma, *pl.* **celiotheliomas, celiotheliomata** A mesothelioma of the abdomen.

cell The fundamental unit of all living tissue. Each cell consists of a nucleus, cytoplasm, and organelles surrounded by a cytoplasmic membrane. Within the nucleus are the nucleolus (containing RNA), and chromatin granules (containing protein and DNA) that develop into chromosomes, the determinants of hereditary characteristics. Organelles within the cytoplasm include the endoplasmic reticulum, ribosomes, the Golgi complex, mitochondria, lysosomes, and the centrosome. The specialized nature of body tissue reflects the specialized structure and function of its constituent cells.

cella, *pl.* **cellae** An enclosed space.

cell biology The science that deals with the structures, living processes, and functions of cells, especially human cells.

cell body The part of a cell that contains the nucleus and surrounding cytoplasm exclusive of any projections or processes, as the axon and dendrites of a neuron or the tail of a spermatozoon. This enlarged area is concerned more with the metabolism of the cell than with a specific function.

cell death 1. Terminal failure of a cell to maintain the essential life functions. **2.** The point in the process of dying at which vital functions have ceased at the cellular level.

cell division The continuous process by which a cell divides in four stages: prophase, metaphase, anaphase, and telophase. Preliminary to prophase the centrosome of the cell divides into two parts, which become oriented at opposite poles of the nucleus. During the prophase, previously dispersed chromatin condenses into chromomeres strung along a threadlike chromonema composed of deoxyribonucleic acid. The chromonema then condenses into compact chromosomes. During metaphase, the chromosomes become oriented in the equatorial plate with a clear area directed toward the two centrosomes. Each chromosome meanwhile has doubled into chromatids attached to each other at the centromere. Each centromere divides during late metaphase and early anaphase. In telophase, the chromosomes form a compact mass, lose their individuality, and disperse into the chromatin of the intermitotic nucleus. Also called **mitosis.**

cell line A colony of animal cells developed as a subculture from a primary culture.

cell-mediated immune response A delayed type IV hypersensitivity reaction, mediated primarily by sensitized T cell lymphocytes as opposed to antibodies. Cell-mediated immune reactions are responsible for defense against certain bacterial, fungal, and viral pathogens, malignant cells, and other foreign protein or tissue.

cell-mediated immunity See **cellular immunity.**

cell membrane The outer covering of a cell, often having projecting microvilli and containing the cellular cytoplasm. The cell membrane is so thin and delicate it is barely visible with a light microscope and can be studied in detail only with an electron microscope. The membrane controls the exchange of materials between the cell and its environment by various processes, as osmosis, phagocytosis, pinocytosis, and secretion. Also called **plasma membrane.**

cell theory The proposition that cells are the basic units of all living substance and that cellular function is the essential process of life.

cellular hypersensitivity reaction Type IV hypersensitivity. See **cell-mediated immune response.**

cellular immunity The mechanism of acquired immunity characterized by the dominant role of small T cell lymphocytes. Cellular immunity is involved in resistance to infectious

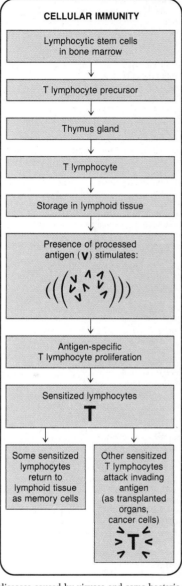

diseases caused by viruses and some bacteria, and in delayed hypersensitivity reactions, some aspects of resistance to cancer, certain autoimmune diseases, graft rejection, and certain allergies. Also called **cell-mediated immunity.** Compare **humoral immunity.**

cellular infiltration The migration and grouping of cells within tissues throughout the body.

cellulitis An infection of the skin characterized most commonly by local heat, redness, pain, and swelling, and occasionally by fever, malaise, chills, and headache. Abscess and tissue destruction usually follow if antibiotics are not taken. Damaged skin, poor circulation, and diabetes mellitus favor the development of cellulitis. Treatment, in addition to appropriate antibiotics, includes warm soaks and avoidance of pressure to the affected areas.

cellulose A colorless, insoluble, nondigestible, transparent solid carbohydrate that is the primary constituent of the skeletal substances of the cell walls of plants. In the diet it provides the bulk necessary for proper gastrointestinal functioning. Rich sources are fruits, as apples and bananas; legumes; bran; and green vegetables, especially celery. See also **dietary fiber.**

cell wall The structure that covers and protects the cell membrane of some kinds of cells, as certain bacteria and all plant cells. The cell walls of plant cells are composed of cellulose.

celom See **coelom.**

celosomia A congenital malformation characterized by a fissure or the absence of the sternum and ribs and protrusion of the viscera.

celosomus A fetus with celosomia.

celothelioma, *pl.* **celotheliomas, celotheliomata** See **mesothelioma.**

Celsius (C) Denoting a temperature scale in which 0° is the freezing point of water and 100° is the boiling point of water at sea level. Also called **centigrade.** Compare **Fahrenheit.**

cement 1. A sticky or mucilaginous substance that helps neighboring tissue cells stick together. **2.** Any of a variety of dental materials used to fill cavities or to hold bridgework or other dental prostheses in place. **3.** A material used in the fixation of a prosthetic joint in adjacent bone, as methyl mathacrylate.

cementifying fibroma A fibrous tumor containing masses of calcified tissue, occurring most frequently in the mandible of older people.

cementoblastoma, *pl.* **cementoblastomas, cementoblastomata** An odontogenic fibrous tumor consisting of cells developing into cementoblasts but containing only a small amount of calcified tissue.

cementoma, *pl.* **cementomas, cementomata** An accumulation of cementum existing free at the apex of a tooth, probably caused by trauma rather than neoplastic growth.

cementum The bonelike connective tissue that covers the roots of the teeth and helps to support them.

cen- A combining form meaning 'common': *cenadelphus, cenesthesia, cenesthopathia.*

cenesthesia, coenesthesia The general sense of existing, derived as the aggregate of all the various stimuli and reactions throughout the body at any specific moment to produce a feeling of health or of illness. Also called **cenesthesis, coenesthesis.**

cenesthesis, coenesthesis See **cenesthesia.**

ceno- A combining form meaning 'new': *cenogenesis, cenophobia, cenopsychic.*

cenogenesis, coenogenesis, caeno- **genesis, kenogenesis** The development of structural characteristics that are absent in earlier forms of a species, as an adaptive response to environmental conditions. Compare **palingenesis. —cenogenetic, coenogenetic, caenogenetic,** *adj.*

cenophobia See **kenophobia.**

censor 1. A person who monitors or evaluates books, newspapers, plays, works of art, speech, or other means of expression in order to suppress certain kinds of information. **2.** In psychoanalysis: a psychic suppression that allows unconscious thoughts to rise to consciousness only if they are heavily disguised.

cente- A combining form meaning 'puncture': *centesis.*

center, centre 1. The middle point of the body or geometric entity, equidistant from points on the periphery. **2.** A group of neurons with a common function, as the accelerating center in the brain which controls the heartbeat.

Centers for Disease Control (CDC) A federal agency of the United States government that provides facilities and services for the investigation, identification, prevention, and control of disease. It is concerned with all aspects of the epidemiology and the laboratory diagnosis of disease. Immunization programs, quarantine regulations and programs, laboratory standards, and community surveillance for disease are among the activities of the CDC, which is located in Atlanta, Georgia. Many state and local health workers and scientists receive training in specific techniques there. Formerly, the Communicable Disease Center, it was concerned only with communicable diseases; today its interests include environmental health, smoking, malnutrition, poisoning, and issues in occupational health.

centesis A perforation or a puncture, as a paracentesis, abdominocentesis, or thoracocentesis.

centi- A combining form meaning 'a hundred or a hundredth': *centibar, centiliter, centipoise.*

centigrade (C) See **Celsius.**

centimeter (cm) The metric unit of measurement equal to one hundredth of a meter, or 0.3937 inches.

centimeter-gram-second system (CGS, cgs) The internationally accepted scientific system of expressing length, mass, and time in basic units of centimeters, grams, and seconds. The CGS system is gradually being replaced by the Système Internationale d'Unites (SI), or the International System of Units, based on the meter, kilogram, and second.

centipede bite A wound produced by the poison claws and the first body segment of a centipede, an elongate arthropod with many pairs of legs. The bite of a few species, including *Scolopendra morsitans* in the southern United States, may cause painful local inflammation, fever, headache, vomiting, and dizziness.

central Of, pertaining to, or situated at a center.

central amaurosis Blindness caused by a

disease of the central nervous system.

central canal of spinal cord The conduit that runs the entire length of the spinal cord and contains most of the 140 ml of cerebrospinal fluid in the body of the average individual. The central canal of the spinal cord lies in the center of the cord between the ventral and the dorsal gray commissures and extends cranialward into the medulla oblongata, where it opens into the fourth ventricle of the brain. Caudalward, the canal runs into the filum terminale after forming a triangular, fusiform dilation about 10 mm (⅜ inch) long in the conus medullaris. Cerebrospinal fluid flows into the canal from the fourth ventricle of the brain, into the subarachnoid space around the spinal cord, and into the subarachnoid space around the brain. Subarachnoid hemorrhage may form blood clots that block drainage of the cerebrospinal fluid from the subarachnoid space. Lumbar puncture, often performed to obtain samples of cerebrospinal fluid for diagnostic purposes, draws fluid from the subarachnoid space around the spinal cord and not from the central canal. See also **lumbar puncture.**

central chondrosarcoma A malignant cartilaginous tumor that forms inside a bone. Also called **enchondrosarcoma.**

central fissure See **central sulcus.**

central implantation See **superficial implantation.**

central lobe One of the five lobes constituting each of the cerebral hemispheres, lying hidden in the depths of the lateral sulcus. The central lobe can be seen only if the lips of the sulcus are parted or cut away. The lips of the lateral sulcus are parts of the frontal, the parietal, and the temporal lobes and are separated by the rami of the lateral sulcus, thus constituting the frontal, the parietal, and the temporal opercula. With the opercula cut away, the insula appears as a triangular area with the limen insulae as the apex. Compare **frontal lobe, occipital lobe, parietal lobe, temporal lobe.**

central nervous system (CNS) One of the two main divisions of the nervous system of the body, consisting of the brain and the spinal cord. The central nervous system processes information to and from the peripheral nervous system and is the main network of coordination and control for the entire body. The brain controls many functions and sensations, as sleep, sexual activity, muscular movement, hunger, thirst, memory, and the emotions. The spinal cord extends various types of nerve fibers from the brain and acts as a switching and relay terminal for the peripheral nervous system. The 12 pairs of cranial nerves emerge directly from the brain. Sensory nerves and motor nerves of the peripheral system leave the spinal cord separately between the vertebrae but unite to form 31 pairs of spinal nerves containing sensory fibers and motor fibers. More than 10 billion neurons constitute but one tenth of the brain cells, the other cells consisting of neuroglia. The neurons and the neuroglia form the soft, jellylike

substance of the brain, which is supported and protected by the skull. The cerebrospinal fluid flows through various cavities of the CNS, as the ventricles of the brain, the subarachnoid spaces of the brain and spinal cord, and the central canal of the spinal cord. This fluid helps to protect surrounding structures and affects the rate of respiration through changes in its content of carbon dioxide. The brain and the spinal cord are composed of gray matter and white matter. The gray matter contains primarily nerve cells and associated processes; the white matter consists of bundles of predominantly unmyelinated nerve fibers. The central nervous system develops from the embryonic neural tube, which first appears as the neural folds in the 3rd week of pregnancy. The cavity of the neural tube is retained after birth in the ventricles of the brain and in the central canal of the spinal cord. Compare **peripheral nervous system.** See also **brain, spinal cord.**

central nervous system depressants Any drug that decreases the function of the central nervous system (CNS), as alcohol, barbiturates, and hypnotics. Such drugs can produce tolerance, physical dependence, and compulsive drug use. The benzodiazepines depress excitable tissue throughout the CNS by stabilizing neuronal membranes, decreasing the amount of transmitter released by the nerve impulse, and generally depressing postsynaptic responsiveness and ion movement. The CNS is more affected by alcohol than any other body system, the effects generally proportional to the concentration of alcohol in the blood. Central nervous system depressants elevate the seizure threshold and can produce physical dependence in a relatively short period of time. All depressants are subject to abuse, and a recent marked increase in the use of illicitly procured depressants has been noted in some adolescent and preadolescent populations. The most abused depressants are the short-acting barbiturates, especially pentobarbital and secobarbital. Glutethimide and methaqualone are also heavily abused.

central nervous system stimulant A substance that quickens the activity of the central nervous system (CNS) by increasing the rate of neuronal discharge or by blocking an inhibitory neurotransmitter. Many natural and synthetic compounds stimulate the CNS, but only a few are used therapeutically. Caffeine, a potent CNS stimulant, is used to help restore mental alertness and overcome respiratory depression, but it may cause nausea, nervousness, tinnitus, tremor, tachycardia, extra systoles, diuresis, and scintillating scotoma. Amphetamines, sympathomimetic amines with CNS-stimulating activity, are employed in treating narcolepsy and obesity, but these drugs have a high potential for abuse and may cause dizziness, restlessness, tachycardia, increased blood pressure, headache, mouth dryness, an unpleasant taste, gastrointestinal symptoms, and urticaria. Various amphetamines and amphetamine analogues, especially methylphenidate and deanol acetami-

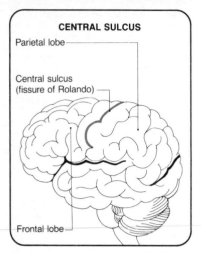

CENTRAL SULCUS

Parietal lobe

Central sulcus
(fissure of Rolando)

Frontal lobe

dobenzoate, a precursor of acetylcholine, are prescribed for the hyperkinetic child syndrome. Doxapram, ethamivan, and nikethamide are used to stimulate the respiratory center and restore consciousness following anesthesia or in the treatment of acute sedative-hypnotic intoxication.

central nervous system syndrome (CNS syndrome) A constellation of neurologic and emotional signs and symptoms that results from a massive whole-body dosage of radiation. The syndrome includes hysteria and disorientation, increasing during the last 24 to 48 hours before death.

central nervous system tumor A neoplasm of the brain or spinal cord that characteristically does not spread beyond the cerebrospinal axis, although it may be highly invasive locally and have widespread effects on body functions. Intracranial neoplasms are about four times more common than those arising in the spinal cord. From 20% to 40% of brain tumors are metastatic lesions from primary cancer in the breast, lung, gastrointestinal tract, kidney, or a site of melanoma. See also **brain tumor, spinal cord tumor.**

central neuritis See **parenchymatous neuritis.**

central placenta previa Placenta previa in which the placenta is implanted in the lower segment of the uterus and completely covers the internal os of the uterine cervix. In labor, as the cervix dilates, the placenta is gradually separated from the underlying blood vessels in the uterine lining, resulting in bleeding that usually begins slowly, is painless, and progresses to hemorrhage that is life-threatening to the mother and the baby. Cesarean section is usually performed to save the mother and the baby. The condition may be discovered before any bleeding occurs by ultrasound visualization or by digital palpation in the normal course of prenatal care.

central processing unit (CPU) In data processing: the group of physical components of a computer system containing the logical, arithmetical, and control circuits for the system. Also called **hardware;** compare **software.**

central scotoma An area of blindness or site of depressed vision involving the macula of the retina.

central stimulant See **central nervous system stimulant.**

central sulcus A cleft separating the frontal from the parietal lobes of the brain. Also called **central fissure, fissure of Rolando.**

central venous pressure (CVP) monitor A device for measuring and recording the venous blood pressure by means of an indwelling catheter and a pressure manometer. It is used to evaluate the right ventricular function, the right atrial filling pressure, and the capacity of the blood vessels.

central vision Vision that results from images falling on the macula of the retina.

centrencephalic Of, pertaining to, or involving the center of the encephalon.

centri- See **centro-.**

centrifugal **1.** Denoting a force that is directed outward, away from a central point or axis, as the force that keeps the moon in its orbit around the earth. **2.** A direction away from the head.

centrifugal current An electric current in the body with the positive pole near the nerve center and the negative pole at the periphery. Also called **descending current.**

centrifuge A device for separating components of different densities contained in liquid by spinning them at high speeds. Centrifugal force causes the heavier components to move to one part of the container, leaving the lighter substances in another. —**centrifugal,** *adj.,* **centrifuge,** *v.*

centrilobular Of, pertaining to, or situated at the center of a lobule.

centriole An intracellular organelle, usually as a component of the centrosome. Usually occurring in pairs, centrioles are associated with cell division and can be closely studied only with an electron microscope. Under a light microscope the centrioles appear as tiny dots, but they are actually tiny cylinders positioned at right angles to each other, with walls consisting of nine bundles of fine tubules, three tubules to a bundle. The centriole measures approximately 150 millimicrons by 300 to 500 millimicrons. Numerous centrioles occur in some large cells, as the giant cells in bone marrow. The precise function of centrioles is still a mystery, but they appear to aid in the formation of the spindle that develops during mitosis.

centripetal **1.** Denoting an afferent direction, as that of a sensory nerve impulse traveling toward the brain. **2.** Denoting the direction of a force pulling an object toward an axis of rotation or constraining an object to a specific curved path.

centripetal current An electric current

passing through the body from a peripheral positive electrode to a negative pole near the nerve center. Also called **ascending current.**

centro-, centri- A combining form meaning 'center': *centrocecal, centrocinesia.*

centromere The specialized, constricted region of the chromosome that joins the two chromatids to each other and attaches to the spindle fiber in mitosis and meiosis. During cell division the centromeres split longitudinally, half going to each of the new daughter chromosomes. The position of the centromere is constant for a specific chromosome and is identified accordingly as acrocentric, metacentric, subcentric, or telocentric. Also called **kinetochore, kinomere, primary constriction. —centromeric,** *adj.*

centrosome A self-propagating cytoplasmic organelle present in animal cells and in those of some lower plants. The structure, which consists of the centrosphere and the centrioles, is located near the nucleus and functions as the dynamic center of the cell, especially during mitosis. Also called **cytocentrum, microcentrum, paranuclear body.**

centrosphere The differentiated, condensed area of cytoplasm surrounding the centrioles in the centrosome of the cell.

centrum, *pl.* **centra** Any kind of center, especially one related to a body structure, as the centrum semiovale of a cerebral hemisphere.

CEO, C.E.O. *abbr* **Chief Executive Officer.**

cephal- See **cephalo.**

cephalad Toward the head, away from the end, or tail. Compare **caudad.**

cephalalgia Headache, often combined with another word to indicate a specific type of headache, as histamine cephalalgia. See **histamine headache.**

cephalexin A cephalosporin antibacterial.

cephalexin monohydrate A cephalosporin antibiotic.

cephalhematoma Swelling owing to subcutaneous bleeding and accumulation of blood. It may begin to form in the scalp of a fetus during labor and enlarge slowly in the first few days after birth. It is usually a result of trauma, often from forceps. Large cephalhematomas may become infected, require surgical drainage, and take several months to resolve. Compare **caput succedaneum, molding.**

-cephalia A combining form meaning '(condition of the) head': *hemicephalia, megacephalia, notancephalia.*

cephalic Of or pertaining to the head.

-cephalic A combining form meaning 'relating to the head': *holocephalic, megalocephalic, postcephalic.*

cephalic presentation A classification of fetal position in which the head of the fetus is at the uterine cervix. Cephalic presentation is usually further qualified by an indication of the part of the head presenting, as the occiput, bregma, or mentum.

cephalic vein One of the four superficial veins of the upper limb. It begins in the dorsal

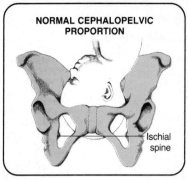

NORMAL CEPHALOPELVIC PROPORTION

Ischial spine

venous network of the hand and winds upward to end in the axillary vein just caudal to the clavicle. It receives deoxygenated blood from the dorsal and the palmar surfaces of the forearm. Just distal to the antecubital fossa, it has a wide anastomosis with the median cubital vein. In the proximal third of the arm, it passes between the pectoralis major and the deltoideus, where it is accompanied by the thoracoacromial artery. Compare **basilic vein, dorsal digital vein, median antebrachial vein.**

cephalo-, cephal- A combining form meaning 'pertaining to the head': *cephalocaudal, cephalocentesis, cephalogenesis.*

cephaloglycin, c. dihydrate Cephalosporin antibiotics.

cephalomelus A deformed individual with a structure resembling an arm or a leg protruding from the head.

cephalometry Scientific measurement of the head, as that performed in dentistry to determine appropriate orthodontic procedures for correcting malocclusions and other abnormal conditions. —**cephalometric,** *adj.*

cephalopagus, *pl.* **cephalopagi** See **craniopagus.**

cephalopelvic disproportion (CPD) An obstetric condition in which an infant's head is too large or the birth canal too small to permit normal labor or birth. In relative cephalopelvic disproportion, the size of the infant's head is within normal limits but larger than average or the size of the birth canal is within normal limits but smaller than average, or both; relative CPD is often overcome by molding of the head, the forces of labor, or by the use of forceps to effect delivery. In absolute cephalopelvic disproportion, the infant's head is markedly or abnormally enlarged or the mother's birth canal is markedly or abnormally contracted, making vaginal delivery impossible.

cephaloridine A cephalosporin antibiotic.

cephalosporin A semisynthetic derivative of an antibiotic originally derived from the microorganism *Cephalosporium acremonium.* Cephalosporins, a family of antibiotics, are similar in structure to penicillins except for a beta-lactam-dihydrothiazine ring in place of beta-lactam-thiazolidin in penicillin.

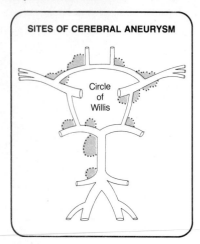

SITES OF CEREBRAL ANEURYSM

Circle of Willis

cephalothin sodium A cephalosporin antibiotic.

cephalothoracoiliopagus See **synadelphus.**

cephalothoracopagus A conjoined twin fetal monster united at the head, neck, and thorax.

-cephaly A combining form meaning a '(specified) condition of the head': *macrencephaly, platycephaly, trochocephaly.* Also **-cephalia.**

cephapirin sodium A cephalosporin antibiotic.

cephradine A cephalosporin antibacterial.

cer- A combining form meaning 'wax': *ceraceous, cerate, cerumen.*

cerato- A combining form meaning 'pertaining to the cornea or to horny tissue': *ceratocricoid, ceratohyal, ceratopharyngeus.* Also **kerato-.**

cercaria, *pl.* **cercariae** A minute, wormlike early developmental form of trematode. It develops in a freshwater snail, is released into the water, and swims toward the sun, rising to the surface of the water in the warmest part of the day. Cercariae enter the body of their next host by ingestion, by direct invasion through the skin, or through a cut or other break in the skin. Some cercariae of the genera *Schistosoma, Chlonorchis, Paragonimus, Fasciolopsis,* and *Fasciola* are known to infect humans. They encyst and complete their development in various organs of the body. Each species tends to migrate to one organ, as *Fasciola hepatica,* which grows to become a liver fluke. See also **fluke, schistosomiasis.**

cerclage **1.** An orthopedic procedure in which the ends of an oblique bone fracture or the chips of a broken patella are bound together with a wire loop or a metal band to hold the bone fragments in position until healed. **2.** A procedure in which a taut silicone band is applied around the sclera to restore contact between the retina and the choroid when the retina is detached. **3.** An obstetric procedure in which a nonabsorbable suture is used for holding the cervix closed to prevent spontaneous abortion in a woman who has an incompetent cervix. The band is usually released when the pregnancy is at full term to allow labor to begin. See also **incompetent cervix.**

cerea flexibilitas A cataleptic state, frequently observed in catatonic schizophrenia, in which the limbs retain for an indefinite period the positions in which they are placed. Also called **flexibilitas cerea, waxy flexibility.** See also **catalepsy.**

cerebellar Of or pertaining to the cerebellum.

cerebellar angioblastoma A tumor in the cerebellum composed of a mass of blood vessels. It may be cystic and is frequently associated with von Hippel-Lindau disease.

cerebellar cortex The superficial gray matter of the cerebellum covering the white substance in the medullary core and consisting of two layers, an external molecular layer and an internal granule cell layer. The layers are separated by an incomplete stratum of Purkinje cells. Also called cortical substance of cerebellum.

cerebellar cortical degeneration See **alcoholic-nutritional cerebellar degeneration.**

cerebellopontine Leading from the cerebellum to the pons varolii.

cerebellospinal Leading from the cerebellum to the spinal cord.

cerebellum, *pl.* **cerebellums, cerebella** The part of the brain located in the posterior cranial fossa behind the brain stem. It consists of two lateral cerebellar hemispheres, or lobes, and a middle section called the vermis. Three pairs of peduncles link it with the brain stem. Its functions are concerned with coordinating voluntary muscular activity.

cerebr- A combining form meaning 'pertaining to the cerebrum': *cerebralgia, cerebrocardiac, cerebropathy.*

cerebral Of or pertaining to the cerebrum.

-cerebral A combining form referring to the brain: *craniocerebral, medicerebral, postcerebral.*

cerebral aneurysm An abnormal localized dilatation of a cerebral artery, most commonly the result of congenital weakness of the media or muscle layer of the vessel wall. Cerebral aneurysms may also be caused by infection, as subacute bacterial endocarditis or syphilis, and by neoplasms, arteriosclerosis, and trauma. The most frequent sites are around the Circle of Willis: the middle cerebral, basilar vertebral, anterior and posterior cerebral, and anterior and posterior communicating arteries, especially at bifurcations of vessels. Cerebral aneurysms may occur in infancy or old age and may be fusiform dilatations of the entire circumference of an artery or saccular outcroppings of the side of a vessel, which may be as small as a pinhead or as large as an orange but are usually the size of a pea. Depending on size and site, an aneurysm may cause headache, drowsiness, confusion, vertigo, facial weakness and pain, tinnitus, visual impairment, neck stiffness, and monoplegia or hemiplegia. Since about half the cases of cerebral aneurysm rupture, the patient is closely monitored for signs of subarachnoid hemorrhage and increased intracranial pressure. Few aneurysms rupture that are less than 1 cm (⅜ inch) in diameter. Antifibrinolytic, analgesic, anticonvulsant, antiemetic, or antihypertensive medication, steroids, and parenteral fluids may be administered.

NURSING CONSIDERATIONS: The pulse, blood pressure, respiration, and neurologic status of the patient are checked frequently. Any sudden change in blood pressure or pupillary response is reported promptly. The patient with a cerebral aneurysm requires intensive care and as little stress as possible. The nurse limits the number of visitors and the length of visits but involves the family in the patient's care and instructions. The patient is almost certain to be anxious about the possibility of rupture of the aneurysm and resultant neurologic problems. This concern may be anticipated by the nurse in order to help the patient express the fear and adapt to the situation.

cerebral angiography   An X-ray procedure for visualizing the vascular system of the brain by injecting a radiopaque contrast material into a carotid, subclavian, brachial, or femoral artery and taking X-rays at specific intervals in a series.

cerebral aqueduct   The narrow conduit, between the third and the fourth ventricles in the midbrain, which conveys the cerebrospinal fluid. Also called **aqueduct of Sylvius.**

cerebral cortex   A thin layer of gray matter on the surface of the cerebral hemisphere, folded into gyri with about two thirds of its area buried in fissures. It integrates higher mental functions, general movement, visceral functions, perception, and behavioral reactions. It has been classified many different ways, according to supposed phylogenetic and ontogenetic differences; structure; cell; and fiber layers; and function areas. Research has described more than 200 areas on the basis of differences in myelinated fiber patterns and has defined 47 separate function areas with different cell designs. The precentral cortex or motor area has received special attention because its stimulation with electrodes causes voluntary muscle contractions. A motor speech area in the frontal operculum is better developed in the left hemisphere of right-handed persons, and its destruction causes motor aphasia or speech defects despite healthy, intact vocal organs. Stimulation of the frontal area affects circulation, respiration, pupillary reaction, and other visceral activity. Also called **pallium.**

cerebral dominance   The specialization of each of the two cerebral hemispheres in the integration and control of different functions. In 90% of the population, the left cerebral hemisphere specializes in or dominates the ability to speak and write and the ability to understand

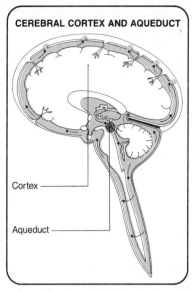

CEREBRAL CORTEX AND AQUEDUCT

Cortex

Aqueduct

spoken and written words. The areas that control these activities are situated in the frontal, parietal, and temporal lobes of the left hemisphere. In the other 10% of the population, either the right hemisphere or both hemispheres dominate the speech and writing abilities. The right cerebral hemisphere dominates the integration of certain sounds other than those associated with speaking, as the sounds of coughing, laughter, crying, and melodies. The right cerebral hemisphere perceives tactual stimuli and visual spatial relationships better than the left cerebral hemisphere. See also **Brodmann's areas.**

cerebral embolism   A cerebrovascular accident caused by an embolus that blocks the flow of blood through the vessels of the cerebrum, resulting in tissue ischemia distal to the occlusion. See also **cerebrovascular accident.**

cerebral gigantism   An abnormal condition characterized by excessive weight and size at birth, accelerated growth during the first 4 or 5 years after birth without any increase in the level of growth hormone, and then reversion to normal growth. Some typical signs of this condition are prognathism, antimongoloid slant, dolichocephalic skull, moderate mental retardation, and impaired coordination.

cerebral hemisphere   One of the halves of the cerebrum. The two cerebral hemispheres are divided by a deep longitudinal fissure and are connected medially at the bottom of the fissure by the corpus callosum. Prominent grooves, subdividing each hemisphere into four lobes, are the central sulcus, the lateral fissure, and the parieto-occipital fissure. Each hemisphere also has a fifth lobe deep in the brain. The central fissure separates the frontal lobe from the parietal lobe. The lateral fissure separates the temporal lobe, which lies below the fissure, from the frontal and parietal lobes, which lie above it. The parieto-occipital fissure separates the occipital lobe from the two parietal lobes. The hemispheres consist of external gray substance, internal white substance, and internal gray substance and are covered by cerebral cortexes at the surface. Recent research indicates that the right hemisphere functions in the perception of certain kinds of sound and may also function better than the left hemisphere at tactual perception and spatial relationships. The left hemisphere contains Broca's area, which controls language functions in most individuals.

cerebral hemorrhage A hemorrhage from a blood vessel in the brain. Three criteria are used to classify cerebral hemorrhages: location (subarachnoid, extradural, subdural), the kind of vessel involved (arterial, venous, capillary), and origin (traumatic, degenerative). Each kind of cerebral hemorrhage has its own clinical characteristics. Most cerebral hemorrhages occur in the region of the basal ganglia and are caused by the rupture of a sclerotic artery as a result of hypertension. Other causes of rupture include congenital aneurysm, cerebrovascular infarction, and head trauma. Bleeding may lead to displacement or destruction of brain tissue and to medullary anemia. Extensive hemorrhage is usually fatal. Recovery from the condition, which occurs more often in men than in women, may be complete. Depending on the extent and the location of the damaged tissue, residual effects may include aphasia, diminished mental function, or disturbance of the function of a special sense. Surgery is often necessary to stop the bleeding in order to prevent death from medullary anemia or from greatly increased intracranial pressure.

NURSING CONSIDERATIONS: Initially, bedside care is directed toward the prevention of recurrence and of the sequelae of prolonged immobility. Special care is taken in the positioning of the head of the patient to avoid flexion of the head on the neck, which might impair circulation to the brain. Fastidious skin care to prevent decubiti and emotional support are required to keep the person comfortable and calm. During convalescence the nurse may be called on to assist the patient in developing self-help capabilities. Physical therapy and speech therapy may be necessary during convalescence. See also **subarachnoid hemorrhage.**

cerebral localization 1. The determination of various areas in the cerebral cortex associated with specific functions, as the 47 areas of Brodmann. 2. The diagnosis of a cerebral condition, as a brain lesion, by determining the area of the brain affected, a determination made by analysis of the signs manifested by the patient and of electroencephalograms.

cerebral nerves See **cranial nerves.**

cerebral palsy A motor function disorder caused by a permanent, nonprogressive brain defect or lesion present at birth or shortly thereafter. The neurologic deficit may result in spastic hemiplegia, monoplegia, diplegia, or quadri-

plegia; athetosis or ataxia; seizures; paresthesia; varying degrees of mental retardation; impaired speech, vision, and hearing. The disorder is usually associated with premature or abnormal birth and intrapartum asphyxia, causing damage to the nervous system. Abnormalities in breathing, sucking, swallowing, and responsiveness are usually apparent soon after birth, but the characteristic stiff, awkward movements of the infant's limbs may be overlooked for several months. Walking is usually delayed and, when attempted, the child manifests a typical scissors gait. The arms may be affected only slightly, but the fingers are often spastic. Deep tendon reflexes are exaggerated, and there may be slurred speech, delay in acquiring sphincter control, and athetotic movements of the face and hands. Early identification of the disorder facilitates the handling of palsied infants and the initiation of an exercise and training program. Treatment is individualized and may include the use of braces, surgical correction of deformities, speech therapy, and various indicated drugs, as muscle relaxants and anticonvulsants. Also called **Little's disease.**

cerebral tabes See **general paresis.**

cerebral thrombosis A clotting of blood in any cerebral vessel, as the middle cerebral artery or the ascending parietal artery.

cerebriform carcinoma See **medullary carcinoma.**

cerebritis 1. Any inflammation of the cerebrum or brain. 2. Bacterial meningitis.

cerebrocerebellar atrophy A deterioration of the cerebellum caused by certain abiotrophic diseases.

cerebroid Resembling the substance of the brain.

cerebroma, *pl.* **cerebromas, cerebromata** Any unusual mass of brain tissue.

cerebromedullary tube See **neural tube.**

cerebropathia psychia toxemia See **Korsakoff's psychosis.**

cerebroretinal angiomatosis A hereditary disease characterized by congenital, tumorlike vascular nodules in the retina and cerebellum. Similar spinal cord lesions, cysts of the pancreas, kidneys, and other viscera, seizures, and mental retardation may be present. Also called **Lindau-von Hippel disease, retinocerebral angiomatosis, von Hippel-Lindau disease.**

cerebrospinal Of, pertaining to, or involving the brain and the spinal cord.

cerebrospinal fluid (CSF) The fluid that flows through and protects the four ventricles of the brain, the subarachnoid space, and the spinal canal. It is composed mainly of secretions of the choroid plexi in the lateral ventricles and in the third and the fourth ventricles of the brain. Openings in the roof of the fourth ventricle allow the fluid to flow into the subarachnoid spaces around the brain and the spinal cord. The flow of fluid is from the blood in the choroid plexi, through the ventricles, the central canal, the subarachnoid spaces, and back into the blood. The volume of cerebrospinal fluid in the adult is about 140 ml, including about 23 ml in the ventricles and 117 ml in the subarachnoid spaces of the brain and the spinal cord. Changes in the carbon dioxide content of CSF affect the respiratory center in the medulla, helping to control breathing. Certain illnesses and various diagnoses may require microscopic examination and chemical analysis of CSF. Samples of the fluid may be removed by lumbar puncture.

cerebrovascular   Of or pertaining to the vascular system and blood supply of the brain.

cerebrovascular accident (CVA)   An abnormal condition of the blood vessels of the brain characterized by occlusion by an embolus or cerebrovascular hemorrhage, resulting in ischemia of the brain tissues normally perfused by the damaged vessels. The sequelae of a cerebrovascular accident depend on the location and extent of ischemia. Paralysis, weakness, speech defect, aphasia, or death may occur. Symptoms remit somewhat after the first few days as brain swelling subsides. Physical therapy and speech therapy may restore much lost function.

cerebrum, *pl.* **cerebrums, cerebra**   The largest and uppermost section of the brain, divided by the longitudinal fissure into the left and the right cerebral hemispheres. At the bottom of the groove the hemispheres are connected by the corpus callosum. The internal structures of the hemispheres merge with those of the diencephalon and further communicate with the brain stem through the cerebral peduncles. Each cerebral hemisphere is composed of the extensive outer cerebral cortex with its gray substance, the underlying semiovale with its white substance, the internal basal ganglia, and certain centrally and medially located structures comprising the rhinencephalon. The surface of the cerebrum is convoluted and lobed, each lobe bearing the name of the bone under which it lies. The cerebrum performs sensory functions, motor functions, and less easily defined integration functions associated with various mental activities. It generates a variety of electrical waves that may be recorded on an electroencephalogram to localize areas of brain dysfunction, to identify altered states of consciousness, or to establish brain death. Memory, speech, writing, and emotional response are also controlled or affected by the cerebrum. See also **cerebral cortex. —cerebral,** *adj.*

cerium (Ce)   A ductile, gray rare-earth element. Its atomic number is 58; its atomic weight is 140.13.

ceroid   A golden, waxy pigment appearing in the cirrhotic livers of some individuals, in the nervous system, and in the muscles. It is an insoluble, acid-fast, sudanophilic pigment.

ceroma, *pl.* **ceromas, ceromata**   A neoplasm that has undergone waxy degeneration.

certificate of need or necessity   A statement or certificate issued by a governmental agency to the effect that a proposed construction or modification of a health facility will be needed

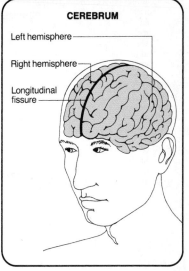

CEREBRUM

Left hemisphere

Right hemisphere

Longitudinal fissure

at the time of its completion. The certificate is issued to the individual or group intending to build or modify the facility.

certification   **1.** A process in which an individual, an institution, or an educational program is evaluated and recognized as meeting certain predetermined standards. Certification is usually made by a nongovernmental agency. The purpose of certification is to assure that the standards met are those necessary for safe and ethical practice of the profession or service.

certification for excellence   See **certification in nursing.**

certification in nursing   One of two processes in which a professional organization formally recognizes the right of a registered nurse to practice a subspecialty of nursing. One process, certification for excellence, bases recognition on professional achievement, advanced training, and superior performance. The second process, entry level certification, bases recognition on advanced training in a program approved by the certifying organization.

certified milk   Raw milk that is obtained, handled, and marketed in compliance with state health laws. The milk must be produced by disease-free cows, which are regularly inspected by a veterinarian and are milked by sterilized equipment in hygienic surroundings, contain less than a specified low bacterial count, and be not older than 36 hours when delivered.

Certified Nurse-Midwife (CNM)   According to the American College of Nurse-Midwives: "an individual educated in the two disciplines of nursing and midwifery, who possesses evidence of certification according to the requirements of the American College of Nurse-Midwives." See also **midwife.**

certified registered nurse anesthetist (CRNA)   See **nurse anesthetist.**

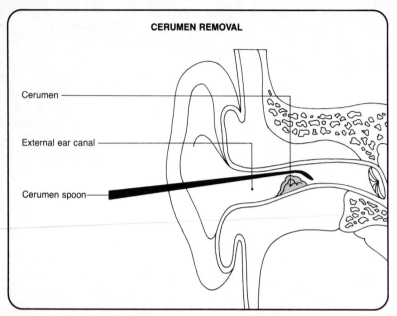

CERUMEN REMOVAL

Cerumen

External ear canal

Cerumen spoon

---

certify   **1.** To guarantee formally that certain requirements have been met based on expert knowledge of significant, pertinent facts. **2.** To attest, by a legal process, that someone is insane. **3.** To attest to the fact of someone's death in writing, usually on a form as required by local authority. **4.** To declare that a person has satisfied certain requirements for membership or acceptance into a professional or other group. See also **board certification.** **—certification,** *n.,* **certifiable,** *adj.*

ceruloplasmin   A glycoprotein in plasma that transports 96% of the plasma copper.

cerumen   Earwax. Cerumen is a yellow or brown waxy secretion produced by vestigial apocrine sweat glands in the external ear canal. Excessive production or impaction of cerumen in the ear canal can cause discomfort, symptoms of hearing loss, and irritation leading to the development of infection. Removal of excess cerumen is accomplished by the local use of a wax-softening agent followed by careful flushing with an ear syringe. A cerumen spoon is sometimes used to scoop out hard collections of old wax.

ceruminosis   Excessive buildup of cerumen in the external auditory canal.

ceruminous gland   One of a number of tiny structures in the external ear canal, believed to be modified sweat glands. They secrete a waxy cerumen instead of watery sweat.

cervic-   A combining form meaning 'pertaining to the neck': *cervicectomy, cervicitis, cervicobrachial.*

cervical   **1.** Of or pertaining to the neck or the region of the neck. **2.** Of or pertaining to the constricted area of a necklike structure, as the neck of a tooth or the cervix of the uterus.

cervical abortion   Spontaneous expulsion of a cervical pregnancy.

cervical adenitis   An abnormal condition characterized by enlarged, tender lymph nodes of the neck. It often occurs in association with acute infections of the throat.

cervical canal   The canal within the uterine cervix, which protrudes into the vagina. The uterine end of the canal is closed at the internal os and, in the nullipara, at the distal end by the external os. The canal is a passageway through which the menstrual flow escapes, sperm travels upward to the uterus and fallopian tubes, and, vastly dilated and effaced by labor, through which the infant must come to be delivered vaginally.

cervical cancer   See **cervical carcinoma.**

cervical cap   A nonsystemic, noninvasive contraceptive device consisting of a small rubber cup fitted over the uterine cervix to prevent spermatozoa from entering the cervical canal. Its effectiveness, even when left in place for days or weeks, may equal or exceed that of the diaphragm, and may be more comfortable. Accurate initial fitting by a trained person is necessary.

cervical carcinoma   A neoplasm of the uterine cervix that can be detected in the early, curable stage by the Papanicolaou test. Factors associated with its development are coitus at an early age, many sexual partners, genital herpesvirus infections, multiparity, and poor obstetric and gynecologic care. Early cervical neoplasia is usually asymptomatic, but there may be a watery vaginal discharge or occasional spotting of blood; advanced lesions may cause a dark, foul-smelling vaginal discharge, leakage from bladder or rectal fistulas, anorexia, weight loss, and back and leg pains. Papanicolaou tests of cervical cells are highly important in screening, but definitive diagnoses are based on colposcopic examination and cytologic study of specimens obtained by biopsy. Suitable sites for biopsy may be indicated by applying 3% acetic acid to the cervix to accentuate characteristic changes in neoplastic epithelium or by using Schiller's test. Cervical dysplasia may regress, persist, or progress to clinical disease, but carcinoma in situ is considered to be a precursor of invasive carcinoma. About 90% of cervical tumors are squamous cell carcinomas, fewer than 10% are adenocarcinomas, and others are mixtures of these kinds, or, in rare cases, sarcomas. Tumors on the surface of the cervix may be huge, polypoid masses while endophytic lesions tend to be small and hard; ulcerative lesions may cause extensive erosion. Cervical carcinoma invades the tissues of adjacent organs and may metastasize through lymphatic channels to distant sites, including the lungs, bone, liver, brain, and para-aortic nodes. Treatment depends on the kind and the extent of the malignancy, the age of the woman, her general health, and her desire to maintain reproductive function. Carcinoma in situ may be treated by excisional conization or cryosurgery. Invasive tumors may be treated with radiotherapy or vaginal or abdominal hysterectomy.

cervical disk syndrome   An abnormal condition characterized by compression or irritation of the cervical nerve roots in or near the intervertebral foramina before the roots divide into the anterior and the posterior rami. Cervical disk syndrome may be caused by ruptured intervertebral disks or degenerative cervical disk disease that produce varying degrees of malalignment, causing nerve root compression; or by cervical injury that involves hyperextension, causing compression because of the anatomic structures involved. Flexion injuries in the cervical area do not result in nerve compression. Edema usually occurs in all cases of cervical disk syndrome. Pain, the most common symptom, usually emanates from the cervical area but may radiate down the arm to the fingers and increase with cervical motion, coughing, sneezing, or any radical movement. Other signs and symptoms may be paresthesia, headache, blurred vision, decreased skeletal function, and weakened hand grip. Nonsurgical intervention, which is usually a successful treatment, may include immobilization of the cervical vertebrae to decrease irritation and to provide rest for the traumatized area. Other treatment may include special exercises, heat therapy, intermittent traction, and mild analgesics. Surgery is usually recommended only when signs and symptoms persist despite nonsurgical treatment. The prognosis is usually good, but recurrence of symptoms is common. Also called **cervical root syndrome.** See also **ruptured intervertebral disk.**

cervical endometritis   An inflammation of the inner lining of the cervix uteri. See also **endometritis.**

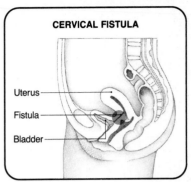

CERVICAL FISTULA

Uterus
Fistula
Bladder

cervical fistula   **1.** See **branchial fistula. 2.** An abnormal passage from the cervix to the vagina or bladder that may be caused by a malignant lesion, radiotherapy, surgical trauma, or injury during childbirth. A cervical fistula communicating with the bladder permits leakage of urine, causing irritation, odor, and embarrassment. When surgical repair is not possible, the patient is advised to take sitz baths, use a deodorizing douche or powder, as sodium borate, and to wear plastic pants or a protective apron.

cervical mucus method of family planning   See **ovulation method of family planning.**

cervical os   **1.** See **external cervical os. 2.** See **internal cervical os.**

cervical plexus   The network of nerves formed by the ventral primary divisions of the first four cervical nerves. Each nerve, except the first, divides into the superior branch and the inferior branch, and both branches unite to form three loops. The plexus is located opposite the cranial aspect of the first four cervical vertebrae, ventrolateral to the levator scapulae and the scalenus medius, and deep to the sternocleidomastoideus. It communicates with certain cranial nerves and numerous muscular and cutaneous branches.

cervical plexus anesthesia   Nerve block at any point below the mastoid process from C_2 to the second cervical vertebra transverse process of the sixth cervical vertebra. This method is used for operations on the area between the jaw and clavicle. Complications may include Horner's syndrome, inadvertent stellate ganglion or brachial plexus block, vertebral artery bleeding, subarachnoid or peridural penetration, phrenic nerve block or palsy, or laryngeal nerve block, manifested by sudden hoarseness.

cervical polyp   An outgrowth of columnar epithelial tissue of the endocervical canal, usually attached to the wall of the canal by a slender pedicle. Often there are no symptoms, but multiple or abraded polyps may cause bleeding, especially with contact during coitus. Polyps are most common in women over 40 years of age. The etiology is not known. Treatment of a symptomatic polyp is removal by simple torsion; scant bleeding and prompt healing usually follow.

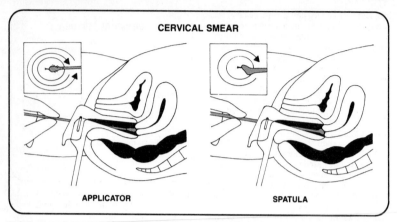

CERVICAL SMEAR

APPLICATOR SPATULA

Pathologic evaluation and histologic examination commonly reveal squamous metaplasia; malignancy is rare. A Papanicolaou test and endometrial biopsy may be performed at the same visit if other pathology is suspected.

cervical smear A small amount of the secretions and superficial cells of the cervix, secured with a sterile applicator or special small wooden or plastic spatula from the external os of the uterine cervix. For a Papanicolaou smear, it is obtained from the squamo-columnar junction of the uterine cervix and from the vaginal vault and endocervical canal. The specimen is spread on a specially labeled glass slide and sent for cytologic examination by a special laboratory. For bacteriologic culture and identification, only the applicator is used; the specimen is spread on a glass slide and stained and examined under a microscope or placed in or on a culture medium and sent to a bacteriologic laboratory for culture and identification.

cervical tenaculum See **tenaculum**.

cervical triangle One of two triangular areas formed in the neck by the oblique course of the sternocleidomastoideus. The anterior triangle is bounded by the midline of the throat anteriorly, the sternocleidomastoideus laterally, and the body of the mandible superiorly. The posterior triangle is bounded by the clavicle inferiorly and by the borders of the sternocleidomastoideus and the trapezius superiorly.

cervical vertebra One of the first seven segments of the vertebral column. They differ from the thoracic and the lumbar vertebrae by the presence of a foramen in each transverse process. The first, second, and seventh cervical vertebrae present exceptional features. The bodies of the four remaining cervical vertebrae are small, oval, and broader than the other three in transverse diameter and contain large, triangular foramens within their tranverse processes. Their spinous processes are short and bifid. The first cervical vertebra has no body, supports the head, and contains a smooth, oval facet for articulation with the dens of the second cervical vertebra. The dens extends from the cranial portion of the body of the second cervical vertebra, which has a very large, strong spinous process with a bifid extremity. The seventh cervical vertebra has a very long, prominent spinous process that is nearly horizontal in direction and is often used as a palpable reference for locating the other cervical spines. Compare **coccygeal vertebra, lumbar vertebra, sacral vertebra, thoracic vertebra**. See also **vertebra**.

cervicitis Acute or chronic inflammation of the uterine cervix. Acute cervicitis is the infection of the cervix marked by redness, edema, and bleeding on contact. Symptoms do not always occur, but may include any or all of the following: copious, foul-smelling discharge from the vagina, pelvic pressure or pain, scant bleeding with intercourse, and itching or burning of the external genitalia. The principle causative organisms are: *Trichomonas, Candida albicans*, and *Hemophilus vaginalis*. Acute cervicitis tends to be a recurrent problem owing to reexposure to the germ, undertreatment, or predisposing factors such as multiple sexual partners or poor nutritional status. **Chronic cervicitis** is a persistent inflammation of the cervix usually occurring among women in their reproductive years. Symptoms include a thick, irritating, malodorous discharge, that may, in severe cases, be accompanied by significant pelvic pain. The cervix looks congested and enlarged, nabothian cysts are often present, there are signs of eversion of the cervix and often old lacerations from childbirth. A Papanicolaou test should be performed prior to treatment. Antibiotic treatment is seldom effective. The symptoms of mild chronic cervicitis may abate with topical treatment, but the underlying inflammatory condition will not change. The most effective treatment is hot or cold cautery. See also *Candida albicans*, **cautery, cervical cancer, cervical polyp, condylomatum accuminatum, nabothian cyst**.

cervico- A combining form meaning 'neck': *cervicodynia, cervicolabial, cervicotomy*.

cervicodynia Pain in the neck. Also called **trachelodynia**.

cervicofacial actinomycosis　See **acti-nomycosis.**

cervicolabial　Of, pertaining to, or situated in the labial area of the neck of an incisor or a canine tooth.

cervicouterine　Of, pertaining to, or situated at the cervix of the uterus.

cervicovesical　Of or pertaining to the cervix of the uterus and the bladder.

cervix　The part of the uterus that protrudes into the cavity of the vagina. The supravaginal portion is separated ventrally from the bladder by the parametrium, which attaches to the sides of the cervix and contains the uterine arteries. The vaginal portion of the cervix projects into the cavity of the vagina and contains the cervical canal and the internal and external os of the canal. The mucous membrane lining the endocervix is broken by numerous oblique ridges, deep glandular follicles, little cysts, and papillae.

ceryl alcohol　A fatty alcohol obtained from spermaceti, used as an emulsifying and stiffening agent.

cesarean hysterectomy　A surgical operation in which the uterus is removed at the time of cesarean section. It is performed most often for complications of cesarean section, usually intractable hemorrhage. Less often it is done to treat preexisting gynecologic disease, as an intraepithelial cervical neoplasia. It is rarely done electively for sterilization because the danger of hemorrhage is greater when both procedures are performed simultaneously.

cesarean section　A surgical procedure in which the abdomen and uterus are incised and a baby is delivered transabdominally. It is performed when abnormal maternal or fetal conditions exist that are judged likely to make vaginal delivery hazardous. Approximately 15% of births in the United States are by cesarean section; the operation is performed less frequently in other countries. The maternal mortality is 0.1% to 0.2%. Maternal indications include hemorrhage from placenta previa or abruptio placentae, severe preeclampsia, and dysfunctional labor. Delivery by cesarean section at a prior parturition is no longer considered an absolute indication for repeating it in future deliveries. Cesarean birth is less traumatic for babies than difficult midforceps delivery. Fetal indications for the operation include fetal distress, cephalopelvic disproportion, and abnormal presentation, as breech and transverse lie. The incision in the skin of the abdomen may be horizontal or vertical, regardless of the kind of internal incision into the uterus. See also **classical cesarean section, extraperitoneal cesarean section, low cervical cesarean section.**

cesium (Cs)　An alkali metal element. Its atomic number is 55; its atomic weight is 132.9. The isotope cesium[137], which has a half-life of 33 years, has been used as a source of gamma rays in medical and industrial radiology.

cesspool fever　*Informal.* Typhoid fever.

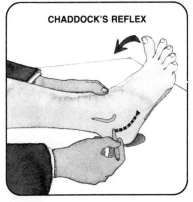

CHADDOCK'S REFLEX

cestode　See **tapeworm.**

cestode infection　See **tapeworm infection.**

cestodiasis　See **tapeworm infection.**

cestoid　Resembling a tapeworm.

cetyl alcohol　A fatty alcohol, derived from spermaceti, used as an emulsifier and stiffening agent. Also called **palmityl alcohol.**

CEU　*abbr* **continuing education unit.**

cevitamic acid　See **ascorbic acid.**

Cf　Symbol for **californium.**

C-F test　*abbr* **complement-fixation test.**

CGS, cgs　*abbr* **centimeter-gram-second (system).**

Ch¹　Symbol for **Christchurch chromosome.**

Chaddock's reflex　**1.** An abnormal variation of Babinski's reflex, elicited by firmly stroking the side of the foot just distal to the lateral malleolus, characterized by extension of the great toe and fanning of the other toes. It is seen in pyramidal tract disease. Also called **Chaddock's sign. 2.** An abnormal reflex, induced by firmly stroking the ulnar surface of the forearm, characterized by flexion of the wrist and extension of the fingers in fanlike position. It is seen on the affected side in hemiplegia. Compare **Gordon reflex, Oppenheim reflex.** See also **Babinski's reflex.**

Chaddock's sign　See **Chaddock's reflex.**

Chadwick's sign　The bluish coloration of the vulva and vagina that develops after the 6th week of pregnancy as a normal result of local venous congestion. It is an early sign of pregnancy.

chafe　An irritation of the skin by friction, as when rough material rubs against an unprotected area of the body.

chafing　Superficial irritation of the skin by friction.

Chagas-Cruz disease　See **Chagas' disease.**

Chagas' disease　A parasitic disease caused by *Trypanosoma cruzi* or by *Schizotrypanum cruzi*, transmitted to man by the bite of bloodsucking insects. The acute form, common in children and rare in adults, is marked by a lesion at the site of the bite, by fever, weakness, en-

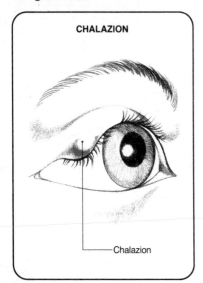

CHALAZION

Chalazion

larged spleen and lymph glands, edema of the face and legs, and tachycardia. It resolves within 4 months unless complications, as encephalitis, develop. The chronic form may be manifested by cardiomyopathy, or by dilatation of the esophagus or colon. Often, infections are asymptomatic. Also called **American trypanosomiasis, Brazilian trypanosomiasis, Chagas-Cruz disease, Cruz trypanosomiasis, South American trypanosomiasis.** See also **trypanosomiasis.**

Chagres fever An arbovirus infection transmitted to humans through the bite of a sandfly. The disease is rarely fatal and is characterized by fever, headache, and muscle pains of the chest or abdomen, and perhaps nausea and vomiting, giddiness, weakness, photophobia, and pain on moving the eyes. The infection subsides within 1 week. Supportive treatment includes analgesics, bed rest, and adequate fluid intake. The disease is most common in Central America.

chain **1.** A length of several units linked together in a linear pattern, as a polypeptide chain of amino acids or a chain of atoms forming a chemical molecule. **2.** A group of individual bacteria linked together, as streptococci formed by a chain of cocci. **3.** The serial relationship of certain structures essential to function, as the chain of ossicles in the middle ear. Each of the small bones moves successively in response to vibration of the tympanic membrane, thus transmitting the auditory stimulus to the oval window. See also **chain ligature.**

chain ligature An interlocking ligature that ties off a pedicle at several places by passing a long thread through the pedicle at different points.

chain reaction **1.** In chemistry: a reaction that produces a compound needed for the reaction to continue, as each product produced in the chain reactions of glycolysis which is essential for each succeeding reaction and the total catabolism of glucose. **2.** In physics: a reaction that perpetuates itself by the proliferating fission of nuclei and the release of atomic particles, which cause more nuclear fissions.

chain reflex A series of reflexes, each stimulated by the preceding one.

chain stitch suture A continuous surgical stitch in which each loop of the suture is secured by the next loop.

chalasia Abnormal relaxation or incompetence of the cardiac sphincter of the stomach, resulting in reflux of the gastric contents into the esophagus with subsequent regurgitation. Conservative treatment in infancy includes feeding several small meals a day to avoid distention of the stomach and holding the baby upright while giving the feeding. The symptoms and treatment are similar to those of a hiatal hernia.

chalazion A small, localized swelling of the eyelid resulting from obstruction and retained secretions of the Meibomian glands. A nonmalignant condition, it often requires surgery for correction. Compare **hordeolum, sty.**

chalice cell See **goblet cell.**

chalkitis An abnormal condition characterized by inflammation of the eyes, caused by rubbing the eyes with the hands after touching or handling brass. Also called **brassy eye.**

chalone Any one of numerous mitotic inhibitors that is elaborated by a tissue and functions within that tissue rather than affecting another tissue.

chamber **1.** A hollow, but not necessarily empty, space or cavity in an organ, as in the anterior and posterior chambers of the eye or the atrial and ventricular chambers of the heart. **2.** A room or closed space used for research or therapeutic purposes, as a decompression chamber or hyperbaric oxygen chamber.

Chamberlain's line A line that extends from the posterior of the hard palate to the dorsum of the foramen magnum.

Chamberlen forceps One of the earliest kinds of obstetric forceps.

chamaeprosopy A facial appearance characterized by a low brow and a broad face with a facial index of 90 or less. —**chamaeprosopic,** *adj.*

CHAMPUS *abbr* **Civilian Health and Medical Programs for Uniformed Services.**

chancr- See **cancr-.**

chancre **1.** A skin lesion of primary syphilis that begins at the site of infection as a papule and develops into a red, bloodless, painless ulcer with a scooped-out appearance. It heals without treatment and leaves no scar. Two or more chancres may develop at the same time, occurring usually in the genital area but sometimes on the hands, face, or other body surface. The chancre teems with *Treponema pallidum* spirochetes and is highly contagious. **2.** A papular lesion or ulcerated area of the skin that marks the point of infection of a nonsyphilitic disease, as tuberculosis. See also **chancroid, syphilis.**

chancroid   A highly contagious, local venereal ulcer caused by infection with a bacillus, *Haemophilus ducreyi.* It characteristically begins as a papule, usually on the skin of the external genitalia; it then grows and ulcerates, other papules form, and, if untreated, the bacillus spreads, causing buboes in the groin. An intradermal skin test is more reliable than smear and culture techniques for diagnosis. Treatment is with sulfa drugs. Because the lesion resembles syphilis and lymphogranuloma venereum, the diagnosis must be made before treatment in order to avoid obscuring simultaneous infections. Compare **chancre.**

channel   A passageway or groove that conveys fluid, as the central channels that connect the arterioles with the venules.

channel ulcer   A rare type of peptic ulcer found in the pyloric canal between the stomach and the duodenum. See also **peptic ulcer.**

chapped   Pertaining to skin that is roughened, cracked, or reddened by exposure to cold or excessive surface evaporation. Stinging or burning sensations often accompany the disorder. Prevention is by protection against exposure to cold and wind. Treatment includes the avoidance of frequent washing, the replacement of soaps and detergents with super-fatted soaps, and the application of emollients. Compare **frostbite. —chap,** *v.*

character   **1.** The integrated composite of traits and behavioral tendencies that enable a person to react in a relatively consistent way to the customs and mores of society. Character, as contrasted with personality, implies volition and morality. Compare **personality. 2.** In data processing: any letter, number, symbol, or space which can be used to represent data.

character analysis   A systematic investigation of the personality of an individual with special attention to psychological defenses and motivations, usually undertaken to improve behavior.

character disorder   A chronic, habitual, maladaptive, and socially unacceptable pattern of behavior and emotional response. The condition is usually accompanied by minimal feelings of anxiety. Also called **character neurosis.** See also **antisocial personality disorder.**

character neurosis   See **character disorder.**

charcoal   See **activated charcoal.**

Charcot-Bouchard aneurysm   A small, round aneurysm of a small artery of the cerebral cortex, which some authorities believe is the cause of massive cerebral hemorrhage. Charcot-Bouchard aneurysms often occur in individuals with very high blood pressure.

Charcot-Leyden crystal   Any one of the crystalline structures shaped like narrow, double pyramids found in the sputum of individuals suffering from bronchial asthma. The Charcot-Leyden crystals are protein compounds and occur in association with the fragmentation of eosinophils. Also called **asthma crystal, leukocytic crystal.**

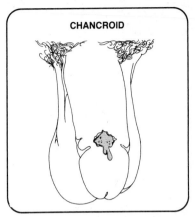

CHANCROID

Charcot-Marie-Tooth atrophy   A progressive hereditary disorder characterized by degeneration of the peroneal muscles of the fibula, resulting in clubfoot, footdrop, and ataxia.

Charcot's fever   A syndrome characterized by a recurrent fever, jaundice, and abdominal pain in the right upper quadrant occurring with inflammation of the bile ducts. It is caused by the intermittent impaction of a stone in the ducts.

Charcot's joint   See **neuropathic joint disease.**

Charles' law   See **Gay-Lussac's law.**

chart   **1.** *Informal.* A patient record. **2.** To note data in a patient record, usually at prescribed intervals.

charta, *pl.* **chartae**   A piece of paper, especially one treated with medicine, as for external application, or with a chemical for a special purpose, as litmus paper.

chauffeur's fracture   Any fracture of the radial styloid, produced by a twisting or a snapping type injury.

Chaussier's areola   An areola of indurated tissue surrounding a malignant pustule.

CHC   *abbr* community health center.

check ligament   See **alar ligament.**

Chediak-Higashi syndrome   A congenital, autosomal disorder, characterized by partial albinism, photophobia, massive leukocytic inclusions, psychomotor abnormalities, recurrent infections, and early death. Antenatal diagnosis can be made by amniocentesis and tissue culture. Treatment includes antibiotics and transfusions.

cheesewasher's lung   A lung disease caused by an allergic reaction to the mold of cheese. Avoiding the causative agent assures prevention. No treatment is necessary.

cheil-   See **cheilo-.**

-cheilia   A combining form meaning '(condition of the) lips': *atelocheilia, dicheilia, xerocheilia.* Also **-chilia.**

cheilitis   An abnormal condition of the lips characterized by inflammation and cracking of the skin. There are several forms, including those caused by excessive exposure to sunlight, al-

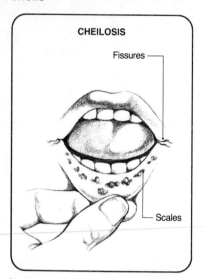

CHEILOSIS

Fissures

Scales

lergic sensitivity to cosmetics, and vitamin deficiency. Compare **cheilosis.**

cheilo-, cheil-   A combining form meaning 'pertaining to the lip': *cheiloangioscopy, cheilocarcinoma, cheiloplasty.*

cheilocarcinoma, *pl.* **cheilocarcinomas, cheilocarcinomata**   A malignant epithelial tumor of the lip.

cheiloplasty   Surgical correction of a defect of the lip.

cheilorraphy   A surgical procedure that sutures the lip, as in the repair of a congenitally cleft lip or a lacerated lip.

cheilosis   A disorder of the lips and mouth characterized by scales and fissures, resulting from a deficiency of riboflavin in the diet. Compare **cheilitis.**

cheir-   See **cheiro-.**

cheiralgia   A pain in the hand, especially the pain associated with arthritis. —**cheiralgic,** *adj.*

-cheiria   See **-chiria.**

cheiro-, cheir-   A combining form meaning 'pertaining to the hand': *cheiragra, cheiromegaly, cheiroplasty.* Also **chir-, chiro-.**

cheiromegaly   An abnormal condition characterized by excessively large hands. —**cheiromegalic,** *adj.*

cheiroplasty   An operation involving plastic surgery of the hand. —**cheiroplastic,** *adj.*

chelate   **1.** Of a metal ion and two or more polar groups of a single molecule: to form a bond, thus creating a ringlike complex. **2.** In medicine: any compound composed of iron ions arranged in ring formations with polar groups of single molecules, used especially in chemotherapeutic treatments for metal poisoning. **3.** Of or pertaining to chelation.

chelating agent   A substance that promotes chelation. Chelating agents are used in the treatment of metal poisoning. See also **chelation.**

chelation   A chemical reaction in which there

is a combination with a metal to form a ring-shaped molecular complex in which the metal is firmly bound and sequestered. See also **chelating agent.**

cheloid   See **keloid.**

cheloidosis   See **keloidosis.**

chemical   **1.** A substance composed of chemical elements or a substance produced by or used in chemical processes. **2.** Pertaining to chemistry.

chemical action   Any process in which natural elements and compounds react with each other to produce a chemical change or a different compound, as hydrogen and oxygen, which combine to produce water.

chemical agent   Any chemical power, active principle, or substance that can produce an effect in the body by interacting with various body substances, as aspirin, which produces an analgesic effect.

chemical antidote   Any substance that reacts chemically with a poison to form a compound that is harmless. There are few true antidotes, and treatment of most poisoning depends largely on eliminating the toxic agent before it can be absorbed by the body.

chemical burn   Tissue damage caused by exposure to a strong acid or alkali, as phenol, creosol, mustard gas, or phosphorus. Emergency treatment includes washing the surface with copious amounts of water to remove the chemical and, if the damage is more than slight and superficial, immediate transport to a medical facility. See also **acid burn, acid poisoning, alkali burn, alkali poisoning.**

chemical cauterization   The corroding or burning of living tissue by a caustic chemical substance, as potassium hydroxide. Also called **chemocautery.**

chemical diabetes   See **latent diabetes.**

chemical equivalence   Of a drug or chemical: containing similar amounts of the same ingredients as another drug or chemical. See also **compendium.**

chemical gastritis   Inflammation of the stomach caused by the ingestion of a chemical compound. Treatment is determined by the substance ingested. Gastric lavage is often advisable, but neither lavage nor emetics are administered in cases involving the most corrosive poisons. Compare **corrosive gastritis, erosive gastritis.**

chemical name   The exact designation of the chemical structure of a drug as determined by the rules of accepted systems of chemical nomenclature. For example, N,N-bis-(2-chloroethyl)-N′-(3-hydroxypropyl) phosphordiamidic acid cyclic acid monohydrate is the chemical name of cyclophosphamide, a drug used in cancer chemotherapy.

chemical warfare   The waging of war with poisonous chemicals and gases.

cheminosis   Any disease caused by a chemical substance.

chemistry   The science dealing with the elements, their compounds, and the chemical structure and interactions of matter. Kinds of chemistry include **inorganic chemistry**, **organic chemistry.**

chemistry, normal values   The amounts of various substances in the normal human body, determined by testing a large sample of people presumed to be healthy. Normal values are expressed in ranges of numbers, and ranges vary among laboratories. Although variations from normal values may be highly significant tools in the diagnoses of certain diseases, in all cases an abnormal result must be cautiously interpreted. See also specific tests.

chemo-   A combining form meaning 'pertaining to a chemical or to chemistry': *chemoantigen, chemobiotic, chemokinesis.*

chemocautery   See **chemical cauterization.**

chemodifferentiation   A stage in embryonic development that precedes and controls specialization and differentiation of the cells into rudimentary organs.

chemoreceptor   A sensory nerve cell activated by chemical stimuli, as a chemoreceptor in the carotid that is sensitive to the Pco_2 in the blood, signaling the respiratory center in the brain to increase or decrease respiration.

chemoreflex   Any reflex initiated by the stimulation of chemical receptors, as the carotid and aortic bodies, which respond to changes in carbon dioxide, hydrogen ion, and oxygen concentrations in the blood. See also **chemoreceptor.**

chemosis   An abnormal edematous swelling of the mucous membrane covering the eyeball and lining the eyelids. Usually the result of local trauma or infection, it may also occur in acute conjunctivitis or in systemic disorders, as angioneurotic edema, anemia, and Bright's disease. An obstruction of normal lymph flow, as from growth of a tumor within the eye socket, is a less common cause. Also called conjunctival edema.

chemostat   A device which assures a steady rate of cell division in bacterial populations by maintaining a constant environment.

chemosurgery   The destruction of malignant, infected, or gangrenous tissue by the application of chemicals. The technique is used successfully to remove skin cancers.

chemotaxis   A response involving movement toward (positive) or away from (negative) a chemical stimulus.

chemotherapeutic index   See **therapeutic index.**

chemotherapy   Treatment of disease by chemical reagents that have a specific toxic effect on a pathogen or that are used to treat neoplasms. Cancer chemotherapy is often used alone to treat such malignancies as leukemia or lymphatic disorders that have no localized focus. Adjuvant chemotherapy is administered after surgery or irradiation of solid tumors to destroy residual cancer cells and prevent local or metastatic recurrence.

chemotherapy (unsealed radioactive)

The oral or parenteral administration of a radioisotope, as iodine 131 (^{131}I) for the treatment of hyperthyroidism or thyroid cancer, phosphorus 32 (^{32}P) for leukemia or polycythemia vera, or gold 198 (^{198}Au) for lung cancer or peritoneal ascites resulting from widely disseminated carcinoma.

NURSING CONSIDERATIONS: Before unsealed radioactive chemotherapy is administered, the patient receives an explanation of the procedure and of the need for isolation during the half-life of the radioisotope (8.1 days for ^{131}I, 14 days for ^{32}P, and 2.7 days for ^{198}Au). The room in which the patient is isolated adjoins a private bathroom. Radioactive tags are posted on the door; individual radioactive badges, kept at the door, are worn by each staff member entering the room to record the amount of radiation exposure; pregnant staff members are not assigned to the patient's care. Family and friends are not allowed to visit in the initial 24 hours of therapy and are thereafter limited to 2-hour visits if the person remains 6 feet or more from the patient. During isolation, the staff member caring for the patient limits the time spent in the room by planning the observations and procedures to be accomplished. Disposable dishes, utensils, and trays are used for the patient. Urine excreted by a patient treated with ^{131}I is collected, directly or via an indwelling catheter, in a lead-lined container, which is sent to the laboratory for assay of the radioisotope. Feces, sputum, and vomitus are placed in the toilet and decontaminated with a dropperful of a saturated solution of potassium iodide before the bowl is flushed. Dressings and bed linen are handled with rubber or plastic gloves; contaminated linens and trash are not removed from the room until monitored with a Geiger-Müller counter. The patient treated with ^{131}I is observed for evidence of neck tenderness, changes in exophthalmia, a transient productive cough, hypoparathyroidism, hypothyroidism, and hyperthyroidism. Similar procedures of care are followed for the patient treated with ^{32}P, but since the beta rays emited by this radionuclide are absorbed by the patient's body, there is no danger of external exposure. If ^{32}P is administered intravenously or injected into the body cavity, no special precautions are needed for disposal of excreta, but dressings and linen contaminated by seepage from wounds are placed in lead-lined containers, as is the vomitus of the patient who is given the radionuclide orally. Additional special precautions are required in caring for the patient treated with radioactive gold, which emits gamma and beta rays. After purple liquid ^{198}Au is injected into the body cavity, the patient is turned with a sheet every 15 minutes for 2 hours so that the radionuclide can spread. Dressings and cleansing tissues contaminated by the purple seepage from wounds are burned immediately; linen in contact with wounds is placed in special containers. The patient injected with ^{198}Au is usually terminally ill, and, if death occurs, a tag is placed on the body to alert the mortician to the presence of the radionuclide.

PATTERNS OF CHEST PAIN IN VARIOUS DISORDERS

	MYOCARDIAL INFARCTION	PERI-CARDITIS	ANGINA	PLEURO-PULMONARY
Onset	Sudden	Sudden	Buildup of intensity (crescendo) or sudden	Gradual or sudden
Location	Substernal, anterior chest; midline	Substernal, to left of midline or precordial only	Substernal, not sharply localized; anterior chest	Over lung fields to side and back
Radiation	Down one or both arms, to jaws, neck, or back	To back or left supraclavicular area	To back, neck, arms, jaws, and occasionally upper abdomen or fingers	Anterior chest, shoulder, neck
Duration	At least 30 min; usually 1 to 2 hr; residual soreness 1 to 3 days	Continuous; may last for days; residual soreness	Usually less than 15 min and not more than 30 min (average: 3 min)	Continuous for hours
Quality-intensity	Severe, stabbing, choking, squeezing; intense pressure, deep sensation	Sharp, stabbing; moderate to severe or only an ache; deep or superficial	Mild to moderate, heavy pressure, squeezing; vague, uniform pattern of attacks, deep sensation, tightness	Sharp ache, not severe; shooting; deep; crushing
Signs and symptoms	Apprehension, nausea, dyspnea, diaphoresis, dizziness, weakness, pulmonary congestion, increased pulse, decreased BP, gallop heart sound, fatigue	Precordial friction rub. Pain increases with muscle movement, inspiration, laughing, coughing or lying on left side; decreases when sitting or leaning forward	Dyspnea, diaphoresis, nausea, desire to void; associated with belching, apprehension, or uneasiness	Dyspnea; tachycardia; apprehension; increasing pain with coughing, on inspiration, and with movement; pain decreases on sitting. Pleural rub; fever

cherry angioma A small, bright-red, clearly circumscribed vascular tumor on the skin. It occurs most often on the trunk but may be found anywhere on the body. The lesion is very common; more than 85% of people over the age of 45 have several cherry angiomas. Also called **capillary angioma, capillary hemangioma, De Morgan's spots, senile angioma.**

cherry red spot An abnormal red circular area of the choroid, seen through the fovea centralis of the eye and surrounded by a contrasting white edema. It is associated with cases of infantile cerebral sphingolipidosis and sometimes appears in the late infantile form of amaurotic familial idiocy. Also called **Tay's spot.**

cherubism An abnormal hereditary condition characterized by progressive bilateral swelling at the angle of the mandible, especially in children. In some cases of cherubism, the entire jaw swells and the eyes turn up, enhancing the cherubic facial appearance. The condition tends to regress during adult life.

chest See **thorax.**

chest binder A broad bandage that encircles the patient's chest, used to apply heat or pressure or to secure dressings.

ESOPHAGO-GASTRIC	MUSCULO-SKELETAL
Gradual or sudden	Gradual or sudden
Substernal, anterior chest; midline	To side of midline
To upper abdomen, back, or shoulder	
Continuous for short or longer intervals, or intermittent	Continuous or intermittent
Squeezing, heartburn	Soreness
Dysphagia, belching, diaphoresis, reflux esophagitis, vomiting; pain decreases on sitting or standing	Pain increases with movement

chest lead 1. An electrocardiographic conductor in which the exploring electrode is placed on the chest or precordium. The indifferent electrode is placed on the patient's back for a CB (chest back) lead, on the front of the chest for a CF (chest front) lead, the left arm for a CL (chest left) lead, and on the right arm for a CR (chest right) lead. 2. *Informal.* The tracing produced by such a lead on an electrocardiograph.

chest pain A physical complaint that requires immediate diagnosis and evaluation. Chest pain may be symptomatic of cardiac disease, as angina pectoris, myocardial infarction, or peri-

carditis, or of disease of the lungs, as pleurisy, pneumonia, or pulmonary embolism or infarction. The source of chest pain may also be musculoskeletal, gastrointestinal, or psychogenic.

chest physiotherapy A group of techniques, including postural drainage, chest percussion and vibration, and coughing and deep-breathing maneuvers, used together to mobilize and help eliminate lung secretions, help reexpand lung tissue, and promote efficient use of respiratory muscles.

chest tube A catheter inserted through the thorax into the chest cavity for removing air or fluid. It is commonly used following chest surgery and lung collapse.

chest wall percussion See **percussion.**

Cheyne-Stokes respiration An abnormal pattern of respiration, characterized by alternating periods of apnea and deep, rapid breathing. The respiratory cycle begins with slow, shallow breaths that gradually increase to abnormal depth and rapidity. Respiration gradually subsides as breathing slows and becomes shallower, climaxing in a 10- to 20-second period without respiration before the cycle is repeated. Each cyclical episode may last from 45 seconds to 3 minutes. The immediate cause of Cheyne-Stokes respiration is a complex alteration in the functioning of the respiratory center in the brain. This may be caused by changes in blood gases, especially an increase in carbon dioxide; a direct reduction in the sensitivity of the respiratory center in the presence of normal blood gas concentrations, as in cerebral vascular disease, tumors of the brain stem, or severe head injury; congestive heart failure, especially in elderly patients with degenerative arterial disease; bronchopneumonia or other respiratory diseases in the elderly; hyperventilation or exposure to high altitudes in an otherwise healthy patient; or an overdose of a narcotic or hypnotic drug. It occurs more frequently during sleep. Compare **Biot's respiration.**

-chezia A combining form meaning '(condition of) defecation, especially involving the discharge of foreign substances': *dyschezia, hematochezia, pyochezia.* Also -chesia.

CHF *abbr* **congestive heart failure.**

Chiari-Frommel syndrome A hormonal disorder that occurs after a pregnancy in which weaning does not spontaneously end lactation. The syndrome is usually the result of a decrease in pituitary gonadotropins and an excess of pituitary prolactin. Treatment includes observation, hormonal therapy, and investigation to confirm or rule out pituitary tumor.

Chiari's syndrome See **Budd-Chiari syndrome.**

chiasm 1. The crossing of two lines or tracts, as the crossing of the optic nerves at the optic chiasm. 2. In genetics: the crossing of two chromatids in the prophase of meiosis. —**chiasmal, chiasmic,** *adj.*

chiasma, *pl.* **chiasmata** In genetics: the visible point of connection between homologous chromosomes during the first meiotic division in gametogenesis. The X-shaped configurations form during the late prophase stage and provide the means by which exchange of genetic material occurs. See also **crossing over.** —**chiasmatic, chiasmic.** *adj.*

chiasmatypy See **crossing over.**

chickenpox An acute, highly contagious viral disease caused by a herpesvirus, varicella zoster virus. It occurs primarily in young children and is characterized by crops of highly pruritic vesicular eruptions on the skin. The disease is transmitted by direct contact with skin lesions or, more commonly, by droplets spread from the respiratory tract of infected persons, usually in the prodromal period or the early stages of the rash. The vesicular fluid and the scabs are infectious until entirely dry. Indirect transmission through uninfected persons or objects is rare. The diagnosis is usually made by physical examination and by the characteristic appearance of the disease. The virus may be identified by culture of the vesicle fluid. The incubation period averages 2 to 3 weeks, followed by slight fever, mild headache, malaise, and anorexia occurring about 24 to 36 hours before the rash begins. The prodromal period is usually mild in children but may be severe in adults. The rash begins as macules and progresses in 1 to 2 days to papules and, finally, to vesicles. Treatment consists of bed rest, antipyretics and topical antipruritics or oral antihistamines plus neomycin-bacitracin for infected vesicles, and systemic antibiotics if the secondary bacterial infection is extensive.

NURSING CONSIDERATIONS: Chickenpox in childhood is usually benign. Few cases require hospitalization. It may be serious or fatal in immunocompromised people, as those receiving chemotherapy or radiotherapy for malignant disease, in those who have undergone organ transplantation, in those with congenital or acquired defects in cell-mediated immunity, or in those receiving high doses of steroids. Common complications are secondary bacterial infections, as abscesses, cellulitis, pneumonia, and sepsis, and hemorrhagic varicella (tiny hemorrhages which may occur in the vesicles or surrounding skin), and, less commonly, encephalitis, Reye's syndrome, thrombocytopenia, and hepatitis. Also called **varicella.**

chiclero's ulcer See **American leishmaniasis.**

chief cell 1. Any one of the columnar epithelial cells or the cuboidal epithelial cells that line the gastric glands and secrete pepsin and the extrinsic factor, which is needed for the absorption of vitamin B_{12} and the normal development of red blood cells. Anemia is caused by the absence of intrinsic factor. Also called **zymogenic cell.** 2. Any one of the epithelioid cells with pale-staining cytoplasm and a large nucleus containing a prominent nucleolus. Cords of such cells form the main substance of the pineal body. 3. Any one of the polyhedral epithelial cells, within the parathyroid glands, which contain pale, clear cytoplasm and a vesicular

nucleus. Also called **principal cell.**

chief complaint A subjective statement made by a patient describing the patient's most significant or serious symptoms or signs of illness or dysfunction.

chief resident A senior resident physician who acts temporarily as the clinical and administrative director of the house staff in a department of the hospital. The period of duty varies depending on the size of the department, the length of the residency, and the number of house staff.

chigger The larva of a mite found in tall grass and weeds. It sticks to the skin and causes irritation and severe itching. Also called **harvest mite.**

chigoe 1. A flea found in tropical and subtropical America and Africa. The pregnant female flea burrows into the skin of the feet, causing an inflammatory condition that may lead to spontaneous amputation of a toe. Also called **burrowing flea, jigger,** *Tunga penetrans.* 2. See **chigger.**

chikungunya encephalitis An arbovirus infection characterized by a high fever that begins abruptly, muscle aches, a rash, and pain in the joints. It is transmitted by the bite of a mosquito and occurs mainly in Africa, Asia, and on some of the Pacific islands, including Guam. The fever may last for 1 week, then rise again after a remission of several days. Pain in the joints may continue after other symptoms have ceased. Supportive nursing care and symptomatic relief are the only treatments.

chilblain Redness and swelling of the skin owing to excessive exposure to cold. Burning, itching, blistering, and ulceration, similar to a thermal burn, may occur. Treatment includes protection against cold and injury, gentle warming, and avoidance of tobacco. Also called **pernio.** Compare **frostbite.**

child abuse The physical, sexual, or emotional maltreatment of a child. It may be overt or covert and often results in permanent physical or psychiatric injury, mental impairment, or, sometimes, death. Child abuse occurs predominantly to children less than 3 years of age and is the result of complex factors involving both parents and child, compounded by various stressful environmental circumstances, as poor socioeconomic conditions, inadequate physical and emotional support within the family, and any major life change or crisis, especially those crises arising from marital strife. Parents at high risk for abuse are characterized as having unsatisfied needs, difficulty in forming adequate interpersonal relationships, unrealistic expectations of the child, and a lack of nurturing experience, often involving neglect or abuse in their own childhoods. Predisposing factors among children include the temperament, personality, and activity level of the child; birth order; sensitivity to parental needs; and a need for special physical or emotional care resulting from illness, premature birth, or congenital or genetic abnormalities. Identification of abused children

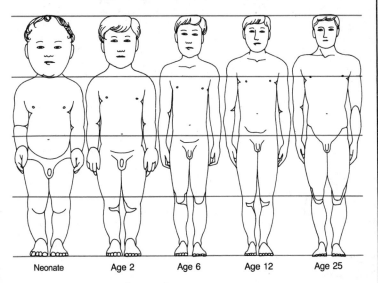

STAGES OF PHYSICAL DEVELOPMENT

Neonate   Age 2   Age 6   Age 12   Age 25

Note: Chart compares the percentage of body parts to total of body area at the different stages of physical development.

or potential child abusers is a major concern for all health-care workers. Physical marks on a child's body, as burns, welts, or bruises, signs of emotional distress or failure to thrive, are common indications of neglect or abuse. Often, X-rays to detect healed or new fractures of the extremities or diagnostic tests to identify sexual molestation are necessary. If abuse is suspected, the nurse is required to make the necessary report. Special counseling services or support groups, as Parents Anonymous, exist to help families in which a child is abused. The nurse can play a significant role in preventing abuse by promoting a positive parent-child relationship, especially in the neonatal period, by teaching parents proper child care and disciplinary techniques, and by explaining normal child development and behavior so that parents can formulate realistic guidelines for discipline. Also called battered child syndrome. Compare **child neglect.**

childbed fever   See **puerperal fever.**

childbirth   See **birth.**

child development   The various stages of physical, social, and psychological growth that occur from birth through adulthood. See also **adolescence, development, growth, infant, neonatal period, psychosexual development, psychosocial development, toddler.**

childhood   1. The period in human development that extends from birth until the onset of puberty. 2. The state or quality of being a child. See also **development, growth.**

childhood polycystic disease (CPD)   See **polycystic kidney disease.**

childhood schizophrenia   A form of schizophrenia, occurring before the onset of puberty, resulting from organic brain damage or from environmental conditions. It is characterized by autistic withdrawal into fantasy, obsessional attachments, failure to communicate verbally, repetitive gestures, emotional unresponsiveness, and a severely impaired sense of identity. Two kinds of childhood schizophrenia are **early infantile autism** and **symbiotic infantile psychotic syndrome.**

child neglect   The failure by parents or guardians to provide the basic needs of a child by physical or emotional deprivation that interferes with normal growth and development or that places the child in jeopardy. Compare **child abuse.** See also **failure to thrive, maternal deprivation syndrome.**

child psychology   The study of the mental, emotional, and behavioral development of infants and children.

child welfare   Any service sponsored by the community or special organizations that provide for the physical, social, or psychological care of children in need of it.

-chilia   See **-cheilia.**

chill   1. The sensation of cold due to exposure to a cold environment. 2. An attack of shivering with pallor and a feeling of coldness, often occurring at the beginning of an infection and accompanied by a rapid rise in temperature.

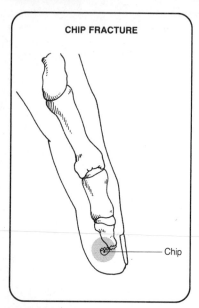

CHIP FRACTURE

Chip

Chilomastix A genus of flagellate protozoa, as *Chilomastix mesnili*, a nonpathogenic intestinal parasite of man.

chimera An organism carrying cell populations derived from different zygotes of the same or of different species. It may be a natural phenomenon, as in a bone marrow graft. Compare **mosaic.**

chimney-sweeps' cancer See **scrotal cancer.**

Chinese restaurant syndrome A syndrome consisting of tingling and burning sensations of the skin, facial pressure, headache, and chest pain that occurs immediately after eating food containing monosodium glutamate, frequently used in Chinese cooking.

chip 1. A relatively small piece of a bone or tooth. 2. To break off or cut away a small piece.

chip fracture Any small fragmental fracture, usually one involving a bony process near a joint.

chir- See **chiro-.**

chirality See **handedness.**

-chiria A combining form meaning: 1. A '(specified) condition involving hands': *acephalochiria, atelochiria, dichiria.* 2. A '(specified) condition involving stimulus and its perception': *allochiria, dyschiria, synchiria.* Also **-cheiria.**

chiro-, chir- See **cheiro-.**

chiropodist See **podiatrist.**

chiropractic A system of therapy based on the theory that the state of a person's health is determined in general by the condition of his nervous system. In most cases, treatment involves the mechanical manipulation of the spinal column. Chiropractors may employ radiology for diagnosis and use physiotherapy and diet in ad-

dition to spinal manipulation, but cannot prescribe drugs or perform surgery. A chiropractor is awarded the degree of Doctor of Chiropractic, or DC, after completing at least 2 years of premedical studies followed by 4 years of training in an approved chiropractic school.

-chirurgia See **-surgery.**

chisel fracture Any fracture in which there is an oblique detachment of a bone fragment from the head of the radius.

chi square (x^2) In statistics: a statistical test for an association between observed data and expected data represented by frequencies. The test yields a statement of the probability of the obtained distribution having occurred by chance alone.

Chlamydia 1. A microorganism of the genus *Chlamydia.* 2. A genus of microorganisms that live as intracellular parasites, have a number of properties in common with gram-negative bacteria, and are currently classified as specialized bacteria. Two species of *Chlamydia* have been recognized; both are pathogenic to humans. **C. trachomatis,** an organism that lives in the conjunctiva of the eye and the epithelium of the urethra and cervix, is responsible for inclusion conjunctivitis, lymphogranuloma venereum, and trachoma. **C. psittaci** is an organism that infects birds and causes a type of pneumonia in humans. See also **psittacosis. —chlamydial,** *adj.*

Chlamydia psittaci See *Chlamydia.*

Chlamydia trachomatis See *Chlamydia.*

chloasma Tan or brown pigmentation, particularly of the forehead, cheeks, and nose, commonly associated with pregnancy or the use of oral contraceptives. The hyperpigmentation may be permanent or may disappear only to recur with subsequent pregnancies or use of oral contraceptives. Also called **mask of pregnancy, melasma.**

chlophedianol hydrochloride A nonnarcotic antitussive agent.

chlor- A combining form meaning 'green': *chloremia, chlorephidrosis, chlorine.*

chloracne A skin condition characterized by small, black follicular plugs and papules on exposed surfaces, especially on the arms, face, and neck of workers in contact with chlorinated compounds, as cutting oils, paints, varnishes, and lacquers. Avoidance of such substances or the use of protective garments prevents the condition.

chloral hydrate A sedative-hypnotic agent.

chlorambucil An alkylating agent used in chemotherapy.

chloramphenicol An antibiotic used as an ophthalmic, otic, and local anti-infective agent.

chloramphenicol palmitate, c. sodium succinate An antibiotic.

chlordane poisoning See **chlorinated organic insecticide poisoning.**

chlordiazepoxide hydrochloride A benzodiazepine antianxiety agent.

chlorhexidine gluconate A disinfectant.

-chloric A combining form meaning 'referring to or containing chlorine': *hydrochloric, hyperchloric, perchloric.*

chloride A compound in which the negative element is chlorine. Chlorides are salts of hydrochloric acid, the most common being sodium chloride (table salt).

chlorinated organic insecticide poisoning Poisoning resulting from the inhalation, ingestion, or absorption of DDT and other insecticides containing chlorophenothane, as heptachlor, dieldrin, and chlordane. It is characterized by vomiting, weakness, malaise, convulsions, tremors, ventricular fibrillation, respiratory failure, and pulmonary edema. Treatment includes control of the neurological and neuromuscular symptoms with phenobarbitol and gastric lavage, instillation of a demulcent and absorbent like sodium sulfate or charcoal in the stomach, parenteral fluids, and supportive therapy as indicated by monitoring vital functions. Also called **DDT poisoning.**

chlorine (Cl) A yellow-green, gaseous element of the halogen group. Its atomic number is 17; its atomic weight is 35.453. It has a strong, distinctive odor, is irritating to the respiratory tract, and is poisonous if ingested or inhaled. It occurs in nature chiefly as a component of sodium chloride in sea water and in salt deposits. It is used as a bleach and as a disinfectant to purify water. Chlorine compounds in general use include many solvents, cleaning fluids, and chloroform.

chlormezanone An antianxiety agent.

chloroform A nonflammable, volatile liquid that was the first inhalation anesthetic to be discovered. Because of ease of administration—often just a medicine dropper and a handkerchief face mask—it is still the principal general anesthetic in many underdeveloped countries, where anesthesia equipment for the newer agents is not available. Chloroform is a dangerous anesthetic drug: a difference of only 10% in drug-plasma levels can result in hypotension, myocardial and respiratory depression, cardiogenic shock, ventricular fibrillation, coma, and death. Delayed poisoning, even weeks after apparently complete recovery, is not unusual, and serious ocular damage is frequently reported.

chloroformism 1. The habit of inhaling chloroform for its narcotic effect. 2. The anesthetic effect of chloroform.

chloroleukemia A kind of myelogenous leukemia in which specific tumor masses are not seen at autopsy but body fluids and organs are green. See also **myelogenous leukemia.**

chlorolymphosarcoma, *pl.* **chlorolymphosarcomas, chlorolymphosarcomata** A greenish neoplasm of myeloid tissue occurring in patients with myelogenous leukemia. The mononuclear cells in the peripheral blood are believed to be lymphocytes rather than myeloblasts, as found with chloroma.

chloroma, *pl.* **chloromas, chloromata** A malignant, green neoplasm of myeloid tissue occurring anywhere in the body in patients with myelogenous leukemia. The green pigment,

primarily myeloperoxidase (verdoperoxidase), has no definite metabolic function. The tumor tissue fluoresces bright red under ultraviolet light. Also called **granulocytic sarcoma, green cancer.**

chloromyeloma See **chloroma.**

chlorophyll A plant pigment capable of absorbing light and converting it to energy for the oxidation and reduction involved in the photosynthesis of carbohydrates. Chlorophylls a and b are found in green plants; chlorophyll c occurs in brown algae, and chlorophyll d occurs in red algae. See also **photosynthesis.**

chlorophyll test See **Boas' test.**

chloroprocaine hydrochloride An ester local anesthetic.

chloroquine hydrochloride, c. phosphate Amebacidic and antimalarial agent.

chlorosis An iron deficiency anemia of young women that is characterized by hypochromic, microcytic erythrocytes and a small reduction in the total number of erythrocytes. See also **anemia.**

chlorothiazide A thiazide diuretic.

chlorotrianisene A synthetic estrogen.

chlorphenesin carbamate A skeletal muscle relaxant.

chlorpheniramine maleate An alkyline antihistamine.

chlorphenoxamine hydrochloride A cholinergic blocking (parasympatholytic) agent.

chlorphentermine hydrochloride An amphetamine-like central nervous system stimulant.

chlorpromazine hydrochloride A phenothiazine tranquilizer and antipsychotic.

chlorpropamide An oral sulfonylurea antidiabetic agent.

chlorprothixene A thioxanthine antipsychotic.

chlortetracycline hydrochloride A local and ophthalmic anti-infective agent.

chlorthalidone A thiazide-like diuretic.

chlorzoxazone A skeletal muscle relaxant.

choana, *pl.* **choanae** 1. A funnel-shaped channel. 2. See **posterior nares.**

choanal atresia A congenital anomaly in which a bony or membranous occlusion blocks the passageway between the nose and pharynx. The condition, which is caused by the failure of the nasopharyngeal septum to rupture during embryonic development, can result in serious ventilation problems in the neonate, requiring an oral airway or endotracheal intubation. The defect is usually repaired surgically shortly after birth.

choke To interrupt respiration by compression or obstruction of larynx or trachea.

choke damp See **damp.**

choked disk *Informal.* Papilledema.

chokes A respiratory condition, occurring in decompression sickness, characterized by shortness of breath, substernal pain, and a nonproductive cough caused by bubbles of gas in the blood vessels of the lungs.

choking The condition in which a respira-

NORMAL I.V. CHOLANGIOGRAM

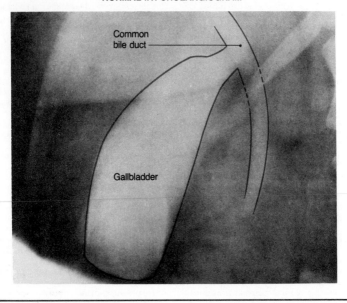

Common bile duct

Gallbladder

tory passage is blocked by constriction of the neck, an obstruction in the trachea, or swelling of the larynx. It is characterized by sudden coughing, a red face that rapidly turns purple, and inability to breathe. Emergency treatment requires removal of the obstruction and resuscitation if necessary. See also **Heimlich maneuver.**

chol- See **chole-.**

cholangeostomy A surgical operation to form an opening in a bile duct.

cholangiogram An X-ray of the biliary duct system obtained after the injection of an appropriate radiopaque material. See also **cholangiography.**

cholangiography The radiographic visualization of the major bile ducts after intravenous injection or direct instillation of a radiopaque contrast material. See also **cholecystography.**

cholangiohepatoma, *pl.* **cholangiohepatomas, cholangiohepatomata** A neoplasm in which there is an abnormal mixture of liver cord cells and bile ducts.

cholangiolitis An abnormal condition characterized by inflammation of the fine tubules of the bile duct system, which may cause cholangiolitic cirrhosis. —**cholangiolitic,** *adj.*

cholangioma, *pl.* **cholangiomas, cholangiomata** A neoplasm of the bile ducts.

cholangitis Inflammation of the bile ducts, caused either by bacterial invasion or by obstruction of the ducts by calculi or a tumor. The condition is characterized by severe right upper quadrant pain, jaundice (if an obstruction is present), and intermittent fever. Blood tests reveal an elevated level of serum bilirubin. Diagnosis is made by oral cholecystogram or intravenous cholangiogram. Treatment is with antibiotics for infection and with surgery for acute obstruction. See also **biliary calculus.**

chole-, chol-, cholo- A combining form meaning 'pertaining to the bile': *cholecystectomy, cholelithotomy, cholesterase.*

cholecalciferol An antirachitic, white, odorless, crystalline, unsaturated alcohol that is the predominant form of vitamin D of animal origin. It is formed from 7-dehydrocholesterol in the skin after exposure to ultraviolet light. It is found in most fish-liver oils, butter, brain, and egg yolk and is formed in the skin, fur, and feathers of animals and birds exposed to sunlight or ultraviolet rays.

cholecystectomy The surgical removal of the gallbladder, performed to treat cholelithiasis and cholecystitis. Surgery may be delayed while the acute inflammation is treated. See also **cholecystitis, cholelithiasis.**

cholecystitis Acute or chronic inflammation of the gallbladder. Acute cholecystitis is usually caused by a gallstone that cannot pass through the cystic duct. Pain is felt in the right upper quadrant of the abdomen, accompanied by nausea, vomiting, eructation, and flatulence. Diagnosis is usually made with an oral cholecystogram, useful in ruling out acute appendicitis, intestinal obstruction, peptic ulcer, and other upper abdominal disorders. Surgery is the preferred mode of treatment. **Chronic cholecystitis,** the more common type, has an insidious onset. Pain, often felt at night, may follow a fatty meal. Complications include biliary calculi, pancreatitis, and carcinoma of the gallbladder. Again, surgery is the preferred treatment. See also **biliary calculus, cholecystectomy, cholelithiasis.**

cholecystogram An X-ray of the gallbladder, made after the ingestion or injection of a radiopaque substance, usually a contrast material containing iodine.

cholecystography An X-ray examination of the gallbladder. The test is useful in the diagnosis of cholecystitis, cholelithiasis, tumors, and the differential diagnosis of a mass in the upper right quadrant of the stomach.

cholecystokinin A hormone, produced by the mucosa of the upper intestine, that stimulates contraction of the gallbladder and the secretion of pancreatic enzymes.

choledocholithiasis See **biliary calculus.**

choledocholithotomy A surgical operation to make an incision in the common bile duct to remove a stone.

cholelithiasis The presence of gallstones in the gallbladder. The condition causes unlocalized abdominal discomfort, eructation, and intolerance to certain foods, or no symptoms at all. In patients with severe attacks, cholecystectomy is recommended to prevent such complications as cholecystitis, cholangitis, and pancreatitis. See also **biliary calculus, cholecystitis.**

cholelithic dyspepsia An abnormal condition characterized by sudden attacks of indigestion associated with the dysfunction of the gallbladder. See also **dyspepsia.**

cholelithotomy A surgical operation to remove gallstones through an incision in the gallbladder.

cholera An acute bacterial infection of the small intestine, characterized by severe diarrhea and vomiting, muscular cramps, dehydration, and depletion of electrolytes. The disease is spread by water and food that have been contaminated by feces of persons previously infected. Complications include circulatory collapse, cyanosis, destruction of kidney tissue, and metabolic acidosis. Mortality is as high as 50% if the infection remains untreated. Treatment includes the administration of antibiotics that destroy the infecting bacteria and the restoration of normal amounts of fluids and electrolytes with intravenous solutions. A cholera vaccine is available for people traveling to areas where the infection is endemic. Other preventive measures include drinking only boiled or bottled water and eating only cooked foods. See also *Vibrio cholerae, Vibrio gastroenteritis.*

choleragen An exotoxin, produced by the cholera bacteria, that stimulates the secretion of electrolytes and water into the small intestine, draining the fluids of the body and weakening the patient.

cholera vaccine An active immunizing agent.

choleretic **1.** Stimulating the production of bile either by cholepoiesis or by hydrocholeresis. **2.** A choleretic agent.

choleric Having a hot temper or an irascible nature.

cholestasis Interruption in the flow of bile through any part of the biliary system, from liver to duodenum. It is essential for the doctor to discover whether the cause is within the liver or outside it. Intrahepatic causes include hepatitis, drug and alcohol use, metastatic carcinoma, and pregnancy. Extrahepatic causes may be an obstructing calculus or tumor in the common bile duct or carcinoma of the pancreas. See also **cholestatic hepatitis. —cholestatic,** *adj.*

cholestatic hepatitis Inflammation of the liver due to hepatitis infection that causes interruption of the flow of bile in the intrahepatic ducts. Signs are persistent jaundice, itching, and elevated alkaline phosphatase. These signs usually abate when the hepatitis remits. See also **cholestasis, hepatitis.**

cholesteatoma A cystic mass composed of epithelial cells and cholesterol that is found in the middle ear and occurs as a congenital defect or as a serious complication of chronic otitis media. The mass may occlude the middle ear, or enzymes produced by it may destroy the adjacent bones, including the ossicles. Surgery is required to remove a cholesteatoma. See also **otitis media.**

cholesteatoma tympani A growth formed by shed squamous epithelial cells in the middle ear. It is associated with chronic infection.

cholesterase An enzyme in the blood and other tissues that forms cholesterol and fatty acids by hydrolyzing cholesterol esters.

cholesteremia See **cholesterolemia.**

cholesterin See **cholesterol.**

cholesterol A fat-soluble crystalline steroid alcohol found in animal fats and oils and egg yolk, and widely distributed in the body, especially in the bile, blood, brain tissue, liver, kidneys, adrenal glands, and myelin sheaths of nerve fibers. It facilitates the absorption and transport of fatty acids, acts for the synthesis of vitamin D at the skin surface, and facilitates the synthesis of various steroid hormones, including sex hormones and adrenal corticoids. Cholesterol is the chief element in most gallstones. Increased levels of serum cholesterol may be associated with the pathogenesis of atherosclerosis. Also called **cholesterin.** See also **cholesterol metabolism, high-density lipoprotein, low-density lipoprotein, vitamin D.**

cholesterolemia **1.** The presence of excessive amounts of cholesterol in the blood. **2.** The abnormal condition of having excessive amounts of cholesterol in the blood. Also called **cholesteremia.**

cholesteroleresis The increased elimination of cholesterol in the bile.

cholesterol metabolism The sum of the anabolic and catabolic processes in the synthesis and degradation of cholesterol in the body. Ingested cholesterol is quickly absorbed. It is also synthesized in the liver and can be synthesized

EFFECTS OF CHOLINERGIC BLOCKING AGENTS		
INNERVATED ORGAN	WHEN BODY NATURALLY RELEASES NEUROHORMONE ACETYLCHOLINE:	WHEN CHOLINERGIC BLOCKERS ARE GIVEN:
Heart	▼	▲
Bronchioles	▲	▼
GI tract	▲	▼
Bladder	▲	▼
Bladder sphincter	▼	▲
Blood vessels	▼	▲
Sweat and salivary glands	▲	▼

KEY: ▼ = relaxes or dilates ▲ = constricts or stimulates

by most other tissues of the body. As more cholesterol is ingested, less is synthesized. Cholesterol is removed from the body by conversion in the liver and excretion in the bile.

cholesterolopoiesis The elaboration of cholesterol by the liver.

cholesterolosis An abnormal condition, found in about 5% of patients with chronic cholecystitis, in which there are deposits of cholesterol within large macrophages in the submucosa of the gallbladder. This produces a spotty appearance, sometimes referred to as a strawberry gallbladder. Cholesterolosis is often associated with gallstones and may be asymptomatic or accompanied by biliary colic. See also **cholecystitis.**

cholestyramine An antilipemic agent.

-cholia A combining form meaning '(condition of the) bile': *albuminocholia, syncholia, uricocholia.* Also **-choly.**

choline A lipotropic substance used to treat disorders of fat metabolism.

choline magnesium salicylate, c.m. trisalicylate Nonnarcotic analgesic and antipyretic agents.

cholinergic 1. Of or pertaining to nerve fibers that liberate acetylcholine at the myoneural junctions. 2. The tendency to transmit or to be stimulated or to stimulate by the elaboration of acetylcholine. Compare **adrenergic.**

cholinergic blocking agent Any agent

that blocks the action of acetylcholine and similar substances, in effect blocking the action of cholinergic nerves.

cholinergic crisis A pronounced muscular weakness and respiratory paralysis caused by excessive acetylcholine, often apparent in patients suffering from myasthenia gravis as a result of overmedication with anticholinesterase drugs.

cholinergic nerve A nerve that transmits impulses by releasing the neurotransmitter acetylcholine at its synapse. The cholinergic nerves include all the preganglionic sympathetic and the preganglionic parasympathetic nerves, the postganglionic parasympathetic nerves, the somatic motor nerves to skeletal muscles, and some nerves to sweat glands and to certain blood vessels.

cholinergic stimulant See **cholinergic.**

cholinergic urticaria An abnormal and usually transient vascular reaction of the skin, often associated with sweating in susceptible individuals subjected to stress, strong exertion, or hot weather. The condition is characterized by small, pale, itchy papules surrounded by reddish areas; it is caused by the action of acetylcholine on mast cells.

cholinesterase An enzyme that acts as a catalyst in the hydrolysis of acetylcholine to choline and acetate.

cholo- See **chole-.**

-choly See **-cholia.**

-chomic See **-chrome**[1].

chondr- See **chondro-.**

chondral Of or pertaining to cartilage.

chondrectomy The surgical excision of a cartilage.

chondri- See **chondro-.**

-chondria A combining form meaning: **1.** A 'condition involving granules in cell composition': *lipochondria, mitochondria, plastochondria.* **2.** An 'abnormal preoccupation with worry about disease': *hypochondria.*

chondriocont A threadlike or rod-shaped mitochondrion.

chondriome, chondrioma The total mitochondria content of a cell, taken as a unit.

chondriomite A single granular mitochondrion or a group of such organelles appearing in a chain formation.

chondriosome See **mitochondrion.**

chondritis Any inflammatory condition affecting the joints.

chondro-, chondr-, chondri- A combining form meaning 'pertaining to cartilage': *chondroangioma, chondroblast, chondroclast, chondrocostal.*

chondroadenoma, *pl.* **chondroadenomas, chondroadenomata** See **adenochondroma.**

chondroangioma, *pl.* **chondroangiomas, chondroangiomata** A benign, mesenchymal tumor containing vascular and cartilaginous elements.

chondroblast A cell that develops from the mesenchyma and forms cartilage. Also called **chondroplast.**

chondroblastoma, *pl.* **chondroblastomas, chondroblastomata** A benign tumor, derived from precursors of cartilage cells, that develops most frequently in epiphyses of the femur and humerus, especially in young men. The lesions may contain scattered areas of calcification and necrosis. Also called **Codman's tumor.**

chondrocalcinosis An arthritic disease in which calcium deposits are found in the peripheral joints. Chondrocalcinosis, which resembles gout, is often found in patients over age 50 who have osteoarthritis or diabetes mellitus. Aspiration of synovial fluid from the affected joints reveals crystals of calcium salts. Inflammation and pain may be relieved by intra-articular injections of hydrocortisone and by anti-inflammatory medications. Also called **pseudogout.** Compare **gout.**

chondrocarcinoma, *pl.* **chondrocarcinomas, chondrocarcinomata** A malignant epithelial tumor in which there is cartilaginous metaplasia.

chondroclast A giant multinucleated cell associated with the resorption of cartilage. — **chondroclastic,** *adj.*

chondrocostal Of or pertaining to the ribs and the costal cartilages.

chondrocyte Any one of the polymorphic cells that form the cartilage of the body. Each chondrocyte contains a nucleus, a relatively large amount of clear cytoplasm, and the common organelles, as mitochondria. —**chondrocytic,** *adj.*

chondrodystrophia calcificans congenita An inherited defect characterized by many small opacities in the epiphyses of the long bones. This sign is present on X-ray films of the newborn. Dwarfism, contractures, cataracts, mental retardation, and short stubby fingers develop as the infant grows into childhood. Also called **chondrodystrophia fetalis calcificans, Conradi's disease.**

chondrodystrophy A group of disorders in which there is abnormal conversion of cartilage to bone, particularly in the epiphyses of the long bones. Patients are dwarfed, with normal trunks and shortened extremities. See also **achondroplasia.**

chondroendothelioma, *pl.* **chondroendotheliomas, chondroendotheliomata** A benign mesenchymal tumor containing cartilaginous and endothelial components.

chondrofibroma, *pl.* **chondrofibromas, chondrofibromata** A fibrous tumor containing cartilaginous components.

chondrogenesis The development of cartilage. —**chondrogenetic,** *adj.*

chondroid Resembling cartilage.

chondrolipoma, *pl.* **chondrolipomas, chondrolipomata** A benign mesenchymal tumor containing fatty and cartilaginous components.

chondroma, *pl.* **chondromas, chondromata** A benign, fairly common tumor of cartilage cells that grows slowly within cartilage (enchondroma) or on the surface (ecchondroma). Kinds of chondromas are **joint chondroma, synovial chondroma.** See also **ecchondroma,** **enchondroma.** —**chondromatous,** *adj.*

-chondroma A combining form meaning a 'benign cartilaginous tumor': *hyaloenchondroma, osteochondroma, sarcoenchondroma.*

chondromalacia A softening of cartilage. **Chondromalacia fetalis** is a lethal congenital form of the condition in which the stillborn infant is born with soft and pliable limbs. **Chondromalacia patellae** occurs in young adults after knee injury and is characterized by swelling and pain and by degenerative changes, which are revealed on examination by X-ray.

chondromalacia fetalis See **chondromalacia.**

chondromalacia patellae See **chondromalacia.**

chondroma sarcomatosum See **chondrosarcoma.**

chondromatosis A condition characterized by the presence of many cartilaginous tumors. A kind of chondromatosis is **synovial chondromatosis.**

chondromere A cartilaginous, embryonic vertebra and its costal component.

chondromyoma, *pl.* **chondromyomas, chondromyomata** A benign mesenchymal tumor containing myomatous and cartilaginous tissue.

chondromyxofibroma A benign tumor that develops from cartilage-forming connective tissue. The lesion, typically a firm, grayish-white, somewhat rubbery mass, tends to occur in the knee and small bones of the foot and may be confused with chondrosarcoma. Also called **chondromyxoid fibroma.**

chondromyxoid Composed of cartilaginous and myxoid elements.

chondromyxoid fibroma See **chondromyxofibroma.**

chondrophyte An abnormal mass of cartilage that may develop at the articular surface of a bone. **—chondrophytic,** *adj.*

chondroplast See **chondroblast.**

chondroplasty The surgical repair of cartilage.

chondrosarcoma, *pl.* **chondrosarcomas, chondrosarcomata** A malignant neoplasm of cartilaginous cells or their precursors that occurs most frequently on long bones, the pelvic girdle, and the scapula. The tumor is a large, smooth, lobulated growth composed of nodules of hyaline cartilage that may show slight to marked calcification. Kinds of chondrosarcomas are **central chondrosarcoma, mesenchymal chondrosarcoma.** Also called **chondroma sarcomatosum. —chondrosarcomatous,** *adj.*

chondrosarcomatosis A condition characterized by multiple, malignant cartilaginous tumors.

chondrosis 1. The development of the cartilage of the body. 2. A cartilaginous tumor.

chondrotomy The surgical division of cartilage.

chord- A combining form meaning 'string, cord': *chordoblastoma, chordoma, chordotomy.*

chordal canal See **notochordal canal.**

chorda spinalis See **spinal cord.**

chorda umbicalis See **umbilical cord.**

chordee A congenital defect of the genitourinary tract resulting in a ventral curvature of the penis, caused by a fibrous band of tissue instead of normal skin along the corpus spongiosum. The condition is often associated with hypospadias and is surgically corrected in early childhood.

chordencephalon The portion of the central nervous system that develops in the early weeks of fetal life from the neural tube and includes the mesencephalon, the rhombencephalon, and the spinal cord. The chordencephalon is segmented and divided into the alar plate, which becomes the sensory portion of the gray substance of the spinal cord, and the basal plate, which becomes the motor portion. **—chordencephalic,** *adj.*

chorditis 1. Inflammation of a spermatic cord. 2. Inflammation of the vocal cords or of the vocal folds.

chordoid Resembling the notocord or notochordal tissue.

chordoma, *pl.* **chordomas, chordomata**

A rare, congenital tumor of the brain developing from the fetal notochord. It is usually located in the midline, behind the sella, and is slow growing but highly invasive. Surgical removal is rarely possible.

chordotomy An operation in which the anterolateral tracts of the spinal cord are surgically divided to relieve pain.

chorea A condition characterized by involuntary, purposeless, rapid motions, as flexing and extending the fingers, raising and lowering the shoulders, or grimacing. In some forms the person is also irritable, emotionally unstable, weak, restless, and fretful. See also **chorea gravidarum, Huntington's chorea, Sydenham's chorea. —choreic,** *adj.*

-chorea A combining form meaning a '(specified) nervous disorder': *hemichorea, monochorea, orthochorea.*

chorea gravidarum A form of chorea occurring during a first pregnancy subsequent to an episode of Sydenham's chorea in childhood. Similar symptoms may develop in a woman taking oral contraceptives.

chorea minor See **Sydenham's chorea.**

choreiform Resembling the rapid jerky movements associated with chorea.

chorio- A combining form meaning 'pertaining to the protective fetal membrane': *chorioblastosis, choriocele, chorioma.*

chorioadenoma, *pl.* **chorioadenomas, chorioadenomata** An epithelial cell tumor of the outermost fetal membrane that is intermediate in the malignant development of a hydatid mole to invasive choriocarcinoma.

chorioadenoma destruens An invasive hydatid mole in which the chorionic villi of the mole penetrate into the myometrium and parametrium of the uterus and metastasize to distant parts of the body, most commonly to the lungs. Also called invasive mole, malignant mole, metastasizing mole.

chorioallantoic graft The grafting of tissue onto the chorioallantoic membrane of the egg of a hen to improve the environment for embryonic growth.

chorioamnionic Of or pertaining to the chorion and the amnion.

chorioblastoma See **choriocarcinoma.**

choriocarcinoma, *pl.* **choriocarcinomas, choriocarcinomata** An epithelial malignancy of fetal origin that develops from the chorionic portion of the products of conception, usually from a hydatid mole, and less frequently following an abortion, during a normal or ectopic pregnancy, or from a genital or extragenital teratoma. The primary tumor usually appears in the uterus, then metastasizes through lymph or blood vessels to form hemorrhagic and necrotic tumors in the vaginal wall, vulva, lymph nodes, lungs, liver, and brain. Urine chorionic gonadotropin often exceeds the level expected in pregnancy, returning to normal after tumor excision. More common in older women, this cancer responds to chemotherapy with cytotoxic drugs. Rarely, a choriocarcinoma arises in a teratoma of the testis, mediastinum, or pineal gland, and chemotherapy is not usually effective. Also called **chorioblastoma, chorioepithelioma, chorionic carcinoma, chorionic epithelioma.**

choriocele   A hernia or protrusion of the tissue of the choroid layer of the eye.

chorioepithelioma   See **choriocarcinoma.**

choriogenesis   The development of the chorion, which is first evident in the first month of pregnancy, after the trophoblast anchors to the uterine tissue and extends primary villi into the intervillous space. The chorion at first contains fluid and loose filaments of extraembryonic mesoderm. As pregnancy proceeds, the amnion grows into the chorionic space and obliterates it. The chorion continues to expand to accommodate the fetus and serves as the outer barrier between the fetus and the uterus. —**choriogenetic,** *adj.*

choriomeningitis   See **lymphocytic choriomeningitis.**

chorion   In biology: the outermost extraembryonic membrane composed of trophoblast lined with mesoderm. It develops villi about 2 weeks after fertilization and is vascularized by allantoic vessels 1 week later. It gives rise to the placenta and persists until birth as the outer of the two layers of membrane containing the amniotic fluid and the fetus.

-chorion   A combining form meaning a 'membrane': *allantochorion, omphalochorion, prochorion.*

chorionic carcinoma   See **choriocarcinoma.**

chorionic epithelioma   See **choriocarcinoma.**

chorionic gonadotropin, human   A gonadotropin used to treat infertility, hypogonadism, and nonobstructive cryptorchidism.

chorionic plate   The part of the fetal placenta that gives rise to chorionic villi, attaching to the uterus during the early stage of formation of the placenta.

chorioretinitis   An inflammatory condition of the choroid and retina of the eye, usually as a result of parasitic or bacterial infection. It is characterized by blurred vision, photophobia, and distorted images.

chorioretinopathy   A noninflammatory process caused by disease involving the choroid and the retina.

choroid   A thin, highly vascular membrane covering the posterior five sixths of the eye between the retina and sclera.

choroidal malignant melanoma   A tumor of the choroid coat that grows into the vitreous humor, causing detachment and degeneration of the overlying retina. Typically mound- or mushroom-shaped, it may break through the sclera and present under the conjunctiva.

choroiditis   An inflammatory condition of the choroid membrane of the eye. See also **chorioretinitis.**

choroidocyclitis   An abnormal condition

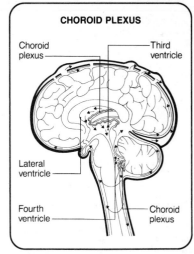

CHOROID PLEXUS

characterized by inflammation of the choroid and the ciliary processes.

choroid plexectomy   A surgical procedure for reducing cerebrospinal fluid production in the ventricles of the brain in hydrocephalus, usually in the newborn. The procedure involves transcortical entry of the lateral ventricles to coagulate or to excise the choroid plexuses and seeks to correct a communicating type of hydrocephalus.

choroid plexus   Any of the tangled masses of tiny blood vessels contained within the third, lateral, and the fourth ventricles of the brain. The choroid plexus of the third ventricle is part of the roof of the anterior commissure of the third ventricle, lying above the interventricular foramen. The choroid plexus of the lateral ventricle is continuous with the choroid plexus of the third ventricle, extending from the interventricular foramen, through the body of the ventricle, to the rostral end of the inferior horn. The choroid plexus of the fourth ventricle, on each side, is an elongated tuft of blood vessels extending through the roof of the ventricle.

Christchurch chromosome (Ch1)   An abnormally small acrocentric chromosome of the G group, involving any members of chromosome pairs 21 or 22, in which the short arms are missing or partially deleted. The aberration is associated with chronic lymphocytic leukemia but has also been found in patients with various other defects. See also **Philadelphia chromosome.**

Christmas disease   See **hemophilia.**
Christmas factor   See **factor IX.**

-chroia   A combining form meaning '(condition of) coloration': *cacochroia, cyanochroia, xanthochroia.*

chrom-   See **chromo-.**

chromaffin   Having an affinity for strong staining with chromium salts, especially strong staining of the cells of the adrenal, the coccygeal,

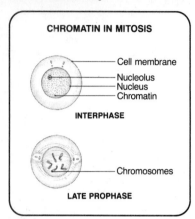

CHROMATIN IN MITOSIS

Cell membrane
Nucleolus
Nucleus
Chromatin

INTERPHASE

Chromosomes

LATE PROPHASE

and the carotid glands, certain cells of the adrenal medulla, and the cells of the paraganglions. Also called **chromaphil.**

chromaffin body See **paraganglion.**

chromaffin cell Any one of the special cells comprising the paraganglia and connected to the ganglia of the celiac, the renal, the suprarenal, the aortic, and the hypogastric plexuses, and sometimes associated with other sympathetic plexuses. The chromaffin cells of the adrenal medulla secrete two catecholamines, epinephrine and norepinephrine, that affect smooth muscle, cardiac muscle, and glands in the same way as sympathetic stimulation, increasing and prolonging sympathetic effects. In response to stress, nerve impulses from the hypothalamus stimulate the chromaffin cells in the adrenal medulla to increase hormonal production, about 80% of which is epinephrine, 20%, norepinephrine.

chromaffinoma See **pheochromocytoma.**

chromaphil See **chromaffin.**

-chromasia 1. A combining form meaning '(condition of) color (as cells, skin)': *allochromasia, hyperchromasia, oligochromasia.* 2. A combining form meaning '(condition of the) stainability of tissues': *amblychromasia, anisochromasia, anochromasia.*

chromatic 1. Of or pertaining to color. 2. Stainable by a dye. 3. Also, chromatinic, of or pertaining to chromatin.

-chromatic A combining form meaning the 'staining properties of tissues and microorganisms': *lithochromatic, orthochromatic, panchromatic.*

chromatic dispersion The splitting of light into its various component wavelengths or frequencies, as with a prism, to separate and study the different colors.

chromatid One of the two identical threadlike filaments of a chromosome. It results from the self-replication of the chromosome during interphase, is held together by a common centromere, and, during mitosis and meiosis, divides longitudinally to form daughter chromosomes.

chromatin The material within the cell nucleus from which the chromosomes are formed. It consists of fine, threadlike strands of deoxyribonucleic acid attached to a protein base, usually histone; it is readily stained with basic dyes; and it occurs in two different forms, euchromatin and heterochromatin, which are distinguishable during the phases of the cell cycle by variant degrees of staining depending on the amount of dispersion or coiling that occurs. During cell division, portions of the chromatin condense and coil to form the chromosomes. A kind of chromatin is **sex chromatin.** Also called **chromoplasm, karyotin.** See also **chromatid, euchromatin, heterochromatin.** —**chromatinic,** *adj.*

chromatin-negative Pertaining to or descriptive of the nuclei of cells that lack sex chromatin, specifically characteristic of the normal male.

chromatin nucleolus See **karyosome.**

chromatin-positive Pertaining to or descriptive of the nuclei of cells that contain sex chromatin, specifically characteristic of the normal female.

chromatism 1. An abnormal condition characterized by hallucinations in which the affected individual sees colored lights.2. Abnormal pigmentation.

chromato-, chromat- 1. A combining form meaning 'pertaining to color': *chromatic, chromatism, chromatogram, chromatopsia.* 2. See **chromo-.**

chromatogram 1. The record produced by the separation of gaseous substances or dissolved chemical substances moving through a column of absorbent material which filters out the various absorbates in different layers. 2. Any graphic record produced by any chromatographic method.

chromatography Any one of several processes for separating and analyzing various gaseous or dissolved chemical materials according to differences in their absorbency with respect to a specific substance and according to their different pigments. Some kinds of chromatography are **column chromatography, gas chromatography, ion-exchange chromatography, paper chromatography.** —**chromatographic,** *adj.*

chromatopsia 1. An abnormal condition characterized by a visual defect that makes colorless objects appear tinged with color. 2. An abnormal condition characterized by the imperfect perception of various colors. It may be caused by a deficiency in one or more of the retinal cones or from defective nerve circuits that convey color-associated impulses to the cerebral cortex. Some color-blind persons may not be able to distinguish red from green or blue from yellow; others cannot perceive any color, seeing everything as gray. Very few individuals are color-blind to blue. Also called **color blindness.** Compare **chromesthesia.**

-chrome[1] A combining form meaning a 'coloring substance within a cell or chemical compound': *cytochrome, hemochrome, serochrome.* Also **-chromatic, -chromic.**

-chrome² A combining form distinguishing 'chromium alloys': *hallachrome, nichrome, nicochrome.*

-chromemia A combining form meaning '(condition of the) hemoglobin in the blood': *hyperchromemia, lipochromemia, polychromemia.*

chromesthesia 1. The color sense that depends on the response of retinal cones to the mixture of wavelengths in the light that enters the eye. Changes in the pigments within the cones affect color vision, and defects in the cones cause various kinds of color blindness. Compare **chromatopsia, color vision. 2.** An abnormal condition characterized by the confusion of other senses, as taste and smell, with imagined sensations of color.

chromhidrosis A rare, functional disorder in which apocrine sweat glands secrete colored sweat. The sweat may be yellow, blue, green, or black and often also fluoresces. A known cause is occupational exposure to copper, catechols, or ferrous oxide. Industrial nurses should be aware of this benign condition.

-chromia A combining form meaning a 'state or condition of pigmentation': *metachromia, normochromia, orthochromia.*

-chromic A combining form meaning: **1.** The '(specified) number of colors seen by the eye': *bichromic, hexachromic, tetrachromic.* **2.** A '(specified) color of the blood indicating the hemoglobin content': *hypochromic, normochromic.* **3.** The 'staining ability of bacteria and tissues': *bathochromic, hemochromic, perchromic.* **4.** A '(specified) skin color as indicative of disease': *heterochromic, pleiochromic, xantochromic.* Also **-chromatic.**

chromic myopia A kind of color blindness that is characterized by the ability to distinguish colors of only those objects which are close to the eye.

chromium (Cr) A hard, brittle, metallic element. Its atomic number is 24; its atomic weight is 51.9. Chromium is used extensively to plate other metals and harden steel, in combination with other elements to form colored compounds, and may be important in human nutrition, especially in carbohydrate metabolism. Workers in chromite mines are susceptible to pneumoconiosis caused by the inhalation of chromite dust particles that lodge in the lung.

chromo-, chrom- A combining form meaning 'pertaining to color': *chromocrinia, chromocyte, chromophilic, chromotrichia.* Also **chromato-.**

chromobacteriosis An extremely rare, usually fatal systemic infection caused by a gram-negative bacillus, *Chromobacterium violaceum*, found in fresh water in tropical and subtropical regions, which enters the body through a break in the skin. The disease is characterized by sepsis, multiple liver abscesses, and severe prostration. Early diagnosis, surgical drainage of abscesses, and the administration of chloram-

phenicol markedly improve the chance of survival.

chromoblastomycosis An infectious skin disease caused by any of a variety of fungi and characterized by the appearance of pruritic, warty nodules that develop in a cut or other break in the skin. What may first appear as a small dull red lesion gradually develops into a large ulcerated growth. Over a period of weeks or months, additional warty growths may appear elsewhere on the skin along the path of lymphatic drainage. Treatment includes surgical excision and, in some cases, topical application of antibiotics. Also called **chromomycosis, verrucous dermatitis.** See also **mycosis**, specific fungal infections.

chromocenter See **karyosome.**

chromolipid, chromolipoid See **lipochrome.**

chromomere 1. Any of the series of beadlike structures that lie along the chromonema of a chromosome during the early stages of cell division. The position of each chromomere is relatively constant for each chromosome and probably reflects the coiling pattern of the DNA molecule for the particular chromosome. Also called **idiomere. 2.** See **granulomere.**

chromomycosis See **chromoblastomycosis.**

chromonema, chromoneme, *pl.* **chromonemata** The coiled filament along which the chromomeres lie that forms the central part of the chromatid of the chromosome during cell division. See also **chromosome. —chromonemal, chromonematic, chromonemic,** *adj.*

chromophilic Denoting a cell, tissue, or microorganism that is easily stained, particularly certain leukocytes. Compare **chromophobic.**

chromophobe adenoma A tumor of the anterior pituitary, composed of cells that are chromophobic and do not stain with acidic or basic dyes. The lesion may be associated with hypopituitarism.

chromophobia 1. The resistance of certain cells and tissues to stains. **2.** A morbid aversion to colors. **—chromophobe,** *n.*

chromophobic Denoting a cell, tissue, or microorganism that is not easily stained, particularly certain cells of the anterior lobe of the pituitary gland. Compare **chromophilic.**

chromophobic adenoma A tumor of the pituitary gland composed of cells that do not stain with acid or basic dyes. Diabetes insipidus and other conditions resulting from deficiency of one or more pituitary hormones are associated with this tumor.

chromoplasm See **chromatin.**

chromosomal aberration Any change in the structure or number of any of the chromosomes for a given species, which can result in anomalies of varying severity, including Down's syndrome, Turner's syndrome, and Klinefelter's syndrome. The incidence for most of the chromosomal disorders is significantly higher than that for the single gene disorders. See also specific trisomy syndromes.

HUMAN CHROMOSOMES

POSITION OF CENTROMERE	GROUP	AUTO-SOMES	SEX CHROMO-SOMES	NUMBER OF CHROMOSOMES Male	Female
Metacentric or submetacentric	A	1, 2, 3		6	6
Submetacentric	B	4, 5		4	4
Metacentric and submetacentric	C	6, 7, 8, 9, 10, 11, 12	X	15	16
Acrocentric (subterminal)	D	13, 14, 15		6	6
Metacentric and submetacentric	E	16, 17, 18		6	6
Metacentric	F	19, 20		4	4
Acrocentric (subterminal)	G	21, 22	Y	5	4
			Total	46	46

chromosomal nomenclature A standard nomenclature that serves to identify the complement of chromosomes in an individual according to the number of chromosomes, sex complement, and the deletion or addition of a specific chromosome or part of a chromosome. Complement in a normal female is recorded as 46,XX and for a normal male, 46,XY. The addition or deletion of a chromosome is identified by number, if it can be identified, as 47,XY, 21 +. If the particular chromosome cannot be identified, the group is recorded, as 47,XY, G +. The short arm of a chromosome is designated 'p,' the long arm is 'q,' and a translocation 't'.

chromosome Any one of the threadlike structures in the nucleus of a cell that functions in the transmission of genetic information. Each consists of a double strand of the nucleoprotein deoxyribonucleic acid (DNA) coiled into a helix formation and attached to a protein base, usually a histone. The genes, which contain the genetic material that controls the inheritance of traits, are arranged in a linear pattern along the entire length of each DNA strand. Chromosomes are readily stainable with basic dyes and can be seen easily during cell division when they are compactly coiled and in their most condensed state. During interphase, the chromosomes disperse into chromatin and undergo self-replication, forming identical chromatids that separate during mitosis so that each new cell receives a full set of chromosomes. Each species has a characteristic number of chromosomes in the so-matic cell, which in humans is 46 and includes 22 homologous pairs of autosomes and one pair of sex chromosomes, with one member of each pair being derived from each parent. Standard nomenclature separates paired autosomes into seven groups lettered A to G, numbered from 1 to 22, and arranged according to decreasing length, followed by the sex chromosome. Chromosomal aberrations are designated by indicating the total chromosomal number, sex complement, and the group or specific chromosome in which the addition or deletion occurs. For example, 47,XX, 21 + indicates a female with an extra chromosome 21, or Down's syndrome. Kinds of chromosomes include **accessory chromosome; Christchurch chromosome; daughter chromosome; gametic chromosome; giant chromosome; homologous chromosomes; Philadelphia chromosome; sex chromosome; somatic chromosome; W chromosome, Z chromosome.** See also **centromere, chromatid, chromatin, Denver classification, gene, karyotype, mitosis.** —**chromosomal,** adj.

chromosome coil The spiral formed by the coiling of two or more chromonemata of the chromatid within the chromosome.

chromosome complement The normal number of chromosomes found in the somatic cell of any given species. In humans it is 46. See **chromosome.**

chromosome puff A band of accumulated chromatic material located at a specific site on a giant chromosome. It is indicative of gene activity, specifically DNA and RNA synthesis, for the particular locus. Such bands appear at certain chromosomal locations within a given tissue at specific developmental stages in insects and are significant for studying the mode of genetic transmission.

chromosome walking The process by which overlapping molecular clones that span large chromosomal intervals are isolated.

chromotrope 1. A component of tissue that stains metachromatically with metachromatic dyes. **2.** Any one of several dyes differentiated by numerical suffixes. —**chromotropic,** *adj.*

chron- See **chrono-.**

-chrone See **-chronia.**

-chronia A combining form meaning: **1.** '(Condition of) processes with respect to time': *isochronia, heterochronia, synchronia.* **2.** '(Condition of) chronaxy between muscle and nerve': *isochronia.* **3.** The 'time of formation of a part or tissue': *heterochronia, synchronia.* Also **-chrone.**

chronic Of a disease or disorder: developing slowly and persisting for a long period of time, often for the remainder of the lifetime of the patient. Glaucoma is an example of a disease that may develop gradually and insidiously or that may occur as an acute disorder marked by sudden severe pain, requiring emergency treatment. Compare **acute.**

chronic alcoholic delirium See **Korsakoff's psychosis.**

chronic alcoholism A pathological condition resulting from the habitual use of alcohol in excessive amounts. Symptoms include anorexia, diarrhea, weight loss, neurological and psychiatric disturbances (most notably depression), and fatty deterioration of the liver, sometimes leading to cirrhosis. Treatment depends on the severity of the disease and resulting complications; it may include hospitalization, nutritional therapy, use of tranquilizers during detoxification, use of disulfiram as an aid to continued abstinence, and psychotherapy. The condition often goes unrecognized in patients admitted to the hospital for care following an accident, or for esophagitis, gastritis, peripheral neuropathy, anemia, or depression, all of which are secondary effects of alcoholism and will persist if alcoholism is not diagnosed and treated. If the patient is to undergo an operation, it is imperative that the anesthesiologist be notified of the alcoholism. Alcoholism is a family disease, and the patient's family should be guided to seek treatment. Long-term support for the alcoholic and the family is offered by such organizations as Alcoholics Anonymous, Al-Anon, Alateen, and rehabilitation facilities for alcoholism. Compare **acute alcoholism.**

chronic appendicitis 1. A type of appendicitis characterized by thickening or scarring of the vermiform appendix, caused by previous inflammation. **2.** An obsolete term formerly used to describe chronic pain in the appendiceal area without any evidence of inflammation.

CHRONIC BRAIN SYNDROME: COMMON TREATABLE CAUSES

Endocrine disorders
• Thyroid, parathyroid, or adrenal dysfunction
• Hypoglycemia

Conditions that cause metabolic disorders
• Hepatic, renal, or pulmonary insufficiency
• Hyponatremia
• Inappropriate antidiuretic hormone secretion
• Porphyria
• Wilson's disease
• Vitamin B deficiencies (pellagra)
• Alcoholism

Toxins
• Drug toxicity (barbiturates, bromides)
• Heavy metal exposure

Vascular disorders
• Postsubarachnoid hemorrhage
• Cerebral anoxia
• Hypertensive encephalopathies
• Anoxic or ischemic vascular derangements
• Vascular stenosis

Inflammation
• General paresis
• Brain abscess
• Meningoencephalitis
• Various types of chronic inflammation
• Postinflammatory arachnoiditis, with hydrocephalus
• Fungal and parasitic infections

Miscellaneous
• Recurrent seizures
• Hematologic disorders
• Occult or communicating hydrocephalus
• Lupus erythematosus
• Trauma (subdural hematoma)
• Neoplasm (brain tumor)

chronic brain syndrome (CBS) An abnormal condition that is caused by impairment of the cerebral tissue function, characterized by loss of memory and disorientation. It may occur in dementia paralytica, cerebral arteriosclerosis, brain trauma, and Huntington's chorea.

chronic bronchitis A very common debilitating respiratory disease, characterized by greatly increased production of mucus by the glands of the trachea and bronchi and resulting in a cough with expectoration for at least 3 months of the year for more than 2 consecutive years. Strongly associated with smoking and occupational and environmental pollutants, and formerly seen almost exclusively in males, the disease is becoming more common in women who smoke. Broad-spectrum antibiotics are usually prescribed during acute exacerbations of symptoms. Bronchodilators as well as sympathomimetic drugs are prescribed to prevent worsening of the condition. Heart failure is managed with sodium restriction, diuretics, and sometimes digitalis.

NURSING CONSIDERATIONS: A major effect should be made to have the patient discontinue smoking and avoid exposure to toxic inhalants, such as hair sprays, aerosol insecticides, and occupational irritants and poisons. Patients with chronic bronchitis should be immunized against influenza and pneumococcal infections. The use of low-flow oxygen in the home, exercise, chest physiotherapy, and postural drainage are often indicated. See also **asthma, chronic obstructive pulmonary disease, cor pulmonale, emphysema, respiratory failure.**

chronic care A pattern of medical and nursing care that focuses on long-term care of people with chronic diseases or conditions, either at home or in a medical facility. It includes care specific to the problem, as well as other measures to encourage self-care, to promote health, and to prevent loss of function.

chronic carrier An individual who acts as host to pathogenic organisms for an extended period of time without displaying any signs of disease.

chronic chorea See **Huntington's chorea.**
chronic cystic mastitis See **fibrocystic disease.**

chronic disease A disease that persists over a long period of time as compared with the course of an acute disease. The symptoms of chronic disease are usually less severe than those of the acute phase of the same disease. Chronic disease may result in complete or partial disability.

chronic glomerulonephritis A noninfectious disease of the glomerulus of the kidney characterized by proteinuria, hematuria, edema, and decreased production of urine. Of unknown cause, it is asymptomatic for years: the symptoms develop slowly, but the disease progresses to kidney failure. Transplantation and dialysis are the only treatments available. See also **acute glomerulonephritis, subacute glomerulonephritis, uremia.**

chronic lingual papillitis An inflammatory disorder of the tongue, sometimes extending to the buccal mucosa and palate, characterized by irregularly scattered red patches, thinning of the lingual papillae, severe burning pain, and shedding of epidermal tissue. The disorder affects middle-aged individuals, especially women, and occurs in attacks alternating with

remissions lasting weeks or months. Also called **Moeller's glossitis.**

chronic lymphocytic leukemia (CLL) A neoplasm of blood-forming tissues, characterized by a proliferation of small, long-lived lymphocytes, chiefly B cells, in bone marrow, blood liver, and in lymphoid organs. CLL is rare under the age of 35, increases in frequency with age, and is more common in men than in women. The disease has an insidious onset and progresses to cause malaise, easy fatigability, anorexia, weight loss, nocturnal sweating, lymphadenopathy, and hepatosplenomegaly. Most patients can continue normal activities for years; 25% die of unrelated diseases. No treatment is curative, but remissions may be induced by chemotherapy with chlorambucil and glucocorticoids or by thymic, splenic, or total-body irradiation.

chronic mucocutaneous candidiasis A rare abnormal condition characterized by large, circular lesions of the skin, mucous membranes, nails, and vagina; viral infections; and recurrent respiratory tract infections. This disease usually occurs during the first year of life but can develop as late as the 20s in both men and women. Associated with an inherited defect of the cell-mediated immune system, it apparently allows autoantibodies to develop against target organs while the humoral immune system functions normally. The onset of infection may precede endocrinopathy.

chronic myelocytic leukemia (CML) A malignant neoplasm of blood-forming tissues, characterized by a proliferation of granular leukocytes and, often, of megakaryocytes. The disease occurs most frequently in older people and begins insidiously. Its progress is marked by malaise, fatigue, heat intolerance, bleeding gums, purpura, skin lesions, weight loss, hyperuricemia, abdominal discomfort, and massive splenomegaly. Differential blood count and bone marrow biopsies aid in the diagnosis. The alkaline phosphate activity of the leukocytes is low, and the Philadelphia chromosome is present in myeloblasts in most patients. Therapy with an oral alkylating agent is usual, but advanced CML is refractory to chemotherapy. Also called **granulocytic leukemia, myelogenous leukemia, myeloid leukemia, splenomedullary leukemia, splenomyelogenous leukemia.**

chronic obstructive pulmonary disease (COPD) A progressive and irreversible condition characterized by diminished inspiratory and expiratory capacity of the lungs. The person complains of dyspnea with physical exertion, of difficulty in inhaling or exhaling deeply, and, sometimes, of a chronic cough. The condition may result from chronic bronchitis, pulmonary emphysema, asthma, or chronic bronchiolitis and is aggravated by cigarette smoking and air pollution. Also called chronic obstructive lung disease (COLD).

chronic pain Pain that continues or recurs over a prolonged period, caused by various diseases or abnormal conditions, as rheumatoid arthritis, and often less intense than acute pain. Chronic pain does not produce increased pulse and rapid respiration because these autonomic reactions to pain cannot be sustained for long periods. Characteristic is the patient's impulse to control the environment, as the patient can't control the disease; the patient's often labeled 'uncooperative' or 'manipulative.' Or the patient may withdraw and concentrate solely on the affliction, ignoring family, friends, and external stimuli. Compare **acute pain.** See also **pain intervention, pain mechanism.**

chronic tuberculous mastitis A rare infection of the breast resulting from extension of tuberculosis of underlying ribs. The condition is also characterized by multiple sinus tracts and tuberculosis elsewhere in the body.

chrono-, chron- A combining form meaning 'pertaining to time': *chronognosis, chronophobia, chronotropism.*

chronograph A device that records small intervals of time, as a stopwatch. —**chronographic,** *adj.*

chronologic, chronological 1. Arranged in time sequence. 2. Of or pertaining to chronology.

chronological age The age of an individual expressed as a period of time that has elapsed since birth. The age of an infant is expressed in hours, days, or months, and the age of children and adults in years.

chrysiasis An abnormal condition characterized by the deposition of gold in the tissues of the body. Also called **auriosis.**

chrysotherapy The treatment of any disease with gold salts. —**chrysotherapeutic,** *adj.*

Churg-Strauss syndrome An allergic disorder marked by granulomatosis, most often of the lungs.

Chvostek's sign An abnormal spasm of the facial muscles elicited by light taps on the facial nerve in patients who are hypocalcemic. It is a sign of tetany.

Chvostek-Weiss sign See **Chvostek's sign.**

chyl- See **chylo-.**

chyle The cloudy liquid products of digestion taken up by the small intestine. Consisting mainly of emulsified fats, chyle passes through fingerlike projections in the small intestine, called lacteals, and into the lymphatic system for transport to the venous circulation at the thoracic duct in the neck. Also called **chylus. chylous,** *adj.*

chyli- See **chylo-.**

-chylia A combining form meaning '(condition of) digestive juices': *dyschylia, euchylia, polychylia.*

chyliform ascites See **chylous ascites.**

chylo-, chyl-, chyli- A combining form meaning 'pertaining to chyle': *chylocyst, chylophonic, chylosis.*

chyloid Resembling the chyle that fills the lacteals of the small intestine during the digestion of fatty foods.

chylomicron The largest of the lipoproteins. Chylomicrons primarily consist of triglycerides with small amounts of cholesterol, phos-

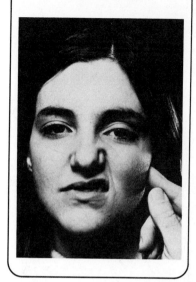

CHVOSTEK'S SIGN

pholipids, and protein. They are synthesized in the gastrointestinal tract and carry dietary glycerides from the intestinal mucosa via the thoracic duct into the plasma and, ultimately, to sites of utilization in the tissues. The remnant chylomicron particles are removed by the liver.

chylosus ascites See **chylous ascites.**

chylothorax The effusion of chyle from the thoracic duct into the pleural space. The cause is usually a traumatic injury to the neck or a tumor that invades the thoracic duct. Treatment is directed at repairing damage to the duct.

chylous ascites An abnormal condition characterized by an accumulation of chyle in the peritoneal cavity. Chylous ascites results from an obstruction of the thoracic duct that may be caused by a tumor or by a destructive lesion resulting in rupture of a lymph vessel. Also called **ascites adiposus, chyliform ascites, chylosus ascites, fatty ascites, milky ascites.** See also **ascites.**

chyluria A condition characterized by the milky appearance of the urine owing to the presence of chyle.

chylus See **chyle.**

chyme The viscous, semifluid contents of the stomach present during digestion of a meal. Chyme then passes through the pylorus into the duodenum, where further digestion occurs.

-chymia A combining form meaning '(condition of) partly digested food in the duodenum': *achymia, ischochymia, oligochymia.* Also **-chymy.**

chymoin See **rennin.**

chymotrypsin 1. An oral or parenterally administered enzyme.

chymotrypsinogen A substance, pro-

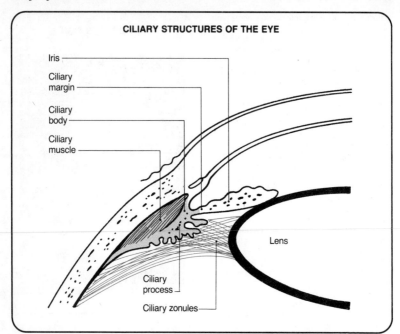

CILIARY STRUCTURES OF THE EYE

Iris

Ciliary
margin

Ciliary
body

Ciliary
muscle

Lens

Ciliary
process

Ciliary zonules

duced in the pancreas, that is the precursor to
the enzyme chymotrypsin. It is converted to chymotrypsin by trypsin.

-chymy See **-chymia.**

Ci *abbr* curie.

CI *abbr* **1.** color index. **2.** *Colour Index.*

cibophobia An abnormal aversion to food
or to eating.

cicatricial ectropion See **ectropion.** See
also **cicatrix.**

cicatricial stenosis Narrowing of a duct
or tube owing to formation of scar tissue.

cicatrix, *pl.* **cicatrices** Scar tissue that is
avascular, pale, contracted, and firm following
the earlier phase of skin-healing characterized
by redness and softness. **—cicatrize,** *v.*

cicutism Poisoning from the root of water
hemlock, *Cicuta maculata* or *C. virosa*, resulting in cyanosis, dilated pupils, convulsions, coma,
and death.

CID *abbr* **cytomegalic inclusion disease.**

-cide A combining element meaning 'killing':
amebicide, herbicide, protozoacide. Also **-cid.**

ciguatera poisoning A nonbacterial food
poisoning that results from eating large fish contaminated with the ciguatera toxin. The cause
of contamination in normally safe fish is unknown. Characteristic of ciguatera poisoning are
vomiting, diarrhea, tingling or numbness of extremities and the skin around the mouth, itching, severe muscle pain, respiratory paralysis,
and death. Cold liquids feel hot to the surfaces
of the mouth and throat. No specific treatment
has been developed.

cili- A combining form meaning: **1.** 'Pertain-

ing to an eyelid': *ciliectomy, ciliretinal, cilios-
cleral.* **2.** 'Pertaining to an eyelash': *ciliary, cilium.* **3.** 'Pertaining to a minute vibratile': *ciliated, ciliogenesis.*

cilia, *sing.* **cilium** **1.** The eyelids or eyelashes.
2. Small, hairlike processes on the outer surfaces
of some cells, aiding metabolism by producing
motion, eddies, or current in a fluid. **—ciliary,**
adj.

ciliary body The thickened part of the vascular tunic of the eye that joins the iris with the
anterior portion of the choroid. It is composed
of the ciliary crown, ciliary processes and folds,
ciliary orbiculus, ciliary muscle, and a basal
lamina.

ciliary canal The spaces of the iridocorneal
angle.

ciliary gland One of the numerous tiny,
modified sweat glands arranged in several rows
near the free margins of the eyelids. The apertures of the glands lie near the attachments of
the eyelashes. Acute localized bacterial infection
of one or more of the ciliary glands causes external sties. Also called **gland of Zeiss.** Compare **tarsal gland.**

ciliary margin The peripheral border of the
iris, continuous with the ciliary body.

ciliary movement The waving motion of
the hairlike processes projecting from the epithelium of the respiratory tract and from certain
microorganisms.

ciliary muscle A semitransparent, circular
band of smooth muscle fibers attached to the
choroid of the eye, the chief agent in adjusting
the eye to view near objects. It draws the ciliary

process centripetally, relaxing the suspensory ligament of the crystalline lens and allowing the lens to become more convex. It consists of meridional fibers and circular fibers and is thickest anteriorly. The circular fibers close to the circumference of the iris are well developed in hypermetropic eyes but are rudimentary or absent in myopic eyes.

ciliary process Any one of about 80 tiny fleshy projections on the posterior surface of the iris, forming a frill around the margin of the crystalline lens of the eye. The larger ciliary processes are about 2.5 cm (1 inch) long and are more regularly arranged than the smaller ones. The processes comprise one of the two zones of the ciliary body of the eye and are formed by infolding of the various layers of the tissue. They are attached anteriorly to the orbicularis ciliaris and posteriorly to the suspensory ligament of the crystalline lens. See also **ciliary body.**

ciliary reflex See **accommodation reflex.**

ciliary ring A small grooved band of tissue, about 4 mm wide, that forms the posterior part of the ciliary body of the eye. It extends from the ora serrata of the retina to the ciliary processes and is thicker near the ciliary processes, owing to the thickness of the ciliary muscle.

ciliary zone An outer circular area on the anterior surface of the iris, separated from the inner circular area by the angular line. The ciliary zone contains the stroma of the iris. Compare **zonula ciliaris.**

Ciliata A class of protozoa of the subphylum Ciliophora, characterized by cilia throughout the life cycle. The class includes the subclasses Euciliata and Protociliata. The only significant ciliate in humans is the intestinal parasite *Balantidium coli.*

ciliate Of or having cilia, as certain epithelial cells of the body or protozoa of the class Ciliata.

ciliated epithelium Any epithelial tissue that projects cilia from its surface, as portions of the epithelium in the respiratory tract.

ciliospinal reflex A normal brain-stem reflex that is initiated by scratching or pinching the skin of the back of the neck, resulting in the dilation of the pupil. Also called **pupillary-skin reflex.**

cimetidine A histamine (H_2)-receptor antagonist used to treat duodenal ulcer and certain pathologic hypersecretory conditions.

Cimex lectularius See **bedbug.**

cinchona The dried bark of the stem or root of species of *Cinchona*, containing the alkaloids quinine and quinidine.

cinchonism A condition resulting from excessive ingestion of cinchona bark or its alkaloid derivatives. Cinchonism is characterized by deafness, headache, ringing in the ears, and signs of cerebral congestion. See also **quinine.**

cine-, kine- A combining form meaning 'pertaining to movement': *cineangiogram, cinefluorography.* Also **kinesio-.**

cineangiocardiogram A radiograph of the cardiovascular system obtained by special instruments that employ a combination of X-ray,

fluoroscopic, and motion-picture techniques.

cineangiocardiography The filming of fluorescent images of the cardiovascular system by using a combination of fluoroscopic, X-ray, and motion-picture techniques. See also **cineradiography.**

cineangiogram A motion-picture record of a blood vessel or of a portion of the cardiovascular system, obtained by injecting a patient with a nontoxic radiopaque medium and filming the action of the vessels through which it courses.

cineangiograph A special movie camera for recording fluorescent images of the cardiovascular system.

cinefluorography See **cineradiography.**

cinematics See **kinematics.**

cineradiography The filming with a movie camera of the images that are made to appear on a fluorescent screen, especially those images of body structures that have been injected with a nontoxic, radiopaque medium for diagnostic purposes. Also called **cinefluorography, cineroentgenofluorography.** See also **cineangiocardiography.**

cineroentgenofluorography See **cineradiography.**

-cinesis See **-kinesis.** Also **-cinesia.**

cingulate 1. Having a zone or a girdle, usually with transverse markings. 2. Of or pertaining to a cingulum.

cingulate sulcus See **callosomarginal fissure.**

cingulectomy The surgical excision of a portion of the cingulate gyrus in the frontal lobe of the brain, and the immediately surrounding tissue.

cingulotomy A procedure in brain surgery to alleviate intractable pain by producing lesions in the tissue of the cingulate gyrus of the frontal lobe. The operation interrupts the fibers of the white matter in the gyrus by the stereotactic application of heat or cold.

cingulum 1. A band of efferent fibers of the cerebral cortex that circles the corpus callosum between the medial margins of the frontal and temporal lobes. 2. The ridge on the lingual surface of incisors, especially upper incisors, near the gum. 3. A structure, part, or band, as of color, that encircles another part.

cinnamon The aromatic inner bark of several species of *Cinnamomum*, a tree native to the East Indies and China. Saigon cinnamon is commonly used as a carminative, an aromatic stimulant, or as a spice. —**cinnamanic,** *adj.*

cinoxacin A urinary tract antiseptic similar to nalidixic acid.

circadian rhythm A pattern based on a 24-hour cycle, especially the repetition of certain physiologic phenomena, as sleeping and eating.

circinate Having ring-shaped outline or formation; annular.

circle In anatomy: a circular or nearly circular structure of the body, as the circle of Willis and circle of Zinn. —**circular,** *adj.*

circle of Carus See **curve of Carus.**

circle of Willis A vascular network at the

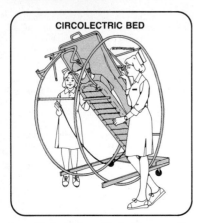

CIRCOLECTRIC BED

base of the brain, formed by the interconnection of the internal carotid, anterior cerebral, posterior cerebral, anterior communicating, and posterior communicating arteries.

CircOlectric (COL) bed A trade name for an electrically controlled bed that can be vertically rotated 210° and permits vertical alteration of the position of the bed patient from prone to supine. This type of bed is used especially in orthopedics and in the treatment of patients with severe burns. The bed consists of a strong aluminum circular frame supporting an anterior and a posterior straight frame between which the patient is "sandwiched" during rotation. Compare **Foster bed, hyperextension bed, Stryker wedge frame.**

circuit A course or pathway, particularly one through which an electrical current passes. Current passes through a closed or continuous circuit and stops if the circuit is open, interrupted, or broken.

circular bandage A bandage wrapped so that each turn completely covers the previous turn. Used to anchor a bandage.

circular fold One of the numerous annular projections in the small intestine. They vary in size and frequency in the duodenum, the jejunum, and the ileum, and are formed by mucous and submucous tissue. Most of the folds make less than a full turn around the inside circumference of the intestine, but others spiral through the lumen, making as many as three turns. Also called **plica circularis, valve of Kerkring.**

circulation Movement of an object or substance through a circular course so it returns to its starting point, as the circulation of blood through the cardiovascular system.

circulation time, normal The time required for blood to flow from one part of the body to another. Timing a particle of blood involves injecting a traceable dye or radioisotope into a vein and timing its reappearance in an artery at the point of injection. Alternatively, a tasteable substance like saccharin can be injected, and the time it takes to travel from the

injection site to the tongue can be noted.

circulatory failure Failure of the cardiovascular system to supply the cells of the body with a volume of blood adequate to meet the metabolic demands of the cells. The condition results from abnormal function of the myocardium, as in myocardial infarction; from an inadequate circulatory volume of blood, as with hemorrhage; or from collapse of the peripheral vascular system, as in gram-negative septicemia. See also **shock.**

circulatory system The network of channels through which the nutrient fluids of the body circulate.

circulus arteriosus minor The small artery encircling the outer circumference of the iris.

circum- A combining form meaning 'around': *circumanal, circumgemmal, circumvascular.*

circumanal Of or pertaining to the area surrounding the anus.

circumcision A surgical procedure in which the prepuce of the penis, or, rarely, the prepuce of the clitoris is excised. Circumcision is widely performed on newborn boys despite the demonstrable lack of medical benefit and the small but significant risk of serious or lethal complications, as hemorrhage, urethral injury, or postoperative infection. These problems occur as often as the penile diseases of uncircumcised adults that circumcision is intended to prevent. The operation is performed on newborns without anesthesia, using one of several kinds of clamps, and sometimes on adult males in the treatment of phymosis and balanitis. Ritual circumcision is required by the religions of approximately one sixth of the world population.

circumduction **1.** The circular movement of a limb or of the eye. **2.** The motion of the head of a bone within an articulating cavity, as the hip joint. The bone circumscribes a conical space, the apex of which is in the cavity and the base of which is described by the distal end of the bone. Circumduction is one of the four basic kinds of motion allowed by various joints of the skeleton and is a combination of abduction, adduction, extension, and flexion. Compare **angular movement, gliding, rotation.** See also **joint.**

circumferential fibrocartilage A structure made of fibrocartilage, in which fibrocartilaginous rims surround the margins of various articular cavities, as the glenoid labra of the hip and the shoulder. The rims deepen such cavities and protect their edges. Compare **connecting fibrocartilage, interarticular fibrocartilage, stratiform cartilage.**

circumferential implantation See **superficial implantation.**

circumoral Of or pertaining to the area of the face around the mouth.

circumscribed scleroderma See **Addison's keloid.**

circumvallate papilla See under **papilla.**

circus movement **1.** An unusual and involuntary rolling or somersaulting, owing to injured neurological mechanisms that control body posture, as the cerebral peduncles or the vestibular apparatus. **2.** An unusual circular gait caused by injury to the brain or to basal nerve centers. **3.** A mechanism associated with the excitatory wave of the atrium of the heart and atrial flutter or fibrillation. The wave travels a circular path characterized by a gap between the refractory and the excitatory tissue, usually resulting in conduction of only a fraction of the impulses to the ventricle.

cirrhosis A chronic degenerative disease of the liver in which the lobes are covered with fibrous tissue, the parenchyma degenerates, and the lobules are infiltrated with fat. Gluconeogenesis, detoxification of drugs and alcohol, bilirubin metabolism, vitamin absorption, gastrointestinal function, hormonal metabolism, and other functions of the liver deteriorate. Blood flow through the liver is obstructed, causing back pressure and leading to portal hypertension and esophageal varices. Unless the cause of the disease is removed, hepatic coma, gastrointestinal hemorrhage, and kidney failure eventually occur. Cirrhosis is most commonly the result of chronic alcohol abuse but can be the result of nutritional deprivation or hepatitis or other infection. Symptoms include nausea, flatulence, anorexia, weight loss, ascites, light-colored stools, weakness, abdominal pain, varicosities, and spider angiomas. Definite diagnosis is made by biopsy, but X-ray, physical examination, and several blood tests of liver function are serially performed to monitor the course of the disease. Treatment usually includes a balanced diet (as rich in protein as can be tolerated), vitamins (especially folic acid), rest, and total abstinence from alcohol. The liver has remarkable ability to regenerate, but recovery may be very slow. Kinds of cirrhosis are **biliary cirrhosis, fatty cirrhosis, posthepatic cirrhosis.** See also **hepatic coma. —cirrhotic,** *adj.*

cirsoid Resembling a varix. An enlarged tortuous vein.

cirsoid aneurysm See **racemose aneurysm.**

cis configuration, cis arrangement, cis position In genetics: **1.** The presence of the dominant alleles of two or more pairs of genes on one chromosome and the recessive alleles on the homologous chromosome. **2.** The presence of the mutant genes of a pair of pseudoalleles on one chromosome and the wild-type genes on the homologous chromosome. Compare **coupling** definition 2, **trans configuration.**

cisplatin, cis-platinum An alkylating agent used in chemotherapy.

cisterna, *pl.* **cisternae** A cavity that serves as a reservoir for lymph or other body fluids. Kinds of cisternae include **cisterna chyli, cisterna subarachnoidea.**

cisterna chyli A dilatation at the beginning of the thoracic duct, situated ventral to the body of the second lumbar vertebra, on the right side of, and dorsal to, the aorta. It receives the two lumbar lymphatic trunks, descending intercos-

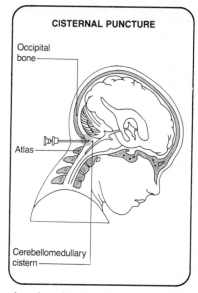

CISTERNAL PUNCTURE

Occipital bone

Atlas

Cerebellomedullary cistern

tal trunk, and the intestinal lymphatic trunk.

cisternal puncture The insertion of a needle into the cerebellomedullary cistern to withdraw cerebrospinal fluid for examination. The puncture is made between the atlas and the occipital bone.

cisterna subarachnoidea Any one of many small subarachnoid spaces that serves as a reservoir for cerebrospinal fluid.

cistron A fragment or portion of DNA that codes for a specific polypeptide. It is the smallest unit functioning as a transmitter of genetic information. Also called **gene. —cistronic,** *adj.*

cisvestitism The practice of wearing attire appropriate to the sex of the individual involved but not suitable to the age, occupation, or status of the wearer, as when a male bookkeeper impersonates a male police officer by wearing a police uniform.

citrate **1.** Any salt or ester of citric acid. **2.** The act of treating with a citrate or citric acid. **—citration,** *n.*

citric acid A white, crystalline, organic acid soluble in water and alcohol. It is extracted from citrus fruits, especially lemons and limes, or obtained by fermentation of sugars and is used as a flavoring agent in foods, carbonated beverages, and certain pharmaceutical products, especially laxatives. It is also used as a preventive of scurvy. See also **ascorbic acid, scurvy.**

citrin A crystalline flavonoid concentrate that is used as a source of bioflavonoid.

citrovorum factor See **folinic acid.**

Civilian Health and Medical Programs for Uniformed Services (CHAMPUS) A health-care insurance system for military dependents and members of the military services when certain kinds of care are not available through the usual military medical service.

CHAMPUS is the first, and one of the few, federal third-party reimbursement systems that will pay for care rendered by nurse-midwives and nurse practitioners.

CJPH abbr **Canadian Journal of Public Health.**

Cl Symbol for **chlorine.**

claims-made policy A professional liability insurance policy that covers the holder for the period in which a claim of malpractice is made. The alleged act of malpractice may have occurred at some previous time, but the policy insures the holder when the claim is made. Compare **occurrence policy.**

clairsentience See **clairvoyance.**

clairvoyance, clairvoyancy The power or ability to perceive or to be aware of objects or events without the use of the physical senses. Also called **clairsentience.** See also **extrasensory perception, parapsychology, telepathy. clairvoyant,** adj., n.

clamp An instrument with serrated tips and locking handles, used for gripping, holding, joining, supporting, or compressing an organ or vessel, as for hemostasis.

clamp forceps See **pedicle clamp.**

clang association, klang association The mental connection between dissociated ideas made because of similarity in the sounds of the words used to describe the ideas. The phenomenon occurs frequently in the manic phase of bipolar disorder.

clapping In massage: the procedure of making percussive movements on the body of a patient by lowering the cupped palms alternately in a series of rapid, stimulating blows, with the movement of the hands from the wrist. Clapping stimulates the circulation and refreshes the skin and is often done to improve the comfort of bedridden patients, especially during the administration of a bed bath.

clarify In chemistry: to clear a turbid liquid by allowing any suspended matter to settle, by adding a substance that precipitates suspended matter, or by heating. —**clarification,** n.

Clark's rule A method of calculating the approximate pediatric dosage of a drug for a child using the formula: [weight (in pounds)/150] × adult dose. See **Cowling's rule.**

clas- A combining form meaning 'a piece broken off': clasmatocyte, clasmatodendrosis, clasmatosis.

-clasia A combining form meaning a '(specified) condition involving crushing or breaking up': aortoclasia, collodoclasia, osteoclasia.

clasmocytic lymphoma See **histiocytic malignant lymphoma.**

clasp 1. In dentistry: a sleevelike fitting that is fastened over a tooth to hold a partial denture in place. 2. In surgery: any device for holding tissues together, especially bones.

clasp-knife reflex An abnormal sign in which a spastic limb resists passive motion and then suddenly gives way, similar to the blade of a jackknife. It is an indication of damage to the pyramidal tract.

classical cesarean section A method for surgically delivering an infant through a vertical midline incision of the upper segment of the uterus. A fast method of cesarean delivery, it produces a weaker scar and, because the upper segment is thicker and more vascular, more bleeding during surgery than does the low cervical cesarean section. Compare **extraperitoneal cesarean section.** See also **cesarean section.**

classical conditioning A form of learning in which a previously neutral stimulus comes to elicit a given response through associative training. Also called **respondent conditioning.** See also **conditioned reflex.**

classic apraxia See **ideomotor apraxia.**

classic typhus See **epidemic typhus.**

classification In research: a process in data collection and analysis in which data are grouped according to previously determined characteristics. —**classify,** v.

-clast A combining form meaning 'something that breaks': angioclast, cranioclast, myeloclast.

-clastic A combining form meaning 'causing disintegration': hemoclastic, histoclastic, lipoclastic.

claudication 1. A lameness or a limping. 2. A complex of symptoms characterized by the absence of pain in a limb at rest, then pain and weakness that intensify during walking, causing limping, until walking is impossible. The pain then subsides after rest.

claustrophobia A morbid fear of being in or becoming trapped in enclosed or narrow places. The phenomenon usually can be traced to some traumatic childhood situation. Treatment consists of psychotherapy to uncover the cause of the phobic reaction, followed by behavior therapy, specifically systematic desensitization or flooding technique.

claustrum, pl. **claustra** 1. A barrier, as a membrane that partially closes an aperture. 2. A thin sheet of gray matter, composed chiefly of spindle cells, situated lateral to the external capsule of the brain and separating the internal capsule from white matter of the insula. Also called claustrum of insula.

clavicle A long, curved, horizontal bone just above the first rib, forming the ventral portion of the shoulder girdle. It articulates medially with the sternum and laterally with the acromion of the scapula and accommodates the attachment of numerous muscles.

clavicular notch One of a pair of oval depressions at the superior end of the sternum. Each clavicular notch is situated on one side of the sternum and articulates with the clavicle from the same side.

clavus See **corn.**

clawfoot See **pes cavus.**

clawhand A hand fixed in a position of acute flexion. Also called **main en griffe.**

claw-type traction frame An orthopedic apparatus that holds various pieces of traction equipment, as the pulleys, the ropes, and the weights by which traction is applied to various parts of the body or by which various parts of the body are suspended. It consists of two metal uprights, one at the head of the bed and the other at the foot, that support an overhead metal bar. Compare **Balkan traction frame, I.V.-type traction frame.**

clearance The removal of a substance from the blood via the kidneys. Kidney function can be tested by measuring the amount of a specific substance excreted in the urine in a given length of time.

clear cell **1.** A type of cell found in the parathyroid gland that does not take on a color with the ordinary tissue stains used for microscopic examination. **2.** The principal cell of most renal-cell carcinomas and, occasionally, of ovarian and parathyroid tumors. **3.** A specific type of epidermal cell, probably of neural origin, that has a dark-staining nucleus but clear cytoplasm with hematoxylin and eosin stain.

clear cell carcinoma **1.** A malignant tumor of the tubular epithelium of the kidney. Characteristically, the malignant cells contain abundant clear cytoplasm. See also **renal cell carcinoma.** **2.** An uncommon ovarian neoplasm characterized by cells with clear cytoplasm.

clear cell carcinoma of the kidney See **renal cell carcinoma.**

clear liquid diet A diet that supplies fluids and provides minimal residue. It consists primarily of dissolved sugar and flavored liquids, as ginger ale, sweetened tea or coffee, fat-free broth, plain gelatin desserts, and strained fruit juices. The diet is nutritionally inadequate and is usually prescribed for a limited amount of time, as 1 day, postoperatively.

cleavage **1.** The series of repeated mitotic cell divisions occurring in the ovum immediately following fertilization to form a mass of cells that transforms the single-celled zygote into a multicellular embryo capable of growth and differentiation. At this initial stage, as the zygote remains uniform in size, the cleavage cells, or blastomeres, become smaller with each division. **2.** The act or process of cleaving or splitting, primarily the splitting of a complex molecule into two or more simpler molecules. Kinds of cleavage include **determinate cleavage, equal cleavage, indeterminate cleavage, partial cleavage, total cleavage, unequal cleavage.**

cleavage cavity See **blastocoele.**

cleavage cell See **blastomere.**

cleavage fracture Any fracture that splits cartilage with the avulsion of a small piece of bone from the distal portion of the lateral condyle of the humerus.

cleavage line Any one of a number of linear striations in the skin that delineate the general structural pattern and tension of the subcutaneous fibrous tissue. They correspond closely to the crease lines on the surface of the skin and are present in all areas of the body but visible only in certain sites, as the palms of the hands and soles of the feet. The lines follow a char-

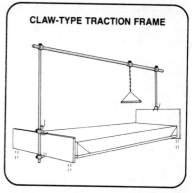

CLAW-TYPE TRACTION FRAME

acteristic pattern for each region of the body, although they vary with body configuration; they are consistent in persons of the same build regardless of age. In general, the lines run obliquely, lying in the direction in which the skin stretches the least. Incisions made parallel to these lines heal with much less scarring than those made perpendicular to them. Also called **Langer's line.**

cleavage nucleus See **segmentation nucleus.**

cleavage plane **1.** The area in a fertilized ovum where cleavage takes place; the axis along which any cell division occurs. **2.** Any plane within the body where organs or structures can be separated with minimal damage to surrounding tissue.

cleft **1.** Divided. **2.** A fissure, especially one that originates in the embryo, as the branchial cleft or the facial cleft.

cleft foot An abnormal condition in which the division between the third and fourth toes extends into the metatarsum of the foot.

cleft lip See **harelip.**

cleft lip repair The surgical correction of a unilateral or bilateral congenital interruption of the upper lip, usually resulting from the embryologic failure of the median nasal and maxillary processes to unite.

cleft palate A congenital defect characterized by a fissure in the midline of the palate, resulting from the failure of the two sides to fuse during embryonic development. The fissure may be complete, extending through both the hard and soft palates into the nasal cavities, or it may show any degree of incomplete or partial cleft, and it is often accompanied by a cleft lip. Feeding is best accomplished with special feeding devices. Surgical repair of the defect is usually not begun until the 1st or 2nd year of life and is usually performed in steps. Care of the child requires a team approach that includes a plastic surgeon, orthodontist, dentist, nurse, speech and hearing therapists, and social workers. Long-term, postoperative problems, including speech impairment and hearing loss, improper tooth development and alignment, chronic respiratory and ear infections, and varying levels of emotional and social maladjustment, may be largely avoided by modern techniques and reconstructive surgery. See also **harelip.**

cleft uvula   An abnormal congenital condition in which the uvula is split into two halves owing to the failure of the posterior palatine folds to unite.

cleido-, cleid-   A combining form meaning 'pertaining to the clavicle': *cleidocostal, cleidocranial, cleidomastoid.*

cleidocranial dysostosis   A rare, abnormal hereditary condition characterized by defective ossification of the cranial bones and by the complete or partial absence of the clavicles. It is transmitted as an autosomal dominant trait. The defective ossification of the cranial bones delays the closing of the cranial sutures and results in large fontanels. The complete or partial absence of the clavicles allows the shoulders to be brought together. This condition also involves dental and vertebral anomalies. Also called **cleidocranial dysplasia.** See also **dysostosis.**

cleidocranial dysplasia   See **cleidocranial dysostosis.**

cleidocranial dystrophia   See **cleidocranial dysostosis.**

clemastine fumarate   An ethanolamine antihistamine.

cleptomania   See **kleptomania.**

click   In cardiology: an extra heart sound that occurs during systole. See also **ejection click, systolic click.**

clidinium bromide   A gastrointestinal anticholinergic agent.

client   **1.** A person who is receiving a professional service. **2.** A patient.

client-centered therapy   A nondirective method of group or individual psychotherapy, originated by Carl Rogers, in which the role of the therapist is to listen to and then reflect or restate without judgment or interpretation the words of the client. The goal of the therapy is personal growth achieved by the client's increased awareness and understanding of his attitudes, feelings, and behavior.

client interview   See **patient interview.**

climacteric   See **menopause.**

climacteric melancholia   See **involutional melancholia.**

clindamycin hydrochloride, c. palmitate hydrochloride, c. phosphate   Antibiotics.

clinic   **1.** A department in a hospital where persons not requiring hospitalization may receive medical care, formerly called a dispensary. **2.** A group practice of doctors, as the Mayo Clinic. **3.** A meeting place for doctors and medical students where instruction can be given at the bedside of a patient or in a similar setting. **4.** A seminar or other scientific medical meeting. **5.** A detailed published report of the diagnosis and treatment of a health care problem.

-clinic   A combining form meaning 'places set aside for medical treatment': *policlinic, polyclinic, psychoclinic.*

clinical   **1.** Of or pertaining to a clinic. **2.** Of or pertaining to direct, bedside medical care.

3. Of or pertaining to materials or equipment used in the care of a sick person.

clinical cytogenetics   The branch of genetics that studies the relationship between chromosomal abnormalities and pathological conditions.

clinical diagnosis   A diagnosis made on the basis of knowledge obtained by medical history and physical examination alone, without benefit of laboratory tests or X-rays.

clinical genetics   A branch of genetics that studies inherited disorders and investigates the possible genetic factors that may influence the occurrence of any pathological condition. Also called **medical genetics.**

clinical laboratory   A laboratory in which tests directly related to the care of patients are performed. Such laboratories use material obtained from patients for testing, as compared with research laboratories where animal and other sources of test material are also used.

clinical nurse specialist (CNS)   A registered nurse who holds a master of science degree in nursing (MSN) and who has acquired advanced knowledge and clinical skills in a specific area of nursing and health care. The CNS, as a practitioner, assumes a leadership role, based on clinical expertise and judgment, in caring for patients, delegating responsibility, teaching other staff members, and influencing and effecting change with respect to the needs of the patient and family and the total health-care delivery system.

clinical-pathological conference   A teaching conference in which a case is presented to a clinician who then demonstrates the process of reasoning that leads to his diagnosis. Often the students suggest a diagnosis based on the same information. A pathologist then presents what is usually the definitive anatomical diagnosis, based on the study of tissue removed at surgery or obtained in autopsy. The conference is the model for the 'case-reports' in the *New England Journal of Medicine* and is a part of the curricula of most medical schools.

clinical pathology   The laboratory study of disease by a pathologist using techniques appropriate to the specimen being studied. Branches include hematology, bacteriology, chemistry, and serology.

clinical pelvimetry   A process for assessing the size of the birth canal by means of the systematic vaginal palpation of specific bony landmarks in the pelvis and an estimation of the distances between them. Internal pelvic diameters are not accessible to direct measurement; they must be inferred. Findings are commonly recorded in terms such as 'adequate,' 'borderline,' or 'inadequate,' rather than in centimeters or inches. Compare **X-ray pelvimetry.** See also **birth canal, cephalopelvic disproportion, contraction, dystocia.**

clinical psychology   The branch of psychology concerned with the diagnosis, treatment, and prevention of personality and behavioral disorders.

clinical research center An organization, often associated with a medical school or a teaching hospital, that studies, analyzes, correlates, and describes medical cases. Such centers usually have extensive laboratory facilities and specialized staffs of doctors and medical technicians. Clinical research centers often offer free or inexpensive diagnoses and treatment for patients participating in various research programs and often produce significant new medical information.

clinical specialist A doctor or nurse having advanced training in a particular field of practice, as a nurse-midwife, pediatrician, or radiologist.

Clinitest A trademark for reagent tablets used to test for the presence of reducing sugars, as glucose, in the urine. The tablets contain copper sulfate, and the procedure is a modified version of Benedict's test.

clino- A combining form meaning 'to bend or make lie down': *clinodactyl, clinostatic, clinostatism.*

clinocephaly, clinocephalism A congenital anomaly of the head in which the upper surface of the skull is concave. **—clinocephalic, clinocephalous,** *adj.*

clinodactyly, clinodactylism A congenital anomaly characterized by abnormal lateral or medial bending of one or more fingers or toes. **—clinodactylic, clinodactylous,** *adj.*

-clinous A combining form meaning 'pertaining to ancestry': *matriclinous, matroclinous, patroclinous.*

clioquinol See **iodochlorhydroxyquin.**

clip A surgical device used for grasping the skin to align the edges of a wound and to stop bleeding, especially of the smaller blood vessels. It is also used in radiography for localization.

clitoris The vulval erectile structure homologous to the corpora cavernosa of the penis. It consists of two corpora cavernosa within a dense layer of fibrous membrane, joined along their inner surfaces by an incomplete fibrous septum. It is situated beneath the anterior commissure, partially hidden between the anterior extremities of the labia minora.

CLL See **chronic lymphocytic leukemia.**

cloaca, *pl.* **cloacae** **1.** In embryology: the end of the hindgut before the developmental division into the rectum, the bladder, and the primitive genital structures. **2.** In pathology: an opening into the sheath of tissue around a necrotic bone.

cloacal membrane A thin sheath that separates the internal and external portions of the cloaca in the developing embryo. It is formed from endoderm and ectoderm and closes the fetal anus during early prenatal development; it later ruptures and is absorbed so that the anal canal becomes continuous with the rectum. Also called **anal membrane.**

cloacal septum See **urorectal septum.**

clocortolone pivalate A topical anti-inflammatory agent.

clofibrate An antilipemic agent.

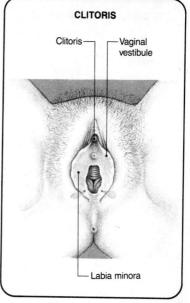

CLITORIS

Clitoris — — Vaginal vestibule

— Labia minora

clomiphene citrate An ovulation inducer.

clomiphene stimulation test A test used to evaluate gonadal function in males who show signs of abnormal pubertal development. Clomiphene, a nonsteroid analog of estrogen, stimulates the hypothalamic-pituitary system to raise FSH and LH levels of the blood. Failure to respond to clomiphene indicates hypothalamic-pituitary disease, possibly a pituitary tumor. See also **gonadotropin.**

clonal selection theory In immunology: a theory of antibody formation proposed by Sir Frank Macfarlane Burnet, stating that preprogrammed, or precommitted, clones of lymphoid cells that are produced in the fetus are capable of interacting with a limited number of antigenic determinants with which the host may come in contact. Any such clones that encounter the specific antigen in utero are destroyed or suppressed so that entire clones are eliminated or inactivated. This removes the cells programmed to become endogenous autoantigens and prevents the development of autoimmune diseases, leaving intact those cells capable of reacting with exogenous antigens.

clonazepam A benzodiazepine anticonvulsant.

clone A group of genetically identical cells or organisms derived from a single common cell or organism through mitosis.

-clonia A combining form meaning '(condition involving) spasms': *logoclonia, myoclonia, polyclonia.*

clonidine hydrochloride A centrally-acting, sympatholytic antihypertensive.

Clonorchis sinensis The Chinese or Oriental liver fluke. Infection occurs in humans

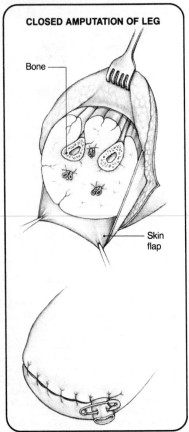

CLOSED AMPUTATION OF LEG

Bone

Skin flap

who eat raw or imperfectly cooked fish, which acts as an intermediate host for the organism. The larvae lie dormant until ingested by a warm-blooded animal, and then produce eggs, which are excreted in the feces of the host, enter water, and repeat the cycle. In human hosts, the liver fluke lives in the bile ducts and gallbladder, causing chronic liver disease with enlargement of the liver, diarrhea, edema, and, eventually, death. Also called *Opisthorchis sinensis.* See also **opisthorchiasis.**

clonus An abnormal pattern of neuromuscular activity, characterized by rapidly alternating involuntary contraction and relaxation of skeletal muscle. Compare **tonus.** **—clonic,** *adj.*

C-loop A surgically formed loop of bowel with a C-shape.

clorazepate dipotassium A benzodiazepine antianxiety agent.

clortermine hydrochloride An amphetamine-like CNS stimulant.

closed amputation A kind of amputation in which one or two broad flaps of muscular and cutaneous tissue are retained to form a cover over the end of the bone. It is only performed

when no infection is present. A rigid dressing may be applied and the patient fitted for a prosthesis immediately after surgery. Compare **open amputation.** See also **amputation.**

closed chain In organic chemistry: of or pertaining to a compound in which the carbon atoms are bonded together to form a closed ring. Also called **carbocyclic.**

closed system In general systems theory: a system closed off from its environment with no exchange of materials, information, or energy.

closed wound suction Any one of several techniques for draining potentially harmful fluids, as blood, pus, serosanguineous fluid, and tissue secretions, from surgical wounds. Such fluids interfere with the healing of wounds and often promote infection. Postoperative drainage aids the healing process by removing dead spaces where extravascular fluids collect and helps draw healing tissues together. Many surgical authorities prefer closed wound suction to other wound drainage methods, as pressure bandages and wicks, because it minimizes danger of infection. Closed wound suction is often an important part of postoperative treatment and may be accomplished with a variety of reliable devices that create a gentle negative pressure to drain away undesirable exudates. The technique is used as an aid to many operations, as mastectomies, augmentations, plastic and reconstructive procedures, and urological and urogenital procedures.

clostridial Of or pertaining to an anaerobic spore-forming bacteria of the genus *Clostridium.*

Clostridium A genus of spore-forming, anaerobic bacteria of the Bacillaceae family: *Clostridium bifermentans* causes gas gangrene and is found in feces and garbage; *C. botulinum* causes botulism; *C. perfringens* causes food poisoning, cellulitis, and wound infections; *C. tetani* is the cause of tetanus.

closure The surgical closing of a wound by suture. See also **flask closure, velopharyngeal closure.**

clot See **blood clot.**

clotrimazole A local anti-infective agent.

clotting See **blood clotting.**

clotting time The time required for blood to form a clot, tested by collecting 4 ml of blood in a glass tube and examining it for clot formation. The first appearance of a clot is noted and timed. This simple test has been used to diagnose hemophilias, but it will not detect mild coagulation disorders. Its chief application is in monitoring anticoagulant therapy. Also called coagulation time.

clove The dried flower bud of *Eugenia caryophyllata.* It contains a volatile oil used as a dental analgesic, germicide, salve, and carminative against nausea, vomiting, and flatulence.

cloverleaf nail A surgical nail shaped in cross section like a cloverleaf, used especially in the repair of fractures of the femur.

cloverleaf skull deformity A congenital

defect characterized by a trilobed skull resulting from premature closure of multiple cranial sutures during embryonic development. The condition is associated with hydrocephalus, facial anomalies, and skeletal deformities. Also called **kleeblattschädel deformity syndrome.**

cloxacillin sodium A penicillin antibiotic.

clubbing An abnormal enlargement of the distal phalanges, usually associated with cyanotic heart disease or advanced chronic pulmonary disease, but sometimes occurring with biliary cirrhosis, colitis, chronic dysentery, and thyrotoxicosis. The mechanism whereby diminished oxygen tension in the blood causes clubbing is not understood. It occurs in all the digits but is most easily seen in the fingers. Advanced clubbing is obvious, but early cases are difficult to diagnose. Clubbing is present if the transverse diameter of the base of the fingernail is greater than the transverse diameter of the most distal joint of the digit. The affected phalange is full, fleshy, quite vascular, and, in late clubbing, may be swollen. The skin may be excoriated. The angle between the nail and nail base may exceed 180° (a 160° angle is normal). The nail thickens and becomes hard, shiny, and curved at the free end.

clubfoot A congenital deformity of the foot, sometimes resulting from intrauterine constriction and characterized by unilateral or bilateral deviation of the metatarsal bones of the forefoot. Most (about 95%) clubfoot deformities are equinovarus, characterized by medial deviation and plantar flexion of the forefoot, but a few are calcaneo valgus, characterized by lateral deviation and dorsiflexion. Treatment depends on the extent and rigidity of the deformity. Splints and casts in infancy may produce complete correction; surgery in several steps may be necessary to achieve normal function. See also **Denis-Browne splint, talipes.**

cluster analysis In statistics: a complex technique of data analysis of numerical scale scores that produces clusters of variables related to one another. The technique is performed using a computer.

cluster headache See **histamine headache.**

cluttering A speech defect characterized by a rapid, confused, nervous delivery with uneven rhythmical patterns and the omission or transposition of various letters or syllables. The condition is commonly associated with other language disorders, as difficulty in learning to speak, read, and spell, and with various personality and behavior problems.

Cm Symbol for **curium.**

CMAJ *abbr* **Canadian Medical Association Journal.**

CMHC *abbr* **community mental health center.**

CML *abbr* **chronic myelocytic leukemia.**

CMV *abbr* **cytomegalovirus.**

CNA *abbr* **Canadian Nurses' Association.**

CNATS *abbr* **Canadian Nurses' Association Testing Service.**

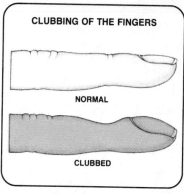

CLUBBING OF THE FINGERS

NORMAL

CLUBBED

-cnemia A combining form meaning '(condition of the) leg below the knee': *bucnemia, cacocnemia, microcnemia.*

CNF *abbr* **Canadian Nurses' Foundation.**

CNM *abbr* **certified nurse-midwife.**

CNP See **community nurse practitioner.**

CNRS *abbr* **Canadian Nurses' Respiratory Society.**

CNS *abbr* **1. central nervous system. 2. clinical nurse specialist.**

CNS syndrome See **central nervous system syndrome.**

Co Symbol for **cobalt.**

co- A combining form meaning 'together, with': *coadaptation, coagulate, coarctate.* Also **col-, com-, con-, cor-.**

CO₂ Symbol for **carbon dioxide.**

coagulase An enzyme produced by bacteria, particularly *Staphylococcus aureus*, that promotes the formation of thrombi.

coagulation See **blood clotting.**

coagulation factor One of 12 factors in the blood, the interactions of which are responsible for the process of blood clotting. The factors, using standardized numerical nomenclature, are factor I, fibrinogen; factor II, prothrombin; factor III, tissue thromboplastin; factor IV, calcium ions; factor V, labile factor; factor VII, stable factor; factor VIII, antihemophilic globulin; factor IX, plasma thromboplastin component (PTC); factor X, Stuart-Prower factor; factor XI, plasma thromboplastin antecedent (PTA); factor XII, Hageman factor; factor XIII, fibrin stabilizing factor. See also **blood clotting, hemophilia.**

coagulopathy A pathological condition affecting the ability of the blood to coagulate.

coal tar See **tars.**

coal worker's pneumoconiosis See **anthracosis.**

coaptation splint A small splint fitted to a fractured limb to prevent overriding of the fragments of bone. A longer splint usually covers the small one to provide for more support and fixation of the entire limb.

coarct The act of narrowing or constricting, especially the lumen of a blood vessel.

coarctation A stricture or contraction of the walls of a vessel, as the aorta.

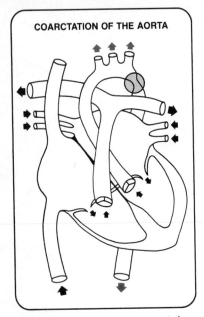

COARCTATION OF THE AORTA

coarctation of the aorta A congenital cardiac anomaly characterized by a localized narrowing of the aorta, which results in increased pressure proximal to the defect and decreased pressure distal to it. Clinical manifestations include dizziness, headaches, fainting, epistaxis, reduced or absent femoral pulses, and muscle cramps in the legs from tissue anoxia during increased exercise. Diagnosis is based on characteristic pressure changes in the upper and lower body and specific radiological findings, including notching of the lower ribs, left ventricular hypertrophy, and dilatation of the aorta proximal to the stricture. A murmur may or may not be present. Surgical repair is recommended for minor defects because of the high incidence of untreated complications, including aortic rupture, hypertension, infective endocarditis, subarachnoid hemorrhage, and congestive heart failure. See also **congenital cardiac anomaly.**

coarse In physiology: involving a wide range of movements, as those associated with tremors and other involuntary movements of the skeletal muscle.

coarse fremitus A rough, loud, tremulous vibration of the chest wall noted on palpation of the chest during a physical examination as the person inhales and exhales. It is most common in pulmonary conditions characterized by consolidation.

coat **1.** A membrane that covers the outside of an organ or part. **2.** One of the layers of a wall of an organ or part, especially a canal or a vessel.

cobalamin A generic term for the vitamin B_{12} group. See also **cyanocobalamin.**

cobalt (Co) A metallic element and component of vitamin B_{12}. Its atomic number is 27; its atomic weight is 58.9. The administration of cobalt in the form of cobaltous chloride has been successful in some patients with certain types of anemia because of the capacity of cobalt to produce polycythemia. Accidental intoxication by cobaltous chloride, especially in children, may produce cyanosis, coma, and death. The only disease for which some experts still advocate the use of cobalt is normochromic, normocytic anemia associated with renal failure.

cobalt 60 (^{60}Co) In radiotherapy: a radioactive isotope of the silver-white metallic element cobalt, with a mass number of 60 and a half-life of 5.2 years. ^{60}Co emits high-energy gamma rays and is the most frequently used radioisotope in radiotherapy. In ^{60}Co machines, the high-energy radioactive source is stored in a position well shielded by lead or uranium.

COBOL In data processing: acronym for Common Business Oriented Language, a computer programing language widely used in business and industry.

coca One of two South American shrubs, native to the Andes. The leaves are dried and chewed for their stimulant effect by some of the people of the region. It is a natural source of cocaine.

cocaine hydrochloride A topical anesthetic applied to the eye, nose, or throat.

cocci-, cocco- A combining form meaning 'seed; pertaining to a sperical bacterial cell': *coccobacillus, coccogenous, coccoid.*

coccidioidomycosis An infectious fungal disease caused by the inhalation of spores of the bacterium *Coccidioides immitis,* which is carried on windborne dust particles. The disease is endemic in hot, dry regions of the southwestern United States and Central and South America. Symptoms of primary infection resemble those of the common cold or influenza. Secondary infection, occurring after a period of remission and lasting for a period of weeks to years, is marked by low-grade fever, anorexia and weight loss, cyanosis, dyspnea, hemoptysis, and arthritic pain in the bones and joints. The diagnosis is made by learning that the patient lived in or visited an endemic area and by identifying *C. immitis* in sputum, exudate, or tissue. Treatment usually employs bed rest and antibiotics. Also called **desert fever, desert rheumatism, San Joaquin fever, valley fever.**

coccidiosis A parasitic disease of tropical and subtropical regions caused by the ingestion of oocysts of the protozoa *Isospora belli* or *I. hominis.* Symptoms include fever, malaise, abdominal discomfort, and watery diarrhea. The infection is usually self-limiting, lasting 1 to 2 weeks, but occasionally it persists, resulting in malabsorption syndrome and, rarely, death. No specific therapy has been found. Compare **coccidioidomycosis.**

cocco- See **cocci-.**

coccus, *pl.* **cocci** A bacterium that is round, spherical, or oval in shape, as gonococcus, pneumococcus, staphylococcus, streptococcus. **—coccal,** *adj.*

COCHLEA

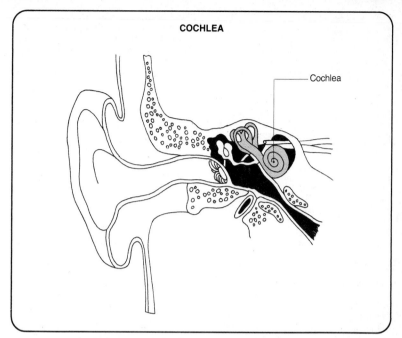

Cochlea

-**coccus** A combining form meaning a 'berry-shaped organism': *dermococcus, enterococcus, pneumonococcus.*

coccyg-, coccygo- A combining form meaning 'coccyx': *coccygeal, coccygectomy, coccygodynia.*

coccygeal vertebra One of the four segments of the vertebral column that fuse in the adult to form the coccyx. They are considered rudimentary vertebrae and have no pedicles, laminae, or spinous processes. Compare **cervical vertebra, lumbar vertebra, sacral vertebra, thoracic vertebra.** See also **coccyx, vertebra.**

coccygeus One of two muscles in the pelvic diaphragm. Stretching across the pelvic cavity like a hammock, it is a triangular sheet of muscle and tendinous fibers, dorsal to the levator ani, arising from the spine of the ischium and from the sacrospinous ligament. It inserts into the coccyx and into the sacrum, is innervated by branches of the pudendal plexus, which contain fibers from the fourth and the fifth sacral nerves, and it acts to draw the coccyx ventrally, helping to support the pelvic floor. Compare **levator ani.**

coccygodynia A pain in the coccygeal area of the body.

coccyx, *pl.* **coccyges** The beaklike bone joined to the sacrum by a disk of fibrocartilage at the base of the vertebral column. It is formed by the union of three to five rudimentary vertebrae. The pieces of the coccyx fuse together in men at an earlier period in life than in women. In men and in women, the coccyx becomes fused with the sacrum by the 6th decade of life. The

coccyx is freely movable on the sacrum during pregnancy. —**coccygeal,** *adj.*

cochineal A red dye prepared from the dried female insects of the species *Coccus cacti* containing young larvae. During the preparation of the dye the larvae are extracted with an aqueous solution of alum, and the resulting dye is used in coloring medicines.

cochlea A conical bony structure of the inner ear, perforated by numerous apertures for passage of the cochlear division of the acoustic nerve. Part of a complex tubular network called the osseous labyrinth, it is a spiral tunnel about 3 cm (1⅕ inches) long with 2¾ turns, resembling a tiny snail shell. —**cochlear,** *adj.*

cochlear canal A bony spiral tunnel within the cochlea, lying along its outer wall between the scala tympani and the scala vestibuli. About 30 mm long, it narrows gradually in diameter as it rises to the apex of the cochlea. Also called **cochlear duct.**

cochlear duct See **cochlear canal.**

cockscomb papilloma A benign, small red lesion that may project from the uterine cervix during pregnancy; it regresses after delivery.

cocktail *Informal.* An unofficial mixture of drugs, usually in solution, combined to achieve a specific purpose. See also **Brompton's cocktail.**

code **1.** In law: a published body of statutes, as a civil code. **2.** A collection of standards and rules of behavior, as a dress code. **3.** A symbolic means of representing information for communication or transfer, as a genetic code. **4.** A system of notation that allows information to be transmitted rapidly, as Morse code, or in secrecy, as a cryptographic code. **5.** *Informal.* A discreet signal used to summon a special team to resuscitate a patient without alarming patients or visitors. See also **no-code.**

codeine, c. phosphate, c. sulfate Narcotic opioid analgesic and antitussive agents.

codes 1. A system of assigned terms designed by a medical institution for quick and accurate communication during emergencies or for patient identification. **2.** Short values of data used to feed commands to a computerized hospital information system.

code team A specially trained and equipped team of doctors, nurses, and technicians that is available to provide cardiopulmonary resuscitation when summoned by a code set by the institution. A code team usually includes a physician, registered nurse, respiratory therapist, and pharmacist. The members may work in any department or unit of the hospital. A schedule is made that ensures a full team on duty at all times.

cod-liver oil A pale yellow, fatty oil extracted from the fresh livers of the codfish and other related species. It is a rich source of vitamins A and D, useful in the treatment of nutritional deficiency of those vitamins or of conditions owing to abnormal absorption of calcium and phosphorus. The oil must be stored in a cool, dark place or it becomes rancid. See also **osteomalacia, rickets, tetany.**

Codman's tumor See **chondroblastoma.**

codominant Of or pertaining to the alleles or to the trait resulting from the full expression of both alleles of a pair in a heterozygote, as the AB or MN blood group antigens. —**codominance,** *n.*

codominant inheritance The transmission of a trait or condition in which both alleles of a pair are given full expression in a heterozygote, as in the AB or MN blood group antigens and the leukocyte antigens.

codon A unit of three adjacent nucleotides along a DNA or messenger RNA molecule that designates a specific amino acid in the polypeptide chain during protein synthesis. Each codon consists of a specific section of the DNA molecule so that the order of the codons along the molecule determines the sequence of the amino acids in each protein. Also called **triplet.** See also **genetic code.**

coefficient A mathematical relationship between factors that can be used to measure or evaluate a characteristic under specified conditions. An example is the oxygen utilization coefficient, which measures the amount of oxygen in a patient's venous blood in terms of the proportion of oxygen in his arterial blood.

coel- A combining form meaning 'pertaining to a cavity or space': *coeloblastula, coelom, coelosomy.*

-coel, -coele See **-cele.**

coelenteron, *pl.* **coelentera** The digestive cavity of those animals having only two germ layers, as the hydra, jellyfish, coral, and sea ane-

mone. See **archenteron.**

coelom, coeloma, coelome, celom, *pl.* **coeloms, coelomata** The body cavity of the developing embryo. It is situated between the layers of mesoderm and in mammals gives rise to the pericardial, pleural, and peritoneal cavities. A kind of coelom is **extraembryonic coelom.** Also called **somatic cavity.** —**coelomic, celomic,** *adj.*

coelosomy A congenital anomaly characterized by the protrusion of the viscera from the body cavity.

coenesthesia See **cenesthesia.**

coenesthesis See **cenesthesis.**

coenogenesis See **cenogenesis.**

coenzyme A nonprotein substance that combines with an apoenzyme to form a complete enzyme or holoenzyme. Coenzymes include some of the vitamins, as B_1 and B_2, and have smaller molecules than enzymes. Coenzymes are dialyzable and heat stable and usually dissociate easily from the protein portions of the enzymes with which they combine. See also **acetylcoenzyme-A.**

coffee The dried and roasted ripe seeds of the tropical *Coffea arabica, C. liberica,* and *C. robusta* trees. Coffee, containing the alkaloid caffeine, is useful in treating the common headache, chronic asthma, and opium poisoning.

coffee ground vomitus Dark brown vomitus the color and consistency of coffee grounds, composed of gastric juices and old blood and indicative of slow upper gastrointestinal bleeding. Compare **hematemesis.**

coffee worker's lung A respiratory condition caused by an allergic reaction to the dust of the coffee bean. See also **organic dust.**

cognition The mental process characterized by knowing, thinking, learning, and judging. Compare **conation.** —**cognitive,** *adj.*

cognitive development The developmental process by which an infant becomes an intelligent person, acquiring, with growth, knowledge and the ability to think, learn, reason, and abstract. Jean Piaget demonstrated the orderly sequence of this process from early infancy through childhood. See also **psychosexual development, psychosocial development.**

cognitive dissonance A state of tension resulting from a discrepancy in a person's emotional and intellectual frame of reference for interpreting and coping with his environment. It usually occurs when new information contradicts existing assumptions or knowledge.

cognitive function An intellectual process by which one becomes aware of, perceives, or comprehends ideas. It involves all aspects of perception, thinking, reasoning, and remembering. Compare **conation.**

cognitive learning Learning that is concerned with acquisition of problem-solving abilities and with intelligence and conscious thought.

cognitive psychology The study of the development of thought, language, and intelligence in infants and children.

cognitive therapy Any of the various methods of treating mental and emotional disorders that help a person change attitudes, perceptions, and patterns of thinking. Therapeutic approaches include behavior therapy, existential therapy, Gestalt therapy, and transactional analysis.

cogwheel rigidity An abnormal rigor in muscle tissue, characterized by jerky movements when the muscle is passively stretched. Some authorities believe cogwheel rigidity masks a muscular tremor that is not evident until the affected muscle is manipulated.

cohere To stick together, as similar molecules of a common substance. —**coherent,** *adj.*

coherence **1.** The property of sticking together, as the molecules within a common substance. **2.** In psychology: the logical pattern of expression and thought evident in the speech of a normal, stable individual.

cohesive termini In molecular genetics: the complementary single-stranded ends projecting from a double-stranded DNA segment that can be joined to introduced fragments. Also called **sticky ends.**

cohort In statistics: a collection or sampling of individuals who share a common characteristic, as the same age or the same sex.

cohort study In research: a study concerning a specific subpopulation, as the children born between December and May in 1975 and the children born in the same months in 1955. See also **prospective study.**

coil *Informal.* See **intrauterine device.**

coiled tubular gland One of the many multicellular glands that contain one coiled, tube-shaped secretory portion, as the sweat glands.

coil spring contraceptive diaphragm A contraceptive diaphragm, in which the flexible metal spring that forms the rim is a coiled, circular spring that is heavier than a flat spring but lighter than an arcing spring. It is available in 10 sizes, with spring type and rim size stamped on the rim, as, for example, 75-mm coil spring. This kind of diaphragm is prescribed when the vaginal musculature offers good support, the uterus is not acutely retroflexed or anteflexed, and the vagina, neither very long nor very short, has a deeper than usual arch behind the symphysis pubis. Compare **arcing spring contraceptive diaphragm, flat spring contraceptive diaphragm.** See also **contraceptive diaphragm fitting.**

coition See **coitus.**

coitus The sexual union of two people of the jopposite sex in which the penis is introduced into the vagina for copulation, typically resulting in mutual excitation and often orgasm. Also called **coition.** —**coital,** *adj.*

coitus interruptus See **withdrawal method.**

col- **1.** A combining form meaning 'pertaining to the colon': *colalgia, colauxe, colectasia.* **2.** See **co-.**

colation The act of filtering or straining, as urine is often strained for medical examination.

COL bed See **CircOlectric (COL) bed.**

colchicine A drug used to treat acute attacks of gout.

cold **1.** The absence of heat. **2.** A contagious viral infection of the upper respiratory tract, usually caused by a strain of rhinovirus. It is characterized by rhinitis, tearing, low-grade fever, and malaise and is treated symptomatically with rest, mild analgesics, decongestants, and an increased intake of fluids. Also called common cold.

cold abscess A site of infection that does not show common signs of heat, redness, and swelling.

cold agglutinin A nonspecific antibody, found on the surface of red blood cells in certain diseases, that may cause clumping of the cells at temperatures below 4°C (39.2°F)and may cause hemolysis. Mycoplasma pneumonia, infectious mononucleosis, and many lymphoproliferative disorders are associated with cold agglutinins.

cold-blooded Unable to regulate body heat, as fishes, reptiles, and amphibians that have internal temperatures that are close to the temperatures of the environments in which they live. Also called **poikilothermic.** Compare **warm-blooded.**

cold cautery See **cryocautery.**

cold hemoglobinuria See **hemoglobinuria.**

cold injury Any of several abnormal and often serious physical conditions caused by exposure to cold temperatures. See also **chilblain, frostbite, hypothermia, immersion foot.**

cold pressor test A test for the tendency to develop essential hypertension. One hand of the individual is immersed in ice water for about 60 seconds. An excessive rise in the blood pressure or an unusual delay in the return of normal blood pressure when the hand is removed from the water is believed to indicate that the individual has a proclivity for hypertension.

cold-sensitive mutation A genetic alteration resulting in a gene that functions at a high temperature and not at a low temperature.

cold sore See **herpes simplex.**

colectomy Surgical excision of part or all of the colon, performed to treat cancer of the colon or severe chronic ulcerative colitis. For several days before surgery, a low residue diet is prescribed. Antibiotics and cleansing enemas are given to reduce the number of bacteria in the bowel. Parenteral fluids and electrolytes are given, and a nasointestinal tube passed. Under general anesthesia the colon is removed. The nurse gives postoperative care as for any abdominal surgery. The tube is connected to suction and remains in place until bowel sounds are heard. See also **abdominal surgery.**

colestipol hydrochloride An antilipemic agent.

colic **1.** Sharp visceral pain resulting from torsion, obstruction, or smooth muscle spasm of a hollow or tubular organ, as a ureter or the intestines. Kinds of colic include **biliary colic, renal colic.** **2.** Of or pertaining to the colon. —**colicky,** *adj.*

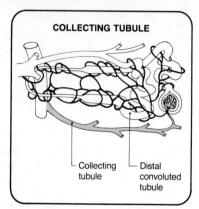

COLLECTING TUBULE

Collecting tubule — Distal convoluted tubule

colicinogen An episome in some strains of *Escherichia coli* that induces secretion of a colicin, a protein lethal to other strains of the bacterium. Specific colicins attach to specific receptors on the cell membrane and impair the synthesis of macromolecules or the production of energy. Also called **colicinogenic factor.**

coliform 1. Of or pertaining to the colonaerogenes group, or the *Escherichia coli* species of microorganisms, constituting most of the intestinal flora in humans and other animals. 2. Having the characteristic of a sieve or cribriform structure, as some of the porous bones of the skull.

colistimethate sodium An antibiotic.

colistin B sulfate An anti-infective otic agent.

colitis An inflammatory condition of the large intestine, either one of the episodic, functional, irritable bowel syndromes or one of the more serious chronic, progressive, inflammatory bowel diseases. Irritable bowel syndrome is characterized by bouts of colicky pain and diarrhea or constipation, often owing to emotional stress. Treatment includes stress reduction and adherence to a diet that may include bland foods and less roughage than in a usual diet. Because individuals with colitis may be irritated by different substances, the diet is individualized to avoid known irritants. Kinds of irritable bowel syndrome are mucous colitis and spastic colon. Inflammatory bowel disease is characterized by abscess formation, severe diarrhea, bleeding, and ulceration of the mucosa of the intestine. Weight loss and pain are significant. Steroids, fluids, electrolytes, antibiotics, and careful attention to diet are the usual modes of therapy. Most of the diseases of this group are of unknown etiology. Kinds of inflammatory bowel disease include **Crohn's disease, ulcerative colitis. —colitic,** *adj.*

collagen A substance consisting of bundles of tiny reticular fibrils, which combine to form the white, glistening, inelastic fibers of the tendons, the ligaments, and the fascia. **—collagenous,** *adj.*

collagenase An enzymatic cleaning and debriding agent that breaks down collagen.

collagen disease Any one of the various abnormal conditions characterized by diffuse immunologic and inflammatory changes in small blood vessels and connective tissue. The cause of most of these diseases is unknown. Hereditary factors and deficiencies, environmental antigens, infections, allergies, and antigen-antibody complexes in various combinations are probably involved. Common features of most of these entities include arthritis, skin lesions, iritis and episcleritis, pericarditis, pleuritis, subcutaneous nodules, myocarditis, vasculitis, and nephritis. Some collagen diseases include polyarteritis nodosa, diseoid and systemic lupus erythematosus, polymyositis, rheumatic fever, and scleroderma. Also called **connective tissue disease.**

collagenoblast A cell that differentiates from a fibroblast and functions in the formation of collagen. It can also transform into cartilage and bone tissue by metaplasia.

collagenous fiber Any one of the tough, white fibers that constitute much of the intercellular substance and the connective tissue of the body. Collagenous fibers contain the protein collagen and are often arranged in bundles that strengthen the tissues in which they are imbedded.

collapse 1. *Nontechnical.* A state of extreme depression or a condition of complete exhaustion owing to physical or to psychosomatic problems. 2. An abnormal condition characterized by shock. 3. The abnormal sagging of an organ or the obliteration of its cavity.

collar Any structure that encircles another, usually around its neck, as the periosteal bone collars that form around the diaphyses of young bones.

collarbone See **clavicle.**

collateral 1. Secondary or accessory. 2. In anatomy: a small branch, as any one of the arterioles or venules in the body.

collateral fissure A fissure separating the subcalcarine and the subcollateral gyri of the cerebral hemisphere.

collecting tubule Any one of the many relatively large straight tubules of the kidney that funnel urine from the distal convoluted tubules in the renal cortex into the renal pelvis. The collecting tubules help maintain fluid balance in the body by allowing water to osmose through their membranes into the interstitial fluid in the renal medulla. Antidiuretic hormone in the blood makes the collecting tubules permeable to water. If no antidiuretic hormone is present in the blood, the membranes of the collecting tubules are practically impermeable to water. See also **Bowman's capsule, kidney.**

collective unconscious In analytic psychology: that portion of the unconscious common to all mankind. Also called **racial unconscious.** See also **analytic psychology.**

collector In medicine: a device with various modifications, used for collecting secretions from the bronchi and the esophagus for bacteriological and cytological examination.

college **1.** An organization of individuals with common professional training and interests, as the American College of Nurse-Midwives, the American College of Cardiology, or the American College of Surgeons. **2.** An institution of higher learning.

Colles' fascia The deep layer of the subcutaneous fascia of the perineum, constituting a distinctive structure in the urogenital region of the body. It is a strong, smooth sheet of tissue containing elastic fibers that give it a characteristic yellow tint. Ventrally, it is continuous with the deep layer of the subcutaneous abdominal fascia and fills a groove between the scrotum and the thigh or between the labium and the thigh; medially, it joins the superficial layer of the subcutaneous perineal fascia to form the dartos tunic of the scrotum or to form the thick fascial sheath of the labium; laterally, it firmly adheres to the ischiopubic ramus; and dorsally, it dips toward the ischiorectal fossa and attaches firmly to deep perineal fascia. In the anal region of the perineum, Colles' fascia adheres to both the superficial layer and the deep layer of the subcutaneous fascia.

Colles' fracture A fracture of the radius at the epiphysis within 1 inch of the joint of the wrist, easily recognized by the dorsal and lateral position of the hand that it causes.

colligative In physical chemistry: of or pertaining to those properties of matter that depend on the number of particles, as molecules and ions, rather than the chemical properties of any substance. One such colligative property is the pressure of a specific volume of gas.

collimator A device for limiting particles of radiation to parallel paths, used to restrict the beam of a radiotherapy machine to a specified area.

colliquation The degeneration of a tissue of the body to a liquid state, usually associated with necrotic tissue.

colliquative Characterized by the profuse discharge of fluid, as suppurating wounds and structures of the body that are infected.

collision tumor A tumor formed as two separate growths, developing close to each other, join. See also **carcinoma.**

collodion, flexible collodion A protectant and wound dressing.

collodion baby An infant whose skin at birth is covered with a scaly, parchmentlike membrane. See also **harlequin fetus, lamellar exfoliation of the newborn.**

colloid A state or division of matter in which large molecules or aggregates of molecules that do not precipitate and that measure between 1 and 100 nm are dispersed in another medium. In a suspension colloid, the particles are insoluble and the medium may be solid, liquid, or gas. In an emulsion colloid, the particles are usually water and the medium is any of several complex hydrophilic, organic substances that become evenly dispersed among the particles of water. Compare **solution, suspension.**

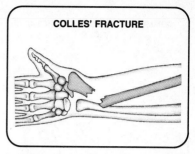

COLLES' FRACTURE

colloid bath A bath taken in water that contains such substances as bran, gelatin, and starch, used to relieve irritation and inflammation. See also **emollient bath.**

colloid carcinoma A former term for mucinous carcinoma.

colloid chemistry The science that deals with the composition and nature of chemical colloids.

colloid goiter A greatly enlarged, soft thyroid gland in which the follicles are distended with colloid.

colo-, colon- A combining form meaning 'pertaining to the colon': *colocolic, colodyspepsia, cololysis.*

coloboma, *pl.* **colobomas, colobomata** A congenital or pathologic defect in the ocular tissue of the body, usually affecting the iris, ciliary body, or choroid by forming a cleft that extends inferiorly. Colobomas are usually the result of the failure of part of the fetal fissure to close. —**colobomatous,** *adj.*

-coloboma A combining form meaning the 'absence or defect of an ocular tissue affecting function, especially of the iris': *blepharocoloboma, iridocoloboma, pseudocoloboma.*

colon The portion of the large intestine extending from the cecum to the rectum. It has four segments: ascending, transverse, descending, and sigmoid colons. —**colonic,** *adj.*

colon- See **colo-.**

-colon A combining form meaning the 'part of the large intestine between the cecum and rectum': *cecocolon, megacolon, paracolon.*

-colonic A combining form meaning 'relating to the colon': *pericolonic, rectocolonic, vesicocolonic.*

colonic fistula An abnormal passage from the colon to the surface of the body or an internal organ or structure. In regional enteritis, chronic inflammation may lead to the formation of a fistula between two adjacent loops of bowel. An external opening from the colon to the surface of the abdomen may be created surgically following the removal of a malignant or severely ulcerated segment of the bowel.

colon stasis See **atonia constipation.**

colony **1.** In bacteriology: a mass of microorganisms in a culture that originates from a single cell. Some kinds of colonies, according to different configurations, are smooth colonies, rough colonies, and dwarf colonies. **2.** In cell

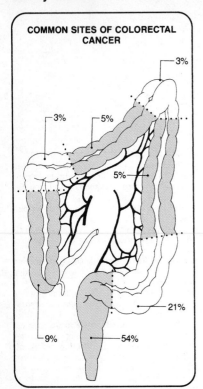

COMMON SITES OF COLORECTAL CANCER

3%
3%
5%
5%
21%
9%
54%

biology: a mass of cells in a culture or in certain experimental tissues, as a spleen colony.

colony counter A device used for counting colonies of bacteria growing in a culture and usually consisting of an illuminated, transparent plate that is divided into sections of known area. Petri dishes containing colonies of bacteria are placed over the plate and the colonies counted according to the number within the areas viewed.

-color A combining form meaning 'hue or hues': *cuticolor, tricolor, versicolor.*

Colorado tick fever A relatively mild, self-limited arbovirus infection transmitted to man by the bite of a tick. It is most prevalent in the spring and summer months throughout the Rocky Mountains, particularly in Colorado. Symptoms, occurring in two phases separated by a period of remission, include chills; fever; headache; pain in the eyes, legs, and back; and sensitivity to light. Treatment is supportive and includes analgesics. Also called American mountain fever. Compare **Rocky Mountain spotted fever.**

color blindness An abnormal condition characterized by an inability to clearly distinguish colors of the spectrum. In most cases it is not a blindness but a weakness in perceiving them distinctly. There are two forms of color blindness. **Daltonism** is the most common form and is characterized by an inability to distinguish reds from greens. It is an inherited, sex-linked disorder. Total color blindness, or achromatic vision, is characterized by an inability to perceive any color at all. Only white, gray, and black are seen. It may be the result of a defect in or the absence of the cones in the retina.

color dysnomia An inability to name colors despite an ability to match and distinguish them. It may be caused by expressive dysphasis.

colorectal cancer A malignant neoplastic disease of the large intestine, characterized by melena, by a change in bowel habits, and by the passing of blood. The diagnosis of colorectal cancer is based on digital rectal examination, testing for blood in the stool, proctosigmoidoscopic examination of the sigmoid, and X-ray studies of the gastrointestinal tract following a barium enema. Malignant tumors of the large bowel usually occur after the age of 50, are slightly more frequent in women than in men, and are almost as common as lung cancer in the United States. The high incidence of colorectal cancer in the western world, as contrasted with the low incidence in Japan and rural Africa, suggests that a diet high in refined carbohydrates and beef and low in roughage may be an etiologic factor. The risk of large bowel cancer is increased in chronic ulcerative colitis, diverticulosis, villous adenomas, and especially in familial polyposis of the colon. People who have inhaled asbestos fibers or who have been irradiated are more likely than others to develop colorectal cancer. In the vermiform appendix, carcinoid is the most common tumor. Most lesions of the large bowel are adenocarcinomas; 54% arise in the rectum, 21% in the sigmoid colon, approximately 9% in the cecum and ascending colon, and the rest in other sites.

colorimetry 1. Measurement of the intensity of color in a fluid or substance. See also **spectrophotometry. 2.** Measurement of color in the blood by use of a colorimeter to determine hemoglobin concentration. The technique is useful only for gross screening purposes, as it is not exact and interpretation is subjective. —**colorimetric,** *adj.*

color index (CI) The ratio between the concentration of hemoglobin and the number of red blood cells in any given sample of blood. The color index is computed by dividing the concentration of hemoglobin, expressed as a percentage of normal concentration, by the approximate number of red blood cells, expressed as a percentage of a normal concentration of 5 million red blood cells per cubic mm. The average color index is about 0.85. Compare *Colour Index.*

color vision A recognition of color as the result of changes in the pigments of the cones in the retina, which react to varying wavelengths of light. The exact mechanisms are not fully understood, but many experts believe they depend on three specialized types of cones, each type responding to red, green, or blue light. Some retinal cones respond to the entire visual spectrum.

colostomate A person who has undergone

any type of a colostomy.

colostomy Surgical creation of an artificial anus on the abdominal wall by incising the colon and bringing it out to the surface, performed for cancer of the colon and benign obstructive tumors. A colostomy may be single-barreled, with one opening; double-barreled, with both distal and proximal loops open onto the abdomen; or a loop colostomy, with a communicating wall between the proximal and distal wall. The colostomy may be located on the ascending, transverse, or sigmoid colon. A temporary colostomy may be done to divert feces from an inflamed area, and repaired when the inflammation subsides. The color of the stoma is checked: a dark blue-black color (rather than bright red) indicates a circulation block, and the surgeon is notified.

colostomy irrigation A procedure used by colostomates to clear the bowel of fecal matter and to help establish an evacuation schedule.

colostrum The fluid secreted by the breast during pregnancy and the first days postpartum before lactation begins, consisting of immunologically active substances and white blood cells, water, protein, fat, and carbohydrates in a thin, yellow, serous fluid.

Colour Index (CI) A publication for dyers, colorists, and textile chemists that specifies all the standard industrial pigments and stains according to five-digit numbers associated with chemical coloring materials, as methylene blue is assigned number 52015. Compare **color index.**

colpo-, colp- A combining form meaning 'pertaining to the vagina': *colpocele, colpocystitis.* Also **kolpo-, kysth-, kystho-.**

columbium Former name for **niobium.**

column chromatography The process of separating and analyzing a group of substances according to the differences in their absorption affinities for a given absorbent as evidenced by pigments deposited during filtration through the same absorbent contained in a glass cylinder or tube. The substances are dissolved in a liquid, which is passed through the absorbent. The absorbates move down the column at different rates and leave behind a band of pigments, which is subsequently washed with a pure solvent to 'develop' discrete pigmented bands that constitute a chromatograph. The cylinder of absorbent is then pushed from the tube, and the individual bands are either separated with a knife or further diluted with the pure solvent and collected in the bottom of the tube for analysis. Compare **gas chromatography, ion-exchange chromatography.**

com- See **co-.**

coma A state of profound unconsciousness, characterized by the absence of spontaneous eye movements, response to painful stimuli, and vocalization. The person cannot be aroused. Coma may be the result of trauma, space-occupying brain tumor, hematoma, toxic condition, acute infectious disease with encephalitis, vascular disease, poisoning, or intoxication. See also

COLOSTOMIES

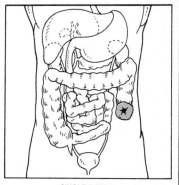

SINGLE-BARREL
COLOSTOMY

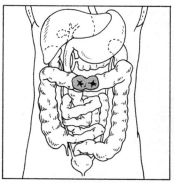

DOUBLE-BARREL
COLOSTOMY

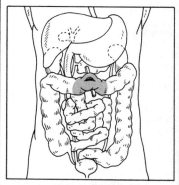

LOOP COLOSTOMY

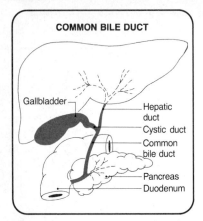

COMMON BILE DUCT

Gallbladder

Hepatic duct

Cystic duct

Common bile duct

Pancreas

Duodenum

Glasgow Coma Scale.

-coma **1.** A combining form meaning '(condition of) profound unconsciousness': *narcoma, semicoma.* **2.** A combining form meaning '(condition of) torpor': *agrypnocoma.*

combat fatigue Any of a variety of psychoneurotic mental disorders, usually temporary but sometimes leading to permanent neurosis, resulting from exhaustion, the stress of combat, or the cumulative emotions and psychological strain of warfare or similar situations. It is characterized by anxiety, depression, irritability, memory and sleep disorders, and various related symptoms. Also called **war neurosis.** See also **posttraumatic stress disorder, shell shock.**

combined anesthesia See **balanced anesthesia.**

combined system disease A disorder of the nervous system caused by a deficiency of vitamin B_{12} that results in pernicious anemia and degeneration of the spinal cord and peripheral nerves, marked by increased difficulty in walking, a feeling of vibration in the legs, and a loss of sense of position. Also known as subacute combined degeneration of the spinal cord. See also **pernicious anemia, cyanocobalamin.**

combining form A component of a word, usually derived from Latin or Greek, that is the base or main stem of the word. It is usually found in combination with a root, prefix, suffix, or all three, as in the words *arthralgia, encephalitis, hepatomegaly,* and *oliguria,* the combining forms are *arthr-, -algia, en-, -cephal-, -itis, hepato-, -megaly,* and *olig-,* and *-uria.*

comedo, *pl.* **comedones** Blackhead, the basic lesion of acne vulgaris, caused by an accumulation of keratin and sebum within the opening of a hair follicle. It is dark owing to the effect of oxygen on sebum, not to the presence of dirt.

comedocarcinoma, *pl.* **comedocarcinomas, comedocarcinomata** A malignant intraductal neoplasm of the breast, in which the central cells degenerate and may be easily

expressed from the cut surface of the tumor. As the growth is confined in the mammary ducts, the prognosis is better than in cases of invasive breast lesions.

comfort, alteration in: pain A nursing diagnosis accepted by the Fifth National Conference on the Classification of Nursing Diagnoses. The etiology of the condition includes injury by biological, chemical, physical, or psychological agents. The defining characteristic is the verbal or nonverbal communication by the client of the presence of pain, including behavior that is self-protective; a narrowed focus that is indicated by an altered time perception, withdrawal from social contact, or impaired thought processes; distraction behavior, marked by moaning, crying, pacing, restlessness, or the seeking out of other people or activities; a facial mask of pain, recognized by eyes that appear dull and lusterless, a 'beaten' look, fixed or scattered facial movements, or grimace; alteration in muscle tone, ranging from listlessness to rigidity; and autonomic responses to increasing pain, including diaphoresis, changes in the blood pressure and pulse rate, pupillary dilatation, and an increased or decreased rate of respiration. See also **nursing diagnosis.**

comfort measure Any action taken to promote comfort of the patient, as a back rub, a change in position, or the prewarming of a stethoscope or a bedpan.

-comma A combining form meaning a 'piece of a structure': *inocomma, myocomma, osteocomma.*

command automatism A condition characterized by an abnormal responsiveness to commands, usually followed without critical judgment, as may be seen in hypnosis and various mental states. See also **automatism.**

commensal Of two different organisms: living together in an arrangement that is not harmful to either and may be beneficial to both. Compare **parasite, synergist.**

comminuted fracture A fracture in which there are several breaks in the bone, creating two or more fragments.

commissurotomy The surgical division of a fibrous band or ring connecting corresponding parts of a body structure. A commissurotomy is commonly performed to separate the thickened, adherent leaves of a stenosed mitral valve.

commitment **1.** The placement or confinement of an individual in a specialized hospital or other institutional facility. See also **institutionalize. 2.** The legal procedure of admitting a mentally ill person to an institution for psychiatric treatment. The process varies from state to state but usually involves judicial or court action based on medical evidence certifying that the person is mentally ill. See also **certification. 3.** A pledge or contract to fulfill some obligation or agreement, used especially in some forms of psychotherapy or marriage counseling.

common bile duct The duct formed by the juncture of the cystic duct and hepatic duct.

common carotid plexus A network of

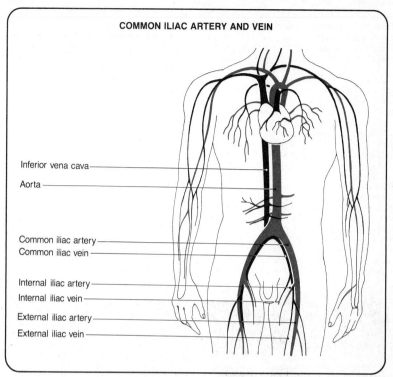

COMMON ILIAC ARTERY AND VEIN

Inferior vena cava

Aorta

Common iliac artery
Common iliac vein

Internal iliac artery
Internal iliac vein

External iliac artery
External iliac vein

nerves on the common carotid artery, supplying sympathetic fibers to the head and the neck, with branches that accompany the cranial blood vessels. The common carotid plexus is formed by the internal and external carotid plexuses and by the cervical ganglia of the sympathetic system. Compare **external carotid plexus, internal carotid plexus.**

common hepatic artery   The visceral branch of the celiac trunk of the abdominal aorta, passing to the pylorus and dividing into five branches, the gastroduodenal, right gastric, right hepatic, left hepatic, and middle hepatic.

common iliac artery   A division of the abdominal aorta, starting to the left of the fourth lumbar vertebra, passing caudally about 5 cm (2 inches), and dividing into external and internal iliac arteries.

common iliac node   A node in one of the seven groups of parietal lymph nodes serving the abdomen and the pelvis. The nodes are arranged in clusters of about five nodes lying along the dorsal aspect of the common iliac artery. They drain the internal and the external iliac nodes and pass their efferents to the lateral aortic nodes. Compare **external iliac node, iliac circumflex node, internal iliac node.** See also **lymph, lymphatic system, lymph node.**

common iliac vein   One of the two veins that are the sources of the inferior vena cava, formed by the union of the internal and the ex-

ternal iliac veins, ventral to the sacroiliac articulation. The right common iliac vein runs almost vertically, ascends dorsal and lateral to its corresponding artery, and is shorter than the left common iliac vein. The left common iliac vein ascends more obliquely, at first to the medial side of the corresponding artery and then dorsal to the right common iliac vein. Each common iliac vein receives the iliolumbar and, in some individuals, the lateral sacral veins. The left common iliac vein also receives the middle sacral vein. Compare **external iliac vein, internal iliac vein.**

communicable disease   Any disease transmitted from one person or animal to another, either directly, by contact with excreta or other discharges from the body; indirectly, via substances or inanimate objects, as contaminated drinking glasses, toys, or water; or via vectors, as flies, mosquitoes, ticks, or other insects. To control a communicable disease it is important to identify the organism, prevent its spread to the environment, protect others against contamination, and treat the infected person. Many communicable diseases, by law, must be reported to the health department. Kinds of communicable diseases include those caused by bacteria, chlamydia, fungi, parasites, rickettsiae, and viruses. Also called **contagious disease.** See also **infectious disease.**

Communicable Disease Center   Former

name of the **Centers for Disease Control.**

communicating hydrocephalus See **hydrocephalus.**

communication Any process in which a message containing information is transferred, especially from one person to another, via any of a number of media. Communication may be verbal or nonverbal; it may occur directly, as in a face-to-face conversation or with the observation of a gesture; or it may occur remotely, spanning space and time, as in writing and reading or in making or playing back a recording.

communication channels In communication theory: any gesture, action, sound, written word, or visual image used in transmitting messages.

communication, impaired verbal A nursing diagnosis accepted by the Fifth National Conference on the Classification of Nursing Diagnoses. The etiology of the condition includes decreased circulation to the brain; a physical barrier to speech, as a brain tumor, laryngectomy, tracheostomy, or intubation; an anatomical deficit, as a cleft palate; a psychological barrier, as a psychosis or lack of stimuli; a cultural difference; or a developmental or age-related factor. The defining characteristics of the condition include slurring, stuttering, difficulty in forming words or sentences, difficulty in expressing thoughts verbally, inappropriate verbalization, dyspnea, or disorientation. The critical defining characteristics, one of which must be present for the diagnosis to be made, are an inability to speak the dominant language of the culture, a difficulty in speaking or verbalizing, or the absence of speech. See also **nursing diagnosis.**

communication theory A theory that describes a model of a system of communication consisting of a source of information (the sender), a transmitter, a communication channel, a source of noise (interference), a receiver, and a purpose for the message.

community health nursing A field of nursing that is a blend of primary health care and nursing practice with public health nursing. The philosophy of care is based on the belief that care directed to the individual, the family, and the group contributes to the health care of the population as a whole. Participation of all consumers of health care is encouraged in the development of community activities that contribute to the promotion, education, and maintenance of good health. These activities require comprehensive health programs that pay special attention to social and ecological influences and specific populations at risk.

community medicine A branch of medicine that is concerned with the health of the members of a community, municipality, or region.

community mental health center (CMHC) A community-based center that provides comprehensive mental health services. The specific services to be provided are specified in an act of Congress, the Community Mental Health Centers Act; these requirements have been updated periodically. The costs of consultation and educational services, instruction, development, and initial operation of the facility are provided by the federal government. The organization, management, and operation of CMHCs are specified by the Act. Consumer representation in each of these areas is required.

community nurse practitioner (CNP) A nurse who has completed a postbaccalaureate program in community nursing.

companionship In psychiatric nursing: the assignment of a staff member or of another patient to stay with a disturbed patient to provide support and to protect the patient from self-harm or the harming of others.

comparative anatomy The study of the morphology and function of all living animals. A comparison of the forms indicates a progression on a scale from the simplest to the most highly specialized animals. See also **applied anatomy, ontogeny, phylogeny.**

comparative embryology The study of the similarities and differences among various organisms during the embryologic period of development.

comparative psychology **1.** The study of human behavior as it relates to or differs from animal behavior. **2.** The study of the psychological and behavioral differences among various peoples.

compatibility **1.** The quality or state of existing together in harmony; congruity. **2.** The orderly, efficient integration of the elements of one system with those of another. **3.** The formation of a stable chemical or biochemical system, specifically in medication, so that two or more drugs can be administered at the same time without producing undesired side effects or without canceling or changing the therapeutic effects of the others. **4.** In immunology: the degree to which the body's defense system will tolerate the presence of foreign material, as transfused blood, grafted tissue, or transplanted organs, without an immune reaction; usually complete compatibility exists between identical twins. **5.** In blood grouping or crossmatching: the lack of reaction between blood groups so that there is no agglutination when the red blood cells of one sample are mixed with the serum of another sample; no reaction from transfused blood. **—compatible,** *adj.*

compendium, *pl.* **compendia** A collected body of information on the standards of strength, purity, and quality of drugs. The official compendia in the United States are the *United States Pharmacopoeia,* the *Homeopathic Pharmacopoeia of the United States,* the *National Formulary,* and their supplements. See also **formulary.**

compensated gluteal gait One of the more common abnormal gaits associated with a weakness of the gluteus medius. It is a variation of the Trendelenburg gait and involves the dropping of the pelvis on the unaffected side of the body during the walking cycle between the moment of heelstrike on the affected side and the moment of heelstrike on the unaffected side. The compensated gluteal gait is also characterized by the dropping of the entire trunk downward and sideways over the affected hip and a short step on the unaffected side.

compensated heart failure   An abnormal cardiac condition in which heart failure is compensated for by normal compensatory mechanisms, as increased sympathetic adrenergic stimulation of the heart, fluid retention with increased venous return, increased end-diastolic ventricular volume and fiber length, and hypertrophy. Compensation may also occur through the administration of digitalis glycosides, with associated improved myocardial function, or by diuresis. However, diuretics may relieve only the symptoms of pulmonary and peripheral congestion and merely appear to compensate for the ventricular function, which remains severely abnormal.

compensating current   An electric current that neutralizes the intensity of a muscle current.

compensation   A complex defense mechanism that allows one to avoid the unpleasant or painful emotional stimuli that result from a feeling of inferiority or inadequacy. This is accomplished by any of several patterns of behavior, for example, one in which an extraordinary effort is spent in overcoming a handicap, one in which the quality lacking is scorned ("sour grapes"), one in which hard work and excellent performance in one field are substituted for a lack of ability in another, or one in which a fantasy of excellence, achievement, or perfection replaces awareness of a weakness or failure. See also **overcompensation.**

compensation neurosis   An unconscious process by which one prolongs the symptoms resulting from an injury or disease in order to receive secondary gains, especially money. Compare **malingering.**

competence   In embryology: the total capacity of an embryonic cell to react to determinative stimuli in various ways of differentiation. A kind of competence is **embryonic competence.** See also **potency.**

competitive antagonist   See **antimetabolite.**

competitive identification   The unconscious modeling of one's personality on that of another as a means of outdoing or bettering the other person. See also **identification.**

complaint   **1.** In law: a pleading by a plaintiff made under oath to initiate a suit. It is a statement of the formal charge and the cause for action against the defendant. For a minor offense, the defendant is tried on the basis of the complaint. A more serious felony prosecution requires an indictment with evidence presented by a state's attorney. **2.** *Informal.* Any ailment, problem, or symptom identified by the client, patient, member of the person's family, or other knowledgeable person. The chief complaint is

often the reason that the person has sought health care.

complement   One of 11 complex, enzymatic, serum proteins. In an antigen-antibody reaction, complement causes lysis. Complement is also involved in other physiological reactions including anaphylaxis and phagocytosis. See also **antibody, antigen, antigen-antibody reaction, immune globulin.**

complement abnormality   An unusual condition characterized by deficiencies or by dysfunctions of any of the nine functional components of the enzymatic proteins of blood serum. The components are labeled C1 through C9. The most common abnormalities are C2 and C3 deficiencies and C5 familial dysfunction. Patients with complement deficiencies or with complement dysfunctions may be more susceptible to infections and to collagen vascular diseases. Studies indicate that primary complement deficiencies may be inherited. Secondary complement deficiencies may stem from immunologic reactions, as drug-induced serum disease, which depletes complement. Complement deficiencies may be associated with other illnesses, as acute streptococcal glomerulonephritis and acute systemic lupus erythematosus. It is difficult and often expensive to diagnose complement abnormalities, but some indications are EKG conduction abnormalities, detection of complement and immunoglobulin in the walls of blood vessels in glomerulonephritis, cerebrospinal fluid pleocytosis, increased erythrocyte sedimentation rate, and the presence in urine of RBCs, RBC casts, and protein. Replacement of complement-fixing antibodies and the control of infection and associated illnesses are part of the standard treatment of complement abnormalities. The patient with complement deficiency or dysfunction commonly receives transfusions of fresh plasma to replace antibodies. Bone marrow transplants and injections of gamma globulin may also be employed. Complement abnormalities may usually be temporarily corrected by replacement therapy, but no permanent cure is yet available.

NURSING CONSIDERATIONS: With plasma infusions, careful matching of leukocytes for HL-A cell types is important to prevent graft-versus-host reaction and other undesirable responses. Bone marrow transplants require close monitoring for transfusion reactions and are usually followed by instructions to the patient for scrupulous hygiene, prompt treatment of the smallest wound, and avoidance of persons with active infection.

complemental inheritance   The acquisition or expression of a trait or condition from the presence of two independent pairs of nonallelic genes. Both of the genes must be present for the characteristic to appear in the phenotype.

complementary gene   Either member of two or more nonallelic gene pairs that interact to produce an effect not expressed in the absence of any of the pairs. Also called **reciprocal gene.**

complement fixation   An immunologic re-

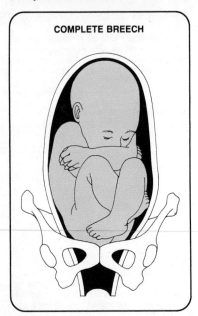

COMPLETE BREECH

action in which an antigen combines with an antibody and its complement, causing the complement factor to become inactive or 'fixed.' The complement fixation reaction can be tested in the laboratory by exposing the patient's serum to antigen, complement, and specially sensitized red blood cells. Complement fixation tests are widely used to detect antibodies for infectious diseases, especially syphilis and viral illnesses. See also **complement, immune system, immunity, Wassermann test.**

complement-fixation test (C-F test) Any serological test in which complement-fixation is detected, indicating the presence of a particular antigen. Specific C-F tests aid diagnosis of amebiasis, Rocky Mountain spotted fever, trypanosomiasis, and typhus.

complete abortion Termination of pregnancy in which the conceptus is expelled or removed in its entirety. Surgical evacuation is not necessary. Compare **incomplete abortion.**

complete blood count (CBC) A determination of the number of red and white blood cells per cubic millimeter of blood. A complete blood count is one of the most routinely performed tests in a clinical laboratory and one of the most valuable screening and diagnostic techniques. The count can be performed manually by staining a smear of blood on a slide and counting the different types of cells under a microscope. Most laboratories use an electronic counter for reporting numbers of red and white blood cells. Platelets are more difficult to count automatically, and many laboratories continue to do this manually. Many electronic blood counters, such as the Coulter counter, also automatically determine hemoglobin or hematocrit

and include this value in the complete blood count. See also **differential white blood cell count, hematocrit, hemoglobin.**

complete breech A fetal presentation in which the fetus presents with the legs folded on the thighs and the thighs on the abdomen. The position of the fetus is the same as in a normal vertex presentation, but upside down.

complete fistula An abnormal passage from an internal organ or structure to the surface of the body or to another internal organ or structure.

complete fracture A bone break that completely disrupts the continuity of osseous tissue across the entire width of the bone involved.

complete health history A health history that includes a history of the present illness, a health history, social history, occupational history, sexual history, and a family health history. See also **health history.**

complete rachischisis A rare congenital fissure of the entire vertebral column and spinal cord resulting from the failure of the embryonic neural tube to close. The condition is characterized by flaccid paralysis and impaired sensations. It is often accompanied by other birth defects, as cleft palate, harelip, and hydrocephalus, and is frequently fatal. Also called **holorachischisis, rachischisis totalis.** See also **spina bifida.**

complex 1. A group of items, as chemical molecules, that are related in structure or function, as the iron and protein portions of hemoglobin or the cobalt and protein portions of vitamin B_{12}. 2. A combination of signs and symptoms of disease that forms a syndrome. 3. In psychology: a group of associated ideas with strong emotional overtones affecting a person's attitudes.

complex fracture A closed fracture in which the soft tissue surrounding the bone is severely damaged.

complex protein A protein that contains a simple protein and at least one molecule of another substance, as a glycoprotein, nucleoprotein, or hemoglobin.

compliance 1. Fulfillment by the patient of the prescribed course of treatment. 2. The quality of yielding to pressure, as in elastic distensibility of an air- or fluid-filled organ, such as the bladder or lung.

component drip set A device used for delivering intravenous fluids, especially whole blood. It includes plastic tubing and a combination drip-chamber and filter. Compare **component syringe set, microaggregate recipient set, straight-line blood set, Y-set.**

component syringe set A device used for delivering intravenous fluids. It includes plastic tubing, two slide clamps, a Y-connector and a syringe. The component syringe set may be used in various procedures, as in the transfusion of platelets and in the transfusion of cryoprecipitates. In such transfusions, the component syringe set is used primarily to avoid clogging the intravenous line. Compare **component drip set,**

235

microaggregate recipient set, straight-line blood set, Y-set.

component therapy A kind of transfusion in which specific blood components are administered instead of whole blood. Packed red cells or platelet-rich plasma suspensions may be transfused in larger quantities than would be possible if whole blood were used. More sophisticated processing provides fibrinogen or antihemophilic globulin solutions for administration in therapeutic amounts in excess of what might be given with conventional blood transfusion therapy. Compare **plasmaphoresis.** See also **packed cells, pooled plasma.**

compound 1. In chemistry: a substance composed of two or more different elements, chemically combined in definite proportions, that cannot be separated by physical means. 2. Any substance composed of two or more different ingredients. 3. To make a substance by combining ingredients, as a pharmaceutical. 4. Denoting an injury characterized by multiple factors, as a compound fracture.

compound aneurysm A localized dilatation of an arterial wall in which some of the layers are distended and others are ruptured or dissected. Also called **mixed aneurysm.**

compound benzoin tincture A demulcent and protectant.

compound fracture A fracture in which the broken end or ends of the bone have torn through the skin. Also called **open fracture.**

compound melanocytoma See **benign juvenile melanoma.**

compound monster A fetus in which some of the parts or organs are duplicated but not fully developed.

compound tubuloalveolar gland One of the many multicellular glands with more than one secretory duct that contains both tube-shaped and sac-shaped portions, as the salivary glands.

comprehensive care See **holistic health care.**

compress A soft pad, usually made of cloth, used to apply heat, cold, or medications to the surface of a body area. A compress also may be applied over a wound to help control bleeding. Compare **dressing.**

compression The act of pressing, squeezing, or otherwise applying pressure to an organ, tissue, or body area. Kinds of pathological compression include **compression fracture,** in which bone surfaces are forced against each other, causing a break, and compression paralysis, marked by paralysis of a body area due to pressure on a nerve.

compression fracture A bone break, especially in a short bone, that disrupts osseous tissue and collapses the affected bone. The bodies of vertebrae are often sites of compression fractures.

compression neuropathy Any of several disorders involving damage to sensory nerve roots or peripheral nerves, caused by mechanical pressure or localized trauma and characterized by paresthesia, weakness, or paralysis. The car-

---

USES OF WHOLE BLOOD COMPONENTS

Whole blood
- To restore an adequate volume of blood in hemorrhaging, trauma, or burn patients

Red blood cells (packed, frozen)
- To correct RBC deficiency and improve oxygen-carrying capacity of blood
- To transfuse organ transplant patients or for patients with repeated febrile transfusion reactions (use frozen-thawed RBCs because the allogeneic leukocytes are destroyed with freezing)

White blood cells (leukocyte concentrate)
- To treat the patient who has life-threatening granulocytopenia from intensive chemotherapy, especially if infections are not responsive to antibiotics

Plasma (fresh, fresh frozen)
- To treat a clotting factor deficiency (when specific concentrates are unavailable or precise deficiency is unknown), hypovolemia, or a patient with a severe hepatic disease who has a limited synthesis of plasma coagulation factors
- To prevent dilutional hypocoagulability

Platelets
- To treat the patient with thrombocytopenia whose bleeding is caused by the following: decreased platelet production, increased platelet destruction, functionally abnormal platelets, or massive transfusions of stored blood (dilutional thrombocytopenia)

Plasma protein fraction
- To treat hypovolemic shock or hypoproteinemia
- For initial treatment of infants in shock or children who are dehydrated or who have electrolyte deficiencies
- May be used cautiously when the patient has congestive heart failure from added fluid and salt load or renal or hepatic failure from added protein load

Albumin 5% (buffered saline)
Albumin 25% (salt-poor)
- To treat shock from burns, trauma, surgery, or infections
- To prevent marked hemoconcentration
- To maintain electrolyte VIII balance
- To treat hypoproteinemia (with or without edema)

Factor VIII (cryoprecipitate concentrate AHF)
- To treat a patient with hemophilia A
- To control bleeding associated with factor deficiency
- To replace fibrinogen or factor XIII

Factors II, VII, IX, X complex
- Before surgery to treat congenital deficiencies of factors II, VII, IX, or X complex and provide a hemostatic level
- To arrest severe hemorrhaging

COMPUTERIZED TOMOGRAPHY SCANNER

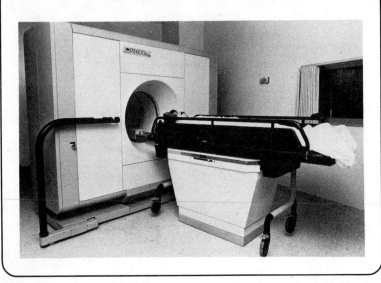

pal, peroneal, radial, and ulnar nerves are most commonly involved. Compare **neuritis.** See also **paresthesia.**

compressor naris The transverse part of the nasalis muscle that serves to depress the cartilage of the nose and to draw the ala toward the septum. Compare **dilatator naris.**

compromised host A person who is less able than normal to resist infection, owing to immunosuppressive therapy, immunologic defect, severe anemia, or concurrent disease or condition.

compulsion An irresistible, repetitive, irrational impulse to perform an act that is usually contrary to one's ordinary judgments or standards yet results in overt anxiety if it is not completed. The impulse is usually the result of an obsession. A kind of compulsion is **repetition compulsion.** See also **obsession. —compulsive,** *adj.*

compulsive personality A type of character structure in which there is a pattern of chronic and obsessive adherence to rigid standards of conduct. The person is usually excessively conscientious and inhibited, is extremely inflexible, has an extraordinary capacity for work, and lacks a normal ability to relax and to relate to other people. The compulsive person is likely to follow repetitive patterns of behavior, as snapping the fingers, crossing the legs, tapping the foot, or refusing to walk on cracks in the sidewalk, and often leads an impoverished emotional life, being dominated by a need for order, cleanliness, punctuality, rules, and systems. See also **obsessive-compulsive neurosis.**

compulsive personality disorder A condition in which an irrational preoccupation

with order, rules, ritual, and detail interferes with everyday functioning and normal behavior. Psychotherapy is the usual treatment and may include behavior therapy with desensitization and flooding in order to reduce maladaptive anxiety. See also **compulsive personality, obsessive-compulsive neurosis.**

compulsive polydipsia See **polydipsia.**

computerized tomography (CT), computerized axial tomography (CAT) In radiology: a technique in which an EMI scanner, comprising an X-ray tube, two scintillation detectors, a line printer, teletyper, and a computer and magnetic disc unit, is used to attain a series of detailed visualizations of the tissues of brain at any depth desired. The procedure is painless, noninvasive, and requires no special preparation. The head is scanned in two planes simultaneously at various angles. The computer calculates tissue absorption, displays a printout of the numerical values, and produces a visualization of the tissues that demonstrates the densities of the various intracranial structures. Tumor masses, infarctions, bone displacement, and accumulations of fluid may be detected. Also called computerized transverse axial tomography, CT scan.

con- See **co-.**

CONA *abbr* **Canadian Orthopedic Nurses' Association.**

conation The mental process characterized by desire, impulse, volition, and striving. Compare **cognition. —conative,** *adj.*

concentrate **1.** To decrease the bulk of a liquid and increase its strength per unit of volume by the removal of inactive ingredients through evaporation or other means. **2.** A substance, particularly a liquid, that has been strengthened and reduced in volume through such means.

concentric Describing two or more circles that share a common center.

concentric fibroma A fibrous tumor surrounding the uterine cavity.

concept A construct or abstract idea or thought that originates and is held within the mind. —**conceptual,** *adj.*

conception 1. The beginning of pregnancy, usually taken to be the instant that a spermatozoon enters an ovum. **2.** The act or process of fertilization. **3.** The act or process of creating an idea or notion. **4.** The idea or notion created; a general impression resulting from the interpretation of a symbol or set of symbols. —**conceptive,** *adj.*

conceptual framework A group of concepts that are broadly defined and systematically organized to provide a focus, a rationale, and a tool for the integration and interpretation of information. Usually expressed abstractly using word models, a conceptual framework is the basis for many theories, as communication theory and general systems theory.

conceptus The products of conception; the fertilized ovum and its enclosing membranes at all stages of intrauterine development, from the time of implantation to birth. See also **embryo, fetus.**

concha A body part or structure that resembles the spiral curvature of a shell, such as the outer ear (pinna); or the turbinate bones of the nasal cavity: the superior, inferior and middle conchae.

concordance In genetics: the expression of one or more specific traits in both members of a pair of twins. Compare **discordance.** —**concordant,** *adj.*

concrete thinking A stage in the development of the cognitive thought processes in the child. During this phase, thought becomes increasingly logical and coherent so that the child is able to classify, sort, order, and organize facts but is incapable of generalizing or dealing in abstractions. Problem solving is accomplished in a concrete, systematic fashion based on what is perceived, keeping to the literal meaning of words, as the word *horse* applying to a particular animal and not to horses in general. In Piaget's classification, this stage occurs between 7 and 11 years of age, is preceded by syncretic thinking, and is followed by abstract thinking.

concurrent nursing audit See **nursing audit.**

concurrent validity Validity of a test or a measurement tool that is established by concurrently applying a previously validated tool or test to the same phenomena or data base and comparing the results. Concurrent validity is achieved if the results are the same or similar at a statistically significant level. See also **validity.**

concussion A violent jarring or shaking, as caused by a blow or an explosion.

condition 1. A state of being, specifically in reference to physical and mental health or well-being. **2.** Anything that is essential for or that restricts or modifies the appearance or occurrence of something else. **3.** To train the body or mind, usually through specific exercises and repeated exposure to a particular state or thing. **4.** In psychology: to subject a person or animal to conditioning or associative learning so that a specific stimulus will always elicit a particular response. See also **classical conditioning.**

conditioned avoidance response A learned reaction that is performed either consciously or unconsciously in order to avoid an unpleasant or painful stimulus or to prevent such stimuli from occurring.

conditioned escape response A learned reaction that is performed either consciously or unconsciously in order to stop or to escape from an aversive stimulus.

conditioned response An automatic reaction to a stimulus that does not normally elicit such response but which has been learned through training. Such responses can be physical or psychological and are produced by repeated association of some physiological function or behavioral pattern with an unrelated stimulus or event. In Pavlov's classic experiments, dogs learned to associate the ringing of a bell with feeding time so that they would salivate at the sound of the bell regardless of whether or not food was given to them. Also called acquired reflex, behavior reflex, conditioned reflex, trained reflex. Compare **unconditioned response.** See also **classical conditioning.**

conditioning A form of learning based on the development of a response or set of responses to a stimulus or series of stimuli. Kinds of conditioning are **classical conditioning, operant conditioning.**

condom A soft, flexible sheath that covers the penis and prevents semen from entering the vagina in sexual intercourse, used to avoid infection and as a contraceptive. Condoms are made of plastic, rubber, or skin. Also called **prophylactic.**

conduction 1. In physics: **a.** A process in which heat is transferred from one substance to another owing to a difference in temperature. **b.** A process in which energy is transmitted through a conductor. **2.** In physiology: the process by which a nerve impulse is transmitted.

conduction anesthesia A loss of sensation, especially pain, in a region of the body, produced by injecting a local anesthetic along the course of a nerve or nerves to inhibit the conduction of impulses to and from the area supplied by that nerve or nerves. Also called **block anesthesia, nerve block anesthesia.**

conduction aphasia A dissociative speech phenomenon in which there is no difficulty in comprehending words seen or heard and in which there is no dysarthria, yet the patient has problems in self-expression. The patient may substitute words similar in sound or meaning to the correct ones, but is unable to repeat from dictation, to spell, and to read aloud. The patient

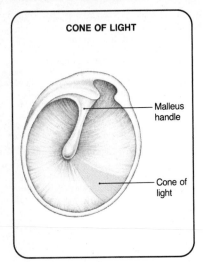

CONE OF LIGHT

Malleus handle

Cone of light

is alert and aware of the deficit. A common cause is an embolus in a branch of the middle cerebral artery. See also **aphasia.**

conductive hearing loss   A form of hearing loss in which sound is inadequately conducted through the external or middle ear to the sensorineural apparatus of the inner ear. Sensitivity to sound is diminished, but clarity (interpretation of the sound) is not changed. If volume is increased to compensate for the loss, hearing is normal. Compare **sensorineural hearing loss.**

condylar fracture   Any fracture of the round end of a hinge joint, usually occurring at the distal end of the humerus or at the distal end of the femur, frequently detaching a small bone fragment that includes the condyle.

condyle   A rounded projection at the end of a bone that anchors muscle ligaments and articulates with adjacent bones.

-condyle   A combining form meaning 'a knucklelike projection on a bone': *entepicondyle, epicondyle, entocondyle.* Also **-condylus.**

condyloid joint   A synovial joint in which a condyle is received into an elliptical cavity, as the wrist joint. A condyloid joint permits no axial rotation but allows flexion, extension, adduction, abduction, and circumduction. Also called **articulatio ellipsoidea.** Compare **pivot joint.**

condyloma, *pl.* **condylomata**   A wartlike growth on the anus, vulva, or glans penis.

condyloma latum, *pl.* **condylomata lata**   A flat, moist, papular growth that appears in secondary syphilis in the coronal sulcus of the perineum or on the glans penis.

condylomatum acuminatum   A soft, wartlike or papillomatous growth common on the warm and moist skin and mucous membrane of the genitalia. It is caused by a virus and is transmitted by sexual contact. Also called **acuminate wart, venereal wart.**

-condylus   See **-condyle.**

cone   **1.** A photoreceptor cell in the retina of the eye that enables a person to visualize colors. There are three kinds of retinal cones, one for each of the colors, blue, green, and red; other colors are seen by stimulation of more than one type of cone. **2.** A cone-shaped device attached to radiological equipment to focus X-rays on a small target of tissue. **3.** See **cone of light.** See also **cone biopsy.** —**conic, conical,** *adj.*

cone biopsy   Surgical removal of a cone-shaped segment of cervix, including both epithelial and endocervical tissue. The cone of tissue is examined microscopically to establish a precise diagnosis, usually to confirm or evaluate a positive Papanicolaou test.

cone of light   **1.** A triangular reflection observed during an ear examination when the light of an otoscope is focused on the image of the malleus. **2.** The group of light rays entering the pupil of the eye and forming an image on the retina.

confabulation   The fabrication of experiences or situations, often recounted in a detailed and plausible way in order to fill in and cover up gaps in the memory. The phenomenon occurs principally as a defense mechanism and is most commonly seen in alcoholics, especially those who have Korsakoff's psychosis. Also called fabrication.

configurationism   See **Gestalt psychology.**

confinement   **1.** A state of being held or restrained within a specific place in order to hinder or minimize activity. **2.** The final phase of pregnancy during which labor and childbirth occur; parturition. See also **puerperium.**

conflict   **1.** A mental struggle, either conscious or unconscious, resulting from the simultaneous presence of opposing or incompatible thoughts, ideas, goals, or emotional forces, as impulses, desires, or drives. **2.** A painful state of consciousness caused by the arousal of such opposing forces and the inability to resolve them; a kind of stress found to a certain degree in every person. **3.** In psychoanalysis: the unconscious emotional struggle between the demands of the id and those of the ego and superego or between the demands of the ego and the restrictions imposed by society. Kinds of conflict include **approach-approach conflict, approach-avoidance conflict, avoidance-avoidance conflict, extrapsychic conflict, intrapsychic conflict.**

confluence of the sinuses   The wide junction of the superior sagittal, the straight, and the occipital sinuses with the two large transverese sinuses of the dura mater. The right tranverse sinus usually receives most of the blood from the superior sagittal sinus, and the left transverse sinus receives the blood from the straight sinus. The confluence is one of six posterior superior sinuses of the dura matter, draining blood from the section and an inner bulging granular section.

confusion   A mental state characterized by

disorientation regarding time, place, or person, causing bewilderment, perplexity, lack of orderly thought, and inability to choose or act decisively. It is usually symptomatic of an organic mental disorder, but it may accompany severe emotional stress and various psychological disorders. —**confusional,** *adj.*

confusional insanity   See **amentia.** See also **Stearns' alcoholic amentia.**

congenital   Present at birth.

congenital absence of sacrum and lumbar vertebrae   An abnormal condition present at birth and characterized by varying degrees of deformity, ranging from the absence of the lower segment of the coccyx to the absence of the entire sacrum and all lumbar vertebrae. Lesser degrees of this anomaly may present so few signs that marked deformities are not present, and the condition may not be diagnosed unless accidentally found on radiographic examination. Signs and symptoms of the more severe kinds may include short stature, flattened buttocks, muscle paralysis to varying degrees, muscle atrophy in the lower extremities, foot deformities, contractures of the hips and the knees, and varying degrees of loss of sensation, especially sensation distal to the knees. The treatment varies greatly for the congenital absence of the sacrum and the lumbar vertebrae and depends on severity. Surgical intervention may be reconstructive or may involve disarticulation procedures at various spinal levels and subsequent fusion of the remaining vertebrae. Depending on the severity, many patients with this anomaly may be surgically provided with enough stability to sit and to walk with assistance. The most severe forms are usually fatal.

congenital adrenal hyperplasia   See **adrenogenital syndrome.**

congenital amputation   The absence of a fetal limb or part at birth, previously attributed to amputation by constricting bands in utero but now regarded as a developmental defect.

congenital anomaly   Any abnormality present at birth, particularly a structural one, which may be inherited genetically, acquired during gestation, or inflicted during parturition. Also called **birth defect.**

congenital cardiac anomaly   Any structural or functional abnormality or defect of the heart or great vessels existing from birth. Congenital heart disease is a major cause of neonatal distress and is the most common cause of death in the newborn other than problems related to prematurity. The incidence of congenital cardiovascular anomalies is 8 to 10 per 1,000 live births, with the mortality rate greatest in the neonatal period. Most defects are probably owing to some interaction between genetic and environmental factors that results in arrested embryonic development. Congenital heart anomalies are classified broadly according to the resulting alteration in circulation, as acyanotic, in which no unoxygenated blood mixes in the systemic system; or cyanotic, in which unoxygenated blood enters the systemic system. The general effects of cardiac malformations on cardiovascular functioning are increased cardiac workload, involving either systolic or diastolic overloading, increased pulmonary vascular resistance, inadequate systemic cardiac output, and decreased oxygen saturation from the shunting of unoxygenated blood directly into the systemic system. The general physical symptoms of these pathophysiological alterations are growth retardation, decreased exercise tolerance, recurrent respiratory infections, dyspnea, tachypnea, tachycardia, cyanosis, tissue hypoxia, and murmurs, all of which vary in severity depending on the type and degree of the defect. Kinds of congenital cardiac anomalies include **aortic stenosis, atrial septal defect, coarctation of the aorta, patent ductus arteriosus, pulmonic stenosis, tetralogy of Fallot, transposition of the great vessels, tricuspid atresia, truncus arteriosus, ventricular septal defect.**

congenital cloaca   See **persistent cloaca.**

congenital dermal sinus   A channel present at birth, extending from the surface of the body and passing between the bodies of two adjacent lumbar vertebrae to the spinal canal.

congenital dislocation of the hip   A congenital orthopedic defect in which the head of the femur does not articulate with the acetabulum, owing to an abnormal shallowness of the acetabulum. Treatment consists of maintaining continuous abduction of the thigh so that the head of the femur presses into the center of the shallow cavity, causing it to deepen. Also called congenital dysplasia of the hip, **congenital subluxation of the hip.** See also **Frejka splint.**

congenital glaucoma   A rare form of glaucoma affecting infants and young children, resulting from a congenital closure of the iridocorneal angle by a membrane that obstructs the flow of aqueous humor and increases the intraorbital pressure. The condition is progressive, usually bilateral, and may damage the optic nerve. It may be corrected surgically. Also called **buphthalmos, hydrophthalmos.**

congenital goiter   An enlargement of the thyroid gland at birth or caused by a congenital deficiency of enzymes required for the production of thyroxine.

congenital heart disease   See **congenital cardiac anomaly.**

congenital hypoplastic anemia   See **Blackfan-Diamond syndrome.**

congenital megacolon   See **Hirschsprung's disease.**

congenital nonspherocytic hemolytic anemia   A large group of blood disorders made up of a number of similar inherited diseases, each with a deficiency of one of the enzymes of red cell glycolysis. Most are associated with varying degrees of hemolysis, but all are less severe than and are to be differentiated from the more serious disorder associated with spherocytosis. Compare **spherocytic anemia.** See also **sickle cell anemia.**

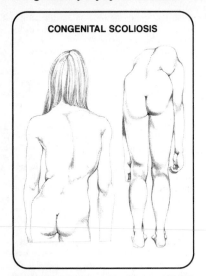

CONGENITAL SCOLIOSIS

congenital polycystic disease (CPD)
See polycystic kidney disease.

congenital pulmonary arteriovenous fistula A direct connection between the arterial and venous systems of the lung present at birth that results in a right-to-left shunt and permits unoxygenated blood to enter systemic circulation. The fistula may be single or multiple and may occur in any part of the lung. Surgical correction is the only effective method of treatment, if it is in an accessible site.

congenital scoliosis An abnormal condition present at birth, characterized by a lateral curvature of the spine, resulting from specific congenital rib and vertebral anomalies. The etiological and the pathological characteristics of congenital scoliosis are divided into six categories. Category I is associated with partial unilateral failure of the formation of a vertebra. Category II is associated with complete unilateral failure of the formation of a vertebra. Category III is associated with bilateral failure of segmentation with the absence of disk space. Category IV is associated with the unilateral failure of segmentation with the unsegmented bar. Category V is associated with the fusion of ribs. Category VI is associated with any condition not covered in the other categories. The degree of obvious deformity caused by congenital scoliosis depends on the cause of the disease. The deformity increases with growth and age, usually progressing slowly during periods of slow growth of the trunk of the body. Diagnosis of the specific congenital anomaly may be confirmed by radiographic examination. Treatment of congenital scoliosis may be surgical or nonsurgical. Some kinds of nonsurgical treatment techniques are exercise programs and the use of orthotic devices. Surgical intervention in this disease may involve an anterior or a posterior spinal fusion.

congenital short neck syndrome A rare congenital malformation of the cervical spine in which the cervical vertebrae are fused, usually in pairs, into one mass of bone, resulting in decreased neck motion and decreased cervical length, sometimes with neurologic involvement. The posterior portion of the laminar arches in the cervical area is not fully developed, resulting in spina bifida in the cervical region, usually involving the lower cervical vertebrae and, in some cases, one or more of the upper thoracic vertebrae. The extreme shortness of the neck is the most common sign of this deformity, which allows only limited motion, lateral bending, and rotation. When the deformity involves nerve root compression, symptoms of peripheral nerve involvement, as pain or a burning sensation, may be evident, accompanied by paralysis, hyperesthesia, or paresthesia. Involvement of the spinal cord may present signs of abnormalities of lower extremities with associated signs of an upper motor lesion. Congenital short neck syndrome may require no treatment. Mild associated symptoms may be alleviated with traction, cast application, or cervical collars. Surgery may be required to relieve neurologic manifestations. Also called **Klippel-Feil syndrome.**

congenital subluxation of the hip See **congenital dislocation of the hip.**

congestion Abnormal accumulation of fluid in an organ or body area. The fluid is usually blood, but it may be bile or mucus.

congestive atelectasis Severe pulmonary congestion characterized by diffuse injury to alveolar-capillary membranes, resulting in hemorrhagic edema, stiffness of the lungs, difficult ventilation, and respiratory failure. Fulminating sepsis, especially when gram-negative organisms are involved, is the most common cause, but congestive atelectasis may occur following trauma, near-drowning, aspiration of gastric acid, paraquat ingestion, inhalation of corrosive chemicals, as chlorine, ammonia, or phosgene, or the use of certain drugs, including barbiturates, chlordiazepoxide, heroin, methadone, propoxyphene, and salicylates. This serious pulmonary disorder may also be caused by diabetic ketoacidosis, fungal infections, high altitudes, pancreatitis, tuberculosis, and uremia. Management of congestive atelectasis consists of treatment of the underlying cause, frequent changes of the patient's position to promote drainage, careful dehydration, assistance with ventilation, and the use of bronchodilators and steroids. Also called **adult respiratory distress syndrome, hemorrhagic lung, pump lung, stiff lung, wet lung.**

congestive heart failure (CHF) An abnormal condition characterized by circulatory congestion caused by cardiac disorders, especially myocardial infarction of the ventricles. This condition usually develops chronically in association with the retention of sodium and water by the kidneys. Humoral agents which significantly affect such retention include renin, angiotensin, aldosterone, vasopressin, estrogen, and norepinephrine. Acute congestive heart failure may develop following myocardial infarction of the left ventricle and cause a significant shift of blood from the systemic to the pulmonary circulation before the typical retention of sodium and water occurs. Pulmonary congestion in this situation may be caused by mechanical obstruction at the left mitral valve or by ventricular failure, impairing the ventilatory function of the lungs. Common symptoms of congestive heart failure include dyspnea, high venous pressure, prolonged circulation time, peripheral edema, and decreased vital capacity. Confirming diagnosis of congestive heart failure often depends on distinguishing this condition from the congested systemic state associated with rapid infusions, severe anemia, and chronic renal insufficiency. Such distinction is often made on the basis of cardiac catheterization, which, in the case of congestive heart failure, reveals an insufficient rise in cardiac output during exercise and a significant rise in cardiac output after the administration of digitalis. Treatment of congestive heart failure includes prolonged rest and the administration of oxygen, digitalis, diuretics, and vasodilators.

Congolian red fever See **murine typhus.**

-conia A combining form meaning 'small particles in the (specified) fluid or part of the body': *chondroconia, otoconia, statoconia.*

conical papilla See **papilla.**

conjoined manipulation The use of both hands in obstetric and gynecological procedures, with one positioned in the vagina, and the other on the abdomen.

conjoined tendon See **inguinal falx.**

conjoined twins Two fetuses developed from the same ovum who are physically united at birth. The defect ranges from a superficial anatomical union of varying extent between equally or nearly equally formed fetuses to one in which only a part of the body is duplicated or in which a small, incompletely developed fetus, or parasite, is attached to a more fully formed one, the autosite. Conjoined twins result when separation of the blastomeres in early embryonic development does not occur until a late cleavage phase and is incomplete, causing the fused condition. Viability depends on the extent of the fusion and the degree of development of the fetuses. See also **Siamese twins.**

conjugated estrogen A mixture of sodium salts of estrogen sulfates, chiefly those of estrone, equilin, and 17-alpha-dihydroequilin, blended to approximate the average composition of estrogenic substances in the urine of pregnant mares.

conjugated protein A compound that contains a protein molecule united to a nonprotein substance.

conjugation In genetics: a form of sexual reproduction in unicellular organisms, such as the Paramecium, in which the gametes temporarily fuse so that genetic material can transfer from the donor male to the recipient female, where it is incorporated, recombined, and then

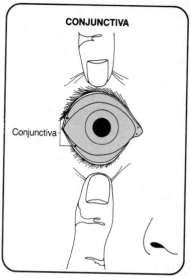

CONJUNCTIVA

Conjunctiva

passed on to the progeny through replication.

conjugon An episome that induces bacterial conjugation.

conjunctiva The mucous membrane lining the inner surfaces of the eyelids and anterior part of the sclera. The **palpebral conjunctiva** lines the inner surface of the eyelids and is thick, opaque, and highly vascular. The **bulbar conjunctiva** is loosely connected, thin, and transparent, covering the sclera of the anterior third of the eye.

conjunctival reflex A protective mechanism for the eye in which the eyelids close whenever the conjunctiva is touched. Compare **corneal reflex.**

conjunctival test A procedure used to identify offending allergens by instilling the eye with a dilute solution of the allergenic extract. A positive reaction in the allergic patient causes tearing and redness of the conjunctiva within 5 to 15 minutes. See also **allergy testing.**

conjunctivitis Inflammation of the conjunctiva, caused by bacterial or viral infection, allergy, or environmental factors. Red eyes, a thick discharge, sticky eyelids in the morning, and inflammation without pain are characteristic. The cause may be found by microscopic examination or bacteriologic culture of a specimen of the discharge. Choice of treatment depends on the causative agent and may include antibacterial agents, antibiotics, or corticosteroids. See also **choroiditis, uveitis.**

connecting fibrocartilage A disk of fibrocartilage found between many joints, especially those with limited mobility, as the spinal vertebrae. Each disk is composed of concentric rings of fibrous tissue separated by cartilaginous laminae. The disk swells outward if it is compressed by the vertebrae above or below. Compare **circumferential fibrocartilage, inter-**

articular fibrocartilage, stratiform fibro-cartilage.

connective tissue Tissue that supports and binds other body tissue and parts. It derives from the mesoderm of the embryo and is dense, containing large numbers of cells and large amounts of intercellular material. The intercellular material is composed of fibers in a matrix or ground substance which may be liquid, gelatinous, or solid, as in bone and cartilage. Connective tissue fibers may be collagenous or elastic. The most common cell in connective tissue is the histiocyte or microphage. Mast cells, plasma cells, and white blood cells are also found in connective tissue throughout different parts of the body. Kinds of connective tissue are **bone, cartilage.**

connective tissue disease See **collagen disease.**

Conn's syndrome A disorder of the adrenal cortex, owing to an adenoma—often unilateral—or, rarely, to adrenal carcinoma or hyperplasia. The resultant hypersecretion of aldosterone may cause hypernatremia, hypervolemia, and hypokalemic alkalosis, with weakness, parathesias, tetany, and transient paralysis.

Conor's disease See **Marseilles fever.**

Conradi's disease See **chondrodystrophia calcificans congenita.**

conscience 1. The moral, self-critical sense of what is right and wrong. 2. In psychoanalysis: the superego.

conscious 1. In neurology: capable of responding to sensory stimuli; awake, alert; aware of one's external environment. 2. In psychiatry: that part of the psyche or mental functioning in which thoughts, ideas, emotions, and other mental content are in the person's complete awareness. Compare **preconscious, unconscious.**

consecutive angiitis An inflammatory condition of blood or lymph vessels resulting from a similar process in surrounding tissues.

consensual A body part capable of being excited by reflex stimulation of its opposite side or of another body part.

consensual reaction to light The constriction of the pupil of one eye when the other eye is illuminated. Stimulation of either optic nerve causes constriction of both pupils. In monocular blindness, the pupil of the blind eye reacts consensually with stimulation of the seeing eye but does not cause constriction of the pupil of either eye. Also called **consensual light reflex.** Compare **direct reaction to light.**

consensus sequence In molecular genetics: a sequence in a strand of RNA nucleotides that is used as a site for the insertion of a splice of an RNA sequence from another source into the segment.

conservation of energy In physics: a law stating that in any closed system the total amount of energy is constant.

conservation of matter In physics: a law stating that matter can neither be created nor destroyed and that the amount of matter in the universe is finite. Also called **conservation of**

mass. See also **conservation of energy.**

conservation principles of nursing A conceptual framework for nursing that is directed toward maintaining the wholeness or integrity of the patient when the normal ability to cope is disturbed or exceeded by stress. Nursing intervention is determined by the patient's need to conserve energy and to maintain structural, personal, and social integrity. Subjective and objective indicators of stress are assessed by the nurse, the stimuli for the stress are identified, and the level of integrity in each area is evaluated.

conservative treatment See **treatment.**

consolidation 1. The combining of separate parts into a single whole. 2. A state of solidification. 3. In medicine: the process of becoming solid, as when the lungs become firm and inelastic in pneumonia.

constipation Difficulty in passing stools or an incomplete or infrequent passage of hard stools. There are many causes, both organic and functional. Among the organic causes are intestinal obstruction, diverticulitis, and tumors. Functional impairment of the colon may occur in elderly or bedridden patients who fail to respond to the urge to defecate. For constipation that is not organically caused, the nurse can encourage a liberal diet of fruits, vegetables, and plenty of water. The patient should be encouraged to exercise moderately, if possible, and to develop regular, unhurried bowel habits. See also **atonia constipation. —constipated,** adj.

constitutional psychology The study of the relationship of individual psychological makeup to body morphology and organic functioning.

constriction ring A band of contracted uterine muscle that forms a stricture around part of the fetus during labor, usually following premature rupture of the membranes and sometimes impeding labor. The uterine wall is thickened in the zone of the ring and is not prone to rupture. Compare **pathologic retraction ring.**

constructional apraxia A form of apraxia characterized by the inability to copy drawings or to manipulate objects to form patterns or designs.

constructive aggression See **aggression.**

construct validity Validity of a test or a measurement tool that is established by demonstrating its ability to identify the variables that it proposes to identify. See also **validity.**

contact 1. The touching or bringing together of two surfaces, as those of upper and lower teeth; often used attributively, as in contact dermatitis and contact lens. 2. The bringing together either directly or indirectly, as through the handling of food or clothing, of two individuals so as to allow the transmission of an infectious organism from one to the other. 3. A person who has been exposed to an infectious disease.

contact dermatitis Skin rash resulting from exposure to a primary irritant or to a sensitizing antigen. In the first, or nonallergic, type, a primary irritant, as an alkaline detergent or an acid, causes a lesion similar to a thermal burn. Emergency treatment is to drench liberally and immediately with water. In the second, or allergic type, sensitizing antigens, on first exposure, result in an immunologic change in certain lymphocytes. Subsequent exposure to the antigen causes the lymphocytes to release irritating chemicals leading to inflammation, edema, and vesiculation. Poison ivy and nickel dermatitis are common examples of this delayed hypersensitivity reaction. The diagnosis can be aided by patch testing with suspected antigens. Treatment includes avoidance of the irritant or sensitizer, topical corticosteroid preparations, and soothing or drying lotions. Also called **dermatitis venenata.** Compare **atopic dermatitis.** See also **cell-mediated immune response.**

contact factor See **factor XII.**

contact hour In continuing education: a term used to express the duration, in hours, of a program or class.

contact lens A small, curved, glass or plastic lens shaped to fit the person's eye and to correct refraction. Contact lenses float on the precorneal tear film and must be inserted, removed, cleaned, and stored as directed to avoid damage or infection to the eyes.

contagious Communicable, as a disease that may be transmitted by direct or indirect contact. **—contagion,** *n.*

contagious disease See **communicable disease.**

content validity Validity of a test or a measurement owing to the use of previously tested items or concepts within the tool. See also **validity.**

context In communications theory: the setting, meaning, and language of a message. If a message is interpreted (decoded) without strict regard for these limits, it will be taken out of context.

continent ileostomy An ileostomy that drains into a surgically created pouch or reservoir in the abdomen. Involuntary discharge of intestinal contents is prevented by a nipple valve created from the ileum. After surgery, the pouch is kept relatively empty by means of a catheter placed in it at surgery. It is removed 1 to 2 weeks afterward, depending on the status of intestinal function and wound healing. Once the indwelling catheter is removed, the pouch is drained by periodically inserting a catheter through the stoma into the pouch through the valve. The length of time allowed to elapse between catheterizations is gradually lengthened as the capacity of the pouch increases to between 500 and 1000 ml (17 to 34 oz). Six months after surgery, drainage may be necessary only 3 to 4 times a day.

NURSING CONSIDERATIONS: A continent ileostomy has several advantages, including the avoidance of unpleasant odors, and the convenience of not having to use a colostomy or ileostomy bag. After surgery, the patient is usually instructed to add

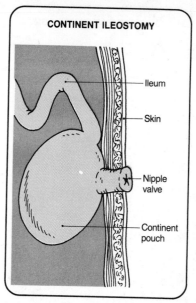

CONTINENT ILEOSTOMY

Ileum

Skin

Nipple valve

Continent pouch

foods one at a time. High-fiber foods and those that cause gas formation are particularly likely to be problematic.

contingency contracting A formal agreement between a psychotherapist and a patient undergoing behavior therapy regarding the consequences of certain actions by both parties.

contingency management Any of a group of techniques used in behavior therapy that attempts to modify a behavioral response by controlling the consequences of that response. Kinds of contingency management include **contingency contracting, shaping, token economy.**

continuing education In nursing: formal, organized, educational programs designed to promote the knowledge, skills, and professional attitudes of nurses. The programs are usually short-term and specific; a certificate may be offered for completion of a course and a number of continuing education units (CEUs) may be conferred. Continuing education is required for relicensure in many states.

continuing education unit (CEU) A point awarded to a professional person by a professional organization for having attended an educational program relevant to the goals of the organization. A value is established for the course, and that number of points is given.

continuous anesthesia A method for maintaining regional nerve block in anesthesia for surgical operations or labor in which an anesthetic solution drips either at intervals or at a low rate of flow. Barbiturates or other central nervous system depressant drugs are used. The procedure is named according to the area infiltrated: continuous spinal, caudal, epidural, peridural, or lumbar. Also called **fractional anesthesia.**

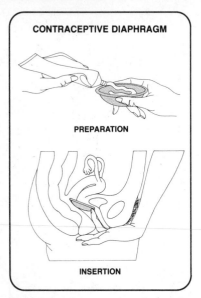

CONTRACEPTIVE DIAPHRAGM

PREPARATION

INSERTION

continuous fever A fever that persists steadily for a prolonged period of time. Compare **intermittent fever.**

continuous positive airway pressure (CPAP) In respiratory therapy: ventilation assisted by a flow of air delivered at a constant pressure throughout the respiratory cycle. It is performed for patients who can initiate their own respirations but who are not able to maintain adequate arterial oxygen levels without assistance. CPAP may be given through an endotracheal tube or through a nasal cannula. Respiratory distress syndrome in the newborn is often treated with CPAP. Also called **continuous positive pressure breathing.** Compare **positive end expiratory pressure.**

continuous positive pressure breathing (CPPB) See **continuous positive airway pressure.**

continuous positive pressure ventilation A pattern of mechanical ventilation in which a positive end-expiratory plateau pressure is maintained during the expiratory phase. See also **positive end-expiratory pressure.**

continuous tremor See **tremor.**

continuous tub bath A therapeutic bath, usually prescribed in the treatment of some dermatologic conditions, in which the patient lies supported in a medicated solution of tepid water. The patient is observed for any febrile reaction, rapid or weak pulse, faintness, or increased severity of symptoms, as itching, burning, or pain.

continuum, *pl.* **continua 1.** A continuous series or whole. **2.** In mathematics: a system of real numbers.

contra- A combining form meaning 'against': *contraception, contralateral, contraparetic.*

contraception A process or technique for

the prevention of pregnancy by means of a medication, device, or method that blocks or alters one or more of the processes of reproduction in such a way that sexual union can occur without impregnation. Kinds of contraception are **cervical cap, condom, diaphragm, intrauterine device, natural family planning, oral contraceptive, spermatocide, sterilization.** Also called **birth control, family planning method, planned parenthood.**

contraceptive diaphragm A contraceptive device consisting of a hemisphere of thin rubber bonded to a flexible ring, inserted in the vagina together with spermaticidal jelly or cream. Fitted between the pubic symphysis and the posterior fornix of the vagina, the diaphragm cups the cervix in a pool of spermaticide so that spermatozoa cannot enter the uterus, thus preventing conception. The rate of failure of the diaphragm method of contraception is approximately 5 to 10 unplanned pregnancies in 100 women using the method properly for 1 year. The principal advantages of the diaphragm are that it has no systemic effects and that it needs to be used only during coitus. The most often reported disadvantages are that it is messy, that it is uncomfortable for some people, and that insertion may interfere with spontaneity or continuity in making love. Diaphragms are manufactured in seven standard sizes from 60 mm (2¼ inches) to 90 mm (3½ inches) in diameter. Kinds of diaphragms are **arcing spring contraceptive diaphragm, coil spring contraceptive diaphragm, flat spring contraceptive diaphragm.** Also called **diaphragm.**

contraceptive diaphragm fitting A procedure, performed in an office or clinic, in which a contraceptive diaphragm is selected according to the clinical assessment of certain anatomical factors specific to the woman being fitted, including the size of the vagina, the position of the uterus, the depth of the arch behind the symphysis pubis, and the degree of support afforded by the muscles surrounding the vagina. See also **arcing spring contraceptive diaphragm, coil spring contraceptive diaphragm, flat spring contraceptive diaphragm.**

contraceptive effectiveness The effectiveness of a method of contraception in preventing pregnancy. It is sometimes represented as a percentage but more accurately as the number of pregnancies per 100 woman-years. The average pregnancy rate for a couple that is sexually active is 90 per 100 woman-years. A contraceptive method that results in a pregnancy rate of less than 10 pregnancies per 100 woman-years is considered highly effective. See also **pregnancy rate, woman-year.**

contract 1. An agreement or a promise that meets certain legal requirements, including competence of both or all parties to the contract, proper lawful subject matter, mutuality of agreement, mutuality of obligation, and consideration (the giving of something of value in payment for the obligation undertaken). **2.** To make such an agreement or promise. **—contractual,** *adj.*

contractile ring dysphagia An abnormal condition characterized by difficulty in swallowing, owing to an overreactive interior esophageal sphincteric mechanism that induces painful sticking sensations under the lower sternum. Compare **dysphagia lusoria, vallecular dysphagia.**

contraction **1.** In labor: a rhythmic tightening of the musculature of the upper uterine segment that begins mildly and becomes very strong late in labor, occurring as frequently as every 2 minutes, and lasting over 1 minute. **2.** Abnormal smallness of the birth canal or part of it, a cause of dystocia. **Inlet contraction** exists if the anteroposterior diameter is 10 cm (4 inches) or less, or if the transverse diameter is 11.5 cm (4½ inches) or less. **Midpelvic contraction** exists if the sum of the measurements in centimeters of the interspinous diameter, normally 10.5 cm (4 inches), and the posterior sagittal diameter, normally 5 cm (2 inches), is 13.5 cm (5¼ inches) or less. **Outlet contraction** exists if the intertuberous diameter is 8 cm (3 inches) or less. See also **pelvimetry.**

contracture An abnormal, usually permanent condition of a joint, characterized by flexion and fixation and caused by atrophy and shortening of muscle fibers or by loss of the normal elasticity of the skin, as from the formation of extensive scar tissue over a joint. See also **Volkmann's contracture.**

contraindication A factor that prohibits the administration of a drug or the performance of a procedure in the care of a specific patient.

contralateral Occurring on or acting with similar parts on an opposite side. See **ipsilateral.**

contrast bath A bath in which the patient alternately immerses a part of the body, usually the hands or feet, in hot and cold water for a specified period of time. The procedure is used to increase the blood flow to a particular area.

contrast enema See **barium enema.**

contrast medium A radiopaque substance injected into the body to facilitate roentgen imaging of internal structures that otherwise are difficult to visualize on X-rays.

contribution In law: a right of a defendant who has been required to pay a judgment to demand that others who are equally liable for the plaintiff's injuries contribute a share of the payment.

control To exercise restraint or maintain influence over a situation, as in self-control, the conscious limitation or suppression of impulses.

control group See **group.**

controlled association **1.** A direct connection of relevant ideas as the result of a specific stimulus. **2.** A process of bringing repressed ideas into the consciousness in response to words spoken by a psychoanalyst. Also called **word association.**

controlled hypotension See **deliberate hypotension.**

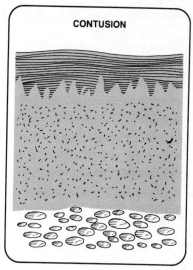

CONTUSION

controlled ventilation The use of an intermittent positive pressure breathing unit or other respirator provided with an automatic cycling device that replaces spontaneous respiration.

contusion An injury that does not break the skin, caused by a blow to the body and characterized by swelling, discoloration, and pain. The immediate application of cold may limit the development of a contusion. Compare **ecchymosis.**

convalescence The period of recovery after an illness, injury, or surgery.

convalescent home See **extended care facility.**

convection In physics: the transfer of heat through a gas or liquid by the circulation of heated particles.

convergent evolution The development of similar structures or functions within widely differing phylogenetic species in response to similar environmental conditions.

convergent strabismus See **esotropia.**

conversion disorder A kind of hysterical neurosis in which emotional conflicts are repressed and converted into sensory, motor, or visceral symptoms having no underlying organic cause, as blindness, anesthesia, hypesthesia, hyperesthesia, parasthesia, involuntary muscular movements (as tics or tremors), paralysis, aphonia, mutism, hallucinations, catalepsy, choking sensations, and respiratory difficulties. Causal factors include a conscious or unconscious desire to escape from or avoid some unpleasant situation or responsibility, or to obtain sympathy or some other secondary gain. Treatment usually consists of psychotherapy. Also called **conversion, hysteria,** conversion reaction.

convulsion A sudden, violent involuntary contraction of a group of muscles that may be paroxysmal and episodic, as in a seizure disorder, or transient and acute, as following a head concussion. A convulsion may be clonic or tonic, focal, unilateral, or bilateral.

Cooley's anemia See **thalassemia.**

cooling Reducing body temperature by the application of a hypothermia blanket, cold moist dressings, ice packs, or an alcohol bath. Subnormal body temperature may be induced to reduce metabolic function before some kinds of surgery. Very high fevers of any etiology may be treated in part by reduction of the fever with cooling techniques. See also **alcohol bath, hypothermia, hypothermia blanket.**

Coombs' test See **antiglobulin test.**

cooperative play Any organized play among a group of children in which activities are planned for the purpose of achieving some goal. It usually occurs among older children. Compare **associative play, parallel play, solitary play.**

coordinated reflex A sequence of muscular actions occurring in a purposeful, orderly progression, as the act of swallowing.

COPD *abbr* **chronic obstructive pulmonary disease.**

coping A process by which a person deals with stress, solves problems, and makes decisions. The process has two components: cognitive and noncognitive. The cognitive component includes the thought and learning necessary to identify the source of the stress. The noncognitive components are automatic and focus on relieving the discomfort.

coping, family: potential for growth A nursing diagnosis accepted by the Fifth National Conference on the Classification of Nursing Diagnoses. The etiology of the problem is the need for self-actualization that occurs when a person's basic needs have been satisfied and the adaptive tasks required by the client's health problem have been mastered. The defining characteristics of the family's potential for growth in this area are the family's expressed wish to discuss the impact of the situation on the client's own life and values, interest in meeting with others in similar situations, and choice of healthful options available to the client. See also **nursing diagnosis.**

coping, ineffective family: compromised A nursing diagnosis accepted by the Fifth National Conference on the Classification of Nursing Diagnoses. The diagnosis refers to a lack or absence of emotional and psychological support for the client that is usually available from a family member or other supportive person, a deficiency that causes further difficulty for the client in coping with the current health problem. The defining characteristics of ineffective compromised family coping include expression by the client that support is lacking or expression by the supportive person that fear, anticipatory grief, anxiety, or other reaction is interfering with the ability to give support to the client. A frank statement of an inadequate understanding of the health problem from the client or supportive person may be made. Objectively, the nurse may observe that the support given is inadequate, that the communication between the parties is limited and unsatisfactory, or that the supportive person offers help that is disproportionate to the need. See also **nursing diagnosis.**

coping, ineffective family: disabling A nursing diagnosis accepted by the Fifth National Conference on the Classification of Nursing Diagnoses. The diagnosis refers to the detrimental attitudes and behavior of a family, a family member, or other person who is important to the client. The etiology of the problem is often the disablement of the significant person by grief, anxiety, guilt, hostility, or despair. The defining characteristics include neglect in the care of the client, intolerance, rejection or abandonment, adoption of the symptoms of the client, disregard of the client's needs, and marked distortion of reality in regard to the client's health problem. See also **nursing diagnosis.**

coping, ineffective individual A nursing diagnosis accepted by the Fifth National Conference on the Classification of Nursing Diagnoses. The defining characteristics include an inability to meet the expectations of a role, an inability to meet one's basic needs, or an alteration in ability to participate in society. The critical defining characteristics, one of which must be present for the diagnosis to be made, are an inability to ask for help, an inability to solve problems, and verbalization of the inability to cope. See also **nursing diagnosis.**

copper (Cu) A malleable, red-brown, metallic element. Its atomic number is 29; its atomic weight is 63.54. Copper occurs in a pure state in nature and in many ores. It is a component of several important enzymes in the body and is essential to good health. Copper deficiency in the body is rare because only 2 to 5 mg daily, easily obtained from various foods, is sufficient for a proper balance. Copper accumulates in individuals with Wilson's disease, primary biliary cirrhosis, and, occasionally, in chronic extrahepatic biliary tract obstruction. See also **ceruloplasmin, hepatolenticular degeneration.**

copperhead A poisonous pit viper found in the southeastern United States. This red-brown, darkly banded snake is responsible for nearly 40% of the snake bites in the United States, though few of its bites are fatal. Pain, swelling, fang marks, and a bruise are usually present. Immediate treatment includes placing a constricting band above the bite, tight enough to prevent lymphatic and superficial venous flow from the wound to the general circulation, but not tight enough to stop deep arterial and venous flow to the limb. The fang marks are incised, the venom is sucked out, and free bleeding is allowed. The victim should be taken to a medical facility and given antivenin if necessary. See also **coral snake, cottonmouth.**

copper oleate solution with tetrahydronaphthalene A pediculicide.

copro-, copr- A combining form meaning 'pertaining to feces': *coprodaeum, coprolalia, coprolith.* Also **kopr-, kopra-.**

coprogogue See **cathartic.**

coproporphyria A rare, hereditary, metabolic disorder in which large quantities of nitrogenous substances, called porphyrins, are excreted in the urine. See also **coproporphyrin, porphyria.**

coproporphyrin Any of the nitrogenous organic substances normally excreted in the feces that are products of the breakdown of bilirubin from hemoglobin decomposition.

cor- See **co-.**

coracoid process The thick, curved extension of the superior border of the scapula, to which the pectoralis minor is attached. Compare **acromion.**

coral snake A poisonous snake with transverse red, black, and yellow bands, native to the southern United States. Bites are rare; pain is not always present, but neuromuscular and respiratory effects may be severe. Coral snake antivenin and oxygen are the usual treatments.

cord Any long, rounded, flexible structure. The body contains many different cords, as the spermatic, vocal, spinal, nerve, umbilical, and hepatic cords. —**cordal,** *adj.*

corditis An abnormal inflammation of the spermatic cord, accompanied by pain in the testis, often caused by an infection originating in the urethra or by tumor, hydrocele, or varicocele. Injury to the groin often causes hematoma of the cord.

core-, coro- A combining form meaning 'pertaining to the pupil of the eye': *coreclisis, corectasis, corectopia.*

-coria¹ A combining form meaning '(condition of the) sense of satiety': *acoria, hypercoria, saccharacoria.*

-coria² A combining form meaning '(condition of the) pupil': *anisocoria, diplocoria, platycoria.*

Cori's disease A rare type of glycogen storage disease, in which a missing enzyme results in abnormally large deposits of glycogen in the liver, skeletal muscles, and heart. Signs are an enlarged liver, hypoglycemia, acidosis, and, occasionally, stunted growth. Symptoms can be controlled by giving the patient frequent, small meals rich in carbohydrate and protein. Also called **Forbes' disease; glycogen storage disease, type III.** See also **glycogen storage disease.**

corium The layer of skin, just below the epidermis, consisting of papillary and reticular layers and containing blood and lymphatic vessels, nerves and nerve endings, glands, and hair follicles.

corkscrew esophagus A neurogenic disorder in which normal peristaltic contractions of the esophagus are replaced by spastic movements occurring spontaneously or with swallowing or gastric acid reflux. Difficulty in swallowing, weight loss, severe pain over the upper chest, and a characteristic corkscrew image on X-ray pictures are the symptoms usually present. Management may include the use of antispasmodic drugs, avoidance of cold fluids, surgical

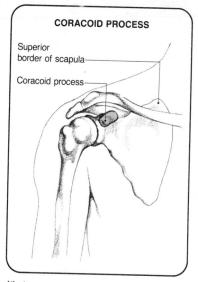

CORACOID PROCESS

Superior border of scapula

Coracoid process

dilation, or myotomy. Compare **achalasia.**

cork worker's lung A lung disease caused by an allergic reaction to cork dust. Also called **suberosis.** See also **organic dust.**

-cormia A combining form meaning an 'abnormal development of the trunk of the body': *camptocormia, nanocormia, schistocormia.* Also **-cormy.**

corn A horny mass of condensed epithelial cells overlying a bony prominence. Corns result from chronic friction and pressure. Treatment includes relief of the mechanical pressure with various pads, and surgical paring or chemical peeling of the excess keratin. Also called **clavus.** Compare **callus.**

cornea The convex, transparent, anterior part of the eye, comprising one sixth of the outermost tunic of the eye bulb. It is a fibrous structure with five layers: the anterior corneal epithelium, continuous with that of the conjunctiva; the anterior limiting layer (Bowman's membrane); the substantia propria; the posterior limiting layer (Descemet's membrane); and the endothelium of the anterior chamber (keratoderma). It is dense, uniform in thickness, nonvascular, and projects like a dome beyond the sclera, which forms the other five sixths of the eye's outermost tunic.

-cornea A combining form meaning 'condition of the cornea': *entocornea, mesocornea, microcornea.*

corneal abrasion The rubbing off of the outer layers of the cornea.

corneal grafting Transplantation of corneal tissue from one human eye to another, done to improve vision in corneal scarring or distortion, or to remove a perforating ulcer. Preoperative preparation includes constricting the pupil with a miotic drug. Under a local anesthetic the affected area is excised; an identical section of clear cornea is cut from the donor eye and

CORONARY ARTERIES

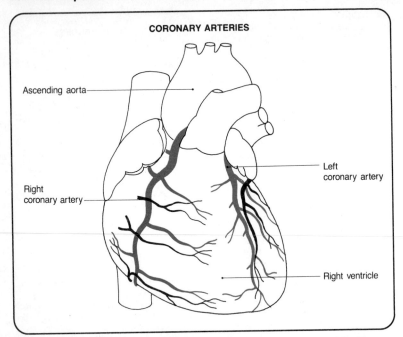

Ascending aorta

Left coronary artery

Right coronary artery

Right ventricle

sutured in place, using an operating microscope. Postoperatively, the eye is covered with a protective metal shield, and the patient is cautioned to avoid coughing, sneezing, sudden movement, or lifting. The dressing is changed daily and antibiotics are instilled. Healing is slow, and the sutures are usually left in place for 1 year. Also called **keratoplasty.**

corneal loupe   In ophthalmology: a loupe designed especially for examining the cornea.

corneal reflex   A protective mechanism for the eye in which the eyelids close when the cornea is touched. This reflex is mediated by the ophthalmic division of the fifth cranial nerve and may be used as a test of integrity of that nerve branch. People who wear contact lenses may have a diminished or absent corneal reflex. Compare **conjunctival reflex.**

cornification   Thickening of the skin by a buildup of dead, keratinized epithelial cells.

corn oil   An energy source.

corn pad   A device that helps relieve the pressure and the pain of a corn by transferring the pressure to surrounding, unaffected areas. Some common kinds of corn pads are the foam toe cap, the foam toe sleeve, the soft corn shield, and the hard corn shield.

cornual pregnancy   An ectopic pregnancy that implants in the portion of the fallopian tube that is within the horn of the uterus. Also called interstitial pregnancy. See also **ectopic pregnancy.**

coro-   See **core-.**

corona   **1.** A crown. **2.** A crownlike projection or encircling structure, as a process ex-

tending from a bone. —**coronoid,** *adj.*

coronal plane   See **frontal plane.**

coronal suture   The serrated transverse suture between the frontal bone and the parietal bone on each side of the skull.

corona radiata, *pl.* **coronae radiatae**   **1.** A network of fibers that weaves through the internal capsule of the cerebral cortex and intermingles with the fibers of the corpus callosum. **2.** An aggregate of cells that surrounds the zona pellucida of the ovum.

coronary   **1.** In anatomy: **a.** Of or pertaining to encircling structures, as the coronary arteries. **b.** Of or pertaining to the heart. **2.** *Nontechnical.* Myocardial infarction or occlusion.

coronary arteriovenous fistula   An unusual congenital abnormality characterized by a direct communication between a coronary artery, usually the right, and the right atrium or ventricle, the coronary sinus, or the vena cava. There may be a left-to-right shunt of small magnitude causing no symptoms, but a large shunt may result in growth failure, limited exercise tolerance, dyspnea, and anginal pain. A loud continuous murmur heard at the lower or midsternal border of the heart suggests a coronary arteriovenous fistula; the diagnosis may be confirmed by coronary arteriography or aortography. Closure of the fistulous tract is a safe surgical procedure with excellent long-term results.

coronary artery   One of a pair of arteries that branch from the aorta, including the left and the right coronary arteries. Coronary arterial anastomoses occur throughout the heart and are especially numerous within the interventricular and interatrial septums, at the apex of the heart, at the crux, over the anterior surface of the right ventricle, and between the sinus node artery and the other atrial arteries. These anastomoses are more numerous and larger in the epicardium than in the endocardium, and they provide important collateral circulation in the recovery of patients who suffer coronary occlusions.

coronary artery disease Any one of the abnormal conditions which may affect the arteries of the heart and produce various pathological effects, especially the reduced flow of oxygen and nutrients to the myocardium. Any of the coronary artery diseases, as coronary atherosclerosis, coronary arteritis, or fibromuscular hyperplasia of the coronary arteries, may produce the common characteristic symptom of angina pectoris, which, however, may also be associated with cardiomyopathy in which the coronary arteries are normal. The most common kind of coronary artery disease is coronary atherosclerosis, which has increased dramatically in the last 50 years and is now the leading cause of death in the Western world. It affects more men than women and occurs more often in Caucasians, the middle-aged, the elderly, and individuals from affluent countries. Coronary atherosclerosis affects more premenopausal women today than in the past. Risk factors associated with coronary artery disease include smoking, stress, obesity, high cholesterol, and hypertension. Diagnosis of coronary artery disease is usually based on patient history, especially a history with characteristic risk factors. Other diagnostic procedures are EKG during angina, treadmill or bicycle exercise tests, coronary angiography, and myocardial perfusion imaging. Treatment of the patient with coronary artery disease concentrates on reducing myocardial oxygen demand or on increasing oxygen supply. Therapy commonly includes the administration of nitrate. Coronary artery bypass surgery may use vein grafts to obviate obstructive lesions. Angioplasty to relieve occlusion by compressing fatty deposits in coronary arteries with no calcification may also be performed.

NURSING CONSIDERATIONS: Nursing care of the pateint with coronary artery disease involves monitoring of blood pressure and heart rate, taking of EKGs during anginal episodes, and administration of nitrate. Meticulous maintenance of pulmonary artery catheters and of I.V. and endotracheal tubes often associated with treatment is important. Nurses should be especially alert to signs of ischemia and arrhythmias and, before the patient is discharged, stress the importance of following the precribed regimens of diet, medication, and exercise.

coronary artery fistula A congenital anomaly characterized by an abnormal communication between a coronary artery and the right side of the heart or the pulmonary artery.

coronary bypass Open-heart surgery in which a prosthesis or a section of a blood vessel is grafted onto one of the coronary arteries and connected to the ascending aorta, bypassing a narrowing or blockage in a coronary artery. The operation is performed in coronary artery disease to improve the blood supply to the heart muscle, reduce the workload of the heart, and relieve anginal pain. Postoperatively, close observation in a coronary intensive care unit or surgical recovery unit is essential to ensure adequate ventilation and cardiac output. The systolic blood pressure is not allowed to drop more than 10 mmHg below the preoperative baseline, nor is it allowed to rise significantly, as hypertension can rupture a graft site. Arrhythmias occur frequently and are treated with lidocaine, procainamide, or digitalis, given intravenously, or by electrical cardioversion. The patient is usually discharged within 10 to 14 days. Nearly 20% of cases are associated with thrombosis within the first year following surgery; 20% to 25% are associated with closure of the graft within the first year, making the surgery controversial.

coronary care unit (CCU) A specially equipped hospital area designed for the treatment of patients with sudden, life-threatening cardiac conditions. Such units contain resuscitation and monitoring equipment and are staffed by personnel especially trained and skilled in recognizing and immediately responding to cardiac emergencies with cardiopulmonary resuscitation techniques, the administration of antiarrhythmic drugs, and other appropriate therapeutic measures.

coronary heart disease (CHD) Damaged myocardium caused by insufficient blood supply from constricted coronary arteries.

coronary occlusion An obstruction of any one of the coronary arteries, usually caused by progressive atherosclerosis and sometimes complicated by thrombosis. In certain heart diseases, arterial spasms may narrow the lumen of a coronary artery, blocking blood flow, and causing the characteristic signs of myocardial infarction, as crushing substernal pain that radiates to the arms, jaw, and neck. Almost half the sudden deaths caused by myocardial infarction occur before the affected individual is hospitalized, often within 1 hour of the onset of symptoms. If treatment begins immediately after the onset of symptoms, the prognosis significantly improves. Occlusion of the circumflex branch of the left coronary artery causes a lateral wall infarction. Occlusion of the anterior descending branch of the left coronary artery causes an infarction of the anterior heart wall. Occlusion of the right coronary artery or one of its branches causes a posterior wall infarction. Occlusions of the sinus node artery and the main coronary artery proximal to the origin of the sinus node branch commonly cause infarctions of the atrium and the sinus node and lead to atrial arrhythmias. Coronary occlusions that produce posterior myocardial infarction cut off the blood supply to the atrioventricular node, resulting in characteristic signs, as fainting and syncope during angina. Treatment of coronary

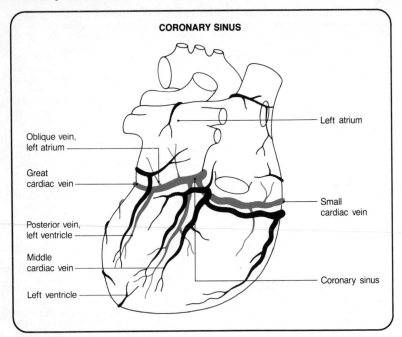

CORONARY SINUS

Oblique vein, left atrium

Great cardiac vein

Posterior vein, left ventricle

Middle cardiac vein

Left ventricle

Left atrium

Small cardiac vein

Coronary sinus

occlusion and associated myocardial infarction often includes administration of lidocaine or other antiarrhythmic drugs, nitroglycerin to relieve pain, oxygen, bed rest, and the implanting of a temporary pacemaker.

coronary sinus The wide venous channel, about 2.25 cm (⅞ inch) long, situated in the coronary sulcus and covered by muscular fibers from the left atrium. It drains five coronary veins through a single semilunar valve. They are the great cardiac vein, small cardiac vein, middle cardiac vein, posterior vein of the left ventricle, and the oblique vein of the left atrium.

coronary thrombosis A development of a thrombus that blocks a coronary artery, often causing myocardial infarction and death. Coronary thromboses commonly develop in segments of arteries with atherosclerotic lesions.

coronary vein One of the veins of the heart that drains blood from the capillary beds of the myocardium through the coronary sinus into the right atrium. A few small coronary veins that collect blood from a small area in the right ventricle drain directly into the right atrium.

coronavirus A member of a family of viruses that includes several types capable of causing acute respiratory illnesses.

coroner A public official who investigates the causes and circumstances of a death occurring within a specific legal jurisdiction or territory, especially a death that may have resulted from unnatural causes. Also called **medical examiner.**

coronoid fossa A small depression in the distal, dorsal surface of the humerus that re-

ceives the coronoid process of the ulna when the forearm is flexed.

coronoid process of mandible A prominence on the anterior surface of the ramus of the mandible to which each temporal muscle attaches.

coronoid process of ulna A wide, flaring projection of the proximal end of the ulna. The proximal surface of the process forms the lower part of the trochlear notch.

corpor- A combining form meaning 'pertaining to the body': *corpora, corporeal, corporic.*

cor pulmonale An abnormal cardiac condition characterized by hypertrophy of the right ventricle of the heart owing to hypertension of the pulmonary circulation. Some of the diseases associated with cor pulmonale include cystic fibrosis, myasthenia gravis, myopathies, and pulmonary arteritis. Approximately 85% of patients with cor pulmonale have chronic obstructive pulmonary disease. Pulmonary capillary destruction and pulmonary vasoconstriction decrease the cross-sectional area of the pulmonary vascular bed, increasing pulmonary vascular resistance and causing pulmonary hypertension. The right ventricle dilates and hypertrophies to compensate for the extra work required in forcing blood through the lungs. To compensate for the low oxygen content associated with cor pulmonale, the bone marrow produces more red blood cells, causing erythrocytosis. Right ventricular failure results when blood viscosity increases and further aggravates pulmonary hypertension, increasing the hemodynamic load on the right ventricle. Cor pulmonale accounts for about 25% of all types of heart failure. Some of the early signs of cor pulmonale include chronic cough, exertional dyspnea, fatigue, wheezing, and weakness. As the disease progresses, dyspnea may become more severe and other signs, as tachypnea, orthopnea, and edema may emerge. Signs of this condition and right ventricular failure may include dependent edema, distended neck veins. hepatojugular reflux, and tachycardia. A weak pulse and hypotension may result from decreased cardiac output, and chest examination may reveal various signs, depending on the cause of the condition. In chronic obstructive pulmonary disease, auscultation may reveal rales, rhonchi, and diminished breath sounds. When cor pulmonale is secondary to obstruction of the upper airway or to damage of CNS respiratory centers, auscultation may reveal a right ventricular lift, a gallop rhythm, and a systolic pulmonic click. A pansystolic murmur, which intensifies on inspiration, may indicate tricuspid insufficiency. The patient with cor pulmonale may also experience fluctuating levels of drowsiness and consciousness. Diagnosis of the condition may be confirmed by measurements of pulmonary artery pressure by pulmonary artery catheterization. The treatment of cor pulmonale seeks to reduce hypoxia, increase exercise tolerance, and correct the functional defect whenever possible. Treatment includes bed rest, the administration of digitalis glycoside, antibiotics to fight any respiratory infection, oxygen therapy, low-salt diet, restricted fluid intake, diuretics, and anticoagulants. Oxygen may be administered by mask or by cannula in concentrations from 24% to 40%, depending on arterial oxygen pressure. Mechanical ventilation may be used in acute cases. A phlebotomy may be performed to reduce red cell mass.

NURSING CONSIDERATIONS: It is important to monitor closely the serum potassium levels of the patient receiving diuretics, since low-serum potassium levels can increase the risk of arrhythmias associated with digitalis. Digitalis toxicity is often a danger. The frequent repositioning of bed patients with cor pulmonale helps to prevent atelectasis. The nursing responsibility also usually includes respiratory care, the periodic measuring of arterial blood gases, and monitoring for signs of respiratory failure, pulse rate changes, labored respirations, and exertional fatigue levels. Before the patient is discharged from the hospital, nurses instruct the patient on personal maintenance, especially the detection of pitting edema of the extremities. The cor pulmonale patient being discharged can also benefit from instructions about breathing exercises, the importance of reporting early signs of infection, the dangers of mingling with crowds, especially during the flu season, and the danger of using nonprescribed medications, especially sedatives that can depress the ventilatory drive.

corpus, pl. **corpora**   See **body.**

corpus cavernosum clitoridis   One of two columns of erectile tissue enclosed in a dense layer of fibrous tissue that fuse together to form the body of the clitoris.

corpus cavernosum penis   One of two columns of erectile tissue surrounded by strong, fibrous tissue that form their junction in the median plane and form the dorsum and the sides of the penis.

corpuscle, corpuscule   In anatomy: **1.** Any cell of the body. **2.** A red or white blood cell. **—corpuscular,** adj.

corpus luteum, pl. **corpora lutea**   An anatomical structure on the surface of the ovary, consisting of a spheroid of yellowish tissue 1 to 2 cm in diameter that grows within the ruptured ovarian follicle following ovulation. During the reproductive years of a woman's life, a corpus luteum forms after every ovulation. It acts as a short-lived endocrine organ that secretes progesterone, which serves to maintain the decidual layer of the endometrium in the richly vascular state necessary for implantation and pregnancy. If conception occurs, the corpus luteum grows and secretes increasing amounts of progesterone. It reaches its maximum function and size (2 to 3 cm) at 10 to 12 weeks of gestation. It persists, slowly diminishing in size and function, until 6 months after the onset of gestation. During the 2 weeks prior to menstruation, the corpus luteum secretes progesterone in decreasing amounts, atrophies, undergoes fibrotic degeneration, and becomes a pale spot (corpus albicans) on the surface of the ovary.

corpus vitreum   See **vitreous humor.**

corrective exercise   A program of physical therapy to restore normal function to diseased, defective, or injured parts of the body. Also called **therapeutic exercise.** See also **exercise, osteopathy.**

correlation   In statistics: a relationship between variables that may be negative (inverse), positive, or curvilinear. Correlation is measured and expressed using numerical scales.

correlative differentiation   In embryology: specialization or diversification of cells or tissues caused by an inductor or other external factor. Also called **dependent differentiation.**

Corrigan's pulse   A bounding pulse in which a great surge is felt followed by a sudden and complete absence of force or fullness in the artery. This kind of pulse occurs in excited emotional states; in various abnormal cardiac conditions, including patent ductus arteriosus; and as a result of systemic arteriosclerosis.

corrosive   **1.** Eating away a substance or tissue, especially by chemical action. **2.** An agent or substance that eats away a substance or tissue. **—corrode,** v., **corrosion,** n.

corrosive gastritis   An acute inflammatory condition of the stomach caused by the ingestion of an acid, alkali, or other corrosive chemical. The amount of tissue destruction and recommended treatment depend on the nature of the corrosive agent and the extent of exposure. Compare **chemical gastritis, erosive gastritis.** See also **acid poisoning, alkali poisoning.**

corrugator supercilii   One of the three

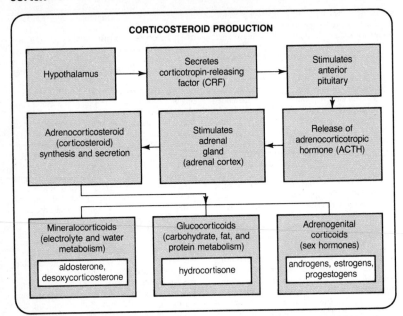

CORTICOSTEROID PRODUCTION

Hypothalamus → Secretes corticotropin-releasing factor (CRF) → Stimulates anterior pituitary

Adrenocorticosteroid (corticosteroid) synthesis and secretion ← Stimulates adrenal gland (adrenal cortex) ← Release of adrenocorticotropic hormone (ACTH)

Mineralocorticoids (electrolyte and water metabolism) — aldosterone, desoxycorticosterone

Glucocorticoids (carbohydrate, fat, and protein metabolism) — hydrocortisone

Adrenogenital corticoids (sex hormones) — androgens, estrogens, progestogens

muscles of the eyelid. Arising from the medial end of the supercilliary arch and inserting into the skin above the orbital arch, it is innervated by temporal and zygomatic branches of the facial nerve and functions to draw the eyebrow downward and inward, as if to frown. Also called **corrugator.** Compare **levator palpebrae superioris, orbicularis oculi.**

cortex, *pl.* **cortices** The outer layer of a body organ or other structure, as distinguished from the internal substance.

cortic- A combining form meaning 'pertaining to the cortex or bark': *corticipetal, corticobulbar, corticothalamic.*

cortical apraxia See **motor apraxia.**

cortical audiometry See **audiometry.**

cortical blindness Blindness that results from a lesion in the visual center of the cerebral cortex of the brain.

cortical fracture Any fracture that involves the cortex of the bone.

corticosteroid Any one of the natural or synthetic hormones associated with the adrenal cortex, which influences or controls key processes of the body, as carbohydrate and protein metabolism, electrolyte and water balance, and the functions of the cardiovascular system, skeletal muscle, kidneys, and other organs. The corticosteroids synthesized by the adrenal glands include the glucocorticoids, the mineralocorticoids, and the adrenogenital corticoids. The principal glucocorticoid is cortisol, also known as hydrocortisone. The only physiologically important mineralocorticoid in humans is aldosterone. The principal adrenogenital corticoids are androgen, estrogen and progestogen. Cortisol and its synthetic analogs can pre-

vent or reduce inflammation by inhibiting edema, leukocytic migration, disposition of collagen, and other complications associated with inflammatory processes. The anti-inflammatory powers of synthetic hormones can be dangerous, however, because they mask the disease process and prevent accurate observation of its progress. Pharmacological doses of glucocorticoids retard bone growth of children and inhibit cell division in various developing structures, as the gastric mucosa, liver, lungs, and brain. Glucocorticoids are absorbed from sites of local application, as synovial spaces, the conjunctival sac, and the skin. When large areas of the skin are involved or when the administration is prolonged, absorption may cause systemic effects, including adrenocortical suppression. Corticosteroids may be administered orally, parenterally, or topically. Toxic effects may result from the too rapid withdrawal of such drugs after prolonged therapy or from the continued use of large doses. Androgens and estrogens replace sex hormones and are administered orally or parenterally. Estrogens and progestogens, used alone or in combination, suppress hormone secretion.

corticotropin (ACTH) See **adrenocorticotropic hormone.**

cortisol See **hydrocortisone.**

cortisone acetate A glucocorticoid agent.

Corti's organ A small, spiral structure within the cochlea of the internal ear, containing hair cells in contact with the acoustic nerve. Also called **spiral organ of Corti.**

Corynebacterium A common genus of rod-shaped, curved bacilli having many species. The most common pathogenic species is *Corynebacterium diphtheriae,* the cause of diphtheria.

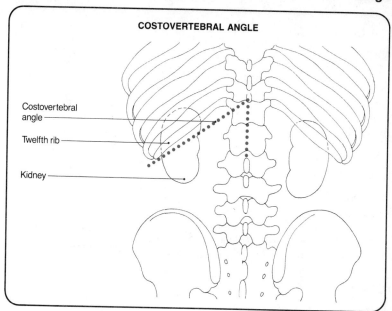

COSTOVERTEBRAL ANGLE

Costovertebral angle

Twelfth rib

Kidney

coryza See **rhinitis.**

coryza spasmodica See **hay fever.**

cosmetic surgery Reconstruction of cutaneous or underlying tissues of the face and neck, performed to correct a structural defect or to remove a scar, birthmark, or some normal evidence of aging. Kinds of cosmetic surgery include **rhinoplasty, rhytidoplasty.** Compare **plastic surgery.**

cosmic radiation High-energy particles with great penetrating power originating in outer space and reaching the earth as normal background radiation. The rays consist partly of high-energy atomic nuclei.

cost- See **costi-.**

costal cartilage See **cartilage.**

cost analysis An analysis of the disbursements of a given activity, agency, department, or program.

cost/benefit ratio A ratio that represents the relationship of the cost of an activity to the benefit of its outcome or product.

cost control The process of monitoring and regulating the expenditure of funds by an agency or institution. Budgets, reports, and cost-accounting procedures are performed to achieve cost control. Also known as cost containment.

cost-effectiveness The extent to which an activity is thought to produce tangible benefits in relation to its expense.

Costen's syndrome See **temporomandibular joint pain-dysfunction syndrome.**

costi-, cost-, costo- A combining form meaning 'pertaining to a rib': *costicartilage, costicervical, costifluous.*

costochondral Of or pertaining to a rib and its cartilage.

costotransverse articulation Any one of 20 gliding joints between the ribs and associated vertebrae, except for the 11th and 12th ribs. The 5 ligaments that associate with each costotransverse joint are the articular capsule, the superior costotransverse ligament, the posterior costotransverse ligament, the ligament of the neck of the rib, and the ligament of the tubercle of the rib.

costovertebral Of or relating to a rib and the vertebral column.

costovertebral angle (CVA) One of two angles that outline a space over the kidneys. The angle is formed by the lateral and downward curve of the lowest rib and the vertical column of the spine. CVA tenderness to percussion is a common finding in pyelonephritis and other infections of the kidney and adjacent structures.

cosyntropin A synthetic form of corticotropin (ACTH).

cot death See **sudden infant death syndrome.**

co-trimoxazole A sulfonamide antibiotic.

cotton-mill fever See **byssinosis.**

cottonmouth A poisonous pit viper commonly found near water and swamps of the southeastern part of the United States. The first symptoms of the bite of a cottonmouth are swelling, edema, and pain. Antivenin and oxygen are the usual treatments. Also called **water moccasin.**

Cotton's fracture A trimalleolar fracture involving medial, lateral, and posterior malleoli.

cotyloid cavity See **acetabulum.**

cough A sudden, audible expulsion of air from the lungs. Coughing is preceded by inspiration, the glottis is partially closed, and the

COUNTERTRACTION

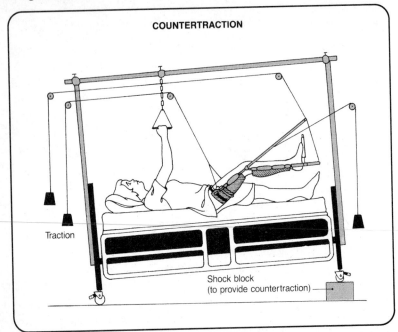

Traction

Shock block
(to provide countertraction)

accessory muscles of expiration contract to expel the air forcibly from the respiratory passages. Coughing is an essential protective response that serves to clear the lungs, bronchi, or trachea of irritants and secretions or to prevent aspiration of foreign material into the lungs. It is a common symptom of diseases of the chest and larynx. Chronic coughing may be indicative of tuberculosis, lung cancer, bronchiectasis, or bronchitis. Otitis medea, subdiaphragmatic irritation, congestive heart failure, and mitral valve disease may be associated with episodes of severe chronic coughing. Coughing is a reflex action which may be induced voluntarily and, to some extent, voluntarily inhibited. Persons with chronic coughs may obtain symptomatic relief through environmental controls that reduce irritants in the air and provide humidification. Medication may be supplied to dilate the bronchi, liquefy secretions, and increase expectoration. Rest, increased fluid intake, and adequate nutrition are necessary. Antitussive medications are sometimes prescribed in the treatment of a cough in the absence of mucus or congestion.

cough fracture   Any fracture of a rib, usually the fifth or the seventh rib, caused by violent coughing.

coulomb   The meter/kilogram/second (mks) unit of electricity equal to the quantity of charge transferred in one second across a conductor in which there is a constant current of one ampere.

Coulomb's law   In physics: a law stating that the force of attraction or repulsion between two electrically charged bodies is directly pro-

portional to the strength of the electrical charges and inversely proportional to the square of the distance between them.

Coulter counter   A trade name for an electrical device that rapidly identifies, sorts, and counts the various kinds of cells present in a small specimen of blood.

coumarin   An anticoagulant. See **warfarin.**

count   A computation of the number of objects or elements present per unit of measurement. Kinds of counts include **Addis count, blood count.**

counterclaim   In law: a claim made by a defendant establishing a cause for action in his favor against the plaintiff. The purpose of a counterclaim is to oppose or detract from the plaintiff's claim or complaint.

countertraction   A force that counteracts the pull of traction, especially in orthopedics, as the force of body weight owing to the pull of gravity. Orthopedic countertraction may also be obtained by altering the angle of the body force in relation to the pull of traction, as by elevating the foot of the bed with shock blocks to attain the Trendelenburg's position. The magnitude of countertraction depends on the amount of force needed to counteract the pull of the traction and is usually developed gradually by methodically changing the position of a patient and by adding or removing weights from weight hangers.

countertransference   The conscious or unconscious emotional response of a psychotherapist or psychoanalyst to a patient. See also **transference.**

coup   Any blow or stroke or the effects of such

a blow to the body, usually used with a French word identifying a type of stroke: **1.** Coup de sabre, a wound resembling a sword cut. **2.** Coup de soleil. See **sunstroke. 3.** Coup sur coup, administration of a drug in small amounts over a short period of time rather than in a single larger dose. **4.** Contre coup, an injury most often associated with a blow to the skull in which the force of the impact is transmitted through the skull bones to the opposite side of the head where the bruise, fracture, or other sign of injury appears.

coupling 1. The act of coming together, joining, or pairing. **2.** In genetics: the situation in linked inheritance in which the nonalleles of two or more mutant genes are located on the same chromosome and are close enough so that they are likely to be inherited together. Compare **repulsion.** See also **cis configuration.**

Courvoisier's law A law stating that the gallbladder is smaller than usual if a gallstone blocks the common bile duct and that it is dilated if the common bile duct is blocked owing to a cause other than a gallstone, as cancer of the pancreas.

Couvelaire uterus A hemorrhagic process in uterine musculature that may accompany severe abruptio placentae. Extravasated blood effuses between the muscle fibrils and under the uterine peritoneum. The uterus takes on a purplish color and does not contract well. Also called **uteroplacental apoplexy.** See also **abruptio placentae.**

Cowling's rule A method of calculating the approximate pediatric dosage of a drug for a child using the formula: (age at next birthday ÷ 24) × adult dose. See **Clark's rule.**

Cowper's gland Either of two round, pea-sized glands embedded in the urethral sphincter of the male. Normally yellow in color, they consist of several lobes with ducts that join and form a single excretory duct. Also called **bulbourethral gland.** Compare **Bartholin's gland.**

cowpox A mild infectious disease characterized by a pustular rash, caused by the vaccinia virus transmitted to humans from infected cattle. Cowpox infection usually confers immunity to smallpox, owing to the similarity of the variola and vaccinia viruses. See also **smallpox, vaccinia.**

coxa, *pl.* **coxae 1.** The head of the femur and the acetabulum of the innominate bone. **2.** The hip joint.

coxal articulation The ball-and-socket joint of the hip, formed by the articulation of the head of the femur into the cup-shaped cavity of the acetabulum. It involves seven ligaments and permits very extensive movements, as flexion, extension, adduction, abduction, circumduction, and rotation. Also called **hip joint.** Compare **shoulder joint.**

coxa magna An abnormal widening of the head and neck of the femur.

coxa plana See **Perthes' disease.**

coxa valga A hip deformity in which the angle formed by the axis of the head and neck

of the femur and the axis of its shaft is significantly increased.

coxa vara A hip deformity in which the angle formed by the axis of the head and neck of the femur and the axis of its shaft is decreased. Also called coxa adducta, coxa flexa.

coxa vara luxans A fissure or crack in the neck of the femur with dislocation of the head, caused by coxa vara.

Coxsackie virus Any of 30 serologically different enteroviruses associated with a variety of symptoms and primarily affecting children during warm weather. The Coxsackie viruses resemble the virus responsible for poliomyelitis, particularly in size; both are picornaviruses. Among the diseases associated with Coxsackie virus infections are herpangina, hand, foot, and mouth disease, epidemic pleurodynia, myocarditis, pericarditis, aseptic meningitis, and several exanthems. There is no known preventive measure except isolation of infected persons, and the treatment is generally directed toward relief of symptoms. See also **viral infection.**

CPAP *abbr* **continuous positive airway pressure.**

CPHA *abbr* the **Canadian Public Health Association.**

CPD *abbr* **1.** **Cephalopelvic disproportion. 2. Childhood polycystic disease.** See **polycystic kidney disease. 3. Congenital polycystic disease.** See **polycystic kidney disease.**

CPK *abbr* creatinine phosphokinase. See **Duchenne's muscular dystrophy.**

CPPB *abbr* **continuous positive pressure breathing.**

CPPV *abbr* **continuous positive pressure ventilation.**

CPR *abbr* **cardiopulmonary resuscitation.**

CPRAM *abbr* controlled partial rebreathing anesthesia method.

CPT *abbr* **current procedural terminology.**

Cr Symbol for **chromium.**

CR *abbr* controlled respiration.

crab louse A species of body louse, *Phthirus pubis,* that infests the hairs of the genital area and is often transmitted between persons by venereal contact. Also called *Pediculus pubis.* See also **pediculosis.**

cradle cap A common seborrheic dermatitis of infants consisting of thick, yellow, greasy scales on the scalp. Treatment includes oil or ointment to soften the scales and frequent shampoos.

cramp 1. A spasmodic and often painful contraction of one or more muscles. **2.** A pain resembling a muscular cramp. Kinds of cramps include cane-cutter's cramp, charley horse, fireman's cramp, miner's cramp, stoker's cramp. See also **dysmenorrhea, heat cramp, torticollis, writer's cramp.**

-crania A combining form meaning '(condition of the) skull or head': *diastematocrania, hemicrania, platycrania.*

cranial arachnoid See **arachnoid membrane.**

CRANIAL NERVES: ORIGIN AND FUNCTION			
NERVE	**ORIGIN**	**TYPE**	**FUNCTION(S)**
I Olfactory	Olfactory bulb	Sensory	Smell
II Optic	Lateral geniculate body	Sensory	Vision
III Oculomotor	Midbrain	Motor	Eye movement (inward, upward), eyelid elevation, pupil constriction, convergence, consensual reaction
IV Trochlear	Midbrain	Motor	Eye movement (downward, outward)
V Trigeminal	Pons	Motor Sensory	Chewing Sensations of the face, scalp, and teeth
VI Abducens	Pons	Motor	Eye movement (lateral)
VII Facial	Pons	Motor Sensory	Facial expressions Taste (anterior two thirds of tongue), salivation, tearing
VIII Acoustic (cochlear, vestibular)	Pons	Sensory	Hearing, equilibrium
IX Glosso-pharyngeal	Medulla	Motor Sensory	Salivation, swallowing Sensations of the throat and tonsils, taste (posterior one third of tongue)
X Vagus	Medulla	Motor Sensory	Swallowing, talking, heart rate, peristalsis Sensations of the throat, larynx, and viscera
XI Spinal accessory	Medulla	Motor	Shoulder movement, head rotation
XII Hypoglossal	Medulla	Motor	Tongue movement

cranial arteritis See **temporal arteritis.**

cranial nerves The 12 pairs of nerves emerging from the cranial cavity through various openings in the skull. Beginning with the most anterior, they are designated by Roman numerals and named (I) olfactory, (II) optic, (III) oculomotor, (IV) trochlear, (V) trigeminal, (VI) abducens, (VII) facial, (VIII) acoustic, (IX) glossopharyngeal, (X) vagus, (XI) spinal accessory, (XII) hypoglossal. Certain cranial nerves, particularly V, VII, and VIII, contain two or more distinct functional components considered as independent nerves by some authorities. In this category the masticatory nerve would be separated from the trigeminal (V), the glosso-palatine from the facial (VII), and the equilibratory from the acoustic (VIII), making 15 pairs in all. Some anatomists also classify the terminal nerve as the first cranial. Also called **cerebral nerves.** See also specific nerves.

cranio- A combining form meaning 'pertaining to the skull or cranium': *craniobuccal, craniognomy, craniosacral.*

craniocele See **encephalocele.**

craniodidymus A two-headed fetal twin monster in which the bodies are fused.

craniofacial dysostosis An abnormal hereditary condition characterized by acrocephaly, exophthalmos, hypertelorism, strabismus, parrot-beaked nose, and hypoplastic maxilla with relative mandibular prognathism. This condition is transmitted as an autosomal dominant trait. See also **dysostosis.**

craniohypophyseal xanthoma A condition in which cholesterol deposits are formed around the hypophyses of the bones.

craniopagus Conjoined twins that are united at the heads. Fusion can occur at either the frontal, occipital, or parietal regions. Also called **cephalopagus.**

craniopharyngeal Of or pertaining to the cranium and the pharynx.

craniopharyngioma, *pl.* **craniopharyngiomas, craniopharyngiomata** A congenital pituitary tumor, appearing most often in children and adolescents, that arises in cells derived from Rathke's pouch or the hypophyseal stalk. The lesion, a solid or cystic body ranging in size from 1 to 8 cm (½ to 3⅛ inches), may expand into the third ventricle or the temporal lobe, commonly becoming calcified. Increased intracranial pressure, severe headaches, vomiting, stunted growth, defective vision, irritability, somnolence, and infantile genitalia are often associated with the lesion in children. Development of the tumor after puberty usually results in amenorrhea in women and loss of libido and potency in men. Also called **ameloblastoma, pituitary adamantinoma, Rathke's pouch tumor.**

craniostenosis A congenital deformity of the skull resulting from premature closure of the sutures between the cranial bones. The severity of the malformation depends on which sutures close, at what point in the developmental process the closure occurred, and the success or failure of the other sutures to compensate by expansion. Impaired brain growth may or may not be involved. The most common form of the condition is permanent closure of the sagittal suture with anteroposterior elongation of the skull. Surgery is generally indicated when multiple sutures are fused in order to relieve cerebral pressure and may be performed for cosmetic reasons. See also **brachycephaly, oxycephaly, plagiocephaly, scaphocephaly.** —**craniostenotic,** *adj.*

craniostosis Premature ossification of the sutures of the skull, often associated with other skeletal defects. The sutures close before or soon after birth. If not surgically corrected, the growth of the skull is inhibited, the head is deformed, and the eyes and brain are often damaged. Also called craniosynostosis.

craniotabes Benign, congenital thinness of the top and back of the skull of a newborn, common because the rate of brain growth exceeds the rate of calcification of the skull during the last month of gestation. The condition disappears with normal nutrition and growth but may persist in infants who develop rickets.

craniotomy Any surgical opening into the skull, done to relieve intracranial pressure, to control bleeding, or to remove a tumor. X-rays of the skull are taken preoperatively and a CT scan or an electroencephalogram is done to establish the diagnosis. Postoperatively, if the cerebral area is involved, the head of the patient's bed is elevated to 45° to reduce the risk of hemorrhage and edema; if the cerebellum or brain stem is affected the patient is kept flat. The dressing is checked frequently for yellowish drainage of cerebrospinal fluid. Any moist areas are reinforced with sterile materials to avoid infection. Frequent observation of neurologic signs, including the level of consciousness, speech, and strength, is essential.

cranium The bony skull that holds the brain.

It is composed of eight bones: frontal, occipital, sphenoid, and ethmoid bones, and paired temporal and parietal bones. —**cranial,** *adj.*

-cranium A combining form meaning 'referring to the skull': *chondrocranium, desmocranium, endocranium.*

crankcase spool catheter A special, elastic catheter stored within a plastic spool to facilitate its insertion, especially for hyperalimentation. Most experts recommend the indirect method of venipuncture for insertion of this kind of catheter, usually into a peripheral vein that connects with the subclavian vein. When fully inserted, the crankcase spool catheter is usually lodged in the subclavian vein. The catheter is highly flexible and each revolution of the crankcase spool feeds about 12.7 cm (5 inches) of the catheter into the vein involved. When the crankcase spool catheter is fully inserted, an X-ray is made of the insertion area to confirm its correct placement.

crash cart A cart carrying emergency equipment, such as medications, antiseptics, suction devices, venipuncture equipment and I.V. supplies, sutures, scalpels, surgical needles, sponges, swabs, retractors, hemostats, forceps, trachea tubes, a cardiac monitor, and often a defibrillator. Hospital emergency rooms and intensive-care units usually have several crash carts equipped according to prescribed specifications. Efficient, effective emergency care often depends on the careful provisioning of crash carts and the precise knowledge of their layouts. Careful daily checks of the cart's equipment and supplies are essential.

-crasia A combining form meaning: **1.** A '(condition of a) mixture, good or bad': *eucrasia, orthocrasia, spermacrasia.* **2.** A '(specified) condition involving loss of control': *copracrasia, uracrasia.*

-cratia A combining form meaning '(condition of) incontinence': *scatacratia, scoracratia, uracratia.*

cravat bandage A triangular bandage, folded lengthwise. It may be used as a circular, figure-eight, or spiral bandage to control bleeding or to tie splints in place.

crawling reflex See **symmetric tonic neck reflex.**

C-reactive protein (CRP) A protein not normally detected in the serum but present in many acute inflammatory conditions and with necrosis. CRP appears in the serum before the erythrocyte sedimentation rate begins to rise, often within 24 to 48 hours of the onset of inflammation. After a myocardial infarction, it is present in 24 hours, begins to fall 3 days later, and is absent after 2 weeks. Acute rheumatic fever is monitored with serial estimations of CRP, as the serum level of the protein is the most sensitive indicator of rheumatic activity. CRP disappears with an inflammatory process is suppressed by salicylates or steroids, or both. Also called **serum C-reactive protein.**

crease An indentation or margin formed by a doubling back of tissue, as the folds or creases on the palm of the hand and sole of the foot.

creat- A combining form meaning 'pertaining to flesh': *creaton, creatorrhea, creatotoxism.*

creatine An important nitrogenous compound produced by metabolic processes in the body. Combined with phosphorus it forms high-energy phosphate. In normal metabolic reactions the phosphorus is yielded to combine with a molecule of adenosine diphosphate to produce a molecule of the very high energy molecule adenosine triphosphate. See also **creatinine.**

creatine kinase An enzyme in muscle, brain, and other tissues that catalyzes the transfer of a phosphate group from adenosine triphosphate to creatine, producing adenosine diphosphate and phosphocreatine.

creatinine A substance formed from the metabolism of creatine, commonly found in blood, urine, and muscle tissue. See also **creatine.**

creatinine phosphokinase (CPK) See **Duchenne's muscular dystrophy.**

Credé's maneuver Manual expulsion of the placenta after birth by pressing the uterus down into the pelvis and compressing it from all sides toward the birth canal. Also, a similar method of expelling urine from the bladder.

Credé's treatment Prevention of ophthalmia neonatorum in the newborn by instillation of 1% to 2% silver nitrate solution into each eye immediately after birth.

creeping eruption A skin lesion characterized by irregular, wandering red lines made by the burrowing larvae of hookworms and certain roundworms. Antiparasitic treatment is specific to the organism. Also called larva migrans.

cremaster A thin, muscular layer spreading out over the spermatic cord in a series of loops. It is a continuation of the obliquus internus. The muscle arises from the inguinal ligament and inserts into the crest of the pubis and into the sheath of the rectus abdominis. It is innervated by the genital branch of the genitofemoral nerve and functions to draw the testis up toward the superficial inguinal ring in response to cold or to stimulation of the nerve.

cremasteric reflex A superficial neural reflex elicited by stroking the skin of the upper inner aspect of the thigh in a male. This normally results in a brisk retraction of the testis on the side of the stimulus. The reflex is lost in diseases of the pyramidal tract above the level of the first lumbar vertebra. See also **superficial reflex.**

crenation The formation of notches or leaflike, scalloped edges on an object. Red blood cells exposed to a hypertonic saline solution acquire a notched, shriveled surface because of the osmotic effect of the solution. —**crenate, crenated,** *adj.*

creosote poisoning See **phenol poisoning.**

crepitus 1. Flatulence or the noisy discharge of fetid gas from the intestine through the anus. 2. A sound that resembles the crackling noise heard when rubbing hair between the fingers or throwing salt on an open fire. Crepitus is associated with gas gangrene, the rubbing of bone fragments, or the rales of a consolidated area of the lung in pneumonia. Also called crepitation.

cresc- A combining form meaning 'to grow': *crescograph.*

CREST syndrome Acronym for **calcinosis, Raynaud's phenomenon, esophageal dysfunction, sclerodactyly,** and **telangiectasis,** which may occur for varying periods of time in patients with scleroderma.

cretin dwarf A person in whom short stature is caused by infantile hypothyroidism and severe deficiency of thyroid hormone. Also called **hypothyroid dwarf.**

cretinism A condition characterized by severe congenital hypothyroidism and often associated with other endocrine abnormalities. Typical signs of cretinism include dwarfism, mental deficiency, puffy facial features, dry skin, a large tongue, umbilical hernia, and muscular incoordination. The disorder usually occurs in areas where the diet is deficient in iodine and where goiter is endemic. Early treatment with thyroid hormone generally promotes normal physical growth but may not prevent mental retardation. —**cretinoid, cretinous,** *adj.,* **cretin,** *n.*

Creutzfeldt-Jakob disease A rare, fatal encephalopathy caused by an as yet unidentified slow virus. The disease occurs in middle age, and symptoms are progressive dementia, dysarthria, muscle wasting, and various involuntary movements, as myoclonus and athetosis. Deterioration is obvious week to week. Death ensues, usually within a year. Transmission between humans is unusual but the disease has been observed years after exposure to needles, instruments, and electrodes previously used in the treatment of a patient with the disease. Isolation is not necessary. Special care in disposal or sterilization of potentially infective items is always necessary. Also called **Jakob-Creutzfeldt disease, spastic pseudoparalysis.**

crib death See **sudden infant death syndrome.**

cribriform carcinoma See **adenocystic carcinoma.**

crico- A combining form meaning 'ring': *cricoderma, cricoid, cricoidectomy.*

cricoid 1. Having a ring shape. 2. A ring-shaped cartilage connected to the thyroid cartilage by the cricothyroid ligament at the level of the sixth cervical vertebra.

cricoid pressure A technique to reduce the risk of the aspiration of stomach contents during induction of general anesthesia. The cricoid cartilage is pushed against the esophagus to prevent passive regurgitation. Cricoid pressure is applied prior to intubation, immediately after injection of the anesthetic drug or muscle relaxant.

cricopharyngeal Of or pertaining to the cricoid cartilage and the pharynx.

cricopharyngeal incoordination A defect in the normal swallowing reflex. The cricopharyngeus muscle ordinarily serves as a sphincter to keep the top of the esophagus closed except when the person is swallowing, vomiting, or belching. The trachea remains open for breathing, but air normally does not enter the esophagus during respiration. In swallowing, the reverse effect occurs and the larynx is closed while food slides past it into the esophagus, which is located immediately behind the larynx. When the somewhat complex series of neuromuscular actions is not properly coordinated as a result of disease or injury, the patient may choke, swallow air, regurgitate fluid into the nose, or experience discomfort in swallowing food. See also **dysphagia.**

cricothyrotomy An emergency incision into the larynx, performed to open the airway in a person who is choking. A small vertical midline cut is made just below the Adam's apple and above the cricoid cartilage. The incision is opened further with a transverse cut through the cricothyroid membrane, and the wound is spread open with a knife handle or other dilator. The new opening must be held open with a tube that is open at both ends to allow air to move in and out until a tracheostomy can be done. Compare **tracheostomy.**

cri du chat syndrome See **cat-cry syndrome.**

Crigler-Najjar syndrome A congenital, familial, autosomal anomaly, in which glucuronide transferase, an enzyme, is deficient or absent. The condition is characterized by nonhemolytic jaundice, an accumulation of unconjugated bilirubin in the blood, and severe disorders of the central nervous system.

Crimean-Congo hemorrhagic fever An arbovirus infection transmitted to humans through the bite of a tick, characterized by fever, dizziness, muscle ache, vomiting, headache, and other neurologic symptoms. After several days, in severe cases, bleeding from the skin and mucous membranes, particularly from the mouth and nose, bloody sputum or vomit, and blood-tinged feces may be seen. Transfusion may be necessary to replace lost blood; otherwise, treatment is symptomatic and supportive. There is no specific medication or therapy available for prevention or cure. It occurs mainly in the U.S.S.R., Asia, and Africa; agricultural workers are most often afflicted. See also **hemorrhagic fever.**

criminal abortion The intentional termination of pregnancy under any condition prohibited by law. See also **induced abortion.**

criminal psychology The study of the mental processes, motivational patterns, and behavior of criminals.

crin- A combining form meaning 'to separate': crinin, crinogenic.

-crinia A combining form meaning '(condition of) endocrine secretion': hemocrinia, hypercrinia, neurocrinia.

-crisia A combining form meaning: **1.** A 'diagnosis': acrisia, urocrisia. **2.** A '(specified) condition of endocrine secretion': hypercrisia,

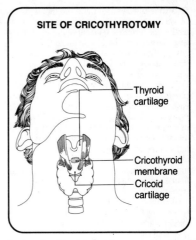

SITE OF CRICOTHYROTOMY

Thyroid cartilage

Cricothyroid membrane

Cricoid cartilage

hyperendocrisia, hypocrisia.

crisis **1.** A turning point for better or worse in the course of a disease, usually indicated by a marked change in the intensity of signs and symptoms. **2.** A turning point in events affecting the emotional state of a person, as death or divorce. **3.** A situation requiring use of problem-solving techniques and coping mechanisms to adapt to or solve the problem. See also **crisis intervention.**

crisis intervention In psychiatry: therapeutic intervention to help resolve a particular and immediate problem. No attempt is made at in-depth analysis. The goal is to restore the person to the level of functioning that existed before the current crisis.

crisis-intervention unit A group trained in emergency medical treatment and in various methods for rendering therapeutic psychiatric assistance to a person or group of persons during a period of crisis. Such networks are found within community hospitals, health-care centers, or as specialized self-contained units, as suicide prevention centers, and operate 24 hours a day.

crisscross inheritance The acquisition of genetic characteristics or conditions from the parent of the opposite sex.

crista supraventricularis The muscular ridge on the interior dorsal wall of the right ventricle of the heart. It defines the limit of the arterial cone and extends toward the pulmonary trunk from the ventral cusp of the atrioventricular ring. Compare **moderator band.**

criteria A set of standard or expected behaviors, conditions, or circumstances established as a basis for making judgments.

critical care See **intensive care.**

critical organs Tissues that are the most sensitive to irradiation, as the gonads, lymphoid organs, and intestines. The skin, cornea, oral cavity, esophagus, vagina, cervix, and optic lens are the next most sensitive organs to irradiation.

CRNA abbr **certified registered nurse anesthetist.** See **nurse anesthetist.**

Crohn's disease A chronic inflammatory bowel disease of unknown etiology, usually affecting the terminal segment of the small intestine, the colon, or both structures. Crohn's disease is characterized by frequent attacks of diarrhea, severe abdominal pain, nausea, fever, chills, weakness, anorexia, and weight loss. Children with the disease often suffer retarded physical growth. The diagnosis of Crohn's disease is based upon clinical signs, X-ray studies using a contrast medium, and endoscopy. The disease is easily confused with ulcerative colitis, an inflammatory bowel disease affecting the colon and rectum. Corticosteroids and antibiotics are used to control symptoms and to attempt to induce remission. In patients who are malnourished because of the disease, intravenous hyperalimentation is used to insure adequate intake of nutrients and to rest the bowel. Surgical removal of the diseased segment of the bowel provides some relief, but recurrence after surgery is likely.
NURSING CONSIDERATIONS: In many cases the inflammation extends to other areas of the bowel or to the stomach or duodenum. Other complications are arthritis, ankylosing spondylitis, kidney and liver disease, and skin and eye disorders. The formation of fistulas from the diseased bowel to the anus, vagina, skin surface, or to other loops of bowel are common. See also **colitis, ileitis.**

cromolyn sodium An adjunct in the treatment of asthma.

Cronkhite-Canada syndrome An abnormal familial condition characterized by gastrointestinal polyposis accompanied by ectodermal defects, as nail atrophy, alopecia, and excessive skin pigmentation. In some individuals it is also accompanied by protein-losing enteropathy, malabsorption, and deficiency of blood calcium, potassium, and magnesium.

cross In genetics: any method of crossbreeding or any individual, organism, or strain produced from crossbreeding. Kinds of crosses include **dihybrid cross, monohybrid cross, polyhybrid cross, trihybrid cross.**

crossbreeding The production of offspring by the mating of individuals from different races or of plants and animals from different varieties, strains, or species; hybridization. See also **inbreeding. —crossbred,** *adj.*

crossed reflex Any neural reflex in which stimulation of one side of the body results in a response on the other side, as the consensual light reflex.

cross-eye See **esophoria.**

cross fertilization **1.** In zoology: the union of gametes from different species or varieties in order to form hybrids. **2.** In botany: the fertilization of the flower of one plant by the pollen from a different plant, as opposed to self-fertilization. Also called **allogamy.**

crossing over The exchange of sections of chromatids between homologous pairs of chromosomes during the prophase stage of the first meiotic division. The process occurs through the formation of chiasmata and results in the recombination of genes. Also called **chiasmatypy.**

crossmatching of blood A procedure used by blood banks to determine compatibility of a donor's blood with that of a recipient after the specimens have been matched for major blood type. Serum from the donor's blood is mixed with red cells from the recipient's blood, and cells from the donor are mixed with serum from the recipient. If agglutination occurs, an antigenic substance is present, and the bloods are not compatible. If no agglutination occurs, the donor's blood may safely be transfused to the recipient. Compare **blood typing.** See also **ABO blood groups, Rh factor, transfusion, transfusion reaction.**

crossover The result of the recombination of genes on homologous pairs of chromosomes during meiosis. See also **crossing over.**

cross-sectional anatomy The study of the relationship of the structures of the body by the examination of cross sections of the tissue or organ. Compare **surface anatomy.**

crotamiton A scabicide.

croup An acute viral infection of the upper and lower respiratory tract that occurs primarily in infants and young children aged 3 months to 3 years, following an upper respiratory tract infection. It is characterized by hoarseness, fever, a distinctive harsh, brassy cough, persistent stridor during inspiration, and varying degrees of respiratory distress resulting from obstruction of the larynx. The most common causative agents are the parainfluenza viruses, especially Type 1, followed by the respiratory syncytial viruses (RSV) and influenza A and B viruses. Transmission occurs by infection with airborne particles or by contact with infected secretions. Onset of the acute stage is rapid, usually occurs at night, and may be precipitated by exposure to cold air. Routine treatment consists of bed rest, adequate fluid intake, and the alleviation of airway obstruction to ensure adequate respiratory exchange. Children with mild infections are usually managed at home with supportive measures, as vaporizers, humidifiers, or steam from hot running water in an enclosed bathroom to reduce the spasm of the laryngeal muscles and to free secretions. Hospitalization is indicated for children with high temperatures, progressive stridor and respiratory distress, and hypoxia, cyanosis, or pallor. Endotracheal intubation and tracheostomy may be necessary. Humidity and oxygen are usually prescribed. Fluids are often given intravenously to reduce physical exertion and the possibility of vomiting, with its attendant increased risk of aspiration. Nebulized racemic epinephrine, administered diluted with water by a face mask aerosol, may provide temporary relief in the acute phase in some children.
NURSING CONSIDERATIONS: The primary focus of nursing care is to ease breathing by providing humidity and to maintain continuous monitoring and surveillance for signs of respiratory dis-

tress and impending airway obstruction, with intubation and tracheostomy equipment kept readily available. To conserve the child's energy and to reduce apprehension, the nurse encourages rest, disturbs the child as little as possible, provides comfort, and encourages parental involvement whenever possible. Fever is usually reduced by the cool atmosphere of the mist tent; antipyretics are given as needed. To prevent chilling, frequent changes of clothing and bed linen are often necessary. The nurse also explains the condition to the parents and discusses appropriate care after discharge. In most children the condition is relatively mild and runs its course in 3 to 7 days. The infection may spread to other areas of the respiratory tract and may cause complications, as bronchiolitis, pneumonia, and otitis media. The most serious complication is laryngeal obstruction, which may cause death. Also called **acute laryngotracheobronchitis, angina trachealis, exudative angina, laryngostasis.** Compare **acute epiglottitis. —croupous, croupy,** *adj.*

Croupette A trade name for a device that provides cool humidification with the administration of oxygen or of compressed air, used especially in the treatment of pediatric patients. The Croupette consists of a nebulizer with attached tubing that connects with a canopy to enclose the patient and contain the humidifying mist. The environment of the patient may be cooled by adding ice to the ice compartment or by using a Croupette with its own refrigeration unit. This device is especially used to relieve hypoxia and liquefy secretions. It is also often used in the treatment of the croup, bronchiolitis, cystic fibrosis, asthma, laryngitis, postoperative dehydration, and hyperpyrexia. The oxygen concentration obtainable is approximately 21% to 60%.

crown 1. The upper part of an organ or structure, as the upper portion of a tooth. 2. An artificial restoration that replaces the natural crown of a tooth.

CRP *abbr* **C-reactive protein.**

CRT In data processing: *abbr* cathode-ray tube, or the display screen on a computer terminal or heart monitor similar to a television screen.

crucial bandage See **T bandage.**

cruciate ligament of the atlas A thin, bandlike ligament attaching the atlas to the base of the occipital bone above and the posterior surface of the body of the axis below.

crude birthrate The number of births/1,000 people in a population during 1 year. Compare **birthrate, refined birthrate, true birthrate.**

crur- A combining form meaning 'pertaining to the leg': *crura, crural, crureus.*

crura anthelicis The two ridges on the external ear marking the superior termination of the anthelix and bounding the triangular fossa. Also called crura of anthelix.

crureus See **vastus intermedius.**

crus, *pl.* **crura 1.** The leg, from knee to foot. **2.** A structure resembling a leg, as crura an-

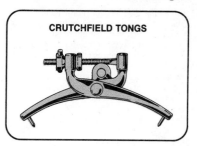

CRUTCHFIELD TONGS

thelicis, crus cerebri, crura ossea.

crus cerebri The ventral part of the cerebral peduncle, composed of the descending fiber tracts passing from the cerebral cortex to form the longitudinal fascicles of the pons. Also called **basis pedunculi cerebri.**

crush syndrome 1. A severe, life-threatening condition caused by extensive crushing trauma, characterized by destruction of muscle and bone tissue, hemorrhage, and fluid loss resulting in hypovolemic shock, hematuria, renal failure, and coma. Massive supportive therapy, including fluids, electrolytes, antibiotics, analgesia, oxygen, and intensive care with close monitoring of all vital functions, is usually necessary. **2.** A severe complication of heroin-induced coma characterized by edema, vascular occlusion, and lymphatic obstruction.

crutch A wooden or metal staff, the most common kind of which reaches from the ground almost to the axilla, to aid a person in walking. A padded, curved surface at the top fits under the arm; a grip in the form of a crossbar is held in the hand at the level of the palms to support the body. Kinds of crutches include axillary crutches, forearm crutches.

Crutchfield tongs An instrument inserted into the skull to hyperextend the head and neck of patients with cervical injuries. The tongs are inserted into small burr holes drilled in each parietal region of the skull; the surrounding skin is sutured and covered with a collodion dressing. A weight of from 10 to 20 lbs is suspended from a rope extending from the center of the tongs, over a pulley attached to the head of the bed allowing the weights to hang freely.

NURSING CONSIDERATIONS: The nurse maintains the patient's body alignment, checks the weight and traction apparatus, administers meticulous skin care, feeds the patient carefully to prevent aspiration, and provides for other care as necessary. A patient may be immobilized by Crutchfield tongs for weeks before surgery is performed; during an operation on the cervical spine and cord, the tongs may be left in place to maintain the proper alignment.

crutch gait A gait achieved by a person on crutches by alternately bearing weight on one or both legs and on the crutches. The gait selected and learned is determined by physical and functional abilities of the patient and by the diagnosis. In a three-point gait, weight is borne on the noninvolved leg, then on both crutches, then on the good leg. Touchdown and progression to full-weight bearing on the involved leg are usual. Four-point gait gives stability but requires bearing weight on both legs. Each leg is used alternately with each crutch. Two-point gait characteristically uses each crutch with the opposing leg. The swing-to and swing-through gaits are often used by paraplegic patients with weight-supporting braces on the legs. Weight is borne on the supported legs; the crutches are placed one stride in front of the person who then swings to that point or through the crutches to a spot in front of them.

Cruz trypanosomiasis   See **Chagas' disease.**

cry   **1.** A sudden, loud, voluntary or automatic vocalization in response to pain, fear, or a startle reflex. **2.** Weeping, because of pain or as an emotional response to depression or grief. **3.** See **cat-cry syndrome.**

cryo-, cry-   A combining form meaning 'pertaining to cold': *cryocautery, cryophilia, cryotolerant.*

cryoanesthesia   The freezing of a part to achieve adequate deadening of neural sensitivity to pain during brief minor surgical procedures.

cryocautery   The application of any substance, as carbon dioxide, that destroys tissue by freezing. Also called **cold cautery.**

cryogen   A chemical that induces freezing, used to destroy diseased tissue without injury to adjacent structures. Kinds of cryogens include carbon dioxide, freon, liquid nitrogen, nitrous oxide. —**cryogenic,** *adj.*

cryoglobulin   An abnormal plasma protein that precipitates and coalesces at low temperatures and dissolves and disperses at body temperature.

cryoglobulinemia   An abnormal condition in which cryoglobulins are present in the blood. Cryoglobulins may be found associated with multiple myeloma and angioneurotic edema.

cryoprecipitate   **1.** Any precipitate formed upon cooling a solution. **2.** A preparation rich in factor VIII needed to restore normal coagulation in hemophilia. It is collected from fresh human plasma that has been frozen and thawed.

cryostat   A device used in surgical pathology that consists of a special microtome used for freezing and slicing sections of tissue for study by a surgical pathologist.

cryosurgery   Use of subfreezing temperature to destroy tissue, as in the destruction of the ganglion of nerve cells in the thalmas in the treatment of Parkinson's disease. The process is also used in ophthalmology to cause the edges of a detached retina to heal and to remove cataracts. The coolant is circulated through a metal probe, chilling it to as low as $-160°C (-256°F)$, depending upon the chemical used. The moist tissues adhere to the cold metal of the probe and freeze. Cells are dehydrated as their membranes burst; they are eventually discarded or absorbed by the body.

cryotherapy   A treatment using cold as a destructive medium. Cutaneous tags, warts,

condylomata acuminatum, actinic keratosis, and dermatofibromas are some of the common skin disorders amenable to cryotherapy. Solid carbon dioxide or liquid nitrogen is applied briefly with a sterile cotton-tipped applicator. A blister forms, followed by necrosis.

crypt   A blind pit or tube on a free surface. Some kinds of crypts are **anal crypt, dental crypt, synovial crypt.**

crypt-   See **crypto-.**

cryptenamine acetate, c. tannate   Sympatholytic veratrine alkaloids used as antihypertensives.

cryptitis   An inflammation of a crypt, usually a perianal crypt, often accompanied by pain, pruritus, and spasm of the sphincter. Treatment may include hot compresses, sitz-baths, antibiotics, or excision.

crypto-, crypt-   A combining form meaning 'hidden': *cryptocephalus, cryptocrystalline, cryptodidymus.* Also **krypto-.**

cryptocephalus   A malformed fetus that has a small, underdeveloped head. —**cryptocephalic, cryptocephalous,** *adj.,* **cryptocephaly,** *n.*

cryptococcosis   An infectious disease caused by a fungus, *Cryptococcus neoformans,* which spreads through the lungs to the brain and central nervous system, skin, skeletal system, and urinary tract. It is characterized by the development of nodules or tumors filled with a gelatinous material in visceral and subcutaneous tissues. Initial symptoms may include coughing or other respiratory effects. After the fungus spreads to the meninges, neurologic symptoms may develop, including headache, blurred vision, and difficulty in speaking. The diagnosis is made by isolation and identification of the fungus in specimens of sputum, pus, or tissue biopsy. Amphotericin B and flucytosine may be administered in order to control the infection. Also called **Buschke's disease, European blastomycosis, torulosis.** See also *Cryptococcus,* specific fungal infections.

Cryptococcus   A genus of yeastlike fungi that reproduces by budding rather than by producing spores. Many nonpathogenic species of *Cryptococcus* are commonly found in the soil and on the skin and mucous membranes of people who are well. Certain pathogenic species exist; *C. neoformans* is the most important. See also **fungus, yeast.**

Cryptococcus neoformans   A species of yeastlike fungus that causes cryptococcosis, a potentially fatal infection which can affect the lungs, skin, and brain.

cryptodidymus   Conjoined twins in which one fetus is small, underdeveloped, and concealed within the body of the other, more fully formed autosite.

crypt of iris   Any one of the small pits in the iris which, along its free margin, is encircled by the circulus arteriosus minor. Also called **crypt of Fuchs.**

cryptomenorrhea   An abnormal condition in which the products of menstruation are retained within the vagina owing to an imperforate hymen or, less often, within the uterus owing to an occlusion of the cervical canal. Cryptomenorrhea is usually accompanied by subjective symptoms of menstruation with scant or absent flow and, sometimes, by severe pain. If the flow is completely obstructed, uterotubal reflux of menstrual flow into the pelvic cavity may cause peritonitis, pain, adhesions, and endometriosis. **—cryptomenorrheal,** *adj.*

cryptophthalmos A developmental anomaly characterized by complete fusion of the eyelids, usually with defective formation or complete lack of the eyes.

cryptorchidism Failure of one or both of the testicles to descend into the scrotum. If spontaneous descent does not occur by the age of 1, hormonal injections may be given. If not successful, surgery, called orchipexy, will likely be performed before the age of 5. Also called **undescended testis.**

crystal A solid inorganic substance, the atoms or molecules of which are arranged in a regular, repeating three-dimensional pattern. **—crystalline,** *adj.*

crystalline lens A transparent biconvex structure of the eye, enclosed in a capsule, situated between the iris and the vitreous humor, and slightly overlapped at its margin by the ciliary processes. The capsule of the lens is a transparent, elastic membrane that touches the free border of the iris anteriorly and is secured by the suspensory ligament of the lens. It is composed of a soft, cortical material, a firm nucleus, and concentric laminae and is covered anteriorly by transparent epithelium. In the fetus, the lens is very soft and has a slightly reddish tint; in the adult it is colorless and firm; in old age it becomes flattened, more dense, slightly opaque, and amber tinted. See also **eye.**

Cs Symbol for **cesium.**

CSF *abbr* **cerebrospinal fluid.**

CSR *abbr* **Cheyne-Stokes respiration.**

CT *abbr* **computerized tomography.** Also called computerized axial tomography.

Cu Symbol for **copper.**

Cuban itch See **alastrim.**

cuboid bone The cuboidal tarsal bone on the lateral side of the foot, proximal to the fourth and fifth metatarsal bones. It articulates with the calcaneus, lateral cuneiform, and fourth and fifth metatarsal bones, and, occasionally, with the navicular. Also called **os cuboideum.**

cuffed endotracheal tube An endotracheal tube with a balloon at one end which may be inflated to tighten the fit of the tube in the lumen of the airway. The balloon forms a cuff that prevents gastric contents from passing along the sides of the tube into the lungs and gas from leaking back from the lungs.

cul-de-sac A blind pouch or cecum, as the conjunctival cul-de-sac and the dural cul-de-sac.

cul-de-sac of Douglas See **rectouterine pouch.**

Cullen's sign The appearance of faint, ir-

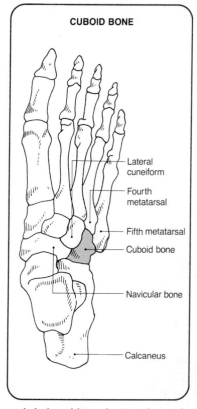

CUBOID BONE

Lateral cuneiform
Fourth metatarsal
Fifth metatarsal
Cuboid bone
Navicular bone
Calcaneus

regularly formed hemorrhagic patches on the skin around the umbilicus. The discolored skin is blue-black and becomes green-brown or yellow. Cullen's sign may appear 1 to 2 days after the onset of anorexia and the severe, poorly localized abdominal pains that are characteristic of acute pancreatitis. Cullen's sign is also present in massive upper gastrointestinal hemorrhage. Compare **Grey Turner's sign.** See also **pancreatitis.**

cult- A combining form meaning 'to tend or cultivate': *cultivation, cultural, culture.*

culture medium See **medium.**

culture procedure In bacteriology: any of several techniques for growing colonies of microorganisms in order to identify a pathogen and to determine which antibiotics are effective in combating the infection caused by the organism.

cumulative Increasing by incremental steps with an eventual total that may exceed the expected result.

cumulative action **1.** The increased activity of a therapeutic measure or agent when administered repeatedly, as the cumulative action of a regular exercise program. **2.** The increased activity demonstrated by a drug when repeated doses accumulate in the body and exert a greater biological effect than the initial dose.

CUP ARTHROPLASTY

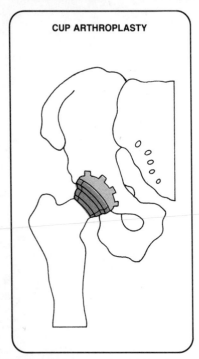

cumulative dose The total dose that accumulates from repeated exposure to radiation or a radiopharmaceutical product.

cumulative gene See **polygene.**

cune- A combining form meaning 'pertaining to a wedge': *cuneate, cuneiform, cuneus.*

cuneate Of tissue: wedge shaped, used especially in describing cells of the nervous system.

cuneiform Of bone and cartilage: wedge-shaped.

cuneiform bone See **triangular bone.**

cup arthroplasty of the hip joint The surgical replacement of the head of the femur by a metal or plastic mold to relieve pain and increase motion in arthritis or to correct a deformity. Under general anesthesia, the damaged or diseased bone is removed, and the acetabulum and the head of the femur are reshaped. A metal Vitallium cup is inserted between the two and becomes the articulating surface of the femur. Postoperatively, the patient's leg is suspended in traction to hold it in a position of abduction and internal rotation to keep the disk in place in the acetabulum. Continued abduction is necessary for 6 weeks. Possible complications include infection, thrombophlebitis, pulmonary embolism, and fat embolism. The patient receives extensive physical therapy; crutches are necessary to avoid bearing of full weight for 6 months, and an exercise program must be followed for several years. Compare **hip replacement.** See also **arthroplasty, knee re-**

placement, osteoarthritis, plastic surgery.

cupping and vibrating The procedures to help remove mucus and fluid from the lungs by the use of percussion and vibration to dislodge and mobilize the secretions. Cupping is performed by the rhythmic percussion of the affected segments of the lungs or bronchi by the cupped hands of the nurse. Cupping is begun gently and is increased in forcefulness as the patient tolerates increased percussion. Vibration is done by placing the nurse's hands over the affected area and shaking the arms from the shoulders, with the shaking sensation produced on the patient's chest comparable to the shaking that accompanies the chill of a fever. See also **postural drainage.**

cupric Of or pertaining to copper in its divalent form, as cupric sulfate.

cupulolithiasis A severe, long-lasting vertigo brought on by movement of the head to certain positions. There are many possible causes, among them otitis media, ear surgery, or injury to the inner ear. In addition to extreme dizziness, signs are nausea, vomiting, and ataxia. There is no treatment except avoidance of the offending head positions. Also called **postural vertigo.**

curare A substance derived from tropical plants of the genus *Stryknos.* It is a potent muscle relaxant that acts by preventing transmission of neural impulses across the myoneural junctions. Large dosage can cause complete paralysis. Pharmacologic preparations of the substance are used as adjuncts to general anesthesia. The use of curare or other neuromuscular blocking agents requires respiratory and ventilatory assistance by a qualified anesthetist or anesthesiologist. See also **tubocurarine chloride.**

curariform In pharmacology: **1.** Chemically similar to curare. **2.** Having the effect of curare.

curative treatment See **treatment.**

cure 1. Restoration to health of a person afflicted with a disease or other disorder. **2.** The favorable outcome of the treatment of a disease or other disorder. **3.** A course of therapy, a medication, a therapeutic measure, or other remedy used in treatment of a medical problem, as faith healing, fasting, rest cure, work cure.

curet 1. A surgical instrument shaped like a spoon or scoop for scraping and removing material or tissue from an organ, cavity, or surface. A curet may be blunt or sharp and is designed in a shape and size appropriate to its use. **2.** To remove tissue or debris with such a device. Kinds of curets include **Hartmann's curet.**

curettage Scraping of material from the wall of a cavity or other surface, performed to remove tumors or other abnormal tissue or to obtain tissue for microscopic examination. Curettage also refers to clearing unwanted material from fistulas and areas of chronic infection. It may be performed with a blunt or a sharp curet or by suction.

curie (Ci, c) A unit of radioactivity equal to 3.70×10^{10} disintegrations per second.

curium (Cm) A radioactive metallic element. Its atomic number is 96; its atomic weight is 247. Curium is an artificial element produced by bombarding plutonium with helium ions in a cyclotron.

Curling's ulcer   A duodenal ulcer that develops in people who have severe burns on the surface of the body. Also called **Curling's stress ulcer.** See also **milk therapy.**

current   **1.** A flowing or streaming movement. **2.** A flow of electrons along a conductor in a closed circuit; an electric current. **3.** Certain physiologic electrical activity and characteristics of blood circulation. Physiologic currents include abnerval current, action current, axial current, centrifugal current, centripetal current, compensating current, demarcation current, electrotonic current.

-current   A combining form meaning 'running, flowing, happening': *concurrent, excurrent, intercurrent.*

current of injury   See **demarcation current.**

Current Procedural Terminology (CPT)   A system developed by the American Medical Association for standardizing the terminology and coding used to describe medical services and procedures.

Curschmann spiral   One of the coiled fibrils of mucus occasionally found in the sputum of persons with bronchial asthma.

cursor   In data processing: a special character used on cathode-ray tube (CRT) screens to mark the spot where the next character will be read to or written from memory. The operator uses cursor control keys to maneuver the cursor on the screen and speed input and output of data.

curvature myopia   A type of nearsightedness caused by refractive errors associated with an excessive curvature of the cornea.

curve   In statistics: a straight or curved line used as a graphic method of demonstrating the distribution of data collected in a study or survey.

curve of Carus   The normal axis of the pelvic outlet. Also called **circle of Carus.**

curvilinear trend   In statistics: a trend in which a graphic representation of the data yields a curved line. The value of the independent variable may be expressed as a polynomial coefficient, by a more complete mathematical expression, as a logistic curve, or by a smoothing process, as a moving average.

cushingoid   Having the habitus and facies characteristic of Cushing's disease: fat pads on the upper back and face, striae on the limbs and trunk, and excess hair on the face.

Cushing's disease   A metabolic disorder characterized by the abnormally increased secretion of adrenocortical steroids caused by increased amounts of adrenocorticotropic hormone (ACTH) secreted by the pituitary, as by a pituitary adenoma. Also called **hyperadrenalism.** Compare **Cushing's syndrome.**

Cushing's syndrome   A metabolic disorder resulting from the chronic and excessive production of adrenocortical hormones or by the

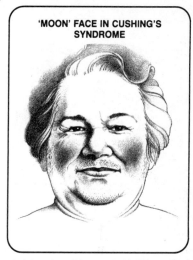

'MOON' FACE IN CUSHING'S SYNDROME

administration of glucocorticoids in large doses for several weeks or longer. The most common cause of the syndrome is a pituitary tumor that causes an increased secretion of ACTH. Less commonly, the syndrome may be due to an adrenal tumor. Characteristically, the patient with Cushing's syndrome has a decreased glucose tolerance, central obesity, round 'moon' face, supraclavicular fat pads, a pendulous, striae-covered pad of fat on the chest and abdomen, oligomenorrhea or decreased testosterone levels, muscular atrophy, edema, hypokalemia, and some degree of emotional change. The skin may be abnormally pigmented and fragile; minor infections may become systemic and long-lasting. Children with the disorder may stop growing. Occasionally, hypertension, kidney stones, and psychosis occur. The objective of all treatment is reduction of the secretion of cortisol. The source of the excess ACTH is discovered by a series of tests that challenge the function of the adrenal and pituitary glands. Most often, as the excess ACTH is the result of an adenoma of the anterior pituitary, X-ray irradiation or surgical excision of the tumor corrects the condition. If the condition is the result of medication, decreasing or changing the medication may alleviate the symptoms.

NURSING CONSIDERATIONS: Some of the medications used for some forms of the condition may cause nausea and anorexia, somnolence, and lethargy, and the patient is informed of this. Weight and electrolyte and fluid balance are monitored; an adequate, balanced diet is urged; and emotional changes are observed with a goal of maintaining emotional equilibrium. Also called hyperadrenocorticism. See also **Addison's disease, Cushing's disease, Nelson's syndrome.**

cusp   **1.** A sharp projection or a rounded eminence that rises from the chewing surface of a tooth, as the two pyramidal cusps that arise from the premolars. **2.** Any one of the small flaps on

cuspids

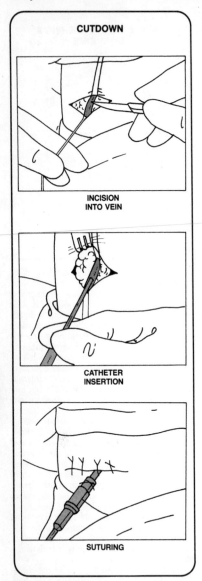

CUTDOWN

INCISION
INTO VEIN

CATHETER
INSERTION

SUTURING

the valves of the heart, as the ventral, dorsal, and medial cusps attached to the right atrioventricular valve.

cuspids The four canine teeth, each having a single cusp or point. See **canine tooth.**

cuspid valve Either of two structures in the heart that control the flow of blood between the atria and the ventricles. The cuspid valves are the mitral, or bicuspid, valve with two flaps between the left atrium and the left ventricle, and the tricuspid valve with three main flaps between the right atrium and the right ventricle.

Also called **atrioventricular valve.**

custodial care Services and care of a nonmedical nature provided on a long-term basis, usually for convalescent and chronically ill individuals. Kinds of custodial care include board, personal assistance.

cut In molecular genetics: a fissure or split in a double strand of DNA, in contrast to a nick in a single strand. See also **nick.**

cut- A combining form meaning 'pertaining to the skin': *cutaneous, cuticle, cuticularization.*

cutaneous Of or pertaining to the skin.

cutaneous absorption The taking up of substances through the skin.

cutaneous anaphylaxis A localized, exaggerated reaction of hypersensitivity in the form of a wheal and flare caused by an antigen injected into the skin of a sensitized individual, generally used as a test of sensitivity to various allergens. Passive cutaneous anaphylaxis, the response to an intradermally injected antibody, is used in studies of antibodies that induce immediate reactions of hypersensitivity.

cutaneous horn A hard, skin-colored projection of the epidermis, usually on the head or face. The lesion may be precancerous and is usually excised.

cutaneous larva migrans A skin condition caused by a hookworm, *Ancylostoma braziliense,* a parasite of cats and dogs. Its ova are deposited in the ground with the feces of infected animals, develop into larvae, and invade the skin of people (particularly those who are barefoot). As the larvae migrate through the epidermis, a trail of inflammation follows the burrow causing severe pruritus. Topical application of a solution of thiabendazole usually eradicates the larvae. Also called **creeping eruption.**

cutaneous leishmaniasis See **oriental sore.**

cutaneous lupus erythematosus See **discoid lupus erythematosus.**

cutaneous papilloma A small brown or flesh-colored outgrowth of skin, occurring most frequently on the neck of an older person. Also called cutaneous tag, skin tag.

cutdown An incision into a vein with insertion of a polyethylene catheter for intravenous infusion. It is performed when an infusion cannot be started by venipuncture and in hyperalimentation therapy, when highly concentrated solutions are given via catheter into the superior vena cava. The skin is cleansed before the procedure; the incision is sutured, and a sterile dressing applied at its conclusion. See also **hyperalimentation, venipuncture.**

cuticle 1. Epidermis. 2. The sheath of a hair follicle. 3. The thin edge of cornified epithelium at the base of a nail.

cutis See **skin.**

cutis laxa Abnormally loose, relaxed skin owing to an absence of elastic fibers in the body, usually a hereditary condition.

cutis marmorata See **livedo.**

CVA *abbr* 1. cerebrovascular accident. 2. costovertebral angle.

CVP monitor See **central venous pressure monitor.**

cyan- See **cyano-.**

cyanide poisoning Poisoning owing to the ingestion or inhalation of cyanide from such substances as bitter almond oil, prussic acid, hydrocyanic acid, or potassium or sodium cyanide. Characterized by tachycardia, drowsiness, convulsion, and headache, cyanide poisoning may result in death within 1 to 15 minutes. Treatment includes gastric lavage, amyl nitrite inhalation, oxygen, and sodium thiosulfate.

cyano-, cyan- A combining form meaning 'blue': *cyanochroia, cyanocrystallin.*

cyanocobalamin A red, crystalline, water-soluble vitamin essential for the metabolism of protein, fats, and carbohydrates, normal blood formation, and neural function. It is the only vitamin that contains essential mineral elements and is the first substance containing cobalt that is found to be vital to life. It cannot be produced synthetically but can be obtained from cultures of *Streptomyces griseus.* Rich dietary sources are liver, kidney, meats, fish, and dairy products. Deficiency also occurs in the absence of intrinsic factor, which is necessary for the absorption of cyanocobalamin from the gastrointestinal tract, and results in pernicious anemia. Symptoms of deficiency include nervousness, neuritis, numbness and tingling in the hands and feet, poor muscular coordination, unpleasant body odor, and menstrual disturbances. Cyanocobalamin is used in the prophylaxis and treatment of pernicious anemia, tropical and nontropical sprue, and other macrocytic and megaloblastic anemias. It is nontoxic, even when administered in amounts greater than those recommended for therapeutic purposes. Also called **antipernicious anemia factor, extrinsic factor, LLD factor, vitamin B₁₂.** See also **intrinsic factor, pernicious anemia.**

cyanomethemoglobin A hemoglobin derivative formed during nitrite therapy for cyanide poisoning.

cyanosis Bluish discoloration of the skin and mucous membranes caused by an excess of deoxygenated hemoglobin in the blood or a structural defect in the hemoglobin molecule, as in methemoglobin. —**cyanotic,** *adj.*

cycl- See **cyclo-.**

cyclacillin A penicillin antibiotic.

cyclamate An artificial, nonnutritive sweetener formerly used in the form of the calcium or sodium salt. It was withdrawn from the market because it caused cancer in laboratory animals.

cyclandelate A peripheral vasodilator.

cyclencephaly A developmental anomaly characterized by the fusion of the two cerebral hemispheres. —**cyclencephalic, cyclencephalous,** *adj.,* **cyclencephalus,** *n.*

cyclic adenosine monophosphate A cyclic nucleotide formed from adenosine triphosphate by the action of adenyl cyclase. This cyclic compound, known as the 'second messenger,' participates in the action of catechol-

amines, vasopressin, adrenocorticotropic hormone, and many other hormones. Also called **adenosine 3′:5′-cyclic phosphate.**

cyclitis Inflammation of the ciliary body causing redness of the sclera adjacent to the cornea of the eye.

cyclizine hydrochloride, c. lactate Antiemetic agents.

cyclo-, cycl- A combining form meaning 'round, recurring'; often with reference to the eye: *cyclodialysis, cycloid, cyclops.*

cyclobenzaprine hydrochloride A skeletal muscle relaxant.

cyclocephaly See **cyclopia.** —**cyclocephalic, cyclocephalous,** *adj.*

cyclopentolate hydrochloride A mydriatic agent.

cyclophosphamide An alkylating agent used in chemotherapy.

cyclopia A developmental anomaly characterized by fusion of the orbits into a single cavity containing one eye. The condition is usually combined with various other head and facial defects. Also called **cyclocephaly, synophthalmia.** —**cyclops,** *n.*

cycloplegia Paralysis of the ciliary muscles, as induced by certain ophthalmic drugs to allow examination of the eye. —**cycloplegic,** *adj., n.*

cycloplegic 1. Of or pertaining to a drug or treatment that causes paralysis of the ciliary muscles of the eye. 2. One of a group of anticholinergic drugs used to paralyze the ciliary muscles of the eye for ophthalmologic examination or surgery. Any of the cycloplegics may cause adverse effects in persons sensitive to anticholinergics.

cyclopropane A highly flammable and explosive potent anesthetic gas that produces good analgesia and skeletal muscle relaxation, with low toxicity, minimal adverse effects, and rapid induction and emergence. It has been largely replaced by the nonflammable halogenated hydrocarbons and is now used for anesthesia only when characteristics of other anesthetic agents contraindicate their use in a specific patient. Also called **trimethylene.**

cycloserine An antitubercular agent.

cyclothiazide A thiazide diuretic.

cyclothymic personality 1. A personality characterized by extreme swings in mood from elation to depression. 2. A person who has this disorder. Also called **bipolar disorder.**

cycrimine hydrochloride A cholinergic blocking (parasympatholytic) agent.

cylindroma, *pl.* **cylindromas, cylindromata** 1. A tumor characterized by cylinders of mucinous tissue in nests of epithelial cells. It may occur in the breast, salivary glands, or mucous glands of the respiratory tract. Also called **adenocystic carcinoma. 2.** A benign neoplasm of the skin, usually of the scalp or face, developing from a hair follicle or sweat gland. Also called **cylindromatous spiradenoma, trichobasalioma hyalinicum.**

cylindromatous carcinoma See **adenocystic carcinoma.**

cylindromatous spiradenoma See **cylindroma,** definition 2.

cyno-, cyn- A combining form meaning 'pertaining to dogs, doglike': *cynobax, cynocephalic, cynophobia.*

cyproheptadine hydrochloride An antihistamine.

Cyprus fever See **brucellosis.**

cyst A closed sac in or under the skin lined with epithelium and containing fluid or semi-solid material, as a **sebaceous cyst.**

cyst- See **cysto-.**

-cyst A combining form meaning a 'pouch or bladder': *enterocyst, microcyst, zoocyst.* Also **-cystis.**

cystadenoma, *pl.* **cystadenomas, cystadenomata 1.** An adenoma associated with a cystoma. **2.** An adenoma containing multiple cystic structures.

cystectomy A surgical procedure in which all or a part of the urinary bladder is removed, as may be required in treating cancer of the bladder.

cysteine An amino acid found in many proteins in the body, including keratin. It is a metabolic precursor of cystine.

cysti- See **cysto-.**

cystic Pertaining to a cyst or to the gallbladder or urinary bladder.

cystic acne See **acne conglobata.**

cystic carcinoma A malignant neoplasm containing cysts or cystlike spaces. Tumors of this kind occur in the breast and ovary.

cystic duct The duct through which bile from the gallbladder passes into the common bile duct.

cysticercosis An infection and infestation by the larval stage of the pork tapeworm *Taenia solium.* The eggs are ingested and hatch in the intestine; the larvae invade the subcutaneous tissue, brain, eye, muscle, heart, liver, lung, and peritoneum. The invasive, early phase of the infection is characterized by fever, malaise, muscle pain, and eosinophilia. Years later, epilepsy and personality change may appear if the brain is affected. Prophylaxis depends on avoiding ingestion of inadequately cooked, infected pork.

cystic fibroma A fibrous tumor in which cystic degeneration has occurred.

cystic fibrosis An inherited disorder of the exocrine glands, causing those glands to produce abnormally thick secretions of mucus. The glands most affected are those in the pancreas, the respiratory system, and the sweat glands. Cystic fibrosis is usually recognized in infancy or early childhood, occurring chiefly among Caucasians. When present in infancy, it may be preceded by meconium ileus, an obstruction of the small bowel by viscid stool. Other early signs are a chronic cough, frequent, foul-smelling stools, and persistent upper respiratory infections. The most reliable diagnostic tool is the sweat test, which shows elevations of both sodium and chloride. Since there is no known cure, treatment is directed at the prevention of respiratory infections, which are the most frequent cause of

death. Mucolytic agents, bronchodilators, and mist tents are used to help liquefy the thick, tenacious mucus. Physical therapy measures, as postural drainage and breathing exercises, can also dislodge secretions. Broad spectrum antibiotics may be used prophylactically.

cystic goiter An enlargement of the thyroid gland containing cysts resulting from mucoid or colloid degeneration.

cystic lymphangioma A cystic growth formed by lymph vessels; usually congenital, it most frequently occurs in the neck, axilla, or groin of children. Also called cystic hygroma, lymphangioma cysticum.

cystic mole See **hydatid mole.**

cystic myxoma A tumor of the connective tissue that has undergone cystic degeneration.

cystic neuroma A neoplasm of nerve tissue that has degenerated and become cystic. Also called **false neuroma.**

cystic tumor A tumor with cavities or sacs containing a semisolid or a liquid material.

cystido- See **cysto-.**

cystine An amino acid found in many proteins in the body, including keratin and insulin. Cystine is a product of the metabolism of cysteine.

cystinosis A congenital disease characterized by glucosuria, proteinuria, cystine deposits in the liver, spleen, bone marrow, and cornea, rickets, excessive amounts of phosphates in the urine, and retardation of growth. Also called cystine storage disease. See also **cystine.**

cystinuria 1. Abnormal presence in the urine of the amino acid cystine. **2.** An inherited defect of the renal tubules, characterized by excessive urinary excretion of cystine and several other amino acids. The disorder is caused by an autosomal recessive trait which impairs cystine reabsorption by the kidney tubules. In high concentration cystine tends to precipitate in the urinary tract and form kidney or bladder stones. Treatment attempts to prevent the formation of stones or to dissolve them by increasing the volume of urine flow, decreasing the pH of the urine, and increasing the solubility of cystine.

-cystis See **-cyst.**

-cystitis A combining form meaning an 'inflammation of the bladder or cyst': *epicystitis, gonecystitis, pericystitis.*

cystitis An inflammatory condition of the urinary bladder and ureters, characterized by pain, urgency, and frequency of urination and by hematuria. It may be caused by a bacterial infection, calculus, or tumor. Depending upon the diagnosis, treatment may include antibiotics, increased fluid intake, bed rest, medications to control bladder wall spasms, and, when necessary, surgery.

cysto-, cyst-, cysti- A combining form meaning 'pertaining to the bladder, or to a cyst or sac': *cystocele, cystodynia, cystomyoma.* Also **cystido-.**

cystocele Herniation of the urinary bladder into the birth canal caused by injury to the vaginal wall during delivery.

CYSTOSCOPY

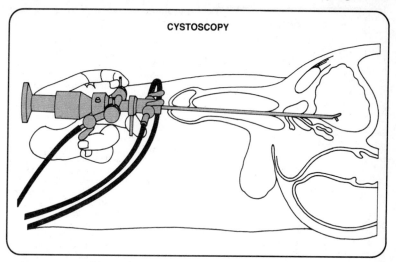

cystogram A graphic record, usually a series of X-ray films, obtained as a part of any excretory urographic procedure, as in retrograde pyelography or retrograde cystoscopy.

cystoma, *pl.* **cystomas, cystomata** Any tumor or growth containing cysts, especially one in or near the ovary.

-cystoma A combining form meaning a 'cystic tumor': *enterocystoma, hydrocystoma, inocystoma.*

cystometry Assessment of the bladder's neuromuscular efficiency by measuring muscle reflex, intravesical pressure and capacity, and reaction to thermal stimulation.

cystoscope An instrument for examining and treating lesions of the urinary bladder, ureter, and kidney. It consists of an outer sheath with a lighting system, a viewing obturator, and a passage for catheters and operative devices. —**cystoscopic,** *adj.*

cystoscopic urography See **retrograde cystoscopy.**

cystoscopy The direct visualization of the urinary tract by means of a cystoscope inserted in the urethra. In addition to visualization, cystoscopy is used for obtaining biopsies of tumors or other growths and for the removal of polyps. After the examination the patient is observed for the common complications of trauma and signs of urinary infection. See also **cystoscope.** —**cystoscopic,** *adj.*

cyt-, cyto- A combining form meaning 'cell' or 'cytoplasm': *cytochrome, cytogenesis, cytosome.*

cytarabine An antimetabolite used in chemotherapy.

-cyte A combining form meaning a 'cell' of a specified type: *gliacyte, hemacyte, plasmacyte.*

-cythemia A combining form meaning a 'condition involving cells in the blood': *achroiocythemia, rhestocythemia, thrombocythe-*mia. Also **-cythaemia.**

cytoarchitecture The typical pattern of cellular arrangement within a particular tissue or organ. —**cytoarchitectural,** *adj.*

cytobiotaxis See **cytoclesis.** —**cytobiotactic,** *adj.*

cytoblast The nucleus of a cell.

cytocentrum See **centrosome.**

cytocerastic See **cytokerastic.**

cytochemism The chemical activity within the living cell, specifically the various reactions to and affinity for chemical substances.

cytochemistry The study of the various chemicals within a living cell and their actions and functions.

cytocide Any substance that is destructive to cells. —**cytocidal,** *adj.*

cytoclesis The influence exerted by one cell on the action of other cells; the vital principle of all living tissue. Also called **cytobiotaxis.** —**cytocletic,** *adj.*

cytoctony The destruction of cells, specifically the killing of cells in culture by viruses.

cytode The simplest type of cell, consisting of a protoplasmic mass without a nucleus, as a bacterium.

cytodieresis, *pl.* **cytodiereses** Cell division, especially the phenomena involving the division of the cytoplasm. See also **meiosis, mitosis.** —**cytodieretic,** *adj.*

cytodifferentiation In embryology: **1.** A process by which embryonic cells acquire biochemical and morphological properties essential for specialization and diversification. **2.** The total and gradual transformation from an undifferentiated to a fully differentiated state.

cytogene A particle within the cytoplasm of a cell that is self-replicating, derived from the genes in the nucleus, and capable of transmitting hereditary information. —**cytogenic,** *adj.*

cytogenesis The origin, development, and differentiation of cells. —**cytogenetic, cyto-**

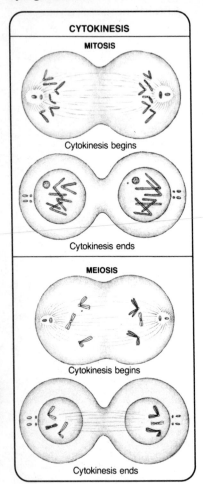

CYTOKINESIS

MITOSIS

Cytokinesis begins

Cytokinesis ends

MEIOSIS

Cytokinesis begins

Cytokinesis ends

genic, *adj.* Also called **cytogeny.**

cytogeneticist One who specializes in cytogenetics.

cytogenetics The branch of genetics that studies the cellular constituents concerned with heredity, primarily the structure, function, and origin of the chromosomes. One kind of cytogenetics is **clinical cytogenetics.** —**cytogenetic,** *adj.*

cytogenic gland A glandular organ that secretes living cells, specifically the testes and ovary.

cytogenic reproduction The formation of a new organism from a unicellular germ cell, either sexually through the fusion of gametes to form a zygote or asexually by means of spores.

cytogeny 1. Cytogenetics. 2. The origin and development of the cell. —**cytogenic, cytogenous,** *adj.*

cytogony Cytogenic reproduction. —**cytogenic,** *adj.*

cytohistogenesis The structural development and formation of cells. —**cytohistogenetic,** *adj.*

cytohyaloplasm See **hyaloplasm.**

cytoid Like or resembling a cell.

cytoid body A small white spot on the retina of each eye that is seen by using an ophthalmoscope in examining the eyes of a patient affected with systemic lupus erythematosus.

cytokerastic, cytocerastic Pertaining to or characteristic of cellular development from a lower to a higher form or from a simple to more complex arrangement.

cytokinesis The division of the cytoplasm, exclusive of nuclear division, that occurs during the final stages of mitosis and meiosis to form daughter cells; the sum total of all the changes that occur in the cytoplasm during mitosis, meiosis, and fertilization. —**cytokinetic,** *adj.*

cytological map The graphic representation of the location of genes on a chromosome, based on correlating genetic recombination test-crossing results with the structural analysis of chromosomes that have undergone such changes as deletions or translocations as detected by banding techniques.

cytologist One who specializes in the study of cells, specifically one who uses cytological techniques in the differential diagnosis of neoplasms.

cytology The study of cells, including their formation, origin, structure, function, biochemical activities, and pathology. Kinds of cytology are **aspiration biopsy cytology, exfoliative cytology.** —**cytologic, cytological,** *adj.*

cytolymph See **hyaloplasm.**

cytolysin An antibody that dissolves antigenic cells. Kinds of cytolysin are **bacteriolysin, hemolysin.**

cytolysis, *pl.* **cytolyses** The destruction or breakdown of the living cell, primarily by the disintegration of the outer membrane. A kind of cytolysis is **immune cytolysis.** —**cytolytic,** *adj.*

cytomegalic inclusion disease (CID) An infection caused by the cytomegalovirus, one of the herpesviruses. It is primarily a congenitally acquired disease of newborn infants and is characterized by microcephaly, retarded growth, hepatosplenomegaly, hemolytic anemia, and pathological fracture of long bones. Also called **cytomegalovirus disease.** See also **TORCH syndrome.**

cytomegalovirus (CMV) disease 1. See **cytomegalic inclusion disease.** 2. A viral infection caused by the cytomegalovirus, characterized by malaise, fever, lymphadenopathy, pneumonia, hepatosplenomegaly, and superinfection with various bacteria and fungi as a result of the depression of immune response characteristic of herpesviruses.

cytometer A device for counting and measuring the number of cells within a given amount of fluid, as blood, urine, or cerebrospinal fluid.

cytometry The counting and measuring of cells, specifically blood cells. —**cytometric,** *adj.*

cytomitome The fibrillary network within

the cytoplasm of a cell, as contrasted with that in the nucleoplasm. See also **karyomitome.**

cytomorphology The study of the various forms of cells and the structures contained within them. —**cytomorphologic, cytomorphological,** *adj.,* **cytomorphologist,** *n.*

cytomorphosis, *pl.* **cytomorphoses** The various changes that occur within a cell during the course of its life cycle, from the earliest undifferentiated stage until destruction.

cyton, cytone The cell body of a neuron or that portion containing the nucleus and its surrounding cytoplasm from which the axon and dendrites are formed.

cytophotometer An instrument for measuring light density through stained portions of cytoplasm, used for locating and identifying chemical substances within cells.

cytophotometry The identification of chemical substances within cells, using a cytophotometer. Also called **microfluorometry.** —**cytophotometric,** *adj.*

cytophysiology The study of the biochemical processes involved in the functioning of an individual cell, as contrasted with the functioning of organs or tissues. —**cytophysiologic, cytophysiological,** *adj.,* **cytophysiologist,** *n.*

cytoplasm All of the substance of a cell other than the nucleus. See also **cell, nucleus.**

cytoplasmic inheritance The acquisition of traits or conditions controlled by self-replicating substances within the cytoplasm, as mitochondria or chloroplasts, rather than by the genes on the chromosomes in the nucleus. The phenomenon occurs in plants and lower animals but has not yet been demonstrated in man.

cytotoxic anaphylaxis An exaggerated reaction of hypersensitivity to an injection of antibodies specific for antigenic substances that occur normally on the surfaces of body cells.

cytotoxic drug Any pharmacological compound that inhibits the proliferation of cells within the body. Such compounds, as the alkylating agents and the antimetabolites, are designed to destroy abnormal cells selectively, while sparing as many normal cells as possible; they are commonly used in chemotherapy. Cytotoxic agents have a potential for producing teratogenesis, mutagenesis, and carcinogenesis.

cytotoxic hypersensitivity An IgG or an IgM complement dependent, immediate-acting hypersensitive humoral response to foreign cells or to alterations of surface antigens on the cells. Direct and immediate destruction of cells occurs, as seen in hemolytic disease of the newborn and in severe transfusion reactions. Also called **type II hypersensitivity.** See also **immune complex hypersensitivity.**

cytotoxin A substance that has a toxic effect on certain cells. —**cytotoxic,** *adj.*

cytotrophoblast The inner layer of cells of the trophoblast of the early mammalian embryo that gives rise to the outer surface and villi of the chorion. Also called **Langhans' layer.** Compare **syncytiotrophoblast.** —**cytotrophoblastic,** *adj.*

D

D   Chemical symbol for **deuterium.**

d   Chemical abbreviation for **dextro-**, a prefix meaning to the right or clockwise.

DA   *abbr* developmental age.

dacarbazine (DTIC)   An alkylating agent used in chemotherapy.

dacry-   See **dacryo-.**

dacryo-, dacry-   A combining form meaning 'pertaining to tears': *dacryocele, dacryolin, dacryorrhea.*

dacryocyst   A lacrimal sac at the medial angle of the eye, a normal anatomical feature.

dacryocystectomy   Partial or total excision of the lacrimal sac.

dacryocystitis   An infection of the lacrimal sac caused by obstruction of the nasolacrimal duct, characterized by tearing and discharge from the eye. In the acute phase, the sac becomes inflamed and painful. The disorder is nearly always unilateral and usually occurs in infants. Systemic administration of antibiotics is usual; local, topical treatment is seldom effective; and, rarely, a dacryocystorhinostomy may be required. Compare **dacryostenosis.**

dacryocystorhinostomy   A surgical procedure for restoring drainage into the nose from the lacrimal sac when the nasolacrimal duct is obstructed.

dacryostenosis   An abnormal stricture of the nasolacrimal duct, occurring either as a congenital condition or as a result of infection or trauma. Dacryocystorhinostomy may be required to correct this condition. Compare **dacryocystitis.**

dactinomycin (actinomycin D)   An antibiotic used in chemotherapy.

dactyl   A digit (finger or toe). —**dactylic,** *adj.*

dactyl-   See **dactylo-.**

-dactyl   A combining form meaning 'digit (finger or toe)': *hermodactyl, pachydactyl, pentadactyl.*

-dactylia   A combining form meaning '(condition of the) fingers or toes': *ankylodactylia, heptadactylia, oligodactylia.* Also **-dactyly.**

dactylo-, dactyl-   A combining form meaning 'pertaining to a finger or toe': *dactylophasia, dactylospasm, dactylosymphysis.*

-dactyly   See **-dactylia.**

Dakin's solution   A formerly used antiseptic solution containing 0.4% to 0.5% of sodium hypochlorite.

daltonism   *Informal.* A form of color blindness characterized by an inability to distinguish the color red. It is genetically transmitted as a sex-linked autosomal recessive trait. Also called **protanopia.**

Dalton's law of partial pressures   In physics: a law stating that the sum of the pressure exerted by a mixture of gases is equal to the total of the partial pressures that could be exerted by the gases if they were separated. See also **Avogadro's law, Boyle's law, Gay-Lussac's law.**

damages   In law: a sum of money awarded to a plaintiff by a court as compensation for any loss, detriment, or injury to the plaintiff's person, property, or rights caused by the malfeasance or negligence of the defendant. **Actual damages** are awarded to reimburse the plaintiff for the loss or injury sustained. **Nominal damages** are awarded to show that a legal wrong has been committed although no recoverable loss can be determined. **Punitive damages** exceed the actual cost of injury or damage and are awarded when the defendant has acted maliciously or in reckless disregard of the plaintiff's rights.

damp   A potentially lethal atmosphere in caves and mines. **Choke damp** (black damp) is caused by absorption of the available oxygen by coal seams. **Fire damp** is composed of methane and other explosive hydrocarbon gases. **White damp** is another name for carbon monoxide.

danazol   An androgenic substance used to treat endometriosis and fibrocystic breast disease.

dance reflex   A normal response in the neonate to simulate walking by a reciprocal flexion and extension of the legs when held in an erect position with the soles touching a hard surface. The reflex disappears by about 3 to 4 weeks of age and is replaced by controlled, deliberate movement. Also called **step reflex.**

D & C   *abbr* dilatation and curettage.

dander   Dry scales shed from the skin or hair of animals or feathers of birds that may cause allergy in some individuals.

dandruff   An excessive amount of scaly material composed of dead, keratinized epithelium shed from the scalp that may be a mild form of seborrheic dermatitis. Treatment with a keratolytic shampoo is usually recommended to soften and remove the scales.

dandy fever   See **dengue.**

Dandy-Walker cyst   A cystic malformation of the fourth ventricle of the brain, resulting from hydrocephalus. Diagnosis of the defect is made with CT scan, with X-rays and, less commonly, with a ventriculogram. See also **hydrocephalus, shunt.**

danthron   A stimulant laxative.

dantrolene sodium   A skeletal muscle relaxant.

dapsone   An antileprotic agent.

Darier's disease   See **keratosis follicularis.**

dark-adapted eye   An eye in which the pupil has dilated, making it more sensitive to dim light.

darkfield illumination   See **darkfield microscopy.**

darkfield microscope   A microscope, with a special condenser and diaphragm, that scatters the light from the observed object, so that the object appears bright against a dark background and is more easily examined.

darkfield microscopy   Examination with a darkfield microscope, in which the specimen is illuminated by a peripheral light source. Organisms in specimens that have been prepared for use with a darkfield microscope appear to glow against a dark background. The technique is used primarily to identify the syphilis spirochete. Also called **darkfield illumination, ultramicroscopy.**

Darwinian theory   The theory postulated by Charles Darwin that organic evolution results from the process of natural selection of those variants of plants and animals best suited to survive in their environmental surroundings. Also called **Darwinism.** Compare **Lamarckism.** —**Darwinian,** *adj., n.*

DASE   *abbr* Denver Articulation Screening Examination.

DAT   *abbr* Dental Aptitude Test. See **dentist.**

data, *sing.* **datum**   Some pieces of information, especially those that are part of a collection of information to be used in an analysis of a problem, as the diagnosis of a health problem.

data analysis   In research: the phase of a study that includes classifying, coding, and tabulating information needed to perform statistical or qualitative analyses according to the research design and appropriate to the data. Data analysis follows data collection and precedes interpretation or application of the data.

data base   A large store or bank of information, especially in a form that can be processed by computer.

data collection   **1.** In research: the phase of a study that includes gathering of information and identification of sampling units as directed by the research design. Data collection precedes data analysis. **2.** In a clinical setting: the gathering of information by observation, interview, examination, and review of records.

daughter chromosome   Either of the paired chromatids that during the anaphase stage of mitosis separate and migrate to opposite ends of the cell prior to division. Each contains the complete genetic information of the original chromosome and was formed during interphase by the duplication of the DNA molecule.

daughter product   See **decay product.**

daunorubicin hydrochloride   An antibiotic used in chemotherapy.

Davidson regimen   A method of treating chronic constipation in children, of developing regular bowel habits, and of identifying those with functional bowel disease or obstructive

disorders. See also **toilet training.**

day-care   A specialized program or facility that provides care for preschool children, usually within a group framework, either as a substitute for or extension of home care, particularly for single parents or for parents who are both employed outside the home. Day-care groups vary in size and function and range from casual neighborhood parent-supervised play groups to formal nursery schools or organized centers run by trained personnel.

db   *abbr* **decibel.**

DD   *abbr* **developmental disability.**

DDS   *abbr* Doctor of Dental Surgery.

DDST   *abbr* **Denver Developmental Screening Test.**

DDT (dichlorodiphenyltrichloroethane)   A water-insoluble chlorinated hydrocarbon used worldwide as a major insecticide, especially in agriculture. In recent years knowledge of its adverse impact on the environment has led to restrictions in its use. In addition, because tolerance in formerly susceptible organisms develops rapidly, DDT has been largely replaced by organophosphate insecticides in the United States. It is still used as a pediculocide where large-scale delousing is justified, as in barracks and refugee camps. Its value as a scabicide is marginal, since scabies and crabs quickly become resistant to it. See also **scabicide.**

DDT poisoning   See **chlorinated organic insecticide poisoning.**

de-   A combining form meaning 'down or from': *deaquation, decartation, dedentition.*

DEA   *abbr* **Drug Enforcement Administration.**

dead-end host   Any animal from which a parasite cannot escape to continue its life cycle. Humans are dead-end hosts for trichinosis, because the larvae encyst in muscle and human flesh is unlikely to be a source of food for other animals susceptible to this parasite. Compare **definitive host, intermediate host, reservoir host.**

dead space   A cavity that remains after the incomplete closure of a surgical or traumatic wound, leaving an area in which blood can collect and delay healing. See also **anatomical dead space, physiological dead space.**

deaf   **1.** Unable to hear; hard of hearing. **2.** People who are unable to hear. —**deafness,** *n.*

deaf-and-dumb   The condition of being unable to hear or speak. See also **deaf-mute.**

deaf-mute   A person who is unable to hear or to speak because of disability of the brain or the organs of hearing and speech. Also called **deaf-and-dumb.**

deafness   A condition characterized by a partial or complete loss of hearing. In assessing deafness the patient's ears are examined for drainage, crusts, accumulation of cerumen, or structural abnormality. It is determined if the deafness is temporary or permanent and if the defect is congenital or a condition acquired in childhood, adolescence, or adulthood. In all cases the degree of loss and the kind of impairment

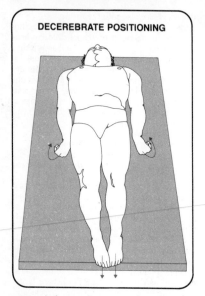

DECEREBRATE POSITIONING

causing the loss are determined. An older person with hearing impairment usually has a sensorineural loss as well as a conductive hearing loss. High sounds are hard to hear and discernment of such letter sounds as 's' and 'f' becomes difficult. Speaking clearly and slowly, allowing the person to lip-read, is helpful, as are visual cues clear with enunciation; shouting is not. The treatment of deafness depends on the cause. Merely removing impacted cerumen from the external auditory canal may significantly improve hearing. Hearing aids, amplification of sound, or lip-reading may be useful. Speech therapy is useful in teaching a person to speak or helping a person to retain the ability to speak. NURSING CONSIDERATIONS: If the patient uses a hearing aid, its placement and operation are checked before the speaker begins to talk; the voice is modulated to a pitch that is comfortable for the patient, and the speaker stands or sits where the lips are visible to the deaf individual. If the patient uses sign language, an interpreter or another means of communication is sought; when a pad and pencil are used, messages are written in short, simple phrases, and adequate time is allowed for the patient to understand and answer. See also **conductive hearing loss, sensorineural hearing loss.**

deanol acetamidobenzoate   A central nervous system stimulant.

death   **1.** Apparent death: the cessation of life as indicated by the absence of heartbeat or respiration. **2.** Legal death: the total absence of activity in the brain and the central nervous, cardiovascular, and respiratory systems, as observed and declared by a physician. See also **cell death, sudden infant death syndrome.**

death trance   A state in which a person appears to be dead.

debility   Feebleness, weakness, or loss of strength. See also **asthenia.**

debride   To remove dirt, foreign objects, damaged tissue, and cellular debris from a wound or a burn in order to prevent infection and to promote healing. In treating a wound, debridement is the first step in cleansing it; debridement also allows thorough examination of the extent of the injury. In treating a burn, debridement of the eschar may be performed in a hydrotherapy bath. —**debridement,** *n.*

dec-   A combining form meaning: **1.** 'Ten': *decagram, decaliter, decipara.* **2.** 'Tenth': *decigram, deciliter, decinormal.*

decalcification   Loss of calcium salts from the teeth and bones caused by malnutrition, malabsorption, or other dietary or physiological factors. See also **calcium, mineral.**

decamethonium bromide   Adjunct to anesthesia to relax skeletal muscle.

decanoic acid   See **capric acid.**

decay product   In radiology: a stable or radioactive nuclide formed directly from the radioactive disintegration of a radionuclide or as a result of successive transformation in a radioactive series. Also called **daughter product.**

deceleration   A decrease in the speed or velocity of an object or reaction. Compare **acceleration.**

deceleration phase   In obstetrics: the latter part of active labor characterized by a decreased rate of dilatation of the cervical os on a Friedman curve.

decerebrate   In research: to remove the higher centers of the brain or render an animal's cerebrum nonfunctional by transection of the spinal cord at the brain stem. Similar brain injuries in man can produce severe neurologic deficit.

decerebrate positioning   A motor response to noxious stimuli, commonly associated with lesions that depress the upper brain stem. In this posture, the patient's head is retracted, and the arms are adducted and extended, with the wrists pronated and the fingers flexed. The legs are stiffly extended, with plantar flexion of the feet. Compare **decorticate positioning.**

decibel (db)   A unit of measure of the intensity of sound. A decibel is one tenth of a bel; an increase of 1 bel is perceived as an approximate doubling of loudness.

decidua   The epithelial tissue of the endometrium lining the uterus, especially that which envelops the conceptus during gestation and is shed in the puerperium, but also that which is shed during menstruation. Kinds of decidua are **decidua basalis, decidua capsularis, decidua vera.**

decidua basalis   The decidua of the endometrium in the uterus that lies beneath the implanted ovum. Also called **decidua serotina.**

decidua capsularis   The decidua of the endometrium of the uterus covering the implanted ovum. Also called **decidua reflexa.**

decidual endometritis   An inflammation or infection of any portion of the decidua during pregnancy. See also **endometritis.**

decidua menstrualis The endometrium shed during menstruation.

decidua parietalis See **decidua vera.**

decidua reflexa See **decidua capsularis.**

decidua serotina See **decidua basalis.**

decidua vera The decidua of the endometrium lining the uterus except for those areas beneath and above the implanted and developing ovum called, respectively, the decidua basalis and the decidua capsularis.

deciduous dentition The eruption of the first teeth, which are later replaced by the permanent teeth. The process usually begins between the 6th and 8th months of life with the appearance of the two lower incisors and is completed between 2 and 3 years of age with a total of 20 teeth. The deciduous teeth are shed in order of appearance and replaced by 32 permanent teeth. Also called **first dentition, primary dentition.** Compare **permanent dentition.** See also **predeciduous dentition, teething.**

deciduous tooth Any 1 of the set of 20 teeth that appear during infancy, consisting of 4 incisors, 2 canines, and 4 molars in each jaw. Deciduous teeth start developing about the 6th week of fetal life as a thickening of the epithelium along the line of the future jaw. During the 7th week the epithelium splits longitudinally into the labial strand and the lingual strand. The labial strand forms the labiodental lamina. The lingual strand becomes the dental lamina, which develops 10 enlargements in each jaw. The enlargements appear about the 9th week and correspond to the future deciduous teeth. The first deciduous tooth erupts about 6 months after birth. Thereafter, 1 or more deciduous teeth erupt about every month until all 20 have appeared. Deciduous teeth are usually shed between the ages of 6 and 13. Also called **milk tooth.** Compare **permanent tooth.** See also **tooth.**

decoic acid See **capric acid.**

decompensation **1.** Failure of the heart to maintain adequate circulation; characterized by dyspnea, venous engorgement, and edema. **2.** Failure of the defense system mechanism as seen in progressive personality disintegration.

decompression sickness A painful, sometimes fatal syndrome caused by the formation of nitrogen bubbles in the tissues of divers, caisson workers, and aviators who move too rapidly from environments of higher pressure to those of lower pressure. Nitrogen breathed in air under pressure dissolves in tissue fluids. When ambient pressure is reduced too rapidly, nitrogen comes out of solution faster than it can be circulated to the lungs for expiration. Gaseous nitrogen then accumulates in the joint spaces and peripheral circulation, impairing tissue oxygenation. Disorientation, severe pain, and syncope follow. Treatment is by rapid return of the patient to an environment of higher pressure followed by gradual decompression. Death is more often caused by accident during syncope than by decompression sickness itself. Also called **the bends, caisson disease.** Compare **barotrauma.**

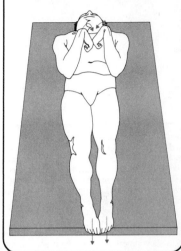

DECORTICATE POSITIONING

decongestant **1.** Of or pertaining to a substance or procedure that eliminates or reduces congestion or swelling. **2.** A decongestant drug. Adrenergic drugs, as epinephrine, ephedrine, and phenylpropanolamine hydrochloride, that cause vasoconstriction of nasal mucosa are used as decongestants. Respiratory tract congestion caused by bacterial infection is usually treated with an antibiotic, and nasal congestion produced by the common cold may be relieved by the inhalation of plain or mentholated steam.

decorticate positioning A motor response to noxious stimuli, associated with lesions of the frontal lobes, internal capsule, or cerebral peduncles. In this posture, the patient's arms are adducted and flexed, with the wrists and fingers flexed on the chest. The legs are stiffly extended and internally rotated, with plantar flexion of the feet. Compare **decerebrate positioning.**

decortication In medicine: the removal of the cortical tissue of an organ or structure, as the kidney, the brain, and the lung. —**decorticate,** *v., adj.*

decubitus A recumbent or horizontal position, as lateral decubitus, which is lying on one side. See also **decubitus care, decubitus ulcer.**

decubitus care The management and prevention of decubitus ulcers that occur most frequently on the sacrum, elbows, heels, outer ankles, inner knees, hips, shoulder blades, and ear rims of immobilized patients, especially those who are obese, elderly, or suffering from paralysis, infections, injuries, or a poor nutritional state. Decubiti may be prevented by repositioning the immobile patient every 2 hours, by keeping the skin dry, and by inspecting pressure areas every 4 to 6 hours for signs of redness. Bed

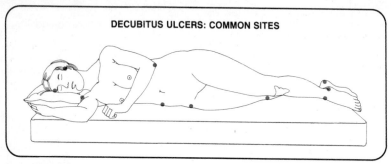

DECUBITUS ULCERS: COMMON SITES

linen is kept dry and wrinkle free; a sheet is used to lift the patient who is moved frequently from the bed but is not allowed to sit in one place for more than 30 minutes. A high-protein diet, vitamins, and iron may be ordered for vulnerable patients, and a prophylactic measure is daily skin care, in which all areas are washed, rinsed, and dried thoroughly, and lotion is gently rubbed on bony prominences. A thin layer of cornstarch or a noncaking powder is applied to areas showing excessive perspiration, and the perineal areas are washed with soap and water after each defecation and urination. Preventive devices include air mattresses, flotation mattresses, sheepskins, silicone pads, foam cushions for wheelchairs, and heel and elbow guards. Decubiti are often resistant to treatment, and large areas of ulceration can be life threatening, especially in a debilitated patient. Prompt and continued care of early lesions can prevent invasion of underlying tissue and promote healing.

decubitus ulcer An inflammation, sore, or ulcer in the skin over a bony prominence. It results from ischemic hypoxia of the tissues owing to prolonged pressure on the part. Decubitus ulcers are most often seen in aged, debilitated, immobilized, or cachectic patients. The sores are graded by stages of severity: Stage I—The skin is red. With massage and relief of pressure, the color of the skin does not return to normal. Stage II—The skin is blistered, peeling, or cracked, though damage is still superficial. Stage III—The skin is broken; a full thickness of skin is lost, subcutaneous tissue may also be damaged, and a serous or bloody drainage may be seen. Stage IV—A deep, craterlike ulcer has formed. The full thickness of skin and the subcutaneous tissues are destroyed. Fascia, connective tissue, bone, or muscle underlying the ulcer are exposed and may be damaged. Prevention of decubitus ulcers is a cardinal aspect of nursing care; treatment is planned specific to the location and the extent of the condition. Decubitus ulcers form most commonly on the skin over the shoulder blades, elbows, sacrum, hips, knees, ankles, and heels. See also **decubitus care.**

decussate To cross in the form of an X, as certain nerve fibers from the retina cross at the optic chiasm. **—decussation,** *n.*

DEd *abbr* Doctor of Education.

deep brachial artery A branch of each of the brachial arteries, arising at the distal border of the teres major, passing deeply into the arm between the long and lateral heads of the triceps brachii, and supplying the humerus and the muscles of the upper arm. It has five branches: the ascending, radial collateral, middle collateral, muscular, and the nutrient. Also called **superior profunda artery.**

deep-breathing and coughing exercises The exercises taught to a person to improve aeration or to maintain respiratory function, especially following prolonged inactivity or after general anesthesia. Incisional pain following surgery in the chest or abdomen inhibits normal respiratory excursion.

NURSING CONSIDERATIONS: The person is assisted to a comfortable position, supine or sitting up. An analgesic is given prior to the exercises if pain is present. Inhalation through the nose and exhalation through the mouth are encouraged. Following a deep inhalation, with the incision supported, the patient is asked to cough. If pain prevents the person from producing a deep, effective cough, a series of short, barklike coughs may be encouraged. When shallow breathing has replaced deep breathing, secretions tend to dry in the respiratory passages, causing damage to the mucous membranes lining the passages. Coughing and deep breathing serve to clear the dried or thick and viscid mucus, to allow moisturized air to enter the bronchi, bronchioles, and alveoli, and to expand the lungs and increase the exchange of gases, thereby improving ventilation. Various devices are available for use in respiratory exercises, as those used in atelectasis to strengthen the muscles used in expiration and to empty the air sacs of retained gas. Postural drainage is commonly performed concurrently with coughing and deep breathing exercises. See also **cupping and vibrating, postural drainage.**

deep fascia The most extensive of three kinds of fascia comprising an intricate series of connective sheets and bands that hold the muscles and other structures in place throughout the body, wrapping the muscles in gray, feltlike membranes. The deep fasciae comprise a continuous system, splitting and fusing in an elaborate network attached to the skeleton and divided into the outer investing layer, the internal investing layer, and the intermediate membranes. Compare **subcutaneous fascia, subserous fascia.**

deep palmar arch The termination of the radial artery, joining the deep palmar branch of the ulnar artery in the palm of the hand.

deep sensation The awareness or perception of pain, pressure, or tension in the deep layers of the skin, the muscles, tendons, or joints. Such sensations are conveyed to the brain via the spinal column. Compare **superficial sensation.**

deep temporal artery One of the branches of the maxillary artery on each side of the head. It branches into the anterior portion and the posterior portion, both rising between the temporalis and the pericranium to supply the temporalis and to anastomose with the middle temporal artery. The anterior branch communicates with the lacrimal artery by small branches that pierce the zygomatic bone and the great wing of the sphenoid. Compare **middle temporal artery, superficial temporal artery.**

deep tendon reflex (DTR) A brisk contraction of a muscle in response to a sudden stretch induced by a sharp tap by a finger or rubber hammer on the tendon of insertion of the muscle. Absence of the reflex may have been caused by damage to the muscle, the peripheral nerve, nerve roots, or the spinal cord at that level. A hyperactive reflex may indicate disease of the pyramidal tract above the level of the reflex arc being tested. Generalized hyperactivity of DTRs may be owing to hyperthyroidism. Kinds of DTRs include **Achilles tendon reflex, biceps reflex, brachioradialis reflex, patellar reflex, triceps reflex.** Also called **myotatic reflex, tendon reflex.** See also **hung-up reflex.**

deep vein One of the many systemic veins that accompany the arteries, usually enclosed in a sheath that wraps both the vein and the associated artery. The larger arteries, as the axillary, the femoral, the popliteal, and the subclavian, are usually accompanied by only one deep vein. The deep veins accompanying the smaller arteries, as the brachial, the peroneal, and the radial, usually occur in pairs, one vein on each side of the artery. Various structures, as the skull, the vertebral column, and the liver, are served by less closely associated arteries and veins. Compare **superficial vein.**

deep X-ray therapy The treatment of internal neoplasms, as Wilms' tumor of the kidney, Hodgkin's disease, and other cancers, with ionizing radiation from an external source. The dose delivered is determined according to the radiosensitivity, size, pathologic grade and differentiation of the tumor, the tolerance of normal surrounding tissue to irradiation, and the condition of the patient. Deep X-ray therapy frequently causes nausea, malaise, diarrhea, and skin reactions, as blanching, erythema, itching, burning, oozing, or desquamation, but with modern techniques the ray is beamed directly to the site, reducing side scatter, and the skin can be spared. Since tumor cells are hypoxic and are more effectively eradicated when they

are well oxygenated, the patient may breathe hyperbaric oxygen or atmospheric oxygen with 5% carbon dioxide during deep X-ray therapy.

deer-fly fever See tularemia.

defamation Any communication, written or spoken, that is untrue and that injures the good name or reputation of another or that in any way brings that person into disrepute.

default judgment In law: a judgment rendered against a defendant because of the defendant's failure to appear in court or to answer the plaintiff's claim within the proper time.

defecation The elimination of feces from the digestive tract through the rectum. See also **constipation, diarrhea, feces. —defecate,** v.

defecation reflex See **rectal reflex.**

defendant In law: the party that is named in a plaintiff's complaint and against whom the plaintiff's allegations are made. The defendant must respond to the allegations.

defense mechanism An unconscious, intrapsychic reaction that offers protection to the self from a stressful situation. Kinds of defense mechanisms include **compensation, conversion, dissociation, displacement, sublimation.** Also called **ego defense mechanism.**

deferent duct The excretory duct of the testis. Also called **ductus deferens.**

deferoxamine mesylate A heavy metal antagonist used to treat iron intoxication or iron overload.

defervescence The diminishing or disappearance of a fever. **—defervescent,** adj.

defibrillation The termination of atrial or ventricular fibrillation, usually accomplished by delivering a direct electrical countershock to the patient's precordium. Defibrillation by electrical countershock is a common emergency measure generally performed by a physician or specially trained nurse or paramedic. The electrode paddles of the defibrillator are covered with a conductive jelly or applied over wet saline sponges. One paddle is placed to the right of the upper sternum below the clavicle and the other is applied to the midaxillary line of the left lower rib cage. In another method, one paddle is placed over the precordium and the other is applied beneath the patient's chest. The defibrillator, usually a condenser discharge system, is set to deliver between 200 and 400 watts per second. Respiratory support is suspended during the shock but is promptly resumed. If one or two shocks fail to cause defibrillation, cardiopulmonary resuscitation (CPR) may be conducted until another shock is attempted. **—defibrillate,** v.

defibrillator A device that delivers an electrical shock at a preset voltage to the myocardium through the chest wall. It is used for restoring the normal cardiac rhythm and rate when the heart has stopped beating or is fibrillating.

deficiency disease A condition resulting from the lack of one or more essential nutrients, from metabolic dysfunction, or from impaired digestion or absorption, excessive excretion, or increased biological requirements. Compare **malnutrition.** See also **avitaminosis.**

definitive 1. Final; clearly established without doubt or question. 2. In embryology: fully formed in the final differentiation of a tissue, structure, or organ. Compare **primitive.** 3. In parasitology: of or pertaining to the host in which the parasite undergoes the sexual phase of its reproductive cycle.

definitive host Any animal in which the reproductive stages of a parasite develop. The female anopheles mosquito is the definitive host for malaria. Humans are definitive hosts for pinworms, schistosomes, and tapeworms. Also called **primary host.** Compare **dead-end host, intermediate host, reservoir host.** See also **host,** definition 1.

definitive treatment Any therapy generally accepted as a specific cure of a disease. Compare **expectant treatment, palliative treatment.** See also **treatment.**

deformity A condition of being distorted, disfigured, flawed, malformed, or misshapen, which may affect the body in general or any part of it and may be the result of disease, injury, or birth defect.

degenerative chorea See **Huntington's chorea.**

degenerative disease Any disease in which there is deterioration of structure or function of tissue. Some kinds of degenerative disease are **arteriosclerosis, cancer, osteoarthritis.**

degenerative joint disease (DJD) See **osteoarthritis.**

deglutition Swallowing.

deglutition apnea The normal absence of respiration during swallowing.

dehydrate 1. To remove or lose water from a substance. 2. To lose excessive water from the body. —**dehydration,** *n.*

dehydrated alcohol A clear, colorless, highly hygroscopic liquid with a burning taste, containing at least 99.5% ethyl alcohol by volume. Also called **absolute alcohol.**

dehydration Excessive loss of water from the body tissues. Dehydration is accompanied by a disturbance in the balance of essential electrolytes, particularly sodium, potassium, and chloride. Dehydration may follow prolonged fever, diarrhea, vomiting, acidosis, and any condition where there is rapid depletion of body fluids. It is of particular concern among infants and young children, since their electrolyte balance is normally precarious. Signs of dehydration include poor skin turgor, flushed dry skin, coated tongue, oliguria, irritability, and confusion. Normal fluid volume and balanced serum electrolyte values are the primary goals of therapy.

dehydration fever A fever that frequently occurs in newborns, thought to be caused by dehydration. Also called **inanition fever.** Compare **inanition, starvation.**

dehydrocholic acid. A digestant used to treat constipation and biliary tract conditions.

déjà vu The sensation or illusion of encountering a set of circumstances or a place previously experienced. The phenomenon, normal in everyone but occuring more frequently or continuously in certain emotional and organic disorders, results from some unconscious emotional connection with the present experience. Compare **jamais vu, paramnesia.**

Dejerine-Sottas disease A rare, congenital spinocerebellar disorder characterized by the development of palpable thickenings along peripheral nerves, degeneration of the peripheral nervous system, pain, paresthesia, ataxia, diminished sensation, and deep tendon reflexes. Diagnosis is made by a histological examination of a peripheral nerve. There is no specific treatment. Also called **interstitial hypertrophic neuropathy.**

delayed dentition See **retarded dentition.**

delayed echolalia A phenomenon, commonly seen in schizophrenia, involving the meaningless, automatic repetition of overheard words and phrases. It occurs hours, days, or even weeks after the original stimulus.

delayed hypersensitivity reaction See **cell-mediated immune response.**

delayed postpartum hemorrhage Hemorrhage occurring later than 24 hours after delivery, characterized by heavy bleeding and signs of impending shock and anemia. The cause is diagnosed and the condition is treated accordingly. A laceration is closed with suture, retained fragments of placenta are removed, infection is treated with antibiotics, or the uterus is caused to contract by the administration of ergotrate or oxytocin.

deletion syndrome Any of a group of congenital autosomal anomalies that result from the loss of chromosomal genetic material, owing to breakage of a chromatid during cell division, as the cat-cry syndrome, which results from the absence of the short arms of chromosome 5.

deliberate hypotension An anesthetic process in which a short-acting hypotensive agent like nitroprusside or trimethaphan is given to reduce blood pressure, thus bleeding, during surgery. The procedure facilitates surgery by making vessels and tissues more visible and reducing blood loss.

delinquency 1. Negligence or failure to fulfill a duty or obligation. 2. An offense, fault, misdemeanor, or misdeed; a tendency to commit such acts. See also **juvenile delinquency.**

delinquent 1. Characterized by neglect of duty or violation of law. 2. One whose behavior is characterized by persistent antisocial, illegal, violent, or criminal acts; a juvenile delinquent.

delirium 1. A state of frenzied excitement or wild enthusiasm. 2. An acute organic mental disorder characterized by confusion, disorientation, restlessness, clouding of the consciousness, incoherence, fear, anxiety, excitement, and often illusions, hallucinations, and, at times, delusions. The condition is caused by disturbances in cerebral functions that may result from metabolic disorders; postpartum or postoperative stress; the ingestion of several types of toxic substances; and any other causes of physical and mental shock or exhaustion. The symptoms are usually of short duration and reversible with treatment of the underlying cause, although in extreme cases, where the toxic condition is extremely severe or prolonged, permanent brain damage may occur. Bed rest in a quiet environment is essential. The delirious patient must be protected from accidents and self-injury. In prolonged cases, dehydration and vitamin deficiency may occur. Sedatives or tranquilizing drugs are often used to relieve excitability. Kinds of delirium include **acute delirium, delirium tremens, exhaustion delirium, senile delirium, traumatic delirium.** Compare **dementia.** —**delirious,** *adj.*

delirium tremens (DTs) An acute and sometimes fatal psychotic reaction caused by excessive intake of alcoholic beverages over a long period of time. The reaction may follow a prolonged alcoholic debauch without an adequate intake of food, occur during a period of abstinence, be precipitated by a head injury or infection, or result from the partial or total withdrawal of alcohol after prolonged drinking. Initial symptoms include loss of appetite, insomnia, and general restlessness, followed by agitation, excitement, disorientation, mental confusion, vivid and often frightening hallucinations, acute fear and anxiety, illusions and delusions, coarse tremors of the hands, feet, legs, and tongue, fever, increased heart rate, extreme perspiration, gastrointestinal distress, and precordial pain. The episode, which usually constitutes a medical emergency, typically lasts from 3 to 6 days and is generally followed by a deep sleep. Treatment includes a quiet, nonstimulating environment in which the person is watched closely and protected from self-injury, not only during the period of delirium but, more importantly, during convalescence when depression and remorse often lead to attempted suicide. Extreme fatigue, pneumonia, respiratory infections, and heart failure are common complications, as are severe dehydration and nutritional deficiencies. Dietary supplements are often given; tube feeding and intravenous fluids may be needed. Sedatives and tranquilizing agents are useful for quieting the person. Compare **alcoholic hallucinosis, Stearns' alcoholic amentia.** See also **Korsakoff's psychosis.**

delivery In obstetrics: the birth of a child; parturition.

delta **1.** The fourth letter of the Greek alphabet, with the symbol Δ or δ. **2.** A triangular space or surface. **3.** The fourth in a series.

delta wave The slowest of the four types of brain waves, characterized by a frequency of 4 Hz and a relatively high voltage. Delta waves are 'deep sleep waves' associated with a dreamless state from which an individual is not easily aroused. Also called delta rhythm. Compare **alpha wave, beta wave, theta wave.**

deltoid **1.** Triangular. **2.** Of or pertaining to the deltoid muscle that covers the shoulder.

deltoid muscle A large, thick triangular muscle that covers the shoulder joint and ab-

DELTOID MUSCLE

Clavicle

Deltoid muscle

ducts, flexes, extends, and rotates the arm. It arises from various surfaces on the clavicle, acromion, and scapula and inserts, with a thick tendon, into the humerus. Also called **deltoideus.**

delusion A persistent, aberrant belief or perception held inviolable by a person even though it is illogical, unique, and probably wrong. Kinds of delusions include **delusion of being controlled, delusion of grandeur, delusion of persecution, nihilistic delusion, somatic delusion.** Compare **illusion.**

delusion of being controlled The false belief that one's feelings, beliefs, thoughts, and acts are governed by some external force, as seen in various forms of schizophrenia. See also **delusion.**

delusion of grandeur The gross exaggeration of one's importance, wealth, power, or talents, as seen in such disorders as megalomania, general paresis, and paranoid schizophrenia. See also **delusion.**

delusion of persecution A morbid belief that one is being mistreated and harassed by unidentified enemies, as seen in paranoia and paranoid schizophrenia. See also **delusion.**

delusion of reference See **idea of reference.**

delusion stupor The state of lethargy and unresponsiveness observed in catatonic schizophrenia.

demarcation current An electric current that flows from an uninjured to an injured end of a muscle. Also called **current of injury.**

deme A small, closely related interbreeding population of organisms or individuals, usually occupying a circumscribed area. Also called **genetic population.**

demecarium bromide A miotic agent.

demeclocycline hydrochloride A tetracycline antibiotic.

dementia A progressive, organic mental disorder characterized by chronic personality disintegration, confusion, disorientation, stupor, deterioration of intellectual capacity and func-

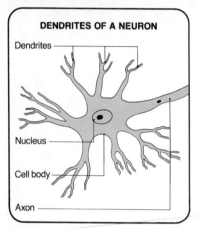

DENDRITES OF A NEURON

Dendrites

Nucleus

Cell body

Axon

tion, and impairment of control of memory, judgment, and impulses. Dementia caused by drug intoxication, hyperthyroidism, pernicious anemia, paresis, subdural hematoma, benign brain tumor, hydrocephalus, insulin shock, and tumor of islet cells of the pancreas can be reversed by treating the condition; Alzheimer's disease, Pick's disease, Huntington's disease, and traumatic injuries to the brain are not currently amenable to treatment. Kinds of dementia include **Alzheimer's disease, dementia praecox, general paresis, secondary dementia, senile psychosis, toxic dementia.**

dementia paralytica See **general paresis.**

dementia praecox Schizophrenia, especially developing in adolescence or early adulthood. See also **schizophrenia.**

-demic A combining form meaning 'relating to disease in a (specified) region': *interedemic, philodemic, prosodemic.*

demigauntlet bandage A glovelike bandage covering only the hand and leaving the fingers free. See also **gauntlet bandage.**

demography The study of human populations, particularly the size, distribution, and characteristics of members of population groups. It is applied in studies of health problems involving ethnic groups, populations of a specific geographic region, and religious groups with special dietary restrictions. Compare **epidemiology.**

De Morgan's spots See **cherry angioma.**

demulcent 1. Any of several oily substances used for soothing and reducing irritation of surfaces that have been abraded or irritated. 2. Soothing, as a counterirritant or balm.

demyelination The process of destruction or removal of the myelin sheath from a nerve or a nerve fiber.

denatured alcohol Ethyl alcohol made unfit for ingestion by the addition of acetone or methanol, used as a solvent and in chemical processes.

dendr- A combining form meaning 'pertaining to a tree or branches': *dendriceptor.*

-dendria A combining form meaning the 'twiglike branching of nerve fibers': *oligodendria, telodendria, zoodendria.*

dendrite A branching process that extends from the cell body of a neuron. Each neuron usually possesses several dendrites, which receive impulses that are conducted to the cell body. Compare **axon.**

dendritic 1. Treelike, with branches that spread toward or into neighboring tissues, as dendritic keratitis. 2. Of or pertaining to a dendrite.

dendritic keratitis A serious infection of the eye, characterized by an ulceration of the surface of the cornea resembling a tree with knobs at the ends of the branches. Photophobia, the sensation of a foreign body in the eye, pain, and conjunctivitis are usual. Treatment includes application of idoxuridine, chemical debridement with an iodine tincture, or surgical removal of the involved layer of corneal tissue cells. Untreated dendritic keratitis may result in permanent scarring of the cornea with impaired vision or blindness.

dendrodendritic synapse A type of synapse in which a dendrite of one neuron comes in contact with a dendrite of another neuron.

-dendron A combining form meaning a 'treelike formation': *neurodendron, telodendron, toxicodendron.*

dengue, dengue fever An acute arbovirus infection transmitted to man by the *Aëdes* mosquito and occurring in tropical and subtropical regions. The disease usually produces a triad of symptoms: fever, rash, and severe head, back, and muscle pain. Manifestations of dengue usually occur in two phases, separated by a day of remission. In the first attack, the patient experiences fever, extreme weakness, headache, sore throat, muscle pains, and edema of the hands and feet. The second attack is marked by a return of fever and by a bright red scarlatinaform rash. Dengue is a self-limited illness, even though it may take patients several weeks to recover. Treatment is symptomatic; analgesics may be given to relieve headache and other pains. Also called **Aden fever, bouquet fever, breakbone fever, dandy fever, solar fever.** See also *Aëdes,* **arbovirus.**

dengue hemorrhagic fever shock syndrome (DHFS) A grave form of dengue fever characterized by shock with collapse or prostration; cold, clammy extremities; a weak, thready pulse; respiratory distress; and all of the symptoms of dengue fever. Hemorrhage, bruises, small reddish spots indicating bleeding from skin capillaries, and bloody vomit, urine, and feces may occur and precede circulatory collapse. Treatment includes fluid and electrolyte replacement and fresh blood, plasma, or platelet transfusions as needed. Oxygen and sedatives may be administered. See also **breakbone fever, dandy fever, dengue.**

denial 1. Refusal or restriction of something requested, claimed, or needed, often resulting in physical or emotional deficiency. 2. An un-

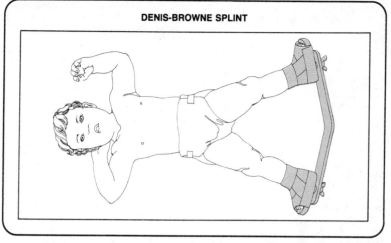

DENIS-BROWNE SPLINT

conscious defense mechanism in which emotional conflict and anxiety are avoided by refusing to acknowledge those thoughts, feelings, desires, impulses, or external facts that are consciously intolerable.

denial and isolation According to Dr. Elisabeth Kübler-Ross, the first stage of dying. The patient in this stage refuses to accept the reality of his impending death. He may visit several doctors, hoping to refute the original diagnosis, or accuse the hospital staff of falsifying or mixing up test reports. Often the patient experiences intense loneliness. See also **anger, bargaining, depression, acceptance.**

Denis-Browne splint A splint that corrects talipes equinovarus (clubfoot) composed of a curved bar attached to the soles of a pair of high-top shoes. Wing nuts allow individualized abduction of each foot. The splint is commonly applied nightly in late infancy after casting and manipulation have reduced the deformity.

Denman's spontaneous evolution A natural, unassisted turning of the fetus from the transverse presentation. The head rotates back and, as the breech descends, the shoulder ascends in the pelvis. The back of the fetus is generally posterior. Also called Denman's method, Denman's spontaneous version.

dens deciduus See **deciduous tooth.**

dense fibrous tissue A fibrous connective tissue consisting of compact, strong, inelastic bundles of parallel collagenous fibers that have a glistening white color. Organized dense fibrous tissue comprises the tendons, the aponeuroses, and the ligaments; unorganized dense fibrous tissue comprises the fascial membranes, the dermis of the skin, the periosteum, and the capsules of organs. Compare **loose fibrous tissue.**

density The amount of mass of a substance in a given volume. The greater the mass in a given volume, the greater the density. See also **mass, volume.**

density gradient The variation of the concentration of a solute in a confined solution.

dens serotinus See **wisdom tooth.**

dent- See **dento-.**

denta- See **dento-.**

dental Of or pertaining to a tooth or teeth.

dental alveolus A tooth socket in the mandible or maxilla.

dental amalgam An alloy of silver, tin, and mercury with small amounts of copper and sometimes zinc, used for filling teeth.

dental anesthesia Any of several anesthetic procedures used in dental surgery. The proliferation of injectable local anesthetics has largely replaced the use of inhalational general anesthesics, especially of nitrous oxide.

dental arch The curving shape formed by the arrangement of a normal set of teeth.

dental assistant A person who assists a dentist in the performance of generalized tasks, including chair-side assistance, clerical work, reception, and some radiography and dental laboratory work.

dental canal See **alveolar canal.**

dental caries An abnormal destructive condition in a tooth, caused by the complex interaction of food, especially starches and sugars, with bacteria that form dental plaque. This material adheres to the surfaces of the teeth and provides the medium for the growth of bacteria and the production of organic acids that then cause breaks in the enamel sheath of the tooth. Enzymes produced by the bacteria then attack the protein component of the tooth. This process, if untreated, ultimately leads to the formation of deep cavities and the bacterial infection of the pulp chamber and nerves. The development of dental caries in a debilitated patient is a concern because of the danger that infections of the teeth or gums might spread to the rest of the body. In addition, missing, decayed, or painful teeth inhibit mastication and lead to dietary changes which may in turn cause nutritional

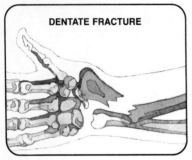

DENTATE FRACTURE

and digestive disorders. Kinds of dental caries include **active dental caries, arrested dental caries, primary dental caries, secondary dental caries.**

dental crypt   The space occupied by a developing tooth.

dental fistula   An abnormal passage from the apical periodontal area of a tooth to the surface of the oral mucous membrane, permitting the discharge of inflammatory or suppurative material. Also called **alveolar fistula.**

dental floss   A waxed or unwaxed thread used to clean tooth surfaces and spaces between the teeth.

dental hygienist   A person with special training to provide dental services under the supervision of a dentist, including dental prophylaxis, radiography, applying medications, and providing dental education.

dental papilla   See under **papilla.**

dental plaque   See **bacterial plaque.**

dental technician   A person who makes dental prostheses and orthodontic appliances as prescribed by a dentist. Kinds of dental prostheses made by dental technicians include full dentures, partial dentures, crowns, bridgework, and other dental restorations.

-dentate   A combining form meaning 'possessing teeth': *edentate, multidentate, tridentate.*

dentate fracture   Any fracture that causes serrated bone ends that fit together like the teeth of gears.

dentin, dentine   The chief material of teeth, surrounding the pulp and situated inside of the enamel and cementum. Harder and denser than bone, it consists of solid organic substratum infiltrated with lime salts.

dentin globule   A small spherical body in peripheral dentin, created by early calcification.

dentinoenamel   Pertaining to both the dentin and the enamel of the teeth.

dentinogenesis   The formation of the dentin of the teeth. —**dentinogenic,** *adj.*

dentinogenesis imperfecta   Hereditary dysplasia of dentin of deciduous and permanent teeth in which brown, opalescent dentin overgrows and obliterates the pulp cavity and the teeth have short roots and wear rapidly. Early restorative dentistry is indicated. The condition is often associated with osteogenesis imperfecta

and other congenital mesodermal dysplasias.

dentist   A person who is qualified by training and licensed by the state to practice dentistry.

dentistry   The art of practicing the prevention and treatment of diseases and disorders of the teeth and surrounding structures of the oral cavity. Responsibilities include the repair and restoration of teeth and replacement of missing teeth, as well as the detection of signs of diseases, as tumors, that require treatment by a physician. In addition to the general practice of dentistry, there are eight recognized specialties, each requiring additional training after graduation from a dental college: endodontics, oral pathology, oral surgery, orthodontics, pedodontics, periodontics, prosthodontics, and public health dentistry.

dentition   **1.** The development and eruption of the teeth. See also **teething. 2.** The arrangement, number, and kind of teeth as they appear in the dental arch of the mouth. **3.** The character of the teeth of an individual or species as determined by their form and arrangement. Kinds of dentition include **deciduous dentition, denture, mixed dentition, natural dentition, permanent dentition, precocious dentition, predeciduous dentition, retarded dentition.**

dento-, dent-, denta-, denti-, dentia-   A combining form meaning 'pertaining to a tooth or the teeth': *dentography, dentoidin, dentonomy.*

dentoalveolar abscess   The formation and accumulation of pus in a tooth socket or the jawbone around the base of a tooth. The pus results from a bacterial infection that is usually secondary to an infection or injury to the tooth or alveolar tissues. Also called **periapical abscess.**

denture   An artificial tooth or a set of artificial teeth not permanently fixed or implanted. Also called artificial dentition. Compare **fixed bridgework.**

denturist   A person who performs the same type of work as a dental technician but without a dentist's prescription, providing dental prostheses directly to clients. Denturists are more likely to be found in Canada than in the United States, where the practice is illegal in many states. See also **dental technician.**

Denver Articulation Screening Examination (DASE)   A test for evaluating the clarity of pronunciation in children between $2^{1}/_{2}$ and 6 years of age. Each child's performance may be compared to a standardized norm for the age.

Denver classification   The system of identifying and classifying human chromosomes according to the criteria established at the Denver (1960), London (1963), and Chicago (1966) conferences of cytogeneticists. Denver classification is based on chromosome size and position of the centromere as determined during mitotic metaphase and is divided into seven major groups, designated A through G, which are arranged according to decreasing length. See also **karyotype.**

Denver Developmental Screening Test

(DDST) A test for evaluating development in children from 1 month to 6 years of age. The developmental level of motor, social, and language skills may be discovered by comparing the child's performance to the average performance of other children. The score, or the developmental age, is expressed as a ratio in which the child's age is the denominator and the age at which the norm possesses skills equal to those of the child being tested is the numerator.

deodorant **1.** Destroying or masking odors. **2.** A substance that destroys or masks odors. Underarm deodorants may contain an antiperspirant, as aluminum chloride, aluminum hydroxyl, aluminum sulfate, or aluminum zirconyl hydroxychloride. These aluminum salts form an obstructive hydroxide gel in sweat ducts. Aluminum salts may produce an allergic reaction in some individuals and hydrolyzed aluminum chloride can cause local tissue necrosis. Also called **antibromic.**

deodorized alcohol A liquid, free of organic impurities, containing 92.5% absolute alcohol.

deoxy-, desoxy- A combining form meaning 'deoxidized or a reduction product of': *deoxygenation, desoxymorphine, desoxyribose.*

deoxyribonucleic acid, desoxyribonucleic acid (DNA) A large nucleic acid molecule, found principally in the chromosomes of the nucleus of a cell, that is the carrier of genetic information in living cells. The genetic information is coded in two nitrogen-containing bases: a purine and a pyramidine. These bases are paired by hydrogen bonds to form two coiled chains, known as the double helix. In DNA, the purines are adenine (A) and guanine (G); the pyramidines, thymine (T) and cytosine (C). See also **nucleic acid, ribonucleic acid.**

dependence The total psychophysical state of one addicted to drugs or alcohol who must receive an increasing amount of the substance to prevent the onset of abstinence symptoms.

dependency needs The sum of the physical and emotional requirements of an infant for survival, including mothering, love, affection, shelter, protection, food, and warmth. Reliance on others to satisfy these needs decreases with age and maturity; continuance in later years, in overt or latent form, is indicative of a pathological emotional disorder. These needs may increase under stress, as during physical illness, in which case they do not reflect a psychopathological condition. Compare **emotional need.**

dependent Of or pertaining to a condition of being reliant upon someone or something else for help, support, favor, and other needs, as a child is dependent on a parent, a narcotics addict is dependent upon a drug, or one variable is dependent on another variable. —**depend,** *v.,* **dependence,** *n.*

dependent differentiation See **correlative differentiation.**

dependent variable In research: a factor that is measured to learn the effect of one or more independent variables, as in a study of the

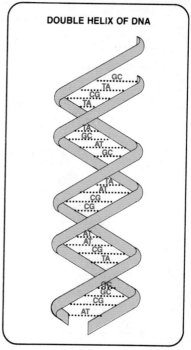

DOUBLE HELIX OF DNA

effect of preoperative nursing intervention on postoperative vomiting, vomiting is the dependent variable measured to determine the effect of the nursing intervention. Compare **independent variable.**

depersonalization A feeling of strangeness or unreality concerning oneself or the environment, often resulting from anxiety and, in severe cases, leading to a neurotic reaction.

depersonalization disorder An emotional disturbance characterized by feelings of strangeness and unreality in which a dreamlike atmosphere pervades the consciousness. The body may not feel like one's own, and dramatic and important events may be watched with equanimity. The reaction is commonly seen in various forms of schizophrenia and in severe depression.

depilation The removal or extraction of hair from the body, either temporarily, by mechanical or chemical means, or permanently, by electrolysis, which destroys the hair follicle. Also called **epilation.** —**depilate,** *v.*

depilatory **1.** Of or pertaining to a substance or procedure that removes hair. **2.** A depilatory agent.

depolarization The neutralization of electrical polarity, as the reduction of ion differential of sodium and potassium across the nerve cells of the neuromuscular junctions. See also **action potential.**

deposition In law: a sworn pretrial testimony given by a witness in response to oral or

DEPRESSED FRACTURE

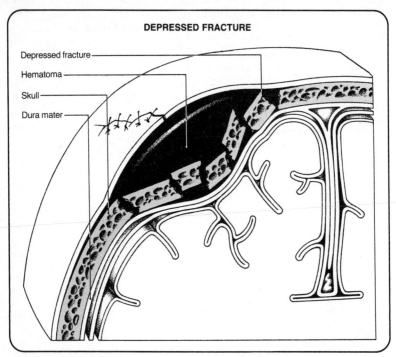

Depressed fracture
Hematoma
Skull
Dura mater

written questions and cross-examination. The deposition is transcribed and may be used for further pretrial investigation. It may also be presented at the trial if the witness cannot be present. Compare **discovery, interrogatories.**

depot   1. Any area of the body in which drugs or other substances are stored and from which they can be distributed. 2. Of a drug: injected or implanted to be slowly absorbed into the circulation.

depressant   1. Of a drug: tending to decrease the function or activity of a system of the body. 2. Such a drug, as a cardiac depressant or a respiratory depressant.

depressed fracture   Any fracture of the skull in which fragments are depressed below the normal surface of the skull.

depression   1. A depressed area, hollow, or fossa; downward or inward displacement. 2. A decrease of vital functional activity. 3. A mood disturbance characterized by feelings of sadness, despair, and discouragement resulting from and proportionate to some personal loss or tragedy. 4. An abnormal emotional state characterized by exaggerated feelings of sadness, melancholy, dejection, worthlessness, emptiness, and hopelessness that are inappropriate and out of proportion to reality. The overt manifestations, which are extremely variable, range from a slight lack of motivation and inability to concentrate to severe physiological alterations of body functions and may represent symptoms of a variety of mental and physical conditions, a syndrome

of related symptoms associated with a particular disease, or a specific mental illness. The condition is neurotic when the precipitating cause is an intrapsychic conflict or a traumatic situation or event that is identifiable, even though the person is unable to explain the overreaction to it. The condition is psychotic when there is severe physical and mental functional impairment owing to some unidentifiable intrapsychic conflict; it is often accompanied by hallucinations, delusions, and confusion concerning time, place, and identity. Kinds of depression include **agitated depression, anaclitic depression, endogenous depression, involutional melancholia, reactive depression, retarded depression.** See also **bipolar disorder. 5.** According to Dr. Elisabeth Kübler-Ross, the fourth stage of dying. The patient in this stage recognizes and mourns silently for his personal loss. He is usually withdrawn and prefers solitude to visits from friends and relatives. This private grieving helps the patient prepare to give up his loved ones and all that has been meaningful to him. See also **anger, bargaining, denial and isolation, acceptance. —depressive,** *adj.*

depressor septi   One of the three muscles of the nose. Arising from the maxilla and inserting into the septum and the posterior aspect of the ala, it lies between the mucous membrane and the muscular structure of the lip and is a direct antagonist of the other muscles of the nose. It is innervated by buccal branches of the facial nerve and serves to draw the ala down, constricting the nostril. Compare **nasalis, procerus.**

depth electroencephalography See **electroencephalography.**

depth perception The ability to judge depth or the relative distance of objects in space and to orient one's position in relation to them. Binocular vision is essential to this ability.

depth psychology Any approach to psychology that emphasizes the study of personality and behavior in relation to unconscious motivation. See also **psychoanalysis.**

de Quervain's fracture Fracture of the navicular bone, with dislocation of the lunar bone.

de Quervain's thyroiditis An inflammatory condition of the thyroid, characterized by swelling and tenderness of the gland, fever, dysphagia, fatigue, and severe pain in the neck, ears, and jaw. The disorder often occurs following a viral infection of the upper respiratory tract and tends to remit spontaneously and to recur several times. The diagnosis may be made by a radiologic scan showing depressed uptake of radioactive iodine in involved areas. Occasionally, a needle biopsy of the thyroid is performed. Treatment may include anti-inflammatory medication, as aspirin, or thyroid hormone, if the condition continues for more than a few days. Corticosteroids are prescribed for prolonged or severe cases. Also called **giant cell thyroiditis, granulomatous thyroiditis, subacute thyroiditis.**

der- A combining form meaning 'pertaining to the neck': *deradelphus, deradenitis, deranencephalia.*

derby hat fracture See **dishpan fracture.**

derived protein A metabolic product of protein hydrolysis, as proteose, peptone, or peptide.

-derm A combining form meaning a 'skin': *angioderm, mucoderm, paraderm.*

-derma A combining form meaning: **1.** A '(specified) skin or covering': *chrysderma, micoderma, sarcoderma.* **2.** A 'skin ailment or skin of a specified type': *pyoderma, rhinoderma, syphiloderma.*

derma- See **dermato-.**

dermabrasion A treatment for the removal of scars on the skin by the use of revolving wire brushes or sandpaper. An aerosol spray is used to freeze the skin for this procedure. Dermabrasion is used to reduce facial scars of severe acne and to remove pigment from undesired tattoos.

dermat- See **dermato-.**

dermatitis An inflammatory condition of the skin, characterized by erythema and pain or pruritus. Various cutaneous eruptions occur and may be unique to a particular allergen, disease, or infection. The condition may be chronic or acute; treatment is specific to the cause. Some kinds of dermatitis are **actinic dermatitis, contact dermatitis, rhus dermatitis, seborrheic dermatitis.** See **dermatosis.**

dermatitis exfoliativa neonatorum See **Ritter's disease, dermatosis.**

dermatitis herpetiformis A chronic, severely pruritic skin disease with symmetrically located groups of red, papulovesicular, vesicular, bullous, or urticarial lesions which leave hyperpigmented spots. It is occasionally associated with a malignancy of an internal organ or with celiac disease, patch, or IgA immunotherapy. Treatment may include a diet free of gluten and the administration of sulfone, dapsone, sulfapyridine, or antipruritic drugs.

dermatitis medicamentosa See **drug eruption.**

dermatitis venenata See **contact dermatitis.**

dermato-, derma-, dermat-, dermo- A combining form meaning 'pertaining to the skin': *dermatobiasis, dermatocele, dermatocyst.*

dermatofibroma, *pl.* **dermatofibromas, dermatofibromata** A cutaneous nodule that is painless, round, firm, gray or red, and elevated. It is most commonly found on the extremities, requires no treatment, and is sometimes associated with systemic lupus erythematosus. Also called **fibrous histiocytoma.**

dermatographia An abnormal skin condition characterized by wheals that develop from tracing on the skin with the fingernail or a blunted instrument. This condition makes the skin especially susceptible to irritation and may be associated with urticaria. Also called **autographism, dermatographism, Ebbecke's reaction.**

dermatographism See **dermatographia.**

dermatologist A physician specializing in disorders of the skin.

dermatology The study of the skin, including anatomy, physiology, and pathology and the diagnosis and treatment of skin disorders.

dermatome **1.** In embryology: the part of the segmented mesodermal layer in the early developing embryo that originates from the somites and gives rise to the dermal layers of the skin. **2.** In neurology: a segmental skin area supplied with sensory nerve fibers by a posterior spinal root. See also **somite.**

dermatomycosis A superficial, fungal infection of the skin, characteristically found on parts that are moist and protected by clothing, as the groin or feet. It is caused by a dermatophyte. See also **dermatophytosis. —dermatomycotic,** *adj.*

dermatomyositis A disease of the connective tissues, characterized by pruritic or eczematous inflammation of the skin and tenderness and weakness of the muscles. Muscle tissue is destroyed and loss is often so severe that the person may become unable to walk or to perform simple tasks. Swelling of the eyelids and face and loss of weight are common manifestations. The cause is unknown, but in 15% of cases the condition develops with an internal malignancy. Viral infection and antibacterial medication are also associated with an increased incidence of dermatomyositis.

DERMATOPHYTOSIS OF THE FOOT

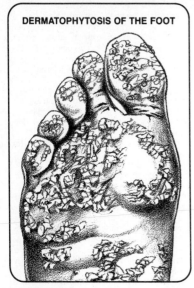

Dermatophagoides farinae A ubiquitous species of household dust mite responsible for allergic reactions in sensitive individuals. Protection against the microscopically small mite includes use of insecticides, vacuum cleaning, and control of the temperature and humidity. The mites thrive on skin scales, hair, pet foods, carpets, and bedding, in addition to ordinary house dust.

dermatophyte Any of several species of fungi that cause parasitic skin disease in human beings. See also **dermatophytid,** specific fungal infections.

dermatophytid An allergic skin reaction characterized by small vesicles and associated with dermatomycosis. The lesions result from sensitization to the infection elsewhere on the skin and do not contain fungi. See also **dermatomycosis, dermatophyte.**

dermatophytosis A superficial fungus infection of the skin, caused by *Microsporum, Epidermophyton,* or *Trichophyton* species of dermatophyte. On the trunk and upper extremities it is commonly called ringworm infection and is characterized by round or oval, scaly patches with slightly raised borders and clearing centers. On the feet small vesicles, cracking, itching, scaling, and often secondary bacterial infections occur and are commonly called athlete's foot. Dermatophytosis is treated with topical antifungal agents. However, fingernails and toenails respond poorly to topical treatment. See also **tinea.**

dermatosis Any disorder of the skin, especially if not associated with inflammation. Compare **dermatitis.**

dermatosis papulosa nigra A common abnormal skin condition in blacks consisting of multiple, tiny, benign, skin-colored or hyperpigmented papules on the cheeks. The lesions are permanent and increase in number with age.

-dermia A combining form meaning a '(specified) skin condition': *allergodermia, carotenodermia, toxidermia.* Also **-derma.**

-dermic A combining form meaning: **1.** 'Related to the skin': *diadermic, epidermic, intradermic.* **2.** 'Related to the variety of skin': *leptodermic, pachydermic, sarcodermic.* **3.** 'Related to skin ailments': *leukodermic, toxicodermic, xerodermic.* **4.** 'Related to a cell division process': *blastodermic, ectodermic, endodermic.*

dermis See **corium.**

-dermis A combining form meaning 'tissue or skin': *hypodermis, endepidermis, osteodermis.*

dermo- See **dermato-.**

dermographism An exaggerated response of the skin to stroking with a blunt instrument. Soon after such mild trauma, a pale, raised wheal with a surrounding erythematous flare appears. Antihistamines may be prescribed to suppress this hypersensitivity.

dermoid **1.** Of or pertaining to the skin. **2.** *Informal.* A dermoid cyst.

dermoid cyst A tumor, derived from embryonal tissues, that consists of a fibrous wall lined with epithelium and a cavity containing fatty material, and, frequently, hair, teeth, bits of bone, and cartilage. More than 10% of all ovarian tumors are dermoid cysts; usually benign, they may cause granulomatous peritonitis if they rupture. Kinds of dermoid cysts are **implantation dermoid cyst, inclusion dermoid cyst, thyroid dermoid cyst, tubal dermoid cyst.** Also called organoid tumor, teratoid tumor. See also **teratoma.**

-dermoma A combining form meaning a 'tumor of the skin layers': *epidermoma, monodermoma, tridermoma.*

DES *abbr* **diethylstilbestrol.**

descending aorta The main portion of the aorta, consisting of the thoracic aorta and the abdominal aorta, that continues from the aortic arch into the trunk of the body and supplies many parts, as the esophagus, lymph glands, ribs, and stomach.

descending colon The segment of the colon that extends from the end of the transverse colon at the splenic flexure on the left side of the abdomen down to the beginning of the sigmoid colon in the pelvis.

descending current See **centrifugal current.**

descending oblique muscle See **obliquus externus abdominis.**

descending urography See **intravenous pyelography.**

descriptive anatomy The study of the morphology and structure of the body by systems, as the vascular system and the nervous system. Each system is composed of similar tissues and organs that are essential to a particular function.

descriptive embryology The study of the changes that occur in cells, tissues, and organs during the progressive stages of prenatal development.

descriptive psychiatry The study of external, readily observable behavior. Compare **dynamic psychiatry.**

desensitization See **systemic desensitization.**

desensitize 1. In immunology: to render an individual insensitive to any of the various antigens. 2. In psychiatry: to relieve an emotionally disturbed person of the stress of phobias and neuroses by encouraging discussion of the anxieties and the stressful experiences that cause the emotional problems involved. 3. In dentistry: to remove or reduce the painful response of vital, exposed dentin to irritating substances and temperature changes.

deserpidine A sympatholytic antihypertensive that acts peripherally.

desert fever See **coccidioidomycosis.**

desert rheumatism A form of coccidioidomycosis characterized by pain in the bones and joints.

desipramine hydrochloride A tricyclic antidepressant.

deslanoside A cardiotonic glycoside used to treat congestive heart failure and some cardiac arrhythmias.

-desma A combining form meaning 'something bridging or connecting': *cytodesma, mesodesma, plasmodesma.*

desmo- A combining form meaning 'pertaining to a ligament': *desmoma, desmorrhexis, desmotomy.*

desmocyte See **fibroblast.** —**desmocytic,** *adj.*

desmoid tumor A neoplasm in skeletal muscle and fascia that may occur in the head, neck, upper arm, abdomen, or lower extremities. The tumor is usually a firm, circumscribed, rubbery mass. Injury may be a factor in the development of this lesion, which is often regarded as overproliferation of scar tissue.

desmopressin acetate An analog of the antidiuretic hormone vasopressin.

desonide A topical anti-inflammatory agent.

desoximetasone A topical anti-inflammatory agent.

desoxy- See **deoxy-.**

desoxycorticosterone A mineralocorticoid that helps regulate water and electrolyte balance.

desoxycorticosterone acetate, d. pivalate A mineralocorticoid.

desoxyribonucleic acid See **deoxyribonucleic acid.**

desquamation A normal process in which the cornified layer of the epidermis is sloughed in fine scales. Certain conditions, injuries, and medications accelerate desquamation and may cause peeling and the loss of deeper layers of the skin. Also called **exfoliation.** —**desquamate,** *v.,* **desquamative,** *adj.*

destructive aggression An act of hostility unnecessary for self-protection or preservation, which is directed toward an external

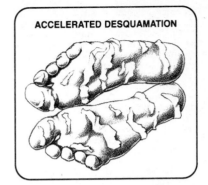

ACCELERATED DESQUAMATION

object or person. See also **aggression.**

detached retina See **retinal detachment.**

detergent 1. A cleansing agent. 2. Cleansing. See also **surfactant.**

determinant evolution The theory that evolution progresses according to a predetermined course. See also **orthogenesis.**

determinate cleavage Mitotic division of the fertilized ovum into blastomeres that are each destined to form a specific part of the embryo. If such cells are isolated, they are incapable of giving rise to an individual, complete embryo. Damage to or destruction of any of these cells results in a malformed organism. Also called **mosaic cleavage.** Compare **indeterminate cleavage.** See also **mosaic development.**

detrusor muscle A complex of longitudinal fibers that form the external layer of the muscular coat of the bladder. These fibers arise from the posterior surface of the pubis, traverse the inferior surface of the bladder, descend along the fundus, and attach to the prostate in men and to the front of the vagina in women. Along the sides of the bladder the fibers pass obliquely and intersect. The detrusor muscle is supplied by branches from the internal iliac artery and innervated by medulled fibers from the third and fourth sacral nerves and by nonmedullated fibers from the hypogastric plexus.

deuterium An isotope of hydrogen, symbol D or ^{2}H, available as a gas or as heavy water and used as a tracer in studies of fat or amino acid metabolism.

deutero-, deuto- A combining form meaning 'second': *deutero-albumose, deuteroconidium, deutero-elastose.*

deuteroplasm See **deutoplasm.**

deuto- See **deutero-.**

deutoplasm, deuteroplasm The inactive elements of the protoplasm, primarily the stored nutritive material contained in the yolk.

DEV *abbr* duck embryo vaccine. See **rabies vaccine.**

development 1. The gradual process of change and differentiation from a simple to a more advanced level of complexity. In humans the physical, mental, and emotional capacities that allow complex adaptation to the environment and the ability to function within society are acquired through growth, maturation, and learning. Kinds of development include **arrested development, mosaic development, psychomotor development, psychosexual development, psychosocial development, regulative development. 2.** In biology: the series of events that occur within an organism from fertilization of the ovum to the adult stage. —**developmental**, *adj.*

developmental age (DA) An expression of a child's developmental progress stated in age and determined by standardized measurements, as of body size and dimensions; by social and psychological functioning; by observations of motor skills; and by the giving of mental and aptitude tests. Compare **achievement age, mental age.**

developmental agraphia A deficiency in a child's ability to learn to form letters and to write. Other learning is normal, and the child usually has no musculoskeletal or neurologic problems.

developmental anatomy The study of the differentiation and the growth of an organism from one cell to birth. Also called **embryology.**

developmental anomaly Any congenital defect that results from the interference with the normal growth and differentiation of the fetus. Such defects can arise at any stage of embryonic development, vary greatly in type and severity, and are caused by a wide variety of determining factors, including genetic mutations, chromosomal aberrations, teratogenic agents, and environmental factors. Developmental anomalies are classified either according to the organ system affected, as congenital heart defects, or according to the way in which the defect occurred, as developmental failure or arrest, failure to atrophy or subdivide, fusion, splitting, incorrect migration, and misplacement. Most developmental defects are apparent at birth, especially any structural malformation, but some, especially those involving the organ systems, do not become evident until days, weeks, or even years later.

developmental arrest See **arrested development.**

developmental crisis Severe, usually transient, stress that occurs when a person is unable to complete the tasks of a psychosocial stage of development and is therefore unable to move on to the next stage. See also **psychosocial development.**

developmental disability (DD) A pathologic condition that starts developing before the age of 18. Most developmental disabilities persist throughout the life of the individual, although many can be effectively treated. See also **congenital condition.**

developmental horizon Any 1 of 25 stages in the development of the human embryo from the one-cell stage at conception to the morphologically and physiologically complex organism at the conclusion of the 7th week of gestation.

developmental idiocy A condition of severe mental retardation resulting from arrest of brain development.

developmental model 1. A conceptual framework devised to be used as a guide in making a diagnosis, in understanding a developmental process, and in forming a prognosis for continued development. **2.** In nursing: a conceptual framework describing four stages of development in the patient during therapy. In the first stage, called orientation, the patient begins a relationship with the nurse and begins to clarify the problem. In the second stage, called identification, the patient develops a sense of closeness and attachment to the nurse. In the third stage, called exploitation, the patient makes full use of the nursing services offered and becomes more independent. During the last stage, called resolution, the therapeutic relationship is terminated; the patient is independent. With this model the nurse may plan interventions appropriate to the developmental level of the patient. In the developmental model, health is viewed as a forward movement of personality development and other ongoing processes. Thus, the focus of nursing is to promote this forward movement by assisting the patient in self-repair and self-renewal.

developmental quotient (DQ) The numerical expression of a child's developmental level as measured by dividing the developmental age by the chronological age and multiplying by 100. Compare **intelligence quotient.** See also **developmental age.**

developmental task A physical or cognitive skill that a child must accomplish during a particular age period to continue developing, as walking, which precedes development of a sense of autonomy in the toddler period.

deviate 1. A person or an act that varies from that which is considered standard, as a social or sexual deviate, or that is within a statistical norm. 2. To vary from that which is considered standard or within a statistical norm. —**deviant**, *adj.*, **deviation**, *n.*

deviated septum A shifted medial partition of the nasal cavity, a condition affecting many adults. The nasal septum more commonly shifts to the left during normal growth, but this deflection may be aggravated by a blow to the nose or by other trauma. A severe deflection of the septum may significantly obstruct the nasal passages and result in infection, sinusitis, shortness of breath, headache, or recurring nosebleeds. Severe septal deviation may be corrected by various surgical procedures, as rhinoplasty or septoplasty. Postoperative care usually includes the maintenance of nasal packing, the administration of sedatives, and the placement of ice packs around the affected area to reduce swelling.

deviation from normal A quality, characteristic, symptom, or clinical finding that is different from what is commonly regarded as normal, as an elevated temperature, multiple gestation, or an extra digit.

device An item other than a drug used directly by, on, or in the patient rather than items, as surgical instruments and other equipment, used by health practitioners for diagnosis and treatment. Devices include orthopedic appliances, crutches, artificial heart valves, pacemakers, prostheses, wheel chairs, cervical collars, hearing aids, and eyeglasses.

devil's grip   See **epidemic pleurodynia.**

dexamethasone, d. acetate, d. sodium phosphate   A topical ophthalmic, otic, oral, and nasal corticosteroid anti-inflammatory agent.

dexchlorpheniramine maleate   An alkylamine antihistamine.

dexpanthenol   A vitamin used to stimulate intestinal peristalsis and as an emollient skin cream. Also called **pantothenic acid.**

dextranomer   A cleaning and debriding agent.

dextrality   See **right-handedness.**

dextran fermentation   The conversion of dextran to dextrose to dextran.

dextran preparation   Any of a group of solutions containing polysaccharides, water, and, in some preparations, electrolytes. These solutions are used as plasma-volume extenders in cases of hypovolemia from hemorrhage, dehydration, or other cause and are available for intravenous administration in several concentrations.

dextro-   A combining form meaning 'right': *dextrocardia, dextrocerebral, dextrogastria.*

dextroamphetamine phosphate, d. sulfate   Amphetamine central nervous system stimulant.

dextromethorphan hydrobromide   A nonnarcotic antitussive.

dextrose and sodium chloride injection   A fluid, nutrient, and electrolyte replenisher. It is available for parenteral use in a variety of concentrations.

dextrose (D-glucose)   Used for fluid replacement and as a caloric supplement.

dextrothyroxine sodium   An antilipemic agent.

DHFS   *abbr* dengue hemorrhagic fever shock syndrome.

dhobie itch   1. A fungal infection of the skin caused by *Tinea cruris* organisms, characterized by ringed lesions in the crural folds of the skin of the thighs, often followed by maceration and secondary infection. Warm, humid climate, tight clothing, and obesity aggravate the infection. 2. A form of contact dermatitis associated with the use of laundry marking fluids. Also called eczema marginatum, jock itch *(informal).* See **Tinea cruris.**

di-   1. A combining form meaning 'two, twice': *diacid, diamide, dimorphic.* 2. A combining form meaning 'apart, through': *diuresia, diactinism.* Also **dia-.** 3. A combining form meaning 'apart, away from': *diffraction, discission, divergent.*

diabetes   1. A clinical condition characterized by the excessive excretion of urine. The excess may be caused by a deficiency of antidiuretic hormone (ADH), as in diabetes insi-

pidus, or it may be the result of the hyperglycemia occurring in diabetes mellitus. **2.** Diabetes mellitus. **—diabetic** *adj., n.*

diabetes insipidus   A metabolic disorder, characterized by extreme polyuria and polydipsia, owing to deficient production or secretion of the antidiuretic hormone (ADH) or an inability of the kidney tubules to respond to ADH. (Rarely, the symptoms are self-induced by an excessive water intake.) The condition may be acquired, familial, idiopathic, or nephrogenic. NURSING CONSIDERATIONS: The onset may be dramatic and sudden, and urinary output may exceed 10 liters in 24 hours. The patient is usually well and comfortable except for the annoyance of frequent urination and a constant need to drink. A person with diabetes insipidus who is unconscious owing to trauma or surgery continues to produce massive quantities of urine. If fluids are not administered in adequate amounts, the patient becomes severely dehydrated and hypernatremic.

diabetes mellitus (DM)   A complex disorder of carbohydrate, fat, and protein metabolism owing primarily to a relative or complete lack of insulin secretion by the beta cells of the pancreas. The disease is often familial but may be acquired, as in Cushing's syndrome, secondary to the administration of excessive glucocorticoid. The onset of diabetes mellitus is sudden in children and usually insidious in adults. Characteristically, the course is progressive and includes polyuria, polydipsia, weight loss, polyphagia, hyperglycemia, and glycosuria. The eyes, kidneys, nervous system, skin, and circulatory system may be affected, infections are common, and atherosclerosis often develops. In childhood and in the brittle, advanced stage of the disease when no endogenous insulin is being secreted, ketoacidosis is a constant danger. The diagnosis is confirmed by glucose tolerance tests, history, and urinalysis. The goal of treatment is to maintain insulin-glucose homeostasis. See also **gestational diabetes, juvenile diabetes.**

diabetic   1. Of or pertaining to diabetes. **2.** Affected with diabetes. **3.** A patient with diabetes mellitus.

diabetic amaurosis   Blindness associated with diabetes, caused by a proliferative, hemorrhagic form of retinopathy that is characterized by capillary microaneurysms and hard or waxy exudates. Cataracts also are common in adult onset diabetes, and, in juvenile onset diabetes, snowflake cataract may progress until the entire lens is milky white.

diabetic coma   A life-threatening condition occurring in diabetic patients, caused by inadequate treatment, failure to take prescribed insulin, or, most frequently, infection, surgery, trauma, or other stress that increases the body's need for insulin. Warning signs of diabetic coma include a dull headache, fatigue, inordinate thirst, excess urination, epigastric pain, nausea, vomiting, parched lips, a flushed face, and sunken eyes. The temperature usually rises and then falls; the systolic blood pressure drops and cir-

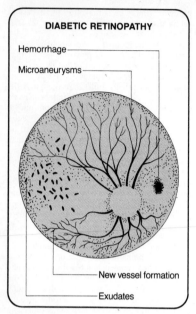

DIABETIC RETINOPATHY

Hemorrhage

Microaneurysms

New vessel formation

Exudates

culatory collapse may occur. Immediate treatment consists of administering insulin and replacing electrolytes and fluids to correct the acidosis and dehydration.

diabetic diet A diet prescribed in the treatment of diabetes mellitus, usually containing limited amounts of sugar or readily available carbohydrates and increased amounts of proteins, complex carbohydrates, and unsaturated fats. Dietary regulation depends on the severity of the disease and on the type and extent of insulin therapy. The diet should be designed to prevent wide fluctuation in the amount of glucose in the blood in order to preserve pancreatic function and to prevent chronic diabetic complications. See also **diabetes mellitus, insulin.**

diabetic ketoacidosis An acute, life-threatening complication of uncontrolled diabetes mellitus in which urinary loss of water, potassium, ammonium, and sodium results in hypovolemia, electrolyte imbalance, extremely high blood sugar levels, and the breakdown of free fatty acids causing acidosis, often with coma. The patient appears flushed; has hot, dry skin; is restless, uncomfortable, agitated, and diaphoretic; and has a fruity odor to the breath. Coma, confusion, and nausea are often noted. Juvenile diabetics and older diabetics who have no endogenous insulin are the most often affected. Untreated, the condition invariably proceeds to coma and death.

NURSING CONSIDERATIONS: The cause for the episode of ketoacidosis is sought. The most common precipitating factors are infection, gastrointestinal upset, alcohol consumption, and the patient's failure to take insulin. In childhood, diabetes characteristically begins suddenly and

progresses rapidly; therefore, the diagnosis of juvenile diabetes is usually made when the child is brought to the hospital in diabetic ketoacidosis. The care of a patient in the hospital after an episode of ketoacidosis is the same as for diabetes mellitus. Compare **insulin shock.**

diabetic retinopathy A disorder of retinal blood vessels characterized by capillary microaneurysms, hemorrhage, exudates, and the formation of new vessels and connective tissue. The disorder occurs most frequently in patients with long-standing, poorly controlled diabetes. Repeated hemorrhage may result in permanent opacity of the vitreous humor, and blindness may eventually result. Photocoagulation of damaged retinal blood vessels by a laser beam may be performed to prevent hemorrhage from the vessels. Rarely, cloudy vitreous humor is surgically removed by vitrectomy.

diabetic treatment Therapy of diabetes mellitus by means of a low carbohydrate diet, insulin injections, or oral hypoglycemic agents.

diabetic xanthoma An eruption of yellow papules or plaques on the skin in uncontrolled mellitus. The lesions disappear as the metabolic functions are stabilized and the disease is brought under control.

diacetic acid See **acetoacetic acid.**

diacondylar fracture Any fracture that runs across the line of a condyle.

Diagnex Blue test A trade name for a test for the presence of hydrochloric acid in gastric secretions. Diagnex Blue tablets, which contain the dye azuresin, are taken by mouth. If the urine appears blue it can be inferred that the stomach is secreting hydrochloric acid. See also **gastric analysis.**

diagnosis, *pl.* **diagnoses** **1.** Identification of a disease or a condition by a scientific evaluation of the physical signs, symptoms, history, laboratory tests, and procedures. **2.** The name of a disease or a condition. Kinds of diagnoses are **clinical diagnosis, nursing diagnosis, physical diagnosis.** —**diagnostic,** *adj.,* **diagnose,** *v.*

diagnostic Pertaining to a diagnosis.

Diagnostic and Statistical Manual of Mental Disorders (DSM) A manual, published by the American Psychiatric Association, listing the official diagnostic classifications of mental disorders. The *DSM* recommends the use of a multiaxial evaluation system as a holistic diagnostic approach consisting of five axes, each of which refers to a different class of information, including both mental and physical data. Axes I and II include all of the mental disorders, classified broadly as clinical syndromes and personality disorders; Axis III contains physical disorders and conditions; and Axes IV and V provide a coded outline of supplemental information on, for instance, psychosocial stressors and adaptive functioning, which may be useful for planning individual treatment and predicting its outcome. Each of the classifications of the mental disorders contains a code that provides a reference to the World Health Organization

(WHO) *Classification of Diseases* and offers such useful diagnostic criteria as essential and associated features of the disorder, age at onset, course, impairment, complications, predisposing factors, prevalence, sex ratio, familial patterns, and differential diagnoses.

diagnostic anesthesia A procedure in which analgesia is induced to a depth that permits patient comfort during performance of moderately painful diagnostic procedures of short duration.

diagnostician A person skilled and trained in making diagnoses.

diagnostic radiopharmaceutical A radioactive drug administered to a patient as a diagnostic tracer to differentiate normal from abnormal anatomic structures or biochemical or physiological functions. Most diagnostic radioactive tracers indicate their position within the body by emitting gamma rays. By monitoring the emissions with a collimated external gamma-ray detector, the concentration of the tracer in different organs can be inferred and low-resolution images of the organs obtained. Tracers prepared with tritium, carbon-14, or phosphorus-32, which do not emit gamma rays, are used diagnostically by analyzing the concentration of the isotope in a metabolic end product in the patient's blood, urine, breath, or, in some cases, biopsy samples. When glucose containing ^{14}C is administered, the subsequent monitoring of $^{14}CO_2$ in the patient's breath can indicate the absorption of the compound, its metabolism, and elimination as a metabolic end product.

diagnostic related group (DRG) A designation in a system that classifies patients by age, diagnosis, and surgical procedure, producing 300 different categories used in predicting the use of hospital resources, including length of stay. The system is being tested for use in anticipating the cost of reimbursement to hospitals by studying the population served to improve the cash flow to the hospital. It is performed using grouped data about how much each particular DRG may be expected to cost in hospital services.

diakinesis The final stage in the first meiotic prophase in gametogenesis in which the chromosomes achieve maximum contraction and are ready to separate. The chiasmata and nucleolus disappear, the nuclear membrane degenerates, and the spindle fibers form in preparation for the formation of dyads. See also **diplotene, leptotene, pachytene, zygotene.**

dialysate A solution used in dialysis.

dialysis 1. The process of separating colloids and crystalline substances in solution by the difference in their rate of diffusion through a semipermeable membrane. 2. A medical procedure for the removal of certain elements from the blood or lymph by virtue of the difference in their rates of diffusion through an external semipermeable membrane or, in the case of peritoneal dialysis, through the peritoneum. Dialysis may be used to remove poisons and excessive amounts of drugs, to correct serious electrolyte and acid-base im-

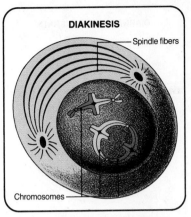

DIAKINESIS
— Spindle fibers
Chromosomes —

balances, and to remove urea, uric acid, and creatinine in patients with chronic end-stage renal disease. Dialysis involves diffusion of particles from an area of high to lower concentration, osmosis of fluid across the membrane from an area of lesser to greater concentration of particles, and the ultrafiltration or movement of the fluid across the membrane as a result of an artificially created pressure differential. See also **hemodialysis, peritoneal dialysis.**

dialyzer 1. A machine used in dialysis. 2. A semipermeable membrane or porous diaphragm in a dialysis machine. See also **hemodialysis, peritoneal dialysis.**

Diamond-Blackfan anemia See **Blackfan-Diamond syndrome.**

diapedesis The passage of blood corpuscles through the walls of the vessels that contain them.

diaper rash A maculopapular and occasionally excoriated eruption in the diaper area of infants caused by irritation from feces, moisture, heat, or ammonia produced by the bacterial decomposition of urine. Secondary infection by monilia is common.

diaper restraint A therapeutic device used especially in orthopedics for countertraction with lower extremity traction when other methods of countertraction are not effective. Diaper restraints are commonly used in treating children with orthopedic diseases and abnormalities and are designed to fit over the pelvic area like a diaper, with rings incorporated at each of four corners. A webbing strap is threaded through the rings and attached to the top side of the bedspring frame. Diaper restraints are used with Russell traction and split Russell traction if additional countertraction is required but are not usually used with other kinds of traction. Compare **jacket restraint, sling restraint.**

diaphanoscopy Examination of an internal structure with a diaphanoscope, an instrument that transilluminates body tissues.

diaphoresis The secretion of sweat, especially the profuse secretion associated with an elevated body temperature, physical exertion, exposure to heat, and mental or emotional stress.

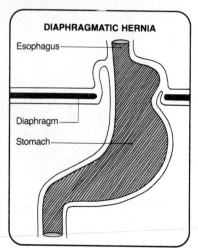

DIAPHRAGMATIC HERNIA

Esophagus

Diaphragm

Stomach

Sweating is centrally controlled by the sympathetic nervous system and is primarily a thermoregulatory mechanism, but the sweat glands on the palms and soles respond to emotional stimuli and do not participate in thermal sweating. Also called **sweating**. —**diaphoretic,** *adj.*

diaphoretic See **sudorific.**

diaphragm **1.** In anatomy: a dome-shaped musculofibrous partition that separates the thoracic and the abdominal cavities. The convex cranial surface of the diaphragm forms the floor of the thoracic cavity, and the concave surface forms the roof of the abdominal cavity. This partition is pierced by various openings through which pass different structures, as the aorta, esophagus, and vena cava. The diaphragm aids respiration by moving up and down. During inspiration it moves down and increases the volume of the thoracic cavity; during expiration it moves up, decreasing the volume. During deep inspiration and expiration the range of diaphragmatic movement in the adult is about 30 mm (1¼ inches) on the right side and about 28 mm (1⅛ inches) on the left side. The height of this structure also varies with the degree of distention of the stomach and the intestines and with the size of the liver. It is innervated by the phrenic nerve from the cervical plexus. **2.** *Informal.* A contraceptive diaphragm. **3.** In optics: an opening that controls the amount of light passing through an optical network. **4.** A thin, membranous partition, as that employed in dialysis. **5.** In radiography: a metal plate with a small opening that limits the diameter of the radiographic beam. —**diaphragmatic,** *adj.*

diaphragmatic hernia The protrusion of part of the stomach through an opening in the diaphragm, most commonly an abnormally enlarged esophageal hiatus. The enlargement of the normal opening for the esophagus may be caused by trauma, congenital weakness, increased abdominal pressure, or relaxation of ligaments of skeletal muscles, and permits part of the stomach to slide into the thorax. Symptoms of diaphragmatic hernia vary but usually include heartburn after meals, when in a supine position, and on exertion, especially when bending forward. There may be regurgitation of food, dysphagia, abdominal distention after eating, belching, rumbling in the intestines, rapid breathing, and a dull epigastric pain radiating to the shoulder. The similarity of some of the symptoms to those of myocardial infarction may make the patient fearful and anxious. The continued reflux of gastric juice into the esophagus may lead to ulceration with bleeding and the formation of fibrous tissue. Gastric contents regurgitated during sleep may be aspirated into the lungs. Rarely, part of the cardiac portion of the stomach becomes incarcerated in the chest. If symptoms are severe and persistent and if they are unrelieved by conservative measures, the hernia may be repaired surgically.

NURSING CONSIDERATIONS: Diaphragmatic hernias are very common, especially among older people who are in the hospital for other indications. The recurrence of the symptoms of diaphragmatic hernia may often be prevented by instructing the patient, before discharge, to have frequent, small, bland meals; to avoid lying down after eating; to lose weight (if indicated); to refrain from smoking; and to avoid constipation. Serious complications and severe discomfort usually may be avoided by the patient if the instructions are observed carefully. Also called **hiatus hernia.**

diaphragmatic node A node in one of three groups of thoracic parietal lymph nodes, situated on the thoracic side of the diaphragm and consisting of the anterior set, the middle set, and the posterior set of nodes. Compare **intercostal node, sternal node.** See also **lymphatic system, lymph node.**

diaphragm pessary See **pessary.**

diaphragm stethoscope An instrument for auscultation of bodily sounds. Originally designed by René Laënnec, it consists of a vibrating disk, or diaphragm, that transmits sound waves through tubing to two ear pieces. Also called **binaural stethoscope.** See also **stethoscope.**

diaphyseal aclasis A relatively rare abnormal condition that affects the skeletal system, characterized by multiple exostoses or bony protrusions. It is hereditary, being transmitted as a dominant trait. Approximately half of the children of an individual with diaphyseal aclasis display varying degrees of its symptoms. The characteristic exostoses are radiographically and microscopically similar to osteochondromas. Evident involvement is diffuse, with the long bones usually affected more severely and more frequently than the short bones. Depending on the specific area involved, various angular or rotational deformities may result. Diaphyseal aclasis is usually bilateral and occurs more frequently in boys than in girls. Although this disease is hereditary, its signs and symptoms are not usually evident until the affected individual is 2 years of age or older. Children of a parent who has the disease are often routinely examined for symptoms. The major signs of the disease are the noticeable protrusions in the areas of the exostoses. Pain is not usually associated with the exostoses and, if present, is usually minimal. Deformities of the extremities may be evident, depending on the severity and the location of the exostoses. Asymptomatic lesions characteristic of diaphyseal aclasis usually require little or no treatment other than continued observation. The lesions located near the joints that interfere with joint motion or impair neurovascular function may be surgically excised. A relatively small number of these lesions may become malignant. Also called **hereditary deforming chondroplasia, multiple cartilaginous exostoses.**

diaphysis   The shaft of a long bone, consisting of a tube of compact bone enclosing the medullary cavity.

diarrhea   The frequent passage of loose, watery stools, generally the result of increased motility in the colon. The stool may also contain mucus, pus, blood, or excessive amounts of fat. Diarrhea is always a symptom of some underlying disorder. Conditions in which diarrhea is an important symptom are dysenteric diseases, malabsorption syndrome, lactose intolerance, irritable bowel syndrome, gastrointestinal tumors, and inflammatory bowel disease. In addition to stool frequency, patients may complain of abdominal cramps and generalized weakness. Untreated, diarrhea may lead to rapid dehydration and electrolyte imbalance and should be treated symptomatically until proper diagnosis can be made. See also **dehydration.** —**diarrheal, diarrheic,** *adj.*

diarthrosis   See **synovial joint.**

diastatic fermentation   The conversion of starch to glucose by the enzyme ptyalin.

diasthesis, *pl.* **diastheses**   An inherited physical constitution predisposing to certain diseases or conditions, many of which are believed associated with the Y chromosome, because males appear to be more susceptible than females.

diastole   The period of time in the cardiac cycle between contractions of the ventricles during which blood enters the relaxed ventricular chambers from the atria. Diastole begins with the onset of the second heart sound and ends with the first heart sound. Compare **systole.** —**diastolic,** *adj.*

-diastole   A combining form referring to 'types and locations of the lower blood pressure measurement': *adiastole, hyperdiastole, prediastole.*

diastrophic dwarf   A person in whom short stature is caused by osteochondrodysplasia. This condition is associated with various deformities of the bones and joints, including scoliosis, clubfoot, micromelia, hand defects, multiple joint contractures and subluxations, ear deformities, and cleft palate. The condition may be genetically related and transmitted as an autosomal recessive trait.

diathermy   A therapeutic procedure that em-

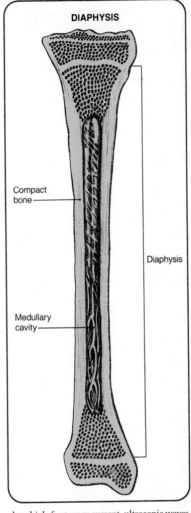

DIAPHYSIS

Compact bone

Diaphysis

Medullary cavity

ploys high-frequency current, ultrasonic waves, or microwaves to slightly raise the temperature of deep tissues.

diazepam   A benzodiazepine anticonvulsant and antianxiety agent.

diazoxide   A vasodilator used as an antihypertensive.

diazoxide, oral   A drug used to treat hypoglycemia.

dibromodulcitol   See **mitolactol.**

dibucaine hydrochloride   An amide antipruritic topical local anesthetic.

DIC   *abbr* **disseminated intravascular coagulation.**

dicephaly   A developmental anomaly in which the fetus has two heads. —**dicephalous, dicephalic,** *adj.*, **dicephalus,** *n.*

dichloracetic acid   A topical caustic agent.

RECOMMENDED DIETARY ALLOWANCES OF VITAMINS AND MINERALS

☐ MALE

☐ FEMALE

ELEMENT	AGES 19 TO 22 154 lb (70 kg) 70" (177 cm)	AGES 23 TO 50 154 lb (70 kg) 70" (177 cm)	AGE 51 + 154 lb (70 kg) 70" (177 cm)	AGES 19 TO 22 120 lb (55 kg) 64" (163 cm)	AGES 23 TO 50 120 lb (55 kg) 64" (163 cm)	AGE 51 + 120 lb (55 kg) 64" (163 cm)
Vitamin A (mcg RE)	1,000	1,000	1,000	800	800	800
Vitamin D (mcg)	7.5	5	5	7.5	5	5
Vitamin E (mg or TE)	10	10	10	8	8	8
Vitamin C (mg)	60	60	60	60	60	60
Thiamine (mg)	1.5	1.4	1.2	1.1	1	1
Riboflavin (mg)	1.7	1.6	1.4	1.3	1.2	1.2
Niacin (mg NE)	19	18	16	14	13	13
Vitamin B_6 (mg)	2.2	2.2	2.2	2	2	2
Folacin (mcg)	400	400	400	400	400	400
Vitamin B_{12} (mcg)	3	3	3	3	3	3
Calcium (mg)	800	800	800	800	800	800
Phosphorus (mg)	800	800	800	800	800	800
Magnesium (mg)	350	350	350	300	300	300
Iron (mg)	10	10	10	18	18	18
Zinc (mg)	15	15	15	15	15	15
Iodine (mcg)	150	150	150	150	150	150

dichlorphenamide   A carbonic anhydrase inhibitor.

dichorial twins, dichorionic twins   See **dizygotic twins.**

dichotomy   A division or separation into two equal parts.

Dick test   A skin test to determine sensitivity to an erythrotoxin produced by the group A streptococci that cause scarlet fever. A skin test dose of the toxin is injected intradermally. An inflammation 1 cm in diameter, appearing within 24 to 48 hours after injection, indicates that the person is not immune, has no antitoxin, and therefore is susceptible to the toxin. Larger doses may then be given to induce immunity. Compare **Shultz-Charlton phenomenon.**

dicloxacillin sodium   A penicillin antibiotic.

dicumarol   An oral anticoagulant of the coumarin type.

dicyclomine hydrochloride   A gastrointestinal anticholinergic agent.

didym-   A combining form meaning 'pertaining to a testis': didymalgia, didymitis, didymodynia.

-didymus   A combining form meaning: **1.** A 'pair of twins joined at a (specified) part of the body': gastrodidymus, thoracodidymus, verte-brodidymus. **2.** A 'fetal monster with supernumerary organ(s)': atlodidymus, opodidymus, pygodidymus.

diecious, dioecious   An animal or plant that is sexually distinct, having either male or female reproductive organs.

diencephalon   The division of the brain between the telencephalon and the mesencephalon. It consists of the hypothalamus, thalamus, metathalamus, and epithalamus and includes most of the third ventricle. Also called betweenbrain, interbrain.

dienestrol   A synthetic estrogen for vaginal application.

diet   **1.** Food and drink considered with regard to their nutritional qualities, composition, and effects on health. **2.** Nutrients prescribed, regulated, or restricted as to kind and amount for therapeutic or other purposes. **3.** The customary allowance of food and drink regularly provided or consumed. Compare **nutrition.** See also specific diets. **—dietetic,** adj.

dietary allowances   The recommended allowances of essential nutrients formulated by the Food and Nutrition Board of the National Research Council to serve as a guide for planning the diet to maintain good nutrition in healthy individuals. In general the recommended allow-

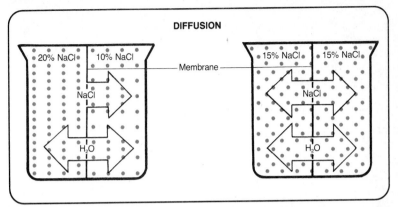

DIFFUSION

20% NaCl | 10% NaCl

—— Membrane ——

15% NaCl | 15% NaCl

NaCl

H_2O

NaCl

H_2O

ances exceed average nutritional requirements and are lower than the amounts needed in disease or deficiency states.

dietary fiber A generic term for the many nondigestible chemical substances found in plant cell walls and surrounding cellular material, each with a different effect on the various gastrointestinal functions, as colon transit time, water absorption, and lipid metabolism. The main dietary fiber components are cellulose, lignin, hemicellulose, pectin, and gums. Also called **bulk, roughage.**

dietetic food **1.** A specially prepared low-calorie food, often containing artificial sweeteners. **2.** A food prepared for any specific dietary need or restriction, as salt-free or vegetarian foods. See also **dietetics.**

dietetics The science of applying nutritional principles to the planning and preparation of foods and regulation of the diet in relation to both health and disease.

diethylcarbamazine citrate An anthelmintic agent.

diethyl ether See **ether.**

diethylpropion hydrochloride An amphetamine-like central nervous system stimulant.

diethylstilbestrol (DES), d. phosphate Synthetic estrogens.

Dietl's crisis A sudden, excruciating pain in the kidney, caused by distention of the renal pelvis, by the rapid ingestion of very large amounts of liquid, or by a kinking of a ureter that produces temporary occlusion of the flow of urine from the kidney. The pain may be accompanied by nausea, vomiting, hematuria, and general collapse. See also **hydronephrosis.**

differential diagnosis See **diagnosis.**

differential growth A comparison of the various increases in size or the different rates of growth of dissimilar organisms, tissues, or structures.

differential white blood cell count An examination and enumeration of the distribution of leukocytes in a stained blood smear. The different kinds of white cells are counted and reported as a percentage of the total examined.

Compare **complete blood count.** See also **hematocrit, hemoglobin.**

differentiation **1.** In embryology: a process in development in which unspecialized cells or tissues are systemically modified and altered to achieve specific and characteristic physical forms, physiologic functions, and chemical properties. Kinds of differentiation are **correlative differentiation, functional differentiation, invisible differentiation, self-differentiation. 2.** Progressive diversification leading to complexity. **3.** The acquisition of functions and forms different from those of the original. **4.** The distinguishing of one thing or disease from another, as in differential diagnosis. —**differentiate,** *v.*

diffraction The bending and scattering of wavelengths of radiation, such as light, as the radiation passes around obstacles in its path. X-ray diffraction is utilized in the study of the internal structure of cells. The X-rays are diffracted by cell parts into patterns that are indicative of chemical and physical structure. See also **refraction.**

diffuse fibrosing alveolitis See **interstitial pneumonia.**

diffuse goiter An enlargement of all parts of the thyroid gland.

diffuse hypersensitivity pneumonia See **hypersensitivity pneumonitis.**

diffuse lipoma See **multiple lipomatosis.**

diffuse lipomatosis See **multiple lipomatosis.**

diffusion The process in which ions and molecules move from an area of greater concentration to an area of lower concentration, resulting in an even distribution of the particles in the fluid.

diffusion of gases A natural process, essential in respiration, in which molecules of a gas pass from an area of higher concentration to one of a lower concentration.

diflorasone diacetate A topical anti-inflammatory agent.

diflunisal A nonnarcotic analgesic and anti-inflammatory agent.

digastricus One of four suprahyoid muscles having two parts, an anterior belly and a pos-

DIGESTIVE SYSTEM

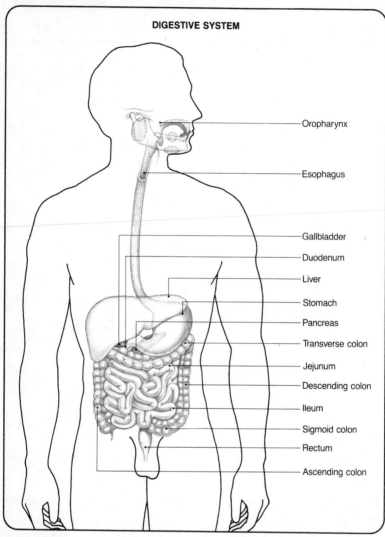

- Oropharynx
- Esophagus
- Gallbladder
- Duodenum
- Liver
- Stomach
- Pancreas
- Transverse colon
- Jejunum
- Descending colon
- Ileum
- Sigmoid colon
- Rectum
- Ascending colon

terior belly. The anterior belly originates in the lower border of the mandible and inserts in the body and great cornu of the hyoid bone. It is innervated by fibers of the mandibular branch of the trigeminal nerve. It acts to open the jaw and to draw the hyoid bone forward. The posterior belly originates in the mastoid notch of the temporal bone and inserts in the body and great cornu of the hyoid bone. It is innervated by fibers of the mandibular branch of the facial nerve and acts to draw back and to raise the hyoid bone. Also called digastric muscle. Compare **geniohyoideus, mylohyoideus, stylohyoideus.**

DiGeorge syndrome A congenital disorder characterized by severe immunodeficiency

and structural abnormalities, including hypertelorism; notched, low-set ears; small mouth; downward-slanting eyes; cardiovascular defects, and the absence of the thymus and parathyroid glands. Death, often from infection, usually occurs before age 2. Rarely, transplantation of a human fetal thymus is performed. Also called **thymic parathyroid aplasia.**

digest 1. To soften by heat and moisture. 2. To break into smaller parts and simpler compounds by mastication, hydrolysis, and the action of intestinal secretions and enzymes, especially in the way the body digests food for the absorption of nutrients required in metabolism. The small intestine digests food by enzymatic actions that produce absorbable amino acids, emulsified fat particles, and monosaccharides. **3.** Any material that results from digestion or hydrolysis.

digestion The conversion of food into absorbable substances in the gastrointestinal tract. Digestion is accomplished through the mechanical and chemical breakdown of food into smaller molecules, with the help of glands located inside and outside the gut. **—digestive,** *adj.*

digestive fever A slight rise in body temperature that normally accompanies the digestive process.

digestive gland Any one of the many structures that secrete reactive agents involved in the breaking down of food into the constituent absorbable substances needed for metabolism. Some kinds of digestive glands are the salivary glands, gastric glands, intestinal glands, liver, and pancreas. Some important secretions produced by different digestive glands are hydrochloric acid, bile, mucus, and various enzymes.

digestive system The organs, structures, and accessory glands of the digestive tube of the body through which food passes from the mouth to the esophagus, stomach, and intestines. The accessory glands secrete the digestive enzymes used by the digestive system to break down food into constituent substances in preparation for absorption into the bloodstream. Waste products are then excreted.

digestive tube A musculomembranous tube, about 9 m (30 feet) long, extending from the mouth to the anus and lined with mucous membrane. Its various portions are the mouth, pharynx, esophagus, stomach, small intestine, and large intestine. The tube is part of the digestive system of the body, which includes numerous accessory organs. Also called **alimentary canal.** See also **digestive system.**

digit- A combining form meaning 'pertaining to a finger or toe': *digitate, digitigrade.*

digital **1.** Of or pertaining to a digit, that is, a finger or toe. **2.** Resembling a finger or toe. See also **digitate.**

digitalis glycoside See **glycoside.**

digitalis leaf A cardiotonic glycoside used to treat congestive heart failure and some cardiac arrhythmias.

digitate wart A fingerlike, horny projection that arises from a pea-shaped base and occurs on the scalp or near the hairline. Like other kinds of warts, it is a benign viral infection of the skin and the adjacent mucous membrane. It may spontaneously disappear as the host individual develops an immune response, or it may require treatment, as by electrodesiccation and curettage.

digitoxin A cardiotonic glycoside used to treat congestive heart failure and some cardiac arrhythmias.

digoxin A cardiotonic glycoside used to treat congestive heart failure and some cardiac arrhythmias.

diGuglielmo's disease See **erythroleukemia.**

diGuglielmo's syndrome See **erythroleukemia.**

dihybrid In genetics: pertaining to or describing a person, organism, or strain that is heterozygous for two specific traits, that is the offspring of parents differing in two specific gene pairs, or that is heterozygous for two particular traits or gene loci under consideration.

dihybrid cross In genetics: the mating of two individuals, organisms, or strains having different gene pairs that determine two specific traits, or in which two particular characteristics or gene loci are being followed.

dihydric alcohol An alcohol containing two hydroxyl groups.

dihydroergotamine mesylate An alpha-adrenergic blocking agent.

dihydrotachysterol (AT-10). A parathyroid-like agent.

dihydroxyaluminum aminoacetate, d. sodium carbonate Antacids.

diiodohydroxyquin An amebicide.

dilatation **1.** Normal physiologic increase in the diameter of a body opening, blood vessel, or tube, as the widening of the pupil of the eye in response to decreased light. **2.** Artificial increase in the diameter of such an opening either by medication, as in the use of cycloplegic eye drops to open the pupil wide for examination of the retina, or by instrumentation, as in the use of a dilator to open the uterine cervix to facilitate curettage. **3.** The diameter of the opening of the cervix in labor as measured on vaginal examination, expressed in centimeters or fingerbreadths, one fingerbreadth being approximately 2.0 cm (¾ inches). At full dilatation the diameter of the cervical opening is 10.0 cm (4 inches). **—dilatate,** *v.*

dilatation and curettage (D & C) Dilatation of the uterine cervix and scraping of the endometrium of the uterus, performed to diagnose disease of the uterus, to correct heavy or prolonged vaginal bleeding, or to remove the products of conception, such as retained placental fragments postpartum or after an incomplete abortion. It is also done to remove tumors, and to find the cause of infertility. Under a light, general anesthesia the cervix is dilated with a series of dilators of increasing size to allow the insertion of a curet into the uterus.

dilatator naris The alar portion of the nasalis muscle that dilates the nostril. Compare **compressor naris.**

dilatator pupillae An involuntary muscle that contracts the iris of the eye and dilates the pupil. It is composed of radiating fibers that converge from the circumference of the iris toward the center and blend with fibers of the sphincter pupillae near the margin of the pupil. The dilatator pupillae is innervated by nerve fibers from the sympathetic system. Compare **sphincter pupillae.**

dimenhydrinate An antiemetic.

dimer A compound formed by the union of two radicals or two molecules of a simpler compound, as a polymer formed from two or more molecules of a monomer.

dimercaprol A heavy metal antagonist used to treat poisoning by lead, gold, arsenic, or mercury.

dimethindene maleate An alkylamine antihistamine.

dimethisoquin hydrochloride An antipruritic and topical anesthetic.

dimethyl carbinol See **isopropyl alcohol.**

dimethyl sulfoxide 50% (DMSO) An anti-inflammatory agent used to treat intestinal cystitis. It has also been used to treat arthritis and other related conditions.

Dimitri disease See **encephalotrigeminal angiomatosis.**

dinoprostone An oxytocic agent.

dinoprost tromethamine An oxytocic agent.

dioctyl calcium sulfosuccinate See **docusate.**

dioctyl sodium sulfosuccinate See **docusate.**

dioecious See **diecious.**

diovular See **binovular.**

diovulatory Routinely releasing two ova during each ovarian cycle. Compare **monovulatory.**

diperodon monohydrate An antipruritic and topical anesthetic.

diphemanil methylsulfate A gastrointestinal anticholinergic agent.

diphenhydramine hydrochloride An ethanolamine antihistamine nonnarcotic antitussive.

diphenidol An antiemetic.

diphenoxylate hydrochloride with atropine sulfate An antidiarrheal agent.

diphenylhydantoin See **phenytoin.**

diphenylpyraline hydrochloride An ethanolamine antihistamine.

diphtheria An acute, contagious disease caused by the bacterium *Corynebacterium diphtheriae,* characterized by the production of a systemic toxin and a false membrane lining of the mucous membrane of the throat. The toxin is particularly damaging to the tissues of the heart and central nervous system, and the dense pseudomembrane in the throat may interfere with eating, drinking, and breathing; the membrane may occur in other body tissues as well. Lymph glands in the neck swell and the neck becomes edematous. Untreated, the disease is often fatal, causing heart and kidney failure. Patients are usually hospitalized in isolation rooms; treatment may include administration of diphtheria antitoxin, antibiotics, bed rest, fluids, and an adequate diet. Tracheostomy is sometimes necessary. Recovery is slow but usually complete. Immunization against diphtheria is available to all children in the United States and is usually given with pertussis and tetanus immunization early in infancy. See also **Schick test.**

diphtheria and tetanus toxoids (DT), adsorbed An active immunizing agent.

diphtheria and tetanus toxoids and

pertussis vaccine (DPT) An active immunizing agent.

diphtheria toxoid, adsorbed An active immunizing agent.

diphtheroid 1. Of or pertaining to diphtheria. 2. Resembling the bacillus *Corynebacterium diphtheriae.*

Diphyllobothrium A genus of large, parasitic, intestinal flatworms having a scolex with two slitlike grooves. The species that most often infects humans is *Diphyllobothrium latum,* the fish tapeworm. See also **tapeworm infection.**

dipivefrin An ophthalmic that is a prodrug of epinephrine.

diplegia Bilateral paralysis of both sides of any part of the body or of like parts on the opposite sides of the body. A kind of diplegia is **facial diplegia.** Compare **hemiplegia. —diplegic,** *adj.*

diplo- A combining form meaning 'double': *diplobacilli, diplococcus, diplokaryon.*

diplococcus, *pl.* **diplococci** A coccus that occurs in pairs.

diploë The loose bony tissue between the two tables of the cranial bones.

diploid 1. Of or pertaining to an individual, organism, strain, or cell that has two complete sets of homologous chromosomes, as normally found in the somatic cells and the primordial germ cells before maturation. In humans the normal diploid number is 46. 2. Diploidic (2n), such an individual, organism, strain, or cell. Compare **haploid, tetraploid, triploid.**

diploidy The state or condition of having two complete sets of homologous chromosomes.

diplokaryon A nucleus that contains twice the diploid number of chromosomes.

diploma program in nursing An educational program that trains nurses in a hospital setting, usually in 2 or 3 years. The recipient of a diploma is eligible to take the national certifying examination to become a registered nurse.

diplomate An individual who has earned a diploma or certificate, especially a doctor who has been certified by a specialty board. See also **board certified.**

diplonema The looplike formation of the chromosomes in the diplotene stage of the first meiotic prophase of gametogenesis.

diplopagus Conjoined twins that are more or less equally developed, although one or several internal organs may be shared.

diplopia Double vision caused by defective function of the extraocular muscles or a disorder of the nerves that innervate the muscles. A transient episode of diplopia is usually of no clinical significance, indicating only a brief relaxation of the fusion mechanism of the central nervous system, which maintains ocular straightness.

-diplopia A combining form meaning '(condition of) double vision': *amphodiplopia, amphoterodiplopia, monodiplopia.*

diplosomatia, diplosomia A congenital anomaly in which fully formed twins are joined at one or more areas of their bodies.

diplotene The fourth stage in the first meiotic

prophase in gametogenesis in which the tetrads exhibit chiasmata between the chromatids of the paired homologous chromosomes and genetic crossing over occurs. The chromosomes then begin to repel each other and separate longitudinally, forming loops. See also **diakinesis, leptotene, pachytene, zygotene.**

dipodia　A developmental anomaly characterized by the duplication of one or both feet.

diprosopus　A malformed fetus that has a double face showing varying degrees of development.

-dipsia　A combining form meaning '(condition of) thirst': *hydroadipsia, oligodipsia, polydipsia.* Also **-dipsy.**

dipsomania　An uncontrollable, often periodic craving for and indulgence in alcoholic beverages; alcoholism.

-dipsy　See **-dipsia.**

dipus　Conjoined twins that have only two feet.

dipygus　A malformed fetus that has a double pelvis, one of which is usually not fully developed.

dipyridamole　A coronary vasodilator.

direct access　The right of a health-care provider and a patient to interact on a professional basis without interference.

direct calorimetry　The measurement of the amount of heat directly generated by any oxidation reaction, especially one involving a living organism. Compare **indirect calorimetry.**

direct contact　Mutual touching of two individuals or organisms. Many communicable diseases may be spread by the direct contact between an infected individual and a healthy person. Some kinds of diseases that may be spread by direct contact are gonorrhea, impetigo, herpes, staphylococcal skin infections, and syphilis. Other infections are transmitted by insect or animal vectors, droplets, or contaminated food.

direct fracture　Any fracture occurring at a specific point of injury that is a direct result of that injury.

direct generation　See **asexual generation.**

direct illumination　See **illumination.**

directive therapy　A psychotherapeutic approach in which the psychotherapist directs the course of therapy by intervening to ask questions and offer interpretations. Compare **nondirective therapy.** See also **psychoanalysis.**

direct lead　**1.** An electrocardiographic conductor in which the exploring electrode is placed directly on the surface of the exposed heart. **2.** *Informal.* A tracing produced by such a lead on an electrocardiograph.

direct patient care　In nursing: care of a patient provided in person by a member of the staff. Direct patient care may involve any aspects of the health care of a patient, including treatments, counseling, self-care, patient education, and administration of medication.

direct reaction to light　The constriction of a pupil receiving increased illumination, as by a flashlight during an ophthalmologic ex-

amination. Compare **consensual reaction to light.**

direct relationship　See **positive relationship.**

dis-　A combining form meaning: **1.** 'Reversal or separation': *disacidify, dischronation, disinfect.* **2.** 'Duplication': *disdiaclast, dissogency, districhiasis.*

disadvantaged　**1.** Any group of people who lack money, education, literacy, or another advantage. **2.** A euphemism for 'poor.'

discharge　**1.** To release a substance or object. Also called **evacuate, excrete, secrete. 2.** To release a patient from a hospital. **3.** To release an electric charge which may be manifested by a spark or surge of electricity from a storage battery, condenser, or other source. **4.** To release a burst of energy from or through a neuron. **5.** A release of emotions, often accompanied by a wide range of voluntary and involuntary reflexes, weeping, rage, or other emotional displays, called affective discharge in psychology. **6.** A substance or object discharged. Also called **evacuation, excretion, secretion.**

discharge planning　The formulation of a program by the patient, his family, the health-care team, and appropriate outside agencies to meet physical and psychological needs after the patient leaves the health-care facility.

disciform keratitis　An inflammatory condition of the eye that often follows an attack of dendritic keratitis and is believed to be an immunologic response to an ocular herpes simplex infection. The condition is characterized by disklike opacities in the cornea, usually with inflammation of the iris. See also **herpes simplex.**

disco-　A combining form meaning 'pertaining to a disk, disk-shaped': *discophorous, discopathy, discoplacenta.*

discoblastula　A blastula formed from the partial cleavage that occurs in a fertilized ovum containing a large amount of yolk. It develops from the blastodisc and consists of a cellular cap, or blastoderm, separated from the uncleaved yolk mass by a small cavity, the blastocoele.

discocyte　A mature, normal, erythrocyte, exhibiting one of its many steady-state configurations. It is a biconcave disk without a nucleus. Compare **burr cell, acanthocyte.**

discoid lupus erythematosus (DLE)　A chronic, recurrent disease, primarily of the skin, characterized by red macules that are covered with scales and extend into follicles. The lesions are typically distributed in a butterfly pattern covering the cheeks and bridge of the nose, but may also occur on other parts of the body. On healing, the lesions atrophy and leave hyperpigmented or hypopigmented scars, and, if hairy areas are involved, alopecia may result. The cause of the disease is not established, but there is evidence that it may be an autoimmune disorder and some cases seem to be induced by certain drugs. It is at least five times more common in women than in men and occurs most

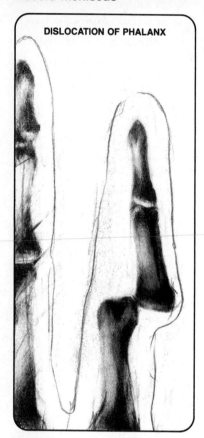

DISLOCATION OF PHALANX

frequently between the ages of 20 to 40. Treatment includes sunscreens, steroids, and systemic antimalarial drugs, as hydroxychloroquinine, and, in severe cases, systemic corticosteroid agents. Also called **cutaneous lupus erythematosus.** See also **systemic lupus erythematosus.**

discoid meniscus An abnormal condition characterized by a discoid rather than semilunar shape of the cartilaginous meniscus of the knee. The lateral meniscus is most often affected, although the medial meniscus may also become involved. A developmental anomaly, asymptomatic in the infant or in the young child, it occurs most frequently in children between the ages of 6 and 8. Common complaints are a clicking in the knee joint or collapse of the knee joint. These characteristics are often associated with a knee injury but also occur without any history of trauma. Examination demonstrates the clicking, usually when the knee is moved from flexion to extension, during the last 15° to 20°.

discordance In genetics: the expression of one or more specific traits in only one member of a pair of twins. Compare **concordance.** —**discordant,** *adj.*

discovery In law: a pretrial procedure allowing one party to examine vital witnesses and documents held exclusively by the adverse party. Discovery is limited to materials, facts, and other resources that could not otherwise be reasonably expected to be discovered and that are necessary to the preparation of the case for trial. Also called **pretrial discovery.** Compare **deposition, interrogatories.**

discus See **disk.**

discus interpubicus See **interpubic disk.**

discus nervi optici See **optic disk.**

disease 1. A condition of abnormal vital function involving any structure, part, or system of an organism. 2. A specific illness or disorder characterized by a recognizable set of signs and symptoms, attributable to heredity, infection, diet, or environment. Compare **condition, diathesis.**

disengagement An obstetrical manipulation in which the presenting part of the baby is dislodged from the maternal pelvis as part of an operative delivery. See also **Kielland rotation, version and extraction.**

dishpan fracture A fracture that depresses the skull. Also called **derby hat fracture.**

disinfection The process of killing pathogenic organisms or of rendering them inert.

disjunction In genetics: the separation of the paired homologous chromosomes during the anaphase stage of the first meiotic division or of the chromatids of a chromosome during the anaphase of mitosis and the second meiotic division. Compare **nondisjunction.**

disk, disc 1. A flat, circular platelike structure, as an articular disk or an optic disk. 2. *Informal.* An intervertebral disk.

dislocation The displacement of any part of the body from its normal position, particularly a bone from its normal articulation with a joint. See also **subluxation.** —**dislocate,** *v.*

dismiss In law: to discharge or dispose of an action, suit, or motion trial. —**dismissal,** *n.*

disodium edetate See **edetate disodium.**

disopyramide, d. phosphate Group I antiarrhythmics.

disorganized schizophrenia A form of schizophrenia characterized by an earlier age of onset, usually at puberty, and a more severe disintegration of the personality than occurs in other forms of the disease. Symptoms include inappropriate laughter and silliness; peculiar mannerisms, as facial grimaces; talking and gesturing to oneself; regressive, bizarre, and often obscene behavior; extreme social withdrawal; and fantastic and unsystematized hallucinations and delusions, which are usually of a sexual, religious, persecutory, or hypochondriacal nature. Also called **hebephrenia, hebephrenic schizophrenia.** See also **schizophrenia.**

disorient To lose awareness or perception of space, time, or personal identity and relationships.

disorientation A state of mental confusion characterized by inadequate or incorrect per-

CAUSES OF DISSEMINATED INTRAVASCULAR COAGULATION

Obstetric:	Amniotic fluid embolism, eclampsia, retained dead fetus, retained placenta, abruptio placentae, and toxemia
Neoplastic:	Sarcoma, metastatic carcinoma, acute leukemia, prostatic cancer, and giant hemangioma
Infectious:	Acute bacteremia; septicemia; rickettsemia; and infection from virus, fungi, or protozoa
Necrotic:	Trauma, destruction of brain tissue, extensive burns, heatstroke, rejection of transplant, and hepatic necrosis
Cardiovascular:	Fat embolism, acute venous thrombosis, cardiopulmonary bypass surgery, hypovolemic shock, cardiac arrest, and hypotension
Other:	Snakebite, cirrhosis, transfusion of incompatible blood, purpura, and glomerulonephritis

ceptions of place, time, or identity. Disorientation may occur in organic mental disorders, in drug and alcohol intoxication, and, less commonly, following severe stress.

dispersing agent A chemical additive used in pharmaceuticals to cause the even distribution of the ingredients throughout the product, as in dermatologic emulsions containing both oil and water. Dispersing agents commonly used in skin creams, lotions, and ointments include glyceryl monostearate, sodium lauryl sulfate, and polyethylene glycol derivatives, as polysorbate 80 and polyoxyl 40 stearate. Any of these agents may cause an allergic reaction or adverse effect.

displaced fracture A traumatic bone break in which two ends of a fractured bone are separated from each other. The ends of broken bones in displaced fractures often pierce surrounding skin, as in an open fracture, or may be contained within the skin, as in a closed fracture.

displacement **1.** The state of being displaced or the act of displacing. **2.** In chemistry: a reaction in which an atom, molecule, or radical is removed from combination and replaced by another. **3.** In physics: the displacing in space of one mass by another, as the weight or volume of a fluid is displaced by a floating or submerged body. **4.** In psychiatry: an unconscious defense mechanism for avoiding emotional conflict and anxiety by transferring emotions, ideas, or wishes from one object to a substitute that is less anxiety-producing. Compare **sublimation.**

dissect To cut apart tissues for visual or microscopic study using a scalpel, probe, or scissors. Compare **bisect. —dissection,** *n.*

dissecting aneurysm A localized dilatation of an artery, most commonly the aorta, characterized by a longitudinal dissection between the outer and middle layers of the vascular wall. Aortic dissecting aneurysms occur most frequently in men between the ages of 40 and 60 and are, in more than 90% of cases, preceded

by hypertension. Blood entering a tear in the intimal lining of the vessel causes a separation of weakened elastic and fibromuscular elements in the medial layer and leads to the formation of cystic spaces filled with ground substance. Dissecting aneurysms in the thoracic aorta may extend into blood vessels of the neck. Rupture of a dissecting aneurysm may be fatal in less than an hour. Treatment consists of resection and replacement of the excised section of aorta with a synthetic prosthesis.

disseminated intravascular coagulation (DIC) A grave coagulopathy resulting from overstimulation of the body's clotting and anticlotting processes in response to disease or injury, as septicemia, acute hypotension, poisonous snake bites, neoplasms, obstetric emergencies, severe trauma, or extensive surgery and hemorrhage. The primary disorder initiates generalized intravascular clotting which, in turn, overstimulates fibrinolytic mechanisms. This initial hypercoagulability is succeeded by a deficiency in clotting factors with hypocoagulability and hemorrhaging. Widespread purpura on the chest and abdomen, reflecting fibrin deposits in capillaries, is a common first sign of DIC and is often followed by the appearance of hemorrhagic bullae, acral cyanosis, and focal gangrene in the skin and mucous membranes. There may be hemorrhages from incisions or catheter or injection sites, gastrointestinal bleeding, hematuria, pulmonary edema, pulmonary embolism, progressive hypotension, tachycardia, an absence of peripheral pulses, restlessness, convulsions, or coma. Treatment of the primary disorder is essential. Heparin may be infused intravenously to prevent clot formation, but, since it may increase bleeding, it is not always used for surgical patients with DIC. Transfusions of whole blood, plasma, platelets, and other blood products replace depleted coagulation factors.

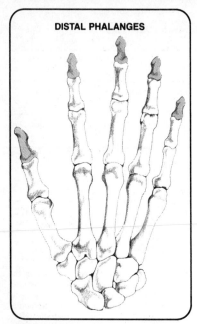

DISTAL PHALANGES

disseminated lupus erythematosus
See systemic lupus erythematosus.

disseminated multiple sclerosis See
multiple sclerosis.

dissent In law: a statement written by a judge
who disagrees with the decision of the majority
of the court. The dissent explicitly states the reasons for the dissenting judge's contrary opinion.
—**dissenting,** *adj.*

dissimilar twins See dizygotic twins.

dissociation **1.** The act of separating into
parts or sections. **2.** In psychoanalysis: an unconscious defense mechanism by which an idea,
thought, emotion, or other mental process is separated from the consciousness and thereby loses
emotional significance. See also **dissociative
disorder, dissociative reaction. —dissociative,** *adj.*

dissociative anesthesia An anesthetic
procedure characterized by analgesia and amnesia without loss of respiratory function or pharyngeal and laryngeal reflexes. This form of
anesthesia may be used to provide analgesia
during brief, superficial operative procedures or
diagnostic processes. It is especially useful for
people who are sensitive to general or local anesthetics or for those who, for other reasons, may
not be safely anesthetized with inhalant gases.
Because the most commonly used drug is the
hallucinogen ketamine hydrochloride, emergence may be accompanied by delirium, excitement, and confusion.

dissociative disorder A type of hysterical
neurosis in which emotional conflicts are so repressed that a separation or split in the personality occurs, resulting in an altered state of con-

sciousness or a confusion in identity. Symptoms
include amnesia, somnambulism, fugue, dream
state, or multiple personality. The disorder is
caused by an inability to cope with severe stress
or conflict and usually occurs suddenly, following a situation catastrophic to the person. Treatment may include hypnosis, especially when
amnesia is the primary symptom, psychotherapy, and antianxiety medication. Compare **conversion disorder.** See also **dissociation, dissociative reaction.**

dissociative reaction A neurotic response to stress or emotional conflict characterized by some degree of personality disorganization with loss of affect and appropriate
emotional response. In extreme cases it may lead
to any of the dissociative disorders, as amnesia,
fugue, or multiple personality. See also **dissociation, dissociative disorder.**

distal **1.** Away from or being the farthest from
a point of origin. **2.** Away from or being the
farthest from the midline or a central point, as
a distal phalanx, which is the bone at the end
of a finger or toe. Compare **proximal.**

distal muscular dystrophy A rare form
of muscular dystrophy, usually affecting adults,
characterized by moderate weakness and by
wasting that begins in the arms and legs and
then extends gradually to the proximal and facial muscles. Also called **Gowers' muscular
dystrophy.**

distal phalanx Any one of the small distal
bones in the third row of phalanges of the hand
or the foot. Each one at the end of the fingers
has a convex dorsal surface and a flat palmar
surface, with a rough elevation at the end of the
palmar surface that supports a fingernail and
its sensitive pulp. Each distal phalanx of the toes
is smaller and more flattened than that of a finger; it also has a rough elevation to support the
toenail and its pulp. Also called **ungual phalanx.**

distal radioulnar articulation The pivotlike articulation of the head of the ulna and
the ulnar notch on the lower end of the radius,
involving two ligaments. The joint allows rotation of the distal end of the radius around an
axis which passes through the center of the head
of the ulna. Also called **inferior radioulnar
joint.** Compare **proximal radioulnar articulation.**

distal renal tubular acidosis (distal RTA)
An abnormal condition characterized by excessive acid accumulation and bicarbonate excretion. It is caused by the inability of the distal
tubules of the kidney to secrete hydrogen ions,
thus decreasing the excretion of titratable acids
and ammonium and increasing the urinary loss
of potassium and bicarbonate. This condition
may result in hypercalciuria and the formation
of kidney stones. Treatment is as for renal tubular acidosis. **Primary distal RTA** occurs
mostly in females, adolescents, older children,
and young adults. It may occur sporadically or
as the result of hereditary defects. **Secondary
distal RTA** is associated with numerous dis-

orders, as cirrhosis of the liver, malnutrition, starvation, and various genetic problems. Compare **proximal renal tubular acidosis.**

distributive analysis and synthesis The system of psychotherapy used by the psychobiological school of psychiatry. It involves an extensive and systematic investigation and analysis of a person's total past experiences in order to discover the emotional factors underlying personality problems and how they can be synthesized into constructive behavioral patterns.

district 1. In hospital nursing: a group of patients in an area of the unit for whom a head nurse or primary nurse is responsible, usually a subdivision of a ward unit. Patients are customarily assigned to a district on the basis of certain shared needs for nursing care. 2. The area of a city or town assigned to a public health nurse.

disulfiram An adjunct used in management of chronic alcoholism.

disuse phenomena The physical and psychologic changes, usually degenerative, that result from the lack of use of a body part or system. Disuse phenomena are associated with confinement and immobility, especially in orthopedics. Some studies have shown that young, healthy individuals confined to bed rest for as little as 3 hours experience disturbances of time sense and memory. Other individuals in similar circumstances have experienced tactile, auditory, and visual hallucinations. Such disorientation is compounded by pain and therapeutic narcotic drugs commonly associated with the treatment of many illnesses and abnormal conditions. In hospitals, many patients become less efficient in remembering, problem solving, and learning. The physical changes often induced by continued bed rest constitute problems affecting the skin, the musculoskeletal system, the gastrointestinal tract, the cardiovascular system, and the respiratory system. The skin of the patient on prolonged bed rest is commonly subjected to abnormal conditions, as pressure exerted by the bed, moisture, friction, and inadequate nutrition. The neurologically impaired patient may feel no pain. This phenomenon, accompanying disuse, may be the first sign of ischemia followed by a rapid breakdown of the skin. Complications also associated with extended bed rest include disuse atrophy of the bones and muscles; contractures; constipation; bone demineralization; osteoporosis; the pooling of respiratory secretions; and cardiovascular problems. Some common therapeutic measures to deal with disuse phenomena are the improvement of diet and nutrition, proper positioning and regular movement of the bed-rest patient, meticulous hygiene, scrupulous skin care, and positive social interaction with the patient.

diuresis Increased formation and secretion of urine. Diuresis is pronounced in conditions such as diabetes mellitus and diabetes insipidus. It is normal in the first 48 hours postpartum. Coffee, tea, certain foods, and diuretic drugs cause diuresis.

diuretic 1. Of a drug or other substance: tending to promote the formation and excretion of urine. 2. A drug that promotes the formation and excretion of urine. The more than 50 diuretic drugs available for prescription in the United States and Canada are classified by chemical structure into several basic pharmacologic groups: thiazides, mercurials, loop diuretics, carbonic anhydrase inhibitors, thiazide-like diuretics, and potassium-sparing diuretics. A diuretic medication may contain drugs from one or more of these groups. Diuretics are prescribed to reduce the volume of extracellular fluid in the treatment of many disorders, including hypertension, congestive heart failure, and edema. The particular drug to be prescribed is selected according to the action desired and the physical status of the patient. Diabetes mellitus may be aggravated by thiazide medications; thus, the presence of a particular condition may prohibit the use of a particular agent. Several adverse reactions are common to all diuretics, including hypovolemia and electrolyte imbalance.

divalent See **bivalent.**

diversional activity, deficit A nursing diagnosis accepted by the Fifth National Conference on the Classification of Nursing Diagnoses. The etiology of the situation includes a lack of diversion in the environment, long-term hospitalization, or frequent or prolonged treatment. See also **nursing diagnosis.**

diverticulitis Inflammation of one or more diverticula. The penetration of fecal matter through the thin-walled diverticula causes inflammation and abcess formation in the tissues surrounding the colon. With repeated inflammation, the lumen of the colon narrows and may become obstructed. During periods of inflammation, the patient will experience crampy pain, particularly over the sigmoid colon, fever, and leukocytosis. Barium enema and proctoscopy are performed to rule out carcinoma of the colon, which exhibits some of the same symptoms. Conservative treatment includes bed rest, intravenous fluids, antibiotics, and nothing by mouth. In acute cases, bowel resection of the affected part greatly reduces mortality and morbidity. Compare **diverticulosis.**

diverticulosis The presence of pouchlike herniations through the muscular layer of the colon, particularly the sigmoid colon. Diverticulosis affects increasing numbers of people over age 50 and may be the result of the modern, highly refined, low-residue diet. Most patients with this condition have few symptoms except for occasional bleeding from the rectum. The doctor must exercise care in ruling out other reasons for bleeding, as carcinoma and inflammatory bowel disease. Barium enema and proctoscopic examination are used in establishing diagnosis. An increase in the dietary fiber can aid in propelling the feces through the colon. Hemorrhage from bleeding diverticula can become quite severe, and the patient may require surgery. Diverticulosis may lead to diverticulitis. See also **diverticulitis.**

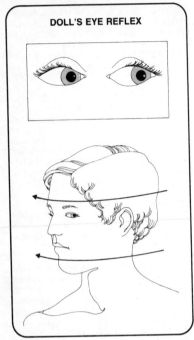

DOLL'S EYE REFLEX

diverticulum, *pl.* **diverticula** A pouchlike herniation through the muscular wall of a tubular organ. A diverticulum may be present in the stomach, small intestine, or, most commonly, in the colon. See also **diverticulitis, diverticulosis, Meckel's diverticulum.** —**diverticular,** *adj.*

diving goiter A large, movable thyroid gland located at times above the sternal notch and at other times below the notch. Also called **plunging goiter, wandering goiter.**

division **1.** An administrative subunit in a hospital, as a division of medical nursing or a division of surgical nursing. **2.** In public health nursing: an area that encompasses several geographical districts.

dizygotic Of or pertaining to twins from two fertilized ova. Compare **monozygotic.** See also **twinning.**

dizygotic twins Two offspring born of the same pregnancy and developed from two ova that were released from the ovary simultaneously and fertilized at the same time. They may be of the same or opposite sex, differ both physically and in genetic constitution, and have two separate and distinct placentas and membranes, both amnion and chorion. Also called **binovular twins, dissimilar twins, false twins, fraternal twins, heterologous twins.** Compare **monozygotic twins.**

dizziness A sensation of faintness or an inability to maintain normal balance in a standing or seated position, sometimes associated with giddiness, mental confusion, nausea, and weak-

ness. A patient who experiences dizziness should be carefully lowered to a safe position on a bed, chair, or floor because of the danger of injury from falling. Compare **syncope, vertigo.**

DLE *abbr* **discoid lupus erythematosus.**

DM *abbr* **diabetes mellitus.**

DMD *abbr* Doctor of Dental Medicine.

DNA *abbr* **deoxyribonucleic acid.**

DNA chimera In molecular genetics: a recombinant molecule of DNA composed of segments from more than one source.

DNA ligase An enzyme that can repair breaks in a strand of DNA by synthesizing a bond between adjoining nucleotides. Under some circumstances the enzyme can join together loose ends of DNA strands, and, in some cases, it can repair breaks in RNA.

DNA nucleotidyltransferase See **DNA polymerase.**

DNA polymerase In molecular genetics: an enzyme that catalyzes the assembly of deoxyribonucleoside triphosphates into DNA, with single-stranded DNA serving as the template.

DNR *abbr* do not resuscitate. See **no code.**

DNSc *abbr* **Doctor of Nursing Science.**

DO *abbr* **Doctor of Osteopathy.**

DOA *abbr* dead on arrival.

Dobie's globule A very small stainable body in the transparent disk of a muscle fiber.

dobutamine hydrochloride A sympathomimetic used to treat refractory heart failure.

doctoral program in nursing An educational program of study that offers preparation for a doctoral degree in the field of nursing, designed to prepare nurses for advanced practice and research. Upon successful completion of the course of study, the degree PhD in nursing or DSN (Doctor of Science in Nursing) is awarded.

Doctor of Medicine (MD) See **physician.**

Doctor of Osteopathy (DO) See **physician.**

docusate calcium, d. potassium, d. sodium Emollient laxatives and stool softeners. Formerly called dioctyl calcium (d. potassium, d. sodium) sulfosuccinate.

Doehle bodies Inclusions in the cytoplasm of some leukocytes in May-Hegglin anomaly.

Döhle-Heller disease See **syphilitic aortitis.**

dolicho- A combining form meaning 'long': *dolichocephaly, dolichocolon, dolichomorphic.*

dolichocephaly See **scaphocephaly.**

doll's eye reflex A normal response in newborns to keep the eyes stationary as the head is moved to the right or left. The reflex disappears as ocular fixation develops but may reappear in an adult with severely decreased levels of consciousness.

DOM *abbr* **dimethoxymethylamphetamine.**

dome fracture Any fracture of the acetabulum involving a weight-bearing surface.

dominance In genetics: a basic principle stating that not all genes determining a given trait operate with equal vigor. If two genes at a given locus produce a different effect, as eye color, they compete for expression. The gene that is manifest is dominant; it masks the effect of the other gene, which is recessive. Compare **codominant.** See also **independent assortment.** —**dominant,** *adj.*

dominant gene One that produces a phenotypic effect regardless of whether its allele is the same or different. Compare **recessive gene.**

Donath-Landsteiner syndrome A rare blood disorder, marked by hemolysis minutes or hours after exposure to cold. Systemic symptoms include the passage of dark urine, severe pain in the back and legs, headache, vomiting, diarrhea, and moderate reticulocytosis. There may be temporary hepatosplenomegaly and mild hyperbilirubinemia following the onset of an attack. The condition may occur with congenital or acquired syphilis, in which case antisyphilitic treatment may be curative. Also called **paroxysmal cold hemoglobinuria.**

donor **1.** A human or other organism that gives living tissue to be used in another body, for example, blood for transfusion or a kidney for transplantation. **2.** A substance or compound that gives part of itself to another substance. Compare **acceptor.** See also **universal donor.**

Donovan bodies Encapsulated gram-negative rods of the species *Calymmato bacterium granulomatis,* present in the cytoplasm of mononuclear phagocytes obtained from the lesions of granuloma inguinale. They may be seen under the microscope in a Wright-stained smear of infected tissue. See also **granuloma inguinale.**

dopamine hydrochloride A sympathomimetic used to treat shock.

dopaminergic Having the effect of dopamine.

dope *Slang.* Morphine, heroin, or another narcotic, or marijuana or other substance illicitly bought, or sold, and often self-administered for sedative, hypnotic, euphoric, or other mood-altering purpose.

Doppler effect The apparent change in frequency of sound or light waves emitted by a source as it moves away from or toward an observer. The frequency increases as the source moves toward the observer and decreases as it moves away, as the rising pitch of the whistle of an approaching train and the falling pitch of a departing train. The Doppler effect is also observed in electromagnetic radiations, as light and radio waves. See also **electromagnetic radiation, ultrasonography, wavelength.**

dorsal Pertaining to the back or posterior. Compare **ventral.** See also **dorsiflect.** —**dorsum,** *n.*

-dorsal A combining form meaning 'the back of something' or 'the back': *predorsal, thoracodorsal, ventrodorsal.*

dorsal carpal ligament See **retinaculum extensorum manus.**

dorsal digital vein One of the communicating veins along the sides of the fingers. The veins from the adjacent sides of the fingers unite to form three dorsal metacarpal veins which end in a dorsal venous network on the back of the hand. Compare **basilic vein, cephalic vein, median antebrachial vein.**

dorsal interventricular artery The arterial branch of the right coronary artery, branching to supply both ventricles. It runs down the dorsal sulcus two thirds of the way to the apex of the heart. Also called **right interventricular artery.**

dorsalis pedis artery The continuation of the anterior tibial artery, starting at the ankle joint, dividing into five branches, and supplying various muscles of the foot and toes. Its branches are the lateral tarsal, medial tarsal, arcuate, first dorsal metatarsal, and deep plantar.

dorsalis pedis pulse The pulse of the dorsalis pedis artery, palpable between the first and second metatarsal bones on the top of the foot, and used to assess peripheral circulation. It can be felt in approximately 90% of people.

dorsal lip The marginal fold of the blastopore during gastrulation in the early stages of embryonic development of many animals. It marks the dorsal limit of the developing embryo, constitutes the primary organizer, gives rise to neural tissue, and corresponds to the primitive node in humans and higher animals.

dorsal scapular nerve One of a pair of supraclavicular branches from the roots of the brachial plexus. It arises from the fifth cervical nerve near the intervertebral foramen, pierces the scalenus medius, and runs dorsally and caudally to the vertebral border of the scapula. It supplies the rhomboideus major and the rhomboideus minor and sends a branch to the levator.

dorsi- See **dorso-.**

dorsiflexion Bending or flexing, as in the upward bending of the hand on the wrist or the foot on the ankle.

dorsiflexor A muscle causing backward flexion of a part of the body, as the hand or foot.

dorsiflexor gait An abnormal gait caused by the weakness of the dorsiflexors of the ankle. It is characterized by footdrop during the entire gait cycle and excessive knee and hip flexion to allow clearance of the involved extremity during the swing phase. The sole of the affected foot also slaps forcibly against the ground at the moment of heelstrike due to the inability of the dorsiflexor to decelerate the body weight as the heel strikes the ground. Compare **Trendelenburg gait.**

dorso-, dorsi- A combining form meaning 'pertaining to a dorsum or to the back': *dorsocephalad, dorsointercostal, dorsomesial, dorsoscapular.*

dorsosacral position See **lithotomy position.**

dosage The regimen governing the size, frequency, and number of doses of a therapeutic agent to be administered to a patient.

dosage compensation In genetics: the mechanism that counterbalances the number of X-linked gene doses in the sex chromosomes so that they are equal in both the male, which has one X chromosome, and the female, which has two. In mammals, this is accomplished by genetic activation of only one of the X chromosomes

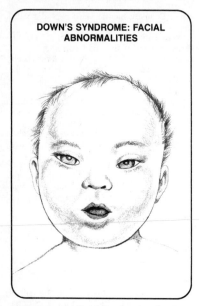

DOWN'S SYNDROME: FACIAL ABNORMALITIES

in the somatic cells of females. See also **Lyon hypothesis.**

dose   The amount of a drug or other substance to be administered at one time.

dose fractionation   See **fractionation,** definition 5.

dose rate   In radiotherapy: the amount of delivered radiation absorbed per unit of time.

dose ratemeter   In radiotherapy: an instrument for measuring the dose rate of radiation.

dose threshold   In radiotherapy: the minimum amount of absorbed radiation that produces a detectable degree of a given effect.

dose to skin   In radiotherapy: the amount of absorbed radiation at the center of the irradiation field on the skin. It is the sum of the dose in the air and the scatter from body parts.

dosimeter   An instrument to detect and measure accumulated radiation exposure. A pencil-sized ionization chamber with a self-reading electrometer monitors exposure.

double-approach conflict   See **approach-approach conflict.**

double-avoidant conflict   See **avoidance-avoidance conflict.**

double-blind study   An experiment designed to test the effect of a treatment or substance using groups of experimental and control subjects in which neither the subjects nor the investigators know which treatment or substance is being administered to which group. In a double-blind test of a new drug, the substance may be identified to the investigators only by a code. The purpose of a double-blind study is to eliminate the risk of prejudgment by the participants, which could distort the results. A double-blind study may be augmented by a **cross-over**

experiment in which experimental subjects unknowingly become control subjects, and vice versa, at some point in the study. See also **control, placebo.**

double-blind technique   An experimental method of studying a drug or other medical treatment in which neither the investigators nor the subjects know which subjects are receiving the experimental drug or procedure and which are serving as controls. Typically, the control group receives a placebo, which is indistinguishable from the substance or procedure being tested. The double-blind technique is designed to eliminate bias in the interpretation of results.

double fracture   A fracture comprising breaks or cracks in two places in a bone, resulting in more than two bone segments.

double gel diffusion   See **immunodiffusion.**

double innervation   Innervation of effector organs by fibers of the sympathetic and parasympathetic divisions of the autonomic nervous system. The pelvic viscera, bronchioles, heart, eyes, and digestive system are all doubly innervated. The fibers of the two divisions operate at cross purposes to achieve a state of balance and to maintain the homeostatic condition of the body. The mode of action of each division varies: in some structures one division is stimulating and the other inhibiting; in others, separate fibers from each division act to stimulate and inhibit complementary function.

double monster   A fetus that has developed from a single ovum but has two heads, trunks, and multiple limbs. Also called **twin monster.**

double quartan fever   A form of malaria in which paroxysms of fever occur in a repeating pattern of 2 consecutive days followed by 1 day of remission. The pattern is usually the result of concurrent infections by two species of the genus *Plasmodium,* one causing paroxysms every 72 hours and the other every 48 hours. Compare **biduotertian fever.**

double setup   A nursing procedure in which an obstetric operating room is prepared for both vaginal delivery and cesarean section. The circulating and scrub nurses lay out the equipment required for both procedures, possibly including a vacuum aspirator, forceps, and cesarean section packs. The scrub nurse remains scrubbed until the infant is delivered but does not participate unless a cesarean section is performed.

double vision   See **diplopia.**

douche   1. A procedure in which 1 liter (1 qt) or more of a solution of a medication or cleansing agent in warm water is introduced into the vagina under low pressure. The woman often performs the procedure herself. Douching may be recommended in the treatment of various pelvic and vaginal infections. 2. To perform a douche.

Down's syndrome   A congenital condition characterized by varying degrees of mental retardation and multiple defects. It is the most common chromosomal abnormality of a generalized syndrome and is caused by the presence of an extra chromosome 21 in the G group or, in a small percentage of cases, by the translocation of chromosomes 14 or 15 in the D group and chromosomes 21 or 22. Down's syndrome occurs in approximately 1 in 600 to 650 live births and is associated with advanced maternal age, particularly ages over 35 years. The incidence is as high as 1 in 80 for offspring of women older than 40 years. In those cases caused by translocation, which is a genetic aberration that is hereditary rather than a chromosomal aberration caused by nondisjunction during cell division, the incidence is not associated with maternal age, and the risk is low: about 1 in 5 if the mother is the carrier and 1 in 20 if the father is the carrier. The condition, which can be diagnosed prenatally by amniocentesis, also occurs as a mosaic variant, in which there is a mixture of trisomy 21 and normal cells. Such patients have fewer physical defects and less severe retardation, depending on the degree of mosaicism. Infants with the syndrome are small, hypotonic, with characteristic microcephaly, brachycephaly, a flattened occiput, and typical facies with a mongoloid slant to the eyes, depressed nasal bridge, low-set ears, and a large, protruding tongue that is furrowed and lacks the central fissure. The hands are short and broad with a transverse palmar or simian crease; the fingers are stubby and show clinodactyly, primarily of the fifth fingers; and the feet are broad and stubby with a wide space between the first and second toes and a prominent plantar crease. Other anomalies associated with the disorder are bowel defects, congenital heart disease, primarily septal defects, chronic respiratory infections, visual problems, abnormalities in tooth development, and susceptibility to acute leukemia. The most significant feature of the syndrome is mental retardation, which varies considerably, although the average IQ is in the range of 50 to 60 so that the child is generally trainable and, in most instances, can be reared at home. The mortality is high within the first few years, especially in those children with cardiac anomalies. Those children who survive tend to be shorter than average, stocky in build, show delayed or incomplete sexual development, and can live to middle or old age, although adults with Down's syndrome are prone to respiratory infections, pneumonia, and lung disease. Also called **mongolism, trisomy 21, trisomy G syndrome.**

doxapram hydrochloride A respiratory stimulant.

doxepin hydrochloride A tricyclic antidepressant.

doxorubicin hydrochloride An antibiotic used in chemotherapy.

doxycycline A tetracycline antibiotic.

doxylamine succinate An ethanolamine antihistamine.

DPT vaccine *abbr* **diphtheria and tetanus toxoids and pertussis vaccine.**

DQ *abbr* **developmental quotient.**

dracontiasis See **dracunculiasis.**

dracunculiasis A parasitic infection caused by infestation by the nematode *Dracunculus medinensis.* It is characterized by ulcerative skin lesions on the legs and feet that are produced by gravid female worms. People are infected by drinking contaminated water or eating contaminated shellfish. It is common in densely populated tropical and subtropical areas of the world. Also called **dracontiasis, guinea worm infection.**

Dracunculus medinensis A parasitic nematode that causes dracunculiasis. Also called **fiery serpent.**

drainage The removal of fluids from a body cavity, wound, or other source of discharge by one or more methods. Closed drainage is a system of tubing and other apparatus attached to the body to remove fluid in an airtight circuit that prevents environmental contaminants from entering the wound or cavity. Open drainage is drainage in which discharge is drained through an open-ended tube into a receptacle. Postural drainage is drainage in which gravity aids in the removal of fluid from the body by the positioning of the patient so discharge flows out, as through the trachea if the fluid source is in the lungs. Suction drainage is drainage in which a pump or other mechanical device is used to assist in extracting a fluid. Tidal drainage is drainage in which a body area is washed out by alternately flooding and then emptying it with the aid of gravity, a technique that may be used in treating a urinary bladder disorder.

drainage tube A heavy-gauge catheter used for the evacuation of air or a fluid from a cavity or wound in the body. The tube may be attached to a suction device or simply allow flow by gravity into a receptacle.

dram A unit of mass equivalent to an apothecaries' measure of 60 gr or ⅛ oz and to 1/16 oz or 27.34 gr avoirdupois.

dramatic play An imitative activity in which a child fantasizes and acts out various domestic and social roles and situations.

drape A sheet of fabric or paper, usually the size of a small bed sheet, for covering all or a part of a person's body during a physical examination or treatment. —**drape,** *v.*

drawing *Informal.* A vague sensation of muscle tension.

dream 1. A symbolically coherent sequence of ideas, thoughts, emotions, or images that pass through the mind during the rapid-eye-movement stage of sleep. 2. Describing the sleeping state in which this process occurs. 3. A visionary creation of the imagination experienced during wakefulness. 4. In psychoanalysis: the expression of thoughts, emotions, memories, or impulses repressed from the consciousness. 5. In analytic psychology: the wishes, emotions, and impulses that reflect the personal unconscious and the archetypes that originate in the collective unconscious. See also **dream analysis, dream state.**

dream analysis A process of gaining access to the unconscious mind by means of examining the content of dreams, usually through the method of free association.

dream association A relationship of thoughts or emotions discovered or experienced as a dream is remembered or analyzed. See also **dream analysis.**

dream state A condition of altered consciousness in which people do not recognize their environment and react in a manner opposed to their usual behavior, as by flight or an act of their violence. The state is seen in epilepsy and certain neuroses. See also **automatism, fugue.**

drepanocytic anemia See **sickle cell anemia.**

dress code The standards set by an institution for the dress of the members of the institution.

dressing A clean or sterile covering applied directly to wounded or diseased tissue for absorption of secretions, protection from trauma, administration of medications, or to stop bleeding. Kinds of dressings include **absorbent dressing, antiseptic dressing, occlusive dressing, pressure dressing, wet dressing.**

dressing forceps A kind of forceps that has a narrow blade and blunt or notched teeth, designed for dressing wounds, removing drainage tubes, or extracting fragments of necrotic tissue.

Dressler's syndrome An autoimmune disorder that may occur several days after acute coronary infarction, characterized by fever, pericarditis, pleurisy, pleural effusions, and joint pain. It results from the body's immunologic response to a damaged myocardium and pericardium. Treatment usually includes intensive aspirin therapy and, in severe cases, corticosteroids. A similar syndrome may occur following cardiac surgery.

DRG *abbr* **diagnostic related group.**

drift 1. Antigenic drift: a change that occurs in a strain of virus so that variations appear periodically with alterations in antigenic qualities. 2. Genetic drift: random variations in gene frequency of a population from one generation to the next. 3. In dentistry: the movement of a tooth from one position in the jaw to another after the loss of a neighboring tooth.

Drinker respirator An airtight respirator consisting of a metal tank that encloses the entire body, except for the head. Used for long-term therapy, it alternates positive and negative air pressure within the tank, providing artificial respiration by contracting and expanding the walls of the chest. Also called **artificial lung, iron lung.**

drip 1. The process of a liquid or moisture forming and falling in drops. Kinds of drip are **nasal drip, postnasal drip. 2.** The slow but continuous infusion of a liquid into the body, as into the stomach or a vein. **3.** To infuse a liquid continuously into the body.

drip system In intravenous therapy: an apparatus for delivering specific volumes of intravenous solutions within predetermined periods and at a specific flow rate. See also **macrodrip, microdrip.**

-drome A combining form meaning 'that which runs' in a specified way: *dermadrome, heterodrome, syndrome.*

dromo- A combining form meaning 'pertaining to running or conduction': *dromonania, dromophobic, dromotropic.*

dromostanolone propionate An antineoplastic that alters hormone balance.

droperidol A phenothiazine used as a preoperative sedative.

drop foot A condition in which the foot is plantar flexed and cannot voluntarily be dorsiflexed. It is usually caused by damage to the peroneal nerve.

droplet infection An infection acquired by the inhalation of pathogenic microorganisms suspended in particles of liquid exhaled, sneezed, or coughed by another infected person or animal. Some diseases spread by droplets are chickenpox, common cold, influenza, and measles.

dropped foot See **footdrop.**

dropsy See **hydrops.**

Drosophila A genus of fly, including *Drosophila melanogaster,* the Mediterranean fruit fly, useful in genetics because of the large chromosomes found in its salivary glands and its sensitivity to environmental effects, as exposure to radiation.

drowning Asphyxiation owing to submersion in a liquid. See also **near-drowning.**

drug 1. Any substance taken by mouth, injected into a muscle, the skin, a blood vessel, or a cavity of the body, or applied topically to treat or prevent a disease or condition. Also called **medicine. 2.** *Informal.* A narcotic substance.

drug abuse The use of a drug for a nontherapeutic effect, especially one for which it was not prescribed or intended. Some of the most commonly abused substances are alcohol, amphetamines, barbiturates, and methaqualone. Drug abuse may lead to organ damage, addiction, and disturbed patterns of behavior. Some illicit drugs, as lysergic acid diethylamide and phencylidine hydrochloride, have no recognized therapeutic effect. Use of these drugs often incurs criminal penalty in addition to the potential for physical, social, and psychological harm. See also **drug addiction.**

drug action The means by which a drug exerts a desired effect. Drugs are usually classified by their actions; for example, a vasodilator, prescribed to decrease the blood pressure, acts by dilating the blood vessels.

drug addiction A condition characterized by an overwhelming desire to continue taking a drug to which one has become habituated through repeated consumption because it produces a particular effect, usually an alteration of mental activity, attitude, or outlook. Addiction is usually accompanied by a compulsion to obtain the drug, a tendency to increase the dose, a psychological or physical dependence, and detrimental consequences for the individual and society. Common addictive drugs are barbiturates, ethanol, and morphine and other narcotics, especially heroin, which has slightly greater euphorigenic properties than other opium derivatives. See also **alcoholism, drug abuse.**

drug allergy Hypersensitivity to a pharmacologic agent, manifested by reactions ranging from a mild rash to anaphylactic shock, depending on the individual, the allergen, and the dose. Allergic responses are frequently produced by contrast media containing iodine, aspirin, phenylbutazone, cephalosporins, penicillin, and other antibiotics, but they may be caused by any drug.

drug dependence A psychological craving for or a physiological reliance on a chemical agent, resulting from habituation, abuse, or addiction. See also **drug abuse, drug addiction.**

drug-drug interaction A modification of the effect of a drug when administered with another drug. The effect may be an increase or a decrease in the action of either substance, or it may be an adverse effect that is not normally associated with either drug. The particular interaction may be the result of a chemical-physical incompatibility of the two drugs or a change in the rate of absorption or the quantity absorbed in the body, the binding ability of either drug, or an alteration in the ability of receptor sites and cell membranes to bind either drug.

Drug Enforcement Administration (DEA) An agency of the federal government, empowered to enforce regulations regarding the import or export of narcotic drugs and certain other substances or the traffic of these substances across state lines.

drug eruption Any skin lesion or rash caused by a drug taken internally. Also called **dermatitis medicamentosa.** See also **fixed drug eruption.**

drug fever A fever caused by the pharmacologic action of a medication, its thermoregulatory action, a local complication of parenteral administration, or, most commonly, an immunologic reaction mediated by drug-induced antibodies. The onset of fever is usually between 7 and 10 days after the medication is begun; a return to normal is seen within 2 days of the discontinuance of the drug. See also **Jarisch-Herxheimer reaction.**

drug monograph A statement that specifies the kinds and amounts of ingredients a drug or class of drugs may contain, the direction for the drug's use, the conditions in which it may be used, and contraindications.

dry catarrh A dry cough, accompanied by almost no expectoration, that occurs in severe coughing spells. It is associated with asthma and emphysema in older people.

dry dressing A plain dressing containing no medication, applied directly to an incision or a wound to prevent contamination or trauma or to absorb secretions.

dry gangrene See **gangrene.**

dry rale An abnormal chest sound produced by air passing through a constricted bronchial tube. Compare **amphoric breath sound,** atelectatic rale, bubbling rale.

Drysdale's corpuscle One of a number of transparent cells in the fluid of some ovarian cysts. Also called **Bennet's small corpuscle.**

dry skin Epidermis lacking moisture or sebum, often characterized by a pattern of fine lines, scaling, and itching. Causes include too frequent bathing, low humidity, decreased production of sebum in aging skin, and ichthyosis. Treatment includes decreased frequency of bathing, increased humidity, bath oils, such emollients as lanolin and glycerin, and hydrophilic ointments. Also called **xerosis.**

dry tooth socket An inflamed condition of a tooth socket (alveolus) after extraction. Normally, a blood clot forms over the alveolar bone at the base of the tooth socket after an extraction. If the clot fails to form properly or becomes dislodged, the bone tissue is exposed to the environment and can become infected, a usually painful condition requiring analgesics and sedatives in addition to treatment to cure the infection. Also called alveolitis sicca dolorosa.

DSM *abbr Diagnostic and Statistical Manual of Mental Disorders.*

DSN *abbr* Doctor of Science in Nursing.

DSR *abbr* **dynamic spatial reconstructor.**

DT See **diphtheria and tetanus toxoids.**

DTR *abbr* **deep tendon reflex.**

DTs *abbr* **delirium tremens.**

DUB 1. See **dysfunctional uterine bleeding.** 2. A genetically determined human blood factor that is associated with immunity to certain diseases, as sickle cell anemia. The blood factors usually are numbered, as DUB-15 or DUB-40, depending on their reactions with an antiserum. 3. A strain of mice used in medical experiments.

Dubin-Johnson syndrome A rare, chronic, hereditary hyperbilirubinemia, characterized by nonhemolytic jaundice, abnormal liver pigmentation, and abnormal function of the gallbladder. It is caused by an inability of the liver to excrete several organic anions.

Duchenne-Erb paralysis See **Erb's palsy.**

Duchenne's disease An eponym, after the French neurologist, for three different neurological conditions: spinal muscular atrophy, bulbar paralysis, and tabes dorsalis. The eponym is also strongly associated with the most common form of muscular dystrophy, pseudohypertrophic muscular dystrophy. See also **muscular dystrophy.**

Duchenne's muscular dystrophy An abnormal congenital condition characterized by progressive symmetric wasting of the leg and pelvic muscles. This disease affects only males and accounts for 50% of all muscular dystrophy diseases. It is an X-linked recessive disease that starts insidiously between the ages of 3 and 5 and spreads from the leg and pelvic muscles to the involuntary muscles. Associated muscle weakness produces a waddling gait and pronounced lordosis. Muscles rapidly deteriorate and calf muscles become firm and enlarged. Affected children develop contractures, have dif-

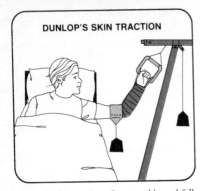

DUNLOP'S SKIN TRACTION

ficulty climbing stairs, often stumble and fall, and display wing scapulae when they raise their arms. Such patients are usually confined to wheelchairs by the age of 12, and progressive weakening of cardiac muscle causes tachycardia and pulmonary problems. There is no correlation between the degree of muscular dystrophy and the severity of cardiac problems, but the electrocardiogram is abnormal in 40% to 90% of the affected patients. The characteristic clinical finding is tachycardia persisting during sleep and often associated with arrhythmia and cardiac enlargement. The patients affected may also have cardiac murmurs, faint heart sounds, and chest pain and suffer arrhythmias or infections that produce overt heart failure. Such complications, especially in the later stages of this disease, can cause sudden death. Duchenne's muscular dystrophy usually results in death within 10 to 15 years of the onset of symptoms. Abnormal cardiac signs may precede recognition of Duchenne's muscular dystrophy and may aid diagnosis based on other abnormalities of gait and voluntary movement. There is no successful treatment of the disease. Orthopedic appliances, exercise, physical therapy, and surgery to correct contractures can help preserve mobility. Splints, braces, grab bars, and overhead slings help the patient to exercise. A wheelchair helps to preserve mobility. Other devices that can increase comfort and help prevent footdrop include footboards, high-topped sneakers, and foot cradles. Nurses encourage the patient to maintain peer relationships and often encourage the parents to keep the child in school as long as possible. Also called pseudohypertrophic muscular dystrophy.

duck embryo vaccine (DEV)   See **rabies vaccine.**

duct   A narrow tubular structure, especially one through which material is secreted or excreted.

duct carcinoma   A neoplasm developed from the epithelium of ducts, especially in the breast or pancreas.

ductless gland   A gland lacking an excretory duct, as an endocrine gland, which secretes hormones into blood or lymph.

duct of Rivinus   One of the minor sublin-

gual ducts. Compare **Bartholin's duct.**

duct of Wirsung   See **pancreatic duct.**

ductus, *pl.* **ductus**   A duct.

ductus arteriosus   A vascular channel in the fetus that joins the pulmonary artery directly to the descending aorta.

ductus deferens   See **deferent duct.**

ductus epididymidis   A tube into which the efferent ductules of the testes empty.

ductus venosus   The vascular channel in the fetus passing through the liver and joining the umbilical vein with the inferior vena cava. Before birth, it carries highly oxygenated blood from the placenta to the fetal circulation. It closes shortly after birth as pulmonary circulation is established and as the vessels in the umbilical cord collapse and become occluded. See also **ductus arteriosus, foramen ovale.**

Duke diet   See **rice diet.**

dumdum fever   See **kala-azar.**

dumping syndrome   The combination of profuse sweating, nausea, dizziness, and weakness experienced by patients who have had a subtotal gastrectomy. Symptoms are felt soon after eating, when the contents of the stomach empty too rapidly into the duodenum. Maintaining a high-protein, high-calorie diet, with small meals taken frequently, should prevent discomfort and ensure adequate nutrition. See also **gastrectomy.**

Dunlop's skeletal traction   An orthopedic mechanism that helps immobilize the upper limb in the treatment of the contracture or the supracondylar fracture of the elbow. The mechanism employs a system of traction weights, pulleys, and ropes. The system is attached to the bone involved with a pin or wire; it may be further secured by adhesive or nonadhesive skin traction components. Dunlop's skeletal traction is usually applied unilaterally but may also be applied bilaterally. Compare **Dunlop's skin traction.**

Dunlop's skin traction   An orthopedic mechanism that helps immobilize the upper limb in the treatment of contracture and supracondylar fracture of the elbow. The mechanism employs a system of traction weights, pulleys, and ropes, usually applied unilaterally but sometimes bilaterally. Dunlop's skin traction may be applied as adhesive skin traction or nonadhesive skin traction. Compare **Dunlop's skeletal traction.**

duodenal   Of or pertaining to the duodenum.

duodenal papilla   See under **papilla.**

duodenal ulcer   An ulcer in the duodenum, the most common type of peptic ulcer. See also **peptic ulcer.**

duodeno-   A combining form meaning 'pertaining to the duodenum': *duodenocolic, duodenohepatic, duodenostomy.*

duodenoscope   An endoscopic instrument, usually fiberoptic, for the visual examination of the duodenum.

duodenoscopy   The visual examination of the duodenum by means of an endoscope, usually a fiberoptic instrument.

duodenum, *pl.* **duodena, duodenums**

The shortest, widest, and most fixed portion of the small intestine, taking an almost circular course from the pyloric valve of the stomach so that its termination is close to its starting point. It is about 25 cm (10 inches) long and is divided into superior, descending, horizontal, and ascending portions. It plays a key role in digestion, because the common bile duct and pancreatic duct empty into it. Compare **ileum, jejunum.**

duplex inheritance See **amphigonous inheritance.**

duplex transmission The passage of a neural impulse in both directions along a nerve fiber.

Dupuytren's contracture A progressive, painless thickening and tightening of subcutaneous tissue of the palm, causing the fingers to bend into the palm and resist extension. The fourth and fifth fingers are most commonly affected. Tendons and nerves are not involved. Although the condition begins in one hand, both will become symmetrically affected. Of unknown cause, it is most frequent in middle-aged males. Early surgical removal of the excess fibrous tissue will restore full use of the hand. Under general anesthesia, an incision is made into the palm, and the thickened tissue is excised carefully to avoid injury to adjacent ligaments.

Dupuytren's fracture See **Galeazzi's fracture.**

dura mater The outermost and most fibrous of the three membranes surrounding the brain and spinal cord. The **dura mater encephali** covers the brain, and the **dura mater spinalis** covers the cord. See also **meninges.**

duress In law: an action compelling another person to do what otherwise would not be done voluntarily. A consent form signed under duress is not valid.

dust Any fine, particulate, dry matter. Kinds of dust are **inorganic dust, organic dust.**

dust fever See **brucellosis.**

Dutton's disease See **Dutton's relapsing fever.**

Dutton's relapsing fever An infection caused by a spirochete, *Borrelia duttoni*, which is transmitted by a soft tick, *Ornithodoros moubata*, found in human dwellings in tropical Africa. The spirochete enters the lesion through the tick bite, characteristically producing a high fever, chills, rapid heartbeat, headache, joint and muscle pain, vomiting, and neurological disorders. The symptoms recur in a pattern of remissions and peaks of fever and other effects. The infection is spread through the community as ticks bite infected people, thereby acquiring the spirochete for inoculation in others. Treatment with tetracycline is usually effective in curing the infection. Also called **Dutton's disease.** See also **relapsing fever.**

duty In law: an obligation owed by one party to another. Duty may be established by statute or other legal process, as by contract or oath supported by statute, or it may be voluntarily undertaken. Every person has a duty of care to

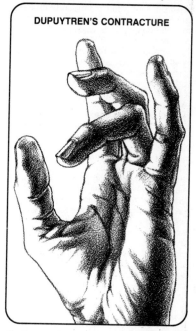

DUPUYTREN'S CONTRACTURE

all other people to avoid causing harm or injury by negligence.

Duverney's fracture Fracture of the ilium just below the anterior superior spine.

dwarf 1. An abnormally short, undersized person, especially one whose bodily parts are not proportional. Kinds of dwarfs include **achondroplastic dwarf, Amsterdam dwarf, asexual dwarf, ateliotic dwarf, bird-headed dwarf, Brissaud's dwarf, cretin dwarf, diastrophic dwarf, phocomelic dwarf, pituitary dwarf, primordial dwarf, rachitic dwarf, renal dwarf, Russell dwarf, sexual dwarf, Silver dwarf, thanatophoric dwarf.** Also called **nanus. 2.** To prevent or retard normal growth.

dwarfism The abnormal underdevelopment of the body, characterized predominantly by extreme shortness of stature, although the condition is associated with numerous other defects and may involve varying degrees of mental retardation. Dwarfism results from multiple causes, including genetic defects; endocrine dysfunction involving either the pituitary or thyroid glands; chronic diseases, as rickets; renal failure; intestinal malabsorption defects; and psychosocial stress, as in the maternal deprivation syndrome. See also **dwarf.**

Dwyer cable instrumentation One of the two most common surgical methods for correcting the spinal curvature associated with scoliosis. The Dwyer cable method uses a mechanical device that assists in obtaining the curvature correction through an anterior approach and is used in association with spinal fusion. The device is inserted to assist in maintaining the corrected curvature while the fusion heals and is not usually removed unless there is postoperative indication of displacement or a pattern of associated symptoms.

Dy Symbol for **dysprosium.**

dyad In genetics: one of the paired homologous chromosomes, which consist of two chromatids, that result from the division of a tetrad in the first meiotic division of gametogenesis. —**dyadic,** *adj.*

dyadic interpersonal communication A process in which two people interact face-to-face as senders and receivers, as in a conversation.

dyclonine hydrochloride An antipruritic and topical anesthetic.

dye 1. To apply coloring matter to a substance. 2. A chemical compound capable of imparting color to a substance to which it is applied. Various dyes are used in medicine as stains for tissues, test reagents, therapeutic agents, and to color pharmaceutical preparations.

-dymia A combining form meaning an 'abnormal condition of anomalous twins joined at part of their bodies': *cephalodymia, prosoposternodymia, sternodymia.*

-dynamia A combining form meaning '(condition of) strength': *ataxiadynamia, hyperdynamia, plastodynamia.* Also **-dynamy.**

dynamic Tending to change or to encourage change, as a dynamic nurse-patient relationship. Compare **static.**

dynamic nurse-patient relationship A conceptual framework in which the interpersonal aspects of the nurse-patient relationship are analyzed. Elements in the process include the behavior of the patient, the reaction of the nurse, and the actions of the nurse that are intended to aid the patient.

dynamic psychiatry The study of motivational, emotional, and biological factors as determinants of human behavior.

dynamic spatial reconstructor (DSR) A kind of roentgenographic machine used in research permitting moving three-dimensional images of human organs to be examined visually from any direction.

dynamo- A combining form meaning 'pertaining to power or strength': *dynamogenesis, dynamometer, dynamophore.*

dynamometer A device for measuring the amount of energy expended in the contraction of a muscle or a group of muscles, as a squeeze dynamometer, which measures the force of the hand when squeezing the device.

-dynamy See **-dynamia.**

dyphylline A respiratory tract spasmolytic agent.

dys- A combining form meaning 'bad, painful, disordered': *dysadrenia, dysbolism, dysmnesia.*

dysadrenia Abnormal adrenal function characterized by decreased production of hormones, as in hypoadrenalism or hypoadrenocorticism, or by increased secretion of the products of the gland, as in hyperadrenalism or hyperadrenocorticism. Also called dysadrenalism.

dysarthria Difficult, poorly articulated speech, resulting from interference in the control over the muscles of speech, usually because of damage to a central or peripheral motor nerve.

dyschondroplasia See **enchondromatosis.**

dyscrasic fracture Any fracture caused by the weakening of a specific bone owing to a debilitating disease.

dysentery An inflammation of the intestine, especially of the colon, that may be caused by chemical irritants, bacteria, protozoa, or parasites. It is characterized by frequent and bloody stools, abdominal pain, and tenesmus. See also **amebic dysentery, shigellosis.**

dysfunctional Of a body organ or system: unable to function normally. —**dysfunction,** *n.*

dysfunctional uterine bleeding (DUB) Uterine bleeding without a recognizable organic lesion, which is usually a result of endocrine imbalance rather than a pathological condition.

dysgenesis, dysgenesia 1. Defective or abnormal formation of an organ or part, primarily during embryonic development. 2. Impairment or loss of the ability to procreate. A kind of dysgenesis is **gonadal dysgenesis.** Compare **agenesis.** —**dysgenic,** *adj.*

dysgenics The study of those factors or situations which are genetically detrimental to the future of a race or species. Compare **eugenics.** —**dysgenic,** *adj.*

dysgenitalism Any condition involving the abnormal development of the genital organs.

dysgraphia An impairment of the ability to write, owing to a pathological disorder. —**dysgraphic,** *adj.*

dyshidrosis A condition in which abnormal sweating occurs. Some kinds of dyshidrosis are **hyperhidrosis, miliaria, pompholyx.** Compare **anhidrosis.** —**dyshidrotic,** *adj.*

dyskeratosis An abnormal or premature keratinization of epithelial cells.

dyskinesia An impairment of the ability to execute voluntary movements. —**dyskinetic,** *adj.*

dyslexia An impairment of the ability to read, owing to a variety of pathological conditions, some of which are associated with the central nervous system. People with this condition often reverse letters and words, cannot adequately distinguish the letter sequences in written words, and have difficulty determining left from right. Some reading experts doubt that dyslexia is a pathological disorder and believe the condition represents a combination of reading problems, such as poor vision, impaired hearing, emotional immaturity, lack of physical development, psychic stress, and inadequate reading instruction. —**dyslexic,** *adj.*

dysmaturity 1. The failure of an organism to develop, ripen, or otherwise achieve maturity in structure or function. 2. The condition of a fetus or newborn being abnormally small or large for its age of gestation. Kinds of dysmaturity are **small-for-gestational-age infant, large-for-**

gestational-age infant. Compare **postmature, premature. —dysmature,** *adj.*

dysmelia An abnormal congenital condition characterized by missing or shortened extremities of the body, associated with abnormalities of the spine in some individuals. It is caused by abnormal metabolism during the development of the embryonic limbs.

dysmenorrhea Pain associated with menstruation. Primary dysmenorrhea is menstrual pain that results from factors intrinsic to the uterus and the process of menstruation; it is extremely common, occurring at least occasionally in almost all women. If the painful episode is mild and brief, it is considered functional and normal and requires no treatment. In approximately 10% of women, dysmenorrhea may cause partial or total disability. The etiology in most cases is poorly understood. Pain occurs typically in the lower abdomen or back and is crampy, coming in successive waves—apparently in conjunction with intense uterine contractions and slight cervical dilatation. Pain usually begins just prior to or at the onset of menstrual flow and lasts a few hours to 1 day or more; but it may persist through the entire period in a few women. Pain is frequently associated with nausea, vomiting, and frequent bowel movements with intestinal cramping. Dizziness, fainting, and pallor may also be observed. Treatment may include antiprostaglandins, oral contraceptive steroids, and, in some cases, potent analgesics or narcotics. Secondary dysmenorrhea is menstrual pain that occurs secondary to specific pelvic abnormalities, as endometriosis, adenomyosis, chronic pelvic infection, chronic pelvic congestion, or degenerating fibroid tumors. Typically, the pain begins earlier in the cycle and lasts longer than the pain of primary dysmenorrhea. Painful bowel or bladder function may accompany the condition, depending on the location of the specific lesions. Diagnosis of the chief cause is made by pelvic examination, ultrasonography, laparoscopy, or laparotomy. Treatment, most often surgical, is directed at the specific organic disease involved.

dysmetria An abnormal condition that prevents the affected individual from properly measuring distances associated with muscular acts and from controlling muscular action. See also **hypermetria, hypometria.**

dysostosis An abnormal condition characterized by defective ossification, especially by defects in the normal ossification of fetal cartilages. Kinds of dysostoses include **cleidocranial dysostosis, craniofacial dysostosis, mandibulofacial dysostosis, metaphyseal dysostosis, Nager's acrofacial dysostosis.**

dyspareunia A condition in women in which sexual intercourse is accompanied by pain. The pain may result from abnormal conditions of the genitalia, dysfunctional psychophysiologic reaction to sexual union, forcible coition, or incomplete sexual arousal. See also **vaginismus.**

dyspepsia A vague feeling of gastric discomfort felt after eating. There is an uncom-

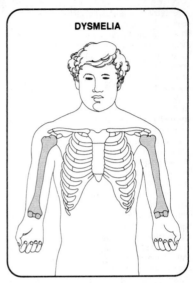

DYSMELIA

fortable feeling of fullness, heartburn, bloating, and nausea. Dyspepsia is not a distinct condition, but it may be a sign of underlying intestinal disorder, as peptic ulcer, gallbladder disease, or chronic appendicitis. —**dyspeptic,** *adj.*

dysphagia Difficulty in swallowing, commonly associated with obstructive or motor disorders of the esophagus. Patients with obstructive disorders, as esophageal tumor or lower esophageal ring, are unable to swallow solids but can tolerate liquids. Persons with motor disorders, as achalasia, are unable to swallow solids or liquids. Diagnosis of the underlying condition is made through barium studies, the observed clinical signs, and evaluation of the patient's symptoms. See also **achalasia, corkscrew esophagus.**

dysphagia lusoria An abnormal condition, characterized by difficulty in swallowing, caused by the compression of the esophagus from an anomalous right subclavian artery that arises from the descending aorta and courses behind the esophagus. Compare **contractile ring dysphagia, vallecular dysphagia.**

dysphasia An impairment of speech, not as severe as aphasia, usually the result of an injury to the speech area in the cerebral cortex of the brain. It may follow a stroke or brain tumor and may be accompanied by other language disorders, as dysgraphia. Compare **dysarthria.**

-dysplasia A combining form meaning '(condition of) abnormal development': *chondrodysplasia, epidermodysplasia, osteomyelodysplasia.*

dyspnea A shortness of breath or a difficulty in breathing that may be caused by certain heart conditions, strenuous exercise, or anxiety. —**dyspneal, dyspneic,** *adj.*

dyspraxia A partial loss of the ability to perform skilled, coordinated movements in the absence of any associated defect in motor or sensory functions. See also **apraxia.**

dysprosium (Dy) A rare-earth metallic element. Its atomic number is 66; its atomic weight is 162.50. Radioactive isotopes of dysprosium are used in radioisotope scanning, particularly in studies of the bones and joints.

dysraphia Failure of a raphe to fuse completely, as in incomplete closure of the neural tube. Also called **status dysraphicus.**

dysreflexia An abnormal neuromuscular condition characterized by abnormal motor response to stimuli that normally produce a specific response. **—dysreflexic,** *adj.*

dyssebacea A skin condition characterized by red, scaly, greasy patches on the nose, eyelids, scrotum, and labia. It results from a deficiency of vitamin B_2 and is most commonly associated with chronic alcoholism, liver disease, chronic diarrhea, and protein malnutrition. Also called shark skin *(informal).*

dystocia Abnormal labor, which occurs for one or more of the following reasons: the uterine expulsive powers are disordered; the birth passage is obstructed or contracted; or the size, shape, or position of the fetal passenger is abnormal. See also **contraction, presentation.**

dystonia musculorum deformans A rare abnormal condition characterized by intense, irregular torsion muscle spasms that contort the body. The muscles of the trunk, shoulder, and pelvis are commonly involved. This disease appears in several forms, generally classified as autosomal recessive or autosomal dominant. The cause of this disorder is not known; a biochemical dysfunction is suspected. The autosomal recessive form appears most often in Ashkenazic Jews and starts between the ages of 5 and 15, causing abnormalities of movement and speech. Muscle power and tone appear normal, but convulsive spasms make the involved muscles relatively useless. The autosomal recessive form of the disease commonly begins with intermittent spasmodic inversion of the foot, so that the affected individual has difficulty in placing the heel on the ground when walking and develops an odd, bowing gait. Lordosis and torsion of pelvis appear as the proximal muscles become more involved. Torticollis is often an early sign if the muscles of the neck and shoulder girdle are involved. The autosomal dominant form of the disease appears in early adult life, generally affects the axial musculature, and progresses more slowly than the autosomal recessive form. Some muscle-relaxing drugs, as the benzodiazepines, have been helpful in treating both forms of the condition. Mild cases have been successfully controlled for long periods with treatments that combine the use of muscle-relaxing drugs and psychotherapy. Some patients have also responded well for long periods to stereotactic thalamotomy, which, however, carries the risk of producing speech disorders.

dystrophy Any abnormal condition caused by defective nutrition. Also called dystrophia. **—dystrophic,** *adj.*

dysuria Painful urination, usually the result of a bacterial infection or obstructive condition in the urinary tract. The patient complains of a burning sensation when passing urine, and laboratory examination may reveal the presence of blood, bacteria, or white blood cells. Dysuria is a symptom of such conditions as cystitis, urethritis, prostatitis, urinary tract tumors, and some gynecological disorders. Compare **hematuria, pyuria.**

E

e- A combining form meaning 'out from': *ebonation, egesta, emollient.*

E Symbol for **expired gas.**

E and GW *abbr* **Economic and General Welfare.**

ear The organ of hearing, consisting of the internal, middle, and external ear.

earache A pain in the ear, sensed as sharp, dull, burning, intermittent, or constant. The cause is not necessarily a disease of the ear since infections and other disorders of the nose, oral cavity, larynx, and temperomandibular joint can produce referred pain in the ear. Also called **otalgia.**

eardrops A topical, liquid form of medication for the local treatment of various conditions of the ear, as inflammation or infection of the lining of the external auditory canal or impacted cerumen.

ear drum See **tympanic membrane.**

Early and Periodic Screening Diagnosis and Treatment (EPSDT) A section of the Medicaid program that requires all states to maintain a program to determine the physical and mental defects of the children under age 21 who are covered by the program and to provide short- and long-range treatment. See also **Medicaid.**

early infantile autism See **infantile autism.**

earwax See **cerumen.**

East African sleeping sickness See **Rhodesian trypanosomiasis.**

Eastern equine encephalitis (EEE) See **equine encephalitis.**

Eaton-agent pneumonia See **mycoplasma pneumonia.**

Ebbecke's reaction See **dermatographia.**

EBP *abbr* **epidural blood patch.**

EBV *abbr* **Epstein-Barr virus.**

ec- A combining form meaning 'out of ': *ecbolic, eccephalosis, ecchondroma.*

eccentric implantation In embryology: the embedding of the blastocyst within a fold or recess of the uterine wall, which then closes off from the main cavity.

ecchondroma A benign cartilaginous tumor that develops on the surface of a cartilage or under the periosteum of bone.

ecchondrosis See **ecchondroma.**

ecchymosis, *pl.* **ecchymoses** Discoloration of an area of the skin or mucous membrane owing to the extravasation of blood into the subcutaneous tissues. Ecchymosis can result from trauma to the underlying blood vessels or fragility of the vessel walls. Also called **bruise.**

Compare **contusion, petechiae.**

eccrine Of or pertaining to a sweat gland that secretes outwardly through a duct to the surface of the skin. Compare **exocrine.**

eccrine gland One of two kinds of sweat glands in the corium of the skin. Such glands promote cooling by evaporation of their secretion, which is clear, has a faint odor, and contains water, sodium chloride, and traces of albumin, urea, and other compounds. Compare **apocrine gland.**

eccyesis See **ectopic pregnancy.**

ECF *abbr* **extracellular fluid.**

ECG *abbr* **1.** electrocardiogram. **2.** electrocardiograph.

-echia A combining form meaning a 'condition of holding': *asynechia, blepharosynechia, synechia.*

echino- A combining form meaning 'pertaining to spines, or spiny': *echinochroma, echinosis, echinostomiasis.*

echinococcosis A tissue infection, usually of the liver, caused by tapeworm larvae of the genus *Echinococcus.* Dogs primarily host the adult worm; sheep, cattle, rodents, and deer host the larvae. Humans, especially children, can become infested with larvae by ingesting eggs shed in the stool of infected dogs or by handling pets that have tapeworm eggs in their hair. The disease is most common in countries where dogs are used to help tend domestic animals. Clinical manifestations and prognoses vary, depending on the tissue invaded and the extent of infestation. Diagnosis is made by skin tests for sensitivity, serologic tests, radiologic evidence of cyst formation, and identification of larval cysts in infected tissue. Surgical excision of the cysts is the only treatment available. The disease can be prevented by avoiding contact with infected dogs, deworming pets, and preventing dogs from eating carcasses of infected intermediate hosts. Also called **hydatid disease, hydatidosis.** See also **cysticerosis, hydatid cyst, tapeworm infection.**

Echinococcus A genus of small tapeworms that infects primarily canines. See also **echinococcosis.**

echinocyte See **burr cell.**

echo **1.** *Informal.* Echoradiography. **2.** In data processing: an automatic response on the display screen, showing the computer's interpretation of input data, which allows the operator to verify entry accuracy. When an entry is made, such as 'CBC' for ordering a laboratory test, the computer prints out, or 'echoes,' the information that the entry code represents in its memory.

echocardiography A diagnostic proce-

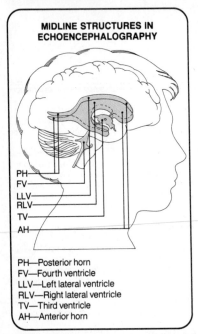

MIDLINE STRUCTURES IN ECHOENCEPHALOGRAPHY

PH—Posterior horn
FV—Fourth ventricle
LLV—Left lateral ventricle
RLV—Right lateral ventricle
TV—Third ventricle
AH—Anterior horn

dure for studying the structure and motion of the heart. Ultrasonic waves directed through the heart reflect backward, or echo, when they pass from one type of tissue to another, as from cardiac muscle to blood. The sound waves are transmitted from and received by a transducer and are recorded on a strip chart. Major diagnostic uses include the detection of atrial tumors and pericardial effusion, the measurement of the ventricular septa and the ventricular chambers, and the determination of mitral valve motion abnormalities and congenital lesions. Also called **ultrasonic cardiography.** See also **phonocardiograph, ultrasonography.**

echoencephalogram A recording produced by an echoencephalograph.

echoencephalography The use of ultrasound to study the intracranial structures of the brain. The technique is useful for showing ventricular dilatation and a major shift of midline structures as a result of an expanding lesion. See also **ultrasonography.** —**echoencephalographic,** *adj.*

echography See **ultrasonography.**

echolalia **1.** In psychiatry: the automatic and meaningless repetition of another's words or phrases, especially as seen in schizophrenia. Also called **echophrasia.** See also **delayed echolalia. 2.** In pediatrics: a child's imitation or repetition of sounds or words produced by others. It occurs normally in early childhood development. —**echolalic,** *adj.*

echophrasia See **echolalia.**

echoradiography A diagnostic procedure using ultrasonography and various devices for

the visualization of internal structures of the body.

echothiophate iodide A miotic agent used to treat glaucoma.

echovirus A picornavirus associated with many clinical syndromes but not identified as the causative organism of any specific disease. There are many echoviruses; most are harmless. Bacterial or viral disease may be complicated by echovirus infection, as seen in aseptic meningitis accompanying some severe bacterial and viral infections.

eclampsia The gravest form of toxemia of pregnancy, characterized by generalized tonic-clonic seizure, coma, hypertension, proteinuria, and edema. Symptoms of impending seizure often include anxiety, epigastric pain, headache, blurred vision, persistent and extremely high blood pressure, and increasingly hyperactive deep-tendon reflexes, or clonus. Seizures may be prevented by bed rest in a quiet, dimly lit room and parenteral administration of magnesium sulfate. The nurse closely monitors the mother's general condition, blood pressure, and urine excretion and the fetal heart rate. Treatment of a seizure must include airway maintenance, protection against self-injury, and administration of medication to check the seizure and decrease blood pressure. Once this is accomplished, delivery is indicated. Seizures rarely occur in the puerperium. Complications of eclampsia include cerebral hemorrhage, pulmonary edema, renal failure, necrosis of the liver, abruptio placentae, hypofibrinogenemia, hemolysis, and retinal hemorrhages, sometimes with temporary blindness. The cause is unknown.

-ecoia A combining form meaning '(condition of the) sense of hearing': *bradyecoia, dysecoia, oxyecoia.*

Economic and General Welfare (E and GW) A unit of the American Nurses' Association that works to upgrade the salaries, benefits, and working conditions of nurses.

ecstasy An emotional state characterized by exultation, rapturous delight, or frenzy. Compare **euphoria, mania.** —**ecstatic,** *adj.*

ECT *abbr* **electroconvulsive therapy.**

-ectasia A combining form meaning '(condition of) dilatation, expansion, or distention of an organ': *esophagectasia, lymphectasia, pharyngectasia.* Also **-ectasis, -ectasy.**

-ectasis See **-ectasia.**

-ectasy See **-ectasia.**

ecthyma A deep, burrowing form of impetigo characterized by large pustules, crusts, and ulcerations surrounded by erythema. Staphylococci and streptococci are the offending bacteria, and the skin of the legs is the most common site. Treatment includes rigorous attention to cleanliness, compresses of cool Burow's solution to soften and remove crusts, and penicillin or erythromycin given systemically. Compare **folliculitis, impetigo.**

ecto- A combining form meaning 'outside': *ectoblast, ectocolon, ectodermal.*

ectoderm The outermost of the three pri-

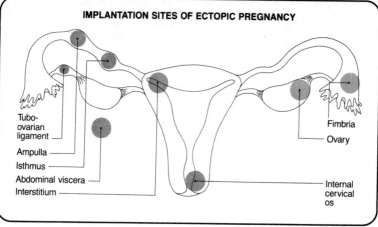

IMPLANTATION SITES OF ECTOPIC PREGNANCY

Tubo-ovarian ligament
Ampulla
Isthmus
Abdominal viscera
Interstitium

Fimbria
Ovary
Internal cervical os

mary cell layers of an embryo. The ectoderm gives rise to the nervous system; the organs of special sense, as the eyes; the epidermis; epidermal tissue, as fingernails and skin glands; and the mucous membranes of the mouth and anus. See also **embryonic layer, endoderm, mesoderm.** —**ectodermal, ectodermic,** *adj.*

ectodermal cloaca A part of the cloaca in the developing embryo that lies external to the cloacal membrane and eventually gives rise to the anus and anal canal. Compare **endodermal cloaca.**

ectomorph A person whose physique is characterized by slenderness, fragility, and a predominance of structures derived from the ectoderm. Compare **endomorph, mesomorph.** See also **asthenic habitus.**

-ectomy A combining form meaning the 'surgical removal of' something specified: *lobectomy, thrombectomy, thyroidectomy.*

ectoparasite In medical parasitology: an organism that lives on the outside of the body of the host, as a louse.

-ectopia A combining form meaning a 'condition in which a (specified) organ or part is out of its normal place': *corectopia, osteectopia, tarsectopia.*

ectopic 1. Of an object or organ: situated in an unusual place, away from its normal location, as an ectopic pregnancy. 2. Of an event: occurring at the wrong time, as a premature heartbeat or premature ventricular contraction.

ectopic myelopoiesis See **extramedullary myelopoiesis.**

ectopic pregnancy An abnormal pregnancy in which the conceptus implants outside the uterine cavity. Kinds of ectopic pregnancy are **abdominal pregnancy, interstitial pregnancy, tubal pregnancy.** Also called **eccyesis.**

ectopic teratism A congenital anomaly in which one or more parts are misplaced, as dextrocardia, palatine teeth, and transposition of the great vessels.

ectotoxin See **exotoxin.**

ectrodactyly, ectrodactylia A congenital anomaly characterized by the absence of part or all of one or more of the fingers or toes. Also called ectrodactylism.

ectrogenic teratism A congenital anomaly caused by developmental failure in which one or more parts or organs are missing.

ectrogeny The congenital absence or defect of any organ or part of the body. —**ectrogenic,** *adj.*

ectromelia The congenital absence or incomplete development of the long bones of one or more of the limbs. Kinds of ectromelia are **amelia, hemimelia, phocomelia.** —**ectromelic,** *adj.,* **ectromelus,** *n.*

ectropion Eversion, most commonly of the eyelid, exposing the conjunctival membrane lining the eyelid and part of the eyeball. The condition may involve only the lower eyelid or both eyelids. The cause may be paralysis of the facial nerve or, in an older person, atrophy of the eyelid tissues. Compare **entropion.**

ectrosyndactyly, ectrosyndactylia A congenital anomaly characterized by the absence of some but not all of the digits, with those that are formed being webbed so as to appear fused.

eczema Superficial dermatitis of unknown cause. In the early stage it may be pruritic, erythematous, papulovesicular, edematous, and exudative. Later it becomes crusted, scaly, thickened, and lichenified. Eczema is not a distinct disease entity. See also **atopic dermatitis, nummular dermatitis.** —**eczematous,** *adj.*

eczema herpeticum A generalized vesiculo-pustular skin disease caused by herpes simplex virus or vaccinia virus infection of a preexisting membrane rash like atopic dermatitis. Hospitalization is advisable because fatalities have occurred with this condition. Also called **Kaposi's varicelliform eruption.**

eczema marginatum See **tinea cruris.**

eczematous conjunctivitis See **phlyctenular keratoconjunctivitis.**

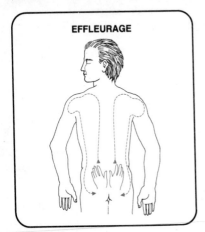
EFFLEURAGE

ED *abbr* **effective dose.**

ED50 Symbol for **median effective dose.**

edaphon The composite of organisms that live in the soil. **—edaphic,** *adj.*

EDC *abbr* **expected date of confinement.**

edema The abnormal accumulation of fluid in interstitial spaces of tissues, in the pericardial sac, intrapleural space, peritoneal cavity, or joint capsules. Edema may be caused by increased capillary fluid pressure; venous obstruction, as in varicosities, thrombophlebitis, or pressure from casts, tight bandages, or garters; congestive heart failure; overloading with parenteral fluids; renal failure; hepatic cirrhosis; hyperaldosteronism, as in Cushing's syndrome; corticosteroid therapy; and inflammatory reactions. Edema may also occur because of loss of serum protein in burns, draining wounds, fistulas, hemorrhage, nephrotic syndrome, or chronic diarrhea; in malnutrition, especially kwashiorkor; in allergic reactions; and in blockage of lymphatic vessels owing to malignant diseases, filariasis, or other disorders. The basic cause is treated, but potassium-sparing diuretics may be administered to promote excretion of sodium and water and care is exercised in protecting edematous parts of the body from prolonged pressure, injury, and temperature extremes. When a limb is edematous because of venous stasis, elevating the extremity and applying an elastic stocking or sleeve facilitates venous return. See also **lymphedema. —edematous, edematose,** *adj.*

-edema A combining form meaning 'swelling resulting from an excessive accumulation of serous fluid in the tissues of the body in (specified) locations': *cephaledema, dactyledema, papilledema.*

edetate calcium disodium, e. disodium Heavy metal antagonists.

edetic acid See **edetate calcium disodium.**

edit In data processing: the process by which the computer is made to examine input data for validity. Incorrect data prompts a warning or error message that usually appears on the screen of the computer imput device.

EDNA *abbr* **Emergency Department Nurses' Association.**

edrophonium chloride A cholinesterase (parasympathomimetic) agent.

Edsall's disease A cramping condition that results from excessive exposure to heat. Also called **heat cramp.**

EDTA *abbr* **edetate calcium disodium.**

educational psychology The application of psychological principles, techniques, and tests to educational problems, as the determination of more effective instructional methods, the assessment of student advancement, and the selection of students for specialized programs.

Edward's syndrome A congenital autosomal disorder, occurring in about 1 in 3,000 births and marked by small size and weight for gestational age; a long, narrow skull with a prominent occiput; flexion deformities of the fingers; cardiovascular abnormalities; and severe mental retardation. Infants with this condition seldom survive longer than a few months. Also called **trisomy E syndrome.**

EEE *abbr* **Eastern equine encephalitis.** See **equine encephalitis.**

EEG *abbr* **1. electroencephalogram. 2. electroencephalography.**

ef- See **ex-.**

effacement The shortening of the vaginal portion of the cervix and thinning of its walls as it is stretched and dilated by the fetus during labor. When the cervix is fully effaced, the constrictive neck of the uterus is obliterated, the cervix being then continuous with the lower uterine segment. The extent of effacement, determined by vaginal examination, is expressed as a percentage of full effacement. See also **cervix, dilatation, station.**

effective dose (ED) The dosage of a drug that may be expected to cause a specific intensity of effect in the patient to whom it is given.

effective half-life In radiotherapy: the time required for a radioactive element in an animal body to be diminished 50% as a result of the combined action of radioactive decay and biological elimination. The effective half-life (ehl) is equal to the product of the biological half-life (bhl) and the radioactive half-life (rhl) divided by the product of the biological half-life and radioactive half-life: $ehl = (bhl \times rhl) \div (bhl + rhl)$. See also **biological half-life.**

efferent Directed away from a center, as certain arteries, veins, nerves, and lymphatics. Compare **afferent.**

efferent duct Any duct through which a gland releases its secretions.

efficacy Of a drug or treatment: the maximum ability of a drug or treatment to produce a result, regardless of dosage. Narcotics have a nearly identical efficacy but require various dosages to obtain the effect. Compare **potency.**

effleurage A technique in massage in which long, light or firm strokes are used, usually over the spine and back. Fingertip effleurage is performed lightly with the fingertips in a circular pattern over one part of the body or in long strokes over the back or an extremity. Fingertip effleurage of the abdomen is commonly used in the Lamaze method of natural childbirth. Compare **pétrissage, rolling effleurage.**

effort syndrome An abnormal condition characterized by chest pain, dizziness, fatigue, and palpitations. This condition is often associated with soldiers in combat but also occurs in other individuals. The symptoms of effort syndrome often mimic angina pectoris but are more closely connected to anxiety states; distinguishing symptoms include cold, moist hands; sighing respiration; and chest pain after, rather than during, exercise. Positive diagnosis may require exercise electrocardiography. Other chest pains that mimic effort syndrome and angina may be caused by musculoskeletal problems, as inflammation of the costochondral junctions, fractured ribs, and cervical spondylosis. Also called **neurocirculatory asthenia.**

effraction A breaking open or weakening.

effusion **1.** The escape of fluid from blood vessels because of rupture or seepage, usually into a body cavity. The condition is usually associated with a circulatory or renal disorder and is often an early sign of congestive heart disease. The term may be associated with an affected body area, as pleural effusion. See also **edema, transudate.** **2.** The outward spread of a bacterial growth.

EFM *abbr* **electronic fetal monitor.**

egest To discharge or evacuate a substance from the body, especially the evacuation of unabsorbed residue of foods from the intestines. —**egesta,** *n. pl.,* **egestive,** *adj.*

ego **1.** The conscious sense of the self; those elements of a person, such as thinking, feeling, willing, and emotions, that distinguish the person as an individual. **2.** In psychoanalysis: the part of the psyche that experiences and maintains conscious contact with reality and that tempers the primitive drives of the id and the demands of the superego with the social and physical needs of society. It represents the rational element of the personality, is the seat of such mental processes as perception and memory, and develops defense mechanisms against anxiety. See also **id, superego.**

ego-alien See **ego-dystonic.**

ego analysis In psychoanalysis: the intensive study of the ego, especially the defense mechanisms.

ego boundary In psychiatry: a sense or awareness that there is a distinction between the self and others. In some psychoses the person does not have an ego boundary and cannot differentiate personal perceptions and feelings from other people's perceptions and feelings.

egocentric **1.** Regarding the self as the center, object, and norm of all experience and having little regard for the needs, interests, ideas, and attitudes of others. **2.** Describing a person possessing these characteristics.

ego defense mechanism See **defense mechanism.**

ego-dystonic Describing those elements of a person's behavior, thoughts, impulses, drives, and attitudes at variance with the standards of the ego and inconsistent with the total personality. Also called **ego-alien, self-alien.** Compare **ego-syntonic.**

ego-dystonic homosexuality A psychosexual disorder in which there is a persistent desire to change sexual orientation from homosexuality to heterosexuality.

ego ideal The image of the self to which one aspires both consciously and unconsciously and against which one measures oneself and one's performance. It is usually based on a positive identification with the significant and influential figures of early childhood years. See also **identification.**

egoism **1.** An overevaluation of the importance of the self expressed as a willingness to gain advantage at the expense of others. Also called **egotism.** **2.** The belief that individual self-interest is or ought to be the basic motive for all conscious behavior.

egoist **1.** One who seeks to satisfy personal interests at the expense of others. **2.** A person who believes in or follows the concept that all conscious action is justifiably motivated by self-interest. Also called egotist. —**egoistic, egoistical,** *adj.*

ego libido In psychoanalysis: concentration of the libido on the self; self-love, narcissism.

egomania A pathological preoccupation with the self and an exaggerated sense of one's own importance.

ego strength In psychotherapy: the ability to maintain the ego by a cluster of traits that together contribute to good mental health. The traits usually considered important include tolerance of the pain of loss, disappointment, shame, or guilt; forgiveness of those who have caused an injury, with feelings of compassion rather than anger and retaliation; acceptance of substitutes and the ability to defer gratification; persistence and perseverance in the pursuit of goals; openness, flexibility, and creativity in learning to adapt; and vitality and power in the activities of life. The psychiatric prognosis for a client correlates positively with ego strength.

ego-syntonic Those elements of a person's behavior, thoughts, impulses, drives, and attitudes that agree with the standards of the ego and are consistent with the total personality. Compare **ego-dystonic.**

egotism See **egoism.**

Egyptian ophthalmia See **trachoma.**

EHD *abbr* **electrohemodynamics.**

Ehlers-Danlos syndrome A hereditary disorder of connective tissue, marked by hyperplasticity of skin, tissue fragility, and hypermotility of joints. Minor trauma may cause a gaping wound with little bleeding. Sprains, joint dislocations, and synovial effusions commonly afflict the patient; life expectancy is usually normal.

eidetic **1.** Pertaining to or characterized by the ability to visualize and reproduce accurately

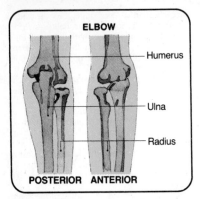

ELBOW

Humerus

Ulna

Radius

POSTERIOR ANTERIOR

the image of objects or events previously seen or imagined. **2.** A person possessing such ability.

eidetic image An unusually vivid, elaborate, and apparently exact mental image resulting from a visual experience and occurring as either a fantasy, dream, or memory. See also **image.**

eighth cranial nerve See **acoustic nerve.**

einsteinium (Es) A man-made transuranic metallic element. Its atomic number is 99; its atomic weight is 254. Einsteinium was first found in the debris from a hydrogen bomb explosion.

ejaculate The semen discharged in a single emission. —**ejaculate,** *v.*

ejaculation The sudden emission of semen from the male urethra, usually occurring during copulation, masturbation, and nocturnal emission. It is a reflex action in two phases: first, sperm, seminal fluid, and prostatic and bulbourethral gland secretions are moved into the urethra; second, strong spasmodic peristaltic contractions force ejaculation. The sensation associated with ejaculation is called orgasm. The fluid volume of the ejaculate is usually between 2 and 5 ml; each ml usually contains 50,000,000 to 150,000,000 spermatozoa. —**ejaculatory,** *adj.*

ejaculatory duct The passage through which semen enters the urethra.

ejection click Sharp clicking sounds from the heart, which may be caused by the sudden swelling of a pulmonary artery, the abrupt dilation of the aorta, or the forceful opening of the aortic cusps. Ejection clicks, often heard during examinations of individuals with septal defects and in cases of patent ductus arteriosis, are associated with high pulmonary resistance and hypertension but are common and of no clinical significance in pregnant women and in many other healthy people.

ejection murmur See **systolic murmur.**

Ekbom syndrome See **restless legs syndrome.**

EKG *abbr* **electrocardiogram.**

elaborate In endocrinology: a process by which a gland synthesizes a complex substance from simpler substances and secretes it, usually under the stimulation of a tropic hormone from the pituitary gland. This process, which is reg-

ulated by a negative feedback system, serves to maintain homeostasis in body function. —**elaboration,** *n.*

elastance **1.** The quality of recoiling or returning to an original form after the removal of pressure. **2.** The degree to which an air-filled or fluid-filled organ, as a lung, bladder, or blood vessel, can return to its original dimensions when a distending or compressing force is removed. **3.** The measurement of the unit volume of change in such an organ per unit of decreased pressure change. Compare **compliance.**

elastic band fixation A method of treatment of fractures of the jaw using rubber bands to connect metal splints or wires that are attached to the maxilla and mandible. The rubber bands produce traction and bring the teeth into occlusion and proper alignment while the fracture is healing. Rubber bands are safer than rigid wires in the event of vomiting. See also **maxillomandibular fixation, nasomandibular fixation.**

elastic bougie A flexible bougie that can be passed through angular or winding channels.

elastic cartilage See **yellow cartilage.**

elasticity The ability of tissue, as muscle tissue, to regain its original shape and size after being stretched, squeezed, or otherwise deformed.

elbow The hinged articulation of the humerus, the ulna, and the radius, covered by a protective capsule associated with three ligaments and an extensive synovial membrane. The elbow joint allows flexion and extension of the forearm and accommodates the radioulnar articulation. It is a common site of inflammation and disorders, as those incurred during participation in various sports. Also called **articulatio cubiti.**

elbow reflex See **triceps reflex.**

elective Of or pertaining to a procedure that is performed by choice but that is not essential, as elective surgery.

elective abortion Induced termination of a pregnancy before the fetus has developed enough to survive outside the uterus, deemed necessary by the woman carrying it and performed at her request. Commonly (but incorrectly) called **therapeutic abortion.** See also **induced abortion, therapeutic abortion.**

electrical burns The tissue damage resulting from heat of up to 5000°C (9032°F) generated by an electrical current. The point of contact on the skin is burnt, and the muscle and subcutaneous tissues may be damaged. In severe burns, circulatory and respiratory failure may occur and are treated before the burn.

electrically stimulated osteogenesis A bone regeneration process induced electrically by surgically implanted electrodes, especially at nonunion fracture sites. The process is effective because of the different electrical potentials within bone tissue. Viable nonstressed bone is electronegative in the metaphyseal regions and over a fracture callus, and electropositive in the diaphyses and other less active regions. The precise mechanisms by which electricity induces osteo-genesis are not understood, but research shows that electrical application of less than 1 volt consumes oxygen at the cathode, producing hydroxyl ions, decreasing the oxygen tension of local tissue, and increasing the alkalinity, thereby encouraging calcification. Electrically stimulated osteogenesis involves percutaneous insertion of cathodes or implantation of electrodes during open surgery. It is contraindicated for pathological fractures owing to benign or malignant tumors; congenital conditions, as congenital pseudarthrosis and osteogenesis imperfecta; in the presence of active systemic infections, clinically active osteomyelitis, patient sensitivity to the nickel or chromium from which the cathode pins are made; and synovial pseudarthrosis, unless the fluid-filled cavity at the nonunion site is excised before the cathodes are inserted.

electric blood warmer An electrical device for heating blood before infusions, especially massive transfusions in which cold blood might put the patient into shock. Authorities warn that the disposable blood warming bag used with the heater must be discarded after one use.

electric cautery See **electrocautery.**

electric shock A traumatic physical state caused by the passage of electric current through the body. It usually involves accidental contact with exposed parts of electrical circuits in home appliances and domestic power supplies but may also result from lightning or contact with high-voltage wires. High-frequency current produces more heat than low-frequency current and can cause burns, coagulation, and necrosis of affected body parts. Low-frequency current can burn tissues if the area of contact is small and concentrated. Severe electrical shock commonly causes unconsciousness, respiratory paralysis, muscle contractions, bone fractures, and cardiac disorders. Even small electrical currents passing through the heart can cause fibrillation. Treatment of this kind of electric shock commonly involves such measures as cardiopulmonary resuscitation, defibrillation, and the intravenous administration of electrolytes to help stabilize vital functions. See also **cardiogenic shock, hypovolemic shock.**

electric shock therapy (EST) See **electroconvulsive therapy.**

electro- A combining form meaning 'pertaining to electricity': *electrobiology, electrocatalysis, electrolepsy.*

electroanalytical chemistry The branch of chemistry concerned with the analysis of compounds using electric current to produce characteristic, observable change in the substance being studied. See also **chemistry.**

electrocardiogram (EKG, ECG) A graphic record produced by an electrocardiograph, showing the electrical current generated by the heartbeat. EKG tracings include P, Q, R, S, T, and U waveforms. The P waveform is produced by excitation of the atria. The Q, R, S waveforms result from excitation of the ventricles. The T waveform indicates ventricular re-

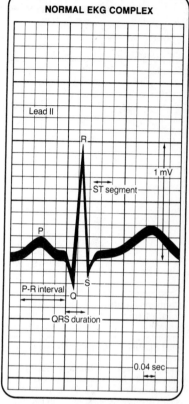

NORMAL EKG COMPLEX

Lead II

R

1 mV

ST segment

P

P-R interval

S

Q

QRS duration

0.04 sec

laxation. The U waveform sometimes follows the T waveform and is of unknown origin.

electrocardiograph (EKG) A device used for recording the electrical activity of the myocardium to detect abnormal transmission of the cardiac impulse through the conductive tissues of the muscle. Electrocardiography allows diagnosis of specific cardiac abnormalities. Leads are affixed to certain anatomic points on the patient's chest, arms, and legs, usually with an adhesive jelly that promotes transmission of the electrical impulse to the recording device. The patient is placed in the supine position on an examining table and asked to lie quietly during the test. —**electrocardiographic,** *adj.*

electrocardiographic-auscultatory syndrome See **Barlow's syndrome.**

electrocardiograph lead 1. A wire connecting an electrocardiograph with an electrode placed on a body part. 2. A record, made by the electrocardiograph, that varies depending on the site of the electrode.

electrocautery The application of a needle or snare heated by electrical current for the destruction of tissue, as for the removal of warts. Also called **electric cautery, galvanic cautery, galvanocautery.** See also **diathermy.**

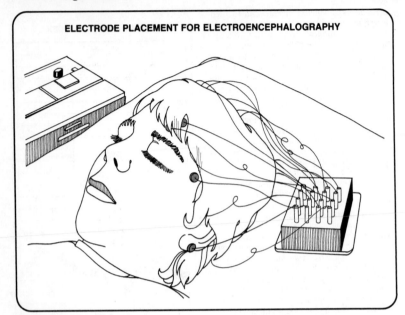

ELECTRODE PLACEMENT FOR ELECTROENCEPHALOGRAPHY

electrocoagulation A therapeutic, destructive form of electrosurgery in which tissue is hardened by the passage of high-frequency current from an electric cautery. Also called **surgical diathermy.** Compare **electrodesiccation.**

electroconvulsive therapy (ECT) The induction of a brief seizure by passing an electric current through the brain for the treatment of affective disorders, especially in patients resistant to psychoactive drug therapy. The patient loses consciousness and undergoes tonic contractions for approximately 10 seconds, followed by a somewhat longer period of clonic seizures accompanied by apnea; on awakening the patient has no memory of the shock. ECT is usually administered three times a week for 2 months and is used primarily for the treatment of acute depression. Once widely used to treat affective psychiatric disorders, ECT has been almost completely replaced by newer, less risky therapeutic measures. Also called **electric shock therapy, electroshock therapy.**

electrocution Death caused by the passage of electric current through the body. See also **electric shock.**

electrodermal audiometry A method of testing hearing in which a harmless electric shock is used to condition the subject to a pure tone; thereafter, the tone, coupled with the anticipation of a shock, elicits a brief electrodermal response, which is recorded, and the lowest intensity of the sound producing the skin response is considered the subject's hearing threshold.

electrodesiccation A form of electrosurgery in which tissue is destroyed by burning with an electric spark. It is used primarily for eliminating small superficial growths but may be used with curettage for eradicating abnormal tissue deeper in the skin, in which case layers of skin may be burnt, then successively debrided. The procedure is performed under local anesthetic. Also called **fulguration.**

electroencephalogram (EEG) A graphic chart on which the electrical potential produced by the brain cells is traced, as detected by electrodes placed on the scalp. The resulting brain waves are called alpha, beta, delta, and theta rhythms, according to the frequencies they produce, which range from 2 to 12 cycles per second with an amplitude of up to 100 microvolts. Variations in brain-wave activity correlate with neurological conditions, psychological states, and levels of consciousness.

electroencephalograph An instrument for performing electroencephalography.

electroencephalography (EEG) The process of recording brain-wave activity by means of electrodes attached to various areas of the patient's head. During the procedure the patient remains quiet, with eyes closed, and refrains from talking or moving, although, in certain cases, prescribed activities may be requested, especially hyperventilation. The test is used to diagnose seizure disorders, brain stem disorders, focal lesions, and impaired consciousness. During neurosurgery, the electrodes can be applied directly to the surface of the brain (intracranial electroencephalography) or placed within the brain tissue (depth electroencephalography) to detect lesions or tumors. —**electroencephalographic,** *adj.*

electrohemodynamics (EHD) A noninvasive technique for measuring the mechanical properties and hemodynamic characteristics of the vascular system, including arterial blood pressure, electrical impedance, blood flow, and resistance to blood flow.

electroimmunodiffusion See **immunodiffusion.**

electrolysis A process in which electrical energy causes a chemical change in a conducting medium, usually a solution or a molten substance, or destruction by passage of an electrical current, as hair follicles. Electrodes induce the flow of electrical energy through the medium. Electrons enter the solution through the cathode and leave the solution through the anode. Negatively charged ions, or anions, are attracted to the anode; positively charged ions, or cations, are attracted to the cathode. Various conducting mediums are used, as solutions of copper, zinc, nickel, lead, and silver. Electrical energy passing through such solutions causes deposition of pure metal at the cathode. Passing electrical energy through solutions of alkali and alkaline-earth salts liberates hydrogen at the cathode. A metal anode causes metal ions to flow from the anode into the solution as the electrical current passes through the medium. An inert electrode, as one of platinum, may liberate an element, as oxygen, at the anode in an aqueous medium. A halogen salt solution liberates free bromine, chlorine, or iodine. Fluorine, which has a high oxidation potential, is not liberated by electrolysis. —**electrolytic,** *adj.*

electrolyte An element or compound that, when melted or dissolved in water or other solvent, dissociates into ions and is able to conduct an electric current. Electrolytes differ in their concentrations in blood plasma, interstitial fluid, and cell fluid and affect the movement of substances between those compartments. Proper quantities of principal electrolytes and balance among them are critical to normal metabolism and function. For example, calcium (Ca^{++}) is necessary for the relaxation of skeletal muscle and contraction of cardiac muscle; potassium (K^+) is required for the contraction of skeletal muscle and relaxation of cardiac muscle. Sodium (Na^+) is essential in maintaining fluid balance. Certain diseases, conditions, and medications may lead to a deficiency of one or more electrolytes and to an imbalance among them, as certain diuretics and a low-sodium diet prescribed in hypertension may cause hypokalemia owing to a loss of potassium. Diarrhea may cause a loss of many electrolytes, leading to hypovolemia and shock, especially in infants. Careful and regular monitoring of electrolytes and intravenous replacement of fluid and electrolytes is part of the acute care in many illnesses. —**electrolytic,** *adj.*

electrolyte balance The equilibrium between electrolytes in the body.

electrolyte solution Any solution containing electrolytes prepared for oral, parenteral, or rectal administration for the replacement or supplementation of specific ions necessary for homeostasis. For example, a solution containing combinations of calcium, sodium, phosphate, chloride, or magnesium may be given to treat acid-base disturbance, as seen in chronic renal dysfunction or diabetic ketoacidosis. Most solutions include various trace minerals.

electromagnetic radiation Every kind of electrical and magnetic radiation, regarded as a continuous spectrum of energy that includes energy with the shortest wavelength (gamma rays, with a wavelength of 0.0011 angstrom) to that with the longest wavelength (long radio waves, with a wavelength of more than 1 million km). The visible part of the electromagnetic spectrum is between 3,800 and 7,600 angstrom. Ultraviolet radiation, having a wavelength of less than 4,000 angstrom, and X-rays, with a wavelength from 0.05 to a few hundred angstrom, occur beyond the short-wave (violet) end of the visible spectrum. Infrared radiation occurs just beyond the long-wave (red) end of the visible spectrum, having a wavelength of 7,000 angstrom or more.

electromyogram (EMG) A record of the intrinsic electrical activity in a skeletal muscle, obtained by applying surface electrodes or by inserting a needle electrode into the muscle and observing electrical activity with an oscilloscope. Helpful in diagnosing neuromuscular problems, electromyograms show abnormalities, as spontaneous electrical potentials within a muscle, help to pinpoint lesions of motor nerves, and measure electrical potentials induced by voluntary muscle contraction. See also **electroneuromyography.**

electron **1.** A negatively charged elementary particle that has a specific charge, mass, and spin. The number of electrons circling the nucleus of an atom is equal to the atomic number of the substance. Electrons may be shared or exchanged by two atoms; after the exchange the atom becomes an ion. **2.** A negative beta particle emitted from a radioactive substance. See also **atom, element, ion, neutron, proton.**

electronarcosis A procedure that produces general anesthesia without the use of anesthetic gases or drugs. Narcosis is produced by passing an electric current through the brain, but adequate control and prevention of undesirable side effects, especially seizures, remain a problem. This procedure is experimental.

electroneuromyography A procedure for testing and recording neuromuscular activity by the electrical stimulation of nerves. The procedure involves the insertion of needle electrodes into any skeletal muscle being studied, applying electrical current to the electrodes, and observing neuromuscular functions by means of an oscilloscope. The procedure helps in studying neuromuscular conduction, the extent of nerve lesions, and reflex responses. See also **electromyogram.**

electronic fetal monitor (EFM) A device that allows observation of fetal heart rate and maternal uterine contractions. Applied externally, it detects the fetal heart by an ultrasound transducer on the abdomen and the uterine con-

ELLIPTOCYTOSIS

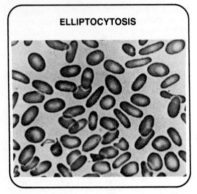

tractions by a pressure sensor on the abdomen. Internal monitoring of the fetal heart rate is accomplished via an electrode clipped to the fetal scalp; the amplitude, frequency, and duration of the uterine contractions are detected by the use of an intrauterine catheter.

electronic thermometer A thermometer that registers temperature rapidly by electronic means.

electron microscope An instrument, similar to but 1,000 times stronger than an optical microscope, that scans cell surfaces with a beam of electrons instead of visible light. Used to study very thin sections of tissue, it creates an image that can be photographed or viewed on a fluorescent screen. Compare **scanning electron microscope.**

electron microscopy A technique, using an electron microscope, for viewing and studying an extremely thin tissue specimen. Also called **transmission electron microscopy.** Compare **scanning electron microscopy.**

electron scanning microscope See **scanning electron microscope.**

electronystagmography A method of assessing and recording eye movements by measuring the electrical activity of the extraocular muscles. See also **electroencephalogram, nystagmus.**

electrophoresis The movement of charged suspended particles through a liquid medium in response to changes in an electric field. Charged particles of a given substance migrate in a predictable direction and at a characteristic speed. The pattern of migration can be recorded in bands on an electrophoretogram. The technique is widely used to separate and identify serum proteins and other biological substances. —**electrophoretic,** *adj.*

electrophoretogram See **electrophoresis.**

electroshock therapy See **electroconvulsive therapy.**

electrosleep therapy A technique designed to induce sleep, especially in psychiatric patients, by administering a low-amplitude pulsating current to the brain. The cathode is placed supraorbitally, and the anode is placed over the mastoid process; the current, which is discharged for 15 to 20 minutes, produces a tingling sensation, but not always sleep. The procedure, repeated from 5 to 30 times, is said to be beneficial for patients with anxiety, depression, gastric distress, insomnia, personality disorders, and schizophrenia, but double-blind studies have yielded contradictory results.

electrosurgery Surgery performed with various electrical instruments that operate on high-frequency electric current. Kinds of electrosurgery include **electrocoagulation, electrodesiccation.**

electrotonic current A current induced in a nerve sheath by an action potential within the nerve or an adjacent nerve.

element One of more than 100 primary, simple substances that cannot be broken down by chemical means into any other substance. Each atom of any element contains a specific number of electrons orbiting the nucleus. The nucleus contains a variable number of neutrons. A **stable element** contains an equal number of neutrons and electrons and does not easily give up neutrons. A **radioactive element** contains an unbalanced number of electrons and neutrons and gives off neutrons readily. See also **atom, compound, molecule.**

element 104 A man-made, radioactive element, the 12th transuranic element, as yet unnamed, and the first beyond the actinide series.

element 105 A man-made element, as yet unnamed; the 13th transuranic element.

eleo- A combining form meaning 'pertaining to oil': *eleoma, eleomyenchysis, eleopten.* Also **oleo-.**

elephantiasis The end-stage lesion of filariasis, characterized by tremendous swelling, usually of the external genitalia and the legs. The overlying skin becomes dark, thick, and coarse. Elephantiasis results from filariasis that has lasted for many years. See also **filariasis.**

elephantoid fever See **elephantiasis, filariasis.**

eleventh nerve See **accessory nerve.**

elimination diet A procedure for identifying a food or foods to which a person is allergic by successively omitting from the diet certain foods in order to detect those responsible for the symptoms.

elixir A clear liquid containing water, alcohol, sweeteners, and flavors, used primarily as a vehicle for the oral administration of a drug.

Elliot forceps See **obstetric forceps.**

Elliot's position A supine posture assumed by the patient on the operating table, with a support placed under the lower costal margin to elevate the chest. The position is used in gallbladder surgery.

elliptocytosis A mild abnormal condition of the blood that is characterized by increased numbers of elliptical or oval erythrocytes with pale centers. Less than 15% of the red cells appear in this form in normal blood; modest increases occur in a variety of anemias, including a rare congenital disorder, hereditary elliptocytosis, which may or may not be associated with a mild hemolytic anemia. Also called **ovalocytosis.** See also **acanthocytosis, congenital nonspherocytic hemolytic anemia, spherocytic anemia, sickle cell anemia.**

em- A combining form meaning 'in, on': *embolism, empasma.* Also **en-.**

emaciation Excessive leanness caused by disease or lack of nutrition.

Embden-Meyerhof pathway A sequence of enzymatic reactions in the anaerobic conversion of glucose to lactic acid, producing energy in the form of adenosine triphosphate.

embolectomy A surgical incision into an artery for the removal of an embolus or clot, performed as emergency treatment for arterial embolism. Thrombi tend to lodge at the juncture of major arteries when the thrombi have broken away from a thrombophlebitis; more than half lodge in the aorta, in arteries of the lower extremities, in the common carotid arteries, or in the pulmonary arteries. The operation is done under a general anesthetic within 4 to 6 hours of the onset of pain, if possible. Preoperatively, anticoagulants are administered, and an arteriogram is done to identify the affected artery. Postoperatively, the blood pressure is maintained close to the preoperative baseline level, as a decrease might predispose to new clot formation. A frequent complication is hemorrhage from small arteries that may have been clogged with the embolus but overlooked while tying larger bleeding vessels.

embolism The obstruction of a blood vessel by an embolus. Symptoms vary with the degree of occlusion; the character of the embolus; and the size, nature, and location of the occluded vessel. Kinds of embolism include **air embolism, fat embolism, blood clot, bone marrow embolism, tumor cell embolism.**

embolus, *pl.* **emboli** A foreign object, a quantity of air or gas, a bit of tissue or tumor, or a piece of a thrombus that circulates in the bloodstream until it becomes lodged in a vessel. Kinds of emboli include **blood clot, bone marrow embolus, tumor cell embolus. —embolic, emboloid,** *adj.*

embryatrics See **fetology.**

embryectomy The surgical removal of an embryo, most commonly in an ectopic pregnancy.

embryo 1. Any organism in the earliest stages of development. 2. In humans, the stage of prenatal development between the time of implantation of the fertilized ovum about 2 weeks after conception until the end of the 7th or 8th week. The period is characterized by rapid growth, differentiation of the major organ systems, and development of the main external features. Compare **fetus, zygote. —embryonal, embryonoid, embryonic,** *adj.*

-embryo A combining form meaning a 'fetus': *embryo, typembryo.*

embryoctony The intentional destruction of the living embryo or fetus in utero. Also called **feticide.** See also **abortion.**

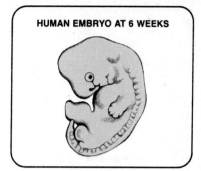

HUMAN EMBRYO AT 6 WEEKS

embryogenesis The process in sexual reproduction in which an embryo forms from the fertilization of an ovum. Also called **embryogeny.** See also **heterogenesis, homogenesis. —embryogenetic, embryogenic.** *adj.*

embryogeny See **embryogenesis.**

embryologic development The various intrauterine stages and processes involved in the growth and differentiation of the conceptus from the time of fertilization of the ovum until the 8th week of gestation. The stages are related to the biological status of the unborn child and are divided into two distinct periods. The first is embryogenesis, or the formation of the embryo, which occurs during the 10 days to 2 weeks following fertilization until implantation. The second period, organogenesis, involves the differentiation of the various cells, tissues, and organ systems and the development of the main external features of the embryo; it occurs from approximately the end of the 2nd week through the 8th week of intrauterine life. By the 4th week of development, the primitive body includes the neural tube, which will develop into the brain, spinal cord, and other neural tissue of the central nervous system; the notochord, which will be replaced by the vertebral column; the somites, which will segment into skeletal and muscle tissue; the nephrotomes, which will form the urogenital system; the gut, which will differentiate into the digestive and respiratory systems; the coelom, which will subdivide into separate cavities for the heart, lungs, and abdominal viscera; and the primitive heart and tiny spaces within the mesoderm that will become the vessels of the circulatory and lymphatic systems. At 8 weeks of development, major differentiation of all the organs has occurred, and the main external features, as the eyes, ears, nose, mouth, and digits, are recognizable. The embryo is now remarkably humanlike in appearance and at this stage is called a fetus. For the remaining 7 months of intrauterine life the primary changes in the fetus are growth, further tissue differentiation, elaboration of structural detail, and specialization of organs and systems. See also **prenatal development.**

embryologist One who specializes in the study of embryology.

embryology The study of the origin, growth,

development, and function of an organism from fertilization to birth. Kinds of embryology include **comparative embryology, descriptive embryology, experimental embryology.** —**embryologic, embryological,** *adj.*

embryomorph Any structure that resembles an embryo, especially a mass of tissue that may represent an aborted conceptus. —**embryomorphous,** *adj.*

embryonal See **embryo.**

embryonal adenomyosarcoma See **Wilms' tumor.**

embryonal adenosarcoma See **Wilms' tumor.**

embryonal carcinoma An extremely malignant neoplasm derived from germinal cells that usually develops in gonads, especially the testes. The tumor—a firm, nodular mass with many hemorrhagic areas—is characterized histologically by large, undifferentiated cells with indistinct borders, eosinophilic cytoplasm, and prominent nucleoli in pleomorphic nuclei. Bodies resembling a 1- or 2-week-old embryo are occasionally seen in these tumors. The neoplasm is relatively resistant to radiation therapy, and, early in its development, it metastasizes by way of lymph channels. Surgery and chemotherapy are usually included in the treatment. See also **choriocarcinoma.**

embryonal leukemia See **stem cell leukemia.**

embryonate 1. Impregnated; containing an embryo. 2. Of, pertaining to, or resembling an embryo.

embryonic See **embryo.**

embryonic abortion 1. Termination of pregnancy before the 20th week of gestation. 2. Expelled products of conception before the 20th week. Compare **fetal abortion.**

embryonic anideus See **anideus.**

embryonic blastoderm The area of the blastoderm that gives rise to the primitive streak from which the embryonic body develops. Compare **extraembryonic blastoderm.**

embryonic competence The ability of an embryonic cell to react normally to the stimulation of an inductor allowing continued, normal growth or differentiation of the embryo.

embryonic disk The thickened plate from which the embryo develops in the 2nd week of pregnancy. Scattered cells from the border of the disk migrate to the space between the trophoblast and yolk sac and become the embryonic mesoderm. The disk develops from the ectoderm and endoderm. Also called **germ disk.**

embryonic layer One of the three layers of the cells in the embryo, the endoderm, the mesoderm, and the ectoderm. From these layers of cells arise all of the structures, organs, and parts of the body. The endoderm is the first to develop, followed by the ectoderm. During the 3rd week of gestation, the mesoderm arises between them.

embryonic stage In embryology: the time interval from the end of the germinal stage (at 10 days of gestation), to the end of the 7th week.

embryoniform Resembling an embryo.

embryopathy Any anomaly occurring in the embryo or fetus as a result of interference with normal intrauterine development. A kind of embryopathy is **rubella embryopathy.**

embryoplastic Of or pertaining to the formation of an embryo, usually used with reference to cells.

embryotome An instrument used in embryotomy.

embryotomy 1. The dismemberment or mutilation of a fetus for removal from the uterus when normal delivery is not possible. 2. The dissection of an embryo for examination and analysis.

embryotroph, embryotrophe The liquefied uterine nutritive material, composed of glandular secretions and degenerative tissue, that nourishes the mammalian embryo until placental circulation is established. Also called **histotroph, histotrophic nutrition.** Compare **hemotroph.**

embryotrophy The nourishment of the embryo. See also **embryotroph, hemotroph.** —**embryotrophic,** *adj.*

embryulcia The surgical removal of the embryo or fetus from the uterus.

emergence A stage in the process of recovery from general anesthesia that includes spontaneous respiration, voluntary swallowing, and consciousness. See also **postoperative care.**

emergency department In a health-care facility: a section of an institution that is staffed and equipped to provide rapid·and varied emergency care, especially for those stricken with sudden and acute illness or those who are the victims of severe trauma.

Emergency Department Nurses' Association (EDNA) A national professional organization of emergency department nurses that defines and promotes emergency nursing practice. The association, headquartered in Chicago, has written and implemented the *Standards of Emergency Nursing Practice.* The association offers a certification examination and awards the designation Certified Emergency Nurse (CEN) to nurses who successfully complete it. EDNA publishes the *Journal of Emergency Nursing (JEN)* and *Continuing Education Core Curriculum of Emergency Nursing Practice.*

emergency doctrine In law: a doctrine that assumes a person's consent to medical treatment when the person is in imminent danger and unable to give informed consent to treatment. Emergency doctrine assumes that the person would consent if able to do so.

Emergency Medical Service (EMS) A network of services coordinated to provide aid and medical assistance from primary response to definitive care, involving personnel trained in the rescue, stabilization, transportation, and advanced treatment of trauma or medical emergency patients. Linked by a communications system that operates on both a local and regional level, EMS is usually initiated by a citizen calling to an emergency number. Stages include the first medical response; involvement of ambulance personnel, medium and heavy rescue equipment, and paramedic units, if necessary; and continued care in the hospital with emergency room nurses, emergency room doctors, specialists, and critical care nurses and physicians. See also **Emergency Medical Technician, Emergency Medical Technician–Advanced Life Support, Emergency Medical Technician–Intravenous, Emergency Medical Technician–Paramedic.**

Emergency Medical Technician (EMT) A person trained in and responsible for the administration of specialized emergency care and the transportation to a medical facility of victims of acute illness or injury. The EMT is trained in basic life support skills, extrication and disentanglement, operation of emergency vehicles, basic anatomy, basic assessment of injury or illness, triage, care for specific injuries and illnesses, environmental emergencies, childbirth, and transport of the patient. EMTs undergo ongoing training in new procedures and must qualify for recertification every 2 years. Kinds of EMTs are **Emergency Medical Technician–Advanced Life Support, Emergency Medical Technician–Intravenous, Emergency Medical Technician–Paramedic.** See also **Emergency Medical Service.**

Emergency Medical Technician–Advanced Life Support (EMT-ALS) A third-level EMT. The EMT-ALS is certified in all the skills of the basic-level EMT and EMT-I.V. and additionally may administer certain medications following the orders of the hospital physician, with whom radio contact is maintained. An EMT-ALS is also trained in the use of advanced life support systems, including electrical defibrillation equipment.

Emergency Medical Technician–Intravenous (EMT-I.V.) A second-level emergency medical technician. The EMT-I.V. is certified in all the skills of the basic-level EMT and also in intravenous therapy, endotracheal intubation, and the use of medical antishock trousers (MAST).

Emergency Medical Technician–Paramedic (EMT-P) An advanced-level emergency medical technician. The EMT-P is certified in all the skills of EMTs of other levels, with additional training in pharmacology and the administration of emergency drugs.

emergency medicine A branch of medicine concerned with the diagnosis and treatment of conditions resulting from trauma or sudden illness. The patient's condition is stabilized, and care of the patient is transferred to the primary physician or to a specialist. Emergency medicine requires a broad interdisciplinary training in the physiology and pathology of all the systems of the body.

emergency nursing Nursing care provided to prevent imminent severe damage or death or to avert serious injury. Activities that exemplify emergency nursing care include basic life support, cardiopulmonary resuscitation, control of hemorrhage and burn care.

emergency room (ER) A hospital area specially designed to receive and initially treat patients suffering from sudden trauma or medical problems, as accidental hemorrhage, poisoning, fracture, heart attack, and respiratory failure.

emergency theory In physiology: a theory stating that when a person is faced with an emergency the adrenal medulla is stimulated by the sympathetic nervous system to release epinephrine, which increases heart rate, raises blood pressure, reduces blood flow to viscera, and mobilizes blood glucose, preparing the body for flight from danger or for the fight to survive. See also **flight or fight reaction.**

emergent evolution The theory that evolution occurs in a series of major changes at certain critical stages and results from the total rearrangement of existing elements so that completely new and unpredictable characteristics appear within the species. See also **saltatory evolution.**

emesis See **vomit.**

emetic 1. Of or pertaining to a substance that causes vomiting. 2. An emetic agent. Apomorphine hydrochloride, acting through the central nervous system, induces vomiting 10 to 15 minutes after parenteral administration. Syrup of ipecac is used in the emergency treatment of drug overdosage and in certain cases of poisoning, but it can be cardiotoxic if it is absorbed and not vomited.

-emetic A combining form meaning 'pertaining to vomiting': *antiemetic, hematemetic, hyperemetic.* Also **-emetical.**

emetine hydrochloride An amebicide.

EMG *abbr* **electromyogram.**

EMG syndrome A hereditary disorder transmitted as an autosomal recessive trait. Clinical manifestations include exophthalmos, macroglossia, and gigantism, often accompanied by visceromegaly, dysplasia of the renal medulla, and enlargement of the cells of the adrenal cortex. Also called **Beckwith-Wiedemann syndrome, exophthalmos-macroglossia-gigantism syndrome.**

EMI *abbr* Electric and Musical Industries. The British manufacturer of the first scanner produced for computerized tomography (CT).

EMI scan See **computerized tomography (CT).**

-emia, -aemia A combining form meaning: 1. A '(specified) blood condition': *hypokinemia, panhyperemia, pyknemia.* 2. A 'blood condition involving a (specified) substance': *calcemia, iodemia, melitemia.* Also **-hemia, -haemia.**

emissary veins The small vessels in the skull that connect the sinuses of the dura with the veins on the exterior of the skull through a series of anastomoses. The major emissary veins are the mastoid emissary vein, the parietal emissary vein, the internal carotid plexus, the rete canalis hypoglossi, the condyloid emissary vein, the rete foraminis ovalis, and the small veins passing through the foramen lacerum to connect

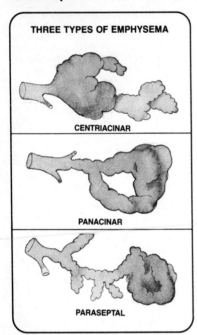

THREE TYPES OF EMPHYSEMA

CENTRIACINAR

PANACINAR

PARASEPTAL

the cavernous sinus with the pterygoid plexus. Also included in the emissary group is a vein passing through the foramen cecum, connecting the superior sagittal sinus with the veins of the nasal cavity.

emmetropia A state of normal vision characterized by the proper relationship between the refractive system of the eyeball and its axial length. This correlation assures that light rays entering the eye parallel to the optic axis are focused exactly on the retina. Compare **amblyopia, hyperopia, myopia. —emmetropic,** *adj.*

emollient A substance that softens tissue, particularly the skin and mucous membranes.

emollient bath A bath taken in water containing an emollient, as bran, to relieve irritation and inflammation. See also **colloid bath.**

emotion The affective aspect of consciousness as compared with volition and cognition. Physiologic alterations often occur with a marked change of emotion regardless of whether the feelings are conscious or unconscious, expressed or unexpressed. See also **emotional need, emotional response.**

emotional amalgam An unconscious effort to deny or counteract anxiety.

emotional care of the dying patient The compassionate, consistent support offered to help the terminally ill patient and the family cope with impending death. See **stages of dying.**

emotional illness See **mental disorder.**

emotional need A psychological or mental requirement of intrapsychic origin, usually centering on such basic feelings as love, fear, anger, sorrow, anxiety, frustration, and depression and involving the understanding, empathy, and support of one person for another. Such needs normally occur in everyone but usually are increased during periods of excessive stress or physical and mental illness and during various stages of life, as infancy, early childhood, and old age. If these needs are not routinely met by appropriate, socially accepted means, they can precipitate psychopathological conditions. Appropriate measures common in nursing for anticipating and satisfying the emotional needs of patients in stress include physical closeness, especially remaining with the person during periods when the feeling is acute; empathic listening as the patient discusses the feeling; encouragement to talk; and planning activities that provide a constructive outlet for the feeling or the situation causing it. Compare **dependency needs.** See also **emotion.**

emotional response A reaction to a particular intrapsychic feeling or feelings, accompanied by physiological changes that may or may not be outwardly manifest but that motivate or precipitate some action or behavioral response.

emotional support The sensitive, understanding approach that helps patients accept and deal with crises, such as their illnesses; communicate their anxieties and fears; derive comfort from a gentle, sympathetic, caring person; and increase their ability to care for themselves. Essential in providing emotional support is recognizing and respecting the individuality, personal preferences, and human needs of each patient. Understanding and appreciating the psychological and physiological effects on the patient of the transition from health to illness is also important.

empathy The ability to recognize and to some extent share the emotions and states of mind of another and to understand the meaning and significance of that person's behavior. Empathy is an essential quality for effective psychotherapy. Compare **sympathy. —empathic,** *adj.,* **empathize,** *v.*

emphysema An abnormal condition of the pulmonary system, characterized by overinflation and destructive changes of alveolar walls, resulting in a loss of lung elasticity and decreased gases. The kinds of emphysema are centriacinar, panacinar, and paraseptal. When emphysema occurs early in life, it is usually related to a rare genetic deficiency of serum $alpha_1$-antitrypsin, which inactivates the enzymes leukocyte collagenase and elastase. Acute emphysema may be caused by the rupture of alveoli by severe respiratory efforts, as in acute bronchopneumonia, suffocation, and whooping cough, and occasionally during labor. Chronic emphysema usually accompanies chronic bronchitis, a major cause of which is cigarette smoking, and may follow asthma or tuberculosis. In old age, the alveolar membranes atrophy and may collapse, resulting in large air-filled spaces with decreased total surface area of the pulmonary membranes. Symptoms include shortness of breath, dyspnea, cough, cyanosis, orthopnea, unequal chest expansion, tachypnea, tachycardia, and an elevated temperature. Anxiety, carbon dioxide narcosis with a decreased pH, increased PCO_2, restlessness, confusion, weakness, anorexia, congestive heart failure, pulmonary edema, and respiratory failure are common in advanced cases. Treatment may include airway maintenance, humidified oxygen, bronchodilators, antibiotics, expectorants, and corticosteroids, postural drainage, cupping and vibration, and IPPB. Sedation is to be avoided, as most sedatives depress respiratory function.

NURSING CONSIDERATIONS: The patient is taught breathing exercises and encouraged to drink between 2,000 and 3,000 ml of fluids daily. Activity is encouraged to the limit of the patient's tolerance. Fatigue, constipation, and upper respiratory tract infection and irritation are to be avoided. Oxygen therapy equipment, such as an IPPB machine, may be prescribed for the patient's use at home.

empiric Of or pertaining to a method of treating disease based on observations and experience without an understanding of the cause or mechanism of the disorder or the way the employed therapeutic agent or procedure effects improvement or cure. The empiric treatment of a new disease may be based on observations and experience gained in the management of analogous disorders. —**empirical,** *adj.*

empiricism A form of therapy based on personal experience and the experience of other practitioners. —**empiric, empirical,** *adj.* —**empiricist,** *n.*

empiric treatment See **treatment.**

emprosthotonos A position of the body characterized by a forward, rigid flexure of the body at the waist. The position is the result of a prolonged, involuntary muscle spasm that is most commonly associated with tetanus infection or strychnine poisoning.

empty-sella syndrome An abnormal enlargement of the sella turcica in which no pituitary tumor is present; the gland may be smaller than normal, or it may be absent. Signs and symptoms of hormonal imbalance may be present, but some patients show no evidence of hypopituitarism or of any other endocrine abnormality. The condition is especially frequent in overweight, middle-aged, multiparous women. The diagnosis may be made by CT skull X-ray, or pneumoencephalography.

empyema An accumulation of pus in a body cavity, especially the pleural space, as a result of bacterial infection, as pleurisy or tuberculosis. It is usually removed by surgical incision, aspiration, and drainage. Antibiotics are administered to correct the underlying infection.

-empyema A combining form meaning an 'accumulation of pus, especially thoracic': *arthroempyema, pneumoempyema, typhloempyema.*

EMS *abbr* Emergency Medical Service.

EMT *abbr* Emergency Medical Technician.

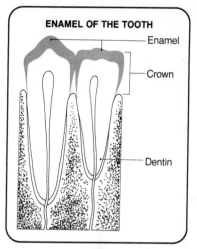

ENAMEL OF THE TOOTH

— Enamel
— Crown
— Dentin

EMT-ALS *abbr* Emergency Medical Technician–Advanced Life Support.

EMT-I.V. *abbr* Emergency Medical Technician–Intravenous.

EMT-P *abbr* Emergency Medical Technician–Paramedic.

emulsify To disperse a liquid into another liquid, making a colloidal suspension. Soaps and detergents emulsify by surrounding small globules of fat, preventing them from settling out. Bile acts as an emulsifying agent in the digestive tract by dispersing ingested fats into small globules. —**emulsification,** *n.*

emulsion A system consisting of two immiscible liquids, one of which is dispersed in the other in the form of small droplets. —**emulsify,** *v.*

en- A combining form meaning 'in, on': *enanthema, encelialgia, enostosis.* Also **em-.**

enamel A hard white substance that covers the dentin of the crown of a tooth.

enamel hypocalcification A hereditary dental defect in which the enamel of the teeth is soft and undercalcified in context yet normal in quantity, caused by defective maturation of the ameloblasts. The teeth are chalky in consistency, the surfaces wear down rapidly, and a yellow-to-brown stain appears as the underlying dentin is exposed. The condition affects both deciduous and permanent teeth. Compare **enamel hypoplasia.** See also **amelogenesis imperfecta.**

enamel hypoplasia A developmental dental defect in which the enamel of the teeth is hard in context but thin and deficient in amount, caused by defective enamel matrix formation with a deficiency in the cementing substance. There is lack of contact between teeth, rapid breakdown of occlusive surfaces, and a yellow-to-brown stain that appears where the dentin is exposed. The condition, which affects both the deciduous and permanent teeth, is transmitted genetically or caused by environmental factors, as vitamin deficiency, fluorosis, exanthematous diseases, congenital syphilis, or injury or trauma to the mouth. Tetracycline use in the second half of pregnancy or during tooth development in the child also causes the condition. Compare **enamel hypocalcification.** See also **amelogenesis imperfecta.**

enanthema An eruptive lesion from the surface of a mucous membrane. Also called enanthem.

enarthrosis See **ball-and-socket joint.**

encapsulated Of arteries, muscles, nerves, and other body parts: enclosed in fibrous or membranous sheaths. See also **fascia bulbi, synovial sheath. —encapsulate,** v.

-encephalia A combining form meaning '(condition of the) brain': *amyelencephalia, rhinencephalia.* Also **-encephaly.**

encephalitis, pl. **encephalitides** An inflammatory condition of the brain. The cause is usually an arbovirus infection transmitted by the bite of an infected mosquito, but it may be the result of lead or other poisoning or of hemorrhage. **Postinfectious encephalitis** occurs as a complication of another infection, as chicken pox, influenza, or measles, or following smallpox vaccination. The condition is characterized by headache, neck pain, fever, nausea, and vomiting. Neurologic disturbances may occur, including seizures, personality change, irritability, lethargy, paralysis, weakness, and coma. The outcome depends on the cause, the age and condition of the person, and the extent of inflammation. Severe inflammation with destruction of nerve tissue may result in a seizure disorder, loss of a special sense or other permanent neurologic problem, or death. Usually, the inflammation involves the spinal cord and brain; hence, in most cases, a more accurate term is encephalomyelitis. See also **encephalomyelitis, equine encephalitis.**

encephalitis lethargica See **epidemic encephalitis.**

encephalocele Protrusion of the brain through a congenital or traumatic defect in the skull; hernia of the brain. Resulting paralysis and hydrocephalus are common. See also **neural tube defect.**

encephalodysplasia Any congenital anomaly of the brain.

encephalogram A radiograph of the brain made during encephalography.

encephalography Radiographic delineation of the structures of the brain containing fluid after the cerebrospinal fluid is withdrawn and replaced by a gas, as air, helium, or oxygen. The procedure is used mainly for indicating the site of cerebrospinal fluid obstruction in hydrocephalus or the structural abnormalities of the posterior fossa. Because of risks involved, it is used only when computerized tomography is not definitive. Kinds of encephalography are **pneumoencephalography, ventriculography.** Also called **air encephalography.** Compare **echoencephalography, electroencephalography. —encephalographic,** adj.

encephaloid carcinoma See **medullary carcinoma.**

encephalomeningocele See **meningoencephalocele.**

encephalomyelitis An inflammatory condition of the brain and the spinal cord characterized by fever, headache, stiff neck, back pain, and vomiting. Depending on the cause, the age and condition of the person, and the extent of the inflammation and irritation to the central nervous system, seizures, paralysis, personality changes, a decreased level of consciousness, coma, or death may occur. Sequelae, such as seizure disorders or decreased mental ability, may occur following severe inflammation that causes extensive damage to the cells and tissues of the nervous system. See also **equine encephalitis.**

encephalomyocarditis An infectious disease of the central nervous system caused by a group of small RNA viruses. Rodents are a major reservoir of the infection. Human illness ranges from asymptomatic infection to severe encephalomyelitis. Myocarditis is not a feature of infection in humans, and most victims recover promptly without sequelae. Treatment is supportive. See also **picornavirus.**

encephalopathy Any abnormal condition of the structure or function of tissues of the brain, especially chronic, destructive, or degenerative conditions, as Wernicke's encephalopathy.

encephalotrigeminal angiomatosis A congenital disorder characterized by a diffuse port wine stain of the face, angiomas of the leptomeninges and choroid, and late glaucoma, often associated with trigeminal nevi, calcified deposits in cerebral or meningeal tissue, mental retardation, epilepsy, and contralateral hemiplegia. Also called **Dimitri disease, Sturge-Weber syndrome.**

-encephaly See **-encephalia.**

enchondroma, pl. **enchondromas, enchondromata** A benign, slowly growing tumor of cartilage cells that arises in the extremity of the shaft of tubular bones, usually in the hands or feet. The growth of the neoplasm, by cell proliferation and the accession of small satellite tumors, may distend the bone. Also called **enchondrosis, true chondroma.**

enchondromatosis A congenital disorder in which cartilage proliferates within the extremity of the shafts of several bones, causing thinning of the cortex and distortion in length. Also called **dyschondroplasia, multiple enchondromatosis, Ollier's disease, skeletal enchondromatosis.** See also **Maffucci's syndrome.**

enchondromatous myxoma A tumor of the connective tissue, characterized by the presence of cartilage between the cells of connective tissue. See also **myxoma.**

enchondrosarcoma See **central chondrosarcoma.**

enchondrosis See **enchondroma.**

enchylema See **hyaloplasm.**

-enchyma A combining form meaning the 'liquid that nourishes tissue, or tissue itself': *karyenchyma, mesenchyma, sclerenchyma.*

encoded message In communication theory: a message as transmitted by a sender to a receiver.

encopresis Fecal incontinence. —**encopretic,** *adj.*

encounter In psychotherapy: the interaction between a patient and a psychotherapist, as occurs in existential therapy, or among several members of a small group, as in encounter or sensitivity-training groups, in which emotional change and personal growth are brought about by the expression of strong feelings by the participants. See also **group therapy, psychotherapy, sensitivity-training group.**

-ency A combining form meaning: **1.** A 'quality or state': *deficiency, dependency*. **2.** A 'person or thing in a state': *latency*. **3.** An 'instance of a quality or state': *emergency*. Also **-ance, -ancy.**

encyst To form a cyst or capsule. See also **cyst.** —**encysted,** *adj.*

end- See **endo-.**

endamebiasis, endamoebiasis See **amebiasis.**

Endamoeba, Endameba See ***Entamoeba.***

endarterectomy A surgical procedure that excises tunica intima of an artery that has become thickened by atherosclerosis.

endarteritis An inflammatory disorder of the inner layer of one or more arteries, which may become partially or completely occluded.

endarteritis obliterans An inflammatory condition of the lining of the arterial walls in which the intima proliferates, narrowing the lumen of the vessels and occluding the smaller vessels.

end bud A mass of undifferentiated cells produced from the remnants of the primitive node and the primitive streak at the caudal end of the developing embryo after the formation of the somites is completed. In lower animals it gives rise to the tail or any other caudal appendage and part of the trunk; in man it forms the caudal portion of the trunk. Also called **tail bud.**

end bulb of Krause See **Krause's corpuscle.**

endemic Of a disease or microorganism: indigenous to a geographic area or population. See also **epidemic, pandemic.**

endemic goiter An enlargement of the thyroid gland caused by the inadequate dietary intake of iodine. Iodine privation leads to diminished production and secretion of thyroid hormone by the gland. The pituitary gland, operating on a negative feedback system, senses the deficiency and secretes increased amounts of thyroid-stimulating hormone, causing hyperplasia and hypertrophy of the thyroid gland. The goiter may grow during the winter months and shrink during the summer months when more iodine-bearing fresh vegetables are eaten. Initially, the goiter is diffuse; later, it becomes multinodular. Endemic goiter occurs occasionally in adolescents at puberty and widely in population groups in geographic areas in which limited amounts of iodine are present in the soil,

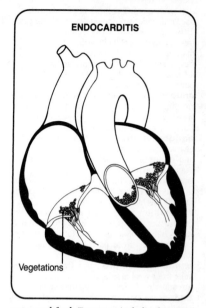

ENDOCARDITIS

Vegetations

water, and food. Treatment includes the use of iodized salt, injection of iodinated poppyseed oil, and dessicated thyroid given orally. A large goiter may cause dysphagia, dyspnea, tracheal deviation, and cosmetic problems.

endemic typhus A rickettsial infection transmitted by the bite of a rat flea infected with *Rickettsia typhi*. The disease, which is endemic to many areas of the world, is similar to epidemic typhus but less severe; the fever and rash last between 10 and 14 days. Permanent immunity follows infection. Treatment includes rest, an adequate intake of fluids, and tetracycline. A vaccine is available for people living in or intending to visit an area in which the disease is endemic. Also called **murine typhus.** Compare **Brill-Zinsser disease, epidemic typhus.**

endo-, end- A combining form meaning 'inward, within': *endobiotic, endocranial, endognathion*. Also **ento-.**

endocardial cushion defect Any cardiac defect resulting from the failure of the endocardial cushions in the embryonic heart to fuse and form the atrial septum. See also **atrial septal defect, congenital cardiac anomaly.**

endocardial fibroelastosis An abnormal condition characterized by hypertrophy of the wall of the left ventricle and the development of a thick, fibroelastic endocardium. This condition often increases the ventricular capacity but sometimes decreases it. Some studies incriminate the mumps virus fibroelastosis, while other studies refute a connection.

endocarditis An abnormal condition that affects the endocardium and the heart valves and is characterized by vegetations on the valves and endocardium produced by fibrin and platelet deposits on infection sites and caused by a variety of diseases. The kinds of endocarditis are bacterial endocarditis, nonbacterial endocarditis, and Libman-Sacks endocarditis. Untreated, all types of endocarditis are rapidly lethal, but they are often successfully treated by various antibacterial and surgical measures. With adequate treatment about 65% to 80% of the patients with endocarditis survive.

endocardium, *pl.* **endocardia** The interior lining of the heart, containing small blood vessels and a few bundles of smooth muscle. Compare **epicardium, myocardium.**

endocervicitis An abnormal condition characterized by inflammation of the epithelium and glands of the canal of the uterine cervix. See also **cervicitis.**

endocervix **1.** The membrane lining the canal of the uterine cervix. **2.** The opening of the cervix into the uterine cavity. —**endocervical,** *adj.*

endocrine **1.** Pertaining to an organ, gland, or structure that secretes a substance, as a hormone, into the blood or lymph for specific effect on another organ or part. **2.** Pertaining to internal secretion; hormonal.

endocrine fracture Any fracture that results from weakness of a specific bone due to an endocrine disorder, as hyperparathyroidism.

endocrine system The network of ductless glands and other structures that elaborate and secrete hormones directly into the blood stream, affecting the function of specific target organs. Glands of the endocrine system include the thyroid and the parathyroid, the anterior pituitary, the posterior pituitary, the pancreas, the suprarenal glands, and the gonads. The pineal gland is also considered an endocrine gland because it is ductless, although its precise endocrine function is not established. The thymus gland, once considered an endocrine gland, is now classified in the lymphatic system. Various other organs have some endocrinologic function. Secretions from the endocrine glands affect various processes throughout the body, as metabolism, growth, and secretions from other organs. See also **exocrine.**

endocrinology The study of the anatomy, physiology, and pathology of the endocrine system and of the treatment of endocrine problems. —**endocrinologist,** *n.*

endoderm In embryology: the innermost of the cell layers that develop from the embryonic disk of the inner cell mass of the blastocyst. From the endoderm arises the epithelium of the trachea, bronchi, lungs, gastrointestinal tract, liver, pancreas, urinary bladder, urachus, pharynx, thyroid, tympanic cavity, tonsils, and parathyroid glands. The endoderm thus comprises the lining of the cavities and passages of the body and the covering for most of the internal organs. Compare **ectoderm, mesoderm.**

endodermal cloaca A part of the cloaca in the developing embryo that lies internal to the cloacal membrane and gives rise to the bladder and urogenital ducts. Compare **ectodermal cloaca.** See also **urogenital sinus.**

endogenous depression A major affective disorder characterized by a persistent dysphoric mood, anxiety, irritability, fear, brooding, appetite and sleep disturbances, weight loss, psychomotor agitation or retardation, decreased energy, feelings of worthlessness or guilt, difficulty in concentrating or thinking, occasional delusions and hallucinations, and thoughts of death or suicide. The disorder may develop over a period of days, weeks, or months; episodes may occur in clusters or singly, separated by several years of normality. The causes of the disorder are multiple and complex and may involve biological, psychological, interpersonal, and sociocultural factors that lead to some unidentifiable intrapsychic conflict. Treatment includes the use of antidepressants and electroconvulsive therapy, followed by long-term psychotherapy. In severe cases, proper nursing care is needed for adequate nutrition, appropriate balance of fluid intake and output, good personal hygiene, and protection of the patient from self-injury. Also called **major depressive episode.** See also **bipolar disorder, depression.**

endogenous obesity Obesity resulting from dysfunction of the endocrine or metabolic systems. Compare **exogenous obesity.** See also **obesity.**

endolymph The fluid in the membranous labyrinth of the internal ear. Compare **perilymph.**

endolymphatic duct A passage joining an endolymphatic sac with a utricle and saccule.

endolymphatic hydrops See **Ménière's disease.**

endometrial **1.** Of or pertaining to the endometrium. **2.** Of or pertaining to the uterine cavity.

endometrial cancer A malignant neoplastic disease of the endometrium of the uterus most often occuring in the 5th or 6th decade of life. Associated factors include a medical history of infertility, anovulation, exogenous estrogen, uterine polyps, and a combination of diabetes, hypertension, and obesity. Abnormal vaginal bleeding, especially in a postmenopausal woman, is the cardinal symptom. Lower abdominal and low back pain may occur. A large, boggy uterus is often a sign of advanced disease. Less than half the patients with endometrial cancer have a positive Papanicolaou (Pap) test of the cervix and vagina, because the tumor cells rarely exfoliate in early stages of the lesion. Diagnosis depends on dilatation and curettage of each section of the uterus, vacuum curettage, or a Pap test of cells obtained from jet washings of the uterine cavity. Adenocarcinomas constitute roughly 90% of all endometrial tumors; mixed carcinomas, sarcomas, and benign adenocanthomas comprise the rest. Endometrial lesions may spread to the cervix but rarely invade the vagina. They metastasize to the broad ligaments, fallopian tubes, and ovaries so frequently that bilateral salpingo-oophorectomy with abdominal hysterectomy is the usual treatment. Radium implant therapy is usually administered pre-

ENDOMETRIOSIS OF THE OVARY, FALLOPIAN TUBE, AND RECTOSIGMOID

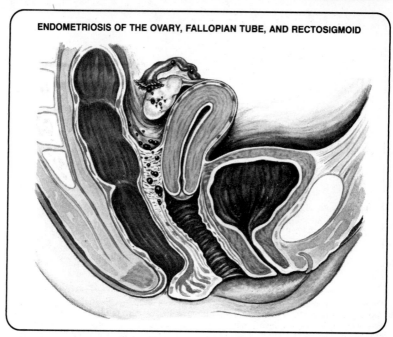

operatively and postoperatively. High doses of a progestogen may be administered for palliation in advanced or inoperable cases.

endometrial hyperplasia An abnormal condition characterized by overgrowth of the endometrium owing to sustained stimulation by estrogen (of endogenous or exogenous origin) that is not opposed by progesterone. Estrogens act as growth hormone for endometrium. Through a complex intercellular mechanism, endometrial cells bind estrogens preferentially and undergo changes characteristic of the proliferative phase of the menstrual cycle. If estrogen stimulation continues for 3 to 6 months without periodic cessation or counteractive progesterone stimulation, as occurs in anovulatory or perimenopausal women or in women receiving replacement estrogen without added progestogen, the endometrium becomes abnormally thickened and glandularized. Unremitting estrogen stimulation eventually causes cystic or adenomatous endometrial hyperplasia, the latter a premalignant lesion that undergoes malignant degeneration in approximately 25% of women having it. The causative relationship between estrogen and endometrial hyperplasia is well established; there is implication but not proof that estrogen also provokes the change from hyperplasia to neoplasia and malignancy. Endometrial hyperplasia often results in abnormal uterine bleeding; such bleeding, particularly in older women, constitutes an indication for biopsy or curettage of the endometrium to establish histopathologic diagnosis and to rule out malignancy. A functioning estrogen-secreting tumor is suspected if the woman is not taking estrogen medication. Progestogen therapy is effective in reversing the abnormal histopathologic changes of endometrial hyperplasia; if the hyperplasia is adenomatous, hysterectomy is commonly performed.

endometrial polyp A pedunculated overgrowth of endometrium, usually benign. Polyps are a common cause of vaginal bleeding in perimenopausal women and are often associated with other uterine abnormalities, as endometrial hyperplasia or fibroids. They may occur singly or in clusters and are usually 1 cm (½ inch) or less in diameter, but they may become much larger and prolapse through the cervix. Treatment for the condition includes surgical dilatation and curettage.

endometriosis An abnormal gynecologic condition characterized by ectopic growth and function of endometrial tissue. Precise incidence of the disease is unknown, but evidence of it is found in approximately 15% of women who undergo pelvic laparotomy for other indications. Women of higher socioeconomic status and women who defer pregnancy are more likely to contract the disease. It is uncommon among black women. Pregnancy has a definite but inconsistent influence in preventing or ameliorating the disease. The etiology of endometriosis is unknown; evidence suggests that the ectopic endometrium of endometriosis develops from vestigial tissue of the Wolffian or Müllerian ducts; other evidence strongly suggests that fragments of endometrium from the lining of the uterus are regurgitated backward during menstruation

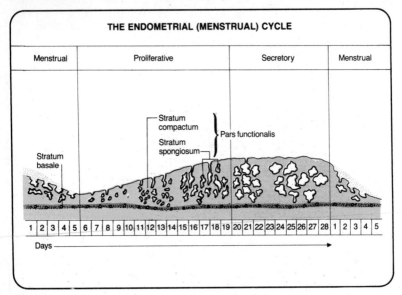

THE ENDOMETRIAL (MENSTRUAL) CYCLE

| Menstrual | Proliferative | Secretory | Menstrual |

Stratum compactum
Stratum spongiosum
Pars functionalis
Stratum basale

1 2 3 4 5 6 7 8 9 10 11 12 13 14 15 16 17 18 19 20 21 22 23 24 25 26 27 28 1 2 3 4 5

Days

through the fallopian tubes into the peritoneal cavity, where they attach, grow, and function. Fragments of this tissue, which is microscopically similar to or identical with endometrium, may be found in the wall of the uterus or on its surface, in or on the tubes, ovaries, rectosigmoid, or pelvic peritoneum, or, occasionally, in remote, extrapelvic areas. When endometriosis occurs in a critical location, it may result in grave dysfunction of the organ involved or, rarely, in death; intestinal obstruction is a common complication. The most characteristic symptom of endometriosis is pain, particularly dysmenorrhea and dyspareunia, but also dysuria, painful defecation, and suprapubic soreness. Pain is not always present, however, and its absence does not rule out the presence of the disease. Other common symptoms include premenstrual vaginal staining of blood, hypermenorrhea, and infertility. On pelvic examination, tender nodularity of the uterosacral ligaments is commonly found. Diagnosis is made by biopsy of lesions. Treatment of milder forms may consist only of medication with analgesics and expectant follow-up, because many women outgrow mild endometriosis or the condition subsides when they become pregnant. With more extensive disease, treatment is hormonal or surgical and is directed at reducing the size and number of lesions, relieving symptoms, and correcting infertility, if present. Prolonged suppression of ovulation may produce a hormonal milieu similar to pregnancy and result in partial or total regression of lesions; this condition of 'pseudopregnancy' may be brought about with administration of estrogen and progestogen separately or in combination or, less often, with an androgen. Among women with endometriosis and infertility who undergo prolonged hormonal therapy, approx-

imately 40% become pregnant subsequent to treatment. Advanced endometriosis often requires surgery, including total abdominal hysterectomy and bilateral salpingo-oophorectomy to remove large lesions and to terminate the cyclic ovarian stimulation on which endometrial growth depends, so that retained lesions atrophy and heal.

endometritis An inflammatory condition of the endometrium, usually caused by bacterial infection, commonly gonococci or hemolytic streptococci. It is characterized by fever, abdominal pain, malodorous discharge, and enlargement of the uterus. It occurs most frequently following childbirth or abortion and in women fitted with an intrauterine contraceptive device. The diagnosis may be made by physical examination, history, laboratory analysis revealing an elevated white blood cell count, ultrasound, and bacteriologic identification of the pathogen. Treatment includes antibiotics, rest, analgesia, an adequate intake of fluids, and, if necessary, surgical drainage of a suppurating abscess, hysterectomy, or salpingo-oophorectomy. Endometritis may be mild and self-limited, chronic, or acute. It may result in sterility owing to scar formation occluding the fallopian tubes.

endometritis dessicans Endometritis characterized by ulceration and shedding of the endometrium of the uterus.

endometrium The mucous membrane lining of the uterus, consisting of the stratum compactum, the stratum spongiosum, and the stratum basale. The endometrium changes in thickness and structure with the menstrual cycle. The stratum compactum and the stratum spongiosum comprise the pars funtionalis and are shed with each menstrual flow. The pars functionalis is known as the decidua during pregnancy, when it underlies the placenta. Compare **parametrium.**

endomorph   A person whose body build is characterized by a soft, round physique with a large trunk and thighs, tapering extremities, an accumulation of fat throughout the body, and a predominance of structures derived from the endoderm. Compare **ectomorph, mesomorph.** See also **pyknic.**

endoparasite   In medical parasitology: an organism that lives within the body of the host, as a tapeworm.

endophthalmitis   An inflammatory condition of the internal eye in which the eye becomes red, swollen, painful, and, sometimes, filled with pus. This condition may blur the vision and cause vomiting, fever, and headache. Endophthalmitis may result from bacterial or fungal infection, trauma, allergy, drug or chemical toxicity, or vascular disease. Depending on the cause, therapy requires surgical intervention or the administration of an antibiotic, atropine, or a corticosteroid. Also called **endophthalmia.**

endophthalmitis phacoanaphylactica   An abnormal condition characterized by an acute autoimmune reaction of the eye. It is caused by hypersensitivity of the eye to the protein of the crystalline lens and commonly occurs after trauma to the crystalline lens or after a cataract operation. Associated symptoms include swelling and inflammation of the eye, severe pain, and blurred vision. The substance of the lens is invaded by polymorphonuclear cells and mononuclear phagocytes. Sensitization of one eye often follows the extracapsular removal of the lens of the other eye. Accurate diagnosis must differentiate between this condition and infectious endophthalmitis. Therapy is supportive and commonly includes the administration of corticosteroids and atropine. Refractory cases may require surgical removal of the lens. Compare **uveitis.**

endophytic   Of or pertaining to the tendency to grow inward, as an endophytic tumor that grows on the inside of an organ or structure.

endoplasmic reticulum   An extensive network of membrane-enclosed tubules in the cytoplasm of cells. The ultramicroscopic organelle, which can be seen only with an electron microscope, is classified as granular or rough-surfaced when ribosomes are attached to the surface of the membrane and agranular or smooth-surfaced when ribosomes are absent. The structure functions in the synthesis of proteins and lipids and in the transport of these metabolites within the cell.

endorphin   Any one of the neuropeptides composed of many amino acids, elaborated by the pituitary gland, and acting on the central and the peripheral nervous systems to reduce pain. Endorphins isolated by researchers are alpha endorphin, beta endorphin, and gamma endorphin, all chemicals producing pharmacological effects similar to morphine. Beta en-

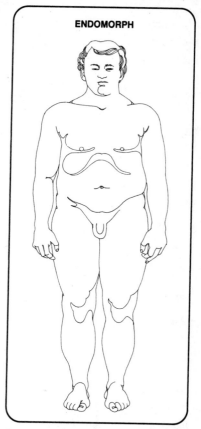

ENDOMORPH

dorphin has been isolated in the brain and in the gastrointestinal tract and seems to be the most potent of the endorphins. Beta endorphin is composed of 31 amino acids that are identical to part of the sequence of 91 amino acids of the hormone beta lipoprotein, also produced by the pituitary gland. Behavioral tests indicate that beta endorphin is a powerful analgesic in humans and animals. Brain-stimulated analgesia in humans releases beta endorphin into the cerebrospinal fluid. Compare **enkephalin.**

endorsement   A statement of recognition of the license of a health practitioner in one state by another state, relieving the health practitioner of going through the full licensing procedure of the state in which practice is to be undertaken.

endoscope   An illuminated optical instrument for the visualization of the interior of a body cavity or organ. Available in varying lengths, it has great flexibility, reaching previously inaccessible areas. Although generally introduced through a natural opening in the body, it may also be inserted through an incision. Other instruments for viewing specific areas of the body include the bronchoscope, cystoscope, gastro-

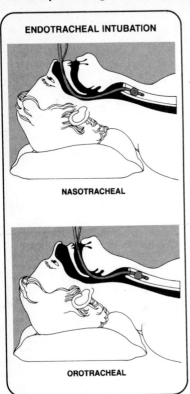

ENDOTRACHEAL INTUBATION

NASOTRACHEAL

OROTRACHEAL

scope, laparoscope, otoscope, and vaginoscope. See also **fiberoptics.** —**endoscopic,** *adj.*

endoscopic retrograde cholangiography In radiology: a diagnostic procedure for outlining the common bile duct. A flexible fiberoptic duodenoscope is placed in the common bile duct, a radiopaque substance is instilled directly into the duct, and serial X-rays are taken. See also **cholangiography.**

endoscopy The visualization of the interior of organs and cavities of the body with an endoscope. The procedure is indicated for the diagnosis of gastric ulcers with atypical radiologic features, to locate the source of upper gastrointestinal bleeding, to establish the presence and extent of varices in the lower esophagus and stomach in patients with liver disease, and to detect any abnormalities of the lower colon. For examination of the lower colon, fecal material is removed by enema, laxative, or suppository. The patient is placed in the knee-chest position for the examination of the lower colon and afterward is observed by the nurse for abdominal pain or rectal bleeding. Endoscopy can also be used to obtain samples for cytological and histological examination and to follow the course of a disease, as the assessment of the healing of gastric and duodenal ulcers. See also **arthroscopy, bronchoscopy, cystoscopy, gastros-**

copy, laparoscopy. —**endoscopic,** *adj.*

endothelial myeloma See **Ewing's sarcoma.**

-endothelioma A combining form meaning 'a tumor of endothelial tissue': *hemendothelioma, lymphendothelioma.*

endothelium The layer of squamous epithelial cells that lines the heart, the blood and the lymph vessels, and the serous cavities of the body. It is highly vascular, heals quickly, and is derived from the mesoderm.

endotoxin A toxin contained in the cell walls of some microorganisms, especially gram-negative bacteria, that is released when the bacterium dies and is broken down in the body. Fever, chills, shock, leukopenia, and a variety of other symptoms result, depending on the particular organism and the condition of the infected person.

endotracheal Within or through the trachea.

endotracheal anesthesia Inhalation anesthesia that is achieved by the passage of an anesthetic gas or mixture of gases through an endotracheal tube into the respiratory tract. General anesthesia is usually obtained by endotracheal anesthesia.

endotracheal intubation The management of the patient with an airway catheter inserted through the mouth or nose into the trachea. An endotracheal tube may be used to maintain a patent airway, to prevent aspiration of material from the digestive tract in the unconscious or paralyzed patient, to permit suctioning of tracheobronchial secretions, or to administer positive pressure ventilation that cannot be given effectively by a mask. Endotracheal tubes may be made of rubber or plastic and usually have an inflatable cuff to maintain a closed system with the ventilator. The endotracheal tube is inserted via the mouth or nose through the larynx into the trachea; if the oral route is used, a bite block or oral airway may be required to keep the patient from biting and obstructing the tube. Breath sounds are auscultated immediately after insertion and every 1 to 2 hours thereafter to make certain the tube is properly positioned and is not obstructing one of the mainstem bronchi. Once the tube is correctly positioned, it is taped securely in place and checked frequently for patency and slippage. The trachea is suctioned as needed and irrigated with normal saline solution, if ordered. The patient is usually on mechanical ventilation with the cuff of the endotracheal tube inflated; if the patient can breathe independently, the trachea and mouth are suctioned, the cuff is deflated, and the respiratory rate and quality are checked hourly. Parenteral fluids are administered as ordered; nothing is given orally; the intake and output of fluids are measured and recorded. The patient's level of consciousness is determined hourly and, if sufficiently conscious, a method of communication is established.

NURSING CONSIDERATIONS: The nurse monitors the position and patency of the endotracheal tube,

ENEMAS

SOLUTION	PREPARATION	PURPOSE
Irrigating enemas		
Harris flush	1,000 ml of tap water	Cleansing
Magnesium sulfate	Add 3 tbsp of magnesium sulfate to 3 tbsp of salt in 1,500 ml of tap water	Therapeutic
Saline	If a commercially prepared solution isn't available, add 2 tsp of salt to 1,000 ml of tap water.	Cleansing
Soap and water	Add 1 packet of mild soap to 1,000 ml of tap water and remove all bubbles before administering	Cleansing
Retention enemas		
Mayo	Dissolve 60 ml of white sugar in 240 ml of warmed tap water. Add 30 ml of sodium bicarbonate to mixture immediately before administration.	Therapeutic
Milk and molasses	Add 175 to 200 ml of hot milk to 175 to 200 ml of molasses. Heat mixture to 71.1°C (160°F) and then cool to 40.5°C (105°F).	Therapeutic
Oil	150 ml of mineral, olive, or cottonseed oil	Cleansing, therapeutic
Olive oil and glycerin	Add 60 ml of olive oil to 60 ml of glycerin	Cleansing, therapeutic
1-2-3	Add 30 ml of magnesium sulfate 50% to 60 ml of glycerin. Add mixture to 90 ml of warm tap water.	Cleansing
Starch	Add 1 tsp of powdered starch to 60 ml of cold tap water and add to 160 ml of boiling tap water or add 30 ml of liquid starch mix to the boiling water. Boil the mixture for 2 minutes and then cool to 40.5°C (105°F).	Therapeutic

performs the necessary suctioning, inflates and deflates the cuff at appropriate times, checks vital signs, and monitors the patient for adequate mechanical ventilation.

endotracheal tube A large-bore catheter inserted through the mouth or nose and into the trachea to a point above the bifurcation of the trachea (carina) proximal to the bronchi. It is used for delivering oxygen when ventilation must be totally controlled and in general anesthetic procedures.

endoxin An endogenous, recently discovered analog of digoxin, occurring naturally in humans. It is a hormone that may regulate the excretion of salt.

-ene A combining form naming hydrocarbons: *ethidene, somnifene, xanthene.*

enema A procedure in which a solution is introduced into the rectum for cleansing or therapeutic purposes. Enemas may be commercially packed disposable units or reusable equipment prepared just prior to use.
NURSING CONSIDERATIONS: The patient is warned that some discomfort may occur because the colon tends to contract when distended by the fluid. The enema is given slowly to avoid sudden distention that would cause peristalsis, or spasm, and increased discomfort. A call bell is kept within reach of the patient during expulsion of the enema, because the procedure and the effort required to expel the enema may cause faintness. The color, consistency, and amount of material evacuated are evaluated. The patient is carefully observed for signs of adverse effects.

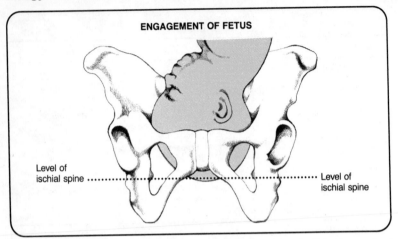

ENGAGEMENT OF FETUS

Level of ischial spine ·· Level of ischial spine

energy The capacity to do work or to perform vigorous activity. Compare **anergy.** —**energetic,** *adj.*

energy-protein malnutrition A condition resulting from a diet deficient in both calories and proteins. Also called protein-calorie malnutrition. See also **marasmic kwashiorkor, marasmus.**

en face French for 'face to face.' A position in which the mother's face and the infant's face are approximately 20 cm (8 inches) apart, as when the mother holds the infant up in front of her face or when she nurses the child. Studies of maternal and infant bonding have shown that the mother seeks eye-to-eye contact with her infant, and, if she is not stopped, she will instinctively move the baby to an en-face position. In addition, infants have been shown to prefer a human face over other visual stimuli and to be best able to focus at a distance of 20 to 25 cm (8 to 10 inches).

enflurane A nonflammable anesthetic gas belonging to the ether family, used for induction and maintenance of general anesthesia in cases in which ethers are the drugs of choice. A halogenated volatile liquid, enflurane is administered through vaporizers specially calibrated for delivery via nitrous oxide or an oxygen-nitrous oxide mixture, permitting close control of dosage. Because excitement may occur on induction, a hypnotic dose of short-acting barbiturate is sometimes used for premedication. Adverse reactions may include seizure activity, muscle fasciculation, hypotension, cardiac arrhythmia, shivering, and elevated white blood cell count. Nausea and vomiting on emergence from anesthesia sometimes occur.

engagement In obstetrics: **1.** Fixation of the presenting part of the fetus in the maternal pelvis. The lowest part of the presenting part is at or below the level of the ischial spines. **2.** Fixation of the fetal head in the maternal pelvis with the biparietal diameter of the head level with the ischial spines.

English position See **lateral recumbent position.**

engrossment See **bonding.**

enkephalin One of two pentapeptides produced in the body that reduce pain. Researchers have isolated enkephalins in the pituitary gland, brain, and gastrointestinal tract. The enkephalins are methionine enkephalin and isoleucine enkephalin, each composed of five amino acids, four of which are identical in both compounds. It is believed that these two neuropeptides can depress neurons throughout the central nervous system. Axon terminals that release enkephalins are concentrated in the posterior horn of the gray matter of the spinal cord, in the central part of the thalamus, and in the amygdala of the limbic system of the cerebrum. Enkephalins inhibit neurotransmitters in the pathway for pain perception, thereby reducing the emotional as well as the physical impact of pain. Although it is not known how these two neuropeptides function, many experts believe the enkephalins are not only natural pain killers, but that they may be involved, with other neuropeptides, in the development of some psychopathological behaviors. Compare **endorphin.**

enomania See **oinomania.**

enophthalmos Backward displacement of the eye in the bony socket, caused by traumatic injury or developmental defect. Ptosis may cause a false impression of enophthalmos. —**enophthalmic,** *adj.*

ensiform process See **xiphoid process.**

entamebiasis, entamoebiasis See **amebiasis.**

Entamoeba, Entameba A genus of intestinal parasite of which several species are pathogenic to humans. See also *Entamoeba histolytica.*

Entamoeba histolytica A pathogenic species of ameba that causes amebic dysentery and hepatic amebiasis in humans. See also **amebiasis, amebic dysentery, hepatic amebiasis.**

enter- See **entero-.**

enteric fever See **typhoid fever.**

enteric infection A disease of the intestine owing to any infection. Symptoms similar to those caused by pathogens may be produced by chemical toxins in ingested foods and by allergic reactions to certain food substances. Among bacteria commonly involved in enteric infections are *Escherichia coli, Vibrio cholerae,* and several species of *Salmonella, Shigella,* and anaerobic streptococci. Enteric infections are characterized by diarrhea, abdominal discomfort, nausea and vomiting, anorexia, and fluid and electrolyte loss as a result of severe vomiting and diarrhea. Treatment may include I.V. replacement of fluids and electrolytes, medication for sedation and relief of abdominal cramps, and antibiotics.Nothing is offered by mouth until vomiting ceases; then a clear liquid diet may be given.

entericoid fever Any febrile disease characterized by intestinal inflammation and dysfunction. See also **enteric infection, typhoid fever.**

enteritis Inflammation of the mucosal lining of the small intestine, resulting from a variety of causes: bacterial, viral, functional, and inflammatory. Involvement of the small and large intestine is called enterocolitis. Compare **gastroenteritis.**

entero-, enter- A combining form meaning 'pertaining to the intestines': *enteric, enterobiliary, enteroptosis.*

Enterobacter aerogenes See *Enterobacter cloacae.*

Enterobacter cloacae A common species of bacterium found in human and animal feces, dairy products, sewage, soil, and water. It is rarely the cause of disease. Also called *Aerobacter aerogenes, Enterobacter aerogenes.*

enterobacterial Of or pertaining to a species of bacterium found in the digestive tract.

Enterobactericae A family of aerobic and anaerobic bacteria that includes both normal and pathogenic enteric microorganisms. Among the significant genera of the family are *Escherichia, Klebsiella, Proteus, Salmonella.*

enterobiasis A parasitic infestation with *Enterobius vermicularis,* the common pinworm. The worms infect the large intestine, and the females deposit eggs in the perianal area, causing pruritis and insomnia. Reinfection commonly occurs by transfer of eggs to the mouth by contaminated fingers. Airborne transmission is possible, as eggs remain viable for 2 or 3 days in contaminated bedclothes. To make the diagnosis, the sticky side of an adhesive cellophane tape swab is pressed against the perianal skin and examined for eggs under a microscope. Therapy for the whole family may be necessary and involves use of anthelmintics. Personal hygiene, including handwashing, is the best preventive measure. There appears to be little benefit from disinfection procedures for the home. Also called **oxyuriasis.**

Enterobius vermicularis A common parasitic nematode that resembles a white thread between 0.5 and 1 cm (¼ and ½ inch) long. Also called **pinworm, seatworm, threadworm.**

enterochromaffin cell See **argentaffin cell.**

enterokinase An intestinal fluid enzyme that activates the proteolytic enzyme in pancreatic fluid by converting trypsinogen to trypsin.

enterolith A stone or concretion found within the intestine. See also **calculus.**

enterolithiasis The presence of enteroliths in the intestine.

enterostomal therapist A registered nurse with at least 2 years of full-time clinical experience, who has completed a continuing education course in the care and teaching of patients with stomas and draining wounds. To be certified by the International Association for Enterostomal Therapy (an advantage but not a requirement for employment as an enterostomal therapist), a nurse must also pass a written examination.

enterostomy A surgical procedure that produces an artificial anus or fistula in the intestine by incision through the abdominal wall. Compare **colostomy.** —**enterostomal,** *adj.*

enterovirus A virus that multiplies primarily in the intestinal tract. Kinds of enteroviruses are **coxsackievirus, echovirus, poliovirus.** —**enteroviral,** *adj.*

ento- See **endo-.**

entoderm See **endoderm.**

entrainment A phenomenon observed in the microanalysis of sound films in which the speaker moves several parts of the body and the listener responds to the sounds by moving in ways that are coordinated with the rhythm of the sounds. Infants have been observed to move in time to the rhythms of adult speech but not to random noises or disconnected words or vowels. Entrainment is thought to be an essential factor in the process of maternal-infant bonding.

entropion Turning inward or turning towards, usually a condition in which the eyelid turns inward toward the eye. **Cicatricial entropion** can occur in either the upper or lower eyelid as a result of scar tissue formation. **Spastic entropion** results from an inflammation of the eyelid or other factor that affects tissue tone. The inflammation may be the result of an infectious disease or irritation from an inverted eyelash. Compare **ectropion.** See also **blepharitis.**

entropy The tendency of a system to go from a state of order to a state of disorder, expressed in physics as a measure of the part of the heat or energy in a thermodynamic system that is not available to perform work. Living organisms tend to go from a state of disorder to a state of order in their development and thus appear to reverse entropy. However, maintaining a living system requires the expenditure of energy, leaving less energy available for work, with the result that the entropy of the universe is increasing.

enucleation **1.** Removal of an organ or tumor in one piece. **2.** Removal of the eyeball,

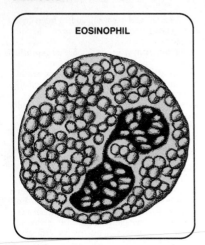

EOSINOPHIL

performed in malignancy, severe infection, extensive trauma, or to control pain in glaucoma. The procedure involves cutting the optic nerve and muscle attachments; if possible, the surrounding layer of fascia is left with the muscles. A ball-shaped implant of silicone, plastic, or tantalum is inserted and the muscles are sutured around it, providing a permanent stump to give support and motion to an artificial eye. Postoperatively, pressure dressings are kept in place for 1 or 2 days to prevent hemorrhage. Other possible complications include thrombosis of nearby blood vessels, which may lead to infection, including meningitis.

enuresis Incontinence of urine, especially in bed at night.

environment All of the many factors, as physical and psychological, that influence or affect the life and survival of a person. See also **biome, climate. —environmental,** *adj.*

environmental carcinogen Any one of many natural and synthetic substances that can cause cancer. Such agents, or oncogens, may be divided into chemical agents, physical agents, and certain hormones and viruses. Some environmental carcinogens are arsenic, asbestos, uranium, vinyl chloride, ionizing radiation, ultraviolet rays, X-rays, and various coal tar derivatives. Carcinogenic effects of chemicals may occur quickly or be delayed as long as 30 years. Most carcinogens are unreactive or secondary carcinogens but are converted to primary carcinogens in the body. Research indicates that numerous factors, as heredity, affect the susceptibilities of different individuals to cancer-causing agents.

enzygotic twins See **monozygotic twins.**

enzyme A protein produced by living cells that catalyzes chemical reactions in organic matter. Most enzymes are produced in minute quantities and catalyze reactions within cells. Digestive enzymes, however, are produced in relatively large quantities and act outside the cells in the lumen of the digestive tube.

eosin A group of red, acidic xanthine dyes, often used in combination with a blue-purple basic dye, as hematoxylin, to stain tissue slides in the laboratory.

eosinophil A granulocytic, bilobed leukocyte, somewhat larger than a neutrophil, characterized by the large number of coarse, refractile, cytoplasmic granules that stain intensely with the acid dye eosin. Eosinophils constitute 1% to 3% of the white blood cells of the body. The total eosinophil count increases with allergy and certain infections and decreases when steroid medications such as cortisone and prednisone are being administered. See also **basophil, neutrophil. —eosinophilic,** *adj.*

eosinophilia An increase in the number of eosinophils in the blood, accompanying many inflammatory conditions. Substantial increases are considered a reflection of an allergic response.

eosinophilic **1.** The tendency of a cell, tissue, or organism to be readily stained by the dye eosin. **2.** Of or pertaining to an eosinophilic leukocyte.

eosinophilic adenoma See **acidophilic adenoma.**

eosinophilic enteropathy A rare form of food allergy that is characterized by nausea, crampy abdominal pain, diarrhea, urticaria, an elevated eosinophil count in the blood, and eosinophilic infiltrates in the intestine. Diagnosis is made by an elimination diet; symptoms usually disappear when the offending food is removed from the diet.

eosinophilic granuloma A growth characterized by numerous eosinophils and histiocytes, occurring as a single or multiple lesion in bone. Eosinophilic granulomas may also develop in the lung and occur most frequently in children and adolescents.

eosinophilic leukemia A malignant neoplasm of leukocytes in which eosinophils are the predominant cells. It resembles chronic myelocytic leukemia but may have an acute course even though there are no blast forms in the peripheral blood.

eosinophilic pneumonia Inflammation of the lungs, characterized by infiltration of the alveoli with eosinophils and large mononuclear cells, pulmonary edema, fever, night sweats, cough, dyspnea, and weight loss. The disease may be caused by a hypersensitivity reaction to spores of fungi, plant fibers, wood dust, bird droppings, porcine, bovine, or piscine proteins, *Bacillus subtilus* enzyme in detergents, or certain drugs. Treatment consists of removal of the offending allergen and symptomatic and supportive therapy.

-eous A combining form meaning 'like something' specified: *anedeous, cutaneous, osseous.*

ep- See **epi-.**

ependyma The lining membrane of the ventricles of the brain and of the central canal of the spinal cord.

ependymal glioma A large, vascular, fairly solid glioma in the brain's fourth ventricle.

ependymoblastoma A malignant neoplasm composed of primitive cells of the ependyma. Also called **malignant ependymoma.**

ependymocytoma See **ependymoma.**

ependymoma A neoplasm composed of differentiated cells of the ependyma. The tumor, which is usually a benign, pale, firm, encapsulated, somewhat nodular mass, commonly arises from the roof of the fourth ventricle and usually grows slowly. It may extend to the spinal cord. Primary lesions may also develop in the spinal cord. Also called **ependymocytoma.**

ephapse A point of lateral contact between nerve fibers across which impulses are transmitted directly by electrical means through the membranes of the cells rather than across the synapse through the action of a neurotransmitter. Compare **synapse. —ephaptic,** *adj.*

ephaptic transmission The passage of a neural impulse from one nerve fiber to another through the nerve membrane by electrical means rather than across a synapse through the action of a neurotransmitter. The mechanism may be a factor in epileptic seizures because of the density of neurons in the brain. Compare **synaptic.**

ephedrine sulfate A sympathomimetic vasoconstrictor often used as a nasal decongestant.

ephemeral fever Any febrile condition lasting only 24 to 48 hours that is uncomplicated and of unknown etiology.

epi-, ep- A combining form meaning 'on, upon': *epicanthus, epicostal, epidural.*

epiblast 1. See **ectoderm.** 2. The primordial outer layer of the blastocyst or blastula, before differentiation of the germ layers, that gives rise to the ectoderm and contains cells capable of forming the endoderm and mesoderm. **—epiblastic,** *adj.*

epicanthus A vertical fold of skin over the angle of the inner canthus of the eye. It may be slight or marked, covering the canthus and the caruncle. It is normal in oriental people and is of no clinical significance. Some infants with Down's syndrome have the folds. Also called epicanthal fold, epicanthic fold. **—epicanthal, epicanthic,** *adj.*

epicardium One of the three layers of tissue that form the wall of the heart. It is composed of a single sheet of squamous epithelial cells overlying delicate connective tissue. The epicardium is the visceral portion of the serous pericardium and folds back upon itself to form the parietal portion of the serous pericardium. Compare **myocardium. —epicardial,** *adj.*

epicondylar fracture Any fracture that involves the medial or the lateral epicondyle of a specific bone, as the humerus.

epicondyle A projection on the surface of a bone above its condyle. **—epicondylar,** *adj.*

epicondylitis A painful and sometimes disabling inflammation of the elbow muscle and surrounding tissue, owing to repeated strain on the forearm near the lateral epicondyle of the humerus, as from violent extension or supination of the wrist against a resisting force. The strain may result from activities, as tennis or golf, twisting a screwdriver, or carrying a heavy load with the arm extended. Treatment usually includes rest, injection of procaine with or without hydrocortisone, and, in some cases, surgery to release part of the muscle from the epicondyle. Also called tennis elbow, lateral humeral epicondylitis.

epicranial aponeurosis A fibrous membrane that covers the cranium between the occipital and frontal muscles of the scalp. Also called **galea aponeurotica.**

epicranium The complete scalp, including the integument, the muscular sheets, and the aponeuroses. Compare **epicranius. —epicranial,** *adj.*

epicranius The broad, muscular, and tendinous layer of tissue covering the top and the sides of the skull from the occipital bone to the eyebrows. It consists of broad, thin muscular bellies, connected by an extensive aponeurosis. Innervation of the epicranius by branches of the facial nerves can draw back the scalp, raise the eyebrows, and move the ears. Compare **epicranium.** See also **galea aponeurotica, occipitofrontalis, temporoparietalis.**

epidemic 1. Affecting a significantly large number of people at the same time. 2. A disease that spreads rapidly through a demographic segment of the human population, as everyone in a given geographic area or everyone of a certain age or sex. 3. A widespread disease that tends to occur periodically. Compare **endemic, epizootic, pandemic.**

epidemic encephalitis Any diffuse inflammation of the brain occurring in epidemic form. Some kinds of epidemic encephalitis are influenzal encephalitis, Japanese B encephalitis, Russian spring-summer encephalitis, St. Louis encephalitis. See also **encephalitis.**

epidemic hemoglobinuria See **hemoglobinuria.**

epidemic hemorrhagic fever A severe viral infection marked by fever and bleeding. The disorder develops rapidly, characterized initially by fever and muscle ache, possibly followed by hemorrhage, peripheral vascular collapse, hypovolemic shock, and acute kidney failure. The arbovirus or other pathogen is believed to be transmitted by mosquitoes, ticks, or mites. The pathophysiology of the hemorrhagic effect is uncertain, although it is assumed the disease organism causes the development of lesions in the lining of the capillaries. Among the various forms of epidemic hemorrhagic fevers are **Argentine hemorrhagic fever, Bolivian hemorrhagic fever, dengue hemorrhagic fever shock syndrome, Lassa fever, yellow fever.** See also specific viral infections.

epidemic myalgia See **epidemic pleurodynia.**

epidemic myositis See **epidemic pleurodynia.**

epidemic parotitis See **mumps.**

epidemic pleurodynia An infection caused by a coxsackievirus, affecting mainly children. It is characterized by severe intermittent pain

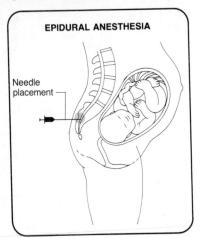

EPIDURAL ANESTHESIA

Needle placement

in the abdomen or lower chest, fever, headache, sore throat, malaise, and extreme myalgia. The symptoms may continue for weeks or subside after a few days and recur for a period of weeks. Treatment is symptomatic; complete recovery is usual. Also called **Bornholm disease, devil's grip, epidemic myositis.** See also **coxsackievirus, viral disease.**

epidemic typhus   An acute, severe rickettsial infection characterized by prolonged high fever, headache, and a dark maculopapular rash that covers most of the body. The causative organism, *Rickettsia prowazekii*, is transmitted indirectly as a result of the bite of the human body louse; the pathogen is contained in feces of the louse and enters the body tissues as the bite is scratched. An intense headache and a fever reaching 40°C (104°F) begin after an incubation period of 10 days to 2 weeks. The rash follows. Complications may include vascular collapse, renal failure, pneumonia, or gangrene. Mortality is high among older patients. Treatment may include chloramphenicol or tetracycline, aspirin, and supportive, symptomatic care. Also called **classic typhus, European typhus, jail fever, louse-borne typhus.** See also **rickettsia, typhus.**

epidemiology   The study of the occurrence, distribution, and causes of health and disease in mankind. —**epidemiologic, epidemiological,** *adj.,* **epidemiologist,** *n.*

epiderm-, epidermo-   A combining form meaning 'of or pertaining to the epidermis': *epidermoid, epidermolysis, epidermolytic.*

epidermis   The superficial, avascular layers of the skin, made up of an outer, dead, cornified portion and a deeper, living, cellular portion. Epidermal cells gradually move outward to the skin surface, undergoing change as they migrate, until they are desquamated as cornified flakes. Cells in various transitional stages make up the basal cell layer, the prickle cell layer, the granular layer, and the cornified layer. Altogether, these layers are between 0.5 mm and 1.1

mm in thickness. Also called **cuticle.** —**epidermal, epidermoid,** *adj.*

epidermoid carcinoma   A malignant neoplasm in which the tumor cells tend to differentiate in the manner of epidermal cells and then form horny cells called prickle cells.

epidermoid cyst   A common, benign, fluctuant, subcutaneous swelling lined by keratinizing epithelium and filled with a cheesy material composed of sebum and epithelial debris. The cyst is movable but attached to the skin by the remains of the duct of a sebaceous gland. Frequently, epidermoid cysts become infected. Treatment is surgical excision. Also called **sebaceous cyst.** Compare **pilar cyst.**

epidermolysis bullosa   A group of rare, hereditary skin diseases in which vesicles and bullae develop, usually at sites of trauma. Severe forms may also involve mucous membranes and may leave scars and contractures on healing. Basal cell and squamous cell carcinomas sometimes develop in the scar tissue. Treatment is symptomatic.

epididymis   One of a pair of long, tightly coiled ducts that carry sperm by the millions from the seminiferous tubules of the testes to the vas deferens.

epididymitis   Acute or chronic inflammation of the epididymis. It may result from venereal disease, urinary tract infection, prostatitis, or prostatectomy. Symptoms include fever and chills, pain in the groin, and a tender, swollen epididymis. Treatment includes bed rest, scrotal support, and antibiotics, as appropriate.

epididymo-orchitis   Inflammation of the epididymis and of the testis. See also **epididymitis, orchitis.**

epidural   Outside the dura mater.

epidural anesthesia   The process of achieving regional anesthesia of the pelvic, abdominal, genital or other area by the injection of a local anesthetic into the epidural space of the spinal column.

epidural blood patch   A patch repairing a tear or a hole in the dura mater around the spinal cord. The tear is usually the result of needle puncture during spinal anesthesia or lumbar puncture. Spinal fluid leaks through the hole, resulting in a spinal headache. To form a seal, 10 to 15 ml of the patient's blood is injected into the epidural space. A clot forms, covering the hole and preventing further loss of fluid. The technique is used to treat persistent or severe spinal headache.

epidural space   The space immediately surrounding the dura mater of the brain or spinal cord, beneath the periosteum of the cranium and the spinal column.

epigastric node   A node in one of the seven groups of parietal lymph nodes serving the abdomen and the pelvis, comprising about four nodes along the caudal portion of the inferior epigastric vessels. See also **lymph, lymphatic system, lymph node.**

epigenesis   In embryology: a theory of development in which the organism grows from a simple to more complex form through the progressive differentiation of an undifferentiated cellular unit. Compare **preformation.** —**epigenesist,** *n.* **epigenetic,** *adj.*

epiglottiditis See **epiglottitis.**

epiglottis The cartilaginous structure that overhangs the larynx like a lid and prevents food from entering the larynx or the trachea while swallowing.

epiglottitis An inflammation of the epiglottis. Acute epiglottitis is a severe form of the condition, affecting primarily children. It is characterized by fever, sore throat, stridor, croupy cough, and an erythematous, swollen epiglottis. The child may become cyanotic and require an emergency tracheostomy to maintain respiration. The causative organism is usually *Haemophilus hemolyticus.* Antibiotics, rest, oxygen, and supportive care are usually included in treatment. Also called **epiglottiditis.**

epilating forceps A kind of small spring forceps, used for removing unwanted hair.

epilation See **depilation.**

epilepsy A group of neurological disorders characterized by various combinations of the following: recurrent episodes of petit mal or convulsive seizures, sensory disturbances, abnormal or repetative behavior, loss of consciousness. Common to all types of epilepsy is an uncontrolled electrical discharge from the nerve cells of the cerebral cortex. Although most epilepsy is of unknown cause (idiopathic), it may sometimes be associated with cerebral trauma, intracranial infection, brain tumor, vascular disturbances, intoxication, or chemical imbalance. The frequency of attacks may range from several times a day to intervals of several years. In predisposed individuals, seizures may occur during sleep or after physical stimulation, as by a flickering light or sudden loud sound. Emotional disturbances also may be significant trigger factors. Some seizures are preceded by an aura, but others have no warning symptoms. Most epileptic attacks are brief. They may be localized or general, with or without clonic movements, and are often followed by drowsiness or confusion. Diagnosis is made by observation of the pattern of seizures and abnormalities or an electroencephalogram. The kind of epilepsy determines the selection of preventive medication. Correctible lesions and metabolic causes are eliminated when possible.

NURSING CONSIDERATIONS: A nurse observing an epileptic attack, in addition to protecting the patient from injury, should carefully note and accurately describe the sequence of seizure activity. The patient and family must be counseled about the disorder, the importance of regularly taking prescribed medication and of never discontinuing treatment without professional advice, the toxic effects of medication, wearing a medical identification tag, and continuing to live as normal a life as possible. Types of epileptic seizures include **absence seizure, generalized tonic-clonic seizure, Jacksonian seizure, psychomotor seizure.** See also **anticonvul-**

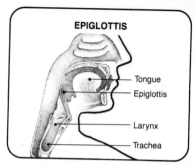

EPIGLOTTIS

Tongue
Epiglottis
Larynx
Trachea

sant, aura, clonus, ictus, tonus. —**epileptic,** *adj., n.*

epileptic mania A mood disorder that is characterized by attacks of violence, which occur immediately preceding, following, or in place of an epileptic seizure. See also **epilepsy, mania.**

epileptic stupor The state of unawareness and unresponsiveness following an epileptic seizure.

epiloia See **tuberous sclerosis.**

epimysium A fibrous sheath that enfolds a muscle and extends between the bundles of muscle fibers, as the perimysium. It is sturdy in some areas but more delicate in others, as those areas where the muscle moves freely under a strong sheet of fascia. The epimysium may also fuse with fascia that attaches a muscle to a bone.

epinephrine, e. bitartrate, e. hydrochloride Sympathomimetic vasoconstrictors used as mydriatic agents and nasal decongestants.

epinephryl borate A mydriatic agent.

epiphora See **tearing.**

epiphyseal fracture A fracture involving the epiphyseal growth plate of a long bone, resulting in separation or in fragmentation of the plate. Also called **Salter fracture.**

epiphysis, *pl.* **epiphyses** The head of a long bone that is separated from the shaft of the bone by the epiphyseal plate until the bone stops growing, the plate is obliterated, and the shaft and the head become united. Compare **diaphysis.** —**epiphyseal,** *adj.*

epiphysis cerebri See **pineal gland.**

epiploic foramen A passage between the peritoneal cavity and the omental bursa. It is lined with peritoneum and is approximately 3 cm (1⅛ inch) in diameter.

epipygus See **pygomelus.**

episcleritis Inflammation of the outermost layers of the sclera and of the tissues overlying the posterior portions of this tough, white outer coat of the eyeball.

episiotomy A surgical procedure in which an incision is made in the perineum to enlarge the vaginal opening for delivery, performed to prevent tearing of the perineum, to hasten or facilitate delivery of the infant, or to prevent stretching of perineal muscles and connective tissue thought to predispose the patient to subsequent abnormalities of pelvic outlet relaxa-

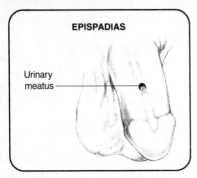

EPISPADIAS

Urinary meatus

tion, as cystocele, rectocele, and uterine prolapse; its prophylactic efficacy is debated. The incision into the vaginal and perineal tissue is closed with absorbable sutures that need not be removed. Deep incisions require closure in two or more layers. Immediate complications include hemorrhage and extension of the incision along the vaginal sulcus or into the anal sphincter or rectum. Delayed complications include hematoma and abscess. Application of cold packs to the perineum for several hours immediately postpartum minimizes swelling. Alternating applications later of heat and cold and warm sitz baths reduce discomfort, but sitz baths longer than 10 minutes soften tissue and prolong healing. A mediolateral episiotomy is an episiotomy cut at an angle of approximately 45° with the midline. Although it affords wide exposure for delivery, it is painful postpartum and is prone to hematoma and infection. A median or midline episiotomy is an incision in the perineum in the midline; although less painful postpartum, it affords less exposure for delivery and may extend into or through the anal sphincter and into the rectum.

episode An incident or event that stands out from the continuity of everyday life, as an episode of illness or a traumatic episode in the course of a child's development. —**episodic,** *adj.*

episodic care A pattern of medical and nursing care in which care is given to a person for a particular problem, without an ongoing relationship being established between the person and health-care professionals. Emergency rooms provide episodic care.

episodic health history An abbreviated form of the health history that is focused on the factors relevant to an illness or complaint that has been previously noted, as in a follow-up visit after a treatment or surgical procedure or in the regular periodic visits for a chronic illness or condition.

episome In bacterial genetics: an extrachromosomal replicating unit that exists autonomously or functions with a chromosome. See also **colicinogen, conjugon, F factor, R factor.**

epispadias A congenital defect in which the urethra opens on the anterior surface of the penis. The condition is most often associated with ex-

trophy of the bladder. Treatment is directed at correcting or managing urinary incontinence, which occurs because the urinary sphincters are defective, and at permitting sexual function. The corresponding defect in women, fissure of the upper wall of the urethra, is quite rare. Compare **hypospadias.**

epistasis In genetics: a type of interaction between genes at different loci on a chromosome in which one is able to mask or suppress the expression of the other. The epistatic effect, which is nonallelic and therefore the opposite of the dominance relationship, may be caused by the presence of homozygous recessives at one gene pair, as occurs in the Bombay phenotype, or by the presence of a dominant allele that counteracts the expression of another dominant gene. Compare **dominance.** —**epistatic,** *adj.*

epistaxis Bleeding from the nose caused by local irritation of mucous membranes, violent sneezing, fragility of the mucous membrane or of the arterial walls, chronic infection, trauma, hypertension, leukemia, vitamin K deficiency, or, most often, by picking of the nose. Epistaxis may result from rupture of tiny vessels in the anterior nasal septum; this occurs most frequently in early childhood and adolescence. In adults, it occurs more commonly in men than in women, may be severe in elderly persons, and may be accompanied by respiratory distress, apprehension, restlessness, vertigo, and nausea and may lead to syncope. The patient suffering epistaxis is instructed to breathe through the mouth, to sit quietly with the head tilted slightly forward in order to prevent blood from entering the pharynx, and to avoid swallowing blood. Bleeding may be controlled by pinching the nose firmly with the fingers, by inserting a cotton ball soaked in a topical vasoconstrictor (as phenylephrine hydrochloride) and applying pressure to both sides of the nose, or by placing an ice compress over the nose. If bleeding continues, the clots may be removed by suction. The nasal mucosa may be anesthetized with topical lidocaine, cauterized with a silver nitrate stick or an electric cautery, and then sprayed with epinephrine. Severe bleeding, especially from the posterior nasal septum, may be treated with packing or a nasal balloon catheter. Persistent or recurrent profuse epistaxis may be treated by ligating an artery supplying the nose, as the external carotid, ethmoid, or internal maxillary.

NURSING CONSIDERATIONS: The nurse checks the patient's blood pressure, pulse, and respiration every half hour until bleeding subsides. Then, as ordered, the nurse limits the patient's activity; encourages expectoration rather than swallowing of blood; reports symptoms of respiratory distress, vertigo, and any bleeding; and provides instruction on the prevention of epistaxis as appropriate. Also called **nosebleed.**

epistropheus See **axis.**

epithalamus One of the five portions of the diencephalon. It includes the trigonum habenulae, the pineal body, and the posterior commissure. Compare **hypothalamus, metathal-**

amus, subthalamus, thalamus. —**epithalamic**, *adj.*

epithelioid leiomyoma   An uncommon neoplasm of smooth muscle in which the cells are polygonal in shape. It usually develops in the stomach. Also called **bizarre leiomyoma, leiomyoblastoma.**

epithelioma   **1.** A neoplasm derived from the epithelium. **2.** Any carcinoma.

-epithelioma   A combining form meaning a 'tumor of epithelial tissue': *inoepithelioma.*

epithelioma adamantinum   See **ameloblastoma.**

epithelioma adenoides cysticum   See **trichoepithelioma.**

epithelium   The covering of the internal and external organs of the body, including the lining of vessels. It consists of cells bound together by connective material and varies in the number of layers and the kinds of cells. Epithelium in different parts of the body is made of simple squamous cells, simple cuboidal cells, and stratified columnar cells. The stratified squamous epithelium of the epidermis comprises five different cellular layers. —**epithelial**, *adj.*

epitope   An antigenic determinant that causes a specific reaction by an immunoglobulin. It consists of a group of amino acids on the surface of the antigen.

epitympanic recess   One of the two areas of the tympanic cavity, the other being the tympanic cavity proper. The recess is cranial to the tympanic membrane and contains the upper half of the malleus and the greater part of the incus.

epizootic   A disease or condition that occurs simultaneously in nearly all of the animals of a species in a geographical area.

epoophorectomy   Surgical removal of the epoophoron.

epoophoron   A structure that is situated in the mesosalpinx between the ovary and the uterine tube. It is composed of a few short tubules. The ends of the tubules converge in one direction toward the ovary and, in the opposite direction, open into a rudimentary duct. The epoophoron is a persistent portion of the embryonic mesonephric duct.

EPSDT   *abbr* **Early and Periodic Screening Diagnosis and Treatment.**

Epsom salt   See **magnesium sulfate.**

Epstein-Barr virus (EBV)   The herpesvirus that causes infectious mononucleosis.

Epstein's pearls   Small, white, pearllike epithelial cysts that occur on both sides of the midline of the hard palate of the neonate. They are normal and usually disappear within a few weeks. Compare **Bednar's aphthae.**

epulis   Any tumor or growth on the gingiva.

equal cleavage   Mitotic division of the fertilized ovum into blastomeres of identical size, as occurs in humans and most mammals. Compare **unequal cleavage.**

equatorial plate   The platelike configuration formed by the chromosomes at the center of the spindle during the metaphase stage of mitosis and meiosis.

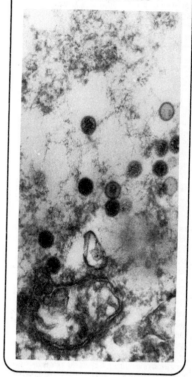

EPSTEIN-BARR VIRUS

equifinality   In general systems theory: a principle stating that the same characteristic state or end result can be achieved in any open system regardless of the starting point; differences in initial conditions or the approach used do not alter the outcome. Compare **general systems theory, multifinality.**

equilibrium   **1.** A state of balance or rest owing to the equal action of opposing forces, such as calcium and phosphorus in the body. **2.** In psychiatry: a state of mental or emotional balance.

equine encephalitis   An arbovirus infection characterized by inflammation of the nerve tissues of the brain and spinal cord, with high fever, headache, nausea, vomiting, myalgia, and neurologic symptoms, as visual disturbances, tremor, lethargy, and disorientation. The virus is transmitted by the bite of an infected mosquito. Horses are the primary host of the particular viruses that cause the infection; humans are a secondary host. **Eastern equine encephalitis (EEE)** is a severe form of the infection. It occurs along the eastern seaboard of the United States and lasts longer and causes more deaths and residual morbidity than **Western equine encephalitis (WEE),** which occurs throughout the United States and results in a mild, brief illness, as does **Venezuelan equine encephalitis (VEE)**, which is common in Central and South America, Florida, and Texas.

Er Symbol for **erbium.**

ER *abbr* **emergency room.**

erbium (Er) A rare-earth, metallic element. Its atomic number is 68; its atomic weight is 167.26.

Erb-Duchenne paralysis See **Erb's palsy.**

Erb's muscular dystrophy A form of muscular dystrophy that first affects the shoulder girdle and, later, often involves the pelvic girdle. It is a progressively crippling disease with onset in childhood or adolescence and is usually inherited as an autosomal recessive trait. It affects both sexes. In males, differential diagnosis between Erb's muscular dystrophy and Duchenne's muscular dystrophy may be difficult.

Erb's palsy A kind of paralysis caused by traumatic injury to the upper brachial plexus, occurring most commonly in childbirth from forcible traction during delivery. The signs of Erb's palsy include loss of sensation in the arm and paralysis and atrophy of the deltoid, the biceps, and the brachialis muscles. The arm on the affected side hangs loosely with the elbow extended and the forearm pronated. Treatment initially requires that the arm and shoulder be immobilized to allow the swelling and inflammation of the associated neuritis to resolve. Physical therapy and splinting may be necessary to improve function of the muscles and to prevent flexion contracture of the elbow. Also called **Erb-Duchenne paralysis.**

erectile Capable of being erected or raised to an erect position, usually applied in the description of spongy tissue of the penis or clitoris that becomes turgid and erectile when filled with blood. It also may be used when referring to the epidermal tissue involved in the appearance of goose bumps (horripilation) in response to fear, anger, cold, or other stimuli.

erectile myxoma An angioma that contains areas of myxomatous tissue.

erectile tumor See **cavernous hemangioma.**

erection The condition of hardness, swelling, and elevation observed in the penis and to a lesser degree in the clitoris, usually due to sexual arousal but also occurring during sleep or as a result of physical stimulation. It occurs as additional blood enters the organ and blood pressure increases and is influenced by psychic and nerve stimulation. It is needed to enable the penis to enter the vagina and to emit semen. See also **ejaculation, nocturnal emission, priapism.**

erector spinae See **sacrospinalis.**

erethistic idiocy Severe mental retardation associated with continuous, purposeless activity and restlessness.

-ergasia A combining form meaning 'interfunctioning of the mind and body': *cacergasia*, *dysergasia*, *orthergasia*.

ergastoplasm A network of cytoplasmic structures that show basophilic-staining properties; granular endoplasmic reticulum. See **endoplasmic reticulum.**

-ergetic See **-ergic.**

-ergic A combining form meaning an 'effect of activity': *allergic, pathergic, telergic.* Also **-ergetic.**

ergo- A combining form meaning 'pertaining to work': *ergodermatosis, ergomaniac, ergotropy.*

ergocalciferol An analog of vitamin D with antirachitic and hypercalcemic activity. It is formed by ultraviolet irradiation of ergosterol, a provitamin D sterol that occurs in yeast, mushrooms, ergot, and other fungi. Also called **vitamin D₂.**

ergonomics A scientific discipline devoted to the study and analysis of human work, especially as it is affected by individual anatomy, psychology, and other human factors. —**ergonomic,** *adj.*

ergonovine maleate An oxytocic agent.

ergosome See **polysome.**

ergosterol An unsaturated hydrocarbon of the vitamin D group isolated from yeast, mushrooms, ergot, and other fungi. When treated with ultraviolet irradiation, it is converted into vitamin D₂. See also **calciferol, viosterol, vitamin D.**

ergot In pharmacology: the food storage body of a fungus, *Claviceps purpura,* which commonly infects rye and other cereal grasses. It contains ergot alkaloids.

ergot alkaloid One of a large group of alkaloids derived from a common fungus that grows on rye and other grains throughout the temperate areas of the world. The alkaloids are divided into three groups: the amino acid alkaloids, typified by ergotamine; the dihydrogenated amino acid alkaloids, as dihydroergotamine; and the amine alkaloids, as ergonovine. Ergotamine and dihydroergotamine are not as effective oxytocics as ergonovine; therefore, ergonovine, given orally or intravenously, is currently used in obstetrics to treat or prevent postpartum uterine atony and to complete an incomplete or missed abortion. Ergotamine is prescribed to relieve migraine headache. It acts by reducing the amplitude of arterial pulsations in the external carotid branches of the cranial arteries. Dihydroergotamine was formerly used to improve cerebral blood flow in elderly patients in order to improve mental function but is no longer thought to be a useful or effective drug for that purpose.

ergotamine tartrate An alpha-adrenergic blocking agent.

ergotherapy The use of physical activity and exercise in the treatment of disease. By extension, the therapy includes any procedure that increases the blood supply to a diseased or injured part, as massage or various types of hot baths. —**ergotherapeutic,** *adj.*

-ergy A combining form meaning: **1.** An 'action': *abioenergy, leukergy, synergy.* **2.** An 'effect or result': *allergy, anabolergy, pathergy.*

erosion The wearing away or gradual destruction of a surface, as of a mucosal or epidermal surface as a result of inflammation, injury, or other effects, usually marked by the appearance of an ulcer. See also **necrosis.**

erosive gastritis An inflammatory condition characterized by multiple erosions of the mucous membrane lining the stomach. Nausea, anorexia, pain, and gastric hemorrhage may occur. Treatment includes removal of the irritating substance, and supportive care includes intravenous fluids, electrolytes, and, if necessary, blood transfusion. See also **chemical gastritis, corrosive gastritis.**

erosive osteoarthritis See **Kellgren's syndrome.**

-erotic A combining form meaning 'pertaining to sexual love or desire': anterotic, homoerotic, hysteroerotic.

eroticism, erotism 1. Sexual impulse or desire. 2. The arousal of or attempt to arouse the sexual instinct by suggestive or symbolic means. 3. The expression of sexual instinct or desire. 4. An abnormally persistent sexual drive. See also **anal eroticism, oral eroticism.**

eroto- A combining form meaning 'pertaining to love or sexual desire': erotogenic, erotopath, erotophobia.

erotomania A psychopathological state characterized by preoccupation with sexuality and sexual behavior.

erotomaniac A person displaying characteristics of erotomania.

ERT abbr **external radiation therapy.**

eructation The act of bringing up air from the stomach with a characteristic sound. Also called **belching.**

eruption The rapid development of a skin lesion, especially of a viral exanthem or of the rash commonly accompanying a drug reaction.

eruptive fever Any disease characterized by fever and a rash.

eruptive xanthoma A skin disorder associated with elevated triglyceride levels in the blood. Erythematous or pale raised papules suddenly appear in large numbers on the trunk, legs, arms, and buttocks.

ERV abbr **expiratory reserve volume.**

erysipelas An infectious skin disease characterized by redness, swelling, vesicles, bullae, fever, pain, and lymphadenopathy. It is caused by a species of group A, beta-hemolytic streptococci. Treatment includes antibiotics, analgesics, and packs or dressings applied locally to the lesions.

erysipeloid An infection of the hands characterized by blue-red nodules or patches and, occasionally, by erythema. It is acquired by handling meat or fish infected with Erysipelothrix rhusiopathiae. The disease is self-limited, lasting about 3 weeks, but will respond to penicillin. Compare **erysipelas.**

erythema Redness or inflammation of the skin or mucous membranes that is the result of dilatation and congestion of superficial capillaries. Examples of erythema are nervous blushes and mild sunburn. See also **erythroderma, rubor. —erythematous,** adj.

erythema chronicum migrans A skin lesion that begins as a small papule and spreads peripherally, extending by a raised, red margin and clearing in the center. It may be associated with **Lyme arthritis,** in which case it is caused by the bite of a small tick.

erythema infectiosum An acute, benign infectious disease, mainly of children, characterized by fever and an erythematous rash beginning on the cheeks and appearing later on the arms, thighs, buttocks, and trunk. As the rash progresses, earlier lesions fade. Sunlight aggravates the eruption, which usually lasts about 10 days. For a period the rash may reappear whenever the skin is irritated. Its cause is unknown, no treatment is necessary, and prognosis is excellent. The isolation of patients is not required. Also called **fifth disease.**

erythema marginatum A variant of **erythema multiforme** seen in acute rheumatic fever, characterized by transient, disk-shaped, nonpruritic, reddened macules with raised margins.

erythema multiforme A hypersensitivity syndrome characterized by polymorphous eruption of skin and mucous membranes. Macules, papules, nodules, vesicles or bullae, and bull's-eye-shaped lesions are evident. Erythema multiforme has been associated with many infections, collagen diseases, drug sensitivities, allergies, and pregnancy. Definitive and preventive treatment depends on finding the specific cause, but topical or systemic corticosteroids are helpful in most cases. A severe form of this condition is known as **Stevens-Johnson syndrome.**

erythema nodosum A hypersensitivity vasculitis characterized by bilateral, reddened, tender, subcutaneous nodules on the shins and, occasionally, on other parts of the body. The nodules last for several days or weeks, never ulcerate, and are often associated with mild fever, malaise, and pains in muscles and joints. This condition may be seen with streptococcal infections, tuberculosis, sarcoid, leprosy, drug sensitivity, ulcerative colitis, and pregnancy. The prognosis is good, given appropriate treatment of the underlying disease. A course of corticosteroids is usually effective in diminishing the symptoms of this condition.

erythema perstans A persistent local redness of the skin, often caused by a fixed drug eruption.

erythema toxicum neonatorum A common skin condition of neonates characterized by a pink papular rash frequently superimposed with vesicles or pustules. The rash appears within 24 to 48 hours after birth; covers the thorax, abdomen, back, and diaper area; and disappears spontaneously after several days. A smear of the papules shows eosinophils rather than neutrophils to differentiate the condition from neonatal pustular melanosis. Also called **toxic erythema of the newborn.**

erythrasma A bacterial skin infection of the axillary or inguinal regions, characterized by irregular, red-brown, raised patches. An

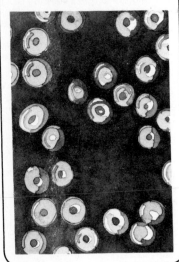

NORMAL ERYTHROCYTES

asymptomatic disease, it is more common in diabetics and responds quickly to oral erythromycin. Compare **intertrigo, tinea cruris.**

erythrityl tetranitrate A coronary vasodilator.

erythro- A combining form meaning 'red': *erythroblast, erythroclast, erythrocyte.*

erythroblastosis fetalis A type of hemolytic anemia that occurs in newborns as a result of maternal-fetal blood group incompatibility, specifically involving the Rh factor and the ABO blood groups. The condition is caused by an antigen-antibody reaction in the bloodstream of the infant resulting from the placental transmission of maternally formed antibodies against the incompatible antigens of the fetal blood. In Rh factor incompatibility, the hemolytic reaction occurs only when the mother is Rh negative and the infant is Rh positive. The isoimmunization process rarely occurs with the first pregnancy, but there is increased risk with each succeeding pregnancy. However, maternal sensitization to the Rh factor can be prevented by injection of a high-titer anti-Rh gamma globulin preparation following delivery or abortion of an Rh-positive fetus. No sensitization may occur in situations in which a strong placental barrier prevents transfer of fetal blood into the maternal circulation. In about 10% to 15% of sensitized mothers, there is no hemolytic reaction in the newborn. Clinical manifestations of the condition include severe anemia, jaundice, and enlargement of the liver and spleen, which, without intervention, can lead to hypoxia, cardiac failure, generalized edema, respiratory distress, and death. Prenatal diagnosis of the disease is confirmed through amniocentesis and analysis of bilirubin levels in amniotic fluid. Higher than normal levels result from the breakdown of hemoglobin from the lysed erythrocytes. Treatment consists of intrauterine transfusion when placental bilirubin levels progressively increase or immediate exchange transfusions following birth. Hemolytic reactions involving the ABO blood groups have similar manifestations but are generally less severe. See also **hydrops fetalis, hyperbilirubinemia of the newborn, Rh factor.**

erythrocyte A biconcave disk about 7 microns in diameter that contains hemoglobin confined within a lipoid membrane. The erythrocyte is the major cellular element of the circulating blood, and its principal function is to transport oxygen. The number of cells per cubic mm of blood is usually maintained between 4.5 and 5.0 million in men and between 4.0 and 4.5 million in women. It varies with age, activity, and environmental conditions. For example, an increase to a level of 8.0 million per cubic mm can normally occur at over 10,000 feet above sea level. An erythrocyte normally lives for 110 to 120 days, at which time it is removed from the bloodstream and broken down by the reticuloendothelial system. New erythrocytes are produced at a rate of slightly more than 1% a day; thus, a constant level is usually maintained. With acute blood loss, hemolytic anemia, or chronic oxygen deprivation, erythrocyte production may increase greatly. Erythrocytes originate in the marrow of the long bones. Maturation proceeds from a stem cell (promegaloblast) through the pronormoblast stage to the normoblast, the last stage before the mature adult cell develops. Kinds of erythrocytes include **discocyte, echinocyte, macrocyte, spherocyte.** Also called **red blood cell, red cell, red corpuscle.** Compare **normoblast, reticulocyte.** See also **erythropoiesis, hemoglobin.**

erythrocyte sedimentation rate (ESR) The rate at which red blood cells settle out in a tube of unclotted blood, expressed in millimeters per hour. Blood is collected in an anticoagulant and allowed to sediment in a calibrated glass column. At the end of one hour, the laboratory technician measures the distance the erythrocytes have fallen in the tube. Elevated sedimentation rates are not specific for any disorder but indicate the presence of inflammation. Inflammation causes an alteration of the blood proteins, which makes the red blood cells aggregate, becoming heavier than normal. The speed with which they fall to the bottom of the tube corresponds to the degree of inflammation. Serial evaluations of erythrocyte sedimentation rate are useful in monitoring the course of inflammatory activity in rheumatic diseases and, when performed with a white blood cell count, can indicate infection. Certain noninflammatory conditions, as pregnancy, are also characterized by high sedimentation rates. Values are higher for women in both methods and vary according to the method used. Also called **sed. rate** (*informal*). See also **inflammation.**

erythrocytosis An abnormal increase in

the number of circulating red cells. See also **polycythemia.**

erythroderma　Any dermatosis associated with abnormal redness of the skin. Compare **erythema, rubor.**

erythroleukemia　A malignant blood disorder characterized by a proliferation of erythropoietic elements in bone marrow; erythroblasts with bizarre, lobulated nuclei; and abnormal myeloblasts in peripheral blood. The disease may have an acute or chronic course. Also called **diGuglielmo's disease, diGuglielmo's syndrome, erythromyeloblastic leukemia.**

erythromelalgia　A rare disorder characterized by a paroxysmal dilatation of the peripheral blood vessels. It occurs bilaterally, usually in the extremities, and is associated with burning, redness of the skin, and pain. —**erythromelalgic,** *adj.*

erythromycin base, e. estolate, e. ethylsuccinate, e. gluceptate, e. lactobionate　Antibiotic local and ophthalmic anti-infective agents.

erythromyeloblastic leukemia　See **erythroleukemia.**

erythrophobia　**1.** An anxiety disorder characterized by an irrational fear of blushing or of displaying embarrassment. **2.** A neurotic symptom manifested by blushing at the slightest provocation. **3.** A morbid fear of or aversion to the color red. —**erythrophobic,** *adj.*

erythroplasia of Queyrat　A premalignant lesion on the glans or corona of the penis. It is a well-circumscribed red patch on the skin. It is usually excised surgically.

erythropoiesis　The process of erythrocyte production involving the maturation of a nucleated precursor into a hemoglobin-filled, nucleus-free erythrocyte that is regulated by erythropoietin, a hormone produced by the kidney. See also **erythropoietin, hemoglobin, leukopoiesis.** —**erythropoietic,** *adj.*

erythropoietic porphyria　See **porphyria.**

erythropoietin　A hormone synthesized in the kidney and released into the bloodstream in response to anoxia. The hormone acts to stimulate and to regulate the production of erythrocytes and is thus able to increase the oxygen-carrying capacity of the blood.

Es　Symbol for **einsteinium.**

escape beat　An automatic beat of the heart that occurs after an interval longer than the duration of the dominant heartbeat cycle. Escape beats function as safety mechanisms, and anything that produces a pause in the prevailing heart cycle may allow an escape to occur. Some kinds of pauses in which escape beats occur are caused by sinoatrial (SA) block, atrioventricular (AV) block, extra systole, and the completion of a paroxysm of tachycardia. In the presence of atrial fibrillation, nodal escape beats present a unique diagnostic problem because fibrillation obviates any dominant heartbeat cycle. In the electrocardiogram, the nodal escape beat commonly presents a QRS-T contour similar to that of the sinus beats but sometimes varies slightly from the dominant beats. Ventricular escape beats are associated with the late rather than the early occurrence of the usual ventricular beat patterns.

-escent　A combining form meaning: **1.** 'Beginning to be': *alkalescent, convalescent, turgescent.* **2.** 'Emitting or reflecting light': *incandescent, iridescent, opalescent.*

eschar　A scab or dry crust resulting from a thermal or chemical burn, infection, or excoriating skin disease. —**escharotic,** *adj.*

escharonodulaire　See **Marseilles fever.**

Escherichia　A genus of bacteria made up of gram-negative, motile or nonmotile short rods, occurring widely in nature, and occasionally pathogenic in humans.

Escherichia coli　A species of coliform bacteria of the family Enterobaccteriacae, normally present in the intestines and common in water, milk, and soil. *Escherichia coli* is the most frequent cause of urinary tract infection and is a serious pathogen in wounds. *E. coli* septicemia may rapidly result in shock and death owing to the action of an endotoxin released from the bacteria.

eserine　See **physostigmine.**

eserine sulfate　See **physostigmine.**

-esis　A combining form meaning an 'action, process, or result of ': *enuresis, oxydesis, synthesis.*

Esmarch's bandage　An elastic bandage wrapped around an elevated limb to force blood out of the limb. It is used prior to certain surgical procedures to create a blood-free field.

eso-　A combining form meaning 'within': *esocataphoria, esogastritis, esotropia.*

esophageal cancer　A malignant neoplastic disease of the esophagus that occurs three times more frequently in men than in women and more often in Asia and Africa than in North America. Risk factors associated with the disease are heavy consumption of alcohol, smoking, betel-nut chewing, Plummer-Vinson syndrome, hiatal hernia, or achalasia. Aflatoxin in moldy grain and peanuts or a dietary deficiency, especially of molybdenum, may be involved. Esophageal cancer does not often cause any symptoms in the early stages but in later stages causes painful dysphagia, anorexia, weight loss, regurgitation, cervical adenopathy, and, in some cases, a persistent cough. Left vocal cord paralysis and hemoptysis indicate an advanced state of the disease. The tumor may spread locally to invade the trachea, bronchi, pericardium, great blood vessels, and thoracic vertebrae or may metastasize to lymph nodes, the lungs, and the liver. Diagnostic measures include X-ray and biopsy. Most esophageal tumors are poorly differentiated squamous cell carcinomas; adenocarcinomas occur less frequently and are usually found in the lower third of the esophagus as extensions of gastric cancer. Surgical treatment may require total or partial esophagectomy with the resected segment replaced by a Dacron graft or a section of the colon. If only the lower third of the esophagus is removed, the proximal end may be anastomosed to the stomach. Patients with inoperable esophageal cancer may be fed by a nasogastric or gastrostomy tube. Radiotherapy may eradicate early local tumors and may effectively palliate the symptoms of advanced lesion. Methotrexate given before irradiation may increase the chances of survival. See also **esophagectomy.**

esophageal lead **1.** An electrocardiographic conductor in which the exploring electrode is placed within the lumen of the esophagus. It is used to detect sizable atrial deflections as an aid in identifying cardiac arrhythmias. **2.** *Informal.* A tracing produced by such a lead on an electrocardiograph.

esophageal varices A complex of longitudinal, tortuous veins at the lower end of the esophagus, enlarged and swollen as the result of portal hypertension. These vessels are especially susceptible to ulceration and hemorrhage.

esophagectomy The surgical removal of all or part of the esophagus, as may be required to treat severe, recurrent, bleeding esophageal varices or esophageal cancer.

esophagitis Inflammation of the mucosal lining of the esophagus, caused by infection, irritation from a nasogastric tube, or, most commonly, backflow of gastric juice from the stomach. See also **gastroesophageal reflux.**

esophagus The muscular canal, about 24 cm (9 inches) long, extending from the pharynx to the stomach. It begins in the neck at the inferior border of the cricoid cartilage, opposite the sixth cervical vertebra, and descends to the cardiac sphincter of the stomach in a vertical path with two slight curves. It is the narrowest part of the digestive tube and is most constricted at its origin and at the point where it passes through the diaphragm. The esophagus is composed of fibrous, muscular, and submucous coats, and is lined with mucous membrane. Also called **gullet.** —**esophageal,** *adj.*

esophoria Deviation of the visual axis of one eye toward that of the other eye in the absence of visual stimuli for fusion. Also called **cross-eye.** Compare **esotropia.** —**esophoric,** *adj.*

esotropia A kind of strabismus characterized by an inward deviation of one eye relative to the other eye. Also called **convergent strabismus, internal strabismus.** Compare **exotropia.** See also **strabismus.** —**esotropic,** *adj.*

ESP *abbr* **extrasensory perception.**

espundia A cutaneous form of American leishmaniasis most common in Brazil, caused by *Leishmania brasilensis.* See also **American leishmaniasis, leishmaniasis.**

ESR *abbr* **erythrocyte sedimentation rate.**

essential amino acid An organic compound not synthesized in the body that is essential for nitrogen equilibrium in adults and for optimal growth in infants and children. Adults require isoleucine, leucine, lysine, methionine, phenylalanine, threonine, tryptophan, and va-

line. Infants need these eight amino acids plus arginine and histidine. Cystine and tyrosine, limited substitutes respectively for methionine and phenylalanine, are considered quasi-essential. See also **amino acid.**

essential crystalline amino acid solution A specialized solution used in management of renal failure.

essential fatty acid A polyunsaturated acid, such as linoleic, linolenic, and arachidonic acids, essential in the diet for the proper growth, maintenance, and functioning of the body. It is a precursor of the prostaglandins and has an important role in fat transport and metabolism and in maintaining the function and integrity of cellular membranes. It is also necessary for the normal functioning of the reproductive and endocrine systems and for the breaking up of cholesterol deposits on arterial walls. The best dietary sources are natural vegetable oils, as safflower, soy, and corn oils; margarines blended with vegetable oils; wheat germ; edible seeds, as pumpkin, sesame, and sunflower seeds; poultry fat; and fish oils, especially cod-liver oil. Deficiency causes changes in cell structure and enzyme function resulting in decreased growth and other disorders. Symptoms include brittle and lusterless hair, nail problems, dandruff, allergic conditions, and dermatoses, especially eczema in infants. Excessive amounts of essential fatty acids may reduce the level of vitamin E in the tissues and cause other metabolic disturbances as well as abnormal weight gain.

essential fever Any fever of unknown etiology.

essential hypertension An elevated systemic arterial pressure for which no cause can be found and which is often the only significant clinical finding. Elevated blood pressure is always considered a risk, and individuals with elevated pressures are at risk for cardiovascular disease. In examining patients with essential hypertension, clinicians consider the normal complex mechanisms that control pressure, as the arterial baroreflex, body fluid regulators, the renin-angiotensin system, and vascular autoregulation. These mechanisms are closely integrated, and it is not precisely clear how their impairment affects normotension and hypertension. Also called **benign hypertension.**

essential nutrient The carbohydrates, proteins, fats, minerals, and vitamins necessary for growth, normal function, and body maintenance. These substances must be supplied by food, since most are not synthesized by the body in the quantities required for health.

essential thrombocythemia See **thrombocytosis.**

essential tremor An involuntary fine shaking of the hand, the head, and the face, especially during routine movements of the body. It is a familial disorder inherited as an autosomal dominant trait and appears during adolescence or in middle age, slowly progressing as a more pronounced disorder. The precise cause of this condition is not known, but it is believed to involve the central nervous system. Essential tremor is aggravated by activity and emotion and can be reduced in some patients by giving alcohol and mild sedatives. Also called **familial tremor.** Compare **Parkinsonism.**

EST *abbr* **electric shock therapy. See electroconvulsive therapy.**

established name The name assigned to a drug by the United States Adopted Names Council (USAN). The established name, generally shorter than the chemical name, is the name by which the drug is known to health practitioners. Also called **generic name.** See also **chemical name.**

ester A class of chemical compound formed by the bonding of an alcohol and one or more organic acids. Fats are esters, formed by the bonding of fatty acids with the alcohol glycerol.

ester-compound local anesthetic Any one of four potent local anesthetics slightly different in chemical structure from the amide group of local anesthetics. Tetracaine is the most commonly used. Kinds of ester-compound local anesthetics are **chloroprocaine hydrochloride, cocaine hydrochloride, procaine hydrochloride, tetracaine hydrochloride.**

esterified estrogens Steroidal (natural) estrogens.

esthesio- A combining form meaning 'pertaining to feeling or to the perceptive faculties': *esthesiogenic, esthesioneure, esthesioscopy.*

-esthetic A combining form meaning 'pertaining to a person's consciousness of something': *cenesthetic, photoesthetic, somatesthetic.* Also **-aesthetic, -esthetical, -aesthetical.**

estradiol, e. cypionate, e. valerate Steroidal (natural) estrogens.

estramustine phosphate sodium An antineoplastic agent that alters hormone balance.

estriol A relatively weak, naturally occurring human estrogen found in high concentrations in urine. See also **estrogen.**

estrogen One of a group of hormonal steroid compounds that promote the development of female secondary sex characteristics. Human estrogen is elaborated in the ovaries, adrenal cortices, testes, and fetoplacental unit. During the menstrual cycle estrogen renders the female genital tract suitable for fertilization, implantation, and nutrition of the early embryo. Pharmaceutical preparations of estrogen are used in oral contraceptives, to palliate postmenopausal breast cancer and prostatic cancer, to inhibit lactation, and to treat threatened abortion, osteoporosis, and ovarian disease. Estrogen is also prescribed to relieve discomforts of menopause, but its long-term, continued use may increase the risk of endometrial carcinoma. Kinds of estrogen are **conjugated estrogen, esterified estrogen, estradiol, estriol, estrone. —estrogenic,** *adj.*

estrone A steroidal (natural) estrogen.

ethacrynate sodium See **ethacrynic acid.**

ethacrynic acid A loop diuretic.

ethambutol hydrochloride An antitubercular agent.

ethanoic acid See **acetic acid.**

ethanol See **alcohol.**

ethaverine hydrochloride A peripheral vasodilator.

ethchlorvynol A sedative-hypnotic agent.

ether A nonhalogenated, volatile liquid used as a general anesthetic. Because ether is generally safe, and because it provides excellent analgesia and profound muscle relaxation, adjuncts to anesthesia, as narcotic analgesics and neuromuscular blocking agents, are often unnecessary. Ether has little depressant effect on the respiratory and cardiovascular systems but may cause hyperglycemia, decreased excretion of urine, decreased intestinal tone and motility, and transient abnormalities in the function of the liver. It has an irritating, pungent odor, is highly flammable and explosive, and frequently causes postoperative nausea and vomiting.

ethical drug A drug available only by prescription and advertised only to physicians and other health professionals. Also called **prescription drug.**

ethinamate A sedative-hypnotic agent.

ethinyl estradiol A steroidal (natural) estrogen.

ethionamide An antitubercular agent.

ethmoidal air cell One of the numerous, small, thin-walled cavities in the ethmoid bone of the skull, rimmed by the frontal maxilla, lacrimal, sphenoidal, and palatine bones. They are lined with mucous membrane continuous with that of the nasal cavity and lie between the upper part of the nasal cavities and the orbits. They are divided bilaterally into anterior, middle, and posterior cavities. The anterior and the middle cavities open into the middle meatus of the nose; the posterior cavities open into the superior meatus. The ethmoidal air cells start to develop at birth. Compare **frontal sinus, maxillary sinus, sphenoidal sinus.**

ethmoid bone The very light and spongy bone at the base of the cranium, forming most of the walls of the superior part of the nasal cavity and consisting of four parts: a horizontal plate, a perpendicular plate, and two lateral labyrinths.

ethnic Pertaining to a group of people who have social customs, language, religion, or physical traits in common.

ethnicity The social, cultural, religious, or racial orientation that influences a person's beliefs, values, customs, and behavior.

ethnocentrism 1. A belief in the inherent superiority of the race or group to which one belongs. 2. A proclivity to consider other ethnic groups in terms of one's own racial origins.

ethoheptazine citrate A non-narcotic analgesic.

ethology 1. In zoology: the scientific study of the behavioral patterns of animals, specifically in their native habitat. 2. In psychology: the empirical study of human behavior, primarily social customs, manners, and mores. —**ethologic, ethological,** *adj.,* **ethologist,** *n.*

ethosuximide A succinimide anticonvul-

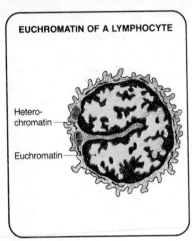

EUCHROMATIN OF A LYMPHOCYTE

Hetero-
chromatin

Euchromatin

sant used in petit mal epilepsy.

ethotoin A hydantoin anticonvulsant.

ethoxazene hydrochloride A urinary tract analgesic.

ethyl alcohol Used as a disinfectant.

ethyl aminobenzoate See benzocaine.

ethyl chloride A topical anesthetic agent.

ethylestrenol An anabolic steroid.

ethylnorepinephrine hydrochloride A sympathomimetic bronchodilating agent.

ethyl oxide A colorless, highly volatile liquid solvent similar to diethyl ether. It is widely used in various pharmaceutical processes.

-etic A combining form used as the equivalent of -ic in forming adjectives: enuretic, genetic, kinetic.

etidocaine hydrochloride An amide local anesthetic.

etidronate disodium A parathyroid-like agent.

etiology **1.** The study of all factors that may be involved in the development of a disease, including susceptibility of the patient, the nature of the disease agent, and the way in which the patient's body is invaded by the agent. **2.** The cause of a disease. Compare **pathogenesis.**

etoposide (VP-16) A podophyllin-derivative drug used in chemotherapy.

eu- A combining form meaning 'well, easily, good': euangiotic, eucrasia, euthyroid.

Eu Symbol for **europium.**

eucaryocyte See **eukaryocyte.**

eucaryon See **eukaryon.**

eucaryosis See **eukaryosis.**

euchromatin That portion of chromosome material that is active in gene expression during cell division. It stains most deeply during mitosis when it is in a coiled, condensed state, and during each division of the cell it passes through a continuous cycle of condensation and dispersion. Compare **heterochromatin.** See also **chromatin.** —euchromatic, adj.

euchromosome See **autosome.**

eugamy The union of those gametes which contain the same haploid number of chromosomes. —eugamic, adj.

eugenics The study of methods for controlling the characteristics of future human populations through selective breeding.

euglobulin A true globulin (a protein insoluble in distilled water). This is only one of a number of different properties that have been used to classify proteins. Compare **albumin, cryoglobulin.** See also **electrophoresis, plasma protein.**

eukaryocyte, eucaryocyte A cell with a true nucleus, found in all higher organisms and in some microorganisms, as amebae, plasmodia, and trypanosomes. Compare **prokaryocyte.** —eukaryotic, adj.

eukaryon, eucaryon **1.** A nucleus that is highly complex, organized, and surrounded by a nuclear membrane, usually characteristic of higher organisms. **2.** An organism containing such a nucleus. Compare **prokaryon.**

eukaryosis, eucaryosis The state of having a highly complex, organized nucleus surrounded by a nuclear membrane and containing organelles, as is characteristic of all organisms except bacteria, viruses, and blue-green algae. Compare **prokaryosis.**

eukaryote, eucaryote An organism having cells that contain a true nucleus. —eukaryotic, eucaryotic, adj.

eunuch A male whose testes have been removed. Symptoms such as a feminine voice and absence of facial hair can stem from the absence of male hormones prior to puberty. See also **secondary sex characteristic.**

eunuchoidism Deficiency of the function of male hormone or of its formation by the testes. The deficiency leads to sterility and to abnormal tallness, small testes, deficient development of secondary sex characteristics and of libido and potency.

euphoretic **1.** Of a substance or event: tending to produce a condition of euphoria. **2.** A substance tending to produce euphoria, as LSD, mescaline, and marijuana.

euphoria **1.** A feeling or state of well-being or elation. **2.** An exaggerated or abnormal sense of physical and emotional well-being not based on reality or truth, disproportionate to its cause, and inappropriate to the situation, as commonly seen in the manic stage of bipolar disorder, in some forms of schizophrenia, in organic mental disorders, and in toxic and drug-induced states. Compare **ecstasy.**

euploid **1.** Of or pertaining to an individual, organism, strain, or cell with a chromosome number that is an exact multiple of the normal, basic haploid number characteristic of the species, as diploid, triploid, tetraploid, or polyploid. Variation occurs through entire sets rather than individual chromosomes, so that there is a balanced number of chromosomes. **2.** Such an individual, organism, strain, or cell. Compare **aneuploid.**

euploidy The state or condition of having a variation in chromosome number that is an ex-

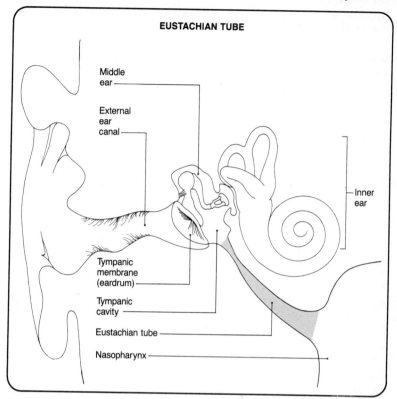

EUSTACHIAN TUBE

Middle ear

External ear canal

Inner ear

Tympanic membrane (eardrum)

Tympanic cavity

Eustachian tube

Nasopharynx

act multiple of the characteristic haploid number. Compare **aneuploidy.**

European blastomycosis See **cryptococcosis.**

European typhus See **epidemic typhus.**

europium (Eu) A rare-earth, metallic element. Its atomic number is 63; its atomic weight is 151.96.

eury- A combining form meaning 'wide, broad': *eurycephalic, eurygnathic, euryopia.*

eustachian tube A tube, lined with mucous membrane, that joins the nasopharynx and the tympanic cavity, allowing equalization of the air pressure in the inner ear with atmospheric pressure. Also called **auditory tube.**

euthanasia Deliberately bringing about the death of a person who is suffering from an incurable disease or condition, either actively, by administering a lethal drug, or passively, by withholding treatment. Also called **mercy killing.**

evacuate 1. To discharge or to remove a substance from a cavity, space, organ, or tract of the body. 2. A substance discharged or removed from the body. **—evacuation,** *n.*

evaluation In five-step nursing process: a category of nursing behavior in which a determination is made and recorded regarding the extent to which the established goals of care have been met. To make this judgment, the nurse estimates the degree of success in meeting the goals, evaluates the implementation of nursing measures, investigates the client's compliance with therapy, and records the client's response to therapy. The nurse evaluates effects of the measures used, the need for change in goals of care, the accuracy of the implementation of nursing measures, and the need for change in the client's environment or in the equipment or procedures used. The impact of the care or treatment on the client, the client's family, and the staff is evaluated, the accuracy of tests and measurements is checked, and the client's and the family's understanding of the information given them is evaluated. The client's expressed and observed response to care is recorded. Although evaluation is the final step of the five-step nursing process, following implementation, in practice, evaluation is integral to effective nursing practice at all steps of the process. See also **assessment, intervention, nursing diagnosis, planning.**

evaporation The change of a substance from a solid or liquid state to a gaseous state. The process of evaporation is hastened by an increase in temperature and a decrease in atmospheric pressure. See also **boiling point. —evaporate,** *v.*

evocation In embryology: a specific morphogenetic change within a developing embryo that occurs as a result of the action of a single evocator. See also **induction.**

evocator A specific chemical substance or hormone that is emitted from the organizer part of the embryonic tissue and acts as a morphogenetic stimulus in the developing embryo.

evoked potential A tracing of a brain wave measured on the surface of the head at various places. The wave, unlike the waves seen on an electroencephalogram, is elicited by a specific stimulus. The stimulus may originate in the visual, auditory, or somatosensory areas normally evoked by the stimulus of the nervous system. The activity and function of the system may be monitored during surgery, while the patient is unconscious. The surgeon is thus able to avoid damage to the nerves during operative procedures. Evoked potentials are also used to diagnose multiple sclerosis and various disorders of hearing and of sight. Kinds of evoked potentials include **brain stem auditory evoked potential, somatosensory evoked potential, visual evoked potential.** See also **brain electrical activity map.**

evolution 1. A gradual, orderly, and continuous process of change and development from one condition or state to another. It encompasses all aspects of life, including physical, psychological, sociological, cultural, and intellectual development, and involves a progressive advancement from a simple to a more complex form or state through the processes of modification, differentiation, and growth. 2. In genetics: the theory of the origin and propagation of all plant and animal species, including man, and their development from lower to more complex forms through the natural selection of variants produced through genetic mutations, hybridization, and inbreeding. Kinds of evolution are **convergent evolution, determinant evolution, emergent evolution, organic evolution, orthogenic evolution, saltatory evolution.** —**evolutionist,** *n.*

Ewing's sarcoma A malignant tumor developing from bone marrow, usually in long bones or the pelvis. It occurs most frequently in adolescent boys and is characterized by pain, swelling, fever, and leukocytosis. The tumor, a soft, crumbly grayish mass that may invade surrounding soft tissues, is difficult to distinguish histologically from a neuroblastoma or a reticulum cell sarcoma. Radiotherapy often produces a dramatic initial response, but relapses are common. Surgical excision, often requiring amputation, may be recommended. Also called **endothelial myeloma, Ewing's tumor.** See also **neuroblastoma.**

Ewing's tumor See **Ewing's sarcoma.**

ex- A combining form meaning 'away from, outside, without': *exacrinous, excoriation, exfoliato.*

exacerbation An increase in the seriousness of a disease or disorder as marked by greater intensity of the patient's signs or symptoms.

exanthem, *pl.* **exanthemata** A skin eruption, as the rash of any common infectious disease of childhood, including chickenpox, measles, roseola infantum, or rubella. Compare **enanthema.** —**exanthematous,** *adj.*

exanthem subitum See **roseola infantum.**

exchange transfusion in the newborn The introduction of whole blood in exchange for 75% to 85% of an infant's circulating blood that is repeatedly withdrawn in small amounts and replaced with equal amounts of donor blood. The procedure is performed to improve the oxygen-carrying capacity of the blood in the treatment of erythroblastosis neonatorum by removing the Rh and the ABO antibodies, sensitized erythrocytes producing hemolysis, and accumulated bilirubin. Prior to exchange transfusion, nothing is administered by mouth for 3 to 4 hours, or the contents of the infant's stomach are aspirated. During the procedure, the patient is observed for bradycardia with less than 100 beats per minute, cyanosis, hypothermia, vomiting, aspiration, apnea, an air embolus, abdominal distention, or cardiac arrest. After the procedure, the infant is observed for signs of tachycardia or bradycardia, tachypnea or bradypnea, hypothermia, lethargy, jitteriness, increasing jaundice, cyanosis, edema, dark urine, bleeding from the cord, convulsions, or such complications as hemorrhage, hypocalcemia, heart failure, hypoglycemia, sepsis, acidosis, hyperkalemia, thrombus formation, or shock. NURSING CONSIDERATIONS: The nurse prepares the equipment and infant for the exchange transfusion, assists the physician in the insertion of the umbilical venous line, and monitors the infant during and after the procedure. The nurse explains the reason for the procedure to the parents. An exchange transfusion is usually administered only to a high-risk infant, but the procedure often effectively counteracts the hemolytic anemia and hyperbilirubinemia associated with erythroblastosis neonatorum.

excise To remove completely, as in the surgical excision of the palatine tonsils. Compare **resect.** —**excision,** *n.*

excision 1. The process of excising. 2. In molecular genetics: the process by which a certain genetic element is removed from a strand of DNA.

exciting eye In sympathetic ophthalmia: the eye that is infected by the sympathizing eye, metastasis being by way of the bloodstream or the lymphatics.

excoriation An injury to the surface of the skin or other part of the body caused by scratching or abrasion.

excrete To evacuate a waste substance from the body, often by means of a normal secretion, as a drug may be excreted in breast milk. —**excretion,** *n.*

excretion The process of eliminating, shedding, or getting rid of substances by body organs or tissues, as part of a natural metabolic activity. Excretion usually begins at the cellular level where water, carbon dioxide, and other waste products of cellular life are emptied into the capillaries. The epidermis excretes dead skin cells by shedding them daily. —**excrete,** *v.*

excretory Relating to the process of excretion, often used in combination with a term to identify an object or procedure associated with excretion, as in excretory urography.

excretory duct A duct that is conductive but not secretory.

excretory urography See **intravenous pyelography.**

exercise **1.** The performance of any physical activity for the purpose of conditioning the body, improving health, or maintaining fitness or as a means of therapy for correcting a deformity or restoring the organs and bodily functions to a state of health. **2.** Any action, skill, or maneuver that exerts the muscles and is performed repeatedly in order to develop or strengthen the body or any of its parts. **3.** To use a muscle or part of the body in a repetitive way in order to maintain or develop its strength. Exercise has a beneficial effect on each of the body systems, although in excess it can lead to the breakdown of tissue and cause injury. Kinds of exercise are **active assisted exercise, active exercise, active resistive exercise, aerobic exercise, anaerobic exercise, corrective exercise, isometric exercise, isotonic exercise, muscle-setting exercise, passive exercise, progressive resistance exercise, range-of-motion exercise.**

exercise electrocardiogram (exercise EKG) A stress test that is important in the diagnosis of coronary artery disease. An exercise electrocardiogram is recorded as a person walks on a treadmill or pedals a stationary bicycle for a given length of time at a specific rate of speed. Abnormal changes in cardiac function that were absent during rest may occur with exercise.

exfoliation Peeling and sloughing off of dead skin layers. This is a normal process that may be exaggerated in certain skin diseases or after severe sunburn. See also **desquamation, exfoliative dermatitis.** —**exfoliative,** *adj.*

exfoliative cytology The microscopic examination of desquamated cells for diagnostic purposes. The cells are obtained from lesions, sputum, secretions, urine, and other material by aspiration, scraping, a smear, or washings of the tissue. Compare **aspiration biopsy cytology.**

exfoliative dermatitis Any inflammatory skin disorder in which there is excessive peeling or shedding of skin. The cause is unknown in about half of the cases. Known causes include drug reactions, scarlet fever, leukemia, lymphoma, and generalized dermatitis. Treatment is individualized, but care is essential to prevent secondary infection, to avoid further irritation, and to maintain fluid balance.

exhalation See **expiration.**

exhale To breathe out or to let out with the breath. —**exhalation,** *n.*

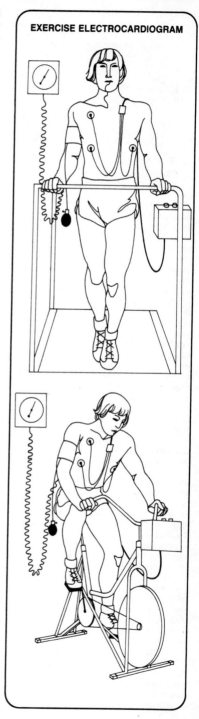

EXERCISE ELECTROCARDIOGRAM

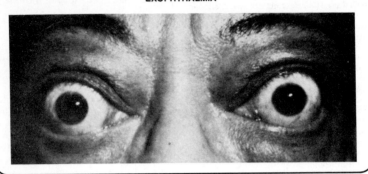

EXOPHTHALMIA

exhaustion delirium A delirium that may result from prolonged physical or emotional stress, fatigue, or shock associated with severe metabolic or nutritional problems. See also **delirium.**

exhibitionism **1.** The flaunting of oneself or one's abilities in order to attract attention. **2.** In psychiatry: a psychosexual disorder occurring in men in which the repetitive act of exposing the genitals to females in socially unacceptable situations is the preferred means of achieving sexual excitement and gratification. See also **paraphilia, scopophilia. —exhibitionist,** *n.*

existential-humanistic psychotherapy See **humanistic-existential therapy.**

existential psychiatry A school of psychiatry based on the philosophy of existentialism that emphasizes an analytical, holistic approach in which mental disorders are viewed as deviations within the total structure of an individual's existence rather than as caused by any biologically or culturally related factors.

existential therapy A kind of psychotherapy that emphasizes the development of a sense of self-direction through choice, awareness, and acceptance of individual responsibility.

exit dose In radiotherapy: the amount of radiation at the surface of the body opposite the surface to which the beam is directed.

exo- A combining form meaning 'outside, outward': *exocataphoria, exohysteropexy.*

exocoelom See **extraembryonic coelom.**

exocrine Of or pertaining to the process of secreting outwardly through a duct to the surface of an organ or tissue or into a vessel, as a gland that secretes through a duct. Compare **endocrine.** See also **eccrine.**

exocrine gland Any one of the two kinds of multicellular glands that open on the surface of the skin through ducts in the epithelium, as the sweat glands and the sebaceous glands. Exocrine glands comprise simple glands having only one duct and compound glands having more than one duct.

exogenous depression See **reactive depression.**

exogenous hyperlipemia See **type I hyperlipoproteinemia.**

exogenous obesity Obesity owing to a caloric intake greater than needed to meet the metabolic needs of the body. Compare **endogenous obesity.** See also **obesity.**

exon In molecular genetics: the part of a DNA molecule that produces the code for the final messenger RNA.

exonuclease In molecular genetics: a nuclease that digests DNA from the ends of the strands.

exophoria Deviation of the visual axis of one eye away from that of the other eye, occurring in the absence of visual stimuli for fusion. Compare **exotropia. —exophoric,** *adj.*

exophthalmia An abnormal condition characterized by marked protrusion of the eyeballs, usually resulting from the increased volume of the orbital contents caused by a tumor; swelling associated with cerebral, intraocular, or intraorbital edema or hemorrhage; paralysis of or trauma to the extraocular muscles; or cavernous sinus thrombosis. It may also be caused by endocrine disorders, as hyperthyroidism and Graves' disease; by varicose veins within the orbit; or by injury to orbital bones. Visual acuity may be impaired in exophthalmia; keratitis, ulceration, infection, and blindness may also occur. Treatment depends on the underlying cause of the condition. The outcome depends on the cause and the stage at which the condition is detected and treatment is begun. Acute advanced exophthalmia is frequently irreversible. Also called **proptosis, protrusio bulbi. —exophthalmic,** *adj.*

exophthalmic goiter Exophthalmos occurring in association with goiter, as in Graves' disease.

exophthalmometer An instrument used for measuring the degree of forward displacement of the eye in exophthalmos. The device allows measurement of the distance from the center of the cornea to the lateral orbital rim. This distance is rarely more than 18 mm (¾ inch). An exophthalmometer is a horizontal calibrated bar with movable carriers on both sides.

exophthalmos, exophthalmus Abnormal protrusion of one or both eyeballs caused by trauma, intracranial lesions, intraorbital disorders, or systemic disease, most commonly hyperthyroidism. Exophthalmos may occur in acromegaly, Cushing's disease, systemic amyloides, Wegener's granulomatosis, or as a result of leukemic infiltration into retrobulbar spaces, nasopharyngeal infection or tumor, or intraorbital inflammatory disease, tumor, or vascular anomaly, as ophthalmic artery aneurysm, arteriovenous malformation, hemangioma, or varices. Dark glasses or shields may be required to protect the cornea from abrasion. Long-standing exophthalmos may lead to drying, infection, or ulceration of the cornea. Treatment may include control of hyperthyroidism, the administration of prednisone, or, as a last resort, decompression of the orbit by lateral orbitotomy, transantral decompression, or transfrontal craniotomy. —**exophthalmic,** *adj.*

exophthalmos - macroglossia - gigantism syndrome See **EMG syndrome.**

exophytic Of or pertaining to the tendency to grow outward, as an exophytic tumor that grows on the surface or exterior portion of an organ or structure.

exophytic carcinoma A malignant, epithelial neoplasm that resembles a papilloma or wart.

exostosis An abnormal, benign growth on the surface of a bone. —**exostosed, exostotic,** *adj.*

exotoxin A toxin that is secreted or excreted by a living microorganism. Compare **endotoxin.**

exotropia Strabismus characterized by the outward deviation of one eye relative to the other. Compare **esotropia.** See also **strabismus.** —**exotropic,** *adj.*

expectant treatment Applying therapeutic measures to relieve symptoms as they arise in the course of a disease rather than treating the cause of the illness itself. Some kinds of expectant treatment are amputations for gangrene in a patient with diabetes, coronary bypass procedures in a patient with generalized atherosclerosis, transplantation of tendons in a patient with severe rheumatoid arthritis. Compare **definitive treatment, palliative treatment.** See also **treatment.**

expectation In nursing: **1.** Anticipation by the staff of a client's behavior based on a knowledge and understanding of the client's abilities and problems. **2.** Anticipation of the performance of the nursing staff, as role expectation.

expectation of life The probable number of years that a person will live after a given age, as determined by the mortality in a specific geographic area. It may be individually qualified by the person's condition, race, sex, age, or other demographic factor. Also called **life expectancy.**

expected date of confinement (EDC) The predicted date of a pregnant woman's delivery. Pregnancy lasts approximately 266 days, or 38 weeks, from the day of fertilization but is considered clinically to last 280 days, or 40 weeks. In the absence of a special calendar or device for calculating the EDC, it is arrived at by counting back 3 months from the 1st day of the last menstrual period and then adding 7 days and 1 year. The expectant mother is advised that the EDC is only an estimate and that the chances are that she will give birth within 2 weeks before or, more commonly, after the calculated date.

expectorant 1. Of or pertaining to a substance that promotes the ejection of mucus or other exudates from the lungs, bronchi, and trachea. **2.** An agent that promotes expectoration by reducing the viscosity of pulmonary secretions or by decreasing the force with which exudates adhere to the lower respiratory tract. —**expectorate,** *v.*

expectoration The ejection of mucus, sputum, or fluids from the trachea and lungs by coughing or spitting.

experience rating 1. A rating system used by an insurance company to set the premium to be paid by the insured, based on the risk to the insurance company of providing the insurance. Experience rating has led to very high malpractice premiums in some specialties and areas, for the insurance company calculates the premium on the basis of settlements made in all malpractice claims during a specified period. Experience rating is also used to set annual membership health maintenance fees in organizations in which the cost of providing the services in a previous accounting period is used to determine the premiums for the next fiscal year. **2.** The rating that is used to calculate an insurance premium.

experimental design In research: a study design used to test cause-and-effect relationships between variables. The classic experimental design specifies an experimental group and a control group. The independent variable is administered to the experimental group and not to the control group, and both groups are measured on the same dependent variable.

experimental embryology The study and analysis through experimental techniques of the factors, mechanisms, and relationships that determine and influence prenatal development.

experimental group See **group.**

experimental medicine A branch of the practice of medicine in which new drugs or treatments are evaluated for safety and efficacy in a clinical laboratory setting by using animals or, in some cases, human subjects.

experimental physiology A branch of the study of physiology in which the functions of various body systems are evaluated in a clinical laboratory setting by using animals or, in some cases, human subjects.

experimental psychology The study of mental processes and phenomena by observation in a controlled environment using various tests, manipulations, and experiments.

experimental variable See **independent variable.**

expert witness A person who has special

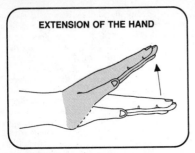

EXTENSION OF THE HAND

knowledge of a subject about which a court requests testimony. Special knowledge may be acquired by experience, education, observation, or study but is not possessed by the average person. An expert witness gives expert testimony or expert evidence. This evidence often serves to educate the court and the jury in the subject under consideration.

expiration Breathing out, normally a passive process, depending on the elastic qualities of lung tissue and the thorax. Also called **exhalation.** Compare **inspiration.** —**expire,** *v.*

expiratory reserve volume (ERV) The maximum volume of gas that can be expired from the resting expiratory level. See also **vital capacity.**

expired gas (E) Any gas exhaled from the lungs.

exposure treatment In burn therapy: method for healing a wound by leaving it open to the air without a dressing, with or without a topical medication. A cradle placed over the patient supports sterile covers to preserve body heat during treatment. The preferred therapy for facial, head, neck, and perineal burns and useful when a large number of casualties require treatment, it produces drying and allows a layer of serum to harden protectively over the wound. If infection occurs, this layer is removed and the wound treated with baths and topical antimicrobials.

expression 1. The indication of a physical or emotional state through facial appearance or vocal intonation. 2. The act of pressing or squeezing in order to expel something, as milk from the breast following pregnancy or the fetus from the uterus by exerting pressure on the abdominal wall. 3. In genetics: the detectable effect or appearance in the phenotype of a particular trait or condition. See also **expressivity.** —**express,** *v.*

expressive aphasia See **motor aphasia.**

expressivity In genetics: the variability with which basic patterns of inheritance are modified, both in degree and in variety, by the effect of a given gene in people of the same genotype. Polydactyly may be expressed as extra toes in one generation and extra fingers in another.

expulsive stage of labor The second stage of labor, during which the mother's uterine contractions are accompanied by a bearing-down reflex. It begins after full dilatation of the cervix

and continues to the complete delivery of the infant.

extended-care facility An institution devoted to providing medical, nursing, or custodial care for an individual over a prolonged period of time, as during the course of a chronic disease or during the rehabilitation phase after an acute illness. Kinds of extended-care facilities are intermediate-care facility, skilled nursing facility. Also called **convalescent home, nursing home.**

extended family A family group consisting of the biological parents, their children, the parents' parents, and other family members. The extended family is the basic family group in many societies. Among its characteristics are increased exchange of information from experienced older members to less experienced younger ones, care of the older family members in the home by the younger ones, and care by the older people of the children of the younger members. Compare **nuclear family.**

extended insulin zinc suspension A long-acting ultralente insulin that is slowly absorbed and slow to act.

extension A movement allowed by certain joints of the skeleton that increases the angle between two adjoining bones. Compare **flexion.**

extensor carpi radialis brevis One of the seven superficial muscles of the posterior forearm. Lying beneath the extensor carpi radialis longus, it arises from the lateral epicondyle of the humerus, from the radial collateral ligament of the elbow joint, and from various intermuscular septa. It inserts into the dorsal surface of the third metacarpal bone. The muscle is innervated by a branch of the radial nerve that contains fibers from the sixth and the seventh cervical nerves, and it functions to extend the hand.

extensor carpi radialis longus One of the seven superficial muscles of the posterior forearm. Arising from the lateral supracondylar ridge of the humerus, it inserts at the base of the second metacarpal bone. It is innervated by a branch of the deep radial nerve that contains fibers from the sixth, seventh, and eighth cervical nerves, and it functions to extend and abduct the hand.

extensor carpi ulnaris One of the seven superficial muscles of the posterior forearm. It arises from the lateral epicondyle of the humerus and dorsal border of the ulnas, and inserts at the base of the fifth metacarpal bone. It is innervated by the deep radial neve and functions to extend and adduct the wrist.

extensor digiti minimi One of the seven superficial muscles of the posterior forearm. Located on the medial side of the extensor digitorum, it is a slender muscle that arises from the common extensor tendon and joins the expansion of the extensor digitorum tendon on the back of the first phalanx of the little finger. The muscle is innervated by a branch of the deep radial nerve that contains fibers from the sixth, seventh, and eighth cervical nerves, and it functions to extend the little finger.

extensor digitorum One of the seven superficial muscles of the posterior forearm. Arising from the lateral epicondyle of the humerus, the intermuscular septa between it and adjacent muscles, and the antebrachial fascia, it divides distally into four tendons that pass through the extensor retinaculum and diverge on the back of the hand, inserting into the second and the third phalanges of the fingers. The muscle is innervated by a branch of the deep radial nerve that contains fibers from the sixth, seventh, and eighth cervical nerves, and it functions to extend the phalanges and, by continued action, the wrist. Also called **extensor digitorum communis.**

extensor digitorum communis See **extensor digitorum.**

extensor digitorum longus A penniform muscle located at the lateral part of the anterior leg. It is one of three anterior crural muscles and arises from the lateral condyle of the tibia, the anterior surface of the fibula, the deep surface of the fascia, and from intermuscular septa. Its distal tendon passes under the extensor retinacula and divides into four slips that insert into the second and third phalanges of the four lesser toes. The muscle is innervated by branches of the deep peroneal nerve containing fibers from the fourth and the fifth lumbar and first sacral nerves. It extends the proximal phalanges of the four small toes and dorsally flexes and pronates the foot. Compare **tibialis anterior.**

extensor retinaculum of the hand See **retinaculum extensorum manus.**

extern, externe A student or recent graduate in medicine, osteopathy, podiatry, or dentistry who is fulfilling an educational requirement by assisting in the medical and surgical care of patients in a health-care facility under the direct supervision of a licensed doctor. Compare **intern, resident.**

external 1. Being on the outside or exterior of the body or an organ. 2. Acting from the outside, as an external influence or exogenous factor. 3. Pertaining to the outward or visible appearance. Compare **internal.**

external absorption The taking up of poisons, drugs, nutrients, or other substances through the mucous membranes or the skin.

external acoustic meatus The S-shaped canal of the external ear, comprised of bone and cartilage, extending from the auricle to the tympanic membrane. Also called **external auditory canal.**

external aperture of aqueduct of vestibule An external opening for the small canal extending from the vestibule of the inner ear, located on the internal surface of the petrous part of the temporal bone, lateral to the opening for the internal acoustic passage.

external aperture of canaliculus of cochlea An external opening of the cochlear channel on the margin of the jugular opening in the temporal bone.

external aperture of tympanic canaliculus The lower opening of the tympanic chan-

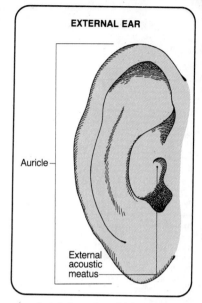

EXTERNAL EAR

Auricle

External acoustic meatus

nel on the inferior surface of the petrous part of the temporal bone.

external auditory canal See **external acoustic meatus.**

external carotid artery One of a pair of arteries with eight major temporal or maxillary branches, rising from the common carotid arteries and supplying various parts and tissues of the head and neck.

external carotid plexus A network of nerves around the external carotid artery, formed by the external carotid nerves from the superior cervical ganglion and supplying sympathetic fibers associated with branches of the external carotid artery. Compare **common carotid plexus, internal carotid plexus.**

external cervical os An external opening of the uterus that leads into the cavity of the cervix. This opening, bounded by the ventral lip and the dorsal lip, is in the center of the rounded extremity of the cervix that projects into the cavity of the vagina. Compare **internal cervical os.**

external conjugate The distance measured with obstetric calipers from the depression below the lowest lumbar vertebra posteriorly to the upper border of the symphysis anteriorly (usually about 21 cm, or 8¼ inches). The external conjugate is roughly 8.5 cm greater than the obstetric conjugate, but the correlation is not consistent, and the measurement is seldom used in modern obstetrics. Also called **Baudelocque's diameter.**

external cuneiform bone See **lateral cuneiform bone.**

external ear The outer structure of the ear, consisting of the auricle and the external acoustic meatus. Sound waves are funneled through

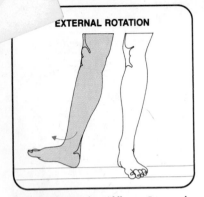

EXTERNAL ROTATION

the external ear to the middle ear. Compare **internal ear, middle ear.**

external fertilization   The union of male and female gametes outside of the bodies from which they originated, as occurs in most fish.

external fistula   An abnormal passage between an internal organ or structure and the cutaneous surface of the body.

external iliac artery   A division of the common iliac artery descending into the thigh and becoming the femoral artery. The external iliac supplies the lower limb and is larger than the internal iliac, except in the fetus, where it is smaller. Compare **internal iliac artery.**

external iliac node   A node in one of the seven groups of parietal nodes serving the lymphatic system in the abdomen and the pelvis. About 10 external iliac nodes, arranged in three groups, lie along the external iliac vessels. Their afferents drain lymph from numerous abdominal and pelvic structures, as the deep abdominal wall, the adductor region of the thigh, the prostate, and the vagina. Compare **common iliac node, iliac circumflex node, internal iliac node.** See also **lymph, lymphatic system, lymph node.**

external iliac vein   One of a pair of veins in the lower body that join the internal iliac vein to form the two common iliac veins. Each external iliac vein begins under the inguinal ligament, ascends along the brim of the lesser pelvis, and ends opposite the sacroiliac articulation by joining the internal iliac vein. In many individuals, it contains at least one valve and sometimes two. It receives the inferior epigastric vein, the deep iliac circumflex vein, and the pubic veins. Compare **internal iliac vein.**

external jugular vein   One of a pair of large vessels in the neck that receive most of the blood from the exterior of the cranium and the deep tissues of the face. Each external jugular vein is formed by the junction of the retromandibular vein with the posterior auricular vein and arises in the parotid gland on a level with the angle of the mandible. It runs perpendicularly down the neck and joins the subclavian vein lateral or ventral to the scalenus anterior. It contains two pairs of valves: the inferior pair at the junc-

tion with the subclavian vein and the superior pair, usually about 4 cm (1½ inches) above the clavicle. A sinus lies between the two sets of valves. Compare **internal jugular vein.**

external oblique muscle   See **obliquus externus abdominis.**

external perimysium   See **epimysium.**

external pin fixation   A method of holding together the fragments of a fractured bone by employing transfixing metal pins through the fragments and a compression device attached to the pins outside the skin surface. Nursing care includes regular cleansing of the skin around the pins and, often, the application of antibiotic solutions or ointments. The pins are removed in a later procedure when the fracture is healed. Compare **internal fixation.**

external pterygoid muscle   See **pterygoideus lateralis.**

external radiation therapy (ERT)   The therapeutic application of ionizing radiation from an external beam from a kilovoltage X-ray machine, a megavoltage cobalt-60 machine, or a supervoltage linear accelerator, cyclotron, or betatron. ERT is used most frequently in the treatment of cancer but may also be applied in the therapy of keloids and some dermatological conditions and in counteracting the body's physiological rejection of transplanted organs.

external rotation   The movement of a body part away from a central axis, as occurs when a ball-and-socket joint, such as the hip, turns a limb outward. Compare **internal rotation.**

external shunt   A device for the passage of a body fluid from one compartment of the body to another, consisting of a tube or catheter or a series of such containers that passes over the surface of the body from one compartment or cavity to another. See also **hemodialysis, hydrocephalus.**

exteroceptive   Pertaining to stimuli that originate from outside of the body or to the sensory receptors that they activate. Compare **interoceptive, proprioception.**

exteroceptor   Any sensory nerve ending, as those located in the skin, mucous membranes, or sense organs, that responds to stimuli originating from outside of the body, as touch, pressure, or sound. Compare **interoceptor, proprioceptor.** See also **chemoreceptor.**

extra-   A combining form meaning 'outside of, beyond, in addition to': *extrabronchial, extradural, extramarginal.*

extrabuccal feeding   The administration of nutrients by means other than the mouth. Also called **extraoral feeding.** See also **gavage, intravenous feeding.**

extracapsular fracture   Any fracture that occurs near a joint but does not directly involve the joint capsule. This type of fracture is extremely common in the hip.

extracellular   Occurring outside a cell or cell tissue, or in cavities or spaces between cell layers or groups of cells. About 40% of the water in a human body is contained in extracellular fluids. See also **cell, edema, interstitial.**

extracellular fluid (ECF) The portion of the body fluid comprising the interstitial fluid and blood plasma. The adult body contains about 11.2 liters of interstitial fluid, constituting about 16% of body weight, and about 2.8 liters of plasma, constituting about 4% of body weight. Plasma and interstitial fluid are very similar chemically and, in conjunction with intracellular fluid, help control the movement of water and electrolytes throughout the body. Some of the important ionized components of extracellular fluid are protein, magnesium, potassium, chlorine, calcium, and certain sulfates.

extradural Outside the dura mater.

extradural anesthesia Anesthetic nerve block achieved by the injection of a local anesthetic solution into the space in the spinal canal outside the dura mater of the spinal cord, as in epidural, caudal, or paravertebral anesthesia.

extradural hemorrhage A hemorrhage of an area surrounding, but outside of, the dura of the brain or spinal cord.

extraembryonic blastoderm The area of the blastoderm that gives rise to the membranes that surround the embryo during gestation. Compare **embryonic blastoderm.** See also **allantois, amnion, chorion, yolk sac.**

extraembryonic coelom A cavity external to the developing embryo that forms between the mesoderm of the chorion and that covering the amniotic cavity and yolk sac. During early prenatal development, there is direct contact with the embryonic coelom at the umbilicus, but this junction is obliterated by the growth of the amnion and the closing of the body wall. Also called **exocoelom.**

extramedullary myeloma A plasma cell tumor that occurs outside of the bone marrow, usually affecting the visceral organs or the nasopharyngeal and oral mucosa. Also called extramedullary plasmacytoma, peripheral plasma cell myeloma, plasma cell tumor. See also **plasmacytoma.**

extramedullary myelopoiesis The formation and development of myeloid tissue outside of the bone marrow. Also called **ectopic myelopoiesis.**

extraocular Outside the eye.

extraocular muscle palsy An abnormal condition characterized by paralysis of the extrinsic muscles of the eye, as the superior, inferior, medial, and lateral rectus muscles and the superior and inferior oblique muscles.

extraoral feeding See **extrabuccal feeding.**

extraperitoneal cesarean section A method for surgically delivering an infant through an incision in the lower uterine segment without entering the peritoneal cavity. The uterus is approached through the paravesicle space. This procedure is performed most often to avoid spread of infection from the uterus into the peritoneal cavity. It is somewhat slower to perform than the low cervical or classic cesarean operations. See also **cesarean section.**

extrapsychic conflict An emotional conflict usually occurring when one's inner needs and desires do not coincide with the restrictions of the environment or society. Compare **intrapsychic conflict.** See also **conflict.**

extrapyramidal **1.** Of or pertaining to the tissues and structures of the brain that are associated with movement of the body, excluding motor neurons, the motor cortex, and the corticospinal and corticobulbar tracts. **2.** Of or pertaining to the function of these tissues and structures.

extrapyramidal disease Any of a large group of conditions characterized by involuntary movement, changes in muscle tone, and abnormal posture, as in tardive dyskinesia, chorea, athetosis, and Parkinson's disease.

extrapyramidal reaction A response to a treatment or a drug characterized by the signs of extrapyramidal disease. The reaction may persist or regress after discontinuation of the treatment or drug.

extrapyramidal system The part of the nervous system that includes the basal ganglia, substantia nigra, subthalamic nucleus, part of the midbrain, and the motor neurons of the spine. The extrapyramidal system controls and coordinates the motor activities required for locomotion and for stasis, body support, and posture. Also called **extrapyramidal tracts.**

extrapyramidal tracts The tracts of motor nerves from the brain to the anterior horns of the spinal cord, except for the fibers of the pyramidal tracts. Within the brain, extrapyramidal tracts comprise various relays of motor neurons between motor areas of the cerebral cortex, the basal ganglia, the thalamus, the cerebellum, and the brain stem. Research into the precise functions of these networks continues, and it is not yet known how some of them work. The extrapyramidal tracts are functional rather than anatomical units, comprising the nuclei and the fibers and excluding the pyramidal tracts. They especially control and coordinate the postural, static, supporting, and locomotor mechanisms and cause contractions of muscle groups in sequence or simultaneously. The extrapyramidal tracts include the corpus striatum, the subthalamic nucleus, the substantia nigra, and the red nucleus, together with their interconnections with the reticular formation, the cerebellum, and the cerebrum. Compare **pyramidal tract.**

extrasensory perception (ESP) Awareness or knowledge acquired without using the physical senses. See also **clairvoyance, parapsychology, telepathy.**

extrasystole A premature atrial, ventricular, or cardiac contraction that does not change the fundamental rhythm of the heart.

extravasation Infiltration into subcutaneous tissues, usually of blood, serum, or lymph, or of a drug or intravenous solution. Compare **bleeding.** See also **exudate, transudate. —extravasate,** *v.*

extraventricular hydrocephalus See **hydrocephalus.**

⌐ See **extroversion.**

⌐⌐⌐⌐ergic alveolitis See **hyper-⌐⌐ity pneumonitis.**

⌐xtrinsic allergic pneumonia See **hypersensitivity pneumonitis.**

extrinsic asthma A form of asthma in which attacks are precipitated primarily by allergens to which the patient is sensitized. The initial onset usually occurs prior to the age of 30 years. Also called **allergic asthma, atopic asthma.** See also **asthma in children.**

extrinsic factor See **cyanocobalamin.**

extroversion, extraversion 1. The tendency to direct one's interests and energies toward external values or things outside the self. 2. The state of being totally or primarily concerned with what is outside the self. Compare **introversion.**

extrovert, extravert 1. A person whose interests are directed away from the self and concerned primarily with external reality and the physical environment rather than with inner feelings and thoughts. This person is usually highly sociable, outgoing, impulsive, and emotionally expressive. 2. A person characterized by extroversion. Compare **introvert. —extroversion,** n.

extrusion reflex A normal response in infants to force the tongue outward when it is touched or depressed. The reflex begins to disappear by about 3 or 4 months of age. Before it fades, food must be placed well back in the mouth to be retained and swallowed. Constant protrusion of a large tongue may be a sign of Down's syndrome.

extubation The process of withdrawing a tube from an orifice or cavity of the body. **—extubate,** v.

exuberant callus See **heterotopic ossification.**

exudate Fluid, cells, or other substances that have been slowly exuded, or discharged, from cells or blood vessels through small pores or breaks in cell membranes. Perspiration is sometimes identified as an exudate.

exudative Relating to the exudation or oozing of fluid and other materials from cells and tissues, usually as a result of inflammation or injury, used in the identification of a disease or disorder marked by signs of exudation, as exudative enteropathy.

exudative angina See **croup.**

exudative enteropathy Diarrhea seen in diseases characterized by inflammation or destruction of intestinal mucosa. Crohn's disease, ulcerative colitis, tuberculosis, and some lymphomas cause an increase of plasma, blood, mucus, and protein to accumulate in the intestine, adding to fecal bulk and frequency. See also **diarrhea.**

eye One of a pair of organs of sight, contained in a bony orbit at the front of the skull, embedded in orbital fat, and innervated by one of a pair of optic nerves from the forebrain. Associated with the eye are certain accessory structures, as the muscles, the fasciae, the eyebrow, the eyelids, the conjunctiva, and the lacrimal gland. The bulb of the eye is composed of segments of two spheres with nearly parallel axes that constitute the outside tunic and one of three fibrous layers enclosing two internal cavities separated by the crystalline lens. The smaller cavity anterior to the lens is divided by the iris into two chambers, both filled with aqueous humor. The posterior chamber is larger than the anterior chamber and contains the jellylike vitreous body, which is divided by the hyaloid canal. The outside tunic of the bulb consists of the transparent cornea anteriorly, constituting one fifth of the tunic, and the opaque sclera posteriorly, constituting five sixths of the tunic. The intermediate vascular, pigmented tunic consists of the choroid, the ciliary body, and the iris. The internal tunic of nervous tissue is the retina. Light waves passing through the lens strike a layer of rods and cones in the retina, creating impulses that are transmitted by the optic nerve to the brain. The transverse and the anteroposterior diameters of the eye bulb are slightly greater than the vertical diameter; the bulb in women is usually smaller than the bulb in men. Also called **bulbus oculi, eyeball.**

eyebrow 1. The supraorbital arch of the frontal bone that separates the orbit of the eye from the forehead. 2. The arch of hairs growing along the ridge formed by the supraorbital arch of the frontal bone.

eyeground The fundus of the eye. See also **funduscopy.**

eye irrigation solutions Substances that stimulate natural tears, used to reduce eye irritation.

eyelash One of many cilia growing in double or triple rows along the border of the eyelids in front of a row of ciliary glands that are in front of a row of Meibomian glands.

eyelid A movable fold of thin skin over the eye, with eyelashes and ciliary and Meibomian glands along its margin. It consists of loose connective tissue containing a thin plate of fibrous tissue lined with mucous membrane. The orbicularis oculi muscle and the oculomotor nerve control the opening and closing of the eyelid. The upper and lower eyelids are separated by the palpebral fissure. Also called **palpebra.**

eye memory See **visual memory.**

F

f **1.** Breaths per unit time. **2.** Symbol for respiratory frequency.

F **1.** Symbol for **fluorine. 2.** *abbr* **farad.**

F₁ In genetics: the symbol for the first filial generation; the heterozygous offspring produced by the mating of two unrelated individuals or by the crossing of a homozygous dominant strain with a homozygous recessive.

F₂ In genetics: the symbol for the second filial generation; the offspring produced by mating two members of the F_1 generation or, broadly, by crossing any two heterozygous strains.

FAAN *abbr* **Fellow of the American Academy of Nursing.**

Fabry's disease, Fabry's syndrome See **angiokeratoma corporis diffusum.**

FACCP *abbr* **Fellow of the American College of Chest Physicians.**

face **1.** The front of the head from the chin to the brow, including the skin, muscles and structures of the forehead, eyes, nose, mouth, cheeks, and jaw. **2.** To direct the face toward something. See also **en face. —facial,** *adj.*

face validity The apparent validity of a test or measurement device used in a particular study. See also **validity.**

facial artery One of a pair of tortuous arteries that arise from the external carotid arteries, divide into four cervical and five facial branches, and supply various organs and tissues in the head. The cervical branches of the facial artery are the ascending palatine, tonsillar, glandular, and the submental. The facial branches are the inferior labial, superior labial, lateral nasal, and the angular.

facial diplegia A rare neuromuscular condition characterized by bilateral paralysis of various facial muscles.

facial muscle One of numerous muscles of the face, seldom remaining distinct over its entire length because of a tendency to merge with a neighboring muscle at its termination or attachment. The five groups of facial muscles include those of the scalp, the extrinsic ear, the nose, and the mouth. The platysma is one of the facial group but is described with the neck muscles. Also called muscle of expression.

facial nerve Either of a pair of mixed sensory and motor cranial nerves that arises from the brain stem at the base of the pons and divides just in front of the ear into its six branches, innervating the scalp, forehead, eyelids, muscles of facial expression, cheeks, and jaw. Also called **seventh cranial nerve.**

facial paralysis An abnormal condition characterized by the partial or total loss of the facial muscle functions or the loss of sensation in the face, caused by disease or trauma. The degree of paralysis depends on the nerves affected. Brain injury above the facial nucleus usually does not block the innervation of the brow and the forehead muscles. Injury to the nucleus of the facial nerve or injury to its peripheral neurons paralyzes all the ipsilateral facial muscles. See also **Bell's palsy.**

facial perception The ability to judge the distance and direction of objects through the sensation felt in the skin of the face. The phenomenon is commonly experienced by those who are blind but rarely experienced in the dark by those with sight. Also called facial vision.

facial vein One of a pair of superficial veins that drain deoxygenated blood from the superficial structures of the face. Each facial vein starts as the angular vein at the union of the frontal and the supraorbital veins and accompanies the facial artery, passing deep to the zygomaticus major and the zygomaticus minor, following the border of the masseter, curving around the mandible into the neck, and communicating with the anterior jugular vein and the external jugular vein to empty into the internal jugular vein. The facial vein anastomoses with the cavernous sinus through various veins. As the vein has no valves that prevent the backflow of blood, infections of the skin near the nose and mouth may cause meningitis, because blood-borne organisms can reach the cavernous sinus through the anastomoses.

facial vision See **facial perception.**

facilitation **1.** The enhancement or reinforcement of any action or function so that it is carried out with increased ease. Compare **inhibition. 2.** In neurology: the phenomenon whereby two or more afferent impulses that individually are not strong enough to elicit a response in a neuron can collectively produce a reflex discharge greater than the sum of the separate responses. See also **summation. 3.** In neurology: the process of lowering the threshold action potential of a neuron by the repeated passage of an impulse along the same pathway. Also called **law of facilitation.**

facio- A combining form meaning 'pertaining to the face': *faciocervical, faciolingual, facioplegia.*

FACOG *abbr* Fellow of the American College of Obstetricians and Gynecologists.

FACS *abbr* **Fellow of the American College of Surgeons.**

FACSM *abbr* Fellow of the American College of Sports Medicine.

-faction A combining form meaning a 'process of making': *bilifaction, liquefaction.*

FACTORS OF BLOOD COAGULATION

FACTOR	SYNONYM	PROFILE	SITE OF SYNTHESIS
I	Fibrinogen	Precursor of fibrin	Liver
II	Prothrombin	Precursor of thrombin	Liver
III	Tissue thromboplastin	Activator of prothrombin	All tissues
IV	Calcium (Ca^{++})	Essential for prothrombin activation and formation of fibrin	From diet
V	Proaccelerin	Accelerates conversion of prothrombin to thrombin	Liver
VII	Serum prothrombin (proconvertin)	Accelerates conversion of prothrombin to thrombin	Liver
VIII	Antihemophilic factor (AHF, hemophilic factor A)	Associated with factors IX, XII, and XI; aids in formation of plasma thromboplastin and conversion of prothrombin to thrombin	Reticuloendothelial system
IX	Christmas factor (hemophilic factor B, plasma thromboplastin component [PTC])	Activated by factor XI; essential to formation of plasma thromboplastin; associated with factors XII, XI, and VIII	Liver
X	Stuart-Prower factor	Triggers prothrombin conversion; requires vitamin K	Liver
XI	Plasma thromboplastin antecedent (PTA)	Activated by factor XII; associated with factors XII, IX, and VIII in formation of plasma thromboplastin	Unknown
XII	Hageman factor	First factor activated in the intrinsic pathway; activates factor XI in formation of plasma thromboplastin	Unknown
XIII	Fibrin stabilizing factor (FSF)	Produces stronger urea-insoluble fibrin clot	Unknown

factitial Artificial or self-induced.

factitial dermatitis A skin rash caused by the patient, usually for secondary gain or as a manifestation of psychiatric illness.

-factive A combining form meaning 'making': *liquefactive, stupefactive, vasofactive.* Also **-fying.**

factor I See **fibrinogen.**

factor II See **prothrombin.**

factor III See **thromboplastin.**

factor IV A designation for calcium as an element in the process of the coagulation of blood.

factor V An unstable procoagulant that occurs in normal plasma but is deficient in the blood of parahemophiliacs. It is needed to rapidly convert prothrombin to thrombin. Some research indicates that during coagulation, factor V changes from an inactive agent to an active prothrombin accelerator. Also called **proaccelerin.**

factor VII A blood procoagulant present in the blood plasma synthesized in the liver by the action of vitamin K. Also called **proconvertin.**

factor VIII A coagulation factor present in normal plasma but deficient in the blood of persons with hemophilia A.

factor IX A coagulation factor present in normal plasma but deficient in the blood of persons with hemophilia B. Also called **Christmas factor.**

factor IX complex A systemic hemostatic used to treat factor IX deficiency.

factor X A coagulation factor present in normal plasma but deficient in some inherited defects in coagulation. Factor X and prothrombin are both synthesized in the liver by vitamin K. Also called **Stuart-Prower factor.**

factor XI A coagulation factor present in normal plasma. Deficiency results in prolonged coagulation time.

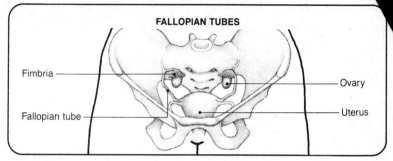

FALLOPIAN TUBES

Fimbria

Ovary

Fallopian tube

Uterus

factor XII A coagulation factor present in normal plasma. It triggers the formation of bradykinin and associated enzymatic reactions. It is required for rapid coagulation in vitro but is apparently not needed for hemostasis in vivo. It can be activated in the laboratory by contact with negatively charged surfaces, which can develop on glass and kaolin or on biological material, as collagen. Also called **activation factor, contact factor, glass factor, Hageman factor.**

factor XIII A coagulation factor present in normal plasma that acts with calcium to produce an insoluble fibrin clot. Also called **fibrinase, fibrin-stabilizing factor.**

factor-searching study In nursing research: a study design that produces a qualitative, narrative description including categories or classifications of phenomena. Factor searching is often a preliminary step in a study at a higher level of inquiry.

facultative Not obligatory; having the ability to adapt to more than one condition.

facultative aerobe An organism able to grow under anaerobic conditions that develops most rapidly in an aerobic environment. Compare **obligate aerobe.** See also **aerobe.**

facultative anaerobe An organism able to grow under aerobic conditions that develops most rapidly in an anaerobic environment. Compare **obligate anaerobe.** See also **anaerobe, anaerobic infection.**

facultative parasite See **parasite.**

faculty 1. An ability to do something specific, as learn languages or remember names. 2. Any mental ability or power, as memory. 3. A department in an institution of learning or the people who teach in a department of such an institution.

faculty practice plan A medical school system by which faculty members can increase income by practicing their specialty of medicine in a departmental practice in a school-controlled organization. Nursing school faculties are beginning to use this system for retrieval of incomes from service.

Faget's sign A falling pulse rate associated with a constant temperature, or a constant pulse associated with a rising temperature. It is an unusual sign found in yellow fever. Also called Faget's law.

fagicladosporic acid A toxin produced by *Cladosporium*, a genus of fungi that cause 'black spot' in stored meat, tinea nigra, and black degeneration of the brain.

Fahrenheit A scale for the measurement of temperature in which the boiling point of water is 212° and the freezing point of water is 32° at sea level. Compare **Celsius.**

failed forceps An attempted midforceps operation that is abandoned because there is a greater degree of resistance to rotation or traction than anticipated, owing to cephalopelvic disproportion. Cesarean section is performed to deliver the infant. Compare **trial forceps.** See also **cephalopelvic disproportion.**

failure to thrive The abnormal retardation of the growth and development of an infant resulting from conditions that interfere with normal metabolism, appetite, and activity. Causative factors include chromosomal abnormalities; major organ system defects that lead to deficiency or malfunction; systemic disease or acute illness; physical deprivation, primarily malnutrition; and various psychosocial factors. Prolonged nutritional deficiency may cause permanent and irreversible retardation of physical, mental, or social development.

faint *Nontechnical.* 1. To lose consciousness. 2. A syncopal attack. See also **syncope.**

falciform body See **sporozoite.**

falciparum malaria The most severe form of malaria, caused by the protozoan *Plasmodium falciparum*, characterized by grave systemic symptoms, mental confusion, enlarged spleen, edema, gastrointestinal symptoms, and anemia. Falciparum malaria does not last as long as other forms of malaria; if treatment is begun promptly, the disease may be mild and the recovery uneventful. Relapses are uncommon, but death may result from dehydration and anemia. The usual treatment is chloroquine, but patients known to have contracted malaria in an area that harbors drug-resistant *P. falciparum* are often treated with a combination of quinine, pyremethamine, and one of the sulfones or sulfonamides. Compare **quartan malaria, tertian malaria.** See also **algid malaria, blackwater fever, malaria.**

fallopian tube One of a pair of ducts opening at one end into the uterus and at the other end into the peritoneal cavity, over the ovary.

the passage through which … to the uterus and through … a move out toward the ovary. … in the upper border of the broad … (the mesosalpinx). Each tube has four … the fimbriae, the infundibulum, the am-…ulla, and the isthmus. The fimbriae drape in fingerlike projections from the infundibulum over the ovary. Just proximal to the infundibulum is the ampulla, the widest portion of the tube. The ampulla is connected to the fundus of the uterus by the isthmus. Also called **oviduct, uterine tube.**

Fallot's syndrome   See **tetralogy of Fallot.**

fallout   The deposition of radioactive debris after a nuclear explosion. The debris from an atmospheric explosion of an atomic bomb may travel thousands of miles over a large geographical area.

false anorexia   See **pseudoanorexia.**

false labor   See **Braxton-Hicks contraction.**

false negative   An incorrect result of a diagnostic test or procedure that falsely indicates the absence of a finding, condition, or disease. As the accuracy and specificity of a test increase, the rate of false negatives decreases. Certain tests are known to yield false negative results at a certain rate. False-negative results are more common than false-positive results, because the person conducting the test is more likely to fail to observe a finding than to report an imaginary finding. Compare **false positive.**

false neuroma   **1.** A neoplasm that does not contain nerve elements. **2.** A cystic neuroma.

false nucleolus   See **karyosome.**

false positive   A test result that wrongly indicates the presence of a disease or other condition the test is designed to reveal.

false rib   See **rib.**

false suture   An immovable fibrous joint in which rough articulating surfaces form the connection between certain bones of the skull. Two kinds of false sutures are **sutura plana, sutura squamosa.** Compare **true suture.**

false twins   See **dizygotic twins.**

false vocal cord   Either of two thick folds of mucous membrane in the larynx separating the ventricle from the vestibule. Each fold encloses a narrow band of fibrous tissue (the ventricular ligament). Compare **vocal cord.**

falx, *pl.* **falces**   **1.** A sickle-shaped structure. **2.** Sickle shaped.

falx cerebelli   A small sickle-shaped process of the dura mater attached to the occipital bone above and projecting into the posterior cerebellar notch between the two cerebellar hemispheres.

falx cerebri   A tough membrane extending into and following the longitudinal fissure of the two hemispheres of the cerebrum.

falx inguinalis   Transverse and internal oblique muscles.

falx ligamentosa   The broad ligament of the liver.

familial cretinism   A rare genetic disorder characterized by hypothyroidism caused by an inborn error of metabolism resulting from a deficiency of the enzyme iodotrysine deiodinase, which interferes with thyroid hormone biosynthesis. Clinical manifestations include lethargy, stunted growth, and mental retardation. The condition, which is transmitted as an autosomal recessive trait, is treated by early administration of thyroid hormone.

familial hypercholesterolemia   An inherited disorder transmitted as a dominant trait and characterized by a high level of serum cholesterol, tendinous xanthomas, and early evidence of atherosclerosis, especially of the coronary arteries. Affected individuals at the age of 50 have 3 to 10 times greater risk of ischemic heart disease than the general population. Cholesterol levels are elevated at birth and increase with age. Xanthomas begin to appear at the age of 20 and occur most frequently on the Achilles tendon, extensor tendons of the hands, elbows, and tibial tuberosities. In Type IIa familial hypercholesterolemia, only low-density lipoprotein (LDL) is elevated, while in Type IIb, LDL and very low-density lipoprotein (VLDL) are increased. The prevalence of the gene in the United States is 1:1000. Treatment consists of a low-cholesterol and low-saturated-fat diet. Cholestyramine may be given to patients with Type IIa familial hypercholesterolemia but not to those with Type IIb. Also called **hypercholesterolemic xanthomatosis, type II hyperlipoproteinemia.**

familial iminoglycinuria   See **iminoglycinuria.**

familial juvenile nephronophthisis   See **medullary cystic disease.**

familial lipoprotein lipase deficiency   See **hyperchylomicronemia.**

familial osteochondrodystrophy   See **Morquio's disease.**

familial spinal muscular atrophy   See **Werdnig-Hoffmann disease.**

familial tremor   See **essential tremor.**

family   **1.** A group of people related by heredity, as parents, children, and siblings. The term is sometimes broadened to include persons living in the same household or those related by marriage. **2.** A group of persons having a common surname, as the Anderson family. **3.** A category of animals or plants situated on a taxonomic scale between order and genus. See also **genetics, heredity. —familial,** *adj.*

family-centered care   Primary health care that includes an assessment of the health of an entire family, identification of actual or potential factors that might influence the health of its members, and implementation of actions to maintain or improve the health of the unit and its members.

family-centered nursing care   Nursing care directed toward improving the potential health of a family or any of its members by assessing individual and family health needs and strengths, by identifying problems influencing the health care of the family as a whole as well as those influencing the individual members, by using family resources, by teaching and counseling, and by evaluating progress toward stated goals.

family ganging An unethical medical practice in which the patient is encouraged or required to involve the entire family in a program of health care even if the other family members do not require such care. Family ganging is often practiced in so-called Medicaid mills. See also **Medicaid.**

family health In a health history: an account of the health of the members of the immediate family. Hereditary and familial diseases are especially noted. The family health history is obtained from the patient or family in the initial interview and becomes a part of the permanent record.

family history An essential portion of a patient's medical history in which the patient is asked about the health of the other members of the family, such as "Has anyone in your family had tuberculosis? diabetes mellitus? breast cancer?," to discover any diseases to which the patient may be particularly vulnerable. Other questions, as those concerning the age, sex, relationships of others in the household, and the marital history of the patient may also be asked.

family medicine The branch of medicine that is concerned with the diagnosis and treatment of health problems in people of either sex and any age. Practitioners of family medicine are often called family practice physicians, family physicians, or, formerly, general practitioners.

family nurse practitioner (FNP) A nurse practitioner possessing skills necessary for the detection and management of acute self-limiting conditions and management of chronic stable conditions. An FNP provides primary, ambulatory care for families, in collaboration with primary care physicians.

family physician **1.** A medical practitioner of the specialty of family medicine. **2.** A general practitioner. **3.** A family practice physician. See also **family medicine.**

family planning See **contraception.**

family practice physician A practitioner of family medicine, usually one who has completed a residency program in the specialty. See also **family medicine.**

family therapy In psychiatry: a therapeutic approach to the care of any one of the members of a family. The entire immediate family may meet together with a therapist.

famine fever See **relapsing fever.**

FANCAP *U.S.* A mnemonic device for helping student nurses learn to assess, provide, and evaluate direct patient care. It stands for *f*luids, *a*eration, *n*utrition, *c*ommunication, *a*ctivity, and *p*ain. Occasionally a variant, FANCAS, is substituted for FANCAP, in which case the 'S' stands for *s*timulation.

Fanconi's syndrome A rare, usually congenital disorder, characterized by aplastic anemia, bone abnormalities, olive-brown skin pig-

mentation, microcephaly, hypogenitalism, cystinosis, and abnormalities of renal tubular function. A form of the syndrome acquired in adulthood is the result of heavy metal poisoning by cadmium, copper, lead, mercury, or uranium; by the ingestion of outdated tetracycline; or by other damage to the renal tubules. The condition may occur with Wilson's disease or follow transplantation of a kidney.

fantasy **1.** The unrestrained free play of the imagination; fancy. **2.** A mental image, usually distorted or grotesque in nature, often the result of the action of drugs or a disease of the central nervous system. **3.** The mental process of transforming undesirable experiences into imagined events or into a sequence of ideas in order to fulfill an unconscious wish, need, or desire, or to give expression to unconscious conflicts, as a daydream.

farad (F) A unit of capacitance that increases the potential difference between the plates of a capacitor by one volt with a charge of one coulomb.

Farber test A microscopic examination of newborn meconium for lanugo and squamous cells. The fetus normally swallows amniotic fluid containing these large proteins, which then pass through the digestive system to be excreted, usually after birth, in the first stools. The absence of hair or skin cells is suggestive of intestinal obstruction or atresia and requires further evaluation.

Far Eastern hemorrhagic fever A form of epidemic hemorrhagic fever, indigenous to Asia, that is transmitted by a virus carried by an Asian rodent. The infection is characterized by chills, fever, headache, abdominal pain, nausea, vomiting, anorexia, and extreme thirst. Hypotensive shock may occur as the fever subsides. Thirst continues into the 2nd week, oliguria develops, and the blood pressure returns to normal. Diuresis follows the oliguric phase, resulting in an output of as much as 8 liters of urine a day and in electrolyte imbalance. Mortality may be as high as 33%. There is no specific treatment.

farmer's lung A respiratory disorder caused by the inhalation of actinomycetes or other organic dusts from moldy hay. It is a form of hypersensitivity pneumonitis, affecting individuals who have developed antibodies to the mold spores, and characterized by coughing, dyspnea, cyanosis, tachycardia, nausea, chills, and fever. Treatment may include cromolyn sodium and a corticosteroid.

far-sightedness See **hyperopia.**

fasci- A combining form meaning 'pertaining to a band or bundle of fibrous tissue': *fasciagram, fascicular.*

fascia, pl. **fasciae** The fibrous connective tissue of the body that may be separated from other specifically organized structures, as the tendons, the aponeuroses, and the ligaments. It varies in thickness and density and in the amounts of fat, collagenous fiber, elastic fiber, and tissue fluid it contains. Kinds of fasciae are **deep fas-**

FASCIA BULBI

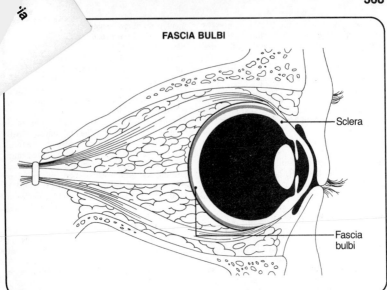

Sclera

Fascia bulbi

cia, **subcutaneous fascia, subserous fascia.**
—fascial, *adj.*

fascia bulbi A thin membranous socket that envelops the eyeball from the optic nerve to the ciliary region and allows the eyeball to move freely. The fascia bulbi has a smooth inner surface, pierced by vessels and nerves, and fuses with the sheath of the optic nerve and with the sclera. The lower part of the membrane thickens into the suspensory ligament, which attaches to the zygomatic arch and the lacrimal bones. Also called **Tenon's capsule.**

fascial cleft A place of cleavage between two contiguous fascial surfaces, as the deep fasciae and the subcutaneous fasciae. A fascial cleft is rich in fluid but poor in traversing fibers; thus, two fascial surfaces may move or be separated from each other easily. Compare **fascial compartment, fascial membrane lamination.**

fascial compartment A part of the body that is walled off by fascial membranes, usually containing a muscle, a group of muscles, or an organ. Compare **fascial cleft, fascial membrane lamination.**

fascial membrane lamination A pad of connective tissue that contains fat and an occasional blood vessel or a lymph node. It is found where a fascial membrane splits into two sheets, as at the division of the outer cervical fascia above the sternum. Compare **fascial cleft, fascial compartment.**

fascia thoracolumbalis The extensive subdivision of the vertebral fascia that sheaths the sacrospinalis muscle. It spreads caudally to become the glistening, white lumbar aponeurosis and the origin of the latissimus dorsi. Medially, the fascia thoracolumbalis attaches to the sacrum, laterally to the ribs and the intercostal fascia, and cranially to the ligamentum nuchae.

Also called **lumbodorsal fascia.**

fascicle A general term for a small bundle of nerve, muscle, or tendon fibers. Also called **fasciculus.**

fascicular neuroma A neoplasm composed of myelinated nerve fibers. Also called **medullated neuroma.**

fasciculation A localized, uncoordinated, uncontrollable twitching of a single muscle group innervated by a single motor nerve fiber or filament that may be palpated and seen under the skin. It results from a variety of drugs as a side effect with normal dosage or from an overdose, or it may be symptomatic of a number of disorders, including dietary deficiency, cerebral palsy, fever, tic, or uremia. Fasciculation of the heart muscle is known as fibrillation. **—fascicular,** *adj.,* **fasciculate,** *v.*

fasciculus, *pl.* **fasciculi** A small bundle of muscle, tendon, or nerve fibers. The arrangement of fasciculi in a muscle is correlated with the power of the muscle and its range of motion. The patterns of muscular fasciculi are penniform, bipenniform, multipenniform, and radiated. **—fascicular,** *adj.*

fascioliasis Infection with the liver fluke *Fasciola hepatica,* characterized by epigastric pain, fever, jaundice, eosinophilia, urticaria, and diarrhea, with fibrosis of the liver a consequence of prolonged infection. It is acquired by ingestion of encysted forms of the fluke found on aquatic plants, as watercress. Bithionol, given orally, is the usual treatment.

fasciolopsiasis An intestinal infection, prevalent in the Far East, caused by the fluke *Fasciolopsis buski.* It is characterized by abdominal pain, diarrhea, constipation, eosinophilia, ascites, and, sometimes, edema. The disease is usually acquired by eating contaminated water plants, as water chestnuts. It is easily treated with anthelmintics.

fascioscapulohumeral dystrophy An abnormal congenital condition and one of the main types of muscular dystrophy. It is characterized by progressive symmetric wasting of the skeletal muscles, especially the muscles of the face, the shoulders, and the upper arms, without any associated neural or sensory disorders. It is not usually fatal but spreads to all the voluntary muscles and commonly produces a pendulous lower lip and the absence of the nasolabial fold. It is an autosomal dominant disease. Fascioscapulohumeral dystrophy usually occurs before age 10 but may also develop during adolescence. Early symptoms include the inability to pucker the lips, abnormal facial movements when laughing or crying, facial flattening, winging of the scapulae, inability to raise the arms over the head, and, in infants, the inability to suckle. Confirming diagnosis is based on muscle biopsy showing abnormal deposits of fat and connective tissue. Electromyography may show attenuated electrical activity, an inconclusive sign when considered alone but helpful in ruling out neurogenic muscle atrophy. No treatment can halt the progression of associated muscle impairment. Some measures that may help preserve mobility are physical therapy, surgery, and the use of orthopedic appliances. NURSING CONSIDERATIONS: Nurses usually help preserve the mobility of the patient by assisting with therapeutic exercises. High-protein, high-fiber diets and the use of stool softeners can help avoid constipation. Nurses often counsel family members who are carriers of the disease about the dangers of transmitting the disorder and refer patients who must learn new job skills to the appropriate agencies. Compare **Duchenne's muscular dystrophy.**

fast **1.** Resistant to change, especially to the action of a specific drug or chemical. **2.** To abstain from all or certain foods. See also **fasting.**

fast-acting insulin One of a group of insulin preparations in which the onset of action is rapid, approximately 1 hour, and the duration of the action is relatively brief, approximately 6 to 14 hours. Kinds of fast-acting insulins include **insulin injection, prompt insulin zinc suspension.**

fastigium **1.** The highest point in the course of a fever, or the most symptomatic point in the course of an illness. **2.** The angle at the top of the roof of the fourth ventricle in the brain.

fasting Abstaining from food for a specific period of time, usually for therapeutic or religious purposes.

fat **1.** A substance composed of lipids or fatty acids and occurring in various forms or consistencies ranging from oil to tallow. **2.** A type of body tissue composed of cells containing stored fat (depot fat). Stored fat is usually identified as white fat, which is found in large cellular vesicles, or brown fat, which consists of lipid droplets. Stored fat contains more than twice as many calories per gram as sugars, and helps cushion

and insulate vital organs. See also **adipose, obesity.**

fatal Resulting in death; pertaining to the actual or imminent cause of death. Compare **lethal.**

fat cell lipoma See **hibernoma.**

fat embolism A serious circulatory condition characterized by the blocking of an artery by an embolus of fat that entered the circulatory system following the fracture of a long bone, or less commonly, after traumatic injury to adipose tissue or to a fatty liver. A systemic condition may occur following extensive trauma, because lipid metabolism is altered by the injury and causes release of free fatty acids resulting in vasculitis with obstruction of many small pulmonary and cerebral arteries. Fat embolism usually occurs suddenly 12 to 36 hours after the injury and is characterized by severe chest pain, pallor, dyspnea, tachycardia, delirium, prostration, and, in some cases, coma. Anemia and thrombocytopenia are common. Classic signs of systemic fat embolism are petechial hemorrhages on the neck, shoulders, axillae, and conjunctivae, appearing 2 or 3 days after the injury. There is no specific therapy; the patient is placed in high-Fowler's position and given oxygen, digitalis, corticosteroids, blood transfusions, respiratory assistance, and other supportive care.

fat emulsions A source of calories used in total parenteral nutrition therapy.

FA test See **fluorescent antibody test.**

father complex *Nontechnical.* A daughter's repressed desire for an incestuous relationship with her father.

father fixation An arrest in female psychosexual development that is characterized by an abnormally persistent, close, and often paralyzing emotional attachment to one's father. Compare **mother fixation.** See also **Freudian fixation.**

fatigue **1.** A state of exhaustion or a loss of strength or endurance, as may follow strenuous physical activity. **2.** Loss of ability of tissues to respond to stimuli that normally evoke muscular contraction or other activity. Muscle cells generally require a refractory or recovery period after activity, during which time cells restore their energy supplies and excrete metabolic waste products. **3.** An emotional state associated with extreme or extended exposure to psychic pressure, as in battle or combat fatigue. See also **lactic acid.**

fatigue fever A benign episode of fever and muscle pain following overexertion, caused by an accumulation of the metabolic waste products of muscle contractions.

fatigue fracture Any fracture that results from excessive physical activity and not from any specific injury, as commonly occurs in the metatarsal bones of runners.

fat metabolism The biochemical process by which fats are broken down and elaborated by the cells of the body. Fats provide more food energy than carbohydrates; the catabolism of 1 g of fat provides 9 kilocalories of heat as com-

alories yielded in the ca-
~ohydrate. Before the final
~abolism can occur, fats must
~nto fatty acids and glycerol. Con-
~ glycerol provides a compound that
~ter the citric acid cycle. Catabolism of
~y acids continues by beta oxidation to produce acetyl-CoA, which also enters the citric
acid cycle. The body synthesizes fats from fatty
acids and glycerol or from compounds derived
from excess glucose or from amino acids. The
body can synthesize only saturated fatty acids.
Essential unsaturated fatty acids can be supplied only by the diet. Certain hormones, as insulin, growth hormone, adrenocorticotropic
hormone, and the glucocorticoids, control fat
metabolism. Fat catabolism is inversely related
to the rate of carbohydrate catabolism, and in
some conditions, as diabetes mellitus, the secretion of these hormones increases to counter
a decrease in carbohydrate catabolism.

fatty acid   Any of several organic acids produced by the hydrolysis of neutral fats. In a living
cell a fatty acid occurs in combination with another molecule rather than in a free state. Essential fatty acids are unsaturated molecules that
cannot be produced by the body and must therefore be included in the diet. Kinds of essential
fatty acids are **arachidonic, linoleic, linolenic.**
See also **saturated fatty acid, unsaturated fatty
acid.**

fatty alcohol   A hydroxide of a hydrocarbon
from the paraffin series.

fatty ascites   See **chylous ascites.**

fatty cirrhosis   See **cirrhosis.**

fatty liver   An accumulation of triglycerides
in the liver. The causes include alcoholic cirrhosis, I.V. administration of such drugs as tetracycline and corticosteroids, and exposure to
toxic substances, as carbon tetrachloride and
yellow phosphorus. Fatty liver is also seen in
kwashiorkor and is a rare complication of unknown etiology in late pregnancy. Its symptoms
are anorexia, hepatomegaly, and abdominal discomfort. This condition is usually reversible. See
also **cirrhosis.**

fauces   The opening of the mouth into the
pharynx. The anterior pillars of the fauces form
the glossopalatine arch, and the posterior pillars
form the pharyngopalatine arch.

favism   An acute hemolytic anemia caused
by ingestion of the beans or inhalation of the
pollen from the *Vicia faba* (fava) plant. Sensitive
individuals show a deficiency of glucose-6-phos-
phate dehydrogenase, usually the result of a hereditary biochemical abnormality of the erythrocytes. Symptoms include dizziness, headache,
vomiting, fever, jaundice, eosinophilia, and, often, diarrhea. The condition is found primarily
in persons of southern Italian extraction and is
treated by blood transfusion and avoidance of
fava beans and pollen. See also **glucose-6-phos-
phate dehydrogenase deficiency.**

favus   A fungal infection of the scalp, more
common in children than adults. It is characterized by thick, yellow crusts with suppuration;

a distinct, "mousy" odor; permanent scars; and
alopecia. Rarely seen in the United States, it is
common in the Middle East and Africa.

FCAP   *abbr* **Fellow of the College of American Pathologists.**

FDA   *abbr* **Food and Drug Administration.**

Fe   Symbol for **iron.**

fear   In nursing: a nursing diagnosis accepted
by the Fifth National Conference on the Classification of Nursing Diagnoses. As a symptom,
fear is analogous to anxiety about, or to dread
of, a specific or real occurrence. The client is
able to identify the object of the fear, which may
itself range from mild apprehension to panic.
See also **nursing diagnosis.**

fear-tension-pain syndrome   A concept
formulated by Grantly Dick-Read, M.D., to explain the pain commonly expected and reported
in childbirth. The concept proposes that mistaken cultural attitudes induce anxiety before
labor and cause fear in labor. This fear causes
muscular and psychological tension that interferes with the natural processes of dilatation and
delivery, resulting in pain. He advocated education, exercise, and warm emotional and physical support in labor to counteract the syndrome,
coining the term "natural childbirth" for a labor
or delivery in which the trained woman, comfortably, and with a calm, cooperative attitude,
participates in the natural experience. Elements
of his method of psychophysical preparation for
childbirth are incorporated into most other
methods of natural childbirth. See also **Bradley
method, Lamaze method.**

febri-   A combining form meaning 'pertaining
to a fever': *febricant, febrifugal, febriphobia.*

febrifuge   See **antipyretic.**

febrile   Pertaining to or characterized by an
elevated body temperature, as a febrile reaction
to an infectious agent. —**febrility,** *n.*

-febrile   A combining form meaning 'pertaining to fever': *afebrile, nonfebrile, subfebrile.*

fecal fistula   An abnormal passage from the
colon to the external surface of the body, dis-
charging feces. Fistulas of this kind are usually
created surgically in operations involving the
removal of malignant or severely ulcerated bowel
segments.

fecal impaction   An accumulation of hardened or inspissated feces in the rectum or sigmoid colon that the individual is unable to move.
Diarrhea may be a sign of fecal impaction since
only liquid material is able to pass the obstruction. Occasionally, fecal impaction may cause
urinary incontinence due to pressure on the
bladder. Treatment includes oil and cleansing
enemas and manual breaking up and removal
of the stool by a gloved finger. Persons who are
dehydrated, nutritionally depleted, on prolonged bed rest, receiving such constipating
medications as iron or opiates, or undergoing
barium X-rays are at risk of developing fecal
impaction. See also **constipation, obstipation.**

fecalith   A hard, impacted mass of feces in
the colon. To allow evacuation, an oil retention
enema is usually administered; if ineffective,

manual removal can be performed. See also **atonia constipation, constipation.**

fecal softener A drug that lowers the surface tension of the fecal mass, allowing the intestinal fluids to penetrate and soften the stool. Also called **stool softener.**

feces Waste or excrement from the digestive tract that is formed in the intestine and expelled through the rectum. Feces consist of water, food residue, bacteria, and secretions of the intestines and liver. Also called **stool.** See also **defecation.** —**fecal,** *adj.*

fecundation Impregnation or fertilization; the act of fertilizing. See also **artificial insemination.** —**fecundate,** *v.*

fecundity The ability to produce offspring, especially in large numbers and rapidly; fertility. —**fecund,** *adj.*

Federation Licensing Examination (FLEX) The standardized licensing examination for state licensure of physicians. Developed by the Federation of State Medical Boards of the United States, the examination is based on National Board of Medical Examiners test materials.

feeblemindedness See **mental retardation.**

feedback **1.** In communication theory: information produced by a receiver and perceived by a sender that informs the sender about the receiver's reaction to the message. Feedback is a cyclic part of the process of communication. **2.** In physiology: the return to the input of part of a system's output, which often modifies the function of the system. This mechanism operates in many body processes; for example, hormone output and enzyme-mediated reactions. See also **negative feedback, positive feedback.**

feeding Taking or giving food or nourishment. Kinds of feeding include **breast-feeding, extrabuccal feeding, forced feeding.**

fee-for-service **1.** A charge made for a professional activity, as for a physical examination. **2.** A system for the payment of professional services in which the practitioner is paid for the particular service rendered, rather than receiving a salary for providing professional services as needed during scheduled hours of work or time on call.

feel life To experience **quickening** *(informal).*

Fehling's solution A solution containing cupric sulfate with sodium hydroxide and potassium sodium tartrate, used for testing for the presence of glucose and other reducing substances in the urine. Also called Fehling's reagent.

Fellow of the American Academy of Nursing (FAAN) A member of the American Academy of Nursing.

Fellow of the American College of Chest Physicians (FACCP) A physician who is a board-certified member of the American College of Chest Physicians.

Fellow of the American College of Surgeons (FACS) A member of the American College of Surgeons, recognized by that professional organization as qualified to practice surgery.

Fellow of the College of American Pathologists (FCAP) A physician who is a member of the College of American Pathologists.

fellowship A grant given to a person for study or training or to allow payment for work on a special project, but not for study toward a degree. It provides a salary and, in some cases, miscellaneous expenses.

felon **1.** A suppurative abscess at the end of a toe or finger. **2.** In law: a person who has committed a felony; a criminal.

felonious assault **1.** See **felony. 2.** See **assault.**

felony In criminal law: a crime declared by statute to be more serious than a misdemeanor and deserving of a more severe penalty. Charges of murder, rape, burglary, and arson are tried as felonies in most cases. Compare **misdemeanor.**

Felty's syndrome Hypersplenism occurring with adult rheumatoid arthritis, characterized by splenomegaly, leukopenia, and frequent infections. Surgical resection of the spleen offers temporary improvement in about half the cases. See **hypersplenism.**

female **1.** Of or pertaining to the sex that bears young or produces ova or eggs. **2.** Feminine.

female catheterization A procedure for removing urine by means of a urinary catheter introduced through the urinary meatus and urethra into the bladder. The procedure is performed to relieve distention if voluntary micturition is not possible (as after trauma or surgery), as a preparation for and during anesthesia, if a specimen of urine from the bladder is required, or if medication is to be instilled into the bladder. A straight catheter or a retention catheter with a balloon may be used. A French size 12 to 16 is usually selected for straight drainage. Catheterization predisposes the urinary tract to infection, and traumatic catheterization increases the risk. Care, gentleness, and asepsis are essential. The indication for catheterization, the age of the patient, and the condition and size of the urethra affect the choice of catheter style and size. Catheterization is needlessly dreaded by many patients; careful explanation may allay the fears. Signs of infection are carefully observed. If a woman is to be catheterized more than twice, an indwelling catheter is usually preferred to a third catheterization.

female reproductive system assessment An evaluation of a patient's genital tract and breasts and an investigation of past and present disorders that may be factors in the individual's current gynecologic condition. See also **pelvic examination.**

feminization **1.** The normal development of female sex characteristics. **2.** The induction of female sex characteristics in a genotypic male. Testicular feminization may be caused by the

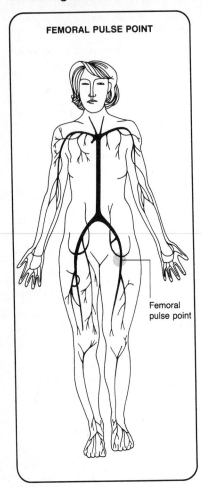

FEMORAL PULSE POINT

Femoral
pulse point

inability of target tissues to respond to endogenous or administered androgen; some cases seem related to an absent or inadequate conversion of testosterone to dihydrotestosterone. Feminization may also be caused by adrenocortical estrogen-secreting tumor; by failure of the liver to inactivate endogenous estrogens, as in advanced alcoholism; or by the administration of estrogen therapy for androgen-dependent neoplasms. Pseudohermaphroditism in males with an X and Y chromosome and a female phenotype may be caused by fetal hypogonadism and is often familial. Individuals with this defect usually have undescended or labial testes; a short, blind vaginal pouch; no uterus; well-developed breasts; sparse or absent axillary and pubic hair; normal plasma levels of testosterone and follicle-stimulating hormone; and increased concentrations of estradiol and luteinizing hormone. Treatment consists of orchiectomy because of the risk of gonadal cancer in these patients. Some testicular

tumors may produce feminizing symptoms, and gynecomastia may be caused by Klinefelter's syndrome and by certain drugs, as reserpine, digitalis, meprobamate, and cimetidine. Compare **virilization.**

feminizing adrenal tumor   A rare neoplasm of the adrenal cortex, characterized in males by gynecomastia, hypertension, diffuse pigmentation, a high level of estrogen in urine, and loss of potency. Testicular atrophy frequently occurs, but the prostate and penis are usually normal in size. Treatment includes surgical resection and chemotherapy with mitotane. In women, these tumors, which are extremely rare, are associated with precocious puberty.

femoral   Of or pertaining to the femur or the thigh.

femoral artery   An extension of the external iliac artery into the lower limb, starting just distal to the inguinal ligament and ending at the junction of the middle and lower third of the thigh. It divides into seven branches and supplies parts of the lower limb and trunk. Its branches are the superficial epigastric, superficial iliac circumflex, superficial external pudendal, deep external pudendal, muscular, profundis femoris, and descending genicular.

femoral hernia   A hernia in which a loop of intestine descends through the femoral canal into the groin. Surgical repair, herniorrhaphy, is the usual treatment. See also **hernia.**

femoral nerve   The largest of the seven branches from the lumbar plexus and the main nerve of the anterior part of the thigh. It arises from the dorsal parts of the ventral primary divisions of the second, third, and fourth lumbar nerves, passes through the lateral, distal fibers of the psoas major, and descends between the psoas major and the iliacus under the cover of the transversalis fascia. Lateral to the femoral artery, it passes under the inguinal ligament, enters the thigh, and breaks into the muscular branches, the anterior cutaneous branches, the intermediate cutaneous nerve, the medial cutaneous nerve, the nerve to the pectineus, the nerve to the sartorius, the saphenous nerve, the branches to the quadriceps femoris, the articular branch to the hip joint, and the articular branches to the knee joint. Also called **anterior crural nerve.**

femoral pulse   The pulse of the femoral artery, palpated in the groin.

femoral torsion   An extreme lateral or a medial twisting rotation of the femur on its longitudinal axis, as may occur owing to the action of the gluteal muscles. Compare **tibial torsion.**

femoral vein   A large vein in the thigh originating in the popliteal vein and accompanying the femoral artery in the proximal two thirds of the thigh. Its distal portion lies lateral to the artery; its proximal portion deeper to the artery. About 4 cm (1½ inches) below the inguinal ligament, it is joined by the deep femoral vein. Near its termination, it is joined by the great saphenous vein. At the inguinal ligament it becomes the external iliac vein. The formal vein has four valves.

femur The thigh bone, which extends from the pelvis to the knee. It is largely cylindrical and is the longest and strongest bone in the body. It has a large, round head that fits the acetabulum of the hip, and it displays a large neck and several prominences and ridges for muscle attachments. In an erect position the femur inclines medially, bringing the knee joint near the line of gravity of the body. Also called **thigh bone.**

fenestra, *pl.* **fenestrae** An aperture, especially in a bandage or cast, that is cut out to relieve pressure or to administer regular skin care.

fenestration **1.** A surgical procedure in which an opening is created to gain access to the cavity within an organ or a bone. **2.** An opening created surgically in a bone or an organ. Also called **window.** —**fenestrate,** *v.*

fenfluramine hydrochloride An amphetamine-like central nervous system stimulant.

fenoprofen calcium A nonsteroidal antiinflammatory agent.

fentanyl citrate A narcotic and opioid analgesic.

fentanyl citrate with droperidol A general anesthetic.

fermentation A chemical change brought about in a substance by the action of an enzyme or microorganism, especially the anaerobic conversion of foodstuffs to certain products. Kinds of fermentation include **acetic fermentation (f.), alcoholic f., ammoniacal f., amylic f., butyric f., caseous f., dextran f., diastatic f., lactic acid f., propionic f., storing f., viscous f.**

fermentative dyspepsia An abnormal condition characterized by impaired digestion associated with the fermentation of digested food. See also **dyspepsia.**

fermium (Fm) A man-made transuranic metallic element. Its atomic number is 100; its atomic weight is 253. Fermium was first detected in the debris from a hydrogen bomb explosion.

-ferous A combining form meaning 'producing or carrying' something specified: *lactiferous, sebiferous, tubiferous.*

ferr- See **ferro-.**

ferri- See **ferro-.**

ferritin An iron compound found in the intestinal mucosa, the spleen, and the liver. It contains over 20% iron and is essential for hematopoiesis.

ferro-, ferr-, ferri- A combining form meaning 'pertaining to iron': *ferrocyanide, ferropectic.*

ferrocholinate A hematinic agent.

ferrous fumarate, f. gluconate, f. sulfate Hematinic agents.

fertile **1.** Capable of reproducing or bearing offspring. **2.** Prolific; fruitful; not sterile. —**fertility,** *n.,* **fertilize,** *v.*

fertile eunuch syndrome A hypogonad-

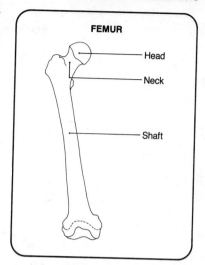

FEMUR

Head

Neck

Shaft

otropic hormonal disorder occurring only in males in which the quantity of testosterone and follicle-stimulating hormone is inadequate for the inducement of spermatogenesis and the development of secondary sexual characteristics. If supplemental hormones are not prescribed, the affected person acquires the appearance of a eunuch.

fertile period The time in the menstrual cycle during which fertilization may occur. Spermatozoa can survive for 48 to 72 hours. An ovum remains viable and capable of being fertilized about 24 hours. The fertile period may be identified by observation of the changes in the quantity and character of cervical mucus or of changes in the basal body temperature, or it may be deduced from a calendar record of six or more menstrual cycles, applying the fact that ovulation usually occurs 14 days prior to menstruation.

fertility factor See **F factor.**

fertilization The union of male and female gametes to form a zygote from which the embryo develops. The process takes place in the fallopian tube of the female when a spermatozoon, carried in the seminal fluid discharged during coitus, comes in contact with and penetrates the ovum. Penetration by the spermatozoon stimulates the completion of the second meiotic division and formation of the pronucleus in the ovum. Fusion and synapsis of the male and female pronuclei restore the diploid number of chromosomes to the germ cell, resulting in the determination of the sex of the zygote and of the characteristics inherited from each parent. Kinds of fertilization include **cross fertilization, external fertilization, internal fertilization.** See also **oogenesis, spermatogenesis.**

fertilization age See **fetal age.**

fertilization membrane A viscous membrane surrounding the fertilized ovum that prevents the penetration of additional spermatozoa.

FETAL CIRCULATION

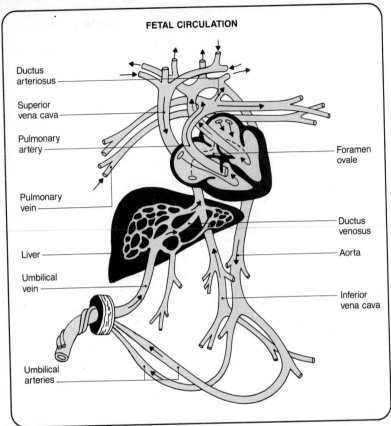

Ductus arteriosus

Superior vena cava

Pulmonary artery

Pulmonary vein

Liver

Umbilical vein

Umbilical arteries

Foramen ovale

Ductus venosus

Aorta

Inferior vena cava

It is formed by granules from the cytoplasm of the fertilized ovum adhering to the vitelline membrane.

fertilizin A glycoprotein found on the plasma membrane of the ovum in various species. See also **acrosomal reaction.**

fetal abortion Termination of pregnancy after the 20th week of gestation but before the fetus has developed enough to live outside of the uterus. Compare **embryonic abortion.**

fetal age The age of the conceptus computed from the time elapsed since fertilization. Also called **fertilization age.** Compare **gestational age.**

fetal attitude The relationship of the fetal parts to each other, as in the "military" attitude, in which the fetal head is not flexed and the chin on chest is as usual but is held straight up. Compare **fetal position, fetal presentation.**

fetal circulation The pathway of blood circulation in the fetus. Oxygenated blood from the placenta travels through the umbilical vein to the liver and the ductus venosus, which carries it to the inferior vena cava and right atrium. The blood enters the right atrium at a pressure sufficient to direct the flow across the atrium and through the foramen ovale into the left atrium; thus, oxygenated blood is available for circulation through the left ventricle to the head and upper extremities. The blood returning from the head and arms enters the right atrium via the superior vena cava. It flows through the atrium at a relatively low pressure; passing the tricuspid valve the blood falls into the right ventricle, from which it is pumped through the pulmonary artery and the ductus arteriosus into the descending aorta for circulation to the lower parts of the body. A small amount of blood in the pulmonary artery is not shunted through the ductus and is carried to the lungs. The blood is returned to the placenta through the umbilical arteries.

fetal distress A compromised condition of the fetus, usually discovered during labor, characterized by an abnormal rate or rhythm of myocardial contraction. Some patterns, as late decelerations of the fetal heart rate seen on records of electronic fetal monitoring, indicate fetal distress. The acid-base balance of the fetal blood is tested. Labor is allowed to continue if the pH is within normal range and if the abnormal pattern does not recur or persist. Cesarean section may be necessary if the fetus is markedly alkalotic or acidotic or if the cause of the distress cannot be corrected. If possible, the fetus is stabilized before being delivered by giving the mother oxygen, increased fluids, or a narcotic antagonist, a vasopressor, or an agent to relax the uterus.

fetal heart rate (FHR)   The number of heartbeats in the fetus occurring in a given unit of time. The FHR varies in cycles of fetal rest and activity and is affected by many factors, including maternal fever, uterine contractions, and many drugs. The normal FHR is 120 to 160 beats per minute.

fetal heart tones (FHT)   The pulsations of the fetal heart heard through the maternal abdomen in pregnancy. The rate, usually between 120 and 160 beats per minute, tends to increase briefly with or just following fetal movement.

fetal hydantoin syndrome (FHS)   A complex of birth defects associated with prenatal maternal ingestion of hydantoin derivatives. Symptoms of FHS include microcephaly, hypoplasia or absence of nails on the fingers or toes, abnormal facies, mental and physical retardation, and cardiac defects. The syndrome occurs to some degree in approximately 10% of infants born of mothers who take this anticonvulsant. Hydantoin may be associated with hemorrhage and, less often, with neural crest tumors in the newborn.

fetal hydrops   Massive edema of the fetus or newborn, as in severe hemolytic disease of the newborn and in other rare hematologic and circulatory disorders of the fetus or newborn. Also called **hydrops fetalis.**

fetal lie   See **presentation.**

fetal lipoma   See **hibernoma.**

fetal monitor   See **electronic fetal monitor.**

fetal position   The relationship of the part of the fetus that presents in the pelvis to four quadrants of the maternal pelvis identified by initial L (left), R (right), A (anterior), and P (posterior). The presenting part is also identified by initial O (occiput), M (mentum), S (sacrum). If a fetus presents with the occiput directed to the posterior aspect of the mother's right side, the fetal position is right occiput posterior (ROP). Compare **fetal attitude, fetal presentation.**

fetal presentation   The part of the fetus that presents in the pelvis. Cephalic presentations include vertex, brow, and chin; breech presentations include frank breech, complete breech, and single- or double-footling breech. Shoulder presentations are rare and require cesarean section or turning before vaginal delivery. Compound presentation involves the entry of more than one part in the true pelvis; most often a hand next to the head. See also **fetal attitude, fetal position.**

fetal stage   In human embryology: the interval of time from the end of the embryonic stage, at the end of the 7th week of gestation, to birth, which occurs 38 to 42 weeks after the first

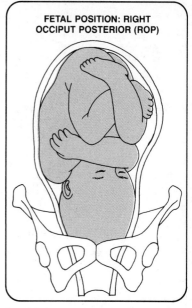

FETAL POSITION: RIGHT OCCIPUT POSTERIOR (ROP)

day of the last menstrual period.

feti-, feto-, foeti-, foeto-   A combining form meaning 'fetus or fetal': *feticide, fetochorionic, fetoscope.*

feticide   See **embryoctony.**

fetish   **1.** Any object or idea given unreasonable or excessive attention or reverence. **2.** In psychology: any inanimate object or any part of the body not of a sexual nature that arouses erotic feelings or fixation. **—fetishism,** *n.*

fetishist   A person who believes in or receives erotic gratification from fetishes.

feto-   See **feti-.**

fetochorionic   Of or pertaining to the fetus and the chorion.

fetography   Roentgenography of the fetus in utero. See also **fetometry.**

fetology   The branch of medicine concerned with the fetus in utero, including the diagnosis of abnormalities, congenital anomalies, the prevention of teratogenic influences, and the treatment of certain disorders. Also called **embryatrics.**

fetometry   The measurement of the size of the fetus, especially the diameter of the head and circumference of the trunk.

fetoplacental   Of or pertaining to the fetus and the placenta.

fetoprotein   An antigen that occurs naturally in fetuses and occasionally in adults as the result of certain diseases. Leukemia, hepatoma, sarcoma, and other neoplasms are associated with **beta fetoprotein** in the blood of adults. An increased amount of **alpha fetoprotein** in the fetus is diagnostic for neural tube defects.

fetoscope   A stethoscope for auscultating the fetal heartbeat through the mother's abdomen.

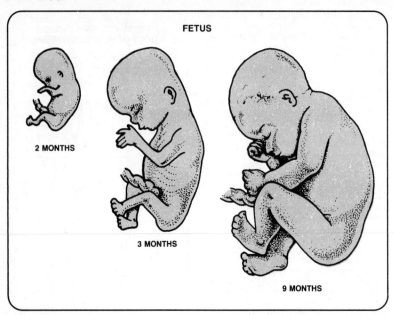

FETUS

2 MONTHS

3 MONTHS

9 MONTHS

fetoscopy A procedure in which a fetus may be directly observed in utero, using a fetoscope introduced through a small incision in the abdomen under a local anesthetic. Photographs of the fetus may be taken and amniotic fluid, fetal cells, or blood may be sampled for prenatal diagnosis of congenital anomalies or genetic defects.

fetus, foetus The unborn offspring of a viviparous animal after it has attained the particular form of the species, more specifically, the human child in utero after the embryonic period and the beginning of the development of the major structural features, usually from the 8th week after fertilization until birth. Kinds of abnormal fetuses include fetus acardiacus, fetus anideus, calcified fetus, mummified fetus, parasitic fetus, sireniform fetus. Compare **embryo.** See also **prenatal development. —fetal, foetal,** *adj.*

fetus acardiacus, fetus acardius See **acardius.**

fetus amorphus A shapeless conceptus in which there are no formed or recognizable parts.

fetus anideus See **anideus.**

fetus in fetu A fetal anomaly in which a small, imperfectly formed twin, incapable of independent existence, is contained within the body of the normal twin, the autosite.

fetus papyraceus A twin fetus that has died in utero early in development and has been pressed flat against the uterine wall by the living fetus. Also called **paper-doll fetus, papyraceous fetus.**

fetus sanguinolentis A fetus that has died in utero and is dark and partly macerated.

FEV *abbr* **forced expiratory volume.**

fever An abnormal elevation of the temperature of the body above 37°C (98.6°F) owing to disease. Fever results from an imbalance between the elimination and the production of heat. Exercise, anxiety, and dehydration may increase the temperature of healthy people. Infection, neurologic disease, malignancy, thromboembolic disease, congestive heart failure, crushing injury, severe trauma, and many drugs may cause fever. No single therapy explains the mechanism whereby the temperature is increased. Fever has no recognized function in conditions other than infection. It increases metabolic activity by 7% per degree centigrade, requiring a greater intake of food. Convulsions may occur in children whose fevers tend to rise abruptly, and delirium is seen with high fevers in adults and in children. Very high temperatures, as in heat stroke, may be fatal. The period of maximum elevation, called the stadium or fastigium, may last for a few days or up to 3 weeks. The fever may resolve suddenly, by crisis, or gradually, by lysis. Also called **hyperpyrexia.** Kinds of fever include **habitual hyperthermia, intermittent fever, relapsing fever.**

fever blister A cold sore caused by herpesvirus I or II. Also called **herpes simplex.**

fever therapy See **artificial fever.**

F factor In bacterial genetics: an episome present in conjugating male bacteria but absent in females. Also called **fertility factor, sex factor.**

FHR *abbr* **fetal heart rate.**

FHS *abbr* **fetal hydantoin syndrome.**

FHT *abbr* **fetal heart tones.**

fiber A slender, elongated thread or filament; a strand of nerve, muscle, or connective tissue.

fiberoptic bronchoscopy The visual examination of the tracheobronchial tree through a fiberoptic bronchoscope. Also called **bronchofibroscopy.** See also **bronchoscopy, fiberoptics.**

fiberoptic duodenoscope An instrument for visualizing the interior of the duodenum, consisting of an eyepiece, a flexible tube incorporating bundles of coated glass or plastic fibers with special optical properties, and a terminal light. When the duodenoscope is introduced into the patient's mouth and threaded through the upper digestive tract to the duodenum, the light illuminates the internal structures and any lesions present.

fiberoptics The technical process by which an internal organ or cavity can be viewed, using glass or plastic fibers to transmit light through a specially designed tube and reflect a magnified image. —**fiberoptic,** adj.

fiberscope A flexible instrument having an inner shaft coated with light-conveying glass or plastic fibers for viewing internal structures. Fiberscopes are specially designed for examining particular organs and cavities of the body and are used in bronchoscopy, endoscopy, and gastroscopy.

fibrillation Involuntary recurrent contraction of a single muscle fiber or of an isolated bundle of nerve fibers. Fibrillation of a heart chamber results in inefficient random contraction of that chamber and disruption of the heart's normal sinus rhythm. Fibrillation is usually described by the part that is contracting abnormally.

fibrin A stringy, insoluble protein, responsible for the semisolid character of a blood clot, that is a product of the action of thrombin on fibrinogen in the clotting process. Compare **fibrinogen.** See also **blood clotting, fibrinolysis, thrombin.**

fibrinase See **factor XIII.**

fibrinogen A plasma protein essential to the blood-clotting process that is converted into fibrin by thrombin in the presence of calcium ions. Compare **fibrin.** See also **afibrinogenemia, blood clotting, fibrinolysis, thrombin.**

fibrinokinase A non–water-soluble enzyme in animal tissue that activates plasminogen. Also called **tissue activator, tissue kinase.**

fibrinolysin A proteolytic enzyme that dissolves fibrin, formed from plasminogen in the blood plasma. Also called **plasmin.** See also **fibrinolysis.**

fibrinolysin and desoxyribonuclease A topically administered enzyme.

fibrinolysis The continual process of fibrin decomposition by fibrinolysis that is the normal mechanism for the removal of small fibrin clots. It is stimulated by anoxia, inflammatory reactions, and other kinds of stress. —**fibrinolytic,** adj.

fibrinopeptide A product of the action of thrombin on fibrinogen. The enzymatic cleavage responsible for the release of this protein fragment produces fibrin as well as the fibrinopep-

tides A and B. The latter consist of short peptides derived from the N-terminal ends of the alpha and beta chains of the fibrinogen molecule. See also **fibrinogen, thrombin.**

fibrin-stabilizing factor See **factor XIII.**

fibro- A combining form meaning 'pertaining to fiber': *fibroadipose, fibroblast, fibrolastosis.*

fibroadenoma, pl. **fibroadenomas, fibroadenomata** A benign tumor of the breast composed of epithelial and fibroblastic tissue. It is nontender, encapsulated, round, movable, and firm. It occurs most frequently in women under 25 years of age and is caused by excessive estrogen. Surgical excision under a local anesthetic and cytologic examination of the mass are usually performed to be sure it is not malignant.

fibroangioma, pl. **fibroangiomas, fibroangiomata** A tumor composed of a mass of blood vessels and fibrous tissue.

fibroareolar tissue See **areolar tissue.**

fibroblast A flat, elongated undifferentiated cell in the connective tissue that gives rise to various precursor cells, as the chondroblast, collagenoblast, and osteoblast, that form the fibrous, binding, and supporting tissue of the body. Also called **desmocyte, fibrocyte.** —**fibroblastic,** adj.

fibroblastoma, pl. **fibroblastomas, fibroblastomata** A tumor derived from a fibroblast, now differentiated as a fibroma or a fibrosarcoma.

fibrocarcinoma See **scirrhous carcinoma.**

fibrocartilage Cartilage that consists of a dense matrix of collagenous fibers. Of the three kinds of cartilage in the body, fibrocartilage has the greatest tensile strength. See also **hyaline cartilage, yellow cartilage.** —**fibrocartilaginous,** adj.

fibrocartilaginous joint See **symphysis.**

fibrocystic disease 1. Of the breast: the presence of single or multiple cysts in the breasts. The cysts are benign and fairly common, yet potentially malignant and must be observed for growth or change. Women with this disease face greater than usual risk of developing breast cancer later in life. The cysts can be aspirated and a biopsy performed. In most cases no treatment is required. The nurse must vigorously counsel women who have this disease to examine their breasts frequently. A woman is shown any cysts present, palpation is taught, and the importance of any change is emphasized. Reassurance should also be given that the condition is very common and usually not associated with cancer. Also called **chronic cystic mastitis.** 2. Of the pancreas: see **cystic fibrosis.**

fibrocyte See **fibroblast.** —**fibrocytic,** adj.

fibroelastic tissue See **fibrous tissue.**

fibroepithelial papilloma A benign epithelial tumor containing extensive fibrous tissue. Also called **fibropapilloma.**

fibroepithelioma, pl. **fibroepitheliomas, fibroepitheliomata** A neoplasm consisting of fibrous and epithelial components, such as **premalignant fibroepithelioma.**

fibroid 1. Having fibers. 2. *Informal.* A fibroma or myoma, particularly of the uterus.

fibroid tumor See **fibroma.**

fibroma, *pl.* **fibromas, fibromata** A benign neoplasm of fibrous or fully developed connective tissue.

-fibroma A combining form meaning a 'benign tumor made up of fibrous tissue': *eulofibroma, hemangiofibroma, lymphangiofibroma.*

fibroma cavernosum A tumor containing large vascular spaces and an excessive amount of fibrous tissue.

fibroma cutis A fibrous tumor of the skin.

fibroma durum See **hard fibroma.**

fibroma molle See **soft fibroma.**

fibroma mucinosum A fibrous tumor in which there is mucoid degeneration.

fibroma myxomatodes See **myxofibroma.**

fibroma pendulum A pendulous fibrous tumor of the skin.

fibroma sarcomatosum See **fibrosarcoma.**

fibroma thecocellulare xanthomatodes See **theca cell tumor.**

fibromyoma uteri See **leiomyoma uteri.**

fibromyositis Any one of a large number of disorders in which the common element is stiffness and joint or muscle pain, accompanied by inflammation of the muscle tissues and of the fibrous connective tissues. Treatment includes rest, heat, massage, administration of salicylates, and, in severe cases, injections of a corticosteroid and procaine. Kinds of fibromyositis include **lumbago, pleurodynia, torticollis.** See also **rheumatism.**

fibropapilloma See **fibroepithelial papilloma.**

fibrosarcoma, *pl.* **fibrosarcomas, fibrosarcomata** A sarcoma that contains connective tissue. It develops suddenly from small nodules on the skin; metastases often occur before the nodules begin to change.

fibrosing alveolitis A severe form of alveolitis characterized by dyspnea and hypoxia, occurring in advanced rheumatoid arthritis and other autoimmune diseases. X-ray films show thickening of the alveolar septa and diffuse pulmonary infiltrates. See also **alveolitis.**

fibrosis 1. A proliferation of fibrous connective tissue. The process occurs normally in the formation of scar tissue to replace normal tissue lost through injury or infection. 2. An abnormal condition in which fibrous connective tissue spreads over or replaces normal smooth muscle or other normal organ tissue. See also **cystic fibrosis, fibrositis.**

fibrositis An inflammation of fibrous connective tissue, usually characterized by a poorly defined set of symptoms, including pain and stiffness of the neck, shoulder, and trunk. Fibrositis usually develops in middle age. Its prevalence in persons who are frequently tense suggests a possible psychogenic etiology. Salicylates, sedatives, tranquilizers, muscle relaxants, and the injection of a local anesthetic may be prescribed. Compare **fibromyositis.**

fibrous Consisting mainly of fibers or fiber-containing materials, as fibrous connective tissue. See also **fibrosis.**

-fibrous A combining form meaning 'composed of fibrous tissue': *cellulofibrous, fibrofibrous, interfibrous.*

fibrous capsule 1. The external layer of an articular capsule. It surrounds the articulation of two adjoining bones. 2. The external, tough membranous envelope surrounding some visceral organs, as the liver. Compare **synovial membrane.**

fibrous dysplasia A condition characterized by fibrous displacement of the osseous tissue within the affected bones. The specific cause is unknown, but indications are that it is developmental or congenital. Kinds of fibrous dysplasia are monostotic fibrous dysplasia, polyostotic fibrous dysplasia, and polyostotic fibrous dysplasia with associated endocrine disorders. All show varying degrees of fibrous replacement of the osseous tissue. The onset of fibrous dysplasia is usually during childhood, progressing beyond puberty and through adulthood, although diagnosis may be delayed until adolescence or early adulthood if symptoms are minimal. The initial signs may be a limp, a pain, or a fracture on the affected side. Girls affected may have an early onset of menses and breast development and early epiphyseal closure. Albright's syndrome is usually diagnosed on the basis of a triad of symptoms: polyostotic fibrous dysplasia, café-au-lait patches on the skin, and precocious puberty. Pathologic fractures are frequently associated with this process. The involved extremity may be shortened, and the classic shepherd's crook deformity is common. Radiographic examination usually reveals a well-circumscribed lesion occupying the shaft of the long bone involved. Pathological fractures in patients with fibrous dysplasia usually heal with conservative treatment, but residual deformities often remain. When symptoms are mild and limited, this disease usually progresses slowly. Biopsies are commonly performed if pain increases or if alterations are seen on radiographic examination.

fibrous goiter An enlargement of the thyroid gland, characterized by hyperplasia of the capsule and connective tissue.

fibrous histiocytoma See **dermatofibroma.**

fibrous joint Any one of many immovable joints, as those of the skull, in which a fibrous tissue or a hyaline cartilage connects the bones. The three kinds of articulation associated with fibrous joints are syndesmosis, satura, and gomphosis. Also called **junctura fibrosa, synarthrosis.** Compare **cartilaginous joint, synovial joint.**

fibrous thyroiditis A disorder characterized by slowly progressive fibrosis of an enlarged thyroid with replacement of normal thyroid tissue by dense fibrous tissue. The gland eventually becomes fixed to the adjacent muscles, nerves, blood vessels, and trachea by this fibrous tissue. The disease occurs most frequently in women and usually after the age of 40. Symptoms include a choking sensation, dyspnea, dysphagia, and hypothyroidism. Treatment includes surgical excision and thyroid hormones. Also called **ligneous thyroiditis, Riedel's struma, Riedel's thyroiditis.**

fibrous tissue The fibrous connective tissue of the body, consisting of closely woven elastic fibers and fluid-filled areolae. Also called **fibroelastic tissue.** Compare **areolar tissue.**

fibula The bone of the leg, lateral to and smaller than the tibia. In proportion to its length, it is the most slender of the long bones and presents three borders and three surfaces, attaching to various muscles, including the peronei longus and brevis and the soleus longus. Also called calf bone.

Fick principle A method for making indirect measurements, based on the law of conservation of mass. It is used to determine cardiac output, in which the amount of oxygen uptake of each unit of blood as it passes through the lungs is equal to the oxygen concentration difference between arterial and mixed venous blood. Cardiac output is calculated by measuring the uptake of oxygen for a given period of time, noted as milliliters per minute, then dividing that ratio by the difference in oxygen saturation of arterial and mixed venous blood samples in milliliters per 100 ml of blood, and multiplying the total by 100.

Fick's Law 1. In chemistry and physics: an observed law stating that the rate at which one substance diffuses through another is directly proportional to the concentration gradient of the diffusing substance. 2. In medicine: an observed law stating that the rate of diffusion across a membrane is directly proportional to the concentration gradient of the substance on the two sides of the membrane and inversely related to the thickness of the membrane.

field In data processing: one unit of data, such as the patient's name or birthdate. A group of related fields forms a record.

field fever A form of leptospirosis caused by *Leptospira grippotyphosa,* affecting primarily agricultural workers, characterized by fever, abdominal pain, diarrhea, vomiting, stupor, and conjunctivitis. Also called **canefield fever, harvest fever.** See also **leptospirosis.**

fiery serpent *Informal. Dracunculus medinesis.* See also **dracunculiasis.**

fifth cranial nerve See **trigeminal nerve.**

fifth disease See **erythema infectiosum.**

fight or flight reaction See **flight or fight reaction.**

FIGLU *abbr* **formiminoglutamic acid.**

figure-eight bandage A bandage with successive laps crossing over and around each other like the figure eight. See also **bandage.**

fila- A combining form meaning 'pertaining to a thread, or threadlike': *filacious, filamentous, filaria.*

filariasis A disease caused by the presence

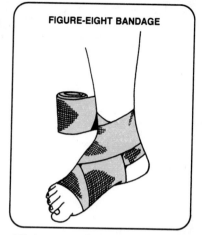

FIGURE-EIGHT BANDAGE

of filariae or microfilariae in body tissues. Filarial worms are round, long, and threadlike and are common in most tropical and subtropical regions. They tend to infest the lymph glands and channels after entering the body as microscopic larvae through the bite of a mosquito or other insect. The infection is characterized by occlusion of the lymphatic vessels, with swelling and pain of the limb distal to the blockage. After many years, the limb may become greatly swollen and the skin coarse and tough. Treatment is largely ineffective. See also **elephantiasis.**

filial generation The offspring produced from a given mating or cross in a genetic sequence. See also F_1, F_2.

filiform bougie An extremely thin bougie for passage through a narrow stricture, as a sinus tract.

filiform catheter A catheter with a slender, threadlike tip that allows the wider portion of the instrument to be passed through canals that are constricted or irregular because of an obstruction or an angulation in the canal.

filiform papilla See under **papilla.**

film badge A photographic film packet, sensitive to ionizing radiation, used for estimating the exposure of personnel working with X-rays and other radioactive sources.

fimbrial tubal pregnancy A kind of tubal pregnancy in which implantation occurs in the fimbriated distal end of one of the fallopian tubes. See also **tubal pregnancy.**

finality In general system theory: a principle of closed systems that states that the end result is wholly determined by the initial conditions.

finger Any of the digits of the hand. The fingers are composed of a metacarpal bone and three bony phalanges. Some anatomists regard the thumb as a finger, since its metacarpal bone ossifies in the same way as a phalange. Other anatomists regard the thumb as being composed of a metacarpal bone and two phalanges. The fingers are numbered 1 to 5, starting with the thumb.

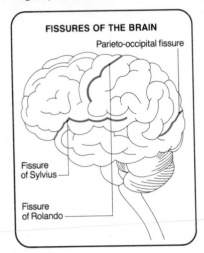

FISSURES OF THE BRAIN

Parieto-occipital fissure

Fissure of Sylvius

Fissure of Rolando

finger percussion   See **percussion**.

Finnish bath   See **Russian bath**.

FIO₂   *abbr* fraction of inspired oxygen; the actual oxygen concentration delivered to the patient.

fire damp   See **damp**.

fireman's cramp   See **heat cramp**.

first aid   The immediate care given to an injured or ill person. It includes self-help and home-care measures if medical assistance isn't readily available. Attention is directed first to the most critical problems: evaluation of the patency of the airway, the presence of bleeding, and the adequacy of cardiac function. The patient is kept warm and as comfortable as possible. See also **cardiopulmonary resuscitation, control of hemorrhage, emergency medicine, emergency nursing**.

first cranial nerve   See **olfactory nerve**.

fish tapeworm infection   An infection caused by the tapeworm *Diphyllobothrium latum* that is transmitted to humans when they eat contaminated raw or undercooked freshwater fish. The infection is common in temperate zones, including the Great Lakes region of the United States. See also *Diphyllobothrium*, **tapeworm infection**.

fiss-   A combining form meaning 'pertaining to a split or cleft': *fissile, fissiparous, fissula*.

fission   **1.** The act or process of splitting or breaking up into parts. **2.** A type of asexual reproduction common in bacteria, protozoa, and other lower forms of life in which the cell divides into two or more equal components, each of which eventually develops into a complete organism. Kinds of fission are **binary fission, multiple fission**. **3.** In physics: the splitting of the nucleus of an atom and subsequent release of energy. Also called **nuclear fission**.

fissiparous   Reproduced by fission.

fissural angioma   A tumor that is composed of a cluster of dilated blood vessels (hemangioma) found in an embryonal fissure, especially on the lip, the face, or the neck.

fissure   **1.** A cleft or a groove on the surface of an organ, often marking division of the organ into parts, as the fissures of the brain. **2.** A crack-like lesion of skin. **3.** A lineal fault on a bony surface occurring during the development of a part, as a fissure in the enamel of a tooth. A fissure is usually deeper than a sulcus, but *fissure* and *sulcus* are often used interchangeably. Also called **fissura**. Compare **sulcus**. —**fissured**, *adj*.

fissure fracture   Any fracture in which a crack extends into the cortex of the bone but not through the entire bone.

fissure of Bichat   See **transverse fissure**.

fissure of Rolando   See **central sulcus**.

fissure of Sylvius   See **lateral cerebral sulcus**.

fistula, *pl.* **fistulas, fistulae**   An abnormal passage from an internal organ to the body surface or between two internal organs, caused by a congenital defect, injury, infection, the spreading of a malignant lesion, radiotherapy of a cancerous growth, or trauma during childbirth. Fistulas may be created for therapeutic purposes or to obtain body secretions for physiologic studies. An arteriovenous fistula is commonly created to gain access to the patient's bloodstream for hemodialysis. Anal fistulas resulting from rupture or drainage of abscesses may be treated by fistulectomy or fistulotomy. —**fistulous, fistular, fistulate**, *adj*.

fistula in ano   See **anal fistula**.

fit   **1.** *Nontechnical.* A paroxysm or seizure. **2.** The sudden onset of an episode of symptoms, as a fit of coughing. **3.** The manner in which one surface is aligned to another.

Fitzgerald treatment   See **zone therapy**.

five-day fever   *Informal.* Trench fever.

five-step nursing process   A nursing process comprising five broad categories of nursing behaviors: assessment, nursing diagnosis, planning, intervention, and evaluation. The nurse gathers information about the patient, formulates nursing diagnoses, develops a plan of care with the patient to meet these diagnoses, implements the plan of care, and evaluates the effects of the intervention. The nurse involves the patient and the patient's family to the greatest extent possible. Implicit in the nursing process is a therapeutic and personal relationship between the nurse, the patient, and the patient's family.

fixating eye   In strabismus: the normal eye that can be focused. Compare **squinting eye**.

fixation   In psychoanalysis: an arrest at a particular stage of psychosexual development, as anal fixation. —**fixate**, *v.*, **fixated**, *adj*.

fixation muscle   A muscle that acts to hold a part of the body in appropriate position. Compare **antagonist, prime mover, synergist**.

fixative   **1.** Any substance used to bind, glue, or stabilize. **2.** Any substance used to preserve gross or histologic specimens of tissue for later examination.

fixed bridgework   A dental device incorporating artificial teeth permanently attached in the upper or the lower jaw.

fixed-combination drug Any of a group of multiple-ingredient preparations that provides concomitant administration of specific amounts of two or more drugs.

fixed coupling An abnormal pulse in which a premature beat follows a normal heart beat in a recurrent, regularly irregular pattern.

fixed dressing A dressing usually made of gauze impregnated with a hardening agent, as plaster of Paris, sodium silicate, starch, or dextrin, applied to support or immobilize a part of the body. The dressing is soaked in water, applied to the part to be immobilized, and allowed to harden. See also **cast.**

fixed drug eruption A circumscribed skin lesion either persisting or recurring in the same location, caused by continuing or repeated exposure to a sensitizing drug.

fixed idea 1. A persistent, obsessional thought or notion. 2. In certain mental disorders, especially obsessive-compulsive neurosis, a delusional idea that dominates mental activity and persists despite contrary evidence or rational refutation. Also called *idée fixe.*

fixed phagocyte See **phagocyte.**

flaccid Weak, soft, and flabby; lacking normal muscle tone, as flaccid muscles. —**flaccidity, flaccidness,** *n.*

flaccid bladder A form of neurogenic bladder caused by interruption of the reflex arc associated with the voiding reflex in the spinal cord. It is marked by continual filling and occasional overfilling of the bladder, absence of bladder sensation, and inability to urinate voluntarily. It is often produced by trauma. Also called **atonic bladder, autonomous bladder, nonreflex bladder.** Compare **spastic bladder.**

flaccid paralysis An abnormal condition characterized by the weakening or the loss of muscle tone. Compare **spastic paralysis.**

flagell- A combining form meaning 'pertaining to a whiplike process, tapping': *flagellation, flagelliform, flagellospore.*

flagellant A person who receives sexual gratification from the practice of flagellation.

flagellate A microorganism that propels itself by waving whiplike filaments or cilia, as *Trypanosoma, Leishmania, Trichomonas,* and *Giardia.* See also **protozoa.**

flagellation 1. The act of whipping, beating, or flogging. 2. A type of massage administered by tapping the body with the fingers. See also **massage.** 3. A type of sexual deviation in which a person is erotically gratified by being whipped or by whipping another. See also **masochism, sadism.** 4. The arrangement of flagella on an organism.

flail chest A thorax in which multiple rib fractures cause instability in part of the chest wall and paradoxical breathing, with the lung underlying the injured area contracting on inspiration and bulging on expiration. The condition, if uncorrected, leads to hypoxia. Flail chest is characterized by sharp pain; uneven chest expansion; shallow, rapid respirations; and decreased breath sounds. Tachycardia and cyanosis may be present. The treatment of choice is internal stabilization of the chest wall through the use of a volume-controlled ventilator with a cuffed tracheostomy tube or endotracheal tube. If the patient breathes against the automatic ventilator, a sedative and muscle relaxant may be ordered to achieve ventilatory control. Chest tubes may be required to remove air or fluid preventing expansion of the affected lung.

NURSING CONSIDERATIONS: The patient with flail chest usually requires a long period of care involving frequent repositioning, scrupulous attention to the patency and cleanliness of the tracheostomy or endotracheal tube, skin care, oral hygiene, and emotional support. The nurse performs passive range-of-motion exercises, explains procedures, and, because the patient can't speak, provides a pad and pencil, a magic slate, or other aid to communication.

flame photometry Measurement of the wavelength of light rays emitted by excited metallic electrons exposed to the heat energy of a flame, used to identify clinical specimens of body fluids. In the clinical laboratory, flame photometry is used to measure sodium, potassium, and lithium levels.

flapping tremor See **asterixis.**

flare 1. A red blush on the skin at the periphery of a urticarial lesion seen in hypersensitivity reactions. 2. An expanding skin flush, spreading from an infective lesion or extending from the site of a reaction to an irritant. 3. The sudden intensification of a disease.

flask closure In dentistry: the joining of two halves of a flask that encloses and forms a denture base. Compare **closure, velopharyngeal closure.**

flat electroencephalogram A graphic chart on which no tracings are recorded during electroencephalography, indicating absence of brain wave activity. Flat readings are indicative of death except in cases of profound hypothermia and central nervous system depression. Also called **isoelectric electroencephalogram.**

flatfoot An abnormal but relatively common condition characterized by the flattening out of the arch of the foot. Also called **pes planus.**

flat spring contraceptive diaphragm A kind of contraceptive diaphragm in which the flexible metal spring that forms the rim is a thin, light, flat band made of stainless steel. The rubber dome is approximately 3.8 cm (1½ inches) deep, and the diameter of the rubber-covered rim is between 5.5 and 10 cm. Ten sizes, in increments of 0.5 cm, allow the clinician to fit the diaphragm individually. This kind of diaphragm is prescribed for a woman whose vaginal musculature provides good support; whose uterus is in the normal position and not acutely retroflexed or anteflexed; and whose vagina, neither very long nor very short, has a shallow arch behind the symphysis pubis. Compare **arcing spring contraceptive diaphragm, coil spring**

FLEXOR MUSCLES

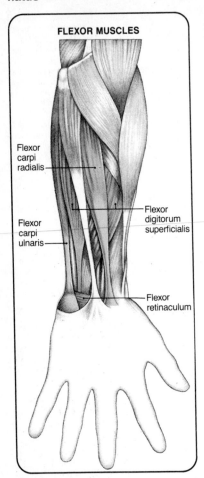

Flexor carpi radialis

Flexor carpi ulnaris

Flexor digitorum superficialis

Flexor retinaculum

contraceptive diaphragm. See also **contraceptive diaphragm fitting.**

flatus Air or gas in the intestine that is passed through the rectum. See also **aerophagy.**

flat wart See **verruca plana.**

flav- A combining form meaning 'yellow': *flavescens, flavin, flavism.*

flavone A colorless, crystalline, flavonoid derivative and component of bioflavonoid that increases capillary resistance.

flavoxate hydrochloride A genitourinary system spasmolytic.

flea A wingless, bloodsucking insect of the order *Siphonaptera*, some species of which transmit arboviruses to humans by acting as host or vector to the organism.

flea bite A small puncture wound produced by a blood-sucking flea. Certain species of fleas transmit plague and murine typhus.

flea-borne typhus See **endemic typhus.**

-flect A combining form meaning 'to bend': *anteflect, circumflect.*

FLEX *abbr* Federation Licensing Examination.

flexibilitas cerea See **cerea flexibilitas.**

flexion A movement allowed by certain joints of the skeleton that decreases the angle between two adjoining bones, as bending the wrist. Compare **extension.**

flexor carpi radialis A slender, superficial muscle of the forearm that lies on the ulnar side of the pronator teres. It arises from the medial epicondyle, the fascia of the forearm, and from several intermuscular septa, and inserts by a long tendon into the base of the second metacarpal bone. It is innervated by a branch of the median nerve and functions to flex and help abduct the hand. Compare **flexor carpi ulnaris, palmaris longus.**

flexor carpi ulnaris A superficial muscle, lying along the ulnar side of the forearm, that arises in a humeral and an ulnar head and inserts in a long tendon into the pisiform bone, extending by ligaments to the hamate and the fifth metacarpal bones. It is innervated by a branch of the ulnar nerve and functions to flex and adduct the hand. Compare **flexor carpi radialis, palmaris longus.**

flexor digitorum sublimis See **flexor digitorum superficialis.**

flexor digitorum superficialis The largest superficial muscle of the forearm, lying on the ulnar side under the palmaris longus, arising by a humeral, an ulnar, and a radial head. The muscle separates into a superficial layer and a deep layer and inserts by four tendons into the second phalanx of the fingers. The flexor digitorum superficialis is innervated by branches of the median nerve. The muscle flexes the second phalanx of each finger and, by continued action, the hand. Also called **flexor digitorum sublimis.** Compare **flexor carpi radialis, flexor carpi ulnaris, palmaris longus, pronator teres.**

flexor retinaculum of the hand See **retinaculum flexorum manus.**

flextime, flexitime A system of staffing that allows flexible work schedules. A person working 7 hours daily might choose to work from 7 to 3, 10 to 5, or other hours. Use of the system tends to improve morale and decrease turnover.

flight into health An abnormal but common reaction to an unpleasant physical sensation or symptom in which the person denies the reality of the feeling or observation, insisting that there is nothing wrong. See also **illness experience.**

flight or fight reaction 1. In physiology: the reaction of the body to stress, in which the sympathetic nervous system and the adrenal medulla act to increase the cardiac output, dilate the pupils of the eyes, increase the rate of the heartbeat, constrict the blood vessels of the skin, increase the glucose and fatty acids in the circulation, and induce an aroused mental state. 2. In psychiatry: a person's reaction to stress by either fleeing from a situation or attempting to deal with it.

floater (muscae volitantes) One or more spots that appear to drift in front of the eye, caused by a shadow cast on the retina by vitreous debris. Most floaters are benign and represent remnants of a network of blood vessels that existed prenatally in the vitreous cavity. The sudden onset of several floaters may indicate serious disease. Hemorrhage into the vitreous humor may cause a large number of big and little shadows and a red discoloration of vision. The cause is often traumatic injury, but spontaneous intraocular hemorrhage is seen in severe diabetes mellitus, hypertension, or increased intracranial pressure. Inflammation of the retina resulting from chorioretinitis may cause entry of inflammatory cells into the vitreous humor. Inflammatory debris may adhere to the vitreous framework in netlike masses that are very disruptive of normal vision. Retinal detachment also causes a sudden appearance of lightninglike floaters and a diminished field of vision as a shower of red cells and pigment is released into the vitreous humor. Ophthalmologic examination is recommended, as each of the pathologic causes can be treated in the early stages and loss of vision can usually be avoided.

floating head Unengaged fetal head. See also **ballottement, engagement.**

floating kidney A kidney that is not securely fixed in the usual anatomic location, owing to congenital malplacement or traumatic injury. Compare **ptotic kidney.**

floating rib See **rib.**

flocculant An agent or substance that causes flocculation.

flocculation test A serologic test in which a positive result depends on the degree of flocculent precipitation produced in the material being tested. Many tests for syphilis are flocculation tests.

flocculent Clumped or tufted, as a cloud, or covered with a woolly, fuzzy surface. —**flocculate,** v., **flocculation, floccule,** n.

flood fever See **typhus.**

flooding A technique used in behavior therapy for the reduction of anxiety associated with various phobias. Repeated exposure to a stimulus that usually provokes anxiety desensitizes a person to that stimulus, thereby reducing fear and anxiety. Also called **implosive therapy.** Compare **systemic desensitization.**

floppy infant syndrome A general term for juvenile spinal muscular atrophies, including Werdnig-Hoffmann disease and Wohlfart-Kugelberg-Welander disease.

flowmeter See **rotameter.**

flow sheet In a patient record: a graphic summary of several changing factors, especially the patient's vital signs and the treatments and medications given to the patient. In labor, the flow sheet displays the progress of labor, including the centimeters of cervical dilatation, the position of the baby's head, the frequency of contractions, the mother's temperature and blood pressure, and any medications given or procedures performed.

floxuridine An antimetabolite drug used in cancer chemotherapy.

flu *Informal.* **1.** Influenza. **2.** Any viral infection, especially of the respiratory or intestinal system.

flucytosine An antifungal agent.

fludrocortisone acetate A mineralocorticoid.

-fluent A combining form meaning 'flowing': *diffluent, ossifluent.*

fluid **1.** A substance, as a liquid or gas, that is able to flow and to adjust its shape to that of a container because it is composed of molecules that are able to change positions with respect to each other without separating from the total mass. **2.** A body fluid, either intracellular or extracellular, that is involved in the transport of electrolytes and other vital chemicals to, through, and from tissue cells. See also **blood, cerebrospinal fluid, lymph.**

fluid dram See **dram.**

fluid ounce A measure of liquid volume in the apothecaries' system, equal to 8 fluidrams or 29.57 ml. See also **apothecaries' measure, metric system.**

fluid volume deficit, actual **1.** A nursing diagnosis accepted by the Fifth National Conference on the Classification of Nursing Diagnoses. The etiology is a failure of the body's homeostatic mechanisms that regulate the retention and excretion of body fluids. The defining characteristics are dilute urine, increased output of urine, and a sudden loss of body weight. Other characteristics may be observed, including hypotension, increased pulse rate, decreased turgor, increased body temperature, hemoconcentration, weakness, and thirst. **2.** A nursing diagnosis accepted by the Fifth National Conference on the Classification of Nursing Diagnoses. The etiology is the active loss of excessive amounts of body fluid. The defining characteristics are decreased output of urine, high specific gravity of the urine, output of urine that is greater than the intake of fluid into the body, a sudden loss of weight, hemoconcentration, and increased serum levels of sodium. Other characteristics are increased thirst, alteration in the mental state, dryness of skin and mucous membranes, elevated temperature, and an increased pulse rate. See also **nursing diagnosis.**

fluke A parasitic flatworm of the class Trematoda, including the genus *Schistosoma.* See also **schistosomiasis.**

flumethasone pivalate A topical anti-inflammatory agent.

flunisolide A corticosteroid administered by nasal inhalation.

fluocinolone acetonide A topical anti-inflammatory agent.

fluocinonide A topical anti-inflammatory agent.

fluorescein sodium A dye used in ophthalmologic procedures.

fluorescence The emission of light of one wavelength (usually ultraviolet) when exposed to light of a different, usually shorter, wavelength, a property possessed by certain substances. Fluorescent substances that simultaneously absorb and emit light appear luminous. **—fluoresce,** *v.,* **fluorescent,** *adj.*

fluorescent antibody test (FA test) A test in which a fluorescent dye is used to stain an antibody to identify clinical specimens. Fluorescent dyes conjugate with immunoglobulins without altering the antibody-antigen reaction, making the dyed organisms glow visibly when examined under a fluorescent microscope. The technique can be used to identify *Mycobacterium tuberculosis* and as a common serologic screening test for syphilis. Kinds of fluorescent antibody tests include the FTA-ABS test. Also called **immunofluorescence test.**

fluorescent microscopy Examination with a fluorescent microscope equipped with a source of ultraviolet light rays, used to study specimens, as tissues, that have been stained with fluorescent dye. Also called **ultraviolet microscopy.** See also **fluorescent antibody test.**

Fluorescent Treponemal Antibody Absorption Test (FTA-ABS test) A serologic test for syphilis. See also **fluorescent antibody test.**

fluoridation The process of adding fluoride, especially to a public water supply, to reduce tooth decay. See also **fluoride.**

fluoride A salt of hydrofluoric acid, introduced into drinking water and applied directly to the teeth to prevent tooth decay.

fluorine (F) An element of the halogen family and the most reactive of the nonmetals. Its atomic number is 9; its atomic weight is 19. It occurs in nature only as a component of substances as fluorspar, cryolite, and phosphate rocks. It is also a component of stable fluorocarbons used in the manufacture of resins and plastics. As a component of fluorides, it is widely distributed throughout the soils of the earth, enters plants, is ingested by humans, and absorbed from the gastrointestinal tract. Small amounts of sodium fluoride are added to the water supply of many communities to harden tooth enamel and decrease dental caries. Excessive amounts of fluoride can mottle tooth enamel and cause osteosclerosis. Acute fluoride poisoning and death can result from the accidental ingestion of insecticides and rodenticides containing fluoride salts.

fluoroacetic acid A colorless, water-soluble, highly toxic compound that blocks the Krebs' citric acid cycle, causing convulsions and ventricular fibrillation. It is derived from a South African tree.

fluorometholone An ophthalmic and topical anti-inflammatory agent.

fluorometry Measurement of fluorescence emitted by compounds when exposed to ultraviolet or other intense radiant energy. The atoms of certain substances produce fluorescence of a characteristic color and wavelength, enabling identification and quantification of several clinically significant compounds in biological specimens. Fluorometry is used to measure urinary estrogens, triglycerides, catecholamines, and other substances. **—fluorometric,** *adj.*

fluoroscope A device used for the immediate projection of an X-ray image on a fluorescent screen for visual examination. **—fluoroscopic,** *adj.*

fluoroscopy A technique in radiology for visually examining a part of the body or the function of an organ using a fluoroscope. The technique offers immediate, serial images in many clinical situations, as in cardiac catheterization.

fluorosis The condition that results from excessive, prolonged ingestion of fluorine. Unusually high concentration of fluorine in drinking water causes mottled discoloration and pitting of the enamel of the permanent and deciduous teeth in children whose teeth developed while maternal intake of fluorinated water was high. Severe chronic fluorine poisoning will lead to osteosclerosis in adults. See also **fluoridation, fluoride.**

fluorouracil An antimetabolite topical chemotherapy drug.

fluoxymesterone An androgenic substance.

fluphenazine decanoate, f. enanthate, f. hydrochloride Phenothiazine antipsychotic drugs.

flurandrenolide A topical anti-inflammatory agent.

flurandrenolone See **flurandrenolide.**

flurazepam hydrochloride A benzodiazepine sedative-hypnotic agent.

flush **1.** A blush or sudden reddening of the face and neck. **2.** A sudden, subjective feeling of heat. **3.** A prolonged reddening of the face such as may be seen with fever, certain drugs, or hyperthyroidism. **4.** A sudden, rapid flow of water or other liquid.

flush device A device for the accurate transmission of a pressure wave from a catheter to a transducer in an I.V. line.

fly A two-winged insect of the order Diptera, some species of which transmit arboviruses to humans.

Fm Symbol for **fermium.**

FMET *abbr* **formylmethionine.**

FMG *abbr* **foreign medical graduate.**

FNP *abbr* **family nurse practitioner.**

foam bath A bath taken in water containing a saporin substance that covers the surface of the liquid and through which air or oxygen is blown to form the foam.

focal illumination See **illumination.**

focal motor seizure See **motor seizure.**

focal seizure A transitory disturbance in motor, sensory, or autonomic function resulting from abnormal neuronal discharges in the brain, most frequently motor or sensory areas adjacent to the fissure of Rolando. These seizures commonly begin as spasmodic movements in the hand, face, or foot and may spread progressively to other muscles to end in a generalized convulsion. Abnormal neuronal discharges in the motor area may be manifested by chewing, lip-smacking, swallowing movements, and by profuse salivation. Seizures originating in the eye-turning area of the brain may begin with a forced turning of the head and eyes away from the side of the focus or lesion. Abnormal electrical activity in the cortex may be evident initially as a numb, prickling, tingling, or crawling feeling, and the neuronal discharge may spread to motor areas. Focal seizures may be caused by localized anoxia or a small brain lesion.

foeti-, foeto-   See **feti-.**

foetus   See **fetus.**

folacin   See **folic acid.**

folate   1. A salt of folic acid. 2. Substances found in some foods and in mammalian cells that act as coenzymes and promote the chemical transfer of carbon units from one molecule to another.

Foley catheter   A rubber catheter with a balloon tip to be filled with air or a sterile liquid after it has been placed in the bladder. This kind of catheter is used when continuous drainage of the bladder is desired, as in surgery, or when repeated urinary catheterization would be necessary if an indwelling catheter were not used. See also **catheterization.**

folic acid   A yellow, crystalline, water-soluble vitamin of the B complex group essential for cell growth and reproduction. It functions as a coenzyme with vitamins B_{12} and C in the breakdown and use of proteins and in the formation of nucleic acids and heme in hemoglobin. It also increases the appetite and stimulates the production of hydrochloric acid in the digestive tract. The vitamin is stored in the liver and may be synthesized by the bacterial flora of the gastrointestinal tract. Deficiency of the vitamin results in poor growth, graying hair, glossitis, stomatitis, gastrointestinal lesions, and diarrhea, and it may lead to megaloblastic anemia. Deficiency is caused by inadequate diet, malabsorption, or metabolic abnormalities. Need for folic acid is increased in pregnancy, infancy, and times of stress. Dietary sources include spinach and other green leafy vegetables, liver, kidney, asparagus, lima beans, nuts, and whole-grain cereals. The nontoxic vitamin may help alleviate menstrual problems and leg ulcers. Also called **folacin.**

folie   A mental disorder; any of a variety of psychopathologic reactions. Kinds of folie include **folie à deux, folie circulaire, folie du doute, folie du pourquoi, folie gemellaire, folie musculaire, folie raisonnante.**

folie à deux   A psychopathological condition characterized by identical manifestations of the same mental disorder, usually ideas, in two closely associated or related persons.

folie circulaire   A major affective disorder characterized by episodes of mania and depression. One or the other phase may be predominant at any given time, one phase may appear alternately with the other, or elements of both phases may be present simultaneously. Characteristics of the manic phase are excessive emotional displays, excitement, euphoria, hyperactivity accompanied by elation, boisterousness,

FOODS HIGH IN FOLIC ACID	
FOOD	**mcg/100 g**
Asparagus spears	109
Beef liver	294
Broccoli spears	54
Collards (cooked)	102
Mushrooms	24
Oatmeal	33
Peanut butter	57
Red beans	180
Wheat germ	305

impaired ability to concentrate, decreased need for sleep, and seemingly unbounded energy, often accompanied by delusions of grandeur. In the depressive phase, marked apathy and underactivity are accompanied by feelings of profound sadness, loneliness, guilt, and lowered self-esteem. Causes of the disorder are multiple and complex, often involving biological, psychological, interpersonal, and social and cultural factors. Treatment includes antidepressants, tranquilizers and antianxiety drugs, or the use of electroconvulsive therapy for persons who present an immediate and serious risk of suicide, followed by long-term psychotherapy. Careful nursing observation is important during depression, particularly during the recovery from depression, because of the possibility of suicide. Also called **bipolar disorder.**

folie du doute   An extreme obsessive-compulsive reaction characterized by persistent doubting, vacillation, repetition of a particular act or behavior, and pathological indecisiveness to the point of being unable to make even the most trifling decision.

folie du pourquoi   A psychopathological condition that is characterized by the persistent tendency to ask questions, usually concerning unrelated topics.

folie gemellaire   A psychotic condition occurring simultaneously in twins, sometimes in those not living together or closely associated at the time.

folie musculaire   Severe chorea.

folie raisonnante   A delusional form of any psychosis.

folinic acid   An active form of folic acid used to treat megaloblastic anemias not caused by vitamin B_{12} deficiency and to counteract the toxic effects of antineoplastic folic acid antagonists, as methotrexate. Also called **citrovorum factor, leucovorin.**

follicle   A pouchlike depression, as the hair follicles within the epidermis. —**follicular,** *adj.*

follicle-stimulating hormone (FSH)   A gonadotropin, secreted by the anterior pituitary gland, that stimulates the growth and maturation of Graafian follicles in the ovary and promotes spermatogenesis in the male. FSH releasing factor produced in the hypothalamus controls the release of FSH by the pituitary. Increasing amounts of FSH are secreted in the postmen-

FONTANELS

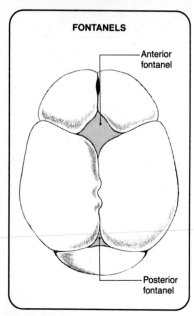

Anterior fontanel

Posterior fontanel

strual or resting phase of the menstrual cycle, causing a primordial follicle to develop into a mature Graafian follicle containing a mature ovum. The Graafian follicle produces estrogen, which reaches a high level before ovulation and suppresses release of FSH. In males, FSH maintains the integrity of the seminiferous tubules and influences all stages of spermatogenesis. It is derived from the urine of postmenopausal women and is called menotropins.

follicular adenocarcinoma A neoplasm characterized by a follicular arrangement of cells that are usually derived from the thyroid gland. It is not especially malignant, but it has a greater tendency to metastasize distantly to the lungs and bones than the more common papillary adenocarcinoma of the thyroid. Surgery is the preferred treatment. See also **medullary carcinoma, papillary adenocarcinoma.**

follicular goiter An enlargement of the thyroid gland characterized by proliferation of the follicles and epithelial tissue.

folliculitis Inflammation of hair follicles, as in sycosis barbae.

folliculoma See **granulosa cell tumor.**

fomentation **1.** A topical treatment with a warm, moist application. **2.** A substance or poultice that is used as a warm, moist application.

fontanel, fontanelle A space covered by tough membranes between the bones of an infant's cranium. The anterior fontanel, roughly diamond-shaped, remains palpable until about 2 years of age. The posterior fontanel, triangular in shape, closes about 2 months after birth. Increased intracranial pressure may cause a fontanel to become tense or bulge. A fontanel may be soft and depressed in the presence of dehydration.

food **1.** Any substance, usually of plant or animal origin, consisting of carbohydrates, proteins, fats, and such supplementary elements as minerals and vitamins, that is ingested and assimilated to provide energy and to promote the growth, repair, and maintenance essential for sustaining life. **2.** Nourishment in solid form as contrasted with liquid form.

food allergy A hypersensitive state resulting from the ingestion of a specific food antigen. Symptoms include allergic rhinitis, bronchial asthma, urticaria, angioneurotic edema, dermatitis, pruritus, headache, labyrinthitis and conjunctivitis, nausea, vomiting, diarrhea, pylorospasm, colic, spastic constipation, mucous colitis, and perianal eczema. Food allergens are predominantly protein in nature. The most common foods causing allergic reactions are wheat, milk, eggs, fish and other seafoods, chocolate, corn, nuts, strawberries, chicken, pork, legumes, tomatoes, cucumbers, garlic, and citrus fruits. Foods that are rarely allergenic are rice, lamb, gelatin, peaches, pears, carrots, lettuce, artichokes, sesame oil, and apples. Diagnosis of a specific food allergy is obtained by a detailed food history, food diary, elimination diet, or cutaneous tests.

Food and Drug Administration (FDA) A federal agency responsible for the enforcement of federal regulations regarding the manufacture and distribution of food, drugs, and cosmetics.

food exchange list A grouping of foods in which the carbohydrate, fat, and protein values are equal for the items listed. The list is used for meal planning in various diseases and deficiency states. The six groups of foods included on the list are milk, vegetables, fruits, bread, meat, and fats. Starchy vegetables are listed as bread exchanges; fish and cheese are meat exchanges.

food poisoning Any of a large group of processes resulting from the ingestion of a food contaminated by toxic substances or by bacteria-containing toxins. Kinds of food poisoning include **bacterial food poisoning, ciguatera poisoning, Minamata disease, mushroom poisoning, shellfish poisoning.** See also **botulism, ergot alkaloid, phalloidine poisoning, toadstool poisoning.**

foot The distal extremity of the leg, consisting of the tarsus, the metatarsus, and the phalanges.

foot-and-mouth disease A common picornavirus disease of farm animals in Europe, Asia, and Africa, which occasionally affects humans exposed to infected stock, hides, meat, or dairy products. Symptoms and signs in humans include headache, fever, malaise, and vesicles on tongue, oral mucous membranes, hands, and feet. Pruritus and painful ulcerations may occur, but the temperature soon falls, the lesions subside in about 1 week, and total healing without scars is complete by 2 or 3 weeks. See also **picornavirus.**

footdrop An abnormal condition of the lower leg and foot characterized by an inability to dorsiflect, or invert, the foot owing to peroneal nerve damage.

-footed A combining form meaning 'having feet' of a specified sort: *clubfooted, flatfooted, splayfooted.*

footling breech An intrauterine position of the fetus in which one or both feet are folded under the buttocks at the inlet of the maternal pelvis, one foot presenting in a single footling breech or both feet in a double footling breech. Compare **frank breech.**

foot-pound A unit for the measurement of work or energy. One foot-pound is the amount of work required to move one pound a distance of one foot in the same direction as that of the applied force.

for- A combining form meaning 'pertaining to an opening': *foramen, foramina, foration.*

foramen, *pl.* **foramina** An opening or aperture in a membranous structure or bone, as the apical dental foramen and the carotid foramen.

foramen magnum A passage in the occipital bone through which the spinal cord enters the spinal column.

foramen of Monro A passage between the lateral and third ventricles of the brain.

foramen ovale An opening in the septum between the right and the left atria in the fetal heart. This opening provides a bypass for blood that would otherwise flow to the fetal lungs. Most of the blood from the inferior vena cava in the fetus flows through the foramen ovale into the left atrium. After birth, the foramen ovale functionally closes when the newborn takes the first breath and full circulation through the lungs begins. See also **ductus arteriosus.**

Forbes-Albright syndrome An endocrine disease characterized by amenorrhea, prolactinemia, and galactorrhea, caused by an adenoma of the anterior pituitary. Diagnosis is made by X-ray of the anterior pituitary and a blood test for prolactin. Surgical resection of the adenoma is usually indicated. See also **galactorrhea, pituitary gland.**

Forbes' disease See **Cori's disease, glycogen storage disease.**

forbidden clone theory A theory, associated with autoimmunity, based on the clonal evolution theory that at birth all the cells of the body that might react against the body have been eliminated, leaving only cells that will react against foreign substances. The forbidden clone theory postulates that certain clone cells that can react against the body persist after birth and can be activated by a viral infection or by some metabolic change. The theory holds that regular cells of the immune system attack only the virus, but clone cells attack the body's tissues. Compare **sequestered antigens theory.**

force Energy applied in such a way that it initiates motion, changes the speed or direction of motion, or alters the size or shape of an object.

forced expiratory volume (FEV) The

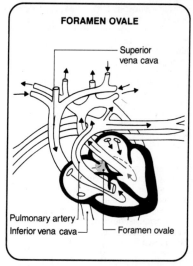

FORAMEN OVALE

Superior vena cava

Pulmonary artery
Inferior vena cava
Foramen ovale

volume of air that can be forcibly expelled in one second following full inspiration. See also **expiratory reserve volume.**

forced feeding The administration of food by force, as nasal feeding, to persons who cannot or will not eat.

forceps A pair of any of a large variety and number of surgical instruments, all of which have two handles or sides, each attached to a blade. The handles may be joined at one end, as a pair of tweezers, or the two sides may be separate to be conjoined in use. Forceps are used to grasp, handle, compress, pull, or join. See specific forceps.

forceps delivery An obstetric operation in which instruments are used to deliver the infant. It is performed to overcome dystocia, to quickly deliver a fetus experiencing distress, or, most often, to shorten normal labor. Prerequisites to forceps delivery include full dilatation of the cervix, engagement of the fetal head, and certain knowledge of the position of the head. Forceps produce marks on an infant's head and face; unless application has been imperfect the marks are usually superficial and disappear in a few days. Kinds of forceps delivery are **high forceps, low forceps, midforceps.** Compare **failed forceps, forceps rotation, trial forceps.** See also **obstetric forceps.**

forceps rotation An obstetric operation in which forceps are used to turn an infant's head that is arrested in transverse or posterior position in the birth canal. Kinds of forceps rotation are **Kielland rotation, Scanzoni rotation.** Compare **forceps delivery, manual rotation.** See also **obstetric forceps.**

forceps tenaculum See **tenaculum.**

fore- A combining form meaning 'front or before': *forearm, foregut, forewaters.*

forebrain See **prosencephalon.**

foregut The cephalic portion of the embryonic alimentary canal. It consists of endodermal tissue and gives rise to the pharynx, esophagus, stomach, liver, pancreas, most of the small intestine, and the respiratory ducts. Compare **hindgut, midgut.**

foreign body   Any object or substance found in an organ or tissue that does not belong there under normal circumstances, as a bolus of food in the trachea.

foreign body obstruction   A disturbance in normal function or a pathologic condition caused by an object lodged in a body orifice, passage, or organ. Most cases occur in children who suddenly inhale or swallow a foreign object or insert it in a body opening. In adults, large boluses of hastily eaten food frequently lodge in the esophagus, causing coughing, choking, and, if the airway is obstructed, asphyxia. Esophageal foreign bodies usually produce an immediate reaction, but occasionally children have a long asymptomatic period before signs of obstruction or infection are evident. Objects may be removed from the larynx, using a grasping forceps through a direct laryngoscope. A foreign body in the trachea may cause wheezing, an audible slap, coughing, and dyspnea; a small object may become lodged in a bronchus, producing coughing, which is often followed by an asymptomatic period before signs of obstruction and inflammation appear. A bronchoscope with suitable forceps and general anesthesia are usually used to remove foreign bodies in the bronchi, but thoracotomy may be required if the object is in the periphery of a lung. Objects that children insert in their nostrils may cause mild discomfort or infection and may be removed by forceps or nasal suction. Needles and hairpins ingested by children often pass through the esophagus and stomach without incident but may become lodged at the turn of the duodenum and require removal by a magnetized nasogastric tube or by laporotomy. Coins, marbles, and closed safety pins usually pass through the digestive tract without creating problems, but bezoars of hair, vegetable fibers, or shellac concretions, sometimes found in the stomach of emotionally disturbed or retarded patients, may cause anorexia, nausea, and vomiting.

foreign medical graduate (FMG)   A physician trained in and graduated from a medical school outside the United States and Canada, including United States citizens.

forensic medicine   A branch of medicine that deals with the legal aspects of health care.

forensic psychiatry   The branch of psychiatry that deals with legal issues relating to mental disorders, especially the legal determination of insanity.

foreskin   A loose fold of skin that covers the end of the penis or clitoris. Its removal constitutes circumcision. Also called **prepuce.**

forest yaws   A cutaneous form of American leishmaniasis, common in South and Central America, caused by the protozoan parasite *Leishmania guyanensis.* See also **American leishmaniasis, leishmaniasis.**

-form   A combining form meaning 'having a (specified) shape or form': *linguiform, toruliform.* Also **-forme.**

formaldehyde   A disinfectant.

formalin   A clear solution of formaldehyde in water. A 37% solution is used for preserving biological specimens for pathologic and histologic examination.

formic acid   A colorless, pungent liquid found in nature in nettles, ants, and other insects. It is prepared commercially from oxalic acid and glycerin and from the oxidation of formaldehyde. Formerly used as a vesicant, it no longer has any therapeutic applications.

formiminoglutamic acid (FIGLU)   A compound formed in the metabolism of histidine, occurring in urine in elevated levels in folic acid deficiency. Increased excretion of FIGLU may indicate folic acid deficiency.

formol   See **formaldehyde.**

formula   A simplified statement, generally using numerals and other symbols, expressing the constituents of a chemical compound, a method for preparing a substance, or a procedure for achieving a desired value or result. **—formulaic,** *adj.*

formulary   A listing intended to include a large enough range of drugs and sufficient information about them to enable health practitioners to prescribe treatment that is medically appropriate. Hospitals maintain formularies which list all drugs commonly stocked in the hospital pharmacy. Third-party organizations, as insurance companies, usually maintain formularies listing drugs for which the company will pay in settlement of claims. See also **compendium,** *United States Pharmacopeia.*

formulation   1. A pharmacologic substance prepared according to a formula. 2. A systematic statement of a problem, a theory, or a method of analysis in research.

formylmethionine (FMET)   In molecular genetics: the first amino acid in a protein sequence.

fornication   In law: sexual intercourse between two people who are not married to each other. The specific legal definition varies among jurisdictions.

fornix, *pl.* **fornices**   An archlike structure or space, as the fornix cerebri, the superior or inferior conjunctival fornices, or the vaginal fornices.

Fort Bragg fever   See **pretibial fever.**

fortified milk   Pasteurized milk enriched with one or more nutrients, usually vitamin D, which has been standardized at 400 International Units/quart. Also called fortified vitamin D milk.

fossa, *pl.* **fossae**   A hollow or depression, especially on the surface of the end of a bone, as the olecranon fossa or the coronoid fossa.

Foster bed   A special bed used in the care and treatment of severely injured patients, especially those with spinal injuries. It consists of two Bradford frames mounted on a castered base and secured with locking bars to the head and foot assemblies. The assembly at each end is

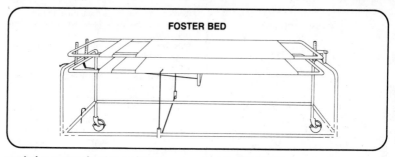

FOSTER BED

attached to a rotary-bearing mechanism, permitting horizontal turning of the patient without moving the spine. The patient can be rotated to supine and prone positions while maintaining proper immobilization and alignment of injured body structures. The Foster bed permits hyperextension and traction at each end of the frame and either end of the bed can be elevated to provide countertraction. It is used in posttraumatic management of patients with spinal instability and in the management of the postoperative patient with multilevel spinal fusion when weight-bearing or ambulation is contraindicated. It is also used in many scoliosis centers for halo-femoral traction, preparatory to spinal procedures with Harrington rods and Dwyer instrumentation. The bed also allows techniques for maintaining continuous cervical traction in flexion for selected patients with unstable cervical neck problems. An outrigger attachment for the bed maintains a constant angle with the patient in the supine or prone position. The bed can be turned by one person, although hospital and nursing officials recommend that two trained hospital staff members perform each turning to ensure the patient's safety. Also, two safety straps are required to guard against slippage. Foster bed patients sometimes display claustrophobia on being 'sandwiched' between frames, and skillful techniques to minimize the 'sandwiching' time are needed to comfort the patient. Frequent sensory stimulation with patient-staff interaction, as discussions and games, and prism glasses that allow the patient to read and watch television increase the person's tolerance of prolonged immobility. Compare **hyperextension bed, Stryker wedge frame.**

foulage   See **pétrissage.**

foundation   A charitable organization usually established to allocate private funds to worthy projects.

four-forty (4-40)   A work schedule in which a person works four 10-hour days each week rather than five 8-hour days.

four-point gait   In patient rehabilitation: a crutch gait in which three points are always in contact with the ground. The patient advances the left crutch, then the right leg, then the right crutch and the left leg, and so on.

four-point restraint   Forcible restraint of a violent or irrational patient by all four extremities.

four-tailed bandage   A narrow piece of cloth with two ties on each end for wrapping a joint, as an elbow or knee, or a prominence, as the nose or chin.

fourth nerve   See **trochlear nerve.**

Fowler's position   The posture assumed by the patient when the head of the bed is raised 18 to 20 inches and the individual's knees are elevated.

Fr   Symbol for **francium.**

fract-   A combining form meaning 'pertaining to a breaking': *fractional, fractography, fracture.*

fractional anesthesia   See **continuous anesthesia.**

fractional dilatation and curettage   A diagnostic technique in which each section of the uterus is examined and curetted to obtain specimens of the endometrium from all parts of the uterus. It is often performed under regional anesthesia to diagnose endometrial cancer.

fractionation   **1.** In neurology: a mechanism within the neural arch of the vertebrae whereby only a portion of the efferent nerves innervating a muscle reacts to a stimulus, even when the reflex requirement is maximal, so that there is a reserve of neurons to respond to additional stimuli. This phenomenon maintains muscle tension. **2.** In chemistry: the separation of a substance into its basic constituents by using such procedures as fractional distillation. **3.** In bacteriology: isolating a pure culture by successive culturing of a small portion of a colony of bacteria. **4.** In histology: isolating the different components of living cells by centrifugation. **5.** In radiology: administering radiation in smaller units over a period of time rather than in a single large dose to minimize tissue damage. Also called **dose fractionation, fractionation radiation.**

fractionation radiation   See **fractionation,** definition 5.

fracture   A traumatic injury in which the continuity of the tissue of the bone is broken. A fracture is classified by the bone involved, the part of that bone, and the nature of the break. Kinds of fracture include **alvulsion fracture, comminuted fracture, compound fracture, dislocation fracture, extracapsular fracture, greenstick fracture, impacted fracture, intracapsular fracture, longitudinal fracture, oblique fracture, simple fracture, and transverse fracture.**

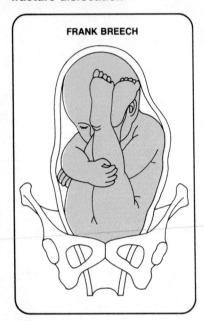

FRANK BREECH

fracture-dislocation A fracture involving the bony structures of any joint, with associated dislocation of the same joint.

fractured rib A break in a bone of the thoracic skeleton caused by a blow or injury or by violent coughing or sneezing. The ribs most commonly broken are the fourth to eighth, and, if the bone is splintered or the fracture is displaced, sharp fragments may pierce the lung, causing hemothorax or pneumothorax. The patient with a fractured rib suffers pain, especially on inspiration, and usually breathes rapidly and shallowly. The site of the break is generally tender to the touch, and the crackling of bone fragments rubbing together may be heard on auscultation. Breath sounds may be absent, decreased, or accompanied by rales and rhonchi. The location and nature of the fracture are determined by chest X-rays, and the patient is observed for signs of hemoptysis, hemothorax, flail chest, atelectasis, pneumothorax, and pneumonia. Fractured ribs may be splinted by applying an elastic belt or bandage or by adhesive strapping. To prevent irritation the area may be shaved and painted with tincture of benzoin before adhesive tape is applied. If hospitalization is required, the patient is placed in semi-Fowler's position. An analgesic may be ordered. The patient is assisted in turning and is instructed in how to deep breathe, to cough, and to perform range-of-motion exercises of extremities. If medication fails to relieve pain, the physician may perform a regional nerve block by infiltrating the intercostal spaces above and below the fracture site with 1% procaine.

NURSING CONSIDERATIONS: The nurse assists in splinting the chest, administers the ordered medication, and helps the patient to turn.

fragilitas ossium See **osteogenesis imperfecta.**

fragmented fracture A fracture that results in multiple bone fragments.

frambesia See **yaws.**

Franceschetti's syndrome A complete form of mandibulofacial dysostosis. See also **Treacher Collins syndrome.**

francium (Fr) A metallic element of the alkali metal group. Its atomic number is 87; its atomic weight is 223. Formed from the decay of actinium, all of its isotopes are radioactive and short-lived.

frank Clinically evident, as the obvious presence of a condition or a disease.

frank breech An intrauterine position of the fetus in which the buttocks present at the maternal pelvic inlet, the legs are straight up in front of the body, and the feet are at the shoulders. Babies born in this position tend to hold their feet near their heads for some days after birth. Compare **complete breech, footling breech.**

Frank-Starling relationship An index for determining cardiac output, based on the length of the myocardial fibers at the onset of contraction. The force exerted per heartbeat is directly proportional to the degree of stretch of the myocardial fiber so that improved performance is the result of a longer initial fiber length or a larger diastolic ventricular volume. Since there are no adequate in vivo methods of measuring fiber length or diastolic volume, end-diastolic pressure is used as an index of volume or stretch. The cardiac output is plotted on a graph against atrial pressure. In congestive heart failure there is a shift in the curve to the right and downward. Also called Frank-Starling mechanism.

fraternal twins See **dizygotic twins.**

fraud In law: the act of intentionally misleading or deceiving another person, resulting in the loss of something valuable or the surrender of a legal right.

FRC *abbr* **functional residual capacity.**

freckle A brown or tan macule on the skin usually resulting from exposure to sunlight. There is an inherited tendency to freckling, most frequently seen in persons with red hair. Compare **lentigo.**

free association **1.** The spontaneous, consciously unrestricted association of ideas, feelings, or mental images. **2.** Spontaneous verbalization of thoughts and emotions entering the consciousness during psychoanalysis.

free clinic A health program, usually located in a neighborhood setting, that provides health care for ambulatory patients at nominal or no cost.

free-floating anxiety A generalized, persistent, pervasive fear that is not attributable to any specific object, event, or source. See also **anxiety, anxiety neurosis.**

free phagocyte See **phagocyte.**

free thyroxine The amount of the unbound, active thyroid hormone, thyroxine (T_4), circulating in the blood. See also **free thyroxine index.**

free thyroxine index   The amount of unbound, physiologically active thyroxine (T_4) in serum, determined by direct assay or calculated on the basis of an in vitro uptake test.

Freiberg's infarction   An abnormal orthopedic condition characterized by the aseptic necrosis of bone tissue, most commonly affecting the head of the second metatarsal.

Frei test   A test performed to confirm a diagnosis of lymphogranuloma venereum. Killed antigen, originally derived from infected patients, is injected in one forearm, and a control material is injected into the other arm. If a red, thickened papule develops at the site of injection of antigen, the test is positive. See also *Chlamydia.*

Frejka splint   A corrective device consisting of a pillow that is belted between the legs of an infant born with dislocated hips to maintain abduction and articulation of the head of the femur with the acetabulum.

fremitus   A tremulous vibration of the chest wall that can be auscultated or palpated during physical examination. Kinds of fremitus include **bronchial fremitus, coarse fremitus, tactile fremitus, vocal fremitus.**

frenulum linguae   See **lingual frenum.**

frenum, *pl.* **frenums, frena**   A restraining portion or structure. Also called frenulum.

frequency   **1.** The number of repetitions of any phenomenon within a fixed period of time, as the number of heartbeats per minute. **2.** In biometry: the proportion of the number of persons having a discrete characteristic to the total number of persons being studied. **3.** In electronics: the number of cycles of a periodic quantity, as alternating current, that occur in a period of 1 second. Electronic frequencies, formerly expressed in cycles per second, are now expressed in hertz (Hz).

Freudian   **1.** Of or pertaining to Sigmund Freud, his theories and doctrines, which stress the formative years of childhood as the basis for later psychoneurotic disorders, primarily through the unconscious repression of instinctual drives and sexual desires, and his system of psychoanalysis for treating such disturbances. **2.** Anything that is interpreted according to the theories of Freud or in psychoanalytic terms. **3.** Of or pertaining to the school of psychiatry based on Freud's teachings. **4.** One who adheres to Freud's school of psychiatry. See also **psychoanalysis.**

Freudian fixation   An arrest in psychosexual development characterized by a firm emotional attachment to another person or object. Some kinds of Freudian fixation are **father fixation, mother fixation.**

Freudianism, Freudism   The school of psychiatry based on the psychoanalytic theories and psychotherapeutic methods developed by Sigmund Freud and his followers. See also **psychoanalysis.**

friction   **1.** The act of rubbing one object against another. See also **attrition. 2.** A type of massage

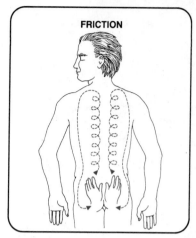

FRICTION

in which deeper tissues are stroked or rubbed, usually through strong circular movements of the hand. See also **massage.**

friction burn   Tissue injury caused by abrasion of the skin. See also **abrasion.**

friction rub   A dry, grating sound heard with a stethoscope during auscultation. It is a normal finding when heard over the liver and splenic areas. A pericardial friction rub auscultated over the pericardial area is suggestive of pericarditis; a pleural friction rub over the lungs may be present in heart or lung disease.

Friedländer's bacillus   A bacterium of the species *Klebsiella pneumoniae,* associated with infection of the respiratory tract, especially lobar pneumonia.

Friedman curve   A graph depicting the progress of labor, prepared by labor attendants to facilitate detection of dysfunctional labor. Observations of cervical dilatation and fetal descent are plotted on the vertical axis against time on the horizontal axis.

Friedreich's ataxia   An abnormal condition characterized by muscular weakness, loss of muscular control, weakness of the lower extremities, and an abnormal gait. Friedreich's ataxia, which may be hereditary, exhibits both dominant and recessive inheritance patterns. The primary pathologic feature of the disease is pronounced sclerosis of the posterior columns of the spinal cord with possible involvement of the spinocerebellar tracts and the corticospinal tracts. Friedreich's ataxia usually affects individuals between the ages of 5 and 20; the highest incidence of onset is at puberty. The characteristically ataxic gait may progress to severe disability, and is caused by a cavus deformity, or clawfoot. The condition may also cause slurred speech, head tremors, tachycardia, and cardiac failure. Thoracic scoliosis is present in approximately 80% to 90% of the patients afflicted. There is no curative treatment for Friedreich's ataxia. Spinal fusion may correct the associated scoliosis. Death in the progression of this disease

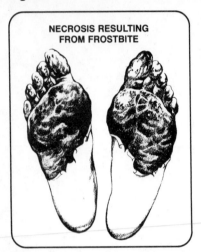

**NECROSIS RESULTING
FROM FROSTBITE**

is usually owing to myocardial failure.

frigid   **1.** Lacking warmth of feeling; unemotional; unimaginative; without passion or ardor and stiff or formal in manner. **2.** A woman who is unresponsive to sexual advances or stimuli, abnormally indifferent or averse to sexual intercourse, or unable to have an orgasm during sexual intercourse. Compare **impotence.** See also **orgasm.** —**frigidity,** *n.*

Fröhlich's syndrome   See **adiposogenital dystrophy.**

frôlement   **1.** The rustling type of sound often heard on auscultating the chest in diseases of the pericardium. **2.** A kind of massage that uses a light brushing stroke with the hand. See also **massage.**

front-   A combining form meaning 'pertaining to the forehead or front': *frontad, frontalis, frontonasal.*

frontal lobe   The largest of five lobes constituting each of the two cerebral hemispheres. It lies beneath the frontal bone; occupies part of the lateral, the medial, and the inferior surfaces of each hemisphere; and extends posteriorly to the central sulcus and inferiorly to the lateral fissure. The frontal lobe significantly influences personality and is associated with the higher mental activities, as planning, judgment, and conceptualizing. Research indicates that the right frontal and the right temporal lobes are associated with the nonverbal, specialized activities of the right cerebral hemisphere and that the left frontal and the left temporal lobes are associated with the verbal activities of the left cerebral hemisphere. Compare **central lobe, occipital lobe, parietal lobe, temporal lobe.**

frontal lobe syndrome   Behavioral and personality changes observed following a neoplastic or traumatic frontal lobe lesion. In some cases, the patient may become sociopathic, boastful, hypomanic, uninhibited, exhibitionistic, and subject to outbursts of irritability or violence; but in others the person may become depressed, apathetic, lacking in initiative, negligent about personal appearance, and inclined to perseverate.

frontal plane   Any one of the vertical planes passing through the body from the head to the feet, perpendicular to the sagittal planes, dividing the body into front and back portions. Also called **coronal plane.** Compare **median plane, transverse plane.**

frontal sinus   One of a pair of small cavities in the frontal bone of the skull that communicates with the nasal cavity. The frontal sinuses, which are rarely symmetrical, are situated behind the superciliary arches. Each sinus measures approximately 3 cm (1¼ inch) in height, 2.5 cm (1 inch) in width, and 2.5 cm in depth and is lined with a mucous membrane that is continuous with that of the nasal cavity. The frontal sinuses are absent at birth, well developed between the 7th and 8th years, and reach their full size after puberty. Compare **ethmoidal air cell, maxillary sinus, sphenoidal sinus.**

frontal vein   One of a pair of superficial veins of the face, arising in the plexus of the forehead. Each frontal vein communicates with the frontal tributaries of the superficial temporal vein and lies near the vein of the opposite side as it courses toward the root of the nose. The two frontal veins communicate by a transverse vessel before joining the supraorbital veins. Compare **angular vein, facial vein.**

frontocortical aphasia   See **motor aphasia.**

frostbite   Traumatic effect of extreme cold on skin and subcutaneous tissues, characterized by distinct pallor of exposed skin surfaces, particularly the nose, ears, fingers, and toes. Vasoconstriction and damage to blood vessels impair local circulation and result in anoxia, edema, vesiculation, and necrosis. Gradual warming is the appropriate first aid treatment. Iatrogenic frostbite is the result of excessive use of ethyl chloride sprays for local anesthesia for the relief of muscle and tendon strains. Compare **chilblain, immersion foot.**

frottage   **1.** See **effleurage. 2.** Sexual gratification obtained by rubbing against the clothing of another person, as can occur in a crowd.

frotteur   A person who obtains sexual gratification by the practice of frottage.

frozen-section method   In surgical pathology: a method used in preparing a selected portion of tissue for pathologic examination. The tissue is moistened and, fixed or unfixed, is rapidly frozen and cut by a microtome in a cryostat.

fructokinase   An enzyme that catalyzes the transfer of a phosphate group from adenosine triphosphate to D-fructose.

fructose   A source of carbohydrate calories.

fructosuria   Presence of the sugar, fructose, in the urine. This harmless and asymptomatic condition is caused by the hereditary absence of the enzyme fructokinase, which normally helps metabolize fructose. Also called **levulosuria.**

fruit sugar   See **fructose.**

FSH *abbr* follicle-stimulating hormone.

FTA-ABS test See Fluorescent Treponemal Antibody Absorption Test.

FTC *abbr* Federal Trade Commission.

fuchsin bodies See Russell's bodies.

fugue A state of dissociative reaction characterized by amnesia and physical flight from an intolerable situation. During the episode, the person appears normal and acts as though consciously aware of what may be very complex activities and behavior, but after the episode, the person has no recollection of the actions or behavior. The syndrome appears to be caused by an inability to cope with a severe conflict or with a chronically stressful life situation. See also **ambulatory automatism, automatism.**

fulcrum The stable point or the position on which a lever, as the ulna and the femur, turns in moving an object. Numerous common movements of the body, as raising the arm and walking, are combinations of lever actions involving fulcrums.

fulguration See **electrodesiccation.**

full bath A bath in which the patient's body is immersed in water up to the neck.

full diet See **regular diet.**

full liquid diet A diet consisting only of liquids and foods that liquefy at body temperature. It includes milk, milk drinks, carbonated beverages, coffee, tea, strained fruit juices, broth, strained cream soup, raw eggs, cream, melted butter or margarine, strained and precooked infant cereals in milk, thin custards, gelatin desserts, ice cream, sherbet, strained vegetables in soup, honey, syrups, sugar, and dry skim milk dissolved in liquids. The diet is prescribed following surgery, in some acute infections of short duration, in the treatment of acute gastrointestinal disorders, and for patients too ill to chew. See also **liquid diet.**

fulminating Of a disease or condition: rapid, sudden, severe, as an infection, fever, or hemorrhage. —**fulminant,** *adj.* **fulminate,** *v.*

fumagillin See **helvolic acid.**

fumigacin See **helvolic acid.**

function 1. An act, process, or series of processes that serve a purpose. 2. To perform an activity or to work properly and normally.

functional contracture See **hypertonic contracture.**

functional differentiation In embryology: specialization or diversification as a result of the particular function of a cell or tissue.

functional disease 1. A disease that affects function or performance. 2. A condition marked by signs or symptoms of an organic disease or disorder although careful examination fails to reveal any evidence of structural or physiological abnormalities. Headache, impotence, certain heart murmurs, and constipation may be symptoms of either organic disease or of functional disease.

functional dyspepsia An abnormal condition characterized by impaired digestion due to an atonic or to a neurologic problem. See also **dyspepsia.**

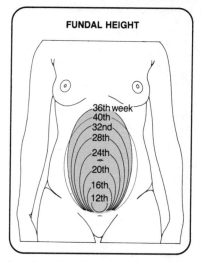

FUNDAL HEIGHT

36th week
40th
32nd
28th
24th
20th
16th
12th

functional imaging In nuclear medicine: a diagnostic procedure in which a sequence of radiographic or scintillation camera images of the distribution of an administered radioactive tracer delineates one or more physiologic processes in the body.

functional impotence See **impotence.**

functional residual capacity In anesthesiology: the volume of gas in the lungs at the end of a normal expiration.

fundal height The height of the fundus, measured in centimeters, from the top of the symphysis pubis to the highest point in the midline at the top of the uterus. Fundal height is measured at each prenatal visit. From the 20th to the 32nd week of pregnancy, the height in centimeters is equal to the gestation in weeks. Two measurements 2 weeks apart showing a deviation of more than 2 cm may indicate that the fetus is large or small for dates, that the estimated gestation is in error, or that the woman is carrying a multiple pregnancy.

fundamental needs of man In nursing education: the 14 basic needs of man, as described in a curriculum for basic nursing. The needs are: respiration; nutrition; elimination; mobility; sleep and rest; clothing; maintenance of normal body temperature; cleanliness; safety; communication; worship, according to the person's faith; work that is satisfying; recreation; learning; and discovery. Recognition and identification of a need precede and serve as the basis for a nurse's plan for care.

fundamentals of nursing The basic principles and practices of nursing as taught in educational programs for nurses, traditionally required in the first semester of the program. The emphasis of this phase of training is on the basic skills of nursing. Currently, nursing educators emphasize the importance of knowledge and understanding of the fundamental needs of man as well as competence in the basic skills as prerequisites to providing comprehensive nursing care.

fundus, *pl.* **fundi** The base or the deepest part of an organ; the portion farthest from the mouth of an organ, as the fundus of the uterus.

funduscope See **ophthalmoscope.**

funduscopy The examination and study of the fundus of the eye by means of an ophthalmoscope. —**fundoscopic, funduscopic,** *adj.*

fundus microscopy Examination of the base of the interior of the eye using an instrument that combines an ophthalmoscope and a lens with high magnifying power for observing minute structures in the cornea and iris.

fundus reflex See **light reflex.**

fungal infection Any inflammatory condition caused by a fungus. Most fungal infections are superficial and mild, though persistent and difficult to eradicate. Some kinds of fungal infections are **aspergillosis, blastomycosis, candidiasis, coccidioidomycosis, histoplasmosis.**

fungemia The presence of fungi in the blood. Compare **bacteremia, parasitemia, viremia.**

fungicide A drug that kills fungi. See also **antifungal,** definition 2. —**fungicidal,** *adj.*

fungiform papilla See under **papilla.**

fungus, *pl.* **fungi** A simple parasitic plant that, lacking chlorophyll, is unable to make its own food and is dependent on other life forms. A simple fungus reproduces by budding; multicellular fungi reproduce by spore formation. Of the 100,000 identified species of fungi, 100 are common in man and 10 are pathogenic. See also **fungal infection.**—**fungal, fungous,** *adj.*

funiculitis Any abnormal inflammatory condition of a cordlike structure of the body, as the spinal cord or spermatic cord.

funiculus umbilicalis See **umbilical cord.**

funnel-feeding A technique in which liquids may be given orally to a patient who cannot move the lips or masticate, as may occur following surgery to the mouth or lips. If the method is used for a weak or young infant, a rubber bulb or a large syringe may be used instead of a funnel.

FUO *abbr* fever of undetermined origin.

furazolidone An antibiotic.

furosemide A loop diuretic.

furuncle A localized, suppurative staphylococcal skin infection originating in a gland or hair follicle, characterized by pain, redness, and swelling. Necrosis deep in the center of the inflamed area forms a core of dead tissue that will be spontaneously extruded, eventually resorbed, or surgically removed. Treatment may include antibiotics, local moist heat, and, when there is definite fluctuation and the hard white core is evident, incision and drainage. Also called **boil.** —**furunculous,** *adj.*

furunculosis An acute skin disease characterized by boils or successive crops of boils that are caused by staphylococci or streptococci.

-fuse A combining form meaning 'to pour or flow': *diffuse, effuse, perfuse.*

fusimotor Pertaining to the motor nerve fibers, or gamma efferent fibers, that innervate the intrafusal fibers of the muscle spindle.

fusion 1. Bringing together into a single entity, as in optical fusion. 2. The act of uniting two or more bones of a joint. 3. The surgical joining together of two or more spinal vertebrae, to stabilize a segment of the spinal column following severe trauma, a herniated disk, or degenerative disease. Postoperative nursing care focuses on strict limitations of motion for the graft site until bony healing occurs.

fusospirochetal disease Any infection characterized by ulcerative lesions in which both a fusiform bacillus and a spirochete are found, as trench mouth.

-fy A combining form meaning 'to make into' something specified: *acidify, decalcify, salify.*

-fying See **-factive.**

G

g *abbr* **gram.**

Ga Symbol for **gallium.**

GA *abbr* **general anesthesia.**

GABA *abbr* **gamma-aminobutyric acid.**

gadolinium (Gd) A rare-earth metallic element. Its atomic number is 64; its atomic weight is 157.25.

gag reflex A normal neural reflex elicited by touching the soft palate or posterior pharynx, the response being elevation of the palate, retraction of the tongue, and contraction of the pharyngeal muscles. The reflex is used as a test of the integrity of the vagus and glossopharyngeal nerves. Also called **pharyngeal reflex.**

gait The manner or style of walking, including rhythm, cadence, and speed.

gait determinant One of the kinetic anatomic factors that govern locomotion. Some authorities have defined pelvic rotation, pelvic tilt, knee and hip flexion, knee and ankle interaction, and lateral pelvic displacement as the main determinants of gait. Such descriptions are often important in analyzing and correcting pathological gaits of individuals afflicted by orthopedic diseases, deformities, or abnormal bone conditions.

-galactia A combining form meaning a 'condition involving secretion of milk': *cacogalactia, dysgalactia.*

galacto-, galact-, galacta- A combining form meaning 'pertaining to milk': *galactochloral, galactogen.*

galactokinase An enzyme that functions in the metabolism of glycogen. Galactokinase catalyzes a metabolic step involving the transfer of a high-energy phosphate group from a donor molecule to a molecule of galactose producing a molecule of D-galactose-1-phosphate.

galactokinase deficiency An inherited disorder of carbohydrate metabolism in which galactokinase is deficient or absent. As a result, dietary galactose is not metabolized, galactose accumulates in the blood, and cataracts usually develop rapidly. Management requires elimination of dietary galactose, as milk and milk products. Compare **lactase deficiency.**

galactophorous duct A passage for milk in the lobes of the breast.

galactorrhea Lactation not associated with childbirth or nursing. It is sometimes a symptom of a pituitary gland tumor. See also **Forbes-Albright syndrome.**

galactose A simple sugar found in the dextrorotatory form in lactose (milk sugar), nerve cell membranes, sugar beets, gums, and seaweed and, in the levorotatory form, in flaxseed mucilage. Prepared galactose, a white crystal-line substance, is less sweet and less soluble in water than glucose but is similar in other properties.

galactosemia An inherited, autosomal recessive disorder of galactose metabolism, characterized by a deficiency of the enzyme galactose-1-phosphate uridyl transferase. Shortly after birth, an intolerance to milk is evident. Hepatosplenomegaly, cataracts, and mental retardation develop. Greater than normal amounts of galactose are present in the blood, the galactose tolerance test is abnormal, and the red blood cells show deficient galactose-1-phosphate uridyl transferase activity. The elimination of galactose from the diet results in the rapid amelioration of all symptoms, except mental retardation. Compare **diabetes mellitus, glycogen storage disease.** See also **galactose, inborn error of metabolism.**

galactosyl ceramide lipidosis A rare, fatal, inherited disorder of lipid metabolism, present at birth. Infants become paralyzed, blind, deaf, increasingly retarded, and eventually die of bulbar paralysis. There is no known treatment for the disorder, but it can be detected in pregnancy by amniocentesis. Also called **globoid leukodystrophy, Krabbe's disease.** Compare **Tay-Sachs disease.**

Galant reflex A normal response in the neonate to move the hips toward the stimulated side when the back is stroked along the spinal cord. It disappears by about 4 weeks of age. Absence of the reflex may indicate spinal cord lesion. Also called **trunk incurvation reflex.**

galea aponeurotica See **epicranial aponeurosis.**

Galeazzi's fracture A fracture of the distal radius accompanied by dislocation of the distal ulnar. Also called **Dupuytren's fracture.**

Galen's bandage A head bandage, consisting of a cloth strip with each end divided into three pieces. The center of the cloth is placed on top of the head; the two strips in front are joined at the back of the neck; the two strips at the back are pulled up and fastened on the forehead; the remaining middle strips are fastened under the chin.

gall See **bile.**

gallamine triethiodide A nondepolarizing neuromuscular blocking agent.

gallbladder A pear-shaped excretory sac lodged in a fossa on the visceral surface of the right lobe of the liver. It serves as a reservoir for bile. About 8 cm (3 inches) long and 2.5 cm (1 inch) wide at its thickest part, it holds about 32 cubic centimeters (2 cubic inches) of bile. During digestion of fats, the gallbladder contracts, ejecting bile through the common bile duct into the duodenum. The gallbladder is divided into a fundus, body, and neck and is covered by the peritoneum. Obstruction of the biliary system by gallstones may lead to jaundice and pain. It is a common condition in overweight, middle-aged women and may require surgical excision.

gallbladder cancer A malignant neoplasm of the bile reservoir, characterized by anorexia, nausea, vomiting, weight loss, progressively severe right upper quadrant pain, and, eventually, jaundice. Tumors of the gallbladder are predominantly adenocarcinomas; often associated with biliary calculi, they are three to four times more common in women than in men and rarely occur before the age of 40. Physical examination reveals an enlarged gallbladder in about half the cases. X-rays may aid diagnosis, but the diagnosis is usually made during a laparotomy. Complete removal of the gallbladder may be curative, but partial hepatectomy may be required, because the liver is often a site of early metastases. Radiotherapy may be palliative; chemotherapy is usually ineffective.

gallium A metallic element. Its atomic number is 31; its atomic weight is 69.72. The melting point of gallium is 29.8°C (85.6°F). Because of its high boiling point (1,983°C, or 3,601°F), it is used in high-temperature thermometers. Radioisotopes of gallium are used in total body scanning procedures. Many of its compounds are poisonous.

gallop In cardiology: a cardiac arrhythmia characterized by a low-pitched extra sound heard in diastole on auscultation of the heart. The rhythm resembles the pattern produced as a horse's hooves strike the ground at a gallop. If the sound is heard early in diastole in a child or a young adult, it is a physiologic third heart sound and is of no clinical significance; in an older person with heart disease it is a ventricular gallop, a pathologic sound. An extra sound late in diastole is an atrial gallop. It indicates increased resistance to ventricular filling.

gallstone See **biliary calculus.**

galvanic cautery See **electrocautery.**

galvanocautery See **electrocautery.**

gam- See **gamo-.**

Gambian trypanosomiasis A usually chronic form of African trypanosomiasis, caused by the parasite *Trypanosoma brucei gambiense.* An infected individual may have relatively mild symptoms for months or years before developing the neurologic symptoms of the terminal stage. Also called **West African sleeping sickness.** Compare **Rhodesian trypanosomiasis.** See also **African trypanosomiasis.**

game In psychology: a psychosocial maneuver consisting of a series of transactions in which the initiator has concealed motivation. The end result is a well-defined bad feeling, as anger or inadequacy.

gamet-, gameto- A combining form meaning 'reproductive cell': *gametocyte, gametophore.*

gamete 1. A mature male or female germ cell that is capable of functioning in fertilization or conjugation and that contains the haploid number of chromosomes of the somatic cell. **2.** The ovum or spermatozoon. See also **meiosis.** —**gametic,** *adj.*

gametic chromosome Any of the chromosomes contained in the haploid cell, specifically the spermatozoon or ovum, as contrasted to those in the diploid, or somatic, cell.

gametocide Any agent destructive to gametes or gametocytes, specifically to the malarial gametocytes. —**gametocidal,** *adj.*

gametocyte In genetics: any cell capable of dividing into, or in the process of developing into, a gamete, specifically an oocyte or spermatocyte.

gametogenesis Maturation of gametes, occurring through the process of meiosis. See also **oogenesis, spermatogenesis.** —**gametogenic, gametogenous,** *adj.*

gamma-aminobutyric acid (GABA) An amino acid found in the brain and in bacteria, yeast, and green plants.

gamma-benzene hexachloride A scabicide and pediculicide.

gamma efferent fiber Any of the motor nerve fibers that transmit impulses from the central nervous system to the intrafusal fibers of the muscle spindle. The gamma efferent fibers are responsible for deep tendon reflexes, spasticity, and rigidity but not for the degree of contractile response. They function in regulating the sensitivity of the spindle and the total tension of the muscle. See also **primary afferent fiber.**

gamma globulin See **immune gamma globulin.**

gamma radiation A very high frequency electromagnetic emission of photons from certain radioactive elements in the course of nuclear transition or from nuclear reactions. Gamma rays are more penetrating than alpha radiation and beta radiation but have less ionizing power and are not deflected in electric and magnetic fields. The wavelengths of gamma rays emitted by radioactive substances are characteristic of the radioisotopes involved and range from about 4×10^{-10} to 5×10^{-13} meters. High-voltage generators can produce X-rays of a wavelength much shorter than that of most gamma rays. The depth to which gamma rays penetrate depends on their wavelengths and energy. Gamma radiation and other forms of radiation can injure, distort, or destroy body cells and tissue, especially cell nuclei, but controlled radiation is used in the diagnosis and treatment of various diseases. Radiation therapy seeks to destroy the nuclei of rapidly dividing cancer cells by bombarding the nuclei with selective doses of radiation that spare normal tissue. Body cells especially sensitive to radiation include lymphoid cells, bone marrow cells, cells that line the alimentary tract, and cells of the testes and the ovaries. Exposure of the entire body to sizable doses of radiation can cause acute radiation sickness. See also **ultraviolet radiation.**

gamma ray An electromagnetic radiation of

short wavelength emitted by the nucleus of an atom during a nuclear reaction. Composed of high-energy photons, gamma rays lack mass and an electric charge and travel at the speed of light. They are usually associated with beta rays (electrons ejected at high velocities from radioactive substances).

gammopathy Abnormal condition characterized by the presence of markedly increased levels of gamma globulin in the blood. **Monoclonal gammopathy** is commonly associated with an electrophoretic pattern showing one sharp, homogenous electrophoretic band in the gamma globulin region. This reflects the presence of excessive amounts of one type of immunoglobulin secreted by a single clone of B cells. **Polyclonal gammopathy** reflects the presence of a diffuse hypergammaglobulinemia in which all immunoglobulin classes are proportionally increased. See also **Bence Jones protein, multiple myeloma.**

gamo-, gam- A combining form meaning 'pertaining to marriage or sexual union': *gamobium, gamont, gamophagia.*

gamogenesis Sexual reproduction occurring through the fusion of gametes. —**gamogenetic,** *adj.*

gamone A chemical substance secreted by the ova and spermatozoa that supposedly attracts the gametes of the opposite sex in order to facilitate union. Kinds of gamones are **androgamone, gynogamone.**

gampsodactyly See **pes cavus.**

-gamy A combining form meaning: **1.** 'A (specified) type of marriage': *endogamy, monogamy, pedogamy.* **2.** 'Possession of organs for reproduction': *cleistogamy, dichogamy, homogamy.* **3.** 'A union for propagation': *hologamy, macrogamy, syngamy.*

gangli-, ganglio- A combining form meaning 'pertaining to a ganglion': *gangliocytoma, ganglioneuroma, ganglioplexus.*

ganglion, *pl.* **ganglia** **1.** A knot, or knotlike mass. **2.** One of the nerve cells, chiefly collected in groups outside the central nervous system. Individual cells and very small groups abound in association with alimentary organs. The two types of ganglia in the body are the sensory ganglia on the dorsal roots of spinal nerves and on the sensory roots of the trigeminal, facial, glossopharyngeal, and vagus nerves and the autonomic ganglia of the sympathetic and parasympathetic systems.

ganglionar neuroma A tumor composed of nerve cells. Also called **ganglionated neuroma, ganglionic neuroma.**

ganglionic blocking agent Any one of a group of drugs prescribed to produce controlled hypotension, as required in certain surgical procedures or in emergency management of hypertensive crisis. These drugs are now generally replaced by vasodilators.

ganglionic crest See **neural crest.**

ganglionic glioma A tumor composed of glial cells and ganglion cells that are nearly mature. See also **neuroblastoma.**

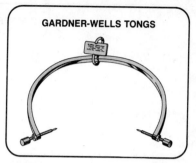

GARDNER-WELLS TONGS

ganglionic neuroma See **ganglionar neuroma.**

ganglionic ridge See **neural crest.**

gangliosidosis type I See **Tay-Sachs disease.**

gangliosidosis type II See **Sandhoff's disease.**

gangrene Tissue necrosis, usually resulting from ischemia, bacterial invasion, and subsequent putrefaction. Gangrene most often affects the extremities, but it can occur in the intestines and gallbladder. Internally, gangrene may be a complication of strangulated hernia, appendicitis, cholecystitis, or thrombosis of the mesenteric arteries to the gut. **Dry gangrene** is a late complication of diabetes mellitus that is already complicated by arteriosclerosis in which the affected extremity becomes cold, dry, and shriveled and eventually turns black. Moist gangrene may follow a crushing injury or an obstruction of blood flow by an embolism, tight bandages, or tourniquet. This form of gangrene has an offensive odor, spreads rapidly, and may result in death in a few days. See also **gas gangrene.** —**gangrenous,** *adj.*

gangrenous necrosis See **necrosis.**

gangrenous stomatitis See **noma.**

ganja *Slang.* See **cannabis.**

gap In molecular genetics: a short, missing segment in one strand of double-stranded DNA.

Gardener's syndrome Familial polyposis of the large bowel, with fibrous dysplasia of the skull, extra teeth, osteomas, fibromas, and epidermal cysts. The condition is inherited as a dominant trait, and malignancies occur more often than usual in families having this syndrome.

Gardner-Diamond syndrome A condition resulting from autoerythrocyte sensitization, marked by large, painful, transient ecchymoses that appear without apparent cause but often accompany emotional upsets, various collagen disorders, and abnormalities of protein metabolism. Treatment includes topical and systemic corticosteriods. Also called **autoerythrocyte sensitization syndrome.**

Gardner-Wells tongs A type of skull tong used to exert traction and immobilize the cervical vertebrae after injury to the cervical spine.

gargle **1.** To hold and agitate a liquid at the back of the throat by tilting the head backward

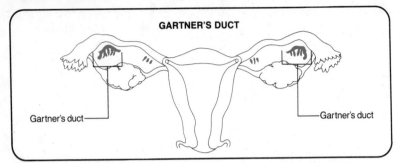

GARTNER'S DUCT

Gartner's duct

Gartner's duct

and forcing air through the solution. The procedure is used for cleansing or medicating the mouth and oropharynx. **2.** A solution used to rinse the mouth and oropharynx.

gargoylism See **Hurler's syndrome.**

Gartner's duct One of two vestigial, closed ducts, each one parallel to a uterine tube.

gas An aeriform fluid possessing complete molecular mobility and the property of indefinite expansion. A gas has no definite shape and its volume is determined by temperature and pressure. Compare **liquid, solid.**

gas chromatography The separation and analysis of different substances according to their different affinities for a standard absorbent. A gaseous mixture of the substances is passed through a glass cylinder containing the absorbent, which may be dampened with a nonvolatile liquid solvent for one or more of the gaseous components. As the mixture passes through the absorbent, each substance is absorbed to a different extent and leaves a characteristic pigment. The bands of different colors left when all the gaseous mixture has moved through the absorbent constitute a chromatograph for analysis. Compare **column chromatography, ion-exchange chromatography.**

gas embolism An occlusion of one or more small blood vessels, especially in the muscles, tendons, and joints, caused by expanding bubbles of gases. Gas emboli can rupture tissue and blood vessels, causing decompression sickness and death. This phenomenon commonly affects deep-sea divers who rise too quickly to the surface without adequate decompression. Gas emboli are most dangerous in the central nervous system because of associated neurologic changes, as syncope, paralysis, and aphasia. Such emboli are extremely painful. The prevention and treatment of gas emboli involves gradual decompression of atmospheric gases, especially nitrogen, that are dissolved in the blood.

gas exchange, impaired A nursing diagnosis accepted by the Fifth National Conference on the Classification of Nursing Diagnoses. The etiology of the condition is an imbalance in ventilatory perfusion. The defining characteristics are confusion, restlessness, irritability, somnolence, hypercapnea, and hypoxia. See also **nursing diagnosis.**

gas gangrene Necrosis accompanied by gas bubbles in soft tissue following surgery or trauma. It is caused by anaerobic organisms, as various species of *Clostridia*, particularly *C. perfringens.* Symptoms include pain, swelling, and tenderness of the wound area, moderate fever, tachycardia, and hypotension. The skin around the wound becomes necrotic and ruptures, revealing necrotic muscle. A characteristic finding is toxic delirium. If untreated, gas gangrene is rapidly fatal. Prompt treatment, including excision of gangrenous tissue and administration of penicillin G intravenously, saves 80% of patients. The disease is prevented by proper wound care. Also called **anaerobic myositis.**

gasoline poisoning See **petroleum distillate poisoning.**

gas scavenging system The equipment and procedures used to eliminate anesthetic gases that escape into the atmosphere of the operating room. See also **trace gas.**

gaster-, gastr- See **gastro-.**

gastrectomy Surgical excision of all or, more commonly, part of the stomach, performed to remove a chronic peptic ulcer, to stop hemorrhage in the perforating ulcer, or to remove a malignancy. Preoperatively, a GI series is done and a nasogastric tube is introduced. Under general anesthesia, one half to two thirds of the stomach is removed, including the ulcer and a large area of acid-secreting mucosa. A gastroenterostomy is then done, joining the remainder of the stomach to the jejunum or duodenum. If a malignant tumor is found, the chest cavity is opened, and the entire stomach is removed, along with the omentum and, usually, the spleen; the jejunum is anastomosed to the esophagus. See also **dumping syndrome, gastroenterostomy, nasogastric tube, peptic ulcer.**

-gastria A combining form meaning '(condition of) possessing a stomach or stomachs': *atretogastria, macrogastria, megalogastria.*

gastric Of or pertaining to the stomach.

-gastric A combining form meaning a 'type of stomach or number of stomachs': *endogastric, paragastric, trigastric.*

gastric analysis Examination of the stomach contents, primarily to determine the quantity of acid and incidentally to detect blood, bile, bacteria, and abnormal cells. A sample of gastric secretion is obtained via a nasogastric tube. The technique used varies according to the infor-

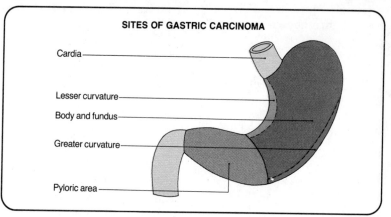

SITES OF GASTRIC CARCINOMA

Cardia

Lesser curvature

Body and fundus

Greater curvature

Pyloric area

mation desired. The total absence of hydrochloric acid is diagnostic of pernicious anemia. Patients with gastric ulcer and gastric cancer may secrete less acid than normal, while patients with duodenal ulcers secrete more. The composition and volume of the secretions may also provide diagnostic information. See also **Diagnex blue test.**

gastric atrophy See **atrophic gastritis.**

gastric cancer A malignancy of the stomach. Dietary factors, as nitrates, smoked and salted fish and meats, and moldy foods containing aflatoxin, are thought to cause gastric cancer, but the etiology remains unknown. The incidence is higher in men than in women and peaks in the 50- to 59-year-old age group. The risk is increased in workers exposed to asbestos and in patients with pernicious anemia. Symptoms of gastric cancer are vague epigastric discomfort, anorexia, weight loss, and unexplained iron-deficiency anemia; but many cases are asymptomatic in the early stages, and metastatic enlargement of the left supraclavicular lymph node may be the first manifestation of a stomach lesion. Approximately 97% of stomach tumors are adenocarcinomas that may be ulcerating, polypoid, diffuse and fibrous, or superficial spreading lesions; less than 3% are lymphomas and leiomyosarcomas. Radical subtotal gastrectomy with excision of contiguous involved tissues and reconstruction by anastomosing the remainder of the stomach to the duodenum or jejunum is usually recommended. Postoperative irradiation is recommended to control microscopic residual tumor; combinations of antineoplastic antimetabolites are used in treating advanced, metastatic gastric cancer.

gastric dyspepsia Gastric discomfort originating in the stomach. See also **dyspepsia.**

gastric fistula An abnormal passage into the stomach, communicating most frequently with an opening on the external surface of the abdomen. A gastric fistula may be created surgically to provide tube feeding for patients with severe esophageal disorders.

gastric intubation A procedure in which

a Levin tube or other small-caliber catheter is passed through the nose into the esophagus and stomach for the introduction into the stomach of liquid formulas to provide nutrition for unconscious patients or for premature or sick newborns. Medication or a contrast medium may be instilled for treatment or for radiologic examination. Gastric intubation is most often performed to remove the contents of the stomach in order to prevent postsurgical gastric distention, to prevent aspiration of gastric contents during general anesthesia, or to remove a poisonous substance and wash the stomach. See also **gastric lavage, Levin tube.**

gastric juice Digestive secretions of the gastric glands in the stomach, consisting chiefly of pepsin, hydrochloric acid, rennin, lipase, and mucin. The pH is strongly acid (0.9 to 1.5). Excessive secretion of gastric juice may lead to mucosal irritation and to peptic ulcer. See also **achlorhydria, gastric analysis, gastric ulcer.**

gastric lavage The washing out of the stomach with sterile water or a saline solution. The procedure is performed before and after surgery to remove irritants or toxic substances and before examinations such as endoscopy or gastroscopy. See also **irrigation.**

gastric motility The spontaneous peristaltic movements of the stomach, which aid in digestion by moving food through the stomach and out through the pyloric sphincter into the duodenum. Excess gastric motility causes pain that is usually treated with antispasmodic medication. Less than normal motility is common in labor, after general anesthesia, and as a side effect of some sedative hypnotics.

gastric node A node in one of three groups of lymph glands associated with the abdominal and pelvic viscera supplied by branches of the celiac artery. The gastric nodes accompany the left gastric artery and are divided into the superior and inferior gastric nodes. Compare **hepatic node, pancreaticolienal node.**

gastric ulcer See **peptic ulcer.**

gastrin A polypeptide hormone, secreted by the pylorus, that stimulates the flow of gastric

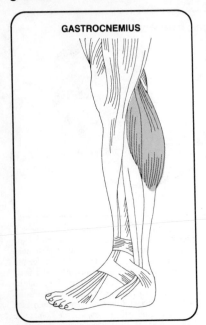

GASTROCNEMIUS

juice and helps stimulate secretion of bile and pancreatic enzymes.

gastritis   An inflammation of the stomach lining. Acute gastritis may be caused by the ingestion of alcohol, aspirin, or other medications or by the presence of viral, bacterial, or chemical toxins. The symptoms, including anorexia, nausea, vomiting, and discomfort after eating, usually abate after the causative agent is removed. Chronic gastritis is usually a sign of underlying disease, as peptic ulcer, stomach cancer, Zollinger-Ellison syndrome, or pernicious anemia. Differential diagnosis is by endoscopy with biopsy. Kinds of gastritis include **antral gastritis, atrophic gastritis, hemorrhagic gastritis, hypertrophic gastritis.** Compare **peptic ulcer.**

gastro-, gaster-, gastr-   A combining form meaning 'pertaining to the stomach or abdomen': *gastroadynamia, gastrocolitis.*

gastrocnemius   The most superficial muscle in the posterior leg. It arises by a lateral head and a medial head and forms the greater part of the calf. The lateral head arises from the lateral condyle of the femur and the capsule of the knee. The medial head arises from the medial condyle of the femur and from the capsule of the knee. The fibers of both heads insert into a broad aponeurosis, which narrows distally to join the tendon of the soleus as part of the tendo calcaneus. Compare **soleus, plantaris.**

gastrocnemius gait   An abnormal gait associated with a weakness of the gastrocnemius. It is characterized by the dropping of the pelvis on the affected side at the last moment of the stance phase in the walking cycle, accompanied by the lagging or the slowness of forward pelvic movement.

gastrocoele   See **archenteron.**

gastrocolic omentum   See **greater omentum.**

gastrocolic reflex   A mass peristaltic movement of the colon that often occurs when food enters the stomach. In infants, it may result in a bowel movement.

gastrodidymus   Conjoined, equally developed twins united at the abdominal region. Also called **omphalodidymus.**

gastrodisk   See **embryonic disk.**

gastroenteritis   Inflammation of the stomach and intestines accompanying numerous gastrointestinal disorders. Symptoms are anorexia, nausea, vomiting, abdominal discomfort, and diarrhea. The condition may be attributed to bacterial enterotoxins, bacterial or viral invasion, chemical toxins, or to miscellaneous conditions, as lactose intolerance. The onset may be slow, but more often it is abrupt and violent, with rapid loss of fluids and electrolytes from persistent vomiting and diarrhea. Hypokalemia and hyponatremia, acidosis, or alkalosis may develop. Treatment is supportive, employing bed rest, sedation, intravenous replacement of electrolytes, and antispasmodic medication to control vomiting and diarrhea.

gastroenterologist   A physician who specializes in gastroenterology.

gastroenterology   The study of diseases affecting the gastrointestinal tract, including the stomach, intestines, gallbladder, and bile duct.

gastroenterostomy   Surgical formation of an artificial opening between the stomach and the small intestine, usually at the jejunum. The operation is performed with a gastrectomy, to route food from the remainder of the stomach into the small intestine, or by itself, for perforating ulcer of the duodenum. Under general anesthesia, the jejunum is pulled up and anastomosed with the stomach. A new opening is then made for food to pass from the stomach directly into the jejunum. Compare **gastrectomy.**

gastroesophageal   Of or pertaining to the stomach and the esophagus.

gastroesophageal hemorrhage   See **Mallory-Weiss syndrome.**

gastroesophageal reflux   A backflow of contents of the stomach into the esophagus that is often the result of incompetence of the lower esophageal sphincter. Gastric juices are acidic and therefore produce burning pain in the esophagus. Repeated episodes of reflux may cause esophagitis, peptic esophageal stricture, or esophageal ulcer. In uncomplicated cases, treatment consists of elevation of the head of the bed, avoidance of acid-stimulating foods, and regular administration of antacids. In complicated cases, surgical repair may provide relief. See also **esophagitis, heartburn, hiatus hernia.**

gastrogavage   See **gastrostomy feeding.**

gastrohepatic omentum   See **lesser omentum.**

gastrointestinal Of or pertaining to the organs of the gastrointestinal tract, from mouth to anus.

gastrointestinal allergy An immediate reaction of hypersensitivity following the ingestion of certain foods or drugs. Gastrointestinal allergy differs from food allergy, which can affect organ systems other than the digestive system. Characteristic symptoms include itching and swelling of the mouth and oral passages, nausea, vomiting, diarrhea (sometimes containing blood), severe abdominal pain, and, if severe, anaphylactic shock. Treatment includes identification and removal of the allergen. In an acute attack, epinephrine may be administered as a stimulant, and muscle relaxants may be given to reduce intestinal spasms. In childhood, gastrointestinal allergy is most often caused by hypersensitivity to cow's milk and is characterized by diarrhea and colicky pain, sometimes with vomiting, eczema, respiratory distress, and thrombocytopenia. See also **lactose intolerance.**

gastrointestinal bleeding Any bleeding from the gastrointestinal tract. The most common underlying conditions are peptic ulcer, esophageal varices, diverticulitis, ulcerative colitis, and carcinoma of the stomach and colon. Vomiting of bright red blood or the passage of coffee ground vomitus indicates upper gastrointestinal bleeding, usually from the esophagus, stomach, or upper duodenum. Tarry, black stools indicate a bleeding source in the upper gastrointestinal tract; bright red blood from the rectum usually indicates bleeding in the distal colon. Gastrointestinal bleeding is treated as a potential emergency. Patients may require transfusions or fluid replacement and are watched carefully for signs of shock and hypovolemia. See also **coffee ground vomitus, hematemesis, hematochezia, melena.**

gastrointestinal obstruction Any obstruction of the passage of intestinal contents, caused by mechanical blockage or failure of motility. Mechanical blockage may be caused by adhesions resulting from surgery or inflammatory bowel disease, an incarcerated hernia, fecal impaction, tumor, intussusception, or volvulus. Failure of motility may follow anesthesia, abdominal surgery, or occlusion of any of the mesenteric arteries to the gut. Symptoms vary with the cause of obstruction but generally include vomiting, abdominal pain, and increasing abdominal distention. The objective of therapy is to remove the obstruction as quickly and safely as possible. A tube is inserted into the stomach or small intestine to aspirate contents and relieve distention. During these procedures, the patient is monitored for proper fluid and electrolyte balance. Surgical intervention may be necessary.

gastrointestinal system assessment An evaluation of the patient's digestive system and symptoms. The nurse conducts the interview, records her observations, and assembles the results of the diagnostic laboratory studies and procedures.

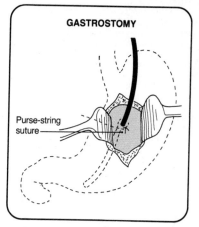

GASTROSTOMY

Purse-string suture

gastropore See **blastopore.**

gastroschisis A congenital defect characterized by incomplete abdominal wall closure and protrusion of the viscera.

gastroscope A fiberoptic instrument for examining the interior of the stomach. See also **fiberoptics. —gastroscopy,** *n.,* **gastroscopic,** *adj.*

gastroscopy Visual inspection of the stomach by means of a gastroscope inserted through the esophagus. The flexible fiberoptic gastroscope has increased the visualization of the prepyloric antrum, but the fundus is not visible. See also **endoscopy, fiberoptics. —gastroscopic,** *adj.*

gastrostomy Surgical creation of an artificial opening into the stomach through the abdominal wall, performed to feed a patient with esophageal cancer or one who is expected to be unconscious for a prolonged period. Under local anesthesia, the anterior wall of the stomach is drawn forward and sutured to the abdominal wall. A Foley catheter or other tube or a special prosthesis is then inserted into an incision in the stomach, and the opening is tightly sutured to prevent leakage of the contents of the stomach. The device is clamped and is opened when food is instilled. Postoperatively, glucose in water may be given; then a warm, blended formula is given every 4 hours. After 2 weeks, the tube is withdrawn after feeding and reinserted before the next meal.

gastrostomy feeding The introduction of a nutrient solution through a tube that has been surgically inserted into the stomach through the abdominal wall. Also called **gastrogavage.**

gastrothoracopagus Conjoined twins that are united at the thorax and abdomen.

gastrula The early embryonic stage formed by the invagination of the blastula. The cup-shaped gastrula consists of an outer layer of ectoderm and an inner layer of mesentoderm. This inner layer later differentiates into the mesoderm and endoderm. See also **blastula, embryonic layer.**

-gastrula A combining form meaning an 'embryonic stage following the blastula': *amphigastrula, discogastrula, paragastrula.*

gastrulation The development of the gastrula in lower animals and the formation of the three germ layers in the embryo of man and higher animals. It is characterized by an extensive series of coordinated morphogenetic movements within the blastula or blastocyst by which the primitive body plan of the organism is established and by which the areas that later differentiate into various structures and organs are in their proper position for development.

Gatch bed A bed that has an adjustable joint, allowing the knees to be flexed and the legs supported.

gate control theory A theory of pain perception which postulates that transmission of pain signals along spinal column nerves is controlled by other nerves that act as 'gates.'

Gaucher's disease A rare, familial disorder of fat metabolism owing to an enzyme deficiency, characterized by widespread reticulum cell hyperplasia in the liver, spleen, lymph nodes, and bone marrow. Beginning in infancy or early childhood, splenomegaly, hepatomegaly, and abnormal bone growth develop. Diagnosis is made through biopsy of the liver, spleen, or bone marrow. Mortality is high, but children who survive adolescence may live for many years. Also called **glucosyl cerebroside lipidosis.**

gauntlet bandage A glovelike bandage covering the hand and the fingers. See also **demigauntlet bandage.**

gauze A transparent fabric of open weave and differing degrees of fineness, most often cotton muslin, used in surgical procedures and for bandages and dressings. It may be sterilized and permeated by an antiseptic or lotion. Kinds of gauze include **absorbable gauze, absorbent gauze, petrolatum gauze.** See also **bandage.**

gavage The process of feeding a patient through a nasogastric tube.

gavage feeding of the newborn A procedure in which a tube passed through the nose or mouth into the stomach is used to feed a newborn infant with weak sucking, uncoordinated sucking and swallowing, respiratory distress, tachypnea, or repeated apneic spells. NURSING CONSIDERATIONS: The nurse administers intermittent gavage feeding to the infant, offers an explanation to the parents of the need for the procedure, and points out that nipple feedings may be instituted when the infant sucks on the gavage tube or pacifier, roots actively, shows good suck and swallow coordination, gains weight, and has a respiratory rate of less than 60 breaths/minute.

gay *Slang.* **1.** Any person who is homosexual. **2.** Of or pertaining to homosexuality.

Gay-Lussac's law In physics: a law stating that the volume of a specific mass of a gas will increase as the temperature is increased at a constant rate, determined by the volume of the gas at 0°C (32°F) if the pressure remains constant. Also called **Charles' law.**

Gay Nurses' Alliance (GNA) A national organization of homosexual nurses.

gaze palsy A partial or complete inability to move the eyes to all directions of gaze. A gaze palsy is often named for the absent direction of gaze, as a right lateral gaze palsy.

GBIA See **Guthrie test.**

gc *Informal. abbr* gonococcus, the causative organism of gonorrhea.

Gd Symbol for **gadolinium.**

Ge Symbol for **germanium.**

Geiger-Müller counter An electronic device that indicates the level of radioactivity of any substance by counting the number of subatomic particles, as electrons, emitted. The counter detects ionizing particles with a Geiger-Müller tube. As ionizing particles cross the tube they ionize the gas within the tube and cause an electrical discharge. Also called Geiger counter.

gel A colloid that is firm even though it contains a large amount of liquid, used in many medicines as a demulcent, a vehicle for other drugs, an antacid, or an astringent, depending on the drug from which it is derived.

gelat- A combining form meaning 'to freeze, congeal': *gelatigenous, gelatinoid, gelatum.*

gelatiniform carcinoma See **mucinous carcinoma.**

gelatinous carcinoma A former term for **mucinous carcinoma.**

gelatin sponge An absorbable local hemostatic.

gel diffusion See **immunodiffusion.**

Gelhorn pessary See **pessary.**

gemellary Of or pertaining to twins.

gemellipara A woman who has given birth to twins.

gemellology The study of twins and the phenomenon of twinning.

gemfibrozil An antilipemic agent.

gemin- A combining form meaning 'pertaining to a twin, or double': *geminate, gemini, geminous.*

gemma, *pl.* **gemmae** **1.** A budlike projection produced by lower forms of life during the budding process of asexual reproduction. **2.** Any budlike or bulblike structure, as a taste bud or end bulb. —**gemmaceous,** *adj.*

gemmate **1.** Having buds or gemmae. **2.** To reproduce by budding.

gemmation In invertebrates, the process of cell reproduction by budding. Also called **gemmulation.**

gemmiferous Having buds or gemmae; gemmiparous.

gemmiform Resembling a bud or gemma.

gemmipara An animal that produces gemmae or reproduces by budding, such as the hydra. —**gemmiparous,** *adj.*

gemmulation See **gemmation.**

gemmule **1.** In genetics: the small, asexual reproductive structure produced by the parent during budding that eventually develops into an independent organism. **2.** According to the early theory of pangenesis, any of the submicroscopic

STAGES OF GENERAL ADAPTATION SYNDROME

ALARM STAGE	RESISTANCE STAGE	EXHAUSTION STAGE
Increased secretion of glucocorticoids and resultant changes	Glucocorticoid secretion returns to normal	Increased glucocorticoid secretion sometimes to higher levels than during alarm reaction
Increased activity of sympathetic nervous system	Sympathetic activity returns to normal	
Increased norepinephrine secretion by adrenal medulla	Norepinephrine secretion returns to normal	
Flight or fight syndrome of changes	Flight or fight syndrome disappears	
Low resistance to stressors	High resistance (adaptation) to stressor	Loss of resistance to stressor; may lead to death
Stress triad (hypertrophied adrenals, atrophied thymus and lymph nodes, bleeding ulcers in stomach and duodenum)		

particles containing hereditary elements that are produced by each somatic cell of the parent, transmitted through the bloodstream to the gametes, and, after fertilization, give rise to cells and tissues that have the exact characteristics of those from which they originated. Compare **biophore.**

gen- A combining form meaning 'to become or produce': *generic, genesiology, genus.*

-gen A combining form meaning: **1.** 'That which generates': *aerogen, proteinogen, venogen.* **2.** 'That which is generated': *immunogen, ionogen, nitrogen.* Also **-gene.**

gender **1.** The classification of the sex of a person into male, female, or intersexual. **2.** The particular sex of a person. See also **sex.**

gender identity The sense or awareness of knowing to which sex one belongs. The process begins in infancy, continues throughout childhood, and is reinforced during adolescence. Also called core gender identity.

gender identity disorder A condition characterized by a persistent feeling of discomfort or inappropriateness concerning one's anatomical sex. The disorder typically begins in childhood with gender identity problems and is manifested in adolescence or adulthood as asexuality, homosexuality, transvestism, or transsexualism.

gender role The expression of a person's gender identity; the image that a person presents to both self and others demonstrating maleness or femaleness.

gene The biological unit of genetic material and inheritance. Since the concept of the gene was introduced with Mendelian genetics, it has undergone considerable modification and change and is still evolving as techniques for studying the molecular components of the cell are refined. The gene is now considered to be a particular nucleic acid sequence within a DNA molecule that occupies a precise locus on a chromosome and is capable of self-replication by coding for a specific polypeptide chain. In diploid organisms, which include humans and other mammals, genes occur as paired alleles and function in numerous capacities, primarily as structural and regulative components in controlling the differentiation of the cells and tissues of the body. Kinds of genes include **complementary genes, dominant gene, lethal gene, mutant gene, operator gene, pleiotropic gene, recessive gene, regulator gene, structural gene, sublethal gene, supplementary gene, wild-type gene.** See also **chromosome, cistron, deoxyribonucleic acid, operon.**

-gene See **-gen.**

gene library In molecular genetics: a collection of all of the genetic information of a specific species, obtained from cloned fragments.

general adaptation syndrome The defense response of the body or the psyche to injury or prolonged stress, as described by Hans Selye. It consists of an initial stage of shock or alarm reaction, followed by a phase of increasing resistance or adaptation, utilizing the various defense mechanisms of the body or mind, and culminating in either a state of adjustment and healing or one of exhaustion and disintegration. Also called **adaptation syndrome.** See also **post-traumatic stress disorder, stress.**

general anesthesia The absence of sensation and consciousness as induced by various anesthetic agents, given primarily by inhalation or intravenous injection. Four kinds of nerve blocks attained by general anesthesia are sensory, voluntary motor, reflex motor, and mental. The depth of anesthesia is planned to allow the surgical procedure to be performed without the patient's experiencing pain or having any recall of the procedure. See also **Guedel's signs.**

generalized anaphylaxis A severe reagin-mediated reaction to an allergen characterized by itching, edema, wheezing respirations, apprehension, cyanosis, dyspnea, pupillary dilation, a rapid, weak pulse, and falling blood pressure, that may rapidly result in shock and death. Systemic anaphylaxis, the most extreme form of hypersensitivity, may be caused by insect stings, proteins in animal sera, food, or certain drugs; parenterally administered penicillin and contrast media containing iodide are frequent causes of anaphylactic shock, especially in individuals with a history of allergies. An anaphylactic reaction is mediated by reaginic antibodies (IgE) that form in response to an initial sensitizing dose of an allergen and render the individual hypersensitive to the allergen by binding it to mast cells and basophils. A subsequent challenging dose of the allergen, causing the cells to degranulate and release histamine, bradykinin, and other vasoactive amines, produces anaphylaxis. Treatment of generalized anaphylaxis includes an immediate subcutaneous or intramuscular injection of 1:1,000 epinephrine hydrochloride, and the administration of an antihistamine and isoproterenol or aminophylline to relieve bronchial spasm. See also **reagin-mediated disorder.**

generalized tonic-clonic seizure An epileptic seizure, frequently preceded by an aura, that begins with a sudden loud cry and loss of consciousness as the patient falls to the ground. The body stiffens (tonic phase), and then alternates between episodes of muscular spasm and relaxation (clonic phase). Tongue-biting, incontinence, labored breathing, apnea, and subsequent cyanosis may also occur. Seizures usually last 2 to 5 minutes. Anticonvulsant therapy, commonly including phenytoin, carbamazepine, phenobarbital, or primidone, prevents generalized tonic-clonic seizures. Formerly called **grand mal seizure.**

generally recognized as effective (GRAE) One of the statutory criteria that must be met by a drug before it can be approved as a 'new drug.' Meeting these criteria relieves the manufacturer of the necessity of obtaining premarket approval as required by the Federal Food, Drug, and Cosmetic Act. To be recognized as effective, the drug must be, according to the Act, considered safe and effective by "experts qualified by scientific training and experience."

general paresis An organic mental disorder resulting from chronic syphilitic infection, characterized by degeneration of the cortical neurons; progressive dementia, tremor, and speech disturbances; muscular weakness; and, ultimately, generalized paralysis. It is often accompanied by periods of exultation and delusions of grandeur. Treatment usually consists of large doses of penicillin without which the outcome is almost invariably progressive deterioration and death. Also called **cerebral tabes, dementia paralytica, paretic dementia, syphilitic meningoencephalitis.**

general practitioner (GP) A family practice physician. See also **family medicine.**

general systems theory The science of wholes; study of the interdisciplinary nature of concepts, models, and principles to provide a possible approach to the unification of science.

generation 1. The act or process of reproduction; procreation. 2. A group of contemporary individuals, animals, or plants that are the same number of life cycles from a common ancestor. 3. The period of time between the birth of one individual or organism and the birth of its offspring. Kinds of generation include **alternate generation, asexual generation, filial generation, parental generation, sexual generation, spontaneous generation.**

generative nursing functions Innovative, rehabilitative, and productive nursing behaviors that help develop new ways to cope with stress.

generic 1. Of or pertaining to a genus. 2. Of or pertaining to a substance, product, or drug that is not protected by trademark. 3. Of or pertaining to the name of a kind of drug that is also the description of the drug, as penicillin or tetracycline.

generic equivalent A drug product sold under its generic name, identical in chemical composition to one or more others sold under a trade name but not, necessarily, equivalent in therapeutic effect.

generic name The official nonproprietary name assigned to a drug. A given drug is licensed under its generic name, and all manufacturers of the drug list it by its generic name. However, a drug is usually marketed under a trade name chosen by the manufacturer. See also **chemical name, established name.**

generic nursing program A program to prepare people with no previous professional nursing experience for entry into the field of nursing, now usually used to distinguish baccalaureate programs from master's programs or practitioner programs.

-genesia, -genesis A combining form meaning: 1. A '(specified) condition concerning information': *agenesia, morphogenesis, paragenesia.* 2. 'The production or procreation of something (specified)': *algogenesia, palingenesia, syngenesia.*

genesis 1. The origin, generation, or developmental evolution of anything. 2. The act of producing or procreating. —**genetic,** *adj.*

gene splicing In molecular genetics: the

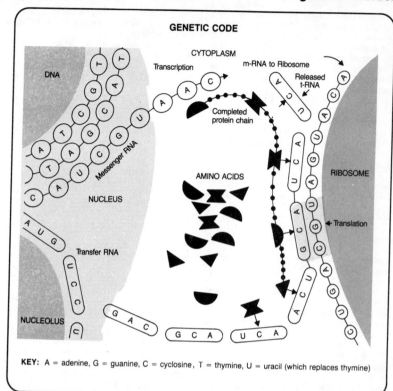

GENETIC CODE

KEY: A = adenine, G = guanine, C = cyclosine, T = thymine, U = uracil (which replaces thymine)

process by which a segment of DNA from one organism is attached to or inserted in a strand of DNA from another organism. In recombinant DNA technology genetic material from humans and other mammals is spliced into bacterial plasmids.

-genetic A combining form meaning: **1.** 'Pertaining to generation by (specified) agents': *gamogenetic, mitogenetic, spermatogenetic.* **2.** 'Generating': *glycogenetic, ovigenetic, ureagenetic.* **3.** 'Pertaining to something generated by a (specified) agent': *biogenetic, ideogenetic, phylogenetic.* Also **-genic, -genous, -geneous.**

genetic **1.** Pertaining to reproduction, birth, or origin. **2.** Pertaining to genetics or heredity. **3.** Pertaining to or produced by a gene; inherited.

genetic affinity Relationship by direct descent.

genetic code The information carried by the DNA molecules that determines the specific amino acids and their arrangement in the polypeptide chain of each protein synthesized by the cell. The genetic code represents the sequence of nucleotides along the DNA molecule of each chromosome in the cell. During transcription, this arrangement is synthesized in messenger RNA and then carried from the nucleus to the cytoplasm of the cell, where it is translated into protein at the site of the ribosomes. A unit of three consecutive nucleotides, called a codon, codes for each amino acid of the protein molecule. See also **transcription, translation.**

genetic colonization The process by which a parasite, such as a bacteriophage, introduces into its host genetic information that induces the host to synthesize products solely for the use of the parasite.

genetic counseling The process of determining the occurrence or risk of occurrence of a genetic disorder within a family and of providing appropriate information and advice about the courses of action that are available, whether care of a child already affected, prenatal diagnosis, termination of a pregnancy, sterilization, or artificial insemination is involved. Effective genetic counseling requires a detailed family history and may require special biochemical or cytogenetic tests. See also **genetic screening, prenatal diagnosis.**

genetic death **1.** The failure of an organism to survive as a result of its genetic makeup. **2.** The removal of a gene or genotype from the gene pool of a population or a given familial descent because of sterility, failure of the individual or organism to reproduce, or death before sexual maturity.

genetic disorder See **inherited disorder.**

genetic drift   The chance fluctuations in gene frequencies that may occur within a given population. The smaller the population, the greater the tendency for variation within each generation, so that eventually small, isolated inbreeding groups become genetically quite different from their ancestors. Also called **drift, random genetic drift.**

genetic engineering   The process of producing recombinant DNA so that the genotype and phenotype of organisms can be altered and controlled. Enzymes are used to break the DNA molecule into fragments so that genes from another organism can be inserted and the nucleotides rearranged in any desired sequence. Through genetic engineering such human proteins as growth hormone, insulin, and interferon have been produced in bacteria. At present, genetic engineering is possible only in microorganisms; but in the future the technique may be applicable to higher organisms, with the possibility of controlling and eliminating genetic disorders and malformations in man.

genetic equilibrium   The state within a population at which the frequency of genes and genotypes does not change from generation to generation. See **Hardy-Weinberg equilibrium principle.**

genetic homeostasis   The maintenance of genetic variability within a population through adaptation to varied or changing environments and conditions of life as a result of shifts or resistance to shifts in gene frequencies.

genetic immunity   See **natural immunity.**

genetic isolate   A group of plants, animals, or individuals that are genetically separated by geographical, racial, social, cultural, or any other barriers that prevent them from interbreeding with those outside of the group. Depending on the size of the group and the amount of inbreeding that occurs, genetic isolates generally show an increased incidence of otherwise rare, inherited defects. Also called **deme.**

geneticist   One who specializes in the study or application of genetics.

genetic load   The average number of accumulated detrimental genes per individual within a population, including those caused by mutation and selection within a recent generation and those inherited from ancestors. Genetic load is measured according to lethal equivalents.

genetic map   The graphic representation of the linear arrangement of genes on a chromosome and the relative distance between them, as expressed in map or morgan units. Also called **linkage map.**

genetic marker   Any specific gene that produces a readily recognizable genetic trait that can be used in family and population studies or in linkage analysis. Also called **marker gene.**

genetic polymorphism   The recurrence within a population of two or more discontinuous genetic variants of a specific trait in such proportions that they cannot be maintained simply by mutation, as the sickle cell trait, the Rh factor, and the blood groups. Compare **balanced polymorphism.**

genetic population   See **deme.**

genetics   **1.** The science that studies the principles and mechanics of heredity, specifically the means by which traits are passed from parents to offspring and the causes of the similarities and differences between related organisms. **2.** The total genetic makeup of a particular individual, family, group, or condition. Kinds of genetics are **clinical genetics, molecular genetics, population genetics.** See also **cytogenetics, Mendel's laws.**

genetic screening   The process of investigating a specific population of persons for the purpose of detecting the presence of disease, either incipient or overt. For example, all neonates are screened for phenylketonuria, for the purpose of identifying those who possess defective genes, gaining information concerning the incidence of a disorder in the population, and providing reproductive information, specifically to those at risk, as the close relatives of persons affected with inborn errors of metabolism or those in certain ethnic groups who have a high incidence of a particular disease, specifically sickle cell anemia in blacks and Tay-Sachs disease in Ashkenazic Jews. See also **genetic counseling.**

Genga's bandage   See **Theden's bandage.**

-genia   A combining form meaning '(condition or development of the) jaw': *microgenia, opisthogenia, progenia.*

-genic   A combining form meaning: **1.** 'Causing, forming, producing': *collagenic, hemorrhagenic, phosphagenic.* **2.** 'Produced by or formed from': *bacillogenic, coccigenic, pituitarigenic.* **3.** 'Related to a gene': *intragenic, polygenic, trigenic.*

geniculate neuralgia   A severe, debilitating, inflammatory condition of the geniculate ganglion of the facial nerve, characterized by pain, loss of the sense of taste, facial paralysis, and a decrease in salivation and lacrimation. It sometimes follows herpes zoster infection. See also **Ramsay Hunt's syndrome.**

geniculate zoster   See **herpes zoster.**

geniohyoideus   One of the four suprahyoid muscles, arising from the symphysis menti of the lower jaw and inserting into the body of the hyoid bone. A narrow muscle, the geniohyoideus is innervated by a branch of the first cervical nerve, and it acts to draw the hyoid bone and the tongue forward. Also called geniohyoid muscle. Compare **digastricus, mylohyoideus, stylohyoideus.**

genital herpes   **1.** See **herpes genitalis.** **2.** See **herpes simplex.**

genital reflex   See **sexual reflex.**

genitals, genitalia   The reproductive organs. —**genital,** *adj.*

genital stage   In psychoanalysis: the final period in psychosexual development, beginning with adolescence and continuing through the adult years when the genitals are the predominant source of pleasurable stimulation. The most significant feature of this stage is direction of sexual interest not just toward self-satisfaction but toward the establishment of a stable and meaningful heterosexual relationship. See also **psychosexual development.**

genitourinary (GU) Referring to the genital and urinary systems of the body, either the organ structures or functions or both. Also called **urogenital.**

genitourinary system See **urogenital system.**

genome The complete set of genes in the chromosomes of each cell of an organism.

genotype 1. The complete genetic constitution of an organism or group, as determined by the particular combination and location of the genes on the chromosomes. 2. The alleles situated at one or more sites on homologous chromosomes. The genetic information carried by a pair of alleles determines a specific characteristic or trait, usually designated by a letter or symbol, as AA when the alleles are identical and Aa when they are different. 3. A group or class of organisms having the same genetic makeup; the type species of a genus. Compare **phenotype. —genotypic,** *adj.*

-genous A combining form meaning 'producing or produced by': *tetanigenous, thyroigenous, tuberculigenous.*

Gensoul's disease See **Ludwig's angina.**

gentamicin sulfate An aminoglycoside antibiotic local and ophthalmic anti-infective agent.

gentian violet (methylrosaniline chloride) A local anti-infective and anthelmintic agent.

gentiotannic acid A form of tannic acid once used as an astringent and in burn treatment but no longer recommended because the compound is hepatotoxic.

genuine issue In law: an issue that is upheld by substantial evidence. It is a real issue, not a false one or one that is subject to interpretation.

genupectoral position Knee-chest position. To assume the genupectoral position, the person kneels so that the weight of the body is supported by the knees and chest, with the abdomen raised. The head is turned to one side and the arms are flexed so that the upper part of the body can be supported in part by the elbows.

genus, *pl.* **genera** A subdivision of a family of animals or plants. A genus usually is composed of several closely related species, but the genus *Homo sapiens* has only one species, humans. See also **family.**

genu valgum A deformity in which the legs are curved inward so that the knees are close together, knocking as the person walks, with the ankles widely separated. Also called **knock-knee.**

genu varum A deformity in which one or both legs are bent outward at the knee. Also called **bowleg.** Compare **genu valgum.**

-geny A combining form meaning 'produc-

tion, generation, origin': *homogeny, hylogeny, morphogeny.*

geo- A combining form meaning 'pertaining to the earth, or soil': *geobiology, geophagia, geotropism.*

geographic tongue A disorder in which small white or yellowish plaques develop on the tongue, gradually enlarge, and desquamate in the center, leaving denuded red patches surrounded by thickened white borders that converge, forming figures with scalloped outlines. The disorder, which may persist for months or years, causes a burning or itching sensation, is aggravated by food, and is often associated with digestive problems, especially in children.

geometric mean See **mean,** definition 3.

geotrichosis An abnormal condition associated with the fungus *Geotrichum candidum,* which may cause oral, bronchial, pharyngeal, and intestinal disorders. *G. candidum,* normally found in healthy individuals, the soil, and in dairy products, is not necessarily pathogenic. Geotrichosis most commonly occurs in immunosuppressed individuals and in diabetics. Bronchopulmonary complications associated with this disorder may produce a cough with thick, bloody sputum. Geotrichosis has produced allergic asthmatic reactions and a type of intestinal disorder.

geriatrician A medical specialist in the field of geriatrics.

geriatrics The branch of medicine dealing with the physiology of aging and the diagnosis and treatment of diseases affecting the aged.

germ 1. Any microorganism, especially one that is pathogenic. 2. A unit of living matter able to develop into a self-sufficient organism, as a seed, spore, or egg. 3. In embryology: the first stage in development, as a spermatozoon or other germ cell.

germanium (Ge) A metallic element with some nonmetallic properties. Its atomic number is 32; its atomic weight is 72.59.

German measles See **rubella.**

germ cell 1. A sexual reproductive cell in any stage of development. 2. An ovum or spermatozoon or any of their preceding forms. 3. Any cell undergoing gametogenesis. Also called **gonoblast, gonocyte.** Compare **somatic cell.**

germ disk See **embryonic disk.**

germicide A drug that kills pathogenic microorganisms. See also **antibacterial,** definition 2, **antifungal,** definition 2, **antiviral,** definition 2. **—germicidal,** *adj.*

germinal Pertaining to or characteristic of a germ cell or to the early stages of development.

germinal disk See **embryonic disk.**

germinal epithelium 1. The epithelial layer covering the genital ridge from which the gonads are derived in early embryonic development. 2. The epithelial covering of the ovary, formerly thought to be the site of the formation of the oogonia. See also **oogenesis.**

germinal membrane See **blastoderm.**

germinal nucleus See **pronucleus.**

germinal pole See **animal pole.**

HOW TO ESTIMATE GESTATIONAL AGE

PHYSICAL TRAITS	LESS THAN 37 WEEKS	37 TO 38 WEEKS	MORE THAN 38 WEEKS
Sole creases	Anterior transverse crease only	Some creases in anterior two thirds	Sole covered with creases
Breast nodule diameter	2 mm	4 mm	7 mm
Scalp hair	Fine and fuzzy	Fine and fuzzy	Coarse and silky
External ear	Pliable, no cartilage	Some cartilage	Stiff, with thick cartilage
Testes and scrotum	Testes in lower canal; scrotum small with few rugae	Testes in intermediate position	Testes pendulous; scrotum full with extensive rugae

germinal spot The nucleolus of a mature oocyte, prior to fertilization. See also **oogenesis, ovum.**

germinal stage In embryology: the time interval from fertilization to implantation during which the ovum undergoes cell division several times, travels to the uterus as a blastocyst, and begins to implant itself in the endometrium. The germinal stage lasts about 10 days.

germinal vesicle The nucleus of a mature oocyte prior to fertilization. Much larger than the nucleus of other cells, it initiates the completion of meiotic division after fertilization. See also **oogenesis, ovum.**

germination 1. The initial growth and development of an organism from the time of fertilization to the formation of the embryo. 2. The sprouting of a spore or the seed of a plant. —**germinate,** *v.*

germ layer One of the three primordial cell layers formed during gastrulation in the early stages of embryonic development from which the entire range of body tissue is derived. Each layer has the potentiality for forming different cellular types that differentiate into the various structures and organs of the body. See also **ectoderm, endoderm, mesoderm.**

germ nucleus See **pronucleus.**

germ plasm 1. The protoplasm of the germ cells containing the basic reproductive and hereditary material; the sum total of the DNA in a particular cell or organism. 2. Germ cells in any stage of development together with the tissues from which they originated. Compare **somatoplasm.** See also **Weismannism.**

germ plasm theory See **Weismannism.**

gero-, geronto- A combining form meaning 'pertaining to old age or the aged': *gerocomia, gerodontology, geromarasmus.*

-gerontic A combining form meaning 'pertaining to old age': *paragerontic, phylogerontic, ungerontic.* Also **-gerontal.**

geronto- See **gero-.**

gerontology The study of the aging process.

-gerous A combining form meaning 'bearing or characterized by' something specified: *calcigerous, ovigerous, setigerous.*

gestalt, *pl.* **gestalts, gestalten** A single physical, psychological, symbolic, or biological configuration or experience, consisting of a number of elements, that has an effect as a whole different from that of the sum of its parts.

Gestalt psychology A school of psychology, originating in Germany, that maintains that a psychological phenomenon is perceived as a total configuration or pattern, rising from the relationships among its constituent elements, rather than as discrete elements possessing attributes of their own, and that the pattern, or gestalt, cannot be derived from the summation of its constituents. Thus, learning is regarded as resulting from insight, defined as a process or reorganization, rather than from association or trial and error. Also called configurationism, Gestaltism. See also **gestalt.**

Gestalt therapy A form of psychotherapy that stresses the unity of self-awareness, behavior, and experience. It incorporates elements of psychoanalytic, behavioristic, and humanistic-existential therapy. See **Gestalt psychology.**

gestate 1. To carry a developing fetus in the womb. 2. To grow and develop slowly toward maturity, as a fetus in the womb.

gestation The length of pregnancy in viviparous animals; the period of time from the fertilization of the ovum until birth. Gestation varies with the species; in humans the average duration is 266 days or approximately 280 days from the onset of the last menstrual period. See also **pregnancy.**

gestational age The age of a fetus or a newborn, usually expressed in weeks dating from the first day of the mother's last menstrual period.

gestational diabetes A disorder characterized by an impaired ability to metabolize carbohydrate, usually caused by a deficiency of insulin, occurring in pregnancy and disappearing after delivery but, in some cases, returning years later. There is evidence that placental lactogen and considerable destruction of insulin by the placenta play a role in precipitating gestational diabetes. Treatment consists of insulin injections, a high-protein diet, and an adequate intake of calcium and iron. See also **diabetes mellitus.**

-geusia A combining form meaning, '(condition of the) sense of taste': *glycogeusia, hemiageusia, parageusia.* Also **-geustia.**

-geustia See **-geusia.**

GH *abbr* **growth hormone.**

GHRF *abbr* **growth hormone releasing factor.**

giant cell arteritis See **temporal arteritis.**

giant cell carcinoma A malignant epithelial neoplasm characteristically containing numerous very large anaplastic cells. A small percentage of adenocarcinomas of the lung and some liver tumors also contain such cells. Also called **carcinoma gigantocellulare.**

giant cell interstitial pneumonia See **interstitial pneumonia.**

giant cell myeloma A bone tumor of multinucleated giant cells that resemble osteoclasts scattered in a matrix of spindle cells. Myelomas of this kind may be benign or malignant and may cause pain, functional disability, and, in some cases, pathologic fractures. Also called **giant cell tumor of bone.**

giant cell thyroiditis See **de Quervain's thyroiditis.**

giant cell tumor of bone See **giant cell myeloma.**

giant chromosome Any of the excessively large chromosomes found in insects and the lower animals, specifically the lampbrush chromosome and polytene chromosome.

giant follicular lymphoma A nodular, well-differentiated, lymphocytic, malignant lymphoma characterized by multiple nodules that distort the normal structure of a lymph node. Also called **Brill-Symmers disease, Symmers' disease.**

giant hypertrophic gastritis A rare disease characterized by large folds of nodular gastric rugae that may cover the wall of the stomach, causing anorexia, nausea, vomiting, and abdominal distress. X-ray or endoscopic examination or surgery may be necessary for diagnosis. The disease is associated with an increased incidence of stomach cancer.

Giardia A common genus of the flagellate protozoans. Many species of *Giardia* normally inhabit the digestive tract, causing inflammation in association with other factors that produce rapid proliferation of the organism. See also **giardiasis.**

giardiasis An inflammatory, intestinal condition caused by overgrowth of the protozoan *Giardia lamblia.* The source of infection is usu-

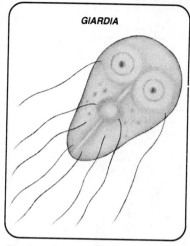

GIARDIA

ally untreated water contaminated with *G. lamblia* cysts. Also called **traveler's diarrhea.**

gibbus **1.** A hump, swelling, or enlargement on a body surface, usually confined to one side. **2.** A convex spinal curvature that may occur after the collapse of a vertebral body, as may result from a fracture or spinal tuberculosis.

Gibraltar fever See **brucellosis.**

Gibson walking splint A kind of Thomas splint that allows ambulation.

Giemsa's stain An azure dye used as a stain in the microscopic examination of the blood for certain protozoan parasites, viral inclusion bodies, rickettsia, and, more routinely, in the preparation of a smear for a differential white cell count.

gigantic acid An antibiotic substance derived from *Aspergillus giganteus,* a species of mold.

gigantism An abnormal condition characterized by excessive size and stature, caused most frequently by hypersecretion of growth hormone (GH) and occurring to a lesser degree in hypogonadism and in certain genetic disorders. Gigantism with normal body proportions and normal sexual development usually results from hypersecretion of GH in early childhood. Hypogonadism, by delaying puberty and closure of the epiphyses, may lead to gigantism. Excessive linear growth often occurs in males with more than one Y chromosome, and it may accompany Klinefelter's syndrome, Marfan's syndrome, and some cases of generalized lipodystrophy. Children with cerebral gigantism are mentally retarded and have a large head and extremities and a clumsy gait. They grow rapidly during their first few years and then at a normal rate. Appropriate gonadal hormones may be administered to control abnormal growth of children with hypogonadism. The treatment of acromegalic gigantism is usually irradiation, but hypophysectomy may be indicated. See also **acromegaly, eunuchoidism.**

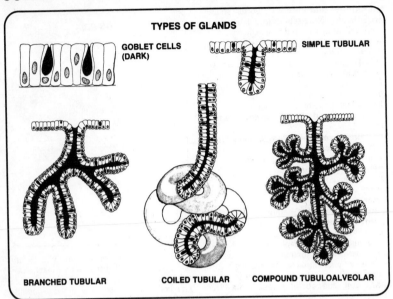

TYPES OF GLANDS

GOBLET CELLS (DARK)

SIMPLE TUBULAR

BRANCHED TUBULAR

COILED TUBULAR

COMPOUND TUBULOALVEOLAR

giganto- A combining form meaning 'huge': *gigantoblast, gigantochromoblast, gigantocyte.*

Gilbert's syndrome A benign, hereditary condition characterized by hyperbilirubinemia and jaundice. No treatment is required. Also called Gilbert's disease.

Gilchrist's disease See **blastomycosis.**

Gilles de la Tourette syndrome An abnormal condition characterized by facial grimaces, tics, and involuntary arm and shoulder movements. In adolescence, the condition worsens; the child may grunt, snort, and shout involuntarily. Coprolalia often develops. In adulthood the condition usually does not worsen; it comes and goes. Recently, treatment with dopamine antagonists has been found to be very effective, demonstrating an organic cause for this syndrome.

gingiva, *pl.* **gingivae** The gum of the mouth, a mucous membrane with supporting fibrous tissue that overlies the crowns of unerupted teeth and encircles the necks of those that have erupted. —**gingival,** *adj.*

gingival hyperplasia Overgrowth of the soft tissue of the gums, often seen in patients treated with phenytoin for epileptic seizures.

gingival papilla See under **papilla.**

gingivectomy Surgical removal of infected and diseased gingival tissue, performed to arrest the development of pyorrhea. Under general anesthesia, all pockets around the teeth are scraped and hypertrophied tissue is removed. The exposed surface of the gum is covered with packing to prevent trauma while eating and to allow new epithelial tissue to cover and fill in the areas. Considerable bleeding and pain are associated with the procedure. The packing is removed 1 week later.

gingivitis A condition in which the gums are red, swollen, and bleeding. Most gingivitis is the result of poor oral hygiene and of the accumulation of bacterial plaque on the teeth, but it may be a sign of another condition. It is common in pregnancy, usually painless, and may be acute or chronic. Compare **Vincent's infection.**

gingivo- A combining form meaning 'pertaining to the gingiva': *gingivoglossitis, gingivolabial, gingivosis.*

gingivostomatitis Multiple, painful ulcers on the gums and mucous membranes of the mouth, the result of a herpesvirus infection. Seen most frequently in infants and young children, the condition usually subsides after a week, but, in rare cases, it may progress to a systemic viral infection. See also **herpes simplex.**

ginglymus joint See **hinge joint.**

Giordano-Giovannetti diet A low-protein, low-fat, high-carbohydrate diet with controlled potassium and sodium intake, used in chronic renal insufficiency and liver failure. Protein is given only in the form of essential amino acids so that the body will use excess blood urea nitrogen to synthesize the nonessential acids for the production of tissue protein. Also called Giovannetti diet. See also **renal diet.**

gitalin A cardiotonic glycoside used to treat congestive heart failure and some cardiac arrhythmias.

glabrous skin Smooth, hairless skin.

gland An organ in the body, comprising specialized cells that secrete or excrete materials not related to their ordinary metabolism. Some glands lubricate; others, like the pituitary gland, produce hormones; hematopoietic glands take part in the production of blood.

GLASGOW COMA SCALE

FACULTY MEASURED	RESPONSE	SCORE
Eye opening	• Spontaneously • To verbal command • To pain • No response	4 3 2 1

Motor response	• To verbal command
	• To painful stimuli (apply knuckle to sternum; observe arms.)
	    Localizes pain
	    Flexes and withdraws
	    Assumes decorticate posture
	    Assumes decerebrate posture
	    No response
		6
		
		5
		4
		3
		2
		1

Verbal response (Arouse patient with painful stimuli, if necessary)	• Oriented and converses • Disoriented and converses • Uses inappropriate words • Makes incomprehensible sounds • No response	5 4 3 2 1
	Total:	3 to 15

Note: The *decorticate posture* may indicate a lesion of the frontal lobes, internal capsule, or cerebral penduncles. The *decerebrate posture* may indicate lesions of the upper brain system. *The patient's use of inappropriate words* may indicate either receptive or expressive aphasia. *Incomprehensible sounds* indicate expressive aphasia.

glanders An infection caused by the bacillus *Pseudomonas mallei*, transmitted to humans from horses and other domestic animals. It is characterized by purulent inflammation of the mucous membranes and the development of skin nodules that ulcerate. If untreated with antibiotics, the infection may spread to the bones, liver, central nervous system, and other tissues and cause death. It is endemic in Africa, Asia, and South America but has been eradicated in Europe and North America.

gland of Montgomery See **areolar gland.**

glands of Zeiss See **ciliary gland.**

glandular carcinoma See **adenocarcinoma.**

glandular fever See **infectious mononucleosis.**

glandula vestibularis major See **Bartholin's gland.**

glans, *pl.* **glandes** **1.** A general term for a small, rounded mass, or glandlike body. **2.** Erectile tissue, as on the ends of the clitoris and the penis.

glans of clitoris The erectile tissue at the end of the clitoris, continuous with the intermediate part of the vaginal vestibular bulbs. It comprises two corpora cavernosa enclosed in a dense, fibrous membrane and connected to the pubis and ischium. Also called glans clitoridis.

glans penis The conical tip of the penis that covers the end of the corpora cavernosa penis and the corpus spongiosom like a cap. The urethral orifice is normally located at the center of the distal tip of the glans penis; the corona glandis, the widest part of the glans penis, is around the base of the proximal portion. A fold of dark, thin, hairless skin forms the foreskin covering the glans penis.

Glanzmann's disease See **thrombasthenia.**

Glasgow Coma Scale A quick, practical, and standardized system for assessing the degree of conscious impairment in the critically ill and for predicting the duration and ultimate outcome of coma, primarily in patients with head injuries. The system involves three determinants: eye opening, verbal response, and motor response, all of which are evaluated independently according to a rank order that indicates the level of consciousness and degree of dysfunction. The degree of consciousness may vary from determinant to determinant and is assessed numerically by the best response. The results are plotted on a graph to provide a visual representation of the improvement, stability, or deterioration of a patient's level of consciousness, which is crucial to predicting the eventual outcome of coma. The results can also be used as

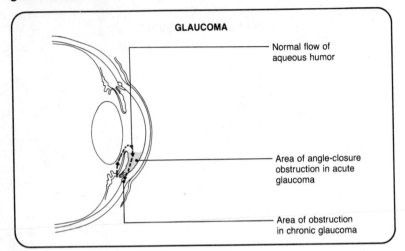

GLAUCOMA

Normal flow of aqueous humor

Area of angle-closure obstruction in acute glaucoma

Area of obstruction in chronic glaucoma

an overall objective measurement. The test score can also function as an indicator for certain diagnostic tests or treatments, as the need for a CT scan, intracranial pressure monitoring, and intubation. Also see **decerebrate posturing** and **decorticate posturing.**

glass factor See **factor XII.**

glaucoma An abnormal condition of elevated pressure within an eye owing to obstruction of the outflow of aqueous humor. **Acute (angle-closure) glaucoma** occurs if the pupil in an eye with a narrow angle between iris and cornea dilates markedly, causing the folded iris to block the exit of aqueous humor from the anterior chamber. **Chronic (open-angle) glaucoma** is more common, often bilateral; it develops slowly and is genetically determined. The obstruction is believed to be within the canal of Schlemm. Acute glaucoma is accompanied by extreme ocular pain, blurred vision, a red eye, and a dilated pupil. Nausea and vomiting may occur. If untreated, acute glaucoma results in complete and permanent blindness within 2 to 5 days. Chronic glaucoma may produce no symptoms except for gradual loss of peripheral vision over a period of years. Sometimes headaches, blurred vision, and dull pain in the eye are present. Cupping of the optic disks may be noted on ophthalmoscopic examination. Halos around lights and central blindness are late manifestations. Both types have elevated intraocular pressure by tonometry. Acute glaucoma is treated with eye drops to constrict the pupil and draw the iris away from the cornea, osmotic agents given systemically to lower intraocular pressure, acetazolamide to reduce fluid formation, and surgical iridectomy to produce a filtration pathway for aqueous humor. Chronic glaucoma can usually be controlled with miotic eye drops. Other treatment includes epinephrine eye drops and timolol eye drops. **—glaucomatous,** *adj.*

-glea A combining form meaning a 'binding

gelatinous medium': *ooglea, mesoglea, zooglea.* Also **-gloea.**

glia See **neuroglia.**

gliadin A protein substance, soluble in diluted alcohol, obtained from wheat and rye.

gliding 1. A smooth, continuous movement. 2. The simplest of the four basic movements allowed by various joints of the skeleton. It is common to all movable joints and allows one surface to move smoothly over an adjacent surface, regardless of shape. Compare **angular movement, circumduction, rotation.**

gliding joint A synovial joint in which articulation of contiguous bones allows only gliding movements, as in the wrist and the ankle. The ligaments or the osseous processes around each gliding joint limit movements of apposed plane surfaces or concavo-convex articulations. Also called **arthrodia, articulatio plana.**

glio- A combining form meaning 'pertaining to the neuroglia, or a gluey substance': *gliococcus, gliosarcoma, gliosome.*

glioblastoma See **spongioblastoma.**

glioblastoma multiforme A malignant, rapidly growing, pulpy or cystic tumor of the cerebrum or, occasionally, of the spinal cord. The lesion spreads with pseudopodlike projections. It is composed of a mixture of monocytes, pyriform cells, immature and mature astrocytes, and neural ectodermal cells with fibrous or protoplasmic processes. Also called **anaplastic astrocytoma, glioma multiforme.**

glioma, *pl.* **gliomas, gliomata** Any of the largest group of primary tumors of the brain, composed of malignant glial cells. Kinds of gliomas are **astrocytoma, ependymoma, glioblastoma multiforme, medulloblastoma, oligodendroglioma.**

-glioma A combining form meaning a 'tumor arising from the neuroglia': *angioglioma, fibroglioma, ganglioma.*

glioma multiforme See **gliobastoma multiforme.**

glioma retinae   See **retinoblastoma.**

glioma sarcomatosum   See **gliosarcoma.**

glioneuroma, *pl.* **glioneuromas, glioneuromata**   A neoplasm composed of nerve cells and elements of their supporting connective tissue.

gliosarcoma, *pl.* **gliosarcomas, gliosarcomata**   A tumor composed of spindle-shaped cells in the delicate supporting connective tissue of nerve cells. Also called **glioblastoma, glioma, spongioblastoma, spongiocytoma.**

gliosarcoma retinae   See **retinoblastoma.**

Glisson's sling   An apparatus with a collar for the neck and chin, which is attached to weights and a pulley and used for traction of the cervical spine.

-globinuria   A combining form meaning '(condition involving) the presence of complex proteins in the urine': *hemoglobinuria, methemoglobinuria, myoglobinuria.*

globoid leukodystrophy   See **galactosyl ceramide lipidosis.**

globule   A small spherical mass. Kinds of globules are **dentin globule, Dobie's globule, milk globule, myelin globule.**

globulin   One of a broad category of simple proteins classified by solubility, electrophoretic mobility, and size. Compare **albumin.** See also **euglobulin, plasma protein.**

globus hystericus   A transitory sensation of a lump in the throat that cannot be swallowed or coughed up, which often accompanies an emotional conflict or acute anxiety. The condition is thought to be due to a functional disturbance of the ninth cranial nerve and spasm of the inferior constrictor muscle that encircles the lower part of the throat. The physical examination tends to be normal, as does the barium esophagram.

globus pallidus   The smaller and more medial part of the lentiform nucleus of the brain, separated from the putamen by the lateral medullary lamina and divided into external and internal portions closely connected to the stratium, thalamus, and mesencephalon.

-gloea   See **-glea.**

glomangioma, *pl.* **glomangiomas, glomangiomatas**   A benign tumor that develops from a cluster of blood cells in the skin. Also called **angiomyoneuroma, angioneuroma.**

glomerular   Of or pertaining to a glomerulus, especially a renal glomerulus.

glomerular capsule   See **Bowman's capsule.**

glomerular disease   Any of a group of diseases affecting the renal glomerulus. Depending on the disease, there may be hyperplasia, atrophy, necrosis, scarring, or deposits in the glomeruli. The symptoms may be abrupt in onset or slowly progressive. See also **glomerulonephritis.**

glomerulonephritis   A noninfectious disease of the glomerulus of the kidney, character-

ized by proteinuria, hematuria, decreased urine production, and edema. Kinds of glomerulonephritis are **acute glomerulonephritis, chronic glomerulonephritis, subacute glomerulonephritis.**

glomerulus, *pl.* **glomeruli**   **1.** A tuft or cluster. **2.** A structure composed of blood vessels or nerve fibers, as a renal glomerulus.

glomus, *pl.* **glomera**   A small group of arterioles connecting directly to veins and having a rich nerve supply.

-glossia   A combining form meaning: **1.** The 'possession of a specified type or condition of tongue': *cacoglossia, megaloglossia.* **2.** The 'possession of a specified number of tongues': *aglossia, diglossia.*

glossitis   Inflammation of the tongue. Acute glossitis, characterized by swelling, intense pain that may be referred to the ears, salivation, fever, and enlarged regional lymph nodes, may develop during an infectious disease or following a burn, bite, or other injury. Glossitis in which there is smooth atrophy of the surface and edges of the tongue is seen in pernicious anemia. Chronic superficial glossitis (Moeller's glossitis), in which irregular, bright red patches appear on the tip or sides of the tongue, occurs chiefly in middle-aged women. The condition causes pain or a burning sensation and sensitivity to hot or spicy foods; it often resists treatment. In congenital glossitis, a flat or slightly elevated patch or plaque appears anterior to the circumvallate papillae in the midline of the dorsal surface of the tongue.

glossitis parasitica   See **parasitic glossitis.**

glossitis rhomboidea mediana   See **median rhomboid glossitis.**

glosso-, gloss-   A combining form meaning 'pertaining to the tongue': *glossocele, glossodynia.*

glossodynia   Pain in the tongue, caused by acute or chronic inflammation, an abscess, or an ulcer.

glossodynia exfoliativa   A form of chronic glossitis, characterized by pain and sensitivity to spicy foods without any evidence of pathology. It occurs primarily in middle-aged women. Also called **Moeller's glossitis.**

glossohyal   Of or pertaining to the tongue and the horseshoe-shaped hyoid bone at the base of the tongue immediately above the thyroid cartilage. Also called **hyoglossal.**

glossolalia   Speech in an unknown language, as speaking in tongues during a state of religious ecstasy when the message being transmitted through the speaker is believed to be from a divine source.

glossoncus   A local swelling or general enlargement of the tongue.

glossopathy   A pathologic condition of the tongue, as acute inflammation caused by a burn, bite, injury, or infectious disease; enlargement resulting from congenital lymphangioma; or a disorder produced by mycotic infection, a malignant lesion, or a congenital anomaly.

glossopexy An adhesion of the tongue to the lip.

glossopharyngeal Of or pertaining to the tongue and pharynx. See also **glossopharyngeal nerve.**

glossopharyngeal nerve Either of a pair of cranial nerves essential to the sense of taste, for sensation in some viscera, and for secretion from certain glands. The nerve has both sensory and motor fibers that pass from the tongue, parotid gland, and pharynx; communicate with the vagus nerve; and connect with two areas in the brain. Also called **nervus glossopharyngeus, ninth cranial nerve.**

glossophytia A condition of the tongue characterized by a blackish patch on the dorsum on which filiform papillae are greatly elongated and thickened like bristly hairs. The usually painless condition may be caused by heavy smoking, the extensive use of broad-spectrum antibiotics, or a mycosis in which *Cryptococcus* grows in symbiosis with *Nocardia.*

glossoplasty A surgical procedure or plastic operation on the tongue performed to correct a congenital anomaly, repair an injury, or restore a measure of function following excision of a malignant lesion.

glossoptosis The retraction or downward displacement of the tongue.

glossopyrosis A burning sensation in the tongue caused by chronic inflammation, by exposure to extremely hot or spicy food, or by psychogenic glossitis.

glossorrhaphy The surgical suturing of a tongue wound.

glossotrichia A condition of the tongue characterized by a hairlike appearance of the papillae. Also called **hairy tongue.**

glott- A combining form meaning 'pertaining to the glottis': *glottic, glottidas, glottis.*

glottis, *pl.* **glottises, glottides** **1.** A slit-like opening between the true vocal cords (plica vocalis). Also called **true glottis, rima glottidis. 2.** The phonation apparatus of the larynx, composed of the true vocal cords and the opening between them (rima glottidis). —**glottal, glottic,** *adj.*

glucagon A hormone, produced by alpha cells in the islets of Langerhans in the pancreas, that stimulates the conversion of glycogen to glucose in the liver. Secretion of glucagon is stimulated by hypoglycemia and by the growth hormone of the anterior pituitary. A preparation of purified, crystallized glucagon is used in the treatment of certain hypoglycemic states. Also called **hyperglycemic-glycogenolytic factor.**

glucagonoma syndrome A disease associated with a glucagon-secreting tumor of the islet cells of the pancreas, characterized by hyperglycemia, stomatitis, anemia, weight loss, and a characteristic rash.

gluco-, glyco- A combining form meaning 'pertaining to sweetness or to glucose': *glucofuranose, glucokinetic, glucosuria.*

glucocorticoid An adrenocortical steroid hormone that increases gluconeogenesis, exerts an anti-inflammatory effect, and influences many body functions. The most important of the three glucocorticoids is cortisol (hydrocortisone); corticosterone is less active, and cortisone is inactive until converted to cortisol. Glucocorticoids promote the release of amino acids from muscle, mobilize fatty acids from fat stores, and increase the ability of skeletal muscles to maintain contractions and avoid fatigue. In vitro, these hormones are known to stabilize mitochondrial and lysosomal membranes, increase the production of adenosine triphosphate, promote the formation of certain key enzymes in the liver, and decrease antibody production and the number of circulating eosinophils. A deficiency of glucocorticoids is characterized by hyperpigmentation of the skin, fasting hypoglycemia, weight loss, and apathy. An excess is associated with impaired glucose tolerance, thinning of the skin, ecchymosis, osteoporosis, poor wound healing, increased susceptibility to infection, and obesity. Glucocorticoid secretion is stimulated by the adrenocorticotropic hormone of the anterior pituitary, which in turn is regulated by the corticotropin-releasing factor of the hypothalamus. Compare **mineralocorticoid.**

gluconeogenesis The formation of carbohydrates from noncarbohydrate molecules, such as amino acids or fatty acids. Also called **glyconeogenesis.**

glucose A simple sugar found in certain foods, especially fruits, and a major energy source occurring in human and animal body fluids. Glucose, when ingested or produced by the digestive hydrolysis of double sugars and starches, is absorbed into the blood from the intestines. Excess circulating glucose is normally polymerized and stored in the liver and muscles as glycogen, which is depolymerized to glucose and liberated as needed. The determination of blood glucose levels is an important diagnostic test in diabetes and other disorders. Pharmaceutical preparations of glucose are widely used in the treatment of many disorders. See also **dextrose, glycogen.**

glucose 1-phosphate An intermediate compound in carbohydrate metabolism.

glucose 6-phosphate An intermediate compound in carbohydrate metabolism.

glucose-6-phosphate dehydrogenase (G-6-PD) deficiency An inherited disorder characterized by red cells partially or completely deficient in glucose-6-phosphate dehydrogenase, a critical enzyme in aerobic glycolysis. The gene for this enzyme is sex-linked, and the defect is fully expressed in affected males despite a heterozygous inheritance pattern. The disorder is associated with acute hemolysis under stress or in response to certain chemicals or drugs. A kind of nonspherocytic hemolytic anemia results. See also **congenital nonspherocytic hemolytic anemia.**

glucose tolerance test A test of the body's ability to metabolize carbohydrates by administering a standard dose of glucose and measuring the blood and urine for glucose at regular intervals. Blood and urine are collected periodically for up to 6 hours. The glucose tolerance test is most often used to aid the diagnosis of diabetes or other disorders affecting carbohydrate metabolism.

glucosuria Abnormal presence of glucose in the urine resulting from the ingestion of large amounts of carbohydrate or from a kidney disease, or a metabolic disease, as diabetes mellitus. See also **glycosuria**. —**glucosuric,** *adj.*

glucosyl cerebroside lipidosis See **Gaucher's disease.**

glue sniffing The practice of inhaling the vapors of toluene, a volatile organic compound used as a solvent in certain glues. The glue is squeezed into a plastic bag, which is placed over the nose and mouth. Intoxication and dizziness result. Prolonged or repeated use may damage a variety of organ systems.

glutamate A salt of glutamic acid.

glutamic acid A nonessential amino acid found widely in some proteins. Preparations of glutamic acid are used as digestive aids.

glutamic acid hydrochloride A digestant.

glutamic-oxaloacetic transaminase (GOT) An enzyme normally present in body serum and in certain body tissues, especially those of the heart and liver. This enzyme affects the intermolecular transfer of amino groups within the myocardium and may increase as the result of myocardial infarction and liver damage. Also called **serum glutamic-oxaloacetic transaminase.** Compare **glutamic-pyruvic transaminase.**

glutamic-pyruvic transaminase (GPT) An enzyme normally present in the serum and tissues of the body, especially the tissues of the liver. This enzyme may increase in persons with acute liver damage. Also called **serum glutamic-pyruvic transaminase.** Compare **glutamic-oxaloacetic transaminase.**

glutaraldehyde A disinfectant.

gluteal gait See **Trendelenburg gait.**

gluteal tuberosity A ridge on the lateral posterior surface of the thigh bone to which is attached the gluteus maximus.

gluten The insoluble protein constituent of wheat and other grains.

gluten enteropathy See **celiac disease.**

glutethimide A sedative-hypnotic agent.

-glycemia A combining form meaning a 'condition of sugar in the blood': *dysglycemia, hyperglycemia.* Also **-glycaemia.**

glycerin, anhydrous An ophthalmic agent that restores transparency to an edematous cornea.

glycerin, glycerine A hyperosmolar laxative and emollient.

glycerol An alcohol that is a component of fats. It is soluble in ethyl alcohol and water. See also **glycerin.**

glycerol kinase An enzyme in the liver and kidneys that catalyzes the transfer of a phosphate group from adenosine triphosphate to form adenosine diphosphate and L-glycerol-3-phosphate.

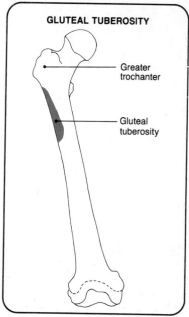

GLUTEAL TUBEROSITY

Greater trochanter

Gluteal tuberosity

glyceryl alcohol See **glycerin.**

glyceryl guaiacolate See **guaifenesin.**

glycine A nonessential amino acid occurring widely as a component of animal and plant proteins. Synthetically produced glycine is used in irrigation solutions to treat muscle diseases, and as an antacid and dietary supplement. See also **amino acid, protein.**

glyco- See **gluco-.**

glycobiarsol An antiamebic agent containing arsenic, formerly used to treat intestinal amebiasis.

glycocoll See **aminoacetic acid.**

glycogen A polysaccharide that is the major carbohydrate stored in animal cells. It is formed from glucose and stored chiefly in the liver. Glycogen is depolymerized to glucose and released into circulation as needed by the body. Also called **animal starch, hepatin, tissue dextrin.** See also **glucose.**

glycogenesis The synthesis of glycogen from glucose.

glycogen storage disease Any of a group of inherited disorders of glycogen metabolism. An enzyme deficiency causes glycogen to accumulate in abnormally large amounts in the body. Biopsy and chemical analysis reveal the missing enzyme. Also called glycogenosis.

glycogen storage disease, type I See **von Gierke's disease.**

glycogen storage disease, type II See **Pompe's disease.**

glycogen storage disease, type III See **Cori's disease.**

glycogen storage disease, type IV See **Andersen's disease.**

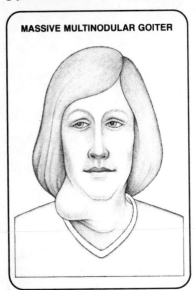

MASSIVE MULTINODULAR GOITER

glycogen storage disease, type V See **McArdle's disease.**

glycogen storage disease, type VI See **Hers' disease.**

glycolic acid A substance in bile, formed by glycine and cholic acid, that aids digestion and fat absorption. Glycolic acid is used as a food additive and an emulsifier.

glycolysis A series of enzymatically catalyzed reactions, occurring within cells, by which glucose and other sugars are broken down to yield lactic acid or pyruvic acid, releasing energy in the form of adenosine triphosphate. **Aerobic glycolysis** yields pyruvic acid in the presence of oxygen. **Anaerobic glycolysis** yields lactic acid without oxygen present. See also **Krebs' citric acid cycle.**

glyconeogenesis See **gluconeogenesis.**

glycopyrrolate A gastrointestinal cholinergic blocking (parasympatholytic) agent.

glycorrhea Any sugary discharge.

glycoside Any of several carbohydrates that yield a sugar and a nonsugar on hydrolysis. *Digitalis purpurea* contains a glycoside used to treat heart diseases.

glycosuria Abnormal presence of a sugar, especially glucose, in the urine. Glycosuria can result from the ingestion of large amounts of carbohydrate, or from endocrine or renal disorders. It is routinely associated with diabetes mellitus. —**glycosuric,** *adj.*

glycosuric acid A compound that is an intermediate product of tyrosine metabolism. It forms a melaninlike stain in the urine of people who have alkaptonuria.

glycyl alcohol See **glycerin.**

GMENAC *abbr* **Graduate Medical Education National Advisory Committee.**

GNA *abbr* **Gay Nurses' Alliance.**

gnath-, gnatho- A combining form meaning 'pertaining to the jaw': *gnathocephalus, gnathodynia.*

-gnathia A combining form meaning a 'condition of the jaw': *brachygnathia, campylognathia, retrognathia.*

gnathic Of or pertaining to the jaw or cheek.

gno- A combining form meaning 'to know or discern': *gnosia, gnosis.*

-gnomonic A combining form meaning 'signs or experience in knowing or judging (a condition)': *pathognomonic, physiognomonic, thanatognomonic.* Also **-gnomonical.**

-gnomy A combining form meaning the 'science or means of judging' something specified: *craniognomy, pathognomy, physiognomy.*

-gnosia A combining form meaning a '(condition of) perceiving or recognizing': *acognosia, hypergnosia.*

-gnosis A combining form meaning 'knowledge': *acrognosis, diagnosis, topognosis.*

goal In nursing: an accomplishment a patient desires to achieve, set within a specific time frame. This may help the patient in realizing a particular need and the nurse in evaluating nursing interventions.

goblet cell One of the many specialized cells that secrete mucus and form glands of the epithelium of the stomach, the intestine, and parts of the respiratory tract. Also called **beaker cell, chalice cell.** See also **gland.**

goiter A hypertrophic thyroid gland, usually evident as a pronounced swelling in the neck. The enlargement may be associated with hyperthyroidism, hypothyroidism, or normal levels of thyroid function. The goiter may be cystic or fibrous, containing nodules or an increased number of follicles; it may surround a large blood vessel, or a part of the enlarged gland may be situated beneath the sternum or in the thoracic cavity. Treatment may include total or subtotal surgical removal, the administration of antithyroid drugs or radioiodine, or the use of thyroid hormone to block the hypothalamic-hypophyseal mechanism that releases thyroid-stimulating hormone. See specific goiter. —**goitrous,** *adj.*

gold (Au) A yellow, soft metallic element that occurs naturally as a free metal and as the telluride $AuAgTe_4$. Its atomic number is 79; its atomic weight is 197. See also **chrysotherapy.**

gold compound A drug containing gold salts, usually administered with other drugs in the treatment of rheumatoid arthritis. Gold is potentially toxic and is administered only under the supervision of a specialist in chrysotherapy. Toxic reactions range from mild dermatoses to lethal poisoning.

gold sodium thiomalate A gold salt used in the treatment of arthritis.

gold therapy See **chrysotherapy.**

Golgi apparatus One of many small membranous structures found in most cells, composed of various elements associated with the formation of carbohydrate side chains of glycoproteins, mucopolysaccharides, and other substances. Saccules within each structure migrate through the cell membrane and release substances associated with external and internal secretion. Also called Golgi body, Golgi complex.

Golgi-Mazzoni corpuscles   Thin capsules enveloping terminal nerve fibrils in the subcutaneous tissue of the fingers. They have thicker cores than Pacini's corpuscles but are similar sensory end-organs. Compare **Pacini's corpuscles, Ruffini's corpuscles.**

gomphosis, *pl.* **gomphoses**   A joint made by the insertion of a conical process into a socket, as a root of a tooth into an alveolus of the mandible. Gomphosis is not a connection between true bones but is considered a type of fibrous joint. Compare **sutura, syndesmosis.**

gon-, gono-   A combining form meaning 'pertaining to semen or seed': *gonococcin, gonophore.*

gonad   A gamete-producing gland, as an ovary or a testis. —**gonadal,** *adj.*

gonadal dysgenesis   A general designation for conditions involving developmental anomalies of the gonads, as Turner's syndrome and gonadal aplasia.

gonadotropin, gonadotrophin   A hormonal substance that stimulates gonadal function. The gonadotropins follicle-stimulating hormone and luteinizing hormone are produced and secreted by the anterior pituitary gland. In early pregnancy, chorionic gonadotropin is produced by the placenta. It acts to sustain the function of the corpus luteum of the ovary, forestalling menstruation and thus maintaining pregnancy. Gonadotropins are prescribed to induce ovulation in infertility caused by inadequate stimulation of the ovary by endogenous gonadotropic hormones. —**gonadotropic, gonadotrophic,** *adj.*

-gonic   A combining form meaning 'agents, processes, or results of generation, reproduction, including the sexual': *dysgonic, endergonic, exergonic.*

gonio-   A combining form meaning 'pertaining to an angle': *goniocraniometry, goniometer.*

goniometry   A system of testing for various labyrinthine diseases that affect the sense of balance. —**goniometric,** *adj.*

gonoblast   See **germ cell.**

gonococcal pyomyositis   An acute inflammatory condition of a muscle caused by infection with a *Neisseria gonorrhoeae,* characterized by abscess formation and pain. It is an unusual form of gonorrhea and must be differentiated from sarcoma. The diagnosis is made by the discovery of the gonococcal diplococci within the abscess when a bacterial culture of a specimen is prepared following exploratory surgery. The person is then usually found to be asymptomatically infected in the urogenital organs. Antibiotic treatment is rapidly effective in curing the infection.

gonococcus, *pl.* **gonococci**   A gram-negative, intracellular diplococcus of the species *Neisseria gonorrhoeae.*

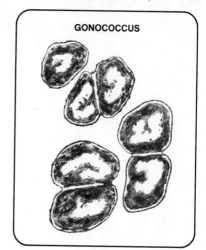

GONOCOCCUS

gonocyte   See **germ cell.**

gonorrhea   A common venereal disease most often affecting the genitourinary tract and, occasionally, the pharynx, conjunctiva, or rectum. The causative organism is *Neisseria gonorrhoeae.* Characteristic symptoms include urethritis; dysuria; purulent, green-yellow urethral or vaginal discharge; red or edematous urethral meatus; and itching, burning, or pain around the vaginal or urethral orifice. Severe disseminated infection is more common in women than in men. Gonorrhea is diagnosed by bacteriologic culture of the organism from a smear obtained from a specimen of exudate. Penicillin is used to treat uncomplicated gonorrhea. Oral treatment with a large, one-time dose of ampicillin is also effective, and erythromycin or tetracycline is sometimes used to treat the infection. The routine instillation of 1% silver nitrate in the eyes of the newborn provides effective prophylaxis against infection. —**gonorrheal, gonorrheic,** *adj.*

gonorrheal conjunctivitis   A destructive form of purulent conjunctivitis caused by *Neisseria gonorrhoeae* organisms. Prompt treatment by the intravenous administration of antibiotics is required to prevent corneal scarring and blindness. Also called **ophthalmia neonatorum.**

gonorrheal salpingitis   **1.** See **pelvic inflammatory disease. 2.** See **gonorrhea.**

gony-, gon-   A combining form meaning 'pertaining to a knee': *gonycampsis, gonyectyposis, gonyoncus.*

-gony   A combining form meaning 'birth or origin': *amphigony, merogony, zoogony.*

Goodell's sign   Softening of the uterine cervix, a probable sign of pregnancy.

Goodpasture's syndrome   A chronic, relapsing pulmonary hemosiderosis, usually associated with glomerulonephritis and characterized by a cough with hemoptysis, dyspnea, anemia, and progressive renal failure. Mild forms

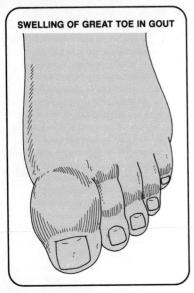

SWELLING OF GREAT TOE IN GOUT

may respond to corticosteroids or immunosuppressive drugs. Severe recurrent cases have a poor prognosis; hemodialysis and kidney transplantation are the only treatments.

gooseflesh See **pilomotor reflex.**

Gordon reflex 1. An abnormal variation of the Babinski reflex, elicited by compressing the calf muscles, characterized by extension of the great toe and fanning of the other toes. It is evidence of disease of the pyramidal tract. **2.** An abnormal reflex, elicited by compressing the forearm muscles, characterized by flexion of the fingers or of the thumb and index finger. It is seen in diseases of the pyramidal tract. Compare **Chaddock reflex, Oppenheim reflex.** See also **Babinski's reflex.**

Gordon's elementary body A particle found in tissues containing eosinophils once thought to be the viral cause of Hodgkin's disease. Also called Gordon's encephalopathic agent.

Gosselin's fracture A V-shaped fracture of the distal tibia, extending to the ankle.

GOT *abbr* **glutamic-oxaloacetic transaminase.**

goundou A condition characterized by bony exostoses of the nasal and maxillary bones, usually occurring as a late sequela of yaws in people of Central and South America.

gout A disease associated with an inborn error of metabolism that increases production or interferes with excretion of uric acid. Excess uric acid is converted to sodium urate crystals that precipitate from the blood and become deposited in joints and other tissues. Men are more often affected than women. The great toe is a common site for the accumulation of urate crystals. The condition can result in exceedingly painful swelling of a joint, accompanied by chills and fever. The symptoms are recurrent; episodes

become longer each year. The disorder is disabling and, if untreated, can progress to the development of tophi and destructive joint changes. Acquired gout is a condition having the signs and symptoms of gout but resulting from another disorder or treatment for a different condition. Diuretic drugs can alter the concentration of uric acid so that uric acid salts precipitate from the blood and are carried to the joints. See also **Lesch-Nyhan syndrome, tophus.**

Gowers' muscular dystrophy See **distal muscular dystrophy.**

G-6-PD deficiency *abbr* **glucose-6-phosphate dehydrogenase deficiency.**

GP *abbr* **general practitioner.**

GPI *abbr* **general paralysis of the insane.** See **general paresis.**

GPT *abbr* **glutamic-pyruvic transaminase.**

gr *abbr* **grain.**

Graafian follicle A mature ovarian vesicle, about 10 to 12 mm in diameter, that ruptures during ovulation to release the ovum. Many primary ovarian follicles, each containing an immature ovum about 35 microns in diameter, are imbedded near the ovarian surface, just below the tunica albuginea. Under the influence of the follicle stimulating hormone, one ovarian follicle ripens into a Graafian follicle during the proliferative phase of each menstrual cycle. Within the follicle the ovum grows to about 100 microns in diameter and, when the follicle ruptures, is swept into the fimbriated opening of the fallopian tube. The cavity of the follicle collapses when the ovum is released, and the remaining follicular cells greatly enlarge to become the corpus luteum. If the ovum is fertilized, the corpus luteum grows and becomes the corpus luteum of pregnancy. As the ovarian follicle ripens into the Graafian follicle, it produces estrogen, which stimulates the proliferation of the endometrium and the enlargement of the uterine glands. If the ovum is not fertilized, the Graafian follicle forms the corpus luteum of menstruation.

gracile Long, slender, and graceful.

gracilis The most superficial of the five medial femoral muscles. A thin, flattened muscle that is broad proximally and narrow distally, it originates in a thin aponeurosis secured on the inferior aspect of the symphysis pubis and the superior half of the pubic arch. The muscle curves around the medial condyle of the tibia and inserts into the body of the tibia, distal to the condyle. It is innervated by a branch of the obturator nerve, which contains fibers from the third and fourth lumbar nerves, and it functions to adduct the thigh and flex the leg and to assist in the medial rotation of the leg after it is flexed. Compare **adductor brevis, adductor longus, adductor magnus, pectineus.**

gradient 1. The rate of increase or decrease of measurable phenomenon, as pressure. **2.** A visual representation of the rate of change of a measurable phenomenon; a curve.

gradient of approach The inverse relationship between the distance from a positive stimulus and the tendency to approach it.

gradient of avoidance The inverse relationship between the distance from a negative stimulus and the tendency to avoid it.

graduated bath A bath in which the water temperature is slowly reduced.

graduated resistance exercise See **progressive resistance exercise.**

graduate medical education Formal medical education pursued after receipt of MD or other professional degree in the medical sciences. Graduate medical education is usually obtained as an intern, resident, or fellow, or in continuing medical education programs.

Graduate Medical Education National Advisory Committee (GMENAC) A committee established by order of the Secretary of the Department of Health, Education and Welfare (now the Department of Health and Human Services) to study the manpower issues in health care. The Committee issued its final report in September 1980.

Graduate Record Examination (GRE) An examination administered to graduates of institutions of higher learning. The scores are used as criteria for admission to masters and doctoral programs in many institutions and areas of specialization, including nursing. The examination tests verbal and mathematical aptitudes and abilities.

GRAE *abbr* **generally recognized as effective.**

graft A tissue or an organ taken from a site or a person and inserted into a new site or person to repair a defect in structure. The graft may be temporary, as an emergency skin transplant for extensive burns, or permanent, as the grafted tissue growing to become a part of the body. Skin, bone, cartilage, blood vessel, nerve, muscle, cornea, and whole organs may be grafted. Preoperative care focuses on a high protein diet and vitamins to ensure optimum physical condition, and on freedom from infection. Rejection is the major complication. Immunosuppressive drugs are given in large doses to suppress antibody production and rejection. Late rejection may occur a year or more after the graft. Also called **transplant.**

graft-versus-host (GVH) reaction A rejection response of certain grafts, especially bone marrow. It involves an incompatibility resulting from an immune response deficiency of some patients and is commonly associated with inadequate immunosuppressive therapy. Characteristic signs may include skin lesions with edema, erythema, ulceration, scaling, and loss of hair. Such reactions may also cause lesions of the joints and the heart and hemolytic anemia with a positive Coombs' reaction. The graft-versus-host reaction is similar to the Type IV reaction in hypersensitive individuals who receive tuberculin injections. Some experts believe that it involves certain immunologically active cells which originate as the result of defective tolerance mechanisms, or as the result of somatic mutation

TYPES OF GRAFTS

GRAFT	SOURCE	COVERAGE
Autograft	The patient's skin	Permanent
Homograft	Skin of the same species	Temporary
Heterograft	Skin of another species	Temporary
Synthetic substitute	Man-made substitute	Temporary

of certain host cells. Also called **homologous disease.**

grain (gr) The smallest unit of mass in avoirdupois, troy, and apothecaries' weights. It is equal to 0.06479891 gram. The troy and apothecaries' ounces contain 480 grains; the avoirdupois ounce, 437.5 grains.

grain itch A skin condition caused by a mite that lives in grain or straw. The lesion consists of an intensely itchy, urticarial papule surmounted by a tiny vesicle.

gram (g) A unit of mass in the metric system equal to 1/1000 of a kilogram, 15.432 grains, and 0.03 ounce avoirdupois.

-gram A combining form meaning: **1.** A 'drawing': *cephalogram, mammogram.* **2.** '1/1,000 kilogram': *centigram, decagram.* Also -**gramme.**

gram calorie See **calorie.**

gram-molecular weight The molecular weight of a substance expressed in grams. See also **mole, molecular weight.**

gram-negative Having the pink color of the counterstain used in Gram's method of staining microorganisms. This property is a primary method of characterizing organisms in microbiology. Some of the most common kinds of gram-negative pathogenic bacteria are *Bacteroides fragilis, Brucella abortus, Escherichia coli, Haemophilus influenzae, Klebsiella pneumoniae, Neisseria gonorrhoeae, Proteus vulgaris, Pseudomonas aeruginosa, Salmonella typhi, Shigella dysenteriae.*

gram-positive Retaining the violet color of the stain used in Gram's method of staining microorganisms. This property is a primary method of characterizing organisms in microbiology. Some of the most common kinds of gram-positive pathogenic bacteria are *Bacillus anthracis, Clostridium, Mycobacterium leprae, Mycobacterium tuberculosis, Staphylococcus aureus, Streptococcus pneumoniae.*

Gram stain The method of staining microorganisms using a violet stain, followed by an iodine solution, decolorizing with an alcohol or acetone solution, and counterstaining with safranin. The retention of either the violet stain or the pink counterstain serves as a primary means of identifying bacteria. Gram-positive organisms appear violet or blue; gram-negative organisms appear rose pink. Also called Gram's method.

grand mal seizure See **generalized tonic-clonic seizure.**

grand rounds A formal conference in which one expert presents a lecture concerning a clinical issue. Charts, tables, films, slides, tapes, and demonstrations are often used in presentation at grand rounds. In some settings grand rounds may be formal teaching rounds conducted by an expert at the bedsides of selected patients.

grant An award given to an institution, a project, or an individual usually consisting of a sum of money. A grant is given by a granting agency, the federal government, a foundation, private enterprise, or institution to provide financial support for research, service, or training. The applicant usually writes a formal application (proposal) for the grant, which is reviewed by the granting agency and compared to other proposals.

granul- A combining form meaning 'pertaining to grains or granules': *granulase, granulocorpuscle, granulocytemia.*

granular 1. Macroscopically looking or feeling like sand. 2. Microscopically appearing to have a few or many particles within or on its surface. —**granularity,** *n.*

granular conjunctivitis See **trachoma.**

granular endoplasmic reticulum See **endoplasmic reticulum.**

granulation tissue Any soft, pink, fleshy projections that form during the healing process in a wound not healing by first intention, consisting of many capillaries surrounded by fibrous collagen. Overgrowth of granulation tissue results in proud flesh growing to protrude above the skin. See also **pyogenic granuloma.**

granulocyte One of a group of leukocytes characterized by the presence of cytoplasmic granules. Kinds of granulocytes are **basophil, eosinophil, neutrophil.** Compare **agranulocyte.**

granulocyte transfusion The use of specially prepared leukocytes for the treatment of severe granulocytopenia and prophylactically for the prevention of serious infection in leukemic patients or those receiving cancer chemotherapy. The procedure has the same risks as a blood transfusion. Also called **buffy coat transfusion.**

granulocytic leukemia See **acute myelocytic leukemia, chronic myelocytic leukemia.**

granulocytic sarcoma See **chloroma.**

granulocytopenia An abnormal blood condition, characterized by a decrease in the total number of granulocytes. Also called **neutropenia.** See also **leukopenia.** —**granulocytopenic,** *adj.*

granuloma, *pl.* **granulomas, granulomata** A mass of nodular granulation tissue resulting from inflammation, injury, or infection. It is composed of capillary buds and growing fibroblasts. Granulomas may resolve spontaneously, become gangrenous, spread, or remain as a focus of infection.

-granuloma A combining form meaning a 'tumor-like mass or nodule of granulation tissue': *paragranuloma, ulcerogranuloma, xanthogranuloma.*

granuloma annulare A self-limited, chronic skin disease of unknown cause, consisting of a ring of reddish papules and nodules and most commonly seen on the distal extremities in children. No treatment is necessary.

granuloma gluteale infantum A neonatal skin condition characterized by large, elevated blue or brown-red nodules on the buttocks, often occurring as a secondary reaction to the prolonged use of strong steroid salves. The lesions routinely disappear several months after discontinuing use of such preparations.

granuloma inguinale A venereal disease characterized by ulcers of the skin and subcutaneous tissues of the groin and genitalia. It is caused by infection with *Calymmatobacterium granulomatis,* a small, gram-negative, rod-shaped bacillus. Diagnosis is made by microscopic identification of characteristic 'safety-pin'-shaped bodies in the cytoplasm of phagocytes taken from a lesion and dyed with Wright's stain. Untreated, the lesions spread, deepen, multiply, and become secondarily infected. Streptomycin is usually an effective treatment. Persons that have or are suspected of having granuloma inguinale are tested for syphilis, since concurrent infection is common.

granulomatosis A condition or disease characterized by the development of granulomas, as **berylliosis, Wegener's granulomatosis.**

granulomatous colitis See **Crohn's disease.**

granulomatous ileitis See **Crohn's disease.**

granulomatous lymphoma See **Hodgkin's disease.**

granulomatous thyroiditis See **de Quervain's thyroiditis.**

granulosa cell tumor A fleshy, yellow-streaked ovarian tumor that originates in primordial membrana granulosa cells and that may grow extremely large. It may be associated with excessive estrogen production, resulting in endometrial hyperplagia and menorrhagia. Also called **granulosa cell carcinoma.**

-graph A combining form meaning: 1. 'Product of drawing or writing': *hemophotograph, micrograph.* 2. 'Machine for producing a drawing': *clonograph, pneumograph.*

-grapher A combining form meaning 'one who writes about' something specified: *nosographer, syphilographer.*

-graphia A combining form meaning a 'psychological abnormality revealed through handwriting': *dysantigraphia, echographia, palingraphia.*

grapho- A combining form meaning 'pertaining to writing': *graphocatharsis, graphomania, graphophobia.*

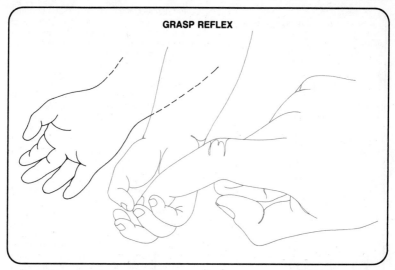

GRASP REFLEX

graphospasm Muscle cramping and pain in the hand and forearm resulting from prolonged writing. Also called **writer's cramp.**

-graphy A combining form meaning a 'kind of printing': *arteriography, cardiagraphy, dermagraphy.*

GRAS *abbr* generally recognized as safe.

grasp reflex A pathological reflex induced by stroking the palm or sole with the result that the fingers or toes flex in a grasping motion. The reflex occurs in diseases of the premotor cortex. In infants the reflex is normal; when an examiner strokes the infant's palms, the examiner's fingers are grasped so firmly that the child can be lifted into the air.

grass *Slang.* See **cannabis.**

Graves' disease A disorder characterized by pronounced hyperthyroidism usually associated with an enlarged thyroid gland and exophthalmos. The etiology is unknown but the disease is familial and may be autoimmune; antibodies to thyroglobulin or to thyroid microsomes are found in more than 60% of patients with the disorder. Graves' disease, which is five times more common in women than in men, occurs most frequently between the ages of 20 and 40 and often arises following an infection or physical or emotional stress. Typical signs are nervousness, a fine tremor of the hands, weight loss, fatigue, breathlessness, palpitations, heat intolerance, increased metabolic rate and gastrointestinal motility. Diagnosis may be established by serum thyroxine and triiodothyronine tests. Radioactive iodine uptake in the gland may be tested. Treatment may include antithyroid drugs and iodine preparations, or subtotal thyroidectomy. In patients with inadequately controlled Graves' disease, infection or stress may precipitate a life-threatening thyroid storm. Also called **exophthalmic goiter, thyrotoxicosis, toxic goiter.**

gravid Pregnant; carrying fertilized eggs or a fetus. —**gravidity, gravidness,** *n.*

gravid- A combining form meaning 'pertaining to pregnancy, or pregnant': *gravida, graviditas, gravidocardiac.*

gravida A pregnant woman. Called gravida I, or primigravida, during the first pregnancy; gravida II, or secundigravida, during the second pregnancy; gravida III, or tertigravida, during the third pregnancy.

-gravida A combining form meaning 'pregnant woman with (specified) number of pregnancies': *nonigravida, plurigravida, unigravida.*

gravity **1.** The force of attraction of all objects toward each other. This force is directly proportional to the product of the objects' masses and inversely proportional to the square of the distance between them. **2.** The tendency of an object to be drawn toward the center of the earth.

gray baby syndrome A toxic condition in neonates, especially premature infants, caused by a reaction to chloramphenicol. Because the body's mechanisms for detoxification and excretion are immature, the infant has limited ability to conjugate and thus eliminate the chloramphenicol. Symptoms include a characteristic ashen-gray cyanosis, accompanied by abdominal distention, hypothermia, vomiting, respiratory distress, and vascular collapse. The condition, which is fatal if the drug is continued, can be prevented by conservative dosages and by restricting use in women during late pregnancy or labor (since chloramphenicol readily crosses the placental barrier) and in lactating mothers.

gray hepatization See **hepatization.**

gray substance The gray tissue that makes up the inner core of the spinal column, arranged in two large lateral masses connected across the

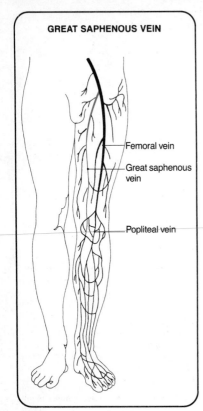

GREAT SAPHENOUS VEIN

Femoral vein

Great saphenous vein

Popliteal vein

midline by a narrow commissure. Each lateral portion of the gray substance splays outward, forming the posterior and anterior horns of the spinal cord. The horns consist primarily of cell bodies of interneurons and cell bodies of motoneurons. The quantity of gray substance varies greatly at different levels of the cord, and its shape is characteristic at each level. In the thoracic region, the gray substance is small in comparison with surrounding white substance; in the cervical and the lumbar regions it is larger; and in the conus medullaris its proportion to the white substance is the greatest. Nuclei in the gray matter of the spinal cord function as centers for all spinal reflexes. Also called gray matter. Compare **white substance.** See also **spinal cord, spinal nerves.**

GRE *abbr* **Graduate Record Examination.**

great auricular nerve One of a pair of cutaneous branches of the cervical plexus, arising from the second and the third cranial nerves. It winds around the border of the sternocleidomastoideus, perforates the deep fascia, and ascends on the surface of the muscle before dividing into the anterior branch and the posterior branch. The anterior branch is distributed to the facial skin over the parotid gland. The posterior branch supplies the skin of the mastoid process

and the back of the auricula. It also communicates with the smaller occipital nerve, the auricular branch of the vagus nerve, and the posterior auricular branch of the facial nerve.

great calorie See **calorie.**

great cardiac vein One of the five tributaries of the coronary sinus, beginning at the apex of the heart and ascending along the anterior interventricular sulcus to the base of the ventricles. It then curves left in the coronary sulcus, reaches the back of the heart, and opens into the left part of the coronary sinus. It receives various tributaries from the left atrium, as the large left marginal vein, which ascends along the left margin of the heart. The great cardiac vein drains the blood through its tributaries from the capillaries of the myocardium. Compare **middle cardiac vein, posterior vein of left ventricle, small cardiac vein.**

greater multangular See **trapezium.**

greater omentum A filmy, transparent extension of the peritoneum, draping the transverse colon and coils of the small intestine. It is attached along the stomach's greater curvature and the first part of the duodenum, and between its two layers contains blood vessels and fat pads. Between the stomach and the colon it forms the gastrocolic ligament, which contains the right and the left gastroepiploic blood vessels near the stomach's greater curvature. The greater omentum is a movable structure that spreads easily into areas of trauma, often sealing hernias and walling off infections that would otherwise cause general peritonitis, as can occur from a ruptured vermiform appendix. Also called **gastrocolic omentum.** Compare **lesser omentum.**

greater trochanter A large projection of the thigh bone to which are attached various muscles, including the gluteus medius, gluteus maximus, and obturator internus. The greater trochanter projects from the angle formed by the neck and the body of the thigh bone.

greater vestibular gland See **Bartholin's gland.**

great saphenous vein One of a pair of the longest veins in the body, containing 10 to 20 valves along its course through the leg and the thigh before ending in the femoral vein. It begins in the medial marginal vein of the dorsum of the foot, ascends anterior to the tibial malleolus and up the medial side of the leg in relation to the saphenous nerve. It runs posterior to the medial condyles of the tibia and the femur and passes through the hiatus saphenus just before joining the femoral vein. It contains more valves in the leg than in the thigh and receives many cutaneous veins and numerous tributaries, as those from the sole of the foot. Near the saphenous hiatus it is joined by the superficial epigastric vein, the superficial epigastric circumflex, and the superficial external pudendal veins. Compare **common iliac vein, femoral vein.**

green cancer See **chloroma.**

Greenough microscope See **stereoscopic microscope.**

greenstick fracture   An incomplete fracture in which the bone is bent but fractured only on the outer arc. Children are likely to have greenstick fractures. Immobilization is usually effective, and healing is rapid. See also **fracture.**

grenade-thrower's fracture   A fracture of the humerus caused by violent muscular contraction.

Grey Turner's sign   Bruising of the skin of the loin in acute hemorrhagic pancreatitis. Also called **Turner's sign.**

grief   A nearly universal pattern of physical and emotional responses to bereavement, separation, or loss. The physical components are similar to those of fear, hunger, rage, and pain. Stimulation of the sympathetic portion of the autonomic nervous system causes increased heart and respiratory rates, dilatation of the pupils, sweating, bristling of the hair, increased flow of blood to the muscles, and increased reserves of energy. Digestion is slowed. The emotional components proceed in stages from alarm to disbelief and denial, to anger and guilt, to developing awareness and, finally, to adjustment to the loss or restitution.

grief reaction   A complex of somatic and psychological symptoms associated with some extreme sorrow or loss, especially the death of a loved one. Somatic symptoms include feelings of tightness in the throat and chest with choking and shortness of breath, abdominal distress, lack of muscular power, and extreme tiredness and lethargy. Psychological reactions involve a generalized awareness of mental anguish and discomfort accompanied by feelings of guilt, anger, hostility, extreme restlessness, inability to concentrate, and the lack of capacity to initiate and maintain organized patterns of activities. Such symptoms may appear immediately following a crisis or they may be delayed, exaggerated, or apparently absent. Appropriate adaptive behavior and normal responses, as sobbing or talking about the dead person or tragedy, are methods of working through the acute grief and lead to successful resolution of the crisis. Most acute grief reactions are resolved within 4 to 6 weeks, although the period varies. Intervention by healthcare professionals is necessary when individuals exhibit maladaptive behavioral patterns that avoid the resolution of grief and can lead to morbid reactions, including such accepted psychosomatic illnesses as asthma and ulcers. Also called grief process. See also **death, parental grief.**

grievance   A complaint voiced to persons in authority with the expectation that it will be acted upon appropriately.

grieving, anticipatory   A nursing diagnosis accepted by the Fifth National Conference on the Classification of Nursing Diagnoses. The defining characteristics of the problem include the potential loss of something or someone important, expressions of distress, denial of potential loss, anger, guilt or sorrow, and changes in eating habits, sleep patterns, activity level,

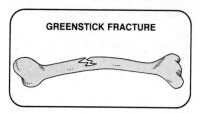

GREENSTICK FRACTURE

libido, and patterns of communication. See also **nursing diagnosis.**

grieving, dysfunctional   A nursing diagnosis accepted by the Fifth National Conference on the Classification of Nursing Diagnoses. The etiology of the problem is an actual or perceived loss of someone or something of great importance. The defining characteristics of the problem include expressions of distress or a denial of the loss; grief, anger, sadness, and weeping; changes in patterns and habits of sleeping, eating, and dreaming; and alterations in libido and activity levels. The lost person or object is idealized, past experience is relived, and concentration and purposeful work are diminished.

griffe des orteils   See **pes cavus.**

grinder's asthma   A condition characterized by asthmatic symptoms caused by inhalation of fine particles produced by industrial grinding processes. Also called grinder's disease. See also **pneumoconiosis.**

grippe   See **influenza.**

griseofulvin   An antifungal agent.

groin   Each of two areas where the abdomen joins the thighs.

Grönblad-Strandberg syndrome   An autosomal recessive disorder of connective tissue characterized by premature aging, skin breakdown, gray or brown retinal streaks, and hemorrhagic arterial degeneration, including retinal bleeding that causes loss of vision. Angina pectoris and hypertension are common; weak pulse, episodic claudication, and fatigue with exertion may affect the extremities. The prognosis depends upon vessel involvement, but life expectancy is shortened. Treatment is symptomatic. Also called **pseudoxanthoma elasticum.**

groove   A shallow, linear depression in various structures throughout the body, as those that form channels for nerves along the bones, those in bones for the insertion of muscles, and those between certain areas of the brain.

gross   **1.** Macroscopic, as gross anatomy, from the study of organs or parts of the body large enough to be seen with the naked eye, or gross pathology, from the study of tissue changes without magnification by a microscope. **2.** Large or obese. Compare **microscopic.**

ground itch   Pruritic macules, papules, and vesicles secondary to penetration of the skin by hookworm larvae, prevalent in tropical and subtropical climates. See also **hookworm.**

ground rules   Rules governing a particular situation that describe legitimate behavior.

ground substance   See **matrix.**

group In research: any set of items or groups of people under study. An **experimental group** is studied to determine the effect of an event, a substance, or a technique. A **control group** serves as a standard or reference for comparison with an experimental group. A control group is similar to the experimental group in number and is identical in specified characteristics, as sex, age, annual income, parity, or other factors.

group therapy The application of psychotherapeutic techniques within a small group of emotionally disturbed persons who, usually under the leadership of a psychotherapist, discuss their problems to promote individual psychological growth and favorable personality change. The procedure provides opportunities for treating a greater number of people in a shorter period of time than would be possible with individual therapy. Group therapy has been found to be particularly effective in the treatment of addictions. A kind of group therapy is **psychodrama.** See also **Gestalt therapy, psychotherapy, self-help group, transactional analysis.**

growing pains *Informal.* **1.** Rheumaticlike pains that occur in the muscles and joints of children or adolescents as a result of fatigue, emotional problems, postural defects, and other causes that are not related to growth and that may be symptoms of various disorders. **2.** Emotional and psychological problems experienced during adolescence.

growth **1.** An increase in the size of an organism or any of its parts, as measured in increments of weight, volume, or linear dimensions, that occurs as a result of hyperplasia or hypertrophy. **2.** The normal progressive anatomical, physiological, psychological, intellectual, social, and cultural development from infancy to adulthood as a result of the gradual and normal processes of accretion and assimilation. The total of the numerous changes that occur during the lifetime of an individual constitute a dynamic and complex process that involves many interrelated components, notably heredity, environment, nutrition, hygiene, and disease, all of which are subject to a variety of influences. In childhood, growth is categorized according to approximate age at which distinctive physical changes usually appear and at which specific developmental tasks are achieved. There are two periods of accelerated growth: the first 12 months, in which the infant triples in weight, grows approximately 50% of the height at birth, and undergoes rapid motor, cognitive, and social development; the second, in the months around puberty, when the child approaches adult height and secondary sexual characteristics emerge. **3.** Any abnormal localized increase of the size or number of cells, as in a tumor or neoplasm. **4.** A proliferation of cells, specifically a bacterial culture or mold. Compare **development, differentiation, maturation.**

growth failure A lack of normal physical and psychological development as a result of genetic, nutritional, pathological, or psychoso-cial factors. See also **failure to thrive, maternal deprivation syndrome.**

growth hormone (GH) A single-chain peptide secreted by the anterior pituitary gland in response to growth hormone releasing factor (GHRF) from the hypothalamus. GH promotes protein synthesis in all cells, increases fat mobilization and use of fatty acids for energy, and decreases utilization of carbohydrate. Growth effects depend on the presence of thyroid hormone, insulin, and carbohydrate. Somatomedins, proteins produced chiefly in the liver, play a vital role in GH-induced skeletal growth, but the hormone cannot cause elongation of long bones after the epiphyses close, so stature does not increase after puberty. GH accelerates the transport of specific amino acids into cells, stimulates the synthesis of messenger RNA and ribosomal RNA, influences the activity of several enzymes, increases the storage of phosphorus and potassium, and promotes a moderate retention of sodium. Somatostatin, an anterior pituitary regulating hormone produced in the hypothalamus, inhibits GH secretion. A deficiency of GH causes dwarfism; an excess results in gigantism or acromegaly. Also called **somatotropic hormone, somatotropin.** See also **acromegaly, dwarfism, gigantism, somatostatin.**

growth hormone–release-inhibiting hormone See **somatostatin.**

growth hormone–releasing factor (GHRF) Somatotropin-releasing factor released by the hypothalamus. Also called **somatoliberin.**

Grünfelder's reflex An involuntary dorsal flexion of the great toe with a fanlike spreading of the other toes, caused by continued pressure on the posterior lateral fontanel. It occurs in children with middle-ear disease.

grunting Abnormal, short, audible gruntlike breaks in exhalation that often accompany severe chest pain. The grunt occurs as the glottis briefly stops the flow of air, halting the movement of the lungs and their surrounding or supporting structures. Grunting is most often heard in pneumonia, pulmonary edema, or fractured or bruised ribs. Atelectasis in the newborn causes grunting owing to the effort required for the baby to fill the lungs.

GU *abbr* genitourinary.

guaiacol poisoning See **phenol poisoning.**

guaifenesin (formerly glyceryl guaiacolate) An expectorant.

guanethidine sulfate A sympatholytic antihypertensive with peripheral action.

guaranine See **caffeine.**

guardian ad litem In law: a person appointed by a court to prosecute or defend a suit for an infant or an incapacitated person. A guardian ad litem is sometimes appointed when a person refuses treatment though his life is in danger.

Guedel's signs A system for describing the stages and planes of anesthesia during an operative procedure. Stage I (amnesia and analgesia) begins with the administration of anesthesia and continues to the loss of consciousness. Respiration is quiet, though sometimes irregular, and reflexes are present. Stage II (delirium or excitement) begins with the loss of consciousness and includes the onset of total anesthesia. During this stage the patient may move his limbs, chatter incoherently, hold his breath, or become violent. Vomiting may occur. No avoidable stimulation is allowed at this stage. Stage III (surgical anesthesia) begins with establishment of a regular pattern of breathing and total loss of consciousness and includes the period during which signs of respiratory or cardiovascular failure first appear. This stage is divided into four planes: At plane 1, all movements cease and respiration is regular and 'automatic.' Eyelid reflexes are lost, but eyeball movements are marked. Pharyngeal reflexes disappear, but laryngeal and peritoneal reflexes are still present. Tonicity of the abdominal muscles can be judged by the tonicity of the extraocular muscles. At plane 2, the eyeballs become fixed centrally, conjunctivae lose their luster, and intercostal muscle activity diminishes. Respiration remains regular, with reduced tidal volume, and does not change in quality or rate in response to incision. Intubation no longer causes laryngospasm. At plane 3, intercostal paralysis occurs, and respiration becomes diaphragmatic. The pupils no longer react to light, and total muscle relaxation occurs. At plane 4, deep anesthesia is achieved, with the cessation of spontaneous respiration and the absence of sensation. Stage IV (premortem) signals danger. This stage is characterized by maximally dilated pupils; cold, ashen skin; extremely low blood pressure; and a feeble or absent brachial pulse. Cardiac arrest is imminent.

Guérin's fracture A fracture of the maxilla. Also called **LeFort I fracture.**

Guillain-Barré syndrome An idiopathic, peripheral polyneuritis occurring between 1 and 3 weeks after a mild fever associated with a viral infection or with immunization. Symmetrical pain and weakness affect the extremities, and paralysis may develop. The neuritis may spread, ascending to the trunk and involving the face, arms, and thoracic muscles. The course of the disease is variable; some people may have minimal symptoms while others may have symptoms severe enough to require critical nursing care, including respiratory assistance and a Circ-O-Lectric bed. The disease resolves itself completely in a few weeks or a few months. The only treatment is supportive care. Also called **acute febrile polyneuritis, acute idiopathic polyneuritis, infectious polyneuritis.**

guilty In criminal law: a court verdict finding beyond reasonable doubt that the defendant committed the crime and is responsible for the offense.

guinea worm infection See **dracunculiasis.**

gullet See **esophagus.**

gum 1. A sticky excretion from certain plants. 2. See **gingiva.**

gumboil An abscess of the gingiva and periosteum resulting from injury, infection, or dental decay. The gum is characteristically red, swollen, and tender. The abscess may rupture spontaneously or require incision. Treatment may include antibiotics and hot mouthwashes. Also called **parulis.**

gum camphor See **camphor.**

gumma, *pl.* **gummas, gummata** 1. A granuloma, characteristic of tertiary syphilis, varying from 1 mm to 1 cm in diameter. It is usually encapsulated and contains a central necrotic mass surrounded by inflammatory and fibrotic zones of tissue. Infectious organisms of the genus *Treponema* may be found in a gumma. The lesion may be localized or diffuse, occurring on the trunk, legs, and face and on various internal organs, especially the liver. A ruptured gumma results in a shallow ulcer that heals slowly. 2. A soft granulomatous lesion sometimes occurring with tuberculosis.

gunshot fracture A fracture caused by a bullet or similar missile.

Gunther's disease A rare congenital disorder of porphyrin metabolism associated with sunlight-induced skin lesions. See also **porphyria.**

gurgling rale An abnormal coarse sound heard during auscultation, especially over large cavities or over a trachea nearly filled with secretions.

gurry *Slang.* The detritus incident to physical trauma or surgery, including body fluids and secretions.

Gurvich radiation See **mitogenetic radiation.**

gustatory organ See **taste bud.**

gut 1. Intestine. 2. *Informal.* Digestive tract. 3. Suture material manufactured from the intestines of sheep.

Guthrie test A screening for phenylketonuria used to detect the abnormal presence of phenylalanine metabolites in the blood. In most states, this test is done on all infants before discharge and again at 2 weeks of age. See also **phenylketonuria.**

guttate psoriasis An acute form of psoriasis consisting of teardrop-shaped, red, scaly patches measuring 3 to 10 mm all over the body. A beta-hemolytic streptococcal pharyngitis or other upper respiratory infection may precipitate this reaction in susceptible individuals. Adequate treatment is essential to prevent a more severe form of psoriasis. Compare **pustular psoriasis.** See also **psoriasis.**

gymno- A combining form meaning 'pertaining to nakedness': *gymnocarpus, gymnocyte, gymnospore.*

gyn *abbr* 1. *Informal.* **gynecology.** 2. **gynecologist.**

gynandrous Describing a man or woman who has some physical characteristics usually attributed to the other sex, as a female pseudohermaphrodite. —**gynandry,** *n.*

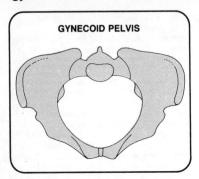

GYNECOID PELVIS

-gyne   A combining form meaning '(specified) female characteristics': *androgyne, epigyne, trichogyne.* Also **-gyn.**

gyneco-, gyn-, gyne-, gyno-   A combining form meaning 'pertaining to a woman or the female sex': *gynecoid, gynecomasia.*

gynecoid pelvis   A type of pelvis characteristic of the normal female and associated with the smallest incidence of fetopelvic disproportion. The inlet is nearly round, the sacrum is parallel to the posterior aspect of the symphysis pubis, the sidewalls are straight, and the ischial spines are blunt and do not encroach on the space in the true pelvis. It is the ideal pelvic type for childbirth.

gynecologic examination   See **pelvic examination.**

gynecologist   A physician specializing in gynecology.

gynecology   A branch of medicine concerned with the health care of women, including their sexual and reproductive function and the diseases of their reproductive organs, except breast diseases requiring surgery. Unlike most specialities in medicine, gynecology encompasses surgical and nonsurgical expertise. It is usually studied and practiced in conjunction with obstetrics. —**gynecologic, gynecological,** *adj.*

gynecomastia, gynecomasty   An abnormal enlargement of one or both breasts in men. The condition is usually temporary and benign. It may be caused by hormonal imbalance, tumor of the testis or pituitary, medication with estrogens or steroidal compounds, or failure of the liver to inactivate circulating estrogen. Less commonly, the gynecomastia may be caused by a hormone-secreting tumor of the breast, lung, or other organ. It tends to remit spontaneously, but, if marked, may be corrected surgically for cosmetic or psychologic reasons. Biopsy may be performed to rule out the presence of cancer. Malignant neoplastic gynecomastia is usually inoperable and only briefly responsive to chemotherapy.

gynephobia   An anxiety disorder characterized by a morbid fear of women. It is an obsessive, phobic phenomenon occurring almost entirely in men and may usually be traced to a frightening childhood experience. Treatment consists of psychotherapy to uncover the causative emotional conflict, followed by behavior therapy, specifically systemic desensitization and flooding to reduce anxiety.

-gynic   A combining form meaning 'relating to the human female': *hologynic, monogynic, polygynic.*

gynogamone   A gamone secreted by the female gamete.

-gynous   A combining form meaning 'pertaining to female characteristics': *androgynous.* Also **-gynic.**

-gyria   A combining form meaning '(condition of the) development of the convolutions of the cerebral cortex': *oculogyria, polymicrogyria, ulegyria.*

gyri cerebri   The convolutions of the outer surface of the cerebral hemisphere, separated from each other by sulci, most of which appear during the 6th or 7th months of fetal life.

gyrus, *pl.* **gyri**   One of the tortuous convolutions of the surface of the brain caused by infolding of the cortex. See also **gyri cerebri.**

H Chemical symbol for **hydrogen.**

habit **1.** A customary or particular practice, manner, or mode of behavior. **2.** An involuntary pattern of behavior or thought. **3.** Appearance or physique. Also called **habitus. 4.** The habitual use of drugs or narcotics.

habit spasm An involuntary twitching or tic usually involving a small muscle group of the face, neck, or shoulders and resulting in movements like spasmodic blinking or rapid jerking of the head to the side. The movements are often generated by emotional conflicts rather than being caused by any organic disorder.

habit training The process of teaching a child how to adjust to the demands of the external world by forming certain habits, primarily those related to eating, sleeping, elimination, and dress.

habitual abortion Spontaneous termination of 3 successive pregnancies before the 20th week of gestation. Habitual abortion can result from chronic infection, abnormalities of the conceptus, maternal hormonal dysfunction, or uterine abnormalities as cervical incompetence. See also **cerclage, incompetent cervix.**

habitual hyperthermia A condition of unknown cause occurring in young females, characterized by body temperatures of 37° to 38°C (99.0° to 100.5°F) regularly or intermittently for years, associated with fatigue, malaise, vague aches and pains, insomnia, bowel disturbances, and headaches. No specific treatment is recommended. Reassurance and psychotherapy offer the best relief. Also called habitual fever.

habituation **1.** An acquired tolerance from repeated exposure to a particular stimulus. **2.** A decline and eventual elimination of a conditioned response by repetition of the conditioned stimulus. Also called **negative adaptation. 3.** Psychological and emotional dependence on a drug, tobacco, or alcohol resulting from the repeated use of the substance but without the addictive, physiological need to increase dosage. Compare **addiction.**

habitus Describing a person's appearance or physique, as an athletic habitus.

Haeckel's law See **recapitulation theory.**

-haemia See **-emia.**

Haemophilus A genus of gram-negative pathogenic bacteria, frequently found in the respiratory tract of humans and some animals. *Haemophilus* species are generally sensitive to tetracyclines and sulfonamides.

Haemophilus influenzae A small, gram-negative, nonmotile, parasitic bacterium that occurs in two forms—encapsulated and nonencapsulated—and in six types—a, b, c, d, e, and f. Almost all infections are caused by encapsulated type b organisms. *Haemophilus influenzae* is found in the throats of 30% of healthy, normal people. In children and in debilitated older people, severe destructive inflammation of the larynx, trachea, and bronchi may result from infection. Subacute bacterial endocarditis and purulent meningitis may also be caused by it. Secondary infection by *H. influenzae* occurs in influenza and in many other respiratory diseases. Immunization is available by inoculation with anti-Haemophilus influenzae serum.

hafnium (Hf) A hard, brittle, silver-gray metallic element of the first transition group. Its atomic number is 72; its atomic weight is 178.49.

Hagedorn needle A flat surgical needle with a cutting edge near its point and a very large eye at the other end.

Hageman factor (HF) See **factor XII.**

hair A filament of keratin consisting of a root and a shaft formed in a specialized follicle in the epidermis. There are two stages of hair development: **anagen,** the active, growing stage, and **telogen,** the resting, or club, stage. Scalp hair grows at an average rate of 1 mm every 3 days; body and eyebrow hair, at a much slower rate. See also **hirsutism, lanugo.**

hair matrix carcinoma See **basal cell carcinoma.**

hair pulling See **trichotillomania.**

hairy-cell leukemia An uncommon neoplasm of blood-forming tissues characterized by pancytopenia, a massively enlarged spleen, and the presence in blood and bone marrow of reticulum cells with many fine projections on their surface. The disease occurs six times more frequently in men than in women, usually appears in the 5th decade with an insidious onset, and runs a variable course marked by anemia, thrombocytopenia, and spontaneous bruising. A tartrate-resistant acid phosphate isoenzyme found in hairy cells may aid in the diagnosis. Splenectomy may control the cytopenia, and some cases may improve with chemotherapy using vincristine and prednisone. Also called **leukemic reticuloendotheliosis.**

hairy tongue A dark, pigmented overgrowth of the filiform papillae of the tongue that is a benign and frequent side effect of some antibiotics. The condition gradually subsides, and no treatment is indicated.

halazepam A benzodiazepene antianxiety agent.

halcinonide A topical anti-inflammatory agent.

half-life, radioactive half-life The time required for a radioactive substance to lose 50%

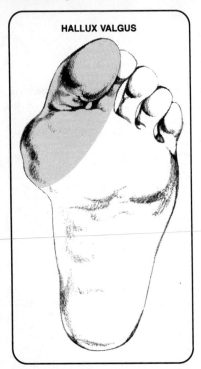

HALLUX VALGUS

of its activity through decay. Each radionuclide has a unique half-life. See also **biological half-life, effective half-life.**

half-sibling One of two or more children who have at least one parent in common; a half brother or half sister. Also called **half-sib.**

halfway house A specialized treatment facility, usually for psychiatric patients who no longer require complete hospitalization but who need some care and time to adjust to living independently.

halitosis Offensive breath resulting from poor oral hygiene; dental or oral infections; the ingestion of certain foods, as garlic or alcohol; use of tobacco; or some systemic diseases, as the odor of acetone, a sign of diabetic ketoacidosis.

Hallpike caloric test A method for evaluating the function of the vestibule of the ear in people with vertigo or hearing loss. Irrigation of the ears with cool and warm water or air mimics the stimulus of turning in the vestibular apparatus, causing nystagmus. Nystagmus can then be evaluated, and specific disorders of the vestibule may be diagnosed. See also **nystagmus.**

hallucination A sensory perception that does not result from an external stimulus. It can occur in any of the senses and is classified accordingly as auditory, gustatory, olfactory, tactile, or visual. Kinds of hallucinations are **hypnagogic hallucination, lilliputian hallucination, stump hallucination. —hallucinate,** *v.*

hallucinogen A substance that causes excitation of the central nervous system, characterized by hallucination; mood change; anxiety; sensory distortion; delusion; depersonalization; increased pulse, temperature, and blood pressure; and dilation of the pupils. Psychic dependence may occur, and depressive or suicidal psychotic states may result from the ingestion of hallucinogenic substances. Some kinds of hallucinogens are **lysergide, mescaline, peyote, phencyclidine, psilocybin.**

hallucinosis A pathological mental state in which awareness consists primarily or exclusively of hallucinations. A kind of hallucinosis is **alcoholic hallucinosis.**

hallux, *pl.* **halluces** The great toe.

hallux rigidus A painful deformity of the great toe, limiting motion at the metatarsophalangeal joint.

hallux valgus A deformity in which the great toe is angulated away from the midline of the body toward the other toes; in some cases the great toe rides over or under the other toes.

halo effect The beneficial effect of an interview or other encounter, as may occur in the course of a research project or a health-care visit. The halo effect cannot be attributed to the content of the interview or to any specific act or treatment; it is the result of indefinable interpersonal factors present in the interaction.

halogenated hydrocarbon A volatile liquid used for general anesthesia, administered in combination with nitrous oxide or oxygen, or both. Nausea, vomiting, laryngospasm, and pharyngeal irritation are less severe and frequent when this anesthesia is used.

haloperidol A butyrophenone antipsychotic agent.

haloprogin A local anti-infective agent.

halothane An inhalation anesthetic.

halo vest An orthopedic device used to help immobilize the neck and head. This device attaches to the trunk by shoulder straps and a vest. It includes an outrigger apparatus that extends from within the vest to secure pins to a band around the skull. The halo vest is used to help the healing of cervical injuries, cervical dislocations, and for postoperative positioning and immobilization following cervical surgery.

Halsted's forceps **1.** A small, pointed hemostatic forceps. Also called **mosquito forceps. 2.** A forceps with slender jaws for grasping arteries and other blood vessels.

hamamelis water See **witch hazel,** definition 2.

hamate bone A carpal bone that rests on the fourth and fifth metacarpal bones and projects a hooklike process, the hamulus, from its palmar surface. Its dorsal surface is rough for ligamentous attachment. Also called **os hamatum, unciform bone.**

Hamman-Rich syndrome Progressive interstitial pulmonary fibrosis of unknown origin, accompanied by right-sided heart disease and cor pulmonale. Anorexia, fatigue, weight loss, and vague chest pains are common symp-

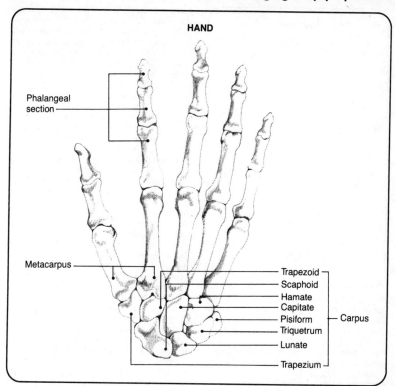

HAND

Phalangeal section

Metacarpus

Trapezoid
Scaphoid
Hamate
Capitate
Pisiform — Carpus
Triquetrum
Lunate
Trapezium

toms. Treatment includes use of corticosteroids, control of infections, and relief of specific symptoms.

hammertoe A foot digit permanently flexed at the midphalangeal joint, resulting in a clawlike appearance. The anomaly may be present in more than one digit but is most common in the second toe.

hamstring muscle Any one of three muscles at the back of the thigh: medially, the semimembranosus and the semitendinosus; laterally, the biceps femoris.

hamstring reflex A normal deep tendon reflex elicited by tapping one of the hamstring tendons behind the knee, resulting in contraction of the tendon and flexion of the knee. The patient should be lying in the supine position with the knee and hip partially flexed and the leg supported by the examiner's hand. An accentuated hamstring reflex may result from a lesion of the pyramidal system above the level of the fourth lumbar nerve root. See also **deep tendon reflex.**

hamstring tendon One of the three tendons from the three hamstring muscles in the back of the thigh. The one lateral and the two medial hamstring tendons connect the hamstring muscles to the knee.

hand The part of the upper limb distal to the forearm. It is the most flexible part of the skeleton

and has a total of 27 bones, 8 forming the carpus, 5 forming the metacarpus, and 14 comprising the phalangeal section. Also called **manus.**

handedness Voluntary or involuntary preference for use of either the left or right hand. The preference is related to cerebral dominance, with left-handedness corresponding to dominance of the right side of the brain and vice versa. Also called **chirality, laterality.**

hand-foot syndrome See **sickle cell crisis.**

handicapped Referring to a person who has a congenital or acquired mental or physical defect that interferes with normal functioning of the body system or the ability to be self-sufficient in modern society.

Hand-Schüller-Christian disease A triad of symptoms, exopthalmos, diabetes insipidus, and bone destruction, which may occur in any of several disorders. See also **eosinophilic granuloma, Letterer-Siwe disease.**

hanging drop preparation A technique used for the examination and identification of certain microorganisms, as spirochetes or trichomonads. The technique requires a special slide that has a central concavity. A specimen suspected of containing the microorganism is diluted with a sterile isotonic solution. A drop of this fluid mixture is placed on a glass cover slip, which is then inverted carefully and placed

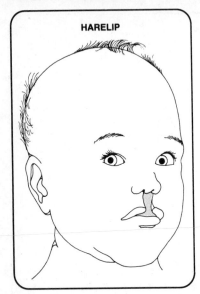

HARELIP

over the slide so that the drop is hanging from the slip into the concavity in the slide. The delicate structures and the method of movement characteristic of the species may then be viewed through the microscope.

hangman's fracture   A fracture of the posterior elements of the cervical vertebrae with dislocation of C2 or C3.

Hankow fever   See **schistosomiasis.**

Hanot's disease   See **biliary cirrhosis.**

Hansen's disease   See **leprosy.**

-haphia   See **-aphia.**

haploid   **1.** Having a single set of unpaired chromosomes, as in mature ova and sperm, or having one set of nonhomologous chromosomes. The haploid number in humans is 23. **2.** A cell or organism with only one member of each pair of homologous chromosomes.

haploidy   The state or condition of having only one complete set of nonhomologous chromosomes.

hapten, haptene   A nonproteinaceous substance that acts as an antigen by combining with particular bonding sites on an antibody. Unlike a true antigen, it does not induce the formation of antibodies. A hapten bonded to a carrier protein may induce an immune response.

haptoglobin   A plasma protein whose only known function is to bind free hemoglobin. The quantity of haptoglobin is increased in certain chronic diseases and inflammatory disorders and is decreased or absent in hemolytic anemia. Compare **transferrin.** See also **hemoglobinemia, hemoglobinuria.**

hardening of the arteries   See **arteriosclerosis.**

hard fibroma   A neoplasm composed of fibrous tissue in which there are few cells. Also called **fibroma durum.**

hard palate   The bony portion of the roof of the mouth, continuous posteriorly with the soft palate and bounded anteriorly and laterally by the alveolar arches and the gums. The palatine process of the maxilla and the horizontal portion of the palatine bone form the bony support for the hard palate, which is covered by periosteum and by the mucous membrane of the mouth. A linear raphe along its middle line ends anteriorly in a small papilla, which corresponds with the incisive canal. On each side and anterior to the raphe, the mucous membrane is thick, pale in color, and corrugated. Posteriorly, the mucous membrane is thin, smooth, and of a deeper color. The hard palate is covered with squamous epithelium and is furnished with numerous palatal glands between the mucous membrane and the underlying surface of the bone. Compare **soft palate.**

hardware   In data processing: the electronic devices and other physical components of a computer. Compare **software.**

Hardy-Weinberg equilibrium principle   The mathematical relationship between the frequency of genes and the resulting genotypes in populations. In a large interbreeding population characterized by random mating, Mendelian inheritance, and the absence of migration, mutation, and selection, the ratio of individuals homozygous for a dominant gene to those heterozygous to those homozygous for a recessive gene is 1:2:1, at which point genetic equilibrium is established. See **genetic equilibrium.**

harelip   A congenital anomaly consisting of one or more clefts in the upper lip, resulting from the failure in the embryo of the maxillary and median nasal processes to close. Treatment is surgical repair in infancy. See also **cleft palate.**

hare's eye   See **lagophthalmos.**

harlequin color   A transient flushing of the skin on the dependent side with pallor of the upward side. Commonly seen in normal young infants, it disappears as the child matures.

harlequin fetus   An infant whose skin at birth is completely covered with thick, horny scales that resemble armor and are divided by deep red fissures. The condition is the most severe form of lamellar exfoliation of the newborn, and the infant is stillborn or dies within a few days of birth. Also called **ichthyosis fetus.**

Harris tube   A tube used for gastric and intestinal decompression. It is a mercury weighted, single lumen tube that is passed through the nose and carried through the alimentary tract by gravity.

Hartmann's curet   A curet used for the removal of adenoids. See also **curet.**

Hartnup disease   A recessive genetic metabolic disorder characterized by pellagralike skin lesions, transient cerebellar ataxia, and hyperaminoaciduria, caused by defects in intestinal absorption and renal reabsorption of neutral amino acids. Bacterial degradation of unabsorbed amino acids in the gut leads to the absorption of breakdown products and their appearance in urine; the unavailability of tryptophan leads to a deficiency of niacin, the antipellagra vitamin. Common symptoms of the disease are dry, scaly, well-circumscribed skin lesions, glossitis, stomatitis, diarrhea, psychiatric problems, and pronounced photosensitivity; brief exposure to the sun may cause erythema, edema, and vesiculation. Treatment consists of oral nicotinamide and a diet containing proteins composed of more easily absorbed small peptides.

Harvard pump A small pump that can be adjusted to deliver small amounts of medication in solution through an intravenous infusion set. Compare **Abbot pump.**

harvest fever See **field fever.**

harvest mite See **chigger.**

Hashimoto's disease An autoimmune thyroid disorder, characterized by the production of antibodies in response to thyroid antigens and the replacement of normal thyroid structures with lymphocytes and lymphoid germinal centers. The thyroid, typically enlarged, pale yellow, and lumpy on the surface, shows dense lymphocytic infiltration, and the remaining thyroid tissue frequently contains small empty follicles. The goiter is usually asymptomatic, but occasionally patients complain of dysphagia and a feeling of local pressure. The thymus is usually enlarged, and regional lymph nodes often show hyperplasia. A definitive diagnosis can be made if a fluorescent scan shows a decrease or absence of thyroid-stable iodine and if a hemagglutination test for thyroid antigens is positive. Replacement therapy with thyroid hormone is indicated for patients with thyroid deficiency and can prevent further enlargement of the goiter. Also called **Hashimoto's struma, Hashimoto's thyroiditis, lymphadenoid goiter, lymphocytic thyroiditis, struma lymphomatosa.**

Hashimoto's struma See **Hashimoto's disease.**

Hashimoto's thyroiditis See **Hashimoto's disease.**

hashish See **cannabis.**

Haverhill fever A febrile disease, caused by infection with *Streptobacillus moniliformis*, transmitted by the bite of a rat. Characteristically, the wound from the bite heals, but within 10 days, fever, chills, vomiting, headache, muscle and joint pain, and a rash appear. Treatment with antibiotics is effective. *S. moniliformis* is identified by laboratory analysis using fluorescent antibody screening. Also called **streptobacillary rat-bite fever.**

Haversian canal One of the many tiny longitudinal canals in bone tissue, averaging about 0.05 mm in diameter. Each contains blood vessels, connective tissue, nerve filaments, and, occasionally, lymphatic vessels. The canals are interconnected and part of an intricate network. See also **Volkmann's canal.**

Haversian canaliculus Any one of the many tiny passages radiating from the lacunae of bone tissue to larger Haversian canals.

Haversian system A circular district of bone tissue, consisting of lamellae in the bone around a central canal. See also **Volkmann's canal.**

Hawthorne effect A general, unintentional, but usually beneficial effect on a person, a group of people, or the function of the system being studied. The Hawthorne effect is the effect of an encounter, as with an investigator or healthcare provider, or of a change in a program or facility, as by painting an office or changing the lighting system. The Hawthorne effect is likely to confound the results of a study or investigation, as it is usually present and difficult to identify.

hay fever *Informal.* An acute, seasonal **allergic rhinitis** stimulated by tree, grass, or weed pollens.

hazard A condition or phenomenon that increases the probability of a loss arising from some danger that may result in injury or illness. —**hazardous,** *adj.*

Hb A *abbr* **hemoglobin A.**

Hb C *abbr* **hemoglobin C.**

Hb F *abbr* **hemoglobin F.**

HBIG *abbr* **hepatitis B immune globulin.**

Hb S *abbr* **hemoglobin S.**

HBsAG *abbr* **hepatitis B surface antigen.** See **Australia antigen.**

Hb S-C *abbr* **hemoglobin S-C.**

HCG *abbr* human chorionic gonadotropin. See **chorionic gonadotropin.**

He Symbol for **helium.**

headache A pain in the head from any cause. Also called **cephalalgia.** Kinds of headaches include **functional headache, migraine, organic headache, sinus headache, tension headache.**

head and neck cancer Any malignant neoplasms of the upper aerodigestive tract, facial features, and structures in the neck, presenting as masses, ulcerations, or flat lesions that usually produce early symptoms. Tumors of the oral cavity, lips, and tongue characteristically begin as a swelling or nonhealing ulcer and are most commonly epidermoid carcinomas that occur in men over age 60; predisposing factors are chronic alcoholism, heavy use of tobacco, poor oral hygiene, syphilis, and Plummer-Vinson syndrome. Nasal and paranasal sinus malignancies, most often epidermoid cancers, cause a bloody discharge, obstruction in breathing, and facial and dental pain. Nasopharyngeal tumors, predominantly squamous cell and undifferentiated carcinomas occurring most frequently in Orientals, are associated with nasal obstruction, serous otitis media, hearing loss, lymphadenopathy, and cranial nerve involvement. Oropharyngeal and tonsillar neoplasms, usually squamous cell carcinomas and less frequently lymphomas, produce dysphagia, pain, dyspnea, and trismus. Most hypopharyngeal and laryngeal tumors are carcinomas that cause hoarseness, dysphagia, dyspnea, coughing, and cervical adenopathy. Salivary gland carcinomas occur most frequently in the parotid gland and may cause facial palsy. Cancer of the mandible, including extremely painful osteosarcoma and, in many patients, painless giant cell tumor, Ewing's sarcoma, and ameloblastoma, may erode through the gingiva, producing an intraoral ulcer, and may cause pathologic fractures. Ear neoplasms involve the auricle in most cases, usually occur in persons over age 50, and are most commonly squamous cell carcinomas that cause pain, deafness, and facial nerve paralysis. Cancers of the lacrimal glands, lacrimal sacs, and parathyroid glands are rare, but hypercalcemia, hypercalcinuria, kidney stones, and renal and bone diseases are associated with parathyroid carcinoma. Tumors of the eye, as malignant melanoma in patients over age 50 and retinoblastoma in children, are also rare. Head and neck tumors are diagnosed by clinical examination, X-rays, tomograms, biopsies, arteriograms, supravital staining of lesions, and cytologic studies. Surgery and radiotherapy are the primary treatment modalities, but their use may cause problems with swallowing and speaking; the effectiveness of chemotherapy is limited by the poor nutritional status of many patients with head or neck lesions. Plastic surgery and various prostheses are often essential in correcting deformities and restoring functions in patients who have undergone the excision or radiotherapy of a head or neck tumor. See also specific cancer.

head, eyes, ears, nose, and throat (HEENT) A specialty in medicine concerned with the anatomy, physiology, and pathology of the head, the eyes, ears, nose, and throat and with the diagnosis and treatment of disorders of those structures.

head injury Any traumatic damage to the head resulting from penetration of the skull or from too rapid inertial acceleration or deceleration of the brain within the skull. See also **concussion.**

head kidney See **pronephros.**

head nurse The clinical and administrative leader of the nurses working in a given geographical division of an institution, usually a floor, ward, or unit. The responsibilities of a head nurse may include directing nursing care activities, scheduling of staff, evaluation of nursing personnel, and hiring, firing, or promoting staff nurses. The head nurse may also be responsible for budget preparation and general clinical leadership.

head process A strand of cells that extends forward from the primitive node in the early stages of embryonic development in vertebrates. It is the precursor of the notochord and forms the primitive axis around which the embryo develops. Also called **notochordal plate.**

Heaf test A tuberculin skin test using a multiple puncture technique. See also **tuberculin test.**

healer 1. A person who cures. 2. A Christian Science practitioner. 3. A person who claims to cure by suggestion.

healing The act or process in which the normal structural and functional characteristics of health are restored to diseased, dysfunctional, or damaged tissues, organs, or systems of the body.

health A condition of physical, mental, and social well-being and the absence of disease or other abnormal condition. It is not a static condition; constant change and adaptation to stress result in homeostasis. See also **high-level wellness, homeostasis.**

health assessment An evaluation of the health status of an individual by performing a physical examination after obtaining a health history. Various laboratory tests may also be ordered to confirm a clinical impression or to screen for dysfunction. A significant part of the health assessment is counseling and education that may explain aspects of anatomy, physiology, and pathophysiology and that introduces or affirms the general tenets of a healthful way of life. The techniques of the health assessment include: palpation, percussion, auscultation, and inspection, including sight, sound, and smell.

health behavior An action taken by a person to maintain, attain, or regain good health and to prevent illness. Some common health behaviors are exercising regularly, eating a balanced diet, and obtaining necessary inoculations.

health belief model A conceptual framework that describes a person's health behavior as an expression of his health beliefs. The model was designed to predict a person's health behavior, including the use of health services, and to justify intervention to alter maladaptive health behavior.

health-care consumer Any actual or potential recipient of health care, as a patient in a hospital, a client in a community mental health center, or a member of a prepaid health maintenance organization.

health-care industry The complex of preventive, remedial, and therapeutic services provided by hospitals and other institutions, nurses, doctors, dentists, government agencies, voluntary agencies, noninstitutional care facilities, pharmaceutical and medical equipment manufacturers, and health insurance companies.

health certificate A statement signed by a health-care provider that attests to the state of a person's health.

health education An educational program directed to the general public that attempts to improve, maintain, and safeguard the health of the community.

health history In nursing and medicine: a collection of information obtained from the client and from other sources concerning the person's physical status and psychological, social, and sexual functions. The history provides a data base upon which a plan for management of the diagnosis, treatment, care, and follow-up of the person may be made. The first part of the history describes the present illness (PI), including its signs and symptoms, onset and character, and any factors or behaviors that aggravate or ameliorate the symptoms. The patient's own words

CROSS SECTION OF THE HEART

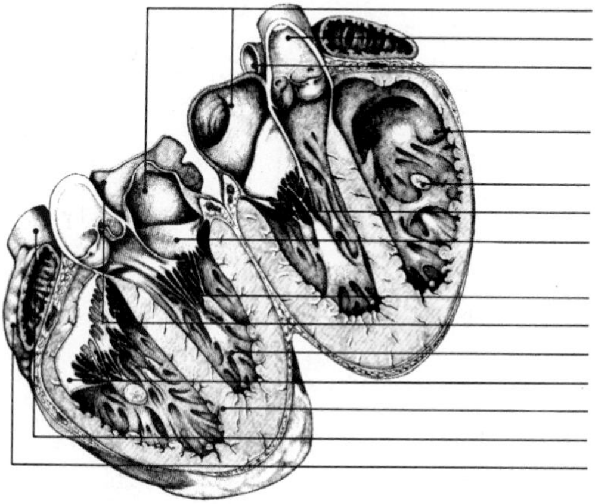

- Left atrium
- Ascending aorta
- Pulmonary trunk
- Right ventricle
- Papillary muscles
- Chordae tendineae
- Mitral valve
- Left ventricle
- Pulmonary vein
- Papillary muscles
- Tricuspid valve
- Interventricular septum
- Superior vena cava
- Right atrium

often serve as the best description and may be quoted. The second part of the history comprises an account of previous illnesses, conditions, allergies, transfusions, immunizations, screening tests, and hospitalizations. An occupational history, describing the person's work and exposure to stress, toxins, radiation, or other occupational hazards, may be included. The effect of the current illness on the person's work is also noted. A social history is taken in which the person's social, cultural, and familial milieux are outlined, focusing on aspects that might have an effect on the current illness. In some instances, a sexual history may be relevant. A review of systems may follow or may be incorporated into the health history. Kinds of history include **complete health history, episodic health history, interval health history.** Also called **medical history.** See also **occupational history, review of systems, sexual history.**

health maintenance   A program or procedure planned to prevent illness, to maintain maximal function, and to promote health. It is central to health care.

Health Maintenance Organization (HMO)   A type of group health-care practice that provides basic and supplemental health maintenance and treatment services to voluntary enrollees who prepay a fixed periodic fee that is set without regard to the amount or kind of services received.

health physics   The study of the effects of ionizing radiation on the body and the methods for protecting people from the undesirable effects of the radiation.

health policy   **1.** A statement of a decision regarding a goal in health care and a plan for achieving that goal, as, in order to prevent an epidemic, a program for inoculating a population is developed and implemented. **2.** A field of study and practice in which the priorities and values underlying health resource allocations are determined.

health professional   Any person who has completed a course of study in a field of health, as a registered nurse. The person is usually licensed by a governmental agency or certified by a professional organization.

health provider   Any individual who provides health services to health-care consumers.

health screening   A program designed to evaluate the health status and potential of an individual person. In the process of evaluation, it may be found that a person has a particular disease or condition or is at greater than normal risk of developing a particular disease or condition.

health supervision   In public health nursing: a visit made to a patient in his home for the purpose of health teaching, counseling, or monitoring the status of the patient's health, rather than for physical care. Compare **care-of-the-sick.**

health systems agency (HSA)   An agency established under the terms of the National Health Planning and Resources Development Act of 1974. Health planning agencies are intended to provide networks of health planning and resource development services in each of several health service areas established by the Act. Health systems agencies are nonprofit and include private organizations, public regional planning bodies, or local governmental agencies and consumers.

hearing aid   A device used to increase the intensity of sound. The most common types available include behind-the-ear aids, eye glass aids, body hearing aids, and in-the-ear aids.

heart   The muscular, cone-shaped organ, about the size of a clenched fist, that pumps blood throughout the body and beats normally about

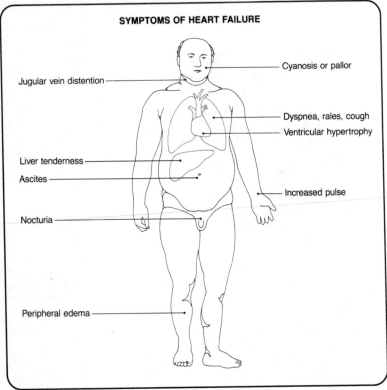

SYMPTOMS OF HEART FAILURE

Jugular vein distention

Cyanosis or pallor

Dyspnea, rales, cough

Ventricular hypertrophy

Liver tenderness

Ascites

Increased pulse

Nocturia

Peripheral edema

70 times per minute by coordinated impulses from the sinoatrial node and muscular contractions. Enclosed in pericardium, the heart rests on the diaphragm between the lower borders of the lungs, occupying the middle of the mediastinum. It is covered ventrally by the sternum and the adjoining parts of the third to the sixth costal cartilages. The organ is about 12 cm (4¾ inches) long, 8 cm (3⅛ inches) wide at its broadest part, and 6 cm (2⅜ inches) thick. The weight of the heart in men averages between 280 and 340 g (17 and 20¾ oz), and in women, between 230 and 280 g (14 and 17 oz). The layers of the heart, starting from the outside, are the epicardium, the myocardium, and the endocardium. The epicardium includes the visceral pericardium and a layer of fibroelastic connective tissue interspersed with fat. The myocardium is composed of layers and bundles of cardiac muscle laced by blood vessels. The endocardium is continuous with the endothelial lining of the blood vessels and is composed of squamous endothelium. The chambers of the heart include two ventricles with thick muscular walls, making up the bulk of the organ, and two atria with thin muscular walls. A septum separates the ventricles and extends between the atria, dividing the heart into the right and the left sides. The left side of the heart pumps oxygenated blood

from the pulmonary veins into the aorta and on to all parts of the body. The right side of the heart pumps deoxygenated blood, received through the venae cavae, into the pulmonary arteries. The sinoatrial node in the right atrium of the heart initiates the cardiac impulse, causing the atria to contract. The atrioventricular node in the septal wall of the right atrium spreads the impulse over the bundle of His, causing the ventricles to contract. The valves of the heart include the tricuspid valve between the right atrium and the right ventricle, the mitral valve between the left atrium and the left ventricle, the aortic valve at the exit of the left ventricle, and the pulmonary valve at the exit of the right ventricle.

heartburn A painful burning sensation in the esophagus just below the sternum. Heartburn is usually caused by the reflux of gastric contents into the esophagus but may be caused by gastric hyperacidity or peptic ulcer. Antacids relieve the symptoms but do not cure the heartburn. Also called **pyrosis.** See also **hiatus hernia.**

heart failure A condition in which the heart cannot pump enough blood in relation to the venous return and the metabolic requirements of body tissues. Extreme exertion may cause heart failure in individuals with normal hearts if there is a discrepancy between the needs of the body and the volume of blood pumped by the heart. Heart failure may be generally classified as cardiac mechanical failure, myocardial failure, and arrhythmic failure. Most forms of heart failure are caused by atrial failure or by ventricular failure, and many patients develop heart failure from more than one cause. Many of the symptoms associated with heart failure are caused by the dysfunction of organs other than the heart, especially the lungs, kidneys, and liver. Ventricular dysfunction is usually the basic disorder in congestive heart failure and often triggers compensatory mechanisms that preserve cardiac output but produce symptoms and signs, as dyspnea, orthopnea, rales, and edema. Heart failure is closely associated with many forms of heart disease and is commonly diagnosed only after the diagnosis of heart disease. Most kinds of heart disease initially affect the left side of the heart, and clinicians commonly divide associated heart failure into left-heart failure and right-heart failure. Peripheral edema occurs in connection with right-heart failure and dyspnea in connection with left-heart failure. The adjustments of the body to heart failure are divided into the acute adjustments, the subacute adjustments, and the chronic adjustments, depending on how long the adjustment takes. The acute adjustments involve numerous complex mechanisms, the most important of which increase autonomic sympathetic excitation to the heart and most of the arteries and veins. The stimulation of the peripheral arteries helps to maintain arterial pressure. The stimulation of the veins helps to increase venous tone and venous pressure. The increased venous pressure aids venous return, ventricular filling, and the diastolic stretching of the ventricular fibers. The subacute adjustments of the body to heart failure mainly involve those mechanisms that cause the kidneys to retain salt and water, resulting in increased blood volume. The localization of edema produced by the excess fluid and salt depends on various hydrostatic factors, as the position of the patient. The main chronic adjustment of the body to heart failure is hypertrophy of the ventricular myocardium, apparently owing to a chronic increase in the tension of the myocardial fibers. Current studies indicate that heart failure in infants and children usually results from congenital heart disease but may also result from myocarditis and ectopic tachycardia. The most frequent cause of congestive heart failure between birth and 1 week of age is aortic atresia. Between the ages of 1 week and 1 month, the most common causes are coarctation of the aorta and transposition of the great vessels, followed in order of causative frequency by endomyocardial disease, ventricular septal defect, and patent ductus arteriosis. Between the ages of 3 and 6 months, endomyocardial disease is the most common cause of cardiac failure, followed in frequency by ventricular septal defect, patent ductus arteriosus, total anomalous pulmonary venous return, coarctation of the

aorta, and transposition of the great vessels. From birth to 6 months of age, paroxysmal atrial tachycardia may cause acute catastrophic heart failure without other evidence of heart disease. The most common causes of heart failure between ages 5 and 15 are acute rheumatic myocarditis, acute glomerulonephritis, and congenital heart disease, especially ventricular septal defect, atrial septal defect, and patent ductus arteriosus. Heart failure during early life is rarely caused by secundum-type atrial septal defect, congenital valve disease, or acquired valve disease. Rheumatic mitral disease and aortic valve disease frequently cause congestive heart failure in young adults. Mitral valve disease, especially mitral stenosis, is the most common cause of heart failure and affects more young women than men. Other heart diseases that may affect young adults are nonrheumatic myocardial disease and congenital heart disease. The common causes of heart failure after the age of 40 are coronary atherosclerosis with myocardial infarction, diastolic hypertension in which the pressure is usually above 110 mmHg, valvular heart disease, pulmonary disease, and diffuse myocardial disease. Some individuals may suffer heart failure caused by a combination of congenital heart disease and acquired disease. After the age of 50, a common cause of heart failure, especially in men, is calcific aortic stenosis. Some of the behavioral and environmental factors that may cause heart failure in asymptomatic patients with heart disease are sudden extraordinary effort, increased work load, excessive dietary intake of sodium, sudden emotional upset, and the administration of excessive volumes of intravenous fluids. Some signs of heart failure based on physical examination may be divided into those signs caused by the effects of cardiac failure on other organs and those signs of cardiac failure that are associated with the heart, the arteries, and the veins. Some of the extracardiac signs are ascites, bronchial wheezing, hydrothorax, edema, enlargement of the liver, moist rales, and splenomegaly. Some of the cardiac signs associated with heart failure are abnormalities in the jugular venous pulsation and the carotid pulse, and abnormal cardiographic tracings of the apex wave. The treatment for heart failure commonly involves the reduction of the work load of the heart; the administration of certain drugs, as digitalis, to increase myocardial contractility and cardiac output; salt-free diets; diuretics; and surgical intervention. Many patients with heart failure, especially elderly patients, become constipated and require laxatives, as mineral oil, milk of magnesia, and cascara sagrada. In acute heart failure, a complex autonomic response and local regulatory mechanisms redistribute the available blood flow, and body tissues receiving less blood than required may use anaerobic metabolism or withdraw more oxygen from each unit of available blood. The sudden onset of acute pulmonary edema associated with some cases of heart failure is a life-threatening condition requiring im-

HEART MURMURS

CONDITION	TIMING	QUALITY	PITCH	LOCATION	RADIATION
Pulmonic stenosis	Midsystolic (systolic ejection)	Harsh, rough	Medium to high	Pulmonic	Toward left shoulder and neck
Aortic stenosis	Midsystolic (systolic ejection)	Harsh, rough	Medium to high	Aortic and suprasternal notch	Toward carotid arteries or apex
Ventricular septal defect	Holosystolic	Harsh	High	Tricuspid	Precordium
Mitral insufficiency	Holosystolic	Blowing	High	Mitral, lower left sternal border	Toward left axilla
Tricuspid insufficiency	Holosystolic	Blowing	High	Tricuspid	Toward apex
Aortic insufficiency	Early diastolic	Blowing	High	Midleft sternal edge (not aortic area)	Toward sternum
Pulmonic insufficiency	Early diastolic	Blowing	High	Pulmonic	Toward sternum
Mitral stenosis	Mid- to late diastolic	Rumbling	Low	Apex	Usually none
Tricuspid stenosis	Mid- to late diastolic	Rumbling	Low	Tricuspid, lower sternal border	Usually none

mediate treatment. Acute pulmonary edema may develop in patients with chronic heart failure owing to atherosclerosis and old infarcts or in patients with normal hearts who develop ectopic tachycardia or pulmonary embolism. Acute pulmonary edema may sometimes be confused with bronchial asthma, and caution is required when giving appropriate drugs. Aminophylline and oxygen are used in therapy for pulmonary edema and acute asthma.

heart-lung machine An apparatus consisting of a pump and an oxygenator that takes over the functions of the heart and lungs, especially during cardiac surgery. The blood is shunted from the venous system through an oxygenator and returned to the arterial circulation.

heart massage See **cardiac massage.**

heart murmur An abnormal sound heard during auscultory examination of the heart, caused by the flow of blood into a chamber or through a valve or by a valve opening or closing. A murmur is classified by the time of its occurrence during the cardiac cycle, the duration, and the intensity of the sound on a scale of I to V. In general, many systolic murmurs are benign and of no significance, but some signal cardiac pathophysiology. Most diastolic murmurs are pathologic.

heart rate The pulse, calculated by counting the number of contractions of the cardiac ventricles per unit of time. Tachycardia is a heart rate of more than 100 beats per minute; bradycardia is a heart rate of fewer than 60 beats per minute. See also **pulse.**

heart sound A noise produced within the heart during the cardiac cycle that can be heard over the precordium and may reveal abnormalities in cardiac structure or function. Cardiac auscultation is performed systematically from apex to base of the heart or from base to apex, using a stethoscope to listen initially with the diaphragm and then with the bell of the instrument. The first heart sound (S_1), a dull, prolonged 'lub,' occurs with the closure of the mitral and tricuspid valves and marks the onset of ventricular systole; the mitral valve sound is loudest at the apex of the heart and that of the tricuspid valve at the left fourth intercostal space. The second heart sound (S_2), a short, sharp 'dup,' occurs with the closing of the aortic and pulmonic valves at the beginning of ventricular diastole; the aortic valve closure is loudest on the right side and that of the pulmonic valve is most distinct on the left side over the second intercostal space. A weak, low-pitched, dull, third heart sound (S_3) is sometimes heard and is thought to be caused by vibrations of the walls of the ventricles when they are suddenly distended by blood from the atria. S_3, which is heard most clearly at the apex of the heart, is called a ventricular or diastolic gallop; it may be normal in children, adolescents, or very thin adults, or it may be a sign of congestive heart failure or hypertension causing left ventricular failure. A fourth heart sound (S_4), which may be heard with a stethoscope's bell at the apex of the heart during expiration, is caused by vibrations of the atria following contraction. Called an atrial or presystolic gallop, S_4 is usually a sign of pathology, as myocardial infarction or impending heart failure from another cause. Asynchronous closure of cardiac valves may result in split heart sounds. An S_1 split occurs in right bundle branch block, mitral stenosis, and tricuspid valve dysfunction associated with pulmonary hypertension. S_2 splits may occur in normal inspiration but may also indicate septal defects, pulmonic stenosis, or other mechanical problems. Brief, periodic endocardial murmurs may indicate various disorders. A murmur characteristic of incompetency of the mitral orifice is loudest at the cardiac apex; a murmur characteristic of tricuspid incompetency is loudest at the ensiform cartilage; and a murmur typical of obstruction of the pulmonic orifice is loudest at the left second intercostal space near the sternum. Systolic and diastolic murmurs that are loudest at the junction of the right second costal cartilage and the sternum indicate problems in the aortic orifice, and a presystolic murmur over the body of the heart may be the result of mitral orifice obstruction. A phonocardiogram recorded simultaneously with the electrocardiogram shows the relationships between heart sounds and electrical events. S_1 begins midway in the QRS complex; during this interval the mitral and the tricuspid valves close, the pulmonic and the aortic valves open, and ejection of blood from the right ventricle begins. Left ventricular ejection occurs between S_1 and S_2, which begins immediately after the T wave and is signaled by closure of the aortic valve, followed by closure of the pulmonic valve and opening of the tricuspid and the mitral valves. S_3 occurs between the T wave and the P wave on the EKG at the end of the rapid-filling phase of the ventricules, and S_4 begins at the peak of the P wave during vibrations of the atria.

heart surgery   Any surgical procedure involving the heart, performed to correct acquired or congenital defects, to replace diseased valves, to open or bypass blocked vessels, or to graft a prosthesis or a transplant in place. Two major types of heart surgery are performed, closed and open. The closed technique is done through a small incision, without using the heart-lung machine. In the open technique, the heart chambers are open and fully visible, and blood is detoured around the surgical field by the heart-lung machine. Preoperative care focuses on the correction of metabolic imbalances and cardiac and pulmonary ailments and on diagnostic and laboratory tests. General anesthesia is used, the chest cavity is opened, and the heart-lung machine is connected. Hypothermia may also be used to reduce the metabolic rate and the need of the tissues for oxygen. The heart is opened and the defect is corrected. Postoperatively, constant observation is required in an intensive care unit for signs of hemorrhage, shock, fibrillation, arrhythmia, sudden chest pain, and pulmonary edema. The blood pressure, all pulses, respirations, and venous and pulmonary artery pressures are monitored. If the blood pressure is high enough to assure cerebral profusion, the head of the patient's bed is lifted to a semi-Fowler's position to encourage chest drainage and lung expansion. Oxygen is given via the endotracheal tube for 18 to 24 hours. The chest tube is cleared hourly to dislodge clots, urinary output and temperature are noted hourly, and intravenous infusions and blood transfusions are often given. Treatment also includes the use of narcotics and antibiotics. The mortality rate is highest during the first 48 hours following surgery. Kinds of heart surgery include **Blalock-Taussig procedure, coronary bypass, endarterectomy, mitral commissurotomy.** See also **arrhythmia, fibrillation, heart-lung machine, hypothermia, pulmonary edema.**

heart valve   One of the four structures within the heart that control the flow of blood by opening and closing with each heartbeat. The valves include two semilunar valves, the mitral valve, and the tricuspid valve. The valves permit the flow of blood in only one direction, and any one of the valves may become defective permitting the backflow associated with heart murmurs. Also called **cardiac valve.** See also **heart.**

heat cramp   Any cramp in the arm, leg, or abdomen caused by depletion in the body of both water and salt owing to heat exhaustion. It usually occurs after vigorous physical exertion in an extremely hot environment or under other conditions that cause profuse sweating and depletion of body fluids and electrolytes. Also called **cane-cutter's cramp, fireman's cramp, miner's cramp, stoker's cramp.** See also **heat exhaustion.**

heated nebulization   A method of inhalation therapy using a heating device with a nebulizer that produces a spray with a higher water content than that of a cold atomizer. The mist may be administered through a mask or in a tent.

heat exhaustion   An abnormal condition characterized by weakness, vertigo, nausea, muscle cramps, and loss of consciousness, caused by depletion of body fluid and electrolytes resulting from exposure to intense heat or the inability to acclimatize to heat. Body temperature is near normal; blood pressure may drop but usually returns to normal as the person is placed in a recumbent position; and the skin is cool, damp, and pale. The person usually recovers with rest and replacement of water and electrolytes. Compare **heat hyperpyrexia.** See also **heat cramp.**

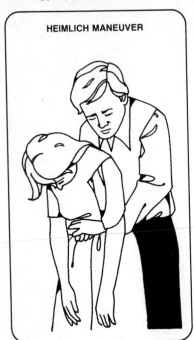

HEIMLICH MANEUVER

heat hyperpyrexia A severe and sometimes fatal condition resulting from the failure of the temperature-regulating capacity of the body, caused by prolonged exposure to the sun or to high temperatures. Reduction or cessation of sweating is an early symptom. Body temperature of 40.5°C (105°F) or higher, tachycardia, hot and dry skin, headache, confusion, unconsciousness, and convulsions may occur. Treatment includes cooling, sedation, and fluid replacement. Also called heatstroke, siriasis, sunstroke. See also **hyperpyrexia.** Compare **heat exhaustion.**

heat labile See **thermolabile.**

heat rash A finely papular or vesicular inflammation of the skin resulting from prolonged exposure to heat and high humidity. Tingling and prickling sensations are common. Prevention and treatment include cool, dry temperatures; ventilation; and absorbent powders. See also **miliaria.**

heaves 1. A chronic respiratory disease of horses, similar to human pulmonary emphysema, characterized by wheezing, coughing, and dyspnea on exertion. The causes of the condition are unknown. 2. *Informal.* Vomiting and retching.

heavy metal A metallic element with a specific gravity five or more times that of water. The heavy metals are cadmium, cerium, chromium, cobalt, copper, gallium, gold, iron, lead, manganese, mercury, nickel, platinum, silver, tellurium, thallium, tin, uranium, vanadium, and zinc. Small amounts of many of these ele-

ments are common and necessary in the diet. Large amounts of any of them may cause poisoning.

heavy metal antagonist A substance that neutralizes or reverses toxic effects of heavy metals by preventing or reversing formation of insoluble metal complexes with organic compounds in the body.

heavy metal poisoning Poisoning caused by the ingestion, inhalation, or absorption of various toxic heavy metals. Kinds of heavy metal poisoning include **antimony poisoning, arsenic poisoning, cadmium poisoning, lead poisoning, mercury poisoning.**

hebephrenia See **disorganized schizophrenia.**

hebephrenic schizophrenia See **disorganized schizophrenia.**

Heberden node An abnormal cartilaginous or bony enlargement of a distal interphalangeal joint of a finger, usually occurring in degenerative diseases of the joints. Compare **Bouchard's node.**

hebetude A state of dullness or lethargy, characteristic of some forms of schizophrenia.

heboid paranoia See **paranoid schizophrenia.**

-hedonia A combining form meaning '(condition of) pleasure, cheerfulness': *anhedonia, hyphedonia, parhedonia.*

-hedron A combining form meaning a 'geometrical figure with (specified) sides': *decahedron, octahedron, polyhedron.*

heel The posterior part of the foot, formed by the largest tarsal bone, the calcaneus.

HEENT *abbr* **head, eyes, ears, nose, and throat.**

Hegar's sign A softening of the isthmus of the uterine cervix early in gestation. It is a probable sign of pregnancy.

height The vertical measurement of a structure, organ, or other object from bottom to top, when it is placed or projected in an upright position.

Heimlich maneuver An emergency procedure for dislodging a bolus of food or other obstruction from the trachea to prevent asphyxiation. The choking person is grasped from behind by the rescuer whose fist is placed thumb side in just below the victim's sternum, with the other hand placed firmly over the fist. The rescuer then pulls his fist firmly and abruptly into the epigastrium forcing the obstruction up the trachea. This procedure can also be done with the unconscious victim in a recumbent position and the rescuer straddling the person's hips. The rescuer positions both hands on the abdomen, above the navel and below the xiphoid process, and presses upward and inward with four quick thrusts.

helium (He) A colorless, odorless, gaseous element; the second lightest element after hydrogen. Its atomic number is 2; its atomic weight is 4. Helium is one of the rare or inert gases and does not usually combine with other elements. Its main physiological and medical uses are in

BASIC FACTS ABOUT COMMON HELMINTH INFECTIONS

CONDITION	CAUSE	SOURCE OF INFECTION
Tapeworm infection	Tapeworm *(Hymenolepis nana, Taenia saginata, Taenia solium, Diphyllobothrium latum)*	Poorly cooked or infected beef, pork, or fish
Enterobiasis	Pinworm *(Enterobius vermicularis)*	Eggs from contaminated objects (books, clothes, toys, wooden objects)
Hookworm infection	Hookworm *(Necator americanus, Ancylostoma duodenale)*	Contaminated feces
Roundworm infection	Roundworm *(Ascaris lumbricoides)*	Contaminated feces
Schistosomiasis (fluke)	Schistosome *(Schistosoma japonicum, Schistosoma mansoni, Schistosoma haematobium)*	Infested water containing larvae from snail vector

respiratory therapy and testing and the prevention of nitrogen narcosis and decompression sickness in hyperbaric environments. A mixture of 80% helium and 20% oxygen is commonly breathed by deep-sea divers to prevent gas embolisms and by patients undergoing treatment to clear obstructed respiratory tracts. Helium is used in pulmonary-function testing to calculate the diffusing and residual capacities of the lungs.

helix   A coiled, spirallike formation characteristic of many organic molecules, such as deoxyribonucleic acid (DNA), which is a double helix.

Hellin's law, Hellin-Zeleny law   A generalized formula for calculating the ratio of multiple births in any population, stating that if twin births occur at the rate of 1:N, then the rate of triplet births is approximately $1:N^2$, quadruplets $1:N^3$, quintuplets $1:N^4$, and so on, with the exponent of N being one less than the number in the multiple set. The constant N varies greatly with population.

helminth   A worm, especially one of the pathogenic parasites of the division Metazoa fluke, including flukes, tapeworms, and roundworms.

-helminth   A combining form meaning 'worm': *nemathelminth, platyhelminth.*

helminthiasis   A parasitic infestation of the body by helminths that may be cutaneous, visceral, or intestinal. Ascariasis, bilharziasis, filariasis, hookworm, and trichinosis are common forms of the disease.

helper T cell   See **T cell.**

helvolic acid   An antibiotic, derived from the mold *Aspergillus fumigatus,* formerly used

as an amebicide. Also called **fumagillin, fumigacin.**

hemadsorption   A process in which a substance or an agent, as certain viruses and bacilli, adheres to the surface of an erythrocyte. The process occurs naturally or it may be induced for laboratory identification of bacteriologic specimens.

hemagglutination   An antigen-antibody reaction resulting in the agglutination of red blood cells. See **ABO blood groups.**

hemangioblastoma, *pl.* **hemangioblastomas, hemangioblastomata**   A brain tumor composed of a proliferation of capillaries and of disorganized clusters of capillary cells or angioblasts.

hemangioendothelioma, *pl.* **hemangioendotheliomas, hemangioendotheliomata**   A tumor, consisting of endothelial cells, that grows around an artery or a vein. It may become malignant. Also called **angioendothelioma.**

hemangioma, *pl.* **hemangiomas, hemangiomata**   A benign tumor consisting of a mass of blood vessels. Kinds of hemangiomas include **capillary hemangioma, cavernous hemangioma, nevus flammeus.**

hemangioma simplex   See **capillary hemangioma.**

hemangiosarcoma, *pl.* **hemangiosarcomas, hemangiosarcomata**   A malignant neoplasm composed of endothelial and fibroblastic tissues that proliferates and eventually surrounds vascular channels. Also called **malignant hemangioendothelioma.**

hematemesis Vomiting of bright, red blood, indicating rapid upper gastrointestinal bleeding, commonly associated with esophageal varices or peptic ulcer. The rate and the source of bleeding are determined by endoscopic examination. Treatment requires replacement of blood by transfusion and administration of intravenous fluids for maintenance of fluid and electrolyte balance. Vasoconstrictors may sometimes be infused at the site of bleeding. Surgery may be necessary. See also **gastrointestinal bleeding.**

hematinic An iron-containing compound used to raise hemoglobin level and red blood cell count.

hematochezia Elimination of bloody stools.

hematocrit A measure of the packed cell volume of red blood cells, expressed as a percentage of the total blood volume. The normal range is between 42% and 54% in men, and between 38% and 46% in women. See also **complete blood count.**

hematolmyelia The appearance of frank blood in the fluid of the spinal cord.

hematologist A medical specialist in the field of hematology.

hematology Scientific medical study of blood and blood-forming tissues. —**hematologic, hematological,** *adj.*

hematoma, *pl.* **hematomas, hematomata** A collection of extravasated blood trapped in the tissues of the skin or in an organ, resulting from trauma or incomplete hemostasis after surgery. A hematoma may be drained early and bleeding arrested with pressure or, if necessary, with surgical ligation of the bleeding vessel. Considerable blood may be lost, and infection is a serious complication.

-hematoma A combining form meaning a 'swelling containing blood': *cephalhematoma, episiohematoma, othematoma.*

hematopoiesis The normal formation and development of blood cells in the bone marrow. In severe anemia and other hematologic disorders, cells may be produced in organs outside the marrow (extramedullary hematopoiesis). See also **erythropoiesis.** —**hematopoietic,** *adj.*

hematuria Abnormal presence of blood in the urine. Hematuria is symptomatic of many renal diseases and disorders of the genitourinary system. —**hematuric,** *adj.*

heme The pigmented, iron-containing, nonprotein portion of the hemoglobin molecule. There are four heme groups in a hemoglobin molecule, each consisting of a cyclic structure of four pyrrole residues, called protoporphyrin, and an atom of iron in the center. Heme binds and carries oxygen in the red blood cells, releasing it to tissues that give off excess amounts of CO_2. Compare **porphobilinogen.** See also **hemoglobin, protoporphyrin.**

hemeralopia An abnormal visual condition in which bright light causes blurring of vision. Hemeralopia is an unpleasant side effect of certain anticonvulsant medications, including trimethadione, which is used in treating children affected with petit mal epilepsy. —**hemeralopic,** *adj.*

-hemia See **-emia.**

hemiacephalus A fetal monster in which the brain and most of the cranium are lacking. See also **anencephaly.**

hemiazygous vein One of the tributaries of the azygous vein of the thorax. It starts in the left ascending lumbar vein, enters the thorax through the left crus of the diaphragm, ascends on the left side of the vertebral column as high as the ninth thoracic vertebra, and passes dorsal to the aorta to enter the azygous. The hemiazygous vein receives about four of the caudal intercostal veins, the left subcostal vein, and some of the esophageal and the mediastinal veins.

hemicellulose Any of a group of polysaccharides that constitute the chief part of the skeletal substances of the cell walls of plants and resemble cellulose but are more soluble and more easily extracted and decomposed. See also **dietary fiber.**

hemicephalia A congenital anomaly characterized by the absence of the cerebrum, caused by severe arrest of brain development in the fetus. The cerebellum and basal ganglia are usually present, at least in rudimentary form.

hemicephalus A fetal monster with congenital absence of the cerebrum.

hemicrania 1. A headache, usually migraine, that affects only one side of the head. 2. A congenital anomaly characterized by the absence of half of the skull in the fetus; incomplete anencephaly.

hemiectromelia A congenital anomaly characterized by the incomplete development of the limbs on one side of the body. —**hemiectromelus,** *n.*

hemignathia A congenital anomaly characterized by incomplete development of the lower jaw on one side of the face. —**hemignathus,** *n.*

hemihyperplasia Overdevelopment or excessive growth of one half of a specific organ or part, or of all the organs and parts on one side of the body.

hemihypoplasia Partial or incomplete development of one half of a specific organ or part, or of all the organs and parts on one side of the body.

hemikaryon A cell nucleus that contains the haploid number of chromosomes, as that of the gametes. Compare **amphikaryon.** —**hemikaryotic,** *adj.*

hemimelia A developmental anomaly characterized by the absence or gross shortening of the lower portion of one or more of the limbs. The condition may involve either or both of the bones of the distal arm or leg and is designated according to whichever bone is absent or defective, as fibular, radial, tibial, or ulnar hemimelia. See also **ectromelia, phocomelia.**

hemipagus Conjoined symmetrical twins who are united at the thorax.

hemiplegia Paralysis of one side of the body. Also called **unilateral paralysis.** Compare **diplegia.** —**hemiplegic,** *adj.*

hemisomus A fetus or individual in which one side of the body is malformed or defective.

hemisphere **1.** One half of a sphere or globe. **2.** The lateral half of the cerebrum or of the cerebellum. —**hemispherical,** *adj.*

hemiteras, *pl.* **hemiterata** **1.** Any individual with a congenital malformation that is not so severe or disabling as to be classified as a monstrous or teratic condition. —**hemiteratic,** *adj.*

hemivertebra An abnormal condition characterized by the congenital failure of a vertebra to develop completely, possibly caused by the complete failure of the growth center of one vertebral body. Usually half of the vertebra involved is completely or partially developed and the other half is absent.

hemizygote An individual, organism, or cell that has only one of a pair of genes for a specific characteristic. Such traits are expressed regardless of whether the genes transmitting them are dominant or recessive, as with the X-linked genes on the single X chromosome in males, which have no alleles on the Y chromosome. —**hemizygosity,** *n.,* **hemizygous, hemizygotic,** *adj.*

hemoblastic leukemia See **stem cell leukemia.**

hemochromatosis A rare disease of iron storage, characterized pathologically by excess iron deposits throughout the body. Hepatomegaly, skin pigmentation, diabetes mellitus, and cardiac failure may occur. The disease most often develops in men over 40 years of age and as a complication of some hemolytic anemias requiring multiple blood transfusions. Compare **hemosiderosis.** See also **iron metabolism.**

hemocytoblastic leukemia See **stem cell leukemia.**

hemodialysis A procedure in which impurities or wastes are removed from the blood, used in treating renal insufficiency and various toxic conditions. The patient's blood is shunted from the body through a machine for diffusion and ultrafiltration and then returned to the patient's circulation. Hemodialysis requires access to the patient's blood stream, a mechanism for the transport of the blood to and from the dialyzer, and a dialyzer. Access may be achieved by an external shunt or an arteriovenous fistula. Either a flat plate, coil, or hollow-fiber type dialyzer may be used. The procedure takes from 3 to 8 hours and may be required daily in acute situations or 2 to 3 times a week in chronic renal failure.

NURSING CONSIDERATIONS: A decrease in the flow of blood through the shunt may result in clotting; therefore, any factor that may result in a slowing of the flow is to be avoided. Some of these factors are systemic hypotension, infection of the shunt or fistula, compression of the shunt or fistula, thrombophlebitis, and prolonged inflation of a blood pressure cuff. Infection is avoided in the area around an external shunt by placing a sterile dressing over the shunt and changing the dressing daily. Headache and nausea are common, especially during the procedure and for a

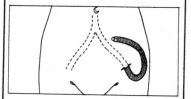

HEMODIALYSIS ACCESS SITES

FEMORAL VEIN CATHETERIZATION

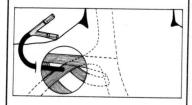

SUBCLAVIAN VEIN CATHETERIZATION

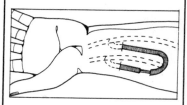

ARTERIOVENOUS SHUNT

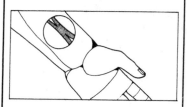

ARTERIOVENOUS FISTULA

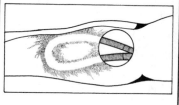

ARTERIOVENOUS VEIN GRAFT

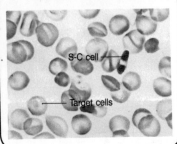

**RED BLOOD CELLS IN
HEMOGLOBIN S-C DISEASE**

S-C cell

Target cells

few hours afterward. Rest, an antiemetic, and a mild analgesic may make the procedure more comfortable. The physical status of the patient is monitored frequently throughout; blood pressure, pulse, and blood tests for electrolyte and acid-base balance are performed. Normal saline solution may be administered to counteract hypotension that occurs as a result of a rapid removal of fluid from the intravascular compartment. The patient is weighed before and after the treatment to determine the amount of fluid lost during the procedure. An anticoagulant is usually given to prevent coagulation of the blood in the dialyzer, cannulas, or catheters; to prevent hemorrhage, protamine sulfate may be given after the procedure to reverse the effect of the anticoagulant. Any treatment that causes tissue trauma, as dental extraction, venipuncture, or intramuscular injection, is not recommended during or immediately following dialysis. See also **arteriovenous fistula, external shunt.**

hemodialyzer See **dialyzer.**

hemoglobin A complex protein-iron compound in the blood that carries oxygen to the cells from the lungs and carbon dioxide away from the cells to the lungs. Each erythrocyte contains between 200 and 300 molecules of hemoglobin, each molecule of hemoglobin contains several molecules of heme, and each molecule of heme can carry one molecule of oxygen. Hemoglobin is normally present in the blood at a concentration within a range of 12 to 16 g/dl in women and 14 to 18 g/dl in men. Hemoglobin then releases the carboxyhemoglobin in the lungs for excretion and more oxygen is picked up for transport to the cells. Hemoglobin has a precise structure consisting of 2 different chains made of 141 and 146 amino acids. The absence, replacement, or addition of only 1 amino acid modifies the properties of the hemoglobin. Such alterations are genetically mediated and may be associated with severe pathology, as in sickle cell disease. See also **carboxyhemoglobin, heme, oxyhemoglobin.**

hemoglobin A (Hb A) A normal hemoglobin. Also called adult hemoglobin. Compare **hemoglobin F.**

hemoglobin C (Hb C) disease A genetic blood disorder characterized by a moderate, chronic hemolytic anemia and associated with the presence of hemoglobin C, an abnormal form of the red cell pigment. Hemoglobin C is inherited as an autosomal codominant gene and, in the homozygous form, is the only kind of hemoglobin found in the blood. In the heterozygous form, hemoglobin C trait, there is no anemia or increased blood hemolysis. Target cells may be seen in microscopic examination of a blood smear. Abnormal hemoglobin C is accompanied by an approximately equal amount of its normal counterpart, hemoglobin A.

hemoglobinemia Presence of free hemoglobin in the blood plasma.

hemoglobin F (Hb F) The normal hemoglobin of the fetus, most of which is broken down in the first days after birth and replaced by hemoglobin A. Small amounts are produced throughout life.

hemoglobinopathy Any of a group of inherited disorders characterized by variation of the structure of the hemoglobin molecule. The alteration appears as the substitution of one or more amino acids in the globin portion of the molecule at selected positions in the two alpha or two beta polypeptide chains. More than 100 variants have been described and identified. Only hemoglobins S, C, and D are seen regularly. The abnormality may occur in the heterozygous or the homozygous form. In the heterozygous form, the normal adult pigment, hemoglobin A, and its variant both appear in the red cell; there may be little or no clinical manifestation of disease. In the homozygous form, only the variant hemoglobin is present, and the characteristic symptoms of that hemoglobinopathy appear. Mixed heterozygous forms are also known to occur. These are characterized by the absence of the normal hemoglobin A and the presence of two or three hemoglobin variants. Kinds of hemoglobinopathies include **hemoglobin C disease, hemoglobin S-C disease, sickle cell anemia.** Compare **thalassemia.** See also **hemoglobin, sickle cell thalassemia, sickle cell trait.**

hemoglobin S (Hb S) An abnormal type of hemoglobin, characterized by the substitution of the amino acid valine for glutamic acid in the B chain of the hemoglobin molecule. As the abnormal molecules become deoxygenated, owing to decreased oxygen tension in the peripheral circulation, they tend to become sickle shaped, to move slowly, to clump together, and to hemolyze. If the proportion of Hb S to Hb A is large, as in sickle cell disease, anemia, local thrombosis, and infarction may occur. See also **sickle cell anemia, sickle cell crisis.**

hemoglobin S-C (Hb S-C) disease A genetic blood disorder in which two different abnormal alleles, one for hemoglobin S and one for hemoglobin C, are inherited. The disorder is characterized by a clinical course considerably less severe than sickle cell anemia despite the absence of the normal hemoglobin. See also

hemoglobin C disease, hemoglobinopathy, sickle cell thalassemia.

hemoglobinuria An abnormal presence in the urine of hemoglobin that is unattached to red blood cells. Hemoglobinuria can result from various autoimmune diseases or episodic hemolytic disorders. It can be diagnosed using a dipstick reagent that is sensitive to free hemoglobin. Kinds of hemoglobinuria include **cold hemoglobinuria, march hemoglobinuria, paroxysmal hemoglobinuria.**

hemoglobin variant Any type of hemoglobin other than hemoglobin A. These variations are genetically determined and, depending on the kind and extent of change, result in altered physical and chemical function of the red blood cells.

hemolysin Any one of the numerous substances which lyse or dissolve red blood cells. Hemolysins are produced by strains of many kinds of bacteria, including some of the staphylococci and streptococci. They are also contained in venoms and in certain vegetables. See also **hemoglobin, hemolysis.**

hemolysis The breakdown of red blood cells and the release of hemoglobin. It occurs normally at the end of the life span of a red blood cell, but it may occur under a variety of other circumstances, including certain antigen-antibody reactions, metabolic abnormalities of the red blood cell that significantly shorten its life span, and mechanical trauma, as in hemodialysis, cardiac prosthesis, or exposure to snake venoms. Dilution of the blood by intravenous administration of excessive amounts of hypotonic solutions, which cause progressive swelling and eventual rupture of the erythrocyte, also results in hemolysis. See also **hemolytic anemia, transfusion reaction. —hemolytic,** adj.

hemolytic anemia A disorder characterized by the premature destruction of red blood cells. Anemia may be minimal or absent, reflecting the ability of the bone marrow to increase production of red blood cells. The condition may occur in association with some infectious diseases, with certain inherited red cell disorders, or as a response to drugs or other toxic agents. Compare **aplastic anemia, congenital nonspherocytic hemolytic anemia, myelophthisic anemia.** See also **anemia, hemolysis, spherocytosis.**

hemolytic uremia syndrome A rare kidney disorder marked by renal failure, microangiopathic hemolytic anemia, and platelet deficiency. This syndrome, of unknown etiology, usually occurs in infancy.

hemophilia An inherited disorder characterized by excessive bleeding. It exists as two distinct but clinically indistinguishable entities, hemophilia A and hemophilia B. Hemophilia A, the classic form, is the result of a deficiency or absence of antihemophilic factor VIII, a trace protein that acts to accelerate the conversion of prothrombin to thrombin through the formation of thromboplastin. Hemophilia B (Christmas disease) represents a deficiency of plasma thromboplastin component, another plasma protein active in the formation of thromboplastin. The clinical severity of the disorder varies markedly with the extent of the deficiency. Greater than usual loss of blood during dental procedures, epistaxis, hematoma, and hemarthrosis are common problems in hemophilia. Severe internal hemorrhage and hematuria are less common. **—hemophiliac,** n., **hemophilic,** adj.

hemophilia A A hereditary blood disorder, transmitted as an X-linked recessive trait, caused by a deficiency of coagulation factor VIII. Hemophilia A is considered the classical type of hemophilia in contrast to hemophilia B and hemophilia C, which may be less severe. See also **coagulation factor, hemophilia.**

hemophilia B A hereditary blood disorder, transmitted as an X-linked recessive trait, caused by a deficiency of factor IX, the plasma thromboplastin component. The condition is clinically similar to but less severe than hemophilia A. Also called Christmas disease. See **coagulation factor, hemophilia.**

hemophilia C A hereditary blood disorder, transmitted as an X-linked recessive trait, caused by a deficiency of factor XI, the plasma thromboplastin antecedent. The condition is clinically similar to but may be less severe than hemophilia A. Also called **Rosenthal's syndrome.** See also **coagulation factor, hemophilia.**

hemoptysis Coughing up of blood from the respiratory tract. Blood-streaked sputum often occurs in minor upper respiratory infections or in bronchitis. More profuse bleeding may indicate *Aspergillus* infection, lung abcess, tuberculosis, or bronchogenic carcinoma. X-ray examination, endoscopy, and bronchoscopy are often used to diagnose hemoptysis. Treatment of significant hemoptysis includes monitoring the patient for signs of shock, preventing asphyxiation, and localizing and stopping the bleeding. Antibiotics and antitussives may be given. Compare **hematemesis.**

hemorrhage A rapid loss of a large amount of blood, either externally or internally. Hemorrhage may be arterial, venous, or capillary. NURSING CONSIDERATIONS: Symptoms of massive hemorrhage are related to hypovolemic shock: rapid, thready pulse; thirst; cold, clammy skin; sighing respirations; dizziness; syncope; pallor; apprehension; restlessness; and hypotension. If bleeding is contained within a cavity or joint, pain will develop as the capsule or cavity is stretched by the rapidly expanding volume of blood. All effort is directed toward stopping the hemorrhage. If hemorrhage is external, pressure is applied directly to the wound or to the appropriate pressure points. The part of the body that is wounded may be elevated. Ice, applied directly to the wound, may slow bleeding by causing vasoconstriction. Body temperature may be maintained by keeping the person covered and flat. If an extremity is wounded, and if the bleeding is severe, a tourniquet may be applied proximal to the wound. A tourniquet is not applied if there is any other way to stanch the flow,

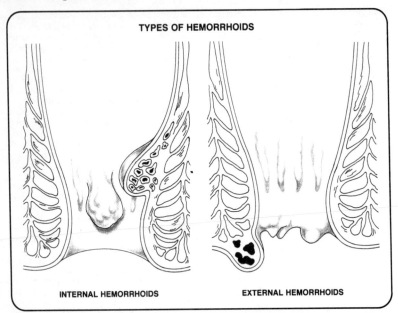

TYPES OF HEMORRHOIDS

INTERNAL HEMORRHOIDS   EXTERNAL HEMORRHOIDS

because the risk is great that the limb will not survive the hypoxia induced by obstruction of the blood supply. The tourniquet is not removed until surgical repair of the wound is possible. Internal bleeding requires prompt medical treatment. The patient is kept warm and quiet, intravenous fluid replacement is begun, and adequate cerebral profusion is attempted until surgical intervention can take place.

hemorrhagic diathesis An inherited predisposition to any one of a number of abnormalities characterized by excessive bleeding. See also **Fanconi's syndrome, hemophilia, von Willebrand's disease.**

hemorrhagic familial angiomatosis See **Osler-Weber-Rendu syndrome.**

hemorrhagic fever An arbovirus infection, characterized by fever, chills, headache, malaise, and respiratory or gastrointestinal symptoms, followed by capillary hemorrhages, and, in severe infection, oliguria, kidney failure, hypotension, and, possibly, death. Many forms of the disease occur in specific geographical areas. Some kinds of hemorrhagic fever are **Argentine hemorrhagic fever, dengue fever, Far Eastern hemorrhagic fever.**

hemorrhagic gastritis A form of acute gastritis usually caused by a toxic agent, as alcohol, aspirin or other drugs, or bacterial toxins that irritate the lining of the stomach. If bleeding is significant, vasoconstrictors and ice water lavage of the stomach may be necessary. Nausea, vomiting, and epigastric distress may persist after the irritant is removed. Treatment is symptomatic.

hemorrhagic lung See **congestive atelectasis.**

hemorrhagic scurvy See **infantile scurvy.**

hemorrhagic shock A state of physical collapse and prostration associated with the sudden and rapid loss of significant amounts of blood. Severe traumatic injuries often cause such blood losses, which, in turn, produce low blood pressure in affected individuals. Death occurs within a relatively short time unless transfusion quickly restores normal blood volume. Hemorrhagic shock often accompanies secondary shock. Compare **primary shock.**

hemorrhoid A varicosity in the lower rectum or anus owing to congestion in the veins of the hemorrhoidal plexus. Internal hemorrhoids originate above the internal sphincter of the anus. If they become large enough to protude from the anus, they become constricted and painful. Small internal hemorrhoids may bleed with defecation. External hemorrhoids appear outside the anal sphincter. They are usually not painful and bleeding does not occur unless a hemorrhoidal vein ruptures or thromboses. Treatment includes local application of a topical medication to lubricate, anesthetize, and shrink the hemorrhoid; sitz baths and cold or hot compresses are also soothing. The hemorrhoids may require sclerosing by injection, ligation, or excision by a surgical procedure. Ligation is increasingly the preferred treatment: it is simple, effective, and does not require anesthesia. In this operation, the hemorrhoid is grasped with a forceps and a rubber band is slipped over the varicosity, causing tissue necrosis and sloughing of the ligated hemorrhoid, which usually occurs within 1 week.

NURSING CONSIDERATIONS: Straining to defecate, constipation, and prolonged sitting contribute to the development of hemorrhoids. As pregnancy is associated with an increased incidence of hemorrhoids, the pregnant woman, in particular, is advised to avoid constipation.

hemosiderin An iron-rich pigment that is a product of red-cell hemolysis. Iron is often stored in this form.

hemosiderosis An abnormal deposition of iron in a variety of tissues, usually in the form of hemosiderin. It is often associated with diseases involving chronic, extensive destruction of red blood cells, as thalassemia major. Compare **hemochromatosis, sideroblastic anemia.** See also **ferritin, iron transport, transferrin.**

hemostasis The termination of bleeding by mechanical or chemical means or by the complex coagulation process of the body, consisting of vasoconstriction, platelet aggregation, and thrombin and fibrin synthesis. See also **platelet, thrombus, vasoconstriction.**

hemostat See **Halsted's forceps.**

hemostatic Of or pertaining to a procedure, device, or substance that arrests the flow of blood. Direct pressure, tourniquets, and surgical clamps are mechanical hemostatic measures. Cold applications are hemostatic and include the use of an ice bag on the abdomen to halt uterine bleeding and irrigation of the stomach with an iced solution to check gastric bleeding. Gelatin sponges, solutions of thrombin, and microfibrillar collagen, which causes the aggregation of platelets and the formation of clots, are used to arrest bleeding in surgical procedures. Aminocaproic acid is administered orally or intravenously in the treatment of excessive bleeding caused by systemic hyperfibrinolysis.

hemostatic forceps See **artery forceps.**

hemothorax An accumulation of blood and fluid in the pleural cavity, between the parietal and visceral pleura, usually the result of trauma. Hemothorax may also be caused by the rupture of small blood vessels owing to inflammation from pneumonia, tuberculosis, or tumors. Shock from hemorrhage, pain, and respiratory failure follows if emergency care is not available.

hemotroph, hemotrophe The total nutritive substances supplied to the embryo from maternal circulation following the development of the placenta. Also called hemotrophic nutrition. Compare **embryotroph. —hemotrophic,** *adj.*

Henle's fissure One of many patches of connective tissue between the muscle fibers of the heart.

Henoch-Schönlein purpura A self-limited hypersensitivity vasculitis, chiefly of children, characterized by purpuric skin lesions that appear predominantly on the lower abdomen, buttocks, and legs, and usually associated with pain in the knees and ankles. Other joint involvement, gastrointestinal bleeding, and hematuria are also common findings. The disease lasts up to 6 weeks and has no sequelae if renal involvement is not severe. Certain immunosuppressive drugs, such as corticosteroids, may help the nephropathy. Also called **anaphylactoid purpura, Schönlein-Henoch purpura.**

Henry's law In physics: a law stating that the solubility of a gas in a liquid is proportional to the pressure of the gas if the temperature is constant and if the gas does not chemically react with the liquid.

Hensen's knot, Hensen's node See **primitive node.**

hen worker's lung See **pigeon breeder's lung.**

heparin A naturally occurring mucopolysaccharide that acts in the body as an antithrombin factor to prevent intravascular clotting. It is produced by basophils and mast cells, which are found in large numbers in the connective tissue surrounding capillaries, particularly in the lungs and liver.

heparin calcium, h. sodium Anticoagulants.

hepat- See **hepato-.**

-hepatia A combining form meaning '(condition of the) liver or its functioning': *anhepatia, dyshepatia, hypohepatia.*

hepatic Of or pertaining to the liver.

hepatic adenoma A rapidly growing liver tumor that may become very large and may rupture, causing a lethal internal hemorrhage. It is sometimes called a 'pill tumor' because of its frequent association with the use of oral contraceptives.

hepatic amebiasis Enlargement and tenderness of the liver that often occurs in association with amebic dysentery, owing to inflammation resulting from infection with *Entamoeba histolytica.* See also **amebiasis,** *Entamoeba histolytica.*

hepatic coma The neurologic manifestation of extensive liver damage owing to chronic or acute liver disease. Either endogenous or exogenous waste toxic to the brain is not neutralized in the liver before being shunted back into the peripheral circulation of the blood, or substances required for cerebral function are not synthesized in the liver and, therefore, are not available to the brain. The condition is characterized by variable consciousness, lethargy, stupor, and coma; a tremor of the hands; personality change; memory loss; hyperreflexia; and hyperventilation. Respiratory alkalosis, mania, convulsions, and death may occur. Treatment in most cases includes administration of neomycin to suppress bacterial flora, preventing them from converting amino acids into ammonia; sorbitol-induced catharsis to produce osmotic diarrhea; administration of lactulose to transfer ammonia from the blood to the colon, where it is then eliminated in the feces; low-protein diet; parenteral hydration with a balanced electrolyte solution; and specific treatment for the underlying cause. Also called **portal-systemic encephalopathy.** See also **cirrhosis, hepatitis.**

hepatic cord A mass of cells, arranged in irregular radiating columns and plates, spreading outward from the central vein of the hepatic lobule. The cells are many-sided and contain one or, sometimes, two distinct nuclei. Many such cords join to form the parenchyma of the lobule. Each cell usually contains granules, some of which are protoplasmic while others consist of glycogen, fat, or an iron compound. Also called **hepatic cells.**

hepatic fistula An abnormal passage from the liver to another organ or body structure.

hepatic node A node in one of three groups of lymph glands associated with the abdominal and the pelvic viscera supplied by branches of the celiac artery. The hepatic nodes are divided into the hepatic and subpyloric groups. Compare **gastric node, pancreaticolienal node.**

hepatico- See **hepato-.**

hepatic porphyria See **porphyria.**

hepatic vein catheterization The introduction of a long, fine catheter into a hepatic venule for the purpose of recording intrahepatic venous pressure. The catheter is inserted through a vein in the arm and is passed through the right atrium, the inferior vena cava, and hepatic vein into the small hepatic vessel.

hepatin See **glycogen.**

hepatitis An inflammatory condition of the liver, characterized by jaundice, hepatomegaly, anorexia, abdominal and gastric discomfort, abnormal liver function, clay-colored stools, and dark urine. The condition may be caused by bacterial or viral infection, parasitic infestation, alcohol, drugs, toxins, or transfusion of incompatible blood. It may be mild and brief or severe, fulminant, and life-threatening. Although the liver can regenerate its tissue, severe hepatitis may lead to cirrhosis and chronic liver dysfunction. See also **viral hepatitis.**

hepatitis A A form of infectious viral hepatitis caused by the hepatitis A virus, characterized by slow onset of signs and symptoms. The virus may be spread by direct contact or through contaminated food or water. The infection most often occurs in young adults and is usually followed by complete recovery. See **viral hepatitis.**

hepatitis B A form of viral hepatitis caused by the hepatitis B virus, characterized by rapid onset of acute symptoms and signs. The virus is transmitted in contaminated serum in blood transfusion or by the use of contaminated needles and instruments. The infection may be severe and result in prolonged illness, destruction of liver cells, cirrhosis, or death. Also called **serum hepatitis.** See **viral hepatitis.**

hepatitis B immune globulin (HBIG) A passive immunizing agent, prescribed for postexposure prophylaxis against infection by the hepatitis B virus.

hepatitis B surface antigen (HBsAG) See **Australia antigen.**

hepatization Transformation of lung tissue into a solid mass resembling the liver, as in early pneumococcal pneumonia in which consolidation and effusion of red blood cells in the alveoli produce red hepatization. In later stages of pneumococcal pneumonia, when white blood cells fill the alveoli, the consolidation becomes **gray hepatization.**

hepato-, hepat- A combining form meaning 'pertaining to the liver': *hepatobiliary, hepatocarcinogenic, hepatocellular.*

hepatocarcinoma See **malignant hepatoma.**

hepatocellular carcinoma See **malignant hepatoma.**

hepatoduodenal ligament The portion of the lesser omentum between the liver and the duodenum, containing the hepatic artery, the common bile duct, the portal vein, lymphatics, and the hepatic plexus of nerves. These structures are enclosed within a fibrous capsule between the two layers of the ligament.

hepatogastric ligament The portion of the lesser omentum lying between the liver and the stomach. Compare **hepatoduodenal ligament.**

hepatojugular reflux An increase in jugular venous pressure when pressure is applied for 30 to 60 seconds over the abdomen, suggestive of right-sided heart failure.

hepatolenticular degeneration See **Wilson's disease.**

hepatoma, *pl.* **hepatomas, hepatomata** A primary malignant tumor of the liver characterized by hepatomegaly, pain, hypoglycemia, weight loss, anorexia, ascites, and the presence of alphafetoprotein in the plasma. It occurs most frequently in association with hepatitis or cirrhosis of the liver and, geographically, in those parts of the world where aflatoxin, a microtoxin, is commonly found.

hepatomegaly Abnormal enlargement of the liver that is usually a sign of liver disease. It is often discovered by percussion and palpation as part of a physical examination: the liver is easily palpable below the ribs and is tender to the touch.

hepatotoxic Potentially destructive of liver cells. —**hepatotoxicity,** *n.*

hepatotoxicity The tendency of an agent, usually a drug or alcohol, to have a destructive effect on the liver. —**hepatotoxic,** *adj.*

hepta-, hept- A combining form meaning 'seven': *heptachromic, heptadactylia, heptavalent.*

heptachlor poisoning See **chlorinated organic insecticide poisoning.**

heptaploid, heptaploidic See **polyploid.**

herald patch See **pityriasis rosea.**

herb bath A medicinal bath taken in water containing a decoction of aromatic herbs.

herbicide poisoning A poisoning caused by the ingestion, inhalation, or absorption of a substance intended for use as a weed killer or defoliant. Most of the commonly used agricultural herbicides, as alachlor, isopropylamine salt of glyphosate, and trifluralin, are only mildly toxic. If ingested, an emetic or gastric lavage is administered. Some herbicides contain extremely toxic substances; poisoning is characterized by dysphagia, burning stomach pain, throat constriction, diarrhea, or other severe symptoms. The substance is identified, the victim is immediately taken to a medical facility, and therapy specific to the poison is promptly instituted.

hereditary   Pertaining to a characteristic, condition, or disease transmitted from parent to offspring; inborn; inherited. Compare **acquired, congenital.**

hereditary ataxia   One of a group of inherited degenerative diseases of the spinal cord, cerebellum, and, often, other parts of the nervous system, characterized by tremor, spasm, wasting of muscle, skeletal change, and sensory disturbances resulting in impaired motor activity. Kinds of hereditary ataxia include **Friedreich's ataxia, spinocerebellar disorder.**

hereditary brown enamel   See **amelogenesis imperfecta.**

hereditary deforming chondroplasia   See **diaphyseal aclasis.**

hereditary disorder, heritable disorder   See **inherited disorder.**

hereditary elliptocytosis   See **elliptocytosis.**

hereditary enamel hypoplasia   See **amelogenesis imperfecta.**

hereditary essential tremor   See **essential tremor.**

hereditary hemorrhagic telangiectasia   See **Osler-Weber-Rendu syndrome.**

hereditary hyperuricemia   See **Lesch-Nyhan syndrome.**

hereditary multiple exostoses   A rare, familial, dyschondroplastic disease in which bony protuberances form on the shafts of the long bones and eventually develop into caps of cartilage covering the ends of the bones. The affected joints lose their mobility and the bones stop growing. The disease begins in childhood and has no cure. Very rarely, a chondrosarcoma may develop from the cap of an exostosis. See also **Ollier's dyschondroplasia.**

hereditary opalescent dentin   See **dentinogenesis imperfecta.**

hereditary protoporphyria   See **porphyria.**

hereditary spherocytosis   See **spherocytic anemia.**

hereditary tyrosinemia   See **tyrosinemia.**

heredity   1. The process by which particular traits or conditions are genetically transmitted from parents to offspring, resulting in resemblance of individuals related by descent. It involves the separation and recombination of genes during meiosis and fertilization and the further interaction of developmental influences and genetic material during embryogenesis. 2. The total genetic constitution of an individual; the sum of the qualities inherited from ancestors and the potentialities of transmitting these qualities to offspring.

heredo-   A combining form meaning 'hereditary': *heredobiologic, heredosyphilitic, heredotrophedema.*

heredofamilial tremor   See **essential tremor.**

Hering-Breuer reflexes   Inhibitory and

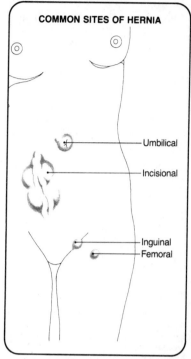

COMMON SITES OF HERNIA

— Umbilical

— Incisional

— Inguinal
— Femoral

excitatory impulses that maintain the rhythm of respiration and prevent the overdistension of alveoli. The impulses originate in stretch receptors of the bronchi and bronchioles, travel via afferent fibers of the vagus nerves to the medullary respiratory centers, and back by motor neurons to the respiratory muscles of the chest. They are stimulated by distension of the airway, increased intratracheal pressures, or pulmonary inflation. The inflation reflex stops inspiration and stimulates expiration; the deflation reflex inhibits expiration and brings on inspiration. These reflexes are hyperactive in conditions of restrictive ventilatory insufficiency.

heritability   The degree to which a given trait is controlled by inheritance.

hermaphroditism   A rare condition in which both male testicular and female ovarian tissue exist in the same person, with the testicular tissue containing seminiferous tubules or spermatozoa and the ovarian tissue containing follicles or corpora albicantia. The condition results from a chromosomal abnormality. Also called hermaphrodism. Compare **pseudohermaphroditism.**

hernia   Protrusion of an organ through an abnormal opening in the muscle wall of the cavity that surrounds it. A hernia may be congenital, may result from the failure of certain structures to close after birth, or may be acquired later in life owing to obesity, muscular weakness, surgery, or illness. Common kinds of hernia include

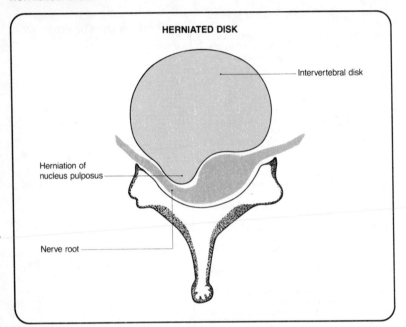

HERNIATED DISK

Intervertebral disk

Herniation of
nucleus pulposus

Nerve root

femoral hernia, hiatal hernia, incisional hernia, inguinal hernia, umbilical hernia. See also **herniorrhaphy.**

herniated disk A rupture of the fibrocartilage surrounding an intervertebral disk. The injury releases the nucleus pulposus that cushions the vertebrae both above and below. The resultant pressure on the spinal nerve roots may cause considerable pain and may damage the nerves. The condition most frequently occurs in the lumbar region. Also called **herniated nucleus pulposus, ruptured intervertebral disk.**

herniation A protrusion of a body organ or portion of an organ through an abnormal opening in a membrane, muscle, or other tissue. See also **hernia, hiatus.**

herniorrhaphy Surgical repair of a hernia.

heroin A morphinelike drug with no currently acceptable medical use in the United States. Heroin is included in Schedule I of the Comprehensive Drug Abuse Prevention and Control Act of 1970. As covered in this legislation, it may not be obtained by prescription, but only for research, instructional use, or for chemical analysis by application to the Drug Enforcement Administration of the Department of Justice. Heroin, like other opium alkaloids, can produce analgesia, respiratory depression, gastrointestinal spasm, and physical dependence. It produces its major effects on the central nervous system (CNS) and the bowel and alters the endocrine and the autonomic nervous systems. The binding sites for heroin are widely distributed in the CNS, especially throughout the limbic system, thalamus, striatum, hypothalamus, midbrain, and spinal cord. Illicitly obtained heroin is commonly used by individuals who become addicted and have a higher death rate than nonaddicts of similar age. Some studies conducted in the United States and England have shown that the majority of herion users are relatively young people who have been introduced to the drug by friends and first start using heroin out of curiosity but continue because of its euphoric effects. Such individuals commonly show similar patterns of behavior, social adjustment, and health impairment. Heroin use in the United States reached epidemic proportions during the 1960s and, in 1971, became a major cause of death in New York City among males between the ages of 15 and 35. The problem abated somewhat during the 1970s but has apparently increased and spread from the larger cities to the smaller communities across the country. Initial street use of the drug commonly involves sniffing powdered heroin, which is absorbed through the mucous membranes of the nasopharynx and the respiratory tract. Other methods of self-administration include subcutaneous injection and intravenous injection. Heroin, which loses much of its analgesic power when taken orally, is more powerful than morphine and acts more rapidly. It is hydrolyzed to morphine by the body and becomes concentrated in the parenchymatous tissues, skeletal muscle, and brain. Heroin administered intravenously is almost immediately effective and produces reactions that last from 3 to 6 hours. Many users liken the initial sensation to a sexual orgasm. Heroin addicts may spend as much as $300 daily for the drug and inject themselves every 3 to 6 hours. Repeated use of this drug produces tolerance to most of the acute narcotic effects; physical dependence develops concurrently with tolerance. Withdrawal from heroin after relatively few exposures commonly produces acute abstinence syndrome. Withdrawal signs are usually observed shortly before the next planned dose and commonly include anxiety, restlessness, irritability, and craving for another dose. Other withdrawal signs that may appear 8 to 15 hours after the last dose include lacrimation, perspiration, yawning, and restless sleep. On awakening from such sleep the severely addicted heroin user may experience withdrawal signs, as vomiting, pain in the bones, diarrhea, convulsions, and cardiovascular collapse. Withdrawal signs usually peak at between 36 and 48 hours and gradually subside during the following 10 days. Associated anxiety and depression may persist for months in many heroin addicts under treatment. Most authorities consider such addiction a complex disease caused by heroin-induced neurochemical disturbances in combination with deep psychological and social factors. A variety of diluents, as quinine, are used to dissolve street heroin for subcutaneous and intravenous injection. Toxic diluents in combination with unhygienic administration and other unhealthy factors are responsible for more than half the fatalities associated with the illegal use of opiates. The most frequent disorders associated with injections of adulterated heroin are tetanus, skin abscesses, cellulitis, and thrombophlebitis. Heroin-connected pulmonary complications may include pneumonia, infarction, and tuberculosis. Neurologic disorders stemming from the use of street heroin may include transverse myelitis, peripheral nerve lesions, and fibrosing chronic myopathy. Women heroin addicts who become pregnant often give birth to premature babies who are highly susceptible to toxemia. Relapses of heroin addicts during withdrawal treatment are common and protracted abstinence signs, as altered blood pressure and pulse rate, anxiety, and depression, may persist for months. Methadone is commonly used as a substitute drug in the treatment of heroin addiction.

herpangina A viral infection, usually of young children, characterized by sore throat, headache, anorexia, and pain in the abdomen, neck, and extremities. Febrile convulsions and vomiting may occur in infants. Papules or vesicles may form in the pharynx and on the tongue, the palate, or the tonsils. The lesions evolve into shallow ulcers which heal spontaneously. The disease usually runs its course in less than 1 week. Treatment is symptomatic. The cause is often infection by a strain of coxsackievirus.

herpes genitalis An infection caused by type 2 herpes simplex virus (HSV-2), usually transmitted by sexual contact, that causes painful vesicular eruptions on the skin and mucous membranes of the genitalia of males and females. When it is acquired during pregnancy, HSV-2 may be transmitted through the placenta to the fetus and to the newborn by direct contact with infected tissue during birth. In the male, herpes genitalis infections may resemble penile ulcers. A small group of vesicular lesions surrounded by erythematous tissue may occur on the glans or prepuce. The lesions erupt into superficial ulcers that often heal in 5 to 7 days, although they also may become the sites of secondary infections. The lesions are painful and are often associated with a burning sensation, urinary dysfunction, fever, malaise, and swelling of the lymph glands in the inguinal area. The female patient may exhibit the same or similar systemic effects, and members of both sexes may complain of painful sexual intercourse. In the female, herpes genitalis lesions are likely to appear as multiple superficial eruptions on the surfaces of the cervix, vagina, or perineum. There may be a discharge from the cervix. Vaginal lesions may appear as mucous patches with gray ulcerations. Laboratory tests from smears of fluid taken from the base of lesions show a positive Tzanck reaction with multiple nucleated giant cells, which distinguishes HSV-2 infections from other venereal diseases. HSV-2 tends to recur. Treatment of uncomplicated herpes genitalis is mainly symptomatic. An attack of the disease is generally self-limiting. Lesions may be cleansed with soap and water, where feasible, to limit the risk of secondary infections, and drying medications may be applied to lesions that rupture or ooze. Secondary infections are treated with appropriate antibiotics. Patients may be referred to the Herpes Resource Center, Box 100, Palo Alto, Calif. 94302 for information on how to cope with the problems associated with this disease.

NURSING CONSIDERATIONS: The nurse exercises extreme caution in contacts with infected patients. Smears for laboratory analysis are obtained by cleansing fresh vesicles with alcohol and removing fluid from the base of lesions with a cotton swab or wooden applicator. Rubber gloves are worn and the hands washed after contact to prevent transfer of virus particles from vesicles to other skin or mucous membranes of the patient or other individuals. Transfer of the virus to the cornea or conjunctiva results in herpetic keratitis. Primary infections that develop in pregnant women may progress to viremia and a marked incidence of fetal mortality and morbidity. Active HSV-2 lesions within 3 weeks of delivery usually require that the infant be delivered by cesarean section to avoid dangerous neonatal herpesvirus infection.

herpes gestationis A generalized, pruritic, vesicular or bullous rash appearing in the second or third trimester of pregnancy and disappearing several weeks postpartum. The lesions often recur with succeeding pregnancies and are associated with premature birth and increased fetal mortality. The disease closely resembles erythema multiforme.

herpes simplex An infection caused by a herpes simplex virus (HSV), which has an affinity for the skin and nervous system and usu-

LESIONS OF HERPES ZOSTER

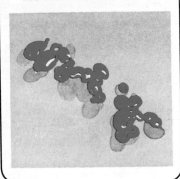

ally produces small, transient, irritating, and sometimes painful fluid-filled blisters on the skin and mucous membranes. HSV-1 (oral herpes, herpes labialis) infections tend to occur in the facial area, particularly around the mouth and nose; HSV-2 (herpes genitalis) infections are usually limited to the genital region. The initial symptoms of a herpes simplex infection usually include burning, tingling, or itching sensations about the edges of the lips or nose within 1 to 2 weeks after contact with an infected person. Several hours later, small red papules develop in the irritated area, followed by the eruption of small vesicles, or fever blisters, filled with fluid. The vesicles generally are associated with itching, pain, or similar discomfort. Other effects often include a mild fever and enlargement of the lymph nodes in the neck. Laboratory analysis of the vesicular fluid usually shows the presence of herpesvirus particles and the absence of pyogenic bacteria. Within 1 week after the onset of symptoms, thin yellow crusts form on the vesicles as healing begins. In skin areas that are moist or protected or in severe cases, healing may be delayed. HSV-2 infections in adolescence are associated with an increased incidence of cervical cancer in adulthood. Treatment of herpes simplex is symptomatic. The lesions may be washed gently with soap and water to reduce the risk of secondary infection. Otherwise, topical applications of drying medications, as camphor or alcohol solutions, may speed healing, but they are very painful. Where secondary infections have begun, appropriate antibiotics are prescribed.

NURSING CONSIDERATIONS: Because herpesviruses are extremely contagious, the nurse follows all appropriate procedures in contacts with patients to avoid acquiring the infection and carrying it to other persons. Once acquired, the virus tends to remain latent in the skin or tissues of the nervous system and may be reactivated by a variety of stimuli, including a febrile illness, physical or emotional stress, exposure to sunlight, or ingestion of certain foods or drugs. The complications of herpetic infections may include encephalitis, herpes simplex keratitis, and gingivostomatitis. In cases involving systemic complications, antibiotics, blood transfusions, I.V. solutions, and other therapeutic measures may be required. In uncomplicated cases, the herpes attack is usually self-limiting and runs its course in 3 weeks or less.

herpesvirus hominis   See **herpes simplex.**

herpes zoster   An acute infection caused by the varicella-zoster virus (V-ZV), affecting mainly adults and characterized by the development of painful vesicular skin eruptions that follow the underlying route of cranial or spinal nerves inflamed by the virus. Distribution of the pain and vesicular eruptions is usually unilateral, although both sides of the body may be involved. Any sensory nerve may be affected, but the virus in most cases tends to invade the posterior root ganglia associated with thoracic and trigeminal nerves. The pain, which may be constant or intermittent, superficial or deep, usually precedes other effects and may mimic other disorders, as appendicitis or pleurisy. Early symptoms may include gastrointestinal disturbances, malaise, fever, and headache. The vesicles usually evolve from small red macules along the path of a nerve, and the skin of the area is hypersensitive. All of the lesions may appear within a period of hours, but they most often develop gradually over a period of several days. The macules vesiculate and, after about 3 days, become turbid with cellular debris. Usually, at the end of the 1st week, the vesicles develop crusts. The symptoms may persist for 3 to 5 weeks, but in most cases they diminish after 2 weeks.

NURSING CONSIDERATIONS: Treatment is primarily symptomatic and includes application of calamine lotion or similar medications to relieve itching and administration of analgesics for pain. Surgical intervention to excise an affected nerve may be advised in cases of severe pain that fail to respond to more conservative treatment. The nurse encourages bed rest during the early stages of zoster infection, when fever and other systemic effects occur. Irritation of the vesicles may be exacerbated by contact with clothing or bed linen. The use of nonadherent dressings and of cradles to prevent direct contact of affected skin areas with irritating fabrics relieves discomfort. An attack of herpes zoster does not confer immunity, but most patients recover without permanent effects except for occasional scarring at sites of severe vesicular lesions. Evidence indicates V-ZV remains latent in the body of a person once infected, and a person lacking varicella immunity can acquire chickenpox from a herpes zoster patient. Also called **shingles.** See also **herpes simplex, varicella-zoster virus.**

herpes zoster oticus   An infection caused by a herpesvirus that involves the eighth nerve ganglia and geniculate ganglion, causing severe pain in the external ear structures and pain or paralysis along the facial nerve. The disease also may result in hearing loss and vertigo. The vertigo is usually transient, but the hearing loss and facial paralysis may be permanent. There may be vesicular eruptions along the external ear canal and ear pinna. Treatment is generally symptomatic, with diazepam administered for vertigo, analgesics for pain, and corticosteroids for other symptoms.

herpes zoster virus (HZV)   See **chickenpox.**

herpetiform   Having clusters of vesicles; resembling the skin lesions of some herpesvirus infections. See also **herpes simplex, herpes zoster.**

Hers' disease   An uncommon metabolic disorder of glycogen storage, characterized by hepatomegaly and an accumulation of abnormally large amounts of glycogen in the liver owing to its inability to break down glycogen. The condition is inherited as an autosomal recessive trait. There is no known treatment. Also called **glycogen storage disease, type VI.** See also **glycogen storage disease.**

hertz (Hz)   A unit of measurement of wave frequency equal to 1 cycle per second (cps).

hesperidin   A crystalline flavone glycoside found in bioflavonoid and occurring in most citrus fruits, especially in the spongy casing of oranges and lemons.

hetacillin, h. potassium   Penicillin antibiotics.

hetastarch   A plasma expander.

heterauxesis   See **allometric growth.**

hetero-, heter-   A combining form meaning 'pertaining to another': *heteroalbumose, heterochronia, heterogamy.*

heteroallele   One of a set of genes located at a specific locus on homologous chromosomes that differs from the other of the pair, resulting in a mutation. —**heteroallelic,** *adj.*

heteroblastic   Developing from different germ layers or kinds of tissue rather than from a single type. Compare **homoblastic.**

heterocephalus   A malformed fetus that has two heads of unequal size. —**heterocephalous, heterocephalic,** *adj.*

heterochromatin   That portion of chromosome material that is inactive in gene expression but may function in controlling metabolic activities, transcription, and cell division. It stains most intensely during the interphase stage and usually remains in a condensed state throughout the cell cycle. It consists of two types, constitutive heterochromatin, which occurs in the centromeric region of the chromosome and is characteristic of the Y chromosome, and facultative heterochromatin, which is present in the inactivated X chromosome of the mammalian female. Compare **euchromatin.** See also **chromatin.** —**heterchromatic,** *adj.*

heterochromatinization   The transformation of genetically active euchromatin into genetically inactive heterochromatin; the inactivation of one of the X chromosomes in the mammalian female during the early stages of embryogenesis. See also **Lyon hypothesis.**

heterochromosome   A sex chromosome.

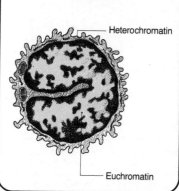

HETEROCHROMATIN OF A LYMPHOCYTE

Heterochromatin

Euchromatin

See also **heterotypical chromosomes.** —**heterochromosomal,** *adj.*

heteroduplex   In molecular genetics: a DNA molecule in which the two strands are derived from different individuals, with the result that some pairs or blocks of base pairs may not match.

heterodymus, heterodidymus   A conjoined twin fetus in which the parasitic element consists of a head, neck, and thorax attached to the thoracic wall of the autosite.

heteroeroticism   Sexual feeling or activity directed toward another individual. Also called alloeroticism, heteroerotism. Compare **autoeroticism.**

heterogamete   A gamete differing markedly in size and structure from one with which it unites, specifically those of higher organisms as opposed to those of lower plants and animals. Compare **anisogamete, isogamete.**

heterogamy   **1.** Sexual reproduction in which there is fusion of dissimilar gametes, usually differing in size and structure. The word is used primarily to denote the reproductive processes of higher organisms as opposed to certain lower plants and animals. Compare **anisogamy, isogamy. 2.** Reproduction by the alternation of sexual and asexual generations; heterogenesis. —**heterogamous,** *adj.*

heterogeneous   **1.** Consisting of dissimilar elements or parts; unlike; incongruous. **2.** Not having a uniform quality throughout. Compare **homogeneous.** —**heterogeneity,** *adj.*

heterogenesis   **1.** Reproduction that differs in successive generations, as the alternation of sexual with asexual reproduction, so that offspring have characteristics different from those of the parents. In the asexual stage, it often involves one or more parthenogenic or hermaphroditic generations, often with various hosts, as in the case of many trematode parasites. Also called heterogeny, heterogony. **2.** A sexual generation. **3.** Abiogenesis. Compare **autogenesis, homogenesis.** See also **metagenesis.** —**heterogenetic, heterogenic,** *adj.*

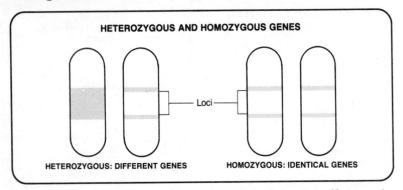

HETEROZYGOUS AND HOMOZYGOUS GENES

Loci

HETEROZYGOUS: DIFFERENT GENES   HOMOZYGOUS: IDENTICAL GENES

heterogenous   Derived or developed from another source or from two different sources.

heterograft   Tissue from another species used as a temporary graft in certain cases, as in treating a severely burned patient when sufficient tissue from the patient or from a tissue bank is not available. It is quickly rejected but provides a cover for the burn for the first few days, reducing the amount of fluid loss from the open wound. Also called zenograft.

heterologous insemination   See **artificial insemination donor.**

heterologous tumor   A neoplasm consisting of tissue different from that of its site.

heterologous twins   See **dizygotic twins.**

heterophil test   A test for the presence of heterophil antibodies in the serum of patients suspected of having infectious mononucleosis, based on an agglutination reaction between heterophil antibodies in a person's serum and heterophil antigen, a normal component of sheep erythrocytes. This antibody eventually appears in the serum of more than 80% of the patients with infectious mononucleosis, hence it is highly diagnostic of the disease. See also **Epstein-Barr virus.**

heteroploid, heteroploidic   1. Of or pertaining to an individual, organism, strain, or cell that has a variation in the number of whole chromosomes characteristic for the somatic cell of the species. The change may involve entire sets of chromosomes or the addition or loss of single whole chromosomes. 2. Such an individual, organism, strain, or cell. See also **aneuploid, euploid.**

heteroploidy   The state or condition of having an abnormal number of chromosomes, either more or less than that characteristic of the somatic cell of the species.

heterosexual   1. A person whose sexual desire or preference is for people of the opposite sex. 2. Of or pertaining to sexual desire or preference for people of the opposite sex. —**heterosexuality,** n.

heterosexual panic   An acute attack of anxiety resulting in the frantic pursuit of heterosexual activity in response to unconscious or latent homosexual impulses. Compare **homosexual panic.**

heterosis   The superiority of first-generation hybrid plants and animals in respect to one or more traits when compared to either of the parent strains or to corresponding inbred strains. Also called **hybrid vigor.**

heterotopic ossification   A nonmalignant overgrowth of bone, frequently occurring after a fracture, that is sometimes confused with certain bone tumors when visualized on X-ray film. Also called **exuberant callus, myositis ossificans.**

heterotypic, heterotypical   Pertaining to or characteristic of a type differing from the usual or the normal, specifically applied to the first meiotic division of germ cells in gametogenesis as distinguished from the second or mitotic division. Compare **homeotypic.**

heterotypical chromosomes   Any unmatched pair of chromosomes, specifically the sex chromosomes.

heterozygosis   1. The formation of a zygote by the union of two gametes that have dissimilar pairs of genes. 2. The production of hybrids through crossbreeding. —**heterozygotic,** adj.

heterozygous   Having two different genes at corresponding loci on homologous chromosomes. An individual who is heterozygous for a particular characteristic has inherited a gene for that characteristic from one parent and the alternative gene from the other parent. A person heterozygous for a genetic disease caused by a dominant gene, as Huntington's chorea, manifests the disorder. An individual heterozygous for a hereditary disorder produced by a recessive gene, as sickle cell anemia, is asymptomatic or exhibits reduced symptoms of the disease. The offspring of a heterozygous carrier of a genetic disorder have a 50% chance of inheriting the gene associated with the trait. Compare **homozygous.**

heuristic   1. Serving to stimulate interest for further investigation. 2. A teaching method in which the student is encouraged to learn through independent research and investigation. 3. A method of argument that postulates what is to be proved.

hex-, hexa-   A combining form meaning 'six': *hexabasic, hexavaccine, hexhydric.*

hexachlorophene   An antiseptic agent.

hexafluorenium bromide A drug that inhibits the enzymatic breakdown of succinylcholine.

hexamethylenamine See **methenamine**.

hexamethylmelamine An experimental antineoplastic that has been used to treat bronchogenic, cervical, and ovarian carcinomas.

hexaploid, hexaploidic See **polyploid**.

hexenmilch See **witch's milk**.

hexobarbital A barbiturate sedative-hypnotic.

hexocyclium methylsulfate A gastrointestinal anticholinergic agent.

hexokinase An enzyme that catalyzes the transfer of a phosphate group from adenosine triphosphate to D-glucose.

Hf Symbol for **hafnium**.

HF *abbr* Hageman factor.

HFPPV *abbr* high-frequency positive-pressure ventilation.

Hg Symbol for **mercury**.

hiatal hernia Protrusion of a portion of the stomach upward through the diaphragm. The condition occurs in about 40% of the population, and most people display few, if any, symptoms. The major difficulty in symptomatic patients is gastroesophageal reflux, the backflow of the acid contents of the stomach into the esophagus. Two types of hiatal hernias are sliding hernia and paraesophageal (rolling) hernia. See also **gastroesophageal reflux, heartburn**.

hiatus A usually normal opening in a membrane or other body tissue. —**hiatal**, *adj*.

hibernoma, *pl*. **hibernomas, hibernomata** A benign tumor, usually on the hips or the back, composed of fat cells that are partly or entirely of fetal origin. Also called **fat cell lipoma, fetal lipoma**.

hiccup, hiccough A characteristic sound that is produced by the involuntary contraction of the diaphragm, followed by rapid closure of the glottis. Hiccups have a variety of causes, including indigestion, rapid eating, certain types of surgery, and epidemic encephalitis. Most episodes of hiccups do not persist longer than a few minutes, but recurrent and prolonged attacks can sometimes occur. Also called **singultus**.

hickory stick fracture See **greenstick fracture**.

hidradenitis See **hydradenitis**.

hidro- A combining form meaning 'pertaining to sweat or a sweat gland': *hidrocystoma, hidrosadenitis, hidroschesis*.

hidrosis Sweat production and secretion. Compare **anhidrosis, dyshidrosis, hyperhidrosis**. —**hidrotic**, *adj*.

hiero-, hier- A combining form meaning 'pertaining to the sacrum, or to religion': *hierolisthesis, hieromania, hierotherapy*.

high blood pressure See **hypertension**.

high-density lipoprotein A plasma protein containing relatively more protein and less cholesterol and triglycerides. It may serve to stabilize very low-density lipoprotein and is also involved in transporting cholesterol and other

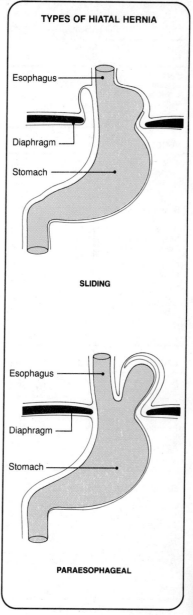

TYPES OF HIATAL HERNIA

Esophagus

Diaphragm

Stomach

SLIDING

Esophagus

Diaphragm

Stomach

PARAESOPHAGEAL

lipids from the plasma to the tissues.

high-energy phosphate compound A chemical compound containing a high-energy bond between phosphoric acid residues and certain organic substances. When the bond is hydrolyzed, a large amount of energy is released. Adenosine triphosphate is the most powerful and ubiquitous of the high energy phosphate com-

DIETARY SOURCES OF POTASSIUM

MEATS	SERVING SIZE	mEq
Beef	4 oz (112 g)	11.2
Chicken	4 oz (112 g)	12.0
Scallops	5 large	30.0
Veal	4 oz (112 g)	15.2

VEGETABLES	SERVING SIZE	mEq
Artichokes	1 large bud	7.7
Asparagus, fresh, frozen, cooked	½ cup	5.5
raw	6 spears	7.7
Beans, dried, cooked	½ cup	10.0
Beans, lima	½ cup	9.5
Broccoli, cooked	½ cup	7.0
Carrots, cooked	½ cup	5.7
raw	1 large	8.8
Mushrooms, raw	4 large	10.6
Potato, baked	1 small	15.4
Spinach, fresh, cooked	½ cup	8.5
Squash, winter, baked	½ cup	12.0
Tomato, raw	1 medium	10.4

FRUITS	SERVING SIZE	mEq
Apricots, dried	4 halves	5.0
fresh	3 small	8.0
Banana	1 medium	12.8
Cantaloupe	½ small	13.0
Figs, dried	7 small	17.5
Peach, fresh	1 medium	6.2
Pear, fresh	1 medium	6.2

BEVERAGES	SERVING SIZE	mEq
Apricot nectar	1 cup (240 ml)	9.0
Grapefruit juice	1 cup (240 ml)	8.2
Orange juice	1 cup (240 ml)	11.4
Pineapple juice	1 cup (240 ml)	9.0
Prune juice	1 cup (240 ml)	14.4
Tomato juice	1 cup (240 ml)	11.6
Milk, whole, skim	1 cup (240 ml)	8.8

pounds found in the body. All of these compounds liberate energy to fuel muscle contraction, active transport across cell membranes, and the synthesis of many substances in the body.

highest intercostal vein One of a pair of veins that drain the blood from the upper two or three intercostal spaces. The right vein descends and opens into the azygous vein. The left vein crosses the arch of the aorta and opens into the left brachiocephalic vein, usually receiving the left bronchial vein.

high forceps An obstetric operation in which forceps are used to deliver a baby whose head is not engaged in the birth canal. The procedure is considered hazardous and is generally condemned. Compare **low forceps, mid forceps.** See also **forceps delivery, obstetric forceps.**

high Fowler's position Placement of the patient in a semisitting position by raising the head of the bed more than 51 cm (20 inches).

high-potassium diet A diet that contains foods rich in potassium, including all leafy green vegetables, brussels sprouts, citrus fruits, bananas, dates, raisins, legumes, meats, and whole grains. It is indicated for any condition resulting in the loss of extracellular fluid, as acute diarrhea, congenital renal alkalosis, aldosteronism, hypokalemia, hypertension, and diabetic coma. It is also indicated for patients receiving thiazide or corticosteroid therapy.

high-protein diet A diet that contains large amounts of protein, consisting largely of meats, fish, milk, legumes, and nuts. It may be indicated in protein depletion from any cause, as a preoperative preparation, in nephrotic syndromes, or in hepatic disorders. It may be contraindicated in liver failure or when function of the kidneys is so impaired that added protein could result in azotemia and acidosis.

high-risk infant Any neonate, regardless of birth weight, size, or gestational age, who, because of preconceptual, prenatal, natal, or postnatal conditions or circumstances that interfere with the normal birth process or impede adjustment to extrauterine growth and development, has a greater than average chance of morbidity or mortality, especially within the first 28 days of life. See also **neonatal period, premature infant.**

high-vitamin diet A dietary regimen that includes a variety of foods that contain therapeutic amounts of all of the vitamins necessary for the metabolic processes of the body. It is often ordered in combination with other therapeutic diets containing larger than usual amounts of protein or calories, especially when treating severe or chronic infection, malnutrition, or vitamin deficiency.

Hill-Burton Act A 1946 amendment to the U.S. Public Health Service Act authorizing grants to states for surveying their hospital and public health center needs and for the planning and construction of additional facilities. Subsequent amendments authorized federal funding for as much as two thirds of the cost of construction projects and broadened the scope of the legislation to include diagnostic and treatment centers, long-term treatment centers, and nursing homes and to aid in modernization of existing hospitals. Also called **Hospital Survey and Construction Act.**

Hill-Burton programs A cluster of programs created by legislation included in the National Health Planning and Resources Development Act of 1974. The programs allow federal monetary assistance for modernization of health facilities, construction of outpatient health centers, construction of inpatient facilities in underserved areas, and the conversion of existing health care facilities for the provision of new health services.

hilus, *pl.* **hili**   A depression or pit at that part of an organ where vessels and nerves enter.

hindgut   The caudal portion of the embryonic alimentary canal. Consisting of endodermal tissue, it is formed by the development of the tail fold and eventually gives rise to part of the small and large intestines, rectum, bladder, and urogenital ducts. Compare **foregut, midgut.** See also **cloaca.**

hind kidney   See **metanephros.**

hinge joint   A synovial joint providing a connection in which articular surfaces are closely molded together in a manner that permits extensive motion in one plane. Also called **ginglymus joint. Compare gliding joint, pivot joint.**

hip   See **coxa.**

hip bath   See **sitz bath.**

hip joint   See **coxal articulation.**

hippocampal fissure   A fissure reaching from the posterior aspect of the corpus callosum to the tip of the temporal lobe.

Hippocratic Oath   An oath, attributed to Hippocrates, that serves as an ethical guide for the medical profession. It is traditionally incorporated into the graduation ceremonies of medical colleges. See also **Æsculapius.**

hip replacement   Replacement of the hip joint with an artificial ball and socket joint, performed to relieve a chronically painful and stiff hip in advanced osteoarthritis, an improperly healed fracture, or degeneration of the joint. A prosthesis of a durable, hard metal alloy or stainless steel is attached to the femur with screws or an acrylic cement; a metal or a plastic acetablum is implanted. Postoperatively, the patient is placed in traction. NURSING CONSIDERATIONS: The affected leg is kept abducted and in straight alignment with pillows; external rotation of the leg must be prevented. The nurse observes nerve function and circulation in the leg frequently during the 1st postoperative day. Support hose may be ordered and anticoagulant therapy begun. The most frequent complications are dislocation or infection requiring removal of the new joint. Ambulation begins gradually, with frequent short walks. Sitting for more than 1 hour is to be avoided, and hip flexion beyond 90° may cause dislocation of the prosthesis. The patient continues an exercise program after discharge to maintain functional motion of the hip joint and to strengthen the abductor muscles.

Hirschsprung's disease   The congenital absence of autonomic ganglia in the smooth-muscle wall of the colon, resulting in poor or absent peristalsis in the involved segment of colon, accumulation of feces, and dilation of the bowel (megacolon). Symptoms include intermittent vomiting, diarrhea, and constipation.

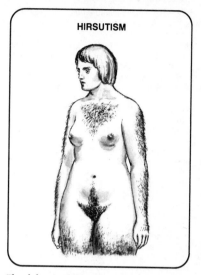

HIRSUTISM

The abdomen may become distended to several times its normal size. The condition is usually diagnosed in infancy, but it may not be recognized until much later in childhood. Diagnosis is confirmed by barium enema; biopsy of the affected tissue shows the absence of ganglia. Surgical repair in early childhood is usually successful. A temporary colostomy is performed and the aganglionic portion of the bowel is resected. The colostomy is almost always reversed a few months later. Also called **congenital megacolon.**

hirsutism   Excessive body hair in a masculine distribution owing to heredity, hormonal dysfunction, porphyria, or medication. Treatment of the specific cause will usually stop growth of more hair. Excess hair may be removed by dermabrasion, electrolysis, chemical depilation, shaving, plucking, or rubbing with pumice. Fine facial hair may be most effectively minimized by bleaching. Also called **hypertrichosis.** —**hirsute,** *adj.*, **hirsuteness,** *n.*

hirsutoid papilloma of the penis   A condition characterized by clusters of small, white papules on the coronal edge of the glans penis. Also called **papillomatosis coronal penis, pearly penile papules.**

His bundle   See **bundle of His.**

hist-   See **histo-.**

histamine   A compound, found in all cells, produced by the breakdown of histidine. It is released in allergic, inflammatory reactions and causes dilation of capillaries, decreased blood pressure, increased secretion of gastric juice, and constriction of smooth muscles of the bronchi and uterus.

histamine headache   A headache associated with the release of histamine from the body tissues and marked by symptoms of dilated carotid arteries, fluid accumulation under the eyes, tearing or lacrimation, and rhinorrhea (runny nose). Symptoms include sudden sharp pain on one side of the head, involving the facial area from the neck to the temple. Treatment includes the use of preparations of antihistamines and ergot that help constrict the arteries. Also called **cluster headache, Horton's histamine cephalalgia.** See also **cephalalgia.**

-histechia A combining form meaning 'a tissue retaining a (specified) substance': *cholesterohistechia, glycohistechia, uratohistechia.*

histiocyte See **macrophage.**

histiocytic leukemia See **monocytic leukemia.**

histiocytic malignant lymphoma A lymphoid neoplasm containing undifferentiated primitive cells or differentiated reticulum cells. Also called **clasmocytic lymphoma, reticulum cell sarcoma.**

histiocytosis X A cluster of conditions encompassing benign eosinophilic granuloma and several malignant lymphomatous diseases.

histiotypic growth The uncontrolled proliferation of cells, as occurs in bacterial cultures and molds. Compare **organotypic growth.**

histo-, hist- A combining form meaning 'pertaining to tissue': *histoclastic, histohematin, histonectomy.*

histocompatibility antigens A group of genetically determined antigens on the surface of many cells. Histocompatibility antigens are the cause of most graft rejections that occur in organ transplantation. See also **isoantigen.**

histocompatibility locus A set of positions on a chromosome that are occupied by a complex of genes that govern several tissue antigens. Together, the loci and the genes comprise the human leukocyte antigen complex.

histogram In research: a graph showing the values of one or more variables plotted against time or against frequency of occurrence. A graph of a patient's temperature, pulse, and respiration is an example of a histogram.

histography The process of describing or of creating visualizations of tissues and cells. —**histographer,** *n.,* **histographic,** *adj.,* **histographically,** *adv.*

histoid neoplasm A growth that resembles the tissues in which it originates. Compare **organoid neoplasm.**

histologist A medical scientist who specializes in the study of **histology.**

histology **1.** The science dealing with the microscopic identification of cells and tissue. **2.** The structure of organ tissues, including the composition of cells and their organization into various body tissues. —**histologic, histological,** *adj.,* **histologically,** *adv.*

histone Any of a group of strongly basic, low molecular weight proteins that are soluble in water, insoluble in dilute ammonia, and combine with nucleic acid to form nucleoproteins. They are found in the cell nucleus, especially of glandular tissue, where they form a complex with deoxyribonucleic acid in the chromatin and function in regulating gene activity. Histones also interfere with coagulation of the blood and

have been isolated from the urine of patients with leukemia and febrile conditions.

Histoplasma capsulatum A dimorphic fungal organism that is a single budding yeast at body temperature and a mold at room temperature. The fungus, spread by airborne spores from soil contaminated with excreta from infected birds, acts as a parasite on the cells of the reticuloendothelial system.

histoplasmosis An infection caused by inhalation of spores of the fungus *Histoplasma capsulatum.* **Primary histoplasmosis** is characterized by fever, malaise, cough, and lymphadenopathy. Spontaneous recovery is usual; small calcifications remain in the lungs and affected lymph glands. **Progressive histoplasmosis,** the sometimes fatal, disseminated form of the infection, is characterized by ulcerating sores in the mouth and nose, enlargement of the spleen, liver, and lymph nodes, and severe and extensive infiltration of the lungs. Infection confers immunity; a histoplasmin skin test may be performed to identify people who may safely work with contaminated soil. The disease is most common in the Mississippi and Ohio Valleys.

history **1.** A record of past events. **2.** A systematic account of the medical and psychosocial occurrences in a patient's life and of factors in family, ancestors, and environment that may have a bearing on the patient's present condition.

history of present illness An account obtained during the interview with the patient of the onset, duration, and character of the present illness as well as of any acts or factors that aggravate or ameliorate the symptoms.

histotroph, histotrophe See **embryotroph.**

histotrophic nutrition See **embryotroph.**

histrionic personality disorder A disorder characterized by dramatic, reactive, and intensely exaggerated behavior, typically self-centered and resulting in severe disturbance in interpersonal relationships that can lead to psychosomatic disorders, depression, alcoholism, and drug dependency. Symptoms include emotional excitability, such as irrational angry outbursts or tantrums; abnormal craving for activity and excitement; overreaction to minor events; manipulative threats and gestures; egocentricity; inconsiderateness; inconsistency; and continuous demand for reassurance because of feelings of helplessness and dependency. A person having this disorder is perceived by others as vain, demanding, superficial, self-centered, and self-indulgent. The disorder is more prevalent in women than in men and is treated by various psychotherapies, depending on the individual and the severity of the condition.

hives *Nontechnical.* Pruritic eruption of the skin, typically consisting of small elevated wheals with a blanched center and surrounding redness. The individual lesions often fade within hours but may recur, as in chronic urticaria. Many cases of hives are precipitated immunologically by certain foods or drugs. Acute hives are characterized by capillary dilation in the dermis, leading to a loss of fluid into the tissues. Treatment includes antihistamines and removal of the stimulus or allergen, if possible. Also called **urticaria.** Compare **angioneurotic edema.**

H₂O See **water.**

HLA See **human leukocyte antigen.**

HLA-A *abbr* human leukocyte antigen A.

HLA-B *abbr* human leukocyte antigen B.

HLA-D *abbr* human leukocyte antigen D.

HLA-L *abbr* human leukocyte antigen L.

HMO See **Health Maintenance Organization.**

Ho Symbol for **holmium.**

H₀ Symbol for **null hypothesis.**

hod- A combining form meaning 'pertaining to pathways': *hodology, hodoneuromare.*

Hodgkin's disease A malignant disorder characterized by painless, progressive enlargement of lymphoid tissue, usually first evident in cervical lymph nodes; splenomegaly; and the presence of Reed-Sternberg cells, large, atypical histiocytes with multiple or hyperlobulated nuclei and prominent nucleoli. Symptoms include anorexia, weight loss, generalized pruritus, low-grade fever, night sweats, anemia, and leukocytosis. The disease is diagnosed in about 7,100 Americans annually, causes approximately 1,700 deaths a year, affects twice as many males as females, and usually develops between the ages of 15 and 35. The diagnosis is established by blood studies, X-rays, lymphangiograms, lymph node biopsies, and ultrasonic and computerized tomographic scans. Total lymphoid radiotherapy, using a covering mantle to protect other organs, is the treatment of choice for early stages of the disease; combination chemotherapy is the treatment for advanced disease. Long-term remissions are achieved in more than half the patients treated, and 60% to 90% of those with localized disease may be cured.

Hoffmann's atrophy See **Werdnig-Hoffmann disease.**

Hoffmann's reflex An abnormal reflex elicited by sudden, forceful flicking of the nail of the index, middle, or ring finger, resulting in flexion of the thumb and of the middle and distal phalanges of one of the other fingers. It is a possible, though not very reliable, sign of pyramidal tract disease above the level of the seventh or eighth cervical and first thoracic vertebra. Also called **Hoffmann's sign.**

hol- See **holo-.**

holandric **1.** Designating genes located on the nonhomologous portion of the Y chromosome. **2.** Of or pertaining to traits or conditions transmitted only through the paternal line. Compare **hologynic.**

holism, wholism A philosophical concept in which an entity is seen as more than the sum of its parts.

holistic health care A system of comprehensive or total patient care that considers the physical, emotional, social, economic, and spiritual needs of the person; the response to the illness; and the impact of the illness on the person's ability to meet self-care needs. Also called **comprehensive care.**

holmium (Ho) A rare-earth metallic element. Its atomic number is 67; its atomic weight is 164.93.

holo-, hol- A combining form meaning 'entire or pertaining to the whole': *holodiastolic, holomastigote, holotonia.*

holoacardius A separate, grossly defective monozygotic twin fetus, usually represented by a shapeless, nonformed mass, in which the heart is absent and the circulation in utero is accomplished totally by the heart of the viable twin through a vascular shunt.

holoacardius acephalus A grossly defective separate twin fetus that lacks a heart, a head, and most of the upper portion of the body.

holoacardius acormus A grossly defective, separate twin fetus in which the trunk is malformed and little more than the head is recognizable.

holoacardius amorphus A malformed separate twin fetus in which there are no recognizable or formed parts.

holoblastic Of or pertaining to an ovum that contains little or no yolk and undergoes total cleavage. Compare **meroblastic.**

holocephalic A malformed fetus in which several parts are deficient although the head is complete.

holodiastolic See **pandiastolic.**

hologynic **1.** Designating genes located on attached X chromosomes. **2.** Of or pertaining to traits or conditions transmitted only through the maternal line. Compare **holandric.**

holoprosencephaly A congenital defect caused by the failure of the prosencephalon to divide into hemispheres during embryonic development. It is characterized by multiple midline facial defects, including cyclopia in severe cases. It can also be caused by an extra chromosome in the 13-15 or D group, manifesting as one of many developmental defects. See also **trisomy 13.** —**holoprosencephalic, holoprosencephalous,** *adj.*

holorachischisis See **complete rachischisis.**

holosystolic See **pansystolic.**

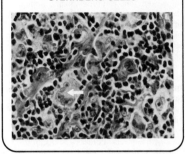

HODGKIN'S DISEASE: REED-STERNBERG CELLS

Holtzman inkblot technique A modification of the Rorschach test in which many more pictures of inkblots are used, the subject is permitted only one response to each design, and the scoring is predominantly objective rather than subjective.

Homan's sign Pain in the calf with dorsiflexion of the foot, indicating thrombophlebitis or thrombosis.

homatropine hydrobromide A mydriatic agent.

homatropine methylbromide A gastrointestinal anticholinergic agent.

home care A health service provided in the client's place of residence for the purpose of promoting, maintaining, or restoring health or minimizing the effects of illness and disability. Service may include such elements as medical, dental, and nursing care, speech and physical therapy, the homemaking services of a home health aide, or the provision of transportation.

home health agency An organization that provides health care in the home. Medicare certification for a home health agency is dependent on the providing of skilled nursing services and of at least one additional therapeutic service.

home maintenance management: impaired A nursing diagnosis accepted by the Fifth National Conference on the Classification of Nursing Diagnoses. This diagnosis describes the situation in which a client is unable to maintain a safe, healthy home environment without help. The etiology may include any of the following: disease or injury of a member of the family or household, disorganization of the family, inadequate finances, lack of knowledge of community or neighborhood resources, impaired or disordered emotional or cognitive function, inadequate support from others, lack of knowledge, or lack of role models competent in home maintenance. Among the defining characteristics reported by the client and other members of the household are difficulty in maintaining the home in a comfortable condition, a need for help from the outside in maintaining the home, and the existence of debt or a financial crisis. Among the defining characteristics that may be observed in the home are disorder, an offensive odor, an inappropriate temperature, lack of necessary equipment or supplies, and the presence of rodents or vermin. The critical defining characteristics, at least one of which must be present for the diagnosis to be made, are unwashed or unavailable cooking utensils, clothes, or linens; the presence of accumulations of dirt, food, waste, and refuse; exhausted or distressed family or household members; and repeated infections and infestations owing to lack of hygiene. See also **nursing diagnosis.**

homeo-, homoeo-, homoio- A combining form meaning 'sameness, similarity': *homeochrome, homeomorphus, homeothermal.*

Homeopathic Pharmacopoeia of the United States One of the three official drug compendia specified in the Federal Food, Drug, and Cosmetic Act. See also **compendium,** *Na-* *tional Formulary, United States Pharmacopoeia.*

homeopathist A physician who practices homeopathy.

homeopathy A system of therapeutics based on the theory that "like cures like." The theory was advanced in the late 18th century by Dr. Samuel Hahnemann, who believed that a large amount of a particular drug may cause symptoms of a disease and moderate dosage may reduce those symptoms; thus, some disease symptoms could be treated by very small doses of medicine. In practice, homeopathists dilute drugs with milk sugar in ratios of 1:10 to achieve the smallest dose of a drug that seems necessary to control the symptoms in a patient and prescribe only one medication at a time. Compare **allopathy. —homeopathic,** *adj.*

homeostasis A relative constancy in the internal environment of the body, naturally maintained by adaptive responses that promote healthy survival. Various sensing, feedback, and control mechanisms function to effect this steady state. Some of the key control mechanisms are the reticular formation in the brain stem and the endocrine glands. Some of the functions controlled by homeostatic mechanisms are the heartbeat, hematopoiesis, blood pressure, body temperature, electrolyte balance, respiration, and glandular secretion. **—homeostatic,** *adj.*

homeotypic, homeotypical Pertaining to or characteristic of the regular or usual type, specifically applied to the second meiotic division of germ cells in gametogenesis as distinguished from the first meiotic division. Compare **heterotypic.**

homo- A combining form meaning: **1.** 'The same' *homocentric, homodont, homolysis.* **2.** 'The addition of one CH_2 group to the main compound': *homocheldonine, homocystine, homoquinine.*

homoblastic Developing from the same germ layer or a single type of tissue. Compare **heteroblastic.**

homochronous inheritance The appearance of traits or conditions in the offspring at the same age as they appeared in the parents.

homocystinuria A rare biochemical abnormality characterized by the abnormal presence of homocystine, an amino acid, in the blood and urine, caused by any of several enzyme deficiencies in the metabolic pathway of methionine to cystine. Inherited as an autosomal recessive trait, the clinical signs of the disease are similar to Marfan's syndrome, including mental retardation, osteoporosis leading to skeletal abnormalities, dislocated lenses, and thromboembolism. Treatment may include a diet low in methionine and supplementation with large doses of vitamin B_6. **—homocystinuric,** *adj.*

homoeo- See **homeo-.**

homogeneous **1.** Consisting of similar elements or parts. **2.** Having a uniform quality throughout. Compare **heterogeneous. —homogeneity,** *adj.*

homogenesis Reproduction by the same

process in succeeding generations so that offspring are similar to the parents. Compare **heterogenesis.**

homogenetic **1.** Of or pertaining to homogenesis. **2.** See **homogenous,** definition 2.

homogenous **1.** Homogeneous. **2.** Having a likeness in form or structure because of a common ancestral origin. Compare **heterogenous. 3.** Homoplasy.

homogentisic acid See **glycosuric acid.**

homogeny **1.** Homogenesis. **2.** A likeness in structure or form owing to a common ancestral origin. Compare **homoplasy.**

homolog, homologue **1.** Any organ that corresponds in function, origin, and structure to another organ (as the flippers of a seal, which correspond to human hands). **2.** In chemistry: one of a series of compounds, each formed by an added common element, as CO, carbon monoxide, is followed by CO_2, carbon dioxide, with the addition of an oxygen atom. —**homologous,** *adj.*

homologous chromosomes Any two chromosomes in the diploid complement of the somatic cell that are identical in size, shape, and gene loci. In man there are 22 pairs of homologous chromosomes and one pair of sex chromosomes, with one member of each pair being derived from the mother and the other from the father.

homologous disease See **graft-versus-host reaction.**

homologous insemination See **artificial insemination husband.**

homologous tumor A neoplasm made up of cells resembling those of the tissue in which it is growing.

homonymous hemianopia Blindness or defective vision in the right or left halves of the visual fields of both eyes.

homoplasy Having a likeness in form or structure acquired through similar environmental conditions or parallel evolution rather than common ancestral origin. Compare **homogeny.** —**homoplastic,** *adj.*

homosexual **1.** Of, pertaining to, or denoting the same sex. **2.** A person who is sexually attracted to members of the same sex. Compare **heterosexual.** See also **lesbian.**

homosexual panic An acute attack of anxiety based on unconscious conflicts concerning gender identity and a fear of being homosexual. Compare **heterosexual panic.**

homovanillic acid A terminal metabolite of dopamine, norepinephrine, and serotonin that occurs in normal urine as a phenolic compound. A high level of homovanillic acid, representing an increased breakdown of its precursors, is found in the cerebrospinal fluid of patients in hepatic coma.

homozygosis **1.** The formation of a zygote by the union of two gametes that have one or more pairs of identical genes. **2.** The production of purebred organisms or strains through the process of inbreeding.

homozygous Having two identical genes at

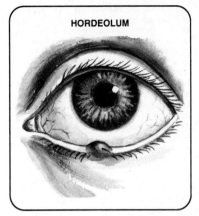

HORDEOLUM

corresponding loci on homologous chromosomes. An individual who is homozygous for a particular characteristic has inherited from each parent one of two identical genes for that characteristic. A person homozygous for a genetic disease caused by a pair of recessive genes, as sickle cell anemia, manifests the disorder, and his or her offspring have a 100% chance of inheriting the gene for the disease. Compare **heterozygous.**

homunculus, *pl.* **homunculi** **1.** A dwarf in which all the body parts are proportionally developed and in which there is no deformity or abnormality. **2.** In early embryological theories of development, primarily preformation: a minute and complete human being contained in each of the germ cells which after fertilization grows from the microscopic to normal size; by extension, the human fetus. **3.** A small anatomical model of the human form; a manikin, specifically, one believed to have been produced by an alchemist and placed in a flask. **4.** In psychiatry: a little man created by the imagination who possesses magical powers.

hookworm *Nontechnical.* A nematode of the genera *Ancylostoma, Necator,* or *Uncinaria.* Most hookworm infections in the Western Hemisphere are caused by the species *Necator americanus.*

hordeolum A furuncle of the margin of the eyelid originating in the sebaceous gland of an eyelash. Treatment includes hot compresses and antibiotic ophthalmic preparations; it occasionally requires incision and drainage. Also called **sty.** Compare **chalazion.**

horizon A specific stage of human embryonic development based on the appearance and ultimate formation of certain anatomical characteristics. The classification comprises 23 stages, each lasting 2 to 3 days, beginning with the fertilization of the ovum and ending 7 to 9 weeks later with the initiation of the fetal period of intrauterine life.

horizontal fissure of the right lung A cleft that marks the separation of the upper and middle lobes of the right lung.

horizontal transmission The spread of an infectious agent from one person or group to another, usually through contact with contaminated material, such as sputum or feces.

horm- A combining form meaning 'to urge or stimulate': *hormesis, hormonal, hormothyrin.*

hormic psychology In psychology: the school that stresses the purposive, goal-oriented nature of human behavior. Also called hormism.

hormone A complex chemical substance produced in one part or organ of the body that initiates or regulates the activity of an organ or a group of cells in another part of the body. Hormones secreted by the endocrine glands are carried through the bloodstream to the target organ. Secretion of these hormones is regulated by other hormones, by neurotransmitters, and by a negative feedback system in which an excess of target organ activity signals a decreased need for the stimulating hormone. Other hormones are released by organs for local effect, most commonly in the digestive tract.

-hormone A combining form meaning: **1.** A 'chemical substance possessing a regulatory effect' classified by source: *necrohormone, phytohormone, zoohormone.* **2.** A 'chemical substance possessing a regulatory effect' classified by activity affected: *cytohormone, neurohormone, parathormone.*

Horner's syndrome A neurologic condition characterized by miotic pupils, ptosis, and facial anhidrosis, resulting from a lesion in the spinal cord, with damage to a cervical nerve.

horny layer See **stratum corneum.**

horripilation See **pilomotor reflex.**

horse serum Immune serum prepared from the blood of a horse, especially tetanus antitoxin. As many people are sensitive to horse serum, a skin test for sensitivity is usually performed prior to immunization. Tetanus immune globulin prepared from human immune serum is preferred.

horseshoe fistula An abnormal, semicircular passage in the perianal area with both openings on the surface of the skin.

Hortega cells See **microglia.**

Horton's arteritis See **temporal arteritis.**

Horton's headache See **migrainous cranial neuralgia.**

Horton's histamine cephalalgia See **histamine headache.**

hospice A system of family-centered care designed to assist the chronically ill person to be comfortable and to maintain a satisfactory life-style through the terminal phases of dying. Hospice care is multidisciplinary and includes home visits, professional medical help available on call, teaching and emotional support of the family, and physical care of the client. Some hospice programs provide care in a center as well as in the home.

hospital-acquired infection See **nosocomial infection.**

hospital information system (HIS) A computer-based information system with multiaccess units to collect, organize, store, and make available data for problem-solving and decision-making.

hospitalism The physical or mental effects of hospitalization or institutionalization on patients, especially infants and children in whom the condition is characterized by social regression, personality disorders, and stunted growth. See also **anaclitic depression.**

Hospital Survey and Construction Act See **Hill-Burton Act.**

host **1.** An organism in which another, usually parasitic organism is nourished and harbored. A **primary,** or **definitive host** is one in which the adult parasite lives and reproduces. A **secondary,** or **intermediate host** is one in which the parasite exists in its nonsexual, larval stage. A **reservoir host** is a primary animal host for organisms that are sometimes parasitic in man and from which humans may become infected. **2.** The recipient of a transplanted organ or tissue. Compare **donor.**

hot bath A bath in which the temperature of the water is gradually raised to about 41°C (106°F).

hot flash A transient sensation of warmth experienced by some women during or after menopause. Hot flashes result from autonomic vasomotor disturbances that accompany changes in the neurohormonal activity of the ovaries, hypothalamus, and pituitary. The exact etiologic mechanism is not known. Hot flashes may be alleviated by cyclic administration of exogenous estrogen.

hot line A means of contacting a trained counselor or specific agency for help with a particular problem, as a rape hot line or a battered-child hot line. The person needing help calls a telephone number and speaks to a counselor who remains anonymous and who offers emotional support, specific recommendations for action, and referral to other medical, social, or community services. Such services are usually maintained by volunteers who answer phones 24 hours a day, 7 days a week.

hot spot In molecular genetics: a site in a gene sequence at which mutations occur with an unusually high frequency.

housemaid's knee A chronic inflammation of the bursa in front of the kneecap, characterized by redness and swelling. It is caused by prolonged and repetitive pressure of the knee on a hard surface.

house physician A physician on call and immediately available in a hospital or other health-care facility.

housewives eczema *Nontechnical.* Contact dermatitis of the hands caused and exacerbated by their frequent immersion in water and by the use of soaps and detergents.

Houston's valves See **plicae transversales recti.**

Howell-Jolly bodies Spherical and granular inclusions in the erythrocytes observed on microscopic examination of stained blood smears. They are most commonly seen in people who have hemolytic or pernicious anemia, leukemia,

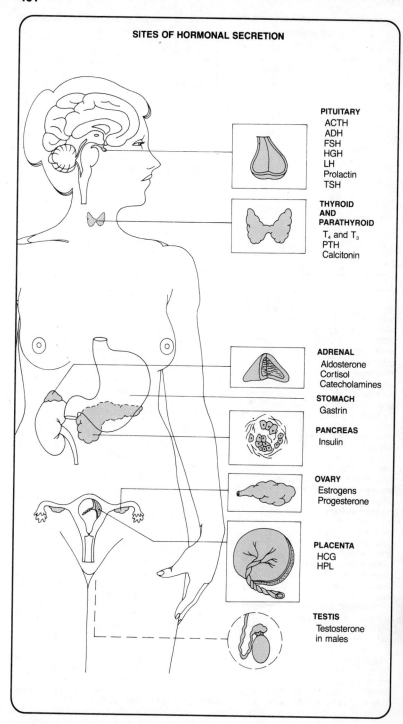

SITES OF HORMONAL SECRETION

PITUITARY
ACTH
ADH
FSH
HGH
LH
Prolactin
TSH

THYROID AND PARATHYROID
T_4 and T_3
PTH
Calcitonin

ADRENAL
Aldosterone
Cortisol
Catecholamines

STOMACH
Gastrin

PANCREAS
Insulin

OVARY
Estrogens
Progesterone

PLACENTA
HCG
HPL

TESTIS
Testosterone
in males

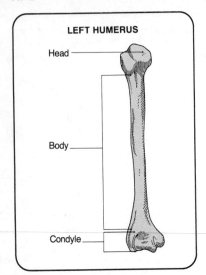

LEFT HUMERUS

Head

Body

Condyle

thalassemia, or congenital absence of the spleen and in those who have had a splenectomy.

HPL *abbr* **human placental lactogen.**

h.s. In prescriptions: *abbr hora somni,* a Latin phrase meaning 'bedtime.'

HSA *abbr* **health systems agency.**

HSV *abbr* herpes simplex virus. See **herpes genitalis, herpes simplex.**

Hubbard tank A large tank in which a patient may be immersed in order to perform underwater exercise. The mechanism provides superficial heat and is generally used for exercising the trunk and lower limbs. See also **whirlpool bath.**

Hüerthle cell tumor A neoplasm of the thyroid gland composed of large cells with granular eosinophilic cytoplasm (Hüerthle cells); it may be benign (Hüerthle cell adenoma) or malignant (Hüerthle cell carcinoma).

human chorionic gonadotropin (HCG) See **chorionic gonadotropin.**

human investigations committee A committee established in a hospital, school, or university to review applications for research involving human subjects to protect the rights of the people to be studied. Also called **human subjects investigation committee.**

humanism A belief in the goodness and value of man, with a committment to work for mankind.

humanistic-existential therapy A kind of psychotherapy that promotes self-awareness and personal growth by stressing current reality and by analyzing and altering specific patterns of response to help realize the potential of a person. Kinds of humanistic-existential psychotherapy are **client-centered therapy, existential therapy, Gestalt therapy.** Also called **existential-humanistic psychotherapy.**

humanistic nursing model A conceptual framework in which the nurse-patient relation-

ship is analyzed as a human-to-human event rather than a nurse-to-client interaction. Four phases are recognized in the development of the therapeutic relationship. The encounter phase is followed by the phase in which the identities of the nurse and patient emerge. The nurse empathizes and then sympathizes with the patient. Nursing intervention proceeds in five steps: observation of the need for intervention; validation of this observation; determination of the ability of the nurse to meet the necessity for referral; formulation of a plan for meeting the need; and evaluation of the degree to which the need was met.

humanistic psychology A branch of psychology that emphasizes a person's struggle to develop and maintain an integrated, harmonious personality as the primary motivational force in human behavior. See also **self-actualization.**

human leukocyte antigen (HLA) Any one of four significant genetic markers identified as specific loci on chromosome 6. They are HLA-A, HLA-B, HLA-L, and HLA-D. Each locus has several genetically determined alleles; each of these is associated with certain diseases or conditions, as HLA-B27 is usually present in people who have ankylosing spondylitis. The HLA system is used to assess tissue compatibility. White blood cells are used for testing. Perfect tissue compatibility exists only between identical twins.

human placental lactogen (HPL) A protein hormone secreted by the placenta that helps to promote growth.

human subjects investigation committee See **human investigations committee.**

humeral articulation See **shoulder joint.**

humerus, *pl.* **humeri** The largest bone of the upper arm, comprising a body, a head, and a condyle. The body is almost cylindrical proximally, prismatic and flattened distally, and has two borders and three surfaces. The nearly hemispherical head articulates with the glenoid cavity of the scapula and has a constriction called the surgical neck, frequently the seat of a fracture. The condyle at the distal end of the bone has several depressions into which articulate the radius and ulna. Also called **arm bone.** —**humeral,** *adj.*

humidifier lung A type of hypersensitivity pneumonitis common among workers involved with refrigeration and air-conditioning equipment. The antigens to which the hypersensitive reaction occurs are genera of the fungi *Micropolyspora* and *Thermoactinomyces.* Symptoms of the acute form of the disease include chills, cough, fever, dyspnea, anorexia, nausea, and vomiting. The chronic form of the disease is characterized by fatigue, chronic cough, weight loss, and dyspnea on exercise. Also called **air conditioner lung.** See also **pneumonitis.**

humoral immunity One of the two forms of immunity that respond to antigens, as bacteria and foreign tissue. Humoral immunity is the result of the development and the continuing presence of circulating antibodies carried in the immunoglobulins IgA, IgB, and IgM. Circulating antibodies are produced by the plasma cells of the reticuloendothelial system. Compare **cellular immunity.**

humoral response One of a broad category of hypersensitivity reactions. Humoral responses are mediated by B cell lymphocytes and occur in type I, type II, and type III hypersensitivity reactions. Compare **cellular immunity.**

hung-up reflex A deep tendon reflex in which, after a stimulus is given and the reflex action takes place, there is a slow return of the limb to its neutral position. This prolonged relaxation phase is characteristic of the reflexes in patients with hypothyroidism. See also **deep tendon reflex.**

Hunner's ulcer See **interstitial cystitis.**

Hunter's canal See **adductor canal.**

Hunter's syndrome A hereditary defect in mucopolysaccharide metabolism affecting only males, characterized by dwarfism, kyphosis, gargoylism, and mental retardation. It is transmitted as an X-linked recessive trait. Females who carry the gene can be identified by biochemical tests. Also called **MPS II.** See also **mucopolysaccharidosis.**

Huntington's chorea A rare, abnormal hereditary condition characterized by chronic, progressive chorea and mental deterioration that terminates in dementia. An individual afflicted with the condition usually shows the first signs in the 4th decade of life and dies about 15 years later. The condition is transmitted as an autosomal trait. Also called **chronic chorea, degenerative chorea.**

Hurler's syndrome A type of mucopolysaccharidosis, transmitted as an autosomal recessive trait, that results in severe mental retardation. The onset of the symptoms of Hurler's syndrome occurs within the first few months of life. Characteristic signs of the disease are enlargement of the liver and the spleen, often with cardiovascular involvement. Facial characteristics of individuals affected by Hurler's syndrome include a low forehead and enlargement of the head, sometimes resulting from hydrocephalus. Corneal clouding is common and the neck is short. Marked kyphosis is apparent at the dorsolumbar level, and the hands and the fingers are short and broad. Flexion contractures are common with this disease. Hurler's syndrome usually results in death during childhood from cardiac complications or pulmonary disorders. Also called **MPS I.** See also **mucopolysaccharidosis.**

Hutchinson's disease See **angioma serpiginosum.**

Hutchinson's freckle A tan patch on the skin that grows slowly, becoming mottled, dark, thick, and nodular. The lesion is usually seen on one side of the face of an elderly person. Local excision is recommended as it often becomes malignant. Also called **lentigo maligna.**

Hutchinson's teeth A characteristic of congenital syphilis in which all the permanent

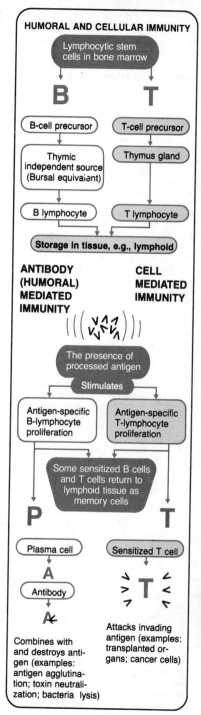

incisor teeth are peg-shaped, widely spaced, and notched at the end with a centrally placed crescent-shaped deformity.

Hutchinson's triad The interstitial keratitis, notched teeth, and deafness characteristic of congenital syphilis.

Hutchison-type neuroblastoma A neuroblastoma that has metastasized to the cranium.

hyaline cartilage The gristly, elastic connective tissue comprised of specialized cells in a translucent, pearly-blue matrix. Hyaline cartilage thinly covers the articulating ends of bones, connects the ribs to the sternum, and supports the nose, trachea, and part of the larynx. Compare **white fibrocartilage, yellow cartilage.**

hyaline membrane disease See **respiratory distress syndrome of the newborn.**

hyaline thrombus A translucent, colorless mass consisting of hemolyzed erythrocytes.

hyalo-, hyal- A combining form meaning 'resembling glass': *hyaloenchondroma, hyaloplasm, hyaloid.*

hyaloid artery An embryonic blood vessel that branches to supply the vitreous body of the eye and develops part of the blood supply to the capsula vasculosa lentis. The hyaloid artery disappears from the fetus in the 9th month of pregnancy, leaving a vestigial remnant that persists in the adult as a narrow passage through the vitreous body from the optic disk to the posterior surface of the crystalline lens.

hyaloplasm The portion of the cytoplasm that is clear and more fluid, as opposed to the granular and reticular part. Also called **cytohyaloplasm, cytolymph, enchylema,** hyalotome, **interfilar mass, interfibrillar mass of Flemming, paramitome, paraplasm.**

hyaluronic acid A mucopolysaccharide formed by the polymerization of acetylglucosamine and glucuronic acid, occurring in vitreous humor, synovial fluids, and various tissues. Known as the cement substance of tissues, it forms a gel in intercellular spaces.

hyaluronidase An enzyme administered parenterally.

hybrid 1. An offspring produced from mating plants or animals from different species, varieties, or genotypes. **2.** Of or pertaining to such a plant or animal.

hybridization 1. The process of producing hybrids by crossbreeding. **2.** In molecular genetics: the process of combining single-stranded nucleic acids whose base composition is identical but whose base sequence is different to form stable double-stranded duplex molecules. The technique involves the fragmentation and separation of the double-stranded molecules by heating, then recombination through cooling. The resulting hybrids can be of a DNA-DNA, DNA-RNA, or RNA-RNA nature.

hybrid vigor See **heterosis.**

hydantoin Any one of a group of anticonvulsant medications, chemically and pharmacologically similar to the barbiturates, that act to limit seizure activity and reduce the spread of the abnormal electrical excitation from the focus of the seizure. A primary drug in the management of almost all forms of epilepsy, the most common hydantoin in current use is phenytoin, formerly known as diphenylhydantoin. Toxic effects of the drug include cardiovascular collapse and central nervous system depression when it is given in excessive dosage intravenously, as may occur in the emergency treatment of status epilepticus. Chronic toxicity, which is related to the dosage and the route of administration, may result in behavioral change, gastrointestinal disturbance, osteomalacia, gingival hyperplasia, or megaloblastic anemia. Hypersensitivity reactions are rare but serious. Frequent observation for the blood concentrations of hydantoin are necessary. Seizures are usually controlled at a level of 10 to 20 micrograms/ml; higher levels of concentration are associated with toxic effects. Phenytoin interacts with many drugs, including chloramphenicol, warfarin, disulfiram, isoniazid, salicylates, phenylbutazone, and some sulfonamides. The interaction usually has the adverse effect of increasing the concentration of phenytoin in the blood, resulting in toxicity. See **barbiturates.**

hydatid A cyst or cystlike structure that usually is filled with fluid, especially the cyst formed around the developing scolex of the dog tapeworm *Echinococcus granulosus.* Humans and sheep can become hosts to the larval stage by ingesting the eggs. See also **hydatid mole, hydatidosis. —hydatidiform,** *adj.*

hydatid cyst A cyst in the liver that contains larvae of the tapeworm *Echinococcus granulosus,* whose eggs are carried from the intestinal tract to the liver via the portal circulation. Patients are generally asymptomatic, except for hepatomegaly and a dull ache over the right upper quadrant of the abdomen. Radiologic tests are employed in diagnosis, and since no medical treatment is available, surgical removal of the cyst is indicated. Compare **hydatid mole.**

hydatid disease See **echinococcosis.**

hydatid mole An intrauterine neoplastic mass of grapelike, enlarged chorionic villi occurring in approximately 1 in 1,500 pregnancies in the United States and 8 times more frequently in some oriental countries. Molar pregnancies are more common in older and younger women than in those between the ages of 20 and 40. The cause of the degenerative disorder is not known. Characteristic signs of the condition are extreme nausea, uterine bleeding, anemia, hyperthyroidism, an unusually large uterus for the length of pregnancy, absence of fetal heart sounds, edema, and high blood pressure. Diagnostic measures include ultrasonography, amniography, and serial bioassay of chorionic gonadotropin in the blood. In most cases the mole is discovered when abortion is threatened or in progress. Oxytocin may be used to stimulate the evacuation of a mole that is not spontaneously aborted, and curettage is usually performed several days later to be certain that no molar tissue remains in the uterus. It is important that pregnancy be avoided for at least 1 year and that assays for chorionic gonadotropin be performed to minimize the risk of developing trophoblastic choriocarcinoma. Also called hydatidiform mole, molar pregnancy. See also **trophoblastic cancer.**

hydatidosis   Infestation with the tapeworm *Echinococcus granulosus*. See also **hydatid cyst.**

hydradenitis, hidradenitis   An infection or inflammation of the sweat glands.

hydralazine hydrochloride   A vasodilator antihypertensive agent.

hydramnios   An abnormal condition of pregnancy characterized by an excess of amniotic fluid. It occurs in less than 1% of pregnancies and is diagnosed by palpation, ultrasonography, or X-ray examination. It is associated with maternal disorders, including toxemia of pregnancy and diabetes mellitus. Some fetal disorders, including anomalies of the gastrointestinal tract, respiratory tract, and cardiovascular system, may interfere with normal exchange of amniotic fluid, resulting in hydramnios. Fetal hydrops and multiple gestation are also associated with the condition. The incidence of premature rupture of the membranes, premature labor, and perinatal mortality are increased. Periodic amniocentesis may be necessary. Also called **polyhydramnios.**

hydrargyrism   See **mercury poisoning.**

hydremic ascites   An abnormal accumulation of fluid within the peritoneal cavity accompanied by hemodilution, as in protein-calorie malnutrition. See also **ascites.**

-hydria   A combining form meaning 'level of fluid in the body': *histohydria, isohydria, oligohydria.*

hydriodic acid   An expectorant.

hydro-, hydr-   A combining form meaning 'pertaining to water or hydrogen': *hydroadipsia, hydrocele, hydropexis.*

hydroa   An unusual vesicular and bullous skin condition of childhood that recurs each summer following exposure to sunlight, sometimes accompanied by itching and lichenification. Treatment includes use of sunscreen preparations and the avoidance of exposure to sunlight.

hydrocarbon   Any one of a large group of organic compounds, the molecules of which are composed of hydrogen and carbon, most of which are derived from petroleum.

hydrocephalus, hydrocephaly   A pathological condition characterized by an abnormal accumulation of cerebrospinal fluid, usually under increased pressure, within the cranial vault and subsequent dilatation of the ventricles. Interference with the normal flow of cerebrospinal fluid may be caused by increased secretion of the fluid, obstruction within the ventricular system (noncommunicating or intraventricular hydrocephalus), or defective reabsorption from the cerebral subarachnoid space (communicating or extraventricular hydrocephalus), resulting from developmental anomalies, infection, trauma, or brain tumors. The con-

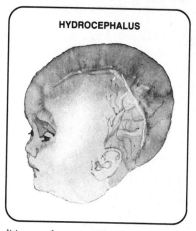

HYDROCEPHALUS

dition may be congenital with rapid onset of symptoms, or it may progress slowly so that neurological manifestations do not appear until early to late childhood or even until early adulthood. In infants, the head grows at an abnormal rate with separation of the sutures, bulging fontanelles, and dilated scalp veins; the face becomes disproportionately small; and the eyes appear depressed within the sockets. Typical behavior includes irritability with lethargy and vomiting, opisthotonos, lower-extremity spasticity, and failure to perform normal reflex actions. If the condition progresses, lower brain stem function is disrupted, the skull becomes enormous, the cortex is destroyed, and the infant displays somnolence, seizures, and cardiopulmonary obstruction, usually not surviving the neonatal period. At later onset, after the cranial sutures have fused and the skull has formed, symptoms are primarily neurological and include headache, edema of the optic disk, strabismus, and loss of muscular coordination. Hydrocephalus in infants is suspected when head growth is observed to be in excess of the normal rate. In all age groups diagnosis is confirmed by such procedures as cerebrospinal fluid examination, computerized axial tomography, air encephalography, arteriography, and echoencephalography. Treatment consists almost exclusively of surgical intervention to correct the ventricular obstruction, reduce the production of cerebrospinal fluid, or shunt the excess fluid by ventricular bypass to the right atrium of the heart or to the peritoneal cavity. Surgically treated hydrocephalus with continued neurosurgical and medical management has a survival rate of approximately 80%, although prognosis depends largely on the cause of the condition. Hydrocephalus is frequently associated with myelomeningocele, in which case there is a less favorable prognosis. NURSING CONSIDERATIONS: Primary care of the child with hydrocephalus consists of maintaining adequate nutrition, proper positioning and support to prevent extra strain on the neck, and assistance with diagnostic evaluation and pro-

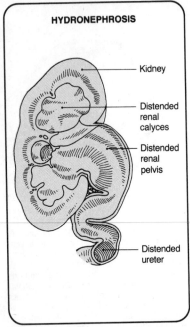

HYDRONEPHROSIS

Kidney

Distended renal calyces

Distended renal pelvis

Distended ureter

cedures. Postoperatively, in addition to routine care and observation to prevent complications, especially infection, the nurse gives support to the parents and teaches them how to care for a child with a functioning shunt, specifically how to recognize signs that indicate shunt malfunction or infection and how to pump the shunt.

hydrochloric acid A compound consisting of hydrogen and chlorine. Hydrochloric acid is secreted in the stomach and is a major component of gastric juice.

hydrochloric acid, dilute A systemic acidifier and digestant.

hydrochlorothiazide A thiazide diuretic.

hydrocodone bitartrate A narcotic antitussive agent.

hydrocortisone, h. acetate, h. sodium phosphate, h. sodium succinate, h. valerate Topical otic, ophthalmic, and systemic anti-inflammatory agents.

hydroflumethiazide A thiazide diuretic.

hydrogen (H) A gaseous, univalent element. Its atomic number is 1; its atomic weight is 1.008. It is the simplest and the lightest of the elements and is normally a colorless, odorless, highly inflammable diatomic gas. Hydrogen is a component of numerous compounds, many of them produced by the body. As a component of water, hydrogen is crucial in the metabolic interaction of acids, bases, and salts within the body and in the fluid balance necessary for the body to survive.

hydrogenation See **reduction.**

hydrogen peroxide A disinfectant.

hydrolysis The chemical alteration or de-

composition of a compound with water.

hydrometer A device that determines the specific gravity or density of a liquid by a comparison of its weight with that of an equal volume of water. A calibrated, hollow glass device is placed in the liquid being examined, and the depth to which the device settles in the liquid is noted.

hydromorphone hydrochloride A narcotic and opioid analgesic, sometimes used as an antitussive.

hydronephrosis Distention of the pelvis and calyces of the kidney by urine that cannot flow past an obstruction in a ureter. Ureteral obstruction may be caused by a tumor, a calculus lodged in the ureter, inflammation of the prostate gland, or edema owing to a urinary tract infection. The person may experience pain in the flank, and, in some cases, hematuria, pyuria, and hyperpyrexia. Intravenous pyelography, cystoscopy, or retrograde pyelography may be used in diagnosis. Surgical repair or removal of the obstruction may be necessary. Prolonged hydronephrosis will result in atrophy and eventual loss of kidney function. See also **urinary calculus.** —**hydronephrotic,** *adj.*

hydrophilic lotion and ointment, h. petrolatum Protectants and emollients.

hydrophobia 1. *Nontechnical.* Rabies. **2.** A morbid, extreme fear of water.

hydrophthalmos See **congenital glaucoma.**

hydrops An abnormal accumulation of clear, watery fluid in a body tissue or cavity, as a joint, Graafian follicle, fallopian tube, or the abdomen or middle ear. Formerly called **dropsy.**

hydrops fetalis Massive edema in the fetus or newborn, usually in association with severe erythroblastosis fetalis. Severe anemia and effusions of the pericardial, pleural, and peritoneal spaces also occur. The condition usually leads to death, even with immediate exchange transfusions following delivery.

hydroquinone An antihyperpigmentation agent.

hydrosalpinx An abnormal condition of the fallopian tube in which the tube is cystically enlarged and filled with clear fluid, the end result of an infection that has previously occluded the tube at both ends. The purulent material produced by the infection undergoes liquefaction during resolution of the acute phase of the inflammatory process.

hydrostatic pressure The pressure exerted by a liquid.

hydrous wool fat See **lanolin.**

hydroxyamphetamine hydrobromide A mydriatic agent.

hydroxybenzene See **carbolic acid.**

hydroxychloroquine sulfate An antimalarial agent.

hydroxyl (OH) A radical compound containing an oxygen atom and a hydrogen atom.

hydroxyprogesterone caproate A progestogen used to treat menstrual disorders and uterine cancer.

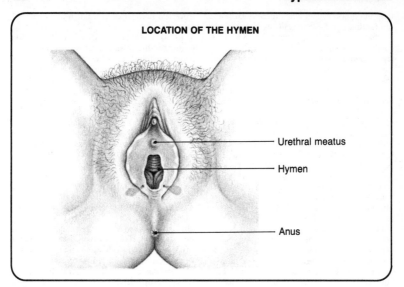

LOCATION OF THE HYMEN

- Urethral meatus
- Hymen
- Anus

hydroxyurea   An antimetabolite used in chemotherapy.

hydroxyzine hydrochloride, h. pamoate   Antianxiety agents.

hygroscopic humidifier   A humidifying device attached to the tubing circuit of a mechanical ventilator or anesthesia gas machine to maintain a constant rate of humidity in the patient's trachea.

hymen   A fold of mucous membrane, skin, and fibrous tissue at the introitus of the vagina. It may be absent, small, thin and pliant, or, rarely, tough and dense, completely occluding the introitus. When the hymen is ruptured, small rounded elevations remain. See also **carunculae hymenales.**

Hymenolepis   A genus of intestinal tapeworms infesting humans, as *Hymenolepis nana*, the dwarf tapeworm, and *H. diminuta.* Heavy infestation by *H. nana* may cause abdominal pain, bloody stools, and disorders of the nervous system, especially in children. Contaminated food spreads the disease, which is endemic in the United States. Quinacrine hydrochloride or hexylresorcinol is used to treat the infestation.

hyoglossal   See **glossohyal.**

hyoid bone   A single bone suspended from the styloid processes of the temporal bones. The body of the hyoid is square and flat, its ventral surface convex and angled cranially. Two greater wings of the bone attach to the lateral thyroid ligaments, and the body of the bone attaches to various muscles, as the hypoglossus and the sternohyoideus. The hyoid is palpable in the neck. Also called **lingual bone, os hyoideum.**

hyoscine   Scopolamine.

hyoscine hydrobromide   See **scopolamine hydrobromide.**

hyoscyamine   See **scopolamine.**

hyper-   A combining form meaning 'exces-

sive, above, or beyond': *hyperacidaminuria, hyperalkalinity, hyperechema.*

hyperactivity   See **attention deficit disorder.**

hyperadrenalism   See **Cushing's disease.**

hyperadrenocorticism   See **Cushing's syndrome.**

hyperaldosteronism   See **aldosteronism.**

hyperalimentation   **1.** Overfeeding or the ingestion or administration of a greater than optimal amount of nutrients in excess of the demands of the appetite. **2.** See **total parenteral nutrition.**

hyperammonemia   Abnormally high levels of ammonia in the blood. Ammonia is produced in the intestine, absorbed into the blood, and detoxified in the liver. If there is an increased production of ammonia or a decreased ability to detoxify it, levels of ammonia in the blood may increase. Untreated, the condition leads to asterixis, vomiting, lethargy, coma, and death.

hyperbetalipoproteinemia   Type II hyperlipoproteinemia, a genetic disorder of lipid metabolism, in which there are abnormally high levels of serum cholesterol, and xanthomas appear on the tendons of the heels, knees, and fingers. There is a marked tendency to develop atherosclerosis and early myocardial infarction, especially among males. Treatment attempts to reduce blood cholesterol levels. The patient is usually counseled to avoid most meats, eggs, milk products, and all saturated fats and is encouraged to eat fish, grains, fruits, vegetables, poultry, and unsaturated fats. See also **cholesterolemia.**

hyperbilirubinemia   Greater than normal amounts of the bile pigment bilirubin in the blood, often characterized by jaundice, anorexia, and malaise. Hyperbilirubinemia is most often associated with liver disease or biliary obstruction, but it also occurs when there is excessive destruction of red blood cells, as in hemolytic anemia. Treatment is specific to the underlying condition. See also **jaundice.**

hyperbilirubinemia of the newborn An excess of bilirubin in the blood of the neonate, resulting from hepatic dysfunction. Commonly known as kernicterus, it is usually caused by a deficiency of an enzyme, owing to physiologic immaturity, or by increased hemolysis, especially from blood group incompatibility, which, in severe cases, can lead to kernicterus. Serum bilirubin levels are elevated in the normal newborn because the concentration of circulating erythrocytes is greater and because infants have a decreased ability to conjugate and excrete bilirubin owing to a lack of the enzyme glucuronyl transferase, to reduced albumin concentration, and to a lack of intestinal bacteria. Jaundice appears when blood levels of bilirubin exceed 5 mg/100 ml, usually not before 24 hours in full-term neonates. Clinically observable jaundice or serum bilirubin levels exceeding 5 mg/100 ml within the first 24 hours of life are abnormal and indicate a pathologic cause of hyperbilirubinemia. Early symptoms of kernicterus are lethargy, poor feeding, and vomiting; followed by severe neurologic excitation or depression, including tremors, twitching, convulsion, opisthotonos, a high-pitched cry, hypotonia, diminished deep-tendon reflexes, and the absence of Moro and sucking reflexes. Brain damage generally does not occur at serum bilirubin levels below 20 mg/100 ml. Factors like metabolic acidosis, lowered albumin levels, hypoxia, hypothermia, free fatty acids, and certain drugs, especially salicylates and sulfonamides, increase the risk at much lower levels. The mortality may reach 50%. Sequelae of kernicterus include mental retardation, minimal brain dysfunction, cerebral palsy, delayed or abnormal motor development, hearing loss, ataxia, athetosis, perceptual problems, and behavioral disorders. Infants with mild jaundice require no treatment, only observation. Phototherapy is the usual treatment for severe or increasing hyperbilirubinemia. If hyperbilirubinemia is caused by increased hemolysis owing to blood group incompatibility, exchange transfusion is the standard procedure. It is usually indicated if laboratory analysis reveals a positive Coombs' test, a hemoglobin concentration of the cord blood below 12 g/100 ml, or a bilirubin level of 20 mg/100 ml or more in a full-term infant or 15 mg/100 ml or more in a premature infant. Phototherapy may be used in conjunction with exchange transfusion, except in Rh incompatibility. If used immediately after the initial exchange tranfusion, phototherapy may remove enough bilirubin from the tissues to make subsequent transfusions unnecessary. Pharmacologic management, as the use of barbiturates to stimulate protein synthesis which, in turn, increases albumin for conjugating bilirubin and promotes hepatic glucuronyl transferase synthesis, is indicated in some instances, although this form of therapy is con-troversial because of the known side effects of the drugs.

NURSING CONSIDERATIONS: An initial concern is to identify high-risk infants who may develop hyperbilirubinemia and kernicterus. The nurse may monitor the serum bilirubin levels and observe for evidence of jaundice, anemia, central nervous system irritability, and such conditions as acidosis, hypoxia, and hypothermia. In erythroblastosis fetalis, exchange transfusion may be necessary. The amounts of blood infused and withdrawn, the vital signs, and any signs of exchange reactions are noted. Resuscitative equipment is kept available. Optimal body temperature is maintained: hypothermia increases oxygen and glucose consumption, causing metabolic acidosis, and hyperthermia damages the donor's erythrocytes, causing an elevation in the amount of free potassium that may lead to infant cardiac arrest. After the procedure, a sterile dressing is applied to the catheter site. Also called **neonatal hyperbilirubinemia.** See also **breast milk jaundice, cholestasis, Crigler-Najjar syndrome, Dubin-Johnson syndrome, erythroblastosis fetalis, Gilbert's syndrome, phototherapy in the newborn, Rotor syndrome.**

hypercalcemia Greater than normal amounts of calcium in the blood, most often resulting from excessive bone resorption and release of calcium, as occurs in hyperparathyroidism, metastatic tumors of bone, Paget's disease, and osteoporosis. Clinically, people with hypercalcemia are confused and have anorexia, abdominal pain, and muscle pain and weakness. Extremely high levels of blood calcium may result in shock, kidney failure, and death. Hypercalciuria is also found in most patients with elevated blood calcium. Prednisone, diuretics, isotonic saline, and other drugs may be used in treatment. —**hypercalcemic,** *adj.*

hypercalciuria The presence of abnormally great amounts of calcium in the urine, resulting from conditions such as sarcoidosis, hyperparathyroidism, or certain types of arthritis, characterized by augmented bone resorption. Immobilized patients are often hypercalciuric. Treatment is directed toward correcting any underlying disease condition and limiting dietary intake of calcium. Also called hypercalcinuria. Compare **hypercalcemia.**

hypercapnia Greater than normal amounts of carbon dioxide in the blood. Also called hypercarbia.

hypercholesterolemia A condition in which greater than normal amounts of cholesterol are present in the blood. High levels of cholesterol and other lipids may lead to the development of atherosclerosis. Hypercholesterolemia may be reduced or prevented by avoiding saturated fats, which are found in red meats, eggs, and dairy products.

hypercholesterolemic xanthomatosis See **familial hypercholesterolemia.**

hyperchromic Having a greater density of color or pigment.

hyperchylomicronemia Type I hyperlipoproteinemia, a rare congenital deficiency of an enzyme essential to fat metabolism. Fat accumulates in the blood as chylomicrons. The condition affects children and young adults, who develop xanthomas (fatty deposits) in the skin, hepatomegaly, and abdominal pain. Strict limitation of dietary fat may allow the person to avoid discomfort and complications. Also called **familial lipoprotein lipase deficiency.**

hypercoagulability A tendency of the blood to coagulate more rapidly than is normal.

hyperdactyly, hyperdactylia, hyperdactylism See **polydactyly.**

hyperdiploid, hyperdiploidic See **hyperploid.**

hyperdynamic syndrome A cluster of symptoms that signal the onset of septic shock, often including a shaking chill, rapid rise in temperature, flushing of the skin, galloping pulse, and alternating rise and fall of the blood pressure. This is a medical emergency that requires expert medical support in a hospital. Emergency measures include keeping the patient warm and elevating the feet to assist venous return. Usually, it is ordered that nothing be given by mouth and that the patient's head be turned to avoid aspiration if there is vomiting. See **septic shock.**

hyperemesis gravidarum An abnormal condition of pregnancy characterized by protracted vomiting, weight loss, and fluid and electrolyte imbalance. If severe and intractable, brain damage, liver and kidney failure, and death may result. The cause of the condition is not known. It occurs in approximately 3 of every 1,000 pregnancies. Dehydration can result in dry mucous membranes, decreased skin elasticity, a rapid pulse, and falling blood pressure. The specific gravity of the urine rises and the volume of urine excreted falls. The hematocrit is elevated because of hemoconcentration. Loss of electrolytes in vomitus leads to metabolic acidosis with hypokalemia, hypochloremia, and hyponatremia. Severe potassium deficit alters myocardial function; the electrocardiogram may show prolonged PR and QT intervals and inverted T waves. In addition to weight loss, undernourishment causes fever, ketosis, and acetonuria. Severe vitamin B deficiency may result in encephalopathy manifested by confusion and, eventually, coma. NURSING CONSIDERATIONS: Effective therapy arrests vomiting, promotes adequate rest, and achieves rehydration, adequate nutrition, and emotional stabilization. Antiemetics safe for the fetus are administered. Fluids, electrolytes, nutrients, and vitamins are given parenterally if the woman is unable to retain fluids by mouth.

hyperemia Increased infusion of blood in part of the body, caused by increased blood flow, as in the inflammatory response, local relaxation of arterioles, or obstruction of blood outflow. Skin overlying a hyperemic area usually becomes reddened and warm. —**hyperemic,** *adj.*

hyperextension Of a joint: a position of maximum extension.

hyperextension bed A bed used in pediatric orthopedics to maintain any correction achieved by suspension of a body part and to increase the range of motion of the hips following an operative muscle-release procedure. The hyperextension bed may be purchased or it may be converted from a regular hospital bed. Removal of the mattress from a regular hospital bed and the addition of three half-mattresses allows sufficient height to permit alternating prone and supine positions and the concomitant alternating flexion and extension of the hips. The bilateral extremities of the patient, in casts, are suspended over the lower half of the bed with rings and traction apparatus. The position of the patient's hips is alternated at 2 hour intervals; abduction and adduction can be controlled by the position of the pulleys. Restraints are required to maintain the child in position so that the horizontal gluteal folds are even with the bottom edge of the stacked mattresses. Also called **Schwartz bed.** Compare **Foster bed, Stryker wedge frame.**

hyperextension suspension An orthopedic procedure used in the postoperative positioning of hip muscles. The procedure uses traction equipment, including metal frames, ropes, and pulleys, to relieve the weight of the lower limbs and to position properly the muscles of the hip without applying traction to the lower limbs involved. Compare **balanced suspension, lower extremity suspension, upper extremity suspension.**

hypergenesis Excessive growth or overdevelopment. The condition may involve the entire body, as in gigantism, or any particular part, or it may result in the formation of extra parts, as the development of additional fingers or toes. —**hypergenetic,** *adj.*

hyperglycemia A greater than normal amount of glucose in the blood. Most frequently associated with diabetes mellitus, the condition may occur in newborns, after the administration of glucocorticoid hormones, and with an excess infusion of intravenous solutions containing glucose, especially in poorly monitored, long-term hyperalimentation. Compare **hypoglycemia.**

hyperglycemic-glycogenolytic factor See **glucagon.**

hyperhidrosis Excessive perspiration, often caused by heat, hyperthyroidism, strong emotion, menopause, or infection. Symptomatic therapy usually includes topical antiperspirants and may involve surgery to remove axillary sweat glands.

hyperkalemia Greater than normal amounts of potassium in the blood. This condition is seen frequently in acute renal failure. Early signs are nausea, diarrhea, and muscle weakness. As potassium levels increase, marked cardiac changes are observed in the EKG. Treatment of severe hyperkalemia includes the intravenous administration of sodium bicarbonate, calcium salts, and dextrose. Hemodialysis is used if these measures fail.

TYPES OF HYPERLIPOPROTEINEMIA

TYPE	CAUSES AND INCIDENCE
I Frederickson's, fat-induced hyperlipemia, idiopathic familial	• Deficient or abnormal lipoprotein lipase, resulting in decreased or absent post–heparin lipolytic activity • Relatively rare
II Familial hyperbetalipoproteinemia, essential familial hypercholesterolemia	• Deficient cell-surface receptor that regulates low-density lipoprotein (LDL) degradation and cholesterol synthesis, resulting in increased levels of plasma LDL over joints and pressure points • Onset between ages 10 and 30
III Familial "broad beta" disease, xanthoma tuberosum	• Unknown underlying defect resulting in deficient conversion of triglyceride-rich very low-density lipoprotein (VLDL) to LDL • Uncommon; usually occurs after age 20 but can occur earlier in men
IV Endogenous hypertriglyceridemia, hyperbetalipoproteinemia	• Usually occurs secondary to obesity, alcoholism, diabetes, or emotional disorders • Relatively common, especially in middle-aged men
V Mixed hypertriglyceridemia, mixed hyperlipidemia	• Defective triglyceride clearance causes pancreatitis; usually secondary to another disorder, such as obesity or nephrosis • Uncommon; usually occurs in late adolescence or early adulthood

hyperkalemic periodic paralysis See **advnamia episodica hereditaria.**

hyperkeratosis 1. Overgrowth and thickening of the cornea. 2. Overgrowth of the cornified epithelial layer of the skin. See also **callus, corn.**

hyperkinesis See **attention deficit disorder.**

hyperkinetic Hyperactive. See **attention deficit disorder.**

hyperlipidemia A general term for an excess of any or all of the lipids in the plasma.

hyperlipoproteinemia Any of a large group of inherited and acquired disorders of lipoprotein metabolism characterized by greater than normal amounts of certain lipoproteins and cholesterol in the blood. The treatment includes diet to control obesity; diet may reduce lipoprotein levels in the blood. Medication and other treatments vary according to the specific metabolic defect, its cause, and its prognosis.

hypermagnesemia A greater than normal amount of magnesium in the plasma, found in people with kidney failure and in those who use a large quantity of drugs containing magnesium, as antacids. Toxic levels of magnesium cause cardiac arrhythmias and depression of deep tendon reflexes and respiration. Treatment often includes intravenous fluids, a diuretic, and hemodialysis.

hypermenorrhea See **menorrhagia.**

hypermetria An abnormal condition, a form of dysmetria, characterized by a dysfunction of the power to control the range of muscular action, resulting in movements which overreach the intended goal of the affected individual. Compare **hypometria.**

hypermetropia, hypermetropy See **hyperopia.**

hypermorph In genetics: a mutant gene that shows an increased activity in the expression of a trait. Compare **amorph, antimorph, hypomorph.**

hypernatremia Greater than normal concentration of sodium in the blood, caused by excessive loss of water and electrolytes owing to polyuria, diarrhea, excessive sweating, or inadequate water intake. People with hypernatremia may become mentally confused, have seizures, and lapse into coma. The treatment is restoration of fluid and electrolyte balance by mouth or by I.V. infusion. In diabetes insipidus, the pituitary hormone vasopressin will control excessive water loss through the kidneys. See also **diabetes insipidus.**

hyperopia Farsightedness, a condition resulting from an error of refraction in which rays of light entering the eye are brought into focus behind the retina. Also called hypermetropia.

hyperparathyroidism An abnormal endocrine condition characterized by hyperactivity of any of the four parathyroid glands with excessive secretion of parathyroid hormone, which results in increased resorption of calcium from the skeletal system and increased absorption of calcium by the kidneys and gastrointestinal system. The condition may be primary, originating in one or more of the parathyroid glands, or secondary, resulting from an abnormal hypocalcemia-producing condition in another part or system of the body, causing a compensatory hyperactivity of the parathyroid glands. Hypercalcemia in primary hyperparathyroidism results in dysfunction of most of the systems of the body. In the kidneys, tissue calcifies, calculi form, and renal failure may ensue. In the bones and joints, osteoporosis develops, causing pain and fragility; fractures, synovitis, and pseudogout often occur. In the gastrointestinal tract chronic, piercing epigastric pain may develop owing to pancreatitis. Hematemesis, anorexia, and nausea may be seen if peptic ulceration occurs. In the neuromuscular system generalized weakness and atrophy develop if the condition is not corrected, and changes in the central nervous system result in alteration of consciousness, coma, psychosis, abnormal behavior, and disturbances of personality. Secondary hyperparathyroidism may result in many of these signs of calcium imbalance and in various abnormalities of the long bones, as in rickets. The diagnosis of primary hyperparathyroidism is made by laboratory findings of increased levels of PTH and calcium in the blood and by the characteristic appearance of the bones on X-ray films. Calcium is present in the blood and urine and chloride and alkaline phosphatase are present in the blood in excessive amounts; phosphorus is present in the serum in less than normal amounts. Primary parathyroidism that is the result of an adenoma of one of the glands is treated by excision of the tumor; other causes of primary disease might require excision of up to one half of the glandular tissue. Dietary intake of calcium may be limited, and diuretics that promote urinary excretion of calcium and sodium may be administered. Secondary hyperparathyroidism is treated by treating the underlying cause of hypertrophy of the gland. Vitamin D is frequently given, and peritoneal dialysis may be necessary to remove excess calcium from the circulation. NURSING CONSIDERATIONS: Frequent laboratory evaluations of blood levels of calcium, phosphorus, potassium, and magnesium are necessary throughout the course of treatment. Because fractures occur easily and are common, great care is taken to avoid trauma to the patient.

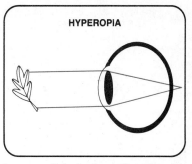

HYPEROPIA

Intravenous hydration is usually performed to dilute the concentration of calcium, and the lungs are auscultated and percussed regularly to detect pulmonary edema in its earliest stages. Tetany is a warning sign of severe hypoglycemia; calcium gluconate is kept available for immediate use postoperatively. Walking and moving about cause pain to the patient but accelerate healing of the affected bones and are therefore encouraged.

hyperphenylalaninemia An abnormally high concentration of phenylalanine in the blood. This symptom may be the result of one of several defects in the metabolic process of breaking down phenylalanine. See also **phenylketonuria.**

hyperphoria The tendency of an eye to deviate upward.

hyperpigmentation Unusual darkening of the skin. Causes include heredity, drugs, exposure to the sun, and adrenal insufficiency. Compare **hypopigmentation.** See also **chloasma, melanocyte-stimulating hormone.**

hyperpituitarism A chronic, progressive disease caused by oversecretion of human growth hormone, which produces changes throughout the body. It occurs before puberty as gigantism or after puberty as acromegaly. See also **acromegaly** and **gigantism.**

hyperplasia An increase in the number of cells. Compare **hypertrophy, hypoplasia.**

hyperploid, hyperploidic 1. Of or pertaining to an individual, an organism, a strain, or a cell that has one or more chromosomes in excess of the basic haploid number or of an exact multiple of the haploid number that is characteristic of the species. The result is unbalanced sets of chromosomes, which are referred to as hyperdiploid, hypertriploid, hypertetraploid, and so on, depending on the number of multiples of the haploid chromosomes they contain. 2. Such an individual, organism, strain, or cell. Compare **hypoploid.** See also **trisomy.** —**hyperploidy,** *n.*

hyperpnea, hyperpnoea A deep, rapid, or labored respiration. It occurs normally with exercise and abnormally with pain, fever, hysteria, or any condition in which the supply of oxygen is inadequate, as cardiac disease and respiratory disease. Compare **dyspnea, hypopnea, orthopnea.** —**hyperpneic, hyperpnoic,** *adj.*

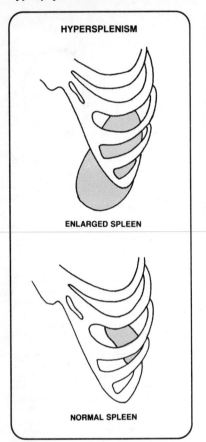

HYPERSPLENISM

ENLARGED SPLEEN

NORMAL SPLEEN

hyperptyalism See **ptyalism.**

hyperpyrexia An extremely elevated temperature, sometimes occurring in acute infectious diseases, especially in young children. Malignant hyperpyrexia, characterized by a rapid rise in temperature, tachycardia, tachypnea, sweating, rigidity, and blotchy cyanosis, occasionally occurs in patients undergoing general anesthesia. A high temperature may be reduced by sponging the body with tepid water and alcohol, by giving a tepid tub bath, hypothermia treatment, or by administering antipyretic medication, as aspirin or acetaminophen. —**hyperpyretic,** adj.

hypersensitivity An abnormal condition characterized by an excessive reaction to a particular stimulus. See also **allergy.** —**hypersensitive,** adj.

hypersensitivity pneumonitis An inflammatory form of interstitial pneumonia that results from an immunologic reaction in a hypersensitive person. The reaction may be provoked by a variety of inhaled organic dusts, often those containing fungal spores. The disease can be prevented by avoiding contact with causative

agents. Its classification rests solely on the type of immune response rather than on clinical manifestations. The hypersensitivity reaction is characterized by infiltration of alveoli with eosinophils and large mononuclear cells, edema, and inflammation of the lungs. Various symptoms may occur, including dyspnea, cough, cyanosis, fever, chills, diaphoresis, malaise, and muscle aches, which usually develop 4 to 6 hours after exposure. Patients with chronic disease may also experience weight loss, cough, and progressive exertional dyspnea. On laboratory examination of the blood, leukocytosis is commonly found. Recovery is usually spontaneous. In an acute attack, corticosteroids may be given to diminish the inflammatory response. Also called alveolitis, allergic alveolitis, allergic interstitial pneumonitis, diffuse hypersensitivity pneumonia, extrinsic allergic alveolitis, extrinsic allergic pneumonia. Some types of hypersensitivity pneumonitis include **bagassosis, cork worker's lung, farmer's lung, humidifier lung, mushroom worker's lung,** and **pigeon breeder's lung.**

hypersensitivity reaction An inappropriate and excessive response of the immune system to a sensitizing antigen. The antigenic stimulant is an allergen. There are several factors that determine the degree of an allergic response: the responsiveness of the host to the allergen, the amount of allergen, the kind of allergen, its route of entrance into the body, the timing of the exposures, and the site of the allergen-immune mediator reaction. Hypersensitivity reactions are classified by the components of the immune system involved in their mediation. Humoral reactions, mediated by the circulating B lymphocytes, are immediate and include three types: anaphylactic hypersensitivity, cytotoxic hypersensitivity, and toxic-complex hypersensitivity. Cellular reactions, mediated by the T lymphocytes, are delayed, cell-mediated hypersensitivity reactions.

hypersomnia 1. Sleep of excessive depth or abnormal duration, usually caused by psychological rather than physical factors and characterized by a state of confusion upon awakening. 2. Extreme drowsiness, often associated with lethargy. 3. A condition characterized by periods of deep, long sleep. Compare **narcolepsy.**

hypersplenism A syndrome consisting of splenomegaly and a deficiency of one or more types of blood cells. The numerous causes of this syndrome include the lymphomas, the hemolytic anemias, malaria, tuberculosis, and various connective tissue and inflammatory diseases. Patients with this syndrome complain of abdominal pain on the left side and often experience fullness after eating very little, because the greatly enlarged spleen is pressing against the stomach. On physical examination, the enlarged spleen is felt and abnormal bruits (vascular sounds) are heard with a stethoscope over the epigastric area. Treatment of the underlying disorder may cure the syndrome. Splenectomy is usually performed only in treating the hemolytic anemias or when splenic enlargement is severe and the danger of vascular accident is significant. See also **splenectomy.**

hypertelorism   A developmental defect characterized by an abnormally wide space between two organs or parts. A kind of hypertelorism is **ocular hypertelorism.** Compare **hypotelorism.**

hypertension   A common, often asymptomatic disorder characterized by elevated blood pressure persistently exceeding 140/90 mmHg. Essential hypertension, the most frequent kind, has no single identifiable cause, but the risk of the disorder is increased by obesity, a high sodium level in serum, hypercholesterolemia, and a family history of high blood pressure. Known causes of hypertension include such adrenal disorders as aldosteronism, Cushing's syndrome, and pheochromocytoma; thyrotoxicosis; toxemia of pregnancy; and chronic glomerulonephritis. The incidence of hypertension is higher in men than in women and is twice as great in blacks as in whites. Persons with mild or moderate hypertension may be asymptomatic or may experience suboccipital headaches, especially on rising; tinnitus; lightheadness; easy fatigability; and palpitations. With sustained hypertension arterial walls become thickened, inelastic, and resistant to blood flow and, as a result, the left ventricle becomes distended and hypertrophied in its efforts to maintain normal circulation. Inadequate blood supply to the coronary arteries may cause angina or myocardial infarction. Left ventricular hypertrophy may lead to congestive heart failure. High blood pressure associated with hypersecretion of catecholamines in pheochromocytoma is often accompanied by anxiety attacks, palpitation, profuse sweating, pallor, nausea, and, in some cases, pulmonary edema. Malignant hypertension, characterized by a diastolic pressure higher than 120 mmHg, severe headaches, blurred vision, and confusion, may result in fatal uremia, myocardial infarction, congestive heart failure, or a cerebral vascular accident. Drugs used to treat hypertension include diuretics; vasodilators; sympathetic nervous system (SNS) depressants, as rauwolfia alkaloids; SNS inhibitors, as guanethidine and methyldopa; and ganglionic blocking agents, as clonidine and propranolol. Patients with high blood pressure are advised to follow a low-sodium, low-saturated fat diet, to reduce calories to control obesity, to exercise, avoid stress, and take adequate rest. See also **blood pressure.**

hypertensive crisis   A sudden severe increase in blood pressure to a level exceeding 200/120 mmHg, occurring most frequently in untreated hypertension and in patients who have stopped taking prescribed antihypertensive medication. Characteristic signs include severe headache, vertigo, diplopia, tinnitus, nosebleed, twitching muscles, tachycardia or other cardiac arrhythmia, distended neck veins, narrowed pulse pressure, nausea, and vomiting. The pa

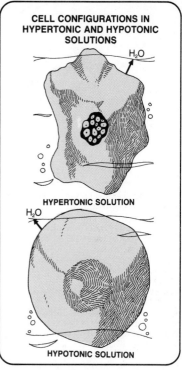

CELL CONFIGURATIONS IN HYPERTONIC AND HYPOTONIC SOLUTIONS

tient may be confused, irritable, or stuporous, and the condition may lead to convulsions, coma, myocardial infarction, renal failure, cardiac arrest, or stroke. Treatment consists of antihypertensive drugs, administered I.V. or I.M., and diuretics and may include the use of anticonvulsants, sedatives, and antiemetics, if indicated.

NURSING CONSIDERATIONS: A major concern in caring for patients who have suffered a hypertensive crisis is observing and reporting any sign of treatment-induced hypotension. In preparation for discharge, the nurse advises the patient to recognize symptoms of any dramatic increase or decrease in blood pressure, to adhere to the prescribed diet and medication, and to avoid fatigue, heavy lifting, smoking, and stressful situations.

hypertetraploid, hypertetraploidic   See **hyperploid.**

hyperthermia   1. A higher than normal body temperature induced therapeutically or iatrogenically. 2. *Nontechnical.* Malignant hyperthermia.

hyperthyroidism   See **Graves' disease.**

hypertonic   Of a solution: having a greater concentration of solute than another solution, hence exerting more osmotic pressure than that solution, as a hypertonic saline solution that contains more salt than is found in intracellular and extracellular fluid. Cells shrink in a hyper

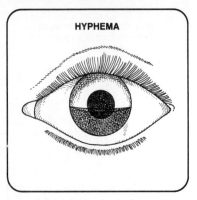

HYPHEMA

tonic solution because of water loss.

hypertonic contracture Prolonged muscle contraction owing to continuous nerve stimulation in spastic paralysis. Anesthesia or sleep eliminates this condition. Also called **functional contracture.**

hypertrichosis See **hirsutism.**

hypertriglyceridemia See **hyperchylomicronemia.**

hypertriploid, hypertriploidic See **hyperploid.**

hypertrophic angioma See **hemangioendothelioma.**

hypertrophic catarrh A chronic condition characterized by inflammation and discharge from a mucous membrane, accompanied by the thickening of the mucosal and submucosal tissue. Compare **atrophic catarrh.** See also **catarrh.**

hypertrophic gastritis An inflammatory condition of the stomach characterized by epigastric pain, nausea, vomiting, and distention. It is differentiated from other forms of gastritis by the presence of prominent rugae (folds), enlarged glands, and nodules on the wall of the stomach. This condition often occurs with peptic ulcer, Zollinger-Ellison syndrome, or gastric hypersecretion. See also **gastritis.**

hypertrophy An increase in the size of a cell or a group of cells and thus, an increase in the size of an organ. Compare **atrophy, hyperplasia.** —**hypertrophic,** *adj.*

hyperuricemia See **gout.**

hyperventilation A pulmonary ventilation rate that is greater than that metabolically necessary for the exchange of respiratory gases. It is the result of an increased frequency of breathing, an increased tidal volume, or a combination of both, and causes excessive intake of oxygen and the blowing off of carbon dioxide. Hypocapnia and respiratory alkalosis then occur, leading to chest pain, dizziness, faintness, numbness of the fingers and toes, and psychomotor impairment. Causes of hyperventilation include asthma or early emphysema; increased metabolism owing to exercise, fever, hyperthyroidism, or infections; lesions of the central nervous system, as in cerebral thrombosis, enceph-

alitis, head injuries, or meningitis; drugs, such as salicylates; difficulties with mechanical respirators; and·psychogenic factors, as acute anxiety or pain. Compare **hypoventilation.**

hypervitaminosis An abnormal condition resulting from excessive intake of toxic amounts of one or more vitamins, especially over a long period of time. Serious effects may result from overdosage of vitamins A, D, E, or K, but rarely from the water-soluble vitamins. Compare **avitaminosis.**

hypesthesia An abnormal weakness of sensation in response to stimulation of the sensory nerves. Also called **hypoesthesia.** —**hypesthetic,** *adj.*

hypha, *pl.* **hyphae** The threadlike structure of the mycelium in a fungus.

hyphema, hyphemia A hemorrhage into the anterior chamber of the eye, usually caused by a blunt or percussive injury. Bed rest and a sedative are indicated. The patient is treated by an ophthalmologist who evaluates the need for evacuation of the blood or the use of mydriatic or miotic medications or a carbonic anhydrase inhibitor.

hypnagogic hallucination One that occurs in the period between wakefulness and sleep. See also **hallucination.**

hypnagogue An agent or substance that tends to induce sleep or the feeling of dreamy sleepiness, as occurs prior to falling asleep. —**hypnagogic,** *adj.*

hypo-, hyp- A combining form meaning 'under, beneath, or deficient': *hypocalcia, hypomastia, hyposynergia.*

hypnoanalysis The use of hypnosis as an adjunct to other techniques in psychoanalysis.

hypnosis A passive, trancelike state that resembles normal sleep, during which perception and memory are altered, resulting in increased responsiveness to suggestion. The condition is usually induced by the monotonous repetition of words and gestures while the subject is completely relaxed. Susceptibility to hypnosis varies from person to person. Hypnosis is used in some forms of psychotherapy and psychoanalysis to gain access to the subconscious, in behavior modification programs to help a person stop smoking or other unwanted behavior, or in medicine to reduce pain and promote relaxation.

hypnotherapy The use of hypnosis as an adjunct to other techniques in psychotherapy.

-hypnotic A combining form meaning 'pertaining to hypnosis': *anhypnotic, autohypnotic, posthypnotic.*

hypnotic trance An artificially induced sleeplike state, as in hypnosis.

hypnotism The study or practice of inducing hypnosis.

hypnotist One who practices hypnotism.

hypnotize 1. To put into a state of hypnosis. 2. To fascinate, entrance, or control through personal charm.

hypo- A combining form meaning 'beneath, deficient,' or, in chemistry, 'lacking oxygen': *hypochlorite, hypodermic, hypodontia.*

hypoacidity An abnormal condition characterized by a decreased secretion of hydrochloric acid. It is usually secondary to another condition, as pernicious anemia or carcinoma of the stomach.

hypoadrenalism See **Addison's disease.**

hypoalimentation A condition of insufficient or inadequate nourishment.

hypobetalipoproteinemia An inherited disorder in which there are less than normal amounts of beta-lipoprotein in the serum. Blood lipids and cholesterol are present at less than the expected levels, regardless of dietary intake of fats. Compare **hyperbetalipoproteinemia.**

hypocalcemia A deficiency of calcium in the serum that may be caused by hypoparathyroidism, vitamin D deficiency, kidney failure, acute pancreatitis, or inadequate plasma magnesium and protein. Although mild hypocalcemia is asymptomatic, severe hypocalcemia is characterized by cardiac arrhythmias and tetany with hyperparesthesia of the hands, feet, lips, and tongue. See also **tetany.** **—hypocalcemic,** *adj.*

hypochlorous acid An unstable compound that decomposes to hydrochloric acid and water. It is used as a bleaching agent and disinfectant.

hypochondriasis, hypochondria 1. A chronic, abnormal concern about the health of the body. 2. A disorder characterized by extreme anxiety, depression, and an unrealistic interpretation of real or imagined physical symptoms as indications of a serious illness or disease despite rational medical evidence that no disorder is present. The condition is caused by some unresolved intrapsychic conflict and may involve a specific organ, as the heart, lungs, or eyes, or several body systems at various times or simultaneously. In severe cases, the distorted body-mind relationship is so strong that actual symptoms and disease may develop. Treatment usually consists of psychotherapy to uncover the underlying emotional conflict. Also called hypochondriacal neurosis. **—hypochondriac,** *adj.*, *n.*, **hypochondriacal,** *adj.*

hypochromic Having less than normal color, usually describing a red blood cell and characterizing anemias associated with decreased synthesis of hemoglobin. Compare **normochromic.**

hypochromic anemia Any of a large group of anemias characterized by a decreased concentration of hemoglobin in the red blood cells. See also **anemia, red cell indices.**

hypocytic leukemia See **subleukemic leukemia.**

hypodermatoclysis See **hypodermoclysis.**

hypodermic Of or pertaining to the area below the skin, as a hypodermic injection.

hypodermic needle A short, thin, hollow needle that attaches to a syringe for injecting a drug or medication under the skin or into vessels and for withdrawing a fluid, as blood, for examination.

hypodermoclysis, hypodermatoclysis The injection of an isotonic or hypotonic solution into subcutaneous tissue to supply the patient with a continuous and large amount of fluid, electrolytes, and nutrients. The procedure is used to replace the loss of or inadequate intake of water and salt during illness or surgery or following shock or hemorrhage and is performed only when the patient is unable to take fluids intravenously, orally, or rectally. The rate of absorption into the circulatory system is increased with the addition to the solution of the enzyme hyaluronidase. The most common sites of administration are the anterior thighs, the abdominal wall along the crest of the ilium, below the breasts in women, and directly over the scapula in children; sites should be changed when multiple infusions are given. The patient is placed in a comfortable position, since the procedure takes a long time. The nurse observes for signs of circulatory collapse, respiratory difficulty, and edema at the site of injection. Also called **interstitial infusion, subcutaneous infusion.**

hypodiploid, hypodiploidic See **hypoploid.**

hypoesthesia See **hypesthesia.** **—hypoesthetic,** *adj.*

hypogammaglobulinemia A less than normal concentration of gamma globulin in the blood, usually the result of increased protein catabolism or the loss of protein in the urine, as in nephrosis. The condition is associated with a decreased resistance to infection. Compare **agammaglobulinemia.**

hypogastric artery See **internal iliac artery.**

hypoglossal nerve Either of a pair of cranial nerves essential for swallowing and for moving the tongue. Each nerve has four major branches, communicates with the vagus nerve, and connects to nucleus XII in the brain. Also called **nervus hypoglossus, twelfth nerve.**

hypoglycemia A less than normal amount of glucose in the blood, usually caused by administration of too much insulin, excessive secretion of insulin by the islet cells of the pancreas, or by dietary deficiency. The condition may result in weakness, headache, hunger, visual disturbances, ataxia, anxiety, personality changes, and, if untreated, delirium, coma, and death. The treatment is the administration of glucose in orange juice by mouth if the person is conscious or in an intravenous glucose solution if the person is unconscious. Compare **diabetic coma.**

hypoglycemic agent Any of a large heterogeneous group of drugs prescribed to decrease the amount of glucose circulating in the blood. Hypoglycemic agents include insulin and the sulfonylureas. Insulin in its various forms is given parenterally and acts by increasing the utilization of carbohydrates and the metabolism of fats and protein. The sulfonylureas, including tolbutamide, tolinamide, chlorpropamide, and acetohexamide, act by stimulating the release of endogenous insulin from the pancreas. The bi-

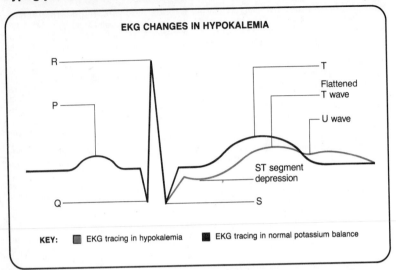

EKG CHANGES IN HYPOKALEMIA

R · P · Q · S · T · Flattened T wave · U wave · ST segment depression

KEY: ▨ EKG tracing in hypokalemia ▪ EKG tracing in normal potassium balance

guanides, of which only phenformin has been recently prescribed, act by potentiating the action of endogenous insulin, augmenting the utilization of glucose by the peripheral cells of the body. Phenformin has been recently removed from the market in the United States, primarily because of its tendency to cause lactic acidosis. The adverse reactions of any hypoglycemic agent and contraindications for its prescription depend on the class of drug and the condition of the patient.

hypoglycemic shock treatment See **insulin-shock treatment.**

hypokalemia A condition in which an inadequate amount of potassium, the major intracellular cation, is found in the circulating blood stream. Hypokalemia is characterized by abnormal EKG, weakness, and flaccid paralysis and may be caused by starvation, treatment of diabetic acidosis, adrenal tumor, or diuretic therapy. Compare **hyperkalemia.** See also **electrolyte balance.**

hypokalemic alkalosis A pathologic condition resulting from the accumulation of base or the loss of acid from the body associated with a low level of serum potassium. The retention of alkali or the loss of acid occurs primarily in extracellular fluid, but the pH of intracellular fluid may also be subnormal. See also **hypokalemia.**

hypolipoproteinemia A group of rare, hereditary defects of lipid metabolism that result in varying complexes of signs. These include abnormal transport of triglycerides in the blood, low levels of high-density lipoproteins, high levels of low-density lipoproteins, and abnormal deposition of lipids in the body, especially in the kidneys and the liver. In some of the syndromes, ocular, intestinal, and neurologic effects are also present. Kinds of hypolipoproteinemias are **abetalipoproteinemia (Bassen-**Kornzweig syndrome), **hypobetalipoproteinemia, Tangier disease.**

hypomagnesemia An abnormally low concentration of magnesium in the blood plasma, resulting in nausea, vomiting, muscle weakness, tremors, tetany, and lethargy. Mild hypomagnesemia is usually the result of inadequate absorption of magnesium in the kidney or intestine, although it is also seen after prolonged parenteral feeding and during lactation. A more severe form is associated with malabsorption syndrome, protein malnutrition, and parathyroid disease. Magnesium salts to correct the deficiency may be given orally or by I.V. infusion.

hypomania A psychopathological state characterized by optimism, excitability, a marked hyperactivity and talkativeness, heightened sexual interest, quick anger and irritability, and a decreased need for sleep. —**hypomaniac,** *n.,* **hypomanic,** *adj.*

hypometria An abnormal condition, a form of dysmetria, characterized by a dysfunction of the power to control the range of muscular action, resulting in movements which fall short of the intended goals of the affected individual. Compare **hypermetria.**

hypomorph In genetics: a mutant allele that has a reduced effect on the expression of a trait but at a level too low to result in abnormal development. Also called **leaky gene.** Compare **amorph, antimorph, hypermorph.**

hyponatremia A less than normal concentration of sodium in the blood, caused by inadequate excretion of water or by excessive water in the circulating bloodstream. In a severe case, the person may develop water intoxication, with confusion and lethargy, leading to muscle excitability, convulsions, and coma. Restoration of fluid and electrolyte balance may be accomplished by I.V. infusion of a balanced solution.

hypopharyngeal 1. Of, pertaining to, or

involving the hypopharynx. **2.** Situated below the pharynx.

hypophosphatasia   Congenital absence of alkaline phosphatase, an enzyme essential to the calcification of bone tissue. Affected newborns vomit and grow slowly; many die in infancy. Children who survive have numerous skeletal abnormalities and are dwarfs. There is no known treatment.

hypophosphatemic rickets   A rare familial disorder in which there is impaired resorption of phosphate in the kidneys and poor absorption of calcium in the small intestine, resulting in osteomalacia, retarded growth, skeletal deformities, and pain. Treatment includes the prescription of phosphate and vitamin D, to be taken by mouth.

hypophyseal cachexia   See **panhypopituitarism.**

hypophyseal dwarf   See **pituitary dwarf.**

hypophysectomy   Surgical removal of the pituitary gland. It may be performed to slow the growth and spread of endocrine-dependent malignant tumors of the breast, ovary, or prostate gland, to halt deterioration of the retina in diabetes, or to excise a pituitary tumor. The gland is removed only if other treatment, as X-ray therapy, radioactive implants, or cryosurgery, fails to destroy all pituitary tissue. Postoperatively, hormone levels, including thyroid stimulating hormone, adrenocorticotropic hormone, and antidiuretic hormone, are monitored, and replacement therapy is begun as needed. Urinary output is measured every 2 hours for several days, and an amount in excess of 300 ml (10 oz) in any 2-hour period is reported. The patient is closely monitored for early signs of thyroid crisis, Addisonian crisis, electrolyte imbalance, hemorrhage, and meningitis. **—hypophysectomize,** *v.*

hypophysis cerebri   See **pituitary gland.**

hypopigmentation   Unusual lack of skin color, seen in albinism or vitiligo. Compare **hyperpigmentation.**

hypoplasia, hypoplasty   Incomplete or underdevelopment of an organ or tissue, usually owing to a decrease in the number of cells. Kinds of hypoplasia are **cartilage-hair hypoplasia, enamel hypoplasia.** Compare **aplasia, hyperplasia.** See also **oligomeganephronia, osteogenesis imperfecta. —hypoplastic,** *adj.*

hypoplasia of the mesenchyme   See **osteogenesis imperfecta.**

hypoplastic anemia   A broad category of anemias characterized by decreased production of red blood cells. Compare **aplastic anemia, polycythemia.** See also **anemia.**

hypoplastic dwarf   See **primordial dwarf.**

hypoploid   **1.** Of or pertaining to an individual, organism, strain, or cell that has fewer than the normal haploid number or an exact multiple of the haploid number of chromosomes characteristic of the species. The result is unbalanced sets of chromosomes, which are referred to as hypodiploid, hypotriploid, hypotetraploid, and so on, depending on the number

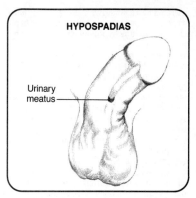

HYPOSPADIAS

Urinary meatus

of multiples of the haploid chromosomes they contain. Also called **hypoploidic. 2.** Such an individual, organism, strain, or cell. Compare **hyperploid.** See also **monosomy. —hypoploidy,** *n.*

hypopnea   Shallow or slow respiration. In well-conditioned athletes, it is normal and is accompanied by a slow pulse; otherwise, it is characteristic of damage to the brain stem, in which case it is accompanied by a rapid, weak pulse and is a grave sign.

hypoproteinemia   A disorder characterized by a decrease in the amount of protein in the blood to an abnormally low level, accompanied by edema, nausea, vomiting, diarrhea, and abdominal pain. It may be caused by an inadequate dietary supply of protein, by intestinal lymphangiectasia, or by renal failure.

hypoprothrombinemia   An abnormal reduction in the amount of prothrombin (factor II) in the circulating blood, characterized by poor clot formation, longer bleeding time, and possible hemorrhage. The condition is usually the result of inadequate synthesis of prothrombin in the liver, most often the result of a deficiency of vitamin K owing to severe liver disease or to anticoagulant therapy with the drug dicoumarol. See also **blood clotting.**

hypoptyalism   A condition in which there is a decrease in the amount of saliva secreted by the salivary glands. Compare **ptyalism.**

hypopyon   An accumulation of pus in the anterior chamber of an eye, appearing as a gray fluid between the cornea and the iris. It may occur as a complication of conjunctivitis, herpetic keratitis, or corneal ulcer.

hyposensitization   See **immunotherapy.**

hypospadias   A congenital defect in which the urinary meatus is on the underside of the penis. The opening may be off-center or anywhere along the underside of the penis or on the perineum. Surgical correction is performed as necessary for cosmetic, urologic, or reproductive indications. A corresponding defect in women is rare but recognized by the location of the urinary meatus in the vagina. Compare **epispadias.**

hypotelorism   A developmental defect characterized by an abnormally decreased distance between two organs or parts. A kind of hypotelorism is **ocular hypotelorism.** Compare **hypertelorism.**

hypotension An abnormal condition in which the blood pressure is not adequate for normal perfusion and oxygenation of the tissues. An expanded intravascular space, a decreased intravascular volume, or a diminished cardiac thrust may be the cause.

hypotensive anesthesia See **deliberate hypotension.**

hypotetraploid, hypotetraploidic See **hypoploid.**

hypothalamic amenorrhea Cessation of menses caused by disorders that inhibit the hypothalamus from initiating the cycle of neurohormonal interactions of the brain, pituitary, and ovary necessary for ovulation and subsequent menstruation. Examples of causes are stress, anxiety, and acute weight loss. See **amenorrhea.**

hypothalamus A portion of the diencephalon of the brain, forming the floor and part of the lateral wall of the third ventricle. It activates, controls, and integrates the peripheral autonomic nervous system, endocrine processes, and many somatic functions, as body temperature, sleep, and appetite. —**hypothalamic,** *adj.*

hypothermia **1.** An abnormal and dangerous condition in which the temperature of the body is below 35°C (95°F), usually owing to prolonged exposure to cold. Respiration is shallow and slow, and the heart rate is faint and slow. The person is very pale and may appear to be dead. Treatment includes slow warming. Hospitalization is necessary for evaluating and treating any metabolic abnormalities that may result from hypothermia. **2.** The deliberate and controlled reduction of body temperature with cooling mattresses or ice as preparation for some surgical procedures.

hypothermia therapy The reduction of a patient's body temperature to counteract high prolonged fever caused by an infectious or neurologic disease or, less frequently, as an adjunct to anesthesia in heart or brain surgery. Hypothermia may be produced by placing crushed ice around the patient, by immersing the body in ice water, by autotransfusing blood after it is circulated through coils submerged in a refrigerant, or, most commonly, by applying hypothermia blankets or vinyl pads containing coils through which cold water and alcohol are circulated by a pump. The cooling unit is placed in an open area; any kinks or twists in the tubing are removed and the blanket is checked for leaks. The patient is wrapped in bath blankets and then covered with the cooling blanket; the patient's temperature, registered by means of a probe inserted in the rectum, is read and recorded before hypothermia is initiated, every 5 minutes until the desired reduction is achieved, and then every 15 minutes. The blood pressure, pulse, respirations, and neurologic status are checked every 5 to 10 minutes until the temperature is stabilized, then every 30 minutes for 2 hours, every 4 hours in the next 24 hours, and subsequently as required. Every 1 to 2 hours the patient is assisted in turning, coughing, and deep breathing. At similar intervals the chest is auscultated for breath sounds, and mouth, nose, and skin care are administered; the skin is lubricated with oil or lotion before and during the procedure. An indwelling catheter is connected to a closed gravity drainage system, as ordered, and fluid intake and output are measured; if less than 30 ml of urine per hour is excreted the physician is notified. If the patient's temperature is less than 32.2°C (90°F), his gag reflex is tested before any oral fluids or foods are administered. Naso-oral suction is performed as indicated; body alignment is maintained, and a passive or active range of motion exercises is performed every 4 hours. Since shivering increases body heat, medication for its prevention, as chlorpromazine hydrochloride, may be ordered.

NURSING CONSIDERATIONS: The patient is observed for medication reactions, decreased blood pressure, bradycardia, arrhythmias, bradypnea, respiratory failure, unequal pupils, increased intracranial pressure, changes in consciousness, intestinal ileus, and frostbite. Any changes in skin color or signs of edema and induration are reported to the physician immediately. At the termination of hypothermia, the cooling blanket is replaced by regular blankets, and the patient usually warms at his own rate. As the patient's temperature approaches normal, the warming blankets are removed, but the temperature probe remains in place until the body temperature is stable. Hypothermia used in the treatment of high fever associated with generalized severe infections reduces body heat by decreasing metabolism and also inhibits the multiplication of the etiologic pathogenic organisms. Patients with a high temperature caused by a neurologic disease, such as meningitis, may be maintained in a state of mild hypothermia (30.6° to 35°C, or 87° to 95°F) for as long as 5 days.

hypothesis In research: a statement derived from a theory that predicts the relationship among variables representing concepts, constructs, or events. Kinds of hypotheses include **causal hypothesis, null hypothesis, predictive hypothesis.**

hypothyroid dwarf See **cretin dwarf.**

hypothyroidism in adults A state of low serum thyroid hormone, resulting from hypothalamic, pituitary, or thyroid insufficiency. Typically, the early clinical features of hypothyroidism are vague: fatigue, forgetfulness, sensitivity to cold, unexplained weight gain, and constipation. As the disorder progresses, characteristic myxedematous symptoms appear: decreasing mental stability; dry, flaky, inelastic skin; puffy face, hands, and feet; hoarseness; periorbital edema; upper eyelid droop; dry, sparse hair; and thick, brittle nails. Cardiovascular involvement leads to decreased cardiac output, slow pulse rate, signs of poor peripheral circulation, and, occasionally, arteriosclerosis and cardiac enlargement. Other common clinical effects of hypothyroidism include anorexia, abdominal distention, menorrhagia, decreased libido, infertility, ataxia, intention tremor, and nystagmus. Reflexes show delayed relaxation time (especially in the Achilles tendon). Progression to myxedema coma is usually gradual, but when stress aggravates severe or prolonged hypothyroidism, coma may develop abruptly. Signs of developing coma include progressive stupor, hypoventilation, hypoglycemia, hyponatremia, hypotension, and hypothermia. Treatment includes thyroid replacement with levothyroxine (T_4), liothyronine (T_3), liotrix, or thyroid USP (desiccated).

hypothyroidism in children See **cretinism.**

hypotonic Of a solution: having a smaller concentration of solute than another solution, hence exerting less osmotic pressure than that solution, as a hypotonic saline solution that contains less salt than is found in intra- or extracellular fluid. Cells expand in a hypotonic solution.

hypotriploid, hypotriploidic See **hypoploid.**

hypoventilation Abnormally reduced rate and depth of respiration. It occurs when the volume of air which enters the alveoli and takes part in gas exchanges is not adequate for the metabolic needs of the body. Hypoventilation may be caused by uneven distribution of inspired air, as in bronchitis, morbid obesity, neuromuscular or skeletal disease affecting the thorax, decreased response of the respiratory center to carbon dioxide, and by reduced functional lung tissue, as in atelectasis, emphysema, and pleural effusion. The result of unresolved hypoventilation is hypoxia, hypercapnia, pulmonary hypertension with cor pulmonale, and respiratory acidosis. Treatment aims to correct the underlying cause.

hypovitaminosis See **avitaminosis.**

hypovolemic shock A state of physical collapse and prostration caused by massive blood loss, circulatory dysfunction, and inadequate tissue perfusion. The loss of about one fifth of total blood volume in the affected individual can produce this condition. The common signs include low blood pressure, feeble pulse, clammy skin, tachycardia, rapid breathing, and reduced urinary output. Disorders that may cause hypovolemic shock are dehydration from excessive perspiration, severe diarrhea, or protracted vomiting, intestinal obstruction, peritonitis, acute pancreatitis, and severe burns, which deplete body fluids. Treatment of hypovolemic shock focuses on prompt replacement of blood and fluid volumes, identification of bleeding sites, and the control of bleeding. Without fast, aggressive treatment, there is further collapse that can cause death. Compare **cardiogenic shock.**

hypoxemia An abnormal deficiency of oxygen in the arterial blood. Symptoms of acute hypoxemia are cyanosis, restlessness, stupor,

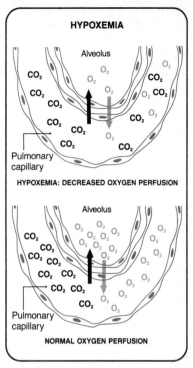

HYPOXEMIA

Alveolus

Pulmonary capillary

HYPOXEMIA: DECREASED OXYGEN PERFUSION

Alveolus

Pulmonary capillary

NORMAL OXYGEN PERFUSION

coma, Cheyne-Stokes breathing, or apnea, increased blood pressure, tachycardia, and an initial increase in cardiac output which later falls, resulting in hypotension and ventricular fibrillation or asystole. Chronic hypoxemia stimulates red cell production by the bone marrow, leading to secondary polycythemia. Hypoxemia caused by decreased alveolar oxygen tension or underventilation improves with the administration of oxygen. Compare **hypoxia.** See also **anoxia, asphyxia.**

hypoxia Oxygen deficiency caused by reduced oxygen-carrying capacity (anemic hypoxia), insufficient oxygen in inspired air (hypoxic hypoxia), impaired tissue utilization of oxygen (histotoxic hypoxia), or inadequate blood flow to transport oxygen (stagnant hypoxia). Compare **hypoxemia.** See also **anoxia, chemoreceptor, hyperventilation, respiratory center, —hypoxic,** *adj.*

hypoxidosis Impairment of cell function due to inadequate oxygenation.

hypsi- A combining form meaning 'high': *hypsicephalia, hypsiconchous, hypsistaphylie.*

hypso- A combining form meaning 'pertaining to height': *hypsonosus, hypsophobia, hypsotherapy.*

hyssibrachycephaly The condition of having a skull that is high with a broad forehead. See also **brachycephaly, oxycephaly. — hyssibrachycephalic,** *adj., n.*

hyssicephaly See **oxycephaly.**

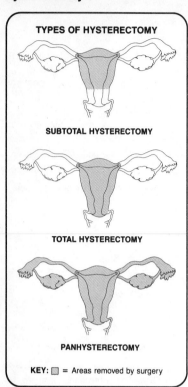

TYPES OF HYSTERECTOMY

SUBTOTAL HYSTERECTOMY

TOTAL HYSTERECTOMY

PANHYSTERECTOMY

KEY: ☐ = Areas removed by surgery

hysterectomy Surgical removal of the uterus, performed to remove fibroid tumors of the uterus and to treat chronic pelvic inflammatory disease, severe recurrent endometrial hyperplasia, uterine hemorrhage, and precancerous and cancerous conditions of the uterus. Types of hysterectomy include total hysterectomy, in which both the uterus and cervix are removed; subtotal hysterectomy, in which the distal portion of the uterus is removed, and the cervix is left intact; radical hysterectomy, in which ovaries, fallopian tubes, lymph nodes, and lymph channels are removed along with the uterus and cervix; and panhysterectomy, in which the uterus, ovaries, fallopian tubes, and cervix are removed. Menstruation ceases after any type of hysterectomy is performed. Under general or spinal anesthesia, the uterus is excised and removed, either through the abdominal wall or, if plastic repair of vaginal structures is needed, through the vagina. Compare **hysterosalpingo-oophorectomy.** —**hysterectomize,** v.

hysteria 1. A general state of tension or excitement in a person or a group, characterized by unmanageable fear and temporary loss of control over the emotions. 2. A psychoneurosis, now commonly called **hysterical neurosis.**

hysterical fever An abnormal rise in body temperature without general symptoms, often seen in hysterical neurosis.

hysterical neurosis A form of psychoneurosis in which extreme excitability and anxiety resulting from an underlying emotional conflict are converted either into physical symptoms having no organic basis or into states of altered consciousness or identity. Kinds of hysterical neurosis are **conversion disorder, dissociative disorder.**

hysterical personality See **histrionic personality disorder.**

hysterical trance A somnambulistic state occurring as a symptom of hysterical neurosis.

hysteric amaurosis Monocular or, more rarely, binocular blindness occurring following an emotional shock and lasting for hours, days, or months.

hysteric apepsia See **anorexia nervosa.**

hysteric lethargy A sleep induced by hypnosis. See also **hypnosis, lethargy.**

hystero-, hyster- A combining form meaning 'pertaining to the uterus': *hysterocleisis, hysterolith.*

hysterolaparotomy Abdominal hysterectomy or hysterotomy.

hysterosalpingogram An X-ray film of the uterus and the fallopian tubes using gas or a radiopaque substance introduced through the cervix. A hysterosalpingogram allows visualization of the cavity of the uterus and the passageway of the tubes. Serial hysterosalpingograms are useful in the diagnosis of the cause of infertility.

hysterosalpingo-oophorectomy Surgical removal of one or both ovaries and oviducts along with the uterus. It is performed most commonly to treat malignant neoplastic disease of the reproductive tract and chronic endometriosis. To avoid the severe symptoms of sudden menopause, a portion of one ovary is left, unless a malignancy is present. With the patient under general anesthesia, the uterus is excised, and one or both oviducts and one or both ovaries are removed. If both ovaries are removed and no malignancy is present, estrogen-replacement therapy is often begun immediately. Compare **hysterectomy.**

hysteroscopy Direct visual inspection of the cervical canal and uterine cavity through a hysteroscope, performed to examine the endometrium, to secure a specimen for biopsy, to remove an intrauterine device, or to excise cervical polyps. The procedure is contraindicated in pregnancy, acute pelvic inflammatory disease, chronic upper genital tract infection, recent uterine perforation, and known or suspected cervical malignancy. —**hysteroscope,** *n.,* **hysteroscopic,** *adj.*

hysterotomy Surgical incision of the uterus, performed as a method of abortion in a pregnancy beyond the first trimester of gestation in which a saline-injection abortion was incomplete or in which a tubal sterilization is to be done with the abortion.

Hz *abbr* **hertz.**

HZV *abbr* herpes zoster virus. See **chickenpox.**

-i A plural-forming element used in native and later scientific Latin words: *bacilli*, and in scientific terms derived through Latin from Greek: *encephali*.

I **1.** Symbol for inspired gas. **2.** Symbol for **iodine.**

-ia A combining form meaning a 'specified condition (disease)': *athrombia, phrenoblabia.*

IADR *abbr* International Association for Dental Research.

IAET *abbr* **International Association for Enterostomal Therapy.**

-iasis A combining form meaning: **1.** A 'disease produced' by something specified: *cestodiasis, myiasis.* **2.** A 'disease producing (specified) characteristics': *elephantiasis, leontiasis.*

-iatria See **-iatry.**

-iatric A combining form meaning 'relating to medical treatment': *neuropsychiatric.* Also **-iatrical.**

-iatrician See **-iatrist.**

-iatrist A combining form meaning a 'physician': *hydriatrist, pediatrist, podiatrist.* Also **-iatrician.**

iatro- A combining form meaning 'pertaining to a physician or to treatment': *iatrogenic, iatrophysics.*

iatrogenic Caused by treatment or diagnostic procedures. An iatrogenic disorder is a condition caused by medical personnel or procedures or through exposure to the environment of a health-care facility. —**iatrogenesis,** *n.*

-iatry A combining form meaning a '(specified) type of medical treatment': *andriatry, pediatry.* Also **-iatria.**

ibuprofen A nonsteroidal anti-inflammatory agent.

-ic, -ac A combining form meaning 'pertaining to, similar to': *allelic, cadaveric.*

IC *abbr* **inspiratory capacity.**

ICCU *abbr* intensive coronary-care unit.

ICD *abbr* **International Classification of Diseases.**

ICD *abbr* intrauterine contraceptive device.

ICDA *abbr* **International Classification of Disease,** adapted for use in the United States.

ichthammol A topical anti-infective used for treating certain skin diseases.

ichthyo- A combining form meaning 'pertaining to fish': *ichthyocolla, ichthyophagy.*

ichthyosis Any of several inherited dermatologic conditions in which the skin is dry, hyperkeratotic, and fissured, resembling fish scales. It usually appears at or shortly after birth and may be part of one of several rare syndromes. Some types of ichthyosis respond to treatment with bath oils, topical retinoic acid,

or propylene glycol. —**ichthyotic,** *adj.*

ichthyosis congenita, ichthyosis fetalis See **lamellar exfoliation of the newborn.**

ichthyosis fetus See **harlequin fetus.**

ichthyosis simplex See **ichthyosis vulgaris.**

ichthyosis vulgaris A hereditary skin disorder characterized by large, dry, dark scales that cover the face, neck, scalp, ears, back, and extensor surfaces but not the flexor surfaces of the body. The condition is transmitted as an autosomal dominant trait; not present at birth, it appears several months to 1 year afterward. Management consists of topical application of emollients and the use of keratolytic agents to remove the scales. Also called **ichthyosis simplex.** See also **sex-linked ichthyosis.**

-ician A combining form meaning a 'specialist in a field': *clinician, pediatrician.*

ICN *abbr* **International Council of Nurses.**

ICP *abbr* intracranial pressure.

-ics A combining form meaning the 'systematic formulation of a body of knowledge': *bionomics, osmics.*

ICS *abbr* **International Congress of Surgeons.**

ICSH *abbr* interstitial cell-stimulating hormone. See **luteinizing hormone.**

icterus Jaundice. See also **hyperbilirubinemia.** —**icteric,** *adj.*

ictus, *pl.* **ictuses, ictus** **1.** A seizure. **2.** A cerebrovascular accident. —**ictal, ictic,** *adj.*

ICU *abbr* **intensive care unit.**

id **1.** In psychoanalysis: the part of the psyche, functioning in the unconscious, that is the source of instinctive energy, impulses, and drives. Based on the pleasure principle, it emphasizes self-preservation. Compare **ego, superego. 2.** The true unconscious.

-id A combining form meaning: **1.** A 'structural element of teeth': *protoconid, talonid.* **2.** A '(specified) body or particle': *cuspid, rhabdoid.*

ID *abbr* identification, immunodiffusion, infective dose, initial dose, intradermal.

-ide A combining form naming binary compounds composed of a metallic and a nonmetallic element: *chloride.*

idea Any thought, concept, intention, or impression that exists in the mind as a result of awareness, understanding, or other mental activity. Kinds of ideas include **autochthonous idea, compulsive idea, dominant idea, fixed idea, idea of influence, idea of persecution, idea of reference.**

idea of influence An obsessive delusion,

I J
K L

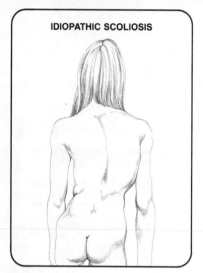

IDIOPATHIC SCOLIOSIS

often seen in paranoid disorders, that external forces or persons are controlling one's thoughts, actions, and feelings.

idea of persecution An obsessive delusion, often seen in paranoid disorders, that one is being threatened, discriminated against, or mistreated by other persons or by external forces.

idea of reference An obsessive delusion that the statements or actions of others refer to oneself, usually taken to be depreciatory, often seen in paranoid disorders. Also called **delusion of reference, referential idea.**

ideational apraxia A condition in which the conceptual process is lost, often owing to a lesion in the submarginal gyrus of the parietal lobe. The individual is unable to formulate a plan of movement and does not know the proper use of an object owing to a lack of perception of its purpose. There is no loss of motor movement, but the reason for the movement is confused. Also called **sensory apraxia.** See also **apraxia.**

idée fixe See **fixed idea.**

identical twins See **monozygotic twins.**

identification An unconscious defense mechanism by which a person patterns his personality on that of another person, assuming the person's qualities, characteristics, and actions. The process is a normal function of personality development and learning, and it contributes to the acquisition of interests and ideals. Kinds of identification are **competitive identification, positive identification.**

identity The characteristics of a person that distinguish his personality; his role in society and his perception of it.

identity crisis A period of disorientation concerning an individual's sense of self and role in society, occurring most frequently in the transition from one stage of life to the next. Identity crises are most common during adolescence,

when a sudden increase in the strength of internal drives combined with greater peer pressure and parents' or society's expectations of more mature behavior often results in conflicts. Although confusion regarding one's identity is usually considered an adolescent problem, it is also widespread among elderly people who lose their status in the community and their position as head of a family.

ideokinetic apraxia See **ideomotor apraxia.**

ideomotor apraxia The inability to translate an idea into motion, resulting from some interference with the transmission of the appropriate impulses from the brain to the motor centers. There is no loss of the ability to perform an action automatically, such as tying the shoelaces, but the action cannot be performed on request. The condition is often associated with diffuse cortical disease. Also called **classic apraxia, ideokinetic apraxia, limb-kinetic apraxia, transcortical apraxia.** See also **apraxia.**

ideophobia An anxiety disorder characterized by the irrational fear or distrust of ideas or reason. See also **phobia.**

idio- A combining form meaning 'pertaining to self or to something separate': *idiocratic, idioneurosis.*

idiomere See **chromomere.**

idiopathic Without a known cause.

idiopathic disease A disease that arises without an apparent or known cause. It may have a recognizable pattern of signs and symptoms, and it may be curable.

idiopathic multiple pigmented hemorrhagic sarcoma See **Kaposi's sarcoma.**

idiopathic scoliosis An abnormal condition characterized by a lateral curvature of the spine. It is the most common type of scoliosis, evident in 70% of all patients with scoliosis and up to 80% of those with structural scoliosis. It may occur at any age, but three types are commonly associated with certain age groups. The infantile type affects 1- to 3-year-olds. The juvenile type affects 3- to 10-year-olds. The adolescent type affects preadolescents and adolescents. The most common is the adolescent type. Early diagnosis is difficult because the associated curvature is often hidden by clothing, and many states have started scoliosis screening programs for the early detection of this condition. The signs commonly associated with scoliosis include unlevel shoulders, a prominent scapula, a prominent breast, a prominent flank area, an unlevel or prominent hip, poor posture, and an obvious curvature. Other signs are occasional transient pain and fatigue and decreased pulmonary function. Nonsurgical intervention commonly employs observation, an exercise program, and a Milwaukee brace. Observation and an exercise program often suffice. The Milwaukee brace, which is usually worn 23 hours a day, is used to control the progress of the curvature. The exercise program is implemented when the adolescent is out of the brace, and additional exercises are performed while in the brace. Surgical intervention may be required if the curvature has progressed to 40° or more at the time of diagnosis or if a slightly lesser degree of curvature exists with a high degree of rotational component or imbalance. Approximately 5% to 10% of patients with idiopathic scoliosis require surgery, which involves fusing of the involved vertebrae to prevent progress of the deformity.

idiopathic thrombocytopenic purpura (ITP) Bleeding into the skin and other organs owing to a deficiency of platelets. **Acute ITP,** a disease of children, may follow a viral infection, lasts a few weeks in and, and usually has no residua. **Chronic ITP,** more common in adolescents and adults, begins more insidiously and lasts longer. Antibodies to platelets have been found in patients with ITP; the condition may be transmitted to the fetus if a pregnant woman develops it. Treatment includes corticosteroids and splenectomy. See also **thrombocytopenia, thrombocytopenic purpura.**

idiopathy Any primary disease that arises without an apparent cause. —**idiopathic,** *adj.*

idiosyncrasy, idiocrasy 1. A physical or behavioral characteristic or manner that is unique to an individual or to a group. 2. An individual's unique hypersensitivity to a particular drug, to a food, or another substance. See also **allergy.** —**idiosyncratic,** *adj.*

idiot A severely retarded person having an intelligence quotient of less than 20, incapable of developing beyond the mental age of 3 or 4 years. Compare **imbecile, moron.** See also **mental retardation.** —**idiocy,** *n.,* **idiotic,** *adj.*

idiot savant, *pl.* **idiots savants** An individual with severe mental retardation who is nonetheless capable of performing certain unusual mental feats, primarily those involving music, puzzle-solving, or the manipulation of numbers.

-idium A noun-forming combining form: *coracidium.*

idoxuridine (IDU) An antiviral agent used to treat ophthalmic herpes simplex virus types I and II.

IFN *abbr* interferon.

-iform A combining form meaning 'in the form of': *amebiform, bulbiform.*

Ig *abbr* immunoglobulin.

IgA *abbr* **immunoglobulin A.**

IgA deficiency A selective lack of immunoglobulin A, the most common type of immunoglobulin deficiency, appearing in about 1 in 400 individuals. Immunoglobulin A is a major protein antibody in the saliva, the mucous membranes of the intestines, and the bronchi. It protects against bacterial and viral infections. A deficiency of immunoglobulin A is associated with autosomal dominant or with autosomal recessive inheritance, and with autoimmune abnormalities. The IgA deficiency is common in patients with rheumatoid arthritis and in patients with systemic lupus erythematosus. Symptoms of IgA deficiency are often lacking in pa-

tients whose humoral immune systems may be compensating for low IgA with extra amounts of IgM to assure adequate defenses. Common symptoms are respiratory allergies associated with chronic sinopulmonary infection; gastrointestinal diseases, as celiac disease and regional enteritis; autoimmune diseases, as rheumatoid arthritis and systemic lupus erythematosus; chronic hepatitis; malignant tumors, as squamous cell carcinoma of the lungs and recticulum cell sarcoma; and thymoma. There is no known cure for selective IgA deficiency; treatment usually involves the effort to control associated diseases, as respiratory and gastrointestinal infections.

NURSING CONSIDERATIONS: The patient with IgA deficiency should not receive gamma globulin because associated sensitization may cause anaphylaxis during administration of blood products. When the IgA deficient patient requires a blood transfusion, the risk of any harmful reaction can be reduced by using washed red blood cells.

IgD *abbr* **immunoglobulin D.**

IgE *abbr* **immunoglobulin E.**

IgG *abbr* **immunoglobulin G.**

IgM *abbr* **immunoglobulin M.**

l-hyoscyamine sulfate A gastrointestinal anticholinergic agent.

Ikwa fever See **trench fever.**

-il A combining form meaning a 'substance related to another': *benzil, uracil, uramil.* Also **-ile.**

-ile See **-il.**

ileitis See **Crohn's disease.**

ileo- A combining form meaning 'pertaining to the ileum': *ileocecum, ileorectostomy, ileotomy.*

ileocecal valve The valve between the ileum of the small intestine and the cecum of the large intestine, consisting of two flaps that project into the lumen of the large intestine, just above the vermiform appendix, allowing the intestine's contents to pass only in a forward direction.

ileocecostomy See **cecoileostomy.**

ileocolic node A node in one of three groups of superior mesenteric lymph glands, forming a chain of approximately 15 nodes around the ileocolic artery. They tend to form in two main groups, one near the duodenum, the other on the lower part of the ileocolic artery. The ileocolic nodes receive afferents from the jejunum, ileum, cecum, vermiform appendix, ascending colon, and transverse colon. Their efferents pass to the preaortic nodes. Compare **mesenteric node, mesocolic node.**

ileostomate A person who has undergone an ileostomy.

ileostomy Surgical formation of an opening of the ileum onto the surface of the abdomen, through which fecal matter is emptied. The operation is performed in advanced or recurrent ulcerative colitis, Crohn's disease, or cancer of the large bowel. The diseased portion of the large bowel is removed in a permanent ileostomy; occasionally, the distal and proximal seg-

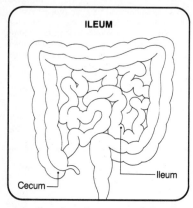

ILEUM

Cecum — Ileum

ments of bowel may be reconnected after ulcerated areas have healed. A loop of the proximal ileum is then brought out onto the abdomen and sutured in place, and a stoma is formed. A pouch may be made with part of the terminal ileum, in which the open end is woven through the rectus muscles to form a valve and then opens onto the abdomen. Postoperatively, the patient wears a temporary disposable bag to collect the semiliquid fecal matter, which begins to drain once peristalsis is restored and the nasogastric tube is removed. Since the secretions contain digestive enzymes which can ulcerate the skin around the stoma, the nurse must provide and teach good peristomal skin care and the use of ileostomy appliances. Compare **colostomy.** See also **enterostomy, ostomy irrigation, stoma.**

ileum The distal portion of the small intestine, extending from the jejunum to the cecum. It has a few small circular folds and numerous clusters of lymph nodes. It ends in the right iliac fossa, opening into the medial side of the large intestine. —**ileac, ileal,** *adj.*

ileus An obstruction of the intestines, as an adynamic ileus caused by immobility of the bowel, or a mechanical ileus in which the intestine is blocked by mechanical means.

-iliac A combining form meaning 'the ilium': *occipitoiliac, subiliac.*

iliac circumflex node A node in one of the seven clusters of parietal lymph nodes of the abdomen. This node is one of a group found along the course of the deep iliac circumflex vessels. Compare **common iliac node, external iliac node, internal iliac node.** See also **lymph, lymphatic system, lymph node.**

iliac fascia The portion of the endoabdominal fascia that is attached with the iliacus to the crest of the ilium and passes under the inguinal ligament into the thigh.

iliacus A flat, triangular muscle that covers the inner curved surface of the iliac fossa. It arises from the inner aspect of the superior iliac crest, from the anterior and the iliolumbar ligaments, and from the sacrum. It joins the psoas major to form the iliopsoas at the inguinal ligament. The iliacus is innervated by branches of the femoral nerve that contain fibers from the second and the third lumbar nerves. It acts to flex and laterally rotate the thigh. Compare **psoas major, psoas minor.**

ilio- A combining form meaning 'of or pertaining to the ilium or flank': *iliocostal.*

iliofemoral Of or pertaining to the ilium and femur.

ilioinguinal Of or pertaining to the hip and inguinal regions.

iliolumbar ligament One of a pair of ligaments forming part of the connection between the vertebral column and the pelvis. Each iliolumbar ligament attaches to a transverse process of the fifth lumbar vertebra and passes to the base of the sacrum.

iliopsoas One of the pair of muscle complexes that flexes the thigh and the lumbar vertebral column. Each complex is comprised of the psoas major, the psoas minor, and the iliacus, although the psoas minor is often absent.

ilium, *pl.* **ilia** One of the three bones that make up the innominate bone. The ilium forms part of the acetabulum and provides attachment for several muscles, including the obturator internus, the gluteals, the iliacus, and the sartorius. The ilium is divided into the body, which forms less than two fifths of the acetabulum, and the ala, which is the large, winglike portion of the greater pelvis. Compare **ischium, pubis.** —**iliac,** *adj.*

illness An abnormal process in which aspects of the social, physical, emotional, or intellectual condition and function of a person are diminished or impaired, compared to that person's previous condition.

illness experience The process of being ill, comprised of five stages: phase I, experiencing a symptom; phase II, assuming a sick role; phase III, making contact for health care; phase IV, being dependent (a patient); and phase V, recovering or being rehabilitated. Each stage is characterized by certain decisions and behaviors. During phase I, the person decides that something is wrong and tries to remedy the situation. During phase II the person decides that the illness is real and that care is necessary. Advice, guidance, and validation are sought. This gives the person permission to act sick and to be excused temporarily from usual obligations. The outcome of this phase is acceptance of the role or denial of its necessity. In phase III professional advice is sought; authoritative declarations identify and validate the illness. The person usually asks for help and negotiates for treatment. Denial may still occur and the patient may 'shop' further for medical care or may accept the illness, the medical authority, and the plan for treatment. In phase IV professional treatment is performed and accepted by the person, who is now perceived as a patient. The patient has a particular need to be informed and to be given emotional support during this phase. During phase V, the patient relinquishes the sick role. The usual tasks and roles are resumed to the greatest degree possible.

illumination The lighting up of a part of the body or object under a microscope for examination. —**illuminate,** *v.*

illusion A false interpretation of an external sensory stimulus, usually visual or auditory, as a mirage in the desert. Compare **delusion, hallucination.**

im- In chemistry: a combining form indicating the bivalent group > NH: *imadyl, imide, imperialine.*

IMA *abbr* **Industrial Medical Association.**

image **1.** A representation or visual reproduction of the likeness of someone or something, as a painting, photograph, or sculpture. **2.** An optical representation of an object, as that produced by refraction or reflection. **3.** A person or thing that closely resembles another; semblance. **4.** A mental picture, representation, idea, or concept of an objective reality. **5.** In psychology: a mental representation of something previously perceived and subsequently modified by other experiences resulting from intrapsychic or extrapsychic stimuli, or both. Kinds of images include **body image, eidetic image, memory image, mental image, motor image, tactile image.**

imagery In psychiatry: the formation of mental concepts, figures: any product of the imagination. In the mentally ill, these images are often bizarre and delusional.

imagination **1.** The ability to form, or the act or process of forming mental images or conscious concepts of things that are not immediately available to the senses. **2.** In psychology: the ability to reproduce images or ideas stored in the memory by the stimulation or suggestion of associated ideas or to regroup former ideas and concepts to form new images and ideas concerned with a particular goal or problem. See also **fantasy.**

imaging **1.** The formation of a mental picture or representation of someone or something using the imagination. See also **fantasy. 2.** The production of clarity, contrast, and detail in images, especially in radiologic and ultrasound images. In diagnostic medicine: imaging includes X-ray, ultrasound, and infrared techniques. In radioisotopic studies of a muscle or organ: imaging produces a detailed picture of areas of blood perfusion.

imago In analytic psychology: an unconscious, usually idealized mental image of a significant individual in a person's early, formative years. See also **identification.**

imbalance **1.** Lack of balance between opposing muscle groups, as in the imbalance of extraocular muscles, leading to strabismus. **2.** An abnormal balance of fluid and electrolytes in the body tissues. **3.** An unequal distribution of subjects in a population group. **4.** Mental abilities that are remarkable in one area but deficient in others, as in an idiot savant.

imbecile A moderately retarded person having an intelligence quotient of 20 to 49, incapable of developing beyond a mental age of 7 or 8 years. Compare **idiot, moron.** See also **mental retar-**dation. —**imbecile, imbecilic,** *adj.,* **imbecility,** *n.*

imbricate To build a surface with overlapping layers of material. Surgeons may imbricate with layers of tissue when closing a wound or another opening in a body part. —**imbrication,** *n.*

imido- A combining form indicating the presence in a chemical compound of the bivalent group > NH: *imidogen.*

imino- A combining form indicating the presence of the bivalent group > NH attached to a nonacid radical: *imino-urea.*

iminoglycinuria A benign familial condition characterized by the abnormal urinary excretion of the amino acids glycine, proline, and hydroxyproline.

imipramine hydrochloride A tricyclic antidepressant.

immediate auscultation A method of examining a patient by placing an ear or stethoscope on the skin directly over the body part being studied.

immediate hypersensitivity An allergic reaction that occurs within minutes after exposure to an allergen.

immediate hypersensitivity reaction See **hypersensitivity reaction.**

immediate posttraumatic automatism A posttraumatic state in which a person acts spontaneously and automatically without any recollection of the behavior.

immersion The placing of a body or an object into water or other liquid so that it is completely covered by the liquid. —**immerse,** *v.*

immersion foot An abnormal condition of the feet characterized by damage to the muscles, nerves, skin and blood vessels, caused by prolonged exposure to dampness or by prolonged immersion in cold water. See also **frostbite.**

imminent abortion See **inevitable abortion.**

immiscible Not capable of being mixed, as oil and water. Compare **miscible.**

immobilize To eliminate motion by cast, splint, or surgical fixation. —**immobilization,** *n.*

immune complex hypersensitivity An IgG or IgM complement-dependent, immediate-acting humoral hypersensitivity to certain soluble antigens. An intradermal skin test results in erythema and edema within 3 to 8 hours and an acute inflammatory reaction with an increase in polymorphonuclear leukocytes. It is seen in serum sickness, Arthus reaction, and glomerulonephritis. Also called **type III hypersensitivity.** Compare **anaphylactic hypersensitivity, cell-mediated immune response, cytotoxic hypersensitivity.**

immune cytolysis Cell destruction mediated by a particular antibody in conjunction with complement.

immune gamma globulin Passive immunizing agents obtained from pooled human plasma. It is prescribed for immunization against measles, poliomyelitis, chickenpox, serum hep-

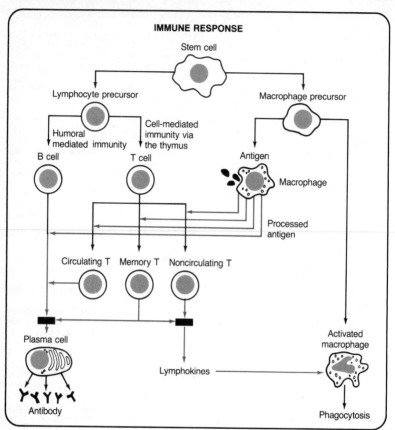

IMMUNE RESPONSE

Stem cell

Lymphocyte precursor

Macrophage precursor

Humoral mediated immunity

Cell-mediated immunity via the thymus

B cell

T cell

Antigen

Macrophage

Processed antigen

Circulating T   Memory T   Noncirculating T

Plasma cell

Lymphokines

Activated macrophage

Antibody

Phagocytosis

atitis following transfusion, hepatitis A, agammaglobulinemia, and hypogammaglobulinemia. See also **immunoglobulin G.**

immune globulin See **immune gamma globulin.**

immune human globulin A sterile solution of globulins, used as a passive immunizing agent, derived from adult human blood.

immune serum See **antiserum.**

immune serum globulin (ISG) **1.** See **chickenpox. 2.** See **immune human globulin. 3.** See **immunoglobulin antibody.**

immune response A defense function of the body that produces antibodies to destroy invading antigens and malignancies. Important components of the immune system and response are immunoglobulins, lymphocytes, phagocytes, complement, properdin, the migratory inhibitory factor, and interferon. Antigens, which are largely foreign protein macromolecules, trigger the immune response during interaction with countless cells of the reticuloendothelial system of the body. The antigen-antibody reaction may transform the toxic antigen into a harmless substance, or it may agglutinate antigens, allowing macrophages and other phagocytes to digest large

numbers of antigens at one time. The antigen-antibody reactions of the humoral immune response also activate the complement in the blood serum, which triggers a nonspecific series of chemical reactions to amplify the humoral immune response. Other proteins associated with the immune response are properdin and interferon. Properdin provides an alternate process for activating complement. Interferon is synthesized by body cells after viral invasion and acts to combat viruses and may retard the growth of cancer cells. Natural immunity, or genetically inherited resistance to specific infectious organisms, is affected by diet, mental health, environment, metabolism, and the virulence of invading pathogens.

immune system A biochemical complex which protects the body against pathogenic organisms and other foreign bodies. The system incorporates the humoral immune response, which produces antibodies to react with specific antigens, and the cell-mediated response, which uses T cells to mobilize tissue macrophages in the presence of a foreign body. The immune system also protects the body from invasion by creating local barriers and inflammation. The humoral response and the cell-mediated response develop if these first-line defenses fail or are inadequate to protect the body. The humoral immune response is especially effective against bacterial and viral invasions and employs B cells that produce appropriate antibodies. The antigen-antibody reactions of the immune system activate the complement system, which removes antigens from the body. The complement system contains several discrete proteins which function to produce lysis of the antigenic cells. The humoral response may begin immediately on invasion by the antigen or may start as long as 48 hours later.

immunity **1.** The quality of being insusceptible to or unaffected by a particular disease or condition. **2.** In civil law: exemption from a duty or an obligation generally required by law, as an exemption from taxation, exemption from penalty for wrongdoing, or protection against liability. —**immune,** *adj.*

immunization A process by which resistance to an infectious disease is induced or augmented.

immunodeficient An abnormal condition of the immune system in which cellular or humoral immunity is inadequate and resistance to infection is decreased. Kinds of immunodeficient conditions are **hypogammaglobulinemia, severe combined immunodeficiency disease.**

immunodiagnosis See **serological diagnosis.**

immunodiagnostic Pertaining to or characterizing a diagnosis based on an antigen-antibody reaction.

immunodiffusion A technique for the identification and quantification of any of the immunoglobulins. It is based on the presence of a visible precipitate that results from an antigen-antibody combination under certain circumstances. **Gel diffusion** involves evaluation of the precipitin reaction in a clear gel, seen when an antigen placed in a hole in the agarose diffuses evenly into the medium. An obvious ring forms where the antigen meets the antibody. **Electroimmunodiffusion** is a gel diffusion to which an electric field is applied, accelerating the reaction. **Double gel diffusion** permits identification of antibodies in mixed specimens. In an agar plate, antigen is placed in one well, antibody in another. Antigen and antibody diffuse out of their wells. In mixed antigen specimens, each antigen-antibody combination forms a separate line; observation of the location, shape, and thickness of a line permits identification and quantification of the antibody.

immunoelectrodiffusion See **immunodiffusion.**

immunoelectrophoresis A technique that combines electrophoresis and immunodiffusion to separate and allow identification of complex proteins. The proteins in the test serum are spread out in agar and separated by electrophoresis. A visible precipitin will form in a series of arcs in the agar when an antigen-antibody reaction

IMMUNODEFICIENCY: CLINICAL SIGNS

Highly suspicious signs
- Chronic infection
- Recurrent infection (more than expected)
- Unusual infecting agents
- Incomplete clearing between episodes of infection or incomplete response to treatment

Moderately suspicious signs
- Skin rash (eczema, candida, etc.)
- Diarrhea (chronic)
- Growth failure
- Hepatosplenomegaly
- Recurrent abscesses
- Recurrent osteomyelitis

Specific rare signs of disorders
- Ataxia
- Telangiectasia
- Short-limbed dwarfism
- Cartilage-hair hypoplasia
- Idiopathic endocrinopathy
- Partial albinism
- Thrombocytopenia
- Eczema
- Tetany

occurs. The shape and location of each arc are specific for known proteins. Unusual arcs are representative of abnormal or unknown protein. Although the density of the precipitation corresponds to the concentration of protein in each electrophoretic band, immunoelectrophoresis does not accurately quantify the amount of protein in the test serum. —**immunoelectrophoretic,** *adj.*

immunofluorescence A technique used for the rapid identification of an antigen by exposing it to known antibodies tagged with the fluorescent dye fluorescein and observing the characteristic antigen-antibody reaction of precipitation. Many of the most common infectious organisms can be identified using this technique. Among them are *Candida albicans, Haemophilus influenzae, Neisseria gonorrhae, Shigella, Staphylococcus aureus,* and several viruses, including rabies virus and many enteroviruses. See also **fluorescent microscopy.** —**immunofluorescent,** *adj.*

immunofluorescence test See **fluorescent antibody test.**

immunofluorescent microscopy See **fluorescent microscopy, immunofluorescence.**

immunogen Any agent or substance capable of provoking an immune response or producing immunity. —**immunogenic,** *adj.*

immunoglobulin A (IgA) One of the five

classes of humoral antibodies produced by the body and one of the most prevalent. It is found in all secretions of the body and is the major antibody in the mucous membrane lining of the intestines and in the bronchi, saliva, and tears. Research indicates that it protects body tissues by seeking out foreign microorganisms and triggering an antigen-antibody reaction. Compare **immunoglobulin D, immunoglobulin E, immunoglobulin G, immunoglobulin M.**

immunoglobulin antibody Any of five structurally and antigenically distinct antibodies present in the serum and external secretions of the body. In response to specific antigens, immunoglobulins are formed in the bone marrow, spleen, and all lymphoid tissue of the body except the thymus. Kinds of immunoglobulins are **immunoglobulin (Ig) A, IgD, IgE, IgG, IgM.** Also called **immune serum globulin.** See also **antibody, antigen, immunity.**

immunoglobulin D (IgD) One of the five classes of humoral antibodies produced by the body. It is a specialized protein found in small amounts in serum tissue. The precise function of IgD is not known, but it increases in quantity during allergic reactions to milk, insulin, penicillin, and various toxins. Compare **immunoglobulin A, immunoglobulin E, immunoglobulin G, immunoglobulin M.**

immunoglobulin E (IgE) One of the five classes of humoral antibodies produced by the body. It is concentrated in the lung, the skin, and the cells of mucous membranes. It provides the primary defense against environmental antigens and is believed to be responsive to immunoglobulin A. IgE reacts with certain antigens to release certain chemical mediators which cause Type I hypersensitivity reactions characterized by wheal and flare. Compare **immunoglobulin A, immunoglobulin D, immunoglobulin G, immunoglobulin M.**

immunoglobulin G (IgG) One of the five classes of humoral antibodies produced by the body. It is a specialized protein synthesized by the body in response to invasions by bacteria, fungi, and viruses. IgG crosses the placenta and protects against red cell antigens and white cell antigens. Compare **immunoglobulin A, immunoglobulin D, immunoglobulin E, immunoglobulin M.**

immunoglobulin M (IgM) One of the five classes of humoral antibodies produced by the body and the largest in molecular structure. It is the first immunoglobulin the body produces when challenged by antigens and is found in circulating fluids. IgM triggers the increased production of immunoglobulin G and the complement fixation required for effective antibody response. It is the dominant antibody in ABO incompatibilities. Compare **immunoglobulin A, immunoglobulin D, immunoglobulin E, immunoglobulin G.**

immunologist A specialist in immunology.
immunology The study of the reaction of tissues of the immune system of the body to antigenic stimulation.

immunomodulator A substance that alters the immune response by augmenting or reducing the ability of the immune system to produce modified serum antibodies or sensitized cells that recognize and react with the antigen that initiated their production. Corticosteroids, cytotoxic agents, thymosin, and the immunoglobulins are among the immunomodulating substances. Some immunomodulating substances are naturally present in the body; some are available in pharmacologic preparations. —**immunomodulation,** *n.*

immunosuppression 1. The administration of agents that significantly interfere with the ability of the immune system to respond to antigenic stimulation by inhibiting cellular and humoral immunity. Corticosteroid hormones given in large amounts, cytotoxic drugs, including antimetabolites and alkylating agents, and irradiation may result in immunosupression. Immunosuppression may be deliberate, as in preparation for bone marrow or other transplantation to prevent rejection by the host of the donor tissue, or incidental, as often results from chemotherapy for the treatment of cancer. 2. An abnormal condition of the immune system characterized by markedly inhibited ability to respond to antigenic stimuli. —**immunosuppressed,** *adj.*

immunosuppressive 1. Of or pertaining to a substance or procedure that lessens or prevents an immune response. 2. An immunosuppresive agent. The immunosuppressive drugs used most frequently to prevent homograft rejection are the cytotoxic purine antimetabolite azathioprine, the alkylating agent cyclophosphamide, and the adrenocoricosteroid prednisone. Methotrexate, cytarabine, dactinomycin, thioguanine, and antilymphocyte globulin are also potent immunosuppressives.

immunotherapy 1. A special treatment of allergic responses which administers increasingly large doses of the offending allergens to gradually develop immunity. Immunotherapy is based on the premise that low doses of the offending allergen will bind with immunoglobulin G (IgG) to prevent an allergic reaction by damping the action of IgE by fostering the synthesis of the blocking IgG antibody. The individual who is exposed to the offending allergen develops an amount of blocking antibody in proportion to the extent of the exposure. The blocking antibody binds to the circulating antigen and seems to decrease the allergic response, or it eliminates the allergic response by producing an immunologic tolerance toward the antigen. 2. In neoplastic diseases: a course of treatment that enhances the patient's immune system in order to restore immunocompetence; to prevent or reverse immunodepression; or to induce or potentiate specific tumor immunity. Also called **hyposensitization.** —**immunotherapeutic,** *adj.*

impacted Tightly or firmly wedged in a limited amount of space. —**impact,** *v.,* **impaction,** *adj.*

impacted fracture A bone break in which the fractured bone's adjacent fragmented ends are mashed together.

impedance audiometry See **audiometry.**

impedance plethysmography A technique for detecting blood vessel occlusion that determines volumetric changes in the limb by measuring changes in its girth as indicated by changes in the electrical impedance of mercury-containing silastic tubes in a pressure cuff. The method is based on the principle that any circumferential rate of change in a limb segment is directly proportional to the volumetric rate of change, which in turn reflects occlusion of venous and arterial blood flow.

imperative conception A thought or impression that appears spontaneously in the mind and cannot be eliminated, as an obsession.

imperforate Lacking a normal opening in a body organ or passageway. An infant may be born with an imperforate anus. Compare **perforate.**

imperforate anus Any of several congenital, developmental malformations of the anorectal portion of the gastrointestinal tract. The most common form is anal agenesis, in which the rectal pouch ends blindly above the surface of the perineum. An anal fistual is present in 80% to 90% of cases. Other forms include anal stenosis, in which the anal aperture is small, and anal membrane atresia, in which the anal membrane covers the aperture creating an obstruction. The defect is usually discovered just after birth, when the nurse attempts to take a rectal temperature during routine newborn assessment. An imperforate anal membrane is excised, and digital dilatation is performed daily as the skin heals. Surgical reconstruction is performed to treat anal agenesis in infants in whom the pouch is below the puborectalis of the levator ani; an anus is created surgically by an anoplasty. Anal atresia in which the pouch at the end of the bowel is high above the perineum may require a colostomy. NURSING CONSIDERATIONS: A newborn who does not pass any stool in the first 24 hours requires further evaluation for the possibility of the defect. The passage of meconium from the vagina or urinary meatus clearly indicates the presence of anal fistula and usually occurs in association with an imperforate anus.

imperforate hymen A completely closed hymen that prevents menstrual flow from the vagina. This condition is treated by surgical incision.

impermeable Of a tissue, membrane, or film: preventing the passage of a substance through it.

impervious See **impermeable.**

impetigo A streptococcal, staphylococcal, or combined infection of the skin beginning as focal erythema and progressing to pruritic vesicles, erosions, and honey-colored crusts. Lesions usually form on the face and spread locally. The disorder is highly contagious by contact with the

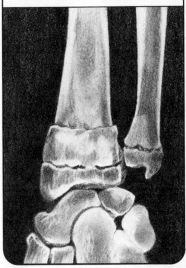

IMPACTED FRACTURE

discharge from the lesions. Treatment includes thorough cleansing with antibacterial soap and water, compresses of Burow's solution, removal of crusts, and topical or oral antibiotics. —**impetiginous,** *adj.*

implant 1. In radiotherapy: an encapsulated radioactive substance embedded in tissue for therapy. Seeds containing iodine 125 (^{125}I) may be implanted permanently in prostate and chest tumors and seeds of iridium 192 (^{192}Ir) in ribbons or wire may be embedded temporarily in head and neck cancers. Patients with radioactive implants are isolated from other patients during treatment. 2. In surgery: material inserted or grafted into an organ or structure of the body. The implant may be of tissue, as in a blood vessel graft, or of an artificial substance, as in a hip prosthesis.

implantation In embryology: the process involving the attachment, penetration, and embedding of the blastocyst in the lining of the uterine wall during the early stages of prenatal development. The degree of invasiveness required for an adequate maternal-fetal exchange varies greatly among species. In man, the process occurs over a period of a few days, beginning about the 7th or 8th day following fertilization. Kinds of implantation include **eccentric implantation, interstitial implantation, superficial implantation.** Also called **nidation.**

implantation dermoid cyst A tumor derived from embryonic tissues, caused by an injury that forces part of the ectoderm into the body.

implementation 1. A deliberate action performed to achieve a goal, as carrying out a plan in caring for a patient. 2. In five-step nursing process: a category of nursing behavior in which the actions necessary for accomplishing the health-care plan are initiated and completed. Implementation includes the performance or assisting in the performance of the client's activities of daily living; counseling and teaching the client or the client's family; giving care to achieve therapeutic goals and to optimize the achievement of health goals by the client; and recording and exchanging information relevant to the client's continued health care. The client may require assistance in performing certain activities of daily living. The nurse helps the client to maintain optimal function, while instituting measures for the client's comfort as necessary. The nurse helps the client and the client's family recognize and manage the emotional and psychological stress of the client's condition. Correct principles, procedures, and techniques of health care are taught, and the client is informed about the current status of his or her health. If necessary, the client or the client's family is referred to a health or social resource in the community. Implementation follows planning and precedes evaluating in the five-step nursing process. See also **analyzing, assessing. —implement,** *v.*

implosion 1. A bursting inward. 2. A psychiatric treatment for people disabled by phobias and anxiety in which the person is desensitized to anxiety-producing stimuli by repeated intense exposure in imagination or reality, until the stimuli are no longer stressful. Also called **flooding. —implode,** *v.*

implosive therapy See **flooding.**

impotence 1. Weakness. 2. Inability of the adult male to achieve penile erection or, less commonly, to ejaculate having achieved an erection. Several forms are recognized. **Anatomic impotence** results from physically defective genitalia. **Atonic impotence** involves disturbed neuromuscular function. Poor health, age, drugs, and fatigue can inhibit normal sexual function. **Functional impotence** has a psychologic basis. Also called **impotency.** Compare **infertile. —impotent,** *adj.*

impotency See **impotence.**

impregnate 1. To inseminate and make pregnant; to fertilize. 2. To saturate or mix with another substance. **—impregnable,** *adj.,* **impregnation,** *n.*

impression 1. In dentistry and prosthetic medicine: a mold of a part of the mouth or other part of the body from which a replacement or prosthesis may be formed. 2. In the medical record: the examiner's diagnosis or assessment of a problem, disease, or condition. 3. A strong sensation or effect on the mind, intellect, or feelings.

imprinting In ethology: a special type of learning that occurs at critical points during the early stages of development in animals. It involves behavioral patterning and social attachment, is characterized by rapid acquisition and irreversibility, and is usually species-specific, although animals exposed to members of a different species during this short period may become attached to and identify with that partic-

ular species instead of their own. The degree to which imprinting occurs in human development has not been determined. See also **bonding.**

impulse 1. In psychology: a sudden, irresistible, often irrational inclination, urge, desire, or action resulting from a particular feeling or mental state. 2. In physiology: the electrochemical process involved in neural transmission. Also called **nerve impulse, neural impulse. —impulsive,** *adj.*

impulsion An abnormal, irrational urge to commit an unlawful or socially unacceptable act.

IMV *abbr* **intermittent mandatory ventilation.**

In Symbol for **indium.**

in- 1. A combining form meaning 'of or pertaining to fibers': *inaxon, inemia.* 2. A combining form meaning 'in, on': *incineration, indigitation.* 3. A combining form meaning 'not': *inaction, inassimilable.*

-in 1. A combining form meaning 'antibiotic': *bacitracin, penicillin.* 2. A combining form meaning 'pharmaceutical product': *aspirin, streptomycin.* 3. A combining form meaning 'chemical compound': *albumin, gelatin.* 4. A combining form meaning 'enzyme': *emulsin, pepsin.* Also **-ine.**

INA *abbr* International Neurological Association.

inactive colon Hypotonicity of the bowel resulting in decreased contractions and propulsive movements and a delay in the normal 12-hour transit time of luminal contents from cecum to anus. Colonic inactivity may be caused by acquired or congential megacolon, aging, anticholinergic drugs, depression, faulty habits of elimination, inadequate fluid intake, lack of exercise, a low-residue or starvation diet, neuroendocrine response to surgical stress, prolonged bed rest, or a neurologic disease, as diabetic visceral neuropathy, multiple sclerosis, parkinsonism, and spinal cord lesions. Treatment of colonic inactivity includes a stimulus-response training program to establish regular bowel habits, the use of stool softeners and hydrophilic colloids to increase fecal bulk, and a diet containing adequate roughage.

inadequate personality A personality characterized by a lack of physical stamina, emotional immaturity, social instability, poor judgment, reduced motivation, ineptness—especially in interpersonal relationships—and an inability to adapt effectively to new or stressful situations.

inanimate Not alive; lacking signs of life.

inanition 1. An exhausted condition resulting from lack of food and water or a defect in assimilation; starvation. 2. A state of lethargy characterized by a loss of vitality in social, moral, and intellectual life.

inanition fever A temporary, mild, febrile condition of the newborn in the first few days after birth, usually caused by dehydration.

inborn Innate; acquired or occurring during intrauterine life, with reference to both normally inherited traits and developmental or genetically transmitted anomalies. See also **congenital, hereditary, inborn error of metabolism.**

inborn error of metabolism   One of many abnormal metabolic conditions caused by an inherited defect of a single enzyme or other protein. Though people with such diseases are each defective in only protein, they generally display a large number of physical signs that are characteristic of the genetic trait. The diseases are rare. Kinds of inborn errors of metabolism include **galactosemia, glucose-6-phosphate dehydrogenase deficiency, Lesch-Nyhan syndrome, phenylketonuria (PKU), Tay-Sachs disease.**

inborn reflex   See **unconditioned response.**

inbreeding   The production of offspring by the mating of closely related individuals, organisms, or plants; self-fertilization is the most extreme form, which normally occurs in certain plants and lower animals. The practice provides a greater chance for recessive genes for both desirable and undesirable traits to become homozygous and to be expressed phenotypically. In humans, the amount of inbreeding in a specific population is largely controlled by tradition and cultural practices. In plants and animals, inbreeding is a standard method for developing desirable genotypes and pure lines. Compare **outbreeding.**

incarcerate   To trap, imprison, or confine, as a loop of intestine in an inguinal hernia. See also **hernia.**

incest   **1.** Sexual intercourse between members of the same family who are so closely related as to be legally prohibited from marrying one another by reason of their consanguinity. **2.** In law: the statutory crime of such acts. —**incestuous,** *adj.*

incidence   **1.** The number of times an event occurs. **2.** In epidemiology: the number of new cases in a particular period of time. Incidence is often expressed as a ratio, in which the number of cases is the numerator and the population at risk is the denominator. See also **rate.**

incipient   Coming into existence; an initial stage; beginning to appear or to become apparent, as a symptom.

incision   The insertion of a sharp instrument, such as a scalpel, into body tissue.

incisor   One of the eight front teeth, four in each dental arch, that first appear as milk teeth during infancy and are replaced by permanent incisors during childhood. Compare **canine tooth, molar, premolar.**

inclusion   **1.** The act of enclosing or the condition of being enclosed. **2.** A structure within another, as inclusions of metabolic wastes, such as oil droplets or crystals, in the cytoplasm of the cells.

inclusion conjunctivitis   An acute, purulent, conjunctival infection caused by *Chlamydia* organisms. It occurs in two forms: bilateral chemosis, redness, and purulent discharge characterize the infection in infants; the adult

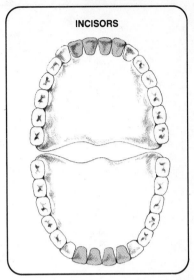

INCISORS

variety is unilateral, less severe, less purulent, and associated with preauricular lymphadenopathy. Local instillation of antibiotics is effective treatment. Also called **swimming pool conjunctivitis.**

inclusion dermoid cyst   A tumor derived from embryonic tissues, caused by the inclusion of a foreign tissue when a developmental cleft closes.

incoherent   **1.** Disordered; without logical connection; disjointed; lacking orderly continuity or relevance; inharmonious. **2.** Unable to express one's thoughts or ideas in an orderly, intelligible manner, usually as a result of emotional stress.

incompatible   Unable to coexist. A tissue transplant may be rejected because recipient and donor antibody factors are incompatible.

incompetence   Lack of ability. Body organs that do not function adequately may be described as incompetent. Kinds of incompetence include aortic incompetence, ileocecal incompetence, valvular incompetence. —**incompetent,** *adj.*

incompetent cervix   In obstetrics: a condition characterized by dilatation of the cervical os of the uterus before term without labor or contractions of the uterus. Miscarriage or premature delivery may result. Incompetent cervix is treated prophylactically by a Shirodkar or other procedure in which the cervix is held closed by a surgically implanted suture.

incomplete abortion   Termination of pregnancy in which the products of conception are not entirely expelled or removed, often causing hemorrhage that may require surgical evacuation by curettage, oxytocics, and blood replacement. Infection is also a frequent complication of incomplete abortion. Compare **complete abortion.**

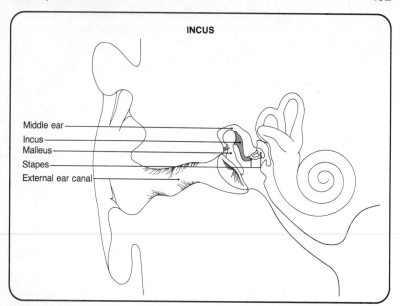

INCUS

Middle ear
Incus
Malleus
Stapes
External ear canal

incomplete fistula   See **blind fistula.**

incomplete fracture   A bone break in which the crack in the osseous tissue does not completely traverse the width of the affected bone but may angle off in one or more directions.

incongruent message   In patient-nurse interaction: communication in which the sender's words are inconsistent with his body language.

incontinence   The inability to control urination or defecation. Urinary incontinence may be caused by cerebral clouding in the aged, infection, lesions in the brain or spinal cord, damage to peripheral nerves of the bladder, or injury to the sphincter or perineal structures, as sometimes occurs in childbirth. Stress incontinence precipitated by coughing, straining, or heavy lifting occurs more often in women than in men and may be treated by exercises involving tightening and relaxing perineal and gluteal muscles. Fecal incontinence may result from relaxation of the anal sphincter or by central nervous system or spinal cord disorders and may be treated by a program of bowel training. See also **bowel training. —incontinent,** *adj.*

increment   **1.** An increase or gain. **2.** The amount of an increase or gain. **—incremental,** *adj.*

increto-   A combining form meaning 'of or pertaining to internal secretions': *incretodiagnosis, incretogenous.*

incrustation   Hardened exudate, scale, or scab.

incubation period   **1.** The time between exposure to a pathogenic organism and the onset of symptoms of a disease. **2.** The time required to induce the development of an embryo in an egg or to induce the development and replication of tissue cells or microorganisms being grown in culture media or other special laboratory environment.

incubator   An apparatus used to provide a controlled environment, especially a particular temperature. Other environmental components, as darkness or light, oxygen, moisture or dryness, may also be provided. Examples of use include the cultivation of eggs or microorganisms in a laboratory or the care of premature infants.

incud-   A combining form meaning 'of or pertaining to an anvil (the incus)': *incudectomy, incudiform.*

incudectomy   Surgical removal of the incus, performed to treat conductive deafness owing to necrosis of the tip of the incus.

incus   One of the three ossicles in the middle ear, resembling an anvil. It communicates sound vibrations from the malleus to the stapes. Compare **malleus, stapes.** See also **middle ear.**

IND   *abbr* **investigational new drug.**

indandione derivative   One of a small group of oral anticoagulants designed for long-term therapeutic use in patients who cannot tolerate other oral anticoagulants. The indandiones are difficult to control and may cause grave adverse effects, including severe renal and hepatic toxicity, agranulocytosis, and leukopenia. Extreme fatigue, sore throat, chills, and fever are signs of impending toxicity and require discontinuation of the drug.

indentation   A notch, pit, or depression in the surface of an object, as toothmarks on the skin. **—indent,** *v.*

independence   **1.** The state or quality of being independent; autonomy; free from the influence, guidance, or control of a person or a group. **2.** A lack of requirement or reliance on another for physical existence or emotional needs. Also called **independency.** —**independent,** *adj.*

independent assortment In genetics: a principle stating that the members of a pair of genes are randomly distributed in the gametes, independent of the distribution of other pairs of genes. See also **dominance, segregation.**

independent practice In nursing: the practice of certain aspects of professional nursing that are encompassed by applicable licensure and law and require no supervision or direction from others. Nurses in independent practice may have an office in which they see patients and charge fees for service. In all nursing settings, state practice acts define aspects of nursing practice that are independent and may define those to be done only under supervision or direction of another individual, usually a doctor.

independent variable In research: a variable that is controlled by the researcher and evaluated by its measurable effect on the dependent variable or variables. For example, in a study of the effect of nursing intervention on postoperative vomiting, nursing intervention is the independent variable evaluated by its effect on the incidence of postoperative vomiting. Also called **experimental variable, predictor variable.** Compare **dependent variable.**

indeterminate cleavage Mitotic division of the fertilized ovum into blastomeres with similar developmental potential that can, if isolated, give rise to a complete individual embryo. Also called **regulative cleavage.** Compare **determinate cleavage.** See also **regulative development.**

index case 1. See **propositus. 2.** In epidemiology: the first case of a disease as contrasted with the appearance of subsequent cases.

Index Medicus An index published monthly by the National Library of Medicine, which lists articles from medical literature from throughout the world by subject and author. An annual edition, the *Cumulative Index Medicus,* contains all 12 issues of the *Index Medicus.*

index myopia A kind of nearsightedness owing to a variation in the index of refraction of the eye's media.

Indian Health Service A bureau within the Department of Health and Human Services for providing public health and medical services to native Americans in the United States.

Indian tick fever See **Marseilles fever.**

indication A reason to prescribe a medication or perform a treatment, as a bacterial infection may be an indication for the prescription of a specific antibiotic. —**indicate,** *v.*

indicator A tape, paper, tablet, or any other substance that is used to test for a particular reaction because it changes in a predictable, visible way. Also called **reagent.** Some kinds of indicators are autoclave indicators, dipsticks, litmus paper.

indigenous Native to or occurring naturally in a specified area or environment, as certain species of bacteria in the human digestive tract.

indigestion See **dyspepsia.**

indigitation See **intussusception** and **invagination.**

indirect anaphylaxis An exaggerated reaction of hypersensitivity to a person's own antigen that occurs because the antigen has been altered in some way.

indirect calorimetry The measurement of the amount of heat generated in an oxidation reaction either by determining the intake or consumption of oxygen or by measuring the amount of carbon dioxide or the amount of nitrogen released, and translating these quantities into a heat equivalent. Compare **direct calorimetry.**

indirect division See **mitosis.**

indirect ophthalmoscope An ophthalmoscope with a biconvex lens that produces a reversed direct image.

indirect percussion See **percussion.**

indium (In) A silvery metallic element with some nonmetallic chemical properties. Its atomic number is 49; its atomic weight is 114.82. It is used in electronic semiconductors.

individual immunity A form of natural immunity not shared by most other members of the race and species. It is rare and probably occurs as the result of an unrecognized infection. Compare **racial immunity, species immunity.**

individual psychology A modified system of psychoanalysis, developed by Alfred Adler, that views maladaptive behavior and personality disorders as resulting from a conflict between the desire to dominate and feelings of inferiority. See also **inferiority complex.**

indoleacetic acid A major terminal metabolite of the amino acid tryptophan, present in tiny amounts in normal urine and excreted in elevated quantities by patients with carcinoid tumors.

indomethacin A nonsteroidal anti-inflammatory agent used to treat arthritis.

induce To cause or stimulate the start of an activity, as an enzyme induces a metabolic activity. See also **induced fever.** —**inducer, induction,** *n.*

induced abortion An intentional termination of pregnancy before the fetus has developed enough to survive outside the uterus. Approximately 20% of pregnancies are terminated deliberately at the request of the mother or for medical indications, during the 1st trimester by curettage or during the 2nd trimester by induction of labor or hysterotomy.

induced fever A deliberate elevation of body temperature by application of heat or inoculation with a fever-producing organism to kill heat-sensitive pathogens.

induced hypotension See **deliberate hypotension.**

induced lethargy A trancelike state produced during hypnosis. See also **hypnosis, lethargy.**

induced trance A somnambulistic state resulting from a hysterical neurosis or hypnotism.

induction In embryology: the process of

stimulating and determining morphogenetic differentiation in a developing embryo through the action of chemical substances transmitted from one to another of the embryonic parts. See also **evocation.**

induction of anesthesia All portions of the anesthetic process that occur prior to attaining the desired level of anesthesia, including premedication with a sedative, hypnotic, tranquilizer, or curariform adjunct to anesthesia; intubation; administration of oxygen; and administration of the anesthetic.

induction of labor An obstetric procedure in which labor is initiated artificially by means of amniotomy or the administration of oxytocics. It is performed electively or for fetal or maternal indications. Elective induction is carried out for the convenience of the mother or the obstetrician, often to avert the possibility of delivery outside of the hospital when labor is judged to be imminent and rapid birth is expected. Elective inductions are performed less often now than in the past. Prerequisites for elective induction are a term gestation, a fetal weight of at least 2,500 g (88.2 oz), a cervix judged ready to dilate, a vertex presentation, and engagement of the presenting part of the fetus in the pelvis. Errors in the estimation of gestational age and fetal weight may result in the delivery of an unexpectedly immature or low–birth-weight infant. Indicated induction is performed when the risk of induction is judged to be less than that of continuing the pregnancy in such conditions as premature rupture of the membranes, severe maternal diabetes, and intractable preeclampsia. Surgical induction is effected by amniotomy, often with stripping of the membranes and digital stretching of the cervix; it is very often carried out in conjunction with medical induction, which is achieved through the administration of oxytocin, almost always by IV infusion, in a carefully controlled manner using an infusion pump. Oxytocin can be administered by subcutaneous or intramuscular injection, but these methods are less controllable and are considered less safe than the IV method. Prostaglandins are now used to induce labor more often than formerly, particularly for therapeutic abortions in the second trimester. Intravenous oxytocin is piggybacked into the most distal Y-injection port of the administration set of the primary IV solution so a keep-open infusion of unmedicated solution can be maintained if oxytocin is stopped. Electronic fetal and uterine monitoring is usually instituted during induction of labor to avoid hyperstimulation of the uterus and fetal distress. If the induction fails to produce effective labor, cesarean section is often required to prevent the adverse sequelae of the procedures used in the induction. For this reason, induction of labor is usually not recommended unless immediate delivery is necessary to avoid severe fetal or maternal morbidity.

inductor In embryology: a tissue or cell that emits a chemical substance that stimulates some morphogenetic effect in the developing embryo.

See also **evocator, organizer.**

induration Hardening of a tissue, particularly the skin, owing to edema, inflammation, or infiltration by a neoplasm. —**indurated,** *adj.*

Industrial Medical Association (IMA) A professional organization whose members are concerned with the identification, prevention, diagnosis, and treatment of disorders associated with technology and industry.

industrial psychology The application of psychological principles and techniques to the problems of business and industry, including selection of personnel, motivation of workers, and development of training programs.

indwelling catheter Any catheter designed to stay in place for a prolonged period. See also **self-retaining catheter.**

-ine A combining form meaning a 'chemical substance': *chlorine, pyrroline.*

inert 1. Not moving or acting, as inert matter. 2. A chemical substance not taking part in a chemical reaction or acting as a catalyst, as neon or other inert gases. 3. A medical ingredient not active pharmacologically; serving only as a bulking, binding, or sweetening agent or other vehicle in a medication.

inert gas A chemically inactive gaseous element. The inert gases are argon, helium, krypton, neon, radon, and xenon. Also called **noble gas.**

inertia 1. The tendency of a body at rest to remain at rest unless acted upon by an outside force, and the tendency of a body in motion to remain at motion in the direction in which it is moving unless acted upon by an outside force. 2. An abnormal condition characterized by a general inactivity or sluggishness, as colonic inertia.

inevitable abortion A condition of pregnancy in which spontaneous termination is imminent and cannot be prevented. It is characterized by bleeding, uterine cramping, dilatation of the cervix, and presentation of the conceptus in the cervical os. If heavy bleeding supervenes, immediate evacuation of the uterus may be required. The point at which an inevitable abortion becomes an incomplete abortion is of medicolegal interest because of the statutory difference between spontaneous and induced abortion. Compare **incomplete abortion, threatened abortion.**

infant 1. A child who is in the earliest stage of extrauterine life, a time extending from birth to approximately 12 months of age, when the baby is able to assume an erect posture; some extend the period to 24 months of age. 2. In law: a person not of full legal age; a minor. 3. Of or pertaining to infancy; in an early stage of development. —**infantile,** *adj.*

infant botulism An intoxication from neurotoxins produced by *Clostridium botulinum* that occurs in children less than 6 months of age. The condition is characterized by severe hypotonicity of all muscles, constipation, lethargy, and feeding difficulties, and it may lead to respiratory insufficiency. The botulism neurotoxin is usually found in the gastrointestinal tract rather than in the blood, indicating that it is probably produced in the gut rather than ingested, although the epidemiology and pathophysiology of the syndrome are not clearly understood. Treatment is supportive, including optimal management of fluids, electrolytes, and nutrition.

infant death   The death of a live-born infant before 1 year of age.

infant feeder   A device for feeding small or weak infants who cannot suck hard enough to nurse from the breast or to get milk from a bottle. The feeder resembles a bulb syringe with a long soft nipple on the end. The bulb is squeezed slowly and gently, permitting the baby to suck and swallow without great effort and preventing the escape of fluid into the infant's trachea.

infant feeding   See **bottle-feeding, breast-feeding.**

infanticide   **1.** The killing of an infant or young child. The act is usually a psychotic reaction often associated with severe depression, as occurs in bipolar disorder and, occasionally, in extreme postpartum disturbances. Infanticide may become a neurotic obsession among mothers who do not want the baby or who do not feel capable of caring for the infant. **2.** One who takes the life of an infant or young child. —**infanticidal,** *adj.*

infantile   **1.** Of, relating to, or characteristic of infants or infancy. **2.** Lacking maturity, sophistication, or reasonableness. **3.** Affected with infantilism. **4.** Being in a very early stage of development.

infantile arteritis   A disorder in infants and young children characterized by inflammation of many arteries in which atherosclerotic lesions are rarely present.

infantile autism   A disability characterized by abnormal emotional, social, and linguistic development, which usually begins at birth. It may result from organic brain dysfunction, in which case it occurs before the age of 3 years, or it may be associated with childhood schizophrenia, in which case the autism occurs later, but before the onset of adolescence. The autistic child remains fixed at one of the consecutive stages through which a normal infant passes as it develops. Such a child withdraws completely from contact with other people, including the mother; develops language disorders; and becomes preoccupied with inanimate objects. Treatment includes psychotherapy, often accompanied by play therapy. Also called early infantile autism.

infantile celiac disease   See **celiac disease.**

infantile cerebral sphingolipidosis   See **Tay-Sachs disease.**

infantile dwarf   A person whose mental and physical development is greatly retarded as a result of various causes, as genetic or developmental defects.

infantile eczema   See **atopic dermatitis.**

infantile paralysis   See **poliomyelitis.**

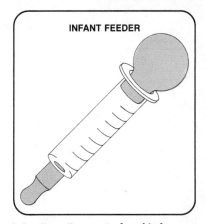

INFANT FEEDER

infantile pellagra   See **kwashiorkor.**

infantile scurvy   A nutritional disease caused by an inadequate dietary supply of vitamin C, most commonly occurring because cow's milk, unfortified with vitamin C, is the principal food in an infant's diet. Families are counseled to feed their children foods rich in vitamin C or to use a formula supplemented with this vitamin. Also called **Barlow's disease, hemorrhagic scurvy.** See also **ascorbic acid, citric acid, scurvy.**

infantile spinal muscular atrophy   See **Werdnig-Hoffmann disease.**

infantilism   **1.** A condition in which various anatomical, physiological, and psychological characteristics of childhood persist in the adult. It is characterized by mental retardation, underdeveloped sexual organs, and, usually, small stature. Compare **progeria. 2.** A condition, usually of psychological rather than organic origin, characterized by speech and voice patterns in an older child or adult that are typical of very young children.

infant mortality   The statistical rate of infant death during the first year after live birth, expressed as the number of such births per 1000 live births in a specific geographical area or institution in a given period of time. Neonatal mortality accounts for 70% of infant mortality.

infant of addicted mother   A newborn infant showing withdrawal symptoms, usually within the first 24 hours of life, most commonly caused by maternal antepartum dependence on heroin, methadone, or alcohol. Characteristic symptoms include tremors, irritability, hyperactive reflexes, increased muscle tone, twitching, increased mucus production, nasal congestion, respiratory distress, excessive sweating, elevated temperature, vomiting, diarrhea, and dehydration.

infant psychiatry   The branch of psychiatry that specializes in the diagnosis, etiology, and treatment of the psychopathological syndromes and symptoms of infants. Such conditons are associated with early pathology, tactile hypersensitivity, and homeostatic disorders and include poor infant-parent attachment, infantile

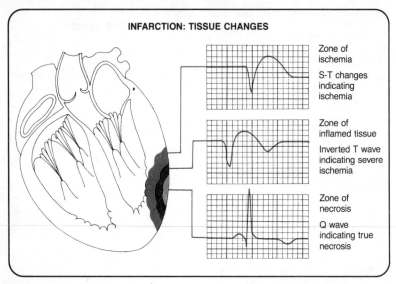

INFARCTION: TISSUE CHANGES

Zone of ischemia
S-T changes indicating ischemia

Zone of inflamed tissue
Inverted T wave indicating severe ischemia

Zone of necrosis
Q wave indicating true necrosis

autism, anaclitic depression, avoidance reaction, persistent stranger and separation anxiety, early signs of aggression, hyperactivity, cyclic vomiting, and disturbances in sleeping, eating, and elimination.

infarct A localized area of necrosis in a tissue, vessel, organ, or part resulting from tissue anoxia caused by an interruption in the blood supply to the area, or, less frequently, by circulatory stasis produced by the occlusion of a vein that ordinarily carries blood away from the area. An infarct may resemble a red swollen bruise, owing to hemorrhage and an accumulation of blood in the area. Some infarcts are pale and white, owing to a lack of circulation to the area. —**infarcted,** *adj.*

infarction 1. The development and formation of an infarct. 2. An infarct.

infect To transmit a pathogen that may induce development of an infectious disease in another person.

infected abortion A spontaneous or induced termination of an immature pregnancy in which the products of conception have become infected, causing fever, and requiring antibiotic therapy and evacuation of the uterus. Compare **septic abortion.**

infection 1. The invasion of the body by pathogenic microorganisms which reproduce and multiply, causing disease by local cellular injury, secretion of a toxin, or antigen-antibody reaction in the host. 2. A disease caused by the invasion of the body by pathogenic microorganisms. Compare **infestation.** —**infectious,** *adj.*

infectious 1. Capable of causing an infection. 2. Caused by an infection.

infectious hepatitis See **hepatitis A.**

infectious mononucleosis An acute herpesvirus infection caused by the Epstein-Barr virus (EBV). It is characterized by fever, sore throat, swollen lymph glands, atypical lymphocytes, splenomegaly, hepatomegaly, abnormal liver function, and bruising. The disease is usually transmitted by droplet infection but is not highly contagious. Young people are most often affected. Treatment is primarily symptomatic, with enforced bed rest to prevent serious complications of the liver or spleen, analgesics to control pain, and saline gargles for throat discomfort. Rupture of the spleen may occur, requiring immediate surgery and blood transfusion. See also **Epstein-Barr virus, viral infection.**

infectious myringitis An inflammatory, contagious condition of the ear drum owing to viral or bacterial infection, characterized by the development of painful vesicles on the drum. Also called **bullous myringitis.**

infectious nucleic acid Viral RNA or, less commonly, DNA that is able to infect the nucleic acid of a cell and to induce the host to produce viruses.

infectious parotitis See **mumps.**

infectious polyneuritis See **Guillain-Barré syndrome.**

infective tubulointerstitial nephritis An acute inflammation of the kidneys caused by an infection by *Escherichia coli* or other pyogenic pathogen. The condition is characterized by chills, fever, nausea and vomiting, flank pain, dysuria, proteinuria, and hematuria. The kidney may become enlarged and portions of the renal cortex may be destroyed. Infection is usually the result of bacterial contamination of a urinary catheter.

inferior 1. Situated below or lower than a given point of reference, as the feet are inferior to the legs. 2. Of poorer quality or value. Compare **superior.**

inferior alveolar artery An artery that descends with the inferior alveolar nerve from the first or mandibular portion of the maxillary artery to the mandibular foramen on the medial surface of the ramus of the mandible. It enters the mandibular canal and runs through to the first premolar tooth where it divides into the mental and incisor branches. Also called **arteria alveolaris inferior.**

inferior aperture of minor pelvis An irregular aperture bounded by the coccyx, the sacrotuberous ligaments, part of the ischium, the sides of the pubic arch, and the symphysis pubis.

inferior aperture of thorax An irregular opening bounded by the 12th thoracic vertebra, the 12th ribs, and the edge of the costal cartilages as they meet the sternum.

inferior conjunctival fornix The space in the fold of conjunctiva created by the reflection of the conjunctiva covering the eyeball and the lining of the lower eyelid.

inferior gastric node A node in one of two groups of gastric lymph glands, lying between the two layers of the lesser omentum along the pyloric half of the greater curvature of the stomach. Compare **hepatic node, superior gastric node.**

inferiority complex **1.** A feeling of fear and resentment resulting from a sense of being physically inadequate, characterized by a variety of abnormal behaviors. **2.** In psychoanalysis: a complex characterized by striving for unrealistic goals owing to an unresolved Oedipus complex. **3.** *Informal.* A feeling of being inferior.

inferior maxillary bone See **mandible.**

inferior mesenteric node A node in one of the three groups of visceral lymph glands serving the viscera of the abdomen and the pelvis. The inferior mesenteric nodes are associated with the branches of the inferior mesenteric artery and are divided into a group of small nodes along the branches of the left colic and sigmoid arteries, another group in the sigmoid mesocolon, and a pararectal group touching the muscular coat of the rectum. The inferior mesenteric nodes drain the descending colon, the iliac and sigmoid parts of the colon, and the upper part of the rectum. Their efferents pass to the preaortic nodes. Compare **gastric node, superior mesenteric node.**

inferior mesenteric vein The vein in the lower body that returns the blood from the rectum, the sigmoid colon, and the descending colon. It begins in the rectum as the superior rectal vein, ascends through the lesser pelvis, and continues upward as the inferior mesenteric vein. It passes dorsal to the pancreas and opens into the lienal vein. Compare **superior mesenteric vein.**

inferior orbital fissure A groove in the inferolateral wall of the orbit that contains the infraorbital and zygomatic nerves and the infraorbital vessels.

inferior phrenic artery A small, visceral branch of the abdominal aorta, arising from the aorta itself, the renal artery, or the celiac artery. It divides into the medial and lateral branches

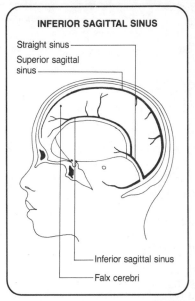

INFERIOR SAGITTAL SINUS

Straight sinus
Superior sagittal sinus
Inferior sagittal sinus
Falx cerebri

and supplies the diaphragm. A few vessels of the inferior vena cava stem from the lateral branch of the right phrenic artery. Some branches of the left phrenic artery supply the esophagus.

inferior radioulnar joint See **distal radioulnar articulation.**

inferior sagittal sinus One of the six venous channels of the posterior dura mater, draining blood from the brain into the internal jugular vein. It is a cylindrical sinus contained in the posterior portion of the free margin of the falx cerebri, increases in size as it courses posteriorly, and ends in the straight sinus. It receives deoxygenated blood from several veins from the falx cerebri and, in some individuals, a few veins from the cerebral hemispheres. Compare **straight sinus, superior sagittal sinus, transverse sinus.**

inferior subscapular nerve One of two small nerves on opposite sides of the back that arise from the posterior cord of the brachial plexus. It supplies the distal part of the subscapularis and ends in the teres major. Compare **superior subscapular nerve.**

inferior thyroid vein One of the few veins that arise in the venous plexus on the thyroid gland and form a plexus ventral to the trachea, under the sternothyroidei. A left vein descends from this plexus to join the left brachiocephalic trunk; a right vein descends obliquely to open into the right brachiocephalic vein at its junction with the superior vena cava. The inferior thyroid veins contain valves at their terminations and receive the esophageal, the tracheal, and the inferior laryngeal veins.

inferior ulnar collateral artery One of a pair of branches of the deep brachial arteries, arising about 5 cm (2 inches) from the elbow,

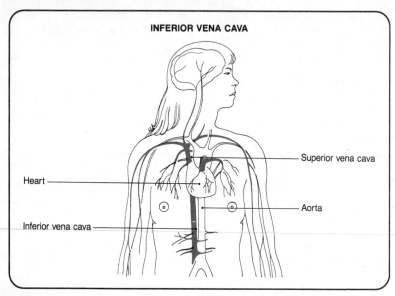

INFERIOR VENA CAVA

Superior vena cava

Heart

Aorta

Inferior vena cava

passing inward to form an arch with the deep brachial artery, and carrying blood to the muscles of the forearm. Compare **superior ulnar collateral artery.**

inferior vena cava The large vein that returns deoxygenated blood to the heart from parts of the body below the diaphragm. It is formed by the junction of the two common iliac veins at the right of the fifth lumbar vertebra and ascends along the vertebral column, pierces the diaphragm and opens into the right atrium of the heart. The inferior vena cava contains a semilunar valve that is rudimentary in the adult but very large and important in the fetus. The vessel receives blood from the two common iliacs, the lumbar veins, and the testicular veins. Compare **superior vena cava.**

infero- A combining form meaning 'low': *inferolateral.*

inferolateral Located below and to the side. Compare **inferomedial.**

inferomedial Located below and toward the center.

infertile 1. Incapable of reproducing or bearing offspring. 2. Sterile.

infertility Inability or diminished ability to reproduce, affecting either the male or female. See **fertile.**

infest To attack, invade, and subsist on the skin or in the internal organs of a host. Compare **infect.**

infestation The presence of animal parasites in the environment or on the skin or in the hair of a host.

inflammation The protective response of the tissues of the body to irritation or injury. Inflammation may be acute or chronic; its cardinal signs are redness (rubor), heat (calor), swelling (tumor), and pain (dolor), accompanied by loss of function. The process begins with a brief increase in vascular permeability. The second stage is prolonged and consists of sustained increase in vascular permeability, exudation of fluids from the vessels, clustering of leukocytes along the vessel walls, phagocytosis of microorganisms, deposition of fibrin in the vessel, disposal of the accumulated debris by macrophages, and, finally, the migration of fibroblasts to the area and the development of new, normal cells. Histimine, kinins, and various other substances mediate the inflammatory process.

inflammatory bowel disease See **ulcerative colitis.**

inflammatory fracture A fracture of bone tissue weakened by inflammation.

influenza A highly contagious infection of the respiratory tract caused by a myxovirus and transmitted by airborne droplet infection. It occurs in isolated cases, epidemics, and pandemics. Symptoms include sore throat, cough, fever, muscle pain, and weakness. The incubation period is brief (from 1 to 3 days), and the onset is usually sudden, with chills, fever, and general malaise. Treatment is symptomatic and usually involves bed rest, aspirin, and drinking of fluids. Fever and constitutional symptoms distinguish influenza from the common cold. Three main strains of influenza virus have been recognized: type A, type B, and type C. New strains of the virus emerge at regular intervals and are named according to their geographic origin. **Asian flu** is a type A influenza. Also called **grippe, la grippe, flu** *(informal).*

influenza virus vaccine An active immunizing agent.

informed consent Permission obtained from a patient to perform a specific test or procedure. Informed consent is required prior to performing most invasive procedures and prior to admitting a patient to a research study. The document used must be written in a language understood by the patient and be dated and signed by the patient and at least one witness. Informed consent is voluntary. By law, informed consent must be obtained more than a given number of days or hours prior to certain procedures, including therapeutic abortion and sterilization, and must always be obtained when the patient is fully competent.

infra- A combining form meaning 'situated, formed, or occurring beneath': *infraclavicular, infracortical.*

infraction fracture A pathologic fracture characterized by a small radiolucent line and most commonly associated with a disorder of metabolism.

infrared radiation Electromagnetic radiation in which the wavelengths are longer than those of visible light waves and shorter than those of radio waves. Infrared radiation striking the body surface is perceived as heat.

infrared therapy Treatment by exposure to various wavelengths of infrared radiation. Hot-water bottles and heating pads of all kinds emit long-wave infrared radiation; incandescent lights emit short-wave infrared radiation. Infrared treatment is performed to relieve pain and to stimulate circulation of blood.

infusion 1. The introduction of a substance, as a fluid, electrolyte, nutrient, or drug, directly into a vein or interstitially by means of gravity flow. Compare **injection, instillation, insufflate.** 2. The substance introduced into the body by infusion. 3. The steeping of a substance, as an herb, in order to extract its medicinal properties. 4. The extract obtained by the steeping process. —**infuse,** *v.*

infusion pump An apparatus designed to deliver measured drugs through injection over a period of time. Some infusion pumps can be implanted surgically.

ingrown hair A hair that fails to follow the normal follicle channel to the surface, with the free end becoming embedded in the skin. The hair then acts like a foreign body, and inflammation and suppuration follow.

ingrown toenail A toenail whose free distal margin grows or is pressed into the skin of the toe, causing an inflammatory reaction. Granulation tissue may develop and secondary infection is common. Treatment includes wider shoes, proper trimming of the nail, and surgical procedures to narrow the nail or to reduce the size of the lateral nail fold.

inguinal Of or pertaining to the groin.

inguinal falx The inferior terminal portion of the common aponeurosis of the obliquus internus abdominis and the transverse abdominis. It is inserted into the crest of the pubis, just under the superficial inguinal ring, and strengthens that part of the anterior abdominal wall. Also called **conjoined tendon.**

inguinal hernia A hernia in which a loop of intestine enters the inguinal canal, sometimes

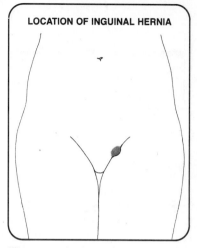

LOCATION OF INGUINAL HERNIA

filling, in a male, the entire scrotal sac. An inguinal hernia is usually repaired surgically to prevent the herniated segment from becoming strangulated, gangrenous, or obstructive, thereby blocking passage of waste through the bowel. Inguinal hernias comprise 75% to 80% of all hernias. See also **hernia.**

inguinal node One of approximately 18 nodes in the group of lymph glands in the upper femoral triangle of the thigh. These nodes are divided into the superficial inguinal nodes and the subinguinal nodes. Compare **anterior tibial node, popliteal node.**

inguino- A combining form meaning 'of or pertaining to the groin': *inguinocrural, inguinodynia.*

inhalation administration of medication The administration of a drug by inhalation of the vapor released from a fragile ampoule packed in a fine mesh that is crushed for immediate administration. The medication is absorbed into circulation through the mucous membrane of the nasal passages. Vaporized medication is also given by inhalation. See also **inhalation therapy.**

inhalation analgesia The occasional administration of anesthetic gas during the second stage of labor to reduce pain. Consciousness is retained to allow the woman to follow instructions and to avoid the adverse effects of general anesthesia.

inhalation anesthesia Surgical narcosis achieved by the administration of an anesthetic gas or a volatile anesthetic liquid via a carrier gas. Although general anesthesia by gas inhalation has been used to permit surgical operations for over a century, the mechanism by which these anesthetics obtund the pain centers of the brain is not yet understood. Administration of an inhalation anesthetic is usually preceded by intravenous or intramuscular administration of a short-acting sedative or hypnotic drug, often a barbiturate. Among the principal inhalation

TYPES OF INJECTIONS

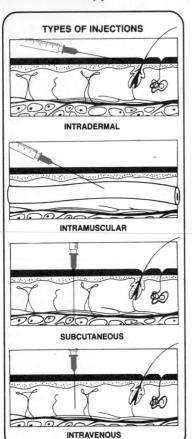

INTRADERMAL

INTRAMUSCULAR

SUBCUTANEOUS

INTRAVENOUS

anesthetics are nitrous oxide, cyclopropane, ethylene, halothane, enflurane, fluroxene, methoxyflurane, trichloroethylene, and isoflurane. Some other inhalation anesthetics, including chloroform, ether, and ethyl chloride, are rarely used in the United States because of adverse effects, potential toxicity, or the possibility of explosion.

inhalation therapy A treatment in which a substance is introduced into the respiratory tract with inspired air. Oxygen, water, and various drugs may be administered using techniques of inhalation therapy. The goals of treatment are varied, as improved strength of respiratory function in a bedridden patient, bronchodilatation in an asthmatic patient, or liquefaction of mucus in a person with chronic obstructive lung disease.

inhale To breathe in or to draw in with the breath. —**inhalation**, n.

inherent Inborn, innate; natural to an environment. Compare **indigenous.**

inheritance In genetics: **1.** The acquisition or expression of traits or conditions by transmission of genetic material from parents to off-

spring. **2.** The sum total of the genetic qualities or traits transmitted from parents to offspring; the total genetic makeup of the fertilized ovum. Kinds of inheritance include **complemental inheritance, cytoplasmic inheritance, hologynic inheritance, homochronous inheritance, maternal inheritance, Mendelism, monofactorial inheritance, multifactorial inheritance, supplemental inheritance.** — **inherited,** adj., **inherit,** v.

inherited disorder Any disease or condition that is genetically determined and involves either a single gene mutation, multifactorial inheritance, or a chromosomal aberration. Also called **genetic disorder.**

inhibiting hormone A chemical substance, produced by the hypothalamus, that inhibits secretion of certain anterior pituitary hormones. Compare **releasing hormone.**

inhibition **1.** The act or state of inhibiting or of being inhibited, restrained, prevented, held back. **2.** In psychology: the unconscious restraint of a behavioral process, usually resulting from the social or cultural forces of the environment; the condition inducing such restraint. **3.** In psychoanalysis: the process in which the superego prevents the conscious expression of an unconscious instinctual drive, thought, or urge. **4.** In physiology: restraining, checking, or arresting the action of an organ or cell or the reducing of a physiological activity by an antagonistic stimulation. **5.** In chemistry: the stopping or slowing down of the rate of a chemical reaction.

inhibitory Tending to stop or slow a process, as a neuron that suppresses a nerve impulse. Compare **induce.**

inio- A combining form meaning 'of or pertaining to the occiput': *iniodymus, iniopagus.*

inion The most prominent point of the back of the head, where the occipital bone protrudes the farthest.

initial contact stance stage One of the five stages in the stance phase of walking or gait, specifically associated with the moment when the foot touches the ground or floor, and the leg prepares to accept the weight of the body. This stage figures in the diagnoses of many abnormal orthopedic conditions and is often correlated with electromyographic studies of the muscles used in walking, as the pretibial muscle and the gluteus maximus. Compare **loading response stance stage, midstance, preswing stance stage, terminal stance.** See also **swing phase of gait.**

initiation codon In molecular genetics: the triplet of nucleotides, usually adenine-uracil-guanine (AUG), or, in some cases, guanine-uracil-guanine (GUG), that code for formylmethionine, the first amino acid in protein sequences. Also called **start codon.**

injection **1.** The act of forcing a liquid into the body by means of a syringe. Injections are designated according to the anatomical site involved; the most common are intra-arterial, intradermal, intramuscular, intravenous, and subcutaneous. Sterile technique is maintained.

Compare **infusion, instillation, insufflate. 2.** The substance injected. **3.** Redness and swelling observed in the physical examination of a part of the body, caused by dilation of the blood vessels secondary to an inflammatory or infectious process. —**inject,** *v,* **injectable,** *adj.*

injection technique See specific injection technique.

injury: potential for A nursing diagnosis accepted by the Fifth National Conference on the Classification of Nursing Diagnoses. The etiology of the condition may be somatic (internal) or environmental (external). The somatic factors may be biological, chemical, physiological, psychological, or developmental; the environmental factors may be biological, chemical, physiological, psychological, or interpersonal. See also **nursing diagnosis.**

inlet contraction See **contraction.**

in loco parentis Latin phrase meaning 'in the place of the parent.' The assumption by a person or institution of the parental obligations of caring for a child without adoption.

innate 1. Existing in or belonging to a person from birth; inborn; hereditary; congenital. **2.** A natural and essential characteristic of something or someone; inherent. **3.** Originating in or produced by the intellect or the mind.

innate immunity See **natural immunity.**

inner cell mass A cluster of cells localized around the animal pole of the blastocyst of placental mammals from which the embryo develops. See also **trophoblast.**

inner ear See **internal ear.**

innervation 1. Distribution and action of the nervous system. **2.** Nerve supply and nerve stimulation of a part.

innervation apraxia See **motor apraxia.**

innidation See nidation. —**innidate,** *v.*

innocent Benign, innocuous, or functional; not malignant, as an innocent heart murmur.

inoculate To introduce a substance (inoculum) into the body to produce or to increase immunity to the disease or condition associated with the substance. It is introduced by making multiple scratches in the skin after placing a drop of the substance on the skin, by puncture of the skin with an implement bearing multiple short tines, or by intradermal, subcutaneous, or intramuscular injection.

inoculum, *pl.* **inocula** A substance introduced into the body to cause or to increase immunity to a specific disease or condition. It may be a toxin; a live, attenuated, or killed virus or bacterium; or an immune serum. Also called inoculant. See also **immune system.**

inorganic In chemistry: pertaining to or composed of chemical compounds that do not contain carbon as the principle element (except carbonates, cyanides, and cyanates).

inorganic acid A compound containing no carbon that is made up of hydrogen and an electronegative element. Examples include hydrochloric, boric, and sulfuric acids. Some inorganic acids, as carbonic acid, contain carbon dioxide.

inorganic chemistry The study of the properties and reactions of all chemical elements and compounds other than hydrocarbons.

inorganic dust Dry, finely powdered particles of an inorganic substance, especially dust, which, when inhaled, can cause abnormal conditions of the lungs. See also **anthracosis, asbestosis, berylliosis, pneumoconiosis, silicosis.**

inosine A nucleoside, derived from animal tissue, especially intestines, originally used in food processing and flavoring and now under investigation in studies of cancer and virology chemotherapy. See also **inosiplex.**

inosiplex A form of inosine that acts as a stimulator of the immune system. It is currently under investigation for use in cancer therapy and in the treatment of herpesvirus and rhinovirus infections.

inositol An isomer of glucose that occurs widely in plant and animal cells. Although inositol has no current therapeutic use, it may be an essential cell constituent.

inotropic Affecting the force of muscular contractions.

inpatient 1. A patient who has been admitted to a hospital or other health-care facility for at least an overnight stay. **2.** Pertaining to the treatment of such a patient or to a health-care facility to which a patient may be admitted for 24-hour care. Compare **outpatient.**

input 1. In data processing: the information entered into a computer; the process of entering information into a computer. **2.** In general systems theory: the information for processing that enters the system.

insanity 1. Any mental disorder. **2.** In law: a mental condition that prevents a person from looking after his own affairs, impairs his ability to distinguish right from wrong, or makes him dangerous to himself or others.

insect bite The bite of any parasitic or venomous arthropod as a louse, flea, mite, tick, or arachnid. Many arthropods inject venom that produces poisoning or severe local reaction, saliva that may contain viruses, or substances that produce mild irritation.

insecticide A chemical agent that kills insects.

insecticide poisoning See **chlorinated organic insecticide poisoning.**

insemination The deposit of seminal fluid into the female genital tract.

insensible perspiration The loss of fluid from the body by evaporation, as normally occurs during respiration. A small amount of perspiration is continually excreted by the sweat glands in the skin; the portion that evaporates before it may be observed also contributes to insensible perspiration. Also called **insensible water loss.**

insensible water loss See **insensible perspiration.**

insertion In anatomy: the place of attachment, as of a muscle to the bone it moves.

in-service education A program of in-

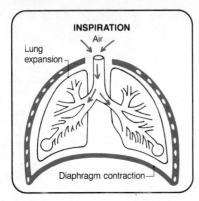

INSPIRATION

Air

Lung expansion

Diaphragm contraction

struction or training that is provided by an agency or institution for its employees. The program is held in the institution or at the agency and is intended to increase the skills and competence of the employees in a specific area.

insidious Of, pertaining to, or describing a development that is gradual, subtle, or imperceptible. Certain chronic diseases, as glaucoma, can develop insidiously with symptoms that are not detected by the patient until the disorder is established. Compare **acute.**

insight 1. The capacity of comprehending the true nature of a situation or of penetrating an underlying truth, primarily through intuitive understanding. 2. In psychology: a type of self-understanding encompassing both an intellectual and emotional awareness of the unconscious nature, origin, and mechanisms of one's attitudes, feelings, and behavior. It is one of the most important goals of psychotherapy and, with integration, leads to modification of maladaptive behavioral patterns. See also **integration.**

in situ 1. In the natural or usual place. 2. Describing a cancer that has not invaded the basement membrane or adjacent tissues, as carcinoma in situ.

insoluble Unable to be dissolved, usually in a specific solvent, as a substance that is insoluble in water.

insomnia Chronic inability to sleep or to remain asleep throughout the night; wakefulness; sleeplessness. The condition is caused by a variety of physical and psychological factors, including emotional stress; physical pain and discomfort; disturbances in cerebral function, like toxic delirium and senile dementia; drug abuse and drug dependence; psychosomatic disorders; neuroses; psychoses; and psychological problems that produce anxiety, irrational fears, and tensions.

insomniac 1. A person with insomnia. 2. Pertaining to, causing, or associated with insomnia. 3. Characteristic of or occurring during a period of sleeplessness.

inspection The act of examining a person to make informed observations. The process involves using the physical senses and clinical knowledge.

inspiration The act of drawing air into the lungs in order to exchange oxygen for carbon dioxide, the end product of tissue metabolism. The major muscle of inspiration is the diaphragm, the contraction of which creates a negative pressure in the chest, causing the lungs to expand and air to flow inward. Additional muscles aiding inspiratory efforts are the external intercostals, scaleni, scapular elevators, and sternocleidomastoids. Lungs at maximal inspiration have an average total capacity of 5,500 to 6,000 ml of air. See also **inspiratory reserve volume.**

inspiratory Of or pertaining to inspiration.

inspiratory capacity The maximum volume of gas that can be inspired from the resting expiratory level; the tidal volume and the inspiratory reserve volume.

inspiratory reserve volume The maximum volume of gas that can be inspired from the end-tidal inspiratory level.

inspissate To thicken or harden a fluid through the absorption or evaporation of the liquid portion, as milk in an inspissated milk duct.

instillation 1. A procedure in which a fluid is slowly introduced into a cavity or passage of the body and allowed to remain for a specific length of time before being drained or withdrawn. It is performed to expose the tissues of the area to the solution, to warmth or cold, or to a drug or substance in the solution. 2. A solution so introduced. Compare **infusion, injection, insufflate. —instill,** v.

instinctive reflex See **unconditioned response.**

institutionalize To place a person in an institution for psychological or physical treatment or for the protection of the person or society. **—institutionalization,** n., **institutionalized,** adj.

institutional licensure A proposed procedure in which licensure for almost all health professions would be abandoned and the responsibility for assessing professional competence would fall to the health-care facility where the health professional is employed. Proponents maintain that health needs would be better and more flexibly served. Opponents maintain that knowledge, judgment, and competency are the products of a good basic education in the profession and that educators cannot teach the profession without a set of standardized expectations, as are now provided by government-controlled licensing procedures and certifying examinations.

institutional review board (IRB) A federally approved committee that reviews all research proposals prior to submission of requests for funding to federal government granting agencies.

instrument A surgical tool or device designed to perform a specific function, as cutting, dissecting, grasping, holding, retracting, or suturing. Surgical instruments are usually made of steel and are specially treated to be durable,

THERAPEUTIC ACTIVITY OF INSULIN

DRUG	ONSET	PEAK	DURATION	REMARKS
Rapid-acting insulins				
prompt insulin zinc suspension (semi-lente)	1 to 2 hr	4 to 7 hr	12 to 16 hr	Glycosuria most likely nocturnally; hypoglycemia most likely 10 A.M. to lunchtime
regular insulin	30 to 60 min	2 to 3 hr	5 to 7 hr	
Intermediate-acting insulins				
insulin zinc suspension (lente)	1 to 2 hr	8 to 12 hr	24 to 28 hr	Glycosuria most likely before lunch; hypoglycemia most likely 3 P.M. to dinnertime
globin zinc insulin	2 hr	8 to 16 hr	18 to 24 hr	
isophane insulin suspension (NPH)	1 to 2 hr	8 to 12 hr	24 to 28 hr	
Long-acting insulins				
extended insulin zinc suspension (ultralente)	4 to 8 hr	18 to 24 hr	> 36 hr	Glycosuria most likely before lunch and at bedtime; hypoglycemia most likely 2 A.M. to breakfast
protamine zinc insulin suspension (PZI)	4 to 8 hr	14 to 24 hr	> 36 hr	

heat-resistant, rust-resistant, and stain-proof. Some kinds of instruments are the **clamp, retractor, speculum.**

instrumental conditioning See **operant conditioning.**

instrumentation The use of instruments for treatment and diagnosis.

insufficiency Inability to perform a necessary function adequately. Some kinds of insufficiency are adrenal insufficiency, aortic insufficiency, ileocecal insufficiency, pulmonary insufficiency, valvular insufficiency.

insufflate To blow gas or powder into a tube, cavity, or organ to allow visual examination, remove an obstruction, or apply medication. See also **Rubin's test.**

insul- A combining form meaning 'of or pertaining to an island, or island-shaped': *insula, insulin.*

insulin 1. A naturally occurring hormone secreted by the beta cells of the islets of Langerhans in the pancreas in response to increased levels of glucose in the blood. The hormone acts to regulate the metabolism of glucose and the processes necessary for the intermediary metabolism of fats, carbohydrates, and proteins. Insulin lowers blood glucose levels and promotes transport and entry of glucose into the muscle cells and other tissues. Inadequate secretion of insulin results in hyperglycemia, hyperlipemia, ketonemia, and azoturia and in the characteristic signs of diabetes mellitus, including polyphagia, polydipsia, and polyuria, and, eventually, lethargy and weight loss. **2.** A pharmacologic preparation of the hormone administered in treating diabetes mellitus. The various preparations of insulin available for prescription vary in promptness, intensity, and duration of action. They are termed rapid-acting, intermediate-acting, and long-acting. Most forms of insulin drugs are given by subcutaneous injection in individualized dosage schedules. Adverse reactions include hypoglycemia and insulin shock from excess dosage and hyperglycemia and diabetic ketoacidosis from inadequate dosage. Fever, stress, infection, pregnancy, surgery, and hyperthyroidism may significantly increase insulin requirements; liver disease, hypothyroidism, vomiting, and renal disease may decrease the need for insulin.

insulin injection This fast-acting insulin is prescribed in the treatment of diabetes mellitus when the desired action is prompt, intense, and short-acting. Insulin injection prepared from zinc insulin crystals is slightly longer-acting than the amorphous noncrystalline form of this type of insulin. Insulin injection is the only form of insulin suitable for intramuscular administration. Also called **regular insulin.**

insulin kinase An enzyme, assumed to be present in the liver, that activates insulin.

insulinogenic Promoting the production and release of insulin by the islets of Langerhans in the pancreas.

insulinoma, *pl.* **insulinomas, insulinomata.** A benign tumor of the insulin-secreting cells of the islets of Langerhans. Surgical resection of the tumor may be possible, thus limiting the development of hypoglycemia. Also called **insuloma, islet cell adenoma.** Compare **islet cell tumor.**

insulin shock Hypoglycemic shock caused by an overdose of insulin, a decreased intake of food, or excessive exercise. It is characterized by sweating, trembling, chilliness, nervousness, irritability, hunger, hallucination, numbness, and pallor. Compare **ketoacidosis.**

insulin-shock treatment (IST) An obsolete therapy involving the injection of large, convulsion-producing doses of insulin, administered as a therapeutic measure in psychoses, especially schizophrenia. Also called **hypoglycemic shock treatment.**

insulin tolerance test A test of the body's ability to use insulin, in which insulin is given and blood glucose is measured at regular intervals. Blood glucose is usually lower but not less than half of the fasting glucose level 30 minutes after the insulin is given. Glucose levels usually return to normal after about 90 minutes.

insuloma, *pl.* **insulomas, insulomata** See **insulinoma.**

intake **1.** In nursing: the amount of food or fluids ingested in a given period of time, measured and noted as milliliters or grams per shift or per 8 or 24 hours. **2.** *Informal.* The process in which a person is admitted to a clinic or hospital or is signed in for an office visit. The reason for the visit and various identifying data about the patient are noted.

integral dose In radiotherapy: the total amount of energy absorbed by a patient or object during exposure to radiation. Also called **volume dose.**

integrating dose meter In radiotherapy: an ionization chamber, usually designed to be placed on the patient's skin, with a measuring system for determining the total radiation administered during an exposure. A device may be included to terminate the exposure when the desired value is reached.

integration **1.** The act or process of unifying or bringing together. **2.** In psychology: the organization of all elements of the personality into a coordinated, functional whole that is in harmony with the environment, one of the primary goals in psychotherapy. It involves the assimilation of insight and the coordination of new and old data, experiences, and emotional reactions so that an effective change can occur in behavior, thinking, or feeling. See also **insight.** —**integrate,** *v.*

integration of self One of the components of high-level wellness. It is a prerequisite for the achievement of maturity and is characterized by the integration of mind, body, and spirit into one harmoniously functioning unit.

integument A covering or skin. —**integumentary,** *adj.*

integumentary system The skin and its appendages, hair, nails, and sweat and sebaceous glands. See also **integument.**

integumentary system assessment An evaluation of the general condition and any abnormalities of a patient's integument and of factors that may contribute to the presence of a dermatologic disorder.

intellect **1.** The power and ability of the mind for knowing and understanding, as contrasted with feeling or with willing. **2.** A person possessing a great capacity for thought and knowledge. —**intellectual,** *adj., n.*

intellectualization In psychiatry: a defense mechanism in which reasoning is used as a means of blocking a confrontation with an unconscious conflict and the emotional stress associated with it.

intelligence **1.** The potential ability and capacity to acquire, retain, and apply experience, understanding, knowledge, reasoning, and judgment. **2.** The manifestation of such ability. See also **intelligence quotient.** —**intelligent,** *adj.*

intelligence quotient (IQ) A numerical expression of a person's intellectual level as measured against the statistical average of his age group. It is determined by dividing the mental age, derived through psychological testing, by the chronological age and multiplying the result by 100. Average IQ is considered to be 100. See also **mental retardation.**

intelligence test Any of a variety of standarized tests designed to determine the mental age of an individual by measuring the relative capacity to absorb information and to solve problems. These tests are routinely used by the medical profession to diagnose and determine degrees of mental retardation. Two kinds of intelligence tests are Stanford-Binet, Wechsler-Bellevue scale. Compare **achievement test, aptitude test, personality test, psychological test.**

intensive care Constant, complex, detailed health care as provided in various acute, life-threatening conditions. Special training is necessary to provide intensive care. Also called **critical care.**

intensive care unit (ICU) A hospital unit in which patients requiring close monitoring and intensive care are housed for as long as needed. An ICU contains highly technical and sophisticated monitoring devices and equipment, and the staff in the unit is educated to give critical care as needed by the patients.

intention A kind of healing process. Healing by **first intention** is the primary union of the edges of a wound, progressing to complete scar formation without granulation; healing by second intention is wound closure in which the edges are separated, granulation tissue develops to fill the gap, and, finally, epithelium grows in over the granulations, producing a larger scar than results from healing by first intention.

intention tremor Fine, rhythmic, purposeless movements that tend to increase during voluntary movements. Compare **continuous tremor.** See also **tremor.**

inter- A combining form meaning 'situated, formed, or occurring between': *interacinar, intercalary.*

interaction processes A component of the theory of effective practice. The processes consist of a series of interactions between a nurse and a client. The series occurs in a sequence of actions and reactions until the client and the nurse both understand what is wanted and the desired behavior or act is achieved. The processes are not used in Canada.

interarticular fibrocartilage One of four kinds of fibrocartilage, consisting of flattened fibrocartilaginous plates between the articular cartilage of the most active joints, as the knee joints. The synovial surfaces extend over the fibrocartilaginous plates and attach to surrounding ligaments. The plates absorb shocks and increase mobility. Compare **circumferential fibrocartilage, connecting fibrocartilage, stratiform fibrocartilage.**

intercalary Occurring between two others, as the absence of the middle part of a bone with the proximal and the distal parts present.

intercalate To insert between adjacent surfaces or structures. —**intercalation,** *n.*

intercapillary glomerulosclerosis An abnormal condition characterized by degeneration of the renal glomeruli. It is associated with diabetes and often produces albuminuria, nephrotic edema, hypertension, and renal insufficiency. Also called **Kimmelstiel-Wilson's disease.**

interchange See **reciprocal translocation.**

interconceptional gynecological care Health care of a woman during her reproductive years, between pregnancies, and after 6 weeks following delivery. Papanicolaou testing for cervical cancer, breast and pelvic examinations, evaluation of general health, and laboratory determination of glucosuria and proteinuria and of the hematocrit or hemoglobin are common and routine aspects of interconceptional care. Testing and treatment for pelvic, vaginal, or genital infections may be required. Interconceptional care is increasingly given by nurse practitioners or nurse midwives who follow protocols for treatment and referral formulated in consultation with a supervising gynecologist.

intercondylar fracture A fracture of the tissue between condyles.

intercostal Pertaining to the space between two ribs.

intercostal bulging The visible bulging of the soft tissues of the intercostal spaces that occurs when increased expiratory effort is needed

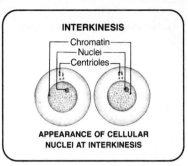

INTERKINESIS
- Chromatin
- Nuclei
- Centrioles

APPEARANCE OF CELLULAR NUCLEI AT INTERKINESIS

to exhale, as in asthma or cystic fibrosis. Compare **retraction of the chest.**

intercostal node A node in one of three groups of thoracic parietal lymph nodes situated near the dorsal parts of the intercostal spaces and associated with lymphatic vessels that drain the posterolateral area of the chest. The efferent vessels from the nodes in the four or five caudal spaces form a descending trunk which opens into the dilated origin of the thoracic duct. The efferents from the nodes in the upper intercostal spaces on the left side connect with the thoracic duct; those on the right side end in the right lymphatic duct. Compare **diaphragmatic node, sternal node.** See also **lymph node.**

intercourse *Informal.* Sexual intercourse. See **coitus.**

intercristal Pertaining to the space between two crests.

intercurrent disease A disease that develops in the course of another disease.

interface In general systems theory: a shared or overlapping boundary between two or more systems or parts within a system.

interferon (IFN) A class of small, soluble proteins produced and released by cells following antigenic stimulation. In noninfected cells, interferons induce the formation of an antiviral protein that prevents viral reproduction. Interferons are species specific. Following viral infection, Type I, or classical, interferon is produced by leukocytes and nonlymphoid cells. Type II, or immune, interferon is induced by certain bacteria and rickettsiae, and by specifically sensitized lymphocytes (T-lymphocytes) following interaction with a specific antigen or antigen-antibody complex. Type II interferon can affect antibody production and cell-mediated immunity. Interferon is also generated by fibroblasts.

interfibrillar mass of Flemming See **hyaloplasm.**

interfilar mass See **hyaloplasm.**

interior mesenteric artery A visceral branch of the abdominal aorta, arising just above the division into the common iliacs and supplying the left half of the transverse colon, all of the descending and iliac colons, and most of the rectum.

interkinesis The interval between the first and second nuclear divisions in meiosis. See also **interphase.**

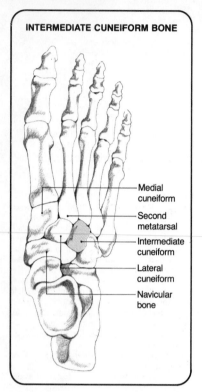

INTERMEDIATE CUNEIFORM BONE

Medial cuneiform

Second metatarsal

Intermediate cuneiform

Lateral cuneiform

Navicular bone

interlobular duct Any duct connecting or draining the lobules of a gland.

interlocked twins, interlocking twins Monozygotic twins so positioned in the uterus that the neck of one becomes entwined with that of the other during presentation so that vaginal delivery is not possible. Such interlocking occurs when one fetus is a breech presentation and the other a vertex presentation.

intermediate-acting insulin A preparation of the antidiabetic principle of beef pancreas or pork pancreas modified by interaction with zinc under specific chemical conditions and having an intermediate range of action. Intermediate-acting preparations begin to act 2 to 4 hours after injection. Neutral protamine Hagedorn insulin (NPH) has a peak action in 8 to 12 hours and a duration of action of 28 to 32 hours, while lente insulin has a similar peak interval and a slightly shorter duration of action. See also **insulin.** Compare **long-acting insulin, short-acting insulin.**

intermediate care A level of medical care for certain chronically ill or disabled individuals in which room and board are provided but skilled nursing care is not.

intermediate cell mass See **nephrotome.**

intermediate cuneiform bone The smallest of the three cuneiform bones of the foot, located between the medial and the lateral cu-

neiform bones. It has six surfaces, is attached to various ligaments, and articulates with the navicular, medial, and lateral cuneiform bones and with the second metatarsal. Also called **middle cuneiform bone, second cuneiform bone.**

intermediate host See **secondary host.**

intermediate mesoderm See **nephrotome.**

intermenstrual Pertaining to the time between menstrual periods.

intermenstrual fever The normal, slight elevation of temperature that marks ovulation, usually occurring about 14 days before the onset of menses.

intermittent Occurring at intervals; alternating between periods of activity and inactivity, as rheumatoid arthritis, which is marked by periods of signs and symptoms followed by periods of remission.

intermittent fever A fever that recurs in cycles of paroxysms and remissions, as in malaria. Kinds of intermittent fever include **biduotertian fever, quartan fever.**

intermittent mandatory ventilation (IMV) A method of respiratory therapy in which the patient is allowed to breathe independently and then at certain prescribed intervals is forced to take a breath by a mechanical ventilator, either under positive pressure or in a measured volume. Compare **continuous positive airway pressure, IPPB.** See also **respiratory therapy.**

intermittent positive pressure breathing See **IPPB.**

intermittent positive pressure breathing unit See **IPPB unit.**

intermittent positive pressure ventilation See **IPPB.**

intern, interne **1.** A physician in the first postgraduate year, learning medical practice under supervision before beginning a residency program. **2.** Any immediate postgraduate trainee in a clinical program. **3.** To work as an intern. Compare **extern, resident.**

internal Within or inside. —**internally,** *adv.*

internal aperture of tympanic canaliculus The upper opening of the tympanic channel in the temporal bone, leading to the tympanum.

internal carotid artery Each of two arteries starting at the bifurcation of the common carotid arteries, opposite the cranial border of the thyroid cartilage, through which blood circulates to many structures and organs in the head. Each artery includes cervical, petrous, cavernous, and cerebral portions and divides into 11 branches.

internal carotid plexus A network of nerves on the internal carotid artery, formed by the internal carotid nerve. The internal carotid plexus supplies sympathetic fibers to the branches of the internal carotid artery, the tympanic plexus, the nerves of the cavernous sinus, and the cranial parasympathetic ganglia through which the fibers pass. Compare **common carotid plexus, external carotid plexus.**

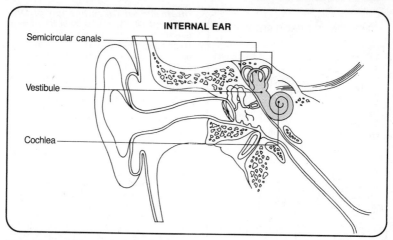

INTERNAL EAR

Semicircular canals

Vestibule

Cochlea

internal cervical os An internal opening of the uterus that corresponds to the slight constriction or isthmus of that organ about midway in its length. The internal cervical os separates the body of the uterus from the cervix. Compare **external cervical os.**

internal cuneiform bone See **medial cuneiform bone.**

internal ear The complex inner structure of the ear, communicating directly with the acoustic nerve, transmitting sound vibrations from the middle ear through the fluid-filled network of three semicircular canals joining at a vestibule connected to the cochlea. It has two parts: the osseous labyrinth and the membranous labyrinth. Also called **inner ear, labyrinth.**

internal fertilization The union of gametes within the body of the female after insemination. See also **artificial insemination.**

internal fistula An abnormal passage between two internal organs or structures.

internal fixation Any method of holding together the fragments of a fractured bone without the use of appliances external to the skin. After open reduction of the fracture, smooth or threaded pins, Kirschner wires, screws, plates attached by screws, or medullary nails may be used to stabilize the fragments. Compare **external pin fixation.**

internal iliac artery A division of the common iliac artery, supplying the walls of the pelvis, the pelvic viscera, the genital organs, and part of the medial thigh. The pattern of its branches is the most variable of any artery in the body. In the fetus, the internal iliac artery is twice as large as the external iliac and is the direct continuation of the common iliac artery. After birth, the internal iliac becomes smaller than the external iliac. Also called **hypogastric artery.** Compare **external iliac artery.**

internal iliac node A node in one of seven groups of parietal lymph nodes serving the abdomen and the pelvis. The internal iliac nodes surround the internal iliac vessels and receive lymphatic vessels corresponding to the branches of the internal iliac artery. Their afferent vessels drain lymph from the pelvic viscera, the buttocks, and dorsal portions of the thighs. Their efferents end in the common iliac nodes. Compare **external iliac node, iliac circumflex node.** See also **lymph, lymphatic system, lymph node.**

internal iliac vein One of the pair of veins in the lower body that join the external iliac vein to form the two common iliac veins. Each internal iliac vein begins at the greater sciatic foramen, ascends dorsally to its corresponding artery, and, at the pelvic brim joins the external iliac vein. Compare **external iliac vein.**

internalization The process of adopting within the self, either unconsciously or consciously through learning and socialization, the attitudes, beliefs, values, and standards of another person or, more generally, of the society or group to which one belongs. See also **socialization.**

internal jugular vein One of a pair of veins in the neck. Each vein collects blood from one side of the brain, the face, and the neck, and both unite with the subclavian vein to form the brachiocephalic vein. The left internal jugular vein is usually smaller than the right, and each vein contains a pair of valves located about 2.5 cm (1 inch) above its termination. Each internal jugular vein is continuous with the transverse sinus in the posterior part of the jugular foramen at the base of the skull where, in some people, the vein forms a jugular bulb. Just above the termination is the inferior bulb. Compare **external jugular vein.**

internal medicine The branch of medicine concerned with the study of the physiology and pathology of the internal organs and with the medical diagnosis and treatment of disorders of these organs.

internal oblique muscle See **obliquus internus abdominis.**

internal podalic version and total breech extraction See **version and extraction.**

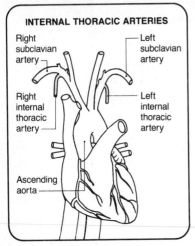

INTERNAL THORACIC ARTERIES

Right subclavian artery

Left subclavian artery

Right internal thoracic artery

Left internal thoracic artery

Ascending aorta

internal pterygoid muscle See **pterygoideus medialis.**

internal respiratory nerve of Bell See **phrenic nerve.**

internal rotation Movement of a body part toward the midline. For example, internal rotation occurs when a ball and socket joint, such as the hip, turns the leg inward. Also called medial rotation. Compare **external rotation.**

internal strabismus See **esotropia.**

internal thoracic artery One of a pair of arteries that arise from the first portions of the subclavian arteries, descend to the margin of the sternum, and divide into the musculophrenic and superior gastric arteries at the level of the sixth intercostal space, supplying the pectoral muscles, the breasts, the pericardium, and the abdominal muscles. Each artery has eight branches.

internal thoracic vein One of a pair of veins that accompanies the internal thoracic artery, receiving tributaries that correspond to those of the artery. It forms a single trunk that runs up on the medial side of the artery and ends in the corresponding brachiocephalic vein. The superior phrenic vein opens into the internal thoracic vein.

International Association for Dental Research (IADR) An international organization concerned with research in dentistry and the exchange of information regarding such research.

International Classification of Disease (ICDA) A classification system adapted for use in the United States by the United States Public Health Service from the parent system developed by the World Health Organization. The system is used in categorizing and indexing hospital records. Each disease is listed as belonging to a major section, as infectious disease or neoplastic disease, and then further coded into major disease categories and subdivisions. The system is updated every 10 years.

International Classification of Diseases (ICD) An official list of categories of diseases, physical and mental, issued by the World Health Organization (WHO). It is used primarily for statistical purposes in the classification of morbidity and mortality data. Any nation belonging to WHO may adjust the classification to meet specific needs, as in the United States, the *ICD-9-CM,* a clinical modification of the 1975 revision, *ICD-9,* was adopted to provide additional data required by clinicians, research workers, epidemiologists, medical record librarians, and administrators of inpatient, outpatient, and community programs. See also *Diagnostic and Statistical Manual of Mental Disorders.*

International Congress of Surgeons (ICS) An international professional organization of surgeons.

International Council of Nurses (ICN) The oldest international health organization. It is a federation of nurses' associations from 93 nations and was one of the first health organizations to develop strict policies of nondiscrimination based on nationality, race, creed, color, politics, sex, or social status. The objectives of the ICN include promotion of national associations of nurses; improvement of standards of nursing and competence of nurses; improvement of the status of nurses within their countries; and provision of an authoritative international voice for nurses. The ICN is active in the World Health Organization (WHO), the United Nations Educational, Scientific, and Cultural Organization (UNESCO), and other international organizations.

International Red Cross Society An international philanthropic organization, based in Geneva, concerned primarily with the humane treatment and welfare of the victims of war and calamity and with the neutrality of hospitals and medical personnel in times of war. See also **American Red Cross.**

International System of Units A system for the standardization of the measurement of certain substances, including some antibiotics, vitamins, enzymes, and hormones. An International Unit (IU) of substance is the amount that produces a specific biological result. Each IU of a substance has the same potency and action as another unit of the same substance.

International Unit (IU, I.U.) A unit of measure in the International System of Units.

internist A physician specializing in internal medicine.

interoceptive Pertaining to stimuli originating from within the body regarding the functioning of the internal organs or to the receptors they activate. Compare **exteroceptive, proprioception.**

interoceptor Any sensory nerve ending located in cells in the viscera that responds to stimuli originating from within the body regarding the function of the internal organs, as digestion, excretion, and blood pressure. Compare **exteroceptor, proprioceptor.**

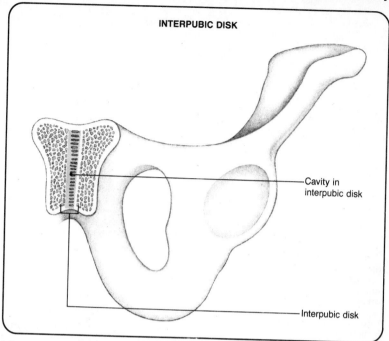

INTERPUBIC DISK

Cavity in
interpubic disk

Interpubic disk

interparietal fissure   See **intraparietal sulcus.**

interperiosteal fracture   An incomplete fracture in which the periosteum is not disrupted.

interpersonal therapy   A kind of psychotherapy that views faulty communications, interactions, and interrelationships as basic factors in maladaptive behavior. A kind of interpersonal therapy is **transactional analysis.**

interphase   The metabolic stage in the cell cycle during which the cell is not dividing, the chromosomes are not individually distinguishable, and such biochemical and physiological activities as DNA synthesis occur. The stage follows telophase of one division and extends to the beginning of prophase of the next division. See also **interkinesis.**

interpubic disk   The fibrocartilaginous plate connecting the opposed surfaces of the pubic bones at the pubic symphysis. Varying in thickness, it is strengthened by interlacing fibers and often contains a cavity that usually appears after the 10th year of life. Also called **discus interpubicus.**

interrogatories   In law: a series of written questions submitted to a witness or other person having information of interest to the court. The answers are transcribed and are sworn to under oath. Compare **discovery, deposition.**

intersex   **1.** Any individual who has anatomical characteristics of both sexes or whose external genitalia are ambiguous or inappropriate

for either the normal male or female. **2.** See **intersexuality.** See also **hermaphroditism, pseudohermaphroditism.**

intersexuality   **1.** The condition in which an individual has both male and female anatomical characteristics to varying degrees or in which the appearance of the external genitalia is ambiguous or differs from the gonadal or genetic sex. **2.** Any disturbance in the normal sequence of sex determination during embryonic development, including sex chromosome aberrations, abnormal differentiation of the gonads or ductal systems, or hormonal imbalance, which may result in situations in which the phenotypic sex differs from the genotypic sex. Those conditions characterized by ambiguous or inappropriate genitalia are apparent at birth, but others, as Turner's syndrome or Klinefelter's syndrome, may not be diagnosed until later as a result of delayed development or infertility. NURSING CONSIDERATIONS: Gender determination of an infant whose sex is doubtful constitutes more of a psychological and social problem than a medical emergency. Such situations are always highly emotional for the parents, who are often overwhelmed by feelings of guilt and shame, and a great deal of support and encouragement are needed. Of special importance is the education of the family about the abnormality, primarily what measures can be undertaken immediately and what will be involved in the long-term management of the condition. See also **hermaphroditism, pseudohermaphroditism. —intersexual,** *adj.*

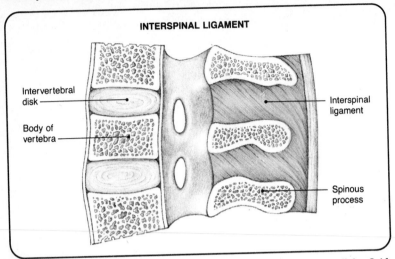

INTERSPINAL LIGAMENT

Intervertebral disk

Body of vertebra

Interspinal ligament

Spinous process

interspace The interval between two similar parts, such as the space between the ribs.

interspinal ligament One of many thin, narrow membranous ligaments that connect adjoining spinous processes and extend from the root of each process to the apex. The interspinal ligaments meet the ligamenta flava ventrally and the supraspinal ligament dorsally and are only slightly developed in the neck.

interspinous Of or pertaining to the space between any spinous processes.

interstitial Of or pertaining to that which occupies the space between tissues, as interstitial fluid.

interstitial cystitis An inflammation of the bladder, believed to be associated with an autoimmune or allergic response. The bladder wall becomes inflamed, ulcerated, and scarred, causing frequent, painful urination. Hematuria often occurs. Treatment may include distention of the bladder and cauterization of the ulcers or weekly lavage of the bladder until the inflammation clears. Both procedures are performed under anesthesia. Corticosteroids are often prescribed to control inflammation. Ulceration is rarely severe enough to require cystectomy with urinary diversion. The condition occurs most often in women of middle age and may resemble the early stages of cancer of the bladder. Cystoscopy and biopsy are required for a diagnosis. Also called **Hunner's ulcer.**

interstitial emphysema A form of emphysema in which air or gas escapes into the interstitial tissues of the lung following a penetrating injury or as the result of a rupture in an alveolar wall. See also **emphysema, pneumothorax.**

interstitial fluid An extracellular fluid that fills the spaces between most of the cells of the body and provides a substantial portion of the liquid environment of the body. Formed by filtration through the blood capillaries, it is drained away as lymph. Compare **intracellular fluid, lymph, plasma.**

interstitial growth An increase in size by hyperplasia or hypertrophy within the interior of a part or structure that is already formed. Compare **appositional growth.**

interstitial hypertrophic neuropathy See **Dejerine-Sottas disease.**

interstitial implantation In embryology: the complete embedding of the blastocyst within the endometrium of the uterine wall.

interstitial infusion See **hypodermoclysis.**

interstitial keratitis An uncommon inflammation within the layers of the cornea. The first symptom is a diffuse haziness. Blood vessels may grow into the area and cause permanent opacities. Its causes are syphilis, tuberculosis, leprosy, and vascular hypersensitivity.

interstitial nephritis Inflammation of the interstitial tissue of the kidney, including the tubules. The condition may be acute or chronic. Acute interstitial nephritis is an immunologic, adverse reaction to certain drugs, often sulfonamide or methicillin. Acute renal failure, fever, rash, and proteinuria are characteristic of this condition. Most people regain normal function of the kidneys when the offending drug is removed. Chronic interstitial nephritis is a syndrome of interstitial inflammation and structural changes, sometimes associated with such conditions as ureteral obstruction, pyelonephritis, exposure of the kidney to a toxin, rejection of a transplant, and certain systemic diseases. Gradually, renal failure, nausea, vomiting, weight loss, fatigue, and anemia develop. Acidosis and hyperkalemia may follow. The nurse watches carefully for signs of electrolyte imbalance, dehydration, and hypovolemia, especially if there is frequent vomiting.

interstitial plasma cell pneumonia See **pneumocystosis.**

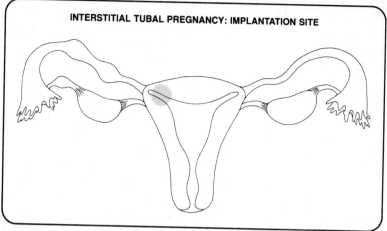

INTERSTITIAL TUBAL PREGNANCY: IMPLANTATION SITE

interstitial pneumonia   A diffuse, chronic inflammation of the lungs beyond the terminal bronchioles, characterized by fibrosis and collagen formation in the alveolar walls and by the presence of large mononuclear cells in the alveolar spaces. The symptoms of this condition are progressive dyspnea, clubbing of the fingers, cyanosis, and fever. The disease may result from a hypersensitive reaction to busulphan, chlorambucil, hexamethonium, or methotrexate. Interstitial pneumonia may also be an autoimmune reaction, since it often accompanies celiac disease, rheumatoid arthritis, Sjögren's syndrome, and systemic sclerosis. X-rays of the lungs show patchy shadows and mottling, as in bronchopneumonia. Later stages of the disease reveal bronchiectasis, dilatation of the bronchi, and shrinkage of the lungs. Treatment of interstitial pneumonia includes bed rest, oxygen therapy, and corticosteroids. Also called **diffuse fibrosing alveolitis, giant cell interstitial pneumonia, Hamman-Rich syndrome.** Compare **bronchopneumonia.**

interstitial pregnancy   See **ectopic pregnancy.**

interstitial tubal pregnancy   A tubal pregnancy in which implantation occurs in the proximal, interstitial portion of one of the fallopian tubes. See also **tubal pregnancy.**

intertransverse ligament   One of many fibrous bands connecting the transverse processes of vertebrae. In the cervical region, intertransverse ligaments consist of a few scattered fibers; in the thoracic region, they are rounded cords connected with the deep muscles of the back.

intertrigo   An erythematous irritation of opposing skin surfaces due to friction. Common sites are the axillae, the folds beneath large or pendulous breasts, and the inner aspects of the thighs. Maceration and monilial infection may occur if the area is warm and moist. —**intertriginous,** *adj.*

intertrochanteric crest   One of a pair of

ridges along the thigh bones, curving obliquely from the greater to the lesser trochanter. Immediately distal to the crest, a slight ridge—the linea quadrata—receives the insertion of the quadratus femoris and a few fibers of the adductor magnus.

intertrochanteric fracture   A fracture characterized by a crack in the tissue of the proximal femur between the greater and the lesser trochanters.

intertrochanteric line   A line that runs across the anterior surface of the thigh bone from the greater to the lesser trochanter, winding around the medial surface, and ending in the linea aspera. The proximal half of the intertrochanteric line is the attachment for the iliofemoral ligament; the distal half holds the vastus medialis muscle.

interval health history   A kind of health history that notes the general condition of a client during the period between visits and is not limited to facts relevant to a particular condition. The interval health history provides an ongoing account of a person's health, serving to bring the data base up to date.

intervention   **1.** Any act performed to prevent harm from occurring to a client or to improve the mental, emotional, or physical function of a client. A physiologic process may be monitored or enhanced, or a pathologic process may be arrested or controlled. **2.** The fourth step of the nursing process. This step includes nursing actions taken to meet patient needs as determined by nursing assessment and diagnosis. See also **nursing intervention.**

intervertebral   Of or pertaining to the space between any two vertebrae, as the fibrocartilaginous disks.

intervertebral disk   One of the fibrous disks found between each of the spinal vertebrae, except the axis and the atlas. The disks vary in size, shape, thickness, and number, depending on the location in the back and on the particular vertebrae they separate.

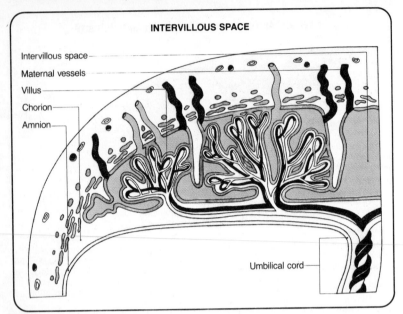

INTERVILLOUS SPACE

Intervillous space
Maternal vessels
Villus
Chorion
Amnion

Umbilical cord

intervertebral fibrocartilage See **intervertebral disk.**

intervertebral foramen Any of the passages between adjacent vertebrae through which the spinal nerves and vessels pass.

intervillous space One of many spaces between the chorionic villi of the endometrium of the gravid uterus, beneath the placenta. The intervillous spaces act as small reservoirs for oxygenated maternal blood from which fetal circulation takes up the nutrients and gases by osmosis, hydrostatic pressure, and diffusion.

intestinal absorption The passage of the products of digestion from the lumen of the small intestine into the blood and lymphatic vessels in the wall of the gut. The surface area of the intestine is greatly increased by the presence of fingerlike projections, called villi, each of which contains capillaries and a lymphatic vessel, or lacteal. Most dissolved nutrients pass quickly into the capillary bed for transport through the portal circulation to the liver.

intestinal amebiasis See **amebic dysentery.**

intestinal angina Chronic vascular insufficiency of the mesentery caused by atherosclerosis and resulting ischemia of the smooth muscle of the small bowel. Abdominal pain or cramping after eating, constipation, melena, malabsorption, and weight loss are characteristic of the condition. Also called **chronic intestinal ischemia.**

intestinal apoplexy The sudden occlusion of one of the three principal arteries to the intestine by an embolism or a thrombus. This condition leads rapidly to necrosis of intestinal tissue and is often fatal. Treatment is usually

surgical: the occlusion is removed, and, often, the affected portion of the bowel is resected. See also **atherosclerosis.**

intestinal dyspepsia An abnormal condition characterized by impaired digestion associated with a problem that originates in the intestines. See also **dyspepsia.**

intestinal fistula An abnormal passage from the intestine to an external abdominal opening or stoma, usually created surgically for the exit of feces following removal of a malignant or severely ulcerated segment of the bowel. See also **colostomy.**

intestinal flu *Informal.* A viral gastroenteritis, usually caused by infection by an enterovirus. It is characterized by abdominal cramps, diarrhea, nausea, and vomiting. Outbreaks may be sporadic or epidemic, and the disease usually is mild and self-limited. Treatment is symptomatic. Control of diarrhea may be achieved with antidiarrheal medication and a diet limited to clear fluids. See also **enteric infection, gastroenteritis.**

intestinal infarction See **intestinal strangulation.**

intestinal juices The secretions of glands lining the intestine.

intestinal lymphangiectasia See **hypoproteinemia.**

intestinal obstruction Any obstruction that results in failure of the contents of the intestine to pass through the lumen of the bowel. The most common cause is a mechanical blockage resulting from adhesions, impacted feces, tumor, hernia, intussusception, volvulus, or the strictures of inflammatory bowel disease. Obstruction may also be the result of paralytic ileus.

INTRA-AORTIC BALLOON PUMP

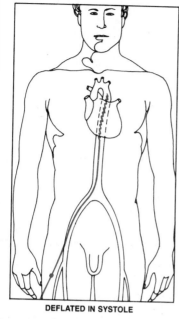

DEFLATED IN SYSTOLE

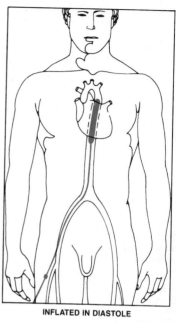

INFLATED IN DIASTOLE

Obstruction of the small bowel may cause severe pain, vomiting of fecal matter, dehydration, and, eventually, a drop in blood pressure. Obstruction of the colon causes less severe pain, marked abdominal distention, and constipation. X-ray examination reveals the level of obstruction and its cause. Treatment includes the evacuation of intestinal contents by means of a nasoenteric decompression tube. Surgical repair is sometimes necessary. Also called **ileus** *(informal).* See also **hernia, intussusception, volvulus.**

intestinal strangulation   The arrest of blood flow to the bowel, resulting in edema, cyanosis, and gangrene of the affected loop of bowel. This condition is usually caused by a hernia, intussusception, or volvulus. Early signs of intestinal strangulation resemble those of intestinal obstruction, but peritonitis, shock, and the presence of a tender mass in the abdomen are important in making a differential diagnosis. Also called **intestinal infarction.**

intestinal tonsil   One of a group of lymphatic nodules forming a single layer in the mucous membrane of the ileum opposite the mesenteric attachment. They are oval patches about 1 cm (⅜ inch) wide and extend for about 4 cm (1½ inches) along the intestine. In most individuals they appear in the distal ileum but also appear in the jejunum of a few individuals Also called **Peyer's patches.** Compare **lingual tonsil, palatine tonsil, pharyngeal tonsil.**

intestine   The portion of the alimentary canal extending from the pyloric opening of the stomach to the anus. It includes the small and large intestines. —**intestinal,** *adj.*

intima, *pl.* **intimae**   The innermost layer of a structure, as the lining membrane of an artery or vein. —**intimal,** *adj.*

intolerance   A condition characterized by an inability to absorb or metabolize a nutrient or medication. Exposure to the substance may cause an adverse reaction, as in lactose intolerance. Compare **allergy, atopic.**

intoxication   **1.** The state of being poisoned by a drug or other toxic substance. **2.** The state of being inebriated owing to an excessive consumption of alcohol. **3.** A state of mental or emotional hyperexcitability, usually euphoric.

intoxication amaurosis   Loss of vision occurring without an apparent ophthalmic lesion, caused by a systemic poison, as alcohol or tobacco.

intra-   A combining form meaning 'situated, formed, or occurring within': *intrabronchial, intracutaneous.*

intra-aortic balloon pump   A counterpulsation device that provides temporary cardiac assist in the management of refractory left ventricular failure, as may follow myocardial infarction or occur in preinfarction angina. The balloon is attached to a catheter inserted in the aorta and is automatically inflated during diastole and deflated during systole. Also called **intra-aortic balloon counterpulsation.**

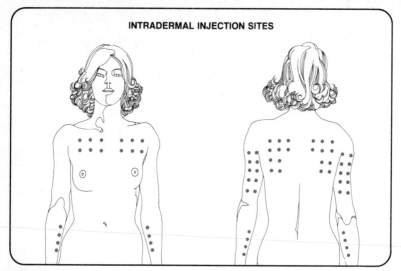

INTRADERMAL INJECTION SITES

intra-articular Within a joint.

intra-articular fracture A fracture involving the articular surfaces of a joint.

intra-articular injection The injection of a medication into a joint space, usually to reduce inflammation, as in bursitis or fibromyostis. Using the same technique, fluid may be withdrawn from the joint space in abnormal, excessive accumulations of fluid in a joint.

intra-articular ligament A ligament that forms part of the joints between 16 of the 24 ribs, dividing the joints into two cavities, each containing a synovial membrane. Each intra-articular ligament consists of a short, flattened band of fibers inside the joint, attached by one extremity to the rib and by the other to the intervertebral disk. Intra-articular ligaments are not present in the joints of the 1st, 10th, 11th, and 12th ribs, each of which has only one synovial cavity. Compare **radiate ligament.**

intra-atrial Within an atrium in the heart.

intra-atrial block Delayed or abnormal conduction within the atria, identified on an electrocardiogram by a prolonged and often notched P wave.

intracanalicular fibroma A breast tumor containing glandular epithelium and fibrous tissue.

intracanicular papilloma A benign warty growth in certain glands, especially the breast glands.

intracapsular fracture A fracture within the capsule of a joint.

intracardiac catheter See **cardiac catheter.**

intracardiac lead **1.** An electrocardiographic conductor in which the exploring electrode is placed within one of the cardiac chambers, usually by means of cardiac catheterization. **2.** *Informal.* A tracing produced by such a lead on an electrocardiograph.

intracartilaginous ossification See **ossification.**

intracatheter A thin, flexible plastic catheter introduced and threaded into a blood vessel to infuse blood, fluid, or medication. Also called **intracath** *(informal).*

intracavitary therapy A kind of radiotherapy in which radioactive sources are placed, usually with the help of an applicator, within a body cavity to irradiate the walls of the cavity or adjacent tissues.

intracellular fluid A fluid within cell membranes throughout most of the body, containing dissolved solutes which are essential to electrolytic balance and to healthy metabolism. Compare **interstitial fluid, lymph, plasma.**

intracerebral Within the tissue of the brain, inside the bony skull.

intracistronic Within a cistron.

intracranial Within the cranium.

intracranial aneurysm Any aneurysm of any of the cerebral arteries. Rupture of an intracranial aneurysm results in mortality approaching 50%, and there is a high risk of recurrence in survivors of a rupture. Characteristics of the condition include sudden severe headache, stiff neck, nausea, vomiting, and, sometimes, loss of consciousness. Kinds of intracranial aneurysms include **berry aneurysm, fusiform aneurysm, mycotic aneurysm.**

intractable Having no relief, as a disease that remains unrelieved by therapy.

intracutaneous Within the layers of the skin.

intracystic papilloma A benign epithelial tumor formed with a cystic adenoma.

intradermal injection Administration of a small amount of solution, usually antigens, between the epidermal and dermal layers of the skin to produce a local effect or to give skin tests for allergy or anergy testing. Intradermal injec-

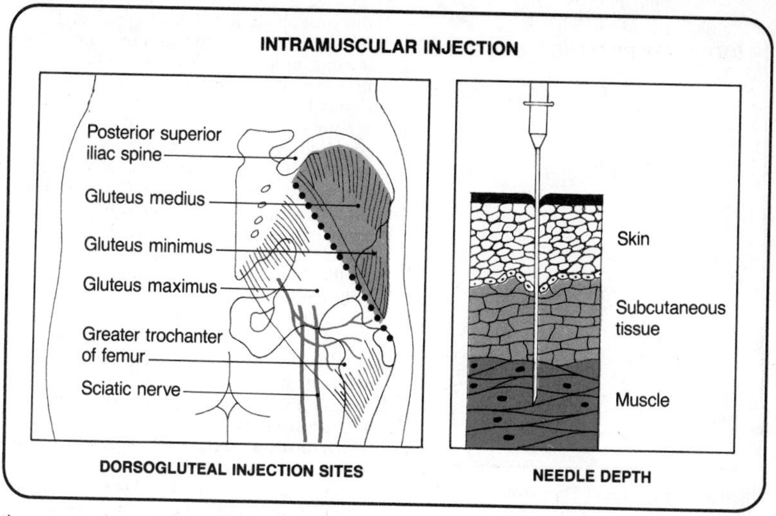

INTRAMUSCULAR INJECTION

Posterior superior iliac spine

Gluteus medius

Gluteus minimus

Gluteus maximus

Greater trochanter of femur

Sciatic nerve

Skin

Subcutaneous tissue

Muscle

DORSOGLUTEAL INJECTION SITES

NEEDLE DEPTH

tions are made most commonly with a 26G or 27G needle, usually on the inner surface of the forearms, the posterior surface of the upper-arms, and the back.

intradermal test A procedure used to identify suspected allergens by intradermally injecting the patient with small amounts of extracts of the suspected allergens. The injections are made at spaced intervals, usually in the forearm or in the scapular region. The patient is concurrently injected with the diluent alone as a control procedure. The test is positive if, within 15 to 30 minutes, the injection of extract produces a wheal surrounded by erythema and the control injection produces no symptoms. Also called subcutaneous test. Compare **patch test, scratch test.** See also **conjunctival test, use test.**

intraductal carcinoma A frequently large neoplasm occuring most often in the breast. The lesion on cross section usually shows well-differentiated tumor cells in calcified and dilated ducts of the breast.

intradural lipoma A fatty tumor in or beneath the dura mater of the spine or sacrum that tends to infiltrate the dorsal column and roots of spinal nerves, causing pain and dysfunction.

intraepidermal carcinoma A neoplasm of squamous epidermal cells that does not proliferate into the basal area and often occurs at many sites simultaneously. The lesions, which enlarge slowly without healing at the center, are resistant to chemotherapy and to radiation. Also called **Bowen's disease, Bowen's precancerous dermatosis, precancerous dermatitis.**

intraepithelial carcinoma See carcinoma in situ.

intramuscular injection The introduction of a sterile needle into a muscle to administer medication. Needle size depends on the viscosity of the medication and the amount of subcutaneous fat over the muscle. The selected site is prepared by cleansing with alcohol or acetone.

NURSING CONSIDERATIONS: If the dorsal gluteal area is chosen, the patient is asked to lie prone with ankles bent and feet curved in so that the toes of each foot are directed toward the opposite foot to relax the gluteal muscles, thus making the injection less painful. Injection in deltoid muscles is more painful than in other sites and is avoided if possible. The ventral gluteal area and the vastus lateralis are the preferred injection sites in infants. Needles and syringes are always disposed of in a safe way; they are usually destroyed. Generally, no more than 3 ml are injected into a muscle since large volumes may result in the formation of a sterile abscess. Not uncommonly, biologicals (serums, vaccines, antigens, antitoxins, and other preparations derived from living organisms) may leave a knot in the muscle that is not painful and that subsides slowly over several weeks or months, though it may cause concern in the patient or the young patients' parents. The lump should not grow larger or become more painful; if it does, it may be assumed that an abscess has formed.

intraocular pressure The internal pressure of the eye, regulated by resistance to the flow of aqueous humor through the fine sieve of the trabecular meshwork. Contraction or relaxation of the longitudinal muscles of the ciliary body affects the size of the apertures in the meshwork. See also **glaucoma.**

intraparietal sulcus An irregular groove on the convex surface of the parietal lobe that marks the division of the inferior and superior parietal lobules. Also called **interparietal fissure.**

intrapartal care Care of a pregnant woman from the onset of labor to the completion of the third stage of labor with the expulsion of the placenta. See also **antepartal care, newborn intrapartal care, postpartal care.**

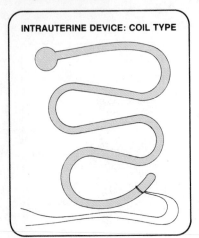

INTRAUTERINE DEVICE: COIL TYPE

intrapartal period The period spanning labor and birth.

intraperiosteal fracture A fracture that does not rupture the periosteum.

intrapsychic conflict An emotional conflict within oneself. See also **conflict.**

intrasocial idiocy A state of mental retardation in which the person is capable of undertaking some form of regular occupation.

intrathecal Of or pertaining to a structure, process, or substance within a sheath, as the cerebrospinal fluid within the theca of the spinal canal.

intrathoracic goiter An enlargement of the thyroid gland that protrudes into the thoracic cavity.

intrauterine contraceptive device (IUCD, ICD) See **intrauterine device.**

intrauterine device (IUD) A contraceptive device consisting of a bent strip of radiopaque plastic with a fine monofilament tail that is inserted and left in the uterine cavity for the purpose of altering the physiology of the uterus and fallopian tubes to prevent pregnancy. The mechanism of action is not known. Also called **coil, intrauterine contraceptive device, loop** (*informal*).

intrauterine fracture A fracture that occurs during fetal life.

intrauterine growth curve A line on a standardized graph representing the mean weight for gestational age through pregnancy to term. It provides a method for classifying infants according to their state of maturity and fetal development.

intrauterine growth retardation An abnormal process in which the development and maturation of the fetus is impeded or delayed by genetic factors, maternal disease, or fetal malnutrition caused by placental insufficiency. See also **small-for-gestational-age infant.**

intravenous Within a vein or veins.

intravenous bolus A dose of medication administered intravenously in a short period of time, usually within 1 to 30 minutes. The intravenous bolus is commonly used when administration of a medication is needed quickly, as in an emergency; when administering drugs that cannot be diluted, as many cancer chemotherapeutic drugs; and when the therapeutic purpose is to achieve a peak drug level in the bloodstream of the patient. The intravenous bolus is not used when the medication involved must be diluted in a large volume of fluid before entering the bloodstream or when the rapid administration of a medication, as potassium chloride, could be life-threatening. The amount of medication to be delivered per minute is determined by dividing the total amount of medication to be injected by the prescribed time for delivery. Depending on the time required for bolus infusion, the venipuncture can be made with either the syringe needle or a winged-tipped needle. Also see **intravenous push.**

intravenous catheter A plastic catheter inserted into a vein used to infuse solutions and drugs. Two main types include **over-the-needle catheter** and **inside-the-needle catheter.**

intravenous cholangiography In diagnostic radiology: a procedure for outlining the major bile ducts. A radiopaque contrast material is injected intravenously and serial X-rays are taken. See also **cholangiography.**

intravenous controller One of several devices that automatically deliver intravenous fluid at selectable flow rates, usually between 1 and 69 drops per minute. The controller is commonly equipped with a rate selector, drop sensor, drop indicator, and a drop alarm. When the infusion does not flow at the prescribed rate, the drop alarm emits a visual and audible signal. The device works by gravity so that the I.V. container must be placed at least 76 cm (30 inches) above the venipuncture site. Compare **intravenous peristaltic pump, intravenous piston pump, intravenous syringe pump.**

intravenous fat emulsion A preparation of 10% or 20% fat administered intravenously to help maintain or increase the weight of an adult patient or the weight and growth of a younger patient. Such fat emulsions are prepared from refined soybean oil and egg yolk phospholipids and may contain such major fatty acids as linoleic, oleic, palmitic, and linolenic acids. The intravenous fat emulsion is isotonic and may be administered into a peripheral vein. Intravenous fat emulsions are often administered simultaneously with hyperalimentation solutions when hyperalimentation is not sufficient to maintain adequate treatment of a patient or when the patient needs calories but cannot tolerate the high percentage of dextrose contained in hyperalimentation solutions. Once the primary intravenous line has been established, intravenous fat emulsions are usually administered with the aid of a volumetric infusion pump to maintain an even flow rate and avoid any fatty-acid overload. Phlebitis occurs less frequently when the fat emulsion is administered simultaneously with the hyperalimentation solution.

SOLUTIONS FOR INTRAVENOUS INFUSION: COMMON ABBREVIATIONS

AA	Amino acids
D	Dextrose solution (percentage unspecified)
D5LR	Dextrose 5% in Ringer's injection, lactated
D5R	Dextrose 5% in Ringer's injection
D-S	Dextrose-saline combinations
D2.5½NS	Dextrose 2.5% in sodium chloride 0.45%
D2.5NS	Dextrose 2.5% in sodium chloride 0.9%
D5¼NS	Dextrose 5% in sodium chloride 0.225%
D5½NS	Dextrose 5% in sodium chloride 0.45%
D5NS	Dextrose 5% in sodium chloride 0.9%
D10NS	Dextrose 10% in sodium chloride 0.9%
D5W	Dextrose 5% in water
D10W	Dextrose 10% in water
DXN-NS	Dextran 6% in sodium chloride 0.9%
IS	Invert sugar
LR	Ringer's injection, lactated
NS	Sodium chloride 0.9%
PH	Protein hydrolysate
R	Ringer's injection
TPN	Total parenteral nutrition
W	Sterile water for injection

intravenous feeding   The administration of nutrients through a vein or veins.

intravenous infusion   **1.** A solution administered intravenously through an infusion set that includes a plastic or glass vacuum bottle or bag containing the solution and tubing connecting the bottle to a catheter or needle in the patient's vein. **2.** The process of administering a solution intravenously. Swelling of the limb around and distal to the site of injection may indicate that the tip of the catheter or needle is in the subcutaneous tissue and not in the vein. The fluid may be infiltrating the tissue spaces. The catheter or needle is withdrawn and the limb is elevated. Redness, swelling, heat, and pain around the vein at the site of injection or proximal to it may indicate thrombophlebitis. See also **venipuncture.**

intravenous infusion filter   Any one of the numerous devices used in helping to ensure the purity of an intravenous solution. Intravenous filters strain the intravenous solution to remove such contaminants as dissolved impurities (detergents, proteins, and polysaccharides), extraneous salts, microorganisms, particles, precipitates, and undissolved drug powders. Some filters are built into the primary intravenous tubing; others must be attached. One of the main criteria for selecting a filter is the assurance that the filter is not too fine for the intravenous solution to be strained. Filters that are too fine will clog. The size of filter membranes varies from 5 microns to 0.22 microns. Filters of 1 to 5 microns will remove most particulate debris but not most fungi or bacteria. Filters that are 0.45 microns or less will remove fungi and most bacteria; filters that are 0.22

microns will remove all fungi and bacteria but will also reduce the flow rate of the intravenous solution, which is crucial when rapid delivery is required. See also **needle filter.**

intravenous infusion technique   The calculations for determining the delivery rate of intravenous fluid for the individual patient and the necessary spiking of the container and priming of the tubing prior to venipuncture and administration of the fluid.

intravenous injection   A hypodermic injection into a vein to instill a single dose of medication, withdraw blood, or begin an intravenous infusion of blood, medication, or a fluid solution, as saline or dextrose in water. See also **venipuncture.**

intravenous peristaltic pump   Any one of several devices for administering intravenous fluids by exerting pressure on the I.V. tubing rather than on the fluid itself. Most peristaltic pumps operate with normal I.V. tubing and deliver fluid at a selectable drop-per-minute rate. This device typically can infuse between 1 and 99 drops of intravenous fluid per minute and is equipped with a drop sensor, rate selector, power switch indicator lamp, and drop indicator and alarm. Compare **intravenous controller, intravenous piston pump, intravenous syringe pump.**

intravenous piston pump   Any one of several devices that accurately control the infusion of intravenous fluids by piston action. Most intravenous piston pumps can be operated by battery as well as by electric current and require special tubing. Some models are portable. Intravenous piston pumps are commonly equipped with controls that allow selectable flow rates and

INTRAVENOUS PYELOGRAPHY

Delayed filling of contrast medium

Normal filling of contrast medium

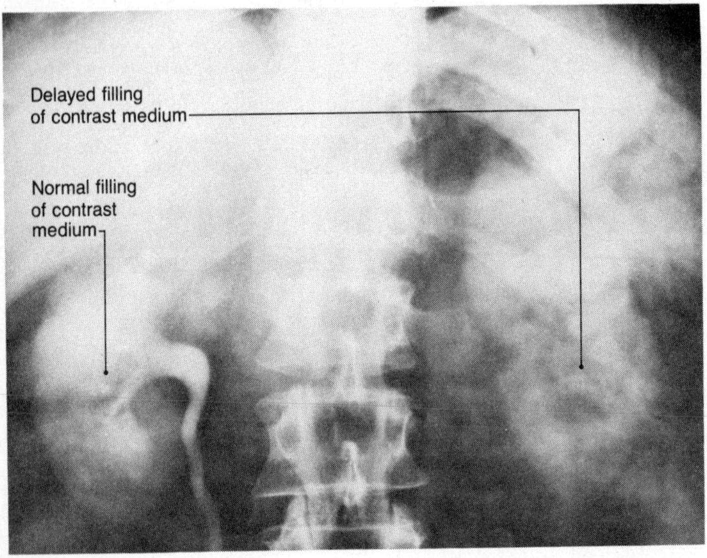

indicators that display flow rates, dose limits, and cumulative fluid volumes. The intravenous piston pump monitors the actual volume of intravenous fluid administered instead of counting drops of fluid. Hence, its accuracy is not affected by drop size, temperature, or fluid viscosity. The pump is designed to reduce the delivery rate to a keep-vein-open rate if the proper flow rate or the dose limit is exceeded. The pump also stops delivery of the intravenous fluid if the I.V. line is clogged or if infiltration is detected. Also called **volumetric infusion pump.** Compare **intravenous controller, intravenous peristaltic pump, intravenous syringe pump.**

intravenous pump   A pump designed to regulate the rate of flow of a fluid given intravenously through an intracatheter or a scalp vein needle.

intravenous push   The rapid administration of a bolus of medication with a syringe. See also **intravenous bolus.**

intravenous pyelography (IVP)   A technique in radiology for examining the structures and evaluating the function of the urinary system. A contrast medium is injected intravenously, and serial X-rays are taken as the medium is cleared from the blood by glomerular filtration. The renal calyces, renal pelvis, ureters, and urinary bladder are all visible on the X-ray films. Tumors, cysts, stones, and many structural and functional abnormalities may be diagnosed using this technique. Also called **descending urography, excretory urography.**

intravenous syringe pump   Any one of several devices that automatically compress a syringe plunger at a controlled rate. Such devices are used with disposable syringes that can deliver blood, medications, or nutrients by intravenous, arterial, or subcutaneous routes. Intravenous syringe pumps can deliver small volumes of fluid at rates as low as 0.01 ml/hour and are often used in the treatment of infants. Small units are usually battery-operated and portable and are especially useful in treating ambulatory patients. Compare **intravenous controller, intravenous peristaltic pump, intravenous piston pump.**

intravenous therapist   A nursing specialist trained and qualified to start and maintain intravenous therapy.

intravenous urography   See **intravenous pyelography (IVP).**

intraventricular   Of or pertaining to the space within a ventricle.

intraventricular heart block   An interruption of the cardiac stimulus as it passes over the ventricles, seen as a prolonged QRS complex on an electrocardiogram. It is usually caused by decreased conduction in the branches of the bundle of His.

intrinsic   A natural or inherent part or quality.

intrinsic asthma   A nonseasonal, nonallergic form of asthma, usually first occurring later in life than allergic asthma, that tends to be chronic and persistent rather than episodic. The precipitating factors include inhalation of irritating pollutants in the atmosphere, as dust particles, smoke, aerosols, strong cooking odors, paint fumes, and other volatile substances.

Bronchospasm may also occur in cold, damp weather, after the sudden inhalation of cold, dry air, and after physical exercise or violent coughing or laughing. Respiratory infections, as the common cold, and psychological factors, as anxiety, may also induce an attack. Compare **allergic asthma.** See also **asthma in children.**

intrinsic factor A substance secreted by the gastric mucosa that is essential for the intestinal absorption of vitamin B_{12}. Intrinsic factor forms a bond with molecules of vitamin B_{12} (cobalamin) and transports them across the membranes of the ileum. A deficiency of intrinsic factor, owing to gastrectomy, myxedema, or atrophy of the gastric mucosa, results in pernicious anemia. See also **pernicious anemia.**

intro- A combining form meaning 'into or within': *introgastric, introjection.*

introitus An entrance or orifice to a cavity or a hollow tubular structure of the body, as the vaginal introitus.

intron In molecular genetics: a sequence of base pairs in DNA that interrupts the continuity of genetic information. Some genes contain a number of long intervening sequences.

introspection The act of examining one's own thoughts and emotions by concentrating on the inner self. —**introspective,** *adj.*

introversion, intraversion **1.** The tendency to direct one's interests, thoughts, and energies inward or toward things concerned only with the self. **2.** The state of being totally or primarily concerned with one's own intrapsychic experience. Compare **extroversion.**

introvert **1.** A person whose interests are directed inward and who is shy, withdrawn, emotionally reserved, and self-absorbed. **2.** To turn inward or to direct one's interests and thoughts toward oneself. Compare **extrovert.** See also **egocentric.** —**introversion,** *n.*

intubation Passage of a tube into a body aperture; specifically, the insertion of a breathing tube through the mouth or nose or into the trachea to ensure a patent airway for the delivery of an anesthetic gas or oxygen. Blind intubation is the insertion of a breathing tube without the use of a laryngoscope. Kinds of intubation are **endotracheal intubation, nasogastric intubation.**

intussusception Prolapse of one segment of bowel into the lumen of another segment. This kind of intestinal obstruction may involve segments of the small intestine, the colon, or the terminal ileum and cecum. It occurs most often in infants and small children and is characterized by abdominal pain, vomiting, and bloody mucus in the stool. Surgery is usually necessary to correct the obstruction. See also **intestinal obstruction.**

inulin A diagnostic aid used in tests of kidney function, specifically glomerular filtration.

inulin clearance A time-consuming, complex, but extremely accurate test of the rate of filtration of a starch, inulin, in the glomerulus of the kidney. Inulin is given intravenously, and the glomerular filtration rate can be estimated

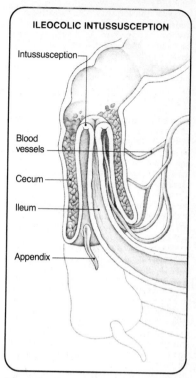

ILEOCOLIC INTUSSUSCEPTION

Intussusception

Blood vessels

Cecum

Ileum

Appendix

from the length of time needed for the inulin to appear in the urine.

inundation fever See **scrub typhus.**

invagination **1.** A condition in which one part of a structure telescopes into another part, as the intestine during peristalsis. If the invagination is extensive or involves a tumor or polyps, it may cause an intestinal obstruction, and surgery is indicated. **2.** Surgery for repair of a hernia by replacing the contents of the hernial sac in the abdominal cavity. See also **hernia, intestinal obstruction, peristalsis.** —**invaginate,** *v.*

invalid **1.** A person who is disabled, particularly one who is chronically ill or confined to a wheelchair or bed. **2.** Unjustified, unsound.

invariable behavior Behavior that results from physiologic response to a stimulus and is not modified by individual experience, as a reflex. Compare **variable behavior.**

invasive Characterized by a tendency to spread, infiltrate, and intrude.

invasive carcinoma A malignant neoplasm composed of epithelial cells that infiltrate and destroy surrounding tissues.

invasive mole See **chorioadenoma destruens.**

inverse anaphylaxis An exaggerated reaction of hypersensitivity induced by an antibody rather than by an antigen. Also called **reverse anaphylaxis.**

inverse relationship See **negative relationship.**

inverse square law In physics: a law stating that the amount of radiation emitted is inversely proportional to the square of the distance between the source and the irradiated surface. For example, a person 2 feet from a patient being treated with radium is exposed to four times more radiation than someone would be exposed to at 4 feet.

inversion 1. An abnormal condition in which an organ is turned inside out, as a uterine inversion. 2. A chromosomal defect in which two or more segments of a chromosome break off and become separated. They rejoin the chromosome in the wrong order, causing the genes carried on one arm of the chromosome to be in a position and sequence different from those on the other arm. 3. The turning inward of a part of the body, such as the hand or foot.

invert 1. To turn inside out or upside down. 2. A homosexual.

invert sugar A nonelectrolyte fluid replacement and source of calories.

investigational new drug (IND) A drug not yet approved for marketing by the Food and Drug Administration and available only for use in experiments to determine its safety and effectiveness. The use of an investigational new drug in human subjects requires a preliminary application that includes reports of animal toxicity tests, descriptions of proposed clinical trials, and a list of the investigators and their qualifications.

invisible differentiation In embryology: a fixed determination for specialization and diversification that exists in embryonic cells but is not yet visibly apparent. See also **chemodifferentiation.**

in vitro A biological reaction occurring in laboratory apparatus. Compare **in vivo.**

in vivo A biological reaction occurring in a living organism. Compare **in vitro.**

in vivo tracer study In nuclear medicine: a diagnostic procedure in which a series of radiograms of an administered radioactive tracer demonstrates normal or abnormal structures or processes as the tracer passes through a compartment in the patient's body. A strip chart recording of an in vivo tracer study, as a radionuclide angiocardiogram, shows the passage of the tracer through the central circulation.

involucrum, *pl.* **involucra** A sheath or coating, as that encasing a sequestrum of necrotic bone.

involuntary Occurring without conscious control or direction. See also **autonomy.**

involuntary muscle See **smooth muscle.**

involuntary nervous system See **visceral nervous system.**

involution 1. A normal process characterized by a decrease in the size of an organ owing to a decrease in the size of its cells, as postpartum involution of the uterus. 2. In embryology: a developmental process in which a group of cells grows over the rim at the border of the organ or part and, rolling inward, rejoins the organ or part to form a tube, as in the heart or bladder.

involutional depression See **involutional melancholia.**

involutional melancholia A state of depression occurring during the climacteric. The disorder begins gradually and is characterized by pessimism, irritability, insomnia, loss of appetite, feelings of anxiety, and an increase in motor activity, ranging from mere restlessness to extreme agitation. Also called **climacteric melancholia, involutional depression, involutional psychosis.** See also **depression.**

involutional psychosis See **involutional melancholia.**

inward aggression Destructive behavior that is directed against oneself. See also **masochism.**

-io A noun-forming combining form: *abrasio, evulsio.*

ioderma, iododerma A skin rash caused by a hypersensitivity to ingested iodides. The lesions may be acneiform, bullous, or fungating.

iodinated glycerol An expectorant.

iodinated ^{125}I **serum albumin** A sterile, buffered isotonic solution containing radioiodinated normal human serum adjusted to provide not more than 1 millicurie of radioactivity per milliliter in diagnostic tests of blood volume and cardiac output.

iodine (I) 1. A nonmetallic element of the halogen group. Its atomic number is 53; its atomic weight, 128.9. Iodine, an essential trace element or micronutrient, is primarily found in the thyroid gland, usually in the form of thyroglobulin. Iodine deficiency can result in goiter or cretinism. 2. A topical disinfectant and thyroid hormone antagonist.

iodize To treat or impregnate with iodine or an iodide. Table salt is iodized to prevent the occurrence of goiter in areas with insufficient iodine in the drinking water.

iodo- A combining form meaning 'of or pertaining to iodine': *iododerma, iodogenic.*

iodochlorhydroxyquin A local anti-infective agent.

iodopsin A photosensitive chemical in the cones of the retina that promotes color vision.

ion An atom or group of atoms that has acquired an electric charge through the gain or loss of an electron or electrons.

-ion 1. A combining form meaning an 'electrically charged particle': *anion, cation.* 2. A noun-forming combining form: *endognation, osteopedion.*

ion-exchange chromatography The process of separating and analyzing different substances according to their affinities for chemically stable but very reactive synthetic exchangers, which are composed largely of polystyrene and cellulose. The process uses an absorbent containing ionizing groups and accommodates the exchange of ions between a solution of substances to be analyzed and the absorbent. Ion-exchange chromatography is often used to separate components of nucleic acids and proteins elaborated by various structures throughout the body. Different ions deposited in the absorbent during the exchange produce bands of different colors, which constitute a chromatograph. Compare **column chromatography, gas chromatography.**

ionization The process in which a neutral atom or molecule gains or loses electrons and thus acquires a negative or positive electric charge. Ionization occurs when atoms or molecules dissociate in solution or when those of gases dissociate in an electric field. Ionizing radiation produces ionization in its passage through matter.

ionize To separate or change into ions. See also **ion. —ionization,** *n*.

ionizing energy The average energy lost by ionizing radiation in producing an ion pair in a gas. In air, the value is approximately 33.73 electron-volts (eV).

ionizing radiation High-energy electromagnetic waves (as X-rays and gamma rays) and particulate rays (as alpha particles, beta rays, electrons, neutrons, positrons, protons, and heavy nuclei) that dissociate substances in their paths into ions. The spatial distribution of the ionization depends on the kind of radiation, its penetrating power, the location of the source, and the nature of the irradiated material. High-energy X-rays penetrate deeply, most beta particles penetrate only a few millimeters, and alpha particles penetrate only a fraction of a millimeter, but they all produce intense ionization along their tracks. Ionizing radiation directly affects living organisms by killing cells or retarding their development; its indirect effects include the production of gene mutations and chromosome breaks.

Iowa trumpet A kind of needle guide used in performing a pudendal block. It consists of a long, thin cylinder through which a needle may be passed. A ring is attached to the proximal end of the guide, allowing the operator to hold it securely.

ipecac syrup An emetic.

IPPB *abbr* **intermittent positive pressure breathing.** The periodic inflation of the lungs with compressed air or oxygen under pressure. Passive exhalation is allowed through a valve, and the cycle begins again as the flow of gas is triggered by inhalation. The use of the IPPB unit involves the combined efforts of the doctor, the respiratory therapist or technician, and the nurse. NURSING CONSIDERATIONS: Secretions may be thinned and cleared, and the passages may be humidified, allowing greater comfort and a better exchange of gases. The patient may require reassurance that the machine will automatically shut off the flow of air at the end of inspiration and encouragement to relax and allow the lungs to be completely filled by the machine. Also called **intermittent positive pressure ventilation.**

IPPB (intermittent positive pressure breathing) unit A machine that provides a flow of air into the lungs at a predetermined

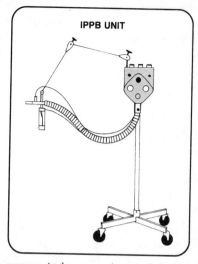

IPPB UNIT

pressure. As the pressure is attained, the flow is stopped, pressure is released, and the patient exhales. The device is used to prevent postoperative atelectasis, to promote full expansion of the lungs, to improve oxygenation, and to administer nebulized medications into the respiratory passages.

IQ *abbr* **intelligence quotient.**

Ir Symbol for **iridium.**

iralgia, iridalgia Any pain or inflammation of the iris. —**iralgic, iridalgic,** *adj*.

IRB *abbr* **institutional review board.**

iridectomy Surgical removal of part of the iris of the eye, performed most often to restore drainage of the aqueous humor in glaucoma or to remove a foreign body or a malignant tumor.

iridium (Ir) A silver-blue metallic element. Its atomic number is 77; its atomic weight is 192.2.

irido- A combining form meaning 'of or pertaining to the iris or to a colored circle': *iridocele, iridokeratitis.*

iridocyclitis Inflammation of the iris and ciliary body.

iridotomy A surgical incision into the iris of the eye, performed to relieve occlusion of the pupil, to enlarge the pupil in cataract extraction, or to treat postoperative glaucoma. See also **iridectomy, iris.**

iris A circular, contractile disk suspended in aqueous humor between the cornea and the crystalline lens of the eye and perforated by a circular pupil. The periphery of the iris is continuous with the ciliary body and is connected to the cornea by the pectinate ligament. The iris divides the space between the lens and the cornea into an anterior and a posterior chamber. In the adult, the two chambers communicate through the pupil but are separated in the fetus, up to the 7th month, by the membrana pupillaris. The involuntary muscle of the iris is composed of circular fibers and radiating fibers.

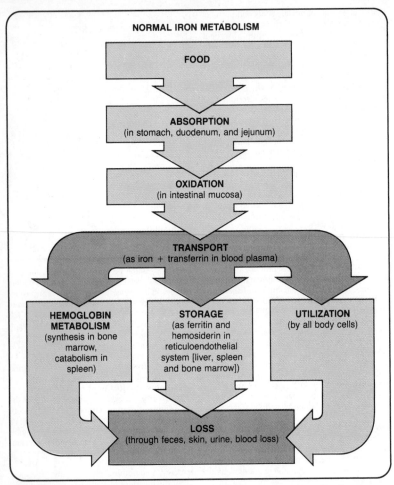

NORMAL IRON METABOLISM

FOOD

ABSORPTION
(in stomach, duodenum, and jejunum)

OXIDATION
(in intestinal mucosa)

TRANSPORT
(as iron + transferrin in blood plasma)

HEMOGLOBIN METABOLISM
(synthesis in bone marrow, catabolism in spleen)

STORAGE
(as ferritin and hemosiderin in reticuloendothelial system [liver, spleen and bone marrow])

UTILIZATION
(by all body cells)

LOSS
(through feces, skin, urine, blood loss)

Dark pigment cells under the translucent tissue of the iris are variously arranged in different people to produce different colored irises. The pigment is absent in albinos. In blue eyes, pigment cells are confined to the posterior surface of the iris; in gray, brown, and black eyes, the pigment cells appear in the anterior epithelium and the stroma. See also **dilatator pupillae, sphincter pupillae. —iridic,** *adj.*

iritis An inflammatory condition of the iris of the eye characterized by pain, lacrimation, photophobia, and diminished visual acuity. On ophthalmic examination, the eye looks cloudy, the iris bulges, and the pupil is contracted. The condition is most often idiopathic. The pupil is dilated, usually with atropine, and a corticosteroid may be prescribed to reduce inflammation. If the inflammation is allowed to continue and the pupil left constricted, permanent scarring may occur, causing an opacity over the lens and diminished vision.

iron (Fe) A common metallic element essential for hemoglobin synthesis. Its atomic number is 26; its atomic weight is 55.847. Iron salts and complexes—such as ferrous sulfate and iron-dextran—are used as hematinics.

iron-deficiency anemia A microcytic, hypochromic anemia caused by inadequate supplies of iron needed to synthesize hemoglobin, characterized by pallor, fatigue, and weakness. Laboratory diagnosis includes hemoglobin, hematocrit, transferrin, and serum iron evaluation. Compare **hemolytic anemia, hypoplastic anemia.** See also **anemia, iron metabolism, red cell indices.**

iron dextran A hematinic agent.

iron lung See **Drinker respirator.**

iron metabolism A series of processes involved in the entry of iron into the body through its absorption, its transport and storage throughout the body, its use for the formation of hemoglobin and other iron compounds, and its eventual excretion. Iron normally enters the body through the epithelium of the intestinal mucosa, being oxidized from ferrous to ferric iron in the process. The rate at which iron enters is modulated by this absorption mechanism. When iron stores are high, iron no longer passes through but, instead, is trapped by the mucosal cells of the intestine to be eliminated upon their death. Once iron enters the blood, it is in a closed system in which, attached to transferrin, it cycles between the plasma and the reticuloendothelial or erythropoietic system. Plasma iron is delivered for hemoglobin synthesis to the normoblast, where it remains up to 4 months, trapped in the hemoglobin molecules of a mature red cell. Senescent red cells then deteriorate and break down. The iron is released from the hemoglobin by the reticuloendothelial system to reenter the transport pool for recycling. The normal iron distribution in a 70-kg (155-lb) man totals approximately 3.7 g, with more than 65% of this in circulating hemoglobin. Another 27% is found in the storage pool as hemosiderin or ferritin. The body normally conserves iron so well that loss, usually only through the feces, is normally limited to about 1 mg/day. This amount is easily provided by a dietary intake of only 10 mg/day. Iron deficiency may follow extended intervals of inadequate iron intake (especially in women) or after excessive blood loss. Iron overload sometimes occurs in disorders in which normal regulation of absorption of iron is impaired. See also **anemia.**

iron-rich food   A nutrient containing a relatively large amount of iron. The best source of dietary iron is liver, with oysters, clams, heart, kidney, lean meat, and tongue as second choices. Leafy green vegetables are the best plant sources. See also **iron, iron-deficiency anemia.**

iron salts poisoning   Poisoning caused by overdosage of ferric or ferrous salts, characterized by vomiting, bloody diarrhea, cyanosis, and gastric and intestinal pain.

iron transport   The process whereby iron is carried from its entry point into the body, the intestinal mucosa, to the various sites of use and storage. Transferrin binds with free iron and shuttles it to storage and use sites. Transferrin becomes attached to exogenous iron entering through the intestinal villi or to iron reentering the plasma from the sinusoids of the spleen. The iron is then released to the normoblasts, and the transferrin is freed for additional transport functions that may, to a small extent, involve iron stored as ferritin or hemosiderin. Compare **transferrin.** See also **hemosiderosis, iron metabolism.**

irradiation   Exposure to any form of radiant energy, as heat, light, or X-ray. Radioactive sources of radiant energy, such as X-rays or isotopes of iodine or cobalt, are used diagnostically to examine internal body structures, using knowledge of the ways in which various tissues absorb or reflect radioactive emissions. The same or similar sources of radioactivity in larger amounts are used to destroy microorganisms or tissue

cells that have become malignant. Infrared or ultraviolet light may be used to produce heat in body tissues to relieve pain and soreness or to treat acne, psoriasis, or other skin ailments. See also **radiation sickness, radioactivity, ultraviolet. —irradiate,** *v.*

irreducible   Unable to be returned to the normal position or condition, as an irreducible hernia. See also **incarcerate.**

irreversible coma   See **brain death.**

irrigation   The process of washing out a body cavity or wounded area with a stream of water or other fluid. It is also used to cleanse a tube or drain inserted into the body, as an indwelling catheter. The procedure is most commonly performed with water, saline, aminoacetic acid, or antiseptic solutions on the eye, ear, throat, vagina, and urinary tract. See also **lavage. —irrigate,** *v.*

irrigator   An apparatus with a flexible tube for flushing or washing out a body cavity.

irritable bowel syndrome   Abnormally increased motility of the small and large intestines, generally associated with emotional stress. Most of those affected are young adults, who complain of diarrhea or small, scanty, hard stools and, occasionally, abdominal pain. The pain is usually relieved by moving the bowels. In the diagnosis of irritable bowel syndrome, more serious conditions (as dysentery, lactose intolerance, and the inflammatory bowel diseases) must be ruled out. Although this is a functional disorder, patients experience pain and discomfort and need emotional support. Also called **mucous colitis, spastic colon.**

IRV   *abbr* inspiratory reserve volume. See **pulmonary function test.**

ischemia   Decreased blood supply to a body organ or part. Some causes of ischemia are arterial embolism, atherosclerosis, thrombosis, and vasoconstriction. Compare **infarction. —ischemic,** *adj.*

ischemic contracture   See **Volkmann's contracture.**

ischemic lumbago   A pain in the lower back and buttocks caused by vascular insufficiency, as in occlusion of the abdominal aorta.

ischemic pain   The unpleasant, often excruciating sensation associated with ischemia, resulting from peripheral vascular disease, from decreased blood flow owing to constricting orthopedic casts, or from insufficient blood flow owing to surgical trauma or accidental injury. Ischemic pain caused by occlusive arterial disease is often severe and may not be relieved, even with narcotics. The individual with peripheral vascular disease may experience ischemic pain only while exercising, because the metabolic demands for oxygen cannot be met by the occluded flow of blood. The ischemic pain of partial arterial occlusion is not as severe as the abrupt, excruciating pain associated with a complete blocking of the artery, as by an embolism. See also **pain intervention, pain mechanism.**

ischio-   A combining form meaning 'of or

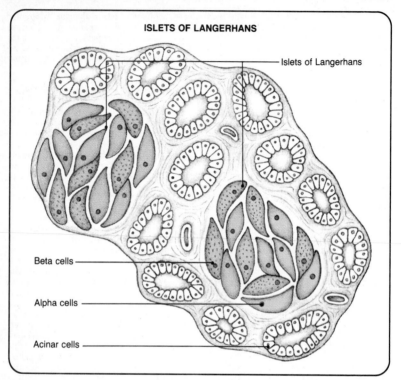

ISLETS OF LANGERHANS

Islets of Langerhans

Beta cells

Alpha cells

Acinar cells

pertaining to the ischium or to the hip': *is-chioanal, ischiodidymus.*

ischium, *pl.* **ischia**   One of the three parts of the hip bone, joining the ilium and the pubis to form the acetabulum. The ischium comprises the dorsal part of the hip bone and is divided into the body of the ischium, which forms two fifths of the acetabulum, and the ramus, which joins the inferior ramus of the pubis. The spine of the ischium provides attachment for various muscles, as the gemellus superior, the coccygeus, and the levator ani. The greater sciatic notch above the spine transmits the superior and the inferior gluteal vessels and various nerves, as gluteal nerves, the sciatic nerve, and the nerves to the obturator internus and the quadratus femoris. A notch below the spine of the ischium transmits various ligaments, vessels, and nerves for other parts. The large dorsal tuberosity of the ischium provides attachment for various muscles, as the adductor longus, the semimembranosus, the biceps femoris, and the semitendinosus. Compare **ilium, pubis.**

ISG   *abbr* **immune serum globulin.**

Ishihara color test   A color vision test using a series of plates on which are printed round dots in a variety of colors and patterns. People with normal color vision are able to discern specific numbers or patterns on the plates; the inability to pick out a given number or shape indicates a deficiency in color perception.

island fever   See **scrub typhus.**

islands of Langerhans   See **islets of Langerhans.**

islet adenoma   See **insulinoma.**

islet cell adenoma   See **insulinoma.**

islet cell tumor   Any tumor of the islets of Langerhans.

islets of Langerhans   Clusters of cells within the pancreas that produce insulin, glucagon, and pancreatic polypeptide. They form the endocrine portion of the gland, and their hormonal secretions released into the bloodstream are balanced, important regulators of sugar metabolism. The islets of Langerhans are scattered throughout the pancreas; the beta cells, which secrete insulin, usually appear in the center of each of the lobules. Alpha cells secrete glucagon, and pancreatic-peptide cells secrete pancreatic peptide. Also called **islands of Langerhans.**

-ism, -ismus   A combining form meaning 'condition of, practice of, theory of': *hyperthyroidism, hypopituitarism.*

iso-   A combining form meaning 'equal': *isobar, isochromatic.*

isoagglutinin   An antibody that causes agglutination of erythrocytes in other members of the same species that carry an isoagglutinogen on their erythrocytes. Also called **isohemagglutinin.** Compare **isoagglutinogen.** See also **ABO blood groups, antibody.**

isoagglutinogen An antigen that causes the agglutination of erythrocytes in others of the same species that carry a corresponding isoagglutinin in their serum. Also called **isohemagglutinin.** Compare **agglutinin.** See also **ABO blood groups.**

isoamyl alcohol See **amyl alcohol.**

isoantibody An antibody to isoantigens found in other members of the same species. See also **autoimmune disease, tissue typing.**

isoantigen An antigen, such as a blood group antigen, that interacts with isoantibodies in other members of the same species. Compare **autoantigen, autoimmune disease.** See also **antigen, isoagglutinogen.**

isobar In nuclear medicine: one of a group of nuclides having the same total number of neutrons and protons in the nucleus but so proportioned as to result in different values of the atomic number.

isobutyl alcohol A clear, colorless liquid that is miscible with ethyl alcohol or ether.

isocarboxazid A monoamine oxidase inhibitor antidepressant.

isodose chart In radiotherapy: a graphic representation of the distribution of radiation in a medium; lines are drawn through points receiving equal doses. Isodose charts are determined for X-rays traversing the body, for radium applicators used in intracavitary or interstitial treatment, and for working areas where X-rays or radionuclides are employed.

isoelectric electroencephalogram See **flat electroencephalogram.**

isoenzyme One of several forms in which an enzyme may exist in tissues. The enzymes share similar catalytic qualities but differ chemically, physically, and immunologically. Special chemical tests separate them from each other. Also called **isozyme.**

isoetharine hydrochloride, i. mesylate Bronchodilator sympathomimetic agents.

isoflurophate A miotic agent.

isogamete A reproductive cell of the same size and structure as the one with which it unites. Compare **anisogamete.** —**isogametic,** *adj.*

isogamy Sexual reproduction in which there is fusion of gametes of the same size and structure, as in certain algae, fungi, and protozoa. Compare **anisogamy, heterogamy.** —**isogamous,** *adj.*

isogenesis, isogeny Development from a common origin and according to similar processes. —**isogenetic, isogenic,** *adj.*

isograft A tissue transplant between genetically identical persons, such as identical twins or highly inbred animals.

isohemagglutinin See **isoagglutinin.**

Isolette A trade name for a self-contained incubator unit that provides a controlled heat, humidity, and oxygen microenvironment for the isolation and care of premature and low-birth-weight neonates. The apparatus is made of a clear plastic material and has a large door and portholes for easy access to the infant with a minimum of heat and oxygen loss.

isoleucine An amino acid, occurring in most dietary proteins, that is essential for proper growth in infants and for nitrogen balance in adults. See also **amino acid, protein.**

isometric Maintaining the same length or dimension.

isometric exercise A form of active exercise that increases muscle tension by applying pressure against stable resistance. This may be accomplished by opposing different muscles in the same individual, as by pressing the hands together or by making a limb push or pull against an immovable object. There is no joint movement, and the length of the muscle remains unchanged, but muscle strength and tone are maintained or improved. Compare **isotonic exercise.** See also **exercise.**

isometric growth An increase in size of different organs or parts of an organism at the same rate. Compare **allometric growth.**

isoniazid (INH) An antitubercular agent.

isopentoic acid See **isovaleric acid.**

isophane insulin suspension (NPH) A modified form of protamine zinc insulin suspension. It is an intermediate-acting insulin that is a stable, commonly prescribed preparation.

isopropamide iodide A gastrointestinal anticholinergic agent.

isopropanol See **isopropyl alcohol.**

isopropylacetic acid See **isovaleric acid.**

isopropyl alcohol A clear, colorless, bitter aromatic liquid that is miscible with water, ether, chloroform, and ethyl alcohol. A solution of approximately 70% isopropyl alcohol in water is used as a rubbing compound. Also called **avantin, dimethyl carbinol, isopropanol.** See also **alcohol.**

isoproterenol hydrochloride, i. sulfate Sympathomimetic agents.

isosmotic See **isotonic.**

isosorbide An ophthalmic osmotic diuretic.

isosorbide dinitrate A coronary vasodilator.

isotonic A solution having the same concentration of solute as another solution, hence exerting the same amount of osmotic pressure as that solution, as an isotonic saline solution that contains an amount of salt equal to that found in the intra- and extracellular fluid. Also called **isosmotic.**

isotonic exercise A form of active exercise in which the muscle contracts and causes movement. Throughout the procedure, there is no significant change in the resistance, so that the force of the contraction remains constant. Such exercise greatly improves joint mobility and helps to improve muscle strength and tonality. Compare **isometric exercise.** See also **exercise.**

isotope One of two or more forms of a chemical element having almost identical properties: they have the same number of protons in the atomic nucleus and the same atomic number, but they differ in the number of their nuclear neutrons and atomic weights. Carbon (^{12}C) has six nuclear neutrons, while its isotope ^{14}C has

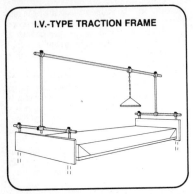

I.V.-TYPE TRACTION FRAME

eight. Many hundreds of radioactive isotopes are used in diagnostic and therapeutic procedures.

isotopic tracer   An isotope or artificial mixture of isotopes of an element incorporated into a sample to permit observation of the course of the element, alone or in combination, through a chemical, physical, or biological process.

isotretinoin   An oral agent used to treat acne vulgaris.

isovaleric acid   A combustible, toxic compound with a disagreeable taste and odor, found in tobacco, valerian, oil of hops, and cheese; in sweat of the feet; and in urine of those with smallpox, typhus, and hepatitis. Commercially produced isovaleric acid is used in perfumes, flavors, and certain drugs. Also called **isopentoic acid, isopropylacetic acid.**

isoxsuprine hydrochloride   A peripheral vasodilator.

-ist   A combining form meaning a 'practitioner of a science': *audiologist, pharmacist.*

isthmus, *pl.* **isthmuses, isthmi**   A narrow connection between two larger bodies or parts, as the isthmus of the auditory tube in the ear, which connects the bony and the cartilaginous parts of the tube.

itch   **1.** To feel a sensation, usually on the skin, that makes one want to scratch. **2.** A tingling, annoying sensation on an area of the skin that may be caused by rhus dermatitis, a mosquito bite, or an allergic reaction. **3.** The pruritic condition of the skin caused by infestation with the parasitic mite *Sarcoptes scabiei.* —**itchy,** *adj.*

-ite   A combining form meaning: **1.** 'Compounds': *nitrite, phosphite.* **2.** A 'body part': *chondriomite, osteite.*

ithy-   A combining form meaning 'straight': *ithylordosis, ithyokyphosis.*

-itic   A combining form meaning 'of or related to something specified': *encephalitic, nephritic.*

-itis   A combining form meaning an 'inflammation of a (specified) organ': *carditis, cecitis.*

ITP   *abbr* **idiopathic thrombocytopenic purpura.**

IU, I.U.   *abbr* **International Unit.**

IUCD   *abbr* **intrauterine contraceptive device.** See **intrauterine device.**

IUD   *abbr* **intrauterine device.**

-ium   A combining form used to name metallic elements: *aluminum, radium.*

I.V.   **1.** *abbr* **intravenous. 2.** *Informal.* Equipment consisting of a bottle of fluid, infusion set with tubing, and an intracatheter, used in intravenous therapy. **3.** Intravenous administration of fluids or medication by injection into a vein.

IVAC pump   A trade name for a portable intravenous pump that electronically regulates and monitors the flow of fluid. It is usually attached to the I.V. stand. See also **intravenous pump.**

ivory bones   See osteopetrosis.

IVP   *abbr* **intravenous pyelography.**

I.V. push   See **intravenous push.**

I.V.-type traction frame   A metal support that holds traction equipment consisting of two metal uprights, one at each end of the bed, that support an overhead metal bar. Each upright is clamped to a horizontal bar that fits into holders inserting at the corners of the bed. Also called basic frame. Compare **claw-type traction frame.** See also **traction frame.**

Ixodes   A genus of parasitic hard-shelled ticks associated with the transmission of a variety of arbovirus infections, as Rocky Mountain spotted fever.

ixodi-   A combining form meaning 'of or pertaining to ticks': *ixodiasis, ixodism.*

ixodid   Of or pertaining to hard ticks of the family Ixodidae.

-ize   A combining form meaning 'do, treat, cause': *anesthetize, canalize.*

J

J Symbol for **joule**.

jacket A supportive or confining therapeutic casing or garment for the torso. Some kinds of jackets are **Minerva jacket, Sayre's jacket.**

jacket restraint An orthopedic device used to help immobilize the trunk of a patient in traction and to discourage the patient from sitting up in bed. The jacket restraint is attached to both sides of the bedspring frame by means of buckled webbing straps that are sewn into the side seams of the restraint. The jacket restraint may be used with most kinds of traction but is not usually used with Dunlop skin traction or Dunlop skeletal traction, Bryant traction, halo-femoral traction, or halo-pelvic traction. Compare **diaper restraint, sling restraint.**

jackknife position A position used for rectal surgery or rectal examination, where the patient is placed face down with the hips flexed. Hip flexion can be accomplished by bending the patient over the edge of the bed or with a specially designed table that bends at hip level.

jacksonian epilepsy Unilateral clonic activity that begins in one group of muscles and 'marches' to adjacent groups. Caused by nerve discharges in the contralateral motor cortex.

Jacob's membrane The outermost of the nine layers of the retina, composed of rods and cones interacting directly with the optic nerve.

Jacquemier's sign A deepening of the color of the vaginal mucosa just below the urethral orifice. It may be noted after the 4th week of pregnancy, but is not a reliable sign of pregnancy.

jact- A combining form meaning 'to throw': *jactatio, jactation, jactitation.*

jail fever See **epidemic typhus**.

Jakob-Creutzfeldt disease See **Creutzfeldt-Jakob disease**.

JAMA *abbr Journal of the American Medical Association.*

jamais vu *French.* The sensation of being a stranger when with a person one knows or when in a familiar place. The phenomenon occurs occasionally in healthy people but more frequently in people who have temporal lobe epilepsy. Compare **déjà vu**.

Janeway lesion A small erythematous or hemorrhagic macule occurring on the palms or soles, sometimes diagnostic of subacute bacterial endocarditis.

janiceps A conjoined, twin fetal monster in which the heads are fused, with the faces looking in opposite directions. The faces and bodies of both twins may be fully formed or one member may be only partially formed and act as a parasite on the more fully developed fetus.

Jansen's disease See **metaphyseal dysostosis**.

Japanese B encephalitis See **Japanese encephalitis**.

Japanese encephalitis A severe epidemic infection of brain tissue seen in East Asia and Japan, characterized by shaking chills, paralysis, and weight loss, and caused by a group of B arboviruses transmitted by mosquitoes. Mortality may be as high as 33%. Various neurologic and psychiatric sequelae are common. There is no specific treatment. Also called **Japanese B encephalitis**.

Japanese flood fever See **scrub typhus**.

Japanese river fever See **scrub typhus**.

JAPHA *abbr Journal of the American Public Health Association.*

Jarisch-Herxheimer reaction A sudden transient fever and exacerbation of skin lesions observed several hours after administration of penicillin or other antibiotics in the treatment of syphilis, leptospirosis, or relapsing fever. The effect lasts less than 24 hours and requires no treatment.

Jarotzky's treatment Therapy of gastric ulcer using a bland diet consisting of egg whites, fresh butter, bread, milk, and noodles.

jaundice A yellow discoloration of the skin, mucous membranes, and sclerae of the eyes, caused by greater than normal amounts of bilirubin in the blood. Persons with jaundice may also experience nausea, vomiting, and abdominal pain and may pass dark urine. Jaundice is a symptom of many disorders, including liver disease, biliary obstruction, and the hemolytic anemias. Newborns commonly develop physiological jaundice, which disappears after a few days. Rarer disorders causing jaundice are Crigler-Najjar syndrome and Gilbert's syndrome. Useful diagnostic procedures include clinical evaluation of the signs and symptoms; tests of liver function; X-ray, CT scan, ultrasonography, endoscopy, or exploratory surgery; and biopsy. Also called **icterus**. See also **hyperbilirubinemia**. **—jaundiced,** *adj.*

jaw One or both bones (mandible and maxilla) that hold the teeth and form the framework of the mouth.

jaw reflex An abnormal reflex elicited by tapping the chin with a rubber hammer while the mouth is half open and the jaw muscles are relaxed. A quick snapping shut of the jaw implies damage to the area of cerebral cortex governing motor activity of the fifth cranial nerve. Also called jaw jerk.

JCAH *abbr* **Joint Commission on Accreditation of Hospitals.**

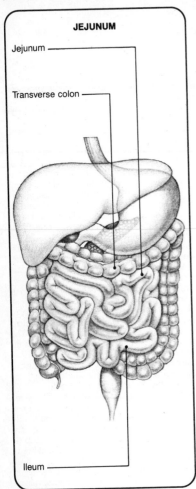

JEJUNUM

Jejunum

Transverse colon

Ileum

jeco- A combining form meaning 'of or pertaining to the liver': *jecolein, jecoral, jecorin.*

Jefferson fracture A fracture characterized by bursting of the ring of the atlas.

jejuno- A combining form meaning 'of or pertaining to the jejunum': *jejunocecostomy, jejunocolostomy, jejunotomy.*

jejunoileitis See **Crohn's disease.**

jejunum, *pl.* **jejuna** One of the three portions of the small intestine, connecting proximally with the duodenum and distally with the ileum. The jejunum has a slightly larger diameter, a deeper color, and a thicker wall than the ileum, and contains heavy, circular folds that are absent in the lower part of the ileum. The jejunum also has larger villi than the ileum. Compare **ileum. —jejunal,** *adj.*

jellyfish sting A wound caused by skin contact with a jellyfish, a sea animal with a bell-shaped gelatinous body and numerous long, sus-

pended tentacles containing stinging structures. In most cases a tender, red welt develops on the affected skin. In some cases, depending on the sensitivity of the person and the particular species of jellyfish, severe localized pain, nausea, weakness, excessive lacrimation, nasal discharge, muscle spasm, perspiration, and dyspnea may occur. Treatment includes carefully removing any tentacles and applying a compress of alcohol, aromatic spirits of ammonia, or Dakin's solution. Calcium gluconate may be administered to control muscle spasms.

Jendrassik's maneuver In neurology: a diagnostic procedure in which the patient hooks the flexed fingers of the two hands together and forcibly tries to pull them apart. While this tension is being exerted, the lower extremity reflexes are tested, particularly the patellar reflex.

jet lag A condition characterized by fatigue, insomnia, and sluggish body functions caused by disruption of the normal circadian rhythm resulting from air travel across several time zones.

jigger See **chigoe.**

Job-Basedow phenomenon Thyrotoxicosis occurring when dietary iodine is given to a patient with endemic goiter in an area of environmental iodine deficiency. It is presumed that iodine deficiency protects some patients with endemic goiter from developing thyrotoxicosis. The phenomenon may also occur when large doses of iodine are given to patients with nontoxic multinodular goiter in areas with sufficient environmental iodine. There is a danger of inducing the phenomenon if iodine containing drugs, as X-ray contrast media, are administered to elderly patients with nontoxic multinodular goiter.

job description A written statement detailing the functions, responsibilities, constraints, and communication pathways of a unit of work or a position.

jock itch See **tinea cruris.**

jogger's heel A painful condition, common among joggers and distance runners. It is characterized by bruising, bursitis, fasciitis, or calcaneal spurs, caused by repeated forceful contact of the heel with the ground. Judicious selection of well-fitting running shoes and avoidance of running on hard surfaces are recommended to avoid occurrence or recurrence of the condition. Rest, heat, or corticosteroid medication or aspirin may be recommended.

joint Any one of the connections between bones. Each is classified according to structure and movability as fibrous, cartilaginous, or synovial. Fibrous joints are immovable, cartilaginous joints slightly movable, and synovial joints freely movable. Typical immovable joints are those connecting most of the bones of the skull with a sutural ligament. Typical slightly movable joints are those connecting the vertebrae and the pubic bones. Most of the joints in the body are freely movable and allow gliding, circumduction, rotation, and angular movement. Also called **articulation.** See also **cartilaginous joint, fibrous joint, synovial joint.**

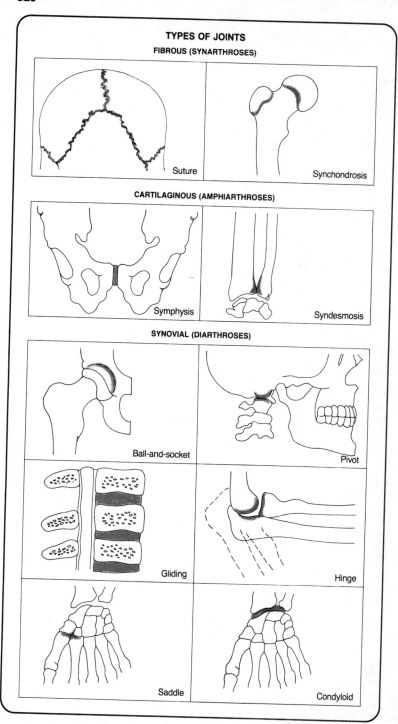

TYPES OF JOINTS

FIBROUS (SYNARTHROSES)

Suture

Synchondrosis

CARTILAGINOUS (AMPHIARTHROSES)

Symphysis

Syndesmosis

SYNOVIAL (DIARTHROSES)

Ball-and-socket

Pivot

Gliding

Hinge

Saddle

Condyloid

**JONES CRITERIA
IN RHEUMATIC FEVER**

Major manifestations
- Carditis
- Polyarthritis
- Chorea
- Erythema marginatum
- Subcutaneous nodules

Minor manifestations
- Fever
- Arthralgia
- Previous rheumatic fever or rheumatic heart disease
- Elevated ESR or positive CRP
- Prolonged P-R interval

In addition, evidence of preceding streptococcal infection includes history of recent scarlet fever, positive throat culture for group A streptococcus, and increased ASO titer or other streptococcal antibodies.

---

joint and several liability In law: a condition in which several persons share the liability for a plaintiff's injury and may be found liable individually or as a group.
joint appointment 1. A faculty appointment to two institutions within a university or system, as to the schools of nursing and medicine of the same university. 2. In academic nursing: the appointment of a member of the faculty of a university to a clinical service of an associated service institution. A psychiatric nurse might hold appointment in a university as an assistant professor and might also be a clinical nurse-specialist in a service institution. The practice of joint appointments is said to have begun at Case Western Reserve University, University Hospital. See also **unification model.**
joint audit See **nursing audit.**
joint chondroma A cartilaginous mass that develops in the synovial membrane of a joint.
Joint Commission on Accreditation of Hospitals (JCAH) A private, nongovernmental agency that establishes guidelines for the operation of hospitals and other health-care facilities, conducts accreditation programs and surveys, and encourages the attainment of high standards of institutional medical care. Members include representatives from the American Medical Association, American College of Physicians, and American College of Surgeons.
joint fracture A fracture of the articular surfaces of the bony structures of a joint.
joint practice 1. The practice of a doctor and a nurse-practitioner, usually private, who work as a team, sharing responsibility for a group of patients. 2. In inpatient nursing: the practice of making joint decisions about patient care by committees of the doctors and nurses working on a division.
Jones criteria A standardized set of guidelines for the diagnosis of rheumatic fever, as recommended by the American Heart Association. See also **rheumatic fever.**
joule The Standard International (SI) unit of energy and heat, intended to replace the **calorie.** The work done by a force of 1 newton acting over a distance of 1 meter.
judgment In law: 1. The final decision of the court regarding the case before it. 2. The reason given by the court for its decision; an opinion. 3. An award, penalty, or other sentence of law given by the court.
jug- A combining form meaning 'yoke': *jugal, jugum.*
jugu- A combining form meaning 'throat or neck': *jugular, jugulation.*
jugular vein See **external jugular vein, internal jugular vein.**
jugular foramen One of a pair of openings between the lateral part of the occipital bone and the petrous part of the temporal bones in the skull. The foramen transmits the inferior petrosal sinus, the transverse sinus, some meningeal branches of the occipital and ascending pharyngeal arteries, and the glossopharyngeal, vagus, and accessory nerves.
juice Any fluid secreted by the tissues of animals or plants. In humans, it usually refers to the secretions of the digestive glands. Kinds of juices include **gastric juice, intestinal juice, pancreatic juice.**
jumping gene In molecular genetics: a unit of genetic information associated with a segment of DNA that can move from one position in the genome to another.
junction nevus A hairless, flat or slightly raised, brown skin blemish arising from pigment cells at the epidermal-dermal junction. A junction nevus may be found anywhere on the surface of the body. All nevi of the palms and soles and all pigmented nevi in early childhood are of this type. Malignant change may be signaled by increase in size, hardness or darkening, bleeding, or the appearance of satellite discoloration around the nevus. Junction nevi undergoing these changes and lesions found in areas subject to trauma should be removed. Also called junctional nevus.
junctura cartilaginea See **cartilaginous joint.**
junctura fibrosa See **fibrous joint.**
junctura synovialis See **synovial joint.**
Jungian psychology See **analytic psychology.**
Junin fever See **arenavirus.**
juvenile 1. A young person; youth; child; youngster. 2. Of, pertaining to, characteristic of, or suitable for a young person; youthful. 3. Physiologically underdeveloped or immature. 4. Denoting psychological or intellectual immaturity; childish.

DIFFERENCES BETWEEN JUVENILE-ONSET AND ADULT-ONSET DIABETES

	JUVENILE TYPE	ADULT TYPE
Type of onset	Abrupt	Gradual
Symptoms	Thirst, urinary frequency, increased appetite, weight loss	Sometimes none
Stability	Wide fluctuations of blood sugar with marked sensitivity to diet, exercise, and insulin	Usually easily controlled if patient adheres to a proper diet
Ketoacidosis	Frequent only if therapy is inadequate	Uncommon except with severe stress, infection, etc.
Hypoglycemia	More frequent	Uncommon
Control of diabetes	Difficult	Less difficult
Endogenous insulin	Absent	Present
Complications	May occur	May occur
Diet	Most important	Most important
Insulin	Needed by all	Needed by 20% to 30%
Oral hypoglycemic agent	Not indicated	Useful for about 40%

juvenile alveolar rhabdomyosarcoma A rapidly growing tumor of striated muscle with a grave prognosis, occurring in children and adolescents, chiefly in the extremities.

juvenile angiofibroma See **nasopharyngeal angiofibroma.**

juvenile delinquency Persistent antisocial, illegal, or criminal behavior by children or adolescents to the degree that it cannot be controlled or corrected by the parents, it endangers others in the community, and it becomes the concern of a law enforcement agency. Such behavioral patterns are characterized by aggressiveness, destructiveness, hostility, and cruelty and occur more frequently in boys than in girls. Causative factors typically involve poor parent-child relationships, especially parental rejection, indifference, and apathy, and unstable family environments where disciplinary methods are lax, erratic, overly strict, or involve harsh physical punishment. Traditional punitive treatments, primarily correctional institutions and reform schools, usually aggravate rather than remedy the situation. More progressive approaches, such as foster-home placement, work and recreational programs, and various community and family counseling services, have been more successful. Behavior therapy and other forms of psychotherapy, often involving the parents as well as the child, are also used as modes of treatment and prevention. See also **antisocial personality disorder, behavior disorder, psychotherapy.**

juvenile diabetes An inability to metabolize carbohydrate caused by an overt insulin deficiency, occurring in children and characterized by polydipsia, polyuria, polyphagia, loss of weight, diminished strength, and marked irritability. The onset is usually rapid, but approximately one third of the patients have a remission within 3 months; this stage may continue for days or years, but diabetes then progresses quickly to a state of total dependence on insulin. Occasionally, the disease is asymptomatic and is discovered only by postprandial hyperglycemia or glucose tolerance tests. Juvenile diabetes tends to be unstable and brittle, with the patients quite sensitive to insulin and physical activity and liable to develop ketoacidosis. Recent evidence suggests that juvenile onset diabetes may be caused by environmental factors, as a virus. See also **diabetes mellitus.**

juvenile kyphosis See **Scheuermann's disease.**

juvenile rheumatoid arthritis See **Still's disease.**

juvenile xanthogranuloma A skin disorder characterized by groups of yellow, red, or brown papules or nodules on the extensor surfaces of the arms and legs, and in some cases on the eyeball, meninges, and testes. The lesions typically appear in infancy or early childhood and usually disappear in a few years.

juxta- A combining form meaning 'near': *juxtaglomerular, juxtangina, juxtaposition, juxtaspinal.*

K Symbol for: **1.** potassium. **2.** the Kelvin temperature scale.

kak- A combining form meaning 'bad': *kakidrosis, kakosmia.*

kakke disease See **beriberi.**

kala-azar A disease caused by the protozoan, *Leishmania donovani,* transmitted to humans, particularly to children, by the bite of the sand fly. Kala-azar occurs primarily in Asia, parts of Africa, several South and Central American countries, and in the Mediterranean region. The liver and spleen are the main sites of infection; signs and symptoms include anemia, hepatomegaly, splenomegaly, irregular fever, and emaciation. Untreated, the disease has an extremely high mortality rate. Treatment includes sodium antimony gluconate, blood transfusions (for anemia), bed rest, and adequate nutrition. Also called **Assam fever, black fever, dumdum fever, ponos, visceral leishmaniasis.** See also **leishmaniasis.**

kali- A combining form meaning 'of or pertaining to potassium': *kaliemia, kaligenous.*

kanamycin sulfate An aminoglycoside antibiotic.

kaodzera See **Rhodesian trypanosomiasis.**

kaolin A claylike powder used in pectin mixtures as an antidiarrheal agent.

Kaposi's sarcoma A malignant, multifocal neoplasm of reticuloendothelial cells that begins as soft, brownish or purple papules on the feet and slowly spreads in the skin, metastasizing to the lymph nodes and viscera. It occurs most often in Jewish, Italian, and black men and is occasionally associated with diabetes or malignant lymphoma. Radiotherapy and chemotherapy are usually recommended. Also called **idiopathic multiple pigmented hemorrhagic sarcoma, multiple idiopathic hemorrhagic sarcoma.**

Kaposi's varicelliform eruption See **eczema herpeticum.**

kaps- See **caps-.**

karaya powder A dried form of *Sterculia urens* or other species of *Sterculia,* used as a bulk cathartic.

karyenchyma See **karyolymph.**

karyo- A combining form meaning 'of or pertaining to a nucleus': *karyochrome, karyokinesis.*

karyogamy The fusion of cell nuclei, as in conjugation and zygosis. —**karyogamic,** *adj.*

karyogenesis The formation and development of the nucleus of a cell. —**karyogenetic,** *adj.*

karyokinesis The division of the nucleus and equal distribution of nuclear material during mitosis and meiosis. The process involves the four stages of prophase, metaphase, anaphase, and telophase, and it precedes the division of the cytoplasm. Also called **karyomitosis.** See also **cytokinesis.** —**karyokinetic,** *adj.*

karyoklasis, karyoclasis 1. The disintegration of the cell nucleus or nuclear membrane. **2.** The interruption of mitosis. —**karyoklastic, karyoclastic,** *adj.*

karyology The branch of cytology that concentrates on the study of the cell nucleus, especially the structure and function of the chromosomes. —**karyologic, karyological,** *adj.,* **karyologist,** *n.*

karyolymph The clear, usually nonstaining, fluid substance of the nucleus. It consists primarily of proteinaceous, colloidal material in which the nucleolus, chromatin, linin, and various submicroscopic particles are dispersed. Also called **karyenchyma, nuclear hyaloplasm, nuclear sap, nucleochyme.** —**karyolymphatic,** *adj.*

karyolysis The dissolution of the cell nucleus. It occurs normally, both as a form of necrobiosis and during the generation of new cells through mitosis and meiosis.

karyolytic 1. Of or pertaining to karyolysis. **2.** That which causes the destruction of the cell nucleus.

karyomere 1. A saclike structure containing an unequal portion of the nuclear material following atypical mitosis. **2.** A segment of the chromosome. See also **chromomere.**

karyometry The measurement of the nucleus of a cell. —**karyometric,** *adj.*

karyomit A single chromatin fibril of the network within the nucleus of a cell.

karyomitome The fibrillar chromatin network within the nucleus of a cell. Also called **karyoreticulum.**

karyomitosis See **karyokinesis.**

karyomorphism The shape or the form of a cell nucleus, especially that of the leukocyte. —**karyomorphic,** *adj.*

karyon The nucleus of a cell. —**karyontic,** *adj.*

karyophage An intracellular protozoan parasite that destroys the nucleus of the cell it infects. —**karyophagic, karyophagous,** *adj.*

karyoplasm See **nucleoplasm.** —**karyoplasmic,** *adj.*

karyoplasmic ratio See **nucleocytoplasmic ratio.**

karyopyknosis The state of a cell in which the nucleus has shrunk and the chromatin has condensed into solid masses, as in cornified cells of stratified squamous epithelium. **—karyopyknotic,** *adj.*

karyoreticulum See **karyomitome.**

karyorrhexis The fragmentation of chromatin and the distribution of it throughout the cytoplasm as a result of nuclear disintegration. **—karyorrhectic,** *adj.*

karyosome A dense irregular mass of chromatin filaments in the cell nucleus. It is often seen during interphase and may be confused with the nucleolus because of similar staining properties. Also called **chromatin nucleolus, chromocenter, false nucleolus, prochromosome.**

karyospherical 1. Of or pertaining to a nucleus that is spherical in shape. **2.** Such a nucleus.

karyostasis The resting stage of the nucleus between mitotic divisions. See also **interphase. —karyostatic,** *adj.*

karyotheca The membrane that encloses a cell nucleus. **—karyothecal,** *adj.*

karyotin See **chromatin.**

karyotype 1. The total morphological characteristics of the somatic chromosome complement of an individual or species, described in terms of number, form, size, and arrangement within the nucleus, as determined by a microphotograph taken during the metaphase stage of mitosis. **2.** A diagrammatic representation of the chromosome complement of an individual or of a species, arranged in pairs in descending order of size and according to the position of the centromere. See also **Denver classification. —karyotypic,** *adj.*

kat- A combining form meaning 'down, against': *katadidymus, katolysis.* Also **kata-, cat-, cata-.**

katadidymus Conjoined twins that are united in the lower portion of the body and separated at the top.

Kawasaki disease See **mucocutaneous lymph node syndrome.**

Kayser-Fleischer ring A gray-green to red-gold pigmented ring at the outer margin of the cornea, pathognomonic of hepatolenticular degeneration, a rare progressive disease caused by a defect in copper metabolism and transmitted as an autosomal recessive trait. The disease is characterized by cerebral degenerative changes, liver cirrhosis, splenomegaly, involuntary movements, muscle rigidity, and dysphagia.

K cell See **null cell.**

Kedani fever See **scrub typhus.**

kefir, kephir A slightly effervescent, acidulous beverage prepared from the milk of cows, sheep, or goats through fermentation by kefir grains, which contain yeasts and lactobacilli. It is an important source of the bacteria necessary in the gastrointestinal tract to synthesize vitamin K.

Kegel exercises See **pubococcygeus exercises.**

Keith-Flack node See **sinoatrial node.**

kel- A combining form meaning 'of or pertaining to a tumor': *kelectome, keloid.*

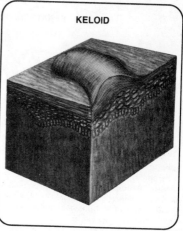

KELOID

Kellgren's syndrome A form of osteoarthritis affecting the proximal and distal interphalangeal joints, the first metatarsophalangeal and carpometacarpal joints, the knees, and the spine. The absence of rheumatoid factor, rheumatoid nodules, and systemic involvement differentiates this syndrome from rheumatoid arthritis. Also called **erosive osteoarthritis.**

Kelly's pad A horseshoe-shaped, inflatable rubber drainage pad used in a bed or on the operating table.

keloid, cheloid Overgrowth of collagenous scar tissue at the site of a wound of the skin. The new tissue is elevated, rounded, and firm, with irregular, clawlike margins. Young women and blacks are particularly susceptible to keloid formation. Most keloids flatten and become less noticeable over a period of years. However, surgery may be indicated to reduce or remove excess scar tissue. Other types of therapy include solid carbon dioxide, liquid nitrogen, intralesional corticosteroid injections, and radiation. **—cheloidal, keloidal,** *adj.*

keloidosis, cheloidosis Habitual or multiple formation of keloids.

Kempner rice-fruit diet See **rice diet.**

Kenny treatment See **Sister Kenny's treatment.**

keno- A combining form meaning 'empty': *kenophobia, kenotoxin.*

kenogenesis See **cenogenesis.**

kenophobia, cenophobia The morbid fear of large and open spaces; also known as agoraphobia.

Kenya fever See **Marseilles fever.**

kera- A combining form meaning 'horn': *keracele, keraphyllocele.*

kerat-, kerato- A combining form meaning: **1.** 'Horny, cornified': *keratolysis, keratoma.* **2.** 'Cornea, corneal': *keratoiritis, keratoleukoma.*

keratectomy Surgical removal of a portion of the cornea, performed to excise a small, superficial lesion that does not warrant a corneal graft.

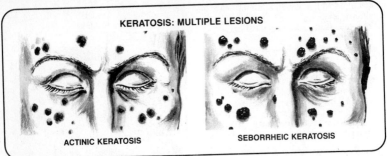

KERATOSIS: MULTIPLE LESIONS

ACTINIC KERATOSIS   SEBORRHEIC KERATOSIS

keratic 1. Of or pertaining to keratin. 2. Of or pertaining to the cornea.

keratic precipitate A group of inflammatory cells deposited on the endothelial surface of the cornea after trauma or inflammation, sometimes obscuring vision.

keratitis Any inflammation of the cornea. Kinds of keratitis include **dendritic keratitis, interstitial keratitis, keratoconjunctivitis sicca,** and **trachoma.** Compare **keratopathy.** —**keratic,** *adj.*

kerato- A combining form meaning 'of or pertaining to the cornea, or to horny tissue': *keratocele, keratocentesis.* Also **cerato-.**

keratoacanthoma, *pl.* **keratoacanthomas, keratoacanthomata** A benign, rapidly growing, flesh-colored papule of the skin with a central plug of keratin. The lesion is most common on the face or the back of the hands and arms. It disappears spontaneously in 4 to 6 months, leaving a slightly depressed scar. Biopsy is often necessary to differentiate it from a squamous carcinoma.

keratoconjunctivitis Any inflammation involving both the cornea and the conjunctiva. Kinds of keratoconjunctivitis include **eczematous conjunctivitis, keratoconjunctivitis sicca.**

keratoconjunctivitis sicca Dryness of the cornea owing to a deficiency of tear secretion in which the corneal surface appears dull and rough, and the eye feels gritty and irritated. The condition may be associated with erythema multiforme, Sjögren's syndrome, trachoma, and vitamin A deficiency.

keratoconus A noninflammatory protrusion of the central part of the cornea. The condition is more common in females, and it may cause marked astigmatism; contact lenses usually restore visual acuity. The cause of the condition is unknown.

keratolytic An agent that promotes softening and dissolution or peeling of the horny layer of the epidermis.

keratomalacia A condition, characterized by xerosis and ulceration of the cornea, resulting from severe vitamin A deficiency. It commonly occurs as a secondary result of diseases that affect vitamin A absorption or storage, as ulcerative colitis, celiac syndrome, cystic fibrosis, or sprue. Also at risk are infants and children who are given dilute formula, who are malnourished, or who are allergic to whole milk and are fed skim milk, which is a poor source of vitamin A. Early symptoms of keratomalacia include night blindness; photophobia; swelling and redness of the eyelids; and drying, roughness, pain, and wrinkling of the conjunctiva. See also **vitamin A.**

keratomycosis linguae See **parasitic glossitis.**

keratopathy Any noninflammatory disease of the cornea. Compare **keratitis.**

keratoplasty A procedure in ophthalmologic surgery in which an opaque portion of the cornea is excised.

keratosis Any skin condition in which there is overgrowth and thickening of the cornified epithelium. Kinds of keratosis are **actinic keratosis** and **seborrheic keratosis.** —**keratotic,** *adj.*

keratosis follicularis An uncommon, hereditary skin disorder characterized by keratotic papules that coalesce to form brown or black, crusted, wartlike patches. These vegetations may spread widely, ulcerate, and become covered with a purulent exudate. Treatment includes large doses of vitamin A orally, topical vitamin A acid cream, and oral or topical corticosteroids. Also called **Darier's disease.**

keratosis seborrheica See **seborrheic keratosis.**

kerauno- A combining form meaning 'of or pertaining to lightning': *keraunoneurosis, keraunophobia.*

kerion An inflamed, boggy granuloma that develops as an immune reaction to a superficial fungus infection in association with *Tinea capitis* of the scalp. The lesion heals within a short time without treatment.

kernicterus An abnormal toxic accumulation of bilirubin in the brain tissues owing to hyperbilirubinemia. See also **hyperbilirubinemia of the newborn.**

kerosene poisoning A toxic condition caused by the ingestion of kerosene or the inhalation of its fumes. Symptoms following ingestion include drowsiness, fever, a rapid heartbeat, tremors, and severe pneumonitis if the fluid is aspirated. Vomiting is not induced. Treatment for ingestion usually includes 30 to 60 ml (1 to 2 oz) of vegetable oil to prevent absorption of

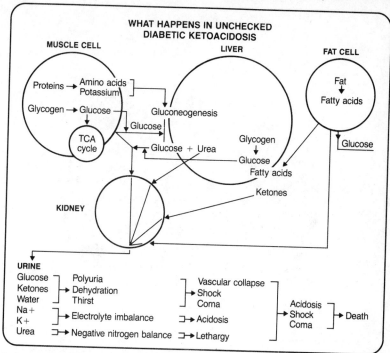

WHAT HAPPENS IN UNCHECKED DIABETIC KETOACIDOSIS

the kerosene in the stomach and gastric lavage with copious amounts of water, a 3% sodium bicarbonate solution, or normal saline solution. Treatment for poisoning by inhalation includes fresh air, oxygen, and respiratory assistance if necessary. See also **petroleum distillate poisoning.**

ketamine hydrochloride A general anesthetic.

keto- A combining form indicating possession of the carbonyl group (C:O): *ketoheptose, ketolysis.*

ketoacidosis Acidosis accompanied by an accumulation of ketones in the body, resulting from faulty carbohydrate metabolism. It occurs primarily as a complication of diabetes mellitus and is characterized by a fruity odor of acetone on the breath, mental confusion, dyspnea, nausea, vomiting, dehydration, weight loss, and, if untreated, coma. Emergency treatment includes the administration of insulin and I.V. fluids and the evaluation and correction of electrolyte imbalance. Nasogastric intubation and bladder catheterization may be required if the patient is comatose. Compare **insulin shock.** See also **diabetes mellitus, ketosis. —ketoacidotic,** *adj.*

ketoaciduria Presence in the urine of excessive amounts of ketone bodies, occurring as a result of uncontrolled diabetes mellitus, starvation, or any other metabolic condition in which fats are rapidly catabolized. The condition can be diagnosed with a dipstick reagent or acetone test tablet. Also called **ketonuria.** See also **Acetest, ketosis. —ketoaciduric,** *adj.*

ketocholanic acids Bile salts used to aid digestion in biliary disorders.

ketoconazole An antifungal agent.

ketone alcohol An alcohol containing the ketone group.

ketone bodies Normal metabolic products, B-hydroxylbutyric acid and aminoacetic acid, from which acetone may arise spontaneously. The two acids are products of lipid pyruvate metabolism, via acetyl-CoA in the liver, and are oxidized by the muscles. Excessive production of these bodies leads to their excretion in urine, as in diabetes mellitus. Also called **acetone bodies.**

ketonuria See **ketoaciduria.**

ketosis The abnormal accumulation of ketones in the body as a result of a deficiency or inadequate use of carbohydrates. Fatty acids are metabolized instead, and the end products, ketones, begin to accumulate. This condition is seen in starvation; occasionally in pregnancy, if the intake of protein and carbohydrates is inadequate; and, most frequently, in diabetes mellitus. It is characterized by ketonuria, loss of potassium in the urine, and a fruity odor of acetone on the breath. Untreated, ketosis may progress to ketoacidosis, coma, and death. See also **diabetes mellitus, ketoacidosis, starvation. —ketotic,** *adj.*

Kew Gardens spotted fever See **rickettsialpox.**

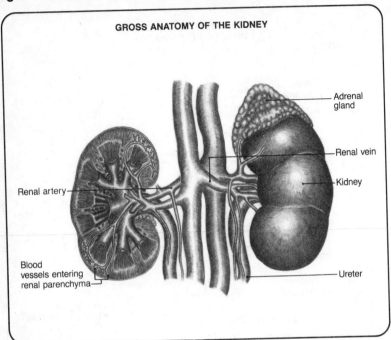

GROSS ANATOMY OF THE KIDNEY

Adrenal gland

Renal vein

Kidney

Renal artery

Blood vessels entering renal parenchyma

Ureter

kidney One of a pair of bean-shaped urinary organs in the dorsal part of the abdomen, one on each side of the vertebral column. In most individuals, the right kidney is more caudal than the left. Each kidney is about 11 cm (4¼ inches) long, 6 cm (2½ inches) wide, and 2.5 cm (1 inch) thick. In men, each kidney weighs from 125 to 170 g (4½ to 6 oz); in women, each kidney weighs from 115 to 155 g (4 to 5 ½ oz). In the newborn, the kidneys are about three times as large in proportion to the body weight as in the adult. The kidneys produce and eliminate urine through a complex filtration network and reabsorption system comprising more than 2 million nephrons. The nephrons are composed of glomeruli and renal tubules that filter blood under high pressure, removing urea, salts, and other soluble wastes from blood plasma and returning the purified filtrate to the blood. More than 1,175 liters (2,500 pints) of blood pass through the kidneys every day, entering the kidneys through the renal arteries and leaving through the renal veins. All the blood in the body passes through the kidneys about 20 times every hour but only about one fifth of the plasma is filtered by the nephrons during that period. The kidneys remove water as urine and return water that has been filtered to the blood plasma, thus helping to maintain the water balance of the body.

kidney cancer A malignant neoplasm of the renal parenchyma or renal pelvis. Factors associated with an increased incidence of disease are exposure to aromatic hydrocarbons or to-bacco smoke and the use of drugs containing phenacetin. A long asymptomatic period may precede the onset of the characteristic symptoms, which include hematuria, flank pain, fever, and the detection of a palpable mass. Adenocarcinoma of the renal parenchyma accounts for 80% of kidney tumors, occurring twice as frequently in men as in women; transitional cell or squamous cell carcinomas in the renal pelvis account for about 15% and are as frequent in men as in women. See also **Wilms' tumor.**

kidney disease Any one of a large group of conditions including infectious, inflammatory, obstructive, vascular, and neoplastic disorders of the kidney. Characteristics of kidney disease are hematuria, persistent proteinuria, pyuria, edema, dysuria, and pain in the flank. Specific symptoms vary with the type of disorder; for example, hematuria with severe, colicky pain suggests obstruction by a kidney stone; hematuria without pain may indicate renal carcinoma; proteinuria is generally a sign of disease in the glomerulus, or filtration unit of the kidney; pyuria indicates infectious disease; and edema is characteristic of the nephrotic syndrome. Treatment depends upon the type of kidney disease diagnosed. Some forms of advanced kidney disease may lead to renal failure, coma, and death unless hemodialysis is started. See also **glomerulonephritis, nephrotic syndrome, renal calculus, renal failure.**

kidney failure *Informal.* Renal failure.

kidney machine 1. See **artificial kidney. 2.** See **dialyzer.**

kidney stone See **urinary calculus.**

Kielland rotation An obstetric operation in which Kielland's forceps are used in turning the head of the fetus from an occiput posterior or occiput transverse position to an occiput anterior position. It is performed most commonly to correct an arrest in the active stage of labor. As it is associated with increased harm to the mother and to the infant, cesarean section is often preferred. See also **forceps delivery, obstetric forceps.**

Kielland's forceps See **obstetric forceps.**

killer cell See **null cell.**

kilo- A combining form meaning '1,000': *kilocalorie, kilogram.*

kilogram (kg) A unit for the measurement of mass in the metric system. One kilogram is equal to 1,000 grams or to 2.2046 pounds avoirdupois.

kilogram calorie See **calorie.**

Kimmelstiel-Wilson's disease See **intercapillary glomerulosclerosis.**

kinase 1. An enzyme that catalyzes the transfer of a phosphate group or another high-energy molecular group to an acceptor molecule. Each of these kinases is named for its receptor, such as acetate kinase, fructokinase, hexokinase. 2. An enzyme that activates a pre-enzyme (zymogen). Each of these kinases is named for its source, such as bacterial kinase, enterokinase, fibrinokinase.

kine- See **kinesio-.**

kinematics In physiology: the geometry of the motion of the body without regard to the forces acting to produce the motion. Kinematics deals with the description and the measurement of body motion and the means of recording it. Kinematics considers the motions of all body parts relative to the segments of the part involved in the motion and not necessarily in relation to the standard anatomical position, as the movements of the fingers are considered in relation to the midline of the hand, not the midline of the body. The most common types of motions studied in kinematics are flexion, extension, adduction, abduction, internal rotation, and external rotation. Also called **cinematics.** Compare **kinetics.**

kinesio- A combining form meaning 'of or pertaining to movement': *kinesiology, kinesioneurosis.* Also **kine-.**

kinesiology The scientific study of muscular activity and of the anatomy, physiology, and mechanics of the movement of body parts.

-kinesis A combining from meaning: **1.** An 'activation': *angiokinesis, lymphokinesis, thrombokinesis.* **2.** 'A division (of cells)': *catakinesis, diakinesis, heterokinesis.* Also **-cinesia, -cinesis, -kinesia.**

kinesthetic memory The recollection of movement, weight, resistance, and position of the body or parts of the body.

-kinetic A combining form meaning: **1.** 'Pertaining to motion': *akinetic, parakinetic.* **2.** 'Pertaining to a (specified) agent causing motion': *chemokinetic, photokinetic.* **3.** 'Referring to ki-

nesis': *astrokinetic, biokinetic.* **4.** 'Referring to activation of a body part by a (specified) agent': *angiokinetic, gametokinetic.* Also **-cinetic, -cinetical, -kinetical.**

kinetics In physiology: the study of the forces that produce, arrest, or modify the motions of the body. Newton's first and third laws of inertia are especially applicable to kinetics. Newton's first law states that bodies at rest tend to stay at rest and bodies in motion tend to keep moving. Newton's third law states that action and reaction are equal in magnitude but opposite in direction. These two laws are applicable to the forces produced by muscles of the body which act on joints. The reaction forces of the muscles contribute to the equilibrium and the motion of the body. Compare **kinematics.**

kineto- A combining form meaning 'movable': *kinetochore, kinetogenic.*

kinetochore See **centromere.**

kinetotherapeutic bath A bath in which underwater exercises are performed in order to strengthen weak or partially paralyzed muscles.

kino- A combining form meaning 'of or pertaining to movement': *kinoplasm, kinosphere.*

kinomere See **centromere.**

kinship-model family group A family unit comprised of the biological parents and their offspring. It is like a nuclear family but is more closely tied to an extended family.

kiono- See **ciono-.**

Kirschner's wire A threaded or smooth metallic wire available in three diameters and 22.86 cm (9 inches) long. The wire is used in internal fixation of fractures or for skeletal traction.

klang association See **clang association.**

Klebsiella A genus of diplococcal bacteria that appear as small, plump rods with rounded ends. Several respiratory diseases, including bronchitis, are caused by infection by species of *Klebsiella.*

Klebs-Loeffler bacillus *Corynebacterium diphtheriae.*

kleeblattschädel deformity syndrome See **cloverleaf skull deformity.**

Kleine-Levine syndrome A disorder of unknown etiology often associated with psychotic conditions, characterized by episodic somnolence, abnormal hunger, and hyperactivity. The episodes of sleep may last for several hours or days and are followed by confusion on awakening. There is no specific treatment. Compare **narcolepsy.**

klepto- A combining form meaning 'of or pertaining to theft or stealing': *kleptolagnia, kleptomania.*

kleptolagnia Sexual excitement or gratification produced by stealing.

kleptomania, cleptomania A neurosis characterized by an abnormal, uncontrollable, and recurrent urge to steal. The objects, taken not for their monetary value or an immediate need for them, but because of a symbolic meaning usually associated with some unconscious emotional conflict, are usually given away, re-

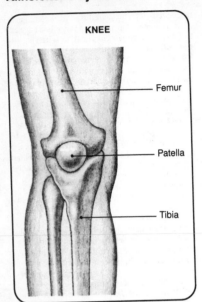

KNEE

Femur

Patella

Tibia

turned surreptitiously, or kept and hidden. People who have the condition experience an increased sense of tension before committing the theft and intense gratification during the act. Afterward, they display signs of depression, guilt, and anxiety over the possibility of being apprehended and losing status in society. In less severe cases, the impulse is expressed by the continuous borrowing of objects without returning them. Treatment usually consists of psychotherapy to uncover the underlying emotional problems. **—kleptomaniac,** *n.*

Klinefelter's syndrome   A syndrome of gonadal defects, appearing in males with an extra X chromosome in at least one cell line. Characteristics are small, firm testes, long legs, gynecomastia, poor social adaptation, subnormal intelligence, chronic pulmonary disease, and varicose veins. The severity of the abnormalities increases with greater numbers of X chromosomes. The most common abnormality is a 47 XXY karyotype.

Klippel-Feil syndrome   See **congenital short neck syndrome.**

kneading   A grasping, rolling, and pressing movement, as is used in massaging the muscles. See also **massage.**

knee   A joint complex that connects the thigh with the lower leg. It consists of 3 condyloid joints, 12 ligaments, 13 bursae, and the patella. Two of the condyloid joints comprising the knee are between the condyles of the femur and the corresponding menisci and condyles of the tibia. The third condyloid joint within the knee is a partially arthrodial joint between the patella and the femur. The motion of this joint is not a simple gliding motion, because the articular surfaces of the bones involved are not mutually adapted

to each other. The ligaments of the knee include the articular capsule, the patellar, the oblique popliteal, the arcuate popliteal, the tibial collateral, the fibular collateral, the anterior cruciate, the posterior cruciate, the medial and the lateral menisci, the transverse ligament, and the coronary ligament. Four of the bursae of the knee are located in front, four laterally, and five medially. The largest bursa is the prepatellar bursa between the patellar ligament and the skin. The painful condition 'housemaid's knee' is caused by inflammation of the prepatellar bursa. The knee is relatively unprotected by surrounding muscles and is often injured by blows, sudden stops, and turns, especially those associated with sports.

knee-ankle interaction   One of the five major kinetic determinants of gait that helps to minimize the displacement of the center of gravity of the body during the walking cycle. The knee and the foot work simultaneously to lower the center of gravity of the body. When the heel of the foot is in contact with the ground, the foot is dorsiflexed and the knee is fully extended so that the associated limb is at its maximum length with the center of gravity at its lower point. Plantar flexion of the foot with the initiation of knee flexion maintains the center of gravity in its forward progression at about the same level, also helping to minimize the vertical displacement of the center of gravity. Compare **knee-hip flexion, lateral pelvic displacement, pelvic rotation, pelvic tilt.**

knee-chest position   See **genupectoral position.**

knee-hip flexion   One of the five major kinematic determinants of gait, which allows the passage of body weight over the supporting extremity during the walking cycle. Knee-hip flexion occurs during the stance and the swing phases of the cycle. The knee first locks into extension as the heel of the weight-bearing limb strikes the ground and is unlocked by final flexion and initiation of the swing phase in the walking cycle. Knee-hip flexion is often a factor in the diagnosis and treatment of various orthopedic diseases, deformities, and abnormal conditions and in the analysis and correction of pathological gaits. Compare **knee-ankle interaction, lateral pelvic displacement, pelvic rotation, pelvic tilt.**

knee-jerk reflex   See **patellar reflex.**

knee joint   The complex, hinged joint at the knee, regarded as three articulations in one, comprising condyloid joints connecting the femur and the tibia and a partly arthrodial joint connecting the patella and the femur. The knee joint and its ligaments permit flexion, extension, and, in certain positions, medial and lateral rotation. It is a common site for sprain and dislocation. Also called **articulatio genus.**

knee replacement   The surgical insertion of a hinged prosthesis, performed to relieve pain and restore motion to a knee severely affected by osteoarthritis, rheumatoid arthritis, or trauma. See also **arthroplasty, hip replacement, os-**

teoarthritis, plastic surgery.

knife needle A slender surgical knife with a needle point, used in the discission of a cataract and in other ophthalmic procedures, as goniotomy and goniopuncture.

knock-knee See **genu valgum.**

knot In surgery: the interlacing of the ends of a ligature or suture so that they remain in place without slipping or becoming detached. The ends of the suture are passed twice around each other before being pulled taut to make a simple surgeon's knot. For additional stability, the ends may be recrossed and a second simple knot made over the first. There are many kinds of knots.

knowledge deficit A nursing diagnosis accepted by the Fifth National Conference on the Classification of Nursing Diagnoses. The etiology of the condition may be a lack of exposure to information, a lack of ability to recall the information, a misinterpretation of the information, a cognitive or perceptual limitation in the ability to learn or to understand the information, a lack of interest in acquiring the information, or an unfamiliarity with the resources necessary to gain the information. The defining characteristics of the knowledge deficit include a statement by the person that the deficit exists, an observed failure on the part of the client to follow through on instructions, the observation of an inadequate performance by the client on a test, or the observation of inappropriate or exaggerated behavior on the part of the client. See also **nursing diagnosis.**

Kocher's forceps A kind of surgical forceps that has notched jaws, interlocking teeth, and thick, curved or straight, powerful handles.

Koch's postulates The prerequisites for establishing that a specific microorganism causes a particular disease. The conditions are: (1) the microorganism must be observed in all cases of the disease; (2) the microorganism must be isolated and grown in pure culture; (3) microorganisms from the pure culture, when inoculated into a susceptible animal, must reproduce the disease; (4) the microorganism must be observed in and recovered from the experimentally diseased animal.

Koebner phenomenon The development of isomorphic lesions at the site of an injury occurring in psoriasis, lichen nitidus, lichen planus, and verruca plana.

koilo- A combining form meaning 'hollow or concave': *koilonychia, koilorrhachic.*

koilonychia Spoon nails; a condition in which nails are thin and concave from side to side. It is usually familial but may occur with iron-deficiency anemia and Raynaud's phenomenon.

koinoni- A combining form meaning 'of or pertaining to a community': *koinonia, koinoniphobia.*

kolpo- See **colpo-.**

koly- A combining form meaning 'to hinder': *kolypeptic, kolyphrenia.*

kon- A combining form meaning 'of or pertaining to dust': *koniocortex, konometer.*

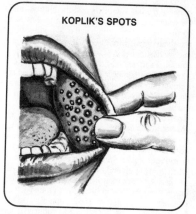

KOPLIK'S SPOTS

Koplik's spots Small red spots with blue-white centers on the lingual and buccal mucosa, characteristic of measles. The rash of measles usually erupts 1 to 2 days after the appearance of Koplik's spots.

kopr- See **copro-.**

kopra- See **copro-.**

Korotkoff sounds Sounds heard during the taking of blood pressure using a sphygmomanometer and stethoscope. As air is released from the cuff, pressure on the brachial artery is reduced, and the blood is heard pulsing through the vessel. See also **blood pressure, diastole, sphygmomanometer, systole.**

Korsakoff's psychosis A form of amnesia often seen in chronic alcoholics, characterized by a loss of short-term memory and an inability to learn new skills. The person is usually disoriented and confabulates to conceal the condition. The cause of the condition can often be traced to degenerative changes in the thalamus owing to a deficiency of B complex vitamins, especially thiamine and B_{12}. Compare **Wernicke's encephalopathy.**

kosher Conforming to or prepared in accordance with the dietary or ceremonial laws of Judaism.

Krabbe's disease See **galactosyl ceramide lipidosis.**

Kraske position An anatomical position in which the patient is prone, with hips flexed and elevated, and head and feet down. The position is used for renal surgery, as it enlarges the costovertebral angle, allowing the surgeon to have optimal access to the kidneys.

kraurosis A thickening and shriveling of the skin. See also **kraurosis vulvae.**

kraurosis vulvae A skin disease of older women characterized by dryness, itching, and atrophy of the external genitalia. It is a condition that exhibits a predisposition to leukoplakia and carcinoma of the vulva. See also **lichen sclerosis et atrophicus.**

Krause's corpuscles A number of sensory end organs in the conjunctiva of the eye, mucous membranes of the lips and tongue, epineurium of nerve trunks, the penis and the clitoris, and the synovial membranes of certain joints. Krause's corpuscles are tiny cylindrical oval bodies with a capsule formed by the expansion of the connective tissue sheath of a medullated fiber. They contain a soft, semifluid core in which the axon terminates either in a bulbous extremity or in a coiled mass. Also called **end bulbs of Krause.** Compare **Golgi-Mazzoni corpuscles, Pacini's corpuscles.**

Krebs' citric acid cycle   A sequence of enzymatic reactions involving the metabolism of carbon chains of sugars, fatty acids, and amino acids to yield carbon dioxide, water, and high-energy phosphate bonds. The cycle is initiated when pyruvate combines with coenzyme A (CoA) to form a two-carbon unit, acetyl-CoA, which enters the cycle by combining with four-carbon oxaloacetic acid to form six-carbon citric acid. In subsequent steps, isocitric acid, produced from citric acid, is oxidized to oxalsuccinic acid, which loses carbon dioxide to form alpha-ketoglutaric acid. Succinic acid, resulting from the oxidative decarboxylation of alpha-ketoglutraic acid, is oxidized to fumaric acid, and its oxidation regenerates oxalacetic acid, which condenses with acetyl-CoA, closing the cycle. The Krebs' cycle provides a major source of adenosine triphosphate energy and also produces intermediate molecules that are starting points for vital metabolic pathways. Also called **tricarboxylic acid cycle.** See also **acetylcoenzyme A.**

Krukenberg's tumor   A neoplasm of the ovary that is a metastasis of a gastrointestinal malignancy, usually stomach cancer. Cytologic examination reveals mucoid degeneration and many large cells shaped like signet rings. Also called **carcinoma mucocellulare.**

krypto-   See **crypto-.**

Kulchitsky-cell carcinoma   See **carcinoid.**

Kulchitsky's cell   See **argentaffin cell.**

Küntscher nail   A stainless steel nail used in orthopedic surgery for the fixation of fractures of the long bones, especially the femur. Also called **Küntscher intramedullary nail.**

Kupffer's cells   Specialized cells of the reticuloendothelial system lining the sinusoids of the liver. The function of Kupffer's cells is to filter bacteria and other small, foreign proteins out of the blood.

kuru   A slow, progressive, fatal viral infection of the central nervous system, seen in the natives of the New Guinea Highlands. The incubation period may be 30 or more years, but death usually occurs within months of the onset of symptoms. Characteristic of kuru are ataxia and decreased coordination progressing to paralysis, dementia, slurring of speech, and visual disturbances. Transmission of the disease is probably the result of cannibalism, as brain tissue from infected people produces the disease when inoculated into laboratory primates, and the disease has declined with the decline of cannibalism.

Kussmaul respirations   Abnormally deep, very rapid sighing respirations, resulting from air hunger, characteristic of diabetic acidosis.

Kveim reaction   A reaction used in a diagnostic test for sarcoidosis, based on an intradermal injection of antigen derived from a lymph node known to be sarcoid. If a noncaseating granuloma appears on the skin at the test site in 4 to 8 weeks, the reaction is said to be positive: evidence that the patient has sarcoidosis.

kwashiorkor   A malnutrition disease, primarily affecting children in undeveloped countries, caused by severe protein deficiency, usually occurring when the child is weaned from the breast. Because calorie-rich starches like breadfruit are available, the child does not lose weight as dramatically and does not look as sick as a marasmic child, who lacks protein and calories. Eventually the following symptoms occur: retarded growth, changes in skin and hair pigmentation, diarrhea, loss of appetite, nervous irritability, edema, anemia, fatty degeneration of the liver, necrosis, dermatoses, and fibrosis, often accompanied by infection and multivitamin deficiencies. Because dietary fats are poorly tolerated in kwashiorkor, a skim-milk formula is used in initial feedings, followed by additional foods, until a full, well-balanced diet is achieved. Also called **infantile pellagra, malignant malnutrition.** See also **marasmic kwashiorkor, marasmus.**

Kyasanur forest disease   An arbovirus infection transmitted by the bite of a tick that is harbored by shrews and other forest animals in western tropical India. Characteristics of the infection include fever, headache, muscle ache, cough, abdominal and eye pain, and photophobia. Treatment is symptomatic.

kymo-   A combining form meaning 'of or pertaining to waves': *kymograph, kymoscope.*

kyno-   A combining form meaning 'of or pertaining to dogs': *kynocephalus, kynophobia.*

kypho-   A combining form meaning 'of or pertaining to a hump': *kyphoscoliosis, kyphosis.*

kyphoscoliosis   An abnormal condition characterized by an anteroposterior curvature and a lateral curvature of the spine. It occurs in both children and adults, often associated with cor pulmonale. Compare **kyphosis, scoliosis. —kyphoscoliotic,** *adj.*

kyphosis   An abnormal condition of the vertebral column, characterized by increased convexity in the curvature of the thoracic spine as viewed from the side. Kyphosis may be caused by rickets or tuberculosis of the spine. Adolescent kyphosis is usually self-limiting and often undiagnosed, but if the curvature progresses, there may be moderate back pain. Conservative treatment consists of spine-stretching exercises and sleeping without a pillow, with a board under the mattress. A modified Milwaukee brace may be used for severe kyphosis, and, rarely, spinal fusion may be required. **—kyphotic,** *adj.*

kysth-   See **colpo-.**

kystho-   See **colpo-.**

kyto-   See **cyt-.**

L Symbol for **lung.**

La Symbol for **lanthanum.**

label In radiology and immunology: **1.** A substance with a special affinity for an organ, tissue, cell, or microorganism in which it may become deposited and fixed. **2.** The process of depositing and fixing a substance in an organ, tissue, cell, or microorganism.

labeled compound A chemical substance in which part of the molecules are labeled with a radionuclide so that observations of the radioactivity or isotopic composition make it possible to follow the compound or its fragments through physical, chemical, or biological processes.

labia, *sing.* **labium** **1.** The fleshy, liplike edges of an organ or tissue. **2.** The folds of skin at the opening of the vagina.

-labial A combining form meaning 'of or pertaining to lips': *alveololabial, glossolabial, maxillolabial.*

labia majora, *sing.* **labium majus** Two long lips of skin, one on each side of the vaginal orifice outside the labia minora. They extend from the anterior labial commissure to the posterior labial commissure and form the lateral boundaries of the pudendal cleft.

labia minora, *sing.* **labium minus** Two folds of skin between the labia majora, extending posteriorly from the clitoris along both sides of the vaginal orifice, ending between it and the labia majora. Anteriorly, each labium divides into an upper and a lower division. The upper divisions pass above the clitoris and meet to form the preputium clitoridis; the lower divisions pass beneath the clitoris and unite to form the frenulum of the clitoris.

labile **1.** Unstable; characterized by a tendency to change or to be altered or modified. **2.** In psychiatry: describing a personality characterized by rapidly shifting or changing emotions, as in bipolar disorder and certain types of schizophrenia; emotionally unstable. —**lability,** *n.*

-labile A combining form meaning 'unstable, subject to change': *frigolabile, siccolabile, thixolabile.*

labio- A combining form meaning 'of or pertaining to the lips, particularly the lips of the mouth': *labiocervical, labiodental, labiomental.*

labioglossolaryngeal paralysis See **bulbar paralysis.**

labor The time and the processes that occur during parturition from the beginning of cervical dilatation to the delivery of the placenta. See also **birth.**

labor, abnormal See **dystocia.**

laboratory **1.** A facility, room, building, or part of a building in which scientific research, experimentation, testing, or other investigative activities are carried out. **2.** Of or pertaining to a laboratory.

laboratory error Any error made by the personnel in a clinical laboratory in the performance of a test, the interpretation of the data, or in reporting or recording the results. Laboratory error must always be considered a possible explanation for findings that are at variance with the composite clinical condition of the patient or that are widely divergent from previous laboratory tests.

laboratory medicine The branch of medicine in which specimens of tissue, fluid, or other body substance is examined outside of the person, usually in the laboratory. Some fields of laboratory medicine are **chemistry, hematology, histology,** and **pathology.**

laboratory test A procedure, usually conducted in a laboratory, that is intended to detect, identify, or quantify one or more significant substances, evaluate organ functions, or establish the nature of a condition or disease. Laboratory tests range from quite simple to extremely sophisticated. In modern medical practice, they are commonly used to help establish or confirm a diagnosis and often aid in the management of disease.

labor coach A person who assists a woman in labor and delivery by closely attending to her emotional needs and by encouraging her to properly use the breathing patterns, concentration techniques, body positions, and massage techniques that were taught in a program of psychophysical preparation for childbirth. Usually, the coach is the father of the baby or a close friend of the mother, but a professional labor coach, often a registered nurse specially trained in a method, may fill the role. See also **monitrice.**

labored breathing Abnormal respiration characterized by evidence of increased effort, including use of the accessory muscles of respiration of the chest wall, stridor, grunting, or nasal flaring.

labyrinth See **internal ear.**

labyrinthitis Inflammation of the labyrinthine canals of the inner ear, resulting in vertigo.

laceration **1.** The act of tearing or lacerating. **2.** A torn, jagged wound. —**lacerate,** *v.,* **lacerated,** *adj.*

lacri-, lachry- A combining form meaning 'of or pertaining to tears': *lacrimalin, lacrimator, lacrimotomy.*

lacrimal, lachrymal Pertaining to tears.

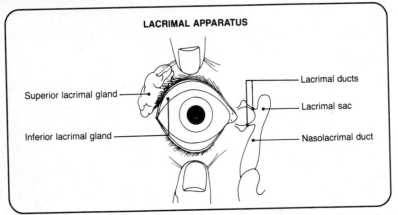

LACRIMAL APPARATUS

Superior lacrimal gland

Inferior lacrimal gland

Lacrimal ducts

Lacrimal sac

Nasolacrimal duct

lacrimal apparatus   A network of structures of the eye that secrete tears and drain them from the surface of the eyeball. These parts include the lacrimal glands, the lacrimal ducts, the lacrimal sacs, and the nasolacrimal ducts.

lacrimal bone   One of the smallest and most fragile bones of the face, located at the anterior part of the medial wall of the orbit. It unites with the maxilla to form the lacrimal fossa, which lodges the lacrimal duct.

lacrimal caruncle   The small, reddish, fleshy protuberance that fills the triangular space between the medial margins of the upper and the lower eyelids. It contains sebaceous and sudoriferous glands and secretes a whitish substance that collects in the corner of the eye.

lacrimal duct   One of two channels through which tears pass from the lacrimal lake to the lacrimal sac of each eye.

lacrimal fistula   An abnormal communication from a tear duct or sac to the surface of the eye or eyelid.

lacrimal gland   One of a pair of glands situated superior and lateral to the eye bulb in the lacrimal fossa. It is an oval structure about the size of an almond and is divided into an orbital part and a palpebral part. The watery secretion from the gland consists of the tears, slightly alkaline and saline, that moisten the conjunctiva.

lacrimal papilla   The small conical elevation on the medial margin of each eyelid, supporting an apex pierced by the punctum lacrimale through which tears emerge to moisten the conjunctiva.

lacrimal sac   The dilated end of each of the two nasolacrimal ducts serving the eyes. Each sac is lodged in a deep groove formed by the lacrimal bone and the frontal process of the maxilla. The sac is oval and about 13 mm (½ inch) long. Its upper end is closed and rounded, its lower end continuous with the nasolacrimal duct. The lacrimal sacs fill with tears, which are secreted by the lacrimal glands and conveyed through the lacrimal ducts.

lacrimation, lachrymation   **1.** The normal continuous secretion of tears by the lacrimal glands. **2.** An excessive amount of tear production, as in crying or weeping.

lact-   See **lacto-**.

lactalbumin   A simple, highly nutritious protein found in milk. It is similar to serum albumin. See also **albumin, serum albumin.**

lactase   An enzyme that catalyzes the hydrolysis of alpha-D-galactoside to D-galactose. Lactase is concentrated in the kidney, liver, and intestinal mucosa. Also called beta-galactosidase.

lactase deficiency   A congenital abnormality in which the amount of the enzyme lactase is deficient, resulting in the inability to digest lactose. The deficiency occurs in infancy in severe form and persists throughout life. In adults, a relative deficiency may appear as a natural process of aging; it occurs more frequently in persons of Asiatic and African heritage. Lactase deficiency may result from subtotal gastrectomy, from any disease of the small intestine in which structural changes occur, as tropical sprue, ulcerative colitis, infectious hepatitis, and kwashiorkor, or from malnutrition. See also **lactose intolerance.**

lactation   The process of the synthesis and secretion of milk from the breasts in the nourishment of an infant or child. See also **breast milk.**

lacteal   Of or pertaining to milk.

lacteal fistula   An abnormal passage opening into a lacteal duct.

lacteal gland   One of the many central lymphatic capillaries in the villi of the small intestine. It opens into the lymphatic vessels in the submucosa. The capillary is filled with chyle that turns milky white during the absorption of fat.

lactic   Referring to milk and milk products. See also **lactic acid, lactose.**

lactic acid   A three-carbon organic acid produced by anaerobic respiration. There are three forms: L-lactic acid in muscle and blood is a product of glucose and glycogen metabolism; D-lactic acid is produced by the fermentation of dextrose by a species of micrococcus; DL-lactic acid is a racemic mixture found in the stomach, in sour milk, and in certain other foods, as sauerkraut, prepared by bacterial fermentation. Also called **alpha-hydroxypropionic acid.** See also **glycolysis.**

lactic acid fermentation   **1.** The production of lactic acid from sugars by various bacteria. **2.** The souring of milk.

lactic dehydrogenase (LDH)   An enzyme that catalyzes the reversible conversion of muscle lactic acid into pyruvic acid. This essential final step in the Embden-Myerhof glycolytic pathway provides the metabolic bridge to the Krebs cycle (citric acid or tricarboxylic acid cycle), ultimately producing cellular energy. Because LDH is present in almost all body tissues, cellular damage causes an elevation of total serum LDH, thus limiting the diagnostic usefulness of LDH. However, five tissue-specific isoenzymes can be identified and measured, using heat inactivation or electrophoresis: two of these isoenzymes, LDH_1 and LDH_2, appear primarily in the heart, red blood cells, and kidneys; LDH_3, primarily in the lungs; and LDH_4 and LDH_5, in the liver and the skeletal muscles. The specificity of LDH isoenzymes and their distribution pattern is useful in diagnosing hepatic, pulmonary, and erythrocytic damage, but the widest clinical application (with other cardiac enzyme tests) is in diagnosing acute myocardial infarction (MI). LDH isoenzyme assay is also useful when creatine phosphokinase (CPK) has not been measured within 24 hours of an acute MI. The myocardial LDH level rises later than CPK (12 to 48 hours after infarction begins), peaks in 2 to 5 days, and drops to normal in 7 to 10 days, if tissue necrosis does not persist.

lactiferous   Of or pertaining to a structure that produces or conveys milk, as the tubules of the breasts.

lactiferous duct   One of many channels carrying milk from the lobes of each breast to the nipple.

lactin   See **lactose.**

lacto-, lact-   A combining form meaning 'of or pertaining to milk': *lactobacillus, lactopeptin, lactotoxin.*

lactobacillus   **1.** An antidiarrheal agent made from processed nonpathogenic bacteria of the genus *Lactobacillus.* **2.** Any one of a group of nonpathogenic, gram-positive rod-shaped bacteria that produce lactic acid from carbohydrates. Many species are normally found in the human intestinal tract and vagina.

lactogen   A drug or other substance that enhances the production and secretion of milk. —**lactogenic,** *adj.*

lactogenic hormone   See **prolactin.**

lacto-ovo-vegetarian   One whose diet consists primarily of foods of vegetable origin and also includes some animal products, as eggs, milk, and cheese but no meat, fish, or poultry. Also called **ovo-lacto-vegetarian.**

lactose   A disaccharide found in milk. On hydrolysis, lactose yields the monosaccharides glucose and galactose. Lactose is used as a lax-

ative, as a diuretic, and as a component of formulas for infants. Also called **lactin, milk sugar.** See also **sugar.**

lactose intolerance   A sensitivity disorder resulting in the inability to digest lactose owing to a deficiency of or defect in the enzyme lactase. Symptoms of the disorder are bloating, flatus, nausea, diarrhea, and abdominal cramps. The diet is adjusted according to the tolerance level, restricting such foods as milk, cheese, butter, margarine, and any products containing milk, as cakes, ice cream, cream soups, and sauces. See **lactase deficiency.**

lactulose   A hyperosmolar laxative also used in management of hepatic encephalopathy.

lacuna, *pl.* **lacunae**   **1.** A small cavity within a structure, especially bony tissue. **2.** A gap, as in the field of vision.

lacus lacrimalis   A triangular space separating the medial ends of the upper and the lower eyelids. It is an extension of the medial canthus and contains the lacrimal caruncle.

Laënnec's catarrh   A form of bronchial asthma characterized by the discharge of small, round, viscous, beadlike bodies of sputum. These bodies, Laënnec's pearls, are formed in the bronchioles and appear in the asthmatic's expectorated bronchial secretions.

Laënnec's cirrhosis   See **cirrhosis.**

Laënnec's pearls   See **Laënnec's catarrh.**

laevo-   See **levo-.**

lagen-   A combining form meaning 'flasklike': *lagena, lageniform.*

-lagnia, -lagny   A combining form meaning a 'sexual predilection': *osmolagnia, pyrolagnia, scoptolagnia.*

lagophthalmos   An abnormal condition in which an eye may not be fully closed owing to a neurologic or muscular disorder. Also called **hare's eye.**

la grippe   See **influenza.**

laked blood   Blood that is clear, red, and homogenous owing to hemolysis of the red blood cells, as may occur in poisoning and severe, extensive burns.

lal-, lalio-, lalo-   A combining form meaning 'talk, babble': *laliatry, lalognosis, lalopathology.*

-lalia   A combining form meaning a 'disorder of speech': *agitolalia, eschrolalia, oxylalia.*

lallation   **1.** Babbling, repetitive, unintelligible utterances, like the babbling of an infant, and the mumbled speech of schizophrenics, alcoholics, and the severely mentally retarded. **2.** A speech disorder characterized by a defective pronunciation of words containing the sound "l" or by the use of the sound "l" in place of the sound "r." Compare **lambdacism, rhotacism.**

Lamarckism   The theory postulated by French naturalist Jean Baptiste de Monet Lamarck that organic evolution results from structural changes in plants and animals that are caused by adaptation to environmental conditions, and that these acquired characteristics are transmitted to offspring. Also called **Lamarckianism, Lamarck's theory.** Compare **Dar-**

LAMBDOIDAL SUTURE OF THE SKULL

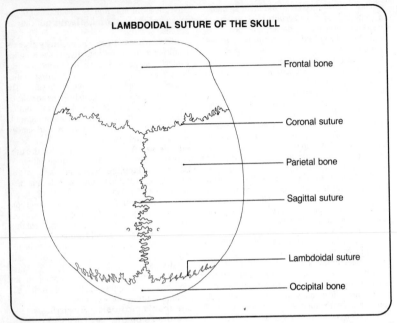

- Frontal bone
- Coronal suture
- Parietal bone
- Sagittal suture
- Lambdoidal suture
- Occipital bone

winian theory. —**Lamarckian,** *adj., n.*

Lamaze method   A method of psychophysical preparation for childbirth developed in the 1950s by a French obstetrician, Fernand Lamaze. The method was popularized in the United States by Marjorie Karmel who wrote the book, *Thank you, Dr. Lamaze,* based on her experience delivering a child in Paris under the care of Dr. Lamaze. The first program was established at Mount Sinai Hospital in New York City under the direction of Marjorie Karmel, Elizabeth Bing, a British physical therapist, and Dr. Alan Guttmacher. In 1960, the American Society for Psychoprophylaxis in Obstetrics was founded. The Lamaze method soon became the most often used method of natural childbirth. It requires classes, practice at home, and coaching during labor and delivery, often by a trained coach called a 'monitrice.' The classes, given during pregnancy, teach the physiology of pregnancy and childbirth, exercises to develop strength in the abdominal muscles and control of isolated muscles of the vagina and perineum, and techniques of breathing and relaxation to promote control and relaxation during labor. The woman is conditioned by repetition and practice to dissociate herself from the source of a stimulus by concentration on a focal point, by consciously relaxing all muscles, and by breathing in a special way at a particular rate, thereby training herself not to pay attention to the stimuli associated with labor. The kind and rate of breathing changes with the advancing stages of labor. Compare **Bradley method, Read method.**

lambdacism   A speech disorder characterized by a defective pronunciation of words containing the sound "l," or by the excessive use of the sound, or by the substitution of the sound "r" for "l." Compare **lallation, rhotacism.**

lambdoidal suture   The serrated connection between the occipital bone and the parietal bones of the skull. It is continuous with the occipitomastoid suture between the occipital and the mastoid portions of the temporal bones.

lamella, *pl.* **lamellae**   **1.** A thin leaf or plate, as of bone. **2.** A medicated disk, prepared from glycerin and an alkaloid, for insertion under the eyelid.

lamellar exfoliation of the newborn   A congenital skin disorder transmitted as an autosomal recessive trait in which a parchment-like, scaly membrane that covers the infant peels off within 24 hours of birth. Complete healing or a progressively less severe process of reforming and shedding of the scales then occurs. Also called **ichthyosis congenita, ichthyosis fetalis, lamellar desquamation of the newborn, lamellar ichthyosis of the newborn.** See also **collodion baby.**

lamin-   A combining form meaning 'layer': *laminagram, laminated, laminotomy.*

lamina, *pl.* **laminae**   A thin, flat plate, as the lamina of the thyroid cartilage that overlays the structure on each side.

laminated thrombus   A thrombus comprised of an aggregation of blood platelets, fibrin, clotting factors, and cellular elements, arranged in layers apparently formed at different times.

laminectomy   Surgical chipping away of the bony arches of one or more vertebrae, performed to relieve compression of the spinal cord, as caused

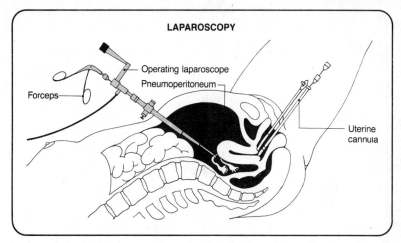

LAPAROSCOPY

Operating laparoscope
Pneumoperitoneum
Forceps
Uterine cannula

by a bone displaced in an injury or as the result of degeneration of a disk, or to reach and remove a displaced intervertebral disk. Spinal fusion may be necessary for stability of the spine if several laminae are removed. —**laminectomize,** *v.*

lampbrush chromosome An excessively large type of chromosome found in the oocytes of many lower animals. It has long, threadlike projecting loops, giving it a hairy, brushlike appearance. See also **giant chromosome.**

lampro- A combining form meaning 'clear': *lamprophonia, lamprophonic.*

lanatoside C A cardiotonic glycoside used to treat congestive heart failure and some cardiac arrhythmias.

lance To incise a furuncle or an abscess to release accumulated pus.

Lancefield's classification A serologic classification of streptococci based on their antigenic characteristics. The bacteria are divided into 13 groups by the identification of their pathologic action. Group A contains most of the streptococci that cause infection in humans. Groups B to T are less pathogenic and are often present without causing disease. Most are hemolytic; of those, the beta subgroup is the most likely to be the cause of infection.

Lancereaux's diabetes A chronic disease of carbohydrate metabolism characterized by marked emaciation. See also **diabetes mellitus.**

lancet **1.** A very small, pointed, surgical knife, sharp on both sides. **2.** A short pointed blade used to obtain a drop of blood for a capillary sample. It has a guard above the blade that prevents deep incision, and it is usually disposable.

lancinating Sharply cutting or tearing, as lancinating pain.

Landau reflex A normal response of infants when held in a horizontal prone position to maintain a convex arc with the head raised and the legs slightly flexed. The reflex is poor in those with floppy-infant syndrome and exaggerated in hypertonic and opisthotonic infants.

landmark position The correct placement of the hands on the chest in cardiopulmonary resuscitation. See also **cardiopulmonary resuscitation.**

Landsteiner's classification The classification of blood groups A, B, AB, and O on the basis of the presence or absence of the two agglutinogens A and B on the erythrocytes in human blood.

Langer's line See **cleavage line.**

Langhans' layer See **cytotrophoblast.**

lano- A combining form meaning 'of or pertaining to wool': *lanolin, lanonol, lanosterol.*

lanolin A fatlike substance from the wool of sheep. It contains about 25% water as a water-in-oil emulsion and is used as an ointment base and an emollient for the skin. Also called **hydrous wool fat.**

lanthanum (La) A rare-earth metallic element. Its atomic number is 57; its atomic weight is 138.91.

lanugo **1.** The soft, downy hair covering a normal fetus, beginning with the fifth month of life and almost entirely shed by the ninth month. **2.** The fine, soft hair covering all parts of the body except palms, soles, and areas where other types of hair are normally found. Also called **vellus hair.** —**lanulous,** *adj.*

laparo- A combining form meaning 'of or pertaining to the loin or flank': *laparocele, laparocolectomy, laparorrhaphy.*

laparoscope A type of endoscope, consisting of an illuminated tube with a fiber-optic system, which is inserted through the abdominal wall for examining the peritoneal cavity. Also called **celioscope, peritoneoscope.** —**laparoscopic,** *adj.,* **laparoscopy,** *v.*

laparoscopy Examination of the abdominal cavity with a laparoscope through a small incision in the abdominal wall. The procedure is also used for examining the ovaries and fallopian tubes and as a gynecologic sterilization technique for oviduct fulguration. Also called **abdominoscopy.** See also **endoscopy.**

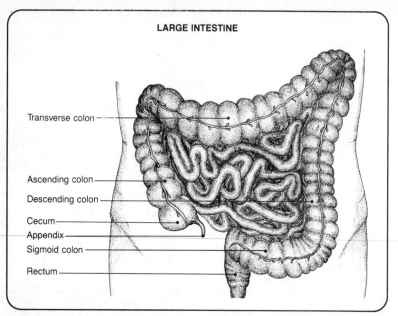

LARGE INTESTINE

Transverse colon

Ascending colon

Descending colon

Cecum

Appendix

Sigmoid colon

Rectum

laparotomy Any surgical incision into the peritoneal cavity, usually performed under general or regional anesthesia, often on an exploratory basis. Some kinds of laparotomy are **appendectomy, cholecystectomy, colostomy.** —**laparotomize,** *v.*

-lapse A combining form meaning 'a slip': *collapse, prolapse, relapse.*

large-for-gestational-age (LGA) infant An infant whose fetal growth was accelerated and whose size and weight at birth fall above the 90th percentile of appropriate-for-gestational-age infants, whether delivered prematurely, at term, or later than term. Factors other than genetic influences that cause accelerated intrauterine growth include maternal diabetes mellitus and Beckwith's syndrome. LGA infants born of diabetic mothers are generally obese and plethoric, with very pink skin and red, shiny cheeks. They are often listless and limp, feed poorly, and become hypoglycemic within the first few hours. A major problem is that preterm LGA infants, because of their size, are not recognized as high-risk neonates with immature organ system development. Often these infants develop respiratory distress syndrome because pulmonary maturation occurs later in gestation. In cases of Beckwith's syndrome, the infant is characterized by gigantism, macroglossia, omphalocele or umbilical hernia, and visceromegaly. Compare **small-for-gestational-age infant.**

large intestine The portion of the digestive tract comprising the cecum; the appendix; the ascending, transverse, and descending colons; and the rectum. The ileocecal valve separates the cecum from the ileum.

larva migrans See **cutaneous larva migrans, visceral larva migrans.**

laryng- See **laryngo-.**

laryngeal cancer A malignant neoplastic disease characterized by a tumor arising from the epithelium of the structures of the larynx. Laryngeal tumors are almost 20 times more common in men than in women and occur most frequently between the ages of 50 and 70. Chronic alcoholism and heavy use of tobacco increase the risk of developing the cancer. Persistent hoarseness is usually the first sign; advanced lesions may cause a sore throat, dyspnea, dysphagia, and unilateral cervical adenopathy. Diagnostic measures include direct laryngoscopy, biopsy, and radiologic examination, including tomographic studies and chest films. Malignant tumors of the larynx are usually epidermoid carcinomas. See also **laryngectomy.**

laryngeal catheterization The insertion of a catheter into the larynx for the purpose of removing secretions or introducing gases.

laryngeal prominence See **Adam's apple.**

laryngectomy Surgical removal of the larynx, performed to treat cancer of the larynx. In a partial laryngectomy only the vocal cords are removed, and a temporary tracheostomy is performed. If the malignancy is extensive the entire larynx is removed, along with the thyroid cartilage and epiglottis, and the tracheostomy is permanent. Compare **neck dissection, radical neck dissection.** —**laryngectomize,** *v.*

laryngitis Inflammation of the mucous membrane lining of the larynx, accompanied by edema of the vocal cords with hoarseness or loss of voice, occurring as an acute disorder caused

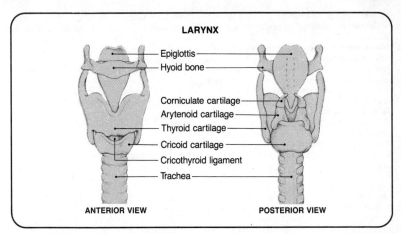

LARYNX

Epiglottis
Hyoid bone

Corniculate cartilage
Arytenoid cartilage
Thyroid cartilage
Cricoid cartilage
Cricothyroid ligament
Trachea

ANTERIOR VIEW   POSTERIOR VIEW

by a respiratory infection, by irritating fumes, by sudden temperature changes, or as a chronic condition resulting from excessive use of the voice, heavy smoking, or exposure to irritating fumes. Acute laryngitis may cause severe respiratory distress in children under the age of 5 because the relatively small larynx of the young child is subject to spasm when irritated or infected and readily becomes partially or totally obstructed. The youngster may develop a hoarse, barking cough and an inspiratory stridor and may become restless, gasping for air. Treatment consists of the administration of copious amounts of vaporized cool mist. Chronic laryngitis may be treated by removal of irritants, avoidance of smoking, voice rest, correction of faulty voice habits, cough medication, steam inhalations, and spraying the throat with an astringent antiseptic.

laryngo-, laryng- A combining form meaning 'of or pertaining to the larynx': *laryngocentesis, laryngograph, laryngometry.*

laryngopharyngitis Inflammation of the larynx and pharynx. See also **laryngitis, pharyngitis.**

laryngopharynx One of the three regions of the throat, extending from the hyoid bone to its termination in the esophagus. Compare **nasopharynx, oropharynx. —laryngopharyngeal,** *adj.*

laryngostasis See **croup.**

laryngotracheobronchitis (LTB) An inflammation of the major respiratory passages, usually causing hoarseness, nonproductive cough, and dyspnea. Among the causes are infection by coxsackieviruses, echoviruses, *Haemophilus influenzae,* and *Corynebacterium diphtheriae.* Treatment includes steam inhalations, cough suppressants, and, for bacterial infections, appropriate antibiotics. See also **croup.**

larynx The organ of voice that is part of the air passage connecting the pharynx with the trachea. It produces a large bump in the neck called the Adam's apple and is larger in men than in women although remaining the same size in men and women until puberty. The larynx forms the caudal portion of the anterior wall of the pharynx and is lined with mucous membrane that is continuous with that of the pharynx and the trachea. It is composed of three single cartilages and three paired cartilages, all connected together by ligaments and moved by various muscles. The single cartilages are the thyroid, cricoid, and epiglottis. The three paired cartilages are the arytenoid, corniculate, and cuneiform. The larynx is broad above and narrow and cylindrical at its caudal extremity. **—laryngeal,** *adj.*

laser Acronym for *light amplification by stimulated emission of radiation.* A source of intense radiation of the visible, ultraviolet, or infrared portions of the spectrum. It is produced by exposing a large number of electrons to a high energy level in a gaseous, solid, or liquid medium. The electrons emit very narrow beams of light, all of one wavelength and parallel to each other. Lasers are used in surgery to divide or cause adhesions or to destroy or fix tissue in place. Also called **optical maser.**

Lassa fever A highly contagious disease caused by a virulent arenavirus. It is characterized by fever, pharyngitis, dysphagia, and ecchymoses. Pleural effusion, edema and renal involvement, mental disorientation, confusion, and death from cardiac failure often ensue. Stringent precautions are taken against the spread of infection. Supportive, symptomatic care is the only treatment available.

late dyspituitary eunuchism See **acromegalic eunuchoidism.**

latency stage In psychoanalysis: a period in psychosexual development occurring between early childhood and puberty when sexual motivation and expression are repressed or transferred through sublimation to the feelings and behavioral patterns expected as typical of the age. The manifestations of this stage are culturally influenced and vary greatly. See also **psychosexual development.**

latent Dormant; existing as a potential, as

tuberculosis may be latent for extended periods of time and become active under certain conditions.

latent carcinoma See **occult carcinoma.**

latent diabetes A mild disorder of carbohydrate metabolism characterized by hyperglycemia or hyperinsulinemia only when stress loads of glucose are administered. Also called **chemical diabetes.** See also **diabetes mellitus.**

latent heart failure An abnormal condition characterized by inadequacy that is not apparent during rest but becomes evident under conditions of increased stress, as produced by exercise, fever, and emotional excitement. During stress situations the heart affected by latent failure is unable to pump an adequate supply of blood in relation to venous return and the metabolic needs of body tissues and structures.

latent period In radiology: an interval of seeming inactivity between the time of exposure to an injurious dose of radiation and the response.

latent phase The early stage of labor that is characterized by irregular, infrequent, and mild contractions and little or no dilatation of the cervix or descent of the fetus. Also called **prodromal labor.** See also **Friedman curve.**

latent schizophrenia A form of schizophrenia characterized by the presence of mild symptoms of the disease. Latent schizophrenics have no previous history of psychotic schizophrenic episodes but do have a preexisting susceptibility to the disease in its overt form. Also called **borderline schizophrenia, pseudoneurotic schizophrenia, pseudopsychopathic schizophrenia.** See also **schizophrenia, schizotypal personality disorder.**

lateral aortic node A lumbar lymph node in any of three clusters of nodes serving the pelvis and abdomen. The right lateral aortic nodes are situated partly ventral to the inferior vena cava, near the termination of the renal vein, and partly dorsal to the inferior vena cava on the right crus of the diaphragm. The left lateral aortic nodes form a chain on the left side of the abdominal aorta, ventral to the origin of the psoas major and ventral to the right crus of the diaphragm. The afferents from both sides drain various structures, as the testes, ovaries, kidneys, and lateral abdominal muscles. Most of the efferents from the lateral aortic nodes converge to form the right and the left lumbar trunks, which join the cisterna chyli. Compare **preaortic node, retroaortic node.**

lateral aperture of the fourth ventricle An opening between the end of each lateral recess of the fourth ventricle and the subarachnoid space.

lateral cerebral sulcus A deep cleft marking the division of the temporal, frontal, and parietal lobes of brain. Also called **fissure of Sylvius.**

lateral cuneiform bone One of the three cuneiform bones of the foot, located in the center of the front row of tarsal bones between the intermediate cuneiform bone medially, the cu-

boid bone laterally, the scaphoid bone posteriorly, and the third metatarsal anteriorly. It also articulates with the second and fourth metatarsals. Also called **external cuneiform bone, third cuneiform bone.**

lateral geniculate body One of two elevations of the lateral posterior thalamus receiving visual impulses from the retina via the optic nerves and tracts and relaying the impulses to the calcarine cortex.

lateral humeral epicondylitis See **epicondylitis.**

laterality See **handedness.**

lateral pectoral nerve One of a pair of branches from the brachial plexus that, with the medial pectoral nerve, supplies the pectoral muscles. It lies lateral to the axillary artery and arises from the lateral cord of the plexus or from the anterior divisions of the superior and the middle trunks just before they unite into the cord. It passes above to the first part of the axillary artery and the axillary vein, gives a filament to the inferior pectoral branch, pierces the clavipectoral fascia, and ends on the deep surface of the clavicular and the cranial sternocostal parts of the pectoralis major. Compare **medial pectoral nerve.**

lateral pelvic displacement One of the five major kinetic determinants of gait that helps to synchronize the rhythmic movements of walking. It is produced by the horizontal shift of the pelvis or by relative hip abduction. It is often a factor in the diagnosis and treatment of various orthopedic diseases, deformities, and abnormal conditions and in the analysis and the correction of dysfunctional gaits. Compare **knee-ankle interaction, knee-hip flexion, pelvic rotation, pelvic tilt.**

lateral recumbent position The posture assumed by the patient lying on the left side with the right thigh and knee drawn up. Also called **English position, obstetrical position.** See also **rotation.**

lateral umbilical fold A fold in the peritoneum produced by a slight protrusion of the inferior epigastric artery and the interfoveolar ligament. The lateral umbilical fold is about 3 cm (1¼ inches) lateral to the middle umbilical fold. Also called **plica umbilicalis lateralis.**

latero- A combining form meaning 'of or pertaining to the side': *laterodeviation, lateroduction, laterotorsion.*

late systolic murmur See **systolic murmur.**

latex fixation test A serologic test used in the diagnosis of rheumatoid arthritis in which antigen-coated latex particles agglutinate with rheumatoid factors in a slide specimen of serum or synovial fluid. If positive, the screening slide test is followed by titration. Also called **RA latex test, RF test.** See also **rheumatoid factor.**

latissimus dorsi One of a pair of large triangular muscles on the thoracic and lumbar areas of the back. The base of the triangle inserts through lumbar aponeuroses to the spines of lumbar and sacral vertebrae and in the supraspinous ligaments, posterior iliac crest, and the lower four ribs. The fibers of the muscle twist as they pass the scapula and converge at the base of the intertubercular groove of the humerus. The latissimus dorsi extends, adducts, and rotates the arm medially, draws the shoulder back and down, and, with the pectoralis major, draws the body up when climbing. It is innervated by the thoracodorsal nerve. Compare **levator scapulae, rhomboideus major, rhomboideus minor, trapezius.**

LATS *abbr* **long-acting thyroid stimulator.**

LATS-P *abbr* long-acting thyroid stimulator protector.

laughing gas *Informal.* Nitrous oxide, a side effect of which is laughter or giggling when administered in less than anesthetizing amounts.

lavage **1.** The process of washing out an organ, usually the bladder, bowel, paranasal sinuses, or stomach for therapeutic purposes. **2.** To perform a lavage. Kinds of lavage are **blood lavage, gastric lavage, peritoneal dialysis.** See also **irrigation.**

law **1.** In a field of study: a rule, standard, or principle that states a fact or a relationship between factors, as Dalton's law regarding partial pressures of gas or Koch's law regarding the specificity of a pathogen. **2. a.** A rule, principle, or regulation established and promulgated by a government to protect or to restrict the people affected. **b.** The field of study concerned with such laws. **c.** The collected body of the laws of a people, derived from custom and from legislation.

law of definite composition In chemistry: a law stating that a given compound is always made of the same elements present in the same proportion.

law of facilitation See **facilitation.**

law of independent assortment See **Mendel's laws.**

law of segregation See Mendel's laws.

law of universal gravitation In physics: a law stating that the force with which bodies are attracted to each other is directly proportional to the masses of the objects and inversely proportional to the square of the distance by which they are separated. See also **gravity, mass.**

lawrencium (Lr) A man-made transuranic metallic element. Its atomic number is 103; its atomic weight is 257.

laxative **1.** Of or pertaining to a substance that causes evacuation of the bowel by a mild action. **2.** A laxative agent that promotes bowel evacuation by increasing the bulk of the feces, by softening the stool, or by lubricating the intestinal wall. Compare **cathartic.**

lazy colon See **atonia constipation.**

LBW *abbr* **low–birth-weight.**

LD *abbr* lethal dose.

LD50 In toxicology: the amount of a substance sufficient to kill one half of the population of test, subjects.

LDH *abbr* **lactic dehydrogenase.**

L-dopa See **levodopa.**

LE *abbr* **lupus erythematosus.** See **systemic lupus erythematosus.**

lead (Pb) A common, soft, blue-gray, metallic element. Its atomic number is 82; its atomic weight is 207.2. In its metallic form, lead is used as a protective shielding against X-rays. Lead is poisonous, a characteristic that has led to a reduction in the use of lead compounds as pigments for paints and inks and as an antiknock additive in gasolines.

lead An electrical connection attached to the body to record electrical activity, especially of the heart or brain. See also **electrocardiograph, electroencephalograph.**

lead equivalent In radiology: the thickness of lead required to achieve the same shielding effect against radiation, under specified conditions, as that provided by a given material.

leader The person who manages patient care and supervises staff who provide this care. A leader assesses care needs, assigns staff to provide care, delegates authority, supervises and evaluates work, teaches patients and staff, and acts as patient-care coordinator.

lead pipe fracture A fracture that compresses the bony tissue at the point of impact and creates a linear fracture on the opposite side of the bone involved.

lead poisoning A toxic condition caused by the ingestion or inhalation of lead or lead compounds. Many children have developed the condition as a result of eating flaked lead-based paint. Poisoning also occurs from the ingestion of water from lead pipes, lead salts in certain foods and wines, the use of pewter or earthenware glazed with a lead glaze, and the use of leaded gasoline for cleaning. Inhalation of lead fumes is common in industry. The acute form of intoxication is characterized by a burning sensation in the mouth and esophagus, colic, constipation or diarrhea, mental disturbances, and paralysis of the extremities, followed in severe cases by convulsions and muscular collapse. Chronic lead poisoning, which is characterized by extreme irritability, anorexia, and anemia, may progress to the acute form. If ingested, treatment commences with gastric lavage with magnesium or sodium sulfate. All cases call for fluid therapy followed by chelation with intramuscular injection of calcium disodium edetate, or for severe cases, British anti-lewisite (BAL). Encephalopathy must be anticipated in children with lead poisoning.

leakage radiation Radiation, exclusive of the primary beam, that is emitted through the housing of equipment used in radiation therapy.

leaky gene See **hypomorph.**

learning **1.** The act or process of acquiring knowledge or some skill by means of study, practice, or experience. **2.** Knowledge, wisdom, or a skill acquired through systematic study or instruction. **3.** In psychology: the modification of behavior through practice, experience, or training. See also **conditioning.**

learning disability An abnormal condition often affecting children of normal or above-av-

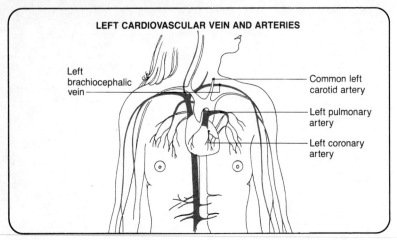

LEFT CARDIOVASCULAR VEIN AND ARTERIES

Left brachiocephalic vein

Common left carotid artery

Left pulmonary artery

Left coronary artery

erage intelligence, characterized by difficulty in learning such fundamental skills as reading, writing, and numerical calculation. The condition may result from psychological or organic causes and is usually related to slow development of perceptual motor skills. See also **attention deficit disorder, dysgraphia, dyslexia.**

Leber's congenital amaurosis A rare kind of blindness or severely impaired vision caused by a defect transmitted as an autosomal recessive trait and occurring at birth or shortly thereafter. The eyes appear normal externally, but pupillary constriction to light is sluggish or absent and retinal pigment is degenerated. Pendular nystagmus, photophobia, cataract, and keratoconus may be present and the ophthalmic disorder may be associated with mental retardation and epilepsy. Also called **amaurosis congenita of Leber.**

Leboyer method of delivery An approach to the delivery of an infant formulated by the French obstetrician, Charles Leboyer. It has four aspects: a gentle, controlled delivery in a quiet, dimly lit room; avoidance of pulling on the head; avoidance of overstimulation of the infant's sensorium; and encouragement of maternal-infant bonding. The goal of the method is to minimize the trauma of birth by gently and pleasantly introducing the newborn to life outside the womb. Following delivery, the baby is gently laid on the mother's abdomen, the back is massaged as the cord stops pulsating, and, when regular spontaneous respirations are established, the baby is gently supported in a warm tub of water. Compare **Bradley method, Lamaze method, Read method.**

lecithin Any of a group of phospholipids common in plants and animals. Lecithins are found in the liver, nerve tissue, semen, and in smaller amounts in bile and blood. They are essential for the metabolism of fats and are used in the processing of foods, pharmaceutical products, cosmetics, and inks. Rich dietary sources are soybeans, egg yolk, and corn. Deficiency leads

to hepatic and renal disorders, high serum cholesterol levels, atherosclerosis, and arteriosclerosis. See also **choline, inositol.**

lecitho- A combining form meaning 'of or pertaining to the yolk of an egg or to the ovum': *lecithoblast, lecithoprotein, lecithovitellin.*

Lee-White test A method of determining the length of time required for a clot to form in a test tube of venous blood. It is not specific for any coagulation disorder but is often used to monitor coagulation during heparin therapy. Because normal values and precise methodology vary, instructions are provided by most laboratories. See also **clotting time.**

Le Fort I fracture See **Guérin's fracture.**

left atrioventricular valve See **mitral valve.**

left brachiocephalic vein A vessel, about 6 cm (2½ inches) long, that starts in the root of the neck at the junction of the internal jugular and the subclavian veins on the left side and runs obliquely across the thorax to join the right brachiocephalic vein and form the superior vena cava. It receives various tributaries, as the vertebral vein, the internal thoracic vein, and the inferior thyroid vein. Also called left innominate vein. Compare **right brachiocephalic vein.**

left common carotid artery The longer of the two common carotid arteries, springing from the aortic arch and having cervical and thoracic portions. The cervical portion passes obliquely from the level of the sternoclavicular articulation to the cranial border of the thyroid cartilage, dividing into the left internal and the left external carotid arteries. Compare **right common carotid artery.**

left coronary artery One of a pair of branches from the ascending aorta, arising in the left posterior aortic sinus, dividing into the left interventricular artery and the circumflex branch, supplying both ventricles and the left atrium. Compare **right coronary artery.**

left-handedness A natural tendency to favor the use of the left hand in performing tasks.

Also called **sinistrality.** See also **cerebral dominance, handedness.**

left-heart failure An abnormal cardiac condition characterized by the impairment of the left side of the heart and by elevated pressure and congestion in the pulmonary veins and capillaries. Left-heart failure is usually related to right-heart failure, because both sides of the heart are part of a circuit and the impairment of one side will eventually affect the other. In "pure" left-heart failure, the body retains significant amounts of sodium and water and consequently develops peripheral edema without clinical evidence of right-heart failure. Also called left-sided failure. Compare **right-heart failure.**

left hepatic duct The duct that drains the bile from the left lobe of the liver into the common bile duct.

left lymphatic duct See **thoracic duct.**

left pulmonary artery The shorter and smaller of two arteries conveying venous blood from the heart to the lungs, rising from the pulmonary trunk, connecting to the left lung, and tending to have more separate branches than the right pulmonary artery. In the fetus it is larger and more important than the right pulmonary artery because it provides the ductus arteriosus. Compare **right pulmonary artery.**

left subclavian artery An artery, divided into three parts, that arises from the aortic arch dorsal to the left common carotid at the level of the fourth thoracic vertebra, ascends to the root of the neck, arches laterally to the scalenus anterior, and forms six main branches to supply the vertebral column, spinal cord, ear, and brain. The short second portion lies dorsal to the scalenus anterior and forms the arch described by the vessel. The third portion runs from the scalenus anterior to the first rib where it becomes the axillary artery. Compare **right subclavian artery.** See also **subclavian artery.**

left ventricle The thick-walled chamber of the heart that pumps blood through the aorta and the systemic arteries, the capillaries, and back through the veins to the right atrium. It has walls about three times thicker than those of the right ventricle and contains a mitral valve with two flaps that controls the flow of blood from the right atrium. The left ventricle occupies about half the diaphragmatic surface of the heart and is longer and more conical than the right ventricle, narrowing caudally to form the apex. The chordae tendinae of the left ventricle are thicker, stronger, and less numerous than those in the right ventricle. See also **heart.**

left ventricular failure Heart failure in which the left ventricle fails to contract forcefully enough to maintain a normal cardiac output and peripheral perfusion. Pulmonary congestion and edema develop from back pressure of accumulated blood in the left ventricle. Signs include breathlessness, pallor, sweating, and peripheral vasoconstriction. The heart is usually enlarged. A prominent third heart sound (gallop), normal in children and young adults, is a sign of left ventricular failure in older adults with heart disease. Hypertension is common and may be a causative factor or a result of pulmonary edema. Treatment includes meperidine or morphine for sedation, diuretics, digitalis, and rest.

legal death See **death.**

leg cylinder cast An orthopedic device of plaster of Paris or fiberglass used to immobilize the leg in treating fractures in the legs from the ankle to the upper thigh. It is used especially for fractures and dislocations of the knee, for soft tissue trauma around the knee, for postoperative positioning and immobilization of the knee, and for correction or maintenance of correction of deformities of the knee.

Legg-Calvé-Perthes' disease See Perthes' disease.

Legionella pneumophila A small, fastidious, gram-negative, rod-shaped bacterium that is the causative agent in **legionnaire's disease.**

legionnaire's disease An acute bacterial pneumonia caused by infection with *Legionella pneumophila* and characterized by an influenzalike illness followed within a week by high fever, chills, muscle aches, and headache. The symptoms may progress to dry cough, pleurisy, and sometimes diarrhea. Usually the disease is self-limited. Contaminated air-conditioning cooling towers and moist soil may be a source of organisms. Person-to-person contagion has not occurred. Treatment includes supportive care and administration of erythromycin. Also called legionellosis.

leio-, lio- A combining form meaning 'smooth': *leiodermia, leiodystonia, leiomyofibroma.*

leiomyoblastoma See **epithelioid leiomyoma.**

leiomyofibroma, *pl.* **leiomyofibromas, leiomyofibromata** A tumor consisting of smooth muscle cells and fibrous connective tissue, commonly occurring in the uterus in middle-aged women. See also **fibroid.**

leiomyoma, *pl.* **leiomyomas, leiomyomata** A benign tumor most commonly occurring in the stomach, esophagus, or small intestine. Surgical resection is necessary only in the rare case in which the tumor undergoes central necrosis, causing sudden and possibly severe hemorrhage.

leiomyoma cutis A neoplasm of the smooth muscles that raise the hair. The lesion is characterized by many small, tender, red nodules.

leiomyoma uteri A benign neoplasm of the smooth muscle of the uterus that is characteristically firm, well-circumscribed, round, and gray-white, and, under the microscope, shows a pattern of whorls. Multiple tumors of this kind develop most often in the myometrium and occur most frequently in women between the ages of 30 and 50. Also called **fibroids** *(informal)*, **fibromyoma uteri, myoma previum.**

leiomyosarcoma A malignant neoplasm of smooth muscle cells, commonly uterine or retroperitoneal.

leipo- See **lip-, lipo-.**

Leishman-Donovan body An intracellular, nonflagellated protozoan parasite that

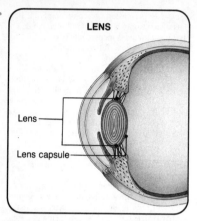

LENS

Lens

Lens capsule

causes visceral and cutaneous leishmaniasis.

leishmaniasis   Infection with any species of protozoan of the genus *Leishmania*, which is transmitted by sand flies. The diseases caused by these organisms may be cutaneous or visceral. Diagnosis is made by microscopic identification of the intracellular, nonflagellated protozoan on a Giemsa-stained smear taken from a cutaneous lesion or visceral biopsy. Kinds of leishmaniasis are **American leishmaniasis, kala-azar, oriental sore. —leishmanial,** *adj.*

-lemma   A combining form meaning a 'confining membrane': *axiolemma, epilemma, neurolemma.*

lemo-   A combining form meaning: **1.** 'Of or pertaining to plague': *lemography, lemology.* **2.** 'Of or pertaining to the gullet': *lemoparalysis, lemostenosis.*

lens   **1.** A curved, transparent piece of plastic or glass that is shaped, molded, or ground to refract light in a specific way, as in eyeglasses, microscopes, or cameras. **2.** The crystalline lens of the eye. —**lenticular,** *adj.*

lens capsule   The clear, thin, elastic capsule that surrounds the lens of the eye. Also called capsule of the lens.

lens implant   An artifical lens of clear polymethylmethacrylate that is usually implanted at the time of cataract extraction but may also be used for patients with extreme myopia, diplopia, ocular albinism, and certain other abnormalities. A high rate of complications is reported in implant surgery, and the procedure is contraindicated for patients with diabetes mellitus or uveitus.

Lente Iletin   A trade name for an antidiabetic (insulin zinc suspension).

Lente Insulin   A trade name for an antidiabetic (insulin zinc suspension).

lentigo, *pl.* **lentigenes**   A tan or brown macule on the skin brought on by sun exposure, usually in a middle-aged or older person. Another variety, called juvenile lentigo, is unrelated to sunlight and appears in children 2 to 5 years of age, before the onset of freckles. The melanin pigment in a lentigo is at a deeper level of the epidermis than in a freckle. Both types are benign and no treatment is necessary. Compare **freckle.**

lentigo maligna   See **Hutchinson's freckle.**

leontiasis ossea   See **macrocephaly.**

lepido-   A combining form meaning 'of or pertaining to a flake or scale': *lepidoma, lepidosis.*

LE prep   *abbr* **lupus erythematosus preparation.**

lepro-   A combining form meaning 'of or pertaining to leprosy': *leprologist, lepromatous, leprosarium.*

lepromin test   A skin sensitivity test used to distinguish between the lepromatous and tuberculoid forms of leprosy. The test consists of an intradermal injection of lepromin, which is prepared from heat-sterilized *Mycobacterium leprae.* The appearance of a palpable nodule in 8 to 10 days is indicative of the tuberculoid form of leprosy. As no nodule appears in the lepromatous form, the test is not diagnostic of leprosy. The test is used only to follow the course of the disease. See also **leprosy.**

leprosy   A chronic, communicable disease, caused by *Mycobacterium leprae,* that may take either of two forms, depending on the degree of immunity of the host. **Tuberculoid leprosy,** seen in those with high resistance, presents as thickening of cutaneous nerves and anesthetic, saucer-shaped skin lesions. Lepromatous leprosy, seen in those with little resistance, involves many systems of the body, with widespread plaques and nodules in the skin, iritis, keratitis, destruction of nasal cartilage and bone, testicular atrophy, peripheral edema, and involvement of the reticuloendothelial system. Blindness may result. Death is rare unless amyloidosis or tuberculosis occur concurrently. Contrary to traditional belief, leprosy is not very contagious, and transmission between individuals requires prolonged, intimate contact. Children are more susceptible than adults. Plastic surgery, physical therapy, and psychotherapy are often necessary. Treatment with sulfones, as dapsone, continued for several years usually results in improvement of skin lesions, but recovery from nerve impairment is limited. The disease is found mostly in underdeveloped tropical and subtropical countries. In the United States, patients may be referred to the U.S. Public Health Service leprosarium in Carville, Louisiana. Bacille Calmette-Guérin (BCG) vaccine may protect against leprosy. Also called **Hansen's disease.** See also *Mycobacterium.*
—**lepromatous, leprotic, leprous,** *adj.*

-lepsia   See **-lepsy.**

-lepsis   See **-lepsy.**

-lepsy   A combining form meaning a 'seizure': *deolepsy, electrolepsy, pyknolepsy.* Also **-lepsia, -lepsis.**

-leptic   A combining form meaning 'pertaining to a (specified) type of seizure': *cataleptic, epileptic, hypnoleptic.*

lepto-   A combining form meaning 'thin, or delicate': *leptocephalia, leptocyte, leptosome.*

leptocyte See **target cell.**

leptocytosis See **thalassemia.**

leptomeninges The arachnoid membrane and the pia mater, two of the three layers covering the spinal cord. Compare **meninges.**

leptonema The threadlike chromosome formation in the leptotene stage in the first meiotic prophase of gametogenesis before the beginning of synapsis.

leptospirosis An acute infectious disease caused by several serotypes of the spirochete *Leptospira interrogans,* transmitted in the urine of wild or domestic animals, especially rats and dogs. Human infections arise directly from contact with an infected animal's urine or tissues or indirectly from contact with contaminated water or soil. Clinical symptoms may include jaundice, hemorrhage into the skin, fever, chills, and muscle pain. The spirochete can be isolated from the urine or blood during the acute stage of the disease, and antibodies can be found in the patient's blood during convalescence. Treatment with antibiotics, usually penicillin or tetracycline, may be effective if they are administered during the first few days of the disease. Fluid and electrolyte replacement is essential if jaundice or other signs of severe illness are present. The disease is usually short-lived and mild, but severe infections can damage the kidneys and the liver. Blood pressure and vital signs should be monitored, and the patient's urine should be disposed of carefully to prevent spread of the organism. The most serious form of the disease is called **Weil's disease.** Also called **autumn fever.** See also **nanukayami.**

leptotene The initial stage in the first meiotic prophase in gametogenesis in which the chromosomes become visible as single thin filaments. See also **diakinesis, diplotene, pachytene, zygotene.**

Leriche syndrome A vascular disorder marked by gradual occlusion of the terminal aorta; intermittent claudication in the buttocks, thighs, or calves; absence of pulsation in femoral arteries; pallor and coldness of the legs; gangrene of the toes; and, in men, impotence. Symptoms are the result of chronic tissue hypoxia owing to inadequate arterial perfusion of the affected areas. Treatment may include endarterectomy, embolectomy, or synthetic bypass graft at the bifurcation of the aorta.

lesbian **1.** A female homosexual. **2.** Of or pertaining to the sexual preference or desire of one woman for another. —**lesbianism,** *n.*

Lesch-Nyhan syndrome A hereditary disorder of purine metabolism, characterized by mental retardation, self-mutilation of the fingers and lips by biting, impaired renal function, and abnormal physical development. It is transmitted as a recessive, sex-linked trait.

lesion Any visible, local abnormality of the tissues of the body, as a wound, sore, rash, or boil. A lesion may be described as benign, cancerous, gross, occult, or primary.

lesser multangular bone See **trapezoid bone.**

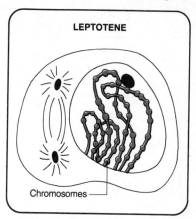

LEPTOTENE

Chromosomes

lesser occipital nerve One of a pair of cutaneous branches of the cervical plexus, arising from the second cervical nerve, curving around the sternocleidomastoideus, and ascending along the side of the head behind the ear to supply the skin. It communicates with the greater occipital and the great auricular nerves and with the posterior auricular branch of the facial nerve.

lesser omentum A membranous extension of the peritoneum from the peritoneal layers covering the ventral and the dorsal surfaces of the stomach and the first part of the duodenum. The lesser omentum extends from the porta of the liver to the diaphragm where the layers separate to enclose the end of the esophagus. It also forms two ligaments, one associated with the liver, the other with the duodenum. Also called **gastrohepatic omentum, small omentum.**

lesser trochanter One of a pair of conical projections at the base of the neck of the femur, providing insertion of the tendon of psoas major. Compare **greater trochanter.**

let-down A sensation in the breasts of lactating women that often occurs as the milk flows into the ducts, as when the infant begins to suck or when the mother hears the baby cry or even thinks of nursing the child.

let-down reflex See **milk-ejection reflex.**

leth- A combining form meaning 'of or pertaining to forgetfulness': *letheomania, letheral, lethologica.*

lethal equivalent Any recessive gene carried in the heterozygous state that, if homozygous, would be lethal and result in the death of the individual or organism before being transmitted. It is estimated that humans carry from three to eight lethal equivalents or any combination of many genes, each with slightly deleterious effects, that are equivalent to three to eight recessive genes.

lethal gene Any gene that produces a phenotypic effect that causes the death of the organism at some stage of development from fertilization of the egg to advanced age. The gene may be dominant, incompletely dominant, or

TYPES OF LEUKEMIA

GENERAL CLASS	SUBCLASS AND CELL TYPE	HISTOCHEMISTRY OR OTHER FEATURES	PROGNOSIS
Acute leukemias	• Subclass: acute lymphatic (ALL) • Cell: lymphoblasts	• Sudan black and PAS +	• Children (2 to 8 years): 50% cured, 90% show response to therapy • Adults: average survival 5 years
	• Subclass: acute myeloblastic (AML) • Cell: myeloblasts	• Peroxidase +	• Adults (15 to 75 years): 50% show response to therapy • Average survival 1 year
	• Subclass: acute monoblastic (monocytic) (AMOL) • Cell: monoblasts	• Muramidase +	• Children: 50% show response to therapy • Adults: average survival 1 year
Chronic leukemias	• Subclass: chronic granulocytic (CGL) • Cell: granulocytic precursors	• Ph¹ chromosome • Low LAP	• After chronic phase: 3 to 4 years • After acute phase: 3 to 6 months
	• Subclass: lymphocytic • Cell: B type	• Immunoglobulin or surface markers	• Average survival 5 years

recessive. In humans, examples of diseases caused by lethal genes are Huntington's chorea, which is transmitted by an autosomal dominant gene, and sickle cell anemia, which shows recessive lethality. Compare **sublethal gene.** See also **lethal equivalent.**

lethargic encephalitis See **epidemic encephalitis.**

lethargy 1. The state or quality of being indifferent, apathetic, or sluggish. **2.** Stupor or coma resulting from disease or hypnosis. Kinds of lethargy include **hysteric lethargy, induced lethargy, lucid lethargy.** —**lethargic,** *adj.*

Letterer-Siwe disease Any of a poorly classified group of malignant neoplastic diseases of unknown etiology, characterized by histiocytic elements. The disease, which is fatal, occurs in infancy and is not familial. Anemia, hemorrhage, splenomegaly, lymphadenopathy, and localized tumefactions over bones are usually present.

leucine A white, crystalline amino acid essential for optimal growth in infants and nitrogen equilibrium in adults. It cannot be synthesized by the body and is obtained by the hydrolysis of protein during pancreatic digestion. An inherited defect in one of the enzymes involved in the process results in a rare disorder called maple syrup urine disease. See also **maple syrup urine disease.**

leucinosis See **maple syrup urine disease.**

leuco- See **leuko-.**

leucovorin calcium An antianemic. See **folinic acid.**

leukemia A malignant neoplasm of blood-forming organs characterized by diffuse replacement of bone marrow with proliferating leukocyte precursors, abnormal numbers and forms of immature white cells in circulation, and infiltration of lymph nodes, the spleen, liver, and other sites. Males are affected twice as frequently as females. The etiology of leukemia is not clear, but it may result from exposure to ionizing radiation, benzene, or other chemicals that are toxic to bone marrow. The risk of the disease is increased in individuals with Down's syndrome, Fanconi's anemia, ataxia-telangiectasia, Bloom's syndrome, or some other forms of congenital aneuploidy, and in an identical twin of a leukemia patient. Leukemia is classified according to the predominant proliferating cells, the clinical course, and the duration of the disease. Also called leukocythemia. See also **acute childhood leukemia, acute lymphocytic leukemia, acute myelocytic leukemia, chronic lymphocytic leukemia, chronic myelocytic leukemia, monocytic leukemia.** —**leukemic, leukemoid,** *adj.*

-leukemia A combining form meaning an

'increased number of leukocytes in the tissues and/or in the blood': *chloroleukemia, erythroleukemia, hypoleukemia.*

leukemia cutis A condition in which yellow-brown, red, or purple nodular lesions and diffuse infiltrations or large accumulations of leukemic cells develop in the skin. It may be general or localized, usually in the skin of the face. Also called **lymphoderma perniciosa.**

leukemic reticuloendotheliosis See **hairy-cell leukemia.**

leukemoid Resembling leukemia.

leukemoid reaction A clinical syndrome resembling leukemia in which the white blood cell count is elevated in response to an allergy, inflammatory disease, infection, poison, hemorrhage, burn, or other causes of severe physical stress. Compare **leukemia.**

leuko- A combining form meaning 'of or pertaining to a white corpuscle, or white': *leukoblast, leukomaine, leukoplakia.* Also **leuco-.**

leukocyte A white blood cell; one of the formed elements of the circulating blood system. There are five types of leukocytes, classified by the presence or absence of granules in the cytoplasm of the cell. The agranulocytes are lymphocytes and monocytes. The granulocytes are neutrophils, basophils, and eosinophils. White cells are able to squeeze through intracellular spaces by diapedesis and migrate by ameboid movements. A cubic mm of normal blood usually contains 5,000 to 12,000 leukocytes. Among the most important functions of the leukocytes are phagocytosis of bacteria, fungi, and viruses; detoxification of toxic proteins that may result from allergic reactions and cellular injury; and the development of immunities. Also called **white blood cell, white corpuscle.** Compare **erythrocyte, platelet.** See also **leukocytosis, leukopenia. —leukocytic,** *adj.*

leukocytic crystal See **Charcot-Leyden crystal.**

leukocytosis An abnormal increase in the number of circulating white blood cells. An increase often accompanies bacterial, but not usually viral infections. The normal range is 5,000 to 10,000 white cells per cubic mm of blood. Leukemia may be associated with a white blood cell count as high as 500,000 to 1 million per cubic mm of blood, the increase being either equally or disproportionately distributed among all types. Kinds of leukocytosis include **basophilia, eosinophilia, neutrophilia.** Compare **leukemia, leukemoid reaction, leukopenia.** See also **leukocyte.**

leukoderma Localized loss of skin pigment owing to any of a number of specific causes. Compare **vitiligo.**

leukoerythroblastic anemia An abnormal condition in which there are large numbers of immature white and red blood cells. It is characteristic of some anemias that occur as a result of the replacement of normal bone marrow with malignant tumor. See also **myeloid metaplasia, myelophthisic anemia.**

leukonychia White spots or streaks on nails,

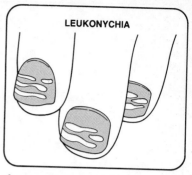

LEUKONYCHIA

often caused by trauma, infection, or systemic illness. A benign condition in which the nails are pure white occurs rarely, and its cause is unknown.

leukopenia An abnormal decrease in the number of white blood cells to fewer than 5,000 cells per cubic mm. Leukopenia may be caused by an adverse drug reaction, radiation poisoning, or other pathological conditions and may affect one or all kinds of white blood cells. Leukopenia may also occur secondary to cancer chemotherapy and/or radiation therapy. The two most common forms of leukopenia are neutrophilic leukopenia and lymphocytic leukopenia. Also called leukocytopenia. Compare **leukocytosis.** See also **aplastic anemia, leukocyte. —leukopenic,** *adj.*

leukopenic leukemia See **subleukemic leukemia.**

leukophlegmasia See **phlegmasia alba dolens.**

leukophoresis A laboratory procedure in which white blood cells are separated by electrophoresis for identification and an evaluation of the types of cells and their proportions.

leukoplakia A precancerous, slowly developing change in a mucous membrane characterized by thickened, white, firmly attached patches that are slightly raised and sharply circumscribed. They may occur on the penis or vulva; those appearing on the lips and buccal mucosa are associated with pipe smoking. Malignant potential is evaluated by microscopic study of biopsied tissue. Compare **lichen planus.** See also **lichen sclerosis et atrophicus.**

leukopoiesis The process by which white blood cells form and develop. Neutrophils, basophils, and eosinophils are produced in myeloid tissue in the bone marrow. Lymphocytes and monocytes are almost all normally derived from hemocytoblasts in lymphoid tissue, but a few develop in the marrow. **—leukopoietic,** *adj.*

leukorrhea A white discharge from the vagina. Normally, vaginal discharge occurs in regular variations of amount and consistency during the course of the menstrual cycle. A greater than usual amount is normal in pregnancy and a decrease is to be expected after delivery, during lactation, and after menopause. An irritating, pruritic, copious, foul-smelling, green or

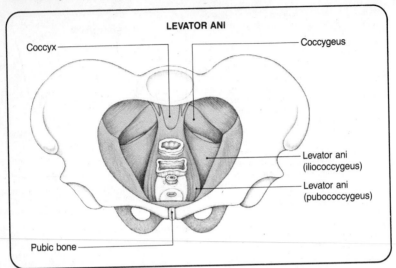

LEVATOR ANI

Coccyx

Coccygeus

Levator ani (iliococcygeus)

Levator ani (pubococcygeus)

Pubic bone

yellow discharge may indicate vaginal or uterine infection or other pathology of gynecologic origin. Leukorrhea is the most common reason why women seek gynecologic care. See also **vaginal discharge.**

leukotomy   See **lobotomy.**

leukotoxin   A substance that can inactivate or destroy leukocytes. —**leukotoxic,** *adj.*

levallorphan tartrate   A narcotic antagonist.

levamisole   A new drug used as an anthelmintic agent against a wide variety of nematodes. It is also under investigation as a stimulant of the immune system that may be effective in the prophylaxis and treatment of bacterial and viral infections.

levarterenol bitartrate   See **norepinephrine injection.**

levator, *pl.* **levators**   **1.** A muscle that raises a structure of the body, as the levator ani raises parts of the pelvic diaphragm. **2.** A surgical instrument used to lift depressed bony fragments in fractures of the skull and other bones.

levator ani   One of a pair of muscles of the pelvic diaphragm that stretches across the bottom of the pelvic cavity like a hammock, supporting the pelvic organs. It is a broad, thin muscle that separates into the pubococcygeus and the iliococcygeus. It originates from the ramus of the pubic bone, the spine of the ischium, and a band of fascia between the pubis and the ischium; it inserts into the last two segments of the coccyx, the anococcygeal raphe, the sphincter ani externus, and the central tendinous point of the perineum. The levator ani is innervated by branches of the pudendal plexus, which contains fibers from the fourth sacral nerve, and it functions to support and slightly raise the pelvic floor. The pubococcygeus draws the anus toward the pubis and constricts it. Compare **coccygeus.**

levator palpebrae superioris   One of the three muscles of the eyelid, also considered a muscle of the eye. It is thin and flat and rises from the small wing of the sphenoid. It splits into three lamellae: the superficial lamella extends to the upper eyelid; the middle lamella inserts into the superior tarsus; and the deep lamella is attached to the conjunctiva. It is innervated by the oculomotor nerve, raises the upper eyelid, and is the antagonist of the orbicularis oculi. Compare **corrugator supercilii, orbicularis oculi.**

levator scapulae   A muscle of the dorsal and lateral aspects of the neck. It arises from the axis and the atlas, and it inserts in the third and fourth cervical vertebrae. It is innervated by the third and fourth cervical nerves and acts to raise the scapula and pull it toward the midline.

LeVeen shunt   A tube that is surgically implanted to connect the peritoneal cavity and the superior vena cava to drain an accumulation of fluid in the peritoneal cavity in cirrhosis of the liver, right-sided heart failure, or cancer of the abdomen. Under anesthesia, a silicone-rubber tube is inserted under the subcutaneous tissue from the peritoneum to the superior vena cava. As the patient inhales, the fluid pressure in the peritoneal cavity rises and that in the blood vessel falls, allowing peritoneal fluid to enter the shunt valve. Excessive dilution of the blood may lead to abnormalities of coagulation.

level of consciousness   The degree of awareness of one's surroundings. This may be affected by a neurologic injury or from nonneurologic causes, such as electrolyte imbalance, hepatic coma, hypoglycemia, hypoxia, or sedative overdose. See **alert, coma, delirium, lethargy, obtund, stupor.**

levels of care   A classification of health-care service levels by the kind of care given, the number of people served, and the people providing the care. Kinds of health-care service levels are **primary health care, secondary health care, tertiary health care.**

lever In physiology: any one of the numerous bones and associated joints of the body that act together as a lever so that force applied to one end of the bone to lift a weight at another point tends to rotate the bone in the direction opposite from that of the applied force.

Levi-Lorain dwarf See **pituitary dwarf.**

Levin tube A plastic catheter, used in gastric intubation, that has a closed, weighted tip and an opening on the side. Compare **Miller-Abbott tube.** See also **gastric intubation.**

levitation In psychiatry: a hallucinatory sensation of floating or of rising in the air. —**levitate,** *v.*

levo- A combining form meaning 'left': *levocardia, levoclination, levotorsion.*

levodopa An antiparkinsonism agent.

levodopa and carbidopa A combination of two antiparkinsonism agents.

levopropoxyphene napsylate A nonnarcotic antitussive.

levorphanol tartrate A narcotic and opioid analgesic.

levothyroxine sodium (T₄ or L-thyroxine sodium) A thyroid hormone.

levulose See **fructose.**

levulosuria See **fructosuria.**

lewisite 2-chlorovinyl arsine; a poisonous gas, used in World War I, that causes irritation of the lungs, dyspnea, damage to the tissues of the respiratory tract, tears, and pain.

-lexia A combining form meaning 'reading': *alexia, bradylexia, dyslexia.*

Leyden-Moebius muscular dystrophy See **pelvifemoral muscular dystrophy.**

Leydig cell tumor A generally benign neoplasm of interstitial cells of a testis that may cause gynecomastia in adults and precocious sexual development if the lesion occurs before puberty. The tumor is usually a circumscribed, lobulated, palpable mass.

Leydig's cells Cells of the interstitial tissue of the testes that secrete testosterone.

LFT *abbr* **liver function test.**

LGA *abbr* **large for gestational age.**

LGV *abbr* **lymphogranuloma venereum.**

LH *abbr* **luteinizing hormone.**

Lhermitte's sign Sudden, transient, electriclike shocks spreading down the body when the head is flexed forward, occurring chiefly in multiple sclerosis but also in compression disorders of the cervical spinal cord.

Li Symbol for **lithium.**

liability 1. Something one is obligated to do or an obligation required to be fulfilled by law, usually financial in nature. 2. The amount of money required to fulfill a financial obligation.

libel A false accusation written, printed, or typewritten, or presented in a picture or a sign that is made with malicious intent to defame the reputation of a living person or the memory of a dead person, resulting in public embarrass-

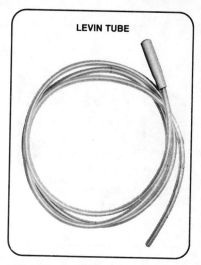

LEVIN TUBE

ment, contempt, ridicule, or hatred.

libidinal development See **psychosexual development.**

libidinous, libidinal 1. Pertaining to or belonging to the libido. 2. Having or characterized by sexual desire. —**libidinize,** *v.*

libido 1. The psychic energy or instinctual drive associated with sexual desire, pleasure, or creativity. 2. In psychoanalysis: the instinctual drives of the id. 3. Lustful desire or striving. Kinds of libido are **bisexual libido, ego libido.**

Libman-Sacks endocarditis An abnormal condition and the most common manifestation of lupus erythematosus, characterized by verrucous lesions that develop near the heart valves but rarely affect valvular action. The lesions are usually dry and granular, with a pink or tawny color, contain basophilic cellular debris, and develop in the angle of the atrioventricular valves and at the base of the mitral valve.

Libman-Sacks syndrome A typical verrucous endocarditis occurring with systemic lupus erythematosus. Also called Libman-Sacks disease.

licensed practical nurse (LPN) *U.S.* A person trained in basic nursing techniques and direct patient care who practices under the supervision of a registered nurse. The course of training usually lasts 1 year. In Canada an LPN is called a nursing assistant. Also called **licensed vocational nurse** *(U.S.).*

licensed psychologist A person who has earned a Ph.D. in psychology from an accredited graduate school and has completed 2 to 3 years of postgraduate training with special emphasis on the diagnosis and treatment of psychological disorders. Also called clinical psychologist. See also **psychotherapist.**

licensed vocational nurse (LVN) See **licensed practical nurse.**

licensure The granting of permission by a competent authority (usually a governmental

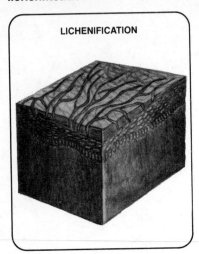

LICHENIFICATION

agency) to an organization or individual to engage in a practice or activity that would otherwise be illegal. Kinds of licensure include the issuing of licenses for general hospitals or nursing homes; for health professionals, as physicians; and for the production or distribution of biological products. Licensure is usually granted on the basis of education and examination rather than performance. It is usually permanent, but a periodic fee, demonstration of competence, or continuing education may be required. Licensure may be revoked by the granting agency for incompetence, criminal acts, or other reasons stipulated in the rules governing the specific area of licensure.

lichenification Thickening and hardening of the skin, often resulting from the irritation caused by repeated scratching of a pruritic lesion. —**lichenified,** *adj.*

lichen nitidus A rare skin disorder characterized by numerous flat, glistening, pale, discrete papules measuring 2 to 3 mm in diameter. Also called **Pinkus' disease.**

lichen planus A nonmalignant, chronic, pruritic skin disease of unknown cause, characterized by small, flat, purplish papules or plaques having fine, gray lines on the surface. Common sites are flexor surfaces of wrists, forearms, ankles, abdomen, and sacrum. On mucous membranes the lesions appear gray and lacy. Nails may have longitudinal ridges. Episodes of disease activity, of which there are numerous variations, may last for months and may recur. Compare **leukoplakia.**

lichen sclerosis et atrophicus A chronic skin disease characterized by white, flat papules with an erythematous halo and black, hard follicular plugs. In advanced cases, the papules tend to coalesce into large, white patches of thin, pruritic skin. Lesions often occur on the torso and in the anogenital regions, in which case the disease is called kraurosis vulvae. Corticosteroids are applied topically to reduce itching.

lichen simplex chronicus A form of neurodermatitis characterized by a patch of pruritic, confluent papules. Psychogenic factors and mechanical trauma, as scratching, contribute to its chronicity. Treatment may include topical or intralesional application of corticosteroids to relieve the pruritis.

licorice See **liquorice.**

lid See **eyelid.**

lidocaine, l. hydrochloride An amide local antipruritic, topical anesthetic and group II antiarrhythmic.

lie detector An electronic device or instrument used to detect lying or anxiety in regard to specific questions. A commonly used lie detector is the polygraph recorder, which senses and records pulse, respiratory rate, blood pressure, and perspiration. Some experts hold that certain patterns indicate the presence of anxiety, guilt, or fear, emotions that are likely to occur when the subject is lying.

lien See **spleen.** —**lienal,** *adj.*

lienal vein A large vein of the lower body that unites with the superior mesenteric vein to form the portal vein. It returns blood from the spleen and arises from about six large tributaries that unite to form the single vessel passing from left to right across the superior, dorsal part of the pancreas. It receives the short gastric veins, the left gastroepiploic vein, the pancreatic veins, and the inferior mesenteric veins. Also called **splenic vein.**

lieno- A combining form meaning 'of or pertaining to the spleen': *lienomalacia, lienomedullary, lienopathy.*

life costs The mortality, morbidity, and suffering associated with a given disease or medical procedure.

life expectancy See **expectation of life.**

life science The study of the laws and properties of living matter. Some kinds of life science are **anatomy, bacteriology, biology.** Compare **physical science.**

ligament 1. One of many predominantly white, shiny, flexible bands of fibrous tissue binding joints together and connecting various bones and cartilages. Such ligaments are slightly elastic and composed of parallel collagenous bundles. When part of the synovial membrane of a joint, they are covered with fibroelastic tissue that blends with surrounding connective tissue. Yellow elastic ligaments, as the ligamenta flava, connect certain parts of adjoining vertebrae. Compare **tendon.** 2. A layer of serous membrane with little or no tensile strength, extending from one visceral organ to another, as the ligaments of the peritoneum. Also called **ligamentum.** See also **broad ligament.** —**ligamentous,** *adj.*

ligamenta flava The bands of yellow elastic tissue connecting the laminae of adjacent vertebrae from the axis to the first segment of the sacrum. They are thin, broad, and long in the cervical region, thicker in the thoracic region, and thickest in the lumbar region. They help to hold the body erect.

ligamental tear   A complete or a partial tear of a ligamentous structure connecting and surrounding the bones of a joint, caused by an injury to the joint, as by a sudden twisting motion or by a forceful blow. Ligamental tears may occur at any joint but are most common in the knees. The pathologic features of ligamental tears of the knee are dependent on the location and severity of the injury. The most common ligaments involved in knee injuries are the medial, lateral, and posterior ligaments and the anterior and posterior cruciate ligaments. Usually, the injury involves more than one structure because of the way in which the structures connect with and support each other. Treatment depends on the severity of the injury. A mild injury may cause little damage, with tenderness, swelling, and pain when stressed. Rest, compression, applications of heat and cold, elevation, and early use are usually recommended. Treatment for a moderate injury in which few fibers have been completely torn is protective. Treatment for a severe, complete tear is restorative. This may be by immobilization followed by physical therapy, or if necessary, by surgical repair.

ligament of the neck of the rib   One of five ligaments of each costotransverse joint, consisting of short, strong fibers passing from the neck of the rib to the transverse process of the adjacent vertebra. Also called **middle costotransverse ligament.**

ligament of the tubercle of the rib   One of the five ligaments of each costotransverse joint, comprised of a short, thick fasciculus passing obliquely from the transverse process of a vertebra to the tubercle of the associated rib. Compare **ligament of the neck of the rib.**

ligamentum, *pl.* **ligamenta**   See **ligament.**
ligamentum latum uteri   See **broad ligament.**

ligamentum nuchae   The fibrous membrane that reaches from the external occipital protuberance and median nuchal line to the spinous process of the seventh vertebra. A fibrous lamina from the ligament attaches to the posterior tubercle of the atlas and to the spinous processes of the cervical vertebrae, forming a septum between muscles on either side of the neck.

ligation   Tying off of a blood vessel or duct with a suture or wire ligature performed to stop or prevent bleeding during surgery, to stop spontaneous or traumatic hemorrhage, or to prevent passage of material through a duct, as in tubal ligation or to treat varicosities. In venous ligation, the saphenous vein is tied above the varicosed portion, and the distal portions are removed. See also **ligature, tubal ligation. — ligate,** *v.*

ligature   **1.** A suture. **2.** A wire, as used in orthodontia.

ligature needle   A long, thin, curved needle used for passing a suture underneath an artery for ligation of the vessel.

light   **1.** Electromagnetic radiation of the wavelength and frequency that stimulates visual

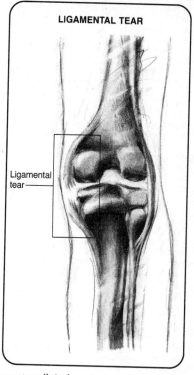

LIGAMENTAL TEAR

Ligamental tear —

receptor cells in the retina to produce nerve impulses that are perceived as vision. **2.** Electromagnetic radiation with wavelengths shorter than ultraviolet light and longer than infrared light, the range of visible light.

light bath   The exposure of uncovered skin to the sun or to actinic light rays from an artificial source for therapeutic purposes.

light diet   A diet suitable for convalescent or bedridden patients taking little or no exercise. It consists of simple, moderate quantities of soft-cooked and easily digested foods.

lightening   A subjective sensation reported by many women late in pregnancy as the fetus settles lower in the pelvis, leaving more space in the upper abdomen. The diaphragm, no longer restricted by the fundus of the uterus beneath it, can move down more fully during inspiration, allowing deeper breaths to be taken. The stomach, too, is less compressed so the woman can comfortably eat more food at a sitting. The profile of the abdomen changes with lightening, as the round, full uterus is visibly lower. The fetus is then said to have 'dropped.'

light reflex   The mechanism by which the pupil of the eye becomes more or less open in response to direct or consensual pupillary stimulation. Also called **pupillary reflex.** See also **consensual reaction to light.**

ligneous thyroiditis   See **fibrous thyroiditis.**

lignin A polysaccharide that with cellulose and hemicellulose forms the chief part of the skeletal substances of the cell walls of plants. It provides bulk in the diet necessary for the proper gastrointestinal functioning. See also **dietary fiber.**

lilliputian hallucination A sensory perception in which things seem smaller than they actually are. See also **hallucination.**

limb 1. An appendage or extremity of the body, as an arm or leg. 2. A branch of an internal organ, as a loop of a nephron.

limb-girdle muscular dystrophy A form of muscular dystrophy transmitted as an autosomal recessive trait. The characteristic weakness and degeneration of the muscles begins in the shoulder girdle or in the pelvic girdle. The condition is progressive, regardless of the area in which it is first manifest. Kinds of limb-girdle muscular dystrophy are **pelvifemoral muscular dystrophy, scapulohumeral muscular dystrophy.**

limbic system A group of structures within the rhinencephalon of the brain that are associated with various emotions and feelings, as anger, fear, sexual arousal, pleasure, and sadness. The structures of the limbic system are the cingulate gyrus, the isthmus, the hippocampal gyrus, the uncas, and the hippocampus. The structures connect with various other parts of the brain, as the septum and the hypothalamus. Unless the limbic system is modulated by other cortical areas, periodic attacks of uncontrollable rage may occur in some individuals. The function of the system is poorly understood.

limb-kinetic apraxia See **ideomotor apraxia.**

lime 1. Any of several oxides and hydroxides of calcium. The various kinds of lime have many uses, including the treatment of sewage, purification of water and refining of sugar, and the manufacture of materials like plaster and fertilizers. 2. A citrus fruit yielding a juice with a high ascorbic acid content. Lime juice was one of the first effective agents to be used in the treatment of scurvy. See also **ascorbic acid, scurvy.**

limo- A combining form meaning 'of or pertaining to hunger': *limophthisis, limosis, limotherapy.*

limp An abnormal pattern of ambulation in which the two phases of gait are markedly asymmetric. See also **stance phase of gait, swing phase of gait.**

lincomycin hydrochloride An antibiotic.

lindane See **gamma benzene hexachloride.**

Lindau-von Hippel disease See **cerebroretinal angiomatosis.**

Lindbergh pump A pump used to preserve an organ of the body by perfusing its tissues with oxygen and other essential nutrients, usually during the transport of an organ from a donor to a recipient. Also called **Carrel-Lindbergh pump.**

linea alba The portion of the anterior abdominal aponeurosis in the middle line of the abdomen, representing the fusion of three aponeuroses into a single tendinous band extending from the xiphoid process to the symphysis pubis. It contains the umbilicus. Compare **linea semilunaris.**

linea arcuata The curved tendinous band in the sheath of the rectus abdominis below the umbilicus. It is usually derived from the aponeurosis of the transversus abdominis or the obliquus internus, or sometimes from both those muscles. It inserts into the linea alba. Compare **linea semilunaris.**

linea aspera The posterior crest of the thigh bone, extending proximally into three ridges to which are attached various muscles, including the gluteus maximus, pectineus, and iliacus.

linear accelerator (LINAC) An apparatus for accelerating charged subatomic particles used in radiotherapy, physics research, and in the production of radionuclides. In a linear accelerator, a pulsed electron beam generated by an electron gun passes through a straight, long vacuum tube containing alternating hollow electrodes. The electrodes are so arranged that when their high-frequency potentials are properly varied, the particles passing through the vacuum-tube waveguide receive successive increments of energy. The electrons are stopped abruptly by a heavy metal target at the end of the waveguide and are directed by a collimator to deliver supervoltage X-rays to the patient receiving radiotherapy.

linear fracture A fracture that extends parallel to the long axis of a bone but does not displace the bone tissue.

linea semilunaris The slightly curved line on the ventral abdominal wall, located approximately parallel to the median line and lying about halfway between the median line and the side of the body. It marks the lateral border of the rectus abdominis and can be seen as a shallow groove when that muscle is tensed. Compare **linea alba.**

line position The official position of an employee in an organizational hierarchy; a position in the direct line of authority.

lingu- A combining form meaning 'of or pertaining to the tongue': *linguiform, lingulectomy, linguodental.*

lingual artery One of a pair of arteries that arises from the external carotid arteries, divides into four branches, and supplies the tongue and surrounding muscles. The branches of the lingual artery are the suprahyoid, dorsal lingual, sublingual, and the deep lingual.

lingual bone See **hyoid bone.**

lingual frenum A band of tissue that extends from the floor of the mouth to the inferior surface of the tongue. Also called **frenulum linguae.**

lingual goiter A tumor at the back of the tongue formed by an enlargement of the primordial thyrolingual duct.

lingual papilla See **papilla.**

lingual tonsil A mass of lymphoid follicles near the root of the tongue. Each follicle forms a rounded eminence containing a small opening leading into a funnel-shaped cavity surrounded by lymphoid tissue.

lingua villosa nigra See **parasitic glossitis.**

liniment A preparation, usually containing an alcoholic, oily, or soapy vehicle, that is rubbed on the skin as a counterirritant.

linitis Inflammation of cellular tissue of the stomach as in linitis plastica, seen frequently in adenocarcinoma of the stomach. The layer of connective tissue of the stomach becomes fibrotic and thick, and the stomach wall becomes shrunken and rigid. Causes of this condition include infiltrating undifferentiated carcinoma, syphilis, and Crohn's disease involving the stomach. Also called **leather-bottle stomach.**

linkage **1.** In genetics: the location of two or more genes on the same chromosome so that they do not segregate independently during meiosis but tend to be transmitted together as a unit. The closer the loci of the genes, the more likely they are to be inherited as a group and associated with a specific trait, while the farther apart they are, the greater the chance that they will be separated by crossing over and carried on homologous chromosomes. The concept of linkage, which opposes the independent assortment theory of Mendelian genetics, led to the foundation of the modern chromosome theory of genetics. See also **synteny.** **2.** In psychology: the association between a stimulus and the response it elicits. **3.** In chemistry: the bond between two atoms or radicals in a chemical compound or the lines used to designate valency connections between the atoms in structural formulas.

linkage group In genetics: a group of genes located on the same chromosome that tends to be inherited as a unit. Theoretically, without crossing over, all of the genes on a given chromosome constitute a linkage group and are equal to the number of autosomes in the haploid cell.

linkage map See **genetic map.**

linked genes Genes that are located on the same chromosome and whose position is close enough so that they tend to be transmitted as a linkage group.

linoleic acid An essential fatty acid with three unsaturated bonds, occurring in linseed and safflower oils.

lio- See **leio-.**

liothyronine sodium A synthetic thyroid hormone.

liotrix A thyroid hormone.

lip-, lipo- A combining form meaning 'fat': *lipase, lipodystrophy, lipoma.*

lipase Any of several enzymes, produced by the organs of the digestive system, that catalyze the breakdown of lipids through the hydrolysis of the linkages between fatty acids and glycerol in triglycerides and phospholipids. See also **fat, fatty acid, glycerol, phospholipid, triglyceride.**

lipectomy An excision of subcutaneous fat, as from the abdominal wall. Also called **adipectomy.**

lipemia A condition in which increased amounts of lipids are present in the blood, a normal occurance after eating.

lipid Any of a class of greasy organic substances insoluble in water but soluble in alcohol, chloroform, ether, and other solvents. Lipids are stored in the body and serve as an energy reserve. Kinds of lipids are **fatty acid, phospholipid.**

lipidosis A general term including several rare familial disorders of fat metabolism. The chief characteristic of these disorders is the accumulation of abnormal levels of certain lipids in the body. Kinds of lipidoses are **Gaucher's disease, Krabbe's disease, Niemann-Pick disease, Tay-Sachs disease.**

lipocele See **adipocele.**

lipochondrodystrophy See **Hurler's syndrome.**

lipochrome Any of the naturally occurring pigments that contain a lipid, as carotene.

lipodystrophia progressiva An abnormal accumulation of fat around the buttocks and thighs and a progressive, symmetrical disappearance of subcutaneous fat from areas above the pelvis and on the face. Also called lipomatosis atrophicans.

lipodystrophy Any abnormality in the metabolism or deposition of fats.

lip of hip fracture A fracture of the posterior lip of the acetabulum, often associated with displacement of the hip.

lipogranuloma, *pl.* **lipogranulomas, lipogranulomata** A nodule of necrotic, fatty tissue associated with granulomatous inflammation or with a foreign-body reaction around a deposit of injected material containing an oily substance.

lipoic acid A bacterial growth factor found in liver and yeast.

lipoid Any substance that resembles a lipid.

lipoma, *pl.* **lipomas, lipomata** A benign tumor consisting of mature fat cells. Also called **adipose tumor.** See also **multiple lipomatosis. —lipomatous,** *adj.*

-lipoma A combining form meaning a 'tumor made up of fatty tissue': *angiolipoma, fibrolipoma, osteolipoma.*

lipoma annulare colli A diffuse, symmetrical accumulation of fat around the neck, but it is not a true lipoma. Also called **Madelung's neck.**

lipoma arborescens A fatty tumor of a joint, characterized by a treelike distribution of fat cells.

lipoma capsulare A benign neoplasm characterized by the abnormal presence of fat cells in the capsule of an organ.

lipoma cavernosum See **angiolipoma.**

lipoma fibrosum A fatty tumor containing masses of fibrous tissue.

lipomatosis A disorder characterized by abnormal tumorlike accumulations of fat in body tissues.

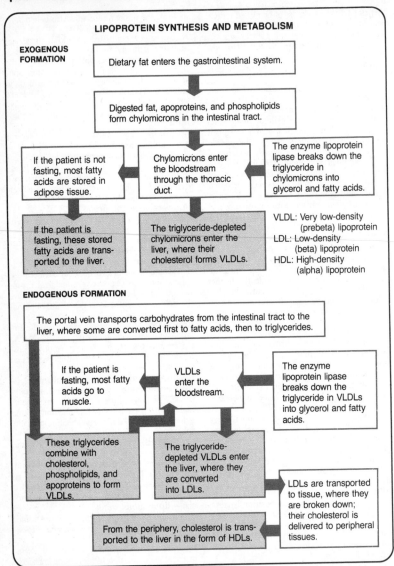

LIPOPROTEIN SYNTHESIS AND METABOLISM

EXOGENOUS FORMATION

Dietary fat enters the gastrointestinal system.

Digested fat, apoproteins, and phospholipids form chylomicrons in the intestinal tract.

If the patient is not fasting, most fatty acids are stored in adipose tissue.

Chylomicrons enter the bloodstream through the thoracic duct.

The enzyme lipoprotein lipase breaks down the triglyceride in chylomicrons into glycerol and fatty acids.

If the patient is fasting, these stored fatty acids are transported to the liver.

The triglyceride-depleted chylomicrons enter the liver, where their cholesterol forms VLDLs.

VLDL: Very low-density (prebeta) lipoprotein
LDL: Low-density (beta) lipoprotein
HDL: High-density (alpha) lipoprotein

ENDOGENOUS FORMATION

The portal vein transports carbohydrates from the intestinal tract to the liver, where some are converted first to fatty acids, then to triglycerides.

If the patient is fasting, most fatty acids go to muscle.

VLDLs enter the bloodstream.

The enzyme lipoprotein lipase breaks down the triglyceride in VLDLs into glycerol and fatty acids.

These triglycerides combine with cholesterol, phospholipids, and apoproteins to form VLDLs.

The triglyceride-depleted VLDLs enter the liver, where they are converted into LDLs.

LDLs are transported to tissue, where they are broken down; their cholesterol is delivered to peripheral tissues.

From the periphery, cholesterol is transported to the liver in the form of HDLs.

lipomatosis dolorosa   A disorder characterized by the abnormal accumulation of painful or tender fat deposits. Also called lipoma dolorosa.

lipomatosis gigantea   A condition characterized by massive deposits of fat.

lipomatous myxoma   A tumor containing fatty tissue that arises in connective tissue.

lipomatous nephritis   A rare condition in which the renal nephrons are replaced by fatty tissue. Kidney failure may result. Also called lipoma diffusum renis, lipomatosis renis.

lipomyxoma, *pl.* **lipomyxomas, lipo-**

myxomata   A myxoma that contains fat cells. Also called lipoma myxomatodes.

lipoprotein   A conjugated protein in which lipids form an integral part of the molecule. They are synthesized primarily in the liver, contain varying amounts of triglycerides, cholesterol, phospholipids, and protein, and are classified according to their composition and density. Practically all of the plasma lipids are present as lipoprotein complexes. Kinds of lipoproteins are **chylomicrons, high-density lipoproteins, low-density lipoproteins, very low-density lipoproteins.** See also **proteolipid.**

liposarcoma, *pl.* **liposarcomas, liposarcomata** A malignant growth composed of primitive fat cells. Also called lipoma sarcomatode.

liposis See **lipomatosis.**

-lipsis, -lipse A combining form meaning 'to leave, fail, omit': *eclipsis, ellipsis, menolipsis.*

liquefaction The process in which a solid or a gas is made liquid.

liquid A state of matter, intermediate between solid and gas, in which the substance flows freely with little application of force and assumes the shape of the vessel in which it is contained. Compare **fluid.** See also **gas, solid.**

liquid diet A diet consisting of foods that can be served in liquid form. It is prescribed in acute infections, in acute inflammatory conditions of the gastrointestinal tract, and for patients unable to consume soft or semifluid foods, usually after surgery. See also **full liquid diet.**

liquid glucose A thick, syrupy, odorless, colorless or yellowish liquid obtained by the incomplete hydrolysis of starch, primarily consisting of dextrose with dextrins, maltose, and water.

liquorice, licorice A dried root of gummy texture from the leguminous plant *Glycyrrhiza glabra.* It has a sweet, astringent taste and is used as a flavoring agent in medicines, especially in cough syrups and laxatives, confectionery, and tobacco.

Lisfranc's fracture A fracture-dislocation of the foot in which one or all of the proximal metatarsals are displaced.

Listeria monocytogenes A common species of gram-positive, motile bacillus that causes listeriosis.

listeriosis, listerosis An infectious disease caused by a genus of gram-positive motile bacteria that are nonsporulating. *Listeria monocytogenes* infects shellfish, birds, spiders, and mammals in all areas of the world, but infection in humans is uncommon. Transmitted by direct contact from infected animals to humans, by inhalation of dust or by contact with mud, sewage, or soil contaminated with the organism, it is characterized by circulatory collapse, shock, endocarditis, hepatosplenomegaly, and a dark red rash over the trunk and the legs. Fever, bacteremia, malaise, and lethargy are commonly seen. Pregnant women characteristically experience a mild, brief episode of illness, but fetal infection acquired through the placental circulation in utero is usually fatal. Infection in the newborn apparently results from exposure to the organism in the birth canal of an infected mother. Meningitis and encephalitis occur in 75% of cases. All secretions from the patient may contain the organism.

Liston's forceps A kind of bone-cutting forceps.

lith See **litho-.**

-lith A combining form meaning 'a calculus': *pneumolith, ptyalith, tonsillolith.*

lithiasis The formation of calculi in the hollow organs or ducts of the body. Calculi are

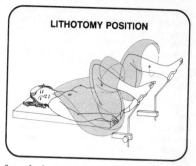

LITHOTOMY POSITION

formed of mineral salts and may irritate, inflame, or obstruct the organ in which they form or lodge. Lithiasis occurs most commonly in the gallbladder, kidney, and lower urinary tract. Lithiasis may be asymptomatic, but more often the condition is extremely painful. Surgery may be necessary if the stones cannot be excreted spontaneously. Lower urinary tract calculi often can be dissolved. See also **biliary calculus, cholelithiasis, renal calculus, urinary calculus.**

lithium (Li) A silvery-white alkali metal occurring in various compounds, as petalite and spodumene. Its atomic number is 3; its atomic weight is 6.940. Lithium is the lightest known metal and one of the most reactive elements. Traces of lithium ion occur in animal tissue, and it abounds in many alkaline mineral-spring waters. Its salts are used in the treatment of manias, but the mechanisms by which these compounds help to stabilize psychological moods are not understood. Lithium carbonate and citrate are the salts approved for psychiatric use in the United States; they have been effective in the prevention of recurrent attacks of manic-depressive illnesses.

lithium carbonate, l. citrate Drugs used to treat manic-depressive illness.

litho-, lith- A combining form meaning 'of or pertaining to a stone or to a calculus': *litholysis, lithomyl, lithophone.*

lithopedion, lithopedium A fetus that has died in utero and has become calcified or ossified. Also called **calcified fetus, ostembryon, osteopedion.**

lithotomy The surgical excision of a calculus, especially one from the urinary tract.

lithotomy forceps A forceps for the extraction of a calculus, usually from the urinary tract.

lithotomy position The posture assumed by the patient lying supine with the hips and the knees flexed and the thighs abducted and rotated externally. Also called **dorsosacral position.**

lithotriptor See **lithotrite.**

lithotrite An instrument for crushing a stone in the urinary bladder. Also called **lithotriptor.** —**lithotrity,** *n.*

litigant In law: a party to a lawsuit. See also **defendant, plaintiff.**

litigate In law: to carry on a suit or to contest.

litigious paranoia A form of paranoia in which the person seeks legal proof or justification for his systematized delusions.

litmus paper Absorbent paper coated with litmus, a blue dye, that is used to determine pH. Acid substances or solutions turn litmus from blue to red. Alkaline substances or solutions do not cause a change in color.

litter A stretcher.

Little's disease See **cerebral palsy**.

Litzmann's obliquity See **asynclitism**.

live birth The birth of an infant, irrespective of the duration of gestation, that exhibits any sign of life, as respiration, heartbeat, umbilical pulsation, or movement of voluntary muscles. Although a live birth is not always a viable birth, it is recorded as a live birth for statistical purposes.

livedo A blue or red mottling of the skin that becomes worse in cold weather, probably owing to arteriolar spasm. One form, livedo reticularis, is characterized by a red-blue, netlike discoloration and may be associated with lupus erythematosus, dermatomyositis, rheumatoid arthritis, or various types of arteritis. **Cutis marmorata** is a transient form of livedo.

livedo vasculitis See **segmented hyalinizing vasculitis**.

liver The largest gland of the body and one of its most complex organs: more than 500 of its functions have been identified. It is divided into four lobes, contains as many as 100,000 lobules, and is served by two distinct blood supplies. The hepatic artery conveys oxygenated blood to the liver, and the hepatic portal vein conveys nutrient-filled blood from the stomach and the intestines. At any given moment, the liver holds about 0.5 liters (1 pint) of blood. Some of the major functions performed by the liver are the production of bile by hepatic cells; the secretion of glucose, proteins, vitamins, fats, and most of the other compounds used by the body; the processing of hemoglobin for vital use of its iron content; and the conversion of poisonous ammonia to urea. Bile from the liver is stored in the gallbladder (which is connected to the liver by connective tissue), in the hepatic duct, and in numerous blood vessels. The liver is located in the cranial, right portion of the abdominal cavity, occupying almost the entire right hypochondrium, the greater part of the epigastrium, and, in many individuals, extending into the left hypochondrium as far as the mammary line. The liver in adult men weighs about 1.5 kg (3¼ lb); in women, about 1.3 kg (2¾ lb). It has a soft, solid consistency, is shaped like an irregular hemisphere, and is dark reddish-brown in color. The right lobe of the liver is much larger than the left lobe or the caudate and the quadrate lobes. The liver attaches to the diaphragm by the coronary and the triangular ligaments. During the descent of the diaphragm in deep breathing, the liver rolls forward, shifting the inferior border downward where it can be felt through the abdominal wall. The tiny lobules of the organ are composed of polyhedral hepatic cells.

These communicate with small ducts that connect with larger ducts to form the left and the right hepatic ducts, which emerge on the caudal surface of the liver. The left and the right hepatic ducts converge to form the single hepatic duct, which conveys the bile to the duodenum and to the gallbladder for storage. The liver cells produce about 0.5 liters (1 pint) of bile daily. They also detoxify numerous ingested substances, as alcohol, nicotine, and other poisons, as well as various toxic substances produced by the intestine. See also **gallbladder**.

liver biopsy A diagnostic procedure in which a special needle is introduced into the liver under local anesthesia to obtain a tissue specimen for pathologic examination.

NURSING CONSIDERATIONS: Results of bleeding, clotting and prothrombin tests should be checked before performing the procedure. The nurse reinforces explanations of the biopsy and its purpose, provides care before and after the procedure, and closely observes the patient for postbiopsy complications, as intraperitoneal hemorrhage, shock, and pneumothorax. A liver biopsy is a valuable aid in establishing a diagnosis of hepatic disease, including primary and metastatic malignant neoplastic disease.

liver breath See **fetor hepaticus**.

liver cancer A malignant neoplastic disease of the liver, occurring most frequently as a metastasis from another malignancy. Primary tumors are 6 to 10 times more prevalent in men than in women, develop most often in the 6th decade of life, and are associated with cirrhosis of the liver in 70% of the cases. Other risk factors include hemochromatosis, schistosomiasis, exposure to vinyl chloride or arsenic, and, possibly, nutritional deficiencies. Alcoholism may be a predisposing factor, but nonalcoholic cirrhosis is a greater risk than alcoholic cirrhosis. Characteristics of liver cancer are abdominal bloating, anorexia, weakness, dull upper abdominal pain, ascites, mild jaundice, and a tender enlarged liver; in some cases tumor nodules are palpable on the liver surface. Diagnostic procedures include radioisotope scan, needle biopsy, and various laboratory studies of liver function. An elevated level of alkaline phosphatase, increased retention of sulfobromophthalein, and the presence of alpha-fetoprotein in the blood suggest liver cancer. All primary liver tumors are adenocarcinomas, classified as hepatomas when derived from hepatic cells and cholangiomas if they originate in cells of the bile duct. They form large single nodules or satellite nodules surrounding a central lesion and are found more often in the right lobe than in the left. Primary lesions spread centrifugally in the liver, invade the portal vein and lymphatic vessels, and metastasize to lymph nodes, the lungs, brain, and other sites. Total hepatic lobectomy is the treatment of choice for primary tumors; because the liver is able to regenerate its cells, 80% of it may be resected without loss of liver function. Systemic chemotherapy or methotrexate and 5-fluorouracil infused through a catheter

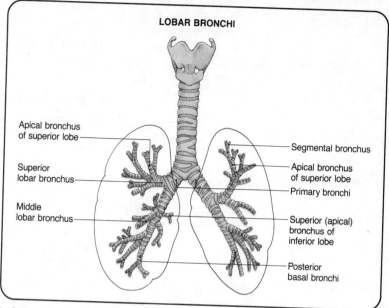

LOBAR BRONCHI

Apical bronchus of superior lobe

Superior lobar bronchus

Middle lobar bronchus

Segmental bronchus

Apical bronchus of superior lobe

Primary bronchi

Superior (apical) bronchus of inferior lobe

Posterior basal bronchi

in the hepatic artery may result in temporary tumor regression. Irradiation is very destructive to liver cells and not very toxic to tumor cells in the liver.

liver cell carcinoma   See **malignant hepatoma.**

liver disease   Any one of a group of disorders of the liver. The most important diseases in this group are cirrhosis, cholestasis, and viral and toxic hepatitis. Characteristics of liver disease are jaundice, anorexia, hepatomegaly, ascites, and impaired consciousness. The exact diagnosis of liver disease is made through a combination of laboratory tests and clinical findings. See also **cholestasis, cirrhosis, hepatitis.**

liver flap   See **asterixis.**

liver function test   A test used to evaluate various functions of the liver; for example, metabolism, storage, filtration, and excretion. Kinds of liver function tests include **alkaline phosphatase, bromsulfalein test, prothrombin time, serum bilirubin, serum glutamic pyruvic transaminase.**

liver scan   A noninvasive technique of visualizing the size, shape, and consistency of the liver by the intravenous injection of a radioactively labeled compound that is readily taken up and trapped in the Kupffer cells of the liver. The radiation emitted by the compound is recorded by a radiation detector and can be photographed with a scintillation camera or filmed with X-ray. Liver scans are most useful for diagnosing three-dimensional lesions, as abscesses or tumors.

liver spot   *Nontechnical.* A senile lentigo or actinic keratosis.

LLD factor   See **cyanocobalamin.**

LMD   *abbr* Local medical doctor, used by house staff or others to distinguish a patient's primary physician from university faculty, attending specialists, physicians, or house staff. Also called PMD, private medical doctor.

LMP   *abbr* last menstrual period.

loading response stance stage   One of the five stages of the stance phase of walking or gait, specifically associated with the moment when the leg reacts to and accepts the weight of the body. The loading response stance stage is one of the factors in the diagnoses of many abnormal orthopedic conditions and is often studied in conjunction with analyses of the electromyographic activity of the muscles used in walking. Compare **initial contact stance stage, midstance, preswing stance stage, terminal stance.**

Loa loa   A species of parasitic nematode worm of Western and Central Africa that causes **loiasis.**

lobar bronchus   A bronchus extending from a primary bronchus to a segmental bronchus into one of the lobes of the right or left lung.

lobar pneumonia   A severe infection of one or more of the five major lobes of the lungs, which, if untreated, eventually results in consolidation of lung tissue. The disease is characterized by fever, chills, cough, rusty sputum, rapid shallow breathing, cyanosis, nausea, vomiting, and pleurisy. *Streptococcus pneumoniae* is the usual cause, but *Klebsiella pneumoniae*, *Haemophilus influenzae*, and other streptococci can produce the disease. Complications include lung abscess, atelectasis, empyema, pericarditis, and pleural effusion. Because the fatality rate in the elderly and those with underlying systemic illness is high, prophylactic polyvalent

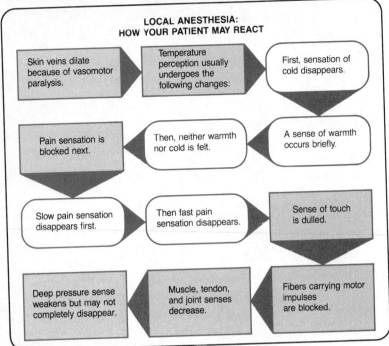

**LOCAL ANESTHESIA:
HOW YOUR PATIENT MAY REACT**

Skin veins dilate because of vasomotor paralysis.

Temperature perception usually undergoes the following changes:

First, sensation of cold disappears.

Pain sensation is blocked next.

Then, neither warmth nor cold is felt.

A sense of warmth occurs briefly.

Slow pain sensation disappears first.

Then fast pain sensation disappears.

Sense of touch is dulled.

Deep pressure sense weakens but may not completely disappear.

Muscle, tendon, and joint senses decrease.

Fibers carrying motor impulses are blocked.

pneumococcal vaccine is recommended for them. Compare **bronchopneumonia.**

lobe **1.** A roundish projection of any structure. **2.** A portion of any organ, demarcated by sulci, fissures, or connective tissue, as the lobes of the brain, liver, and lungs. —**lobar, lobular,** *adj.*

-lobe A combining form meaning a 'rounded prominence': *gonilobe, multilobe, sublobe.*

lobectomy A type of chest surgery in which a lobe of a lung is excised, performed to remove a malignant tumor and to treat uncontrolled bronchiectasis, trauma with hemorrhage, or intractable tuberculosis. The chest cavity is entered through a long back-to-front incision, and the diseased lobe is removed. A large caliber tube remains in the wound and is connected to a water-sealed drainage system. Oxygen is given to the patient during the first 24 hours after surgery. The vital signs are closely monitored, coughing and deep breathing are encouraged hourly, a blood transfusion may be given, and I.V. fluids are continued. Care is taken that the chest tube remain open and that the drainage system be sealed and functional. The chest tube is removed 2 to 3 days after surgery. Some compensatory emphysema is expected as the remaining lung tissue overexpands to fill the new space. —**lobectomize,** *v.*

lobotomy A neurosurgical procedure in which the nerve fibers in the bundle of white matter in the frontal lobe of the brain are severed to interrupt the transmission of various affective responses. Severe intractable depression and pain are among the indications for this procedure. It is rarely performed because it has many unpredictable and undesirable effects. A cannula is passed through the bony orbit of the eye and a wire loop is inserted through the cannula to the cingulum. The nerve fibers are severed with the wire loop. Also called **leukotomy.**

lobster-claw deformity See **bidactyly.**

lobular carcinoma A neoplasm that often forms a diffuse mass and accounts for a small percentage of breast tumors.

lobule A small lobe, as the soft, lower, pendulous part of the external ear. —**lobular,** *adj.*

LOC *abbr* **level of consciousness.**

loc- A combining form meaning 'place': *locomotor, locum, locus.*

local **1.** Of or pertaining to a small circumscribed area of the body. **2.** Of or pertaining to a treatment or drug applied locally. **3.** *Informal.* A local anesthetic.

local anesthesia The direct administration of an anesthetic agent to induce the absence of sensation in a small area of the body. Brief surgical or dental procedures are the most common indications for local anesthesia. The anesthetic may be applied topically to the surface of the skin or membrane or injected subcutaneously through an intradermal weal. The principal drawbacks to the use of local anesthesia are the incidence of allergic reactions to certain agents, especially the '-caine' drugs, and the occasional difficulty encountered in achieving adequate anesthesia. The advantages include low cost, ease of administration, low toxicity, and safety; a conscious patient can cooperate and does not require respiratory support or intubation. To avoid general anesthesia, major surgical procedures are occasionally performed under local anesthesia. The tissues are anesthetized layer by layer, as the surgeon approaches the deeper structures of the body. Regional anesthesia has largely replaced this procedure. In all cases, the recommended dosage of any anesthetic agent is the smallest possible to achieve the desired effect. Compare **general anesthesia, regional anesthesia, topical anesthesia.**

local anesthetic   A substance used to reduce or eliminate neural sensation, specifically pain, in a limited area of the body. Local anesthetics act by blocking transmission of nerve impulses. More than 100 drugs are available for local anesthesia; they are classified as members of the alcohol-ester or the amineamide family. Principal representatives of the alcohol-ester group are phenols and benzyl, ethyl, and salicylic alcohol; these have generally been replaced by the less toxic esters (chloroprocaine, cocaine, procaine, tetracaine) and the amides (dibucaine, bupivacaine, lidocaine, mepivacaine, prilocaine, etidocaine). Any substance sufficiently potent to induce local anesthesia has potential for causing adverse side effects, ranging from easily reversible dermatitis to lethal anaphylaxis or simultaneous respiratory and cardiac arrest. Among the factors that influence an adverse reaction to a local anesthetic are hypersensitivity to the drug, the vascularity of the injection site, the speed with which the drug is given, the rapidity of action of the drug, and the presence of epinephrine in the solution. Serious adverse results have occurred when the operator has failed to notice that the local anesthetic contains epinephrine in solution. A person might be able to tolerate the local agent without adverse reaction but might be dangerously hypersensitive to the epinephrine. Some people who are sensitive to local anesthetics of the amide group, which are broken down in the liver, can tolerate local anesthetics of the ester group, which are broken down in the plasma. Vasopressors should also be at hand in case of hypotension or other forms of circulatory depression.

localization audiometry   See **audiometry.**

localization film   In radiotherapy: a diagnostic film taken to confirm a treatment portal or to view the position of an intracavitary or interstitial implant, especially for the purpose of computing the dose delivered.

localized scleroderma   See **Addison's keloid.**

lochia   The discharge that flows from the vagina following childbirth. During the first 3 or 4 days postpartum, the lochia is red (lochia rubra) and is made up of blood, endometrial decidua, and fetal lanugo, vernix, and sometimes meconium, small shreds of placental tissue and membranes. After the 3rd day, the amount of blood diminishes, the placental site exudes serous material and lymph, and the lochia becomes darker and thinner (lochia fusca), and then serous (lochia serosa) as evacuation of particulate material is completed. During the 2nd week, white blood cells and bacteria appear in large numbers along with fatty, mucinous decidual material, causing the lochia to appear yellow (lochia flava or purulenta). During the 3rd week and thereafter, as endometrial epithelialization progresses, the amount of lochia decreases markedly and takes on a seromucinous consistency and a gray-white color (lochia alba). Cessation of the flow of lochia at about 6 weeks is usual. —**lochial,** adj.

locked twins   See **interlocked twins.**

lockjaw   Informal. Tetanus.

locomotor ataxia   See **tabes dorsalis.**

loculate   Divided into small spaces or cavities.

loculus   A small chamber, pocket, or cavity, as the interior of a polyp.

locum tenens   A temporary substitute for a physician who is away from his practice.

locus   A specific place or position, as the locus of a particular gene on a chromosome.

locus of infection   A site in the body where an infection originates.

Löffler's syndrome   A benign, idiopathic disorder marked by episodes of pulmonary eosinophilia, transient opacities in the lungs, anorexia, breathlessness, fever, and weight loss. Recovery is spontaneous and prompt.

log-, logo-   A combining form meaning 'word, speech, thought': logagnosia, logopathy, logorrhea.

loga-   A combining form meaning 'of or pertaining to the whites of the eyes': logadectomy, logaditis, logadoblennorrhea.

-logia   See **-logy.**

logo-   A combining form meaning 'of or pertaining to words or speech': logomania, logoneurosis, logopathy.

logroll   A maneuver used to turn a reclining patient from one side to the other or completely over without flexing the spinal column. The arms of the patient are folded across the chest and the legs extended. A draw sheet under the patient is manipulated by attending nursing personnel to facilitate the procedure.

-logy   A combining form meaning 'a science': mammalogy, metabology. Also **-logia.**

loiasis   A form of filariasis caused by the worm *Loa loa*, which may migrate for 10 to 15 years in subcutaneous tissue, producing localized inflammation known as **Calabar swellings.** Occasionally, the migrating worms may be visible beneath the conjunctiva. The disease is acquired through the bite of an infected African deerfly. See also **filariasis, onchocerciasis.**

loin   A part of the body on each side of the spinal column between the false ribs and the hip bones.

lomustine (CCNU)   An alkylating agent used in cancer chemotherapy.

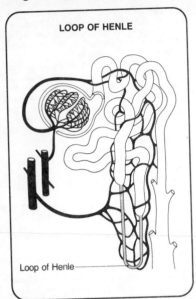

LOOP OF HENLE

Loop of Henle

long-acting drug   A pharmacologic agent with a prolonged effect owing to a formulation resulting in the slow release of the active principle or the continued absorption of small amounts of the dosage of the drug over an extended period.

long-acting insulin   A preparation of the antidiabetic principle of beef pancreas or pork pancreas modified by an interaction with zinc under specific chemical conditions and supplied as a suspension with a prolonged action. An injection of the preparation takes effect within 8 hours, reaches a peak of action in 16 to 24 hours, and has a duration of action of more than 36 hours. Also called **slow-acting insulin.** See also **insulin.** Compare **intermediate-acting insulin, short-acting insulin.**

long-acting thyroid stimulator (LATS)   An immunoglobulin, probably an autoantibody, that exerts a prolonged stimulatory effect on the thyroid gland, causing rapid growth of the gland and excess activity of thyroid function, resulting in hyperthyroidism. It is found circulating in the blood of 50% of people affected with Graves' disease.

long arm cast   An orthopedic cast applied to immobilize upper extremities from the hand to the upper arm. It is used in the treatment of fractures of the forearm, elbow, and humerus; for postoperative positioning of the distal arm, the elbow, or the upper arm; and for correction or for maintenance of correction of deformities of the distal arm, the wrist, or the elbow. Compare **short arm cast.**

long leg cast   An orthopedic cast applied to immobilize the leg from the toes to the upper thigh. It is used in treating fractures and dislocations of the knee; for postoperative posi-

tioning and immobilization of the knee, distal leg, and ankle; and for correction or for maintenance of correction of the foot, distal leg, and knee. The cast sometimes includes a rubber walker, allowing the patient to walk while the leg is encased in the cast and when weight-bearing ambulation is allowed. Compare **short leg cast.**

long-term memory   The ability to recall sensations, events, ideas, and other information for long periods of time without apparent effort.

long thoracic nerve   One of a pair of supraclavicular branches from the roots of the brachial plexus. It arises by three roots, from the fifth, the sixth, and the seventh cervical nerves. Its fibers from the fifth and the sixth cervical nerves join just after they pierce the scalenus medius and are united with its fibers from the seventh cervical nerve at the level of the first rib. Compare **phrenic nerve.**

loop   *Informal.* See **intrauterine device.**

loop diuretic   See **diuretic.**

loop of Henle   The U-shaped portion of a renal tubule, consisting of a thin descending limb and a thick ascending limb.

loose fibrous tissue   A constrictive, pliable fibrous connective tissue consisting of interwoven elastic and collagenous fibers, interspersed with fluid-filled areolae. It is found in adipose tissue, areolar tissue, reticular tissue, and fibroelastic tissue. Compare **dense fibrous tissue.**

loperamide, l. hydrochloride   Antidiarrheal agents.

loph-   A combining form meaning 'of or pertaining to a ridge': *lophius, lophodont, lophotrichous.*

lorazepam   A benzodiazepine antianxiety agent.

lordosis   **1.** The normal curvature of the lumbar and cervical spine, seen as an anterior concavity if a person is observed from the side. **2.** An abnormal, increased degree of curvature of any part of the back.

LOS   *abbr* length of stay.

lotion   A liquid preparation applied externally to protect the skin or to treat a dermatologic disorder.

loupe   A magnifying lens mounted in a frame worn on the head, as used to examine the eyes.

louse, *pl.* **lice**   A small, wingless, parasitic insect that is the carrier of such diseases as relapsing fever and typhus. Lice are common parasites on the skin and may cause intense pruritus. See also **pediculosis.**

louse bite   A minute puncture wound produced by a louse, which may transmit typhus, trench fever, and relapsing fever. Secondary infection may result from scratching the affected area. Head and body lice are the most common and are frequently found among school children. Washing and bathing, application of an insecticide, and the washing of clothes and bed linens are recommended for treatment and prophylaxis against spread of the infestation. See also **pediculosis.**

louse-borne typhus See **epidemic typhus.**

low back pain Local or referred pain at the base of the spine caused by a sprain, strain, osteoarthritis, ankylosing spondylitis, a neoplasm, or a prolapsed intervertebral disk. Low back pain is a common complaint and is often associated with poor posture, obesity, sagging abdominal muscles, or prolonged periods of sitting. Pain may be localized and static; it may be accompanied by muscle weakness or spasms; or it may radiate down the back of one or both legs, as in sciatica. To guard against the pain, the person may decrease the range of motion of the spine. If an intervertebral disk is prolapsed, deep pressure over the interspace generally causes pain, and flexion of the hip elicits sciatic pain when the knee is extended but not when the knee is flexed (Lasègue's sign). The patient is placed in semi-Fowler's position on a firm mattress with the knees flexed and supported. Analgesics, muscle relaxants, and tranquilizers may be administered, and dry or moist heat is applied. Diagnostic X-rays, pelvic traction, physiotherapy, and a myelogram may be performed if a herniated disk is suspected. When the acute pain subsides, the patient may increase activity as tolerated; fatigue is avoided; and a corset or back brace may be ordered. The patient is instructed to use a straight-backed chair, not to sit with legs crossed or extended on a footstool, and to sleep on the side or back with knees flexed and a small pillow under the head. Before discharge, the patient is advised to maintain a normal weight, to follow the ordered exercise program, to wear flat-heeled shoes, and to avoid constipation by using natural laxatives, if required.

low–birth-weight (LBW) infant An infant whose weight at birth is less than 2,500 g (5½ lb), regardless of gestational age. These infants are at risk for the development of hypoxia during labor, hypoglycemia after birth, and growth retardation in childhood, especially if the condition is the result of prolonged placental insufficiency, maternal malnutrition, or drug addiction. Many low–birth-weight infants have no problems and develop normally.

low-calcium diet A diet that restricts calcium use and eliminates most of the dairy foods, all breads made with milk or dry skim milk, and deep green leafy vegetables. It is prescribed for people who form renal calculi. Meats, poultry, fish, vegetables, legumes, and fruits are recommended.

low-caloric diet A diet prescribed to limit the intake of calories, usually to reduce body weight. Such diets may be designated as 800 calorie, 1,000 calorie, or other specific numbers of calories. Exchange lists may be used to allow the patient to select preferred foods from groups of foods categorized as carbohydrate, protein, and fat.

low cervical cesarean section A method for surgically delivering an infant through a transverse incision in the thin supracervical

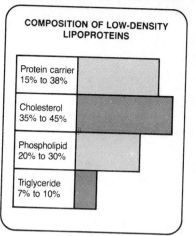

COMPOSITION OF LOW-DENSITY
LIPOPROTEINS

Protein carrier
15% to 38%

Cholesterol
35% to 45%

Phospholipid
20% to 30%

Triglyceride
7% to 10%

portion of the lower uterine segment, behind the bladder and the bladder flap. This incision bleeds less during surgery and heals with a stronger scar than the higher vertical scar of the classic cesarean section. Compare **extraperitoneal cesarean section.** See also **cesarean section.**

low-cholesterol diet A diet that restricts foods containing animal fats and saturated fatty acids and concentrates on poultry, fish, vegetables, fruits, cottage cheese, and polyunsaturated fats. The diet is indicated for persons with high–serum cholesterol levels, cardiovascular disorders, obesity, hyperlipidemia, hypercholesterolemia, or hyperlipoproteinemia. Also called **low–saturated-fat diet.**

low-density lipoprotein (LDL) A plasma protein containing relatively more cholesterol and triglycerides than protein. It is derived in part, if not completely, from the intravascular breakdown of the very low-density lipoproteins. The high cholesterol content may account for its greater atherogenic potential as compared to the very low-density lipoproteins and chylomicrons.

lower extremity suspension An orthopedic procedure used to treat bone fractures and correct orthopedic abnormalities of the lower limbs. The procedure uses traction equipment to relieve the weight of the lower limb rather than to exert traction pull. Lower extremity suspension may be either unilateral or bilateral and is used in the postoperative, posttraumatic, or postreduction control of edema. Compare **balanced suspension, hyperextension suspension, upper extremity suspension.**

lower motor neuron paralysis An injury or lesion in the spinal cord that damages the cell bodies or axons, or both, of the lower motor neurons, located in the anterior horn cells and the spinal and peripheral nerves. In complete transection of the spinal cord, voluntary muscle control is totally lost. In partial transection, function is altered in varying degrees, depending on the areas innervated by the nerves involved. In lower motor neuron paralysis, the

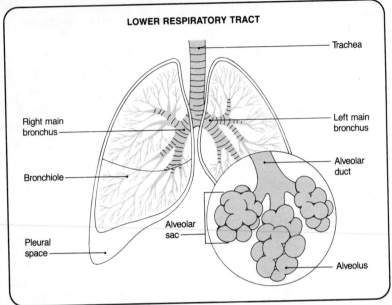

LOWER RESPIRATORY TRACT

Trachea

Right main bronchus

Left main bronchus

Alveolar duct

Bronchiole

Alveolar sac

Pleural space

Alveolus

reflex arcs are permanently damaged, causing decreased muscle tone and flaccidity, diminished or absent reflexes, absence of pathological reflexes, local twitching of muscle groups, and progressive atrophy of the atonic muscles. Compare **upper motor neuron paralysis.**

lower respiratory infection   See **respiratory tract infection.**

lower respiratory tract   One of the two divisions of the respiratory system. The lower respiratory tract includes the trachea, the left and the right bronchi, and the lungs. The bronchi divide into smaller bronchioles in the lungs, the bronchioles divide into alveolar ducts, the ducts into alveolar sacs, and the sacs into alveoli. The exchange of oxygen and carbon dioxide occurs between the most internal alveolar surface and the tiny capillaries surrounding the external alveolar wall. The lower respiratory tract is a common site of infections, obstructive conditions, and neoplastic disease. Compare **upper respiratory tract.** See also **lung.**

low-fat diet   A diet containing limited amounts of fat and consisting chiefly of easily digestible foods of high carbohydrate content. The diet may be indicated in gallbladder disease and malabsorption syndromes.

low-fat milk   Milk containing 1% to 2% fat, making it an intermediate in fat content between whole and skim milk.

low forceps   An obstetric operation in which forceps are used to deliver a fetus whose head is on the pelvic floor. It is performed most often as an elective procedure to shorten normal labor and to control delivery, usually in conjunction with anesthesia and episiotomy. It is commonly required for mothers whose expulsive powers

have been weakened by analgesia, anesthesia, or fatigue. Also called **outlet forceps, prophylactic forceps.** Compare **high forceps, midforceps, natural childbirth, spontaneous delivery.** See also **forceps delivery, obstetric forceps.**

low-grade fever   A temperature that is above 37°C (98.6°F) but below 38°C (100.4°F) for 24 hours.

Lown-Ganong-Levine syndrome   A disorder of the atrioventricular (AV) conduction system, marked by ventricular preexcitation. Part or all of the AV nodal connection is bypassed by an abnormal AV connection from the atrial muscle to the bundle of His. The condition may be discovered by routine EKG or may be seen in association with paroxysmal atrial arrhythmias, supraventricular tachycardia, atrial flutter, and fibrillation. Treatments include the use of antiarrhythmic drugs, surgical interruption of the abnormal AV pathway, and implantation of a pacemaker. Compare **Wolff-Parkinson-White syndrome.**

low-residue diet   A diet that will leave a minimal residue in the lower intestinal tract after digestion and absorption. The diet is prescribed in cases of diverticulosis and diverticulitis, gastrointestinal irritability or inflammation, and before and after gastrointestinal surgery. Since it is lacking in calcium, iron, and vitamins, it should be used only for a limited period of time.

low–saturated-fat diet   See **low-cholesterol diet.**

low-sodium diet   A diet that restricts the use of sodium chloride and other sodium compounds, as baking powder or soda. It is indicated in hypertension, edematous states (especially when associated with cardiovascular disease), renal or liver disease, and therapy with corticosteroids. The degree of sodium restriction depends on the severity of the condition. Many flavoring extracts, spices, and herbs can be used to add taste to the diet. Foods to be avoided include fresh or canned shellfish, ham, bacon, frankfurters, luncheon meats, sausage, cheese, salted butter or margarine, any breads or cereals made with salt, beets, carrots, celery, sauerkraut, spinach, and most canned or frozen foods unless prepared without sodium. Also to be avoided are many drugs, as laxatives, sedatives, and alkalizers, which contain sodium, and drinking water from a source using a water softener, since this appliance adds sodium to the water. Also called **salt-free diet, sodium-restricted diet.**

loxapine succinate   A dibenzoxazepine antipsychotic agent.

loxo-   A combining form meaning 'oblique': *loxophthalmus, loxotic, loxotomy.*

lozenge   See **troche.**

LP   *abbr* **lumbar puncture.**

LPN   *abbr* **licensed practical nurse.**

LTB   *abbr* laryngotracheobronchitis. See **croup.**

Lu   Symbol for **lutetium.**

luc-   A combining form meaning 'of or pertaining to light': *lucifugal, lucipetal, lucotherapy.*

-lucent   A combining form meaning 'light-admitting': *radiolucent, roentgenolucent, translucent.*

lucid   Clear, rational, and able to be understood.

lucid interval   A period of relative mental clarity between periods of irrationality, especially in organic mental disorders, as delirium and dementia.

lucid lethargy   A mental state characterized by a loss of will even though the person is conscious and intellectual function is normal. See also **lethargy.**

Ludwig's angina   Acute streptococcal cellulitis of the floor of the mouth. It is treated with penicillin.

lue-   A combining form meaning 'of or pertaining to syphilis': *luetic, luetin, luetism.*

Luer-Lok syringe   A syringe for injection having a simple lock mechanism that securely holds the needle in place.

lues   See **syphilis.**

-luetic, -luic   A combining form meaning 'pertaining to syphilis': *antiluetic, heredoluetic, paraluetic.*

luetic aortitis   See **syphilitic aortitis.**

Lugol's solution   An aqueous solution of iodine (5%) and potassium iodide (10%); a thyroid hormone antagonist.

lukewarm bath   A bath in which the temperature of the water is between 32.2° and 35.5°C (90° and 96°F).

lumbago   Pain in the lumbar region caused by a muscle strain, rheumatoid arthritis, os-

teoarthritis, or a herniated intravertebral disk. Ischemic lumbago, characterized by pain in the lower back and buttocks, is caused by vascular insufficiency. See also **low back pain.**

lumbar   Of or pertaining to the part of the body between the thorax and the pelvis.

lumbar nerves   The five pairs of spinal nerves rising in the lumbar region. They become increasingly large the more caudal their location and pass laterally and downward under the cover of the psoas major or between its fasciculi. The first three lumbar nerves and the larger part of the fourth are connected by communicating loops and, in many individuals, communicate with the twelfth thoracic nerve, forming the lumbar plexus. The ventral primary divisions of the lumbar nerves give rise to muscular branches, which supply the psoas major and the quadratus lumborum before the nerves enter the lumbar plexus. The smaller section of the fourth lumbar nerve joins the fifth lumbar nerve to form the lumbosacral trunk, which comprises part of the sacral plexus. Only the first two lumbar nerves extend white rami to the sympathetic trunk. All lumbar nerves receive gray rami. The lumbar ganglia follow no fixed pattern, and massive fusions of ganglia are common. When occurring independently, the lumbar ganglia lie on the corresponding vertebrae or intervertebral disks caudally. The ganglion on the second lumbar vertebra is the largest, the most constant, and the most easily palpated.

lumbar node   A node in one of the seven groups of parietal lymph nodes serving the abdomen and the pelvis. The lumbar nodes are very numerous and are divided into the lateral aortic nodes, the preaortic nodes, and the retroaortic nodes. Compare **sacral node.** See also **lymph, lymphatic system, lymph node.**

lumbar plexus   A network of nerves formed by the ventral primary divisions of the first three and the greater part of the fourth lumbar nerves. It is located on the inside of the posterior abdominal wall, either dorsal to the psoas major or among its fibers and ventral to the transverse processes of the lumbar vertebrae. The plexus develops from the splitting of various lumbar nerves. The first lumbar nerve splits into the cranial and the caudal branches. The cranial branch forms the iliohypogastric and the ilioinguinal nerves. The caudal branch unites with a branch from the second lumbar nerve to form the genitofemoral nerve. The rest of the second nerve and the third and the fourth nerves each split into a small ventral and a large dorsal section. The ventral portions unite to form the obturator nerve. The dorsal portions of the second and the third nerves each divide into two smaller branches to form the lateral femoral cutaneous nerve and two larger branches that join the dorsal portion of the fourth lumbar nerve to form the femoral nerve. Part of the fourth lumbar nerve joins the fifth lumbar nerve in the lumbosacral trunk. The branches of the lumbar plexus are the iliohypogastric nerve, the ilioinguinal nerve, the genitofemoral nerve, the lateral femoral cu-

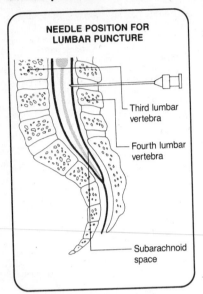

**NEEDLE POSITION FOR
LUMBAR PUNCTURE**

Third lumbar
vertebra

Fourth lumbar
vertebra

Subarachnoid
space

taneous nerve, the obturator nerve, the accessory obturator nerve, and the femoral nerve. The iliohypogastric, the ilioinguinal, and the genitofemoral nerves supply the caudal part of the abdominal wall. The lateral femoral cutaneous, the obturator, the accessory obturator, and the femoral nerves supply the anterior thigh and the middle of the leg. The accessory obturator nerve is present in only 20% of individuals and comes from the third and the fourth lumbar nerves. Compare **sacral plexus.**

lumbar puncture (LP) The introduction of a hollow needle and stylet into the subarachnoid space of the lumbar portion of the spinal canal, usually between the third and fourth lumbar space. Using strict sterile technique, it is performed in various therapeutic and diagnostic procedures. Diagnostic indications include measuring of cerebrospinal fluid (CSF) pressure, obtaining CSF for laboratory analysis, evaluating the canal for the pressure of a tumor, and injecting air, oxygen, or a radiopaque substance for radiographic visualization of the structures of the nervous system of the spinal canal, the meninges, and the brain. Therapeutic indications for lumbar puncture include removing blood or pus from the subarachnoid space, injecting sera or drugs, withdrawing CSF to reduce intracranial pressure, introducing a local anesthetic to induce spinal anesthesia, and placing a small amount of the patient's blood in the subarachnoid space to form a clot to patch a rent or hole in the dura in order to prevent leakage of CSF into the epidural space.

lumbar subarachnoid peritoneostomy
A surgical procedure for draining cerebrospinal fluid in hydrocephalus, usually in the newborn. It spares the kidney but is a somewhat less effective method than a lumbar subarachnoid ur-

eterostomy. It may be used when a temporary shunt is needed. First a lumbar laminectomy is performed; then a tube is passed from the subarachnoid space around the flank and into the peritoneum. It is performed to correct a communicating type of hydrocephalus.

lumbar subarachnoid ureterostomy
A surgical procedure for draining excess cerebrospinal fluid though the ureter to the bladder in hydrocephalus, usually in the newborn. It first completes a lumbar laminectomy and a left nephrectomy, after which a polyethylene tube is passed from the lumbar subarachnoid space through the paraspinal muscles and into the free ureter. It is performed to correct a communicating type of hydrocephalus.

lumbar veins Four pairs of veins that collect blood by dorsal tributaries from the loins and by abdominal tributaries from the walls of the abdomen. They receive veins from the vertebral plexus, pass ventrally around the vertebrae, dorsal to the psoas major, and end in the inferior vena cava. The left lumbar veins are longer than the right and pass dorsal to the aorta. The lumbar veins are connected by the ascending lumbar vein, which runs ventral to the transverse processes of the lumbar vertebrae.

lumbar vertebra One of the five largest segments of the movable part of the vertebral column, distinguished by the absence of a foramen in the transverse process and by vertebral bodies without facets. The body of each lumbar vertebra is flattened or slightly concave superiorly and inferiorly and is deeply constricted ventrally at the sides. The spinous process of each is thick, broad, and somewhat quadrilateral. The body of the fifth lumbar vertebra is much deeper ventrally than dorsally. Compare **cervical vertebra, coccygeal vertebra, sacral vertebra, thoracic vertebra.**

lumbo- A combining form meaning 'of or pertaining to the loins': *lumbocolostomy, lumbocostal, lumbosacral.*

lumbodorsal fascia See **fascia thoracolumbalis.**

lumbosacral plexus The combination of all the ventral primary divisions of the lumbar, the sacral, and the coccygeal nerves. The lumbar and the sacral plexuses supply the lower limb. The sacral nerves also supply the perineum through the pudendal plexus and the coccygeal area through the coccygeal plexus. See also **lumbar plexus, sacral plexus.**

lumen, *pl.* **lumina, lumens. 1.** A cavity or the channel within any organ or structure of the body. **2.** A unit of luminous flux that equals the flux emitted in a unit solid angle by a point source of one candle intensity. —**lumenal, luminal,** *adj.*

lumin- A combining form meaning 'of or pertaining to light': *luminescence, luminiferous, luminophore.*

lumpectomy Surgical excision of a tumor without removal of large amounts of surrounding tissue or lymph nodes.

lun- A combining form meaning 'of or per-

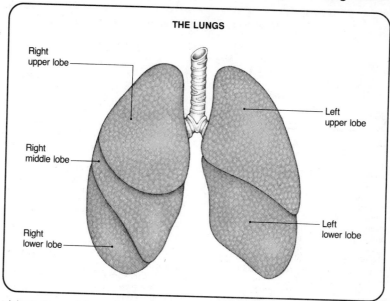

THE LUNGS

Right upper lobe

Left upper lobe

Right middle lobe

Right lower lobe

Left lower lobe

taining to the moon': *lunacy, lunate, lunatism.*

lunate bone The carpal bone in the center of the proximal row of carpal bones between the scaphoid and triangular bones. It articulates with five bones: the radius proximally, the capitate and the hamate distally, the scaphoid laterally, and the triangular medially. Also called **os lunatum, semilunar bone.**

lung One of a pair of light, spongy organs in the thorax, constituting the main component of the respiratory system. The two highly elastic lungs are the main mechanisms in the body for inspiring air from which oxygen is extracted for the arterial blood system and for exhaling carbon dioxide dispersed from the venous system. The lungs are composed of lobes that are smooth and shiny on their surface. The right lung contains three lobes; the left lung two lobes. Each lung is composed of an external serous coat, a subserous layer of areolar tissue, and the parenchyma. The serous coat comprises the thin, visceral pleura. The subserous areolar tissue contains many elastic fibers and invests the entire surface of the organ. The parenchyma is composed of secondary lobules divided into primary lobules, each of which consists of blood vessels, lymphatics, nerves, and an alveolar duct connecting with air spaces. The lungs of men are usually heavier than the lungs of women and usually have a greater capacity. The quantity of air that can be exhaled from the lungs after the deepest inspiration averages 3,700 cc. Each lung is conical and has an apex, a base, three borders, and two surfaces. The apex is rounded and extends into the root of the neck about 4 cm (1½ inches) above the first rib. The base of the lung is broad and concave, rests upon the convex surface of the diaphragm, and, with the diaphragm, moves up during expiration and down during inspiration. The surfaces of the lungs are partially concave, with a cardiac impression that cradles the heart. The bronchial arteries supply blood to nourish the lungs and are derived from the ventral side of the thoracic aorta or from the aortic intercostal arteries. The bronchial vein is formed at the root of the lung. Most of the blood supplied by the bronchial arteries is returned by the pulmonary veins.

lung cancer A pulmonary malignancy attributable to cigarette smoking in 75% of cases. Other predisposing factors are exposure to asbestos, acronitrile, arsenic, beryllium, chromium, chloromethyl ether, coal products, ionizing radiation, iron oxide, mustard gas, nickel, petroleum, uranium, and vinyl chloride. Lung cancer develops most often in scarred or chronically diseased lungs and is usually far advanced when detected. Symptoms of lung cancer include persistent cough, dyspnea, purulent or blood-streaked sputum, chest pain, and repeated attacks of bronchitis or pneumonia. Diagnostic measures include X-rays, fluoroscopy, tomography, bronchoscopy, angiography, cytologic studies of sputum, bronchial washings or brushings, and needle biopsy. Epidermoid cancers and adenocarcinomas each account for approximately 30% of lung tumors, about 25% are small- or oat-cell carcinomas, and 15% are large-cell anaplastic cancers. Epidermoid tumors tend to remain in the thorax, but other lung lesions metastasize widely. Surgery is the treatment of choice for primary lung cancer without evidence of distant metastases; for primary lung cancer with small-cell carcinoma, however, radiation or chemotherapy are generally used. Radiation, perhaps in conjunction with chemotherapy, is often used for more advanced primary tumors of all cell types. See also **oat-cell carcinoma.**

LUTEAL PHASE OF MENSTRUAL CYCLE

Luteal phase

OVARIAN FOLLICLE DEVELOPMENT

lung compliance A measure of the ease of expansion by the lungs and thorax during respiratory movements. It is determined by pulmonary volume and elasticity: a high degree of compliance indicates a loss of elastic recoil of the lungs, as in old age or emphysema. Decreased compliance of the lungs occurs in conditions when greater pressure is needed for changes of volume, as in atelectasis, edema, fibrosis, pneumonia, or absence of surfactant. Dyspnea on exertion is the main symptom of diminished lung compliance. See also **expiratory reserve volume, residual volume, respiration, vital capacity.**

lupoid hepatitis See **hepatitis.**

lupus 1. *Nontechnical.* Lupus erythematosus. **2.** Any chronic skin condition in which ulcerative lesions spread over the body over a long period of time. —**lupoid,** *adj.*

lupus erythematosus (LE) See **systemic lupus erythematosus.**

lupus erythematosus preparation (LE prep) A laboratory test for lupus erythematosus in which normal neutrophils are incubated with a specimen of the patient's serum, resulting in the appearance of large, spherical, phagocytized inclusions within the neutrophils if the patient has lupus erythematosus.

lupus vulgaris A rare cutaneous form of tuberculosis in which areas of the skin become ulcerated and heal slowly, leaving deeply scarred tissue.

lusus naturae A congenital anomaly; teratism.

luteal Of or pertaining to the corpus luteum or its functions or effects.

luteal phase Of the menstrual cycle: the second half of the cycle during which the corpus luteum is stimulated by luteinizing hormone to produce progesterone. This hormone causes the endometrium to develop from the proliferative to the secretory state, becoming a rich, dense wall suitable for nidation by a fertilized ovum. If fertilization does not occur, progesterone secretion slowly diminishes until, approximately 14 days after ovulation, the amount is not adequate for maintenance of the endometrium, and menstruation occurs.

lutein A yellow-red, crystalline, carotenoid pigment found in plants with carotenes and chlorophylls and in animal fats, egg yolk, the corpus luteum, or any lipochrome.

luteinizing hormone (LH) A glycoprotein hormone, produced by the anterior pituitary, that stimulates the secretion of sex hormones by the ovaries and the testes and is involved in the maturation of spermatozoa and ova. In men, it induces testosterone secretion by the interstitial cells of the testes. Testosterone, together with follicle stimulating hormone (FSH), induces the maturation of seminiferous tubules and stimulates them to produce sperm. In women, LH, working together with FSH, stimulates the growing follicle in the ovary to secrete estrogen. High concentrations of estrogen stimulate the release of a surge of LH, which stimulates ovulation. LH then induces the development of the ruptured follicle into the corpus luteum, which continues to secrete estrogen and progesterone. See also **menstrual cycle.**

luteoma, *pl.* **luteomas, luteomata 1.** A granulosa-theca-cell tumor whose cells resemble those of the corpus luteum. **2.** A unilateral or bilateral nodular hyperplasia of ovarian lutein cells, occasionally developing during the last trimester of pregnancy. Also called pregnancy luteoma.

luteotropin See **prolactin.**

lutetium (Lu) A rare-earth metallic element. Its atomic number is 71; its atomic weight is 174.97.

LVN *abbr* licensed vocational nurse. See **licensed practical nurse.**

lyco- A combining form meaning 'of or pertaining to a wolf ': *lycomania, lycorexia.*

lycopene A red, crystalline, unsaturated hydrocarbon that is the carotenoid pigment in tomatoes and various berries and fruits. It is considered the primary substance from which all natural carotenoid pigments are derived.

lying-in 1. Designating the time before, during, and after childbirth. **2.** Designating a hospital that provides care for women in childbirth and the puerperium. **3.** The condition of being in confinement or childbed.

Lyme arthritis An acute, recurrent inflammatory disease, involving one or a few joints, believed to be transmitted by an unidentified tickborne virus. The condition has been reported in parts of the northeastern United States and, sporadically, in other countries. Knees, other large joints, and temperomandibular joints are most commonly involved, with local heat and swelling. Chills, fever, headache, malaise, and erythema chronicum migrans, an expanding annular, erythematous skin eruption, often precede the joint manifestations. Occasionally, cardiac conduction abnormalities, aseptic meningitis, or Bell's palsy are associated conditions. Symptoms appear in recurrent episodes, lasting usually about 1 week, at intervals of from 1 to several weeks, declining in severity over a 2- or 3-year period. There is no significant permanent joint damage. Treatment includes salicylates for joint symptoms and corticosteroids to reduce cardiac and neurological manifestations.

lymph A thin opalescent fluid originating in many organs and tissues that is circulated through the lymphatic vessels and filtered by the lymph nodes. Lymph enters the blood stream at the junction of the internal jugular and subclavian veins. It contains chyle, a few erythrocytes, and variable numbers of leukocytes, most of which are lymphocytes. It is otherwise similar to plasma. See also **chyle.**

lymph- See **lympho-.**

-lymph A combining form meaning a 'clear body fluid': *hemolymph, neurolymph, perilymph.*

lymphadenitis An inflammatory condition of the lymph nodes, usually the result of systemic neoplastic disease or bacterial infection or other inflammatory condition. The nodes may be enlarged, hard, smooth or irregular, red, and may feel hot. The location of the affected node is indicative of the site or origin of disease.

lymphadenoid goiter See **Hashimoto's disease.**

lymphangiectasia Dilatation of lymphatic vessels, characterized by diarrhea, steatorrhea, and protein malabsorption. It usually results from obstruction, as in pelvic tuberculosis, mesenteric node metastases, and certain protozoan diseases.

lymphangioma, *pl.* **lymphangiomas, lymphangiomata** A benign, yellow-tan tumor on the skin, composed of a mass of dilated lymph vessels. It is often removed for cosmetic reasons by excision or electrocoagulation. Also called **angioma lymphaticum.** See also **angioma.**

lymphangioma cavernosum A tumor formed by dilated lymphatic vessels and filled with lymph that is often mixed with coagulated blood. The lesion, which is often congenital, may cause extensive enlargement of the affected tissue, especially of the tongue and lips. Also called **cavernous lymphangioma.**

lymphangioma circumscriptum A benign skin lesion developing from superficial hypertrophic lymph vessels. Most common in young children, it is characteristically pigmented and may grow to several centimeters in diameter.

lymphangioma cysticum See **cystic lymphangioma.**

lymphangioma simplex A growth formed by moderately dilated lymph vessels in a circumscribed area, chiefly on the skin.

lymphangitis An inflammation of one or more lymphatic vessels, usually resulting from an acute streptococcal infection of one of the extremities. It is characterized by fine red streaks extending from the infected area to the axilla or groin and by fever, chills, headache, and myalgia. The infection may spread to the bloodstream. Penicillin and hot soaks are usually prescribed.

lymphatic 1. Of or pertaining to the lymphatic system of the body, consisting of a vast network of tubes transporting lymph. 2. Any one of the vessels associated with the lymphatic network.

lymphatic capillary plexus One of the numerous networks of lymphatic capillaries that collect lymph from the intercellular fluid and constitute the beginning of the lymphatic system. The lymphatic vessels arise from the capillary plexuses, which vary in size and number in different regions and organs of the body. The capillary networks do not contain lymphatic valves, unlike the vessels. The plexuses are especially abundant in the dermis of the skin but also lace many other areas, as the mucous membranes of the repiratory and digestive systems, testes, ovaries, liver, kidneys and heart. See also **lymphatic system.**

lymphatic leukemia See **acute lymphocytic leukemia, chronic lymphocytic leukemia.**

lymphatic nodule See **Malpighian body.**

lymphatic system A vast, complex network of capillaries, thin vessels, valves, ducts, nodes, and organs that helps to protect and maintain the internal fluid environment of the body by producing, filtering, and conveying lymph and by producing various blood cells. The lymphatic network also transports fats, proteins, and other substances to the blood system and restores 60% of the fluid that filters out of the blood capillaries into interstitial spaces during normal metabolism. The peripheral parts of the lymphatic complex do not directly communicate with the venous system into which the lymph flows, but the endothelium of the veins at the junction of the blood and the lymphatic networks is continuous with the endothelium of the lymphatic vessels. Small semilunar valves throughout the lymphatic network help to control the flow of lymph and, at the junction with the venous system, prevent venous blood from flowing into the lymphatic vessels. The lymph collected drains into the blood through two ducts situated in the neck. Various body dynamics, as respiratory pressure changes, muscular contractions, and movements of organs surrounding lymphatic vessels, combine to pump the lymph through the lymphatic system. The thoracic duct that rises into the left side of the neck is the major vessel of the lymphatic system and conveys lymph from the whole body, except for the right quadrant, which is served by the right lymphatic duct. Lymphatics have a beaded appearance because of sinuses associated with the many valves in the vessels. The lymphatic capillaries, which are the beginning of the system, abound in the dermis of the skin, forming a continuous network over the entire body, except for the cornea. The system also includes specialized lymphatic organs, as the tonsils, the thymus, and the spleen.

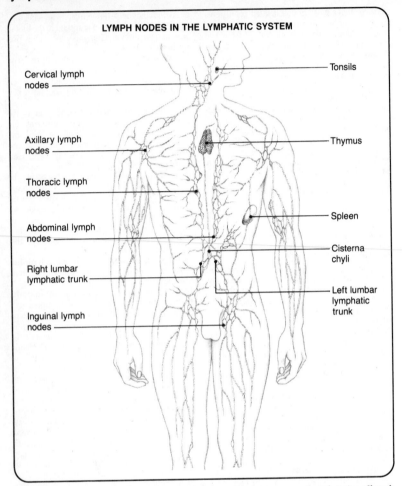

LYMPH NODES IN THE LYMPHATIC SYSTEM

Cervical lymph nodes — Tonsils

Axillary lymph nodes — Thymus

Thoracic lymph nodes

Abdominal lymph nodes — Spleen

Right lumbar lymphatic trunk — Cisterna chyli

Inguinal lymph nodes — Left lumbar lymphatic trunk

The lymphatics of the intestine contain a special substance, especially during the digestion of fatty foods. Lymph flows into the general circulation through the thoracic duct at a rate of about 125 ml/hour (4¼ oz/hour) during routine exertion. The rate may jump to as high as 1,800 ml/hour (61 oz/hour) during vigorous exercise. See also **lymph, lymph node, spleen, thymus.**

lymphedema A primary or secondary disorder characterized by the accumulation of lymph in soft tissue and swelling, caused by inflammation, obstruction, or removal of lymph channels. Congenital lymphedema is a hereditary disorder characterized by chronic lymphatic obstruction. Lymphedema praecox occurs in adolescence, chiefly in females, and causes puffiness and swelling of the lower limbs, apparently because of hyperplastic development of lymph vessels. Secondary lymphedema may follow surgical removal of lymph channels in mastectomy, obstruction of lymph drainage caused by malignant tumors, or the infestation of lymph vessels with adult filarial parasites. Lymphedema of the lower extremities begins with mild swelling of the foot, gradually extends to the entire limb, and is aggravated by prolonged standing, pregnancy, obesity, warm weather, and the menstrual period. There is no cure for the disorder, but lymph drainage from the extremity can be improved if the patient sleeps with the foot of the bed elevated 10.2 to 20.3 cm (4 to 8 inches), wears an elastic stocking, and takes moderate exercise regularly. Surgery may be performed to remove hypertrophied lymph channels and disfiguring tissue. **—lymphedematous, lymphedematose,** *adj.*

lymph node One of the many small, oval structures that filter the lymph, fight infection, and in which are formed lymphocytes, monocytes, and plasma cells. The lymph nodes are of different sizes, some as small as pinheads, others as large as lima beans. Each node is enclosed in a capsule, is composed of a lighter colored cortical portion and a darker medullary portion, and consists of closely packed lymphocytes, reticular connective tissue laced by trabeculae, and three kinds of sinuses: subcapsular, cortical, and medullary. Lymph flows into the node through afferent lymphatic vessels that open into the subcapsular sinuses. Efferent lymphatic vessels arise from the medullary sinuses of the node and emerge through a small peripheral hilum that also receives blood vessels. The sinuses and meshes of reticular fibers retard the flow of lymph, to which lymphocytes are added from germinal centers within the node. Most lymph nodes are clustered in areas, as the mouth, the neck, the lower arm, the axilla, and the groin. Also called lymph gland.

lympho-, lymph- A combining form meaning 'of or pertaining to the lymph': *lymphoduct*.

lymphoblastic lymphoma, lymphosarcoma, lymphoblastoma See **poorly differentiated lymphocytic malignant lymphoma.**

lymphocyte One of two kinds of small, agranulocytic leukocytes, originating from stem cells and developing in the bone marrow. Lymphocytes normally comprise 25% of the total white blood cell count but increase in number in response to infection. They occur in two forms: **B cells** and **T cells.** B cells circulate in an immature form and synthesize antibodies for insertion into their own cytoplasmic membranes. They reproduce mitotically, each of the clones displaying identical antibodies on their surface membranes. When an immature B cell is exposed to a specific antigen, the cell is activated, traveling to the spleen or to the lymph nodes, differentiating, and rapidly producing **plasma cells** and **memory cells.** Plasma cells synthesize and secrete copious amounts of antibody. Memory cells do not secrete antibody, but if reexposure to the specific antigen occurs, they develop into antibody-secreting plasma cells. The function of the B cell is to search out, identify, and bind with specific antigens. T cells are lymphocytes that have circulated through the thymus gland and have differentiated to become thymocytes. When exposed to an antigen, they divide rapidly and produce large numbers of new T cells sensitized to that antigen. T cells are often called killer cells because they secrete immunologically essential chemical compounds and assist B cells in destroying foreign protein. T cells also appear to play a significant role in the body's resistance to the proliferation of cancer cells. See also **lymphokine.**

lymphocytic choriomeningitis An arenavirus infection of the meninges and cerebrospinal fluid, caused by the lymphocytic choriomeningitis virus and characterized by fever, headache, and stiff neck. The infection occurs mainly in young adults, most often in the fall and winter.

lymphocytic leukemia See **acute lymphocytic leukemia, chronic lymphocytic leukemia.**

lymphocytic lymphoma, lymphosarcoma See **well-differentiated lymphocytic malignant lymphoma.**

lymphocytic thyroiditis See **Hashimoto's disease.**

lymphocytoma See **well-differentiated lymphocytic malignant lymphoma.**

lymphocytopenia A smaller than normal number of lymphocytes in the peripheral circulation, occurring as a primary hematologic disorder or in association with nutritional deficiency, malignancy, or infectious mononucleosis. See also **agranulocyte.**

lymphoderma perniciosa See **leukemia cutis.**

lymphoepithelial carcinoma See **lymphoepithelioma.**

lymphoepithelioma A poorly differentiated neoplasm developing from the epithelium overlying lymphoid tissue in the nasopharynx. This skin disorder occurs most frequently in young Orientals. Also called **lymphoepithelial carcinoma.**

lymphogenous leukemia See **acute lymphocytic leukemia, chronic lymphocytic leukemia.**

lymphogranuloma venereum (LGV) An infection caused by a strain of the bacterium *Chlamydia trachomatis*. It is characterized by ulcerative genital lesions, marked swelling of the lymph nodes in the groin, headache, fever, and malaise. Ulcerations of the rectal wall occur less commonly. The disease is transmitted by coitus and is diagnosed by isolating the organism from an infected node, demonstrating LGV antibodies by serologic blood test or by a Frei intradermal test. Tetracycline is usually prescribed. Also called **lymphopathia venereum.** See also *Chlamydia*.

lymphoid leukemia See **acute lymphocytic leukemia, chronic lymphocytic leukemia.**

lymphoidocytic leukemia See **stem cell leukemia.**

lymphokine A chemical factor produced and released by T-lymphocytes that attracts macrophages to the site of infection or inflammation and prepares them for attack. Kinds of lymphokines include **lymphotoxin, mitogenic factor.**

lympholysis Cellular destruction of lymphocytes, especially of certain lymphocytes in the process of an immune response. —**lympholytic,** *adj.*

lymphoma, *pl.* **lymphomas, lymphomata** A neoplasm of lymphoid tissue that is usually malignant but, rarely, may be benign. The various lymphomas differ in degree of cellular differentiation and content. Men are more likely than women to develop lymphoid tumors. Treatment for lymphoma includes intensive radiotherapy and chemotherapy. Kinds of lymphoma include **Burkitt's lymphoma, giant follicular lymphoma, histiocytic malignant lymphoma, Hodgkin's disease, mixed-cell malignant lymphoma.** —**lymphomatoid,** *adj.*

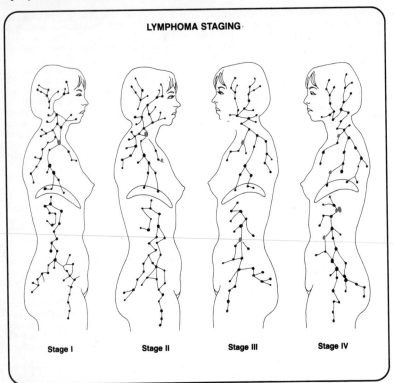

LYMPHOMA STAGING

Stage I　　　　Stage II　　　　Stage III　　　　Stage IV

-lymphoma　　A combining form meaning 'a tumor or neoplastic disorder of lymphoid tissue': *adenolymphoma, angiolymphoma, cystadenolymphoma.*

lymphoma staging　　A system for classifying lymphomas according to the stage of the disease. Stage I is characterized by the involvement of a single lymph node region or one extralymphatic organ or site and Stage II by the involvement of two or more lymph node regions on the same side of the diaphragm or a localized involvement of an extralymphatic organ or site plus one or more node regions on the same side of the diaphragm. In Stage III, lymph nodes on both sides of the diaphragm are affected, and there may be involvement of the spleen or localized involvement of an extralymphatic organ or site. Stage IV is typified by diffuse or disseminated involvement of one or more extralymphatic organs or sites with or without associated lymph node involvement.

lymphopathia venereum　　See **lymphogranuloma venereum.**

lymphopenia　　See **lymphocytopenia.**

lymphoreticulosis　　Subacute granulomatous inflammation of lymphoid tissue with proliferation of reticuloendothelial cells, resulting most often from a cat scratch. No causative agent is known. The disorder is characterized by ulcerated papule formation at the scratch site and by fever and tender lymphadenopathy, sometimes progressing to suppuration. Also called **cat-scratch fever.**

lymphosarcoma, *pl.* **lymphosarcomas, lymphosarcomata**　　See **non-Hodgkin's lymphoma.**

lymphosarcoma cell leukemia　　A malignancy of blood-forming tissues characterized by many lymphosarcoma cells in the peripheral circulation that tend to infiltrate surrounding tissues. These cells are extremely immature and larger and more reticulated than lymphocytes. The disease may accompany lymphoma or exist separately, with more bone marrow involvement than in lymphoma.

lyo-　　A combining form meaning 'dissolved': *lyogel, lyophobe, lyotropic.*

Lyon hypothesis　　In genetics: a hypothesis stating that only one of the two X chromosomes in a female is functional, the other having become inactive early in development. A female is mosaic in regard to X chromosomes: some are from her father, some from her mother. Sex-linked genes may therefore appear on some of her cells and not on others.

lypressin　　An analog of the antidiuretic hormone vasopressin.

-lysin　　A combining form meaning 'a cell-dissolving antibody': *antilysin, betalysin, paralysin.*

lysine An essential amino acid needed for proper growth in infants and for maintenance of nitrogen balance in adults. See also **amino acid, protein.**

lysine intolerance A congenital disorder resulting in the inability to use the essential amino acid lysine owing to an enzyme deficiency or defect. The disorder is characterized by weakness, vomiting, and coma and is treated by adjusting the protein content of the diet, restricting those foods especially high in lysine.

lysinemia A condition caused by an inborn error of metabolism and resulting in the inability to utilize the essential amino acid lysine, owing to an enzyme defect or deficiency. It is characterized by muscle weakness and mental retardation. Treatment consists of a diet that controls the intake of lysine by reducing proteins and including such foods as fruits, vegetables, and rice.

lysine monohydrochloride A salt of the amino acid lysine, used as a dietary supplement to increase the utilization of vegetable proteins, as corn, rice, and wheat.

lysis **1.** Destruction or dissolution of a cell or molecule through the action of a specific agent. Cell lysis is frequently caused by a lysin. **2.** Gradual diminution in the symptoms of a disease. Compare **crisis.**

-lysis A combining form meaning 'a breaking down or detachment': *cytolysis, dialysis, osteolysis.*

lyso- A combining form meaning 'of or pertaining to dissolution': *lysocephalin, lysotype.*

lysosome A cytoplasmic, membrane-bound particle that contains hydrolytic enzymes that function in intracellular digestive processes. The organelles are found in most cells but are particularly prominent in leukocytes and in the cells of the liver and kidney. If the hydrolytic enzymes are released into the cytoplasm, they cause self-digestion of the cell so that lysosomes may play an important role in certain self-destructive diseases characterized by the wasting of tissue, as muscular dystrophy.

lysso- A combining form meaning 'of or pertaining to rabies or hydrophobia': *lyssoderis, lyssoid, lyssophobia.*

-lyte A combining form meaning 'a substance capable of or resulting from decomposition': *ampholyte, cytolyte.*

lytes *Informal.* Electrolytes, especially the levels of potassium, sodium, phosphorus, magnesium, and calcium in the blood, as determined by laboratory testing.

-lytic A combining form meaning 'pertaining to or effecting decomposition': *fibrillolytic, leukolytic, myelolytic.*

lytic cocktail An informal name for an anesthetic compound of chlorpromazine, meperidine, and promethazine that blocks the autonomic nervous system, depresses the circulatory system, and induces neuroplegia.

-lyze, -lyse A combining form meaning 'to produce decomposition': *bacteriolyze, hemolyze, paralyze.*

M

m *abbr* **meter.**

M **1.** Symbol for **molar solution. 2.** *abbr* **metastasis** in the TNM system for staging malignant neoplastic disease. See also **cancer staging.**

ma *abbr* **milliampere.**

MA *abbr* **mental age.**

M.A. *abbr* **Master of Arts.**

MAC *abbr* **1. minimum alveolar concentration. 2.** maximum allowable concentration.

macerate To soften something solid by soaking. **—maceration,** *n.*

machupo See **Bolivian hemorrhagic fever.**

macrencephaly, macroencephaly Congenital anomaly marked by abnormal largeness of the brain. See also **macrocephaly. —macrencephalic, macroencephalic,** *adj., n.*

macro- A combining form meaning 'large, or abnormal size': *macrobiosis, macrocardius.*

macroblepharia The condition of having abnormally large eyelids.

macrocephaly, macrocephalia A congenital anomaly characterized by abnormal largeness of the head and brain in relation to the rest of the body, resulting in some degree of mental and growth retardation. The head is more than two standard deviations above the average circumference size with excessively wide fontanelles; the facial features are usually normal. The condition may be caused by some defect in formation during embryonic development, or it may be the result of progressively degenerative processes, as Schilder's disease. In macrocephaly there is symmetrical overgrowth at the head without increased intracranial pressure, as differentiated from hydrocephalus in which the lateral, asymmetrical growth of the head is caused by excessive accumulation of cerebrospinal fluid, usually under increased pressure. Treatment is primarily symptomatic. Also called **megalocephaly.** Compare **microcephaly.** See also **hydrocephalus. —macrocephalic, macrocephalous,** *adj.,* **macrocephalus,** *n.*

macrocyte An abnormally large, mature erythrocyte usually exceeding 9 microns in diameter. It is most commonly seen in megaloblastic anemia. Compare **microcyte.** See also **macrocytic anemia. —macrocytic,** *adj.*

macrocytic Of a cell: larger than normal, as the erythrocytes in macrocytic anemia.

macrocytic anemia A disorder of the blood characterized by impaired erythropoiesis and the abnormal presence of large, fragile red blood cells in the circulation. Macrocytic anemia is most often the result of a deficiency of folic acid and vitamin B_{12}.

macrocytosis An abnormal proliferation of macrocytes in the peripheral blood.

macrodrip In intravenous therapy: an apparatus that is used to deliver measured amounts of intravenous solutions at specific flow rates based on the size of drops of the solution. The size of the drops is controlled by the fixed diameter of a plastic delivery tube. The drops delivered by a macrodrip are larger than those delivered by a microdrip. Different macrodrip systems deliver from 10 to 20 drops/ml of solution. Macrodrips are not usually used to deliver a small amount of intravenous solution or to keep a vein open, because the time between drips is so long that a clot may form at the tip of the intravenous catheter. Compare **microdrip.**

macroelement See **macronutrient.**

macroencephaly See **macrencephaly.**

macrogamete A large, nonmotile female gamete of certain thallophytes and sporozoa, specifically the malarial parasite *Plasmodium.* It corresponds to the ovum of the higher animals and is fertilized by the smaller, motile male gamete. See also **microgamete.**

macrogametocyte An enlarged merozoite that undergoes meiosis to form the mature female gamete during the sexual phase of the life cycle of certain thallophytes and sporozoa, specifically the malarial parasite *Plasmodium.* Macrogametocytes are found in the red blood cells of a person infected with the malarial parasite.

macrogenitosomia A congenital condition in which the genitalia are abnormal owing to an excess of androgen during fetal development. It is characterized in boys by enlarged external genitalia and in girls by pseudohermaphroditism.

macroglobulinemia A form of monoclonal gammopathy in which a large immunoglobulin (IgM) is vastly overproduced by the clones of a plasma B cell in response to an antigenic signal. Increased viscosity of the blood may result in circulatory impairment, weakness, neurologic disorders, and fatigue. Normal immunoglobulin synthesis is decreased and the person is susceptible to infection. Also called **Waldenström's macroglobulinemia.** See also **multiple myeloma.**

macroglossia A congenital anomaly characterized by excessive size of the tongue, as seen in certain syndromes of congenital defects, including Down's syndrome.

macrognathia An abnormally large growth of the jaw. Compare **micrognathia. —macrognathic,** *adj.*

macronucleus **1.** A large nucleus. **2.** In

protozoa: the larger of two nuclei in each cell; it governs cell metabolism and growth as opposed to the micronucleus, which functions in sexual reproduction.

macronutrient A chemical element required in relatively large quantities for the normal physiological processes of the body. Macronutrients include carbon, hydrogen, oxygen, nitrogen, potassium, sodium, calcium, chloride, magnesium, phosphorus, and sulfur. Also called **macroelement, major element.** Compare **micronutrient.**

macrophage Any phagocytic cell of the reticuloendothelial system including Kupffer cell in the liver, splenocyte in the spleen, and histocyte in the loose connective tissue. See also **phagocyte, reticuloendothelial system.**

macrosomia See **gigantism.**

macula, *pl.* **maculae** A small, pigmented area or a spot that appears separate or different from the surrounding tissue.

macula cerulea *pl.* **maculae cerulea.** See **blue spot,** definition 1.

macula lutea An oval yellow spot at the center of the retina 2 mm from the optic nerve. It contains a pit, no blood vessels, and the fovea centralis. Central vision occurs when an image is focused directly on the fovea centralis of the macula lutea. Also called **macula** *(informal).*

macule **1.** A small, flat blemish or discoloration that is flush with the skin surface. Examples are the rashes of measles and roseola. Compare **papule. 2.** A gray scar on the cornea that is visible without magnification. —**macular,** *adj.*

maculopapular Consisting of or relating to a skin eruption with thickened or discolored areas that are flush with the surface (**macules**) as well as small, solid, raised lesions (**papules**).

Madelung's neck See **lipoma annulare colli.**

mad hatter's disease See **mercury poisoning.**

Madura foot A progressive, destructive, tropical fungal infection of the foot. Also called maduromycosis.

maduromycosis See **Madura foot.**

mafenide acetate A local anti-infective agent.

magaldrate An antacid.

Maffucci's syndrome A condition characterized by enchondromatosis and multiple cutaneous or visceral hemangiomas.

Magendie's law See **Bell's law.**

magic bullet approach **1.** A therapeutic or diagnostic method that makes use of a specific mechanistic connection between a drug and a disease or organ. **2.** In clinical medicine: the administration of a specific drug to cure or ameliorate a given disease or condition. **3.** In traditional diagnostic radiology: the administration of a dye to aid X-ray of a given organ, as the intravenous injection of a specific dye for renal studies. **4.** In nuclear medicine: the administration of a specific radioactive isotope, tagged to an appropriate carrier, to provide a

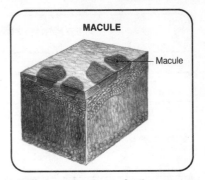

MACULE

Macule

scintillation camera image of a given organ or structure, as the use of a substance containing phosphate and technetium for bone scanning.

magnesia magma (MOM) An antacid.

magnesium (Mg) A silver-white mineral element. Its atomic number is 12; its atomic weight is 24.32. Magnesium occurs abundantly in nature, always in combination with other elements, in seawater, bones, seeds, the chlorophyll in the green parts of plants, and in minerals, as magnesite. Magnesium is the second most abundant cation of the intracellular fluids in the body and is essential for many enzyme activities. It is also important to neurochemical transmissions and muscular excitability. Very little is known about the exchange of magnesium between the plasma, the intracellular capsule, and the bone. About 30% of the magnesium in the skeleton represents an exchangeable pool. The average adult in the United States ingests between 20 to 40 mEq of magnesium daily, and about 33% of the quantity ingested is absorbed from the gastrointestinal tract. Magnesium is excreted mainly by the kidneys, and 3% to 5% of the magnesium is excreted in the urine. Small amounts of magnesium are excreted in milk and in the saliva. The element influences many enzymes in the body and is a cofactor of all enzymes participating in phosphate transfer reactions involving adenosine triphosphate and other nucleotide triphosphates as substrates. It is also essential to the interaction of intracellular particles and the binding of macromolecules to subcellular organelles, as the binding of messenger RNA to ribosomes. Magnesium affects the central nervous, neuromuscular, and cardiovascular systems.

magnesium carbonate An antacid and laxative agent.

magnesium salicylate A salicylate nonnarcotic analgesic and antipyretic.

magnesium salts A hyperosmolar laxative.

magnesium sulfate An anticonvulsant and electrolyte source.

magnesium trisilicate An antacid.

magnet reflex A pathologic reflex seen in an animal that has had its cerebellum removed. If the animal is placed on its back and its head is strongly flexed, all four limbs will flex. Light

MNO

MAJOR AFFECTIVE DISORDERS

DEPRESSIVE DISORDER

SYMPTOMS	MILD-SEVERE BUT NOT PSYCHOTIC	SEVERE AND PSYCHOTIC
Anxiety	• Mild, moderate, or severe	• Severe, especially in agitated form
Depression	• Mild, moderate, or severe	• Severe, with or without precipitating environmental factors • Worst in early morning • Flat affect, inactive, hopeless
Problems in relating to others	• Dependent on others • Marginally able to meet commitments	• Speaks infrequently in groups • Poor self-image • Severely withdrawn
Anger, aggression, hostility	• Mild to severe; turned inward • Contemplates and may attempt suicide	• Feels anger toward self but usually doesn't have energy to act on feelings
Disruption in thought processes	• Remains in contact with reality (aware of behavior but can't stop it) • Can't concentrate	• Delusions of sinfulness, disease, or impending doom • Severely impaired judgment

BIPOLAR AFFECTIVE DISORDER

SYMPTOMS	MANIC PHASE	DEPRESSIVE PHASE
Anxiety	• Severe, manifested by increased activity	• Variable
Depression	• Symptoms of mania to ward off depression • Labile affect (happy/tearful)	• Severe • May show signs and symptoms of other depressions
Problems in relating to others	• Overinvolved in activities of others; manipulative • Dresses and uses makeup inappropriately and bizarrely • Lacks normal inhibitions	• Loses interest in activities • Becomes isolated • May show signs and symptoms of other depressions
Anger, aggression, hostility	• May be angry and irritable, especially when behavior is controlled • May become violent	• Hates self; thinks frequently of death; may attempt suicide • May show signs and symptoms of other depressions
Disruption in thought processes	• Rhymes, plays with words • Pressured speech • Delusions of grandeur and persecution • Flight of ideas	• Delusions • Decreased thinking ability • May show signs and symptoms of other depressions

pressure by a finger on a toepad then causes contraction of limb extensor muscles so that if the finger is slowly removed the limb appears to follow the finger.

main en griffe See **clawhand.**

Majocchi's granuloma A rare type of tinea corporis, mainly affecting the lower legs. It is caused by the fungus *Trichophyton*, which infects the hairs of the affected site and raises spongy granulomas. The lesions persist for 3 to 4 months and are gradually absorbed, or they necrose, often leaving deep scars. Also called **trichophytic granuloma.**

major affective disorder Any of a group

of psychotic disorders characterized by severe and inappropriate emotional responses, by prolonged and persistent disturbances of mood and related thought distortions, and by other symptoms associated with either depressed or manic states, as occur in bipolar disorder, depression, and involutional melancholia. The disorder is usually episodic but may be chronic or cyclical. It is not caused by any organic dysfunction of the brain.

major depressive episode See **endogenous depression.**

major element See **macronutrient.**

major medical insurance Insurance coverage designed to offset the costs of prolonged or catastrophic illness and injury. Most major medical insurance policies are written to pay a certain percentage of costs up to a predetermined figure. Many require the insured person to pay in full a specified initial or deductible amount.

makro- See **macro-.**

mal French. An illness or disease, as grand mal.

mal- A combining form meaning 'abnormal': maladjustment, malignant.

malabsorption Impaired absorption of nutrients from the gastrointestinal tract. It occurs in celiac disease, sprue, dysentery, diarrhea, and other disorders and may result from an inborn error of metabolism, malnutrition, or any chemical or anatomic condition of the digestive system that prevents normal absorption. See **inborn error of metabolism, malnutrition.**

malabsorption syndrome A complex of symptoms resulting from disorders in the intestinal absorption of nutrients, characterized by anorexia, weight loss, bloating of the abdomen, muscle cramps, bone pain, and steatorrhea. Anemia, weakness, and fatigue occur because iron, folic acid, and vitamin B_{12} are not absorbed in sufficient amounts. Among the many conditions causing this syndrome are gastric or small-bowel resection, celiac disease, tropical sprue, Whipple's disease, intestinal lymphangiectasia, and cystic fibrosis. See also **celiac disease, cystic fibrosis, hypoproteinemia, tropical sprue.**

malacia 1. A morbid softening or a sponginess in any part or any tissue of the body. 2. A craving for spicy foods, as mustard, hot peppers, or pickles. **—malacic,** adj.

-malacia A combining form meaning the 'softening of tissue': cardiomalacia, esophagomalacia.

malaco- A combining form meaning 'a condition of abnormal softness': malacoplakia, malacosarcosis.

maladaptation Faulty intrapersonal adaptation to stress or change. It may involve a failure to make necessary changes in desires, values, needs, and attitudes or an inability to make necessary adjustments in the external world. Illness often provokes maladaptive behavior that increases the problems accompanying the illness.

malaise A vague feeling of bodily weakness or discomfort, often marking the onset of disease.

malar Of or pertaining to the cheek or the cheek bone.

malaria A serious infectious illness caused by four species of the protozoan genus Plasmodium, characterized by chills, fever, anemia, an enlarged spleen, and a tendency to recur. The disease is transmitted from human to human by a bite from an infected Anopheles mosquito. Malarial infection can also be spread by blood transfusion from an infected patient or by the use of an infected hypodermic needle. Although the endemic disease is limited largely to tropical areas of South and Central America, Africa, and Asia, a number of new cases have been brought to the U.S. in recent years by refugees, military personnel returning from Southeast Asia, and travelers to malarial areas. Plasmodium parasites penetrate the erythrocytes of the human host, where they mature, reproduce, and burst out periodically. Because the life cycle of the infecting parasite varies according to species, the clinical patterns of chills and fever differ as do the course and severity of the disease. Bouts of malaria usually last from 1 to 4 weeks. Relapse is common, and the disease can persist for years. Diagnosis is made by demonstrating the Plasmodium parasite in a blood smear. Chloroquine, given orally or intramuscularly, is the drug of choice for all but those strains of Plasmodium resistant to chloroquine, which are treated with a combination of quinine, pyrimethamine, and one of the sulfonamides or sulfones. Modern antimalarial drugs can suppress symptoms or cure malaria completely. Symptoms of headache, nausea, muscle ache, and high fever can be relieved with cold compresses, aspirin, and fluids. Prophylaxis with antimalarial drugs is still important for those visiting endemic areas. The use of netting and mosquito repellent is also encouraged. See also **blackwater fever, falciparum malaria, quartan malaria, tertian malaria. —malarial,** adj.

malarial hemoglobinuria See **blackwater fever.**

malathion poisoning A toxic condition caused by the ingestion or absorption through the skin of malathion, an organophosphorus insecticide. Symptoms include vomiting, nausea, abdominal cramps, headache, dizziness, weakness, confusion, convulsions, and respiratory difficulties. Treatment includes immediate intravenous administration of atropine, followed by pralidoxime chloride, gastric lavage, a saline cathartic, respiratory assistance, and oxygen. Malathion is the only organophosphorus insecticide approved for household use.

malaxation See **pétrissage.**

Malayan pit viper venom See **ancrod.**

mal del pinto See **pinta.**

male 1. a. Of or pertaining to the sex that fertilizes the female to beget offspring. b. Masculine. 2. A male person.

male reproductive system assessment An evaluation of the condition of the patient's

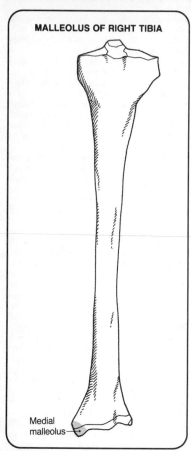

MALLEOLUS OF RIGHT TIBIA

Medial
malleolus—

genitalia, reproductive history, and past and present genitourinary infections and disorders.

male sexual dysfunction Impaired or inadequate ability of a man to carry on his sex life to his own satisfaction. Symptoms, often psychologic in origin, include difficulties in starting and maintaining an erection, premature ejaculation, inability to ejaculate, and even loss of desire. Men are often so ashamed of the problem that they ask the physician to treat a "prostate problem." See also **sexuality.**

malfeasance Performance of an unlawful, wrongful act. Compare **misfeasance, nonfeasance.**

malformation An anomalous structure in the body. See also **congenital anomaly.**

malgaigne of pelvis Trauma involving multiple pelvic fractures, including fracture of the wing of the ilium or sacrum and of the ipsilateral pubic rami.

malignant 1. Tending to become worse and cause death. Also called **virulent.** 2. Describing a cancer that is invasive and metastatic. —**malignancy,** n.

malignant ependymoma See **ependymoblastoma.**

malignant hemangioendothelioma See **hemangiosarcoma.**

malignant hepatoma A malignant tumor of the liver. Relatively rare in the United States, its occurrence is 80% higher in Africa and the Far East. The only effective treatment is surgical excision of the tumor. This is often not feasible, as the tumors grow rapidly and spread through both lobes of the liver. The prognosis is poor. Also called **hepatocarcinoma, hepatocellular carcinoma, liver cell carcinoma.**

malignant hypertension An abnormal condition and the most lethal form of both essential hypertension and secondary hypertension. It is a fulminating condition, characterized by severely elevated blood pressure, that commonly damages the intima of small vessels, the brain, retina, heart, and kidneys. It affects more blacks than whites and may be caused by a variety of factors, as stress, genetic predisposition, high intake of sodium chloride, a sedentary life-style, and aging. Many patients with this condition exhibit signs of hypokalemia, alkalosis, and aldosterone secretion rates even higher than those associated with primary aldosteronism.

malignant hyperthermia (MH) An autosomal dominant trait characterized by often fatal hyperthermia with rigidity of the muscles occurring in affected people exposed to certain anesthetic agents, particularly halothane, succinylcholine, and methoxyflurane. Treatment includes the administration of dantrolene or 100% oxygen, cooling procedures, and the correction of acidosis and hyperkalemia.

malignant malnutrition See **kwashiorkor.**

malignant mesenchymoma A sarcoma that contains two or more cellular elements, not including fibrous elements; a mixed cell sarcoma.

malignant mole See **chorioadenoma destruens.**

malignant neoplasm A tumor that tends to grow, invade, and metastasize. It usually has an irregular shape and is composed of poorly differentiated cells. If untreated it can kill the organism. The degree to which a neoplasm is malignant varies with the kind of tumor and the condition of the patient.

malignant neuroma See **neurosarcoma.**

malignant pustule See **anthrax.**

malignant tumor A neoplasm that characteristically invades surrounding tissue, metastasizes to distant sites, and contains anaplastic cells. A malignant tumor may be expected to result in the death of the host if remission or treatment does not intervene.

malingering A willful and deliberate feigning of the symptoms of a disease or injury to gain some consciously desired end. Compare **compensation neurosis. —malinger,** v., **malingerer,** n.

malleolus, pl. **malleoli** A rounded bony

process, as the protuberance on each side of the ankle.

mallet fracture Avulsion fracture of the dorsal base of a distal phalanx of the hand or foot, involving the associated extensor apparatus and causing dropped flexion of the distal segment.

malleus One of the three ossicles in the middle ear, resembling a hammer with a head, a neck, and three processes. It is connected to the tympanic membrane and transmits sound vibrations to the incus. Compare **incus, stapes.** See also **middle ear.**

Mallory-Weiss syndrome A condition characterized by massive bleeding following a tear in the mucous membrane at the junction of the esophagus and the stomach. The laceration is usually caused by protracted vomiting, most commonly in alcoholics or in persons whose pylorus is obstructed. The esophageal tear is located by esophagoscopy or arteriography. Surgery is usually necessary to stop the bleeding.

malnutrition Any disorder concerning nutrition. It may result from an unbalanced, insufficient, or excessive diet or from the impaired absorption, assimilation, or utilization of foods. Compare **deficiency disease.**

malocclusion Abnormal contact of the teeth of the upper jaw with the teeth of the lower jaw. See also **occlusion.**

malonic acid A white, crystalline, highly toxic substance used as an intermediate compound in the production of barbiturates.

malpighian body **1.** The renal corpuscle, which includes a glomerulus with Bowman's capsule. **2.** Lymphoid tissue surrounding the arteries of the spleen. Also called **lymphatic nodule.**

malpighian corpuscle One of a number of small, round, deep-red bodies in the cortex of the kidney, each communicating with a renal tubule. They average about 0.2 mm in diameter, each capsule composed of two parts: a central glomerulus and a glomerular capsule. The corpuscles are thought to be part of a filter system through which nonprotein components of blood plasma enter the tubules for urinary excretion. Also called **malpighian body, renal corpuscle.**

malpractice In law: professional negligence that is the proximate cause of injury or harm to a patient, resulting from a lack of professional knowledge, experience, or skill that can be expected in others in the profession or from a failure to exercise reasonable judgment in the application of professional knowledge, experience, or skill.

Malta fever See **brucellosis.**

malt worker's lung A respiratory disorder acquired by occupational exposure to fungi-laden particles of moldy barley grain or malt. See also **organic dust.**

malunion An imperfect union of previously fragmented bone or other tissue.

mamm- A combining form meaning 'of or pertaining to the breast': *mammectomy, mammogram.*

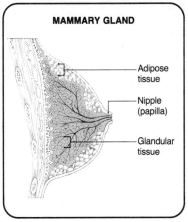

MAMMARY GLAND

Adipose tissue

Nipple (papilla)

Glandular tissue

mammary duct See **lactiferous duct.**

mammary gland One of two discoid, hemispherical glands on the chest of mature females, and present in rudimentary form in children and in males. Glandular tissue forms a radius of lobes containing alveoli, each lobe having a system of ducts for the passage of milk from the alveoli to the nipple during lactation. The left breast is usually larger than the right. Also called **breast.** See also **lactation.**

mammary papilla See **nipple.**

mammillary body Either of the two small round masses of gray matter in the hypothalamus located close to one another in the interpeduncular space.

mammogram An X-ray film of the breast's soft tissues.

mammography Radiography of the soft tissues of the breast to allow identification of various benign and malignant neoplastic processes.

mammoplasty Plastic reshaping of the breasts, performed to reduce or lift enlarged or sagging breasts, to enlarge small breasts, or to reconstruct a breast after removal of a tumor. To reduce the size of the breasts and raise them, excess tissue is removed from the underside of the breasts; the breast is then lifted and the nipple brought through an opening in an overhanging skin flap. To enlarge a breast, a thin plastic sac of silicone fluid is inserted in a pouch formed beneath the breast on the chest wall. The complications after surgery are infection and, with the use of implants, rejection reaction of tissues to the foreign body. The nurse observes the nipples for signs of vascular insufficiency or congestion, applies a firm supporting breast binder, and instructs the patient not to use her arms to lift herself. The patient stays supine in semi-Fowler's position, with elbows at her sides. Some patients experience severe pain in the first days after surgery.

mammothermography A diagnostic procedure which uses thermography to examine the breast for abnormal growths. Compare **mammography.** See also **thermography.**

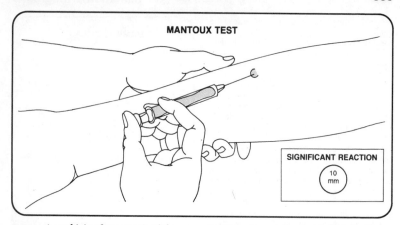

MANTOUX TEST

SIGNIFICANT REACTION

10 mm

man- A combining form meaning 'of or referring to the hand': *manoptoscope, manual.*

management by objectives A system for attaining effective organization that hinges on the joint effort of management and labor to define job functions, set realistic goals, and outline ways to achieve such goals.

-mancy A combining form meaning 'divination in, through, or by': *labiomancy, uromancy.* Also **-mantia.**

mandible A large bone constituting the lower jaw. It contains the lower teeth and consists of a horizontal portion, a body, and two perpendicular rami that join the body at almost right angles. The body of the mandible is curved, somewhat resembling a horseshoe, and has two surfaces and two borders. The external surface is marked by the symphysis menti, indicating the junction of the two halves of the mandible in the fetus. The superior border of the mandible contains sockets for the 16 lower teeth. The mandible and its rami provide attachment for various muscles, as the masseter, temporalis, pterygoideus lateralis, and digastricus. Also called **inferior maxillary bone.** Compare **maxilla.** —**mandibular,** *adj.*

mandibulofacial dysostosis An abnormal hereditary condition characterized by antimongoloid slant of the palpebral fissures, colomboma of the lower lid, micrognathia and hypoplasia of the zygomatic arches, and microtia. Evidence indicates that this disorder is transmitted as an autosomal dominant trait. The condition occurs in the complete form as Franceschetti's syndrome and in the incomplete form as Treacher Collins' syndrome. See also **dysostosis.**

maneuver 1. An adroit or skillful manipulation or procedure. 2. In obstetrics: a manipulation of the fetus performed to aid in delivery.

manganese (Mn) A common metallic element found in trace amounts in tissues of the body. Its atomic number is 25; its atomic weight is 54.938.

mani- A combining form meaning 'mental aberration': *mania, maniaphobia.*

mania A mood disorder characterized by an expansive emotional state, extreme excitement, excessive elation, hyperactivity, agitation, overtalkativeness, flight of ideas, increased psychomotor activity, fleeting attention, and sometimes violent, destructive, or self-destructive behavior. It is manifested in major affective disorders, and in certain organic mental disorders, as delirium. Kinds of mania include **Bell's mania, epileptic mania, hysterical mania, periodical mania, puerperal mania, transitory mania.** —**maniac,** *n., adj.,* **maniacal,** *adj.*

-mania A combining form meaning a '(specified) state of mental disorder': *desanimania, tristimania.*

-maniac 1. A combining form meaning a 'person exhibiting a type of psychosis': *kleptomaniac, narcomaniac.* 2. A combining form meaning a 'person revealing an inordinate interest in something': *ergomaniac, nymphomaniac.*

-manic 1. A combining form meaning a '(specified) psychosis': *choromanic, melomanic.* 2. A combining form meaning a 'mental state like mania': *hyomanic, submanic.*

manic depressive A person with or exhibiting the symptoms of bipolar disorder.

manic-depressive psychosis See **bipolar disorder.**

manipulation The skillful use of the hands in therapeutic or diagnostic procedures, as palpation, reducing a dislocation, turning the position of the fetus, or various treatments in physical therapy and osteopathy. A kind of manipulation is **conjoined manipulation.** See also **massage.**

mannitol An osmotic diuretic.

mannitol hexanitrate A coronary vasodilator.

manometer A device for measuring the pressure of a fluid, consisting of a tube that is marked with a scale and contains a relatively incompressible fluid.

-mantia See **-mancy.**

Mantoux test A tuberculin skin test that consists of intradermal injection of a purified protein derivative of the tubercle bacillus. An indurated area of 10 mm or more appearing 24 to 72 hours after injection is a significant reaction. This method is the most reliable means of testing tuberculin sensitivity. See also **tuberculin test.**

manual rotation   An obstetric maneuver to facilitate delivery by turning the fetal head by hand from a transverse to an antero-posterior position in the birth canal. Compare **forceps rotation.**

manubriosternal articulation   The fibrocartilaginous connection between the manubrium and the sternum, which usually closes by age 25. Compare **xiphisternal articulation.**

manubrium   One of the three bones of the sternum, presenting a broad quadrangular shape which narrows caudally at its articulation with the superior end of the body of the sternum. The pectoralis major and the sternocleidomastoideus are attached to the manubrium. Compare **xiphoid process. —manubrial,** *adj.*

manus, *pl.* **manus**   See **hand.**

many-tailed binder   A broad, evenly shaped binder with both ends split into strips of equal size and number. As the binder is placed on the abdomen, chest, or limb, the ends may be overlapped. See also **scultetus binder.**

MAO   *abbr* **monoamine oxidase.**

MAO inhibitor   See **monoamine oxidase inhibitor.**

MAP   *abbr* **mean arterial pressure.**

map distance   See **map unit.**

maple bark disease   A hypersensitivity pneumonitis caused by exposure to the mold *Cryptostroma corticale,* found in the bark of maple trees. In the susceptible person, the condition may be acute, accompanied by fever, cough, dyspnea, and vomiting, or it may be chronic, characterized also by fatigue and weight loss. In an acute or severe case, a short course of prednisone may be used to control the symptoms; avoiding exposure to the bark prevents further reaction.

maple syrup urine disease   An inherited metabolic disorder in which an enzyme necessary for the breakdown of the amino acids lysine, leucine, and isoleucine is lacking. The disease is usually diagnosed in infancy, being recognized by the characteristic maple-syrup odor of the urine and by hyperreflexia. Stress, fever, infection, and the ingestion of lysine, leucine, or isoleucine aggravate the condition. Treatment includes a diet avoiding these amino acids and, rarely, dialysis or transfusion.

mapping   **1.** In genetics: the process of locating the relative position of genes on a chromosome through the analysis of genetic recombination. Distances between genes in a linkage group are expressed in map or morgan units. Also called chromosome mapping. **2.** *Informal.* In neurology: documentation of sensory innervation testing for pain, temperature, and touch on a dermatome chart.

maprotiline hydrochloride   A tetracyclic antidepressant.

map unit   In genetics: an arbitrary unit of measure used to designate the distance between genes on a chromosome. The measurement is accurate only for small distances, since double crossovers do not appear as new recombinations. Also called **map distance.** See also **morgan.**

marasmic kwashiorkor   A malnutrition disease, primarily affecting children, resulting from the deficiency of both calories and protein. The condition is characterized by severe tissue wasting, dehydration, loss of subcutaneous fat, lethargy, and growth retardation.

marasmic thrombus   An aggregation of blood platelets, fibrin, clotting factors, and cellular elements formed in infants with marasmus. Marasmic thrombus is often a terminal event in cachexia.

marasmus   A condition of extreme malnutrition and emaciation, occurring chiefly in young children, characterized by progressive wasting of subcutaneous tissue and muscle. It results from a lack of adequate calories and proteins and is seen in failure-to-thrive children and in starvation. Less commonly, marasmus occurs as a result of an inability to assimilate or use protein owing to a metabolism defect. Care involves the reestablishment of fluid and electrolyte balance, followed by the slow and gradual addition of foods as they are tolerated. Stimulation appropriate to the developmental age should be provided. See also **failure to thrive, kwashiorkor.**

marble bones   See **osteopetrosis.**

Marburg-Ebola virus disease   A serious febrile disease characterized by rash and severe gastrointestinal hemorrhages. An epidemic in Marburg, Germany, in 1967, was apparently contracted from imported monkeys. In 1976, in the Ebola River District of Zaire and Sudan, an explosive epidemic occurred that had a mortality of 85%. This disease may be transmitted to hospital personnel by improper handling of contaminated needles or from contact with hemorrhagic lesions of patients. The diagnosis is made by serologic abnormalities. There is no effective treatment. Also called Marburg virus disease.

march foot   An abnormal condition of the foot owing to excessive use, as in a long march. The forefoot is swollen and painful, and one or more of the metatarsal bones may be broken. See also **metatarsal stress fracture.**

march fracture   See **metatarsal stress fracture.**

march hemoglobinuria   A rare, abnormal condition, characterized by the presence of hemoglobin in the urine, that occurs following strenuous physical exertion or prolonged exercise, as marching or distance running. See also **hemolysis.**

Marchiafava-Micheli disease   A rare disorder of unknown etiology characterized by episodic hemoglobinuria, occurring usually, but not always, at night.

Marchi's method   A laboratory staining

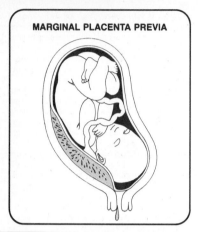

MARGINAL PLACENTA PREVIA

procedure for demonstrating degenerated nerve fibers. The tissue specimen is first fixed in a solution of potassium bichromate, which prevents normal nerve fibers from being stained with osmic acid; osmic acid is then applied as a definitive stain for abnormal nerve fibers.

Marcus Gunn pupil sign Paradoxical dilation of the pupils in an ophthalmologic examination in response to afferent visual stimuli. In a dark room a beam of light is moved from one eye to the other. Normal miosis is caused by the consensual pupil reaction when the normal eye is illuminated; but as the light is moved to the opposite, abnormal eye, the direct reaction to light is weaker than the consensual reaction; hence both pupils dilate.

Marfan's syndrome An abnormal condition characterized by elongation of the bones, often with associated abnormalities of the eyes and the cardiovascular system. Marfan's syndrome is inherited as an autosomal dominant trait. The disease causes major pathologic musculoskeletal disturbances, such as muscular underdevelopment, ligamentous laxity, joint hypermobility, and bone elongation. With this syndrome, pathologic alterations of the cardiovascular system appear to produce fragmentation of the elastic fibers in the media of the aorta, which may lead to aneurysm. Ocular changes associated with the disease include a variety of disorders, including dislocation of the lens. The skulls of affected patients are usually asymmetric. Pectus excavatum is common, and a lateral curvature of the spine may develop and increase during the years of rapid vertebral growth with kyphoscoliosis developing to varying degrees. Observation of the severe ligamental laxity and the joint hypermobility associated with Marfan's syndrome is possible through radiographic examination. These conditions often result in pes valgus and genu recurvatum. No specific treatment is advocated, and symptomatic management of the associated problems is the usual alternative. Resulting deformities, as kyphoscoliosis, may be treated with orthoses or other surgical procedures. Also called **arachnodactyly.**

marginal peptic ulcer An ulcer that develops postoperatively at the surgical anastomosis of the stomach and jejunum. See also **peptic ulcer.**

marginal placenta previa Placenta previa in which the placenta is implanted in the lower uterine segment, with its margin touching or spreading to some degree over the internal os of the uterine cervix. During labor, as the cervix dilates, bleeding may occur from the separation of the edge of the placenta from the uterus beneath it. In some cases severe hemorrhage may occur, but the pressure of the presenting part of the baby is often sufficient to act as a tamponade, arresting the hemorrhage. Diagnosis of marginal placenta previa may be suggested by the location of the placenta on ultrasonic visualization. Cesarean section is not usually necessary. See also **placenta previa.**

marginal rale See **atelectatic rale.**

Marie-Strumpell disease See **ankylosing spondylitis.**

marijuana See **cannabis.**

mark Any nevus or birthmark.

marker gene See **genetic marker.**

marrow See **bone marrow.**

Marseilles fever A disease endemic around the Mediterranean, in Africa, in the Crimea, and in India, caused by *Rickettsia conorii* transmitted by the brown dog tick *(Rhipicephalus sanguineus).* Symptoms are chills, fever, an ulcer covered with a black crust at the site of the tick bite, and a rash appearing on the 2nd to 4th day. Also called **boutonneuse fever, Bruch's disease, Conor's disease, escharonodulaire, Indian tick fever, Kenya fever.**

marsupialize To form a pouch surgically in order to treat a cyst when simple removal would not be effective, as in a pancreatic or a pilonidal cyst. The cyst sac is opened and emptied; its edges are sutured to adjacent tissues; and a drain is left in place. Secretions decrease over a period of several months and granulation tissue closes the wound.

Martorell's disease See **aortic arch syndrome.**

Martorell's syndrome See **Takayasu's arteritis.**

masculine Having the characteristics of a male. —**masculinization,** *n.,* **masculinize,** *v.*

masculinization See **adrenal virilism, virilization.**

mask **1.** To obscure, as symptomatic treatment that may mask the development of a disease. **2.** To cover, as a skin-toned cosmetic that may mask a pigmented nevus. **3.** A cover worn over the nose and mouth to prevent inhalation of toxic or irritating materials, to control delivery of oxygen or anesthetic gas, or (by medical personnel) to shield a patient during aseptic procedures from pathogenic organisms exhaled from the respiratory tract.

masking **1.** The covering or concealing of a disorder by a second condition, as when a per-

MASLOW'S HIERARCHY OF NEED

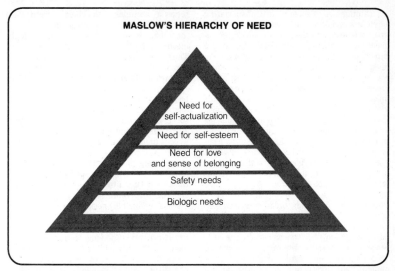

Need for
self-actualization

Need for self-esteem

Need for love
and sense of belonging

Safety needs

Biologic needs

son begins a weight-loss diet while an undiagnosed disease such as cancer has developed. **2.** The unconscious display of a personality trait that conceals a behavioral aberration.

masking agent A cosmetic preparation for covering nevi, surgical scars, and other blemishes. Masking agents are generally composed of a flesh-colored pigment in a lotion or cream base.

mask of pregnancy See **chloasma**.

Maslow's hierarchy of need In sociology: a hierarchical categorization of the basic needs of man. The most basic needs on the scale are the physiologic or biologic, as the need for air. Of second priority are the safety needs, including protection and freedom from fear. Next in the progression are the need to belong, to love, and to be loved; the need for self-esteem; and ultimately, the need for self-actualization. To progress from one need to another the more basic need must first be satisfied.

masochism Pleasure or gratification derived from receiving physical, mental, or emotional abuse. The maltreatment may be inflicted by another person or by oneself. Compare **sadism**. —**masochist**, *n.*, **masochistic**, *adj.*

masochist A person deriving pleasure or gratification from masochistic acts or abuse. See also **masochism**.

mass **1.** The physical property of matter that gives it weight and inertia. **2.** In pharmacy: a mixture from which pills are formed. **3.** An aggregate of cells clumped together, as a tumor. Compare **weight**. See also **inertia**.

massage The manipulation of the soft tissue of the body through stroking, rubbing, kneading, or tapping, to increase circulation, improve muscle tone, and relax the patient. The procedure is performed either with the bare hands or through some mechanical means, as a vibrator. The most common sites for massage are the back, knees, elbows, and heels. Care is taken not to massage inflamed areas, particularly of the extremities, because of the danger of loosening blood clots. Kinds of massage are **effleurage, flagellation, friction, frôlement, pétrissage, tapotement, vibration**.

-massage A combining form meaning a 'therapeutic kneading of the body': *electromassage, hydromassage*.

masseter The thick, rectangular muscle in the cheek that functions to close the jaw. It is one of the four muscles of mastication and consists of a superficial portion and a deep portion, each arising from the zygomatic arch and inserting into the mandible. The deep portion is the smaller and more muscular of the two parts. The masseter is innervated by the masseteric nerve from the mandibular division of the trigeminal nerve.

mass reflex An abnormal condition, seen in patients with transection of the spinal cord, characterized by a widespread nerve discharge, resulting in flexor muscle spasms, incontinence of urine and feces, priapism, hypertension, and profuse sweating. A mass reflex may be triggered by scratching or other painful stimulus to the skin, overdistention of the bladder or intestines, cold weather, prolonged sitting, or emotional stress. Muscle spasms may be so violent as to throw the patient off a bed or stretcher. Medications to reduce mass reflexes include diazepam, dantraline, chlordiazepoxide, and meprobamate. Hubbard baths and exercises in warm water also help. Occasionally, chordotomy, rhizotomy, peripheral nerve transaction, or tenotomy may be necessary.

NURSING CONSIDERATIONS: It is important to prevent decubitus ulcers and bladder infections in paraplegic and quadriplegic patients as they may also serve as triggers to initiate mass reflexes. Side rails should be kept up on the bed and restraining straps secured to transportation stretchers and Stryker frames.

mass spectrometer An analytic instrument for identifying a substance by sorting a stream of charged particles (ions) according to their mass. The mass spectrometer, a noninvasive monitoring system, can be used at the patient's bedside, especially in intensive care, or in a laboratory. Its bedside purposes include determination of optimal ventilator settings, assessment of patient weaning, and monitoring of unstable nonintubated or intubated patients.

mass spectrometry In chemistry: a technique for the analysis of a substance in which the constituents are identified and quantified using a mass spectrometer. See also **spectrometry, spectrophotometry.**

mast- See **masto-.**

mastalgia Pain in the breast caused by congestion or 'caking' during lactation, an infection, fibrocystic disease, especially during or prior to menstruation, or advanced cancer. The early stages of breast cancer are rarely accompanied by pain. Frequent, regular breast-feeding or pumping will prevent or alleviate mastalgia associated with lactation. —**mastalgic,** *adj.*

mast cell A constituent of connective tissue containing large basophilic granules that bear heparin, serotonin, bradykinin, and histamine. These substances are freed from the mast cell in response to injury and infection.

mast cell leukemia A malignant neoplasm of leukocytes characterized by many connective tissue mast cells in circulating blood.

mastectomy The surgical removal of one or both breasts, performed to remove a malignant tumor. In a simple mastectomy, only breast tissue is removed. In a radical mastectomy, some of the muscles of the chest and all lymph nodes in the axilla are removed with the breast. In a modified radical mastectomy, the large muscles of the chest that move the arm are preserved. If a biopsy specimen shows a malignancy, the tumor and adjacent tissues are removed in one piece. After surgery, a drainage catheter is placed in the wound. The nurse inspects the wound for swelling or excessive bleeding and encourages the patient to take deep breaths and to cough at frequent intervals. The affected arm is positioned with the hand pointed upwards or on pillows so that the hand is higher than the lower arm, with the lower arm above heart level. Hand and wrist movements and flexion and extension of the elbow are begun within 24 hours and performed regularly. No abduction or external rotation of the upper arm is permitted before the 10th day. An elastic bandage and, later, a pressure gradient elastic sleeve are used to reduce edema of the arm. The patient is fitted with a prosthesis when the wound is completely healed. Emotional support and counseling are essential. See also **modified radical mastectomy, radical mastectomy, simple mastectomy.** —**mastectomize,** *v.*

master problem list In a problem-oriented medical record: a list of a client's problems that serves as an index to the client's record. Each problem, the date the problem was first noted, the treatment, and the outcome are added to the master problem list as each becomes known. Thus, the list provides an ongoing guide for reviewing the client's status and health care.

master's degree program in nursing A postgraduate program in a school of nursing, based in a university setting, that grants the degree Master of Science in Nursing (MSN) to successful candidates. Nurses with this degree often work in leadership roles in clinical nursing, as consultants in various settings, and in faculty positions in schools of nursing. Some programs also prepare the nurse to function as a nurse-practitioner in a specific specialty.

Master's two-step test A standardized, electrocardiographic test for coronary artery disease in which the patient repeatedly ascends and descends two 9-inch steps.

-mastia See **-mazia.**

mastication Chewing, tearing, or grinding food with the teeth while it becomes mixed with saliva. See also **bolus, digestion, ptyalin.**

mastitis An inflammatory condition of the breast, usually caused by streptococcal or staphylococcal infection and infrequent breast-feeding. Acute mastitis, most common in the first 2 months of lactation, is characterized by pain, swelling, redness, axillary lymphadenopathy, fever, and malaise. If untreated or inadequately treated, abscesses may form. Antibiotics, rest, analgesia, and warm soaks are usually prescribed. Usually, breast-feeding may continue. Regular, frequent breast-feeding often prevents this condition. **Chronic tuberculous mastitis** is rare; when it occurs it represents extension of tuberculosis from the lungs and ribs beneath the breast.

masto-, mast- A combining form meaning 'of or pertaining to the breast': *mastochondroma, mastologist.*

mastocytosis Local or systemic overproduction of mast cells, which, in rare instances, may infiltrate liver, spleen, bones, the gastrointestinal system, and skin. Systemic mastocytosis may precede mast cell leukemia.

mastoid **1.** Of or pertaining to the mastoid process of the temporal bone. **2.** Breast-shaped.

mastoidectomy Surgical excision of a portion of the mastoid part of the temporal bone, performed to treat chronic suppurative otitis media or mastoiditis when antibiotics are ineffective. In a simple mastoidectomy, infected bone cells are removed and the eardrum is incised to drain the middle ear. Topical antibiotics are then instilled in the ear. In a radical procedure, the eardrum and most middle ear structures are removed; the stapes is left intact so a hearing aid may be used. The opening to the eustachian tube is plugged. In a modified radical procedure, the eardrum and the middle ear structures are saved, and the patient will hear better than after a radical mastoidectomy. After surgery any bright red blood on the dressing may indicate hemorrhage. A stiff neck or dis-

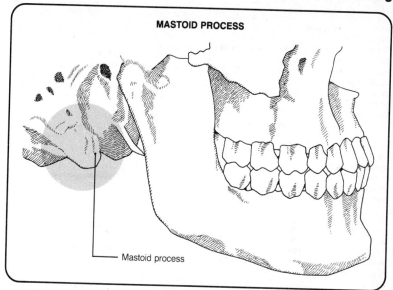

MASTOID PROCESS

Mastoid process

orientation may signal the onset of meningitis. Dizziness is usual and may be expected to last for several days.

mastoiditis An infection of one of the mastoid bones, usually an extension of a middle ear infection, characterized by earache, fever, headache, and malaise. The infection is difficult to treat, often requiring antibiotics administered intravenously for several days. Children are most often affected. Residual hearing loss may follow.

mastoid process The conical projection of the caudal, posterior portion of the temporal bone, serving as the attachment for various muscles, including the sternocleidomastoideus and splenius capitis. A hollow section of the process contains air cells which are distinguished from a large, irregular tympanic antrum in the superior anterior portion of the process. See also **temporal bone.**

masturbation Sexual activity in which the penis or clitoris is stimulated, usually to orgasm, by means other than coitus. It is performed, at least occasionally, by most people and is considered to be normal and harmless. Also called, in men, onanism. —**masturbate,** *v.,* **masturbatic, masturbatory,** *adj.*

-masty See **-mazia.**

materia medica 1. The study of drugs and other substances used in medicine, their origins, preparation, uses, and effects. **2.** A substance or a drug used in medical treatment.

maternal and child health (MCH) services Various facilities and programs organized for the purpose of providing medical and social services for mothers and children. Medical services include prenatal, postnatal, family-planning care, and pediatric care in infancy.

maternal-child attachment See **maternal-infant bonding.**

maternal-child separation syndrome See **separation anxiety.**

maternal deprivation syndrome A condition characterized by developmental retardation that occurs as a result of physical or emotional deprivation. It is seen primarily in infants. Typical symptoms include lack of physical growth, with weight below the third percentile for age and size; malnutrition; pronounced withdrawal, silence, apathy, and irritability; and a characteristic posture and body language, featuring unnatural stiffness and rigidity with a slow response reaction to others. Causes of the syndrome are usually multiple and complex, involving such factors as parental indifference; emotional instability or insecurity of the mother; unrealistic expectations or disappointment concerning the sex, appearance, or adaptability of the child; or unfavorable socioeconomic conditions within the family. Treatment often requires hospitalization, especially in cases of severe malnutrition. Care includes assessment of the family situation, and treatment often involves psychotherapy, counseling, or special nursing instruction to help the parents learn to deal with and provide for the child. Emotionally deprived children often remain below normal in intellectual development, fail to learn acceptable social behavior, and are unable to form trusting, meaningful relationships with others. In severe cases of early and prolonged deprivation, the damage to an infant may be irreversible. See also **failure to thrive.**

maternal effect See **maternal inheritance.**

maternal-infant bonding The complex process of attachment of a mother to her newborn. Disastrous effects of the disruption or absence of this attachment have long been known.

The specific steps in its development and the factors that disturb or encourage it have been identified and described by anthropologists, pediatricians, nurses, midwives, and sociologists. In the first minutes and hours after birth, a sensitive period occurs during which the infant and the mother become intimately involved with each other. They move in turn to the voice and sounds of the other, a process known as entrainment; it can be likened to a dance. The infant's movements constitute a response to the mother's voice, and she is encouraged to continue the process. The secretion of oxytocin and prolactin by the maternal pituitary gland is stimulated by the newborn's sucking or licking of the mother's breasts; T and B lymphocytes and macrophages are given to the infant in the mother's milk, promoting resistance to infection. The child is also colonized by the normal flora of the mother's skin and nasal passages, improving the ability to fend off infection. Physically, the mother provides her body heat for the newborn's warmth and comfort. Thus, the extended contact in the newborn period satisfies physical as well as emotional needs of the mother and child. After birth, silver nitrate drops are not placed in the newborn's eyes until the mother and child have had time to be together, with eye contact, for an extended period of time, as the drops cause a film to form over the eyes, dimming vision. Ideally, during the 1st hour after birth, the parents and the infant are not separated and are given as much privacy as possible. Skin-to-skin contact is encouraged; various methods may be used to maintain an ambient temperature adequate to maintain the infant's body temperature. On the postpartum unit the mother and the child are kept together for at least 5 hours a day, but optimally for 24 hours a day in a 24-hour rooming-in unit. The entire family is allowed to visit. The mother has responsibility for the care of her child, with consultation available from a midwife or a nurse.

maternal inheritance The transmission of traits or conditions controlled by cytoplasmic factors within the ovum that are not self-replicating and are determined by genes within the nucleus. Also called maternal effect.

maternity cycle The antepartal, intrapartal, and postpartal periods of pregnancy and the puerperium, from conception to 6 weeks after birth.

maternity nursing Nursing care of women and their families during pregnancy, parturition, and through the first days of the puerperium. Increasingly, postpartum maternity nursing includes the supervision of the mothers' care of their newborns in rooming-in units and may include care of normal newborns in the nursery when they are not with their mothers. Maternity nursing requires extensive instruction of the mothers in the usual behavior and needs of a newborn, expected patterns of growth and development of the infant during the first week, and in details of care needed by the mother during the first weeks after birth. Breast-feeding,

bottle-feeding, baby baths, perineal care, nutrition, and danger signs of the puerperium are usually taught by the maternity nurse. Observation for abnormal conditions, as thrombophlebitis, mastitis and other infections, and preeclampsia are daily ongoing concerns of the maternity nurse on the postpartum unit. Intrapartum maternity nursing involves the care of mothers in labor and delivery, as well as high-risk technical nursing, emotional support in labor and delivery, and the customary ongoing observation for abnormal signs or symptoms. Often, pregnant women with medical problems associated with pregnancy are cared for on a special high-risk antepartum unit by specially trained maternity nurses.

matrix 1. An intercellular substance. 2. A basic substance from which a specific organ or kind of tissue develops. Also called **ground substance**. 3. A form used in shaping a tooth surface in dental procedures.

matter 1. Anything that has mass and occupies space. 2. Any substance not otherwise identified as to its constituents, as gray matter or pus.

maturation 1. The process or condition of attaining complete development. In humans, the unfolding of full physical, emotional, and intellectual capacities that enable a person to function at a higher level of competency and adaptability within the environment. 2. The final stages in the meiotic formation of germ cells in which the number of chromosomes in each cell is reduced to the haploid number characteristic of the species. See also **meiosis, oogenesis, spermatogenesis**. 3. Suppuration. —**maturate**, v.

mature To become fully developed; to ripen.

mature cell leukemia See **polymorphocytic leukemia**.

maturity 1. A state of complete growth or development, usually designated as the period of life between adolescence and old age. 2. The stage at which an organism is capable of reproduction.

maturity-onset diabetes Diabetes mellitus arising in adults, usually after the age of 50. See also **diabetes mellitus**.

maxilla, pl. **maxillae** One of a pair of large bones that form the upper jaw, consisting of a pyramidal body and four processes: the zygomatic, frontal, alveolar, and palatine.

-maxilla A combining form meaning the 'upper jaw or the bones composing it': *intermaxilla, submaxilla*.

maxillary artery Either of two larger terminal branches of the external carotid arteries that rise from the neck of the mandible near the parotid gland and divide into three branches, supplying the deep structures of the face.

maxillary sinus One of the pair of large air cells forming a pyramidal cavity in the body of the maxilla. The apex of each sinus extends into the zygomatic arch, and its floor, formed by the aveolar process, is usually 1 mm to 10 mm below the floor of the nose. In the adult the volume of the sinus averages 14.75 cubic cm (1 cubic inch).

The mucous membrane of the sinus is continuous with that of the nasal cavity; an opening in the medial wall of the sinus communicates with the middle meatus. Compare **ethmoidal air cell, frontal sinus, sphenoidal sinus.**

maxillary vein One of a pair of deep veins of the face, accompanying the maxillary artery and passing between the condyle of the mandible and the sphenomandibular ligament. Each maxillary vein is formed by the confluence of veins in the pterygoid plexus and joins the superficial temporal vein to form the retromandibular vein. Each maxillary vein is a tributary of the internal jugular and the external jugular veins.

maxillofacial prosthesis A prosthetic replacement for part, or all, of the upper jaw, nose, or cheek. It is applied when surgical repair alone is inadequate.

maxillomandibular fixation Stabilization of face or jaw fractures by temporarily connecting the maxilla and mandible by wires, elastic bands, or metal splints. See also **elastic band fixation, nasomandibular fixation.**

maximal breathing capacity The amount of gas exchanged per minute with maximal rate and depth of respiration.

maximal expiratory flow rate (MEFR) The rate of the most rapid flow of gas from the lungs during the expiratory phase of respiration.

maximum inspiratory pressure (MIP) The maximum pressure within the alveoli of the lungs that occurs during the inspiratory phase of respiration.

maximum permissible dose equivalent In radiotherapy: the greatest amount of radiation that a person or a specific body part is allowed to receive in a given period of time.

Mayer's reflex A normal reflex elicited by grasping the ring finger and flexing it at the metacarpalphalangeal joint of a subject whose hand is relaxed with thumb abducted. The normal response is adduction and apposition of the thumb. The reflex is absent in disease of the pyramidal system.

May-Hegglin anomaly An inherited hematologic condition characterized by leukopenia, giant platelets, and Döhle bodies. The condition is usually benign but may be associated with a decreased ability of the blood to coagulate. Compare **Pelger-Huët anomaly.**

Mayo scissors See **scissors.**

-mazia A combining form meaning '(condition of the) breasts': *macromazia, pleomazia.* Also **-mastia, -masty.**

mazindol An amphetaminelike central nervous system stimulant.

mazo- A combining form meaning 'of or pertaining to the breast': *mazodynia, mazopexy.*

MBC *abbr* **maximal breathing capacity.**

MBD *abbr* **minimal brain dysfunction.** See also **attention deficit disorder.**

mc *abbr* **millicurie.**

mC *abbr* **millicoulomb.**

Mc *abbr* megacurie, a unit of one million curies, which is a measure of radioactivity.

McArdle's disease An inherited metabolic

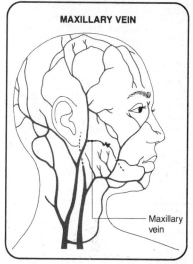

MAXILLARY VEIN

Maxillary vein

disease in which abnormally large amounts of glycogen accumulate in skeletal muscle. It is characterized only by muscle weakness and cramping after exercise. There is no known treatment. Also called **glycogen storage disease, type V.** See also **glycogen storage disease.**

MCAT *abbr* **Medical College Aptitude Test.**

McBurney's point A site of extreme sensitivity in acute appendicitis, situated in the normal area of the appendix about 5 cm (2 inches) below the right anterior superior spine of the ilium, on a line between that spine and the umbilicus.

McBurney's sign A reaction of the patient indicating severe pain and extreme tenderness when McBurney's point is palpated. Such a reaction indicates appendicitis.

mcg *abbr* **microgram.**

MCH *abbr* **1. mean corpuscular hemoglobin. 2. maternal and child health.**

MCHC *abbr* **mean corpuscular hemoglobin concentration.**

mCi *abbr* **millicurie.**

McMurray's sign A click heard when rotating the tibia on the femur, indicating meniscal structure injury.

MCTD *abbr* **mixed connective tissue disease.**

MCV *abbr* **mean corpuscular volume.**

MD *abbr* Doctor of Medicine. See **physician.**

mean **1.** Occupying a position midway between two extremes of a set of values or data. **2.** Arithmetic mean, a value that is derived by dividing the total of a set of values by the number of items in the set. **3.** Geometric mean, a value that is between the first and last of a set of values organized in a geometric progression.

mean arterial pressure (MAP) The arithmetic mean of blood pressure in arterial portion of circulation.

MEASLES, MUMPS, RUBELLA VACCINATIONS IN IMMUNIZATION SEQUENCE	
AGE	**IMMUNIZATION**
2 months	First dose: diptheria/tetanus/pertussis vaccine; polio vaccine
4 months	Second dose: diphtheria/tetanus/pertussis vaccine; polio vaccine
6 months	Third dose: diphtheria/tetanus/pertussis vaccine
15 months	Measles vaccine; mumps; rubella
18 months	Diphtheria/tetanus/pertussis; polio vaccine (third)
4 to 5 years	Diphtheria/tetanus/pertussis; polio vaccine

mean corpuscular hemoglobin (MCH)
An estimate of the amount of hemoglobin in an average erythrocyte, derived from the ratio between the amount of hemoglobin and the number of erythrocytes present in a specimen. The normal MCH is between 28 and 32 picograms of hemoglobin per red blood cell. See also **hypochromic anemia, iron-deficiency anemia.**
mean corpuscular hemoglobin concentration (MCHC) An estimation of the concentration of hemoglobin in grams per 100 ml (3¾ oz) of packed red blood cells, derived from the ratio of the hemoglobin to the hematocrit. The normal MCHC is between 32% and 36%.
mean corpuscular volume (MCV) An evaluation of the average volume of each red blood cell, derived from the ratio of the volume of packed red blood cells (the hematocrit) to the total number of red blood cells. The normal MCV is between 82 and 92 cubic microns.
measles An acute, highly contagious, viral disease involving the respiratory tract and characterized by a spreading maculopapular cutaneous rash. It occurs primarily in young children who have not been immunized. Measles is caused by a paramyxovirus and is transmitted by direct contact with droplets spread from the nose, throat, and mouth of infected persons. Diagnosis is confirmed by the identification of Koplik spots on the buccal mucosa and by bacteriologic culture or serologic examination. An incubation period of 7 to 14 days is followed by the prodromal stage, characterized by fever, malaise, coryza, cough, conjunctivitis, photophobia, anorexia, and the pathognomonic Koplik's spots, which appear 1 to 2 days before onset of the rash.

Pharyngitis and inflammation of the laryngeal and tracheobronchial mucosa develop, the temperature may rise to 39.5°C (103°F) or 40°C (104°F), and there is marked granulocytic leukopenia. The papules of the rash first appear as irregular brown-pink spots around the hairline, the ears, and the neck, then spread rapidly, within 24 to 48 hours, to the trunk and extremities, becoming red, maculopapular, and dense, giving a blotchy appearance. Within 3 to 5 days, the fever subsides, and the lesions flatten and begin to fade. Routine treatment consists of bed rest, antipyretics, the administration of antibiotics to control secondary bacterial infection, and, when necessary, the application of calamine lotion, corn starch solution, or cool water to relieve itching. Preventive measures include active immunization with measles virus vaccine after the infant is 1 year old.
NURSING CONSIDERATIONS: Bed rest, isolation, and quiet activity are recommended as long as fever and rash persist. Aspirin, fluids, cool sponge baths, nose drops, and cough medication may be necessary to counteract fever and respiratory symptoms. Bright sunlight may be irritating to the eyes. Special attention is given to the care and cleansing of the eyes and skin, especially in cases of severe papular eruption. Complications sometimes occur, including otitis media, pneumonia, bronchiolitis, obstructive laryngitis, laryngotracheitis, and, occasionally, encephalitis and appendicitis. Rarely, but most gravely, the measles virus causes subacute sclerosing panencephalitis several years after the acute infection. Also called **morbilli, rubeola.** See also **roseola infantum, rubella.**
measles and rubella virus vaccine, live An active immunizing agent. It is prescribed for immunization against measles and rubella. Immunosuppression, concomitant administration of corticosteroids, tuberculosis, known or suspected pregnancy, hypersensitivity to neomycin, neoplasms of the lymphatic system or bone marrow, or active infection prohibits its use. It should not be given for 3 months following the use of whole blood, plasma, or immune serume globulin, or for 1 month before or after immunization with other live virus vaccines, except mumps vaccine. The most serious adverse reaction is anaphylaxis.
measles, mumps, and rubella virus vaccine, live An active immunizing agent that is prescribed for simultaneous immunization against the measles, mumps, and rubella. Immunosuppression, the concomitant administration of corticosteroids, tuberculosis, hypersensitivity to neomycin, neoplasms of the lymphatic system or of the bone marrow, known or suspected pregnancy, or acute infection prohibits its use. The vaccine should not be given for 3 months following the administration of whole blood, plasma, or immune serum globulin, and it should not be given for 1 month before or after immunization with other live virus vaccines. The most serious adverse reaction is anaphylaxis.

measurement The determination, expressed numerically, of the extent or quantity of a substance, energy, or time. See also **International Unit, metric system.**

meatorrhaphy The suturing of the cut end of the urethra to the glans penis after surgery to enlarge the urethral meatus.

meatoscopy The visual examination of any meatus, especially the urethra, usually performed with the aid of a speculum.

meatus, *pl.* **meatuses, meatus** An opening or tunnel through any part of the body, as the external acoustic meatus that leads from the external ear to the tympanic membrane.

mebendazole An anthelmintic agent.

mecamylamine hydrochloride A sympatholytic antihypertensive that is a ganglionic blocking agent.

mechanical advantage In physiology: the ratio of the output force developed by the muscles to the input force applied to the body structures that the muscles move, especially the ratio of these forces associated with the body structures that act as levers. Variations in the sizes of muscles and the lengths of bones in different individuals partially account for the different mechanical advantages from one body type to another.

mechanical vector See **vector.**

mechanism of labor See **cardinal movements of labor.**

mechano- A combining form meaning 'mechanical': *mechanochemistry, mechanocyte, mechanotherapy.*

mechanoreceptor Any sensory nerve ending that responds to mechanical stimuli, as touch, pressure, and muscular contractions. See also **proprioceptor.**

mechlorethamine hydrochloride (nitrogen mustard) An alkylating agent used in chemotherapy.

Meckel's diverticulum An anomalous sac protruding from the wall of the ileum between 30 and 90 cm (11¾ and 35½ inches) from the ileocecal sphincter. It is congenital, resulting from the incomplete closure of the yolk stalk, and occurs in 1% to 2% of the population. The diverticulum is usually asymptomatic, but the condition is suggested by signs of appendicitis in infancy, by sudden and painless bleeding, usually in childhood, or by symptoms of intestinal obstruction. Symptomatic diverticula are most commonly resected. Surgical resection of asymptomatic diverticula is also recommended to avoid diverticulitis, obstruction, and blood loss.

meclizine hydrochloride An antiemetic agent.

meclocycline sulfosalicylate A local anti-infective agent.

meclofenamate A nonsteroidal anti-inflammatory agent.

mecocephaly See **scaphocephaly.**

meconium A material that collects in the intestines of a fetus and forms the first stools of a newborn. It is thick and sticky in consistency, usually green to black in color, and composed

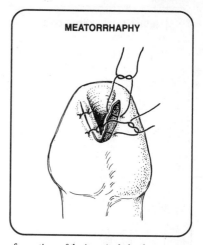

MEATORRHAPHY

of secretions of the intestinal glands, some amniotic fluid, and intrauterine debris, as bile pigments and fatty acids. With ingestion of breast milk or formula and the proper functioning of the gastrointestinal tract, the color, consistency, and frequency of the stools change by the third or fourth day after the initiation of feedings. The presence of meconium in the amniotic fluid during labor may indicate fetal distress.

meconium ileus Obstruction of the small intestine in the newborn caused by impaction of thick, dry, tenacious meconium, usually at or near the ileocecal valve. Symptoms include abdominal distention, vomiting, failure to pass meconium within the first 24 to 48 hours after birth, and rapid dehydration with associated electrolyte imbalance. The condition results from a deficiency in pancreatic enzymes and is the earliest manifestation of cystic fibrosis. In uncomplicated cases in which perforation, volvulus, or atresia does not occur, the obstruction may be relieved by giving enemas with a contrast medium under fluoroscopy. Fluid loss is replaced intravenously to prevent dehydration. If two to three enemas do not dislodge the obstruction, surgery is necessary. See also **meconium plug syndrome.**

meconium plug syndrome Obstruction of the large intestine in the newborn caused by thick, rubbery meconium that may fill the entire colon and part of the terminal ileum. Symptoms include failure to pass meconium within the first 24 to 48 hours following birth, abdominal distention, and vomiting if complete intestinal blockage occurs. A barium enema will indicate the plug and in most cases will dislodge it from the bowel wall. Subsequent gentle saline enemas may be needed to expel the plug. The condition may be an indication of Hirschsprung's disease or cystic fibrosis. See also **meconium ileus.**

MED *abbr* minimal effective dose or minimal erythema dose.

MEDEX 1. An educational program accredited by the AMA for training military personnel

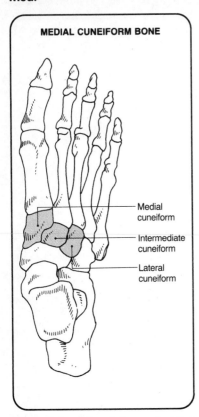

MEDIAL CUNEIFORM BONE

Medial cuneiform

Intermediate cuneiform

Lateral cuneiform

with medical experience to become physician's assistants. **2.** A physician's assistant who has gained medical experience during military service.

medi- A combining form meaning 'middle': *medialecithal, mediotarsal.*

medial **1.** Situated or oriented toward the midline of the body. **2.** Pertaining to the media, the middle layer of a blood vessel wall. Also called **mesial.**

medial antebrachial cutaneous nerve A nerve of the arm that arises from the medial cord of the brachial plexus, medial to the axillary artery. Near the axilla it passes a filament to supply the skin over the biceps almost as far as the elbow. It descends on the ulnar side of the arm medial to the brachial artery, pierces the deep fascia with the basilic vein about the middle of the arm, and divides into the anterior branch and the ulnar branch. Compare **medial brachial cutaneous nerve.**

medial arteriosclerosis See **Monckeberg's atherosclerosis.**

medial brachial cutaneous nerve A nerve of the arm arising from the medial cord of the brachial plexus and distributed to the medial side of the arm. It passes through the axilla, pierces the deep fascia in the middle of

the arm, and supplies the skin of the arm as far as the olecranon. Compare **medial antebrachial cutaneous nerve.**

medial cuneiform bone The largest of three cuneiform bones of the foot, situated on the medial side of the tarsus, between the scaphoid bone and the first metatarsal. It serves as the attachment for various ligaments, the tendons of the tibialis anterior, and the peroneus longus. Also called **internal cuneiform bone.**

medial geniculate body Either of the two areas on the posterior dorsal thalamus, relaying auditory impulses from the lateral lemniscus to the auditory cortex.

medial pectoral nerve A branch of the brachial plexus, that, with the lateral pectoral nerve, supplies the pectoral muscles. It arises from the medial cord of the plexus, medial to the axillary artery, passes between the axillary artery and the axillary vein, and joins the lateral pectoral nerve to form a loop around the artery before ending deep in the pectoralis minor. The loop branches to supply the pectoralis minor and the pectoralis major. Compare **lateral pectoral nerve.**

medial rotation See **lateral rotation.**

median In statistics: the number representing the middle value of the scores in a sample. In an odd number of scores arrayed in ascending order, it is the middle score; in an even number of scores so arrayed, it is the average between the two central scores.

median antebrachial vein One of the superficial veins of the upper limb that drains the venous plexus on the palmar surface of the hand. It ascends on the ulnar side of the anterior forearm and, at its terminus, joins the median cubital vein. In many individuals it divides into two vessels, one joining the basilic vein, the other joining the cephalic vein distal to the elbow. One of the veins of the median cubital complex commonly anastomoses with the deep veins of the forearm. The anastomosis holds the superficial vein in place and makes it a practical choice for venipuncture. Compare **basilic vein, cephalic vein, dorsal digital vein.**

median aperture of fourth ventricle An opening between the lower part of the roof of the fourth ventricle and the subarachnoid space.

median atlantoaxial joint One of three points of articulation of the atlas and the axis. It is a pivot articulation between the dens and ring of the atlas and involves five ligaments. It allows rotation of the axis and the skull, the extent of rotation limited by the alar ligaments.

median basilic vein One of the superficial veins of the upper limb, often formed as one of two branches from the median cubital vein. The median basilic vein courses across the palmar surface of the forearm near the elbow and is commonly used for venipuncture, phlebotomy, or intravenous infusion. Compare **basilic vein.**

median effective dose (ED50) The dosage of a drug that may be expected to cause a specific intensity of effect in one half of the subjects to whom it is given.

median glossitis See **median rhomboid glossitis.**

median lethal dose (MLD) In radiotherapy: the amount of radiation that kills 50% of the individuals in a large group of animals or organisms within a specified period of time. Also called **LD50.**

median nerve One of the terminal branches of the brachial plexus that extends along the radial portions of the forearm and the hand and supplies various muscles and the skin of these parts. It arises from the brachial plexus by two large roots, one from the lateral and one from the medial cord. The roots unite to form the trunk of the nerve that courses down the arm with the brachial artery. In the forearm it passes between the two heads of the pronator teres and passes through the flexor retinaculum into the palm of the hand, where it is covered only by the skin and the palmar aponeurosis. Emerging from the retinaculum it is enlarged and flattened and splits into digital and muscular branches. Compare **musculocutaneous nerve, radial nerve, ulnar nerve.**

median palatine suture The line of junction between the horizontal portions of the palatine bones that extends from both sides of the skull to form the posterior part of the hard palate.

median plane A vertical plane that divides the body into right and left halves and passes approximately through the sagittal suture of the skull. Compare **frontal plane, sagittal plane, transverse plane.**

median rhomboid glossitis A red, depressed, diamond-shaped area on the dorsum of the tongue, frequently irritated by alcohol, hot drinks, or spicy foods. The condition is most often seen in adult males and may be caused by candidiasis.

median toxic dose (TD50) The dosage that may be expected to cause a toxic effect in one half of the subjects to whom it is given.

mediastinum, *pl.* **mediastina** A portion of the thoracic cavity in the middle of the thorax, between the pleural sacs containing the two lungs. It extends from the sternum to the vertebral column and contains all the thoracic viscera, except the lungs. It is enclosed in a thick extension of the thoracic subserous fascia and is divided into the cranial portion and the caudal portion by a plane extending from the sternal angle to the caudal border of the fourth thoracic vertebra. —**mediastinal,** *adj.*

mediate 1. To cause a change to occur, as in stimulation by a hormone. 2. To settle a dispute, as in collective bargaining. 3. Situated between two places, things, parts, or terms. 4. In psychology: an event that follows upon one process or event and precedes another, as, in the process of cognition, perception follows stimulation and precedes thinking. —**mediating,** *adj.,* **mediator,** *n.*

mediate percussion See **percussion.**

Medicaid A federally funded, state-operated program of medical assistance to people with

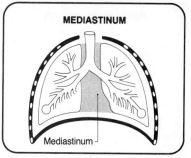

MEDIASTINUM

Mediastinum

low incomes, authorized by the Social Security Act. Under broad federal guidelines, the individual states determine benefits, eligibility, rates of payment, and methods of administration.

Medicaid mill *Informal.* A health program or facility that solely or primarily serves persons eligible for Medicaid. Such facilities are found mainly in economically depressed areas where there are few other health services.

medical center 1. A health-care facility. 2. A hospital, especially one staffed and equipped to care for many patients and for a large number of kinds of diseases.

Medical College Aptitude Test (MCAT) An examination taken by persons applying to medical school, the score on this examination being an important criteria for acceptance.

medical examiner See **coroner.**

medical genetics See **clinical genetics.**

medical history See **health history.**

medical indigency The lack of financial reserves adequate to pay for medical care, especially in a person or family able to manage other expenses.

medical induction of labor See **induction of labor.**

medical model The traditional approach to the diagnosis and treatment of illness as practiced by doctors in the western world since the time of Koch and Pasteur. The doctor focuses on the defect, or dysfunction, within the person, using a problem-solving approach. The medical history and the physical examination and diagnostic tests provide the basis for the identification and treatment of a specific illness. The medical model is thus focused on the physical and biological aspects of specific diseases and conditions. Nursing differs from the medical model in that the patient is perceived primarily as a social person relating to the environment; nursing care is formulated on the basis of a nursing assessment that assumes multiple causes for the person's problems.

medical staff All doctors, dentists, and health professionals responsible for providing health care in a hospital or other health-care facility. Medical staff personnel may be full-time or part-time, employed by the facility, or simply affiliated, that is, not employees.

medical-surgical nursing The nursing care of people whose conditions or disorders are

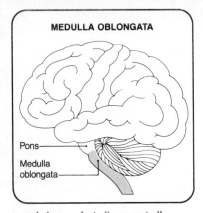

MEDULLA OBLONGATA

Pons

Medulla
oblongata

treated pharmacologically or surgically.

Medical Women's International Association (MWIA)   An international professional organization of women doctors.

Medicare   Federally funded national health insurance for certain persons age 65 or older. The program is administered in two parts. Part A provides basic protection against costs of medical, surgical, and psychiatric hospital care. Part B is a voluntary medical insurance program financed in part from federal funds and in part from premiums contributed by persons enrolled in the program. Medicare enrollment is offered to persons age 65 or older who are entitled to receive Social Security or Railroad Retirement benefits. Other persons age 65 or older, as federal employees and aliens, may not be eligible. Medicare was authorized by the Social Security Act.

medicated tub bath   A therapeutic bath in which medication is dispersed in water, usually in the treatment of dermatologic disorders.

medication   1. A drug or other substance that is used as a medicine. 2. The administration of a medicine.

medicinal treatment   Therapy of disorders based chiefly on the use of appropriate pharmacologic agents.

medicine   1. A drug or a remedy for illness. 2. The art and science of the diagnosis, treatment, and prevention of disease and the maintenance of good health. 3. The art or technique of treating disease without surgery. Two major divisions of medicine are academic medicine and clinical medicine. Some of the many branches of medicine include **family medicine, forensic medicine, internal medicine. —medical,** *adj.*

medicolegal   Of or pertaining to both medicine and law. Medicolegal considerations are a significant part of the process of making many patient-care decisions and in determining definitions and policies regarding the treatment of mentally incompetent people and minors, the performance of sterilization or therapeutic abortion, and the care of terminally ill patients. Medicolegal considerations, decisions, definitions, and policies provide the framework for informed

consent, professional liability, and many other aspects of health-care practice.

Mediterranean anemia   See **thalassemia.**

Mediterranean fever   See **brucellosis.**

medium, *pl.* **media**   A substance through which something moves or through which it acts. A **contrast medium** is a substance that has a density different from that of body tissues, permitting visual comparison of structures when used with imaging techniques such as X-ray. A culture medium is a substance that provides a nutritional environment for the growth of microorganisms or cells. A dispersion medium is the substance in which a colloid is dispersed. The refracting media are the transparent tissues and fluid of the eye that refract light.

medium-chain triglycerides   Oral calorie sources for treating fat malabsorption.

MEDLARS   A computerized literature retrieval service of the National Library of Medicine in Bethesda, Maryland. MEDLARS contains more than 4,500,000 references to medical articles found in professional journals and books published since 1966. The references are made available on request to more than 1,000 hospitals, universities, and government agencies throughout the world by means of a network of computer terminals. The references are filed in 15 data bases, including MEDLINE, TOXLINE, CHEMLINE, RTECS, CANCERLIT, and EPILEPSYLINE. See also **MEDLINE.**

MEDLINE   A National Library of Medicine computer data base that covers approximately 600,000 references to biomedical journal articles published in the current and 2 preceding years. The files duplicate the contents of the monthly and annual volumes of the *Unabridged Index Medicus,* also published by the National Library, which indexes medical reports from 3,000 professional journals in more than 70 countries. See also **MEDLARS.**

medroxyprogesterone acetate   A progestogen.

medrysone   An ophthalmic anti-inflammatory agent.

medulla, *pl.* **medullas, medullae**   1. The most internal part of a structure or organ, as the spinal medulla. See also **marrow.** 2. *Informal.* **Medulla oblongata.**

medulla oblongata   The most vital part of the brain, continuing as the bulbous portion of the spinal cord just above the foramen magnum and separated from the pons by a horizontal groove. It is one of three parts of the brain stem and contains mostly white substance with some mixture of gray substance. The medulla contains the cardiac, the vasomotor, and the respiratory centers of the brain, and medullary injury or disease often proves fatal. Compare **mesencephalon, pons.**

medullary, medullar   1. Of or pertaining to the medulla of the brain. 2. Of or pertaining to the bone marrow. 3. Of or pertaining to the spinal cord and central nervous system.

medullary carcinoma   A soft, malignant neoplasm of the epithelium containing little or no fibrous tissue. A small percentage of breast and thyroid tumors are medullary carcinomas. Also called **carcinoma medullare, carcinoma molle, encephaloid carcinoma.**

medullary cystic disease   A chronic familial disease of the kidney, characterized by the slow onset of uremia. The disease appears in young children or adolescents, who pass large volumes of dilute urine with greater than normal amounts of sodium. Hemodialysis is the usual treatment as the uremia becomes severe. See also **uremia.**

medullary fold   See **neural fold.**

medullary groove   See **neural groove.**

medullary plate   See **neural plate.**

medullary sponge kidney   A congenital defect of the kidney, leading to cystic dilatation of the collecting tubules. Persons with this defect often develop a kidney stone or an infection of the kidney owing to urinary stasis. Treatment includes drugs to acidify the urine and a diet low in calcium and high in fluids to discourage formation of stones.

medullary tube   See **neural tube.**

medulla spinalis   See **spinal cord.**

medullated neuroma   See **fascicular neuroma.**

medulloblastoma   A poorly differentiated, malignant neoplasm that is composed of tightly packed cells of spongioblastic and neuroblastic lineage. The tumor usually arises in the cerebellum, occurs most frequently between the ages of 5 and 9 years, and affects more boys than girls. Although medulloblastomas are extremely radiosensitive, they grow rapidly, and radiotherapy usually prolongs life for only 1 or 2 years.

medulloepithelioma   See **neurocytoma.**

mefenamic acid   A nonsteroidal anti-inflammatory agent.

MEFR   *abbr* **maximal expiratory flow rate.**

mega-, megalo-, mego-   A combining form meaning 'great or huge': *megacardia, megacoccus.*

megabladder   See **megalocystis.**

megacaryocyte   An extremely large bone marrow cell measuring between 35 and 160 cubic microns in diameter and having a nucleus with many lobes. Megacaryocytes are essential for the production and proliferation of platelets in the marrow. See also **platelet. —megacaryocytic,** *adj.*

megacolon   Massive, abnormal dilatation of the colon that may be congenital, toxic, or acquired. Congenital megacolon (Hirschsprung's disease) is caused by the absence of autonomic ganglia in the smooth-muscle wall of the colon. Toxic megacolon is a grave complication of ulcerative colitis and may result in perforation of the colon, septicemia, and death. Surgery is the usual treatment for toxic and congenital megacolon. Acquired megacolon is the result of a chronic refusal to defecate, usually occurring in children who are psychotic or mentally retarded. The colon becomes dilated by an accumulation of impacted feces. Laxatives, enemas, and psychiatric treatment are often necessary. See also

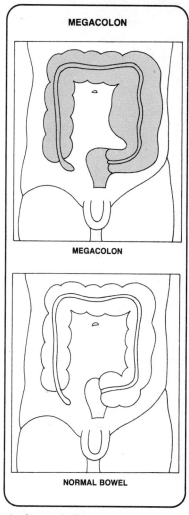

MEGACOLON

MEGACOLON

NORMAL BOWEL

Hirschsprung's disease.

megaesophagus   Abnormal dilatation of the lower segments of the esophagus owing to distention from the failure of the cardiac sphincter to relax and allow the passage of food into the stomach. See also **achalasia.**

megakaryocytic leukemia   A rare malignancy of blood-forming tissue in which megakaryocytes proliferate abnormally in the bone marrow and circulate in the blood in relatively large numbers.

megalencephaly   A condition characterized by pathologic overgrowth of the head and brain. In some cases, generalized cerebral hyperplasia is associated with mental retardation or a brain disorder, as epilepsy. Also called **macrencephaly, macroencephaly. —megalencephalic, megalencephalous,** *adj.*

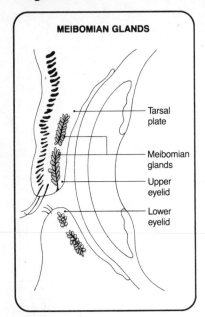

MEIBOMIAN GLANDS

Tarsal plate

Meibomian glands

Upper eyelid

Lower eyelid

-megalia See **-megaly.**

megalo- See **mega-.**

megaloblast An abnormally large nucleated immature erythrocyte that develops in large numbers in the bone marrow and is plentiful in the circulation in many anemias owing to deficiency of vitamin B$_{12}$, folic acid, or intrinsic factor. —**megaloblastic,** *adj.*

megaloblastic anemia A hematologic disorder characterized by the production and peripheral proliferation of immature, large, and dysfunctional erythrocytes. Megaloblasts are usually associated with severe pernicious anemia or folic acid deficiency anemia.

megalocephaly See **macrocephaly.**

megalocystis An abnormal condition occurring primarily in female children, characterized by an enlarged and thin-walled bladder. Reduction of the size of the bladder or diversion of the flow of urine through the ileum may be surgically performed to correct this condition. Also called **megabladder.**

megalomania An abnormal mental state characterized by delusions of grandeur in which one believes oneself to be a person of great importance, power, fame, or wealth. See also **mania.**

megaloureter An abnormal condition characterized by dilatation of one or both ureters, resulting from dysfunctional peristaltic action of the smooth muscle in the ureters. Treatment may include surgical resection.

-megaly A combining form meaning an 'enlargement of a (specified) body part': *cardiomegaly, gastromegaly.* Also **-megalia.**

megestrol acetate An antineoplastic agent that alters hormone balance.

mego- See **mega-.**

megrim See **migraine.**

Meibomian cyst See **chalazion.**

Meibomian gland One of several sebaceous glands that secrete sebum from their ducts on the posterior margin of each eyelid. The glands are embedded in the tarsal plate of each eyelid. Also called **palpebral gland, tarsal gland.**

Meigs' syndrome Ascites and hydrothorax associated with ovary fibroma or other pelvic tumor.

meio- See **mio-.**

meiocyte Any cell undergoing meiosis.

meiogenic Producing or causing meiosis.

meiosis A type of cell division that occurs in the maturation of sperm and ova and results in four daughter cells with half the number of chromosomes characteristic of the species. Compare **mitosis.** —**meiotic,** *adj.*

meiotic division See **meiosis.**

Meissner's corpuscle See **tactile corpuscle.**

mel- A combining form meaning 'limb, member': *melalgia, melomelus.*

melancholia **1.** Extreme sadness; melancholy. **2.** The major affective depressive disorder. See also **bipolar disorder, depression.**

melancholia agitata A state of depression in which psychomotor excitement is a prominent symptom. See also **agitated depression, bipolar disorder.**

melancholia simplex A mild state of depression. See also **bipolar disorder.**

melancholia stuporosa A state of depression in which stupor in varying degrees is often accompanied by hallucinations. See also **bipolar disorder, stupor.**

melanin A black or dark brown pigment that occurs naturally in the hair, skin, and in the iris and choroid of the eye. See also **melanocyte.**

melano- A combining form meaning 'black' or '(related to) melanin': *melanoderm, melanoleukoderma.*

melanocyte A body cell capable of producing melanin. Such cells are distributed throughout the basal cell layer of the epidermis and form melanin pigment from tyrosine, an amino acid. Melanin granules are then transferred to adjacent basal cells and to hair. Melanocyte-stimulating hormone from the pituitary controls the amount of melanin produced.

melanocyte-stimulating hormone (MSH) A polypeptide hormone secreted by the pituitary gland. It controls the intensity of pigmentation in pigmented cells. It is synthesized on the same precursor polypeptide as adrenocorticotrophic hormone and the enkephalins.

melanoderma Any abnormal darkening of the skin caused by increased deposits of melanin or by the salts of iron or silver.

melanoma Any of a group of malignant neoplasms, primarily of the skin, that are composed of melanocytes. Most melanomas develop from a pigmented nevus over a period of several months or years and occur most commonly in fair-skinned people having light-colored eyes. Any black or

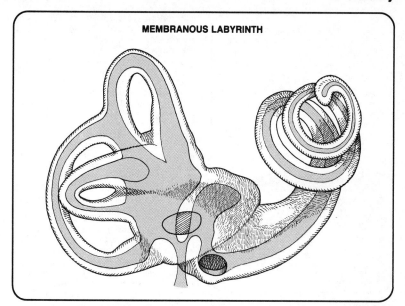

MEMBRANOUS LABYRINTH

brown spot having an irregular border, pigment appearing to radiate beyond that border, a red, black, and blue coloration observable upon close examination, or a nodular surface is suggestive of melanoma and is usually excised for biopsy. Kinds of melanoma are **amelanotic melanoma, benign juvenile melanoma, nodular melanoma, primary cutaneous melanoma, superficial spreading melanoma.**

melanotrichia linguae   See **parasitic glossitis.**

melasma   See **chloasma.**

melatonin   The only hormone secreted into the bloodstream by the pineal gland. It has marked diurnal rhythm; blood levels are up to 10 times greater at night than during the day. The hormone appears to inhibit numerous endocrine functions, including the gonadotropic hormones, and to decrease the pigmentation of the skin. When injected, exogenous melatonin causes drowsiness. Decreased secretion of melatonin occurs when calcification or tumor formation destroys or damages the pineal gland. A marked decrease results in precocious puberty, especially in boys, and in diabetes insipidus, hypogonadism, and optic atrophy.

melena   Abnormal, black, tarry stool containing digested blood. It usually results from bleeding in the upper gastrointestinal tract and is often a sign of peptic ulcer or small bowel disease. See also **gastrointestinal bleeding.**

meli-   A combining form meaning 'sweet or related to honey': *melitagra, melitoptyalism.*

-melia   A combining form meaning '(condition of the) limbs': *acromelia, dolichomelia.*

melioidosis   An uncommon infection of humans caused by the gram-negative bacillus *Malleomyces pseudomallei.* Acute melioidosis is ful-

minant and usually characterized by pneumonia, empyema, lung abscess, septicemia, and liver or spleen involvement. Chronic melioidosis is associated with osteomyelitis, multiple abscesses of the internal organs, and the development of fistulas from the abscesses. The disease, most commonly seen in China and Southeast Asia, is acquired by direct contact with infected animals. Treatment using chloramphenicol, sulfonamides, or tetracycline is usually successful.

melphalan   An alkylating agent used in cancer chemotherapy.

membrana tectoria   The broad, strong ligament covering the dens and helping to connect the axis to the occipital bone of the skull. Also called **occipitoaxial ligament.** Compare **alar ligament, apical dental ligament.**

membrana tympani   See **tympanic membrane.**

membrane   A thin layer of tissue that covers a surface, lines a cavity, or divides a space, as the abdominal membrane that lines the abdominal wall. The principal kinds of membranes are **cutaneous membrane, mucous membrane, serous membrane, synovial membrane.**

membranous labyrinth   A network of three fluid-filled, membranous, semicircular ducts suspended within the bony semicircular canals of the inner ear, associated with the sense of balance. The ducts, which contain endolymph, follow the contours of the bony canals.

membranous stomatitis   See **pseudomembranous stomatitis.**

memory   1. The mental faculty or power that enables one to retain and to recall, through unconscious associative processes, previously experienced sensations, impressions, ideas, concepts, and all information that has been

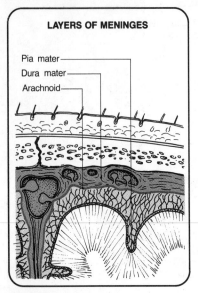

LAYERS OF MENINGES

Pia mater
Dura mater
Arachnoid

consciously learned. **2.** The reservoir of all past experiences and knowledge that may be recollected or recalled at will. Kinds of memory include **affect memory, anterograde memory, kinesthetic memory, long-term memory, screen memory, short-term memory, visual memory.** See also **amnesia, déjà vu.**

memory cell See under **lymphocyte.**

memory image A sensation, impression, or sense perception as it is recalled in the memory.

-men A combining form meaning a 'condition or result of a (specified) action': *lumen, semen.*

menadiol sodium diphosphate A water-soluble analog of vitamin K. See **menadione.**

menadione An analog of vitamin K. It is prescribed in the treatment of vitamin K deficiency and hypoprothrombinemia (other than the hereditary type). It is not indicated in pregnancy, for anticoagulant overdose, or to counteract heparin. Known hypersensitivity to this drug prohibits its use. Among the most serious adverse reactions are kernicterus in the newborn and hemolytic anemia in glucose-6-phosphate dehydrogenase deficient individuals. Gastrointestinal upset, rashes, and headaches also may occur.

menadione sodium bisulfite A water-soluble analog of vitamin K. See **menadione.**

menaphthone See **menadione.**

menarche The first menstruation and the commencement of cyclic menstrual function. It usually occurs between the ages of 9 and 17. See also **pubarche.**

mendelevium (Mv) A man-made element in the actinide group. Its atomic number is 101. The atomic weight of its most stable isotope is 256.

Mendelian genetics See **Mendel's laws.**

Mendelism, Mendelianism The concept of inheritance derived from the application of Mendel's laws. **—Mendelian,** *adj.*

Mendel's laws, Mendelian laws The basic principles of inheritance based on the breeding experiments of garden peas by the 19th-century Austrian monk Gregor Mendel. These are usually stated as two laws, commonly called the law of segregation and the law of independent assortment. According to the first, each characteristic of a species is represented in the somatic cells by a pair of units, now known as genes, which separate during meiosis so that each gamete receives only one gene for each trait. In any monohybrid crossing, the possible ratio for the phenotypic expression of a particular dominant characteristic is 3:1, while the ratio of pure dominants to dominant hybrids to pure recessives is 1:2:1. According to the second law, the members of a gene pair on different chromosomes segregate independently from other pairs during meiosis, so that the gametes show all possible combinations of factors. Genes on the same chromosome are affected by linkage and segregate in blocks according to the amount of crossing over that occurs, a discovery made after Mendel. Also called **Mendelian genetics.** See also **chromosome, crossing over, dominant gene, linkage, meiosis, recessive gene.**

Mendelson's syndrome A respiratory condition caused by the chemical pneumonia resulting from the aspiration of acidic gastric contents into the lungs. It usually occurs when a person vomits when inebriated, when stuporous from anesthesia, or when unconscious, as during a seizure.

Ménétrier's disease See **giant hypertrophic gastritis.**

-menia A combining form meaning '(condition of) menstrual activity': *catamenia, ischomenia.*

Ménière's disease A chronic disease of the inner ear characterized by recurrent episodes of vertigo, progressive unilateral nerve deafness, and tinnitus. The cause is unknown, although occasionally the condition follows middle ear infection or trauma to the head. There also may be associated nausea, vomiting, and profuse sweating. Attacks last from a few minutes to several hours. Treatment includes a low-salt diet and the administration of dimenhydrinate, diphenhydramine, or atropine sulfate. In severe cases, surgery may be necessary.

NURSING CONSIDERATIONS: Since sudden movements often aggravate the vertigo, the patient will usually prefer to move at a self-determined rate, although walking without assistance should not be undertaken. Siderails should be in place on the bed at all times. Also called **Ménière's syndrome, paroxysmal labyrinthine vertigo.**

meningeal hydrops See **pseudotumor cerebri.**

meninges, *sing.* **meninx** The three membranes that enclose the brain and the spinal cord, comprising the dura mater, the pia mater, and the arachnoid. The pia mater and the arachnoid can become inflamed by bacterial meningitis, causing serious complications, which may be life-threatening. —**meningeal,** *adj.*

meningioma, *pl.* **meningiomas, meningiomata** A mesenchymal fibroblastic tumor of the membranes enveloping the brain and spinal cord. Meningiomas often grow slowly, are usually vascular, and occur most commonly near the superior longitudinal transverse and cavernous sinuses of the dura mater of the brain. The tumors may be nodular, plaquelike, or diffuse lesions that invade the skull, causing bone erosion and compression of brain tissue. Meningiomas usually occur in adults, in some cases following a head injury.

meningism An abnormal condition characterized by irritation of the brain and the spinal cord and by symptoms that mimic those of meningitis. In meningism, however, there is no actual inflammation of the meninges.

meningitis Any infection or inflammation of the membranes covering the brain and spinal cord. It is usually purulent and involves the fluid in the subarachnoid space. It is characterized by severe headache, vomiting, and pain and stiffness in the neck. The most common causes are bacterial infection with *Streptococcus pneumoniae, Neisseria meningitides,* or *Haemophilus influenzae.* Aseptic meningitis may be caused by other kinds of bacteria, by chemical irritation, neoplasm, or by viruses. Many of these diseases are benign and self-limited. Others are more severe, as those involving herpesviruses. Yeasts, as *Candida,* and fungi, as *Cryptococcus,* may cause a severe, often fatal, meningitis. Tuberculous meningitis, invariably fatal if untreated, may result in a variety of neurological abnormalities, even with the best treatment available. Bacterial meningitis is treated promptly with antibiotics. Except for adenine arabinoside, recommended for herpes simplex meningitis, there is no specific therapy available for viral infections of the meninges. Antifungal medications, as amphotericin B, may prevent death from fungal meningitis, but serious neurological sequelae may occur. NURSING CONSIDERATIONS: Constant nursing attention is necessary to ensure early recognition of rising intracranial pressure, to prevent aspiration in the event of convulsive seizures, and to avoid airway obstruction. Except for the first 1 or 2 days of meningococcal disease, strict isolation procedures are unnecessary. Intravenous fluids and nasogastric tube feeding may be necessary for a prolonged period. Compare **encephalitis.**

meningo- A combining form meaning 'pertaining to membranes covering the brain or spinal cord or to other membranes': *meningocele, meningococcus.*

meningocele A saclike protrusion of either the cerebral or spinal meninges through a congenital defect in the skull or the vertebral column. It forms a hernial cyst that is filled with cerebrospinal fluid but does not contain neural

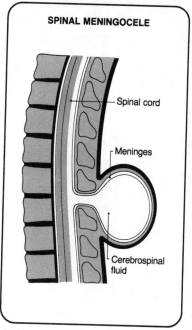

SPINAL MENINGOCELE

- Spinal cord
- Meninges
- Cerebrospinal fluid

tissue. The anomaly is designated a cranial meningocele or spinal meningocele, depending on the site of the defect; it can be easily repaired by surgery. See also **myelomeningocele, neural tube defect.**

meningococcal polysaccharide vaccine Either of two active immunizing agents against group A, C, Y, and W-135 meningococcal organisms. It is prescribed for immunization against meningococcal meningitis. Immunosuppression or acute infection prohibits its use. The most serious adverse reaction is anaphylaxis.

meningococcemia See **Rocky Mountain spotted fever.**

meningococcus, *pl.* **meningococci** A bacterium of the species *Neisseria meningitidis,* a nonmotile, gram-negative diplococcus, frequently found in the nasopharynx of asymptomatic carriers, that may cause septicemia or epidemic cerebrospinal meningitis. Meningococcal infections are not highly communicable; however, crowded conditions, as may be found in army camps, concentrate the number of carriers and reduce individual resistance to the organism. Hemorrhagic skin lesions are significant clues to the diagnosis. Early treatment with appropriate antibiotics, as penicillin G, is essential for cure. Several meningococcal vaccines are available. See also **meningitis.** —**meningococcal,** *adj.*

meningoencephalocele A saclike cyst containing brain tissue, cerebrospinal fluid, and meninges that protrudes through a congenital defect in the skull. The anomaly is commonly

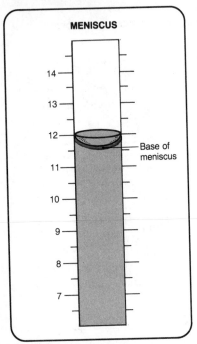

MENISCUS

14
13
12 — Base of meniscus
11
10
9
8
7

associated with defects in the brain. Also called **encephalomeningocele.** See also **neural tube defect.**

meningomyelocele   See **myelomeningocele.**

meniscectomy   Surgical excision of one of the crescent-shaped cartilages of the knee joint, performed when a torn cartilage results in chronic pain and in instability or locking of the joint. Under low-spinal or general anesthesia, the torn cartilage is freed and removed, and an elastic compression bandage is applied. After surgery, the leg is kept elevated to reduce swelling, and exercises are performed to maintain muscle strength. Crutch walking usually begins about the 4th day and full ambulation about the 12th day.

meniscocystosis   See **sickle cell anemia.**

meniscus   1. The crescent shape of fluid located at the interface between a liquid and air. Liquid measurements should be read from the base of the meniscus. 2. A lens with both convex and concave aspects. 3. A curved, fibrous cartilage in the knees and other joints.

Menke's kinky hair syndrome   A familial disorder caused by a defect in intestinal copper absorption and characterized by the growth of sparse, kinky hair. Infants with the syndrome suffer cerebral degeneration, retarded growth, and early death. Early diagnosis and intravenous administration of copper may prevent irreversible damage.

meno-   A combining form meaning 'of or relating to the menses': *menopause, menorrhea.*

menometrorrhagia   Excessive menstrual and uterine bleeding other than that caused by menstruation. It is a combination of metrorrhagia and menorrhagia and may be a sign of a urogenital malignancy.

menopause   Strictly, the cessation of menses, but commonly used to refer to the period of the female climacteric. Menses stop naturally with the decline of cyclic hormonal production and function between the ages of 45 and 60 but may stop earlier in life as a result of illness or the surgical removal of the uterus or both ovaries. As the production of ovarian estrogen and pituitary gonadotropins decreases, ovulation and menstruation become less frequent and eventually stop. Hot flashes are the only nearly universal symptom of the menopause. They can often be controlled with estrogen but are seldom so severe as to require therapy and cease in time without hormonal treatment. Occasionally, heavy irregular bleeding occurs at this time, usually associated with myomata (fibroids) or other uterine pathology. Estrogens given in large parenteral doses may be effective, but hysterectomy is sometimes required for control of the bleeding. Formerly—and incorrectly—emotional and psychological turmoil was expected with the menopause and attributed to it. Symptoms of this sort that are coincidental with the cessation of the menses are unusual and are not attributable to it.

menorrhagia   Abnormally heavy or long menstrual periods. Menorrhagia occurs occasionally during the reproductive years of most women's lives. If the condition becomes chronic, anemia from recurrent excessive blood loss may result. Abnormal bleeding following menopause always warrants investigation to rule out malignancy. Menorrhagia is a relatively common complication of benign uterine fibromyomata; it may be so severe or intractable as to require hysterectomy. Also called **hypermenorrhea.** Compare **metrorrhagia, oligomenorrhea.** **—menorrhagic,** *adj.*

menostasis   An abnormal condition in which the products of menstruation cannot escape the uterus or vagina owing to stenosis, an occlusion of the cervix, or the introitus of the vagina. An imperforate hymen is a rare cause of menostasis. **—menostatic,** *adj.*

menotropins   A gonadotropin.

menses   The normal flow of blood and decidua that occurs during menstruation. The 1st day of the flow of the menses is the 1st day of the menstrual cycle.

menstrual cycle   The recurring cycle of change in the endometrium during which the decidual layer of the endometrium is shed, then regrows, proliferates, is maintained for several days, and sheds again at menstruation. The average duration of menstruation is 5 days; the average length of the cycle, from the 1st day of bleeding of one cycle to the 1st of another, is 28 days. The length, duration, and character vary greatly among women. Menstrual cycles begin at menarche and end with menopause.

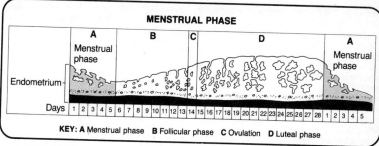

MENSTRUAL PHASE

KEY: **A** Menstrual phase **B** Follicular phase **C** Ovulation **D** Luteal phase

menstrual phase The final of the four phases of the menstrual cycle, the one in which menstruation occurs. The necrotic mucosa of the endometrium is shed, leaving the stratum basale; bleeding, primarily from spiral arteries, occurs. The average blood loss is 30 ml (1 oz). Compare **luteal phase, secretory phase.**

ment- A combining form meaning 'mind': *mental.*

mental **1.** Of, relating to, or characteristic of the mind or psyche. **2.** Existing in the mind; that which is performed or accomplished by the mind. **3.** Of, relating to, or characterized by a disorder of the mind. **4.** Of or pertaining to the chin.

mental age (MA) The age level at which one functions intellectually, as determined by standardized psychological and intelligence tests and expressed as the age at which that level is average. Compare **achievement age.** See also **developmental age.**

mental deficiency See **mental retardation.**

mental disorder Any disturbance of emotional equilibrium, manifested in maladaptive behavior and impaired functioning, caused by genetic, physical, chemical, biological, psychological, social, or cultural factors. Also called **emotional illness, mental illness, psychiatric disorder.**

mental handicap Any mental defect or characteristic resulting from a congenital abnormality, traumatic injury, or disease that impairs normal intellectual functioning and prevents a person from participating normally in activities appropriate for the person's particular age group. See also **mental retardation.**

mental health A relative state of mind in which a person who is healthy is able to cope with and adjust to the recurrent stresses of everyday living in an acceptable way.

Mental Health Association (MHA) A voluntary, nonprofessional agency dedicated to the improvement of mental health facilities and services in community clinics and hospitals, the recruitment and training of volunteers, and the promotion of mental health legislation. Formerly called the **National Association for Mental Health.**

mental health nursing See **psychiatric nursing.**

mental health service Any one of a group

of government, professional, or lay organizations operating at a community, state, national, or international level to aid in the prevention and treatment of mental disorders. See also **community mental health center.**

mental hygiene The study concerned with the development of healthy mental and emotional habits, attitudes, and behavior and with the prevention of mental illness. Also called **psychophylaxis.**

mental illness See **mental disorder.**

mental image Any concept or sensation produced in the mind through memory or imagination.

mentality **1.** The functional power and the capacity of the mind. **2.** Intellectual character.

mental retardation A disorder characterized by subaverage general intellectual function with deficits or impairments in the ability to learn and to adapt socially. The disorder, which is twice as prevalent among men as women, is classified according to the intelligence quotient as: borderline, IQ 71 to 84; mild, IQ 50 to 70; moderate, IQ 35 to 49; severe, IQ 20 to 34; and profound, IQ below 20. Treatment consists of educational programs and training specific to the level of retardation. Also called **mental deficiency.** See also **Down's syndrome, Hurler's syndrome, phenylketonuria, Tay-Sachs disease.**

mental status The degree of competence shown by a person in intellectual, emotional, psychological, and personality functioning as measured by psychological testing with reference to a statistical norm. See also **mental status examination.**

mental status examination A diagnostic procedure for determining the mental status of a person. The trained interviewer poses certain questions in a carefully standardized manner and evaluates the verbal responses and behavioral reactions.

mentation Any mental activity, including conscious and unconscious processes.

menthol A topical antipruritic agent.

-mentia A combining form meaning '(condition of the) mind': *dementia, moramentia, pseudodementia.*

mentum The chin, especially of the fetus.

menu In computer science: the list of available functions that appears on the CRT (cathode-ray tube) or screen. When the user inputs the symbol for the desired function, the computer retrieves the corresponding program.

mepenzolate bromide A gastrointestinal anticholinergic agent.

meperidine hydrochloride A narcotic and opioid analgesic.

mephentermine sulfate A sympathomimetic agent.

mephenytoin An hydantoin anticonvulsant.

mephobarbital A barbiturate sedative-hypnotic anticonvulsant.

mepivacaine hydrochloride An amide local anesthetic.

meprobamate An antianxiety agent.

mEq *abbr* **milliequivalent.**

-mer, -mere A combining form meaning 'part, portion': *isomer, monomer.*

meralgia The presence of pain in the thigh.

meralgia paresthetica A condition characterized by pain, paresthesia, and numbness on the lateral surface of the thigh in the region supplied by the lateral femoral cutaneous nerve. The cause of the condition is ischemia of the nerve owing to its entrapped position in the inguinal ligament.

merbromin An antiseptic agent.

mercaptopurine An antimetabolite used in cancer chemotherapy.

mercurial **1.** Of or pertaining to mercury, particularly a medicine containing the element mercury. **2.** An adverse effect associated with the administration of a mercurial medication, as a mercurial tremor owing to mercury poisoning.

mercurial diuretic Any one of several diuretic agents that contain mercury in an organic chemical form. Mercurial diuretics inhibit tubular reabsorption of sodium and chloride and the excretion of potassium but do not produce diuresis in patients who are in metabolic alkalosis. The principal use for the drugs is in treating edema of cardiac origin, ascites associated with cirrhosis, or oliguria in the nephrotic stage of glomerulonephritis. Response usually begins within 1 to 2 hours and lasts for 12 hours. Immediate fatal reactions have occurred, usually owing to ventricular failure following intravascular injection and transient high concentration of mercury in the blood. Flushing, urticaria, fever, nausea, and vomiting are common side effects. Thrombocytopenia, neutropenia, agranulocytosis, systemic mercury poisoning, and severe hypersensitivity reactions are among the more serious adverse effects of the mercurial diuretics; the drugs are contraindicated for use in the presence of renal insufficiency or acute nephritis. Because of their toxicity, these drugs are considered obsolete. Current practice usually recommends their replacement with more convenient and less toxic diuretics, as furosemide or ethacrynic acid.

mercurialism See **mercury poisoning.**

-mercuric A combining form meaning 'molecules of bivalent mercury or its compounds': *phenylmercuric, potassiomercuric.*

mercury (Hg) A metallic element. Its atomic number is 80; its atomic weight is 200.6. It is the only common metal that is liquid at room temperature, and it occurs in nature almost entirely in the form of its sulfide, cinnabar. Mercury is produced commercially and is used in thermometers, barometers, and other measuring instruments. It forms many poisonous compounds. The major toxic forms of this metal are mercury vapor, mercuric salts, and organic mercurials. Elemental mercury is only mildly toxic when ingested, because it is poorly absorbed. The vapor of elemental mercury, however, is readily absorbed through the lungs and enters the brain before it is oxidized. The kidneys retain mercury longer than any of the other body tissues.

mercury poisoning A toxic condition caused by the ingestion or inhalation of mercury or a mercury compound. The chronic form, resulting from inhalation of the vapors or dust of mercurial compounds or from repeated ingestion of very small amounts, is characterized by irritability, excessive salivation, loosened teeth, gum disorders, slurred speech, tremors, and staggering. Symptoms of acute mercury poisoning appear in a few to 30 minutes and include a metallic taste in the mouth, thirst, nausea, vomiting, severe abdominal pain, bloody diarrhea, and renal failure that may result in death. The presence of mercury in the body is determined by a urine test. Treatment may include gastric lavage with milk and egg white or sodium bicarbonate, chelation with British antilewisite (BAL), and fluid therapy. Mercury compounds are found in agricultural fungicides and in certain antiseptics and pigments. Industrial wastes containing mercury have been identified in some areas, and seafood from contaminated waters has caused serious public health problems. Also called **hydrargyrism, mad hatter's disease, mercurialism.** See also **Minamata disease.**

mercy killing See **euthanasia.**

merergasia A mild mental incapacity characterized by some emotional instability and some anxiety. —**merergastic,** *adj.*

-meria A combining form meaning '(condition of) parts': *platymeria, polymeria.*

merisis An increase in size as a result of cell division and the addition of new material rather than of cell expansion. Also called **multiplicative growth.** Compare **auxesis.** See also **hyperplasia.**

mero- A combining form meaning 'part': *meroacrania, meropia.*

meroblastic Pertaining to or characterizing an ovum that contains a large amount of yolk and in which cleavage is restricted to a part of the cytoplasm. Compare **holoblastic.**

meromelia A general designation for the congenital absence of any part of a limb. It is used in reference to such conditions as adactyly or hemimelia. Compare **amelia.**

merozoite An organism produced from segmentation of a schizont during the asexual reproductive phase of the life cycle of a sporozoan, specifically the malarial parasite *Plasmodium.* See also *Plasmodium.*

mescaline   A psychoactive, poisonous alkaloid derived from a colorless alkaline oil in the flowering heads of the cactus *Lophophora williamsii.* Related chemically to epinephrine, mescaline causes heart palpitations, diaphoresis, pupillary dilation, and anxiety. The drug, taken in capsules or dissolved in a drink, produces visual hallucinations, as color patterns and spatial distortions, but it does not ordinarily induce disorientation. North American Indians used mescaline in ceremonial feasts to produce euphoria and a feeling of ecstasy. Also called **peyote.**

mesencephalon   One of the three parts of the brain stem, lying just below the cerebrum and just above the pons. It consists primarily of white substance with some gray substance around the cerebral aqueduct. A red nucleus lies within the reticular formation of the mesencephalon and contains the terminations of fibers from the cerebellum and the frontal lobe of the cerebral cortex. The ventral part of the mesencephalon is formed by the cerebral peduncles; the dorsal part is formed by the corpora quadrigemina. Deep within the mesencephalon are nuclei of the third and fourth cranial nerves and the anterior part of the fifth cranial nerve. The mesencephalon also contains nuclei for certain auditory and certain visual reflexes. Also called **midbrain. —mesencephalic,** *adj.*

mesenchymal chondrosarcoma   A malignant cartilaginous tumor that develops in many sites.

mesenchymoma   A mixed mesenchymal neoplasm composed of two or more cellular elements, not usually associated, and fibrous tissue. See also **benign mesenchymoma, malignant mesenchymoma.**

mesenteric adenitis   See **adenitis.**

mesenteric node   A node in one of three groups of superior mesenteric lymph glands serving parts of the intestine. An average of 125 mesenteric nodes in three different groups lie between the layers of the mesentery. The first group lies close to the wall of the small intestine, among the terminal twigs of the superior mesenteric artery. The second group is located in relation to the loops and primary branches of the artery. The third group lies along the trunk of the artery. The mesenteric nodes receive afferents from the jejunum, ileum, cecum, vermiform appendix, ascending colon, and transverse colon. Compare **ileocolic node, mesocolic node.**

mesentery   A peritoneal fold that attaches the stomach, small intestine, pancreas, and other abdominal organs to the dorsal body wall. Commonly, the term refers to the membranous folds which invest the small intestine.

mesentery proper   A broad, fan-shaped fold of peritoneum connecting the jejunum and the ileum with the dorsal wall of the abdomen. The root of the mesentery proper is about 15 cm

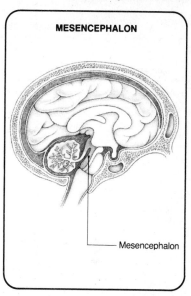

MESENCEPHALON

Mesencephalon

(6 inches) long and is connected to certain structures ventral to the vertebral column. The intestinal border of the mesentery proper is about 6 m (19¾ feet) long and separates to enclose the intestine. The central part of the mesentery proper is narrow, but it widens to about 20 cm (7 ⅞ inches) and suspends the small intestine and various nerves and arteries. Also called mesentery of the small intestine. Compare **sigmoid mesocolon, transverse mesocolon.**

mesial   See **medial.**

meso-   A combining form meaning: **1.** 'Middle': *mesocardium, mesocecum.* **2.** 'Inactive or without effect on polarized light': *mesomerism, meson.*

mesocolic node   A node in one of three groups of superior mesenteric lymph glands, proliferating between the layers of the transverse mesocolon, close to the transverse colon. They are best developed near the right and the left colic flexures. Compare **mesenteric node.**

mesocolopexy   Suspension or fixation of the mesocolon.

mesoderm   In embryology: the middle of the three cell layers of the developing embryo. It lies between the ectoderm and the endoderm.

mesoglia   See **microglia.**

mesometritis   See **myometritis.**

mesomorph   A person whose physique is characterized by a predominance of muscle, bone, and connective tissue, structures which develop from the mesodermal layer of the embryo. Compare **ectomorph, endomorph.**

mesonephric duct   In embryology: a duct that, in the male, gives rise to the ducts of the reproductive system (ejaculatory duct). In the female, it persists vestigially as **Gartner's duct.** Also called **Wolffian duct.**

mesonephric tubule   Any of the embry-

METABOLIC ACIDOSIS AND ALKALOSIS

CONDITION	POSSIBLE CAUSES	SYMPTOMS
Metabolic acidosis (primary bicarbonate deficit)	Renal disease, starvation, diabetic ketosis, lactic acidosis, severe diarrhea, biliary fistulas, ingestion of substances such as methyl alcohol, salicylates, paraldehyde, or ethylene glycol	Kussmaul's respiration, restlessness, disorientation, stupor
Metabolic alkalosis (primary bicarbonate excess)	Vomiting, diuretics, hyperadrenocorticism, hyperaldosteronism, nasogastric suction, ingestion of sodium bicarbonate or other alkali	Weakness, apathy, leg cramps, paresthesias, paralysis, polyuria

KEY: ⇓ = decreased ⇑ = increased. Shaded arrows indicate the primary abnormality.

onic renal tubules comprising the mesonephros. They function as excretory structures during the early embryonic development of humans and other mammals but are later incorporated into the reproductive system.
mesonephron, *pl.* **mesonephra** See **mesonephros.**
mesonephros, mesonephron, *pl.* **mesonephroi, mesonephra** The second type of excretory organ to develop in the vertebrate embryo. This organ consists of a series of twisting tubules that arise from the nephrogenic cord and lie caudal to the pronephros. At one end, the tubules form the glomerulus, and at the other end they connect with the excretory mesonephric duct. The organ is the permanent kidney in the lower animals, but in humans and various other mammals the mesonephros is functional only during early embryonic development and is later replaced by the metanephros, although the duct system is retained and incorporated into the male reproductive system. Also called **middle kidney, Wolffian body.** See also **metanephros, pronephros.** —**mesonephric, mesonephroid,** *adj.*
mesoridazine besylate A phenothiozine antipsychotic agent.
mesosalpinx Cephalic, free border of the broad ligament in which uterine tubes lie.

mesothelioma, *pl.* **mesotheliomas, mesotheliomata** A rare, malignant tumor of the mesothelium of the pleura or peritoneum, associated with earlier exposure to asbestos. The lesion, composed of spindle cells or fibrous tissue, may form thick sheets covering the viscera. The prognosis is poor. Also called **celothelioma.**
messenger RNA (mRNA) In molecular genetics: an RNA fraction that transmits information from DNA to the protein-synthesizing ribosomes of cells.
mestranol An estrogen prescribed as an oral contraceptive, always in fixed-combination drugs with a progestin.
MET *abbr* **metabolic equivalent.**
meta- A combining form meaning: **1.** 'Change or exchange': *metabasis, metallaxis.* **2.** 'After or next': *metachemical, metapneumonic.* **3.** 'The 1,3 position in derivative of benzine': *metacetone, metacresol.*
metabolic Of or pertaining to **metabolism.**
metabolic acidosis A condition resulting from excessive absorption or retention of acid or, excessive excretion of bicarbonate. In starvation and in uncontrolled diabetes mellitus, glucose is not present or is not available for oxidation for cellular nutrition. The plasma bicarbonate of the body is used up in neutralizing

SIGNS	BLOOD GAS LEVELS			NURSING CONSIDERATIONS
	pH	HCO₃₋	Paco₂	
Shock, coma, tachypnea, almond odor from mouth	< 7.35			• Treatment is directed at underlying disorder. • In patients with diabetes, expect a drop in blood pressure, stupor, and possible coma. Monitor vital signs carefully. Draw blood glucose immediately. • Secondary or compensatory metabolic alkalosis can result from the body's compensatory mechanisms to increase bicarbonate levels.
Signs of potassium depletion, tetany, respiratory depression, arrhythmias possibly leading to cardiac arrest	> 7.45			• Treatment is directed at underlying condition. • Volume and potassium depletion should be corrected. • This condition, most commonly seen after acute vomiting or nasogastric suctioning, is the result of hydrogen ion loss from the hydrochloric acid of digestive juices. • Can also occur in patients who ingest sodium bicarbonate regularly (for example, to relieve acid stomach). • Monitor heart for arrhythmias due to potassium loss through body compensatory mechanisms.

the ketones produced by the breakdown of body fat for energy that occurs in compensation for the lack of glucose. Metabolic acidosis also occurs when oxidation takes place without adequate oxygen, as in heart failure or shock. Severe diarrhea, renal failure, and lactic acidosis may also result in metabolic acidosis. Signs of metabolic acidosis include shock, coma, tachypnea, and almond breath odor. Hyperkalemia often accompanies the condition.

metabolic alkalosis An abnormal condition characterized by the significant loss of acid in the body or by increased levels of base bicarbonate. The reduction of acid may be caused by excessive vomiting, insufficient replacement of electrolytes, hyperadrenocorticism, and Cushing's disease. A decrease in base bicarbonate may be caused by various problems, as the ingestion of excessive bicarbonate of soda and other antacids during the treatment of peptic ulcers, and by the administration of excessive intravenous fluids containing high concentrations of bicarbonate. Severe, untreated metabolic alkalosis can lead to coma and death. Signs and symptoms of metabolic alkalosis may include apnea, headache, lethargy, irritability, nausea, vomiting, and atrial tachycardia. Confirmation of the diagnosis is commonly based on laboratory findings that show a blood pH level greater than 7.45, a carbonic acid concentration greater than 29 mEq/liter, and alkaline urine. The patient with this condition may have tachycardia. Treatment may include the intravenous administration of ammonium chloride to release hydrogen chloride and restore chloride levels. Potassium chloride and normal saline solutions usually replace fluid losses from gastric drainage but are contraindicated in patients with associated congestive heart failure.

NURSING CONSIDERATIONS: Nurses administer any prescribed intravenous solutions. The intravenous administration of ammonium chloride is usually contraindicated in patients with liver or kidney disease. Too rapid infusion of ammonium chloride may hemolyze the red blood cells, and excessive dosage may overcorrect alkalosis and cause acidosis. Decreased respiratory rate indicates an effort to compensate for alkalosis. Compare **respiratory alkalosis.** See also **metabolic acidosis, respiratory acidosis.**

metabolic disorder Any pathophysiologic dysfunction that results in a loss of metabolic control of homeostasis in the body.

metabolic equivalent (MET) The amount of oxygen consumed per kilogram of body weight per minute when at rest.

metabolic rate The amount of energy expended in a given unit of time. Energy is stored

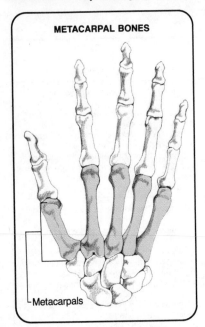

METACARPAL BONES

Metacarpals

in the body in energy-rich phosphate compounds and in proteins, fats, and complex carbohydrates. See also **basal metabolic rate.**

metabolic respiratory quotient (R) The ratio of production of carbon dioxide to the corresponding consumption of oxygen. The values of R change according to the fuel being burned; thus, as fat contains relatively little oxygen compared with glucose, the R of fat is lower than that of glucose, while the R of protein is between that of glucose and fat.

metabolism The aggregate of all chemical processes that take place in living organisms, resulting in growth, generation of energy, elimination of wastes, and other bodily functions as they relate to the distribution of nutrients in the blood after digestion. Metabolism takes place in two steps: anabolism, the constructive phase, in which smaller molecules (as amino acids) are converted to larger molecules (as proteins); and catabolism, the destructive phase, in which larger molecules (as glycogen) are converted to smaller molecules (as pyruvic acid). The metabolic rate is customarily expressed (in calories) as the heat liberated in the course of metabolism. See also **acid-base metabolism, anabolism, basal metabolism, catabolism. —metabolic,** *adj.*

metabolite A substance produced by metabolic action or necessary for a metabolic process.

metacarpus The middle portion of the hand, consisting of five slender bones numbered from the thumb side, metacarpals I through V. Each metacarpal consists of a body and two extremities. **—metacarpal,** *adj., n.*

metacentric Pertaining to a chromosome in

which the centromere is located near the center so that the arms of the chromatids are of approximately equal length. Compare **acrocentric, submetacentric, telocentric.**

metagenesis The regular alternation of sexual with asexual methods of reproduction within the same species. **—metagenetic, metagenic,** *adj.*

metal Any element that conducts heat and electricity, is malleable and ductile, and forms positively charged ions (cations) in solution.

metal fume fever An occupational disorder caused by the inhalation of fumes of metallic oxides and characterized by symptoms similar to those of influenza. The condition occurs among workers engaged in welding and other occupations dealing with the manipulation of metals. Access to fresh air and treatment of the symptoms usually alleviate the condition. Also called **brassfounder's ague, zinc chill.** Compare **siderosis.**

metamorphopsia A defect in vision in which objects are seen as distorted in shape, resulting from disease of the retina or imperfection of the media.

metamorphosis A change in shape or structure, especially a change from one stage of development to another, as the transition from the larval to the adult stage.

metamyelocyte A stage in the development of the granulocyte series of leukocytes. It is intermediate between the myelocyte stage and the mature granulocyte. See also **leukocyte, myeloblast, myelocyte.**

metanephrine One of the two principal urinary metabolites of epinephrine and norepinephrine in the urine, the other being vanillylmandelic acid. The 24-hour normal value for total metanephrine is < 1.3 mg. Normally, less than 1.3 mg of metanephrine is excreted in 24 hours.

metanephrogenic Capable of forming the metanephros, or fetal kidney.

metanephron, *pl.* **metanephra** See **metanephros.**

metanephros, metanephron, *pl.* **metanephroi, metanephra** The third and permanent, excretory organ to develop in the vertebrate embryo. It consists of a complex structure of secretory and collecting tubules that develop into the kidney and are formed later than the mesonephros from the caudal end of the nephrogenic cord and the mesonephric duct. Also called **hind kidney.** See also **kidney, mesonephros, pronephros.**

metaphase The second of the four stages of nuclear division in mitosis and in each of the two divisions of meiosis, during which the chromosomes become arranged in the equatorial plane of the spindle to form the equatorial plate, with the centromeres attached to the spindle fibers in preparation for separation. See also **anaphase, interphase, meiosis, mitosis, prophase, telophase.**

metaphyseal dysostosis An abnormal condition that affects the skeletal system and is characterized by a disturbance of the mineralization of the metaphyseal area of the bones, resulting in dwarfism. Metaphyseal dysostosis is classified as the Gansen type, Schmidt type, Spahar-Hartmann type, or cartilage-hair hypoplasia. The Gansen type is characterized by metaphyseal alterations similar to those of achondroplasia but not involving the skull or the epiphyses of the long bones. The Schmidt type is characterized by changes from the weight-bearing age to approximately 5 years. The metaphyseal alterations associated with the Schmidt type are similar to those of achondroplasia, resulting in moderate dwarfism. The Spahar-Hartmann type is characterized by skeletal changes and severe genu varum. Cartilage-hair hypoplasia is characterized by severe dwarfism and hair that is sparse, short, and brittle. Mental retardation is not usually associated with metaphyseal dysostosis. Radiographic examination of all types of the disease reveals characteristic widening of the metaphyses of the tubular bones, with normal diaphyseal and epiphyseal ossification centers. Treatment is supportive and symptomatic.

metaphyseal dysplasia An abnormal condition characterized by disordered modeling of the cylindrical bones. The involvement of this disease is limited to the long bones and displays a characteristic radiographic image of the Erlenmeyer flask deformity in which the metaphyseal circumference is enlarged and the medullary area of the affected bone is reduced. Metaphyseal dysplasia most often affects the distal femur or the proximal tibia.

metaproterenol sulfate A sympathomimetic bronchodilator.

metaraminol bitartrate A sympathomimetic agent.

metastasis, *pl.* **metastases** The process by which tumor cells are spread to distant parts of the body. Because malignant tumors have no enclosing capsule, cells may escape, become emboli, and be transported by the lymphatic circulation or the bloodstream to implant on lymph nodes, the skeleton, or other organs far from the primary tumor. —**metastatic,** *adj.,* **metastasize,** *v.*

metastasizing mole See **chorioadenoma destruens.**

metastatic ophthalmia See **sympathetic ophthalmia.**

metatarsal 1. Of or pertaining to the metatarsus of the foot. 2. Any one of the five bones comprising the metatarsus.

metatarsalgia A painful condition involving the metatarsal bones caused by a structural abnormality of the foot or recalcification of degenerated heads of metatarsal bones. Also called **Morton's foot, Morton's neuroma, Morton's toe.**

metatarsal stress fracture A break or rupture of a metatarsal bone, resulting from prolonged running or walking. The condition is often difficult to diagnose with X-ray films. Also called **fatigue fracture, march fracture.**

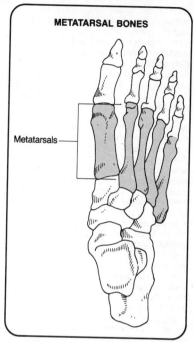

METATARSAL BONES

Metatarsals

metatarsus A part of the foot, consisting of five bones numbered I to V, from the medial side. Each bone has a long, slender body; a wedge-shaped proximal end; a convex distal end; and flattened, grooved sides for the attachment of ligaments. —**metatarsal,** *adj.*

metathalamus One of five parts of the diencephalon, composed of a medial geniculate body and a lateral geniculate body on each side. The medial geniculate body acts as a relay station for nerve impulses between the inferior brachium and the auditory cortex. The lateral geniculate body is an oval bulge at the posterior end of the thalamus, which accommodates the terminal ends of the fibers of the optic tract. Compare **epithalamus, hypothalamus, subthalamus.** —**metathalamic,** *adj.*

metaxalone A skeletal muscle relaxant.

Metchnikoff theory A theory that living cells ingest microorganisms. The theory proved correct, as seen in the process of phagocytosis.

meteorism Accumulation of gas in the abdomen or the intestine.

meteorotropism A reaction to meteorological influences shown by various biological occurrences, as angina. —**meteorotropic,** *adj.*

-meter, -metre A combining form meaning a 'measuring instrument': *anesthesimeter, scopometer.*

meter (m) A metric unit of length equal to 39.37 inches.

methacycline hydrochloride A tetracycline antibiotic.

methadone hydrochloride A parenteral

and oral narcotic and opioid analgesic.

methamphetamine hydrochloride An amphetamine central nervous system stimulant.

methampyrone See **dipyrone**.

methandrostenolone An androgen.

methanol A clear, colorless, toxic, liquid distillate of wood miscible with water, alcohol, and ether, widely used as a solvent and in making formaldehyde. Ingestion paralyzes the optic nerve and may cause death. Also called **wood alcohol**.

methanol-extractable residue (MER) An immunotherapeutic substance, prepared from a methanol-extracted fraction of the bacillus Calmette-Guérin (BCG). It is given to prevent or delay recurrences of Stage II malignant melanoma after surgery and to prolong drug-induced remissions in acute myelocytic leukemia.

methantheline bromide A gastrointestinal anticholinergic agent.

methaqualone A sedative-hypnotic agent.

metharbital A barbiturate anticonvulsant.

methazolamide A carbonic anhydrase inhibitor.

methdilazine hydrochloride A phenothiazine antihistamine.

methemoglobin A form of hemoglobin in which the iron component has been oxidized from the ferrous to the ferric state. Methemoglobin cannot carry oxygen and so contributes nothing to the oxygen-transporting capacity of the blood. Methemoglobin is a product of the various oxidative reactions that constitute normal metabolic activity. It is present in only trace amounts (about 1%) in the blood. See also **hemoglobin**.

methenamine hippurate, m. mandelate Urinary tract antiseptics.

methicillin sodium A penicillin antibiotic.

methimazole A thyroid hormone antagonist.

methixene hydrochloride A gastrointestinal anticholinergic agent.

methocarbamol A skeletal muscle relaxant.

method A technique or procedure for producing a desired effect, as a surgical procedure or a laboratory test.

methodology 1. The system of principles or methods of procedure in any discipline, as education, research, diagnosis, or treatment. 2. The section of a research proposal in which the methods to be used are described. —**methodological**, *adj.*

methohexital sodium A general anesthetic.

methotrexate, m. sodium Antimetabolites used in cancer chemothery.

methotrimeprazine, m. hydrochloride Nonnarcotic phenothiazine derivatives used as preanesthetic sedative-hypnotics and analgesics.

methoxamine hydrochloride An adrenergic that acts as a vasoconstrictor.

methoxsalen A skin pigmentation enhancing agent.

methscopolamine bromide A gastrointestinal anticholinergic agent.

methsuximide A succinimide anticonvulsant agent.

methyclothiazide A thiazide diuretic.

methyl alcohol See **methanol**.

methylcellulose A bulk-forming laxative.

methyldopa A sympatholytic antihypertensive that is centrally acting.

methylene blue A urinary tract antiseptic.

methylergonovine maleate An oxytocic agent.

methylphenidate hydrochloride A central nervous system stimulant.

methylprednisolone, m. acetate, m. disodium phosphate, m. sodium succinate Topical otic glucocorticoid anti-inflammatory agents.

methylrosaniline chloride See **gentian violet**.

methyl salicylate A counterirritant.

methyltestosterone An androgen substance.

methyprylon A sedative-hypnotic agent.

methysergide maleate A serotonin antagonist.

metoclopramide hydrochloride A drug that stimulates upper gastrointestinal tract motility.

metocurine iodide A nondepolarizing neuromuscular blocking agent.

metolazone A thiazide-like diuretic.

'me-too' drug *Informal.* A drug product that is similar, identical, or closely related to an already available drug for which a manufacturer has obtained a new drug application. The original drug is marketed by a company or companies other than the holder of the new drug application. On the assumption that the new drug has been recognized as safe and effective, clinical trials required of the original manufacturer are not required of the new supplier, but information regarding manufacture, bioavailability, and labeling is required to complete the abbreviated procedure for approval by the Food and Drug Administration.

metopic Of or pertaining to the forehead.

metopo- A combining form meaning 'of or related to the forehead': *metopodynia, metopopagus, metopoplasty.*

metoprolol tartrate A sympatholytic antihypertensive beta-adrenergic blocking agent.

metr- A combining form meaning 'measure': *metric.*

metra- See **metro-**.

metralgia Tenderness or pain in the uterus. Also called **metrodynia.**

-metria[1] A combining form meaning '(condition of the) ability to measure muscular acts': *dysmetria, hypermetria.*

-metria[2] A combining form meaning '(condition of the) uterus': *ametria, dimetria.*

metric Of or pertaining to a system of measurement that uses the meter as a basis. See also **metric system.**

metric equivalent Any value in metric units

METRIC SYSTEM PREFIXES, MULTIPLES, SUBMULTIPLES			
PREFIX	SYMBOL	POWER	MULTIPLE, SUBMULTIPLE
tera	T	10^{12}	1,000,000,000,000
giga	G	10^9	1,000,000,000
mega	M	10^6	1,000,000
kilo	k	10^3	1,000
hecto	h	10^2	100
deca	da	10^1	10
(single unit)			1
deci	d	10^{-1}	0.1
centi	c	10^{-2}	0.01
milli	m	10^{-3}	0.001
micro	μ	10^{-6}	0.000001
nano	n	10^{-9}	0.000000001
pico	p	10^{-12}	0.000000000001
femto	f	10^{-15}	0.000000000000001
atto	a	10^{-18}	0.000000000000000001

of measurement that equals the same value in English units, as 2.54 centimeters equal 1 inch or 1 liter equals 1.0567 quarts.

metric system A decimal system of measurement based on the meter (39.37 inches) as the unit of length, on the gram (15.432 grains) as the unit of weight or mass, and, as a derived unit, on the liter (0.908 U.S. dry quart or 1.0567 U.S. liquid quarts) as the unit of volume.

metritis Inflammation of the walls of the uterus. Also called **uteritis.** Kinds of metritis are **endometritis, parametritis.** See also **puerperal fever.**

metro-, metra- A combining form meaning 'of or related to the uterus': *metrocele, metrofibroma.*

metrodynia Tenderness or pain in the uterus. Also called **metralgia.**

metronidazole, m. hydrochloride Trichomonocides and amebicides.

-metropia A combining form meaning '(condition of the) refraction of the eye': *allometropia, isometropia.* Also **-metropy.**

metrorrhagia Uterine bleeding other than that caused by menstruation. It may be caused by uterine lesions and a sign of a urogenital malignancy.

-metry A combining form meaning the 'process of measuring something' specified: *pelvimetry, symmetry.* Also **-metria.**

metyrosine An antihypertensive that is an enzyme inhibitor.

Metzenbaum scissors See **scissors.**

Meuse fever See **trench fever.**

MeV, mev *abbr* million electron volts, the equivalent of 3.82 × 10^{-14} small calories, or 1.6 × 10^{-6} ergs.

mevalonate kinase An enzyme in the liver and in yeast that catalyzes the transfer of a phos-

phate group from adenosine triphosphate to produce adenosine diphosphate and 5-phosphomevalonate.

Meynet's node Any one of the numerous nodules that may develop within the capsules surrounding joints and in tendons affected by rheumatic diseases, especially in children.

mezlocillin sodium A penicillin antibiotic.

mfd *abbr* microfarad.

MFD *abbr* minimal fatal dose.

mg *abbr* milligram.

Mg Symbol for **magnesium.**

MH *abbr* malignant hyperthermia.

MHA *abbr* Mental Health Association.

MI *abbr* myocardial infarction.

miconazole, m. nitrate 2% Local anti-infective and antifungal agents.

micr- See **micro-.**

micrencephalon 1. An abnormally small brain. See also **microcephaly. 2.** The cerebellum. —**micrencephalic,** *adj., n.*

micrencephaly, micrencephalia See **microcephaly.**

micro-, micr- A combining form meaning 'small': *microadenopathy, microanalysis.* Also **mikro-.**

microaerotonometer An instrument for measuring the volume of gases in the blood.

microaggregate recipient set A device composed of plastic components for the intra-venous delivery of large volumes of stored whole blood or of packed blood cells. The components of the set include the plastic tubing, the roller clamp, and the special filter that prevents the microaggregates or deteriorated red blood cells of stored whole blood from entering and clogging the circulatory system of the patient. The plastic tubing of this device has a larger lumen

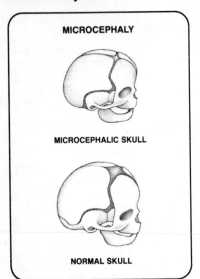

MICROCEPHALY

MICROCEPHALIC SKULL

NORMAL SKULL

than the tubing of most other intravenous sets, thus allowing the blood to be delivered more rapidly. Compare **component drip set, component syringe set, straight-line blood set, Y set.**

microaneurysm A microscopic aneurysm characteristic of thrombotic purpura.

microangiopathy A disease of the small blood vessels, as diabetic microangiopathy, in which the basement membrane of capillaries thickens.

microbe A pathogenic microorganism. —**microbial,** *adj.*

-microbe A combining form meaning a 'small living organism': *aeromicrobe, ultramicrobe.*

-microbic A combining form meaning 'referring to or consisting of microbes': *amicrobic, monomicrobic.*

microbiology The branch of biology concerned with the study of microorganisms.

microbrachia A developmental defect characterized by abnormal smallness of the arms. —**microbrachius,** *n.*

microcentrum See **centrosome.**

microcephaly, microcephalia, microcephalism A congenital anomaly characterized by abnormal smallness of the head in relation to the rest of the body and by underdevelopment of the brain, resulting in some degree of mental retardation. The head is more than two standard deviations below the average circumference size for age, sex, race, and period of gestation, and it has a narrow, receding forehead, a flattened occiput, and a pointed vertex. The condition may be caused by an autosomal recessive disorder; a chromosomal abnormality; a toxic stimulus, as irradiation, chemical agents, or maternal infection during prenatal development; or any trauma, especially during the third trimester of pregnancy or early infancy. There

is no treatment, and nursing care is primarily supportive. Compare **macrocephaly.** —**microcephalic, microcephalous,** *adj.,* **microcephalic, microcephalus,** *n.*

microcheiria, microchiria A developmental defect characterized by abnormal smallness of the hands. The condition is usually associated with other congenital malformations or with bone and muscle disorders.

microcirculation The flow of blood throughout the system of smaller vessels (those with a diameter of 100 microns or less) of the body.

microcurie (μCi, μc) A unit of radiation equal to one millionth (10^{-6}) of a curie.

microcyte An abnormally small erythrocyte with a mean corpuscular volume of less than 80 microns, often occurring in iron deficiency and other anemias.

microcytic Of a cell: smaller than normal, as the erythrocytes in microcytic anemia.

microcytic anemia A hematologic disorder characterized by abnormally small erythrocytes, usually associated with chronic blood loss or a nutritional anemia, as iron deficiency anemia. Compare **macrocytic anemia.**

microcytosis A hematologic condition characterized by erythrocytes that are smaller than normal. Microcytosis and hypochromatosis is usual in iron deficiency anemia. —**microcytic,** *adj.*

microdactyly A developmental defect characterized by abnormal smallness of the fingers and toes. The condition is usually associated with bone and muscle disorders, as progressive myositis ossificans.

microdrip In intravenous therapy: an apparatus for delivering relatively small, measured amounts of intravenous solutions at specific flow rates. The microdrip device usually consists of plastic tubing designed to allow small drops of solution to pass into the primary intravenous tubing through a clear plastic housing. Compare **macrodrip.**

microelement See **micronutrient.**

microencapsulation A laboratory technique used in the bioassay of hormones in which certain antibodies are encapsulated with a perforated membrane, resembling a whiffle ball. The technique is used for encapsulating unstable enzymes and in the preparation of some drugs in slow- or timed-release forms.

microfibrillar collagen hemostat A local hemostatic agent.

microfilaria, *pl.* **microfilariae** The prelarval form of any filarial worm. Certain bloodsucking insects ingest these forms from an infected host, and the microfilariae then develop in the body of the insect and become infective larvae. See also **dracunculiasis, filariasis, loiasis, onchocerciasis, Wuchereria.**

microfluorometry See **cytophotometry.** —**microfluorometric,** *adj.*

microgamete The small, motile male gamete of certain thallophytes and sporozoa, specifically the malarial parasite *Plasmodium*. See also **macrogamete, *plasmodium.***

microgametocyte An enlarged merozoite that undergoes meiosis to form the mature male gamete during the sexual phase of the life cycle of certain thallophytes and sporozoa, specifically the malarial parasite *Plasmodium*. Microgametocytes are found in the red blood cells of a person infected with the malarial parasite.

microgenitalia A condition characterized by abnormally small external genitalia.

microglia Small migratory interstitial cells that form part of the central nervous system. They have various forms and slender, branched processes. Microglia serve as phagocytes that collect waste products of the nerve tissue of the body. Also called **Hortega cells, mesoglia.**

micrognathia Underdevelopment of the jaw, especially the mandible. Compare **macrognathia. —micrognathic,** *adj.*

microgram (mgm, μgm) A measurement of mass equal to one millionth (10^{-6}) of a gram. See also **gram.**

microgyria A developmental defect of the brain in which the convolutions are abnormally small, resulting in structural malformation of the cortex. The condition is usually associated with mental retardation and physical defects. Also called **polymicrogyria.**

microgyrus, *pl.* **microgyri** An underdeveloped, malformed convolution of the brain.

microhm A unit of electrical resistance equal to one millionth (10^{-6}) of an ohm.

microinvasive carcinoma A squamous epithelial neoplasm that has penetrated the basement membrane, the first stage in invasive cancer. It is most frequently diagnosed in the uterine cervix, but the lesion is difficult to demonstrate. Some oncologists often prefer to designate the lesion as either invasive or in situ. See also **carcinoma in situ.**

microliter (μl) A unit of liquid volume equal to one millionth (10^{-6}) of a liter.

microlith A small, rounded mass of mineral matter or calcified stone.

micromelic dwarf A dwarf whose limbs are abnormally short.

micrometer **1.** An instrument used for measuring small angles or distances on objects being observed through a microscope or telescope. **2.** A unit of measurement, commonly referred to as a *micron*, that is one thousandth (10^{-3}) of a millimeter.

micromicro- (μμ) A combining form meaning '10^{-12}': *micromicron.*

micromyeloblastic leukemia A malignant neoplasm of blood-forming tissues, characterized by the proliferation of small myeloblasts distinguishable from lymphocytes only by special staining techniques and microscopic examination.

micron (μ, mu) **1.** A metric unit of length equal to one millionth (10^{-6}) of a meter. **2.** In physical chemistry: a colloidal particle with a diameter of between 0.2 and 10 microns.

micronucleus **1.** A small or minute nucleus. **2.** In protozoa: the smaller of two nuclei

in each cell; it functions in sexual reproduction. **3.** See **nucleolus.**

micronutrient An organic compound, as a vitamin, or a chemical element, as zinc or iodine, essential only in minute amounts for the normal physiological processes of the body. Also called **microelement, minor element, trace element.**

microorganism Any microscopic entity capable of carrying on living processes. It may be pathogenic. Kinds of microorganisms include **bacteria, fungi, protozoa, viruses.**

micropenis See **microphallus.**

microphage A neutrophil capable of ingesting small things, as bacteria. Compare **macrophage. —microphagic,** *adj.*

microphallus An abnormally small penis. When observed in the newborn the nurse examines the child for other signs of ambiguous genitalia. Also called **micropenis.** See also **ambiguous genitalia.**

microphthalmos, microphthalmia A developmental anomaly characterized by abnormal smallness of one or both eyes. When the condition occurs in the absence of other ocular defects, it is called pure microphthalmos or nanophthalmos. **—microphthalmic,** *adj.,* **microphthalmus,** *n.*

microplasia See **dwarfism.**

micropodia A developmental anomaly characterized by abnormal smallness of the feet, often associated with other congenital malformations or bone disorders.

microprosopus A fetus in which the face is abnormally small or underdeveloped.

micropsia A condition of vision by which a person perceives objects smaller than they really are. **—microptic,** *adj.*

microscopic **1.** Of or pertaining to a microscope. **2.** Very small; visible only when magnified.

microscopic anatomy The study of the microscopic structure of the tissues and cells. Kinds of microscopic anatomy are **cytology, histology.**

microscopy A technique for observing minute materials using a microscope. Kinds of microscopy include **darkfield microscopy, electron microscopy.**

microsomia The condition of having an abnormally small and underdeveloped yet otherwise perfectly formed body with normal proportionate relationships of the various parts. See also **primordial dwarf.**

microtome A device that cuts specimens of tissue prepared in paraffin blocks into extremely thin slices for microscopic study.

micturate See **urination.**

micturition See **urination.**

micturition reflex A normal reaction to a rise in pressure within the bladder, resulting in contraction of the bladder wall and relaxation of the urethral sphincter. Voluntary inhibition normally prevents incontinence, with urination occurring on withdrawal of this inhibition.

midbrain See **mesencephalon.**

MIDCLAVICULAR LINES

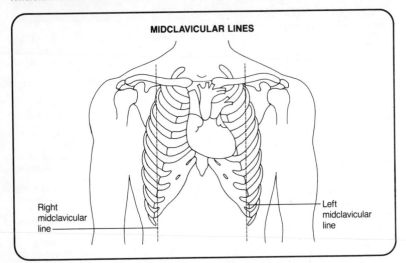

Right midclavicular line

Left midclavicular line

midclavicular line In anatomy: an imaginary line that extends downward over the trunk from the midpoint of the clavicle, dividing each side of the anterior chest into two parts. The left midclavicular line is an important marker in describing the location of various cardiac phenomena.

middle cardiac vein One of the five tributaries of the coronary sinus that drains blood from the capillary bed of the myocardium. It starts at the apex of the heart, rises in the posterior interventricular sulcus, receives tributaries from both ventricles, and ends in the right extremity of the coronary sinus. Compare **great cardiac vein, small cardiac vein.**

middle costotransverse ligament See **ligament of the neck of the rib.**

middle cuneiform bone See **intermediate cuneiform bone.**

middle ear The tympanic cavity and the auditory ossicles contained in an irregular space in the temporal bone. The auditory tube carries air from the posterior pharynx into the middle ear.

middle kidney See **mesonephros.**

middle lobe syndrome Localized atelectasis of the middle lobe of the right lung, characterized by chronic infection, cough, dyspnea, wheezing, and obstructive pneumonitis. Asymptomatic obstruction of the bronchus may occur. The condition is caused by enlargement of the surrounding cuff of lymphatic glands, owing to nonspecific or tuberculous inflammation during childhood. Treatment includes antituberculosis chemotherapy, corticosteroids, or surgical excision. See also **atelectasis.**

middle mediastinum The widest part of the mediastinum containing the heart, ascending aorta, lower half of the superior vena cava, pulmonary trunk, and phrenic nerves. It is one of three caudal portions of the mediastinum. Compare **anterior mediastinum, posterior mediastinum, superior mediastinum.**

middle plate See **nephrotome.**

middle sacral artery A small, visceral branch of the abdominal aorta, descending to the fourth and fifth lumbar vertebrae, the sacrum, and the coccyx. Minute branches supply the posterior surface of the rectum.

middle suprarenal artery One of a pair of small, visceral branches of the abdominal aorta supplying the suprarenal gland.

middle temporal artery One of the branches of the superficial temporal artery on each side of the head. It arises just above the zygomatic arch, pierces the temporal fascia, branches to the temporalis, and anastomoses with the deep temporal branches of the maxillary artery. Compare **deep temporal artery, superficial temporal artery.**

middle umbilical fold The fold of peritoneum over the urachal remnant within the abdomen. The lateral umbilical fold is approximately 3 cm (1¼ inches) lateral to the middle umbilical fold. Between the lateral and the middle folds is the medial umbilical fold. Also called **plica umbilicalis mediana.**

midforceps An obstetric procedure in which forceps are applied to the fetal head when it has reached the midplane of the mother's pelvis. An episiotomy is usually performed. In some cases, as in severe fetal distress, midforceps may be the most rapid and safest means of delivery. Difficult midforceps delivery is likely to produce more fetal and maternal trauma than cesarean section. Compare **high forceps, low forceps.** See also **failed forceps, forceps delivery, obstetric forceps, trial forceps.**

midgut The middle portion of the embryonic alimentary canal. It consists of endodermal tissue, is connected to the yolk sac during early prenatal development, and eventually gives rise to some of the small intestine and part of the large intestine. Compare **foregut, hindgut.**

MIGRAINE HEADACHES

TYPE	SIGNS AND SYMPTOMS
Common migraine *(most prevalent)* Usually occurs on weekends and holidays	• Prodromal symptoms (fatigue, nausea and vomiting, and fluid imbalance) precede headache by about 1 day. • Sensitivity to light and noise (most prominent feature) • Headache pain (unilateral or bilateral, aching or throbbing)
Classic migraine Usually occurs in compulsive personalities and within families	• Prodromal symptoms include visual disturbances, such as zigzag lines and bright lights (most common), sensory disturbances (tingling of face, lips, and hands), or motor disturbances (staggering gait). • Recurrent and periodic headaches
Hemiplegic and ophthalmoplegic migraine *(rare)* Usually occurs in young adults	• Severe, unilateral pain • Extraocular muscle palsies (involving third cranial nerve) and ptosis • With repeated headaches, possible permanent third cranial nerve injury • In hemiplegic migraine, neurologic deficits (hemiparesis, hemiplegia) may persist after headache subsides.
Basilar artery migraine Occurs in young women before their menstrual periods	• Prodromal symptoms usually include partial vision loss followed by vertigo; ataxia; dysarthria; tinnitus; and sometimes tingling of fingers and toes, lasting from several minutes to almost 1 hour. • Headache pain, severe occipital throbbing, vomiting

midline episiotomy See **episiotomy.**

midpelvic contraction See **contraction.**

midsagittal plane See **cardinal sagittal plane.**

midstance One of the five stages in the stance phase of walking, or gait, directly associated with the period of single-leg support of body weight or the period during which the body advances over the stationary foot. During midstance the tibialis posterior and the flexor hallucis longus display their greatest activity. The midstance phase is considered in the diagnosis of many abnormal orthopedic conditions and in the analysis of the associated weaknesses of certain muscles and muscle groups. Compare **initial contact stance stage, loading response stance stage, preswing stance stage, terminal stance.** See also **swing phase of gait.**

midwife **1.** In traditional use: a person who assists women in childbirth. **2.** According to the International Confederation of Midwives, World Health Organization, and Federation of International Gynecologists and Obstetricians "a person who, having been regularly admitted to a midwifery educational program fully recognized in the country in which it is located, has successfully completed the prescribed course of studies in midwifery and has acquired the requisite qualifications to be registered and/or legally licensed to practice midwifery." Among the responsibilities of the midwife are supervision of pregnancy, labor, delivery, and puerperium. The midwife conducts the delivery independently, cares for the newborn, procures medical assistance when necessary, executes emergency measures as required, and may practice in a hospital, clinic, maternity home, or in a woman's home. **3.** A lay-midwife. **4.** A nurse-midwife or Certified Nurse Midwife.

migraine Recurring vascular headache characterized by a prodromal aura, unilateral onset, and severe pain, photophobia, and autonomic disturbances during the acute phase, which may last for hours or days. The disorder occurs more frequently in women than in men and a predisposition to migraine may be inherited. The exact cause is not known. Allergic reactions, excess carbohydrates, iodine-rich foods, alcohol, bright lights, or loud noises may trigger attacks, which often occur during a period of relaxation following physical or psychic stress. An impending attack may be heralded by visual disturbances, as flashing lights or wavy lines; by a strange taste or odor; numbness; tingling; vertigo; tinnitus; or a feeling that part of the body is distorted in size or shape. The acute phase may be accompanied by nausea, vomiting, chills, polyuria, sweating, facial edema, irritability, and extreme fatigue. After an attack the individual often has dull head and neck pains and a great need for sleep. Aspirin seldom provides relief during an attack, but ergotamine tartrate preparations that constrict cranial arteries can usually prevent the headache from developing fully if administered soon after onset as an injection, suppository, or tablet. Migraine patients unable to tolerate ergot preparations may use other analgesics, including acetaminophen, phenacetin, and propoxyphene. Drugs such as propranolol are also used to prevent attacks. Also called **hemicrania, megrim.**

migrainous cranial neuralgia A variant of migraine, characterized by closely spaced episodes of excruciating, throbbing, unilateral headaches often accompanied by dilation of temporal blood vessels, flushing, sweating, lacrimation, nasal congestion or rhinorrhea, ptosis, and facial edema. Repeated episodes usually occur in clusters within a few days or weeks and may be followed by a relatively long remission period. Histamine diphosphate injected subcutaneously in persons subject to these headaches produces symptoms identical to those occurring in a spontaneous attack. The pain may be relieved by antihistamines, and ergotamine tartrate preparations may be helpful if administered at the onset of an attack. Also called **cluster headache, histamine headache, Horton's headache.** See also **migraine.**

migratory gonorrheal polyarthritis See **migratory polyarthritis.**

migratory ophthalmia See **sympathetic ophthalmia.**

migratory polyarthritis Arthritis progressively affecting a number of joints and finally settling in one or more, occurring in patients with gonorrhea and developing a few days to a few weeks following the onset of gonorrheal urethritis. The patient usually has a moderate fever and 1 to 5 days of migratory polyarthralgia with variable signs of inflammation. Treatment with penicillin or tetracycline generally produces some response in 24 to 72 hours. Also called **migratory gonorrheal polyarthritis.**

migratory thrombophlebitis An abnormal condition in which multiple thromboses appear in both superficial and deep veins. It may be associated with malignancy, especially cancer of the pancreas, often preceding other evidence of cancer by several months. Also called **thrombophlebitis migrans.** See also **thrombophlebitis.**

mikro- See **micro-.**

Mikulicz's syndrome An abnormal bilateral enlargement of the salivary and lacrimal glands, found in a variety of diseases, including leukemia, tuberculosis, and sarcoidosis. Also called **Mikulicz's disease.**

mild A quality of gentleness, subtlety, or low intensity.

milia Minute, white cysts of the epidermis caused by obstruction of hair follicles and eccrine sweat glands. One variety is seen in newborn infants and disappears within a few weeks. Another type is found primarily on the faces of middle-aged women. Milia may be treated with an abrasive cleanser or by incision and drainage. Compare **miliaria.**

milia neonatorum A normal dermatologic condition characterized by minute epidermal cysts consisting of keratinous debris that occur on the face and, occasionally, the trunk of the newborn. They are eliminated by normal desquamation of the skin within a few weeks following birth and leave no scars.

miliaria Minute vesicles and papules, often with surrounding erythema, caused by occlusion of sweat ducts. Back-up pressure may cause sweat to escape into adjacent tissue producing itching and prickling. Prevention and treatment include cool environment, ventilation, colloidal baths, and dusting powders. Also called **prickly heat.** Compare **milia.**

miliary Describing a condition marked by the appearance of very small lesions the size of millet seeds, as miliary tuberculosis.

miliary carcinosis A condition characterized by the presence of numerous cancerous nodules resembling miliary tubercles.

miliary tuberculosis Extensive dissemination by the bloodstream of tubercle bacilli. In children it is associated with high fever, night sweats, and, often, meningitis, pleural effusions, or peritonitis. A similar illness may occur in adults but with a less abrupt onset and, occasionally, with weeks or months of nonspecific symptoms, as weight loss, weakness, and low-grade fever. The tuberculin test may be negative, and diagnosis is made by biopsy of the infected tissue or organ. Combined drug therapy with isoniazid and rifampin or with isoniazid and streptomycin is usually successful if the diagnosis is not delayed. See also *Mycobacterium,* **tuberculosis.**

milieu, *pl.* **milieus, milieux** *French.* The environment, surroundings, or setting. Kinds of milieus are **milieu extérieur, milieu intérieur.**

milieu extérieur *French.* The external or physical surroundings of an organism, including such social environments as the home, that play a dominant role in personality development.

milieu intérieur *French.* The basic concept in physiology, originated by Claude Bernard, that multicellular organisms exist in an aqueous internal environment composed of blood, lymph, and interstitial fluid that bathes all cells and provides a medium for the elementary exchange of nutrients and waste material. All fundamental processes necessary for the maintenance and life of the tissue elements are dependent on the stability and balance of this environment.

milieu therapy A type of psychotherapy in which the total environment is used in treating mental and behavioral disorders. It is primarily conducted in a hospital or other institutional setting where the entire facility acts as a therapeutic community. The emphasis is on providing pleasant physical surroundings, structured activities, and a stable social environment where behavior modification and personal growth are promoted through patient-group interaction, staff support and understanding, and a total, humanistic approach. Also called **situation therapy.**

milk A liquid secreted by the mammary glands or udders of animals that suckle their young. Humans consume cow's milk as well as that of many other animals, including goats, camels, and yaks. Milk is a basic food containing carbohydrate (in the form of lactose), protein (mainly casein, with small amounts of lactalbumin and lactoglobulin), suspended fat, the minerals calcium and phosphorous, the vitamins riboflavin, niacin, thiamine, A, and, when the milk is fortified, vitamin D. It is a valuable nutrient for adults and a complete food for infants, especially breast milk. Some individuals show a sensitivity reaction to milk owing to a deficiency of the enzyme lactase. See also **breast milk.**

milk baby   An infant with iron-deficiency anemia caused by ingestion of excessive amounts of milk and the delayed or inadequate addition of iron-rich foods to the diet. Milk babies are overweight, have pale skin and poor muscle development, and are highly susceptible to infection. See also **anemia.**

milk bath   A bath taken in milk for cosmetic or emollient reasons.

milk-ejection reflex   A normal reflex in a lactating woman elicited by tactile stimulation of the nipple, resulting in release of milk from the glands of the breast. Also called **let-down reflex.** See also **oxytocin.**

milker's nodule   A smooth, brownish-red papilloma of the fingers or palm that begins as a macule and progresses through a vesicular stage to become a nodule. The disease is acquired from pustular lesions on the udder of a cow infected with poxvirus. No treatment is necessary because immunity is produced after primary infection.

milk fever   *Nontechnical.* Postpartum fever that begins with the onset of lactation. It was formerly considered a normal reaction to lactation. Maternal temperature during the puerperium does not normally exceed 37.2°C (99°F).

milk globule   A spherical droplet of fat in milk that tends to separate out as cream.

milking   A procedure used to express the contents of a duct or tube, to test for tenderness, or to obtain a specimen for study. The examiner compresses the structure with a finger and moves the finger firmly along the duct or tube to its opening. Also called **stripping.**

milk leg   See **phlegmasia alba dolens.**

milk of magnesia   An antacid.

milkpox   See **alastrim.**

milk sugar   See **lactose.**

milk therapy   A nutritional treatment used in the therapy of Curling's ulcer in patients who have been severely burned. Cool, homogenized milk is administered in doses of 30 to 60 ml (1 to 2 oz) every hour through a nasogastric tube. After instillation the tube is clamped for 5 minutes and then unclamped. Milk remaining in the stomach is allowed to flow into a basin. As the milk is better absorbed and tolerated, feedings are increased to 150 ml of milk/kg (about 2¼ oz/lb) of body weight daily, and the interval between the feedings lengthened to 4 hours.

milk tooth   See **deciduous tooth.**

milky ascites   See **chylous ascites.**

Miller-Abbott tube   A long, small-caliber, double-lumen catheter, used in intestinal intu-

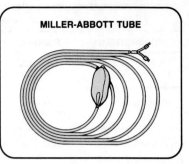

MILLER-ABBOTT TUBE

bation for decompression. It has several openings on the side of its tip and a balloon above the tip. Compare **Harris tube.** See also **gastric intubation.**

Miller analogy test   A requirement for admission to some graduate nursing schools, this test evaluates reasoning ability by having the person being tested provide the missing terms in a series of proportions.

milli-   A combining form meaning '1/1,000th part': *milliampere, millibar, milliliter.*

milliampere (ma)   A unit of electrical current that is one thousandth (10^{-3}) of an ampere.

millicoulomb (mC)   A unit of electrical charge that is one thousandth (10^{-3}) of a coulomb.

millicurie (mCi, mc)   A unit of radioactivity that is equal to one thousandth (10^{-3}) of a curie, or 3.7×10^7 disintegrations/second.

milliequivalent (mEq)   The number of grams of solute dissolved in 1 ml of a normal solution.

milligram (mg)   A metric unit of weight equal to one thousandth (10^{-3}) of a gram.

milliliter (ml)   A metric unit of volume that is one thousandth (10^{-3}) of a liter.

millimeter (mm)   A metric unit of length equal to one thousandth (10^{-3}) of a meter.

millimicrogram (mμg)   One thousandth (10^{-3}) of a microgram, or one billionth (10^{-9}) of a gram. Also called **nanogram.**

millimole (mmol)   A unit of metric measurement of mass that is equal to one thousandth (10^{-3}) of a mole (also called a gram molecule).

milliosmol   A unit of measure representing the concentration of an ion in a solution, expressed in milligrams per liter divided by atomic weight. See also **osmol, osmolality, osmolarity. —milliosmolar,** *adj.*

millipede   A many-legged, wormlike arthropod. Certain species squirt irritating fluids that may cause dermatitis.

millirad   One thousandth (10^{-3}) of a rad, a unit of measurement of absorbed dose of ionizing radiation.

milliroentgen (mR, mr)   A unit of radiation that is equal to one thousandth (10^{-3}) of a roentgen.

millivolt (mV, mv)   A unit of electromotive force equal to one thousandth (10^{-3}) of a volt.

Milwaukee brace   An orthotic device that

MINERALS

MICRONUTRIENT	FOOD SOURCES	DISORDERS
Sodium	Table salt, beef, pork, sardines, cheese, milk, eggs	**Toxicity:** hypernatremia **Deficiency:** hyponatremia
Chloride	Table salt, seafood, milk, meat, eggs	**Toxicity:** hyperchloremia **Deficiency:** hypochloremia
Potassium	Milk, dates, meat, fish, bananas	**Toxicity:** hyperkalemia **Deficiency:** hypokalemia
Calcium	Milk, milk products, meat, fish, eggs, cereals, beans, fruit, vegetables	**Toxicity:** hypercalcemia **Deficiency:** hypocalcemia
Phosphorus	Milk, cheese, meat, poultry, fish, whole-grain cereals, nuts, legumes	**Toxicity:** hyperphosphatemia **Deficiency:** hypophosphatemia
Magnesium	Seafood, soybeans, nuts, cocoa, whole-grain cereals, peas, dried beans, meat, milk	**Toxicity:** hypermagnesemia **Deficiency:** hypomagnesemia
Iron	Liver, meat, egg yolks, beans, clams, peaches, whole or enriched grains, legumes	**Toxicity:** hemochromatosis **Deficiency:** anemia

helps to immobilize the torso and the neck of a patient in the treatment or correction of spinal scoliosis, lordosis, or kyphosis. It is usually constructed of strong, light, metal and fiberglass supports lined with rubber to protect against abrasion. They commonly connect cervical supports, rib supports, and hip supports with rigid bars of metal that hold the trunk and the neck erect while controlling cervical flexion and hip movements.

-mimesis A combining form meaning 'simulation, imitation': *necromimesis, pathomimesis.*

-mimetic A combining form meaning 'pertaining to simulation of (specified) effects': *andromimetic, neuromimetic.*

-mimia A combining form meaning '(condition of) ability to express thought through gestures': *macromimia.*

mimic spasm Involuntary, stereotyped movements of a small group of muscles, as of the face. The spasm is usually psychogenic and may be aggravated by stress or anxiety but is generally controllable momentarily. Also called **tic.**

min *abbr* minim.

Minamata disease A severe, degenerative, neurologic disorder caused by the ingestion of seed grain heated with alkyl compounds of mercury or of seafood taken from waters polluted with industrial wastes contaminated by soluble mercuric salts. It is most often seen in those Japanese who eat seafood from Minamata Bay. Mercury passes the placental barrier, causing the congenital form of the disease. Symptoms may not appear for several weeks or months, and include paresthesia of the mouth and extremities; tunnel vision; difficulties with speech, hearing, muscular coordination, and concentration; weakness; emotional instability; and stupor. Continued ingestion causes serious damage to the renal tubules and corrosion of the gastrointestinal tract. Acute cases may result in coma and death. See also **mercury poisoning.**

mind **1.** The part of the brain that is the seat of mental activity and that enables one to know, reason, understand, remember, think, feel, and adapt to surroundings and all external and internal stimuli. **2.** The totality of all conscious and unconscious processes of the individual that influence and direct mental and physical behavior. **3.** The faculty of the intellect or understanding in contrast to emotion and will. See also **brain, intellect, psyche.**

mine damp See **damp.**

mineral **1.** An inorganic substance occurring naturally in the earth's crust, having a characteristic chemical composition and (usually)

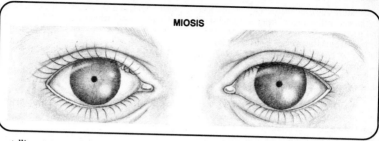

MIOSIS

crystalline structure. **2.** In nutrition: a mineral is usually referred to by the name of a metal, nonmetal, radical, or phosphate rather than by the name of the compound of which it is a part, and it is ingested as a compound, like sodium chloride (table salt), rather than as a free element. Minerals play a vital role in regulating many bodily functions.

mineral deficiency The inability to utilize one or more of the mineral elements essential in human nutrition because of a genetic defect, a malabsorption dysfunction, or the lack of that mineral in the diet. Minerals, which are constituents of all the body tissues and fluids, are important factors in maintaining physiological processes. They act as catalysts in nerve response and muscle contraction. In addition, they aid in the metabolism of nutrients in foods, regulate electrolyte balance and hormonal production, and strengthen skeletal structures. See also specific minerals.

mineralization The addition of any mineral to the body.

mineralocorticoid A hormone, secreted by the adrenal cortex, that maintains normal blood volume, promotes sodium and water retention, and increases urinary excretion of potassium and hydrogen ions. Aldosterone, the most potent mineralocorticoid in regard to electrolyte balance, and corticosterone, a glucocorticoid as well as mineralocorticoid, act on the distal tubules of the kidneys to enhance the reabsorption of sodium into the plasma. Trauma and stress increase mineralocorticoid secretion. The synthetic mineralocorticoids desoxycorticosterone, which does not influence carbohydrate metabolism, and fluorocortisone, which also has glucocorticoid activity, are used in treating the salt-losing, adrenogenital syndrome and the severe corticoid deficiency characteristic of Addison's disease. See also **glucocorticoid.**

mineral oil A lubricant laxative.

miner's cramp See **heat cramp.**

miner's elbow An inflammation of the olecranon bursa, caused by resting the weight of the body on the elbow, as in hewing for coal. The condition is sometimes seen in schoolchildren who lean on their elbows. Compare **lateral humeral epicondylitis.** See also **bursitis.**

miner's pneumoconiosis See **anthracosis.**

Minerva cast An orthopedic cast applied to the trunk and the head, with spaces cut out for the face area and the ears. The section encasing the trunk extends to the sternum and the distal rib border anteriorly and across the distal rib border posteriorly. The cast is used for immobilizing the head and part of the trunk in the treatment of torticollis, cervical injuries, and cervical spinal infections.

Minerva jacket A cast extending from the chin to the hips, applied for support and immobilization of the cervical and thoracic spine, especially after a fracture.

minim (min) A measurement of volume in the apothecaries' system, originally one drop (of water). Sixty minims equal one fluid dram (about 0.06 ml).

minimal brain dysfunction (MBD) See **attention deficit disorder.**

minimum alveolar concentration (MAC) The smallest amount of a gas detected and measured in the lung's alveoli.

minocycline hydrochloride A tetracycline antibiotic.

minor In law: a person not of legal age; beneath the age of majority. Minors usually cannot consent to their own medical treatment unless they are substantially independent from their parents, are married, support themselves, or satisfy other requirements as provided by statute.

minor element See **micronutrient.**

minor renal calyx See **renal calyx.**

minoxidil A vasodilator antihypertensive.

mio-, meio- A combining form meaning 'less': miolecithal, mioplasmia, miosphygmia.

miosis Contraction of the sphincter muscle of the iris, causing the pupil to become smaller. Certain drugs and stimulation of the pupillary light reflex by an increase in light result in miosis. Compare **mydriasis. —miotic,** adj.

miotic 1. Of or pertaining to miosis. **2.** Causing constriction of the pupil of the eye. **3.** Any substance or pharmaceutical, as pilocarpine, that causes constriction of the pupil of the eye. Such agents are used in the treatment of glaucoma. **—miosis,** n.

MIP abbr **maximum inspiratory pressure.**

miracidium, pl. **miracidia** The ciliated larva of a parasitic trematode that hatches from an egg and can survive only by penetrating and further developing within a host snail, whereupon the larva further develops into a maternal sporocyte that produces more larvae.

mirage An optical illusion caused by the refraction of light through air layers of different temperatures, as the illusionary sheets of water that seem to shimmer over stretches of hot sand and pavement. This phenomenon is caused by horizontal light waves being bent upwards from the layer of heated air directly over the hot surface. Individuals under severe stress are especially susceptible to interpreting these optical phenomena in bizarre, unrealistic ways.

miscarriage See **spontaneous abortion.**

miscible Able to be mixed or mingled with another substance. Compare **immiscible.**

misdemeanor In criminal law: an offense that is considered less serious than a felony and carries with it a lesser penalty, usually a fine or imprisonment for less than 1 year.

misfeasance An improper performance of a lawful act, especially in a way that might cause damage or injury. Compare **malfeasance, nonfeasance.**

miso- A combining form meaning 'hatred of': *misocainia, misogyny.*

misogamy An aversion to marriage. —**misogamic, misogamous,** *adj.,* **misogamist,** *n.*

misogyny An aversion to women. —**misogynist,** *n.,* **misogamic,** *adj.*

misopedia An aversion to children. —**misopedic,** *adj.,* **misopedist,** *n.*

missed abortion A condition in which a dead, immature embryo or fetus is not expelled from the uterus for 2 or more months. The uterus diminishes in size and symptoms of pregnancy abate; infection and disorders of the clotting of the mother's blood may follow. The fetus and placenta may become necrotic or, less commonly, the fetus becomes calcified.

missile fracture A penetration fracture caused by a projectile, as a bullet or a piece of shrapnel.

mist tent See **Croupette, tent.**

mite A minute arachnid with a flat, almost transparent body. Many species of these relatives of ticks and spiders are parasitic, including the chigger and *Sarcoptes scabei,* which cause localized pruritus and inflammation. See also **scabies.**

mite typhus See **scrub typhus.**

mithramycin An antibiotic used in cancer chemotherapy.

mithridatism See **tachyphylaxis.**

mito- A combining form meaning 'threadlike': *mitochondria, mitokinetic, mitoplasm.*

mitochondrion, *pl.* **mitochondria** A small rodlike, threadlike, or granular organelle within the cytoplasm that functions in cellular metabolism and respiration. It occurs in varying numbers in all living cells except bacteria, viruses, blue-green algae, and mature erythrocytes. It consists of two sets of membranes, a smooth outer one and a convoluted inner one. Mitochondria provide the principal source of cellular energy through oxidative phosphorylation and adenosine triphosphate synthesis. They also contain the enzymes involved with electron transport and the citric and fatty acid cycles. Mitochondria are self-replicating and contain an extranuclear source of DNA, RNA polymerase,

transfer RNA, and ribosomes. Also called **chondriosome.** —**mitochondrial,** *adj.*

mitogen An agent that triggers mitosis. —**mitogenic,** *adj.*

mitogenesia The production by or formation resulting from mitosis.

mitogenesis The induction of mitosis in a cell. —**mitogenetic,** *adj.*

mitogenetic radiation, mitogenic radiation The force or specific energy that is supposedly given off by cells undergoing division. It may, in turn, stimulate the process of mitosis in other cells. Also called **Gurvich radiation.**

mitogenic factor A kind of lymphokine that is released from activated T lymphocytes and stimulates the production of normal unsensitized lymphocytes.

mitolactol An antineoplastic currently used investigationally for a variety of neoplasms, including Hodgkin's disease. Also called **dibromodulcitol.**

mitome The reticular network found within the cell's cytoplasm and nucleoplasm. See also **cytomitome, karyomitome.**

mitomycin An antibiotic used in cancer chemotherapy.

mitosis A type of cell division that occurs in somatic cells and results in the formation of two genetically identical daughter cells containing the diploid number of chromosomes characteristic of the species. It consists of the division of the nucleus, during which the two chromatids of the chromosomes separate and migrate to opposite ends of the cell, followed by the division of the cytoplasm. Mitosis is the process by which the body produces new cells for both growth and repair of injured tissue. Kinds of mitosis are **heterotypic mitosis, homeotypic mitosis, multipolar mitosis, pathologic mitosis.** Also called **indirect division.** Compare **meiosis.** See also **interphase.** —**mitotic,** *adj.*

mitotane An antineoplastic agent that alters hormone balance.

mitotic figure Any chromosome or chromosome aggregation during any of the stages of mitosis.

mitotic index The number of cells per unit (usually 1,000) undergoing mitosis in a given time, used to estimate the rate of tissue growth.

mitral 1. Of or pertaining to the mitral valve of the heart. 2. Shaped like a miter.

mitral gradient The difference in pressure in the left atrium and left ventricle during diastole.

mitral stenosis See **mitral valve stenosis, valvular heart disease.**

mitral valve One of the four valves of the heart, situated between the left atrium and the left ventricle; the only valve with two, rather than three flaps. The mitral valve allows blood to flow from the left atrium into the left ventricle but prevents blood from flowing back into the atrium. Ventricular contraction in systole forces the blood against the valve, closing the two flaps and assuring the flow of blood from the ventricle into the pulmonary artery and the aorta. Also called **bicuspid valve, left atrioventricular valve.** Compare **semilunar valve, tricuspid valve.**

mitral valve stenosis An obstructive lesion in the mitral valve of the heart caused by adhesions on the leaflets of the valve, usually the result of recurrent episodes of rheumatic endocarditis. Hypertrophy of the left atrium develops and may be followed by right-sided heart failure and pulmonary edema (cor pulmonale). Reduced cardiac output characteristically produces fatigue, dyspnea, orthopnea, and cyanosis. Surgical correction of the defective valve may be necessary.

mittelschmerz Abdominal pain in the region of an ovary during ovulation. Present in many women, mittelschmerz is useful for identifying ovulation, thus pinpointing the fertile period of the cycle.

mixed anesthesia See **balanced anesthesia.**

mixed aneurysm See **compound aneurysm.**

mixed-cell malignant lymphoma A lymphoid neoplasm containing lymphocytes and histiocytes (macrophages).

mixed-cell sarcoma A tumor consisting of two or more cellular elements, excluding fibrous tissue. Also called **malignant mesenchymoma.**

mixed connective tissue disease (MCTD) A systemic disease characterized by the combined symptoms of various collagen diseases, as synovitis. This condition involves a high concentration of antibodies of ribonucleoprotein and may produce arthralgia, inflammation of the muscles, nondeforming arthritis, swollen hands, esophageal hypomotility, and reduced diffusing capacity of the lungs. Treatment often includes the administration of corticosteroids.

mixed dentition A phase of dentition during which some of the teeth are permanent and some are deciduous.

mixed glioma A tumor, composed of glial cells, that contains more than one kind of cell, the most common being nonneural cells of ectodermal origin.

mixed leukemia A malignancy of blood-forming tissues characterized by the proliferation of eosinophilic, neutrophilic, and basophilic granulocytes, in contrast to one predominant cell line.

mixed-lymphocyte culture (MLC) reaction An assay of the function of the T cell lymphocytes, primarily used for histocompatibility testing prior to grafting.

mixed porphyria See **variegate porphyria.**

mixed tumor A growth composed of more than one kind of neoplastic tissue, especially a complex embryonal tumor of local origin.

-mixia See **-mixis.**

-mixis A combining form meaning a '(specified) means of conjugation': *automixis, endomixis.* Also **-mixia, -mixie, -mixy.**

mixture 1. A substance composed of ingredients that are not chemically combined and do not necessarily occur in a fixed proportion. 2. In pharmacology: a liquid containing one or more medications in suspension. Compare **compound, solution.**

-mixy See **-mixis.**

ml *abbr* milliliter.

MLC *abbr* mixed lymphocyte culture. See **mixed-lymphocyte culture reaction.**

MLD *abbr* median lethal dose.

mm *abbr* millimeter.

MMEF *abbr* maximal midexpiratory flow.

mmol *abbr* millimole.

Mn Symbol for **manganese.**

mne- A combining form meaning 'of or pertaining to memory': *mnemic, mnemonic.*

-mnesia A combining form meaning '(condition or type of) memory': *ecmnesia, logamnesia.*

-mnestic A combining form meaning 'pertaining to memory': *anamnestic, catamnestic.* Also **-mnesic.**

Mo Symbol for **molybdenum.**

mobility, impaired physical A nursing diagnosis accepted by the Fifth National Conference on the Classification of Nursing Diagnoses. The etiology may be a decrease in the person's strength or endurance, the presence of pain or discomfort, impaired cognition or perception, depression or severe anxiety, or impaired neuromuscular or musculoskeletal function. The defining characteristics include an inability to achieve a functional level of mobility, a reluctance to move, a limited range of motion of the limbs or extremities, a decrease in the strength or control of the musculoskeletal system, abnormal or impaired ability to coordinate movements, or any of imposed restrictions on movement. It is suggested that the limitation of injury be ranked from '0' (completely independent) to '4' (dependent, does not participate in any activity). See also **nursing diagnosis.**

-mobility See **-motility.**

Mobitz I heart block Second degree or partial atrioventricular (AV) block in which the PR interval increases progressively until the propagation of an atrial impulse does not occur and the corresponding ventricular beat drops out. Symptoms include fatigue, dizziness, and, in some cases, syncope. Mobitz I block is often caused by abnormal conduction of the cardiac impulse at the AV junction proximal to the bundle of His and may be precipitated by increased vagal tone, occurring spontaneously; after carotid sinus pressure; or following digitalis toxicity. It may be a complication of inferior myocardial infarction but is usually a transitory condition requiring no treatment. Also called **Wenckebach heart block.**

Mobitz II heart block Second degree or partial atrioventricular block, characterized by the sudden nonconduction of an atrial impulse and a periodic dropped beat without prior lengthening of the PR interval. This kind of block usually results from impaired conduction in the

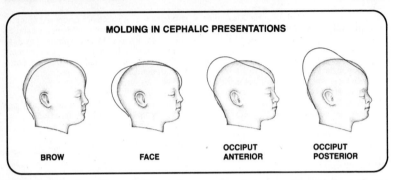

MOLDING IN CEPHALIC PRESENTATIONS

BROW   FACE   OCCIPUT ANTERIOR   OCCIPUT POSTERIOR

bundle of His and may be caused by anterior myocardial infarction, myocarditis, digitalis toxicity, electrolyte disturbances, rheumatoid nodules, and degenerative diseases. Syncopal attacks, occurring without warning, are common in Mobitz II block, which may be transient or suddenly progress to complete block. Long-term therapy requires the implantation of a pacemaker.

mode A value or term in a set of data that occurs more frequently than other values or terms.

model In nursing research: a symbolic representation of the interrelations exhibited by the phenomena within a system or a process. The model is presented as a conceptual framework or a theory that explains the phenomena and allows predictions to be made about a patient or a process.

modeling A behavior therapy technique in which a person learns a desired response by observing it.

moderator band A thick bundle of muscle in the central part of the right ventricle of the heart. It varies in size or can be absent among individuals. It usually contains part of the atrioventricular conduction bundle. Also called **trabecula septomarginalis.**

modified milk Cow's milk in which the protein content has been reduced and the fat content increased to correspond to the composition of human breast milk. See also **formula, infant.**

modified radical mastectomy A surgical procedure in which a breast is completely removed with the underlying pectoralis minor and some of the adjacent lymph nodes. The pectoralis major is not excised. The operation is performed in treating early and well-localized malignant neoplasms of the breast. Compare **radical mastectomy, simple mastectomy.**

Moeller's glossitis A form of chronic glossitis, characterized by burning or pain in the tongue and an increased sensitivity to hot or spicy foods. Also called **glossodynia exfoliativa.** See also **glossitis.**

mogi- A combining form meaning 'difficult, or with difficulty': *mogigraphia, mogilalia.*

molety A part of a molecule that exhibits a particular set of chemical and pharmacological characteristics.

mol See **mole².**

molar 1. Any one of the 12 molar teeth, 6 in each dental arch, 3 located posterior to the premolar teeth. 2. Of or pertaining to the gram molecular weight of a substance. See also **mole².**

molar pregnancy Pregnancy in which a hydatid mole develops from the trophoblastic tissue of the early embryonic stage of development. The signs of pregnancy are all exaggerated: the uterus grows more rapidly than is normal, morning sickness is often severe and constant, blood pressure is likely to be elevated, and blood levels of chorionic gonadotropins are extremely high. The uterus must be evacuated, as the mole may develop into choriocarcinoma. See also **hydatid mole.**

molar solution (M) A solution that contains one mole of solute per liter of solution.

mold 1. A fungus. 2. A growth of fungi. 3. A hollow form for casting or shaping an object, as a prosthesis.

molding The natural process by which a baby's head is shaped during labor as it is squeezed into and through the birth passage by the forces of labor. The head often becomes quite elongated, and the bones of the skull may be caused to overlap slightly at the suture lines. Most of the changes caused by molding resolve themselves during the first few days of life. Compare **caput succedaneum.** See also **cephalhematoma.**

mole¹ *Informal.* 1. A pigmented nevus. 2. In obstetrics: a hydatid mole.

mole², mol The standard unit used to measure the amount of a substance. A mole of a substance is the amount containing the same number of elementary particles as there are atoms in 0.012 kg of carbon 12. Also called gram molecule, gram-molecular weight. **—molar,** *adj.*

molecular genetics The branch of genetics that focuses on the chemical structure and the functions, replication, and mutations of the molecules involved in the transmission of genetic information, as DNA and RNA. Molecular genetics is concerned with the arrangement of genes on DNA, the double helix molecule's replication and transcription into RNA, and the way RNA directs the formation of proteins. See also **recombinant DNA.**

molecular weight The total of the atomic weights of the atoms in a molecule. See also atom, atomic weight, molecule.

molecule The smallest unit of matter that can exist alone and exhibit the characteristic chemical properties of an element or compound. A molecule is composed of two or more atoms held together by chemical forces. See also **atom, compound.**

molindone hydrochloride A dihydroindole antipsychotic agent.

molluscum Any skin disease having soft, rounded masses or nodules. See also **molluscum contagiosum.**

molluscum contagiosum A disease of the skin and mucous membranes, caused by a poxvirus and found all over the world. It is characterized by scattered white papules. The disease most frequently occurs in children and in adults with an impaired immune response. It lasts up to 3 years, although individual lesions persist for only 6 to 8 weeks. Diagnosis is easily made by electron microscopy. Curettage or electrical or chemical dessication helps to clear the lesions, but untreated lesions eventually resolve spontaneously without scarring.

molybdenum (Mo) A grayish metallic element. Its atomic number is 42; its atomic weight is 95.94. Molybdenum is poisonous if ingested in large quantities.

Mönckeberg's arteriosclerosis A form of arteriosclerosis in which extensive calcium deposits are found in the media of the artery with little obstruction of the lumen. Also called **medial arteriosclerosis.**

Monday morning fever See **byssinosis.**

Mongolian spot A benign, blue-black macule, between 2 and 8 cm ($\frac{3}{4}$ and $3\frac{1}{4}$ inches), occurring over the sacrum and on the buttocks of some newborns. It is common in blacks, American Indians, southern Europeans, and Orientals and usually disappears during early childhood.

mongolism See **Down's syndrome.**

mongoloid idiocy See **Down's syndrome.**

Monilia See ***Candida albicans.*** —**monilial,** *adj.*

monilial vulvovaginitis See **candidiasis.**

moniliasis See **candidiasis.**

monitor 1. To observe and evaluate a function of the body closely and constantly. 2. A mechanical device that provides a visual or audible signal or a graphic record of a particular function, as a cardiac monitor or an intracranial pressure monitor.

monitrice A labor coach, usually a registered nurse, who is specially trained in the Lamaze method of childbirth. The coach provides emotional support and leads the mother through labor and delivery, using the specific techniques for breathing, concentration, and massage taught by the Lamaze method.

mono- A combining form meaning 'one': *monobacillary.*

monoamine An amine containing one amine group.

monoamine oxidase (MAO) An enzyme that catalyzes the oxidation of amines. Also called

amino oxidase. See also **monoamine oxidase inhibitor.**

monoamine oxidase (MAO) inhibitor Any of a chemically heterogeneous group of drugs used primarily in the treatment of depression. These drugs also exert an antianxiety effect, especially anxiety associated with phobia. The effects of the drugs vary greatly, and their specific actions leading to clinical benefits are poorly understood. Among the most common adverse effects are drowsiness, dry mouth, orthostatic hypotension, and constipation. Overdosage may cause tremor, euphoria, or manic behavior. MAO inhibitors interact with many drugs and with foods containing large amounts of the amino acid tyramine. Ingestion of these foods by a person taking a MAO inhibitor is likely to cause a severe hypertensive episode associated with headache, palpitations, and nausea. Among the drugs that interact with MAO inhibitors are dopamine, meperidine, and the indirectly acting sympathomimetics, one of which, ephedrine, is an ingredient in many common cold remedies. MAO inhibitors are also sometimes used to treat migraine headache and hypertension.

monobasic acid An acid with only one replaceable hydrogen atom, as hydrochloric acid (HCl).

monobenzone A depigmenting agent.

monoblast A large, immature monocyte. Certain of the leukemias are characterized by greatly increased production of monoblasts in the marrow and by the abnormal presence of these forms in the peripheral circulation. Compare **megaloblast, myeloblast.** See also **bone marrow, leukocyte.** —**monoblastic,** *adj.*

monoblastic leukemia A progressive malignancy of blood-forming organs, characterized by the proliferation of monoblasts and monocytes. The disease occurs in children and adults and develops late in the course of a small but significant number of cases of plasma cell myeloma. Also called **monocytic leukemia, Schilling's leukemia.**

monocephalus See **syncephalus.**

monochorial twins, monochorionic twins See **monozygotic twins.**

monoclonal Of, pertaining to, or designating a group of identical cells or organisms derived from a single cell.

monoclonal gammopathy See **gammopathy.**

monocyte A large mononuclear leukocyte, 13 to 25 microns in diameter, with an ovoid or kidney-shaped nucleus, and containing lacy, linear chromatin material and abundant gray-blue cytoplasm filled with fine, reddish, and azurophilic granules. See also **monocytosis.**

monocytic leukemia A malignancy of blood-forming tissues in which the predominant cells are monocytes. The disease has an erratic course characterized by malaise, fatigue, fever, anorexia, weight loss, splenomegaly, bleeding gums, dermal petechiae, anemia, and unresponsiveness to therapy. There are two forms: **Schilling's leukemia,** in which most of the cells

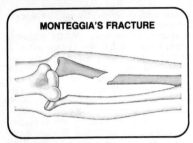

MONTEGGIA'S FRACTURE

are monocytes that probably arise from the reticuloendothelial system, and the more common **Naegeli's leukemia,** in which a large number of the cells resemble myeloblasts. Also called **histiocytic leukemia.**

monocytosis An increased proportion of monocytic white blood cells in the circulation.

monofactorial inheritance The acquisition or expression of a trait or condition that is dependent on the transmission of a single specific gene. Compare **multifactorial inheritance.**

monohybrid Pertaining to or describing an individual, organism, or strain that is heterozygous for the single trait or gene locus under consideration.

monohybrid cross The mating of two individuals, organisms, or strains that have different gene pairs for only one specific trait or in which only one particular characteristic or gene locus is being followed.

monohydric alcohol An alcohol containing one hydroxyl group.

monomer A molecule that repeats itself to form a polymer. —**monomeric,** *adj.*

monomphalus Conjoined twins that are united at the umbilicus. Also called **omphalopagus.**

mononeuritis multiplex See **multiple mononeuropathy.**

mononeuropathy Any disease or disorder that affects a single nerve trunk. Some common causes of such disorders are electrical shock, radiation, and fractured bones that may compress or lacerate nerve fibers. Accidental injection of penicillin and other medications into the sciatic nerve can seriously injure the nerve, especially if the injected medication is an oil-based drug. The peripheral nerve trunks are especially vulnerable to compression and entrapment.

mononucleosis **1.** An abnormal increase in the number of mononuclear leukocytes in the blood. **2.** See **infectious mononucleosis.**

monophasic Having one phase, part, aspect, or stage.

monoploid, monoploidic See **haploid.**

monopodial symmelia See **sympus monopus.**

monopus A fetus or individual with the congenital absence of a foot or leg.

monorchid A man who has monorchism.

monorchidism See **monorchism.**

monorchism A condition in which only one

testicle has descended into the scrotum. Also called **monorchidism.** See also **cryptorchidism.** —**monorchidic,** *adj.*

monosodium glutamate See **sodium glutamate.**

monosome **1.** The unpaired sex chromosome. **2.** The single, unpaired chromosome in monosomy.

monosomy A chromosomal aberration characterized by the absence of one chromosome from the normal diploid complement. In humans, the monosomic cell contains 45 chromosomes and is designated $2n - 1$, as occurs in the XO condition in Turner's syndrome. Compare **trisomy.** —**monosomic,** *adj.*

monosomy X See **Turner's syndrome.**

monotropy A concept named by J. Bowlby, describing the phenomenon in which a mother appears to be able to bond with only one infant at a time. The concept is used in studies of maternal-infant bonding in mothers of twins. When one twin is taken home from the hospital earlier than the other, the mother often reports that she does not feel that the infant discharged later is hers. The second twin is much more likely to fail to thrive or to be neglected or abused. Monotropy may also explain a mother's common tendency to dress twins alike, in effect making them one. —**monotropic,** *adj.*

monounsaturated fatty acid See **unsaturated fatty acid.**

monovular, mono-ovular See **uniovular.**

monovulatory Routinely releasing one ovum during each ovarian cycle. Compare **diovulatory.**

monozygotic (MZ) Pertaining to a single fertilized ovum, or zygote, as occurs in identical twins. Compare **dizygotic.** —**monozygosity,** *n.,* **monozygous,** *adj.*

monozygotic twins Two offspring born of the same pregnancy and developed from a single fertilized ovum that splits into equal halves during an early cleavage phase in embryonic development, giving rise to separate fetuses. Such twins are always of the same sex, have the same genetic constitution, possess identical blood groups, and closely resemble each other in physical, psychological, and mental characteristics. Also called **enzygotic twins, identical twins, true twins, uniovular twins.** Compare **dizygotic twins.** See also **Siamese twins.**

monster A fetus that is grossly malformed and usually nonviable. Kinds of monsters include **compound monster, double monster, single monster.**

monstrosity **1.** The state or condition of having severe congenital defects. **2.** Anything that deviates greatly from the normal; a monster or teras.

Monteggia's fracture Fracture of the proximal third of the proximal half of the ulna, associated with radial dislocation or rupture of the annular ligament and resulting in the angulation or overriding of ulnar fragments.

Montercaux fracture A fracture of the neck

MORO REFLEX

of the fibula associated with the diastasis of the ankle mortise.

Montgomery's gland See **areolar gland**.

Montgomery's tubercle One of several sebaceous glands on the areolae of the breasts. The tubercles normally enlarge during pregnancy.

moon face A condition characterized by a rounded, puffy face, occurring in people treated with large doses of corticosteroids, as those with rheumatoid arthritis or acute childhood leukemia. The features return to normal when the medication is stopped.

moor bath A bath taken in water containing earth from a swamp.

Moore's fracture A fracture of the distal radius with associated dislocation of the ulnar head.

MOPP An acronym for a combination drug regimen used in the treatment of cancer, containing three antineoplastics—Mustargen (mechlorethamine), Oncovin (vincristine sulfate), and procarbazine hydrochloride (Matulane)—and prednisone (a glucocorticoid). MOPP is prescribed in the treatment of Hodgkin's disease.

morbid anatomy See **pathological anatomy**.

morbidity 1. An illness or an abnormal condition. 2. In statistics: **a.** The rate at which an illness or abnormality occurs, calculated by dividing the entire number of people in a group by the number in that group who are affected with the illness or abnormality. **b.** The rate at which an illness occurs in a particular area or population.

morbilli See **measles**.

morbilliform Describing a skin condition that resembles the erythematous, maculopapular rash of measles.

Morgagni's globule A minute, opaque sphere that may form between the eye lens and its capsule, especially in cataract.

Morgagni's tubercle One of several small, soft nodules on the surface of each of the areolae in women. The tubercles are produced by large sebaceous glands just under the surface of the areolae. They secrete a bacteriostatic, lubricating substance during pregnancy and lactation.

morgan In genetics: a unit of measure used in mapping the relative distances between genes on a chromosome. The measurement, named after the biologist Thomas Hunt Morgan, uses the total crossover value as the basic unit so that one morgan equals 100% crossing over or one centimorgan equals 1% recombination.

-moria A combining form meaning '(condition of) dementia': *monomoria, phantasmatomoria.*

morning-after pill *Informal.* A large dose of an estrogen given orally, over a short period of time, to a woman within 24-72 hours after sexual intercourse to prevent conception, most commonly in an emergency situation such as rape or incest. The woman is warned that the medication may cause the formation of clots, severe nausea and vomiting, and carcinogenic effects on the fetus if pregnancy already exists. See also **diethystilbestrol**.

morning sickness *Nontechnical.* See **nausea and vomiting of pregnancy**.

moron A retarded person having an IQ between 50 and 70 and incapable of developing beyond the mental age of 12 years. Compare **idiot, imbecile**. See also **mental retardation**.

moronism, moronity The condition of being a moron.

Moro reflex A normal mass reflex in a young infant elicited by a sudden loud noise or by striking the table on which the infant lies, resulting in flexion of the legs, an embracing posture of the arms, and usually a brief cry. Also called **startle reflex**.

morph- A combining form meaning 'form or shape': *morphallaxis, morphea.*

-morph A combining form meaning 'something possessing a (specified) form': *endomorph, hypomorph.*

morphea Localized scleroderma consisting of patches of yellowish or ivory-colored, rigid, dry, smooth skin. It is more common in females and rarely progresses to a generalized or systemic form of sclerosis.

-morphia A combining form meaning a 'condition of form': *pantamorphia, theromorphia.* Also **-morphy**.

morphine sulfate A narcotic and opioid

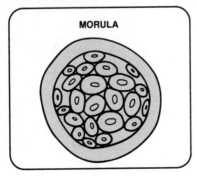

MORULA

analgesic used for severe pain.

-morphism A combining form meaning the 'condition of having a (specified) shape': *amorphism, isomorphism.*

morphogenesis, morphogeny The development and differentiation of the structures and the form of an organism, specifically the changes that occur in the cells and tissue during embryonic development.

morphogenetic, morphogenic In embryology: of or pertaining to a substance or hormone that acts as an evocator in differentiation.

morphogeny See **morphogenesis.**

morphology The study of the physical shape and size of a specimen, a plant, or an animal. —**morphologic,** *adj.*

-morphosis A combining form meaning a 'development or change': *chemomorphosis, epimorphosis.*

Morquio's disease A familial form of mucopolysaccharidosis that results in abnormal musculoskeletal development in childhood. Dwarfism, hunchback, enlarged sternum, and knock-knees may occur. The disease may first be evident as the child, learning to walk, displays an abnormal, waddling gait.

morrhuate sodium injection A sclerosing agent.

mortality **1.** The condition of being subject to death. **2.** The death rate, which reflects the number of deaths per unit of population in any specific region, age group, disease, or other classification, usually expressed as deaths per 1,000, 10,000, or 100,000.

mortar A cup-shaped vessel in which materials are ground or crushed by a pestle in the preparation of drugs.

Morton's foot See **metatarsalgia.**

Morton's neuroma See **metatarsalgia.**

Morton's plantar neuralgia A severe throbbing pain that affects the anastomotic nerve branch between the medial and the lateral plantar nerves. Also called **Morton's plantar neuroma.**

Morton's plantar neuroma See **Morton's plantar neuralgia.**

Morton's toe See **metatarsalgia.**

morula, *pl.* **morulas, morulae** A solid, spherical mass of cells resulting from the cleavage of the fertilized ovum in the early stages of embryonic development. It represents an intermediate stage between the zygote and the blastocyst. —**morular,** *adj.*

-morula A combining form meaning a 'clump of blastomeres formed by cleavage of a fertilized ovum': *amphimorula, archimorula.*

mosaic **1.** In genetics: an individual or organism that developed from a single zygote but that has two or more kinds of cell populations in regard to genetic constitution. Such a condition results from a mutation, crossing-over, or, more commonly in humans, nondisjunction of the chromosomes during early embryogenesis, which causes a variation in the number of chromosomes in the cells. The degree of clinical involvement depends on the type of tissue containing the abnormality and may vary from near normal to full manifestation of a syndrome, as Down's syndrome or Turner's syndrome. Compare **chimera.** See also **monosomy, sex chromosome mosaic, trisomy. 2.** In embryology: a fertilized ovum that undergoes determinate cleavage. See also **mosaic development.**

mosaic bone Bone tissue appearing to be made up of many tiny pieces cemented together, as seen upon microscopic examination of an X-ray film of the affected bone. It is characteristic of Paget's disease of the bone.

mosaic cleavage See **determinate cleavage.**

mosaic development A kind of embryonic development occurring in the blastocyst. The fertilized ovum undergoes determinate cleavage, developing according to a precise, unalterable plan. Damage to or destruction of these cells results in a defective organism. Compare **regulative development.**

mosaicism In genetics: a condition in which an individual or an organism that develops from a single zygote has two or more cell populations that differ in genetic constitution. Most commonly seen in humans is a variation in the number of cell chromosomes, which may involve either a particular autosome, as in Down's syndrome, or the sex chromosomes, as in Turner's syndrome and Kleinfelter's syndrome. See also **mosaic, sex chromosome mosaic.**

mosaic wart A group of contiguous plantar warts.

mosquito bite A bite of a bloodsucking arthropod of the subfamily Culicidae that may result in a systemic allergic reaction in a hypersensitive person, an infection, or, most often, a pruritic wheal.

mosquito forceps See **Halsted's forceps,** definition 1.

Mössbauer spectrometer An instrument that can detect small changes between an atomic nucleus and its environment, as caused by changes in temperature, pressure, or chemical state. The device is used in chemical and physical research with applications in medicine.

mot- A combining form meaning 'of or related to movement': *motoneuron, motorgraphic.*

mother fixation An arrest in psychosexual development characterized by an abnormally

MOTOR END PLATE

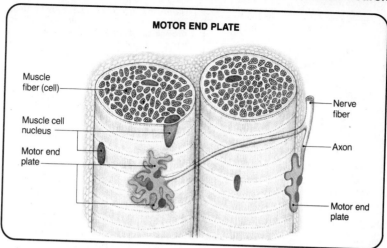

Muscle fiber (cell)

Muscle cell nucleus

Motor end plate

Nerve fiber

Axon

Motor end plate

persistent, close, and often paralyzing emotional attachment to one's mother. Compare **father fixation.** See also **Freudian fixation.**

motile Capable of spontaneous but unconscious or involuntary movement. —**motility,** *n.*

-motility A combining form meaning the 'condition of being capable of movement': *cardiomotility, hypermotility.* Also **-mobility.**

motion sickness A condition caused by erratic or rhythmic motions in any combination of directions, as in a boat or a car. Severe cases are characterized by nausea, vomiting, vertigo, and headache; mild cases by headache and general discomfort. Various antihistamines are used prophylactically. Kinds of motion sickness are air sickness, car sickness, seasickness *(mal de mer).*

motivation In psychology: any positive, negative, or indirect inducement or force that directs behavior toward satisfying needs or achieving goals.

motivational conflict A conflict resulting from the arousal of two or more motives that direct behavior toward incompatible goals. Kinds of motivational conflict include **approach-approach conflict, approach-avoidance conflict, avoidance-avoidance conflict.** See also **motivation.**

motor 1. Of or pertaining to motion, the body apparatus involved in movement, or the brain functions that direct purposeful activities. 2. Of or pertaining to a muscle, nerve, or brain center that produces or subserves motion.

-motor A combining form meaning 'pertaining to the effects of activity in a body part': *nervimotor, psychomotor.*

motor aphasia The inability to utter remembered words, owing to a cerebral lesion in the inferior frontal gyrus (Broca's motor speech area) of the left hemisphere in right-handed individuals. The condition most commonly is the result of a stroke. The patient knows what to say but cannot articulate the words. Also called

ataxic aphasia, expressive aphasia, frontocortical aphasia, verbal aphasia.

motor apraxia The inability to carry out planned movements or to handle small objects, although the proper use of the object is recognized. The condition results from a lesion in the premotor frontal cortex on the opposite side of the affected limb. Also called **cortical apraxia, innervation apraxia.** See also **apraxia.**

motor area A portion of the cerebral cortex that includes the precentral gyrus and the posterior part of the frontal gyri and which is responsible for the contraction of the voluntary muscles upon stimulation with electrodes. It corresponds to Brodmann's areas IV and VI. It contains the giant pyramidal cells of Betz in layer V. Normal voluntary activity requires associations between the motor area and other parts of the cortex; removal of the motor area from one cerebral hemisphere causes paralysis of voluntary muscles, especially of the opposite side of the body. Various parts of the motor area are associated with different body structures, as the lower limb, the face, and the hand. The parts associated with more complicated movements are larger than those associated with more general movements.

motor end plate A broad band of terminal fibers of the motor nerves of the voluntary muscles. Motor nerves derived from the cranial and spinal nerves enter the sheaths of striated muscle fibers, lose their myelin sheaths, and ramify like the roots of a tree.

motor fiber One of the fibers in the spinal nerves that transmit impulses to muscle fibers.

motor image A visual concept of one's bodily movements, real or imagined.

motor nerve A nerve consisting of efferent fibers that conduct impulses away from the brain or the spinal cord to one of the muscles or one of the organs. Compare **sensory nerve.** See also **nervous system.**

motor neuron, motoneuron One of var-

MOUTH

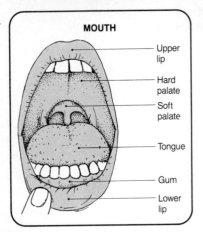

- Upper lip
- Hard palate
- Soft palate
- Tongue
- Gum
- Lower lip

ious kinds of nerve cells that transmit nerve impulses from the brain or from the spinal cord to muscular or glandular tissue. According to location, motor neurons are the peripheral motor neurons and the upper motor neurons.

motor neuron paralysis An injury to the spinal cord that causes damage to the motor neurons and results in various degrees of functional impairment depending on the site of the lesion. See **lower motor neuron paralysis, upper motor neuron paralysis.**

motor point 1. A point at which a motor nerve enters the muscle it innervates. 2. A point at which electrical stimulation will cause contraction of a muscle. Compare **motor end plate.** See also **motor nerve, nervous system.**

motor seizure A transitory disturbance in brain function caused by abnormal neuronal discharges that arise initially in a localized motor area of the cerebral cortex. The manifestations depend on the site of the abnormal electrical activity, as tonic contractures of the thumb, caused by excessive discharges in the motor area of the cortex controlling the first digit. The disturbance may spread, or it may end in a shower of clonic movements or a generalized convulsion. Also called **focal motor seizure.**

motor sense The feeling or perception enabling a person to accomplish a purposeful movement. This is presumably achieved by evocation of a sensory engram or memory of the pattern for that specific movement; proprioceptive signals transmitted by feedback pathways through the cerebellum and sensory areas of the motor cortex are compared with the engram and modify the movement. Experiments with animals show that a movement cannot be performed if the corresponding sensory area of the brain is removed.

motor unit A functional structure consisting of a motor neuron and the muscle fibers it innervates.

mountain fever 1. See **brucellosis.** 2. See **Colorado tick fever.** 3. See **Rocky Mountain spotted fever.**

mountain tick fever 1. See **Rocky Mountain spotted fever.** 2. See **Colorado tick fever.**

mouse-tooth forceps A kind of dressing forceps that has one or more fine sharp points on the tip of each blade. The tips turn in, and the delicate teeth interlock.

mouth 1. The nearly oval oral cavity at the anterior end of the digestive tube, bounded anteriorly by the lips and containing the tongue and the teeth. It consists of the vestibule and the mouth cavity proper. 2. An orifice.

mouth-to-mouth resuscitation A procedure in artificial resuscitation, performed most often with cardiac massage. The victim's nose is sealed by pinching the nostrils closed, the head is extended, and air is breathed by the rescuer through the mouth into the lungs. See also **cardiopulmonary resuscitation.**

mouth-to-nose resuscitation A procedure in artificial resuscitation in which the mouth of the victim is held closed and air is breathed through the victim's nose into the lungs. See also **mouth-to-mouth resuscitation.**

moxalactam disodium A cephalosporin antibiotic.

moxibustion Cauterization by means of a cylinder or cone of cotton wool, called a moxa, placed on the skin and fired at the top. It is used to produce counterirritation.

MPD *abbr* **maximum permissible dose.**

MPH *abbr* Master of Public Health.

MPS *abbr* **mucopolysaccharidosis.**

MPS I *abbr* mucopolysaccharidosis I. See **Hurler's syndrome.**

MPS II *abbr* mucopolysaccharidosis II. See **Hunter's syndrome.**

mR, mr *abbr* **milliroentgen.**

MS *abbr* **multiple sclerosis.**

MS *abbr* 1. Master of Science. 2. Master of Surgery.

MSH *abbr* **melanocyte-stimulating hormone.**

MSN *abbr* Master of Science in Nursing. See **master's degree program in nursing.**

MT *abbr* Medical Technologist.

mu, μ Symbol for **micron.**

Much's granules Granules and rods, found in tuberculosis sputum, that stain with gram stain but not as for acid-fast bacilli.

mucin A mucopolysaccharide, the chief ingredient in mucus, present in most glands that secrete mucus and the lubricant protecting body surfaces from friction and erosion.

mucinous adenocarcinoma See **mucinous carcinoma.**

mucinous carcinoma An epithelial neoplasm with a sticky gelatinous consistency owing to the copious mucin secreted by its cells. Also called **colloid carcinoma, gelatiniform carcinoma, gelatinous carcinoma.**

mucocutaneous Of or pertaining to the mucous membrane and skin.

mucocutaneous leishmaniasis See **American leishmaniasis.**

mucocutaneous lymph node syndrome An acute, febrile illness, primarily of

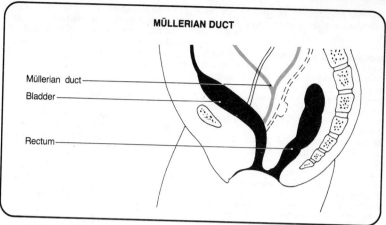

MÜLLERIAN DUCT

Müllerian duct

Bladder

Rectum

young children, which is characterized by inflamed mucous membranes of the mouth, 'strawberry tongue,' cervical lymphadenopathy, polymorphous rash on the trunk, and edema, erythema, and desquamation of the skin on the extremities. The cause is unknown. Salicylate therapy may be useful in suppressing fever and discomfort of the disease. Also called **Kawasaki disease.**

mucoepidermoid carcinoma A malignant neoplasm of glandular tissues, especially the ducts of the salivary glands. The tumor contains mucinous and epidermoid squamous cells.

mucoid 1. Resembling mucus. Also called myxoid. **2.** Any one of a group of mucuslike proteins derived from an animal source. The mucoids differ from the mucins in solubility; they are precipitated by acetic acid. Kinds of mucoids are **colloid, ovomucoid.**

mucolytic Capable of dissolving mucus.

mucomembranous Of or pertaining to a mucous membrane, as that of the small intestine.

mucopolysaccharidosis (MPS), *pl.* **mucopolysaccharidoses** One of a group of genetic disorders characterized by greater than normal accumulations of mucopolysaccharides in the tissues. The disorders are numbered MPS I through MPS VII, and each type has a specific eponym. In all types, there is pronounced skeletal deformity (especially of the face), mental and physical retardation, and decreased life expectancy. The disorders may be detected before birth by testing fetal cells present in amniotic fluid. After birth, diagnosis is established through urine testing, skeletal changes observed on X-ray, and family history. There is no successful treatment. Kinds of mucopolysaccharidosis include **Hunter's syndrome (MPS II), Hurler's syndrome (MPS I).**

mucoprotein A compound, present in connective and supporting tissue, that contains mucopolysaccharides as prosthetic groups and is resistant to denaturation.

mucopurulent Characteristic of a combination of mucus and pus.

mucormycosis See **zygomycosis.**

mucosa *pl.* **mucosae** Mucous membrane. **—mucosal,** *adj.*

mucous Of or pertaining to mucus.

-mucous A combining form meaning 'containing or composed of mucus': *fibromucous, puromucous.*

mucous colitis See **irritable bowel syndrome.**

mucous membrane Any one of four major kinds of thin sheets of tissue that cover or line various parts of the body. They line cavities or canals of the body that open to the outside, as the linings of the mouth. They consist of a surface layer of epithelial tissue covering a deeper layer of connective tissue and protect the underlying structure, secrete mucus, and absorb water, salts, and other solutes. Compare **serous membrane, skin, synovial membrane.**

mucous plug In obstetrics: a collection of thick mucus in the uterine cervix that is often expelled at the onset of dilatation of the cervix, just before labor begins or in its early hours.

mucous shreds See **shreds.**

mucous tumor See **myxoma.**

mucoviscidosis See **cystic fibrosis.**

mucus The viscous, slippery secretions of the mucous membranes and glands, containing mucin, white blood cells, water, inorganic salts, and exfoliated cells. **—mucoid,** *adj.,* **mucous,** *adj.*

mud bath The application of warm mud to the body for therapeutic purposes.

Müllerian Of or pertaining to the Müllerian ducts, named for Johannes Peter Müller.

Müllerian duct One of a pair of embryonic ducts that become the fallopian tubes, uterus, and vagina in females and that atrophy in males.

multi- A combining form meaning 'many': *multicapsular.*

multicentric mitosis See **multipolar mitosis.**

multifactorial Of, pertaining to, or characteristic of any condition or disease resulting from the interaction of many factors, specifically of several genes, usually polygenes. Many disorders, as spina bifida, neural tube defects, and Hirschsprung's disease, are considered to be multifactorial.

multifactorial inheritance The tendency to develop a characteristic, disease, or condition that is genetic and environmental, as neural tube defect.

multifinality In general systems theory: a principle stating that the choice of means shapes the end result, with different means achieving dissimilar end results.

multi-infarct dementia A form of organic brain disease characterized by the rapid deterioration of intellectual functioning, caused by vascular disease. Symptoms include emotional lability; disturbances in memory, abstract thinking, judgment, and impulse control; and focal neurological impairment, such as gait abnormalities, pseudobulbar palsy, and paresthesia. The condition is more prevalent in men than in women and may be caused by a cerebrovascular accident. See also **dementia, senile psychosis.**

multipenniform Of a bodily structure: having a shape resembling a pattern of many feathers, especially that of the muscular fasciculi that converge to several tendons. Compare **bipenniform, penniform.**

multiphasic screening A technique of screening populations for diseases in which there is combined use of a battery of screening tests.

multiple benign cystic epithelioma See **trichoepithelioma.**

multiple cartilaginous exostoses See **diaphyseal aclasis.**

multiple enchondromatosis See **enchondromatosis.**

multiple endocrine adenomatosis See **adenomatosis.**

multiple factor See **polygene.**

multiple fission Cell division in which the nucleus first divides into several equal parts followed by the division of the cytoplasm into as many cells as there are nuclei. It is the common form of asexual reproduction in certain unicellular organisms. Compare **binary fission.**

multiple fracture **1.** A fracture extending several fracture lines in one bone. **2.** The fracture of several bones at one time or from the same injury.

multiple gene See **polygene.**

multiple idiopathic hemorrhagic sarcoma See **Kaposi's sarcoma.**

multiple lipomatosis A rare, inherited disorder characterized by discrete, localized, subcutaneous deposits of fat in the tissues of the body. This fat is not available for metabolic use, even in starvation.

multiple mononeuropathy An abnormal condition characterized by dysfunction of several individual nerve trunks. It may be caused by various diseases, as necrotizing angiopathy and some immunologic disorders. Also called **mononeuritis multiplex.**

multiple myeloma A malignant neoplasm of the bone marrow. The tumor, composed of plasma cells, destroys osseous tissue, especially in flat bones, causing pain, fractures, and skeletal deformities. Characteristically, there are abnormal proteins in the plasma and urine, anemia, weight loss, pulmonary complications secondary to rib fractures, and kidney failure. Also called **multiple plasmacytoma of bone, myelomatosis, plasma cell myeloma.**

multiple myositis See **polymyositis.**

multiple neuroma See **neuromatosis.**

multiple peripheral neuritis Acute or subacute disseminated inflammation or degeneration of symmetrically distributed peripheral nerves, characterized initially by numbness, tingling in the extremities, hot and cold sensations, and slight fever, progressing to pain, weakness, diminished reflexes, and in some cases flaccid paralysis. The disorder may be caused by toxic substances, as antimony, arsenic, carbon monoxide, copper, lead, mercury, nitrobenzol, organophosphates, and thallium, or various drugs, including diphenylhydantoin, isoniazid, nitrofurantoin, thalidomide, and vincristine. Therapy consists of removal of the toxic agent or treatment of the causative disease, rest, and medication for pain. Guillain-Barré syndrome sometimes occurs following an influenza vaccination. Also called **peripheral polyneuritis.** See also **Guillain-Barré syndrome.**

multiple personality An abnormal condition in which the organization of the personality is fragmented. It is characterized by the presence of two or more distinct subpersonalities. Also called **split personality.**

multiple personality disorder A dissociative disorder characterized by the existence of two or more distinct, clearly differentiated personality structures within the same individual, any of which may dominate at a particular time. Each personality is a complex unit with separate, well-developed emotional and thought processes, behavior patterns, and social relationships. The various subpersonalities are usually dramatically different from one another and may or may not be aware of the existence of the others. Often, complex interrelationships exist between the personalities. Transition from one subpersonality to another is usually sudden and associated with psychosocial stress. The condition, most often diagnosed in female adolescents or young adults, primarily results from intrapsychic conflicts that are so deep-seated that the only solution is to separate the conflicting parts of the psyche into autonomous personality systems. Treatment may include hypnosis or psychotropic medication and long-term psychotherapy aimed at uncovering the emotional conflicts that precipitated the development and maintenance of the various subpersonalities. See also **dissociative disorder, hysterical neurosis.**

multiple plasmacytoma of bone See **multiple myeloma.**

multiple sclerosis (MS) A progressive disease characterized by disseminated demyelination of nerve fibers of the brain and spinal cord. It begins slowly, usually in young adulthood, and continues throughout life with periods of exacerbation and remission. The first signs are paresthesias, or abnormal sensations in the extremities or on one side of the face. Other early signs are muscle weakness, vertigo, and visual disturbances, as nystagmus, diplopia (double vision), and partial blindness. Because many other conditions affect the nervous system and produce similar symptoms, diagnosing MS is difficult. A history of recurring exacerbation and remission of symptoms and the presence of greater than normal amounts of protein in cerebrospinal fluid are characteristic. As the disease progresses, the intervals between exacerbations grow shorter, and disability becomes greater. There is no specific treatment for the disease; corticosteroids and other drugs are used to treat the symptoms accompanying acute episodes. Physical therapy may help to postpone or prevent specific disabilities. Also called **disseminated multiple sclerosis.**

multiple self-healing squamous epithelioma   See keratoacanthoma.

multiplicative growth   See merisis.

multipolar mitosis   A type of cell division in which the spindle has three or more poles, resulting in the formation of a corresponding number of daughter cells. Also called **multicentric mitosis, pluripolar mitosis.** See also **trisomy.**

multisource drug   A drug that can be purchased under any of several trade names from different manufacturers or distributors. See also **generic equivalent, generic name.**

multivalent   1. In chemistry: an ion or radial with more than one valency. 2. In immunology: able to act against more than one strain of organism. Also called polyvalent. Compare **valence.**

mummified fetus   A fetus that has died in utero and has shriveled and dried up.

mumps   An acute viral disease, characterized by a swelling of the parotid glands, caused by a paramyxovirus. It is most likely to affect children between 5 and 15 years of age, but it may occur at any age. In adulthood the infection may be severe. The incidence of mumps is highest during late winter and early spring. The mumps paramyxovirus lives in the saliva of the affected individual and is transmitted in droplets or by direct contact. The time of maximum communicability is believed to be the 48-hour period immediately preceding the start of parotid swelling. The prognosis in mumps is good, but the disease sometimes involves complications, as arthritis, pancreatitis, myocarditis, oophoritis, nephritis, and orchitis. About half of the men with mumps-induced orchitis suffer some atrophy of the testicles, but sterility rarely results. The common symptoms of mumps usually last for about 24 hours and include anorexia, headache, malaise, and low-grade fever. These signs are commonly followed by earache, parotid gland swelling, and a temperature of 38.3°C

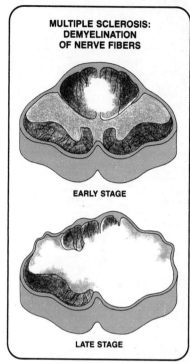

MULTIPLE SCLEROSIS: DEMYELINATION OF NERVE FIBERS

EARLY STAGE

LATE STAGE

to 40°C (101°F to 104°F). The patient also experiences pain when drinking acidic liquids or when chewing. The salivary glands may also become swollen. Complications, as epididymoorchitis and mumps meningitis, may develop. About 25% of the postpubertal males who contract mumps develop epididymo-orchitis with associated testicular swelling and tenderness that may persist for several weeks. Mumps meningitis develops in 10% of the patients with mumps and occurs in three to five times as many males as females. Diagnosis of mumps is usually based on typical symptoms, especially parotid gland swelling. If the parotid gland is not swollen, confirming diagnosis may be based on serologic antibody tests. Treatment commonly includes bed rest, respiratory isolation of the patient, and the administration of analgesics, antipyretics, and a fluid intake adequate to prevent dehydration associated with fever and anorexia. Intravenous fluids may be administered to patients who can't swallow.

NURSING CONSIDERATIONS: During the acute phase of the disease, the nurse is especially alert to any signs of central nervous system involvement, as nuchal rigidity. All cases of mumps are routinely reported to local health authorities. Nurses aid public health education by stressing the importance of immunization. Immunization within 24 hours of exposure may prevent the disease or may minimize its effects. Also called **epidemic parotitis, infectious parotitis.**

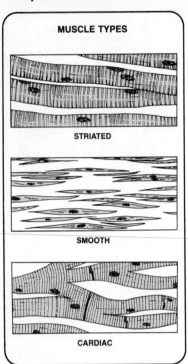

MUSCLE TYPES

STRIATED

SMOOTH

CARDIAC

mumps virus vaccine live An active immunizing agent prescribed for immunization against mumps. Immmunosuppression, concomitant use of corticosteroids, acute infection, pregnancy, or known hypersensitivity to chicken proteins, neomycin, or this drug prohibits its use. Among the most serious effects are fevers, parotitis, and allergic reactions.

Munchausen's syndrome An unusual personality disorder characterized by habitual pleas for treatment and hospitalization for dramatic but false symptoms. The person may convincingly present the symptoms and history of a real disease or simulate acute illness. Upon discovery of the real nature of his symptoms, the patient commonly leaves without notice and moves on to another hospital. Also called **pathomimicry.**

Murchison fever See **Pel-Ebstein fever.**

murine typhus An acute arbovirus infection caused by *Rickettsia typhi* and transmitted by the bite of an infected flea. It is characterized by headache, chills, myalgia, rash, and a fever that lasts about 12 days. A dull-red, maculopapular rash, mainly on the trunk, appears about the 5th day and lasts for 4 to 8 days. Recovery is usually rapid and complete, but death has occurred in elderly or debilitated people. Weil-Felix and complement fixation tests aid in the diagnosis. Chloramphenicol or tetracycline is usually prescribed in treatment. Prevention involves the elimination of the rodents that are the

natural host of the organism and the use of appropriate insecticides to control fleas. Also called **endemic typhus, flea-borne typhus, new world typhus, rat typhus, urban typhus.** Compare **epidemic typhus, Rocky Mountain spotted fever.**

murmur A low-pitched fluttering or humming sound, as a heart murmur.

Murray Valley encephalitis An acute inflammatory disease of the brain, once epidemic in Australia's Murray Valley, characterized by convulsions, muscle rigidity, high fever, mental confusion, and coma. It is considered identical to Australian X disease, which is caused by a neurotropic herpeslike virus.

muscae volitantes See **floater.**

muscarinic Stimulating the postganglionic parasympathetic receptor.

muscle A kind of tissue comprised of fibers that are able to contract, causing and allowing movement of the parts and organs of the body. Muscle fibers are richly vascular, irritable, conductive, and elastic. There are two basic kinds, striated muscle and smooth muscle. Striated muscle, which comprises all skeletal muscles except for the myocardium, is long and voluntary. Smooth muscle, which comprises all visceral muscles, is short and involuntary. The myocardium is sometimes classified as a third (cardiac) kind of muscle, but it is basically a striated muscle. See also **cardiac muscle, smooth muscle, striated muscle.**

muscle albumin Albumin present in muscle.

muscle relaxant A drug that reduces the contractility of muscle fibers. Curare derivatives and succinylcholine compete with acetylcholine and block neural transmission at the myoneural junction. These drugs are used during anesthesia, in the management of patients undergoing mechanical ventilation, and in shock therapy, to reduce muscle contractions in pharmacologically or electrically induced seizures. Several drugs that relieve muscle spasms act at various levels in the central nervous system: baclofen inhibits monosynaptic and polysynaptic reflexes at the spinal level; cyclobenzaprine acts primarily in the brain stem.

muscle-setting exercise A method of maintaining muscle strength and tonality by alternately contracting and relaxing a skeletal muscle or any group of muscles without moving the associated part of the body. Such activity is useful in preventing atrophy of the muscles.

muscular 1. Of or pertaining to a muscle. 2. Characteristic of well-developed musculature.

muscular branch of the deep brachial artery One of several similar branches of the deep brachial artery, supplying certain arm muscles, as the coracobrachialis.

muscular dystrophy A group of genetically transmitted diseases characterized by progressive atrophy of skeletal muscles without evidence of involvement or degeneration of neural tissue. In all forms of muscular dystrophy there is an insidious loss of strength with increasing disability and deformity, although each type differs in the groups of muscles affected, the age of onset, the rate of progression, and the mode of genetic inheritance. The basic etiology is unknown but appears to be an inborn error of metabolism. Serum creatine phosphokinase is increased in affected individuals and acts as a diagnostic aid, especially in asymptomatic children in families at risk. Diagnostic confirmation is made by muscle biopsy, electromyography, and genetic pedigree. Treatment consists primarily of supportive measures, as physical therapy. The main types of the disease are pseudohypertrophic (Duchenne) muscular dystrophy, limb-girdle muscular dystrophy, and facioscapulohumeral (Landouzy-Dejerine) muscular dystrophy. Rarer forms include Becker's muscular dystrophy, distal muscular dystrophy, myotonic muscular dystrophy, and ocular myopathy. See also **myotonic myopathy.**

muscular sarcoidosis   Sarcoidosis of the skeletal muscles in which there is interstitial inflammation, fibrosis, atrophy, and damage of the muscle fibers, as sarcoid tubercles form within and replace normal muscle cells. See also **sarcoidosis.**

muscular tumor   See **myoma.**

musculocutaneous nerve   One of the terminal branches of the brachial plexus. It is formed on each side by division of the lateral cord of the plexus into two branches. It pierces the coracobrachialis and crosses to the lateral side of the arm, where it pierces the deep fascia just above the elbow and continues into the forearm as the lateral antebrachial cutaneous nerve. Compare **median nerve, radial nerve, ulnar nerve.**

musculoskeletal   Of or pertaining to the muscles and the skeleton.

musculoskeletal system assessment An evaluation of the condition and functioning of the patient's muscles, joints, and bones and of factors which may contribute to abnormalities in these body structures.

musculospiral nerve   See **radial nerve.**

mushroom   The fruiting body of the fungus of the class *Basidomycetes*, especially those of the edible order Agaricales, commonly known as field or meadow mushrooms. Although mushrooms contain some protein and minerals, they are of limited nutritional value. Fungal poisoning is caused by ingestion of mushrooms of the genus *Amanita*, in particular *A. muscaria* and *A. phalloides*. Some mushrooms, especially *Psilocybe mexicana*, contain substances that produce hallucinatory states.

mushroom poisoning   A toxic condition caused by the ingestion of certain mushrooms, particularly two species of the genus *Amanita*. Muscarine in *A. muscaria* produces intoxication in a few to 120 minutes. Symptoms include lacrimation, salivation, sweating, vomiting, labored breathing, abdominal cramps, diarrhea, and, in severe cases, convulsions, coma, and circulatory failure. Atropine is usually admin-

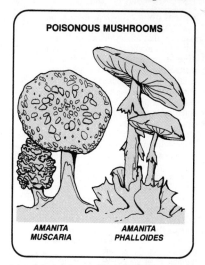

POISONOUS MUSHROOMS

AMANITA MUSCARIA   *AMANITA PHALLOIDES*

istered in treatment. More deadly but slower acting phalloidine in *A. phalloides* and *A. verna* causes similar symptoms as well as liver damage, renal failure, and death in 30% to 50% of the cases. Treatment includes emptying the stomach by gastric lavage with a weak solution of tannic acid or of potassium permanganate, followed by a saline purgative. Intensive care, as for kidney or liver failure, and hemodialysis may reduce mortality. In some people, the consumption of alcohol complicates mushroom poisoning and the combination has the effect of disulfiram.

mushroom worker's lung   A type of hypersensitivity pneumonitis common among workers in the mushroom-growing industry. The antigens to which the hypersensitive reactions occur are fungi of the genera *Micropolyspora* and *Thermoactinomyces*. Spores of these fungi are found in the postspawning compost used to grow mushrooms. Symptoms of the acute form of the disease include chills, cough, fever, dyspnea, anorexia, nausea, and vomiting. The chronic form of the disease is characterized by fatigue, chronic cough, weight loss, and dyspnea on exertion.

music therapy   A form of adjunctive psychotherapy in which music is used as a means of recreation and communication, especially with autistic children, and as a means to elevate the mood of depressed and psychotic patients.

mustard gas   A poisonous gas used in chemical warfare during World War I. It causes corrosive destruction of the skin and mucous membranes, often resulting in permanent respiratory damage and death.

mutagen   Any chemical or physical environmental agent that induces a genetic mutation or increases the mutation rate. —**mutagenic,** *adj.,* **mutagenicity,** *n.*

mutagenesis   The induction or occurrence of a genetic mutation. See also **teratogenesis.**

mutant gene Any gene that has undergone a change, as the loss, gain, or exchange of genetic material, that affects the normal transmission and expression of a trait. See also **amorph, antimorph, hypermorph, hypomorph.**

mutation An unusual change in genetic material occurring spontaneously or by induction. The alteration changes the original expression of the gene. Genes are stable units, but when a mutation occurs it is transmitted to future generations. —**mutate,** v., **mutational,** adj.

mutism The inability or refusal to speak. The condition may result from an unconscious response to emotional conflict and confusion and is commonly observed in patients who are catatonic, stuporous, hysterical, or depressed. A kind of mutism is **akinetic mutism.**

muton In molecular genetics: the smallest DNA segment whose alteration can result in a mutation.

mutually exclusive categories Categories on a research instrument that are sufficiently precise to allow each subject, factor, or variable to be classified in only one category.

mV, mv abbr **millivolt.**

Mv Symbol for **mendelevium.**

mVO₂ Symbol for myocardial oxygen consumption.

MVV abbr maximal voluntary ventilation. See **maximal breathing capacity.**

MWIA abbr **Medical Women's International Association.**

my- See **myo-.**

myalgia Diffuse muscle pain, usually accompanied by malaise, occurring in many infectious diseases, as brucellosis, dengue, influenza, leptospirosis, measles, and poliomyelitis. Myalgia occurs in arteriosclerosis obliterans, fibrositis, fibromyositis, Guillain-Barré syndrome, hyperparathyroidism, hypoglycemia, hypothyroidism, muscle tumor, myoglobinuria, myositis, and renal tubular acidosis. Various drugs that may cause myalgia include amphotericin B, carbenoxolone, chloroquinine, clofibrate, and corticosteroids. See also **epidemic myalgia.** —**myalgic,** adj.

myalgic asthenia A condition characterized by a general feeling of fatigue and muscular pain, often resulting from or associated with psychological stress.

myasthenia A condition characterized by an abnormal weakness of a muscle or a group of muscles that may be the result of a systemic myoneural disturbance, as in myasthenia gravis, or of a local circulatory inadequacy, as in intermittent claudication. —**myasthenic,** adj.

myasthenia gravis An abnormal condition characterized by the chronic fatigability and weakness of muscles, especially in the face and throat, as a result of a defect in the conduction of nerve impulses at the myoneural junction. It is caused by the inability of receptors at the myoneural junction to depolarize because of a deficiency of acetylcholine; hence, the diagnosis may be made by administering an anticholinesterase drug and observing improved muscle strength and stamina. The onset of symptoms is usually gradual, with ptosis of the upper eyelids, diplopia, and weakness of the facial muscles. Muscular exertion aggravates the symptoms, which typically vary over the course of the day. The disease occurs in younger women more often than in older women and in men over 60 years of age more often than in younger men. Anticholinesterase drugs are given. The Tensilon test is used to determine the optimal maintenance dose. Neostigmine or pyridostigmine is the drug most often used.

NURSING CONSIDERATIONS: Physical activity is restricted and bed rest encouraged. Anticholinesterase drugs are usually administered before meals, and the patient is monitored for toxic side effects. Myasthenic crisis may require emergency respiratory assistance.

myasthenia gravis crisis Acute exacerbation of the muscular weakness characterizing the disease, triggered by infection, surgery, emotional stress, or an overdose or insufficiency of anticholinesterase medication. Typical signs and symptoms include respiratory distress progressing to periods of apnea, extreme fatigue, increased muscular weakness, dysphagia, dysarthria, and fever. The patient may be anxious, restless, irritable, unable to move the jaws or to raise one or both eyelids. If the condition is caused by anticholinesterase toxicity, there may be anorexia, nausea, vomiting, abdominal cramps, diarrhea, excessive salivation, sweating, lacrimation, blurred vision, vertigo, and muscle cramps and spasms, as well as general weakness, dysarthria, and respiratory distress. Initial treatment is directed to maintaining patency of the airway. Oxygen with assisted or controlled ventilation is administered. The withdrawal or reduction of anticholinergic drugs may be ordered, or they may be given to differentiate the kind of crisis. Parenteral fluids, antibiotics, nasogastric tube feeding, and the insertion of an indwelling catheter with closed gravity drainage may be ordered. The patient is turned every 2 hours and given mouth and skin care; the lips are kept well lubricated and decubiti are avoided by using an air mattress or sheepskin and by keeping the skin dry at all times. If an eyelid is affected, the eye may be covered with a moist patch; crusts are removed whenever required, and lubricating eyedrops or ointment may be administered. To enable the patient to communicate, the call bell and a pad and pencil or magic slate are placed within reach. Walking and other activities are planned at the time of the maximum effect of medication. Active or passive range-of-motion exercises are performed, but rest periods are maintained to avoid relapse.

NURSING CONSIDERATIONS: The patient is instructed on the importance of taking the prescribed medication and of reporting toxic side effects and symptoms of recurrent or progressive disease. The nurse points out the need to maintain a regular diet, to exercise to tolerance, to rest, and to avoid infections and exposure to hot or cold weather as well as the use of alcohol and tobacco.

myc- See **myco-**.

mycelium, *pl.* **mycelia** A mass of interwoven, branched, threadlike filaments, called hyphae, which make up most fungi.

mycetismus Mushroom poisoning.

myceto- See **myco-**.

mycetoma A serious fungal infection involving skin, subcutaneous tissue, fascia, and bone. One kind of mycetoma is **Madura foot**.

myco-, myc- A combining form meaning 'related to fungus': *mycophage.* Also **myceto-, myko-**.

mycobacteria Acid-fast microorganisms belonging to the genus *Mycobacterium.* —**mycobacterial,** *adj.*

mycobacteriosis A tuberculosislike disease caused by mycobacteria other than *Mycobacterium tuberculosis.*

Mycobacterium A genus of rod-shaped, acid-fast bacteria having two significant pathogenic species: *Mycobacterium leprae* causes leprosy; *M. tuberculosis* causes tuberculosis.

mycology The study of fungi and fungoid diseases. —**mycologic, mycological,** *adj.,* **mycologist,** *n.*

mycomyringitis See **myringomycosis**.

mycophenolic acid A bacteriostatic and fungistatic crystalline antibiotic obtained from *Pencillium brevi compactum* and related species.

Mycoplasma A genus of ultramicroscopic organisms lacking rigid cell walls and considered to be the smallest free-living organisms. Some are saprophytes, some are parasites, and many are pathogens. One species is a cause of mycoplasma pneumonia. Also called **pleuropneumonia-like organism**.

mycoplasma pneumonia A contagious disease of children and young adults caused by *Mycoplasma pneumoniae,* characterized by a 9- to 12-day incubation period and followed by symptoms of an upper respiratory infection, dry cough, and fever. Harsh or diminished breath sounds and fine inspiratory rales are frequently heard. Pulmonary infiltrates visible on chest X-ray may resemble bacterial or viral pneumonia and may persist for 3 weeks in untreated cases. Rarely, complications, as sinusitis, pleurisy, polyneuritis, myocarditis, or Stevens-Johnson syndrome, may follow the pneumonia. In untreated adults prolonged cough, weakness, and malaise are common. Diagnosis is suggested by observation of elevated cold agglutinins and is confirmed by a complement fixation test. Prognosis is favorable. Antibiotics, bed rest, a high-protein diet, and an adequate intake of fluids are recommended. Also called **Eaton-agent pneumonia, primary atypical pneumonia, viral pneumonia, walking pneumonia.** See also **cold agglutinin.**

mycosis Any disease caused by a fungus. Some kinds of mycoses are **candidiasis, coccidioidomycosis, tinea.** —**mycotic,** *adj.*

mycosis fungoides A rare, chronic, lym-

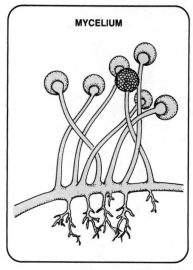

MYCELIUM

phomatous skin malignancy resembling eczema or a cutaneous tumor that is followed by microabscesses in the epidermis and lesions simulating those of Hodgkin's disease in lymph nodes and viscera. The condition is considered a distinctive entity by some specialists and a cutaneous manifestation of a malignant lymphoma by others.

mycotic aneurysm A localized dilatation in the wall of a blood vessel caused by the growth of a fungus, usually occurring as a complication of bacterial endocarditis. Also called **bacterial aneurysm.**

mydriasis **1.** Dilation of the pupil of the eye caused by contraction of the dilator muscle of the iris. With a decrease in light or the pharmacologic action of certain drugs the dilator acts to pull the iris outward, enlarging the pupil. **2.** An abnormal condition characterized by contraction of the dilator muscle, resulting in widely dilated pupils. Compare **miosis**. —**mydriatic,** *adj.*

mydriatic cycloplegic agent Any one of several ophthalmic topical preparations that dilate the pupil and paralyze the ocular muscles of accommodation. These drugs are used in diagnostic ophthalmoscopic and refractive examination of the eye, before and after various procedures in eye surgery, in some tests for glaucoma, in the treatment of anterior uveitis, and in treating certain kinds of glaucoma. Blurred vision, thirst, flushing, fever, and rash may occur. In children and elderly people, ataxia, somnolence, delirium, and hallucination may occur but are rare. Among these drugs are atropine, cyclopentolate, homatropine, scopolamine and tropicamide.

myel- See **myelo-**.

myelacephalus A fetal monster, usually a separate monozygotic twin, whose form and parts are barely recognizable. —**myelacephalous,** *adj.*

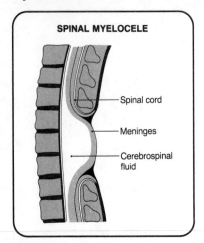

SPINAL MYELOCELE

Spinal cord

Meninges

Cerebrospinal fluid

myelatelia Any developmental defect involving the spinal cord.

myelauxe A developmental anomaly characterized by hypertrophy of the spinal cord.

-myelia A combining form meaning '(condition of the) spinal cord': atelomyelia, hydromyelia.

myelin A substance constituting the sheaths of various nerve fibers throughout the body. It is largely composed of fat, which gives the fibers a white, creamy color. —myelinic, adj.

myelinated Of a nerve: having a myelin sheath.

myelination The process of furnishing or taking on myelin.

myelin globule A fatlike droplet found in some sputum.

myelinic Of or pertaining to myelin.

myelinic neuroma A neuroma neoplasm composed of myelinated nerve fibers.

myelinization Development of the myelin sheath around a nerve fiber.

myelinogenesis See **myelinization.** —myelinogenetic, adj.

myelinolysis A pathological process that dissolves the myelin sheaths around certain nerve fibers, as those of the pons in patients with alcoholism.

myelin sheath A segmented, fatty lamination composed of myelin that wraps the axons of many nerves in the body. In myelinated peripheral nerves, the sheaths are composed of Schwann cells. The myelin sheaths around the central nerve fibers are composed of oligodendroglia. Their lipoid content gives these coverings a whitish appearance. The usual thickness of the myelin sheath is between 2 and 10 microns. Various diseases, as multiple sclerosis, can destroy these myelin wrappings.

myelitis An abnormal condition characterized by inflammation of the spinal cord with motor or sensory dysfunction. Some kinds of myelitis are **acute transverse myelitis, poliomyelitis.** —myelitic, adj.

myelo-, myel- A combining form meaning 'related to marrow': myelocyte, myelomenia.

myeloblast One of the earliest precursors of the granulocytic leukocytes. The cytoplasm appears light blue, scanty, and nongranular when seen in a stained blood smear through a microscope. In certain leukemias, a marked increase in myeloblasts is observed in the marrow and in the peripheral blood. Compare **megaloblast, myelocyte, normoblast.** See also **myelocytic leukemia.** —myeloblastic, adj.

myeloblastemia See **myeloblastosis.**

myeloblastic leukemia A malignant neoplasm of blood-forming tissues, characterized by many myeloblasts in the circulating blood and tissues. The disease may be a terminal event in chronic granulocytic leukemia.

myeloblastomatosis Abnormal, localized clusters of myeloblasts in the peripheral circulation.

myeloblastosis The abnormal presence of myeloblasts in the circulation.

myelocele A saclike protrusion of the spinal cord through a congenital defect in the vertebral column. See also **myelomeningocele, neural tube defect.**

myeloclast A cell that breaks down the myelin sheaths of nerves of the central nervous system.

myelocyst Any benign cyst that is formed from the rudimentary medullary canals that give rise to the vertebral canal during embryonic development.

myelocystocele A protrusion of a cystic tumor containing spinal cord substance through a defect in the vertebral column. See also **myelomeningocele, neural tube defect, spina bifida.**

myelocystomeningocele A protrusion of a cystic tumor containing both spinal cord substance and meninges through a defect in the vertebral column. See also **myelomeningocele, neural tube defect, spina bifida.**

myelocyte An immature white blood cell normally found in the bone marrow, being the first of the maturation stages of the granulocytic leukocytes. When microscopically examined, granules typical of the granulocytic series are seen in the cytoplasm. The nuclear material of the myelocyte is denser than that of the myeloblast, but it lacks a definable membrane. These cells appear in the circulating blood only in certain forms of leukemia. Compare **myeloblast.** See also **myelocytic leukemia.**

myelocythemia An abnormal presence of myelocytes in the circulating blood, as in myelocytic leukemia.

myelocytic leukemia A disorder characterized by the unregulated and excessive production of myelocytes of the granulocytic series. As many as several hundred thousand per cubic mm may be seen. Also called **granulocytic leukemia, myelogenous leukemia.** Compare **leukemoid reaction, lymphatic leukemia.** See also **leukocytosis.**

myelocytoma A localized cluster of mye-

NORMAL SPINAL MYELOGRAMS

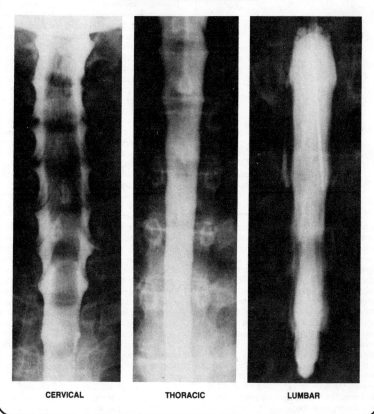

CERVICAL   THORACIC   LUMBAR

locytes in the peripheral vasculature that may occur in myelocytic leukemia.

myelocytosis See **myelocythemia.**

myelodiastasis Disintegration and necrosis of the spinal cord.

myelodysplasia A general designation for the defective development of any part of the spinal cord. The term is used primarily to describe abnormalities without gross superficial defects, specifically spina bifida occulta.

myelofibrosis See **myeloid metaplasia.**

myelogenesis **1.** The formation and differentiation of the nervous system during prenatal development, in particular the brain and spinal cord. See also **neural tube formation. 2.** The development of the myelin sheath around the nerve fiber. See also **myelinization.**

myelogenous Pertaining to the cells produced in bone marrow or to the tissue from which such cells originate. —**myelogenetic, myelogenic,** *adj.*

myelogenous leukemia See **acute myelocytic leukemia, chronic myelocytic leukemia.**

myelogeny The formation and differentiation of the myelin sheaths of nerve fibers during the prenatal development of the central nervous system.

myelogram **1.** An X-ray taken following the injection of a radiopaque medium into the subarachnoid space to demonstrate any distortions of the spinal cord, spinal nerve roots, and the subarachnoid space. **2.** A graphic representation of a count of the different kinds of cells in a stained preparation of bone marrow.

myelography A radiographic process by which the spinal cord and the spinal subarachnoid space are viewed and photographed after the introduction of a contrast medium. It is used to identify and study spinal lesions caused by trauma or disease. —**myelographic,** *adj.*

myeloid **1.** Of or pertaining to the bone marrow. **2.** Of or pertaining to the spinal cord. **3.** Of or pertaining to myelocytic forms that do not necessarily originate in the bone marrow.

myeloid leukemia See **acute myelocytic leukemia, chronic myelocytic leukemia.**

myeloid metaplasia A disorder in which

SPINAL MYELOMENINGOCELE

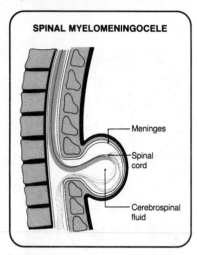

Meninges

Spinal cord

Cerebrospinal fluid

bone marrow tissue develops in abnormal sites. Characteristics are anemia, splenomegaly, immature blood cells in the circulation, and hematopoesis occurring in the liver and spleen. Myeloid metaplasia may be secondary to carcinoma, leukemia, polycythemia vera, or tuberculosis. The primary form is also called **agnogenic myeloid metaplasia, myelofibrosis.**

myeloidosis An abnormal condition characterized by general hyperplasia of the myeloid tissue. See also **Hodgkin's disease, multiple myeloma.**

myeloma An osteolytic neoplasm consisting of a profusion of cells typical of the bone marrow. It may develop simultaneously in many sites, causing extensive areas of patchy destruction of the bone. The tumor, which is usually grayish-red, occurs most frequently in the ribs, vertebrae, pelvic bones, and flat bones of the skull. Intense pain and spontaneous fractures are common. The tumor is radiosensitive and local lesions are curable. Kinds of myeloma are **endothelial myeloma, extramedullary myeloma, giant cell myeloma, multiple myeloma, osteogenic myeloma.**

-myeloma A combining form meaning a 'tumor composed of cells normally found in bone marrow': *globomyeloma, lymphomyeloma.*

myelomalacia Abnormal softening of the spinal cord, caused primarily by inadequate blood supply.

myelomatosis See **multiple myeloma.**

myelomeningocele A developmental defect of the central nervous system in which a hernial sac containing a portion of the spinal cord, its meninges, and cerebrospinal fluid protrudes through a congenital cleft in the vertebral column. The condition is caused primarily by the failure of the neural tube to close during embryonic development, although it may result from the reopening of the tube from an abnormal increase in cerebrospinal fluid pressure. The defect, which occurs in approximately 2 in every

1,000 live births, is apparent and easily diagnosed at birth. Although the opening may be located at any point along the spinal column, it characteristically occurs in the lumbar, low thoracic, or sacral region and extends for three to six vertebral segments. The saclike structure may be covered with a thin layer of skin or with a fine membrane that can be easily ruptured, increasing the risk of meningeal infection. The severity of neurological dysfunction is directly related to the amount of neural tissue involved, which can be roughly estimated by the degree of the transillumination of the mass. Usually the condition is accompanied by varying degrees of paralysis of the lower extremities; by musculoskeletal defects, as clubfoot, flexion and joint deformities, or hip dysplasia; and by anal and bladder sphincter dysfunction, which can lead to serious genitourinary disorders. Hydrocephalus, frequently related to the Arnold-Chiari malformation, is the most common anomaly associated with myelomeningocele and occurs in approximately 90% of the cases in which the spinal lesion is located in the lumbosacral region. In most cases, hydrocephalus is apparent at birth, although it may appear shortly afterward. Supplementary diagnostic procedures include X-rays of the spine, skull, and chest; a computerized axial tomographic scan of the brain to establish the ventricular size and the presence of any structural congenital anomalies; and laboratory examinations, especially urine analysis, culture, blood urea nitrogen evaluation, and creatinine clearance determination. Supportive care and surgery are the only treatments for myelomeningocele, and they require a multidisciplinary approach involving specialists from neurology, neurosurgery, urology, pediatrics, orthopedics, rehabilitation, and physical therapy, as well as intensive nursing care. Initial treatment involves prevention of infection and assessment of neurological involvement. Immediate surgical repair is essential if the defect is leaking cerebrospinal fluid. Although improved surgical techniques and other treatment modalities have significantly increased the survival rate, these procedures cannot alter the major physical disability and deformity, mental retardation, and chronic urinary tract and pulmonary infections that afflict these children for life. Prognosis is determined by the severity of neurologic involvement and the number of associated anomalies. With proper care and long-term maintenance, most children can survive and do well.

NURSING CONSIDERATIONS: Care of the child with a spinal defect entails the prevention of local infection and trauma by careful handling and positioning of the infant, applying sterile moist dressings to the membranous sac, avoiding fecal contamination and breakdown of sensitive skin areas, and maintaining adequate hydration and electrolyte balance. Gentle range-of-motion exercises are carried out to prevent or minimize hip and lower extremity deformity. An important function of the nurse is to involve the parents

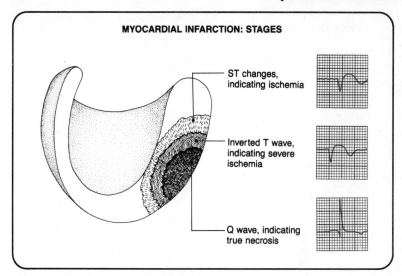

MYOCARDIAL INFARCTION: STAGES

ST changes, indicating ischemia

Inverted T wave, indicating severe ischemia

Q wave, indicating true necrosis

in the care of the infant as soon as possible and to teach them the essential procedures for adequate home care. Also called **meningomyelocele.** See also **neural tube defect, spina bifida.**

myelomere Any of the embryonic segments of the brain or spinal cord during prenatal development.

myelomonocytic leukemia See **monocytic leukemia.**

myelopathic anemia See **myelophthisic anemia.**

myelopathy 1. Any disease of the spinal cord. 2. Any disease of the myelopoietic tissues.

myelophthisic anemia A disorder attributed to several pathological processes that displace the hemopoietic tissues of the bone marrow. It is characterized by anemia and the appearance of immature granulocytes and nucleated erythroid elements in the peripheral blood. Also called **myelopathic anemia.** Compare **leukoerythroblastic anemia.**

myelopoiesis The formation and development of the bone marrow or the cells that originate from it. A kind of myelopoiesis is **extramedullary myelopoiesis. —myelopoietic,** *adj.*

myeloradiculodysplasia Any developmental abnormality of the spinal cord and spinal nerve roots. See also **myelomeningocele, neural tube defect.**

myeloschisis A developmental defect characterized by a cleft spinal cord that results from the failure of the neural plate to fuse and form a complete neural tube. See also **neural tube defect, neural tube formation, myelomeningocele, spina bifida.**

myesthesia Perception of any sensation in a muscle, as touch or proprioception.

myiasis Infection or infestation of the body by the larvae of flies, usually through a wound or an ulcer.

myitis See **myositis.**

myko- See **myco-.**

mylohyoideus One of a pair of flat triangular muscles that form the floor of the cavity of the mouth. One of the four suprahyoid muscles, immediately superior to the digastricus, the mylohyoideus arises from the whole length of the mylohyoid line of the mandible and inserts into the hyoid bone. Also called **mylohyoid muscle.** Compare **digastricus, geniohyoideus, stylohyoideus.**

myo-, my- A combining form meaning 'relating to muscle': *myocardia, myocele.*

myocardial infarction (MI) An occlusion of a coronary artery, which is caused by either atherosclerosis or an embolus and which results in a necrotic area in the vasculature myocardium. The onset of MI is characterized by a crushing, viselike chest pain that may radiate to the left arm, neck, or epigastrium and sometimes simulates the sensation of acute indigestion. The patient usually becomes ashen, clammy, short of breath, faint, and anxious and often feels that death is imminent. Typical signs are tachycardia, a barely perceptible pulse, low blood pressure, an elevated temperature, cardiac arrhythmia, and electrocardiographic evidence of ST segment elevation, T wave inversion, and a prominent Q wave. Laboratory studies usually show an increased sedimentation rate, leukocytosis, and elevated serum levels of creatine phosphokinase, lactic dehydrogenase, and glutamic-oxaloacetic transaminase. Potential complications in MI are pulmonary or systemic embolism, pulmonary edema, shock, and cardiac arrest. Emergency treatment may require cardiopulmonary resuscitation before the patient is admitted to an intensive cardiac care unit and placed on a cardiac monitor. In the acute phase oxygen, cardiotonic drugs, antiarrhythmic agents, and anticoagulants are usually administered and

TYPES OF UTERINE MYOMA

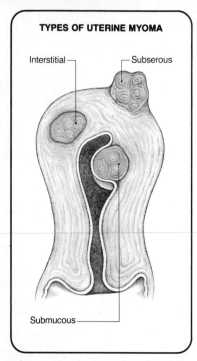

Interstitial — Subserous

Submucous —

sedatives and analgesics may be indicated. Parenteral fluids may be administered; iced drinks and cold foods are avoided and the patient is usually served a low-sodium, low cholesterol diet. Stool softeners and laxatives may be indicated to prevent straining during defecation. NURSING CONSIDERATIONS: Nursing care is directed toward detecting complications, preventing further myocardial damage, and promoting comfort, rest, and emotional well-being, as well as preparing the patient for discharge. The nurse instructs the patient and family regarding the need to adhere to the prescribed diet, medications, and exercise regime. The patient is counseled in regard to resuming sexual activity, as well as the need to avoid smoking and emotional stress.

myocardiopathy Any disease of the myocardium. Also called **cardiomyopathy.**

myocarditis Inflammation of the myocardium caused by viral, bacterial, or fungal infection, serum sickness, rheumatic fever, a chemical agent, or as a complication of a collagen disease. It most frequently occurs in an acute viral form and is self-limited but may lead to acute heart failure. Management includes treatment of the cause, analgesia, oxygen, anti-inflammatory agents, constant monitoring, and rest to prevent heart failure.

myocardium A thick, contractile, middle layer of uniquely constructed and arranged muscle cells that forms the bulk of the heart wall. The myocardium contains a minimum of other tissue, except for the blood vessels, and is covered interiorly by the endocardium. The contractile tissue of the myocardium is composed of fibers with the characteristic cross striations of muscular tissue. The fibers, which are about one third as large in diameter as those of skeletal muscle and which contain more sarcoplasm, branch frequently and are interconnected to form a network that is continuous except where the bundles and the laminae are attached at their origins and insertions into the fibrous trigone of the heart. Myocardial muscle fibers contain characteristic intercalated disks. Electron microscope studies reveal that these disks represent cell boundries and may cross an entire fiber in a straight line or may be arranged in a steplike configuration. Myocardial muscle contains less connective tissue than skeletal muscle. The fibers of the connective tissue are covered by a delicate fibrillar net with few elastic fibers. Collagenous fibers run between the muscular bundles and the associated blood vessels. Specially modified fibers of myocardial muscle constitute the conduction system of the heart, including the sinoatrial node, the atrioventricular node, the atrioventricular bundle, and the Purkinje fibers. Most of the myocardial fibers function to contract the heart. The metabolic processes of the myocardium are almost exclusively aerobic. The heart uses free fatty acids as its predominant fuel as well as important quantities of glucose, lactate, pyruvate, and ketone bodies and a very small amount of amino acids. Oxygen, which significantly affects contractibility, is the most important metabolic nutrient for the myocardium, which consumes from 6.5 to 10 ml/100 g of tissue per minute. Without this oxygen supply, myocardial contractions decrease in a few minutes. The heart normally extracts about 70% of the oxygen reaching it by the coronary arteries. This leaves only about 30% in coronary sinus blood and limits the amount of additional oxygen the heart can extract from its blood supply. —**myocardial,** adj.

myoclonus A spasm of a muscle or a group of muscles. —**myoclonic,** adj.

myodiastasis An abnormal condition in which there is separation of a muscle.

myoedema, pl. **myoedemas, myoedemata** Muscle edema. Compare **myxedema.**

myofacial pain-dysfunction syndrome See **temporomandibular joint pain-dysfunction syndrome.**

myogelosis A condition in which there are hardened areas or nodules within muscles, especially the gluteal muscles. There are no serious consequences of this condition and no treatment is necessary.

myoglobin A ferrous globin complex consisting of one heme molecule containing one iron molecule attached to a single globin chain. Myoglobin is found in muscle and is responsible for its red color and its ability to store oxygen.

myokinase See **adenylate kinase.**

myoma, pl. **myomas, myomata** A common, benign fibroid tumor on the uterine mus-

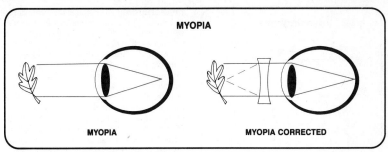

MYOPIA

MYOPIA   MYOPIA CORRECTED

cle. It develops most frequently after the age of 30 in women, especially black women, who have never been pregnant. Menorrhagia, backache, constipation, dysmenorrhea, dyspareunia, and other symptoms develop. Obstruction of a ureter may result. A myoma may be associated with sterility if it blocks the fallopian tube, with abortion if it interferes with fetal growth, or with difficult childbirth and hemorrhage if it is in or near the cervix. Also called **fibroid** (*informal*).

myoma previum See **leiomyoma uteri.**

myoma striocellulare See **rhabdomyoma.**

myomeningocele An abnormal saclike protrusion from the spine of a segment of the meninges and the spinal cord caused by the defective closure of the neural tube during the first trimester of pregnancy. The sac commonly protrudes from the lumbosacral area and, less frequently, from the sacral, thoracic, or cervical area. Depending on the level of protrusion, the myomeningocele may cause permanent neurologic defects, including paralysis and incontinence. Associated problems may include cyanosis, ulceration, clubfoot, and knee contractions. About 90% of the affected patients develop hydrocephalus. Others may develop Arnold-Chiari syndrome, spinal curvature, and mental retardation. Myomeningocele is usually obvious on examination and is easily distinguished from meningocele. The sac of myomeningocele does not transilluminate; the sac of meningocele does. Sensory and motor function can usually be determined by neurologic examination. Prenatal amniocentesis can detect myomeningocele, and it is recommended for all pregnant women who have delivered a child with a neural tube defect. Surgical closure of the sac is the common treatment. A shunt is often required to relieve associated hydrocephalus. Surgery can place the myomeningocele tissues back inside the spinal column but usually cannot repair neurologic damage already sustained. Urinary and fecal incontinence are common.

NURSING CONSIDERATIONS: Emotional support and counseling are necessary in helping the parents adjust to the diagnoses and procedures. The patient is handled carefully to avoid exerting pressure on the myomeningocele sac and is placed in the prone position. The head circumference is measured daily and meticulous skin care to the lesion, the buttocks, and the genitalia is per-

formed to prevent infection. The bladder is emptied at regular intervals. Glycerin suppositories and manual pressure on the abdomen are common aids to prevent bowel obstruction. For more information about spinal disorders the patients may be referred to the Spina Bifida Association of America. Compare **meningocele, spina bifida.**

myomere See **myotome.** —**myomeric,** *adj.*

myometritis An inflammation or infection of the myometrium of the uterus.

myometrium, *pl.* **myometria** The muscular layer of the wall of the uterus. The fibers of the myometrium course around the uterus.

myonecrosis The death of muscle fibers. Progressive, or clostridial, myonecrosis is caused by the anaerobic bacteria of the genus *Clostridium.* Seen in deep wound infections, progressive myonecrosis is accompanied by pain, tenderness, a brown serous exudate, and a rapid accumulation of gas within the tissue of the muscle. The affected muscle turns black-green. Treatment includes thorough wound debridement, I.V. administration of penicillin, and the use of hyperbaric oxygen therapy to destroy the anaerobe and to promote healing.

myoneural Of or pertaining to a muscle and its associated nerve, especially to nerve endings in muscles.

myoneural junction See **neuromuscular junction.**

myopathy An abnormal condition of skeletal muscle characterized by muscle weakness, wasting, and histiologic changes within muscle tissue, as seen in any of the muscular dystrophies. A myopathy is distinct from a muscle disorder caused by nerve dysfunction. The specific diagnosis of any myopathy is made using tests of serum enzymes, electromyography, and muscle biopsy. See also **muscular dystrophy.** —**myopathic,** *adj.*

myope An individual who is nearsighted.

myophosphorylase deficiency glycogenosis See **McArdle's disease.**

myopia A condition of nearsightedness caused by the elongation of the eyeball or by an error in refraction so that parallel rays are focused in front of the retina. Some kinds of myopia are **curvature myopia, index myopia, pathologic myopia.** Also called **short sight.** See also **second sight.** —**myopic,** *adj.*

myorrhaphy Suturing of a muscle wound.

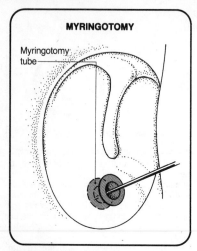

MYRINGOTOMY

Myringotomy tube

myorrhexis A tearing in any muscle. —**myorrhectic,** *adj.*

myosarcoma A malignant tumor of muscular tissue.

myosin A protein that makes up close to half of the proteins that occur in muscle tissue. The interaction of myosin and actin is essential for muscle contraction.

myositis Inflammation of muscle tissue, usually of the voluntary muscles. Causes of myositis include infection, trauma, and infestation by parasites. Kinds of myositis include **epidemic pleurodynia, polymyositis, traumatic myositis.** Also called **myitis.** Compare **fibrositis.**

myositis fibrosa An inflammation of the muscles, characterized by abnormal formation of connective tissue. Also called **interstitial myositis.** See also **myositis.**

myositis ossificans A rare, inherited disease in which muscle tissue is replaced by bone. It begins in childhood with stiffness in the neck and back and progresses to rigidity of the spine, trunk, and limbs. Diphosphonates may prevent the abnormal deposition of bone, but there is no cure. Compare **myositis.**

myositis purulenta Any bacterial infection of muscle tissue. This condition may result in the formation of an abscess or multiple abscesses.

myositis trichinosa Inflammation of the muscles resulting from infection by the parasite *Trichinella spiralis.* See also **trichinosis.**

myostasis An abnormal condition of weakened muscle in which there is a relatively fixed length of muscle fibers in the relaxed state. In normal muscle the force of contraction is greatest at the resting length of the muscle; in myostasis the resting length is shorter than normal, and there is a shorter acting length in which the contractile force can work. —**myostatic,** *adj.*

myostroma Framework of muscle tissue.

myotatic reflex See **deep tendon reflex.**

myotenotomy Division of the whole or part of a muscle by cutting through its main tendon.

myotome 1. The muscle plate of an embryonic somite that develops into a voluntary muscle. Also called **myomere.** 2. A group of muscles innervated by a single spinal segment. 3. An instrument for cutting a muscle.

myotomic muscle Any of the numerous muscles of the trunk of the body, derived from the myotomes and divided into the deep muscles of the back and the thoracicoabdominal muscles.

myotomy The cutting of a muscle, performed to gain access to underlying tissues or to relieve constriction in a sphincter, as in severe esophagitis. See also **abdominal surgery.**

myotonia Any condition in which a muscle or a group of muscles do not readily relax after contracting. —**myotonic** *adj.*

myotonia atrophica See **myotonic muscular dystrophy.**

myotonia congenita A rare, mild, and nonprogressive form of myotonic myopathy evident early in life. The only effects of the disorder are hypertrophy and stiffness of the muscles. Also called **Thomsen's disease.**

myotonic muscular dystrophy A severe form of muscular dystrophy marked by ptosis, facial weakness, and dysarthria. Weakness of the hands and feet precedes that in the shoulders and hips. Myotonia of the hands is usually present. Electromyography is helpful in establishing the diagnosis. Although there is no specific treatment, active and passive exercises are used to alleviate symptoms. Also called **myotonia atrophica, Steinert's disease.**

myotonic myopathy Any of a group of disorders characterized by increased skeletal muscle tone and decreased relaxation of muscle after contraction. Kinds of myotonic myopathy include **myotonia congenita, myotonic muscular dystrophy.**

myria- A combining form meaning 'a great number': *myriapod.*

myringa See **tympanic membrane.**

myringectomy Excision of the tympanic membrane.

myringitis Inflammation or infection of the tympanic membrane.

myringo- A combining form meaning 'related to the tympanic membrane': *myringodectomy, myringoplasty, myringoscope.*

myringomycosis A fungal infection of the tympanic membrane. Also called **mycomyringitis.**

myringoplasty Surgical repair of perforations of the eardrum with a tissue graft, performed to correct hearing loss. The openings in the eardrum are enlarged, and the grafting material is sutured over them. After surgery, an antihistamine with an ephedrine derivitive is given. The nurse keeps the outer ear clean and dry. Debris is removed by gentle suctioning about 12 days after surgery. See also **myringotomy.**

myringotomy Surgical incision of the eardrum, performed to relieve pressure and release fluid or purulent material from the middle ear.

Antibiotics are given before surgery and continued afterward. The drum is incised and cultures are taken; fluid is gently suctioned from the middle ear. Small tubes may be inserted to allow continued drainage for several months. These tubes are expelled within 6 months, and the incision then heals. The nurse cautions against putting cotton in the canal, since the ear must drain freely. The outer ear is kept clean and dry. If pain increases, the procedure may have to be repeated. Severe headache or disorientation must be reported. See also **myringoplasty.**

mysophobia, misophobia An anxiety disorder characterized by an overreaction to uncleanliness or by an irrational fear of dirt or defilement. —**mysophobic, misophobic,** *adj.*

myxedema A condition resulting from advanced hypothyroidism and marked by dry, waxy swelling (nonpitting edema), with abnormal deposits of mucin in the skin (mucinosis) and other tissues. Swollen lips and a thickened nose are characteristic facial changes. Also called adult **hypothyroidism.** —**myxedematous,** *adj.*

myxo- A combining form meaning 'relating to mucus': *myxoblastoma, myxocyte, myxoma.*

myxofibroma A fibrous tumor that contains myxomatous tissue.

myxoma A neoplasm of the connective tissue, composed of stellate cells in a loose mucoid matrix crossed by delicate reticulum fibers. These tumors may grow to enormous size and are usually pale gray, soft, and jellylike; they may occur under the skin but are also found in bones, the genitourinary tract, and the retroperitoneal area. Some have exceeded 30 cm (12 inches) in diameter. —**myxomatous,** *adj.*

-myxoma A combining form meaning a 'soft tumor made up of primitive connective tissues': *adenomyxoma.*

myxoma fibrosum See **myxofibroma.**

myxoma sarcomatosum See **myxosarcoma.**

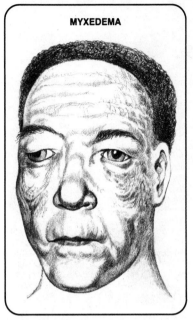

MYXEDEMA

myxopoiesis The production of mucus.

myxosarcoma A sarcoma that contains some myxomatous tissue. Also called **myxoma sarcomatosum.**

myxovirus Any of a group of medium-sized RNA viruses that are further divided into orthomyxoviruses and paramyxoviruses. Infection with these viruses is usually transmitted by the respiratory secretions of an infected host. Some kinds of myxoviruses are those that cause influenza, mumps, and parainfluenza.

MZ *abbr* monozygotic.

N

n, 2n, 3n, 4n   Symbols for the haploid, diploid, triploid, and tetraploid number of chromosomes in a cell, organism, strain, or individual.

N   1. Symbol for **normal.** 2. *abbr* **node** in the TNM system for staging malignant neoplastic disease. See also **cancer staging.** 3. Symbol for **nitrogen.**

Na   Chemical symbol for **sodium.**

N₂O   Symbol for **nitrous oxide.**

NAACOG   *abbr* **Nurses Association of the American College of Obstetrics and Gynecology.**

Nabothian cyst   A cyst formed in a Nabothian gland of the uterine cervix. It is a common finding on routine pelvic examination of women of reproductive age, especially in women who have borne children. The cyst, which is pearly white and firm, seldom results in adverse or pathologic effects.

Nabothian gland   One of many small, mucus-secreting glands of the uterine cervix.

nadir   The lowest point on a curve or scale, often related to blood counts, as in "Cancer chemotherapy produces a *nadir* in the leukocyte count after several days."

nadolol   A sympatholytic antihypertensive that is a beta-adrenergic blocking agent.

Naegeli's leukemia   See **monocytic leukemia.**

nafcillin sodium   A penicillin antibiotic.

Nägele's obliquity   See **asynclitism.**

Nägele's rule   A method for calculating the estimated date of delivery based on a mean length of gestation. Three months are subtracted from the 1st day of the last normal menstrual period, and 7 days are added to that date. See also **expected date of confinement.**

Nager's acrofacial dysostosis   An abnormal congenital condition characterized by limb deformities, as radioulnar synostosis, hypoplasia, and the absence of the radius or of the thumbs. Compare **cleidocranial dysostosis, craniofacial dysostosis, mandibulofacial dysostosis.**

Nahrungs Einheit Milch (nem)   A nutritional unit in Pirquet's system of feeding that is equivalent to 1 g of breast milk.

nail   A flattened, elastic structure with a horny texture at the end of a finger or a toe. Each nail consists of a root, body, and free edge at the distal extremity. The root fastens the nail to the finger or toe by fitting into a groove in the skin and is closely molded to the surface of the corium. The nail matrix beneath the body and the root projects longitudinal vascular ridges, which are easily visible through the translucent tissue of the body. The matrix firmly attaches the body of the nail to the underlying connective tissue. The whitish lunula near the root contains irregularly arranged papillae, which are less firmly attached to the connective tissue than the rest of the matrix. The cuticle is attached to the nail surface just ahead of the root. The superficial horny part of the nail consists of the thick stratum lucidum, the thin stratum corneum, which forms the eponychium overlapping the lunula, and the stratum mucosum. The nails grow longer by cell proliferation in the stratum germinativum at the root. They grow thicker from proliferation of that part of the stratum germinativum underlying the lunula. Also called **unguis.**

nalbuphine hydrochloride   A narcotic analgesic with narcotic antagonist activity.

nalidixic acid   A urinary tract antiseptic.

naloxone   A narcotic antagonist.

NAMH   *abbr* National Association for Mental Health. See **Mental Health Association.**

NANB   *abbr* **non-A, non-B hepatitis.**

nandrolone decanoate, n. phenpropionate   Anabolic steroids.

nanism   An abnormal smallness or underdevelopment of the body; dwarfism. Kinds of nanism are **mulibrey nanism, Paltauf's nanism, pituitary nanism, renal nanism, senile nanism, symptomatic nanism.** Also called nanosomia. —**nanus,** *n.*

nano-   A combining form meaning 'small, or related to smallness or dwarfism': *nanocephalia, nanocormia, nanomelia.*

nanocephalic dwarf   See **bird-headed dwarf.**

nanocephaly, nanocephalia, nanocephalism   A developmental defect characterized by abnormal smallness of the head. —**nanocephalous,** *adj.,* **nanocephalus,** *n.*

nanocormia   A developmental defect characterized by abnormal and disproportionate smallness of the trunk of the body in comparison to the head and limbs. —**nanocormus,** *n.*

nanocurie (nC, nc)   A unit of radiation equal to one billionth of a curie.

nanogram   See **millimicrogram.**

nanomelia   A developmental defect characterized by abnormally small limbs in comparison to the size of the head and trunk. —**nanomelous,** *adj.,* **nanomelus,** *n.*

nanophthalmos, nanophthalmia   The condition in which one or both eyes are abnormally small, although other ocular defects are not present. See also **microphthalmos.**

nanosomus   A person of extremely short stature; a dwarf.

nanukayami   An acute, infectious disease

caused by one of the serotypes of the spirochete *Leptospira* that is indigenous to Japan. See also **leptospirosis.**

nanus   **1.** A dwarf. **2.** A pygmy. —**nanoid,** *adj.*

nape   The back of the neck.

naphazoline hydrochloride   A sympathomimetic vasoconstrictor used as a nasal decongestant and ophthalmic vasoconstrictor.

naphthalene poisoning   A toxic condition, caused by the ingestion of naphthalene or paradichlorobenzene, that may cause nausea, vomiting, headache, abdominal pain, spasm, and convulsions. Treatment may include induced emesis, lavage, a saline cathartic, and sodium bicarbonate. Blood transfusion and fluid replacement may be necessary. Diazepam is indicated for the control of involuntary muscular contractions. Naphthalene and paradichlorobenzene are common ingredients in mothballs and moth crystals; paradichlorobenzene is also used as an insecticide in agriculture.

naphthol camphor   A syrupy mixture of two parts of camphor and one part betanaphthol, used externally as an antiseptic.

naphthol poisoning   See **phenol poisoning.**

napkin-ring tumor   A tumor that encircles a tubular structure of the body, usually impairing its function and constricting its lumen to some degree. These tumors are typical of colorectal cancer of the sigmoid colon.

NAP-NAP   *abbr* **National Association of Pediatric Nurse Associates/Practitioners.**

NAPNES   *abbr* **National Association for Practical Nurse Education and Services.**

naproxen, n. sodium   Nonsteroidal antiinflammatory agents.

narcissism   **1.** An abnormal interest in oneself, especially in one's own body and sexual characteristics; self-love. **2.** In psychoanalysis: sexual self-interest that is a normal characteristic of the phallic stage of psychosexual development, occurring as the infantile ego acquires a libido. Narcissism in the adult is abnormal, representing fixation at this stage of development or regression to it. Compare **egotism.** See also **narcissistic personality disorder.**

narcissistic personality disorder   A condition characterized by an exaggerated sense of self-importance and uniqueness, an abnormal need for attention and admiration, preoccupation with grandiose fantasies concerning the self, and disturbances in interpersonal relationships, usually involving the exploitation of others and a lack of empathy for them. Symptoms include depression, egocentricity, self-consciousness, inconsiderateness, inconsistency, preoccupation with grooming and remaining youthful, and intense concern with psychosomatic pains and illnesses. Treatment depends on the individual and the severity of the condition. See also **histrionic personality disorder.**

narco-   A combining form meaning 'related to stupor or a stuporous state': *narcolepsy, narcomania, narcotic.*

narcoanesthesia   See **basal anesthesia.**

narcolepsy   A syndrome characterized by sudden sleep attacks, cataplexy, sleep paralysis, and visual or auditory hallucinations that occur at the onset of sleep. The syndrome begins in adolescence or young adulthood and persists throughout life. Its cause is unknown, and no pathological lesions are found in the brain. Persons with narcolepsy experience an uncontrollable desire to sleep, sometimes many times in one day. Episodes may last from a few minutes to several hours. Momentary loss of muscle tone occurs during waking hours (cataplexy), or while the person is asleep. Narcolepsy may be difficult to diagnose because all persons with the disorder do not experience all four symptoms. EEG or other brain studies may be necessary to distinguish narcolepsy from disorders such as an intracranial mass or encephalitis. Amphetamines and other stimulant drugs are prescribed effectively to prevent the attacks. —**narcoleptic,** *adj.*

narcoleptic   **1.** Of or pertaining to a condition or substance that causes an uncontrollable desire for sleep. **2.** A narcoleptic drug. **3.** A person suffering from narcolepsy.

narcosis   A state of insensibility or stupor that is caused by narcotic drugs. See also **narcotic.**

narcotic   In pharmacology: **1.** Of or pertaining to a substance that produces insensibility or stupor. **2.** A narcotic drug. Narcotic analgesics, derived from opium or produced synthetically, alter perception of pain; induce euphoria, mood changes, mental clouding, and deep sleep; depress respiration and the cough reflex; constrict the pupils; and cause smooth muscle spasm, decreased peristalsis, emesis, and nausea.

-narcotic   A combining form meaning 'pertaining to analgesic or soporific drugs': *antinarcotic, prenarcotic.* Also **-narcotical.**

narcotic agonist-antagonist   A drug that acts both as a narcotic and a narcotic antagonist. Such drugs are thought to depress the central nervous system less than narcotics. Examples are nalbuphine hydrochloride and butorphanol tartrate.

narcotic analgesic   See **analgesic.**

narcotic antagonist   A drug that is used primarily in the treatment of narcotic-induced respiratory depression. The narcotic antagonists levallorphan and naloxone are usually administered parenterally. See also **antagonist drug.**

narcotic antitussive   See **antitussive.**

nares, *sing.* **naris**   The pairs of anterior and posterior openings in the nose that allow the passage of air from the nose to the pharynx and the lungs during respiration. See also **anterior nares, posterior nares.**

nasal   Of or pertaining to the nose and the nasal cavity. —**nasally,** *adv.*

nasal cavity   One of a pair of cavities that open on the face through the pear-shaped anterior nasal aperture and communicate with the pharynx.

nasal decongestant   A drug that provides

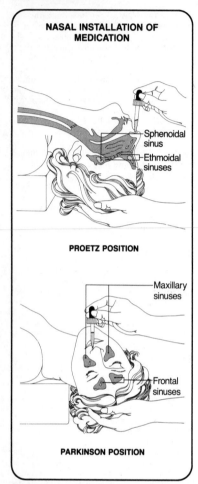

NASAL INSTALLATION OF MEDICATION

Sphenoidal sinus

Ethmoidal sinuses

PROETZ POSITION

Maxillary sinuses

Frontal sinuses

PARKINSON POSITION

ferior nasal conchae. The olfactory region is located in the most superior part of the fossa and contains olfactory cells, olfactory nerves, and olfactory hairs. The respiratory region is lined with mucous membrane, numerous glands, nerves, a plexus of dilated veins, and blood spaces. The plexus is easily irritated, causing the membrane to swell, blocking the meatuses and the openings of sinuses.

nasal glioma A neoplasm characterized by the ectopic growth of neural tissue in the nasal cavity.

nasal instillation of medication The instillation of a medicated solution into the nostrils by drops from a dropper or by an atomized spray from a squeeze bottle.

nasalis One of the three muscles of the nose, divided into a transverse part and an alar part. The transverse part arises from the maxilla and covers the bridge of the nose; the alar part attaches at one end to the greater alar cartilage and at the other end to the skin at the end of the nose. The transverse part serves to depress the cartilaginous portion of the nose and to draw the alar toward the septum. The alar part serves to dilate the nostril. The nasalis is innervated by buccal branches of the facial nerve. Compare **depressor septi, procerus.**

nasal septum The partition dividing the nostrils. It is composed of bone and cartilage covered by mucous membrane.

nasal sinus Any one of the numerous cavities in various bones of the skull, lined with ciliated mucous membrane continuous with that of the nasal cavity. The membrane is very sensitive; easily irritated, it may cause swelling that blocks the sinuses. The nasal sinuses are divided into frontal sinuses, ethmoidal air cells, sphenoidal sinuses, and maxillary sinuses. Also called **air cells of the nose.**

nascent **1.** Just born; beginning to exist; incipient. **2.** In chemistry: pertaining to any substance liberated during a chemical reaction, which, because of its uncombined state, is more reactive.

nasion **1.** The anthropometric reference point at the front of the skull where the midsagittal plane intersects a horizontal line tangential to the highest points in the superior palpebral sulci. **2.** The depression at the root of the nose that indicates the frontonasal suture.

naso-, nas- A combining form meaning 'of or pertaining to the nose': *nasociliary, nasolabial, nasonnement.*

nasogastric feeding The process of introducing nutrients in a liquid form directly into the stomach via a nasogastric tube. Also called **gavage feeding.** See also **nasogastric intubation.**

nasogastric intubation The placement of a nasogastric tube through the nose into the stomach in order to relieve gastric distention by removing gas, gastric secretions, or food; to instill medication, food, or fluids; or to obtain a specimen for laboratory analysis. After surgery and in any condition in which the person is able

temporary relief of nasal symptoms in acute and chronic rhinitis and sinusitis. Most are over-the-counter products compounded with a small amount of vasoconstrictor, as ephedrine or phenylephrine. An antihistamine may enhance the value of a nasal decongestant in allergic rhinitis, and a corticosteroid may reduce inflammation. Prolonged use or dosage greater than recommended on the package label may cause rebound vasodilatation and severe congestion.

nasal fossa One of the pair of approximately equal chambers of the nasal cavity, which are separated by the nasal septum and open externally through the nostrils and internally into the nasopharynx through the choanae. Each fossa is divided into an olfactory region, consisting of the superior nasal concha and part of the septum and a respiratory region, constituting the rest of the chamber. Overhanging the three meatuses of each fossa on the lateral wall are the corresponding superior, middle, and into digest food but not eat it, the tube may be introduced and left in place for tube feeding until the ability to eat normally is restored.

nasogastric tube Any tube passed into the stomach through the nose. See **nasogastric intubation.**

nasolabial reflex A sudden backward movement of the head, arching of the back, and extension and stretching of the limbs that occurs in infants in response to a light touch to the tip of the nose with an upward sweeping motion. The reflex disappears by about 5 months of age.

nasolacrimal Of or pertaining to the nasal cavity and associated lacrimal ducts.

nasolacrimal duct A channel that carries tears from the lacrimal sac to the nasal cavity.

nasomandibular fixation A type of maxillomandibular fixation to stabilize fractures of the jaw by using maxillomandibular splints connected to a wire through a hole drilled in the anterior nasal spine of the maxillary bone. It has been used particularly in edentulous patients. See also **maxillomandibular fixation.**

nasopharyngeal angiofibroma A benign tumor of the nasopharynx, consisting of fibrous connective tissue with many vascular spaces. The tumor usually arises in puberty and is more common in boys than in girls. Typical signs are nasal and eustachian tube obstruction, adenoidal speech, and dysphagia. Also called **juvenile angiofibroma.**

nasopharyngeal cancer A malignant neoplastic disease of the nasopharynx. Depending on the site of a nasopharyngeal tumor, there may be nasal obstruction, otitis media, hearing loss, sensory or motor nerve damage, bony destruction of the skull, or deep cervical lymphadenopathy. Diagnostic measures include nasopharyngoscopy, biopsy, and radiologic examination of the skull with tomographic studies. Squamous cell and undifferentiated carcinomas are the most common lesions. Radiation is the most effective therapy, and 5-fluorouracil and adriamycin are also used.

nasopharyngoscopy A technique in physical examination in which the nose and throat are visually examined using a laryngoscope, a fiberoptic device, a flashlight, and a dilator for the nares. —**nasopharyngoscopic,** *adj.*

nasopharynx One of the three regions of the throat, situated behind the nose and extending from the posterior nares to the level of the soft palate. On the posterior wall of the nasopharynx, opposite the posterior nares, are the pharyngeal tonsils. Compare **laryngopharynx, oropharynx.** See also **tonsil.** —**nasopharyngeal,** *adj.*

nasotracheal tube A catheter inserted into the trachea through the nasal cavity and the pharynx. It is commonly used to administer oxygen and in other respiratory therapy.

natal 1. Of or pertaining to birth. **2.** Of or pertaining to the nates, or buttocks.

natamycin An ophthalmic anti-infective agent.

nates, *sing.* **natis** The large fleshy protu-

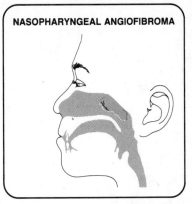

NASOPHARYNGEAL ANGIOFIBROMA

berances at the lower posterior portion of the torso comprising fat and the gluteal muscles. Also called **buttocks.**

National Association for Mental Health See **Mental Health Association.**

National Association for Practical Nurse Education and Services (NAPNES) A national professional organization concerned with the education of practical nurses and with the services provided by licensed practical nurses.

National Association of Pediatric Nurse Associates/Practitioners (NAP-NAP) A national organization of nurses who are prepared by training or experience to give primary care to pediatric patients. NAP-NAP works in conjunction with the American Academy of Pediatrics.

National Bureau of Standards (NBS) A federal agency in the Department of Commerce that sets accurate measurement standards for commerce, industry, and science in the United States. The NBS compares and coordinates its standards with those of other countries and provides research and technical service to improve computer science, materials technology, building construction, and consumer product safety.

National Eye Institute (NEI) A division of the National Institutes of Health. NEI was established in 1968 to support research in the normal functioning of the human eye and visual system, the pathology of visual disorders, and the rehabilitation of the visually handicapped. See also **eye, vision.**

National Formulary (NF) A publication containing the official standards for the preparation of various pharmaceuticals not listed in the *United States Pharmacopoeia.*

National Health Service Corps (NHSC) A program of the United States Public Health Service (USPHS) in which health-care personnel are placed in areas that are underserved. Nurses, physicians, and dentists serve in rural and urban areas, usually as employees of local health-care agencies. The USPHS pays most of the salary of each corps member.

National Institute of Child Health and Human Development (NICHHD) The

NATURAL DENTITION

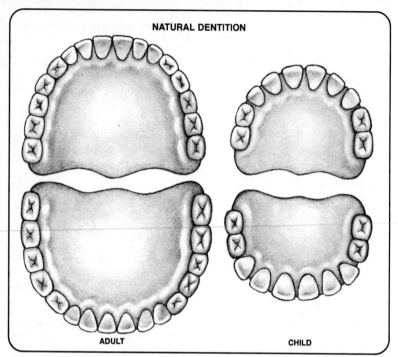

ADULT   CHILD

Institute in the National Institutes of Health that is concerned with all aspects of the growth, development, and health of the children of the United States.

National Institutes of Health (NIH) An agency within the United States Public Health Service made up of several institutions and constituent divisions, including the Bureau of Health Manpower Education, the National Library of Medicine, the National Cancer Institute, National Institute on Aging, and several research institutes and divisions.

National League for Nursing (NLN) An organization concerned with the improvement of nursing education, nursing service, and the delivery of health care in the United States. Among its many activities are accreditation of nursing programs at all levels, preadmission and achievement tests for nursing students, and compilation of statistical data on nursing manpower and on trends in health-care delivery. It acts as the testing service for the State Board Test Pool Examinations for registered and practical nurse licensure. A monthly refereed journal, *Nursing and Health Care*, is the official publication of the organization.

National Male Nurses' Association (NMNA) A national organization that promotes the interests and practice of male nurses.

National Student Nurses' Association (NSNA) A national organization of students in the field of nursing. Among its purposes are the improvement of nursing education to improve health care, to aid in the development of the student nurse, and to encourage optimal achievement in the professional role of the nurse and the health care of people. It publishes a journal, *Imprint*, five times a year, participates in legislative activities at all levels, and gives scholarships, awards, and career workshops.

natriuresis The excretion of greater-than-normal amounts of sodium in the urine, as from the administration of natriuretic diuretic drugs or from various metabolic or endocrine disorders. —**natriuretic,** *adj.*

natriuretic 1. Of or pertaining to the process of natriuresis. **2.** A substance that inhibits the resorption of sodium ions from the glomerular filtrate in the kidneys, thus allowing more sodium to be excreted with the urine.

natural childbirth Labor and parturition accomplished by a mother with little or no medical intervention. It is generally considered the optimal way of giving birth and being born: safest for the baby and most satisfying for the mother. Prerequisites include normal gestation, an adequate birth canal, strong maternal motivation, physical and emotional preparation, and constant and intensive support of the mother during labor and birth. Also called prepared childbirth. See also **Bradley method, Lamaze method, Read method.**

natural dentition The entire array of natural teeth in the dental arch, consisting of deciduous or permanent teeth or a mixture of the two. See also **tooth.**

natural family-planning method Any one of several methods of family planning that does not rely on a medication or a device for effectiveness in avoiding pregnancy. Some of the methods are also used to pinpoint the time of ovulation in order to increase the chance of fertilization when artificial insemination or extraction of an oocyte for in vitro fertilization is to be performed. Natural family-planning methods require thorough instruction, the cooperation and self-motivation of the couple, and the diligent, accurate observation and recording of the data relevant to the method. Kinds of natural family planning include **basal body temperature method of family planning, calendar method of family planning, ovulation method of family planning, symptothermal method of family planning.** Also called rhythm method.

natural immunity A usually innate and permanent form of immunity to a specific disease. Kinds of natural immunity include **individual immunity, racial immunity, species immunity.** Also called **genetic immunity, innate immunity.**

naturally acquired immunity See **acquired immunity.**

natural network In psychiatric nursing: a patient's contacts in the community, including church and social groups, friends, family, and occupation, that support the person's function outside the treatment environment.

natural selection The natural evolutionary processes by which those organisms best suited for adaptation to the environment tend to survive and propagate the species while those unfit are eliminated. Compare **artificial selection.**

naturopathy A system of therapeutics based on natural foods, regular exercise, and the avoidance of medications. Advocates believe that illness can be healed by the natural processes of the body.

Nauheim bath A bath taken in water through which carbon dioxide is bubbled, followed by systematic exercises, used in the treatment of cardiac conditions.

nausea A sensation often leading to the urge to vomit. Common causes are sea- and motion sickness, early pregnancy, intense pain, emotional stress, gallbladder disease, food poisoning, and various enteroviruses. —**nauseate,** v., **nauseous,** adj.

nausea and vomiting of pregnancy A common condition of early pregnancy characterized by recurrent or persistent nausea, often in the morning, that may result in vomiting, weight loss, anorexia, general weakness, and malaise. It usually does not begin before the 6th week after the last menstrual period and ends by the 12th to the 14th week of pregnancy. Symptomatic relief is often obtained by eating small, easily digested meals frequently and by not allowing the stomach to be empty. In the past, antiemetic drugs were routinely prescribed for this complaint, but this practice is currently reserved for severe cases. Nausea and vomiting after the 16th week is an unusual complication

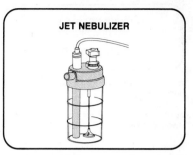

JET NEBULIZER

of pregnancy, called persistent nausea and vomiting of pregnancy. If severe and intractable, hyperemesis gravidarum may ensue. Also called **morning sickness.**

navel The depression in the abdomen at the point of insertion of the umbilical cord in the fetus. It interrupts the linea alba about halfway between the infrasternal notch and the pubic symphysis.

navicular Having the shape of a boat.

navicular bone See **scaphoid bone.**

Nb Symbol for **niobium.**

NBS abbr **National Bureau of Standards.**

NBS standard In nuclear medicine: a radioactive source standardized or certified, or both, by the National Bureau of Standards.

nC, nc abbr **nanocurie.**

N-CAP abbr **Nurses Coalition for Action in Politics.**

NCH abbr nursing care home.

NCI abbr National Cancer Institute. See **National Institutes of Health.**

Nd abbr **neodymium.**

ne- See **neo-.**

Ne Symbol for **neon.**

near-drowning A pathological state in which the victim has survived exposure to circumstances that usually cause drowning. Cardiopulmonary resuscitation is performed immediately; hospitalization is always indicated. The return of consciousness does not necessarily assure recovery. Intensive supportive therapy may be required for up to several days. Compare **drowning.** See also **hypothermia.**

nearest-neighbor analysis In molecular genetics: a biochemical method used to estimate the frequency with which pairs of bases are located next to one another.

nearsightedness See **myopia.**

nebula, pl. **nebulae. 1.** A slight corneal opacity or scar that seldom obstructs vision and that can be seen only by oblique illumination. **2.** A murkiness in the urine. **3.** An oily concoction that is applied with an atomizer.

nebulize To vaporize or disperse a liquid in a fine spray.

nebulizer A device that uses a baffle to produce a fine aerosol spray consisting of particles less than 30 micrometers in diameter. Kinds of nebulizers include jet nebulizer and ultrasonic nebulizer.

NEC abbr **necrotizing enterocolitis.**

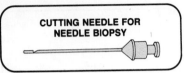

CUTTING NEEDLE FOR NEEDLE BIOPSY

neck A constricted section, as the part of the body that connects the head with the trunk. Other such constrictions are the neck of the humerus and the neck of the femur.

neck dissection Surgical removal of the cervical lymph nodes, performed to prevent the spread of malignant tumors of the head and neck. Compare **radical neck dissection.**

neck-righting reflex **1.** An involuntary, normal neonatal response in which turning the head to one side while the neonate is supine causes rotation of the shoulders and trunk in the same direction. The reflex enables the infant to roll over from the supine to prone position. Absence of the reflex or persistence beyond about 10 months of age may indicate central nervous system damage. **2.** Any tonic reflex associated with the neck that maintains body orientation in relation to the head.

necro- A combining form meaning 'of or pertaining to death or a corpse': *necrobiosis, necronectomy.*

necrobiosis lipoidica A skin disease characterized by thin, shiny, yellow to red plaques on the shins or forearms. Telangiectases, crusting, and ulceration of these plaques may occur. Necrobiosis lipoidica is usually associated with diabetes mellitus. Treatment includes precise control of the diabetes and, possibly, intralesional application of corticosteroids.

necrolysis Disintegration or exfoliation of dead tissue. Compare **necrosis. —necrolytic,** *adj.*

necrophilia **1.** A morbid obsession with and usually sexual attraction for dead bodies. **2.** The sexual violation of a corpse. **—necrophile, necrophiliac,** *n.*

necropsy See **autopsy.**

necroscopy See **autopsy.**

necrosis Localized tissue death that occurs in groups of cells in response to disease or injury. In **coagulation necrosis,** blood clots block the flow of blood, causing tissue ischemia distal to the clot; in **gangrenous necrosis,** ischemia combined with bacterial action causes putrefaction to set in. See also **gangrene.**

necrotizing angiitis See **periarteritis nodosa.**

necrotizing enteritis Acute inflammation of the small and the large intestine by the bacterium *Clostridium perfringens,* characterized by severe abdominal pain, bloody diarrhea, and vomiting. Some people recover completely, some survive with chronic bowel obstruction, and some die of perforation of the intestine, dehydration, peritonitis, or septicemia.

necrotizing enterocolitis (NEC) An acute inflammatory bowel disorder that occurs primarily in preterm or low-birth-weight neonates. It is characterized by ischemic necrosis of the gastrointestinal mucosa that may lead to perforation and peritonitis. The cause of the disorder is unknown, although it appears to be a defect in host defenses with infection resulting from normal gastrointestinal flora rather than from invading organisms. Initial symptoms, which usually develop after several days of life, include temperature instability (usually hypothermia), lethargy, poor feeding, vomiting of bile, abdominal distention, blood in the stools, and decreased or absent bowel sounds. Signs of deterioration are apnea, pallor, hyperbilirubinemia, oliguria, abdominal tenderness, erythema and edema of the anterior abdominal wall or palpable masses, with eventual respiratory failure leading to death. Diagnosis is confirmed by X-ray visualization of the intestine or by the presence of increased peritoneal fluid or pneumoperitoneum. Treatment includes discontinuing oral feeding, beginning intravenous infusion, abdominial decompression by nasogastric suction, hydration, plasma or whole blood transfusion, and administration of antibiotics (usually ampicillin, gentamicin, or kanamycin).

NURSING CONSIDERATIONS: The primary concern of the nurse is to observe high-risk, formula-fed infants for early symptoms of necrotizing enterocolitis, especially for difficulty in feeding, bile-stained regurgitation, bloody stools, temperature variations, or a distended, shiny abdomen. Once the diagnosis is confirmed, the nurse initiates nasogastric intubation for abdominal decompression and continues to monitor the infant constantly for dehydration and electrolyte balance. In addition to the ordered laboratory tests, daily weight is taken. Infants who are unable to take fluids by mouth require special oral care. Glycerin and lemon swabs reduce dryness, and a pacifier or a nipple stuffed with gauze helps to meet the infant's need to suck. Parents are encouraged to visit and are helped to meet the emotional needs of the infant and to provide tactile, auditory, and visual stimulation. The nurse explains the usual course of the disease and the medical and nursing procedures, and keeps the parents informed of the infant's progress. Frequent visits to the care unit facilitate family-infant relationships, and provide the nurse with an opportunity to teach proper care techniques prior to discharge. Also called **pseudomembranous enterocolitis.** See also **enteritis.**

necrotizing vasculitis An inflammatory condition of blood vessels, characterized by necrosis, fibrosis, and proliferation of the inner layer of the vascular wall, in some cases resulting in occlusion and infarction. Necrotizing vasculitis may occur in rheumatoid arthritis and is common in systemic lupus erythematosus, periarteritis nodosa, and progressive systemic sclerosis. The condition is usually treated with corticosteroids.

needle biopsy The removal of a segment of living tissue for microscopic examination by inserting a hollow needle through the skin or the external surface of an organ or tumor and rotating it within the underlying cellular layers. See also **aspiration biopsy.**

needle filter A device, usually made of plastic, used for filtering medications that are drawn into a syringe before administration. Some syringe needles are equipped with built-in filters; other filters are separate units that are attached to the needle before use.

negative **1.** Of a laboratory test: indicating that a substance or a reaction is not present. **2.** Of a sign: indicating on physical examination that a finding is not present, often meaning that there is no pathologic change. **3.** Of a substance: tending to carry or carrying a negative chemical charge.

negative adaptation See **habituation.**

negative anxiety In psychology: an emotional and psychological condition in which anxiety prevents a person's normal functioning and interrupts the person's ability to perform the usual activities of daily living.

negative catalysis A decrease in the rate of any chemical reaction caused by a substance that is neither part of the process itself nor consumed nor affected by the reaction. Compare **catalysis.** See also **catalyst.**

negative feedback **1.** In physiology: a decrease in function in response to a stimulus, as the secretion of follicle-stimulating hormone decreases as the amount of circulating estrogen increases. **2.** *Informal.* A critical, derogatory, or otherwise negative response.

negative pi meson (pion) A form of electromagnetic radiation emitted from a proton linear accelerator. In the treatment of certain tumors, negative pi meson particles are beamed at the tumor; the atomic nuclei of malignant cells take in the radioactive particles and explode, scattering intensely radioactive subatomic particles through the adjacent malignant tissue.

negative pi meson (pion) radiotherapy A form of radiotherapy using a negative pi meson beam emitted by a proton linear accelerator. Pion radiotherapy requires fewer rad and has a 60% greater biologic effect than conventional, X-radiation techniques. Some locally advanced neoplasms, especially those of the prostate, are destroyed. Gliomas and advanced cancers of the head and neck may also be well controlled with pion radiotherapy.

negative pressure Less-than-ambient atmospheric pressure, as in a vacuum, at an altitude above sea level, or in a hypobaric chamber. Some ventilators have a negative cycle that may help stimulate or cycle exhalation in controlled ventilation in IPPB therapy.

negative relationship In research: an inverse relationship between two variables; as one variable increases the other decreases. Also called **inverse relationship.** Compare **positive relationship.**

negativism A behavioral attitude characterized by opposition, resistance, the refusal to cooperate with even the most reasonable request, and the tendency to act in a contrary man-

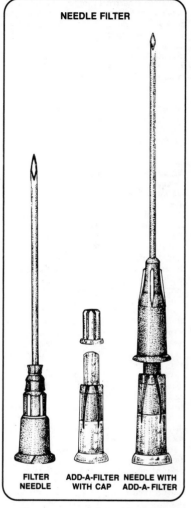

NEEDLE FILTER

FILTER NEEDLE   ADD-A-FILTER WITH CAP   NEEDLE WITH ADD-A-FILTER

ner. The response may be passive, as the immobile, rigid postures observed in catatonic schizophrenia, or active, as in a belligerent, impulsive, or capricious act, such as lowering the arms when asked to raise them.

negatol A local hemostatic agent.

negligence In law: the commission of an act that a prudent person would not have done or the omission of a duty that a prudent person would have fulfilled, resulting in injury or harm to another person. In particular, in a malpractice suit, a professional person is negligent if harm to a client results from such an act or such failure to act, but it must be proved that other prudent persons of the same profession would ordinarily have acted differently under the same circumstances.

negligence per se In law: a finding of

negligence rendered in judgment of a professional action or inaction in violation of a statute or so at odds with common sense that, beyond any doubt, no prudent person would have been guilty of it.

negotiation The process of resolving a conflict by arriving at a mutually acceptable solution through conference, discussion, and compromise.

NEI *abbr* **National Eye Institute.**

Neisseria gonorrhoeae A gram-negative, nonmotile, diplococcal bacterium usually seen microscopically as flattened pairs within the cytoplasm of neutrophils. It is the causative organism of gonorrhea. Also called **gonococcus.**

Neisseria meningitidis See **meningococcus.**

NEJM abbr New England Journal of Medicine.

Nelson's syndrome An endocrine disorder that may follow adrenalectomy for Cushing's disease. It is characterized by a marked increase in the secretion of ACTH and MSH by the pituitary gland. Treatment includes irradiation to decrease pituitary function and, in some cases, hypophysectomy. See also **Cushing's disease.**

nem *abbr* **Nahrungs Einheit Milch** (German for 'nutritional unit milk').

-nema A combining form meaning a 'threadlike stage in the development of chromosomes': *chromonema, plasmonema, uronema.*

nemato- A combining form meaning 'pertaining to a nematode, or to a threadlike structure': *nematoblast, nematocide, nematodiasis.*

nematode A multicellular, parasitic animal of the phylum Nematoda. All roundworms belong to the phylum, including *Ancylostoma duodenale, Ascaris lumbricoides, Enterobius vermicularis, Necator americanus, Strongyloides stercoralis,* and several other species.

-nemia See **-anemia.**

neo-, ne- A combining form meaning 'new': *neobiogenesis, neocyte, neonatal.*

neoantigen A new specific antigen that develops in a cell infected by oncogenic virus.

neobehaviorism A school of psychology based on the general principles of behaviorism but broader and more flexible in concept. It stresses experimental research and laboratory analyses in the study of overt behavior and in various subjective phenomena that cannot be directly observed and measured, as fantasies, love, stress, empathy, trust, and personality. See also **behaviorism.**

neoblastic Of or pertaining to a new tissue or development within a new tissue.

neodymium (Nd) A rare earth element. Its atomic number is 60; its atomic weight is 144.27.

neologism 1. A newly coined word or term. 2. In psychiatry: a word coined by a psychotic or a delirious patient that is meaningful only to the patient.

neomycin sulfate An aminoglycoside antibiotic, also used as an ophthalmic, otic, and local anti-infective agent.

neon (Ne) A colorless, odorless gaseous element and one of the inert gases. Its atomic number is 10; its atomic weight is 20.2. Neon has no compounds and occurs in the atmosphere in the ratio of about 18 parts per million. Some minerals and meteorites contain traces of this element. It is prepared commercially by the fractional distillation of liquefied air and is one of the first components to boil off. Neon is an excellent conductor of electricity, which ionizes the gas and causes it to emit a reddish-orange glow; this characteristic makes neon useful in devices to warn against electric current overload.

Neonatal Behavior Assessment Scale A scale for evaluating and assessing an infant's alertness, motor maturity, irritability, consolability, and interaction with people. It is used as a tool for the evaluation of the neurologic condition as well as the behavior of a newborn infant. Using the scale, the individuality of an infant may be demonstrated for parents, and some researchers theorize that the quality of the parent-child relationship may be predicted.

neonatal breathing Respiration in newborn infants, which begins when pulmonary fluid in the lungs is expelled by mechanical compression of the thorax during delivery and by resorption from the alveoli into the bloodstream and lymphatics. As air enters the lungs, the chest and lungs recoil to a resting position, but forceful inspirations are necessary to keep the lungs inflated. These forces come from changes in blood gas tension, strong Hering-Breuer reflexes, temperature, and tactile stimuli. Irregular fetal breathing movements, which occur during rapideye-movement sleep, may be observed as early as 13 weeks of gestation. At birth, the peripheral and central chemoreceptors are very active, and newborns are highly sensitive to carbon dioxide during the first weeks. However, control of rhythm is not fully developed at birth.

neonatal developmental profile An evaluation of the developmental status of a newborn infant based on three examinations: a gestational age inventory, a neurologic examination, and a Neonatal Behavior Assessment score.

neonatal hyperbilirubinemia See **hyperbilirubinemia of the newborn.**

neonatal intensive care unit (NICU) A hospital unit containing a variety of sophisticated mechanical devices and special equipment for the management and care of premature and seriously ill newborn infants. The unit is staffed by a team of nurses and neonatologists who are highly trained in the pathophysiology of the newborn.

neonatal mortality The statistical rate of infant death during the first 28 days after live birth, expressed as the number of such deaths per 1,000 live births in a specific geographic area or institution in a given period of time.

neonatal period The interval from birth to 28 days of age. It represents the time of the greatest risk to the infant; approximately 65% of all deaths that occur in the 1st year of life happen during this period.

ESSENTIAL DIFFERENCES BETWEEN BENIGN AND MALIGNANT NEOPLASMS

TRAITS	BENIGN	MALIGNANT
Growth	Slow expansion; push aside surrounding tissue but do not infiltrate	Usually infiltrate surrounding tissues rapidly, expanding in all directions
Limitation	Frequently encapsulated	Seldom encapsulated; often poorly delineated
Recurrence	Rare after surgical removal	When removed surgically, frequently recur due to infiltration into surrounding tissues
Morphology	Cells closely resemble cells of tissue of origin	Cells may differ considerably from those of tissue of origin
Differentiation	Well differentiated	Poor or no differentiation
Mitotic activity	Slight	Extensive
Tissue destruction	Usually slight	Extensive due to infiltration and metastatic lesion
Spread	No metastasis	Spread via blood and/or lymph systems; establish secondary tumors
Effect on body	Cachexia rare; usually not fatal but may obstruct vital organs, exert pressure, produce excess hormones; can become malignant	Cachexia typical—anemia, loss of weight, weakness, etc.; fatal if untreated

neonatal pustular melanosis A transient skin condition of the neonate characterized by vesicles present at birth that become pustular. The lesions contain neutrophils rather than eosinophils as seen in erythema toxicum neonatorum, and they disappear within 72 hours, leaving dark spots that fade by about 3 months of age.

neonatal thermoregulation The regulation of the body temperature of a newborn infant, which may be affected by evaporation, conduction, radiation, and convection.

neonatal tyrosinemia See **tyrosinemia.**

neonate An infant from birth to 4 weeks of age. —**neonatal,** adj.

neonatology The branch of medicine that concentrates on the care of the neonate and specializes in the diagnosis and treatment of disorders of the newborn infant. —**neonatologic, neonatological,** adj., **neonatologist,** n.

neoplasm Any abnormal growth of new tissue, benign or malignant. See also **benign, malignant.** —**neoplastic, neoplasia,** adj.

neoplastic fracture A fracture resulting from weakened bone tissue caused by neoplasm or by a malignant growth. Also called **pathologic fracture.**

neostigmine bromide, n. methylsulfate Cholinergic (parasympathomimetic) agents.

neoteny The attainment of sexual maturity during the larval stage of development, as in certain amphibians, especially salamanders.

nephelometer An apparatus used to determine the concentration of solids suspended in a liquid or a gas, as may be used to determine the number of bacteria in a specimen. —**nephelometry,** n.

nephr- See **nephro-.**

nephrectomy The surgical removal of a kidney, performed to remove a tumor, drain an abcess, or treat hydronephrosis.

NURSING CONSIDERATIONS: Postoperatively, the nurse observes carefully for rapid pulse, restlessness, sweating, and a drop in blood pressure. The urinary output is measured hourly, and fluid intake and body weight are closely monitored. Deep breathing is difficult because the incision is close to the diaphragm; intermittent positive pressure breathing apparatus is used to drain secretions. The nurse reports at once any sudden shortness of breath, a sign of spontaneous pneumothorax that may occur if the pleura was accidentally nicked during surgery.

-nephric A combining form meaning 'of or referring to the kidneys': archinephric, cardionephric, splenonephric.

nephritis Any one of a large group of diseases of the kidney characterized by inflammation and abnormal function.

nephro-, nephr- A combining form mean-

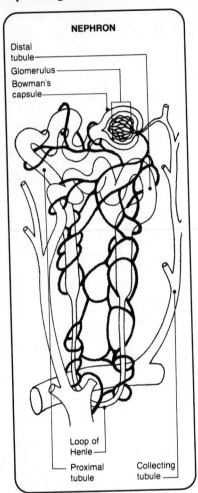

NEPHRON

Distal tubule
Glomerulus
Bowman's capsule
Loop of Henle
Proximal tubule
Collecting tubule

ing 'of or related to the kidneys': *nephroblastoma, nephrogram, nephrorrhagia.*

nephroangiosclerosis Necrosis of the renal arterioles, associated with hypertension. Early signs of the condition are headaches, blurring of vision, and a diastolic blood pressure greater than 120 mmHg. Examination of the retina reveals hemorrhages, vascular exudates, and papilledema. The heart is usually enlarged, especially the left ventricle. Proteins and red blood cells are found in the urine. Heart failure and kidney failure may occur if the disease remains untreated. Treatment includes measures to lower blood pressure using diet and antihypertensive medications. Hemodialysis is used when preventive measures have failed. Also called **malignant hypertension.** See also **hypertension, renal failure.**

nephroblastoma See **Wilms' tumor.**

nephrocalcinosis An abnormal condition of the kidneys in which deposits of calcium form in the parenchyma at the site of previous inflammation or degenerative change. Infection, hematuria, renal colic, and decreased function of the kidney may occur.

nephrogenic **1.** Generating kidney tissue. **2.** Originating in the kidney.

nephrogenic ascites The abnormal presence of fluid in the peritoneal cavity of persons undergoing hemodialysis for renal failure. The cause of this type of ascites is unknown. See also **ascites.**

nephrogenic cord Either of the paired longitudinal ridges of tissue that lie along the dorsal surface of the coelom in the early developing vertebrate embryo. It is formed from the fusion of the nephrotome tissue and gives rise to the structures comprising the embryonic urogenital system. See also **mesonephros, metanephros, pronephros.**

nephrogenic diabetes insipidus An abnormal condition in which the kidneys do not concentrate the urine, resulting in polyuria, polydipsia, and very dilute urine. The secretion of antidiuretic hormone (ADH) by the pituitary is normal, and all kidney function is normal except that there is no response to ADH. See also **diabetes insipidus.**

nephrogenous Of or pertaining to the formation and development of the kidneys.

nephrolith A calculus formed in a kidney. —**nephrolithic,** *adj.*

nephrolithiasis A disorder characterized by the presence of calculi in the kidney. See also **urinary calculus.**

nephrology The study of the anatomy, physiology, and pathology of the kidney. —**nephrologic, nephrological,** *adj.*

nephrolytic Of or pertaining to the destruction of the structure and function of a kidney.

-nephroma A combining form meaning a 'tumor of the kidney or area of the kidney': *epinephroma, paranephroma.*

nephromere See **nephrotome.**

nephron, nephrone A structural and functional unit of the kidney, resembling a microscopic funnel with a long stem and two convoluted sections. Each kidney contains about 1.25 million nephrons, each consisting of the renal corpuscle, the loop of Henle, and the renal tubules. Each renal corpuscle consists of the glomerulus of renal capillaries enclosed within Bowman's capsule. The renal corpuscles and the convoluted portions of the renal tubules are located in the cortex of the kidney. The renal medulla contains the loops of Henle and the collecting tubules. Urine is formed in the renal corpuscles and in the renal tubules by filtration, reabsorption, and secretion. See also **kidney.**

nephronophthisis See **medullary cystic disease.**

nephropathy Any disorder of the kidney, including inflammatory, degenerative, and sclerotic conditions. See also **kidney disease.**

nephropexy A surgical operation to fixate a floating or ptotic kidney.

nephroptosis A downward displacement or dropping of a kidney.

nephrorrhaphy An operation that sutures a floating kidney in place.

nephrosclerosis See **nephroangiosclerosis.**

nephrosis See **nephrotic syndrome.**

nephrostoma, nephrostome, *pl.* **nephrostomata, nephrostomes** The funnel-shaped ciliated opening of the excretory tubules into the coelom of the early developing vertebrate embryo. —**nephrostomic,** *adj.*

nephrotic syndrome An abnormal condition of the kidney characterized by marked proteinuria, hypoalbuminemia, and edema. It occurs in glomerular disease, thrombosis of a renal vein, and as a complication of many systemic diseases, as diabetes mellitus, amyloidosis, systemic lupus erythematosus, and multiple myeloma. Patients with primary nephrotic syndrome usually respond favorably to corticosteroids. Diuretics are used to control edema, and dialysis may be necessary. Also called **nephrosis.**

nephrotome A zone of segmented mesodermal tissue in the developing vertebrate embryo lying along each side of the body dorsal to the abdominal cavity between the somite-forming dorsal mesoderm and the unsegmented lateral-plate mesoderm. It is the primordial tissue for the urogenital system and gives rise to the nephrogenic cord. Also called **intermediate cell mass, intermediate mesoderm, middle plate, nephromere.** See also **mesonephros, metanephros, pronephros.**

nephrotomy A surgical procedure in which an incision is made in the kidney.

nephrotoxic Toxic or destructive to a kidney.

nephrotoxin A toxin with specific destructive properties for the kidneys.

neptunium (Np) A transuranic, metallic element. Its atomic number is 93; its atomic weight is 237. Although neptunium is considered a man-made element, traces of natural neptunium have been found in uranium ores.

nerve One or more bundles of fibers outside the central nervous system that connect the brain and the spinal cord with other parts of the body. Nerves transmit afferent impulses from receptor organs toward the brain and the spinal cord and efferent impulses peripherally to the effector organs. Each nerve consists of an epineurium enclosing fasciculi of nerve fibers, each fasciculus surrounded by its own sheath of connective tissue. Individual nerve fibers, which are microscopic, consist of formed elements within a matrix of protoplasm and are wrapped in a neurilemmal sheath. Inside the neurilemma are nerve fibers, also enclosed in a myelin sheath, derived from the neurilemmal cells. See also **axon, dendrite, neuroglia, neuron.**

nerve accommodation The ability of nerve tissue to adjust to a constant source and intensity of stimulation so that some change in either intensity or duration of the stimulus is necessary

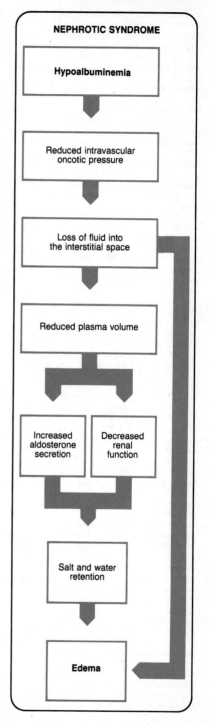

NEPHROTIC SYNDROME

Hypoalbuminemia

↓

Reduced intravascular oncotic pressure

↓

Loss of fluid into the interstitial space

↓

Reduced plasma volume

↓

Increased aldosterone secretion   Decreased renal function

↓

Salt and water retention

↓

Edema

in order to elicit a response beyond the initial reaction. Accommodation is probably owing to reduced sodium ion permeability, which causes an increased threshold intensity and subsequent stabilization of the resting membrane potential.

nerve block anesthesia See **conduction anesthesia.**

nerve compression A pathological event that causes harmful pressure on one or more nerve trunks, resulting in nerve damage and muscle weakness or atrophy. Any nerve that passes over a rigid prominence is vulnerable, and the degree of damage depends on the magnitude and the duration of the compressive force. Various factors may contribute to susceptibility, as inherited predisposition, malnutrition, trauma, and disease. Various activities associated with routine occupations may unduly compress especially vulnerable nerves, as the median nerve, the radial nerve, the femoral nerve, and the plantar nerves. Rest and the cessation or modification of causative activities often heal nerve damage owing to compression. Surgery may be required to correct more severe cases.

nerve entrapment An abnormal condition and type of mononeuropathy, characterized by nerve damage and muscle weakness or atrophy. The peripheral nerve trunks of the body are especially vulnerable to entrapment in which repeated compression results in significant impairment. Nerves that pass over rigid prominences or through narrow bony and fascial canals are particularly prone to entrapment. The common signs of this disorder are pain and muscular weakness. Nerve damage by entrapment occurs more often when adjacent joints are affected by swelling and inflammation, as in rheumatoid arthritis, pregnancy, and acromegaly. Signs of nerve entrapment may also develop after repeated bruising of certain nerves by various activities involving repeated motions, as those associated with knitting and prolonged walking. One of the most common types of entrapment is **carpal tunnel syndrome.**

nerve growth factor (NGF) A protein resembling insulin whose hormonelike action affects differentiation, growth, and maintenance of neurons.

nerve impulse See **impulse.**

nervous breakdown *Informal.* Any mental condition that markedly interferes with and disrupts normal functioning.

nervous system The extensive, intricate network of structures that activates, coordinates, and controls all the functions of the body. It is divided into the central nervous system, composed of the brain and the spinal cord, and the peripheral nervous system, which includes the cranial nerves and the spinal nerves. These morphological subdivisions combine and communicate to innervate the somatic and the visceral parts of the body with the afferent and the efferent nerve fibers. Afferent fibers carry sensory impulses to the central nervous system; efferent fibers carry motor impulses from the central nervous system to the muscles and other

organs. The somatic fibers are associated with the bones, the muscles, and the skin. The visceral fibers are associated with the internal organs, the blood vessels, and the mucous membranes. Various functions throughout the nervous system are coordinated through a vast complex of tiny structures, as neurons, axons, dendrites, and ganglia. Compare **autonomic nervous system, visceral nervous system.**

nervus abducens See **abducent nerve.**

nervus accessorius See **accessory nerve.**

nervus facialis See **facial nerve.**

nervus glossopharyngeus See **glossopharyngeal nerve.**

nervus hypoglossus See **hypoglossal nerve.**

nervus oculomotorius See **oculomotor nerve.**

nervus olfactorius See **olfactory nerve.**

nervus opticus See **optic nerve.**

nervus terminalis See **terminal nerve.**

nervus trigeminus See **trigeminal nerve.**

nervus trochlearis See **trochlear nerve.**

nervus vagus See **vagus nerve.**

nettle rash A fine, urticarial eruption resulting from skin contact with nettle, a common weed. It is characterized by stinging and itching that lasts from a few minutes to several hours.

networking **1.** In psychiatric nursing: the process of developing a set of agencies and professional personnel that are able to create a system of communication and support for psychiatric patients, usually those newly discharged from inpatient psychiatric facilities. Kinds of networks include **natural network, professional network. 2.** A network of supportive contacts or services, as the Women's Health Network.

Neufeld nail An orthopedic nail with a V-shaped tip and shank used for fixating an intertrochanteric fracture. The nail is driven into the neck of the femur until it reaches a round metal plate screwed onto the side of the femur. The nail is secured to a receptacle on the plate. Also called Neufeld angled nail.

neur- See **neuro-.**

neural Of or pertaining to nerve cells and their processes.

-neural, -neuric A combining form meaning 'of or relating to a nerve or nerves': *epineural, epithelioneural, myoneural.*

neural canal See **neurocoele.**

neural crest The band of ectodermally derived cells that lies along the outer surface of each side of the neural tube in the early stages of embryonic development. The cells migrate laterally throughout the embryo and give rise to certain spinal, cranial, and sympathetic ganglia. Also called **ganglionic crest, ganglionic ridge.** See also **neural tube formation.**

neural ectoderm The part of the embryonic ectoderm that develops into the neural tube. Also called neuroderm. See also **neural tube formation.**

neural fold Either of the paired longitudinal elevations resulting from the invagination of the

NEURAL TUBE FORMATION

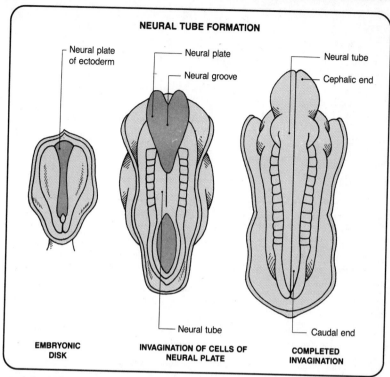

Neural plate of ectoderm — Neural plate — Neural tube

Neural groove — Cephalic end

Neural tube — Caudal end

EMBRYONIC DISK — **INVAGINATION OF CELLS OF NEURAL PLATE** — **COMPLETED INVAGINATION**

neural plate in the early developing embryo. Also called **medullary fold.** See also **neural tube formation.**

neuralgia An abnormal condition characterized by severe stabbing pain, caused by a variety of disorders affecting the nervous system. —**neuralgic,** *adj.*

neural groove The longitudinal depression that occurs between the neural folds during the invagination of the neural plate to form the neural tube in the early stages of embryonic development. Also called **medullary groove.** See also **neural tube formation.**

neural impulse See **impulse.**

neural plate A thick layer of ectodermal tissue that lies along the central longitudinal axis of the early developing embryo and gives rise to the neural tube and subsequently to the brain, spinal cord, and other tissues of the central nervous system. Also called **medullary plate.** See also **neural tube formation.**

neural tube The longitudinal tube, lying along the central axis of the early developing embryo, that gives rise to the brain, spinal cord, and other neural tissue of the central nervous system. Also called **cerebromedullary tube, medullary tube.** See also **neural tube defect, neural tube formation.**

neural tube defect Any of a group of congenital malformations involving defects in the skull and spinal column that are caused primarily by the failure of the neural tube to close during embryonic development. The defect may occur at any point along the neural axis or extend the entire length of the spinal column, as in holorachischisis. The amount of deformity and disability depends on the degree of neural involvement, the most severe defect being complete cranioschisis, or the total absence of the skull and defective brain development. Other cerebral dysplasias resulting from the failure of the cranial end of the neural tube to fuse are meningoencephalocele and cranial meningocele. Most neural tube malformations are caused by incomplete fusion of one or more laminae of the vertebral column, with varying degrees of tissue protrusion and neural involvement. Such anomalies include rachischisis, spinal bifida, myelocele, myelomeningocele, and meningocele. In all of these conditions, there is constant risk of rupture of the saclike protrusion and danger of meningeal infection. Often, immediate surgical repair is necessary. Many of the major neural tube defects can be determined prenatally by ultrasonic scanning of the uterus and by the presence of elevated concentrations of alpha-fetoprotein levels in the amniotic fluid.

neural tube formation The various processes and stages involved in the embryonic development of the neural tube. The primitive tube originates from a flat, single layer of ectodermal tissue that extends longitudinally along the mid-

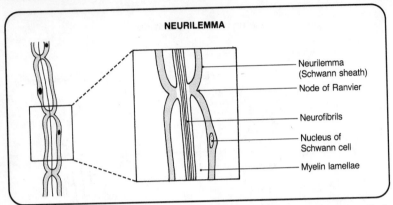

NEURILEMMA

- Neurilemma (Schwann sheath)
- Node of Ranvier
- Neurofibrils
- Nucleus of Schwann cell
- Myelin lamellae

dorsal line of the embryonic disk from the area of the primitive streak forward to the cephalic extremity. This tissue, called the neural plate, grows rapidly and becomes striated and thickened. The rate of growth is greater along the midplane than at the margin, resulting in the invagination of the cells and formation of a hollow groove, the neural groove, bounded on either side by the elevated neural folds. With continued cell division, the groove becomes deeper and the folds thicken so that they eventually meet and fuse, converting the neural groove into the neural tube. The closing of the neural tube occurs first at the midpoint and progresses toward both the caudal and the cephalic regions. At the cephalic end, the tube expands into a large vesicle with three subdivisions that differentiate into the forebrain (prosencephalon), the midbrain (mesencephalon), and the hindbrain (rhombencephalon). The epithelium of the wall of the tube develops into the various tissues of the nervous system. The caudal portion of the tube subsequently forms the spinal cord. Failure of any part of the neural tube to close during early embryonic development results in a number of congenital defects. See also **neural tube defect.**

neurasthenia **1.** An abnormal condition characterized by nervous exhaustion and a vague functional fatigue that often follows depression. **2.** In psychiatry: a stage in the recovery from a schizophrenic experience during which the patient is listless and is apparently unable to cope with routine activities and relationships. —**neurasthenic,** *adj.*

-neure A combining form meaning a 'nerve cell': *ganglioneure, myoneure, sporadoneure.* Also **-neuron.**

neurenteric canal A tubular passage between the posterior part of the neural tube and the archenteron in the early embryonic development of lower animals. It corresponds to the notochordal canal in humans and higher animals. Also called **archenteric canal, blastoporic canal, Braun's canal.**

-neuria A combining form meaning a '(specified) condition involving nerves': *acystineuria, ovariodysneuria.*

neurilemma, neurolemma A layer of cells composed of one or more Schwann cells that encloses the segmented myelin sheaths of peripheral nerve fibers. Each myelinated nerve fiber has a neurilemma cell for each internodal segment between the nodes of Ranvier. The cell nucleus is a flattened oval that lies in a small depression in the myelin. Also called Schwann's sheath. —**neurilemmal, neurilemmatic, neurilemmatous,** *adj.*

neurilemoma See **schwannoma.**

neurinoma, *pl.* **neurinomas, neurinomata** **1.** A tumor of the nerve sheath. It is usually benign but may undergo malignant change. A kind of neurinoma is acoustic neurinoma. See also **schwannoma. 2.** A neuroma.

neuritis, *pl.* **neuritides** An abnormal condition characterized by inflammation of a nerve. Some of the signs of this condition are neuralgia, hyperthesia, anesthesia, paralysis, muscular atrophy, and defective reflexes.

neuro-, neur- A combining form meaning 'of or pertaining to nerves': *neuroclonic, neurohormone, neuromast.*

neuroblast Any embryonic cell that develops into a functional neuron; an immature nerve cell. —**neuroblastic,** *adj.*

neuroblastoma, *pl.* **neuroblastomas, neuroblastomata** A highly malignant tumor composed of primitive ectodermal cells derived from the neural plate during embryonic life. The tumor may originate in any part of the sympathetic nervous system, but it is most common in the adrenal medulla of young children. Neuroblastomas metastasize early and widely to lymph nodes, liver, lung, and bone. Symptoms may include an abdominal mass, respiratory distress, and anemia, depending on the site of the primary tumor and metastases, and hormonally active adrenal lesions may cause irritability, flushing, sweating, hypertension, and tachycardia. Prior to metastasis, treatment with radical surgery, deep irradiation, and chemotherapy are often successful. Remissions may occur with the tumor undergoing maturation and forming a benign ganglioneuroma. A kind of neuroblastoma is **Pepper syndrome.**

NEURO CHECK

LEVEL OF CONSCIOUSNESS	CHARACTERISTIC RESPONSES
Alert	• Awake • Responds appropriately to auditory, tactile, and visual stimuli; oriented to person, place, and time
Lethargic	• Sleeps often • Arouses easily; responds appropriately
Obtunded	• Aroused by shaking or shouting; responds appropriately • Returns to sleep
Stuporous	• Responds only to painful stimulus • Withdraws finger or pushes your hand away (purposeful movement) • Not completely awake during stimulation
Semicomatose	• Responds only to painful stimulus • Performs reflex movement, such as decerebrate posturing
Comatose	• Shows no response; shows no reflexes • Exhibits flaccid muscle tone in arms and legs

neurocele   See **neurocoele.**

neurocentral   Pertaining to the centrum and the developing vertebrae in the early stages of embryology.

neurocentrum   The embryonic mesodermal tissue that subsequently gives rise to the vertebrae. See also **sclerotome.**

neuro check   *Informal.* A brief neurologic assessment, usually performed in the triage treatment of patients in an emergency situation or on admission to an emergency service. First, the level of consciousness is evaluated. Then, the movements of the extremities are determined to be voluntary or involuntary. The color, temperature, and turgor of the skin are noted. The pupils of the eyes are observed for equality of dilatation, reactivity to light, and ability to accommodate. Finally, routine vital signs are measured. See also **Glasgow Coma Scale, neurologic assessment.**

neurocirculatory asthenia   A psychosomatic disorder characterized by nervous and circulatory irregularities, including dyspnea, palpitation, giddiness, vertigo, tremor, precordial pain, and increased susceptibility to fatigue.

neurocoele, neurocele, neurocoel   A system of cavities in the central nervous system of man and other vertebrate animals. It consists of the ventricles of the brain and the central canal of the spinal cord, which originate from the neural tube during early embryonic development. Also called **neural canal.**

neurocytoma   A tumor composed of undifferentiated nerve cells that are usually ganglionic. Also called **neuroma.**

neuroderm   See **neuroectoderm. —neurodermal,** *adj.*

neurodermatitis   A nonspecific, pruritic skin disorder seen in anxious, nervous individuals. Excoriations and lichenification are found on easily accessible, exposed areas of the body, as the forearms and forehead. Sometimes loosely (and incorrectly) applied to **atopic dermatitis.**

neuroectoderm   The part of the embryonic ectoderm that gives rise to the central and peripheral nervous systems, including some glial cells. **—neuroectodermal,** *adj.*

neuroepithelioma   An uncommon neoplasm of neuroepithelium in a sensory nerve. Also called **neuroepithelial tumor.**

neurofibroma, *pl.* **neurofibromas, neurofibromata**   A fibrous tumor of nerve tissue resulting from the abnormal proliferation of Schwann cells. Multiple growths of this type in the peripheral nervous system are often associated with extensive abnormalities in other tissues.

neurofibromatosis   A congenital condition transmitted as an autosomal dominant trait, characterized by numerous neurofibromas of the nerves and skin, by café-au-lait spots on the skin, and, in some cases, by developmental anomalies of the muscles, bones, and viscera. Many large, pedunculated soft-tissue tumors may develop, as exemplified by the 'Elephant Man.' Bone changes may result in skeletal deformities, especially curvature of the spine. Neurofibromas may develop in the alimentary tract, bladder, endocrine glands, and cranial nerves. The disorder occurs in 1 of 2,500 to 3,000 live births. Also called **multiple neuroma, neuromatosis, von Recklinghausen's disease.**

neurogen   1. See **neurotransmitter.** 2. A substance within the early developing embryo that stimulates the primary organizer to initiate the formation of the neural plate, which gives rise to the primary axis of the body.

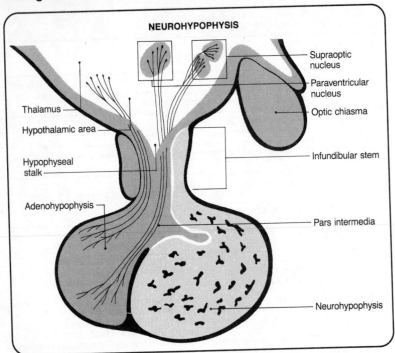

NEUROHYPOPHYSIS

Supraoptic nucleus

Paraventricular nucleus

Optic chiasma

Thalamus

Hypothalamic area

Hypophyseal stalk

Adenohypophysis

Infundibular stem

Pars intermedia

Neurohypophysis

neurogenesis The development of the tissue of the nervous system. —**neurogenetic,** *adj.*

neurogenic arthropathy An abnormal condition associated with neural damage, characterized by the gradual and usually painless degeneration of a joint. One of the major causes of this condition is believed to be a minor injury that is disregarded by the affected individual because of a lack of sensation in the injured tissue. Inadequate rest and care aggravate such injuries and prevent proper healing.

neurogenic bladder Dysfunctional urinary bladder caused by a lesion of the nervous system. Treatment is aimed at enabling the bladder to empty completely and regularly, preventing infection, controlling incontinence, and preserving kidney function. Kinds of neurogenic bladder are **flaccid bladder, spastic bladder.** Also called **neuropathic bladder.**

neurogenic fracture A fracture resulting from the destruction of the nerve supply to a specific bone.

neuroglia One of the two main kinds of cells comprising the nervous system. It performs the less specialized functions of the nerve network. Compare **neuron.** —**neuroglial,** *adj.*

neurohormonal regulation Regulation of the function of an organ or a gland by the combined effect of neurological and hormonal activity.

neurohumor One of the chemical substances, formed and transmitted by a neuron, that is essential for the activity of adjacent neurons or nearby organs or muscles. Kinds of neurohumoral substances are **acetylcholine, dopamine, epinephrine, norepinephrine, serotonin.** —**neurohumoral,** *adj.*

neurohypophysis The posterior lobe of the pituitary gland that is the source of antidiuretic hormone (ADH) and oxytocin. Nervous stimulation controls the release of both substances into the blood. The neurohypophysis releases ADH when stimulated by the hypothalamus by an increase in the osmotic pressure of extracellular fluid in the body. The hormone acts on the cells in the distal and the collecting tubules of the kidneys, making them more permeable to water and reducing the volume of urine. The neurohypophysis releases oxytocin under appropriate stimulation from the hypothalamus. Oxytocin produces powerful contractions of the pregnant uterus and causes milk to flow from lactating breasts. Stimulation of the nipples of the breast by a nursing infant triggers the release of this hormone. Also called posterior pituitary gland. Compare **adenohypophysis.** See also **antidiuretic hormone, oxytocin.** —**neurohypophyseal,** *adj.*

neurolemma See **neurilemma.**

neurolepsis An altered state of consciousness characterized by quiescence, reduced motor activity and anxiety, and indifference to the surroundings. Sleep may occur, but usually the person can be roused and can respond to commands.

neurolept See **neuroleptic.**

neurolept analgesia A form of analgesia achieved by the concurrent administration of a neuroleptic and an analgesic. Anxiety, motor activity, and sensitivity to painful stimuli are reduced; the person is quiet and indifferent to the environment and surroundings. Sleep may or may not occur, but the patient is not unconscious and is able to respond to commands. If nitrous oxide in oxygen is also administered, neurolept analgesia can be converted to neurolept anesthesia.

neurolept anesthesia A form of anesthesia achieved by the administration of a neuroleptic agent, a narcotic analgesic, and nitrous oxide in oxygen. Induction of anesthesia is slow, but consciousness returns quickly after the inhalation of nitrous oxide is stopped.

neuroleptic, neurolept 1. Of or pertaining to neurolepsis. 2. A drug that causes neurolepsis, as droperidol.

neurologic assessment An evaluation of the patient's neurologic status and symptoms. See **Glasgow Coma Scale, neuro check.**

neurologic examination A systematic examination of the nervous system, including an assessment of mental status, the function of each of the cranial nerves, sensory and neuromuscular function, the reflexes, and proprioception and other cerebellar functions.

neurology The field of medicine dealing with the nervous system and its disorders. —**neurologic, neurological,** adj. **neurologist,** n.

neuroma, pl. **neuromas, neuromata** A benign neoplasm composed chiefly of neurons and nerve fibers, usually arising from a nerve tissue. Pain radiating from the lesion to the periphery of the affected nerve is usually intermittent but may become continuous and severe. Kinds of neuromas include **acoustic neuroma, cystic neuroma, false neuroma, myelinic neuroma, neuroma cutis, nevoid neuroma, traumatic neuroma.**

-neuroma A combining form meaning a 'tumor made up of nerve cells and fibers': *angiomyoneuroma, ioneuroma, myoneuroma.*

neuroma cutis A neoplasm in the skin that contains nerve tissue and that may be extremely sensitive to painful stimuli.

neuroma telangiectodes See **nevoid neuroma.**

neuromatosis A neoplastic disease characterized by numerous neuromas. Also called **multiple neuroma.** See also **neurofibromatosis.**

neuromuscular Of or pertaining to the nerves and the muscles.

neuromuscular blocking agent A chemical substance that interferes locally with the transmission or reception of impulses from motor nerves to skeletal muscles. Nondepolarizing agents, as metocurine, pancuronium, and tubocurarine, competitively block the transmitter action of acetylcholine at the postjunctional membrane. Depolarizing blocking agents, as succinylcholine chloride, compete with acetylcholine for cholinergic receptors of the motor

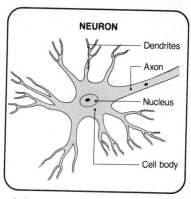

NEURON
— Dendrites
— Axon
— Nucleus
— Cell body

end plate. Neuromuscular blocking agents are used to induce muscle relaxation in anesthesia, endotracheal intubation, and electroshock therapy and as adjuncts in the treatment of tetanus, encephalitis, and poliomyelitis. Neuromuscular blocking drugs can cause bronchospasm, hyperthermia, hypotension, or respiratory paralysis and are used with caution, especially in patients with myasthenia gravis; renal, hepatic, or pulmonary impairment; and in elderly and debilitated individuals. See also **muscle relaxant.**

neuromuscular junction The area of contact between the ends of a large myelinated nerve fiber and a fiber of skeletal muscle. Also called **myoneural junction.** See also **motor end plate, myelin, nerve.**

neuromuscular spindle Any one of a number of small bundles of delicate muscular fibers, enclosed by a capsule, in which sensory nerve fibers terminate. The spindles vary in length from 0.8 to 5 mm, accommodating as many as four large myelinated nerve fibers, which pierce the capsule and lose their myelin sheaths. The nerve fibers end as naked axons encircling the intrafusal fibers with flattened expansions or ovoid disks.

neuromyal transmission The passage of excitation from a motor neuron to a muscle fiber at the myoneural junction.

neuromyelitis An abnormal condition characterized by inflammation of the spinal cord and peripheral nerves.

neuron, neurone The basic nerve cell of the nervous system, containing a nucleus within a cell body and extending one or more processes. Neurons are classified according to the direction in which they conduct impulses and according to the number of processes they extend. Sensory neurons transmit nerve impulses to the spinal cord and the brain. Motor neurons transmit nerve impulses from the brain and the spinal cord to the muscles and the glandular tissue. Multipolar neurons, the bipolar neurons, and the unipolar neurons are classified according to the number of processes they extend to the different kinds of neurons. Multipolar neurons have one axon and several dendrites, as do most of the neurons in the brain and the spinal cord. Bipolar neurons, which are less numerous than the other types, have only one axon and one dendrite. Unipolar neurons are embryonic structures that originate as bipolar bodies but fuse dendrites and axons into a single fiber that stretches for a short distance from the cell body before separating again into the two processes. All neurons have at least one axon and one or more dendrites and have a slightly gray color when clustered, as in the brain and the spinal cord. As the carriers of nerve impulses, neurons function according to electrochemical processes involving positively charged sodium and potassium ions and the changing electrical potential of the extracellular and the intracellular fluid of the neuron.

-neuron See **-neure.**

neuronitis An abnormal condition characterized by inflammation of a nerve or a nerve cell, especially the cells and the roots of the spinal nerves.

neuropathic bladder See **neurogenic bladder.**

neuropathic joint disease A chronic, progressive, degenerative disease of one or more joints, characterized by swelling, instability of the joint, hemorrhage, heat, and atrophic and hypertrophic changes in the bone. The disease is the result of an underlying neurologic disorder, as tabes dorsalis from syphilis, diabetic neuropathy, leprosy, or congenital absence or depression of pain sensation. Early recognition of the disease and prophylactic protection of the joint may prevent further damage in some cases. Surgical reconstruction is not usually effective, because healing is slow. Amputation may be necessary. Also called **Charcot's joint.**

neuropathy Any abnormal condition characterized by inflammation and degeneration of the peripheral nerves. **—neuropathic,** *adj.*

neuroplegia Nerve paralysis owing to disease, injury, or the effect of neuroleptic drugs. See also **lytic cocktail.**

neuropore The opening at each end of the neural tube during early embryonic development. The closure of these apertures as the tube grows and differentiates occurs with such precision that they are used to indicate horizons XI and XII in the systematic anatomical charting of human embryonic development. Kinds of neuropores are **anterior neuropore, posterior neuropore.** See also **horizon, neural tube formation.**

neurosarcoma A malignant neoplasm composed of nerve tissue, connective tissue, and vascular tissue. Also called **malignant neuroma.**

neurosis 1. Any faulty or inefficient way of coping with anxiety or inner conflict, which may ultimately lead to a neurotic disorder. 2. *Informal.* An emotional disturbance other than psychosis. See also **neurotic disorder, neurotic process.**

-neurosis A combining form meaning a 'disease of the nerves' or a 'mental disorder': *angioneurosis, psychoneurosis, synneurosis.*

neurosurgery Any surgery involving the brain, spinal cord, or peripheral nerves. Brain surgery is performed to treat a wound, remove a tumor or foreign body, relieve pressure in intracranial hemorrhage, excise an abcess, treat parkinsonism, or relieve pain. After surgery, the nurse carefully observes vital signs and changes in the level of consciousness, speech, and strength. Any yellowish drainage from the wound may be cerebrospinal fluid and is reported immediately. Sterile dressing technique is essential. Kinds of brain surgery include craniotomy, lobotomy, and hypophysectomy. Surgery of the spine is performed to correct a defect, remove a tumor, repair a ruptured intervertebral disk, or relieve pain. After surgery, the nurse keeps the bed flat and the patient's spine in good alignment. Return of sensation and motor function are monitored carefully. Kinds of spinal surgery include fusion and laminectomy. Surgery on the peripheral nerves is performed to remove a tumor, relieve pain, or reconnect a severed nerve. Local anesthesia is usually used. After surgery, the nurse observes closely the return of sensation to the area. One kind of nerve surgery is **sympathectomy.**

neurosyphilis An infection of the central nervous system by syphilis organisms, which may invade the meninges and cerebrovascular system. If the brain tissue is affected by the disease, general paresis may result; if the spinal cord is infected, tabes dorsalis may result. See also **syphilis,** *Treponema pallidum.* **—neurosyphiltic,** *adj.*

neurotendinous spindle A capsule containing enlarged tendon fibers, found chiefly near the junctions of tendons and muscles. One or more nerve fibers pierce the side of the capsule and lose their medullary sheaths; the axons subdivide and terminate between the tendon fibers in irregular disks or varicosities. Also called **organ of Golgi.**

neurotic 1. Of or pertaining to neurosis or to a neurotic disorder. 2. Pertaining to the nerves. 3. One who is afflicted with a neurosis. 4. *Informal.* An emotionally unstable person.

-neurotic A combining form meaning: 1. 'Pertaining to a (specified) abnormal condition of the nerves': *angioneurotic, aponeurotic, vasoneurotic.* 2. 'Pertaining to (psycho)neurosis': *hyperneurotic, psychoneurotic, unneurotic.*

neurotic disorder Any mental disorder characterized by a symptom or group of symptoms that a person finds distressing, unacceptable, and alien to the person's personality, as severe anxiety, obsessional thoughts, and compulsive acts, and that produces psychological pain or discomfort disproportionate to the reality of the situation. Although one's ability to function may be markedly impaired, one's behavior generally remains within acceptable social norms and one's perception of reality is unaffected. There is no proof of organic cause. The disturbance is relatively long lasting, cannot be considered simply a reaction to stress, and may recur if untreated. Kinds of neurotic disorders include **anxiety neurosis, obsessive-compulsive neurosis, psychosexual disorder, somatoform disorder.**

neurotic process In psychology: a process in which unconscious conflicts lead to feelings of anxiety. Defense mechanisms are employed to avoid these uncomfortable feelings, and personality disturbance and the symptoms of neurosis ensue.

neurotoxic Having a poisonous effect on nerves and nerve cells.

neurotoxin A toxin that acts directly on the tissues of the central nervous system, traveling along the axis cylinders of the motor nerves to the brain. The toxin may be secreted in the venom of certain snakes, or it may be present on the spines of a shell or in the flesh of fish or shellfish; it may be produced by certain bacteria or by the cellular disintegration of certain bacteria.

neurotransmitter Any one of numerous chemicals that modify or result in the transmission of nerve impulses between synapses. Neurotransmitters are released from synaptic knobs into synaptic clefts and bridge the gap between presynaptic and postsynaptic neurons. Each vesicle within a synaptic knob stores as many as 10,000 neurotransmitter molecules. When a nerve impulse reaches a synaptic knob, thousands of neurotransmitter molecules squirt into the synaptic cleft and bind to specific receptors. This flow allows an associated diffusion of potassium and sodium ions, which causes an action potential. Excitatory neurotransmitters decrease the negativity of postsynaptic membrane potentials; inhibitory neurotransmitters increase such potentials. Kinds of neurotransmitters include **acetylcholine, gamma-aminobutyric acid, norepinephrine.**

neurula, *pl.* **neurulas, neurulae** An early embryo during the period of neurulation when the nervous system tissue begins to differentiate. The embryo at this level of growth represents a third stage in embryonic development, following the morula and blastocyst stages in man and the higher animals and the blastula and gastrula stages in lower animals. In man, the neurula stage occurs from about 19 to 26 days after fertilization.

neutral The state exactly between two opposing values, qualities, or properties, as, in electricity, a neutral state is one in which there is neither a positive nor a negative charge or, in chemistry, a neutral state is one in which a substance is neither acid nor alkaline.

neutralization The interaction between an acid and a base that produces a solution that is neither acidic nor basic. The usual products of neutralization are a salt and water.

neutral thermal environment An environment created by any method or apparatus to maintain the normal body temperature in order to minimize oxygen consumption and caloric expenditure. See also **incubator, Isolette.**

neutron In physics: an elementary particle that is a constituent of the nuclei of all elements except hydrogen. It has no electrical charge and

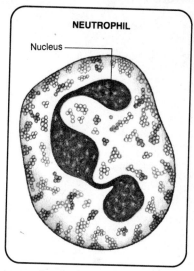

NEUTROPHIL

Nucleus

is approximately the same size as a proton.

neutron activation analysis The analysis of elements in a specimen, performed by exposing it to neutron irradiation to convert many elements to a radioactive form in which they can be identified by measuring their emissions of radiation.

neutropenia An abnormal decrease in the number of neutrophils in the blood. Neutropenia is associated with acute leukemia, infection, rheumatoid arthritis, vitamin B_{12} deficiency, and chronic splenomegaly. Compare **leukopenia.**

neutrophil A polymorphonuclear granular leukocyte that stains easily with neutral dyes. Neutrophils are the circulating white blood cells essential for phagocytosis and proteolysis in which bacteria, cellular debris, and solid particles are removed and destroyed. An increase in neutrophils is the most common form of leukocytosis and may result from many causes, including acute infection, intoxication, hemorrhage, and malignant neoplastic disease. See also **granulocyte, polymorphonuclear leukocyte.**

neutrophilia An increase in the number of neutrophil leukocytes in the blood. This form of leukocytosis may result from many causes, among them acute infections, hemorrhage, and rapidly growing malignant neoplasms.

neutrophilic leukemia See **polymorphocytic leukemia.**

nevoid amentia See **Sturge-Weber syndrome.**

nevoid neuroma A tumor of nerve tissue that contains numerous small blood vessels. Also called **neuroma telangiectodes.**

nevus A pigmented, congenital skin blemish, usually benign but, rarely, may become cancerous. Changes in color, size, or texture, or bleeding or itching of a nevus deserves investigation. Also called **birthmark, mole.** See also **blue nevus, junction nevus, nevus flammeus.**

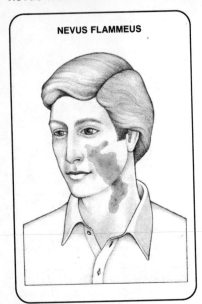

NEVUS FLAMMEUS

nevus flammeus A flat, capillary hemangioma that is present at birth and that varies in color from pale red to deep red-purple. It is most commonly seen on the occiput and rarely causes any problems. If the lesion appears on any other part of the body, it tends to be dark in color and, unlike the scalp lesions, does not regress spontaneously. These lesions are most often seen on the face, where they persist and develop a thick, verrucous nodular surface. Nevus flammeus is usually unilateral, following the distribution of a cutaneous nerve. If the lesion appears on the middle of the face, congenital Sturge-Weber syndrome is suspected. Cosmetic creams are often used to cover the lesion and electrodessication or cryotherapy is sometimes performed, especially to improve the verrucous surface appearance. Also called **port-wine stain.**

newborn 1. Recently born. **2.** A recently born infant; neonate.

newborn intrapartal care Care of the newborn in the delivery area during the time after birth before the mother and infant are transferred to the postpartum unit.

NURSING CONSIDERATIONS: Most newborns are healthy and normal; if abnormal function is observed, expert assistance may be summoned as emergency measures, including tracheal suction with a deLee mucous trap and administration of oxygen by ventilator or mask, are initiated. If there are no problems the nurse may instill silver nitrate drops in the conjunctival sacs of the eyes, clamp and trim the umbilical cord, administer an injection of vitamin K, obtain footprints for identification, and diaper and wrap the baby.

new drug A drug for which the Food and Drug Administration requires premarketing approval. A new drug is generally regarded as one for which safety and effectiveness has not yet been demonstrated for its prescribed use.

New England Journal of Medicine (NEJM) A professional medical journal that publishes findings of medical research and articles about political and ethical issues in the practice of medicine.

New World leishmaniasis See **American leishmaniasis.**

New World typhus See **murine typhus.**

Nezelof's syndrome An abnormal condition characterized by absent T cell function, deficient B cell function, fairly normal immunoglobulin levels, and little or no specific antibody production. The cause of Nezelof's syndrome is unknown. It affects both male and female siblings, indicating the possibility of a genetic disorder transmitted as an autosomal recessive trait, but not all individuals with this disease have a positive family history. The disease may be caused by a cytogenic dysfunction of the stem cells, resulting in deficiencies of T cells and B cells. Another theory is that the disorder is caused by underdevelopment of the thymus gland and the consequent inhibition of T cell development. Still another holds that the disease results from the failure to produce or to secrete thymic humoral factors, especially thymosin. Initial supportive treatment of Nezelof's syndrome may include monthly injections of gamma globulin or monthly infusions of fresh frozen plasma and the heavy use of antibiotics to fight infection. Cell-mediated immune function associated with T cells can usually be temporarily restored within weeks by a fetal thymus transplant. Repeated transplants are required to maintain the immunity. Cell-mediated immunity can be only partially restored with either transfer factor therapy or repeated injection of thymosin. Histocompatible bone marrow transplants have been used in treating this disease, but effective evaluation of this treatment method is incomplete.

NURSING CONSIDERATIONS: The injection site for gamma globulin in a large muscle mass is massaged after the injection, and injection sites are rotated and recorded to prevent tissue damage. Gamma globulin doses greater than 1.5 ml are divided and injected into more than one site.

NF abbr **National Formulary.**

NGF abbr **nerve growth factor.**

NGU abbr **nongonococcal urethritis.**

NHSC abbr **National Health Service Corps.**

Ni Symbol for **nickel.**

niacin A B-complex vitamin with antilipemic and vasodilator activity. Also called vitamin B_3, nicotinic acid.

NICHHD abbr **National Institute of Child Health and Human Development.**

nick In molecular genetics: a fissure or split in a single strand of DNA that can be made with the enzyme deoxyribonuclease or with ethidium bromide.

nickel (Ni) A silvery-white metallic element. Its atomic number is 28; its atomic weight is

58.71. Large numbers of people are allergic to nickel.

nickel dermatitis An allergic contact dermatitis owing to the metal nickel. Exposure comes usually from jewelry, wristwatches, metal clasps, and coins. Sweating increases the severity of the rash. Treatment includes avoidance of exposure to nickel and reduction of perspiration.

nick translation A method of labeling DNA in the laboratory by using the enzyme DNA polymerase.

niclosamide An anthelmintic agent.

nicotinamide See **niacinamide.**

nicotine A colorless, rapidly acting toxic substance in tobacco that is one of the major contributors to the ill effects of smoking. It is used as an insecticide in agriculture and as a parasiticide in veterinary medicine. Ingestion of large amounts causes salivation, nausea, vomiting, diarrhea, headache, vertigo, slowing of the heartbeat and, in acute cases, paralysis of respiratory muscles. Treatment includes gastric lavage with a weak solution of potassium permanganate, followed by activated charcoal, and the administration of artificial respiration and oxygen, as needed. Pentobarbitol is used to control convulsions, ephedrine for hypotension, and autonomic blocking agents to control visceral symptoms.

nicotine poisoning Poisoning from intake of nicotine. Nicotine poisoning is characterized by stimulation of the central and autonomic nervous systems followed by depression of these systems. In fatal cases, death occurs from respiratory failure.

nicotinic acid See **niacin.**

nicotinyl alcohol A peripheral vasodilator.

NICU *abbr* **neonatal intensive care unit.**

nidation The process by which an embryo burrows into the endometrium of the uterus. Also called **implantation.** See also **placenta, uterus.**

Niemann-Pick disease An autosomal recessive disorder of lipid metabolism in which there are accumulations of sphingomyelin in the bone marrow, the spleen, and the lymph nodes. The disease, which in the United States and Canada is most common among Jewish people, begins in infancy or childhood and is characterized by enlargement of the liver and the spleen, anemia, lymphadenopathy, and progressive mental and physical deterioration. There is no effective treatment, and children with the disease usually die within a few years of the onset of symptons.

nifedipine A group V antiarrhythmic and antiangina agent.

night blindness An abnormal reduction in vision in darkness, resulting from a decreased synthesis of rhodopsin, vitamin A deficiency, retinal degeneration, or a congenital defect. Also called **nyctalopia.**

Nightingale, Florence (1820–1910) The founder of modern nursing. After limited formal training in nursing in Germany and Paris, she became superintendent in 1853 of a small hospital in London. Her outstanding success in reorganizing the hospital led to a request by the British government to head a mission to the Crimea, where Britain was fighting a war with Russia. She arrived in November 1854 with 38 nurses to find 5,000 men lacking adequate food and medical supplies, crowded into dilapidated buildings that were filthy and mostly without beds. Through superhuman efforts, often working 20 hours on the wards and then sending off a stream of letters to England to obtain money and supplies and to mobilize the government to act, she brought order out of chaos. After her return to England in 1856 she wrote *Notes on Hospitals* and *Notes on Nursing* and founded a training school for nurses at St. Thomas' Hospital, where she attracted well-educated, dedicated women. She carried on her work on the sanitary reform of India, conducted a study of midwifery, helped to establish visiting nurse service, and worked for the reform of the poor laws in which she proposed separate institutions for the sick, the insane, the incurable, and children. After Longfellow wrote *Santa Filomena,* she became known as 'The Lady with the Lamp,' and the Nightingale Pledge, named for her, embodies her ideals and has inspired thousands of young graduating nurses.

Nightingale ward A kind of hospital ward, designed by Florence Nightingale, that revolutionized hospital design. The number of beds allowed in a ward of given size was limited to permit the circulation of air and for general cleanliness and the comfort of patients. Although multiple-bed wards are now obsolete in hospital design, the concerns and the benefits that impelled Miss Nightingale to create them remain central to hospital planning.

nightmare A dream occurring during rapid eye movement sleep that arouses feelings of intense, inescapable fear, terror, distress, or extreme anxiety and that usually awakens the sleeper. Compare **pavor nocturnus, sleep terror disorder.**

night vision A capacity to see dimly lit objects. The retinal rods contain the highly light-sensitive chemical rhodopsin, or visual purple, which is essential for the conduction of optic impulses in subdued light. Night vision may be diminished by a deficiency of vitamin A, an important component of rhodopsin.

nigrites linguae See **parasitic glossitis.**

NIH *abbr* **National Institutes of Health.**

nihilistic delusion A persistent denial of the existence of particular things or of everything, including oneself, as seen in various forms of schizophrenia. A person who has such a delusion may believe that he lives in a limbo world or that he died several years ago and that only his spirit, in a vaporous form, really exists. See also **delusion.**

nikethamide A respiratory stimulant.

Nikolsky's sign Easy separation of the epidermis from the basal cell layer by rubbing apparently normal skin areas; found in pemphigus and a few other bullous diseases.

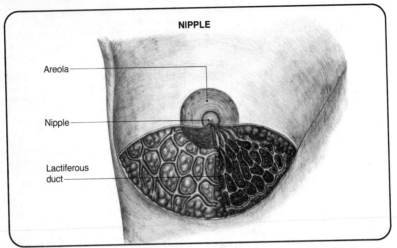

NIPPLE

Areola

Nipple

Lactiferous
duct

90-90 traction   See **traction, 90-90.**

ninth cranial nerve   See **glossopharyn-geal nerve.**

niobium (Nb)   A silver-gray metallic element. Its atomic number is 41; its atomic weight is 92.906. Formerly called **columbium.**

nipple   A small cylindrical, pigmented structure that projects just below the center of each breast. The tip of the nipple has about 20 tiny openings to the lactiferous ducts. The skin of the nipple is surrounded by the lighter pigmented skin of the areola. In pregnancy, the skin of the nipple darkens but loses some of this pigmentation when lactation is completed. Stimulation of the nipple in men and women causes the structure to become erect through the contraction of radiating smooth muscle bundles in the surrounding areola.

nipple cancer   An inflammatory malignant neoplasm of the nipple and areola that is usually associated with carcinoma in deeper breast structures. It represents only a small percentage of breast cancers and usually begins in the nipple and spreads to the areola. Also called **Paget's disease of the nipple.**

nipple discharge   Spontaneous exudation of material from the nipple that may be normal, as colostrum in pregnancy, or that may be a sign of endocrinologic, neoplastic, or infectious disease.

nipple shield   A device to protect the nipples of a lactating woman. The shield is usually made of soft latex, is 4 or 5 cm (1½ or 2 inches) wide, and has a tab on one side with which the mother may hold it. The infant nurses from a nipple at the center of the shield. It is most often used to allow sore or cracked nipples to heal while maintaining lactation. Also called nipple protector.

niridazole   An antischistosomal drug available only from the Centers for Disease Control.

Nissl body   Any one of the large granular structures in the cytoplasm of nerve cells that stains with basic dyes and contains ribonucleoprotein.

nit   The egg of a parasitic insect, particularly a louse. It may be found attached to human or animal hair or to clothing fiber. See also **pediculosis.**

nitric acid   A colorless, highly corrosive liquid that may give off suffocating brown fumes of nitrogen dioxide on exposure to air. Traces of nitric acid are found in rain water during a thunderstorm. Commercially prepared nitric acid is a powerful oxidizing agent used in photoengraving and metallurgy; in the manufacture of explosives, fertilizers, dyes, and drugs; and, occasionally, as a cauterizing agent for the removal of warts.

nitrite   An ester or salt of nitrous acid, used as a vasodilator and antispasmodic. Among the most widely used nitrites in medicine are amyl, ethyl, potassium, and sodium nitrite.

nitro-   A combining form indicating presence of the group $-NO_2$: *nitrobenzol, nitrofuran, nitromethane.*

nitrobenzene poisoning   A toxic condition caused by the absorption into the body of nitrobenzene, a pale yellow, oily liquid used in the manufacture of aniline, shoe dyes, soap, perfume, and artificial flavors. Nitrobenzene, especially its vapors, is extremely toxic. Symptoms of acute poisoning include headache, drowsiness, nausea, ataxia, cyanosis, and in extreme cases respiratory failure. Contaminated clothing is removed and the skin is washed with vinegar, followed by soap and water. Oxygen, blood transfusion, and, in severe cases, hemodialysis may be required. Ingestion is treated with gastric lavage with weak acetic acid, followed by the administration of liquid petrolatum, a saline cathartic, and oxygen and blood transfusion if indicated. Chronic exposure to nitrobenzene may cause headache, fatigue, loss of appetite, and anemia.

nitrofuran   One of a group of synthetic antimicrobials used to treat infections caused by protozoa or by certain gram-positive or gram-negative bacteria.

nitrofurantoin, n. macrocrystals Urinary tract antiseptics.

nitrofurazone A local anti-infective agent.

nitrogen (N) A gaseous nonmetallic element. Its atomic number is 7; its atomic weight is 14.007. Nitrogen constitutes approximately 78% of the atmosphere and is a component of all proteins and a major component of most organic substances. Nitrogen is found in mineral compounds, as saltpeter, and is the 17th most abundant element in the earth's crust. Compounds of nitrogen are essential constituents of all living organisms, the proteins and the nucleic acids being especially basic to all life forms. Nitrogen forms a series of oxides and oxyacids, the most important of which is nitric acid. It also unites with hydrogen to form ammonia and with many metallic elements to form nitrides.

nitrogen balance The relationship between the nitrogen taken into the body, usually as food, and the nitrogen excreted from the body in urine and feces. Most of the body's nitrogen is incorporated into protein. Positive nitrogen balance, which occurs when the intake of nitrogen is greater than its excretion, implies tissue formation. Negative nitrogen balance, which occurs when more nitrogen is excreted than is taken in, indicates wasting or destruction of tissue.

nitrogen fixation The process by which free nitrogen in the atmosphere is converted by biological or chemical means to ammonia and to other forms usable by plants and animals.

nitrogen mustard See **mechlorethamine hydrochloride.**

nitroglycerin A coronary vasodilator.

nitromersal A disinfectant.

nitroprusside sodium A potent vasodilator and antihypertensive.

nitroso- A combining form indicating presence of the group -N:O: *nitrosobacteria, nitrososubstitution.*

nitrosourea One of a group of alkylating drugs used as an antineoplastic drug in the chemotherapy of brain tumors, multiple myeloma, Hodgkin's disease, chronic leukemias, lymphomas, myelomas, and cancers of the breast and ovaries. They have been less successful in therapy for cancers of the lungs, head, neck, and gastrointestinal tract. Like other alkylating agents, they have severe toxic effects, including bone marrow depression. Nausea and vomiting are almost always present. Safe use during pregnancy has not been established, and animal studies have generally shown teratogenicity and embryotoxicity. Carmustine and lomustine are typical examples of this group.

nitrous oxide (N_2O) A gas used as an anesthetic in dentistry, surgery, and childbirth. It provides light anesthesia and is delivered in various concentrations with oxygen. Nitrous oxide alone does not provide deep enough anesthesia for major surgery, for which it is supplemented

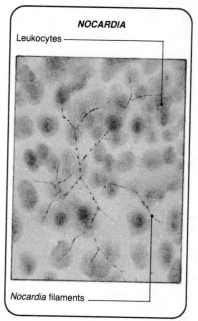

NOCARDIA

Leukocytes

Nocardia filaments

with other anesthetic agents. It is often given for induction of anesthesia, preceded by the administration of a barbiturate or an analgesic narcotic. Nitrous oxide is neither explosive nor flammable, and recovery is rapid. It is not administered to patients with hypoxemia, respiratory disease, or intestinal occlusion. Also known as **laughing gas.**

NLN *abbr* **National League for Nursing.**

NMNA *abbr* **National Male Nurses' Association.**

NMR *abbr* **nuclear magnetic resonance.**

No Symbol for **nobelium.**

nobelium (No) A man-made, transuranic metallic element. Its atomic number is 102; its atomic weight is 254.

noble gas See **inert gas.**

Nocardia A genus of gram-positive aerobic bacteria, some species of which are pathogenic, as *Nocardia asteroides,* which causes maduromycosis. See also **nocardiosis.**

nocardiosis Infection with *Nocardia asteroides,* an aerobic gram-positive species of actinomycetes, characterized by pneumonia, often with cavitation, and by chronic abcesses in the brain and subcutaneous tissues. The organism enters via the respiratory tract and spreads by the bloodstream, especially in Cushing's syndrome. Surgical drainage of abscesses and sulfonamide therapy for 12 to 18 months cures 50% to 60% of the cases treated.

no-code A note written in the patient record and signed by a qualified (usually senior or attending) physician, instructing the staff of the institution not to attempt to resuscitate a particular patient in the event of cardiac or respi-

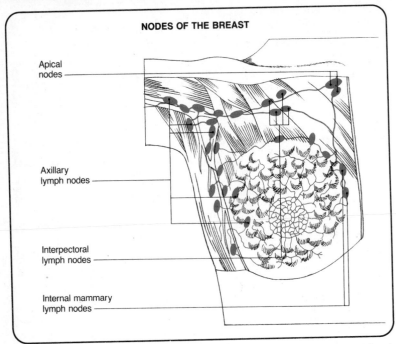

NODES OF THE BREAST

Apical nodes

Axillary lymph nodes

Interpectoral lymph nodes

Internal mammary lymph nodes

ratory failure. This instruction is usually given only when a person is so gravely ill that death is imminent and inevitable. Also called **DNR.** See also **code,** definition 5.

noctambulation See **somnambulism.**

nocturia Particularly excessive urination at night. While it may be a symptom of renal disease, it may occur in the absence of disease in persons who drink excessive amounts of fluids, particularly alcohol or coffee, before bedtime or in those with prostatic disease. It may occur in older patients, who may have excess fluids that are mobilized by lying down at night. Also called **nycturia.** Compare **enuresis.**

nocturnal **1.** Pertaining to or occurring during the night. **2.** Describing an individual or animal that is active at night and sleeps during the day.

nocturnal emission Involuntary emission of semen during sleep, usually in association with an erotic dream. Also called **wet dream.**

nocturnal paroxysmal dyspnea An abnormal condition of the respiratory system, characterized by sudden attacks of shortness of breath, profuse sweating, tachycardia, and wheezing that awakens the person from sleep. The paroxysms may be induced by nightmares, noises, or coughing. The condition is usually associated with heart failure or pulmonary edema. Characteristically, the attack is relieved by an upright posture. See also **dyspnea.**

nod- A combining form meaning 'knot': *nodal, nodose, nodulus.*

nodal bradycardia See **bradycardia.**

node **1.** A small rounded mass. **2.** A lymph node.

nodular Of a structure or mass: small, firm, and knotty. See also **node, nodule.**

nodular circumscribed lipomatosis A condition in which many circumscribed, encapsulated lipomas are distributed around the neck symmetrically, randomly, or like a collar. The adipose deposits may be painful and tender.

nodular cutaneous angiitis An inflammatory condition of small arteries accompanied by lesions of the skin.

nodular melanoma A melanoma that is uniformly pigmented, usually bluish-black and sometimes surrounded by an irregular halo of pale, unpigmented skin. The lesion is always raised and may be dome-shaped or polypoid.

nodule **1.** A small node. **2.** A small nodelike structure.

-noia A combining form meaning '(condition of the) mind or will': *aponoia, hypernoia, hyponoia.*

noma An acute, necrotizing ulcerative process involving mucous membranes of the mouth or genitalia. The condition is most commonly seen in children with poor nutrition and hygiene. There is rapid-spreading and painless destruction of bone and soft tissue accompanied by a putrid odor. Fusospirochetal organisms have been implicated. Healing eventually occurs but often with disfiguring defects. Also called **acute necrotizing ulcerative mucositis, gangrenous stomatitis.**

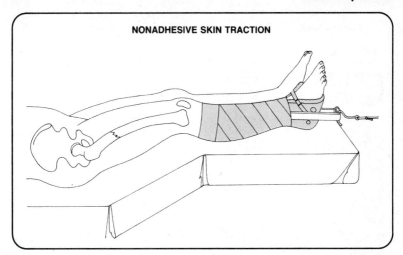

NONADHESIVE SKIN TRACTION

-noma A combining form meaning a 'spreading, invasive gangrene': *müllerianoma, pelidnoma.*

nomenclature A consistent, systematic method of naming used in a scientific discipline to denote classifications and to avoid ambiguities in names, as binomial nomenclature in biology and chemical nomenclature in chemistry.

-nomia A combining form meaning 'aphasia involving names or naming ability': *anomia, paranomia, dysnomia.*

Nomina Anatomica The book of official international nomenclature for anatomy as designated by the International Congress of Anatomists.

nominal damages See **damages.**

nomo- A combining form meaning 'of or relating to usage or law': *nomogenesis, nomogram, nomotopic.*

nomogram 1. A graphic representation of a numerical relationship. 2. A graph on which a number of variables is plotted so that the value of a dependent variable can be read on the appropriate line when the values of the other variables are given.

-nomy A combining form meaning 'received knowledge in a field': *pathonomy, physionomy, psychonomy.*

non- A combining form meaning 'nine': *nonan, nonigravida, nonipara.*

non-A, non-B (NANB) hepatitis Viral hepatitis that is caused by a virus antigenically separate from the serologic strains that cause hepatitis A or hepatitis B. It accounts for more than 90% of the cases of posttransfusion hepatitis in the United States, occurring primarily in people receiving multiple transfusions. NANB hepatitis is usually milder than types A or B but is otherwise clinically indistinguishable from them. The treatment is the same as for other forms of viral hepatitis.

nonadhesive skin traction One of two kinds of skin traction in which the therapeutic pull of traction weights is applied with foambacked traction straps that do not stick to the skin over the body structure involved. Nonadhesive skin traction straps may be easily removed to facilitate skin care and are usually used when continuous traction is not required. The straps spread the traction pull over a wide area of skin surface, thus decreasing the vulnerability of the patient to skin breakdown. Compare **adhesive skin traction.**

nonbacterial thrombic endocarditis One of the three main types of endocarditis, characterized by various kinds of lesions that affect the heart valves. This disease equally affects men and women between the ages of 18 and 90, causes heart murmurs in about 30% of the cases, and most often affects the valves on the left side of the heart. There is no successful treatment. See also **Libman-Sacks endocarditis.**

noncommunicating hydrocephalus See **hydrocephalus.**

noncompliance A nursing diagnosis accepted by the Fifth National Conference on the Classification of Nursing Diagnoses. The specific nature of the noncompliance is to be specified, as noncompliance: medications. The etiology of noncompliance is an informed decision on the part of the client not to adhere to a therapeutic suggestion owing to a health belief, a cultural or spiritual value, or a problem in the relationship between the provider of the recommendation and the client. The defining characteristics of noncompliance include objective tests that show noncompliance, observation of physical or psychological signs that demonstrate lack of compliance, or a failure to keep appointments. The critical defining characteristic is an observation of the client's failure to adhere to a recommendation or a statement by the client or other knowledgeable person that the recommendations are not being followed. See also **nursing diagnosis.**

NONOSTEOGENIC FIBROMA

Nonosteogenic fibroma

urethritis by microscopic examination and bacteriologic culture of the exudate. Untreated NGU may result in urethral stricture, epididymitis, proctitis, and chronic inflammation of the urethra. Women exposed to the exudate during coitus may develop a hypertrophic erosion of the cervix and purulent cervical mucus. An infant in passing through the cervix and vagina of a mother infected with *C. trachomatis* may develop conjunctivitis and nasopharyngeal infection in the first few days after birth and pneumonia at 3 to 4 months. Most cases of NGU are successfully treated with tetracycline or erythromycin. Sexual contacts are treated whether or not they are symptomatic. Nearly 50% of all cases of urethritis are nongonococcal.

non-Hodgkin's lymphoma Any kind of malignant lymphoma except Hodgkin's disease. Also called **lymphosarcoma.**

noninvasive In health care: of or pertaining to a diagnostic or therapeutic technique that does not require the skin to be broken or a cavity or organ of the body to be entered, as obtaining a blood pressure reading by auscultation with a stethoscope and sphygmomanometer.

nonosteogenic fibroma A common bone lesion in which there is degeneration and proliferation of the medullary and cortical tissue, usually near the ends of the diaphyses of the large long bones, especially those of the lower extremities. Frequently it does not cause any symptoms and is only discovered during X-rays of the skeleton for other reasons.

nonparametric test of significance In statistics: one of several tests that use a qualitative approach to analyze rank order data and incidence data that cannot be assumed to have a normal distribution.

nonproductive cough A sudden, noisy expulsion of air from the lungs that may be caused by irritation or inflammation and does not remove sputum from the respiratory tract. Expectorants increase respiratory tract secretions and may result in productive coughing when administered to patients with respiratory infections. If suppression of coughing is required, antitussives that depress the cough reflex may be prescribed. Intratracheal suctioning may be necessary when secretions cause severe respiratory difficulty and coughing is unproductive. Compare **productive cough.**

nonrapid eye movement (NREM) See **sleep.**

nonreflex bladder See **flaccid bladder.**

nonsense mutation See **amber mutation.**

nonsexual generation See **asexual generation.**

nonspecific urethritis (NSU) Inflammation of the urethra not known to be caused by a specific organism. Onset of symptoms is often related to sexual intercourse. Its acute phase is seldom seen in women, but its chronic phase is a common urologic difficulty among them. The condition is noted by urethral discharge in men and by reddening of the urethral mucosa

nondirective therapy A psychotherapeutic approach in which the psychotherapist refrains from offering the client advice or interpretation. In the process of nondirective therapy, clients are helped to identify their conflicts and to clarify and understand their feelings and values. Compare **directive therapy.** See also **client-centered therapy.**

nondisjunction Failure of homologous pairs of chromosomes to separate during the first meiotic division or of the two chromatids of a chromosome to split during anaphase of mitosis or the second meiotic division. The result is an abnormal number of chromosomes in the daughter cells. Compare **disjunction.** See also **monosomy, trisomy.**

nonfeasance In law: a failure to perform a task, duty, or undertaking that one has agreed to perform or that one had a legal duty to perform. Compare **malfeasance, misfeasance.** See also **negligence.**

nongonococcal urethritis (NGU) An infectious condition of the urethra that is characterized by mild dysuria and a scanty to moderate amount of penile discharge. The discharge may be white or clear, thin or mucoid, or, less often, purulent. The infection is often caused by the obligate intracellular parasite *Chlamydia trachomatis.* The diagnosis of NGU is made by excluding a diagnosis of gonococcal

in women. Treatment with antibiotics is not often successful. See also **nongonococcal urethritis.**

nontoxic   Not poisonous. Also called **atoxic.**

nontropical sprue   A malabsorption syndrome resulting from an inborn inability to digest foods that contain gluten. See also **celiac disease.**

nonulcerative blepharitis   A form of blepharitis characterized by greasy scales on the margins of the eyelids around the lashes and hyperemia and thickening of the skin. Nonulcerative blepharitis is often associated with seborrhea of the scalp, eyebrows, and the skin behind the ears.

nonverbal communication   The transmission of information by means other than language, such as behavior, facial expression, body carriage or position. The message conveyed may conflict with verbal information.

Noonan's syndrome   A hypergonadotropic disorder, occurring only in males, characterized by short stature, low-set ears, webbing of the neck, and cubitus valgus. Testicular function may be normal, but fertility is often decreased. The number and morphology of the chromosomes are normal. The cause is unknown. See also **Turner's syndrome.**

norepinephrine   An adrenergic hormone that acts to increase blood pressure by vasoconstriction but does not affect cardiac output. It is synthesized naturally by the adrenal medulla but is also available as a drug given to maintain the blood pressure in acute hypotension secondary to trauma, heart disease, or vascular collapse.

norepinephrine injection   A sympathomimetic agent. (Formerly levarterenol bitartrate.)

norethindrone, n. acetate   Progestogens.

norgestrel   A progestogen.

norm   A measure of a phenomenon generally accepted as the ideal standard performance against which other measures of the phenomenon may be measured.

norma basalis   The inferior surface of the base of the skull with the mandible removed, formed by the palatine bones, the vomer, the pterygoid processes, and parts of the sphenoid and temporal bones.

normal   **1.** Describing a standard, average, or typical example of a set of objects or values. **2.** Describing a chemical solution in which 1 liter contains 1 g of a substance or the equivalent in replaceable hydrogen ions.

-normal   A combining form meaning 'relating to a norm': *centinormal, decanormal, prenormal.*

normal dwarf   See **primordial dwarf.**

normal human serum albumin   An isotonic preparation of pooled human serum albumin for treating hypoproteinemia, hypovolemia, and threatened or existing shock.

normoblast   A nucleated cell that is the normal precursor of the adult circulating erythrocyte. The developmental stages include the pronormoblast, the basophilic normoblast, the

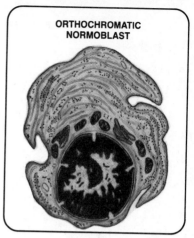

ORTHOCHROMATIC NORMOBLAST

polychromatic normoblast, and the orthochromatic normoblast. After the extrusion of the nucleus of the normoblast, the young erythrocyte becomes known as a reticulocyte. See also **reticulocyte.** —**normoblastic,** *adj.*

normochromic   Of a blood cell: having normal color, usually because it contains an adequate amount of hemoglobin. Compare **hypochromic.** See also **red cell indices.**

normocyte   A normal, adult red blood cell of average size having a diameter of 7 microns. Compare **macrocyte, microcyte.** —**normocytic,** *adj.*

normotensive   Of or pertaining to the condition of having normal blood pressure. —**normotension,** *n.*

North American blastomycosis   An infection caused by inhaling the fungus *Blastomyces dermatitidis.* It may resemble bacterial pneumonia, and X-ray films of the chest may show cavities. Painless, well-demarcated, verrucous or ulcerated skin lesions occur on the face and hands. The disease may progress to involve bones and the brain; many viscera are infected in fatal cases. Diagnosis is made by microscopic examination of body secretions. Treatment is amphotericin B, given intravenously, or, in severe cases, a combination of amphotericin B and sulfonamides. Compare **paracoccidioidomycosis.**

North Asian tick-borne rickettsiosis   An infection, acquired in the Eastern Hemisphere, caused by *Rickettsia siberica,* transmitted by ticks and resembling Rocky Mountain spotted fever. Usual findings include a generalized maculopapular rash involving palms and soles, fever, and lymph node enlargement. It is rarely fatal and responds quickly to treatment with chloramphenicol. No vaccine is available; prevention depends on avoidance of tick bites.

North Asian tick typhus   See **Siberian tick typhus.**

nortriptyline hydrochloride   A tricyclic antidepressant.

NOSE: INTERNAL STRUCTURES

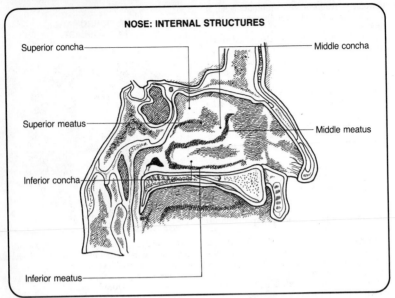

Superior concha — Middle concha
Superior meatus — Middle meatus
Inferior concha —
Inferior meatus —

noscapine hydrochloride A nonnarcotic antitussive.

nose The structure that protrudes from the anterior portion of the skull and serves as a passageway for air to and from the lungs. The nose filters the air, warming, moistening, and chemically examining it for impurities that might irritate the mucous lining of the respiratory tract. The nose also serves as the organ of smell, and it aids the faculty of speech. It consists of an internal portion and an external portion. The external portion, which protrudes from the face, is considerably smaller than the internal portion, which lies over the roof of the mouth. The hollow interior portion is separated into a right cavity and a left cavity by a septum. Each cavity is divided into the superior, middle, and inferior meati by the projection of nasal conchae. The external portion of the nose is perforated by two nostrils and the internal portion by two posterior nares. The pairs of sinuses that drain into the nose are the frontal, maxillary, ethmoidal, and sphenoidal sinuses. Ciliated mucous membrane lines the nose, closely adhering to the periosteum. The mucous membrane is continuous with the skin through the nares and with the mucous membrane of the nasal part of the pharynx through the choanae. The mucous membrane contains the olfactory cells, which connect with the olfactory nerves.

nosebleed Abnormal hemorrhage from the nose. Emergency responses to nosebleed include seating the patient upright with the head thrust forward to prevent swallowing of blood. Pressure with both thumbs directly under the nostril and above the lips may block the main artery supplying blood to the nose. Alternatively, pressure with both forefingers on each side of the nostril often slows bleeding by blocking the main arteries as well as their branches. Continued bleeding may require the insertion of cotton or other absorbent material into the nostril and reapplication of pressure. Cold compresses on the nose, lips, and the back of the head may help control hemorrhage. Also called **epistaxis.**

noso- A combining form meaning 'of or relating to disease': *nosochthonography, nosogeny, nosophobe.*

nosocomial Of or pertaining to a hospital.

nosocomial infection An infection acquired during hospitalization, often caused by *Candida albicans, Escherichia coli,* hepatitis viruses, herpes zoster virus, *Pseudomonas,* or *Staphylococcus.* Also called **hospital-acquired infection.**

nosology The science of classifying diseases. See also **nomenclature.**

nostrils See **anterior nares.**

notch An indentation or a depression in a bone or other organ, as the auricular notch or the cardiac notch.

noto- A combining form meaning 'of or relating to the back': *notochord, notogenesis, notomyelitis.*

notochord An elongated strip of mesodermal tissue that originates from the primitive node and extends along the dorsal surface of the developing embryo beneath the neural tube, forming the primary longitudinal skeletal axis of the body of all chordates. In humans and other vertebrate animals, the structure is replaced by vertebrae, although a remnant of it remains as part of the nucleus pulposus of the intervertebral disks. See also **neural tube. —notochordal,** *adj.*

notochordal canal A tubular passage that

extends from the primitive pit into the head process during the early stages of embryonic development in mammals. It perforates the splanchnopleure layer, so that there is a temporary connection between the yolk sac and the amnion. Also called **chordal canal.**

notochordal plate See **head process.**

notogenesis The formation of the notochord. —**notogenetic,** *adj.*

notomelus A congenital malformation in which one or more accessory limbs are attached to the back.

nourish To furnish or supply the essential foods or nutrients for maintaining life. —**nourishment,** *n.*

novobiocin calcium, n. sodium Antibiotics.

noxious Harmful, injurious, or detrimental to health.

Np Symbol for **neptunium.**

NPO *abbr nil per os,* a Latin phrase meaning 'nothing by mouth.'

N-propyl alcohol A clear, colorless liquid used as a solvent for resins.

NREM *abbr* **nonrapid eye movement.** See **sleep.**

NSNA *abbr* **National Student Nurses' Association.**

NSU *abbr* **nonspecific urethritis.**

nucha, *pl.* **nuchae** The nape, or back of the neck. —**nuchal,** *adj.*

nuchal cord An abnormal but common condition in which the umbilical cord is wrapped around the neck of the fetus in utero or during delivery. It is usually possible to slip the loop or loops of cord gently over the infant's head. If the cord is too tight for this maneuver, it may be clamped in two places and cut with sterile, blunt-tipped scissors.

nuchal rigidity An involuntary muscle stiffening at the nape of the neck that usually accompanies cervical spine injury, meningeal irritation, or subarachnoid bleeding after a head injury; a characteristic sign of meningitis. Efforts to move the head provoke pain and muscle spasm.

nucle- See **nucleo-.**

-nuclear A combining form meaning 'of or referring to the nucleus': *circumnuclear, endonuclear.*

nuclear family A family unit consisting of the biologic parents and their offspring. The nuclear family is a relatively recent product of western society. The nuclear family unit is less efficient than an extended family unit in providing information and vital services to family members, as child rearing, child care, and care of older family members. Compare **extended family.**

nuclear fission See **fission.**

nuclear hyaloplasm See **karyolymph.**

nuclear isomer One of two or more nuclides with the same number of neutrons and protons in the nucleus (the same atomic number, or Z, and the same atomic mass, or A) but existing in different energy states.

nuclear magnetic resonance Spectra emitted by phosphorus in body tissues as measured and imaged on phosphorus nuclear magnetic resonance instruments.

nuclear sap See **karyolymph.**

nucleic acid A polymeric compound of high molecular weight composed of nucleotides, each consisting of a purine or pyrimidine base, a ribose or deoxyribose sugar, and a phosphate group. Nucleic acids are involved in energy storage and release and in the determination and transmission of genetic characteristics. Kinds of nucleic acid are **deoxyribonucleic acid, ribonucleic acid.**

nucleo-, nucle- A combining form meaning 'of or related to a nucleus': *nucleochylema, nucleokeratin, nucleolus.*

nucleocapsid A viral enclosure consisting of a capsid or protein coat that encloses nucleic acid. Some viruses consist solely of bare nucleocapsids; others have more complex enclosures.

nucleochylema The ground substance of the nucleus, as distinguished from that of the cytoplasm.

nucleochyme See **karyolymph.**

nucleocytoplasmic Of or relating to the nucleus and cytoplasm of a cell.

nucleocytoplasmic ratio The ratio of the volume of a nucleus of a cell to the volume of the cytoplasm. The proportion is usually constant for a specific cell type and an increase is indicative of malignant neoplasms. Also called **karyoplasmic ratio, nucleoplasmic ratio.**

nucleohistone A complex nucleoprotein that consists of deoxyribonucleic acid and a histone. It is the basic constituent of the chromatin in the cell nucleus.

nucleolar organizer A part of the nucleus of the cell, thought to consist of heterochromatin, that is responsible for the formation of the nucleolus. Also called **nucleolus organizer.**

nucleolus, *pl.* **nucleoli** Any one of the small, dense structures composed largely of ribonucleic acid and situated within the cytoplasm of cells. Nucleoli are essential in the formation of ribosomes, which synthesize cell proteins.

nucleolus organizer See **nucleolar organizer.**

nucleoplasm The protoplasm composing the nucleus as contrasted with that of the cell. Also called **karyoplasm.** Compare **cytoplasm.** —**nucleoplasmic,** *adj.*

nucleoplasmic ratio See **nucleocytoplasmic ratio.**

nucleoside monophosphate kinase A liver enzyme that catalyzes the transfer of a phosphate group from adenosine triphosphate, producing adenosine diphosphate and a nucleoside diphosphate.

nucleosome Any one of the repeating nucleoprotein units consisting of histones forming a complex with deoxyribonucleic acid that appear as the beadlike structures at distinct intervals along the chromosome.

nucleotide Any one of the compounds into

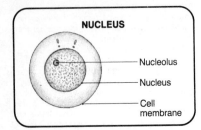

NUCLEUS

- Nucleolus
- Nucleus
- Cell membrane

which nucleic acid is split by the action of nuclease. A nucleotide consists of a phosphate group, a pentose sugar, and a nitrogenous base. Chains of such structures form deoxyribonucleic acid molecules essential for life.

nucleus 1. The central controlling body within a living cell, usually a spherical unit enclosed in a membrane and containing genetic codes for maintaining life systems of the organism and for issuing commands for growth and reproduction. 2. A group of nerve cells of the central nervous system having a common function, as supporting the sense of hearing or smell. 3. The center of an atom around which electrons revolve. 4. The central element in an organic chemical compound or in a class of compounds. —**nuclear,** *adj.*

nucleus pulposus The central portion of each intervertebral disk, consisting of a pulpy elastic substance that loses some of its resiliency with age.

nuclide A species of atom characterized by the number of protons and neutrons, energy content, and mass of its nucleus, capable of existing for a measurable time, generally greater than 10^{10} seconds.

null cell A lymphocyte that develops in the bone marrow, and lacks the characteristic surface markers of the B and T lymphocytes. It represents a small proportion of the lymphocyte population. Stimulated by the presence of an antibody, cells of this kind can apparently attack certain cellular targets directly and are known as 'killer,' or K cells. Compare **B cell, T cell.** See also **cytotoxin.**

null hypothesis (H₀) In research: a hypothesis that predicts that no difference or relationship exists among the variables studied that could not have occurred by chance alone.

nullipara, *pl.* **nulliparae** A woman who has not delivered a viable infant. On the chart, the designation 'para O' indicates nulliparity. —**nulliparity,** *n.,* **nulliparous,** *adj.*

numbness A partial or total lack of sensation in a part of the body, resulting from any factor that interrupts the transmission of impulses from the sensory nerve fibers.

nummular dermatitis A skin disease characterized by coin-shaped, vesicular, or scaling eczemalike lesions on the forearms and the front of the calves. The cause is unknown.

nurse 1. A person educated and licensed in the practice of nursing. The practice of the nurse includes data collection, diagnosis, planning,

treatment, and evaluation within the framework of the nurse's singular concern with the person's response to the problem, rather than to the problem itself. The nurse acts to promote, maintain, or restore the health of the person; wellness is the goal. The nurse may be a generalist or a specialist and, as a professional, is ethically and legally accountable for the nursing activities performed and for the actions of others to whom the nurse has delegated responsibility. 2. To provide nursing care. See also **five-step nursing process, nursing, registered nurse.** 3. To breast-feed an infant.

nurse anesthetist A registered nurse qualified by advanced training in an accredited program in the speciality of nurse anesthetist to manage the anesthetic care of the patient in certain surgical situations.

nurse-client interaction Any process in which a nurse and a client exchange or share information, verbally or nonverbally. It is fundamental to communication and is an essential component of the nursing assessment.

nurse-client relationship A therapeutic relationship between a nurse and a client built on a series of interactions and developing over time. All interactions do not develop into relationships but may nonetheless be therapeutic. The relationship differs from a social relationship in that it is designed to meet the needs only of the patient. Its structure varies with the context, the client's needs, and the goals of the nurse and the client. Its nature varies with the context, including the setting, the kind of nursing, and the needs of the patient. The relationship is dynamic and uses cognitive and affective levels of interaction. It is time-limited and goal-oriented and has three phases. During the first phase, the phase of establishment, the nurse establishes the structure, purpose, timing, and context of the relationship and expresses an interest in discussing this initial structure with the client. Data collection for the nursing-care plan continues, and basic goals for the relationship are stated. During the middle, developmental phase of the relationship, the nurse and the client get to know each other better and test the structure of the relationship in order to be able to trust one another. Plans may be devised for improved ways of coping with problems and achieving goals. The last phase, termination, ideally occurs when the goals of the relationship have been accomplished, when both the client and the nurse feel a sense of resolution and satisfaction.

nurse clinician A nurse who is prepared to identify and diagnose problems of clients by using the expanded knowledge and skills gained by advanced study in a specific area of nursing practice. The specialist may function independently within standing orders or protocols and collaborates with associates to implement a plan of care that is focused on the client.

Nurse Corps The branch within each of the armed services comprised of the nurses within that service, as the Army Nurse Corps. In each of the armed services, the members of the Nurse

Corps have the rank, title, responsibilities, and status of officers.

nurse educator A registered nurse whose primary area of interest, competence, and professional practice is the education of nurses.

nurse practice act A statute enacted by the legislature of any of the states or by the appropriate officers of the districts or possessions. The act delineates the legal scope of the practice of nursing within the geographical boundaries of the jurisdiction.

nurse practitioner A nurse who, by advanced training and clinical experience in a branch of nursing, as in a master's degree program in nursing, has acquired expert knowledge in a specialized branch of practice.

nursery diarrhea Diarrhea of the neonate. In nurseries, outbreaks of diarrhea caused by *Escherichia coli, Salmonella*, echoviruses, or adenoviruses are potentially life threatening to the neonate. Infection can occur at the time of birth from organisms in the mother's stool or later from organisms spread by the hands of hospital personnel. Fluid loss is the most serious aspect of the disease, leading to dehydration and electrolyte imbalance. Good hand-washing technique, use of disposable nursing bottles and nipples, and early isolation of infected neonates reduce the possibility of such outbreaks.

nurse's aide A person who is employed to carry out basic nonspecialized tasks in the care of a patient, as bathing and feeding, making beds, and transporting patients.

Nurses' Association of the American College of Obstetrics and Gynecology (NAACOG) A national organization of nurses who work in obstetrics and gynecology.

Nurses' Coalition for Action in Politics (N-CAP) An organization that works in association with the American Nurses' Association. It raises funds for political contributions to candidates for public office at the state and national levels.

nurse's registry An employment agency or listing service for nurses who wish to work in a specific area of nursing, usually for a short period of time or on a per diem basis.

nurses' station An area in a clinic, unit, or ward in a health-care facility that serves as the administrative center for nursing care for a particular group of patients. It is usually centrally located and may be staffed by a ward secretary or clerk who assists with paperwork and the telephone and other communication. Before going on duty, nurses usually meet there to receive daily assignments, to review the patients' charts, and to update the Cardex. The nurses' station is equipped appropriately for the care of patients in that area or unit.

nurse-therapist model In psychiatric nursing research: a theoretical framework to clarify the role of the mental-health nurse. Techniques from traditional and contemporary modes of treatment, including transactional analysis and crisis intervention, may be used singly or in various combinations. The nurse therapist chooses the technique or techniques after using the model to examine the nurse-client interaction, the feedback, and the goal of the interaction.

nursing 1. The professional practice of a nurse. **2.** The process of acting as a nurse, of providing care that encourages and promotes the health of the person being served. **3.** Breastfeeding an infant. See also **nurse.**

nursing assessment An identification by a nurse of the needs, preferences, and abilities of a patient. Assessment follows an interview with and observation of a patient by the nurse and considers the symptoms and signs of the condition, the patient's verbal and nonverbal communication, medical and social history, and any other information available. Among the physical aspects assessed are vital signs, skin color and condition, motor and sensory nerve function, nutrition, rest, sleep, activity, elimination, and conciousness. Among the social and emotional factors assessed are religion, occupation, attitude toward hospital and health care, mood, emotional tone, and family ties and responsibilities.

nursing assistant *Canada.* A person trained in basic nursing techniques and direct patient care who practices under the supervision of a registered nurse.

nursing audit A thorough investigation designed to identify, examine, or verify the performance of certain specified aspects of nursing care using established criteria. A concurrent nursing audit is performed during ongoing nursing care. A retrospective nursing audit is performed after discharge from the care facility, using the patient's record. Often, a nursing audit and a medical audit are performed collaboratively, resulting in a joint audit.

nursing-bottle caries A dental condition that occurs in children between the ages of 18 months and 3 years as a result of being given a bottle at bedtime, resulting in prolonged exposure of the teeth to milk or juice. Caries are formed because pools of milk or juice in the mouth break down to lactic acid and other decay-causing substances. Preventive measures include elimination of the bedtime feeding or substitution of water for milk or juice in the nighttime bottle. Also called **bottle-mouth syndrome.**

nursing-care plan A plan that is based on a nursing assessment and a nursing diagnosis, devised by a nurse. It has four essential components: the identification of the nursing care problems and a statement of the nursing approach to solve those problems; the statement of the expected benefit to the patient; the statement of the specific actions taken by the nurse that reflect the nursing approach and the achievement of the goals specified; and the evaluation of the patient's response to nursing care and the readjustment of that care as required. The nursing-care plan is begun when the patient is admitted to the health service, and, following the initial nursing assessment, a diagnosis is formulated, and nursing orders are developed.

NURSING DIAGNOSES

activity intolerance

airway clearance, ineffective

anxiety

bowel elimination, alteration in: constipation

bowel elimination, alteration in: diarrhea

bowel elimination, alteration in: incontinence

breathing pattern, ineffective

cardiac output, alteration in: decreased

comfort, alteration in: pain

communication, impaired verbal

coping, family: potential for growth

coping, ineffective family: compromised

coping, ineffective family: disabling

coping, ineffective individual

diversional activity, deficit

family processes, alteration in

fear

fluid volume, alteration in: excess

fluid volume deficit, actual

fluid volume deficit, potential

gas exchange, impaired

grieving, anticipatory

grieving, dysfunctional

health maintenance, alteration in

home maintenance management: impaired

injury: potential for

knowledge deficit

mobility, impaired physical

noncompliance

nutrition, alteration in: less than body requirements

nutrition, alteration in: more than body requirements

nutrition, alteration in: potential for more than body requirements

oral mucous membrane, alterations in

parenting, alteration in: actual or potential

powerlessness

rape-trauma syndrome

self-care deficit: feeding, bathing/hygiene, dressing/grooming, toileting

self-concept, disturbance in: body image, self-esteem, role performance, personal identity

sensory perceptual alteration: visual, auditory, kinesthetic, gustatory, tactile, olfactory

sexual dysfunction

skin integrity, impairment of: actual

skin integrity, impairment of: potential

sleep pattern disturbance

social isolation

spiritual distress (distress of the human spirit)

thought processes, alteration in

tissue perfusion, alteration in: cerebral, cardiopulmonary, renal, gastrointestinal, peripheral

urinary elimination, alteration in patterns

violence, potential for: self-directed or directed at others

The goal of the process is to ensure that nursing care is consistent with the patient's needs and progress toward self-care. A written nursing-care plan should be a part of every patient's chart; an abbreviated form should be available for quick reference, as in a Rand or Cardex file. See also **diagnosis, nursing assessment, nursing orders.**

nursing diagnosis A descriptive interpretation of collected and categorized data indicating the patient's problems or needs that can be affected by nursing care. Four steps are required in the formulation of a nursing diagnosis. A data base is established by collecting information from all available sources, including interviews with the client and the client's family, a review of any existing records of the client's health, observation of the response of the client to any alterations in health status, a physical assessment, and a conference or consultation with others concerned in the care of the client. The data base is continually updated. The second step includes an analysis of the client's responses to the problems, healthy or unhealthy, and a classification of those responses as psychological, physiological, spiritual, or sociological. The third step is the organization of the data so that a tentative diagnostic statement can be made that

summarizes the pattern of problems discovered. The last step is the confirmation of the sufficiency and accuracy of the data base by evaluation of the appropriateness of the diagnosis to nursing intervention and by the assurance that, given the same information, most other qualified practitioners would arrive at the same nursing diagnosis. In use, each diagnostic category has three parts: the term that concisely describes the problem, the probable etiology of the problem, and the defining characteristics of the problem. A number of nursing diagnoses have been identified and are listed as accepted by the National Group on the Classification of Nursing Diagnoses, updated and refined at periodic meetings of the group. The nursing diagnoses accepted at the Fifth National Conference are listed in the chart above.

nursing goal A general goal of nursing involving activities that are desirable but difficult to measure, as self-care, good nutrition, and relaxation. Compare **nursing objective.**

nursing history The compilation of data from a nursing assessment, used to devise a comprehensive nursing-care plan and including aspects of the patient's medical background; education; financial situation; daily activities; physical, emotional, and intellectual develop-

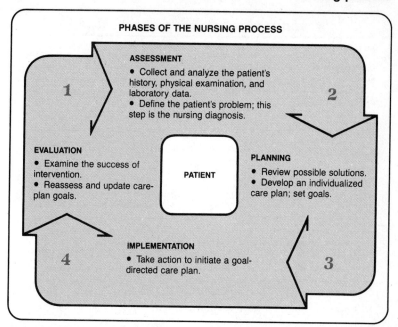

PHASES OF THE NURSING PROCESS

1

ASSESSMENT
- Collect and analyze the patient's history, physical examination, and laboratory data.
- Define the patient's problem; this step is the nursing diagnosis.

2

EVALUATION
- Examine the success of intervention.
- Reassess and update care-plan goals.

PATIENT

PLANNING
- Review possible solutions.
- Develop an individualized care plan; set goals.

4

IMPLEMENTATION
- Take action to initiate a goal-directed care plan.

3

ment; and social and cultural orientation.

nursing home See **extended-care facility.**

nursing intervention Any act by a nurse that implements the nursing-care plan or any specific objective of that plan, as turning a comatose patient to avoid the development of decubitus ulcers or teaching injection technique to a person with diabetes before discharge from the hospital. The patient may require intervention in the form of support, limitation, medication, or treatment for the current condition or to prevent the development of further stress.

nursing-intervention model In nursing research: a conceptual framework used to determine appropriate nursing interventions. The client's physiological, psychological, sociocultural, and developmental status, the stressors and ability to react to them, and the levels and patterns of available health care are observed. The goal is to learn what nursing interventions would be most effective for the particular problem within the available health-care system.

nursing objective A specific aim planned by a nurse to decrease a person's stress or improve the ability to adapt, or both. A nursing objective may be physical, emotional, social, or cultural and may involve the person's family and friends and other patients. It is the purpose of any specific nursing order or nursing intervention. Some common nursing objectives are adequate understanding by the patient of certain details of the condition, adequate and comfortable daily elimination, a certain amount of rest, a balanced diet. Nursing objectives, contrasted with nursing goals, can be measured. Compare **nursing goal.**

nursing observation An objective, holistic evaluation made by a nurse of the various aspects of a client's condition. It includes the person's general appearance, emotional affect, and nutritional status, habits, and preferences, as well as body temperature, skin condition, and any obvious abnormal processes, including those complained of by the client. The client's religious preference, ethnic background, and familial relationships are also noted. Compare **nursing assessment, nursing intervention.**

nursing orders Specific instructions for implementing the nursing-care plan, including the patient's preferences, timing of activities, details of health education that are necessary for the particular patient, role of the family, and plans for care after discharge. Nursing orders must be signed by the professional nurse who writes them. Nursing orders should not duplicate the orders of the medical staff or of other members of the health team.

nursing process The process that serves as an organizational framework for the practice of nursing. It encompasses all of the steps taken by the nurse in caring for a patient: data collection or assessment, diagnosis, planning, intervention, and evaluation. The rationale for each step is founded in nursing theory. The process requires a systematic approach to a nursing assessment of the person's situation, including an evaluation and reconciliation of the perceptions by the person, the person's family, and the nurse. A plan for the nursing actions to be taken may then be made and, with the participation of the person and the person's family, the plan may be set. The plan developed with the person

ESSENTIAL NUTRIENTS AND THEIR FUNCTIONS

NUTRIENTS	FUNCTIONS
Carbohydrates	• Energy source
Fats and essential fatty acids	• Energy source; essential for growth, normal skin, and membranes
Proteins and amino acids	• Synthesis of all body proteins, growth, and tissue maintenance

Water-soluble vitamins:

• Ascorbic acid (C)	• Collagen synthesis, wound healing, antioxidation
• Thiamine (B_1)	• Coenzyme in carbohydrate (CHO) metabolism
• Riboflavin (B_2)	• Coenzyme in energy metabolism
• Niacin	• Coenzyme in CHO, fat, energy metabolism, and tissue metabolism
• Vitamin B_{12}	• DNA and RNA synthesis; erythrocyte formation
• Folic acid	• Coenzyme in amino acid metabolism; heme and hemoglobin formation

Fat-soluble vitamins:

• Vitamin A	• Vision in dim light, mucosal epithelium integrity, tooth development, endocrine function
• Vitamin D	• Regulation of calcium and phosphate absorption and metabolism; renal phosphate clearance
• Vitamin E	• Antioxidation; essential for muscle, liver, and RBC integrity
• Vitamin K	• Blood clotting (catalyzes synthesis of prothrombin by liver)

and the person's family is then implemented. Evaluation of the outcome is performed with the person and the person's family. The steps follow each other at the start of the process but may need to be taken concurrently in some situations. The process does not reach completion with evaluation; the steps are begun again, allowing recurrent evaluation of the assessment, plan, goals, and actions. See also **five-step nursing process, nursing.**

nursing-process model A conceptual framework in which the nurse-patient relationship is the basis of the nursing process. The nursing process is represented as dynamic and interpersonal, the nurse and the patient being affected by each other's behavior and by the environment around them. Each successful two-way communication is termed a 'transaction' and can be analyzed to discover the factors that promote transactions. The constraints that the various systems in the environment (personal, interpersonal, and social) place on the development of the relationship are also examined.

nursing research A detailed process in which a systematic study of a problem in the field of nursing is performed. One basic approach requires the following steps: formulation of the problem; review of the literature; formation of a hypothesis or hypotheses; definition of variables; determination of a method for weighting and counting variables; selection of a research design; choice of a population; plan for the analysis of the data; determination of interpretation; development of a theory; and plan for promulgation of the results. Nursing research is practice or discipline oriented and is essential for the continued development of the scientific aspects of professional nursing.

Nursing Research A bimonthly refereed journal containing papers and other materials concerning nursing research.

nursing rounds Chart rounds, walking rounds, teaching rounds, or grand rounds that are held specifically for nurses and that focus on nursing-care problems. See also **rounds.**

nursing skills The cognitive, affective, and psychomotor abilities a nurse uses in delivering nursing care.

nursing specialty A nurse's particular professional field of practice, as surgical, pediatric, obstetric, or psychiatric nursing. Compare **subspecialty.**

nursing supervisor A nurse whose function is the administrative and clinical leadership of the nursing service of a division of a health-care facility, as a nursing supervisor of maternal and infant-care nurses.

nutation The act of nodding, especially involuntary nodding as occurs in some neurologic disorders.

nutri- A combining form meaning 'of or relating to nourishment': *nutriceptor, nutrient, nutritorium.*

nutrient A substance that provides nourishment and affects the nutritive and metabolic processes of the body.

nutrient artery of the humerus One of a pair of branches of the deep brachial arteries, arising near the middle of the arm and entering the nutrient canal of the humerus.

nutriment Any substance that nourishes and aids the growth and the development of the body. See also **food.**

nutrition 1. Nourishment. 2. The sum of the processes involved in the taking in of nutrients and in their assimilation and utilization for proper body functioning and maintenance of health. The successive stages include ingestion, digestion, absorption, assimilation, and excretion. 3. The study of food and drink as related to the growth and maintenance of living organisms. —**nutritionist,** *n.*

nutritional-alcoholic cerebellar degeneration See **alcoholic-nutritional cerebellar degeneration.**

nutritional anemia A disorder characterized by the inadequate production of hemoglobin or erythrocytes owing to nutritional deficiency of iron, folic acid, or vitamin B_{12} or other nutritional disorders. See also **iron deficiency anemia, megaloblastic anemia, pernicious anemia.**

nutritional care The substances, procedures, and setting involved in assuring the proper intake and assimilation of nutriments, especially for the hospitalized patient.

NURSING CONSIDERATIONS: Patients who are unable to feed themselves are assisted, and abnormal intake of food is recorded and reported. Supplemental nourishment, when indicated, and fluids are offered between meals. The nutritional assessment includes observations of the patient's appetite, food preferences, height, weight, measurements of the head, arms, abdomen, and skinfold thickness, the skin color and turgor, and the condition of the mouth, eyes, and hair. Any cutaneous lesions, thyroid enlargement, dental caries, loose teeth, ill-fitting dentures, gum problems, nausea, vomiting, dehydration, diarrhea, or constipation are noted. The nurse sees that food is presented attractively, offers a washcloth and mouthwash before and after meals, and, when necessary, feeds the patient to maintain an adequate intake. If indicated, as in obese patients or those with disorders requiring a highly restricted diet, the nurse restricts the intake of food as ordered. Tube feedings are administered as ordered.

nutrition, alteration in: less than body requirements A nursing diagnosis accepted by the Fifth National Conference on the Classification of Nursing Diagnoses. The etiology of the condition is an inability, based on psychological, biological, or economic factors, to ingest or digest food or to absorb nutrients in sufficient quantity for the maintenance of normal health. The defining characteristics of the condition may include loss of weight, reported intake of less food than is recommended, evidence or report of a lack of food, lack of interest in food, aversion to eating, alteration in the taste of food, feelings of fullness immediately after eating small quantities, abdominal pain with no other explanation, sores in the mouth, diarrhea or steatorrhea, pallor, weakness, and loss of hair. See also **nursing diagnosis.**

NUTRITIONAL CARE: REQUIREMENTS

Protein
1 to 3 g/kg/day

Carbohydrates
Enough to supply necessary calories and, in combination with fat, to supply 20 to 50 nonprotein calories for every gram of protein.

Fats
1 to 4 g/kg/day to provide necessary calories in combination with carbohydrates. If patient's fat intake is restricted, supply 2% to 4% of the calories as linoleic acid to prevent essential fatty acid deficiency.

Electrolytes
Sodium . . . . 3 to 4 mEq/kg/day
Potassium . . . . 2 to 3 mEq/kg/day
Chloride . . . . 2 to 4 mEq/kg/day
Acetate . . . . 1 to 1.5 mEq/kg/day

Vitamins
Folic acid . . . . 50 to 75 mcg/kg/day
Vitamin B_{12} . . . . 5 to 10 mcg/kg/day
Vitamin K . . . . . . .150 to 200 mcg/kg/day
MVI . . . . 0.5 ml/kg/day

Minerals
Phosphate . . . . . 1 to 3 millimoles/kg/day
Calcium . . . 300 to 800 mg/kg/day as the gluconate salt
Magnesium . . . . 0.25 to 0.5 mEq/kg/day

Trace elements
Zinc . . . . .300 mcg/kg/day in infants less than 3 kg; 100 mcg/kg/day over 3 kg
Chromium . . . . .0.14 mcg/kg/day
Manganese . . . . 2 mcg/kg/day
Copper . . . . 20 mcg/kg/day

---

nutrition, alteration in: more than body requirements A nursing diagnosis accepted by the Fifth National Conference on the Classification of Nursing Diagnoses. The etiology of the condition is an excessive intake of food in relation to the metabolic needs of the body. The defining characteristics of the condition include overweight, sedentary activity level, and dysfunctional eating habits, including eating in response to internal cues other than hunger. See also **nursing diagnosis.**

nutrition, alteration in: potential for more than body requirements A nursing diagnosis accepted by the Fifth National Conference on the Classification of Nursing Diagnoses. The etiology of the condition may be an inherited or familial predisposition to overweight, an excessive intake of calories during adolescence and other periods of rapid growth, frequent, closely spaced pregnancies, dysfunctional psychological conditioning in regard to food, or membership in a lower socioeconomic group. Definition of the problem may include the use of solid foods as a significant part of the diet before the age of 5 months, the use of food as a reward, an observed increase in the baseline weight at the onset of each pregnancy, or dysfunctional eating patterns, as eating in response to external cues, such as social situations or the time of day. The critical defining characteristics include reported or observed obesity in one or both parents and rapidly increasing percentiles in measurement of the infant's or child's weight as compared to others of the same age. See also **nursing diagnosis.**

nyctalopia Poor vision at night or in dim light, associated with vitamin A deficiency and pigmentary degeneration of the retina. Also called **night blindness. —nyctalopic,** *adj.*

nycto- A combining form meaning 'pertaining to night or darkness': *nyctohemeral, nyctophilia, nyctophobia.*

nyctophobia An anxiety reaction characterized by an obsessive, irrational fear of darkness.

nycturia See **nocturia.**

nylidrin hydrochloride A peripheral vasodilator.

nympho- A combining form meaning 'of or pertaining to the labia minora': *nymphocaruncular, nymphohymeneal, nymphoncus.*

nymphomania A psychosexual disorder of women characterized by an insatiable desire for sexual satisfaction, often resulting from an unconscious conflict concerning personal adequacy. Compare **satyriasis.** See also **psychosexual disorder.**

nymphomaniac **1.** A person with or displaying the characteristics of nymphomania. **2.** Of, pertaining to, or exhibiting nymphomania.

—nymphomaniacal, *adj.*

nystagmus Involuntary, rhythmic movements of the eyes; the oscillations may be horizontal, vertical, rotary, or mixed. Jerking nystagmus, characterized by faster movements in one direction than in the opposite direction, is more common than pendular nystagmus, in which the oscillations are approximately equal in rate in both directions. Jerking nystagmus occurs normally when an individual watches a moving object, but, on other occasions, it may be a sign of barbiturate intoxication or of labyrinthine-vestibular, vascular, or neurologic disease. Labyrinthine-vestibular nystagmus, most frequently rotary, is usually accompanied by vertigo and nausea. Vertical nystagmus is considered pathognomonic of disease of the brain stem's tegmentum, and nystagmus occurring only in the abducting eye is said to be a sign of multiple sclerosis. Seesaw nystagmus, in which one eye moves up and the other down, may be seen in bilateral hemianopia. Pendular nystagmus occurs in albinism, various diseases of the retina and refractive media, and in miners, following many years of working in darkness. In miners, the eye movements are very rapid, increase on upward gaze, and are often associated with vertigo, head tremor, and photophobia. Electronystagmography, used in testing for vestibular disease and in evaluating patients with vertigo, hearing loss, or tinnitus, records changes in the electrical field around the eyes when nystagmus is induced by douching cold or warm water into the external auditory canal; this test causes nystagmus in normal individuals and a diminished or absent reaction in patients with labyrinth disorder. Also called **nystaxis. —nystagmic,** *adj.*

nystatin An antifungal agent.

nystaxis See **nystagmus.**

O Symbol for **oxygen.**

O₂ Symbol for molecular oxygen.

OASDHI *abbr* **Old Age, Survivors, Disability and Health Insurance program,** as provided by the Social Security Act.

oat cell carcinoma A malignant, usually bronchogenic epithelial neoplasm consisting of small, tightly packed round, oval, or spindle-shaped epithelial cells that stain darkly and contain neurosecretory granules and little or no cytoplasm. Tumors produced by these cells do not form bulky masses but usually spread along submucosal lymphatics. One third of all malignant tumors of the lung are of this type. Surgical resection is usually not possible, and chemotherapy and radiation therapy are usually not effective; thus, the prognosis is poor. Also called **small-cell carcinoma.**

OB *abbr* **1. Obstetrics. 2. Obstetrician.**

ob- A combining form meaning 'against, in front of': *obdormition, obduction, obtuse.* Also **oc-.**

obesity An abnormal increase in the proportion of fat cells in the subcutaneous tissues of the body. Obesity may be exogenous or endogenous.

objective 1. A goal. **2.** Of or pertaining to a phenomenon or clinical finding that is observed; not subjective.

objective data collection The process in which data relating to the client's problem are obtained by an observer through direct physical examination, including observation, palpation, and auscultation, and by laboratory analyses and radiologic and other studies. Compare **subjective data collection.**

obligate Characterized by the ability to survive only in a particular set of environmental conditions, as an obligate parasite, which can survive only within the host organism. Compare **facultative.**

obligate aerobe An organism that cannot grow in the absence of oxygen. Compare **facultative aerobe.** See also **aerobe.**

obligate anaerobe An organism that cannot grow in the presence of oxygen. Compare **facultative anaerobe.** See also **anaerobe, anaerobic infection.**

obligate parasite See **parasite.**

oblique A slanting direction or any variation from the perpendicular or the horizontal.

oblique bandage A circular bandage applied spirally in slanting turns, usually to a limb.

oblique fissure of the lung 1. The groove that marks the division between the lower and the middle lobes in the right lung. **2.** The groove that marks the division between the upper and the lower lobes in the left lung.

oblique fracture A fracture that cracks a bone at an oblique angle.

oblique illumination See **illumination.**

obliquus externus abdominis One of a pair of muscles that are the largest and the most superficial of the five anterolateral muscles of the abdomen. A broad, thin, four-sided muscle that arises by eight fleshy digitations from the lower eight ribs and by the broad abdominal aponeurosis, it inserts in the iliac crest and the linea alba. It is innervated by branches of the 8th through the 12th intercostal nerves and by the iliohypogastric and ilioinguinal nerves. It acts to compress the contents of the abdomen and assists in micturition, defecation, emesis, parturition, and forced expiration. Both sides acting together serve to flex the vertebral column, drawing the pubis toward the xiphoid process. One side alone functions to bend the vertebral column laterally and to rotate it, drawing the shoulder of the same side forward. Also called **descending oblique muscle, external oblique muscle.** Compare **obliquus internus abdominis, pyramidalis, rectus abdominis, transversus abdominis.**

obliquus internus abdominis One of a pair of anterolateral muscles of the abdomen, lying under the obliquus externus abdominis in the lateral and ventral part of the abdominal wall. Smaller and thinner than the obliquus externus abdominis, it arises from the inguinal ligament, the iliac crest, and the lower portion of the lumbar aponeurosis. It inserts into the last three or four ribs and into the linea alba. The obliquus internus abdominis compresses the abdominal contents and assists in micturition, defecation, emesis, parturition, and forced expiration. Both sides acting together serve to flex the vertebral column, drawing the costal cartilages toward the pubis. One side acting alone acts to bend the vertebral column laterally and rotate it, drawing the shoulder of the opposite side downward. Also called **ascending oblique muscle, internal oblique muscle.** Compare **obliquus externus abdominis, pyramidalis, rectus abdominis, transversus abdominis.**

observation 1. The act of watching carefully and attentively. **2.** A report of what is seen or noticed, as a **nursing observation.**

obsession A persistent thought or idea with which the mind is continually and involuntarily preoccupied and which suggests an irrational act. The thought cannot be eliminated by reason and usually gives rise to a compulsion. See also **compulsion, obsessive-compulsive neurosis. —obsessive,** *adj.*

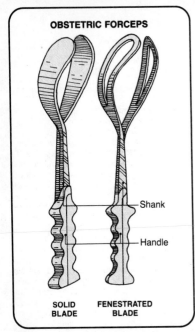

OBSTETRIC FORCEPS

— Shank

— Handle

SOLID BLADE   **FENESTRATED BLADE**

This behavior is manifested in many forms and may range from mildly stylized personal habits, as repeating certain words or phrases before undertaking a particular act, to more serious compulsive acts, as the continuous washing of hands or changing of clothes. A person with this kind of personality is usually orderly, meticulous, punctual, dependable, and scrupulous, though with a tendency to be rigid, stubborn, and pedantic. When the acts or rituals become irrational and exaggerated, they reduce the flexibility of behavior and interfere with everyday functioning in society, becoming neurotic reactions.

obsessive-compulsive reaction   See **obsessive-compulsive neurosis.**

obstetrical position   See **lateral recumbent position.**

obstetric anesthesia   Any of various procedures used to provide anesthesia for childbirth, including local anesthesia for episiotomy or episiotomy repair; regional anesthesia for labor or delivery, as by paracervical block or pudendal block; or, for a wider block, epidural, caudal, or saddle block. Anesthesia for cesarean section may be achieved with an epidural block or by general anesthesia. Light inhalation anesthesia with a mixture of nitrous oxide and oxygen is commonly given when forceps are required or when a difficult vaginal delivery is expected.

obstetric forceps   Forceps used to assist delivery of the fetal head. They vary in weight, length, shape, and mechanism of action, but all consist of a pair of instruments comprising a handle, a shank, and a blade. The blade is curved and, sometimes, fenestrated. The shank is long enough to allow the blade to reach the fetal head. The several styles of forceps are designed to assist in various clinical situations. Kinds of obstetric forceps include **Barton forceps, Elliot forceps, Kielland's forceps, Simpson's forceps.** See also **forceps delivery.**

obstetrician   A doctor who specializes in obstetrics.

obstetrics   The branch of medicine concerned with pregnancy and childbirth, including the study of the physiologic and pathologic function of the female reproductive tract and the care of the mother and fetus throughout pregnancy, childbirth, and the immediate postpartum period. —**obstetric, obstetrical,** *adj.*

obstipation   1. A condition of extreme and persistent constipation caused by intestinal or eliminatory obstruction. See also **constipation.** 2. A process of blocking. —**obstipant,** *n.,* **obstipate,** *v.*

obstruction   1. Something that blocks or impedes. 2. The act of blocking or preventing passage. 3. The condition of being obstructed. —**obstruct,** *v.,* **obstructive,** *adj.*

obstructive anuria   A urologic condition characterized by an almost total absence of urination and caused by a urinary tract obstruction. See also **anuria.**

obstructive jaundice   See **cholestasis.**

obsessional personality   A type of personality in which persistent, intrusive, irrational, uncontrollable, and unwanted thoughts lead to compulsive actions. The thoughts may consist of single words, simple ideas or desires, images, ruminations, or, more commonly, a complex train of ideas referring to past events and completed actions or to anticipated events and future actions. A person with an obsessional personality is punctual, orderly, meticulous, and dependable; dominated by feelings of inadequacy, insecurity, and guilt; and highly vulnerable to threat, worry, indecision, overscrupulousness, and excessive anxiety.

obsessive-compulsive   1. Characterized by or relating to the tendency to perform repetitive acts or rituals, usually as a means of releasing tension or relieving anxiety. 2. Describing a person who has an obsessive-compulsive neurosis.

obsessive-compulsive neurosis   A neurotic condition characterized by the inability to resist or stop the intrusion of persistent, irrational, and uncontrollable urges, ideas, thoughts, or fears contrary to the person's standards or judgments. The disorder usually appears after adolescence, resulting from fear, guilt, and anticipation of punishment. Treatment may consist of psychotherapy to uncover the basic fears and to help the person distinguish objective from imagined dangers. Also called **obsessive-compulsive reaction, psychasthenia.**

obsessive-compulsive personality   A type of personality in which there is an uncontrollable need to perform certain acts or rituals.

obtund **1.** To deaden pain. **2.** To render insensitive to unpleasant or painful stimuli by reducing the level of consciousness, as by anesthesia. —**obtundation, obtundity,** *n.,* **obtunded, obtundent,** *adj.*

obtundation The use of an agent that soothes and reduces irritation or pain by blocking sensibility at some level of the central nervous system, as in the preoperative use of general or local anesthesia.

obturator **1.** A device used to block a passage or a canal or to fill in a space, as a prosthesis implanted to bridge the gap in the roof of the mouth in a cleft palate. **2.** *Nontechnical.* An obturator muscle or membrane.

obturator externus The flat, triangular muscle covering the outer surface of the anterior pelvic wall. It arises in several pelvic structures, including the rami of the pubis and the ramus of each ischium, and inserts into the trochanteric fossa of the femur. The obturator externus is innervated by a branch of the obturator nerve, and it functions to rotate the thigh laterally. Compare **obturator internus.**

obturator foramen A large opening on each side of the lower portion of the innominate bone, formed posteriorly by the ischium, superiorly by the illium, and anteriorly by the pubis.

obturator internus A muscle that covers a large area of the inferior aspect of the lesser pelvis, where it surrounds the obturator foramen. It arises from the superior and the inferior rami of the pubis, the ischium, and the obturator membrane and inserts into the greater trochanter of the femur. It is innervated by a special nerve from the sacral plexus and functions to rotate the thigh laterally and to extend and abduct the thigh when it is flexed. Compare **obturator externus, piriformis.**

obturator membrane A tough fibrous membrane that covers the obturator foramen of each side of the pelvis.

obturator muscle A muscle of the pelvis and upper leg that acts to rotate the leg laterally.

oc- See **ob-.**

occipital **1.** Of or pertaining to the occiput. **2.** Situated near the occipital bone.

occipital artery One of a pair of tortuous branches from the external carotid arteries that divides into six branches and supplies parts of the head and scalp. Each terminal portion at the vertex of the skull is accompanied by the greater occipital nerve.

occipital bone The cuplike bone at the back of the skull, pierced by a large opening called the foramen magnum, that communicates with the vertebral canal. Its inner surface is divided into four fossae. The occipital bone articulates with the two parietal bones, the two temporal bones, the sphenoid, and the atlas.

occipital lobe One of the five lobes of each cerebral hemisphere, occupying a relatively small pyramidal portion of the occipital pole. The occipital lobe lies beneath the occipital bone and presents medial, lateral, and inferior surfaces. The medial surface is bounded anteriorly by the

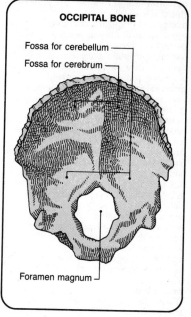

OCCIPITAL BONE

Fossa for cerebellum —

Fossa for cerebrum —

Foramen magnum ⌐

pareito-occipital sulcus and the preoccipital notch and is divided by the posterior calcarine sulcus into the wedge-shaped cuneus and the lingual gyrus. The lateral surface of the lobe is divided by the lateral sulcus into the superior and the inferior occipital gyri. An imaginary transverse line across the preoccipital notch limits the inferior surface. Compare **central lobe, frontal lobe, parietal lobe, temporal lobe.**

occipital sinus The smallest of the cranial sinuses and one of six posterior superior venous channels associated with the dura mater. It is located in the attached margin of the falx cerebelli, courses around the foramen magnum by several small channels, communicates with the posterior internal vertebral venous plexuses, and ends in the confluence of the sinuses. Compare **inferior sagittal sinus, straight sinus, superior sagittal sinus.**

occipitoaxial ligament See **membrana tectoria.**

occipitobregmatic Of or pertaining to the occiput and the bregma.

occipitofrontal Of or pertaining to the occiput and the frontal bone of the skull.

occipitofrontalis One of a pair of thin, broad muscles covering the top of the skull, consisting of an occipital and a frontal belly connected by an extensive aponeurosis. The frontal belly originates at the galea aponeurotica and inserts in the skin of the eyebrows and nose. The occipital belly originates in the superior nuchal line of the occipital bone and inserts at the galea aponeurotica. The occipitofrontalis is innervated by the facial nerve. It draws the scalp and raises the eyebrows. Compare **temporoparietalis.**

occipitoparietal fissure See **parieto-occipital sulcus.**

occiput, *pl.* **occiputs, occipita** The back part of the head. Also called **occiput cranii.**

occlusal Pertaining to the closure of an opening; specifically, to the relation of the contacting surfaces of the maxillary and mandibular teeth when brought together in a bite.

occlusal trauma Injury to a tooth and surrounding structures caused by malocclusive stresses.

occlusion A blockage in a canal, vessel, or passage of the body. —**occlude,** *v.,* **occlusive,** *adj.*

occlusion rim An artificial dental structure on which occluding surfaces are attached to temporary or permanent denture bases. The structure used to record the relation of the maxilla to the mandible and to position the teeth. Also called **bite block.**

occlusive dressing A dressing that prevents air from reaching a wound or lesion. It may be a thin plastic sheet affixed with transparent tape. See also **dressing.**

occult Hidden or difficult to observe directly, as occult prolapse of the umbilical cord or occult blood.

occult blood A minute or hidden quantity of blood that can be detected only by a chemical test or a microscopic or spectroscopic examination. Occult blood is often present in the stools of patients with gastrointestinal lesions.

occult carcinoma A small carcinoma that does not cause overt symptoms. It may remain localized and be discovered only incidentally at autopsy following death owing to another cause, or it may metastasize and be discovered in the diagnostic study of the resulting metastatic disease. Also called **latent carcinoma.**

occult fracture A fracture that cannot be initially detected by radiography but may be evident radiographically weeks later. It is accompanied by the usual signs of pain and trauma and may produce soft tissue edema.

occupational accident An accidental injury to an employee that occurs in the workplace. Occupational accidents account for over 95% of occupational disabilities.

occupational asthma An abnormal respiratory condition resulting from exposure in the workplace to allergenic or other irritating substances. The condition is most common among persons working with detergents, Western red cedar, cotton, flax, hemp, grain, flour, and stone. See also **asthma, byssinosis, occupational lung disease.**

occupational disability A condition in which a worker is unable to perform a job satisfactorily, owing to an occupational disease or accident.

occupational disease A disease that results from a particular employment, usually from the effects of long-term exposure to specific substances or of continuous or repetitive physical acts.

occupational history A portion of the health history in which questions are asked about the person's occupation, source of income, effects of the work on the worker's health, the duration of the job, and to what degree the occupation satisfies the person. Any adverse effects known to be associated with the occupation or the place of work are investigated by the interviewer.

occupational lung disease Any one of a group of abnormal lung conditions caused by the inhalation of dusts, fumes, gases, or vapors in the workplace. See also **chronic obstructive pulmonary disease, metal fume fever, occupational asthma, silo fillers' disease.**

occupational neurosis A neurotic disorder in which various symptoms occur that prevent the activities required by the occupation, as in writer's block. The symptoms are not caused by the occupation; rather, they serve as an expression of a neurotic conflict.

occupational therapist A person who practices occupational therapy and who may be licensed, registered, certified, or otherwise regulated by law.

occupational therapy A subdivision of physical medicine in which handicapped or convalescing patients are trained in vocational skills and activities of daily life through a program designed to satisfy the specific needs of the patient while providing diversion and exercise.

occurrence policy A professional liability insurance policy that covers the holder during the period an alleged act of malpractice occurred. Because the statute of limitations on malpractice allegations is unlimited, an individual could be sued years after an event. An occurrence malpractice policy provides protection against such a suit.

ochre mutation See **amber mutation.**

ochronosis A condition characterized by the deposition of brown-black pigment in connective tissue and cartilage, often caused by alkaptonuria or poisoning with phenol. Blue macules may be noted on the sclera, fingers, ears, nose, genitalia, buccal mucosa, and axillae. The urine may be dark. See also **alkaptonuria.**

octaploid, octaploidic See **polyploid.**

ocular 1. Of or pertaining to the eye. 2. An eyepiece of an optical instrument.

ocular hypertelorism A developmental defect involving the frontal region of the cranium, characterized by an abnormally widened bridge of the nose and increased distance between the eyes. The condition is often associated with other cranial and facial deformities and some degree of mental retardation. Also called **orbital hypertelorism.**

ocular hypotelorism A developmental defect involving the frontal region of the cranium, characterized by a narrowing of the bridge of the nose and an abnormal decrease in the distance between the eyes, with resulting convergent strabismus. The condition is often associated with other cranial and facial deformities, primarily microcephaly and trigonocephaly, and

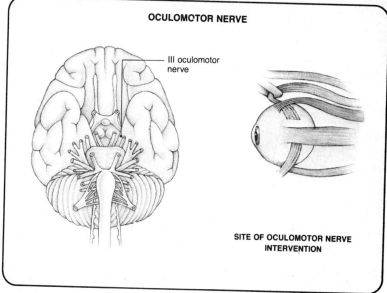

OCULOMOTOR NERVE

III oculomotor nerve

SITE OF OCULOMOTOR NERVE INTERVENTION

some degree of mental retardation. Also called **orbital hypotelorism.**

ocular myopathy   Slowly progressive weakness of ocular muscles, characterized by decreased eye mobility and drooping of the upper lid. It may be unilateral or bilateral and may be the result of damage to the oculomotor nerve, an intracranial tumor, or a neuromuscular disease.

ocular spot   An abnormal opacity in the eye. A shower of red and black dots may be seen in the eye after hemorrhage of a retinal vessel; opacities in the crystalline lens are characteristic in cataracts. In asteroid hyalitis, often associated with diabetes, small, white spherical and stellate opacities are found in the vitreous humor.

oculo-   A combining form meaning 'of or pertaining to the eye': *oculofacial, oculomycosis, oculopathy.*

oculogyric crisis   A paroxysm in which the eyes are held in a fixed position, usually up and sideways, for minutes or several hours, often occurring in postencephalitic patients with signs of parkinsonism. In some cases the eyes are held down or sideways, and there may be spasm or closing of the lids. The crisis may result from emotional stress.

oculomotor nerve   Either of a pair of cranial nerves essential for eye movements, supplying certain extrinsic and intrinsic eye muscles. They pass through the superior orbital fissure, connecting to the brain in nucleus III. Also called **nervus oculomotorius, third nerve.**

O.D.   *abbr oculus dexter,* Latin for 'right eye.'

-ode   A combining form meaning: **1.** A 'type of (specified) electrical conductor': *anode, cathode, electrode.* **2.** 'Like in form' of something

specified: *cytode, sarcode.*

odont-, ondonto-   A combining form meaning 'of or pertaining to the teeth': *odontoblast, odontopathy.*

-odontia   A combining form meaning a 'form, condition, or mode of treatment of the teeth': *periodontia, prosthodontia, radiodontia.*

odontiasis   The process of cutting teeth; teething.

-odontic   A combining form meaning: **1.** 'Pertaining to the size of teeth': *isodontic, macrodontic, mesodontic.* **2.** 'Pertaining to a type of dental treatment': *gerodontic, orthodontic, pedodontic.*

odontitis   Abnormal enlargement of a tooth, usually resulting from an inflammation of the odontoblasts. It may be caused by infection, tumor, or trauma.

odontogenesis imperfecta   See **dentinogenesis imperfecta.**

odontogenic   **1.** Generating teeth. **2.** Developing in tissues that produce teeth.

odontogenic fibroma   A benign neoplasm of the jaw derived from the embryonic part of the tooth germ, dental follicle, or dental papilla or developing later from the periodontal membrane.

odontogenic fibrosarcoma   A malignant neoplasm of the jaw that develops in a mesenchymal component of a tooth or tooth germ.

odontogenic myxoma   A rare tumor of the jaw that seems to develop from the mesenchyme of the tooth germ.

odontoid ligament   See **alar ligament.**

odontoid vertebra   See **axis.**

odontology   The scientific study of the anatomy and physiology of the teeth and of the structures of the oral cavity.

OLECRANON OF THE ULNA

- Olecranon

- Trochlear notch

---

odor A scent or smell. The sense of smell is activated when airborne molecules stimulate the first cranial nerve.

-odyne A combining form meaning 'referring to, treating pain': *acesodyne, anodyne, biodyne.*

-odynia A combining form meaning a 'state of pain in a (specified) location': *coccyodynia, odontodynia, uterodynia.*

odyno- A combining form meaning 'pain': *odynolysis, odynophagia, odynopoeia.*

odynophagia A severe sensation of burning, squeezing pain while swallowing, caused by irritation of the mucosa or a muscular disorder of the esophagus.

Oedipus complex The unconscious attachment of a child to the parent of the opposite sex, accompanied by hostility toward the parent of the same sex. It originally referred to the son's attachment to the mother.

oenomania See **oinomania.**

OH Symbol for **hydroxyl.**

OHF *abbr* **Omsk hemorrhagic fever.**

ohm A unit of measurement of electrical resistance. One ohm is the resistance of a conductor in which an electrical potential of 1 volt produces a current of 1 ampere.

-oi A plural-forming element in borrowings from Greek: *auloi, catanephroi, mesonephroi.* Also **-i.**

-oid A combining form meaning: **1.** 'Resembling' something specified: *alkaloid, trochoid.* **2.** 'Having the form or appearance of': *cuboid, ovoid.*

oiko- A combining form meaning 'house': *oikofugic, oikology, oikophobia.*

oil Any of a large number of greasy liquid substances not miscible in water. Oil may be fixed or volatile and is derived from animal, vegetable, or mineral matter.

oinomania, enomania, oenomania 1. A periodic, irresistible craving for alcohol. **2.** Delirium tremens.

ointment A semisolid, externally applied preparation, usually containing a drug. Various ointments are used as local analgesic, anesthetic, anti-infective, astringent, depigmenting, irritant, and keratolytic agents. Also called **salve, unction, unguent.**

-ol, -ole 1. A combining form designating a member of the alcohol group: *ethanol, methanol, naphthol.* **2.** A combining form meaning an 'oil': *benzol, furol, petrol.*

-ola A combining form meaning a 'singular

diminutive of the noun named': *arteriola, neurovariola, taeniola.*

Old Age, Survivors, Disability and Health Insurance (OASDHI) program A benefit program, administered by the Social Security Administration, that provides cash benefits to workers who are retired or disabled, their dependents, and survivors. This part of the program is commonly referred to as Social Security. The program also provides health insurance benefits for people over 65 and for disabled people under 65. This part of the program is commonly referred to as Medicare. See also **Medicare.**

Old World leishmaniasis See **oriental sore.**

oleandomycin See **troleandomycin.**

olecranon A proximal projection of the ulna that forms the point of the elbow and fits into the olecranon fossa of the humerus when the forearm is extended. The anterior surface of the olecranon forms part of the trochlear notch that articulates with the humerus. Also called **olecranon process.**

olecranon bursa The bursa of the elbow.

olecranon fossa The depression in the posterior surface of the humerus that receives the olecranon of the ulna when the forearm is extended. Compare **coronoid fossa.**

olecranon process See **olecranon.**

oleic acid A colorless, liquid, monounsaturated fatty acid occurring in almost all natural fats.

oleo- A combining form meaning 'of or pertaining to oil': *oleocreosote, oleodistearin, oleoresin.* Also **eleo-.**

oleometer A device for measuring the purity of oils.

oleovitamin A preparation of fish-liver oil or edible vegetable oil that contains one or more of the fat-soluble vitamins or their derivatives.

oleovitamin A A preparation, usually containing fish-liver oil and the natural or synthetic form of vitamin A. See also **vitamin A.**

oleovitamin D$_2$ See **calciferol.**

olfactory Of or pertaining to the sense of smell. —**olfaction,** *n.*

olfactory anesthesia See **anosmia.**

olfactory center The part of the brain responsible for the subjective appreciation of odors, a complex group of neurons located near the junction of the temporal and parietal lobes.

olfactory foramen One of several openings in the cribriform plate of the ethmoid bone.

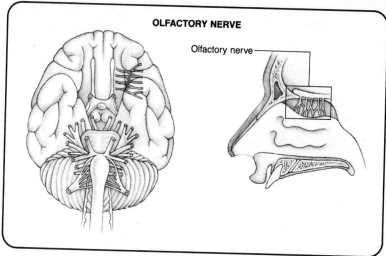

OLFACTORY NERVE

Olfactory nerve

olfactory nerve One of a pair of nerves associated with the sense of smell. The olfactory nerve is cranial nerve I and is composed of numerous fine filaments that ramify in the mucous membrane of the olfactory area. The fibers of the olfactory nerve are nonmedullated and unite into fasciculi which form a plexus under the mucous membrane and rise in grooves or canals in the ethmoid bone. The fibers pass into the skull and form synapses with the dendrites of the mitral cells. The area in which the olfactory nerves arise is situated in the most superior portion of the mucous membrane that covers the superior nasal concha. The olfactory nerves connect with the olfactory bulb and the olfactory tract, which are components of the portion of the brain associated with the sense of smell.

oligo-, olig- A combining form meaning 'few, little': *oligocholia, oligodontia, oligosialia.*

oligodactyly, oligodactylism, oligodactylia A congenital anomaly characterized by the absence of one or more of the fingers or toes. **—oligodactylic,** *adj.*

oligodendroglioma, *pl.* **oligodendrogliomas, oligodendrogliomata** An uncommon brain tumor composed of nonneural ectodermal cells that usually form part of the supporting connective tissue around nerve cells. The lesion, a firm, red-gray mass with calcified spots and a distinct margin, may grow to a large size. It often develops in frontal, parietal, and paraventricular sites but may occur in the cerebellum. Also called oligodendroblastoma.

oligodontia A genetically determined dental defect characterized by the development of fewer than the normal number of teeth.

oligogenic Of or pertaining to hereditary characteristics produced by one or only a few genes.

oligomeganephronia A type of congenital renal hypoplasia associated with chronic renal failure in children and characterized by a decreased number of functioning nephrons and hypertrophy of other renal elements without the presence of aberrant tissue. Also called oligomeganephronic renal hypoplasia. **—oligomeganephronic,** *adj.*

oligomenorrhea Abnormally light or infrequent menstruation. **—oligomenorrheic,** *adj.*

oligopnea, oligopnoea See **hypopnea.** **—oligopneic, oligopnoic,** *adj.*

oligospermia Insufficient spermatozoa in the semen. Compare **azoospermia.**

oliguria A diminished capacity to form and pass urine so that the metabolic end products cannot be excreted efficiently. It is usually caused by body fluid and electrolyte imbalances, renal lesions, or urinary tract obstruction. Also called oliguresis. Compare **anuria. —oliguric,** *adj.*

olivopontocerebellar Of or pertaining to the olivae, the middle peduncles, and the cerebellum.

Ollier's disease See **enchondromatosis.**

Ollier's dyschondroplasia A rare disorder in which the epiphyseal tissue responsible for growth spreads through the bones, causing abnormal irregular growth and, eventually, deformity. The long bones and the ilia are most often affected. Orthopedic procedures to correct deformities may be helpful, but invalidism is the usual prognosis. A kind of dyschondroplasia is **hereditary multiple exostoses.** Also called **multiple enchondromatosis.**

oma-, omo- A combining form meaning 'of or pertaining to the shoulder': *omoclavicular, omohyoid.*

-oma A combining form meaning a 'tumor': *capsuloma, lymphadenoma, neurinoma.*

omental bursa A cavity in the peritoneum behind the stomach, the lesser omentum, and the lower border of the liver and in front of the pancreas and duodenum.

omentum, *pl.* **omenta, omentums** An extension of the peritoneum that enfolds one or

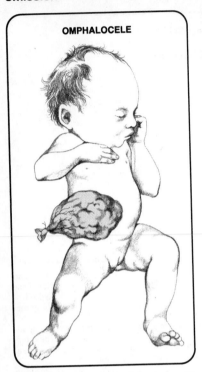

OMPHALOCELE

more adjacent organs in the abdominal cavity. See also **greater omentum, lesser omentum.** —**omental,** *adj.*

omission In law: intentional or unintentional neglect to fulfill a duty required by law.

omphalo-, omphal- A combining form meaning 'of or related to the navel': *omphalocele, omphaloma.*

omphaloangiopagus See **allantoidoangiopagus.**

omphalocele Congenital herniation of intra-abdominal viscera through a defect in the abdominal wall around the umbilicus. The defect is usually closed surgically soon after birth.

omphalodidymus See **gastrodidymus.**

omphalogenesis The umbilicus or yolk sac formation during embryonic development. —**omphalogenetic,** *adj.*

omphalomesenteric artery See **vitelline artery.**

omphalomesenteric circulation See **vitelline circulation.**

omphalomesenteric duct See **yolk stalk.**

omphalomesenteric vein See **vitelline vein.**

omphalopagus See **monomphalus.**

omphalosite The underdeveloped parasitic member of unequal conjoined twins united by the vessels of the umbilical cord. The omphalosite has no heart, derives its blood supply from the placenta of the autosite, and is incapable of independent existence after birth.

OMS *abbr* **Organisation Mondiale de la Santé.** See **World Health Organization.**

Omsk hemorrhagic fever (OHF) An acute infection, seen in regions of the U.S.S.R., caused by an arbovirus transmitted by the bite of an infected tick or by handling infected muskrats. The disease is characterized by fever, headache, epistaxis, gastrointestinal and uterine bleeding, and other hemorrhagic manifestations.

-on A combining form meaning: **1.** An 'elementary atomic particle': *electron, proton.* **2.** A 'unit': *magneton, photon.* **3.** A '(nonmetallic) chemical element': *carbon, krypton.*

onanism See **masturbation.**

onchocerciasis A form of filariasis common in Central and South America and in Africa, characterized by subcutaneous nodules, pruritic rash, and eye lesions. It is transmitted by the bites of black flies that deposit microfilariae under the skin. The microfilariae migrate to the subcutaneous tissue and eyes, and fibrous nodules develop around the developing adult worms. Hypersensitive reactions to the dying microfilariae include extreme pruritus, a cellulitislike rash, lichenification, and depigmentation. Involvement of the eye may include keratitis, iridocyclitis, and, rarely, blindness from choroidoretinitis. Diagnosis is made by demonstrating microfilariae by skin biopsy or in the eye by slit lamp. Treatment is diethylcarbamazine for the microfilariae and surgical excision of nodules to remove adult worms. Also called **river blindness.**

onco- A combining form meaning 'of or pertaining to a swelling, tumor, or mass': *oncogenesis, oncograph.*

oncogenesis The process initiating and promoting the development of a neoplasm. Compare **sarcomagenesis, tumorigenesis.** —**oncogenic,** *adj.*

oncogenic virus A virus able to cause the development of a malignant neoplastic disease. Over one hundred oncogenic viruses have been identified. In the laboratory, oncogenic viruses have been inoculated and grown in all major groups of animals, including primates. Many, especially the slow viruses, are thought to cause cancer in humans, but this is not yet proven.

oncologist A doctor who specializes in the study and treatment of neoplastic diseases, particularly cancer.

oncology The branch of medicine concerned with the study of tumors.

Oncology Nursing Society (ONS) An organization of nurses interested or specialized in nursing of the patient with cancer. The national publication of the ONS is *Oncology Nursing Forum.*

oncovirus A member of a family of viruses associated with leukemia and sarcoma in animals and, possibly, in humans.

Ondine's curse An eponym for apnea owing to loss of automatic control of respiration. The term refers to a syndrome in patients with marked sensitivity to retained carbon dioxide.

A defect in the central chemoreceptor responsiveness to carbon dioxide leaves the patient with hypercapnia and hypoxemia, but able to breathe voluntarily. This condition may result in the Pickwickian syndrome or sleep-apnea syndrome, and it may be a cause of sudden infant death syndrome. Ondine's curse may occur as a result of drug overdose, after bulbar poliomyelitis or encephalitis, or after surgery involving the brain stem or the higher segments of cervical cord, as in cervical cordotomy.

-one A combining form designating organic compounds: *acetone, ketone, quinone.*

one-and-a-half spica cast An orthopedic cast used for immobilizing the trunk of the body cranially to the nipple line, one leg caudally as far as the toes, and the other leg caudally as far as the knee. For stability, a diagonal crossbar connects the parts of the cast encasing the legs. This type of cast is used for immobilization during convalescence after healing of surgical hip repair or a fractured femur and for the correction and the maintenance of correction of a hip deformity. Compare **bilateral long-leg spica cast, unilateral long-leg spica cast.**

oneiro- A combining form meaning 'of or related to a dream': *oneirodynia, oneirology, oneiroscopy.*

ontogenetic, ontogenic 1. Of, relating to, or acquired during ontogeny. 2. An association based on visible morphological characteristics and not necessarily indicative of a natural evolutionary relationship.

ontogeny The life history of one organism from a single-celled ovum to the time of birth, including all phases of differentiation and growth. Compare **phylogeny.** Also called ontogenesis. — **ontogenetic,** *adj.*

onych-, onycho- A combining form meaning 'of or related to the nails': *onychogenic, onychohelcosis.*

onychia Inflammation of the nail bed. Compare **paronychia.**

-onychia A combining form meaning a 'condition of the fingernails or toenails': *celonychia, melanonychia.*

onychogryphosis Thickened, curved, clawlike overgrowth of fingernails or toenails.

onycholysis Separation of a nail from its bed, beginning at the free margin, commonly associated with psoriasis.

onychomycosis Any fungus infection of the nails.

oo- A combining form meaning 'of or pertaining to an egg or ovum': *ooblast, oocytase.*

ooblast The primodial germ cell from which the mature ovum is developed.

oocenter See **ovocenter.**

oocyst A stage in the development of any sporozoan in which, after fertilization, a zygote is produced that develops about itself an enclosing cyst wall. Oocysts of malarial parasites are found in the stomachs of infected mosquitoes. Compare **oocyte.**

oocyte A primordial or incompletely developed ovum.

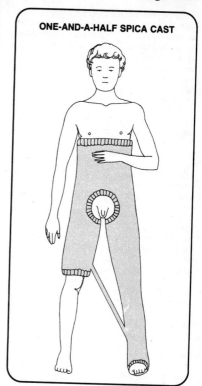

ONE-AND-A-HALF SPICA CAST

oocytin The substance in a spermatozoon that stimulates the formation of the fertilization membrane after penetration of an ovum.

oogamy 1. Sexual reproduction by the fertilization of a large, nonmotile female gamete by a smaller, actively motile male gamete, as occurs in certain algae and the malarial parasite *Plasmodium.* 2. Heterogamy. Compare **isogamy.** —**oogamous,** *adj.*

oogenesis The process of the growth and maturation of the female gametes, or ova. Development begins during intrauterine life when the primordial germ cells within the epithelium of the fetal ovarian cortex give rise to precursor oogonia. By the time of birth, the oogonia have multiplied and developed into primary oocytes, each surrounded by a layer of epithelial cells that together form the primordial follicle. These have entered the prophase stage of the first meiotic division and remain suspended in this state until sexual maturity is reached. Then, at monthly intervals, one or sometimes two of the primary oocytes are stimulated simultaneously by the anterior pituitary hormones and the maturation of the follicle to continue meiotic division, forming a large secondary oocyte and a much smaller nonfunctional first polar body. The second meiotic division begins at about the time of ovulation and remains suspended in the prophase stage until fertilization stimulates the completion of the process, resulting in one large mature ovum, or ootid, and either one or three smaller secondary polar bodies that soon disintegrate. The ootid contains a pronucleus with the haploid number of maternal chromosomes that will fuse with the pronucleus of the spermatozoon to form the zygote. If fertilization does not occur, the ovum disintegrates and is discharged with the menses. The female infant is born with the entire number of primary oocytes that will function throughout reproductive life. Only a fraction of these survive until puberty and only a small percentage will be ovulated. Follicles containing the primary oocytes are found in varying stages of development in the ovary of the sexually mature woman. Also called **ovogenesis.** Compare **spermatogenesis.** See also **meiosis, menstrual cycle, ovulation. —oogenetic,** *adj.*

oogonium, *pl.* **oogonia**   The precursor cell from which an oocyte develops in the fetus during intrauterine life. Also called **ovogonium.** See also **oogenesis.**

ookinesis, ookinesia   The mitotic phenomena occurring in the nucleus of the egg cell during maturation and fertilization. See also **oogenesis. —ookinetic,** *adj.*

ookinete   The motile elongated zygote that is formed by the fertilization of the macrogamete during the sexual reproductive phase of the life cycle of a sporozoan, specifically the malarial parasite *Plasmodium*. It penetrates the lining of the stomach of the female *Anopheles* mosquito and attaches to the outer wall, where it forms an oocyst and gives rise to sporozoites.

oolemma   See **zona pellucida.**

oophor-, oophoro-, ootheco-   A combining form meaning 'of or pertaining to the ovary': *oophorocytosis, oophorogenous.*

oophorectomy   The surgical removal of one or both ovaries, performed to remove a cyst or tumor, excise an abcess, treat endometriosis, or, in breast cancer, to remove the source of estrogen, which stimulates some kinds of cancer. If both ovaries are removed, sterility results and menopause is abruptly induced; in premenopausal women one ovary or a portion of one may be left intact unless a malignancy is present. The operation often accompanies a hysterectomy. Unless a malignancy is present, estrogen may be given to treat the unpleasant side effects of the abrupt onset of menopause. Also called **ovariectomy.**

oophoritis   An inflammatory condition of one or both ovaries, usually occurring with salpingitis.

oophorosalpingectomy   The surgical removal of one or both ovaries and the corresponding oviducts, performed to remove a cyst or tumor, excise an abcess, or treat the condition of endometriosis. In a bilateral procedure the patient becomes sterile and menopause is induced. Estrogen therapy may be started after bilateral surgery unless a malignancy is present to relieve the side effects of the abrupt onset of menopause.

ooplasm   The cytoplasm of the egg, or ovum, including the yolk in lower animals. Also called **ovoplasm.**

oosperm   A fertilized egg; the cell resulting from the union of the pronuclei of the spermatozoon and the ovum following fertilization; a zygote.

ootid   The mature ovum after penetration by the spermatozoon and completion of the second meiotic division but prior to the fusion of the pronuclei to form the zygote. It is one of the four cells resulting from oogenesis, the other three being nonfunctional secondary polar bodies, and corresponds to the four spermatid cells derived from spermatogenesis. See also **meiosis, oogenesis.**

opaque   **1.** Of or pertaining to a substance or surface that neither transmits nor allows the passage of light. **2.** Neither transparent nor translucent.

-ope   A combining form meaning a 'person having an eye defect': *asthenope, hyperope, protanope.*

open-air treatment   See **exposure treatment.**

open amputation   A kind of amputation in which a straight, guillotine cut is made without skin flaps. Open amputation is performed if an infection is probable, developing, or recurrent. The cross section is left open for drainage, and skin traction is applied to prevent retraction. Antibiotic therapy is begun, and surgical closure is completed when the infection clears. Compare **closed amputation.** See also **amputation, gangrene.**

open drainage   See **drainage.**

open-drop anesthesia   The oldest and simplest anesthetic technique. A volatile liquid anesthetic agent is dripped, a drop at a time, onto a porous cloth or mask held over the patient's face. Chloroform and ether are the major general anesthetics used. Some psychologists believe that open-drop anesthesia can be a traumatic experience to a child. It is not currently used in developed countries.

open-ended question or statement   In a dialogue, a message that indicates the nurse's interest in the patient's messages. Such a message adds no content to the dialogue, but encourages the patient to elaborate on the subject in his own words.

open fracture   See **compound fracture.**

operant   Any act or response occurring without an identifiable stimulus. The result of the act or response determines whether or not it is repeated.

operant conditioning   A form of learning used in behavior therapy in which the person undergoing therapy is rewarded for the correct response and punished for the incorrect response. Also called instrumental conditioning.

operating microscope   A binocular microscope used in delicate surgery, especially eye or ear surgery. The standing type of operating microscope has a motorized zoom system operated by a foot pedal that changes the magni-

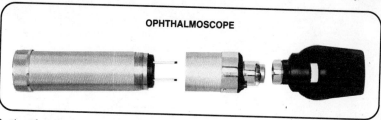

OPHTHALMOSCOPE

fication. The operating microscope that attaches to a surgeon's head has interchangeable oculars for different magnifications. Also called surgical microscope.

operating room (OR) **1.** A room in a health-care facility in which surgical procedures requiring anesthesia are performed. **2.** *Informal.* A suite of rooms or an area in a health-care facility in which patients are prepared for surgery, undergo surgical procedures, and recover from the anesthetic procedures required for the surgery.

operation Any surgical procedure, as an appendectomy.

operative cholangiography In diagnostic radiology: a procedure for outlining the major bile ducts. It is performed during surgery by injecting a radio-opaque contrast material directly into these ducts. It is usually performed to detect residual calculi in the biliary tract. See also **cholangiography.**

operator gene In molecular genetics: a genetic unit that regulates the transcription of structural genes in its operon. The operator gene serves as the starting point in the coding sequence and interacts with a repressor protein in controlling the activity of structural genes.

operculum, *pl.* **opercula, operculums** A lid or covering, as the mucous plug that blocks the cervix of the gravid uterus. —**opercular,** *adj.*

operon In molecular biology: a segment of DNA consisting of an operator gene and one or more structural genes with related functions controlled by the operator gene in conjunction with a regulatory gene. See also **operator gene, regulatory gene.**

-ophidia A combining form meaning 'venomous snakes': *thanatophidia, toxicophidia.*

ophthalm- See **ophthalmo-.**

ophthalmia Severe inflammation of the conjunctiva or of the deeper parts of the eye. Some kinds of ophthalmia are **ophthalmia neonatorum, sympathetic ophthalmia.**

-ophthalmia A combining form meaning a 'pathological or anatomical condition of the eye': *allophthalmia, echinophthalmia, polemophthalmia.*

ophthalmia neonatorum A purulent gonococcal conjunctivitis and keratitis of the newborn resulting from exposure of the eyes to infected maternal secretions during passage through the vagina at birth. Routine prophylaxis by the topical instillation of a 1% solution of silver nitrate or an antibiotic ointment in the conjunctival

sac of every newborn has largely eradicated the infection. When necessary, intravenous antibiotic therapy given in the hospital for several days is effective, and recovery is usually complete.

ophthalmic Of or pertaining to the eye.

-ophthalmic A combining form meaning 'referring to, near, or for the eye': *exophthalmic, periophthalmic.*

ophthalmic administration of medication The administration of a drug by instillation of a cream, ointment, or drops of a liquid preparation in the conjunctival sac.

ophthalmic herpes zoster See **herpes zoster.**

ophthalmo-, ophthalm- A combining form meaning 'of or pertaining to the eye': *ophthalmodynia, ophthalmolith.*

ophthalmologist A physician who specializes in ophthalmology.

ophthalmology The branch of medicine concerned with the study of the physiology, anatomy, and pathology of the eye and the diagnosis and treatment of disorders of the eye. —**ophthalmologic, ophthalmological,** *adj.*

ophthalmoplegia An abnormal condition characterized by paralysis of the motor nerves of the eye. Bilateral ophthalmoplegia of rapid onset is associated with acute myasthenia gravis, acute thiamin deficiency, botulism, and acute inflammatory cranial polyneuropathy. These diseases are potentially very destructive and require prompt attention. In some patients with myopathic ophthalmoplegia, structural abnormalities and biochemical disorders may be evident in limb muscles. Ophthalmoplegia is also associated with ocular dystrophy.

ophthalmoscope A device for examining the interior of the eye. It includes a light, a mirror with a single hole through which the examiner may look, and a dial holding several lenses of varying strengths. The lenses are selected to allow clear visualization of the structures of the eye at any depth.

ophthalmoscopy The technique of using an ophthalmoscope.

-opia A combining form meaning a '(specified) visual condition': *boopia, senopia.* Also **-opy, -opsia, -opsy.**

opiate **1.** A narcotic drug containing opium, its derivatives, or any of several semisynthetic or synthetic drugs with opiumlike activity. **2.** *Informal.* Any soporific or narcotic drug. **3.** Of or pertaining to a substance that causes sleep or relief of pain. Also called **opioid.**

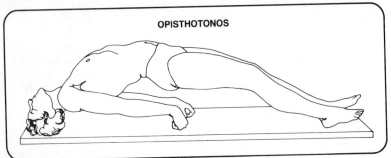

OPISTHOTONOS

-opic, -opical A combining form meaning 'kind of vision or visual defect': *cyclopic, hemeralopic, nyctalopic.*

opinion In law: **1.** A statement by the court, usually in writing, of the reasoning for its decision or judgment in a case. **2.** A statement prepared for a client by an attorney that represents the attorney's understanding of the law as it pertains to a legal question posed by the client.

opistho- A combining form meaning 'backward or relating to the back': *opisthognathism, opisthoporeia.*

opisthorchiasis Infection with one of two species of liver flukes commonly found in the Philippines, India, Thailand, and Laos. Symptoms and signs are similar to those caused by *Clonorchis sinensis.* Treatment is unsatisfactory. The disease is prevented by avoiding ingestion of raw or inadequately cooked freshwater fish.

Opisthorchis sinensis See *Clonorchis sinensis.*

opisthotonos A prolonged severe spasm of the muscles causing the back to arch acutely, the head to bend back on the neck, the heels to bend back on the legs, and the arms and hands to flex rigidly at the joints.

opium A milky exudate from the unripe capsules of *Papaver somniferum* and *Papaver album* yielding 9.5% or more of anhydrous morphine. It is a narcotic analgesic, a hypnotic, and an astringent. Opium contains several alkaloids, including codeine, morphine, and papaverine. See also **codeine, morphine sulfate, opium tincture, papaverine hydrochloride, paregoric.**

opium alkaloid One of several alkaloids isolated from the milky exudate of the unripe seed pods of *Papaver somniferum,* a species of poppy indigenous to the Near East. Morphine (an opium alkaloid) is the standard against which the analgesic effect of newer drugs for relief of pain is measured. The opium alkaloids and their semisynthetic derivatives, including heroin, act on the central nervous system, producing analgesia, change in mood, drowsiness, and mental slowness. The effects in a person who has pain are usually pleasant; euphoria and pain-free sleep are not uncommon, but nausea and vomiting sometimes occur. In usual doses, the anal-

gesic effects are achieved without loss of consciousness. Morphine and its surrogates appear to relieve the discomfort of the original sensation and the person's reaction to the sensation; thus the actual pain diminishes, and what remains of it is less distressing to the patient.

opium tincture An analgesic and antidiarrheal.

Oppenheim reflex A variation of Babinski's reflex, elicited by firmly stroking downward on the anterior and medial surfaces of the tibia, characterized by extension of the great toe and fanning of other toes. It is a sign of pyramidal tract disease. Compare **Chaddock reflex, Gordon reflex.** See also **Babinski's reflex.**

Oppenheim's disease A rare congenital disease of infants, characterized by flabby, atonic muscles, especially in the legs, and absent or very sluggish deep reflexes. The infant seems paralyzed during the first few months of life and almost a third do not survive beyond the first year. Compare **amyotonia congenita, myotonia congenita.**

opportunistic infection **1.** An infection caused by normally nonpathogenic organisms in a host whose resistance has been decreased by such disorders as diabetes mellitus, cancer, or by a surgical procedure, as a cerebrospinal fluid shunt. **2.** An unusual infection with a common pathogen, as cellulitis, meningitis, or otitis media.

-opsia See **-opia.**

opsonin An antibody or complement split product that, on attaching to a foreign material, microorganism, or other antigen, enhances phagocytosis of that substance by leukocytes and other macrophages. **—opsonize,** *v.*

opsonization The process by which opsonins render bacteria more susceptible to phagocytosis by leukocytes.

-opter A combining form referring to 'measurement of vision': *myodiopter, oxyopter, phoropter.*

optic Of or pertaining to the eyes or to sight. **—optical,** *adj.*

-optic A combining form meaning 'pertaining to vision': *bioptic, panoptic, preoptic.*

optical maser See **laser.**

optic atrophy Wasting of the optic disk resulting from degeneration of fibers of the optic nerve and optic tract. In primary optic atrophy

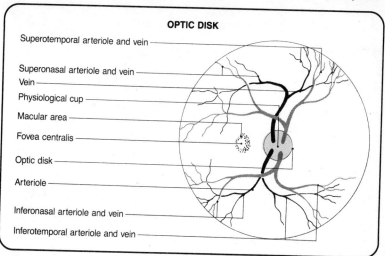

OPTIC DISK

Superotemporal arteriole and vein

Superonasal arteriole and vein

Vein

Physiological cup

Macular area

Fovea centralis

Optic disk

Arteriole

Inferonasal arteriole and vein

Inferotemporal arteriole and vein

the disk is white and sharply margined, the central depression (physiologic cup) is enlarged, and the optic foramen of the sclera is clearly seen. In secondary atrophy the disk is gray, its margins are blurred, the depression is filled in, and the foramen is difficult to detect. Optic atrophy may be caused by a congenital defect; inflammation; occlusion of the central retinal artery or internal carotid artery; or by alcohol, arsenic, lead, tobacco, or other toxic substances. Degeneration of the disk may accompany arteriosclerosis, diabetes, glaucoma, hydrocephalus, pernicious anemia, and various neurologic disorders.

optic cup   A two-layered embryonic cavity that develops in early pregnancy. The optic cup is completed by the 7th week with the closing of the choroidal fissure. The cup initially develops from the infolding of the optic vesicle after the vesicle separates from the embryonic ectoderm. The cells of the optic cup differentiate to form the retina that first develops its layers of rods and cones in the central portion of the cup, growing as the layer gradually spreads toward the cup margin. The outer layer of the cup persists as the pigmented layer of the retina; the inner layer develops the nervous elements and the supporting fibers of the retina. Compare **optic stalk.**

optic disk   The small blind spot on the surface of the retina, located about 3 mm to the nasal side of the macula. It is the only part of the retina which is insensitive to light. At its center the porus opticus marks the point of entrance of the central artery of the retina. Also called **blind spot** (*informal*), **discus nervi optici.**

optic glioma   A tumor of glial cells. It develops slowly on the optic nerve or in the optic chiasm, causing loss of vision, and is often accompanied by secondary strabismus, exophthalmos, and ocular paralysis.

optician   A person who grinds, fits, and dispenses eyeglass lenses, contact lenses, and ophthalmic accessories by prescription. To become an optician, a person must complete a 4- or 5-year apprenticeship.

optic nerve   Either of a pair of cranial nerves consisting mainly of coarse, myelinated fibers that arise in the retinal ganglionic layer, traverse the thalamus, and connect with the visual cortex. At the optic chiasm the fibers from the inner or nasal half of the retina cross to the optic tract of the opposite side. The remaining fibers from the temporal or outer half of each retina pass to the visual cortex on the same side. The visual cortex functions in the perception of light, shade, and objects. Optic radiations conduct impulses from the geniculate bodies in the cerebral hemispheres to the visual cortices. The optic nerve is divided into portions within the bulb, orbit, optic canal, and cranial cavity. The intraocular portion of the nerve is about 1 mm long and contains unmyelinated fibers which become myelinated after passing through the lamina cribosa. The orbital portion of the nerve, about 3.5 mm (⅛ inch) in diameter and about 25 mm (1 inch) long, is invested by sheaths derived from the dura, the arachnoid, and the pia mater. The portion of the nerve within the optic canal lies superior to the ophthalmic artery, and the three sheaths are fused to each other, to the nerve, and to the periosteum of the bone, securing the nerve and preventing it from being forced back and forth in the foramen. The intracranial portion of the nerve rests on the anterior portion of the cranial sinus in close proximity to the internal carotid artery. The optic nerve is cranial nerve II and develops from a diverticulum of the laterial portion of the forebrain. The optic nerve fibers therefore correspond to a tract of fibers within the brain rather than to the other cranial nerves.

optico-, opto-   A combining form meaning

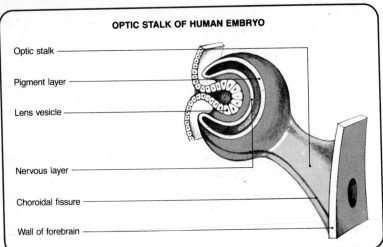

OPTIC STALK OF HUMAN EMBRYO

Optic stalk

Pigment layer

Lens vesicle

Nervous layer

Choroidal fissure

Wall of forebrain

'visible, or pertaining to vision or sight': *opto-blast, optometer*. Also *opti-*.

optic papilla See **papilla.**

optics 1. In physics: a field of study dealing with electromagnetic radiation of wavelengths shorter than radio waves but longer than X-rays. **2.** In physiology: a field of study dealing with vision and the process by which the functions of the eye and the brain are integrated. **—optic, optical,** *adj.*

optic stalk One of a pair of slender embryonic structures that become the optic nerve. In the embryo the optic stalk develops during the 2nd week and attaches the optic vesicle to the wall of the brain. The stalk becomes complete during the 7th week of pregnancy when the choroidal fissure closes and is later converted into the optic nerve when nerve fibers fill the cavity of the stalk. Most of the fibers are centripetal and grow backward into the stalk from the nerve cells of the retina. A few fibers grow into the stalk from the brain. About the 10th week after birth the fibers of the optic nerve receive their myelin sheaths. Compare **optic cup.**

optic system assessment An evaluation of the patient's eyes, vision, and current and past disorders or injuries that may be responsible for abnormalities in the individual's optic system. The patient is interviewed to determine if vision is blurred, double, decreased, or absent in one or both eyes, or diminished peripherally at night or in bright light. The interviewer asks if halos or lights are seen; if the patient collides with unfamiliar objects; is unable to distinguish objects held too close or too far; if the eyes water, itch, feel tender, painful, or fatigued; and if an injury to the eye, face, or head has occurred. Observations are made of the patient's general appearance, vital signs, kind of eyeglasses or contact lenses worn, the amount of tearing, ability to blink, tendency to rub the eyes, and visual acuity. Evidence is recorded of conjunctivitis,

drainage, optic hemorrhage, edema or ptosis of the eyelids, exophthalmos, strabismus, nystagmus, scleral edema, chalazion, lacerations, contusions, or a foreign body in the eye. Carefully noted are signs of aging, glaucoma, cataract, retinal detachment, and the presence of multiple sclerosis, diabetes mellitus, myasthenia gravis, gonorrhea, thyroid dysfunction, sinus problems, or cerebral trauma or tumors. The patient's report of previous eye operations or treatments, head or face trauma, arteriosclerosis, glomerulonephritis, retinal degeneration, episodes of coma, therapy with oxygen, and drug misuse are investigated, as well as a family history of glaucoma or diabetes. Also explored are the possibility that the patient has a hazardous job or recreation, and note is made of any safety precautions taken, the individual's misuse of alcohol, and use of medication, especially antibiotics, antiemetics, miotics, mydriatics, and acetazolamide. Diagnostic aids for the evaluation include a test of visual fields, X-rays of the orbit and skull, an ophthalmoscopic examination, tonometry, brain scan, and microscopic studies of conjunctival scrapings.

NURSING CONSIDERATIONS: The nurse conducts an interview, makes the observations of the patient, and assembles the pertinent background data and the results of the diagnostic procedures. A careful assessment of the patient's eyes, vision, and of certain aspects of the medical, family, and social history is a significant aid in establishing the diagnosis of an optic system disorder.

optometrist A person who practices optometry. An optometrist is awarded the degree of Doctor of Optometry (OD) after completing at least 2 years of college and 4 years in an approved college of optometry. A state examination and license are also required. See also **optician, optometry.**

optometry The practice of testing the eyes

for visual acuity, prescribing corrective lenses, and recommending eye exercises. See also **optician.**

OPV *abbr* oral poliovirus vaccine.

O.R., OR *abbr* **operating room.**

oral Of or pertaining to the mouth. Compare **buccal, parenteral.**

oral administration of medication The administration of a tablet, a capsule, an elixir, or a solution or other liquid form of medication by mouth.

oral airway A curved tubular device of rubber, plastic, or metal placed in the oropharynx during general anesthesia to maintain free passage of air and keep the tongue from obstructing the trachea. The artificial airway is not removed until the patient begins to awaken and regains pharyngeal, cough, and swallowing reflexes.

oral cancer A malignant neoplasm on the lip or in the mouth, occurring at an average age of 60 with a frequency eight times higher in men than in women. Predisposing factors in the etiology of the disease are alcoholism, heavy use of tobacco, poor oral hygiene, ill-fitting dentures, syphilis, Plummer-Vinson syndrome, betel nut chewing, and, in lip cancer, pipe smoking and overexposure to sun and wind. Premalignant leukoplakia, erythroplasia, or a painless, nonhealing ulcer may be the first sign of oral cancer; localized pain usually appears later, but lymph nodes may be involved early in the course. Diagnostic measures include digital examination, biopsy, exfoliative cytology, X-rays of the mandible, and chest films to detect metastatic lung lesions. Almost all oral tumors are epidermoid carcinomas; adenocarcinomas occur occasionally. Small primary lesions may be treated by excision or irradiation and more extensive oral tumors by surgery, with removal of involved lymph nodes and preoperative or postoperative radiotherapy. Among chemotherapeutic agents administered palliatively for inoperable or recurrent lesions are methotrexate, 5-fluorouracil, bleomycin, and adriamycin.

oral character In psychoanalysis: a kind of personality exhibiting patterns of behavior originating in the oral phase of infancy, characterized either by optimism, self-confidence, and carefree generosity reflecting the pleasurable aspects of the stage; or by pessimism, futility, anxiety, and sadism as manifestations of frustrations or conflicts that occurred during the period. See also **oral stage, psychosexual development.**

oral contraceptive See **contraception.**

oral eroticism, oral erotism In psychoanalysis: libidinal fixation at or regression to the oral stage of psychosexual development, often reflected in such personality traits as passivity, insecurity, and oversensitivity. Compare **anal eroticism.** See also **oral character.**

oral herpes See **herpes simplex.**

oral hygiene The condition or practice of maintaining the tissues and structures of the mouth. Oral hygiene includes brushing the teeth; massaging the gums with a tooth brush, dental

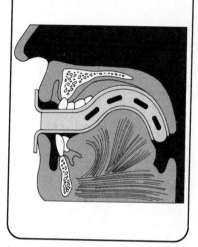

ORAL AIRWAY

floss, or water irrigator; and cleansing dentures and ensuring their proper fit. Oral hygiene for dependent or unconcious patients includes lubricating the lips; cleaning the inside of the cheeks, the roof of the mouth, and the tongue; and checking for loose teeth that might be swallowed or aspirated.

oral poliovirus vaccine (OPV) An attenuated preparation of live poliovirus that confers immunity to poliomyelitis. Also called **Sabin vaccine.**

oral sadism In psychoanalysis: a sadistic form of oral eroticism, manifested by such behavior as biting, chewing, and other aggressive impulses associated with eating habits. Compare **anal sadism.**

oral stage In psychoanalysis: the initial stage of psychosexual development, occurring in the first 12 to 18 months of life when the feeding experience and other oral activities are the predominant source of pleasurable stimulation. Experiences during this stage greatly determine later attitudes concerning food, love, acceptance and rejection, and many other aspects of interpersonal relationships and behavioral patterns. Pleasurable experiences associated with suckling may lead to oral eroticism in adulthood. Unpleasant experiences may lead to extreme aggression and such patterns as smoking, overeating, excessive talking, or sarcasm, and may be a pervasive influence or underlying determinant in addictive disorders. See also **oral character, psychosexual development.**

orbicularis ciliaris One of the two zones of the ciliary body of the eye, extending from the ora serrata of the retina to the ciliary processes at the margin of the iris. The orbicularis ciliaris is about 4 millimeters wide and increases in thickness as it approaches the ciliary processes.

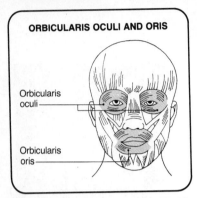

ORBICULARIS OCULI AND ORIS

Orbicularis oculi

Orbicularis oris

orbicularis oculi The muscular body of the eyelid comprising the palpebral, orbital, and lacrimal muscles. It arises from the nasal part of the frontal bone, from the frontal process of the maxilla in front of the lacrimal groove, and from the anterior surface of the medial palpebral ligament. The palpebral muscle functions to close the eyelid gently; the orbital muscle functions to close it more energetically, as in winking. Also called orbicularis palpebrarum. Compare **corrugator, levator palpebrae superioris.**

orbicularis oris The muscle surrounding the mouth, consisting partly of fibers derived from other facial muscles, as the buccinator, that are inserted into the lips, and partly of fibers proper to the lips. It is innervated by buccal branches of the facial nerve and serves to close and purse the lips.

orbicularis pupillary reflex A normal phenomenon elicited by forceful closure of the eyelids or attempting to close them while they are held apart, resulting first in constriction and then dilatation of the pupil.

orbit One of a pair of bony, conical cavities in the skull that accommodate the eyeballs and associated structures. The medial walls of the orbits are approximately parallel with each other and with the middle line, but the lateral walls diverge widely. The roof of each orbit is formed by the orbital plate of the frontal bone and the small wing of the sphenoid bones. The trochlear fovea of the orbital roof accommodates the cartilaginous pulley of the obliquus superior oculi, and the lacrimal fossa in the roof cradles the lacrimal gland. The superior orbital fissure between the roof and the lateral wall of the orbit admits various nerves.The openings that communicate with each orbit are the optic foramen, the superior and the inferior orbital fissures, the supraorbital foramen, the infraorbital canal, the anterior and the posterior ethmoidal foramina, the zygomatic foramen, and the canal for the nasolacrimal duct. —**orbital,** *adj.*

orbital aperture An opening in the cranium to the orbit of the eye.

orbital fat A semifluid cushion of fat that lines the bony orbit supporting the eye. Traumatic loss of the fat causes a sunken appearance

of the eye. Replacement of the fat by tumor or abnormal tissue may be discovered on ophthalmologic examination.

orbital hypertelorism See **ocular hypertelorism.**

orbital hypotelorism See **ocular hypotelorism.**

orbital pseudotumor A specific inflammatory reaction of the orbital tissues of the eye, characterized by exophthalmos and edematous congestion of the eyelids. The etiology is unknown.

orchi-, orchio- A combining form meaning 'of or pertaining to the testes': *orchiocatabasis, orchipathy, orchioscirrhus.*

orchidectomy Surgical removal of one or both testes. It may be indicated for serious disease or injury or to control cancer of the prostate by removing a source of androgenic hormones. Also called orchiectomy.

orchiopexy An operation to mobilize an undescended testis, bring it into the scrotum, and attach it so that it will not retract. Sometimes a suture is attached to the lower scrotum and taped to the inner thigh.

orchis See **testis.**

orchitis Inflammation of one or both of the testes, characterized by swelling and pain, and often caused by mumps, syphilis, or tuberculosis. —**orchitic,** *adj.*

orciprenaline sulfate See **metaproterenol sulfate.**

-orexia A combining form meaning '(condition of the) appetite': *cynorexia, dysorexia, hyperorexia.*

orexigenic A substance that increases or stimulates the appetite.

oreximania A condition characterized by a greatly increased appetite and excessive eating resulting from an unrealistic or exaggerated fear of becoming thin. Compare **anorexia nervosa.**

orexis 1. Desire, appetite. 2. The aspect of the mind involving feeling and striving as contrasted with the intellectual aspect.

orf A viral skin disease acquired from sheep, characterized by painless vesicles which may progress to red, weeping nodules and, finally, to crusting and healing. Treatment is not necessary because the condition is self-limited, and active infection results in immunity.

organ A structural part of a body system, comprised of tissues and cells that enable it to perform a particular function, as the liver or spleen. Each one of the paired organs can function independently of the other. Also called organon, organum. —**organic,** *adj.*

organ albumin Albumin characteristic of a particular organ.

organelle, organella 1. Any one of various particles of living substance bound within most cells, as the mitochondria, the lysosomes, and the centrioles. 2. Any one of the tiny organs of protozoa associated with locomotion, metabolism, and other processes.

organic 1. Any chemical compound containing carbon. Compare **inorganic.** 2. Pertaining to substances derived from living organisms. **3.** Of or pertaining to an organ.

-organic A combining form meaning 'related to the internal organs of the body': *enorganic, homorganic.*

organic chemistry The branch of chemistry concerned with the composition, properties, and reactions of chemical compounds containing carbon.

organic dust Dried particles of plants, animals, fungi, or bacteria that are fine enough to be windborne. Many kinds of organic dust cause various respiratory disorders if inhaled. See also **asthma, bagassosis, byssinosis, hay fever, rose fever.**

organic evolution The theory of the origin and perpetuation of species, which states that all existing forms of animal and plant life have descended with modification from previous, simpler forms or from a single cell.

organic headache See **headache.**

organic mental disorder Any psychological or behavioral abnormality associated with transient or permanent brain dysfunction caused by a disturbance of the physiological functioning of brain tissue, as may occur with many pathologic conditions. Also called organic brain syndrome.

organic motivation See **physiological motivation.**

Organisation Mondiale de la Santé (OMS) See **World Health Organization.**

organism An individual living animal or plant able to carry on life functions through mutually dependent organs or organelles.

organization center A focal point within the developing embryo from which the organism grows and differentiates. In vertebrates this point is the chordamesoderm of the dorsal lip of the blastopore.

organizer In embryology: any part of the embryo that induces morphologic differentiation in some other part. Those parts that are formed and in turn give rise to other parts are classified as organizers of the second degree, third degree, and so on as the embryo develops in complexity. Kinds of organizers include **nucleolar organizer, primary organizer.**

organo- A combining form meaning 'of or pertaining to an organ or organs': *organofaction, organogenesis.*

organ of Giraldes See **paradidymis.**

organ of Golgi See **neurotendinous spindle.**

organogenesis In embryology: the formation and differentiation of organs and organ systems during embryonic development. In humans the period extends from approximately the end of the 2nd week through the 8th week of gestation, when the embryo undergoes rapid growth and differentiation and is extremely vulnerable to environmental hazards and toxic substances. Any interference with the sequential processes involved with organogenesis causes an arrest in development and results in one or more congenital anomalies. Also called organ-

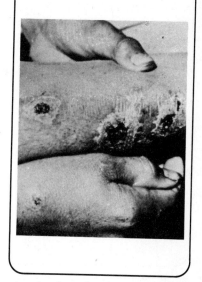

ORIENTAL SORE

ogeny. See also **embryologic development, prenatal development.** —**organogenetic,** *adj.*

organoid **1.** Resembling an organ. **2.** Any structure that resembles an organ in appearance or function, specifically an abnormal tumor mass. **3.** See **organelle.**

organoid neoplasm A growth that resembles a body organ. Compare **histoid neoplasm.**

organoid tumor See **teratoma.**

organotherapy The treatment of disease by administering animal endocrine glands or their extracts. Whole glands are no longer implanted, but substances derived from animal organs are widely used. Also called **Brown-Séquard's treatment.** —**organotherapeutic,** *adj.*

organotypic growth The controlled reproduction of cells, as occurs in the normal growth of tissues and organs. Compare **histiotypic growth.**

orgasm Sexual climax. A series of strong, involuntary contractions of the muscles of the genitalia experienced as exceedingly pleasurable, orgasm is set off by sexual excitation of critical intensity. —**orgasmic,** *adj.*

orient **1.** To make someone aware of new surroundings, including people and their roles, the layout of a facility, and its routines, rules, and services. **2.** To help a person become aware of a situation or simply of reality, as when a patient recovers from anesthesia. —**orientation,** *n.,* **oriented,** *adj.*

oriental sore A dermatologic disease caused by the parasite *Leishmania tropica,* transmitted to humans by the bite of the sand fly. This form of leishmaniasis, characterized by ulcerative lesions, occurs primarily in Africa, Asia, and some

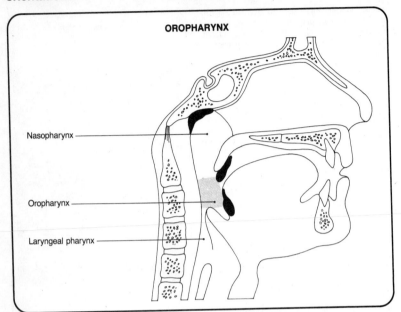

OROPHARYNX

Nasopharynx

Oropharynx

Laryngeal pharynx

Mediterranean countries. It causes no systemic symptoms, but the sores are susceptible to secondary infections. Treatment options include infrared therapy and injection of ulcers with sodium antimony gluconate. Also called Aleppo boil, cutaneous leishmaniasis, Delhi boil, Old World leishmaniasis, tropical sore. See also **leishmaniasis.**

orientation   In molecular genetics: the insertion of a fragment of genetic material into a vector so that the placement of the fragment is in the same direction as the genetic map of the vector (the n orientation) or in the opposite direction (the u orientation).

orifice   The entrance or the outlet of any cavity in the body. Also called ostium. —**orificial,** *adj.*

ori gene   In molecular genetics: the site or region in which DNA replication starts.

origin   The more fixed end of a muscle attachment. Compare **insertion.**

Ornithodoros   A genus of ticks, some species of which are vectors for the spirochetes of relapsing fevers.

ornithosis   See **psittacosis.**

oro-   1. A combining form meaning 'of or pertaining to the mouth': *orolingual, oromaxillary, oropharynx.*

oropharynx   One of the three anatomical divisions of the pharynx. It extends behind the mouth from the soft palate above to the level of the hyoid bone below and contains the palatine tonsils and the lingual tonsils. Compare **laryngopharynx, nasopharynx.** —**oropharyngeal,** *adj.*

Oroya fever   See **bartonellosis.**

orphenadrine citrate   A skeletal muscle relaxant.

orphenadrine hydrochloride   An anticholinergic and antihistaminic agent.

orrho-   A combining form meaning 'of or pertaining to serum': *orrhomeningitis, orrhoreaction, orrhorrhea.*

ortho-   A combining form meaning 'straight, normal, correct': *orthobiosis, orthodontist, orthotopic.*

orthoboric acid   See **boric acid.**

orthodontics   The specialty of dentistry concerned with the diagnosis and treatment of malocclusion and irregularities of the teeth. Also called orthodontia.

orthodromic conduction   The conduction of a neural impulse in the normal direction, from a synaptic junction or a receptor forward along an axon to its termination with depolarization.

orthogenesis   The theory that evolution is controlled by intrinsic factors within the organism and progresses according to a predetermined course rather than in several directions as a result of natural selection and other environmental factors. —**orthogenetic,** *adj.*

orthogenic   1. Of or pertaining to orthogenesis; orthogenetic. 2. Of or pertaining to the treatment and rehabilitation of children who are mentally or emotionally disturbed. See also **orthopsychiatry.**

orthogenic evolution   Change within an animal or plant induced solely by an intrinsic factor. Also called bathmic evolution.

orthomyxovirus   A member of a family of viruses that includes several organisms responsible for human influenza infection.

orthopantogram   An X-ray showing a panoramic view of the entire dentition, alveolar bone, and other contiguous structures on a single film, taken extraorally.

orthopedic nurse   A nurse whose primary area of interest, competence, and professional practice is in orthopedic nursing.

orthopedics   The branch of medicine devoted to the study and treatment of the skeletal system, its joints, muscles, and associated structures.

orthopedic traction   A procedure in which a patient is maintained in a device attached by ropes and pulleys to weights that exert a pulling force on an extremity or body part while countertraction is maintained. Traction is applied most often to reduce and immobilize fractures, but it also is used to overcome muscle spasm, to stretch adhesions, to correct certain deformities, and to help release arthritic contractures. Traction may be applied directly to the skin by attaching the rope-pulley-weight system to bands of adhesive, moleskin, or foam rubber, or to a splint affixed to the affected limb; side-arm traction is a kind of skin traction used to align a fractured humerus following open reduction. Skeletal traction is exerted directly on a bone in which a wire or pin is inserted under anesthesia in the open reduction of a fracture; the ends of the pin protruding through the skin on both sides of the bone are covered with corks and attached to a metal U-shaped spreader or bow, which in turn is attached to the traction rope. Skin or skeletal traction applied to a lower extremity by a balanced suspension apparatus, as the Thomas splint and Pearson's attachment, permits the patient to move more freely in bed since the leg is balanced with countertraction and any slack in traction caused by the patient's movements is taken up by the suspension apparatus. Bryant's traction for treating fractures of the femur shaft in young children uses a suspension apparatus to hold the child's legs at right angles to the body. A girdle that fits over the iliac crests and pelvis is used in the application of traction to relieve low back pain and a cervical halter is employed in applying traction to reduce neck pain; cervical traction may also be used when a fracture of the cervical spine is suspected. To maintain the required constant pull, the traction ropes are kept taut, free to ride over the pulleys, and securely tied to the weights that hang free—away from the bed and off the floor. Countertraction is maintained by elevating the patient's bed under the body part to which traction is applied and by a pull exerted in the opposite direction; a chest restraint sheet may be applied to the patient in side-arm traction for countertraction if necessary.

NURSING CONSIDERATIONS: During the initial stages of traction, the involved extremity is checked every 2 hours for quality of the distal pulse, color, warmth, motion, sensation, and swelling. Blood pressure, temperature, pulse, and respirations are recorded every 4 hours until stable. Pain is controlled and the patient is positioned as ordered. If the patient is in balanced suspension, abduction of the leg and a 20°

angle between the thigh and bed are maintained; the heel is kept free of the sling under the calf. A harness restraint is used to prevent a child in Bryant's traction from turning over, and the child's buttocks are raised slightly from the mattress. Bed linen is changed only as necessary and an air mattress is used when required. Every 2 hours the patient is helped to cough and deep-breathe; bony prominences are massaged, but vigorous rubbing is avoided. Lotion is applied to the skin, which is periodically inspected for signs of redness, abrasions, blisters, dryness, itching, excoriation, and pressure areas; special attention is given to the pin insertion sites of the patient in skeletal traction. The patient is observed every 4 hours for neurologic signs, as tingling, numbness, and loss of sensation or motion; for thrombophlebitis in the involved extremity; and for evidence of a pulmonary blood clot or fat embolus, as indicated by decreased breath sounds, fever, tachypnea, diaphoresis, pallor, bloody or purulent sputum, and tachycardia. Oral hygiene is administered every 4 hours and, unless contraindicated, a daily intake of 2,500 to 3,000 ml of fluids is encouraged. As the patient's condition improves, the position is changed every 4 hours; if the kind of traction permits and if the upper extremities are not involved, a trapeze is added to the bed. The patient is taught to perform range of motion exercises with the uninvolved extremities, dorsiflexion and plantar flexion of the ankles, and isometric exercises, as gluteal and abdominal contraction. A high-protein, low-carbohydrate diet is served, and vitamin and iron therapy may be ordered. The immobilized patient uses a flat, fracture bedpan and usually requires stool softeners or a mild laxative. The patient in traction often needs extensive physical care and emotional support. The person is encouraged to verbalize feelings and concerns about prolonged hospitalization and absence from work or school. To the greatest degree possible, the nurse encourages the patient to participate in self-care and to engage in diversions, as handicrafts, reading, watching television, and listening to the radio. The healthy young adult or adolescent in traction for the treatment of a fracture usually has an uneventful recovery, but diligent attention and nursing care are necessary to avoid the formation of decubitus ulcers, infection, constipation, and other sequelae of immobility. See specific devices and specific kinds of traction.

orthopedist   A specialist in orthopedics. Also called orthopod (*informal*).

orthopnea   An abnormal condition in which a person must sit or stand in order to breathe deeply or comfortably. It occurs in many cardiac and respiratory disorders, as asthma, pulmonary edema, emphysema, pneumonia, and angina pectoris. See also **dyspnea. —orthopneic,** *adj.*

orthopsychiatry   The branch of psychiatry that specializes in correcting incipient and borderline mental and behavioral disorders, espe-

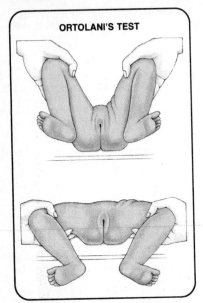

ORTOLANI'S TEST

cially in children, and in developing preventive techniques to promote mental health and emotional growth and development. See also **mental hygiene.**

orthoptic **1.** Of or pertaining to normal binocular vision. **2.** Of or pertaining to a procedure or technique for correcting the visual axes of eyes improperly coordinated for binocular vision.

orthoptic examination An ophthalmoscopic examination of the binocular function of the eyes. A stereoscopic instrument presents a slightly different picture to each eye. The examiner notes the degree to which the pictures are combined by the normal process of fusion. If the person has diplopia separate pictures are seen. If the person has suppression amblyopia only one picture is seen.

orthosis A force system designed to control, correct, or compensate for a bone deformity, deforming forces, or forces absent from the body. Orthosis often involves the use of special braces. **—orthotic,** *adj., n.*

orthostatic hypotension Abnormally low blood pressure occurring when an individual assumes a standing posture. Also called postural hypotension.

orthostatic proteinuria Presence of protein in the urine of some people, especially teenagers, who have been standing. It disappears when they recline and is of no pathologic significance. The condition is also called orthostatic albuminuria, postural albuminuria, postural proteinuria.

orthotonos A straight, rigid posture of the body caused by a tetanic spasm, usually owing to strychnine poisoning or tetanus infection. The neck and all other body parts are in a position

of extension but not as severely as in opisthotonos. Compare **emprosthotonos.**

Ortolani's test A procedure used to evaluate the stability of the hip joints in newborns and infants. The infant is placed in the supine position and the hips and knees are flexed at right angles and abducted until the lateral aspects of the knees are touching the table. The examiner's fingers are extended along the outside of the thighs, with the thumbs grasping the insides of the knees. Internal and external rotation are attempted, and symmetry of mobility is evaluated. A click or a popping sensation (Ortolani's sign) may be felt if the joint is unstable, because the head of the femur moves out of the acetabulum under pressure from the examiner's hands during rotation and abduction. See also **congenital dislocation of the hip.**

os See **bone.**

-os A combining form signaling singular nouns: *biologos, hepatomphalos, megophthalmos.*

Os Symbol for **osmium.**

O.S. *abbr oculus sinister,* Latin for 'left eye.'

os calcis See **calcaneus.**

os capitatum See **capitate bone.**

oscheo- A combining form meaning 'of or pertaining to the scrotum': *oscheocele, oscheolith, oscheoma.*

os cuboideum See **cuboid bone.**

-ose A combining form meaning: **1.** A 'carbohydrate': *cellulose, lactose, sucrose.* **2.** A 'primary product of hydrolysis': *albumose, nucleose.*

Osgood's disease See **Osgood-Schlatter disease.**

Osgood-Schlatter disease Inflammation or partial separation of the tibial tubercle caused by chronic irritation, usually secondary to overuse of the quadriceps muscle. The condition is seen primarily in muscular, athletic adolescent boys and is characterized by swelling and tenderness over the tibial tubercle that increase with exercise or any activity that extends the leg. Treatment consists primarily of preventing further irritation during the healing process and may necessitate complete immobilization of the knee in a cast. Any residual nonunion of a proximal fragment after healing may require surgical excision. Also called Osgood's disease, Schlatter's disease, Schlatter-Osgood disease.

os hamatum See **hamate bone.**

os hyoideum See **hyoid bone.**

-osis A combining form meaning: **1.** A '(specified) action, process, or result': *homeosis, narcosis, zygosis.* **2.** A 'pathological condition': *calcicosis, psittacosis, varicosis.*

Osler's disease See **Osler-Weber-Rendu syndrome.**

Osler's nodes Tender, reddish or purplish subcutaneous nodules of the soft tissue on the ends of fingers or toes, seen in subacute bacterial endocarditis and usually lasting only one or two days.

Osler-Weber-Rendu syndrome A vascular anomaly, inherited as an autosomal dom-

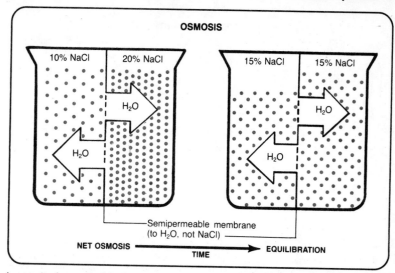

OSMOSIS

| 10% NaCl | 20% NaCl | | 15% NaCl | 15% NaCl |

H_2O

H_2O

H_2O

H_2O

Semipermeable membrane
(to H_2O, not NaCl)

NET OSMOSIS ⟶ EQUILIBRATION

TIME

inant trait, characterized by hemorrhagic tel-angiectasia of skin and mucosa. Small red-to-violet lesions are found on the lips, the oral and nasal mucosa, the tongue, and the tips of fingers and toes. The thin, dilated vessels may bleed spontaneously or as a result of only minor trauma, and this condition becomes progressively more severe. Bleeding from superficial lesions is often profuse and may result in severe anemia. No specific treatment is known, but accessible, bleeding lesions may be treated with pressure, styptics, and topical hemostatics. Transfusions may be indicated for acute hemorrhage, and iron deficiency anemia may require continuous treatment. Also called hemorrhagic familial angiomatosis, hereditary hemorrhagic telangiectasia, Rendu-Osler-Weber syndrome.

os lunatum   See **lunate bone.**

os magnum   See **capitate bone.**

-osmia   A combining form meaning '(condition of the) sense of smell': *dysosmia, hemianosmia, merosmia.*

osmium (Os)   A hard, gray, pungent-smelling metallic element. Its atomic number is 76; its atomic weight is 190.2. It is highly toxic.

osmo-   A combining form meaning: **1.** 'Of or pertaining to odors': *osmoceptor, osmodysphoria, osmonosology.* **2.** 'Pertaining to an impulse, or to osmosis': *osmophilic, osmosology, osmotaxis.*

osmol   The quantity of a substance in solution in the form of molecules or ions or both (usually expressed in grams) that has the same osmotic pressure as one mole of an ideal nonelectrolyte. **—osmolal,** *adj.*

osmolality   The osmotic pressure of a solution expressed in osmols or milliosmols per kilogram of water. Compare **osmolarity.**

osmolar   Of or pertaining to the osmotic characteristics of a solution of one or more molecular substances or ionic substances or both,

expressed in osmols or milliosmols.

osmolarity   The osmotic pressure of a solution expressed in osmols or milliosmols per kilogram of the solution. Compare **osmolality.**

osmometry   A field of study that deals with the phenomenon of osmosis and the measurement of osmotic forces. **—osmometric,** *adj.*

osmosis   The movement of a pure solvent, as water, through a semipermeable membrane from a solution that has a lower solute concentration to one that has a higher solute concentration. The membrane is impermeable to the solute but is permeable to the solvent. The rate of osmosis depends on the concentration of solute, the temperature of the solution, the electrical charge of the solute, and the difference between the osmotic pressures exerted by the solutions. Movement across the membrane continues until the concentrations of the solutions equalize.

osmotic diuresis   Diuresis owing to the presence of certain nonabsorbable substances in renal tubules, as mannitol, urea, or glucose.

osmotic fragility   A sensitivity to change in osmotic pressure characteristic of red blood cells. Exposed to a hypotonic concentration of sodium in a solution, red cells take in increasing quantities of water, swell until the capacity of the cell membrane is exceeded, and burst. Exposed to a hypertonic concentration of sodium in a solution, red cells give up intracellular fluid, shrink, and break up. Laboratory findings of exceptional fragility or resistance may be diagnostic of certain conditions.

osmotic pressure   **1.** The pressure exerted on a semipermeable membrane separating a solution from a solvent, the membrane being impermeable to the solutes in the solution and permeable only to the solvent. **2.** The pressure exerted on a semipermeable membrane by a solution containing one or more solutes that cannot

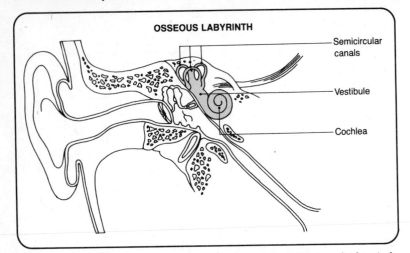

OSSEOUS LABYRINTH

Semicircular canals

Vestibule

Cochlea

penetrate the membrane, which is permeable only by the solvent surrounding it. See also **osmosis.**

os naviculares pedis See **scaphoid bone.**

-osphresia A combining form meaning 'a condition of the sense of smell': *anosphresia, hyperosphresia, oxyosphresia.* Also -osphrasia.

osphresio- A combining form meaning 'of or pertaining to odors': *osphresiolagnia, osphresiology, osphresiophilia.*

oss- A combining form meaning 'of or pertaining to bone': *osseocartilaginous, ossicle, ossific.*

osseous labyrinth The bony portion of the internal ear, composed of three cavities: the vestibule, the semicircular canals, and the cochlea, transmitting sound vibrations from the middle ear to the acoustic nerve. All three cavities contain perilymph, in which a membranous labyrinth is suspended. Also called **labyrinthus osseus.** Compare **membranous labyrinth.**

ossicle A small bone, as the malleus, the incus, or the stapes, the ossicles of the inner ear. **—ossicular,** *adj.*

ossification The development of bone. Intramembranous ossification is that preceded by membrane, as in the process initially forming the roof and the sides of the skull. **Intracartilaginous ossification** is that preceded by rods of cartilage, as that forming the bones of the limbs.

ossifying fibroma A slow-growing, benign neoplasm of bone, occurring most often in the jaws, especially the mandible. The tumor is composed of bone that develops within fibrous connective tissue.

ostealgia Any pain associated with an abnormal condition within a bone, as osteomyelitis. **—ostealgic,** *adj.*

osteanagenesis See **osteoanagenesis.**

osteitis An inflammation of bone, caused by infection, degeneration, or trauma. Swelling, tenderness, dull aching pain, and redness in the skin over the affected bone are characteristic of the condition. Some kinds of osteitis are **osteitis deformans, osteitis fibrosa cystica.** See also **osteomyelitis, Paget's disease.**

osteitis deformans See **Paget's disease.**

osteitis fibrosa cystica An inflammatory degenerative condition in which normal bone is replaced by cysts and fibrous tissue. It is usually associated with hyperparathyroidism.

osteitis fibrosa disseminata See **Albright's syndrome.**

ostembryon See **lithopedion.**

osteo- A combining form meaning 'of or pertaining to bone': *osteoanesthesia, osteocele, osteopathy.*

osteoanagenesis, osteanagenesis The regeneration or formation of bone tissue.

osteoarthritis The most common form of arthritis, in which one or many joints undergo degenerative changes, including subchondral bony sclerosis, loss of articular cartilage, and proliferation of bone and cartilage in the joint, forming osteophytes. Inflammation of the synovial membrane of the joint is common late in the disease. Its cause is unknown. Emotional stress often aggravates the condition. Usually, it begins with pain after exercise or use of the joint. Stiffness, tenderness to the touch, crepitus, and enlargement develop, and deformity, subluxation, and synovial effusion may eventually occur. Involvement of the hip, knee, or the spine causes more disability than osteoarthritis of other areas. Treatment includes rest of the involved joints, heat, and anti-inflammatory drugs. Intraarticular injections of corticosteroids may give relief. Surgical treatment is sometimes necessary and may reduce pain and greatly improve joint function. Compare **rheumatoid arthritis.**

osteoblast A cell that originates in the embryonic mesenchyme and, during the early development of the skeleton, differentiates from a fibroblast to function in the formation of bone tissue. Osteoblasts synthesize the collagen and glycoproteins to form the matrix and, with growth, develop into osteocytes. Also called **osteoplast.** See also **ossification. —osteoblastic,** *adj.*

osteoblastoma, *pl.* **osteoblastomas, osteoblastomata** A small, benign, fairly vascular tumor of poorly formed bone and fibrous tissue, occurring most frequently in a vertebra, femur, tibia, or upper extremity bone in children and young adults. The lesion causes pain, erosion, and resorption of native bone. When feasible, excision is the preferred treatment. Also called **osteoid osteoma.**

osteochondrodystrophy See **Morquio's disease.**

osteochondroma A benign tumor made of bone and cartilage.

osteochondrosis A disease affecting the ossification centers of bone in children, initially characterized by degeneration and necrosis, followed by regeneration and recalcification. Kinds of osteochondrosis include **Legg-Calvé-Perthe's disease, Osgood-Schlatter disease, Scheuermann's disease.**

osteoclasia 1. The destruction and absorption of bony tissue by osteoclasts, as during growth or the healing of fractures. 2. The degeneration of bone through disease. See also **osteolysis.**

osteoclasis The surgical fracture of a bone to correct a deformity. Also called osteoclasty. **—osteoclastic,** *adj.*

osteoclast 1. A large type of multinucleated bone cell that functions in the development and periods of growth or repair, as the breakdown and resorption of osseous tissue. During bone healing of fractures, or during certain disease processes, osteoclasts excavate passages through the surrounding tissue by enzymatic action. Osteoclasts become activated in the presence of parathyroid hormone and also in a lymphokine substance produced by lymphocytes in such diseases as multiple myeloma and malignant lymphomas. Also called **osteophage.** See also **ossification.** 2. A surgical instrument used in the fracturing or refracturing of bones for therapeutic purposes.

osteoclastic 1. Pertaining to or of the nature of osteoclasts. 2. Destructive to bone.

osteoclastoma, *pl.* **osteoclastomas, osteoclastomata** A giant cell tumor of the bone, occurring most frequently at the end of a long bone and appearing as a mass surrounded by a thin shell of new, periosteal bone. The lesion may be benign but is more often malignant. It causes local pain, loss of function, and, in some cases, weakness followed by pathologic fracture. Also called **giant cell myeloma, giant cell tumor of bone.**

osteocyte A bone cell; a mature osteoblast embedded in the bone matrix. It occupies a small cavity and sends out protoplasmic projections that anastomose with those of other osteoblasts to form a system of minute canals within the bone matrix. **—osteocytic,** *adj.*

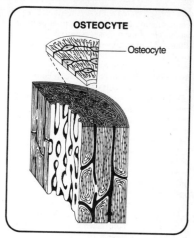

OSTEOCYTE

Osteocyte

osteodystrophy Any generalized defect in bone development, usually associated with disturbances in calcium and phosphorus metabolism and renal insufficiency, as in renal osteodystrophy. Also called osteodystrophia.

osteogenesis, osteogeny The origin and development of bone tissue. See also **ossification. —osteogenetic, osteogenic,** *adj.*

osteogenesis imperfecta A genetic disorder involving defective development of the connective tissue. It is inherited as an autosomal dominant trait and is characterized by abnormally brittle and fragile bones that are easily fractured by the slightest trauma. In its most severe form, the disease may be apparent at birth, when it is known as osteogenesis imperfecta congenita. The newborn has multiple fractures that have occurred in utero and is usually severely deformed, owing to imperfect formation and mineralization of bone. Most infants with this disorder die shortly after birth, although a few survive as deformed dwarfs with normal mental development if no head trauma has occurred. If the disease has a later onset, it is called osteogenesis imperfecta tarda and usually runs a milder course. Symptoms generally appear when the child begins to walk, but they become less severe with age, and the tendency to fracture decreases and disappears after puberty. Other manifestations of the condition include blue sclerae, translucent skin, hyperextensibility of ligaments, hypoplasia of the teeth, recurrent epistaxis, excessive diaphoresis, mild hyperpyrexia, and a tendency to bruise easily and to develop otosclerosis with hearing loss. The number and extent of pathological features may range from minimal to severe involvement. There is no known cure for the disease. Treatment is predominantly supportive; extreme care must be taken in handling patients, especially infants who are severely affected, to prevent fractures. In many children, oral administration of magnesium oxide may decrease the fracture rate, as well as the diaphoresis, hyperpyrexia, and constipation associated with the condition. The primary function of the nurse is to educate the parents about the disease, especially the extent of the child's limitations, and to help them plan suitable activities that will promote optimum growth and development and, at the same time, protect the child from harm. Genetic counseling is also one of the goals of long-term care. Also called **fragilitas ossium, hypoplasia of the mesenchyme, osteopsathyrosis.**

osteogenic, osteogenous Composed of or originating from any tissue involved in the development, growth, or repair of bone.

osteogenic sarcoma See **osteosarcoma.**

osteogeny See **osteogenesis.**

osteoid Of, pertaining to, or resembling bone.

osteoid osteoma See **osteoblastoma.**

osteolysis The degeneration and dissolution of bone, caused by disease, infection, or ischemia. The condition commonly affects the terminal bones of the hands and feet, as in acroosteolysis, and is seen in disorders involving blood vessels, as in Raynaud's disease. —**osteolytic,** adj.

osteoma, pl. **osteomas, osteomata** A tumor of bone tissue.

-osteoma A combining form meaning 'a tumor composed of bone tissue, usually benign': endosteoma, myosteoma, periosteoma.

osteomalacia An abnormal condition of the lamellar bone, characterized by a loss of calcification of the matrix, resulting in softening of the bone and accompanied by weakness, fracture, pain, anorexia, and weight loss. The condition is the result of an inadequate amount of phosphorus and calcium available in the blood for mineralization of the bones. This deficiency may be caused by a diet lacking these minerals or vitamin D, by a lack of exposure to sunlight, or by a metabolic disorder causing malabsorption. Osteomalacia results from and also complicates many diseases and conditions. Treatment usually includes the administration of the necessary vitamins and minerals and therapy for the underlying disorder. See also **hyperparathyroidism, Paget's disease, rickets.**

osteomyelitis Local or generalized infection of bone and bone marrow, usually caused by bacteria introduced by trauma or surgery, by direct extension from a nearby infection, or via the bloodstream. Staphylococci are the most common causative agents. The long bones in children and the vertebrae in adults are the commonest sites of infection as a result of hematogenous spread. Persistent, severe, and increasing bone pain, tenderness, guarding on movement, regional muscle spasm, and fever suggest this diagnosis. Draining sinus tracts may accompany posttraumatic osteomyelitis or osteomyelitis from a contiguous infection. Specific diagnosis and selection of therapy depend on bacterial examination of bone, tissue, or pus. Treatment includes bed rest and parenteral antibiotics for several weeks. Surgery may be necessary to remove necrotic bone and tissue, to obliterate cavities, to remove infected prosthetic appliances,

and to apply prostheses to stabilize affected parts. NURSING CONSIDERATIONS: Any drainage is disposed of with the usual precautions against contamination. Absolute rest of the affected part may be necessary, with careful positioning using pillows and sandbags for good alignment. During the early phase of infection, pain is extremely severe, and extraordinary gentleness in moving and manipulating the infected part is essential. —**osteomyelitic,** adj.

osteon The basic structural unit of compact bone, consisting of the haversian canal and its concentric rings of 4 to 20 lamellae. Most of the units run with the long axis of the bone.

-osteon A combining form meaning 'bone': melacosteon, otosteon, pleurosteon. Also **-osteum.**

osteonecrosis The destruction and death of bone tissue, as from ischemia, infection, malignant neoplastic disease, or trauma. —**osteonecrotic,** adj.

osteopath, osteopathist A physician specialized in osteopathy.

osteopathy A therapeutic approach to the practice of medicine that utilizes all the usual forms of medical therapy and diagnosis, but that places greater emphasis on the role of the relationship of the organs and the musculoskeletal system than is done in medicine. Osteopathic physicians recognize and correct structural problems using manipulation. See also **Doctor of Osteopathy.** —**osteopathic,** adj.

osteopedion See **lithopedion.**

osteopetrosis An inherited disorder characterized by a generalized increase in bone density, probably caused by faulty bone resorption from a deficiency of osteoclasts. In its most severe form, transmitted as an autosomal recessive condition, there is obliteration of the bone marrow cavity, causing severe anemia, marked deformities of the skull, and compression of the cranial nerves, which may result in deafness and blindness and lead to early death. A milder, benign form, transmitted as an autosomal dominant trait, is characterized by short stature, fragile bones, and a proneness to develop osteomyelitis. Also called **Albers-Schönberg disease, ivory bones, marble bones.** —**osteopetrotic,** adj.

osteophage See **osteoclast.**

osteoplast See **osteoblast.**

osteopoikilosis An inherited condition of the bones, transmitted as an autosomal dominant trait, characterized by multiple areas of dense calcification throughout the osseous tissue, producing a mottled appearance on X-ray examination. It is a benign condition, usually without symptoms and of unknown cause. Also called osteosclerosis fragilis congenita. —**osteopoikilotic,** adj.

osteoporosis A disorder characterized by abnormal rarefaction of bone, occurring most frequently in postmenopausal women, in sedentary or immobilized individuals, and in patients on long-term steroid or heparin therapy. The disorder may cause pain, especially in the

OSTOMIES FOR URINARY DIVERSION

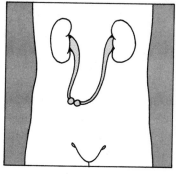

DOUBLE-BARREL URETEROSTOMY

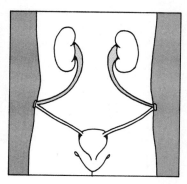

FLANK LOOP URETEROSTOMY

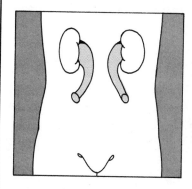

BILATERAL URETEROSTOMY

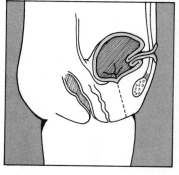

CONTINENT VESICOSTOMY

lower back, pathologic fractures, loss of stature, and various deformities. Osteoporosis may be idiopathic or secondary to other disorders, as thyrotoxicosis or the bone demineralization caused by hyperparathyroidism. Estrogen therapy is often used for the prevention and management of postmenopausal osteoporosis, but use of the hormone carries the risk of endometrial cancer.

osteopsathyrosis See **osteogenesis imperfecta.**

osteosarcoma A malignant bone tumor composed of anaplastic cells derived from mesenchyme. Also called **osteogenic sarcoma.**

osteosclerosis An abnormal increase in the density of bone tissue. The condition occurs in a variety of disease states, is commonly associated with ischemia, chronic infection, and tumor formation, and may be caused by faulty bone resorption as a result of some abnormality involving the osteoclasts. See also **achondro-**

plasia, osteopetrosis, osteopoikilosis. —**osteosclerotic,** *adj.*

-osteum See **-osteon.**

ostium, *pl.* **ostia** See **orifice.** —**ostial,** *adj.*

ostium primum defect See **atrial septal defect.**

ostium secundum defect See **atrial septal defect.**

ostomate A person who has undergone an ostomy.

ostomy *Informal.* A surgical procedure in which an opening is made to allow the passage of urine from the bladder or of intestinal contents from the bowel to an incision or stoma surgically created in the abdominal wall. An ostomy procedure may be performed to correct an anatomic defect or relieve a urinary or intestional obstruction. Each procedure is named for the anatomic location of the ostomy, as colostomy or cystostomy.

ostomy care The management and support

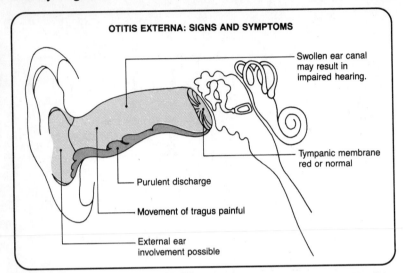

OTITIS EXTERNA: SIGNS AND SYMPTOMS

Swollen ear canal may result in impaired hearing.

Tympanic membrane red or normal

Purulent discharge

Movement of tragus painful

External ear involvement possible

of a patient with a surgical opening created in the bladder, ileum, or colon for the temporary or permanent passage of urine or feces, necessitated by carcinoma, intestinal obstruction, trauma, or severe ulceration distal to the site of the incision. In most cases, the opening is covered with a temporary disposable bag in the operating room.

NURSING CONSIDERATIONS: Before discharge, each step in the care of the stoma and surrounding skin is rehearsed with the patient, using the equipment that will be available at home. Appropriate dietary instruction is provided, emphasizing the need to eat adequate meals regularly, to chew slowly, and to avoid extremely hot and cold food. The patient is urged to establish a regular pattern of evacuation and to report any signs of wound infection or obstruction, as nausea, vomiting, decreased drainage from the stoma, abdominal distention, and cramps. Normal daily activity is encouraged.

ostomy irrigation A procedure for cleansing, stimulating, and regulating evacuation of an artificially created orifice. Fluids used in irrigation include tap water and saline or medicated solutions. Loop and double-barrel colostomies require a sequential irrigation of the proximal loop, distal loop, and rectum in order to prevent the accumulation of discharge.

os trapezium See **trapezium.**

os trapezoideum See **trapezoid bone.**

os triquetrum See **triangular bone.**

ot- See **oto-.**

otalgia Pain in the ear. Also called **otodynia, otoneuralgia.**

OTC *abbr* **over-the-counter,** describing a drug available without a prescription.

Othello syndrome A psychopathological condition, characterized by suspicion of a spouse's infidelity and by morbid jealousy. It may be accompanied by rage and violence and is frequently associated with paranoia.

-otia A combining form meaning '(condition of the) ear': *melotia, microtia, synotia.*

otic Of or pertaining to the ear. Also called **auricular.**

-otic A combining form meaning: **1.** 'Pertaining to part of the ear': *entotic, epitotic, prootic.* **2.** 'Pertaining to an area spatially related to the ear': *opisthotic, parotic, periotic.* **3.** 'Pertaining to a bone spatially related to the ear': *basiotic, prootic, sphenotic.* **4.** 'Pertaining to a (specified) action or condition': *antidotic, biotic, osmotic.* **5.** 'Pertaining to a disease condition': *anthracotic, mycotic, neurotic.* **6.** 'Pertaining to an increase (of something specified)': *hematotic, morphotic, zymotic.*

otics A group of drugs used locally to treat external ear canal inflammation or to remove excess cerumen.

otitic barotrauma See **barotrauma.**

otitis Inflammation or infection of the ear. Kinds of otitis are **otitis externa, otitis media.**

otitis externa Inflammation or infection of the external canal or auricle. Major causes are allergy, bacteria, fungi, viruses, and trauma. Allergy to nickel or chromium in earrings, chemicals in hair sprays, cosmetics, hearing-aids, and medications, particularly sulfonamides and neomycin, is common. *Staphylococcus aureus, Pseudomonas aeruginosa,* and *Streptococcus pyogenes* are common bacterial causes. Herpes simplex and herpes zoster viruses are frequently implicated. Eczema, psoriasis, and seborrheic dermatitis also may affect the external ear. Abrasions of the ear canal may become infected, and excessive swimming may wash out protective cerumen, remove skin lipids, and lead to secondary infection. Otitis externa is more prevalent during hot, humid weather. Folliculitis is particularly painful in the external auditory meatus and is a common occupational hazard in nurses, owing to irritation by the earpieces of stethoscopes. Treatment includes oral anal-

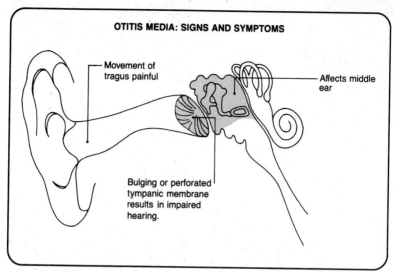

OTITIS MEDIA: SIGNS AND SYMPTOMS

Movement of tragus painful

Affects middle ear

Bulging or perforated tympanic membrane results in impaired hearing.

gesics, thorough local cleansing, topical antimicrobials to treat infection, or topical corticosteroids to reduce inflammation.

otitis interna   See **labyrinthitis.**

otitis media   Inflammation or infection of the middle ear, a common affliction of childhood. Acute otitis media is most often caused by *Haemophilus influenzae* or *Streptococcus pneumoniae.* Chronic otitis media is usually caused by gram-negative bacteria, as *Proteus, Klebsiella,* and *Pseudomonas.* Allergy, *Mycoplasma,* and several viruses also may be etiologic factors. Otitis media is often preceded by an upper respiratory infection. Organisms gain entry to the middle ear through the eustachian tube. The small diameter and horizontal orientation of the tube in infants predisposes them to infection. Obstruction of the eustachian tube and accumulation of exudate may increase pressure within the middle ear, forcing infection into the mastoid bone or rupturing the tympanic membrane. Symptoms of acute otitis media include a sense of fullness in the ear, diminished hearing, pain, and fever. Usually, only one ear is affected. Squamous epithelium may grow in the middle ear through a rupture in the tympanic membrane, and development of a cholesteatoma and deafness may occur if repeated infections cause an opening to persist. Pneumoccoccal otitis media may spread to the meninges. Diagnosis of the causative microorganism is important for selection of effective antimicrobial therapy. Other types of treatment include analgesics, local heat, nasal decongestants, needle aspiration of secretions that have collected behind the membrane, and myringotomy.

NURSING CONSIDERATIONS: Parents are taught to recognize and watch for the early warning signs of otitis media. The use of vaporizers and oral or nasal decongestants is often recommended during an upper respiratory tract infection as prophylaxis against otitis media.

oto-, ot-   A combining form meaning 'of or pertaining to the ear': *otoantritis, otoblennorrhea, otocyst.*

otocephalus   A fetus with otocephaly.

otocephaly   A congenital malformation characterized by the absence of the lower jaw, defective mouth formation, and union or close approximation of the ears on the front of the neck. See also **agnathocephaly. —otocephalic, otocephalous,** *adj.*

otodynia   See **otalgia.**

otolith-righting reflex   An involuntary tilting of the body in newborns that, when the infant is erect, causes the head to return to the upright position. The reflex enables the infant to raise the head and is important for development of later gross motor skills. Absence of the reflex may indicate central nervous system damage.

otoneuralgia   See **otalgia.**

otoplasty   A common procedure in reconstructive plastic surgery in which, for cosmetic reasons, some of the cartilage in the ears is removed to bring the auricle and pinna closer to the head.

otorrhea   Any discharge from the external ear. Otorrhea resulting from external or middle ear infections may be serous, sanguineous, or purulent. Otorrhea may also result from fracture of the temporal bone, due to escape of cerebrospinal fluid through the external auditory meatus. **—otorrheal, otorrheic, otorrhetic,** *adj.*

otosclerosis   A hereditary condition of unknown cause in which irregular ossification in the bony labyrinth of the inner ear, especially of the stapes, occurs, causing tinnitus, then deafness. The deafness is usually first noticed between the ages of 11 and 30. Women are affected twice as often as men. The condition may worsen in pregnancy. Stapedectomy can usually restore hearing. Also called otospongiosis.

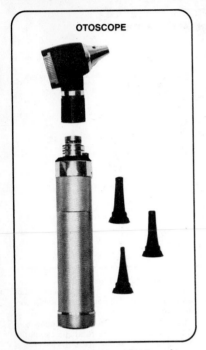

OTOSCOPE

otoscope An instrument that is used to examine the external ear, the eardrum, and, through the eardrum, the ossicles of the middle ear. The otoscope consists of a light, a magnifying lens, and a device for insufflation.

ototoxic Of a substance: having a harmful effect on the eighth cranial nerve or the organs of hearing and balance. Common ototoxic drugs include the aminoglycoside antibiotics, aspirin, furosemide, and quinine.

O.U. *abbr oculus uterque,* Latin for 'each eye.'

ouabain A cardiotonic glycoside used to treat congestive heart failure and some cardiac arrhythmias.

ounce (oz) A unit of weight equal to 1/16 of a pound avoirdupois.

-ous A combining form meaning an 'element or compound with a valence lower than the corresponding one ending in *-ic*': *cuprous, ferrous, hypochlorous.* Also **-eous.**

outbreeding The production of offspring by the mating of unrelated individuals, organisms, or plants, which can lead to superior hybrid traits or strains. Compare **inbreeding.** See also **heterosis.**

outcome data Data collected to evaluate the capacity of a client to function at a level described in the outcome statement of a nursing-care plan or in standards for client care.

outcome measure A measure of the quality of medical care, the standard on which is made the assessment of the expected end result of the intervention employed.

outlet contraction See **contraction.**

outlet contracture An abnormally small pelvic outlet. It may be anteroposterior or transverse and is of significance in childbirth, as it may impede or prevent fetal passage through the birth canal. Anteroposterior contracture owing to fixation of the coccyx may sometimes be overcome by the force of labor, freeing the bones and allowing them to move back. Significant narrowing of the space between the ischial tuberosities is unlikely to be overcome and is most commonly associated with a heavy, android type of pelvis.

outlet forceps See **low forceps.**

outpatient 1. A patient, not hospitalized, who is being treated in an office, clinic, or other ambulatory care facility. 2. Of or pertaining to a health-care facility for patients who are not hospitalized or to the treatment or care of such a patient. Compare **inpatient.**

ovale malaria See **tertian malaria.**

ovalocytosis See **elliptocytosis.**

ovari-, ovario A combining form meaning 'of or pertaining to the ovary: *ovariocentesis, ovariosteresis, ovariotubal.* Also **oario-, ootheco-.**

-ovaria A combining form meaning '(condition of the) ovary or ovarial activity': *anovaria, hyperovaria.*

ovarian Of or pertaining to the ovary.

ovarian artery A slender branch of the abdominal aorta, arising caudal to the renal arteries, and supplying an ovary. Compare **testicular artery.**

ovarian cancer A malignant neoplastic disease of the ovary, occurring most frequently in women between the ages of 40 and 60 and occasionally in young adolescents. Risk factors in adults are a history of infertility, endometriosis, nulliparity or low parity, repeated spontaneous abortion, delayed childbearing, a family history of ovarian cancer, Peutz-Jeghers syndrome, previous irradiation of the pelvic organs, and exposure to chemical carcinogens. Ovarian tumors are usually advanced before any symptoms appear. Regular yearly pelvic examinations after the age of 40 contribute significantly to early diagnosis and the possibility of curative treatment. Characteristic of the disease as it advances are abdominal swelling and discomfort, abnormal vaginal bleeding, weight loss, dysuria or abnormal frequency of urination, constipation, and a palpable ovarian mass, especially in postmenopausal women. Ultrasonography and computerized tomography are useful in the diagnosis, but laparotomy and surgical exploration are required to determine the extent and character of the tumor. Many kinds of tumors may arise in the ovary. About 85% are epithelial in origin, with papillary serous tumors the most common, followed by mucinous, endometroid, and undifferentiated solid cancers. The surgery recommended for ovarian cancer is total abdominal hysterectomy and bilateral salpingo-oophorectomy with omentectomy. Postoperative radiotherapy is used to control residual tumor, and antineoplastic agents are used to treat met-

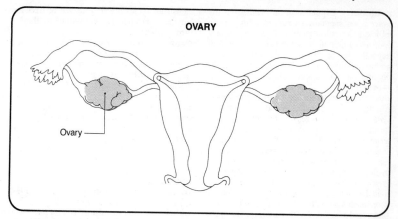

OVARY

Ovary

are used to treat metastatic lesions.

ovarian carcinoma See **ovarian cancer.**

ovarian cyst A globular sac filled with fluid or semisolid material that develops in or on the ovary. It may be transient and physiologic or pathologic. Kinds of ovarian cysts include chocolate cyst, corpus luteum cyst.

ovarian varicocele A varicose swelling of the veins of the uterine broad ligament. Also called **pelvic varicocele.**

ovarian vein One of a pair of veins that emerge from convoluted plexuses in the broad ligament near the ovaries and the uterine tubes. The veins from each plexus ascend and unite to form single veins. The right ovarian vein opens into the inferior vena cava, the left ovarian vein into the renal vein. In some individuals, the ovarian veins contain valves and greatly enlarge during pregnancy. Compare **testicular vein.**

ovariectomy See **oophorectomy.**

ovary One of the pair of female gonads found on each side of the lower abdomen, beside the uterus, in a fold of the broad ligament. At ovulation, an egg is extruded from a follicle on the surface of the ovary under the stimulation of the follicle-stimulating hormone and luteinizing hormone. The mature ovarian follicle secretes estrogen and progesterone to regulate the menstrual cycle by a negative feedback system. Each ovary is normally firm and smooth and resembles an almond in size and shape. The ovaries are homologous to the testes.

overcompensation An exaggerated attempt, either conscious or unconscious, to overcome a real or imagined physical or psychological deficit. See also **compensation.**

overload **1.** A burden greater than the capacity of the system designed to move or process it. **2.** In physiology: any factor or influence that stresses the body beyond its natural limits and impairs its health.

overoxygenation An abnormal condition in which the oxygen concentration in the blood and other tissues of the body is greater than normal, and the carbon dioxide concentration is less than normal. The condition is character-ized by a fall in blood pressure, decreased vital capacity, fatigue, errors in judgment, paresthesia of the hands and feet, anorexia, nausea and vomiting, and hyperemia.

over-the-counter (OTC) Of a drug: available without a prescription.

overweight More than normal in body weight after adjustment for height, body build, and age.

ovi-, ovo- A combining form meaning 'of or pertaining to an egg or to ova': *ovoglobulin, ovoplasm, ovotestis.*

oviduct See **fallopian tube.**

oviferous Bearing or capable of producing ova.

oviparous Giving birth to young by laying eggs. Compare **ovoviviparous, viviparous.**

oviposition The act of laying or depositing eggs by the female member of oviparous animals.

ovipositor A specialized organ, found primarily in insects, for depositing eggs on plants or in the soil.

ovocenter The centrosome of a fertilized ovum. Also called **oocenter.**

ovoflavin A riboflavin derived from the yolk of eggs.

ovogenesis See **oogenesis.** —**ovogenetic, ovogenic,** *adj.*

ovoglobulin A globulin derived from the white of eggs.

ovogonium See **oogonium.**

ovo-lacto-vegetarian See **lacto-ovo-vegetarian.**

ovomucin A glycoprotein derived from the white of eggs.

ovomucoid Of or pertaining to a glycoprotein, similar to mucin, derived from the white of eggs.

ovoplasm See **ooplasm.**

ovotestis A gonad with both ovarian and testicular tissue; a hermaphroditic gonad. —**ovotesticular,** *adj.*

ovovitellin See **vitellin.**

ovoviviparous Bearing young in eggs that are hatched within the body, as some reptiles and fishes. Compare **oviparous, viviparous.**

ovulation Expulsion of an ovum from the ovary upon spontaneous rupture of a mature follicle, as a result of cyclic ovarian and pituitary endocrine function. It usually occurs on the 14th day following the 1st day of the last menstrual period and often causes brief, sharp lower abdominal pain on the side of the ovulating ovary. —**ovulate,** *v.*

ovulation method of family planning A natural method of family planning that uses observation of changes in the character and quantity of cervical mucus as a means of determining the time of ovulation during the menstrual cycle. As pregnancy occurs with fertilization of an ovum extruded from the ovary at ovulation, the method is used to increase or decrease the woman's chance of becoming pregnant by causing or avoiding insemination by spontaneous or artificial means during the fertile period associated with ovulation. The cyclic changes in gonadotropic hormones, especially estrogen, cause changes in the quantity and character of cervical mucus. In the first days after menstruation, scant thick mucus is secreted by the cervix. These 'dry days' are 'safe days,' with ovulation several days away. The quantity of mucus then increases; it is pearly-white and sticky, becoming clearer and less sticky as ovulation approaches; these 'wet days' are 'unsafe days.' During and just after ovulation, the mucus is clear, slippery, and elastic; it resembles the uncooked white of an egg. The day on which this sign is most apparent is the 'peak day,' probably the day preceding ovulation. The 4 days following the 'peak day' are 'unsafe': fertilization might occur. By the end of the 4 days, the mucus becomes pearly-white and sticky again and progressively decreases in quantity until menstruation supervenes to begin a new cycle. Essential to the effectiveness of this method are thorough instruction by a family-planning counselor and strong self-motivation in the couple. During the first cycle, abstinence may be necessary to allow observation of the mucus without the confusing addition of semen or contraceptive foam, cream, or jelly, if being used. Daily close monitoring of the mucus is necessary even after several cycles because the length of the 'safe' and 'unsafe' periods and the time of ovulation vary from cycle to cycle, as they do from woman to woman. Postpartally and during lactation, the method is not effective until the menses have become regular. Effectiveness of the method in identifying the most fertile days of the cycle is augmented by using the basal body temperature method. This combined method is called the symptothermal method of planning. Proponents of the ovulation method claim the benefits of low cost, naturalness, and effectiveness. Detractors emphasize a limited public health application of the method, stating that it requires extensive teaching and self-motivation and that is effectiveness is limited by the ability of the user to observe correctly and diligently the changes in the cervical mucus. Abstinence may be necessary for up to 10 days by a woman whose menstrual cycles are long or are of irregular length. Also called **cervical mucus method of family planning.**

ovum, *pl.* **ova** 1. An egg. 2. A female germ cell extruded from the ovary at ovulation.

oxacillin sodium A penicillin antibiotic.

oxaluric acid A compound derived from uric acid or from parabonic acid, which occurs in normal urine.

oxamniquine An anthelmintic agent.

oxandrolone An anabolic steroid.

oxazepam A benzodiazepine antianxiety agent.

-oxemia A combining form meaning 'a (specified) state of oxygen in the blood': *anoxemia, hyperoxemia.*

oxethazaine An antacid.

-oxia A combining form meaning '(condition of) oxygenation': *anoxia, asthenoxia, hypoxia.*

oxidation In chemistry: 1. Any process in which the oxygen content of a compound is increased. 2. Any reaction in which the positive valence of a compound or a radical is increased owing to a loss of electrons. —**oxidize,** *v.*

oxidize Of an element or compound: to combine or cause to combine with oxygen, to remove hydrogen, or to increase the valence of an element through the loss of electrons. —**oxidation,** *n.,* **oxidizing,** *adj.*

oxidized cellulose A local hemostatic agent.

oxidizing agent A compound that readily gives up oxygen and attracts hydrogen from another compound. In chemical reactions, an oxidizing agent acts as an acceptor of electrons, thereby increasing the valence of an element.

oxtriphylline A respiratory tract spasmolytic.

oxy- 1. A combining form meaning 'sharp, quick, or sour': *oxyblepsia, oxycephalia, oxyecoia.* 2. A combining form indicating the presence of oxygen in a compound: *oxyacanthine, oxycamphor, oxyquinoline.*

oxybenzene See **carbolic acid.**

oxybutynin chloride A genitourinary system spasmolytic agent.

oxycephaly, oxycephalia A congenital malformation in which premature closure of the coronal and sagittal sutures results in accelerated upward growth of the head, giving it a long, narrow appearance with the top pointed or conical in shape. Also called **acrocephaly, hyssicephaly, steeple head, tower head, tower skull, turricephaly.** See also **craniostenosis.** —**oxycephalus,** *n.,* **oxycephalous,** *adj.*

oxychlorosene calcium, o. sodium Antiseptic agents.

oxycodone hydrochloride A narcotic and opioid analgesic.

oxygen (O) A tasteless, odorless, colorless gas essential for human respiration. In anesthesia, oxygen functions as a carrier gas for the delivery of anesthetic agents to the tissues of the body. In respiratory therapy, oxygen is administered to increase the amount of oxygen and thus decrease the amount of other gases circulating in the blood. Overdose of oxygen can cause

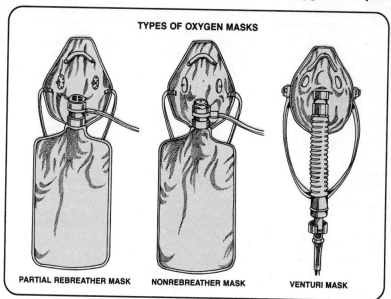

TYPES OF OXYGEN MASKS

PARTIAL REBREATHER MASK   NONREBREATHER MASK   VENTURI MASK

irreversible toxicity in people with pulmonary abnormalities, especially when complicated by chronic carbon dioxide retention. Prolonged administration of high concentrations of oxygen may cause irreversible damage to infants' eyes. Oxygen itself is not flammable or explosive, but because an oxygen-rich environment is favorable to fire and explosion, flame or electric spark must be avoided when oxygen is being administered.

oxygenation The process of combining or treating with oxygen. —**oxygenate,** *v.*

oxygen mask A device used to administer oxygen. It is shaped to fit snugly over the mouth and nose and may be secured in place with a strap or held with the hand. The mask has inspiratory and expiratory valves allowing oxygen to be inhaled or pumped into the respiratory tract and carbon dioxide to be exhaled into the environment. Oxygen flows at a prescribed rate through a tubing to the mask. Types of oxygen masks include simple mask, partial rebreathing mask, nonrebreathing mask, and Venturi mask.

oxygen tension The force with which oxygen molecules that are physically dissolved in blood are constantly trying to escape, expressed as partial pressure (PO_2). The tension at any instant is related to the amount of oxygen physically dissolved in plasma; the larger amount carried in chemical combination with hemoglobin serves as a reservoir that releases oxygen molecules to physical solution when the tension decreases and that stores additional molecules of the gas when the tension increases.

oxygen therapy Any procedure in which oxygen is administered to relieve hypoxia. Of the many methods for providing oxygen therapy, the one selected depends upon the condition of the patient and the cause of hypoxia. Low or moderate amounts of oxygen may be supplied to postoperative patients by a nasal catheter or cannula. Low concentrations, precisely measured, may be delivered to patients with chronic obstructive lung disease by a Venturi mask. If hypoxia is the result of impaired cardiac function, a high concentration of oxygen may be delivered by a nonrebreathing or partial rebreathing mask. Humidity and drugs in aerosol form may be given with oxygen using a variety of devices, as a Croupette, aerosol face mask, or T-piece. Oxygen therapy may be used in the treatment of any condition that results in hypoxia. Although there are several kinds of hypoxia, all result in hypoxemia. The administration of oxygen may relieve hypotension, cardiac arrythmias, tachypnea, headache, disorientation, nausea, and agitation characteristic of hypoxia, as well as restore the ability of the cells of the body to carry on normal metabolic function. Thorough and careful observation of the patient's need for oxygen and his response to therapy are important. The concentration of oxygen received by the patient must not be assumed by the rate and concentration at which it is delivered: a person whose respirations are rapid and shallow receives more oxygen than does a person breathing deeply and slowly. The adverse effects of oxygen therapy include respiratory depression, absorption atelectasis, alveolar collapse, alveolar edema, pulmonary congestion, intra-alveolar collapse, alveolar edema, pulmonary congestion, intra-alveolar hemorrhage, hyaline membrane formation, pain, retrolental fibroplasia, and disturbance of the central nervous system with seizures and, possibly, death.

oxygen transport The process by which

oxygen in the lungs is absorbed by the hemoglobin and carried to the peripheral tissues. This process is made possible by a special characteristic of hemoglobin: the ability to combine with large quantities of oxygen present at a high concentration, as in the lungs, and to release this oxygen when the concentration is low, as in the peripheral tissues. See also **hemoglobin.**

oxyhemoglobin The product of the combining of hemoglobin with oxygen. It is a loosely bound complex that dissociates easily when there is a low concentration of oxygen.

oxymetazoline hydrochloride A sympathomimetic vasoconstrictor used as a nasal decongestant.

oxymetholone An anabolic steroid.

oxymorphone hydrochloride A narcotic and opioid analgesic.

oxyopia, oxyopy Unusual acuteness of vision. A person with oxyopia has better than 20/20 vision.

oxyphenbutazone A nonsteroidal anti-inflammatory agent.

oxyphencyclimine hydrochloride A gastrointestinal anticholinergic agent.

oxyphenonium bromide A gastrointestinal anticholinergic agent.

oxytetracycline hydrochloride A tetracycline antibiotic.

oxytocic 1. Of or pertaining to a substance that is similar to the hormone oxytocin. 2. Any one of numerous drugs that stimulate the smooth muscle of the uterus to contract. These drugs are often used to initiate labor at term. Oxytocic agents commonly used include oxytocin, certain prostaglandins, and the ergot alkaloids. These drugs are used to induce or augment labor, control postpartum hemorrhage, correct postpartum uterine atony, produce uterine contractions after cesarean section or other uterine surgery, and induce therapeutic abortion. The United States Food and Drug Administration has ruled that oxytocin is not indicated for elective termination of pregnancy and should be used only in cases where continued pregnancy is seen as a greater risk to the mother or to the fetus than the risk of drug-induced labor.

oxytocin An oxytocic agent given by nasal inhalation or injection.

oxytocin challenge test A stress test for the assessment of intrauterine function of the fetus and the placenta. It is performed to evaluate the ability of the fetus to tolerate continuation of pregnancy or the anticipated stress of labor and delivery. A dilute intravenous infusion of oxytocin is begun, monitored by a meter or regulated by an infusion pump. The uterine activity is monitored with a tocodynamometer, and the fetal heart rate is monitored with an ultrasonic sensor, as the uterus is stimulated to contract by the oxytocin. The amount of solution infused is increased as necessary to cause the uterus to contract for 30 to 40 seconds three times every 10 minutes. The fetal heart rate is observed for variability and for the timing of any marked variation from the normal in relation to uterine contractions. Decelerations of the fetal heart rate in certain repeating patterns may indicate fetal distress. One quarter of the infants diagnosed by this method as being in distress are normal; therefore, other tests of fetal well-being are recommended before performing an emergency cesarean section or induction of labor.

oxyuriasis See **enterobiasis.**

Oxyuris vermicularis See *Enterobius vermicularis.*

ozena A condition characterized by atrophy of the nasal chonchae and mucous membranes. Symptoms include crusting of nasal secretions, discharge, and, especially, a very offensive odor. Ozena may follow chronic inflammation of the nasal mucosa.

ozone (O_3) A form of oxygen characterized by molecules having three atoms. Ozone is formed when oxygen is electrically charged, as might occur in a lightning storm.

ozone shield The layer of ozone that hangs in the atmosphere from 20 to 40 miles above the surface of the earth and that protects the earth from excessive ultraviolet radiation. Some experts warn that the manufacture of various chemicals, such as chlorofluorocarbons used as propellants in aerosol sprays, and the effects of high-flying jet aircraft are destroying this protective layer and allowing excessive amounts of ultraviolet radiation to penetrate the earth's atmosphere, consequently subjecting humans to increased dangers of skin cancer and other health problems. Some chemistry experts and federal health officials warn that an additional threat comes from the nitrous oxide found in nitrogenous fertilizers, which rises into the atmosphere and reacts unfavorably with the ozone shield. Other experts say that the depletion of the ozone layer by chlorofluorocarbons may be offset by the release of carbon dioxide into the atmosphere from the combustion of fuels. One study indicates that ozone concentration has actually increased 6% since monitoring was begun more than 50 years ago. The ozone shield is implicated in certain health problems that affect some air travelers. See also **ozone sickness.**

ozone sickness An abnormal condition caused by the inhalation of ozone that may seep into jet aircraft at altitudes over 12,192 m (40,000 feet). It is characterized by headaches, chest pains, itchy eyes, and sleepiness. Exactly why and how ozone causes this condition is not known. It is more prevalent early in the year and occurs more often over the Pacific Ocean.

P

P 1. Symbol for gas partial pressure. See **partial pressure.** 2. Symbol for **phosphorus.** 3. *abbr* position, posterior, postpartum, probability (in statistics), pulse, pupil.

P₁ In genetics: symbol for **parental generation.**

PA *abbr* **physician's assistant.**

PABA *abbr* **para-aminobenzoic acid.**

pabulum Any substance that is food or nutrient.

pacemaker An electrical apparatus used for maintaining a normal sinus rhythm of myocardial contraction by electrically stimulating the heart muscle. A pacemaker may be fixed rate, emitting the stimulus at a constant rate, or it may fire only on demand, when the heart does not spontaneously contract at a minimum rate. Pacemakers can be permanent or temporary. Also called cardiac pacemaker.

pachometer See **pachymeter.**

pachy- A combining form meaning 'thick': *pachyaria, pachycephaly.*

pachycephaly An abnormal thickness of the skull, as in acromegaly. Also called **pachycephalia.—pachycephalic, pachycephalous,** *adj.*

pachydactyly An abnormal thickening of the fingers or the toes. —**pachydactylic, pachydactylous,** *adj.*

pachymeter An instrument used to measure thickness, especially of thin structures, as a membrane or a tissue. Also called **pachometer.**

pachynema The postsynaptic tetradic chromosome formation that occurs in the pachytene stage of the first meiotic prophase of gametogenesis.

pachyonychia congenita A congenital deformity characterized by abnormally thickened and raised fingernails and toenails and hyperkeratosis of the palms of the hands and the soles of the feet. The papillae of the tongue also atrophy, causing a whitish coating over the lingual surface.

pachytene The third stage in the first meiotic prophase of gametogenesis in which the paired homologous chromosomes form tetrads. The bivalent pairs become short and thick and intertwine so that four chromatids are visible. See also **diakinesis, diplotene, leptotene, zygotene.**

pacifier 1. An agent that soothes or comforts. 2. A nipple-shaped object used by infants and children for sucking. Such devices can be dangerous if they are too small or poorly constructed, as the entire object or part of it can be aspirated or lodged in the pharynx or trachea, causing obstruction of the airway.

pacing Regulation of the rate of an event, such as the heartbeat.

Pacini's corpuscles A number of special sensory end organs resembling tiny white bulbs, each attached to the end of a single nerve fiber in the subcutaneous, submucous, and subserous connective tissue of many parts of the body, especially the palm of the hand, sole of the foot, genital organs, joints, and in the pancreas. They average about 3 mm in diameter, contain numerous concentric layers around a central core, and in cross section resemble an onion. Also called Pacinian corpuscles. Compare **Golgi-Mazzoni corpuscles, Krause's corpuscles.**

pack 1. A treatment in which the entire body or a portion of it is wrapped in wet or dry towels or in ice for various therapeutic purposes, as with cold packs for the reduction of high temperatures and swellings or for inducing hypothermia during certain surgical procedures, especially heart surgery and organ transplants. 2. A tampon. 3. In dentistry: the act of applying a dressing or cement to a surgical wound. 4. In dentistry: a surgical dressing to cover a wound or to fill the cavity left from a tooth extraction, especially an extraction of a wisdom tooth.

package insert A leaflet that, by order of the FDA, must be placed inside the package of every prescription drug. In it, the manufacturer is required to describe the drug, to state its generic name, and to give the approved indications, contraindications, warnings, precautions, adverse effects, form, dosage, and administration.

packed cells A preparation of blood cells separated from liquid plasma, often administered in severe anemia to restore adequate levels of hemoglobin and red blood cells without overloading the vascular system with excess fluids. See also **bank blood, pooled plasma.**

packing 1. The process of filling a cavity or wound with absorbent material. 2. The material used for filling a cavity or wound; for example, gauze, sponges, or pads.

pad 1. A mass of soft material used to cushion shock, prevent wear, or absorb moisture, as the abdominal pads used to absorb discharges from abdominal wounds or to separate viscera and improve accessibility during abdominal surgery. 2. In anatomy: a mass of fat that cushions various structures, as the infrapatellar pad lying below the patella between the patellar ligament, the head of the tibia, and the femoral condyles.

paedogenesis See **pedogenesis.**

PAF *abbr* platelet-activating factor.

Paget's disease A common, nonmetabolic disease of bone of unknown cause, usually affecting middle-aged and elderly people, characterized by excessive bone destruction and unorganized bone repair. Most cases are asymptomatic or mild; however, bone pain may be the first symptom. Bowed tibias (saber shins), kyphosis, and frequent fractures result from the soft, abnormal bone in this condition. Enlargement of the head, headaches, and warmth over involved areas from increased vascularity are additional features. The serum alkaline phosphatase is often markedly elevated and there is increased urinary calcium and hydroxyproline. The X-ray picture of areas of decreased bone density adjacent to sites of increased density is characteristic. Radioactive bone scans help locate regions of active disease. Complications include fractures, kidney stones if the patient is immobilized, heart failure, deafness or blindness owing to pressure from bony overgrowth, and osteosarcoma. No treatment is necessary for mild cases. A high-protein, high-calcium diet, unless the patient is immobilized, is recommended. Parenteral synthetic salmon calcitonin may help the patient temporarily. Diphosphonates and mithramycin are also effective but require close monitoring for side effects. NURSING CONSIDERATIONS: Immobilization of the patient is avoided, if possible, to prevent hypercalcemia and kidney stones. Observation for neurological signs and symptoms and reporting of changes may help to avert irreversible nerve damage. Also called **osteitis deformans.**

Paget's disease of the nipple See **nipple cancer.**

pagophagia An abnormal condition characterized by a craving to eat enormous quantities of ice. This condition is associated with a lack of nutrient iron. —**pagophagic, pagophagous,** adj.

-pagus A combining form meaning 'conjoined twins': craniopagus, pyropagus.

pain An unpleasant sensation caused by noxious stimulation of the sensory nerve endings. It is a cardinal symptom of inflammation and is valuable in the diagnosis of many disorders. Pain may be mild or severe, chronic or acute, lancinating, burning, dull or sharp, precisely or poorly localized, or referred. See also **referred pain.**

pain and suffering In law: an element in a claim for damages that allows recovery for the mental and physical distress and trauma that an individual has endured as a result of injury.

pain assessment An evaluation of the factors that alleviate or exacerbate a patient's pain. The patient is asked to describe the cause of the pain, if known, its intensity, location, and duration, the events preceding it, and the pattern usually followed for handling pain. Severe pain causes pallor, cold perspiration, piloerection, dilated pupils, and increases in the pulse and respiratory rate, blood pressure, and muscle tension. When brief, intense pain subsides, the pulse rate may be slower and the blood pressure lower than before the pain began. If pain occurs frequently or is prolonged, the pulse rate and blood pressure may not increase markedly, and, if pain persists for many days, there may be an increased production of eosinophils and 17-ketosteroids and greater susceptibility to infections. The patient's statements regarding pain, the tone of voice, speed of speech, cries, groans, or other vocalizations, facial expressions, body movements, or tendency to withdraw are all noted. Pertinent background information in the assessment includes a record of the patient's chronic conditions, previous surgery, and any illnesses that caused pain, the patient's experiences with relatives and friends in pain, the role or position of the patient in the family structure, and the patient's use of alcohol and medications. NURSING CONSIDERATIONS: The nurse teaches the person about pain and how to modify the anxiety associated with it. Analgesics ordered for the patient are administered by the nurse before the pain becomes intense, for this increases their effectiveness. In addition to helping promote rest and relaxation, the nurse helps to distract the patient by using guided imagery, walking, watching television, or reading. If the patient believes that certain acceptable measures alleviate pain, the nurse uses them. Dramatic relief of intense or chronic pain is often difficult to accomplish, but the patient can be helped to learn to handle pain effectively and to function fairly normally.

pain evaluation The clinical assessment of the pain experienced by an individual, used as an aid in the diagnosis and the treatment of disease and trauma. Responses to pain vary widely among individuals and depend on many different physical and psychological factors, as specific diseases and injuries, the health, pain threshold, fear and anxiety, and cultural background of the individual involved, as well as the way different individuals express their pain experiences. Some important factors in pain evaluation are nonverbal expressions of pain, as wincing, grimacing, moaning and groaning, the clenching of fists, and the rubbing of painful areas. Other evaluation factors are the intensity, the location, the duration, and the pattern of pain. Key aspects in evaluating pain intensity are the size of the pain area, the tenderness within the pain area, and the effects of movement and pressure on the pain. Duration of pain is considered in terms of hours, days, weeks, months, or years. Pain patterns are associated with various sensations as burning, pricking, aching, rhythmic throbbing, and the effects on the sympathetic and the parasympathetic nervous systems. Also considered in pain evaluation are the past experiences of the individual experiencing the pain, especially any distinction between sudden, new pain and chronic pain. Evaluation includes the meanings that the individual may attach to pain, such as a test of character, a penance, or a sign of worsening illness. Such interpretations may affect the intensity of pain and may even mask its significance. Also called **pain assessment.** See also **pain intervention, pain mechanism.**

pain intervention The relief of the painful sensations experienced in suffering the physiologic and the psychologic effects of disease and trauma. Effective pain intervention depends on proper evaluation of the type of pain the patient is experiencing, the physical and the psychological origins of the pain, and the behavioral patterns commonly associated with different kinds of pain. The most common method of pain intervention is the administration of narcotics, as morphine, but many authorities believe that the exclusive use of painkilling drugs without consideration and implementation of psychological aids is too narrow an approach. Methods of pain intervention for acute pain are different from those for chronic pain. Acute pain, occurring in the first 24 to 48 hours after surgery, is often difficult to relieve, and narcotics are seldom fully effective. The type of pain intervention usually depends on the description of the pain by the individual experiencing it. Mild pain may best be relieved by comfort measures and the distraction afforded by television, visitors, reading, and other passive activities. Moderate pain may best be relieved by a combination of comfort measures and mild nonnarcotic analgesics. Cognitive dissonance, often employed to dampen moderate pain, encourages the patient to reflect on pleasant experiences and describe them to health-care personnel. Intervention to relieve severe pain often includes the administration of potentially addictive opioids, such as morphine. Opioid analgesics administered for the relief of pain, cough, or diarrhea provide only symptomatic treatment and are used cautiously in the care of patients with acute or chronic diseases. Opioids may obscure the symptoms or the progress of the disease, and repeated daily administration of any opioid will eventually produce some tolerance to the therapeutic effects of the drug as well as some physical dependence on the dosage. The risk of developing psychological and physical dependency on any drug is always present, especially with opioids. In usual doses, opioids relieve suffering by altering the emotional component of the painful experience as well as by effecting analgesia. Some care-givers are so concerned about the addictive dangers of opioids that they tend to prescribe initial doses that are too low or too infrequent to alleviate pain. In severe pain, treatment may also include purposeful interaction between the patient and attending hospital personnel; reduction of environmental stimuli; increased comfort measures; and 'waking imagined analgesia,' in which the patient is encouraged to concentrate on and become distracted by former pleasant experiences, as relaxing on a beach surrounded by cool ocean water. In the alleviation of all types of pain, dampening or decreasing stimuli that create pain is the chief goal. Pain often increases in a cold room because the patient's muscles tend to contract; but the local application of cold, as with an ice pack, often alleviates pain by reducing swelling. Pain intervention seeks to reduce the effects of other factors that compound

pain, as fatigue and anxiety. Sensory restriction may increase pain, because it blocks otherwise effective distraction; overstimulation may cause fatigue and anxiety, thus increasing pain. Religious beliefs may be effective in helping the patient to decrease pain or increase tolerance if the pain is viewed by the patient as requiring self-discipline or as a catharsis for past transgressions. Religious beliefs, however, may increase pain if the patient interprets the pain as punishment and relates the severity of the pain to the gravity of transgressions or faults. Morphine and related opioids may produce unwanted side effects, as nausea, vomiting, dizziness, and constipation. Rarely, a patient treated with an opioid may become delirious. Some patients may also develop increased sensitivity to pain after the opioid has worn off. Patients with reduced blood volume are more susceptible to the hypotensive effect of morphine and related drugs. Opioids are used with extreme caution in obese patients and in those with head injuries, emphysema, or other problems associated with decreased respiratory function. In patients with prostatic hypertrophy, morphine may cause acute urinary retention, requiring repeated catheterization. Pain intervention in the treatment of terminal illnesses employs numerous drugs that relieve pain and produce euphoria and tranquility in patients who would otherwise suffer greatly. Nerve block by the injection of alcohol, chordotomy, and other neurosurgical interventions may sometimes be employed. See also **pain evaluation.**

pain mechanism The psychosomatic network that communicates unpleasant sensations and the perceptions of noxious stimuli throughout the body, most commonly in association with physical disease and trauma involving tissue damage. One of the biggest problems in pain research is that the actual cause of pain originating at the peripheral level is poorly understood. Some authorities believe that bradykinin and histamine, two chemical substances elaborated by the body, cause pain. Recently discovered painkillers produced naturally by the body are the enkephalins and the endorphins. Some studies indicate that the enkephalins are 10 times as potent as morphine in reducing pain. It is known that once histamine and some other naturally occurring chemical substances are released in the body, pain sensations travel along fast-conducting nerve fibers and slow-conducting nerve fibers. These pain-transmitting neuropathways communicate the pain sensation to the dorsal root ganglia of the spinal cord and synapse with certain neurons in the posterior horns of the gray matter. The pain sensation is then transmitted to the reticular formation and the thalamus by neurons that form the anterolateral spinothalamic tract and is conveyed to various areas of the brain, as the cortex and the hypothalamus, by synapses at the thalamus. The immediate reaction to pain is transmitted over the reflex arc by sensory fibers in the dorsal horn of the spinal cord and by synapsing motor neu-

PAIN RECEPTORS AND NEUROPATHWAYS FOR PAIN PERCEPTION

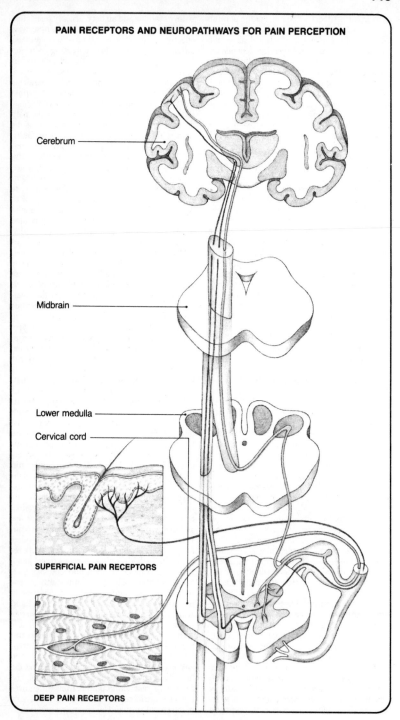

Cerebrum

Midbrain

Lower medulla

Cervical cord

SUPERFICIAL PAIN RECEPTORS

DEEP PAIN RECEPTORS

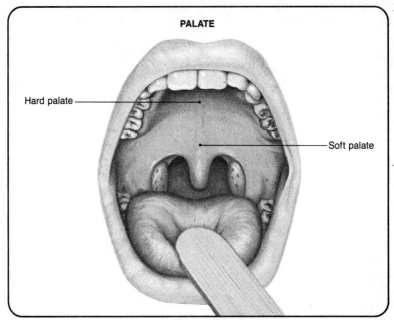

PALATE

Hard palate

Soft palate

rons in the anterior horn. This anatomic pattern of sensory and motor neurons allows the individual to move quickly at the touch of some harmful stimulus, as extreme heat. Nerve impulses alerting the individual to move away from such stimuli are simultaneously sent along efferent nerve fibers from the brain. Past experiences, anxiety, and motivations greatly affect the pain sensations of everyone, and the fear of pain is second only to the fear of death for most people. Fear and anxiety often intensify pain.

pain receptor Any one of the many free nerve endings throughout the body that warn of potentially harmful changes in the environment, as excessive pressure or temperature. The free nerve endings constituting most of the pain receptors occur chiefly in the epidermis and in the epithelial covering of certain mucous membranes. They also appear in the stratified squamous epithelium of the cornea, in the root sheaths and in the papillae of the hairs, and around the bodies of sudoriferous glands. The terminal ends of pain receptors consist of unmyelinated nerve fibers, which often anastomose into small knobs between the epithelial cells. Any kind of stimulus, if it is intense enough, can stimulate the pain receptors in the skin and the mucosa, but only radical changes in pressure and certain chemicals can stimulate the pain receptors in the viscera. Referred pain results only from stimulation of pain receptors located in deep structures, as the viscera and the joints, but never from pain receptors in the skin.

paint 1. To apply a medicated solution to the skin, usually over a wide area. 2. A medicated solution that is applied in this way. Kinds of paint include **antiseptic, germicide, sporicide.** See also **Castellani's paint.**

pain threshold The point at which a stimulus, usually one associated with pressure or temperature, activates pain receptors and produces a sensation of pain. Individuals with low pain thresholds experience pain much sooner and faster than individuals with higher pain thresholds.

palatal 1. Of or pertaining to the palate. 2. Of or pertaining to the lingual surface of a maxillary tooth.

palate A structure that forms the roof of the mouth. It is divided into the hard palate and the soft palate. —**palatal, palatine,** *adj.*

palatine Of or pertaining to the palate.

palatine arch The vault-shaped muscular structure forming the soft palate between the mouth and the nasopharynx. An opening in the arch connects the mouth with the oropharynx; the uvula is suspended from the middle of the posterior border of the arch.

palatine bone One of a pair of bones of the skull, forming the posterior part of the hard palate, part of the nasal cavity, and the floor of the orbit of the eye. It resembles a capital L and consists of horizontal and vertical parts and three processes.

palatine ridge Any one of the four to six transverse ridges on the anterior surface of the hard palate.

palatine suture One of a number of thin, wavy lines marking the joining of the palatine processes that form the hard palate. See also **median palatine suture, transverse palatine suture.**

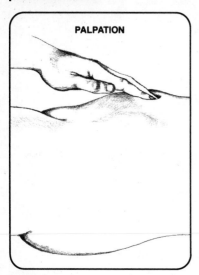

PALPATION

palatine tonsil One of a pair of almond-shaped masses of lymphoid tissue between the palatoglossal and the palatopharyngeal arches on each side of the fauces. They are covered with mucous membrane and contain numerous lymph follicles and various crypts.

palatitis An inflammation of the hard palate.

palato- A combining form meaning 'of or pertaining to the palate': *palatoglossal, palatography.*

palato- A combining form meaning 'of the palate': *palatoproximal, palatoschisis.*

palatomaxillary Of or pertaining to the palate and the maxilla.

palatonasal Of or pertaining to the palate and the nose.

paleo- A combining form meaning 'old': *paleocerebellar.*

paleogenesis See **palingenesis.**

paleogenetic **1.** A trait or structure of an organism or species that originated in a previous generation. **2.** Relating to the development of such a trait or structure.

pali- See **palin-.**

palilalia An abnormal condition characterized by the increasingly rapid repetition of the same word or phrase.

palin-, pali- A combining form meaning 'again': *palindromia, palingenesis.*

palindrome In molecular genetics: a segment of DNA in which identical or almost identical sequences of bases run in opposite directions.

palingenesis **1.** The regeneration of a lost part. **2.** The hereditary transmission of ancestral structural characteristics, especially abnormalities, in successive generations. Also called **paleogenesis.** Compare **cenogenesis.** —**palingenetic, palingenic,** *adj.*

palladium (Pd) A hard, silvery metallic element. Its atomic number is 46; its atomic weight

is 106.4. Highly resistant to tarnish and corrosion, palladium is used in high-grade surgical instruments and in dental inlays, bridgework, and orthodontic appliances.

palliate To soothe or relieve. —**palliation,** *n.,* **palliative,** *adj.*

palliative treatment Therapy designed to relieve or reduce intensity of uncomfortable symptoms but not to produce a cure. Some kinds of palliative treatment are the use of narcotics to relieve pain in advanced cancer and the creation of a colostomy to bypass an inoperable obstructing bowel lesion. Compare **definitive treatment, expectant treatment.**

pallidum See **globus pallidus.**

pallium See **cerebral cortex.**

pallor An unnatural paleness or absence of color in the skin.

palm The lower side of the hand, between the wrist and the bases of the fingers, when the hand is held horizontal with the thumb in medial position. —**palmar,** *adj.*

palmar aponeurosis Fascia surrounding the muscles of the palm. Also called **palmar fascia.**

palmar crease A normal groove across the palm of the hand.

palmar fascia See **palmar aponeurosis.**

palmaris longus A long, slender, superficial, fusiform muscle of the forearm, lying on the medial side of the flexor carpi radialis. It arises from the medial epicondyle of the humerus by a tendon from the intermuscular septa between it and the adjacent muscles and from the antebrachial fascia. A tendinous slip of the muscle is often found extending to the thumb. The palmaris longus is innervated by a branch of the median nerve, which contains fibers from the sixth and the seventh cervical nerves, and it functions to flex the hand. Compare **flexor carpi radialis, flexor carpi ulnaris.**

palmar metacarpal artery One of several arteries arising from the deep palmar arch, supplying the fingers.

palmar reflex A reflex that curls the fingers when the palm of the hand is tickled.

palmature An abnormal condition in which the fingers are webbed.

palm-chin reflex See **palmomental reflex.**

palmityl alcohol See **cetyl alcohol.**

palmomental reflex An abnormal neurological sign, elicited by scratching the palm at the base of the thumb, characterized by contraction of the muscles of the chin and corner of the mouth on the same side of the body as the stimulus. It is occasionally seen in normal individuals but an exaggerated reflex may be seen in pyramidal tract disease, latent tetany, increased intracranial pressure, and central facial paresis. Also called **palm-chin reflex.**

palpable Perceivable by touch.

palpation A technique used in physical examination in which the examiner feels the texture, size, consistency, and location of certain parts of the body with the hands. —**palpable,** *adj.,* **palpate,** *v.*

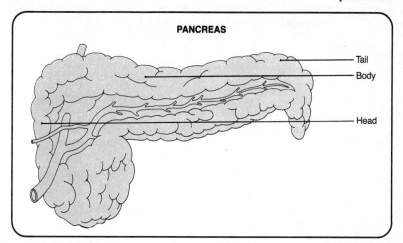

PANCREAS

- Tail
- Body
- Head

palpatory percussion A technique in physical examination in which the vibrations produced by percussion are evaluated by using light pressure of the flat of the examiner's hand.

palpebra, *pl.* **palpebrae** See **eyelid.**

palpebral commissure See **canthus.**

palpebral fissure The opening between the margins of the upper and lower eyelids.

palpebral gland See **Meibomian gland.**

palpebra superior, *pl.* **palpebrae superiores** The upper eyelid, larger and more movable than the lower eyelid and furnished with an elevator muscle.

palpebrate 1. To wink or blink. 2. Having eyelids.

palpeleral conjunctiva See **conjunctiva.**

palpitate To pulsate rapidly, as in the unusually fast beating of the heart under various conditions of stress and in patients with certain heart problems.

palpitation A pounding or racing of the heart, associated with normal emotional responses or with certain heart disorders. Some people may complain of pounding hearts and display no evidence of heart disease, while others, with serious heart disorders, may not detect associated abnormal palpitations. Some patients complain of palpitations after receiving digitalis medication, because it increases the force of heart contractions. Many healthy individuals become concerned and describe as palpitations the normal sounds of their hearts against their pillows when they lie down to sleep.

palsy An abnormal condition characterized by paralysis. Some kinds of palsy are **Bell's palsy, cerebral palsy.**

Paltauf's dwarf See **pituitary dwarf.**

Paltauf's nanism Dwarfism associated with excessive production or growth of lymphoid tissue.

paludism Malaria.

PAMP *abbr* pulmonary arterial mean pressure.

pampiniform Having the shape of a tendril.

pampiniform body See **epoophoron.**

pan- A combining form meaning 'all': *panacea, pandemic.*

panacea 1. A universal remedy. 2. An ancient name for an herb or a liquid potion with healing properties.

panacinar emphysema A form of emphysema that affects all lung areas by causing dilatation and atrophy of the alveoli and by destroying the vascular bed of the lung. Also called **panlobular emphysema.**

panarthritis An abnormal condition characterized by the inflammation of many body joints. —**panarthritic,** *adj.*

pancake kidney A congenital anomaly in which the left and right kidneys are fused into a single mass in the pelvis. The fused kidney has two collecting systems and two ureters and frequently becomes obstructed because of its abnormal position.

pancarditis An abnormal condition characterized by inflammation of the entire heart, including the endocardium, myocardium, and pericardium.

Pancoast's syndrome 1. A combination of various signs associated with a tumor in the apex of the lung. The signs include neuritic pain in the arm, an X-ray shadow at the apex of the lung, atrophy of the muscles of the arm and the hand, and Horner's syndrome. The signs are caused by the damaging effects of the tumor on the brachial plexus. 2. An abnormal condition caused by osteolysis in the posterior part of one or more ribs, sometimes involving associated vertebrae.

Pancoast's tumor See **pulmonary sulcus tumor.**

pancolectomy The excision of the entire colon, also requiring an ileostomy.

pancreas A fish-shaped, grayish-pink gland that stretches transversely across the posterior abdominal wall in the epigastric and hypochondriac regions of the body and secretes various substances, as digestive enzymes, insulin,

CHARACTERISTICS OF PANCREATIC CANCER

PATHOLOGY	CLINICAL FEATURES
Head of pancreas • Often obstructs ampulla of Vater and common bile duct • Directly metastasizes to duodenum • Adhesions anchor tumor to spine, stomach, and intestines.	• Jaundice (predominant symptom)—slowly progressive, unremitting; may cause skin (especially of the face and genitals) to turn olive green or black • Pruritus—often severe • Weight loss—rapid and severe (as great as 13.6 kg, or 30 lb); may lead to emaciation, weakness, and muscle atrophy • Slowed digestion, gastric distention, nausea, diarrhea, and steatorrhea with clay-colored stools • Liver and gallbladder enlargement from lymph node metastasis to biliary tract and duct wall results in compression and obstruction; gallbladder may be palpable (Courvoisier's sign). • Dull, nondescript, continuous abdominal pain radiating to upper right quadrant; relieved by the patient bending forward • GI hemorrhage and biliary infection common
Body and tail of pancreas • Large nodular masses become fixed to retropancreatic tissues and spine. • Direct invasion of spleen, left kidney, suprarenal gland, diaphragm • Involvement of celiac plexus results in thrombosis of splenic vein and spleen infarction.	**Body** • Pain (predominant symptom)—usually epigastric; develops slowly and radiates to back; relieved by bending forward or sitting up; intensified by lying supine; most intense 3 to 4 hours after eating; when celiac plexus is involved, pain is more intense and lasts longer • Venous thrombosis and thrombophlebitis—frequent; may precede other symptoms by months • Splenomegaly (from infarction), hepatomegaly (occasionally), and jaundice (rarely) **Tail** Symptoms result from metastasis: • Abdominal tumor (most common finding) produces a palpable abdominal mass; abdominal pain radiates to left hypochondrium and left chest. • Anorexia leads to weight loss, emaciation, and weakness. • Splenomegaly and upper GI bleeding

and glucagon. It is divided into a head, a body, and a tail. The head of the gland, divided from the body by a small constriction, is tucked into the curve of the duodenum. The tapered left extremity of the organ forms the tail. In adults, the pancreas is about 13 cm (5 inches) long and weighs more in men than in women. A compound racemose gland composed of exocrine and endocrine tissue, it contains a main duct that runs the length of the organ, draining smaller ducts and emptying into the duodenum at the major duodenal papilla, the same site that accommodates the exit of the common bile duct. About 1 million cellular islets of Langerhans are embedded between the exocrine units of the pancreas. Beta cells of the islets secrete insulin, which helps control carbohydrate metabolism. Alpha cells of the islets secrete glucagon, which counters the action of insulin. The acinar units of the pancreas secrete digestive enzymes.

pancreatectomy The surgical removal of all or part of the pancreas, performed to remove a cyst or tumor, treat pancreatitis, or repair trauma. During surgery, the gastrointestinal tract is reconstructed, usually with an anastomosis between the common bile duct and the upper jejunum. Drains are left in the wound. After surgery, the patient is given a low-sugar, low-fat diet. If the entire pancreas is removed, a brittle type of diabetes develops, requiring precise management of both diet and insulin dosage. A frequent complication is the formation of a fistula in the pancreatic bile duct, allowing digestive enzymes to contact adjacent tissues.

-pancreatic A combining form meaning the 'pancreas or a condition of the pancreas or adjacent organs': *hepaticopancreatic, splenopancreatic.*

pancreatic cancer A malignant neoplastic disease of the pancreas, characterized by anorexia, flatulence, weakness, dramatic weight loss, epigastric or back pain, jaundice, pruritus, a palpable abdominal mass, the recent onset of diabetes, and clay-colored stools if the pancreatic ducts are obstructed. Insulin-secreting tumors of islet cells cause hypoglycemia, especially in the morning. Nonfunctioning islet-cell lesions produce gastrin, causing symptoms of peptic ulcer or, in some cases, acute diarrhea, hypokalemia, and achlorhydria, the result of the lesion's elaboration of secretin. Exploratory laparotomy is often required for a definitive diag-

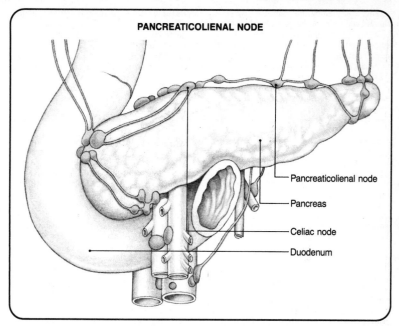

PANCREATICOLIENAL NODE

Pancreaticolienal node
Pancreas
Celiac node
Duodenum

nosis. About 90% of pancreatic tumors are adenocarcinomas; two thirds are in the head of the pancreas. Most tumors are not resectable at the time of diagnosis, but localized cancers may be treated by partial or total pancreatectomy with excision of the common bile duct, duodenum, and distal part of the stomach. Functioning islet-cell lesions may be excised or treated with streptozotocin, an antibiotic toxic to beta cells of the pancreas. Total gastrectomy is recommended for nonfunctioning islet-cell tumors that are accompanied by peptic ulcer disease. Radiotherapy or chemotherapy with 5-fluorouracil or mitomycin-C may offer temporary palliation, but cancer of the pancreas has a poor prognosis: few people survive longer than 1 year after diagnosis. Pancreatic cancer occurs three to four times more often in men than in women. Though uncommon, it is increasing in incidence in the industrialized areas of the world. People who smoke more than 20 cigarettes a day, who have diabetes mellitus, or who have been exposed to polychlorinated biphenyl compounds are at increased risk of developing it.

pancreatic diverticulum   One of a pair of membranous pouches arising from the embryonic duodenum. These two diverticula later form the pancreas and its ducts.

pancreatic duct   The primary secretory channel of the pancreas. Also called **duct of Wirsung.**

pancreatic enzyme   Any one of the enzymes secreted by the pancreas in the process of digestion. The most important are trypsin, chymotrypsin, steapsin, and amylopsin. See also **pancreatic juice.**

pancreatic hormone   Any one of several chemical compounds secreted by the pancreas, associated with the regulation of cellular metabolism. Major hormones secreted by the pancreas are insulin, glucagon, and pancreatic polypeptide. Insulin and glucagon are secreted by different types of cells within the alpha and beta cells of the islets of Langerhans; pancreatic polypeptide is secreted by a group of glandular cells arranged in a halo around each islet of Langerhans.

pancreatic insufficiency   A condition characterized by inadequate production and secretion of pancreatic hormones or enzymes, usually occurring secondary to a disease process destructive of pancreatic tissue. Nutritional malabsorption, anorexia, poorly localized upper abdominal or epigastric pain, malaise, and severe weight loss often occur. Alcohol-induced pancreatitis is the most common form of the condition. Replacement or augmentation of the absent or lacking substances is usually recommended as therapy.

pancreatic juice   The fluid secretion of the pancreas, produced by the stimulation of food in the duodenum. Pancreatic juice contains water, protein, inorganic salts, and enzymes. The juice is essential in breaking down proteins into their amino acid components, in reducing dietary fats to glycerol and fatty acids, and in converting starch to simple sugars.

pancreaticolienal node   A node in one of three groups of lymph glands associated with branches of the abdominal and the pelvic viscera that are supplied by branches of the celiac artery. The pancreaticolienal nodes accompany the splenic artery along the posterior surface and the upper border of the pancreas. Their afferents, which originate from the stomach, the spleen, and the pancreas, join the celiac group of preaortic nodes. Also called **splenic gland.** Compare **gastric node, hepatic node.**

pancreatin A substance containing pancreatic enzymes, used as an aid to digestion.

pancreatitis An inflammatory condition of the pancreas that may be acute or chronic. Acute pancreatitis is generally the result of damage to the biliary tract, as by alcohol, trauma, infectious disease, or certain drugs. It is characterized by severe abdominal pain radiating to the back, fever, anorexia, nausea, and vomiting. There may be jaundice if the common bile duct is obstructed. The development of pseudocysts or abscesses in pancreatic tissue is a serious complication. Treatment includes nasogastric suction to remove gastric secretions. To prevent any stimulation of the pancreas, nothing is given by mouth. Intravenous fluids and electrolytes are administered, and nonmorphine derivatives are given to relieve pain. Acute pancreatitis is associated with a mortality of 50%. The causes of chronic pancreatitis are similar to those of the acute form. When the cause is alcohol abuse, there may be calcification and scarring of the smaller pancreatic ducts. There is abdominal pain, nausea, and vomiting, as well as steatorrhea and creatorrhea, owing to the diminished output of pancreatic enzymes. Pancreatic insulin production may be diminished, and some patients develop diabetes mellitus. Treatment includes analgesics for pain and subtotal pancreatectomy when pain is intractable. A pancreatic extract is given orally to replace the missing enzymes; vitamin supplements are essential. Both forms of pancreatitis are diagnosed by history, physical examination, radiologic studies, endoscopy, and laboratory analysis of the amount of pancreatic enzymes in the blood.

pancreatoduodenectomy A surgical procedure in which the head of the pancreas and the loop of duodenum that surrounds it are excised. The operation is performed to remove the periampullary masses occurring in certain forms of biliary tract cancer.

pancreatography Visualization of the pancreas or its ducts by means of X-rays and contrast media injected into the ducts at surgery or via an endoscope or by means of ultrasonography, computerized tomography, or radionuclide imaging.

pancreatolith A stone or calculus in the pancreas.

pancrelipase A pancreatic substance used as an aid to digestion.

pancuronium bromide A nondepolarizing neuromuscular blocking agent.

pancytopenia An abnormal condition characterized by a marked reduction in the number of all of the cellular elements of the blood—the red blood cells, white blood cells, and platelets. See also **anemia, aplasia. —pancytopenic,** *adj.*

p and a *abbr* percussion and auscultation, as noted in the patient's chart following physical examination of the chest. See **auscultation, percussion.**

pandemic Of a disease: occurring throughout the population of a country, a people, or the world.

pandiastolic Of or pertaining to the complete diastole. Also called **holodiastolic.**

panencephalitis Inflammation of the entire brain, characterized by an insidious onset, a progressive course with deterioration of motor and mental functions, and evidence of a viral etiology. Subacute sclerosing panencephalitis is an uncommon childhood disease thought to be caused by a 'slow' latent measles virus following recovery from a previous infection. Most of the patients are younger than 11 and many more boys than girls are affected. The disease results in ataxia, myoclonus, atrophy, cortical blindness, and mental deterioration. Antiviral drugs, immunosuppressants, and interferon inducers are sometimes administered, but the disease is usually fatal. Rubella panencephalitis, a rare disease of adolescents, follows a chronic progressive course marked by motor and mental deterioration and sometimes resembles juvenile paresis.

panendoscope A cystoscope that allows a wide view of the interior of the bladder.

panesthesia The total of all sensations experienced by an individual at one time. Compare **cenesthesia.**

pangenesis A Darwinian theory that every cell and particle of a parent reproduces itself in progeny.

panhypopituitarism Generalized insufficiency of pituitary hormones, resulting from damage to or deficiency of the gland. **Prepubertal panhypopituitarism,** a rare disorder usually associated with a suprasellar cyst or craniopharyngioma, is characterized by dwarfism with normal body proportions, subnormal sexual development, and insufficient thyroid and adrenal function. Diabetes insipidus is frequently present; there may be bitemporal hemianopia or complete blindness; skin is often yellow and wrinkled, but mentality is usually unimpaired. The condition is treated with cortisone, thyroid and sex hormones, and, if available, human growth hormone. **Postpubertal panhypopituitarism** may be caused by postpartum pituitary necrosis, resulting from thrombosis of pituitary circulation during or after delivery. Characteristic signs of the disorder are failure to lactate, amenorrhea, weakness, cold intolerance, lethargy, loss of libido and of axillary and pubic hair. There may be bradycardia or hypotension, and progression of the disorder leads to premature wrinkling of the skin and atrophy of the thyroid and adrenal glands. Treatment consists of the administration of ACTH, thyroid-stimulating hormone, and hormones of the target organs. Also called **hypophyseal cachexia, pituitary cachexia, pituitary dwarf, Simmonds' disease.**

panhysterectomy Complete surgical removal of the uterus, cervix, fallopian tubes, and ovaries. See also **hysterectomy.**

panic An intense, sudden, and overwhelming fear or feeling of anxiety that produces terror and immediate physiological changes that result in paralysislike immobility or senseless, hysterical behavior.

panic disorder See **anxiety neurosis.**

panivorous Of or pertaining to the practice of subsisting exclusively on bread products. — **panivore,** *n.*

panlobular emphysema See **panacinar emphysema.**

panniculus, *pl.* **panniculi** A membranous layer; the many sheets of fascia covering various structures in the body.

pannus An inflamed lymphatic gland that is not suppurating.

panophthalmitis An inflammation of the entire eye, usually caused by virulent pyogenic organisms, as strains of meningococci, pneumococci, streptococci, anthrax bacilli, and clostradia. Initial symptoms are pain, fever, headache, drowsiness, edema, and swelling. As the infection progresses, the iris appears muddy and gray, the aqueous humor becomes turbid, and precipitates form on the cornea's posterior surface. Treatment consists of systemic and local antibiotic therapy; evisceration of the globe or excision of the eye may be required, but excision is contraindicated if surrounding tissues are infected.

panphobia, panophobia, pantophobia An anxiety disorder characterized by an irrational, vague fear or apprehension of some pervading or unknown evil; a generalized feeling of fear. —**panophobic,** *adj.*

panphobic melancholia A state of depression characterized by an irrational dread or pervading fear of everything. See also **bipolar disorder, phobia.**

pansystolic Of or pertaining to the entire systole. Also called **holosystolic.**

pansystolic murmur See **systolic murmur.**

pant- See **panto-.**

panthenol An alcohol converted in the body to pantothenic acid, a vitamin in the B complex.

panto-, pant- A combining form meaning 'all, the whole': *pantophobia, pantoscopic, pantosomatous.*

pantograph A jointed device for copying a plane figure to any desired scale.

pantothenic acid A member of the vitamin B complex. It is widely distributed in plant and animal tissues and may be an important element in human nutrition. See **dexpanthenol.**

pantothenyl alcohol See **panthenol.**

PaO₂ Symbol for arterial partial pressure of oxygen.

papain An enzyme from the fruit of *Carica papaya,* the tropical melon tree, prescribed for enzymatic debridement of wounds and promotion of healing.

Papanicolaou test A simple smear method

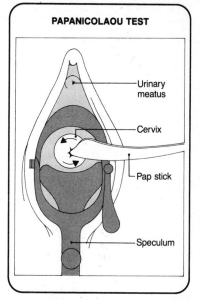

PAPANICOLAOU TEST

of examining stained exfoliative cells. It is used most commonly to detect cancers of the cervix, but it may be used for tissue specimens from any organ. A smear is usually obtained during a pelvic examination. The technique permits early diagnosis of cancer and has contributed to a lower death rate from cervical cancer. The findings may be reported descriptively or grouped into the following classes: Class I, absence of atypical or abnormal cells; Class II, atypical cells but no evidence of malignancy; Class III, suggestive of, but inconclusive for, malignancy; Class IV, strongly suggestive of malignancy; Class V, conclusive for malignancy. Also called **Pap test** *(informal).*

papaverine hydrochloride An opium alkaloid used as a coronary vasodilator.

paper chromatography The analysis of a substance by dissolving it in a solvent and filtering it through a strip of special paper.

paper-doll fetus See **fetus papyraceus.**

papilla, *pl.* **papillae** A small nipple-shaped projection, as the conoid papillae of the tongue, and the papillae of the corium that extend from collagen fibers, the capillary blood vessels, and sometimes the nerves of the dermis. —**papillary,** *adj.*

papilla of Vater The duodenal end of the drainage systems of the pancreatic and common bile ducts.

papillary Of or pertaining to a papilla.

papillary adenocarcinoma A malignant neoplasm characterized by small papillae of vascular connective tissue covered by neoplastic epithelium that project into follicles, glands, or cysts. The tumor is most common in the ovaries and thyroid gland. Also called **polypoid adenocarcinoma.**

PAPILLARY MUSCLES OF THE HEART

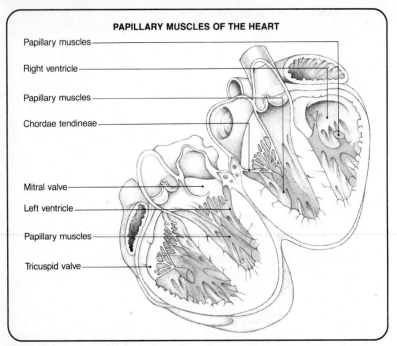

Papillary muscles

Right ventricle

Papillary muscles

Chordae tendineae

Mitral valve

Left ventricle

Papillary muscles

Tricuspid valve

papillary adenocystoma lymphomatosum An unusual tumor, consisting of epithelial and lymphoid tissues, that develops in the area of the parotid and submaxillary glands. Also called **adenolymphoma, Warthin's tumor.**

papillary adenoma A benign epithelial tumor in which the membrane lining the glandular tissue forms papillary processes that project into the alveoli or grow out of the surface of a cavity.

papillary carcinoma A malignant neoplasm characterized by many fingerlike projections. It is the most common thyroid tumor.

papillary duct Any one of the thousands of straight collecting renal tubules that descend through the medulla of the kidney and join with others to form the common ducts opening into the renal papillae. See also **kidney.**

papillary muscle Any one of the rounded or conical muscular projections attached to the chordae tendineae in the ventricles of the heart. The papillary muscles vary in number, but the two main ones are the anterior papillary muscle and the posterior papillary muscle. The papillary muscles are associated with the atrioventricular valves, which they help to open and close. Compare **trabecula carnea.**

papillary tumor See **papilloma.**

papillate Marked by papillae or nipplelike prominences.

papilledema, *pl.* **papilledemas, papilledemata** Swelling of the optic disk, visible on ophthalmoscopic examination of the fundus of the eye, caused by increased intracranial pressure. The meningeal sheaths that surround the optic nerves from the optic disk are continuous with the meninges of the brain; therefore, increased intracranial pressure is transmitted forward from the brain to the optic disk in the eye to cause the swelling.

papilliform Shaped like a papilla.

papillitis **1.** An abnormal condition characterized by the inflammation of a papilla, as the lacrimal papilla. **2.** An abnormal condition characterized by the inflammation of a renal papilla.

papilloma A benign epithelial neoplasm characterized by a branching or lobular tumor. Kinds of papilloma are **basal cell papilloma, cockscomb papilloma, cutaneous papilloma, fibroepithelial papilloma, hirsutoid papilloma of the penis, intracanalicular papilloma, intracystic papilloma, villous papilloma.** Also called **papillary tumor.**

-papilloma A combining form meaning an 'epithelial tumor': *fibropapilloma, myxopapilloma.*

papillomatosis An abnormal condition in which there is widespread development of nipplelike growths.

papillomatosis coronal penis See **hirsutoid papilloma of the penis.**

papillomavirus The virus that causes warts in humans; belongs to the papovavirus family.

papovavirus One of a group of small DNA viruses, some of which may be potentially cancer producing. The human wart is caused by a kind of papovavirus, but it very rarely undergoes malignant transformation. Kinds of papoviruses are papilloma papovavirus, polyoma papovavirus, SV-40 papovavirus.

pappataci See **phlebotomus fever.**

pappus The first growth of beard, characterized by downy hairs.

Pap smear *Informal.* A specimen of exfoliated epithelial cells and cervical mucus collected during a pelvic examination for cytologic evaluation according to the Papanicolaou cytologic classification.

Pap test *Informal.* See **Papanicolaou test.**

papular scaling disease Any of a group of skin disorders in which there are discrete, raised, dry, scaling lesions. Also called **papulosquamous disease.** Some kinds of papular scaling diseases are **lichen planus, pityriasis rosea, psoriasis.**

papulation The development of papules.

papule A small, solid, raised skin lesion less than 1 cm (⅜ inch) in diameter, as the lesions of lichen planus and nonpustular acne. Compare **macule. —papular,** *adj.*

papulosquamous disease See **papular scaling disease.**

papyraceous Having a paperlike quality.

papyraceous fetus See **fetus papyraceus.**

Paquelin's cautery A cauterizing device consisting of a platinum loop through which a heated hydrocarbon is passed.

par A pair, specifically a pair of cranial nerves, as the par nonum or the ninth pair.

PAR *abbr* **pulmonary arteriolar resistance.**

par- A combining form meaning 'aside, beyond, apart from, against': *parabacteria, parotid.*

para-, par- A combining form meaning 'similar, beside': *paronchia, parasympathetic.*

-para A combining form meaning: **1.** A 'woman who has given birth to children in a number of pregnancies': *bipara, nonipara.* **2.** A 'female of any species producing a number or type of egg or offspring': *nymphipara, ovovipara.*

para-aminobenzoic acid (PABA) A topical sunscreen.

para-aminosalicylic acid (PAS, PASA) An antitubercular agent.

paracentesis A procedure in which fluid is withdrawn from a cavity of the body. An incision is made in the skin and a hollow trocar, cannula, or catheter is passed through the incision into the cavity to allow outflow of fluid into a collecting device. Paracentesis is commonly performed to remove excessive ascitic fluid from the abdomen.

paracervical block A form of regional anesthesia in which a local anesthetic is injected into the area on each side of the uterine cervix that contains the plexus of nerves innervating the uterine cervix. Effective anesthesia for active labor is often achieved. The duration of the anesthetic effect depends on the agent used. Transient maternal hypotension sometimes occurs

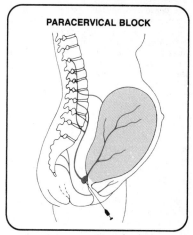

PARACERVICAL BLOCK

following paracervical block, usually owing to inadvertent intravascular injection of the anesthetic.

paracoccidiodal granuloma See **paracoccidioidomycosis.**

paracoccidioidomycosis A chronic, occasionally fatal, fungous infection caused by *Paracoccidioides brasiliensis,* characterized by ulcers of the oral cavity, larynx, and nose; large, draining lymph nodes; cough; dyspnea; weight loss; and skin, genital, and intestinal lesions. The disease occurs only in Mexico and Central and South America and is acquired by inhalation of spores of the fungus. The diagnosis is made by microscopic examination of a smear prepared from a lesion. Treatment requires several years of sulfonamides or, in severe cases, intravenous amphotericin B followed by oral sulfonamides. Also called **paracoccidioidal granuloma, South American blastomycosis.** Compare **North American blastomycosis.**

paradichlorobenzene poisoning See **naphthalene poisoning.**

paradidymal **1.** Pertaining to the paradidymis. **2.** Beside the testis.

paradidymis, *pl.* **paradidymides** A rudimentary structure in the male, situated on the spermatic cord of the epididymis, that consists of vestigial remains of the caudal part of the embryonic mesonephric tubules. A similar vestigial structure, the paroophoron, is found in the female. Also called **organ of Giraldes, parepididymis.** See also **aberrant ductule, appendix epididymis.**

paraffin bath The application of heat to a specific area of the body through the use of paraffin. The technique is effective for heating traumatized or inflamed areas, especially the hands, feet, and wrists, and is used primarily for patients with arthritis and rheumatism or any joint condition. Also called **wax bath.**

paraffin method In surgical pathology: a method used in preparing a selected portion of tissue for pathologic examination. The tissue is fixed, dehydrated, and infiltrated and embedded in paraffin, forming a block that is sliced with a microtome for microscopic examination. This method, which is more commonly used than the frozen-section method, is slower and therefore not used during surgery.

paraganglion, *pl.* **paraganglia.** Any one of the small groups of chromaffin cells associated with the ganglia of the sympathetic nerve trunk and situated outside the adrenal medulla, most often near the sympathetic ganglia along the aorta and its branches. The paraganglia are also connected with the ganglia of the celiac, renal, suprarenal, aortic, and hypogastric plexuses. The paraganglia secrete the hormones epinephrine and norepinephrine. Also called **chromaffin body.** See also **chromaffin cell.**

paragonimiasis Chronic infection with the lung fluke *Paragonimus westermani,* occurring most commonly in Asia. It is characterized by hemoptysis, bronchitis, and, occasionally, abdominal masses, pain and diarrhea, or cerebral involvement with paralysis, ocular pathology, or seizures. The disease is acquired by ingesting cysts in infected freshwater crabs or crayfish, the intermediate hosts. Adequate cooking of shellfish prevents the disease. Bithionol, given orally, is the usual treatment.

parainfluenza virus A myxovirus with four serotypes, causing respiratory infections in infants and young children, and, less commonly, in adults. Compare **influenza.**

paraldehyde A sedative-hypnotic and anticonvulsant agent.

parallel play A form of play among a group of children, primarily toddlers, in which each one engages in an independent activity that is similar to but not influenced by or shared with the others. Compare **cooperative play.** See also **associative play, solitary play.**

paralysis, *pl.* **paralyses.** An abnormal condition characterized by the loss of muscle function or the loss of sensation. It may be caused by a variety of problems, as trauma, disease, and poisoning. Paralyses may be classified according to etiology, muscle tone, distribution, or the part of the body affected. See also **flaccid paralysis, spastic paralysis. —paralytic,** *adj.*

paralysis agitans See **Parkinson's disease.**

-paralytic A combining form meaning 'pertaining to paralysis': *antiparalytic, subparalytic.*

paralytic dementia See **paresis,** definition 2.

paralytic ileus A decrease in or absence of intestinal peristalsis that may occur following abdominal surgery or peritoneal injury or in connection with severe pyelonephritis; ureteral calculus; fractured ribs; myocardial infarction; extensive intestinal ulceration; heavy metal poisoning; porphyria; retroperitoneal hematomas, especially those associated with fractured vertebrae; or any severe metabolic disease. The most common cause of intestinal obstruction, it is mediated by a hormonal component of the sym-

pathoadrenal system. Treatment includes keeping the patient in bed in low Fowler's position with nothing given orally. A nasoenteric tube is inserted into the duodenum and connected to intermittent suction; it is not taped to the nose and the patient is positioned to facilitate the advancement of the tube, which is checked every 30 to 60 minutes.

NURSING CONSIDERATIONS: The character of gastrointestinal drainage is monitored every 2 to 4 hours, and any increase or decrease in the amount or changes in the color or consistency is reported. Bowel sounds and vital signs are checked every 2 to 4 hours and rectal temperature every 4 hours. Abdominal girth is measured every 2 hours and report is made of any increase. Parenteral fluids with electrolytes and medication to promote peristalsis are administered, as ordered; intake and output are measured and, if less than 30 ml of urine is excreted per hour, the physician is informed. When bowel sounds return or flatus is passed, the intestinal tube may be clamped and small amounts of warm tea or a carbonated beverage may be given. If pain, distention, or cramps do not recur, the intestinal tube may be removed but a rectal tube or an enema may be ordered to relieve distention.

paralytic shellfish poisoning See **shellfish poisoning.**

paramedic A person who acts as an assistant to a physician or in place of a physician, especially a person in the military, trained in emergency medical procedures. **—paramedical,** *adj.*

paramedical personnel Health-care workers other than physicians, dentists, podiatrists, and nurses who have special training in the performance of supportive health-care tasks. Kinds of paramedical personnel are ambulance attendants, audiologists, X-ray technologists.

paramesonephric duct One of a pair of embryonic ducts that develops into the uterus and the uterine tubes. Also called **Müllerian duct.**

parameter 1. A value or constant used to describe or measure a set of data representing a physiological function or system, as in the use of acid-base relationships of the blood as parameters for evaluating the function of a patient's respiratory system. 2. A statistical value of a population group. 3. *Informal.* **a.** Any standard against which something is measured. **b.** Limits or boundary.

paramethadione An oxazolidone anticonvulsant.

paramethasone acetate A glucocorticoid anti-inflammatory agent.

parametric imaging In nuclear medicine: a diagnostic procedure in which an image of an administered radioactive tracer is derived according to a mathematical rule, as by the division of one image by another.

parametritis An inflammatory condition of the tissue of the structures around the uterus. See also **pelvic inflammatory disease.**

parametrium, *pl.* **parametria** The lateral

extension of the uterine subserous connective tissue into the broad ligament. Compare **endometrium, myometrium.**

paramitome See **hyaloplasm.**

paramnesia **1.** A perversion of memory in which one remembers events and circumstances that never actually occurred. Compare **déjà vu. 2.** A condition in which words are remembered and used without the comprehension of their meaning.

paramyxovirus A member of a family of viruses that includes the organisms that cause parainfluenza, measles, mumps, and some respiratory infections.

paranasal Situated near or alongside the nose, as the paranasal sinuses.

paranasal sinuses The air cavities in various bones around the nose, as the frontal sinus in the frontal bone lying deep to the medial part of the superciliary ridge and the maxillary sinus within the maxilla between the orbit, the nasal cavity, and the upper teeth. Compare **confluence of the sinuses, occipital sinus.**

parangi See **yaws.**

paranoia, paranoea In psychiatry: a disorder characterized by delusions of persecution and grandeur usually centered on one major theme, such as a job situation or an unfaithful spouse. The delusional system develops progressively over months or years, becoming intricate, logical, and highly organized. The person appears perfectly normal in his conduct, conversation, thinking patterns, and emotional responses aside from the delusions. Associated symptoms include suspiciousness, seclusion, stubbornness, resentfulness, aloofness, hostility, aggressiveness, dominating or grandiose attitudes, and unrealistic expectations. Paranoia may result from inadequate socialization during childhood, poor development of interpersonal relationships, and sexual maladjustment, and does not involve genetic or biochemical alterations. Persons with the disorder are highly resistant to available methods of treatment, although individual or group psychotherapy and behavior therapy may be effective in the early stages. Kinds of paranoia include **acute hallucinatory paranoia, alcoholic paranoia, litigious paranoia, querulous paranoia.** Compare **paranoid schizophrenia.**

paranoiac, paranoeac A person afflicted with or exhibiting characteristics of paranoia.

paranoia hallucinatoria See **acute hallucinatory paranoia.**

paranoia quaerula See **querulous paranoia.**

paranoid **1.** Pertaining to or resembling paranoia. **2.** A person afflicted with a paranoid disorder. **3.** *Informal.* A person who is overly suspicious or exhibits persecutory trends or attitudes.

paranoid disorder Any of a group of mental disorders characterized by an impaired sense of reality and persistent delusions. Kinds of paranoid disorders include **acute paranoid disorder, paranoia, shared paranoid disorder.**

paranoid ideation An exaggerated belief or suspicion, usually not of a delusional nature, that one is being harassed, persecuted, or treated unfairly.

paranoid personality disorder A disorder characterized by extreme suspiciousness and distrust of others to the degree that one blames them for one's mistakes and failures and goes to abnormal lengths to validate prejudices, attitudes, or biases. Symptoms include hypersensitivity, rigidity, hostility, stubbornness, envy, exaggerated self-importance, extreme argumentativeness, tenseness, and lack of passive, sentimental, or tender feelings. The condition is more commonly diagnosed in men than in women. The disorganization of the personality in this condition is less severe than in paranoid schizophrenia.

paranoid reaction A psychopathological condition of the aged, characterized by the gradual formation of delusions, usually of a persecutory nature and often accompanied by related hallucinations. Other manifestations of senile degeneration, as memory loss and confusion, do not usually accompany the reaction, and the individual maintains orientation for time, place, and person.

paranoid schizophrenia A form of schizophrenia characterized by persistent preoccupation with illogical, absurd, and changeable delusions, usually of a persecutory, grandiose, or jealous nature, accompanied by related hallucinations. The symptoms include extreme anxiety, exaggerated suspiciousness, aggressiveness, anger, argumentativeness, hostility, and violence. The condition occurs most frequently during middle age. Current therapy is not usually effective. Also called **heboid paranoia.** Compare **paranoia.** See also **schizophrenia.**

paranoid state A transitory abnormal mental condition characterized by illogical thought processes and generalized suspicion and distrust, with a tendency toward persecutory ideas or delusions.

paranuclear body See **centrosome.**

parapertussis An acute bacterial respiratory infection caused by *Bordetella parapertussis*, having symptoms closely resembling those of pertussis. It is usually milder than pertussis, although it can be fatal. It is possible to be infected with both *B. parapertussis* and *B. pertussis* at the same time. A parapertussis vaccine is available and may be given in combination with pertussis vaccine.

parapharyngeal abscess A suppurative infection of tissues adjacent to the pharynx, usually a complication of acute pharyngitis or tonsillitis. Infection may spread to the jugular vein where it may cause thrombophlebitis and septic emboli. Systemic antibiotics and surgical drainage may be required. Also called parapharyngeal space abscess. Compare **peritonsillar abscess, retropharyngeal abscess.** See also **tonsillitis.**

paraphilia Sexual perversion or deviation; a

condition in which the sexual instinct is expressed in biologically undesirable or socially unacceptable ways, such as the use of an inanimate object for sexual arousal. Kinds of paraphilia include **exhibitionism, fetish, pedophilia, voyeurism, zoophilia. —paraphiliac,** *adj., n.*

paraphimosis A condition characterized by an inability to replace the foreskin in its normal position after it has been retracted behind the glans penis. Caused by a narrow or inflamed foreskin, the condition may lead to gangrene. Circumcision may be required. Compare **phimosis.**

paraplasm 1. See **hyaloplasm.** 2. Any abnormal growth or malformation. **—paraplasmic,** *adj.*

paraplastic 1. Misshapen or malformed. 2. Showing abnormal formative power; of the nature of a paraplasm.

paraplegia An abnormal condition characterized by motor or sensory loss in the lower limbs. This condition may or may not involve the back and abdominal muscles and may cause either complete or incomplete paralysis. The signs and symptoms of paraplegia may develop immediately from trauma and include the loss of sensation, motion, and reflexes below the level of the lesion. Depending on the level of the lesion and whether damage to the spinal cord is complete or incomplete, the patient may lose bladder and bowel control and develop sexual dysfunctions. An incomplete spinal cord injury does not usually inhibit circumanal sensation, voluntary toe flexion, or sphincter control. A complete spinal cord injury destroys sensation and voluntary muscle control and usually causes the permanent loss of muscle function distal to the injury. Diagnosis is based on clinical history, neurologic examination, and X-rays. The treatment of paraplegia seeks to restore proper spine alignment, stabilize the injured spinal area, decompress any involved neurologic structures, and rehabilitate the patient as quickly as possible. A laminectomy may be performed if bone fragments are pressing on the spinal cord. Drugs may be administered to relieve any muscle spasms associated with dysfunction of the upper motor neurons. Other treatment may include the administration of a high-bulk diet and suppositories to prevent constipation.

NURSING CONSIDERATIONS: Nursing care in paraplegic cases commonly includes the proper positioning and maintenance of the patient on a Stryker frame or a CircOlectric bed; proper wound care following a laminectomy; meticulous monitoring of intake and output; catheter care, if applicable; and skin care. When the paraplegic patient progresses from bed rest to a wheelchair, the nurse is alert to any signs of orthostatic hypotension.

parapsoriasis A group of chronic skin diseases resembling psoriasis, characterized by maculopapular, erythematous, scaly eruptions without systemic symptoms. Parapsoriasis is resistant to all treatment.

parapsychology A branch of psychology concerned with the study of psychic phenomena, as clairvoyance, extrasensory perception, and telepathy.

paraquat poisoning A toxic condition caused by the ingestion of paraquat dichloride, a highly poisonous pesticide. Characteristically, progressive pulmonary fibrosis and damage to the esophagus, kidneys, and liver develop several days following ingestion. Once fibrosis begins, death is inevitable, usually within 3 weeks. The mechanism of action of the poison is unknown. Most often, poisoning results from accidental occupational exposure. There is considerable concern that the inhalation of the smoke of marijuana treated with the herbicide may cause intoxication, but no clinical syndrome resulting from such exposure has been documented.

parasite 1. An organism living in or on and obtaining nourishment from another organism. A **facultative parasite** may live on a host but is capable of living independently. An **obligate parasite** is one that depends entirely on its host for survival. 2. In conjoined twins, the less complete twin who derives support from the more complete twin. **—parasitic,** *adj.*

parasitemia The presence of parasites in the blood. Compare **bacteremia, fungemia, viremia.**

parasitic fetus The smaller, usually malformed member of conjoined, unequal, or asymmetrical twins that is attached to and dependent upon the more normal fetus for growth and development. Compare **autosite.**

parasitic fibroma A pedunculated uterine fibroid deriving part of its blood supply from the omentum.

parasitic thrombus An aggregation of bodies and spores of malarial parasites formed in the vessels of the brain in cerebral malaria.

parasympathetic Of or pertaining to the craniosacral division of the autonomic nervous system, consisting of the oculomotor, facial, glossopharyngeal, vagus, and pelvic nerves. The actions of the parasympathetic division are mediated by the release of acetylcholine and primarily involve the protection, conservation, and restoration of body resources. Preganglionic parasympathetic fibers, which emerge from the hypothalamus, other brain areas, and sacral segments of the spinal cord, form synapses in ganglia located near or in the walls of the organs to be innervated. Parasympathetic fibers slow the heart; stimulate peristalsis; promote the secretion of lacrimal, salivary, and digestive glands; induce bile and insulin release; dilate peripheral and visceral blood vessels; constrict the pupils, esophagus, and bronchioles; and relax sphincters during micturition and defecation. Postganglionic parasympathetic fibers extend to the uterus, vagina, oviducts, and ovaries in females, and to the prostate, seminal vesicles, and external genitalia in males, innervating blood vessels of pelvic organs in both sexes; stimulation of these nerves causes vasodilation in the clitoris and labia minora and erection of the penis.

parasympathetic nervous system   See **autonomic nervous system.**
parasympatholytic   See **anticholinergic.**
parasympatholytic drug   See **anticholinergic.**
parasympathomimetic   **1.** Of or pertaining to a substance producing effects similar to those caused by stimulation of a parasympathetic nerve. **2.** An agent whose effects mimic those resulting from stimulation of parasympathetic nerves, especially the effects produced by acetylcholine. The parasympathomimetic drugs include bethanecol chloride, neostigmine bromide, neostigmine methylsulfate, and pyridostigmine bromide, variously used to treat myasthenia gravis, acute postoperative and postpartum nonobstructional urinary retention, and to reverse or antagonize the action of nondepolarizing muscle relaxants. Also called **cholinergic.**
parasympathomimetic drug   See **cholinergic.**
parasystole   An arrhythmia caused by the presence of two foci that independently initiate regular cardiac impulses. The sinoatrial node, the normal pacemaker of the heart, and an ectopic focus, usually in the ventricle, are responsible for this cardiac irregularity.
parataxic distortion   A defense mechanism in which current interpersonal relationships are perceived and judged according to a mode of reference established by an earlier experience. See also **transference.**
parathion poisoning   A toxic condition caused by the ingestion, inhalation, or absorption through the skin of the highly toxic organophosphorus insecticide parathion. Symptoms include nausea, vomiting, abdominal cramps, confusion, headache, lack of muscle control, convulsions, and dyspnea. Treatment calls for immediate intravenous administration of atropine, followed by administration of pralidoxime chloride and oxygen.
parathyroid gland   One of several small structures, usually four in number, attached to the dorsal surfaces of the lateral lobes of the thyroid gland. The parathyroid glands secrete parathyroid hormone, which helps to maintain the level of blood calcium concentration and assures normal neuromuscular irritability, blood clotting, and cell membrane permeability. Each parathyroid gland has the appearance of an oval, brown-red disk and measures about 4 mm by 6 mm. The parathyroids are divided, according to their location, into the superior parathyroids and the inferior parathyroids. The superior parathyroids, usually two in number, are commonly situated, one on each side, on the caudal border of the cricoid cartilage beside the junction of the pharynx and the esophagus. The inferior parathyroids, also usually two in number, may be situated on the caudal edge of the lateral lobes of the thyroid gland, just caudal to the gland, or adjacent to one of the inferior thyroid veins. Parathyroid hypofunction usually causes tetany, which can be treated with calcium salts

PARATHYROID GLANDS

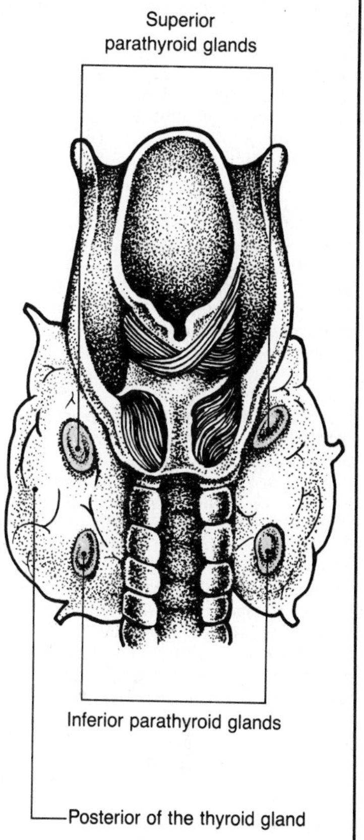

Superior parathyroid glands

Inferior parathyroid glands

Posterior of the thyroid gland

or parathyroid extracts.
parathyroid hormone (PTH)   A hormone secreted by the parathyroid glands that acts to maintain a constant concentration of calcium in the extracellular fluid. The hormone regulates absorption of calcium from the gastrointestinal tract, mobilization of calcium from the bones, deposition of calcium in the bones, and excretion of calcium in the breast milk, feces, sweat, and urine. Surgical removal of the parathyroid glands, as may inadvertently occur in thyroidectomy, results in hypocalcemia, leading to anorexia, tetany, seizures, and death if not corrected.
paratrooper fracture   A fracture of the distal tibia and its malleolus, commonly occurring when an individual jumps from an elevated platform, as the back of a truck, or parachutes from an airplane and lands feet first on the ground, subjecting the ankles to extreme force.

paratyphoid fever A bacterial infection, caused by any *Salmonella* species other than *S. typhi*, characterized by symptoms resembling typhoid fever, although somewhat milder. See also **rose spots, *Salmonella*, salmonellosis, typhoid fever.**

paraurethral duct One of two ducts that drain the bulbourethral glands into the vestibule of the vagina. Also called **Skene's duct.**

paravaccinia See **milker's nodule.**

parenchyma The tissue of an organ as distinguished from supporting or connective tissue.

parenchymatous neuritis Any inflammation affecting the substance, axons, or myelin of the nerve. Also called **axial neuritis, central neuritis.** See also **neuritis.**

parent A mother or father; one who bears offspring. **—parental,** *adj.*

parental generation (P_1) The initial cross between two varieties in a genetic sequence; the parents of any individual, organism, or plant belonging to an F_1 generation.

parental grief The behavioral reactions that characterize the grieving process and result in the resolution of the loss of a child from expected or unexpected death. All persons who survive the loss of a loved one normally experience symptoms of both somatic and psychological distress, as feelings of guilt and hostility accompanied by changes in usual patterns of conduct. In terminal illness, there is time for anticipatory grieving, so that parents can evaluate their relationship with the child, set priorities, and prepare for the death of the child. In such cases, parental grieving begins with the diagnosis of a life-threatening condition. The immediate reaction is shock and disbelief, followed by acute grief. Periods of depression, anger, hope, fear, and anxiety alternate during induction therapy, remission, and maintenance of the disease. Heightened anticipatory grieving recurs during episodes of relapse and the parents experience increased fear, depression, and the final acceptance of death during the terminal stages of the illness. At the time of death there is a period of acute grief, when parents need to express their sorrow and anger. Extended mourning follows, with the eventual resolution of grief and integration into society. In sudden, unexpected death, parents usually have extreme feelings of guilt and remorse. The function of the nurse during all phases of parental grief is primarily supportive. Nurses can act directly, or they can help to find other potential sources of support for the parents, as extended family members, other parents who have lost children, or specific community services or agencies. See also **death, grief reaction.**

parent-child relationship See **maternal-infant bonding.**

parenteral Not in or through the digestive system. **—parenterally,** *adv.*

parenteral absorption The taking up of substances by body structures other than the digestive tract.

parenteral nutrition The administration of nutrients by a route other than through the alimentary canal, as subcutaneously, intravenously, intramuscularly, or intradermally. The parenteral fluids usually consist of physiological saline with glucose, amino acids, electrolytes, vitamins, and medications. They are not nutritionally complete but maintain fluid and electrolyte balance during the immediate postoperative period and in other conditions, as shock, coma, malnutrition, and chronic renal and hepatic failures. See also **total parenteral nutrition.**

parent figure 1. A parent or a substitute parent or guardian who cares for a child, providing the physical, social, and emotional requirements necessary for normal growth and development. 2. A person who symbolically represents an ideal parent, having those attributes which may be desirable or which one conceptualizes as necessary for forming the perfect parent-child relationship.

parent image A conscious and unconscious concept that a child forms concerning the roles and characteristics of the personality of the mother and father. See also **imago, primordial image.**

parenting, alteration in: actual or potential A nursing diagnosis accepted by the Fifth National Conference on the Classification of Nursing Diagnoses. This diagnosis includes any maladjustment or marked potential for maladjustment of a mother or father to the role of parent. The etiology of the problem may involve several factors, as lack of an available role model; lack of support; interruption of the process of bonding in the newborn period; unrealistic expectations for the self, the infant, or the partner; mental or physical illness; the presence of financial, legal, or cultural stressors; a lack of knowledge; limited cognitive ability; multiple pregnancies; or a death in the family concurrent with the birth or early infancy of the new baby. The critical defining characteristics, at least one of which must be present to make the diagnosis, include an observed lack of actions that demonstrate attachment to the child; inattentiveness to the needs of the child; inappropriate caretaking behavior, especially in toilet training and in sleep and feeding patterns; and a history of abuse or abandonment of the child. See also **nursing diagnosis.**

Parents Anonymous A self-help group for parents who have abused their children or who feel that they are prone to maltreat them. See also **child abuse.**

parepididymis, *pl.* **parepididymides** See **paradidymis.**

paresis 1. Slight or partial paralysis related in some cases to local neuritis. 2. A late manifestation of neurosyphilis, characterized by generalized paralysis, tremulous incoordination, transient seizures, Argyll Robertson pupils, and progressive dementia caused by degeneration of cortical neurons. Paresis resulting from untreated syphilis usually develops in the 3rd to 5th decades but may occur at an early

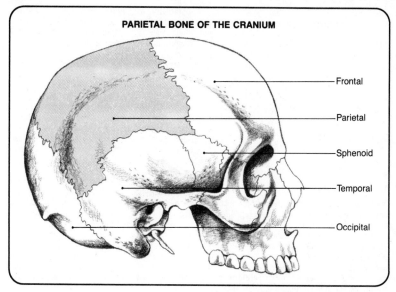

PARIETAL BONE OF THE CRANIUM

Frontal
Parietal
Sphenoid
Temporal
Occipital

age in patients with congenital syphilis. Also called **general paresis, paralytic dementia.** —**paretic,** *adj.*

paresthesia Abnormal sensations, such as numbness, prickling and tingling, that occur without apparent cause; heightened sensitivity.

paretic dementia See **general paresis.**

pareunia See **coitus.**

pargyline hydrochloride An antihypertensive with enzyme-inhibiting action.

paries, *pl.* **parietes** The wall of an organ or cavity in the body. —**parietal,** *adj.*

parietal **1.** Of or pertaining to the outer wall of a cavity. **2.** Of or pertaining to the parietal bone of the skull, such as the parietal lobe of the brain.

parietal bone One of a pair of bones that form the sides of the cranium. Each parietal bone has two surfaces, four borders, and four angles and articulates with five bones: the opposite parietal, occipital, frontal, temporal, and sphenoid.

parietal lobe A portion of each cerebral hemisphere that occupies the parts of the lateral and the medial surfaces that are covered by the parietal bone. On the lateral surface of the hemisphere the parietal lobe is separated from the frontal lobe by the central sulcus and from the temporal lobe by an imaginary line that extends from the posterior ramus of the lateral sulcus toward the occipital pole. On the parietal lobe the postcentral sulcus runs parallel with the central sulcus, so that the postcentral gyrus lies between them. The part of the parietal lobe posterior to the postcentral sulcus is divided by the horizontal intraparietal sulcus into the superior and the inferior parietal lobules. On the medial surface of the hemisphere the parieto-occipital sulcus separates the parietal and the occipital

lobes. Compare **central lobe, frontal lobe, occipital lobe, temporal lobe.**

parietal lymph node One of the small oval glands that filter the lymph coursing through the lymphatic vessels in the walls of the thorax or through the lymphatic vessels associated with the larger blood vessels of the abdomen and the pelvis. The parietal lymph nodes of the thorax include the sternal nodes, intercostal nodes, and diaphragmatic nodes. The parietal lymph nodes of the abdomen and pelvis include the common iliac nodes, epigastric nodes, external iliac nodes, iliac circumflex nodes, internal iliac nodes, lumbar nodes, and sacral nodes. See also **lymph, lymphatic system, lymph node.**

parietal pain A sharp sensation of distress in the parietal pleura, aggravated by respiration and thoracic movements and caused by pneumonia, empyema, pneumothorax, asbestosis, tuberculosis, neoplasm, or fluid accumulation from heart, liver, or kidney disease. Noxious stimuli do not cause pain in visceral pleura.

parietal peritoneum The portion of the largest serous membrane in the body that lines the abdominal wall. Compare **visceral peritoneum.** See also **peritoneal cavity.**

parietal pleura The serous membrane that lines the internal surface of the thoracic cavity. See also **visceral pleura.**

parieto-occipital Of or pertaining to the parietal and the occipital bones or lobes.

parieto-occipital sulcus A groove on each cerebral hemisphere marking the division of the parietal and occipital lobes of the brain. Also called **occipitoparietal fissure.**

Parinaud's syndrome A term often used to refer to conjunctivitis that is usually unilateral, follicular, and followed by enlargement of the preauricular lymph nodes and tenderness.

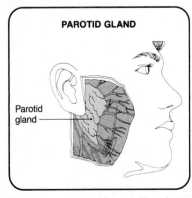

PAROTID GLAND

Parotid gland

The syndrome is frequently caused by infection with a species of the microorganism *Leptothrix*. It may also be associated with other infections, as tularemia, cat-scratch fever, and lymphogranuloma venereum. Also called **ophthalmoplegia.**

parity 1. In obstetrics: the classification of a woman by the number of live-born children and still-births she has delivered at more than 28 weeks of gestation. Commonly, parity is noted with the total number of pregnancies and represented by the letter P or the word para. A para 4 (P4) gravida 5 (G5) has had four deliveries after 28 weeks and one abortion or miscarriage before 28 weeks. Currently, a more complete system is in use in which the total number of pregnancies is followed by the number of deliveries at term, the number of premature infants, the number of abortions or miscarriages before 28 weeks' gestation, and the number of children living at present. This system may be written as TPAL. 2. In epidemiology: the classification of a woman by the number of live-born children she has delivered.

parkinsonism A neurologic disorder characterized by tremor; muscle rigidity; hypokinesia; a slow, shuffling gait; and difficulty in chewing, swallowing, and speaking, caused by various lesions in the extrapyramidal motor system. Signs and symptoms of parkinsonism resemble those of idiopathic Parkinson's disease and may develop during or following acute encephalitis and in syphilis, malaria, and poliomyelitis. Parkinsonism frequently occurs in patients treated with antipsychotic drugs. See also **Parkinson's disease.**

Parkinson's disease A slowly progressive, degenerative, neurologic disorder characterized by resting tremor, pill rolling of the fingers, a masklike facies, shuffling gait, forward flexion of the trunk, and muscle rigidity and weakness. It is usually an idiopathic disease of persons over the age of 60, though it may occur in younger persons, especially following acute encephalitis or carbon dioxide, metallic, or other poisoning. Signs and symptoms of Parkinson's disease, which include drooling, increased appetite, intolerance to heat, oily skin, emotional

instability, and defective judgment, are increased by fatigue, excitement, and frustration. Intelligence is rarely impaired. Palliative and symptomatic treatment of the disease focuses on correcting the imbalance between depleted dopamine and abundant acetylcholine in the striatum, since dopamine normally appears to inhibit excitatory cholinergic activity in this brain area. Treatment includes administration of drugs, such as levodopa, carbidopa-levadopa, amantadine, and anticholinergics. Patients with the disease are encouraged to continue to work and remain active as long as possible and to prevent the spine from bending forward by lying prone on a firm mattress and by walking with the hands folded behind the back. Hand tremor is less apparent if the patient grasps the arms of the chair when seated. Surgery may be performed to destroy portions of the globus pallidus to relieve rigidity or of the thalamus to alleviate tremor. Also called **paralysis agitans.**

paromomycin sulfate An amebicide.

paronychia An infection of the fold of skin at the margin of a nail. Treatment includes hot compresses or soaks, antibiotics, and, possibly, surgical incision and drainage. Compare **onychia.**

paroophoritis 1. Inflammation of the paroophoron. 2. Inflammation of the tissues surrounding the ovary.

paroophoron A small vestigial remnant of the mesonephros, consisting of a few rudimentary tubules lying in the broad ligament between the epoophoron and the uterus. It is most evident in very young girls. Compare **epoophoron.**

parotid duct A tubular canal, about 7 cm (2¾ inches) long, that extends from the anterior part of the parotid gland to the mouth. It crosses the masseter after leaving the parotid gland, pierces the buccinator, runs for a short distance obliquely forward between the buccinator and the mucous membrane of the mouth, and opens on the oral surface of the cheek through a small opening opposite the second upper molar tooth. As the parotid duct crosses the masseter, it receives the duct from the accessory portion of the parotid gland. The duct, which has a thick wall, is about 4 mm in diameter over most of its length but narrows considerably at the opening into the mouth. Also called **Stensen's duct.** See also **parotid gland.**

parotid gland One of the largest pair of salivary glands that lie at the side of the face just below and in front of the external ear. The main part of the gland is superficial, somewhat flattened and quadrilateral, and lies between the ramus of the mandible, the mastoid process, and the sternocleidomastoideus. It is wide superiorly and reaches nearly to the zygomatic arch, inferiorly tapering near the angle of the mandible. The rest of the gland is wedge-shaped and extends deeply toward the pharyngeal wall. It is enclosed in a capsule continuous with the deep cervical fascia. The parotid duct starts at the anterior part of the gland and opens on the inside of the cheek opposite the second upper molar.

Compare **sublingual gland, submandibular gland.** See also **salivary gland.**

parotitis   Inflammation or infection of one or both parotid salivary glands. See also **mumps.**

-parous   A combining form meaning 'pertaining to the quantity of offspring produced simultaneously or to the method of gestation': *quadriparous, viviparous.*

parovarium   See **epoophoron.**

paroxysm   **1.** A marked, usually episodic increase in symptoms. **2.** A convulsion, fit, seizure, or spasm. —**paroxysmal,** *adj.*

paroxysmal cold hemoglobinuria (PCH) A rare autoimmune disorder characterized by hemolysis and hematuria, associated with exposure to cold.

paroxysmal hemoglobinuria   The sudden passage of hemoglobin in urine, occurring following exposure to low temperatures, as in paroxysmal cold hemoglobinuria. See also **Marchiafava-Micheli disease.**

paroxysmal labyrinthine vertigo   See **Ménière's disease.**

paroxysmal nocturnal dyspnea (PND) A disorder characterized by sudden attacks of respiratory distress, usually occurring after several hours of sleep in a reclining position, most commonly caused by pulmonary edema resulting from congestive heart failure. The attacks are often accompanied by coughing, a feeling of suffocation, cold sweat, and tachycardia with a gallop rhythm. Sleeping with the head propped up on pillows may prevent dyspneic paroxysms at night, but treatment of the underlying cause is required to prevent fluid from accumulating in the lungs.

paroxysmal nocturnal hemoglobinuria (PNH)   A disorder characterized by intravascular hemolysis and hemoglobinuria. It occurs in irregular episodes of several days duration, especially at night. The basic defect in the red blood cell is an unusual sensitivity to lysis by complement or a deficiency or absence of acetylcholinesterase. The etiology of the condition is unknown, but it is associated with abnormal function of the bone marrow. Occurring predominantly in adults between 25 and 45 years of age, it is characterized by abdominal pain, back pain, and headache. Its course may be complicated by thrombotic episodes and by iron deficiency, owing to excessive loss of hemoglobin. Therapy includes blood transfusion and the oral or parenteral administration of iron. Corticosteroids are sometimes employed and found useful; treatment of thromboses may require anticoagulant therapy.

parrot fever   See **psittacosis.**

parry fracture   See **Monteggia's fracture.**

pars   A part, as the pars abdominalis esophagi. Also called **part.**

part   A portion of a larger area, as the condylar part of the occipital bone. Also called **pars.**

part-   A combining form meaning 'of or related to childbirth': *parturient, parturifacient.*

parthenogenesis   A type of nonsexual reproduction in which an organism develops from

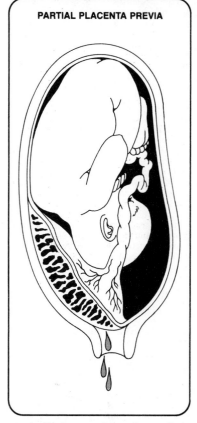

PARTIAL PLACENTA PREVIA

an unfertilized ovum, as in many lower animals. Initiation of the development of the unfertilized ovum may be artificially induced through mechanical or chemical stimulation. —**parthenogenetic, parthenogenic,** *adj.*

partial breech extraction   See **assisted breech.**

partial cleavage   Mitotic division of only part of a fertilized ovum into blastomeres, usually the activated cytoplasmic portion surrounding the nucleus; restricted division. Compare **total cleavage.** See also **meroblastic.**

partial placenta previa   Placenta previa in which the placenta is implanted in the lower uterine segment and partially covers the internal os of the uterine cervix. As the cervix dilates in labor, the portion of the placenta that lies over the cervix is separated, causing bleeding from the villous spaces of the uterine wall. Depending on the degree of separation, the bleeding may be scant or severe, resulting in hemorrhage that is life-threatening to the mother and the fetus. Treatment may require cesarean section. Diagnosis may be made by ultrasonic visualization or digital palpation in the course of prenatal examination. See also **placenta previa.**

partial pressure The pressure exerted by any single gas in a mixture of gases.

partial thromboplastin time (PTT) A test for detecting coagulation defects of the intrinsic system by adding activated partial thromboplastin to a sample of test plasma and to a control sample of normal plasma. The time required for the formation of a clot in test plasma is compared with that in the normal plasma. A delayed clotting time suggests an abnormality in one or more factors of the intrinsic system. If indicated, specific factor abnormalities can be identified by exposing the test plasma to a series of plasma samples with known factor deficiencies and observing for coagulation, which occurs only if the test plasma provides the missing clotting factors. Partial thromboplastin time is one of the basic tests used to measure specific factor activity and to detect hemophilias. It can also be used to monitor the activity of the anticoagulant, heparin. Also called PTT; activated partial thromboplastin time, APTT. Compare **prothrombin time.** See also **hemostasis.**

particle **1.** A minute quantity of material. **2.** A subatomic component of the nucleus of radioactive elements; for example, alpha and beta particles.

particulate Composed of **particles.**

-partite A combining form meaning 'having the (specified) number of parts': *bipartite, tripartite.*

parturition The process of giving birth.

parulis See **gumboil.**

PAS, PASA *abbr* para-aminosalicylic acid.

Pascal's principle In physics: a law stating that a confined liquid transmits pressure applied to it from an external source equally in all directions. Pascal's principle provides the basis for all hydraulic devices.

passive-aggressive personality A personality characterized by passivity and aggression in which forceful actions or attitudes are expressed in an indirect, nonviolent manner, such as pouting, obstructionism, procrastination, inefficiency, stubbornness, and forgetfulness. Compare **aggressive personality, passive-dependent personality.** See also **passive-aggressive personality disorder.**

passive-aggressive personality disorder A disorder characterized by the indirect expression of resistance to occupational or social demands, resulting in persistent, pervasive ineffectiveness, lack of self-confidence, poor interpersonal relationships, and pessimism that can lead, in severe cases, to major depression, alcoholism, or drug dependence. The behavior often reflects an unexpressed hostility or resentment stemming from a frustrating interpersonal or institutional relationship on which an individual is overdependent. Treatment may consist of behavior therapy or any of the various psychotherapeutic procedures.

passive algolagnia See **masochism.**

passive anaphylaxis See **antiserum anaphylaxis.**

passive-dependent personality A personality characterized by helplessness, indecisiveness, and a tendency to cling to and seek support from others. Compare **aggressive personality, passive-aggressive personality.**

passive euthanasia The practice of allowing terminally ill and mortally injured individuals to die without taking exceptional or heroic measures to prolong their lives, as connecting their organic systems to artificial devices, which may sustain heartbeats and brain waves but offer no hope for natural survival.

passive exercise Repetitive movement of a part of the body as a result of an externally applied force or the voluntary effort of the muscles controlling another part of the body. Compare **active exercise.** See also **aerobic exercise, anaerobic exercise.**

passive immunity A form of acquired immunity resulting from antibodies that are transmitted naturally through the placenta to a fetus or through the colostrum to an infant, or artificially by injection of antiserum for treatment or prophylaxis. It is not permanent and does not last as long as active immunity.

passive movement The moving of parts of the body by an outside force without voluntary action or resistance by the individual. Compare **active movement.**

passive play Play in which a person does not participate actively. For younger children such activity may include watching and listening to other children or adults, observing animals, listening to stories, or looking at pictures. Older children are passively entertained by watching television or by activities that require concentration and intellectual skill, as chess, reading, and listening to music. Compare **active play.**

passive smoking The inhalation by nonsmokers of the smoke from other people's cigarettes, pipes, and cigars. The amount of such smoke is small compared with that inhaled by tobacco users, but research provides increasing evidence that passive smoking can aggravate respiratory illnesses and contribute to more serious illnesses, as cancer, and can injure the health of nonsmoking spouses and of infants and unborn babies.

passive transfer test See **Prausnitz-Küstner test.**

passive transport The movement of small molecules across the membrane of a cell by diffusion. Passive transport occurs when the chemicals outside a cell become concentrated and start moving into the cell, changing the intracellular equilibrium. Passive transport is essential to various processes of metabolism, as the intake of digestive products by the cells lining the intestines. Compare **active transport, osmosis.**

passive tremor An involuntary trembling occurring when the person is at rest, one of the signs of Parkinson's disease. Also called **resting tremor.**

Pasteurella A genus of gram-negative bacilli or coccobacilli, including species pathogenic to man and domestic animals. The plague bacillus, *Pasteurella pestis*, is now called *Yer-*

sinia pestis. P. tularensis, which causes tularemia, is now called *Francisella tularensis.* Pasteurella infections may be transmitted to man by animal bites.

pasteurization The process of applying heat, usually to milk or cheese, for a specified period of time for the purpose of killing or retarding the development of pathogenic bacteria. —**pasteurize,** *v.*

pasteurized milk Milk that has been treated by heat to destroy pathogenic bacteria. By law, pasteurization requires a temperature of 62.8°C to 65.6°C (145°F to 150°F) for not less than 30 minutes, followed by a temperature of 71.7°C (161°F) for 15 seconds, followed by immediate cooling.

past health In a health history: an overall summary of the person's general health to date, including past injuries, allergies, surgical procedures, immunizations, hospitalizations, and obstetric and psychiatric history. It is obtained from the person or the person's family at the initial interview and becomes part of the permanent record.

Patau's syndrome A complex of birth defects owing to trisomy of chromosome 13 and occurring in approximately 1 in 5,000 births. Affected newborns are tiny, prone to apneic spells, severely mentally retarded, and have a variety of physical abnormalities, as cleft lip, cleft palate, deafness, and cardiovascular and brain anomalies. Approximately 70% die before reaching the age of 6 months, and fewer than 20% survive beyond the 1st year. Also called **trisomy D syndrome.**

patch test A skin test for identifying allergens, especially those causing contact dermatitis. The suspected substance (food, pollen, animal fur, etc.), is applied to an adhesive patch that is placed on the patient's skin. Another patch, with nothing on it, serves as a control. After a certain period of time (usually 24 to 48 hours), both patches are removed. If the skin under the suspect patch is red and swollen and the control area is not, the test is said to be positive, and the subject is probably allergic to that substance. Compare **Prausnitz-Küstner test, radioallergosorbent test.**

patek See **yaws.**

patella A flat, triangular bone at the front of the knee joint, having a pointed apex that attaches to the ligamentum patellae. The convex, anterior surface of the bone is perforated for the passage of nutrient vessels and covered by an expansion from the tendon of the quadriceps femoris. Also called kneecap.

patellar ligament The central portion of the common tendon of the quadriceps femoris. The ligament is a strong, flat, ligamentous band, about 8 cm (3⅛ inch) long, attached proximally to the apex and the adjoining margins of the patella and distally to the tuberosity of the tibia.

patellar reflex A deep tendon reflex, elicited by a sharp tap on the tendon just distal to the patella, normally characterized by contraction of the quadriceps muscle and extension of the

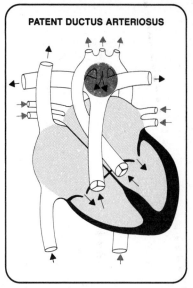

PATENT DUCTUS ARTERIOSUS

leg at the knee. The reflex is hyperactive in disease of the pyramidal tract above the level of the second lumbar vertebra. Also called **knee-jerk reflex, quadriceps reflex.** See also **deep tendon reflex.**

patent The condition of being open and unblocked, as a patent airway or a patent anus.

patent ductus arteriosus (PDA) An abnormal opening between the pulmonary artery and the aorta caused by failure of the fetal ductus arteriosus to close after birth. The defect, which is seen primarily in premature infants, allows blood from the aorta to flow into the pulmonary artery and to recirculate through the lungs, where it is reoxygenated and returned to the left atrium and left ventricle, causing an increased workload on the left side of the heart and increased pulmonary vascular congestion and resistance. Clinical manifestations include cardiomegaly, especially of the left atrium and left ventricle, dilated ascending aorta, bounding pulses from increased systolic pressure, tachycardia, and a typical machinery-like murmur that is heard during all of systole and most of diastole. Correction is delayed until the child is old enough to tolerate surgery and to allow time for spontaneous closure. Complications include congestive heart failure, pulmonary vascular disease, calcification of the ductal site, and infective endocarditis. See also **congenital cardiac anomaly.**

Paterson-Kelly syndrome A condition of the digestive system associated with iron deficiency anemia, characterized by the development of esophageal webs in the upper esophagus, making swallowing of solids difficult. The webs are easily ruptured during esophagoscopy and tube feeding and can produce hemorrhage. When the hemoglobin count is improved, the

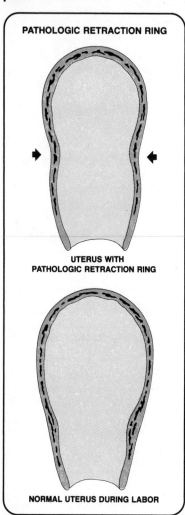

PATHOLOGIC RETRACTION RING

UTERUS WITH
PATHOLOGIC RETRACTION RING

NORMAL UTERUS DURING LABOR

webs disappear. Also called **Plummer-Vinson syndrome.**

path- See **patho-.**

-path A combining form meaning: **1.** 'One suffering from a (specified) illness': *cardiopath, neuropath.* **2.** 'One who treats illness by a (specified) system': *dermopath, naprapath, naturopath.*

-pathetic A combining form meaning 'pertaining to emotions': *antipathetic, sympathetic.* Also -pathetical.

-pathic A combining form meaning: **1.** 'Referring to an illness or affected part of the body': *angiopathic, encephalopathic.* **2.** 'Referring to a form or system of treatment': *homeopathic.*

patho-, path- A combining form meaning 'of or related to disease': *pathocrinia, pathoformic.*

pathogen Any microorganism capable of producing disease. —**pathogenic,** *adj.*

pathogenesis The source or cause of an illness or abnormal condition.

pathognomonic Of a sign or symptom: specific to a disease or condition, as Koplik's spots on the buccal and lingual musosa, which are indicative of measles.

pathognomonic symptom See **symptom.**

pathologic **1.** Pertaining to that branch of medicine that studies the nature and cause of disease. **2.** Indicative of or caused by disease.

pathologic absorption The taking up by the blood of an excretory or morbid substance.

pathological anatomy In applied anatomy: the study of the structure and morphology of the tissues and cells of the body as related to disease. Also called **morbid anatomy.**

pathological diagnosis A diagnosis by examining the substance and function of body tissues, especially of the abnormal developmental changes in tissues by histologic techniques.

pathologic fracture See **neoplastic fracture.**

pathologic mitosis Any cell division that is atypical, asymmetrical, or multipolar and results in an unequal number of chromosomes in the nuclei of the daughter cells. It is indicative of malignancy, as occurs in cancer.

pathologic myopia A type of progressive nearsightedness characterized by changes in the fundus of the eye, posterior staphyloma, and deficient corrected acuity.

pathologic retraction ring A ridge that may form around the uterus at the junction of the upper and lower uterine segments during the prolonged second stage of an obstructed labor. The lower segment is abnormally distended and thin, while the upper segment is abnormally thick. The ring, which may be seen and felt abdominally, is a warning of impending uterine rupture. Also called **Bandl's ring.** Compare **physiologic retraction ring, constriction ring.**

pathologist A physician who specializes in the study of disease, usually in a hospital, school of medicine, or research institute or laboratory. A pathologist usually specializes in autopsy, clinical pathology, or surgical pathology.

pathology **1.** The study of the characteristics, causes, and effects of disease, as observed in the structure and function of the body. **2.** Cellular pathology: the study of cellular changes in disease. **3.** Clinical pathology: the study of disease by the use of laboratory tests and methods. —**pathologic,** *adj.*

pathomimicry See **Munchausen's syndrome.**

pathophysiology The study of the biological and physical manifestations of disease as they correlate with the underlying abnormalities and physiologic disturbances. Pathophysiology does not deal directly with the treatment of disease; rather, it explains the processes within the body that result in the signs and symptoms of a disease. —**pathophysiologic,** *adj.*

pathway **1.** A network of neurons that provides a transmission route for nerve impulses from any part of the body to the spinal cord and the cerebral cortex or from the central nervous system to the muscles and organs. Neural pathways in the body are the somatic sensory pathways and the somatic motor pathways. **2.** A chain of chemical reactions that produces various compounds in critical sequence, as the Embden-Meyerhof pathway.

-pathy A combining form meaning: **1.** A 'suffering or illness' of a specified sort: *gynecopathy.* **2.** A 'therapy for suffering': *homeopathy.*

patient **1.** A health-care recipient who is ill or hospitalized. **2.** A client in a health-care service.

patient day (PD) A unit in a system of accounting used by health-care facilities and health-care planners. Each day represents a unit of time during which the services of the institution or facility were used by a patient, thus 50 patients in a hospital for 1 day would represent 50 patient days.

patient interview A systematic interview of a patient to obtain information that can be used to develop an individualized plan for care. Also called **client interview.**

patient mix **1.** The distribution of demographic variables in a patient population, often represented by the percentage of a given race, age, sex, or ethnic derivation. **2.** The distribution of indications for admission in a patient population, such as surgical, maternity, or trauma indications.

patient record A collection of documents that provides a record of each time a person visited or sought treatment and received care or a referral for care from a health-care facility. This confidential record is usually held by the facility, and the information in it is released only to the person, or with the person's written permission. It contains the initial assessment, health history, laboratory reports, and notes by nurses, physicians, and consultants, as well as order sheets, medication sheets, admission records, discharge summaries, and other pertinent data. A problem-oriented medical record also contains a master problem list. The patient record is often a collection of papers held in a folder, but, increasingly, hospitals are computerizing the records after every discharge, making the past record available on visual display terminals. Also called **chart** *(informal).*

Patient's Bill of Rights A list of patient's rights promulgated by the American Hospital Association. It offers some guidance and protection to patients by stating the responsibilities that a hospital and its staff have toward patients and their families during hospitalization, but it is not a legally binding document.

Paul's tube A large-bore glass drainage tube with a projecting rim, used in performing an enterostomy. Also called **Paul-Mixter tube.**

Pautrier microabscess An accumulation of intensely staining mononuclear cells in the epidermis, characterizing malignant lymphoma of the skin, especially mycosis fungoides. See also **mycosis fungoides.**

Pauwel's fracture A fracture of the proximal femoral neck with varying degrees of angulation.

pavor A reaction to a frightening stimulus characterized by excessive terror. Kinds of pavor are **pavor diurnus, pavor nocturnus.**

pavor diurnus A sleep disorder occurring in children during daytime sleep in which they cry out in alarm and awaken in fear and panic. See also **sleep terror disorder.**

pavor nocturnus A sleep disorder occurring in children during nighttime sleep that causes them to cry out in alarm and awaken in fear and panic. See also **nightmare, sleep terror disorder.**

Payr's clamp A clamp used in gastrointestinal surgery.

Pb Symbol for **lead.**

PBI *abbr* **protein-bound iodine.**

p.c. *abbr* Latin *post cibum*, after meals.

PCH *abbr* **paroxysmal cold hemoglobinuria.**

PCO_2 Symbol for partial pressure of carbon dioxide. See **partial pressure.**

PCP *abbr* **phencyclidine hydrochloride.**

PCWP *abbr* **pulmonary capillary wedge pressure.**

Pd Symbol for **palladium.**

PD *abbr* **patient day.**

PDA *abbr* **patent ductus arteriosus.**

PDR *abbr* **Physician's Desk Reference.**

PE *abbr* **pulmonary embolism.**

Péan's forceps A basic hemostatic clamp.

pearly penile papules See **hirsutoid papilloma of the penis.**

pearly tumor See **cholesteatoma.**

Pearson's product movement correlation In statistics: a statistical test of the relationship between two variables measured in interval or ratio scales. Correlations computed fall between $+1.00$ and -1.00.

pecilo- See **poikilo-.**

pectin A gelatinous substance found in fruits and succulent vegetables that is used as the setting agent for jams and jellies and as an emulsifier and stabilizer in many foods. It also adds to the diet bulk necessary for proper gastrointestinal functioning. See also **dietary fiber.**

pectineus The most anterior of the five medial femoral muscles. It arises from the pectineal line and inserts in a rough line on the femur extending distally and caudally from the lesser trochanter to the linea aspera. The muscle functions to flex and adduct the thigh and to rotate it medially. Compare **adductor brevis, adductor longus, adductor magnus, gracilis.**

pector- A combining form meaning 'of or pertaining to the breast': *pectoralgia, pectorophony.*

pectoralis major A large muscle of the upper chest wall that acts on the joint of the shoulder. Thick and fan-shaped, it arises from the clavicle, the sternum, the cartilages of the second to the sixth ribs, and the aponeurosis of the obliquus externus abdominis. It inserts by a flat wide tendon into the crest of the greater tubercle of the humerus. The pectoralis major serves to flex, adduct, and medially rotate the arm in the shoulder joint.

pectoralis minor A thin, triangular muscle of the upper chest wall beneath the pectoralis major. The base arises from the third, fourth, and fifth ribs on their upper, outer surfaces. It inserts as a flat tendon into the corocoid process of the scapula. It functions to rotate the scapula, to draw it downward and forward, and to raise the third, fourth, and fifth ribs in forced inspiration. Compare **pectoralis major, subclavius.**

pectoriloquy (P) The transmission of vocal sounds through the chest wall on auscultation over the lung, indicating **cavitation** or **consolidation.** Softly spoken words can be heard in whispering pectoriloquy.

ped- See **pedo-.**

-ped A combining form meaning: **1.** A 'creature possessing feet of a (specified) sort or quantity': *biped, quadruped.* **2.** 'Possessing feet of a (specified) sort or quantity': *taliped.* Also **-pede.**

-pedal See **-pedic².**

pederosis, paederosis See **pedophilia.**

pedia-, ped-, pedo- A combining form meaning 'of or pertaining to a child': *pediatric, pediatrics.*

-pedia A combining form meaning 'compendium of knowledge': *orthopedia, logopedia.* Also **-paedia.**

pediatric anesthesia A subspecialty of anesthesiology dealing with the anesthesia of neonates, infants, and children up to age 12.

pediatric dosage The determination of the correct amount, frequency, and total number of doses of a medication to be administered to a child or infant. Such variables as age, weight, body surface area, and the ability of the child to absorb, metabolize, and excrete the medication must be considered as well as the expected action of the drug, possible side effects, and potential toxicity. Various formulas have been devised to calculate pediatric dosage from a standard adult dose, although the most reliable method is to use the proportional amount of body surface area to body weight, based on one of the formulas. See also **Clark's rule, Cowling's rule, Young's rule.**

pediatric hospitalization The confinement of a child or infant in a hospital for diagnostic testing or therapeutic treatment. Hospitalization constitutes a major crisis in the life of a child, and the emotional trauma elicits various behavioral reactions that the nurse must recognize and be prepared to cope with in order to facilitate recovery. The dominant factors influencing stress, which vary according to the child's developmental age, previous experience with illness, and the seriousness of the condition, include separation from the parents and familiar environment, disruption of routine patterns of daily life, loss of independence, and worry about bodily injury or painful experiences. The nurse can minimize stress by preparing the child and family through prehospital counseling; by encouraging active parental participation in the care of the child through rooming-in facilities or frequent visits; by maintaining as normal a daily routine as possible, especially with eating, sleeping, hygiene, and play activities; by explaining all hospital procedures and the immediate and long-term prognosis in terms that the child can easily understand; and by providing support and guidance for parents and siblings. The nurse may also use the hospital experience to foster an improved parent-child relationship and to teach other members of the family about proper health care. Emergency admission greatly increases the emotional trauma of hospitalization, making the role of the nurse in counteracting negative reactions even more significant.

pediatrician, pediatrist A physician who specializes in pediatrics.

pediatric nurse practitioner (PNP) A nurse practitioner who, by advanced study and clinical practice, has gained expert knowledge in the nursing care of infants and children. See also **pediatric nursing.**

pediatric nursing The branch of nursing concerned with the care of infants and children. Pediatric nursing requires knowledge of normal psychomotor, psychosocial, and cognitive growth and development as well as of the health problems and needs of people in this age group. Preventive care and anticipatory guidance are integral to the practice of pediatric nursing. See also **pediatric nurse practitioner.**

pediatric nutrition The maintenance of a proper, well-balanced diet, consisting of the essential nutrients and the adequate caloric intake necessary to promote growth and sustain the physiological requirements at the various stages of development. Directly related to the rate of growth, nutritional needs vary considerably with age, level of activity, and environmental conditions. In the prenatal period, growth is totally dependent on adequate maternal nutrition. During infancy the need for calories, especially in the form of protein, is greater than at any postnatal period because of the rapid increase in both height and weight. From the toddler through the preschool and middle childhood years, growth is uneven and occurs in spurts, with a subsequent fluctuation in appetite and calorie consumption. In general, the average child expends 55% of energy on metabolic maintenance, 25% on activities, 12% on growth, and 8% on excretion. The accelerated growth phase during adolescence demands greater nutritional requirements, although food habits are often influenced by emotional factors, peer pressure, and fad diets. Inadequate nutrition, especially during critical periods of growth, results in retarded development or illness, as anemia from deficiency of iron or scurvy from deficiency of vitamin C. An important function of the nurse is to give nutritional guidance and teach good eating habits. A special problem is overfeeding in the early childhood years, which may lead to obesity or hypervitaminosis. See also **dietary allowances,** specific vitamins.

pediatrics A branch of medicine concerned with the development and care of children. Its specialties are the particular diseases of children and their treatment and prevention. **—pediatric,** *adj.*

pediatric surgery The special preparation and care of the child undergoing surgical procedures for injuries, deformities, or disease. In addition to the usual fears and emotional trauma of illness and hospitalization, the child is especially concerned about being anesthetized. Younger children worry more about what will happen to them and how they will feel after awakening from anesthesia, whereas the older child fears the operation itself and possible death, the loss of control while under anesthesia, and any change in body image or mutilation of parts. The role of the nurse is to prepare the child psychologically and physically for the particular surgical procedure and any postoperative reactions; to offer support to the parents and involve them as much as possible in the care, both before and after surgery; and to explain immediate and long-term prognoses. See also **pediatric hospitalization.**

-pedic¹ A combining form meaning 'of or pertaining to children or their treatment': *gymnopedic, orthopedic.* Also -paedic.

-pedic² A combining form meaning 'referring or pertaining to the feet': *talipedic, velocepedic.* Also -pedal.

pedicle 1. The narrow basal part that connects a nonsessile tumor to the adjacent normal tissue. 2. Any slender stemlike structure or narrow connection; for example, the pedicle of a vertebra.

pedicle clamp A locking surgical forceps used for compressing blood vessels or pedicles of tumors during surgery. Also called **clamp forceps.**

pediculicide Any of a group of drugs that kill lice.

pediculosis Infestation with bloodsucking lice. **Pediculosis capitis** is infestation of the scalp with lice. **Pediculosis corporis** is infestation of the skin of the body with lice. **Pediculosis palpebrae** is infestation of the eyelids and eyelashes with lice. **Pediculosis pubis** is infestation of the pubic hair region with lice. Infestation with lice causes intense itching, often resulting in excoriation of the skin and secondary bacterial infection. Frequently, only the eggs of the lice may be seen. Body lice lay eggs in the seams of clothing; crab and head lice attach their eggs to hairs. Lice are spread by direct contact with infested clothing, people, or toilet seats. Body lice may transmit certain diseases, among them relapsing fever, typhus, and trench fever. Treatment includes the topical use of 1% lindane as shampoo, lotion, or cream, or of malathion 0.5% lotion. After applying the pediculocide, the eggs are combed out of the hair with a fine-toothed comb. Lice and eggs on the eyelashes

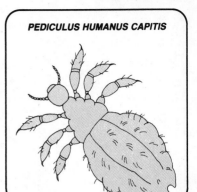

PEDICULUS HUMANUS CAPITIS

require topical treatment with an ophthalmic ointment containing 0.25% physostigmine. Infestation sometimes may be prevented by avoiding contact with the organism and by washing and ironing any clothing or bedding that may be infested. See also **crab louse, louse.**

Pediculus humanus capitis The head louse.

pedigree 1. Line of descent; lineage; ancestry. 2. In genetics: a chart that shows the genetic makeup of a person's ancestors, used in the Mendelian analysis of an inherited characteristic or disease in a particular family. See also **Punnett square.**

pedo-¹ A combining form meaning 'of or related to a child': *pedodontics, pedogenesis.*

pedo-², ped-, pedia- A combining form meaning 'of or pertaining to the foot': *pedodynamometer, pedograph.*

pedodontics A field of dentistry devoted to the diagnosis and the treatment of dental problems of children.

pedogenesis, paedogenesis The production of offspring by young or larval forms of animals, often by parthenogenesis, as in certain amphibians. **—pedogenetic,** *adj.*

pedophilia, paedophilia 1. An abnormal interest in children. 2. In psychiatry: a psychosexual disorder in which the fantasy or act of engaging in sexual activity with prepubertal children is the preferred or exclusive means of achieving sexual excitement and gratification. It may be heterosexual or homosexual. Also called **pederosis.** See also **paraphilia. —paedophilic, pedophilic,** *adj.*

peds *Informal.* Pediatrics.

peduncle A stemlike connecting part, as the pineal peduncle. **—peduncular, pedunculate,** *adj.*

PEEP *abbr* **positive end expiratory pressure.**

peer review In nursing: an appraisal by professional coworkers of equal status of the way an individual nurse conducts practice, education, or research. See also **Professional Standards Review Organization.**

Pel-Ebstein fever A recurrent feve

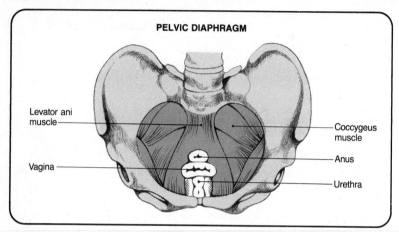

PELVIC DIAPHRAGM

Levator ani muscle

Vagina

Coccygeus muscle

Anus

Urethra

curring in cycles of several days or weeks, characteristic of Hodgkin's disease or malignant lymphoma. Also called **Murchison fever.**

Pelger-Huët anomaly An inherited disorder characterized by granulocytes with unusually coarse nuclear material and a dumbbell-shaped or peanut-shaped nucleus. Normal nuclear segmentation does not seem to occur, but there are no associated findings. See also **band.**

pell- A combining form meaning 'of or pertaining to the skin': *pellagra, pellicle.*

pellagra A disease resulting from a deficiency of niacin or tryptophan or a metabolic defect that interferes with the conversion of the precursor tryptophan to niacin. It is frequently seen in individuals whose diet consists primarily of maize, which is deficient in tryptophan. It is characterized by scaly dermatitis, especially of the skin exposed to the sun, glossitis, inflammation of the mucous membranes, diarrhea, and mental disturbances, including depression, confusion, disorientation, hallucination, and delirium. Treatment and prophylaxis consist of administration of niacin and tryptophan, usually in conjunction with other vitamins, particularly thiamine and riboflavin, and a well-balanced diet containing foods rich in these nutrients, as liver, eggs, milk, and meat. Kinds of pellagra are **pellagra sine pellagra, typhoid pellagra.** Compare **kwashiorkor. —pellagrous,** *adj.*

pellagra sine pellagra A form of pellagra in which the characteristic dermatitis is not present. See **pellagra.**

pelo- A combining form meaning 'of or pertaining to mud': *pelohemia, pelology.*

pelvic Of or pertaining to the pelvis.

pelvic brim The curved top of the bones of the hip extending from the anterior superior iliac crest in front on one side around and past the sacrum to the crest on the other side. Below the brim is the pelvis.

pelvic cellulitis Bacterial infection of the parametrium, occurring after childbirth or spontaneous therapeutic abortion. It represents an extension of infection via the blood vessels and lymphatics from a primary wound infection in the external genitalia, perineum, vagina, cervix, or uterus. It is characterized by fever, uterine subinvolution, chills and sweats, abdominal pain that spreads laterally, and, if untreated, by the formation of a large abscess and by signs of peritonitis. It is seen most commonly between the 3rd and the 9th days after delivery or abortion. Treatment includes an antibiotic, bed rest, intravenous fluids, and drainage of any abscess that forms. Oxytocics may be given to augment involution.

pelvic classification 1. A process in which the anatomic and spatial relationships of the bones of the pelvis are evaluated, usually to assess the adequacy of the pelvic structures for vaginal delivery. Caldwell-Moloy's system of classification is the one most commonly used. 2. One of the types in a classification system of the pelvis.

pelvic congestion syndrome An abnormal gynecologic condition characterized by chronic low back pain, dysuria, dysmenorrhea, vague lower abdominal pain, vaginal discharge, and dyspareunia. The cause is not understood; formerly it was thought that the vascular bed of the area was distended with blood, but this has not been demonstrated. Women between 25 and 45 are most often affected.

pelvic diaphragm The caudal aspect of the body wall, stretched like a hammock across the pelvic cavity and comprised of the levator ani and the coccygeus muscles. It holds the abdominal contents, supports the pelvic viscera, and is pierced by the anal canal, the urethra, and the vagina. It is reinforced by fasciae and muscles associated with these structures and with the perineum.

pelvic examination A diagnostic procedure in which the external and internal genitalia are physically examined using inspection, palpation, percussion, and auscultation. It should be performed regularly throughout a woman's life, usually every 1 to 3 years. The woman empties her bladder, disrobes, and puts on an examining gown. She is made as comfortable as possible in the dorsal lithotomy position, her feet in stirrups and her buttocks at the very edge of the foot of the examining table, and is then draped. Breast examination is often carried out at this point, prior to the pelvic examination, and the lower abdomen is palpated. Particular attention is paid to the suprapubic area to detect any masses extending from the pelvis above the symphysis and to the groin to detect inguinal lymphadenopathy or hernia. If a mass is felt, percussion may be performed to delineate it. If pregnancy is suspected, palpation and percussion of the uterus and auscultation of fetal heart tones are attempted. The examiner then moves to the stool at the foot of the table between the patient's legs. The labia majora are spread apart to permit inspection of the clitoris, the urethral meatus, the labia minora, and the vaginal vestibule. Any swelling, discoloration, lesion, scar, cyst, discharge, or bleeding is noted. Skene's and Bartholin's glands and ducts are palpated and milked, and any secretions expressed are evaluated and a specimen is spread on culture media. The tone of the perineal and paravaginal musculature is assessed. Cystocele, rectocele, or varying degrees of uterine descensus may be observed as the woman is asked to bear down. Because lubricating jelly interferes with cytologic and bacteriologic studies, the speculum examination is usually performed without using the jelly. The speculum is warmed, lubricated with warm water, and introduced gradually. The examiner is careful to direct the speculum along the axis of the vagina, which is at an angle of approximately 45° to the axis of the table if the woman is lying flat. The speculum may need to be moved lightly from side to side in order to slip it over the vaginal rugae. The woman is advised that she may feel a stretching sensation; the speculum is gently opened and its position is adjusted to hold the vaginal folds out of the way to reveal the cervix. The color and condition of the vaginal epithelium are observed and the position, size, and quality of the superficial epithelium are evaluated. Specimens for bacteriologic study are obtained before the Papanicolaou (Pap) test. For the Pap test, scrapings of the endocevix and the cervix and a sample of the vaginal secretions are secured on a Pap stick and an applicator and lightly spread on labeled glass slides. The slides are immediately sprayed with a fixative or dipped in it. The speculum is then closed, rotated slightly, removed from the vagina and rinsed or placed directly in a germicidal solution. In the bimanual part of the examination, two gloved fingers are well lubricated and inserted slowly and gently into the vagina. The examiner uses the opposite hand to apply pressure to the lower abdomen in several positions and directions to bring the uterus, tubes, and ovaries into positions in which they may be felt. The size, shape, position, mobility, and consistency of the organs and tissues are evaluated, and any tenderness or discomfort is noted. Rectal or rectovaginal examination is then performed. Prior to the insertion of a finger in the anus, lateral pressure is applied to the sphincter and the woman is urged to bear down lightly to relax the muscle and minimize discomfort. Pelvic examination may demonstrate many pelvic abnormalities and diseases. Cytologic and bacteriologic specimens are conveniently obtained. A pelvic examination cannot be satisfactorily performed without the cooperation of the woman being examined; inadequate relaxation, obesity, extensive scarring, pelvic tenderness, and heavy vaginal discharge may also preclude an adequate examination.

NURSING CONSIDERATIONS: Instruments, culture materials, a light, drapes, and a gown are all made ready beforehand. The table, instruments, and drapes are clean and warm. The woman is forewarned of what to expect at each step of the examination. Gentleness and quietness are exercised. Upon completion of the examination the woman is helped to slide well back on the table before sitting up. Syncope following pelvic examination is uncommon but not rare; there is risk of injury should the patient faint and fall from the examining table. The woman is observed briefly after sitting up before being left alone. She is then given tissues, a sanitary napkin or tampon, and a private area in which to dress.

pelvic inferior aperture See **pelvic outlet.**

pelvic inflammatory disease (PID) Any inflammatory condition of the female pelvic organs, especially one caused by bacterial infection. Characteristics of the condition include fever, foul-smelling vaginal discharge, pain in the lower abdomen, abnormal uterine bleeding, pain with coitus, and tenderness or pain in the uterus, affected ovary, or fallopian tube on bimanual pelvic examination. If an abscess has already developed, a soft, tender, fluid-filled mass may be palpated. Bed rest and antibiotics are usually prescribed, but surgical drainage of an abscess may be required. Severe, fulminating PID may necessitate hysterectomy to avoid fatal septicemia. If the cause is infection by gonococci or chlamydiae, the woman's sexual partners are also treated with antibiotics. PID may become chronic and recurrent. Severe PID is usually very painful: the woman may be prostrate and require narcotic analgesia. Recurrent or severe PID often results in scarring of the fallopian tubes, obstruction, and infertility.

pelvic inlet In obstetrics: the inlet to the true pelvis, bounded by the sacral promontory, the horizontal rami of the pubic bones, and the top of the symphysis pubis. As the fetus must pass through the inlet to enter the true pelvis and to be born vaginally, the anteroposterior, transverse, and oblique dimensions of the inlet are important measurements to be made in assessing the pelvis in pregnancy. There are three anteroposterior diameters: the true conjugate, the obstetric conjugate, and the diagonal conjugate. The true conjugate, measured only on X-ray, extends from the sacral promontory to the top of the symphysis pubis. Its normal measurement is

PELVIC OUTLET

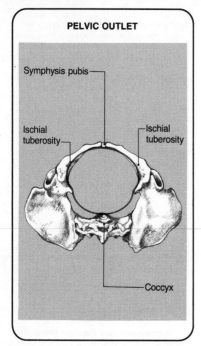

Symphysis pubis

Ischial tuberosity

Ischial tuberosity

Coccyx

11 cm (4¼ inches) or more. The obstetric conjugate is the shortest of the three, as it extends from the sacral promontory to the thickest part of the pubic bone. It measures 10 cm (4 inches) or more. The diagonal conjugate is the most easily and commonly assessed, as it extends from the lower border of the symphysis pubis to the sacral promontory. It normally measures 11.5 cm (4½ inches) or more. The inlet is said to be contracted when any of these diameters is smaller than normal. The transverse diameter of the inlet is bounded by the inferior border of the walls of the iliac bones and is measured at the widest point. It is normally close to 13.5 cm (5¼ inches) but may be less in the small gynecoid pelvis and anthropoid pelvis. The oblique diameters of the pelvis extend from the juncture of the sacrum and ilium to the eminence on the ilium on the opposite side of the pelvis. Each oblique diameter measures nearly 13 cm (5⅛ inches). This dimension is smaller than normal in the small gynecoid and platypelloid pelves. See also **android pelvis, anthropoid pelvis, gynecoid pelvis, platypelloid pelvis.**

pelvic kidney See ptotic kidney.

pelvic minilaparotomy A surgical procedure in which the lower abdomen is entered through a small, suprapubic incision, performed most often for tubal sterilization but also for diagnosis and treatment of eccyesis, ovarian cyst, endometriosis, and infertility. It may be performed as an alternative to laparoscopy, often on an outpatient basis.

NURSING CONSIDERATIONS: As incisional pain in the postoperative period may mask the pain of intraperitoneal bleeding, vital signs are monitored frequently. Tachycardia and hypotension that are not alleviated by analgesia may be signs of hemorrhage or injury to the bowel. Prior to discharge, outpatients are carefully instructed in the postoperative danger signs and in the proper care of the incision at home. Compare **laparoscopy.** See also **tubal ligation, sterilization.**

pelvic outlet The space surrounded by the bones of the lower portion of the true pelvis. In men, the shape of the pelvic outlet is narrower than in women, but this is of no clinical significance. In women, the shape and size of the pelvis varies and is of importance in childbirth. The shapes are classified by the length of the diameters as compared to each other and by the thickness of the bones. The diameters of the outlet are the anteroposterior, from the symphysis pubis to the coccyx, and the intertuberous, laterally from one to the other ischial tuberosity. See also **pelvic classification.**

pelvic pain Pain in the pelvis, as occurs in appendicitis. The character and onset of pelvic pain and any factors that alleviate or aggravate it are significant in diagnosis.

pelvic pole The end of the axis at which the breech of the fetus is located.

pelvic rotation One of the five major kinematic determinants of gait, involving the alternate rotation of the pelvis to the right and the left of the central axis of the body. The usual pelvic rotation occurring at each hip joint in most healthy individuals is approximately 4° to each side of the central axis. Pelvic rotation occurs during the stance phase of gait and involves a medial-to-lateral circular motion. With normal locomotion or walking, considered a progressive sinusoidal movement, pelvic rotation serves to minimize the vertical displacement of the center of gravity of the body during the act of walking. Analysis of pelvic rotation is a factor in diagnosing various orthopedic diseases and deformities and in the correction of pathological gaits. Compare **knee-ankle interaction, knee-hip flexion, lateral pelvic displacement, pelvic tilt.**

pelvic tilt One of the five major kinematic determinants of gait that lowers the pelvis on the side of the swinging lower limb during the walking cycle. Through the action of the hip joint, the pelvis tilts laterally downward, adducting the lower limb in the stance phase of gait and abducting the opposite extremity in the swing phase of gait. The knee joint of the nonweight-bearing limb flexes during its swing phase to allow the pelvic tilt, which helps minimize the vertical displacement of the center of gravity of the body, thus conserving energy during walking. Pelvic tilt is a factor in the diagnosis of various orthopedic diseases and deformities and in the correction of pathological gaits. Compare **knee-ankle interaction, knee-hip flexion, lateral pelvic displacement, pelvic rotation.**

pelvic varicocele See ovarian varicocele.

BONES OF THE PELVIS

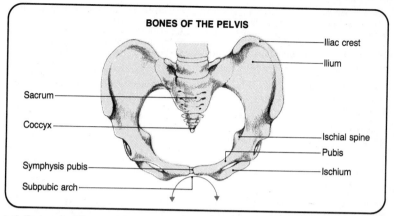

Iliac crest — Ilium — Sacrum — Coccyx — Symphysis pubis — Subpubic arch — Ischial spine — Pubis — Ischium

pelvifemoral Of or pertaining to the structures of the hip joint, especially the muscles and the area around the bony pelvis and the head of the femur that make up the pelvic girdle.

pelvifemoral muscular dystrophy A form of limb-girdle muscular dystrophy that begins in the pelvic girdle. Also called **Leyden-Moebius muscular dystrophy.**

pelvimetry The act or process of determining the dimensions of the bony birth canal. Kinds of pelvimetry are **clinical pelvimetry, X-ray pelvimetry.**

pelvis, *pl.* **pelves** The lower portion of the trunk of the body, composed of four bones: the two innominate bones laterally and ventrally and the sacrum and coccyx posteriorly. It is divided into the greater, or false, pelvis and the lesser, or true, pelvis by an oblique plane passing through the sacrum and the pubic symphysis. The greater pelvis is the expanded portion of the cavity situated cranially and ventral to the pelvic brim. The lesser pelvis is situated distal to the pelvic brim, and its bony walls are more complete than those of the greater pelvis. The inlet and outlet of the pelvis have three important diameters: anteroposterior, oblique, and transverse. The pelvis of a woman is usually less massive but is wider and more circular than that of a man. —**pelvic,** *adj.*

pemoline A central nervous system stimulant.

pemphigoid A bullous disease resembling pemphigus, distinguished by thicker-walled bullae arising from erythematous macules or urticarial bases. Oral lesions are uncommon. It may rarely be associated with an internal malignancy. Spontaneous remission occasionally occurs after several years. Treatment is usually with oral corticosteroids. Compare **pemphigus.**

pemphigus An uncommon, serious disease of the skin and mucous membranes, characterized by thin-walled bullae arising from apparently normal skin or mucous membrane. The bullae rupture easily, leaving raw patches. The person loses weight, becomes weak, and is sub-

ject to major infections. Treatment with corticosteroids and other immunosuppressive medications has changed the prognosis of this disease from an almost universally fatal one to a controllable problem compatible with a nearly normal life. The cause is unknown. Compare **pemphigoid.**

pendular nystagmus An undulating involuntary movement of the eyeball.

penetrance In genetics: a variable factor that modifies basic patterns of inheritance. It is the regularity with which an inherited trait is manifest in the person who carries the gene. If a gene always produces its effect on the phenotype, it is fully and completely penetrant. Achondroplasia is caused by a fully penetrant gene; if the gene is present, achondroplasia results. If a gene produces its effect less frequently than 100% of the time, it is not fully penetrant. Retinoblastoma develops in 90% of the children carrying the gene; in 10% of the children, the gene is nonpenetrant. —**penetrant,** *adj.*

penfluridol An investigational antipsychotic drug, chemically similar to pimozide.

penicillamine See **D-penicillamine.**

penicillic acid An antibiotic compound isolated from various species of the fungus *Penicillium.*

penicillin Any one of a group of antibiotics derived from cultures of species of the fungus *Penicillium* or produced semisynthetically. Various penicillins administered for the treatment of bacterial infections exert their antimicrobial action by inhibiting the biosynthesis of cell wall mucopeptides during active multiplication of the organisms. Penicillin G (benzylpenicillin), a widely used therapeutic agent for meningococcal, pneumococcal, and streptococcal infections, syphilis, and a number of other diseases, is rapidly absorbed when injected intramuscularly or subcutaneously, but it is inactivated by gastric acid and hydrolyzed by penicillinase produced by most strains of *Staphylococcus aureus.* Penicillin V (phenethicillin) is also active against gram-positive cocci, with the exception of penicillinase-producing staphylococci, and, since it is resistant to gastric acid, it is effective when administered orally. Penicillins resistant to the action of the enzyme penicillinase (beta-lactamase) are cloxacillin, dicloxacillin, methicillin, nafcillin, and oxacillin. Ampicillin, amoxicillin, carbenicillin, and hetacillin are broad-spectrum penicillins that are active against gram-negative organizations, including *Escherichia coli, Hemophilus influenzae, Neisseria gonorrhoeae, Proteus mirabilis,*and species of *Pseudomonas.* Hypersensitivity reactions are common in patients receiving penicillin and may appear in the absence of prior exposure to the drug. The most common hypersensitivity reactions are rash, fever, and bronchospasm, followed in frequency by vasculitis, serum sickness, and exfoliative dermatitis. Some patients develop severe erythema multiforme accompanied by headache, fever, arthralgia, and conjunctivitis (Stevens-Johnson syndrome); the most frequent cause of anaphylactic shock is an injection of penicillin.

penicillinase An enzyme elaborated by certain bacteria, including many strains of staphylococci, which inactivates penicillin and thereby promotes resistance to the antibiotic. A purified preparation of penicillinase, derived from cultures of saprophytic, spore-forming *Bacillus cereus,* is used in the treatment of adverse reactions to penicillin. Also called beta-lactamase.

penicillinase-producing staphylococci Strains of staphylococcal organisms that elaborate the penicillin inactivating enzyme penicillinase (beta-lactamase) and thereby resist the bacteriocidal action of the antibiotic.

penicillinase-resistant antibiotic An antimicrobial agent that is not rendered inactive by penicillinase, an enzyme produced by certain bacteria, especially by strains of staphylococci. The semisynthetic penicillins—as cloxacillin sodium, dicloxacillin sodium, methicillin sodium, nafcillin sodium, and oxacillin sodium—resist the action of penicillinase and are used in treating infections caused by staphylococci that elaborate the enzyme.

penicillinase-resistant penicillin One of the semisynthetic penicillins derived from *Penicillium,* a genus of mold. Among these drugs are cloxacillin sodium, dicloxacillin sodium, methicillin sodium, nafcillin sodium, and oxacillin sodium. They are not inactivated by penicillinase, which is produced by certain strains of staphylococci. These resistant antibiotics are used in treating infections caused by organisms that elaborate the enzyme.

penicillin G benzathine, p.G. potassium, p.G. procaine, p.G. sodium Penicillin antibiotics.

penicillin phenoxymethyl See **penicillin V.**

penicillin V, p.V. potassium Penicillin antibiotics.

penicilliosis Pulmonary infection caused by fungi of the genus *Penicillium.*

Penicillium A genus of fungi, some species of which have been tentatively linked to disease in humans. Penicillin G is obtained from *Penicillium chrysogenum* and *P. notatum.*

penile cancer A rare malignancy of the penis occurring in uncircumcised men and associated with genital herpesvirus infection and poor personal hygiene. Smegma may be a causative factor, but the specific substances and mechanisms are unknown. Leukoplakia or the flat-topped papules of balanitis xerotica obliterans may be premalignant lesions, and the velvety, red, painful papules of Queyrat's erythroplasia are penile squamous cell carcinoma in situ. Cancer of the penis is characterized by a bleeding ulcer and metastasizes early in its course. Surgical treatment involves partial or total amputation of the penis and excision of inguinal nodes and adjacent tissue when necessary. Radiotherapy is often used preoperatively and postoperatively. Methotrexate or bleomycin may also be administered, especially in metastatic disease.

penis The external reproductive organ of a man, homologous with the clitoris of a woman. It is attached with ligaments to the front and sides of the pubic arch and is composed of three cylindrical masses of cavernous tissue covered with skin. The corpora cavernosa penis surround a median mass called the corpus spongiosum penis, which contains the greater part of the urethra. The subcutaneous fascia of the penis is directly continuous with that of the scrotum, which contains the testes.

-pennate A combining form meaning 'having feathers': *bipennate, pennate.*

penniform Of or pertaining to the shape of a feather, especially the patterns of muscular fasciculi that correlate with the range of motion and the power of muscles. Penniform fasciculi converge on one side of certain tendons. Compare **bipenniform, multipenniform.**

pent-, penta- A combining form meaning 'five': *pentaploid, pentose, pentoside.*

pentaerythritol tetranitrate A coronary vasodilator.

pentamidine An antiprotozoal that is available only from the Centers for Disease Control. It is sometimes prescribed in the treatment of trypanosomiasis and leishmaniasis, but, owing to its extreme toxicity, other agents are usually prescribed.

pentaploid, pentaploidic See **polyploid.**

pentazocine hydrochloride, p. lactate Narcotic analgesics that have narcotic antagonist activity.

pentobarbital, p. sodium Barbiturate sedative-hypnotics.

pentose A monosaccharide with five carbon atoms ($C_5H_{10}O_5$); for example, ribose and xylose.

pentosuria A rare condition in which pentose is found in the urine, caused by a genetically transmitted error of metabolism.

pentylenetetrazol A respiratory stimulant.

Pepper syndrome A neuroblastoma of the right adrenal gland that usually metastasizes to the liver.

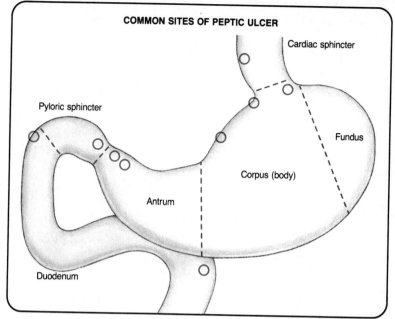

COMMON SITES OF PEPTIC ULCER

Cardiac sphincter

Pyloric sphincter

Fundus

Corpus (body)

Antrum

Duodenum

peps- A combining form meaning 'of or pertaining to digestion': *pepsin, pepsiniferous.* Also **pept-.**

-pepsia, -pepsy A combining form meaning a 'state of the digestion': *anapepsia, colodyspepsia.*

pepsin An enzyme secreted in the stomach that catalyzes the hydrolysis of protein. Preparations of pepsin obtained from pork and beef stomachs are sometimes used as digestive aids. See also **enzyme, hydrolysis.**

pept- See **peps-.**

peptic Of or pertaining to digestion or to the enzymes and secretions essential to digestion.

-peptic A combining form meaning: **1.** 'Pertaining to digestion': *apeptic, kolypeptic.* **2.** 'Pertaining to a (specified) condition of digestion': *dyspeptic, hyperpeptic.*

peptic ulcer A sharply circumscribed loss of the mucous membrane of the stomach, duodenum, or of any other part of the gastrointestinal system exposed to gastric juices containing acid and pepsin. Peptic ulcers may be acute or chronic. Acute lesions are almost always multiple and superficial. They may be totally asymptomatic and usually heal without scarring. Chronic ulcers are deep, single, persistent, and symptomatic; the muscular coat of the wall of the organ does not regenerate; a scar forms, marking the site, and the mucosa may heal completely. Characteristically, ulcers cause a gnawing pain in the epigastrium that has a temporal pattern that mimics the diurnal rhythm of gastric acidity. Symptomatic relief is provided with antacids and frequent, small, bland meals. The underlying cause is treated if known. Cimeti-

dine is an effective drug that blocks the formation of gastric acid, but it is associated with serious adverse effects. Anticholinergic medications may slow gastric motility and diminish pain in some patients. Hemorrhage owing to perforation of the muscle and blood vessels may require surgical resection of the damaged area. NURSING CONSIDERATIONS: The patient is reassured that in most cases the ulcers heal completely and that the pain may be controlled with simple measures. The nurse emphasizes the correct use of antacids and other prescribed medications. It is usually recommended that the patient eat frequent small meals of nonirritating foods; fatty, highly spiced, heavy, or fibrous foods often provoke pain. The use of tobacco and alcohol is discouraged. Also called **gastric ulcer.**

peptide A compound composed of two or more amino acids joined by peptide bonds. See also **amino acid, polypeptide, protein.**

per- A combining form meaning: **1.** 'Throughout, or completely': *peracephalus, perfuse.* **2.** 'A large amount (in chemical terms)' or to designate a combination of an element in its highest valence: *peracetate, perhydride.*

perceived severity In health-belief model: a person's perception of the seriousness of the consequences of contracting a disease. Compare **perceived susceptibility.**

perceived susceptibility In health-belief model: a person's perception of the likelihood of contracting a disease. Compare **perceived severity.**

percentage depth dose In radiotherapy: the amount of radiation delivered at a specified dose, expressed as a percentage of the skin dose.

INSERTION SITE IN PERCUTANEOUS TRANSHEPATIC CHOLANGIOGRAPHY

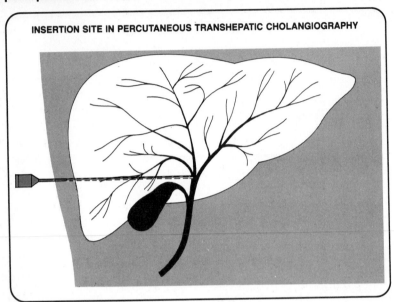

percephalus, *pl.* **percephali** A fetus or individual with a malformed head.

percept The mental impression of an object that is perceived through the use of the senses.

perception **1.** The conscious recognition and interpretation of sensory stimuli through unconscious associations, especially memory, that serve as a basis for understanding, learning, and knowing or for the motivation of a particular action or reaction. **2.** The end result or product of perceiving. Kinds of perception include **depth perception, extrasensory perception, facial perception, stereognostic perception.** **—perceptive, perceptual,** *adj.*

perceptivity The ability to receive sense impressions; perceptiveness.

perceptual defect Any of a broad group of disorders or dysfunctions of the central nervous system that interfere with the conscious mental recognition of sensory stimuli. Such conditions are caused by lesions at specific sites in the cerebral cortex that may result from any illness or trauma affecting the brain at any age or stage of development. Impairment of mental activity, cognitive processes, and emotional responses may be diffuse, as occurs in organic mental disorders, as the psychoses, delirium, and dementia, and in attention deficit disorder, or they may be manifested focally, as in aphasia, apraxia, epilepsy, disorders of memory, cerebrovascular disorders, and various intercranial neoplasms.

perchloromethane See **carbon tetrachloride.**

percolation **1.** The act of filtering any liquid through a porous medium. **2.** In pharmocology: the removal of the soluble parts of a crude drug by passing a liquid solvent through it.

percussion A technique in physical examination used to evaluate the size, borders, and consistency of some of the internal organs and to discover the presence and evaluate the amount of fluid in a cavity of the body. Direct or immediate percussion refers to percussion performed by striking the fingers directly on the body surface; finger, indirect, or mediate percussion involves striking a finger of one hand on a finger of the other hand as it is placed over the organ. See also **pleximeter. —percuss,** *v.,* **percussable,** *adj.*

percussor A small, hammerlike diagnostic tool having a rubber head that is used to tap the body lightly in percussion. Also called plexor. See also **percussion.**

percutaneous Of a procedure: performed through the skin, as the aspiration of fluid from a space below the skin using a needle, catheter, and syringe or the instillation of a fluid in a cavity or space by similar means.

percutaneous catheter placement In arteriography: the technique in which an intracatheter is introduced through the skin into an artery and placed at the place or structure to be studied. Selective angiography and other diagnostic procedures are performed using this technique.

percutaneous transhepatic cholangiography In diagnostic radiology: a procedure for outlining the major bile ducts. A radiopaque contrast material is injected or a catheter introduced through the skin into the liver.

percutaneous transluminal coronary angioplasty (PTCA) A technique in the treatment of atherosclerotic coronary heart disease and angina pectoris in which one or more plaques in the arteries of the heart are flattened

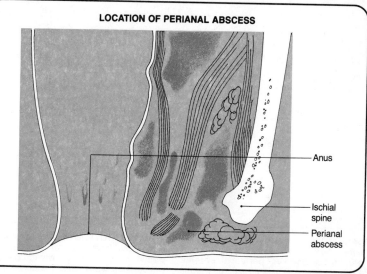

LOCATION OF PERIANAL ABSCESS

- Anus
- Ischial spine
- Perianal abscess

against the arterial walls, resulting in improved circulation. The procedure involves threading a catheter through the vessel to the atherosclerotic plaque and inflating and deflating a small balloon at the tip of the catheter several times, then removing the catheter. The procedure is performed under X-ray or ultrasonic visualization. When it is successful, the plaques remain compressed and the symptoms of heart disease, including the pain of angina, are decreased. The alternative to this treatment is coronary bypass surgery, which is more expensive and dangerous and requires longer hospitalization.

Perez reflex   The normal response of an infant to cry, flex the limbs, and elevate the head and pelvis when supported in a prone position with a finger pressed along the spine from the sacrum to the neck. Persistence of the reflex beyond the age of 6 months may indicate brain damage.

perforate   **1.** To pierce, punch, puncture, or otherwise make a hole. **2.** Riddled with small holes. **3.** Of the anus: having a normal opening. **—perforation,** *n.*

perforating fracture   An open fracture caused by a projectile, making a small surface wound.

peri-   A combining form meaning 'around': *periaxial, pericardial.*

perianal abscess   A focal, purulent, subcutaneous infection in the region of the anus. Treatment includes hot soaks, antibiotics, and, possibly, incision and drainage. If a rectal fistula or sinus track is the cause of recurrent perianal abscesses, surgical excision is usually performed.

periapical   Of or pertaining to the tissues around the apex of a tooth, including the periodontal membrane and the alveolar bone.

periapical abscess   An infection around

the root of a tooth, usually a result of spread from dental caries. The abscess may extend into nearby bone, causing osteomyelitis; more often, it may spread to soft tissues, causing cellulitis and a swollen face, or it may perforate into the oral cavity or maxillary sinus. There may be associated fever, malaise, and nausea. Treatment includes drilling into the pulp of the tooth to establish drainage and relieve pain, followed by antibiotics and, later, root canal therapy or tooth extraction.

periapical infection   Infection surrounding the root of a tooth, often accompanied by toothache.

periarteritis   An inflammatory condition of the outer coat of one or more arteries and the tissue surrounding the vessel. Kinds of periarteritis are **periarteritis nodosa, syphilitic periarteritis.**

periarteritis gummosa   See **syphilitic periarteritis.**

periarteritis nodosa   A progressive, polymorphic disease of the connective tissue that is characterized by numerous large and palpable or visible nodules in clusters along segments of middle-sized arteries, particularly near points of bifurcation. This process causes occlusion of the vessel, resulting in regional ischemia, hemorrhage, necrosis, and pain. The early signs of the disease include tachycardia, fever, weight loss, and pain in the viscera. Kidney, lung, and intestinal involvement are common. Other systems and organs of the body may also be affected. Periarteritis nodosa is treated with corticosteroid medication and sometimes with cytotoxic drugs. The rate of survival 4 years after diagnosis is approximately 50%.

pericardial artery   One of several small vessels branching from the thoracic aorta, supplying the dorsal surface of the pericardium.

PERICARDIUM: GROSS ANATOMY

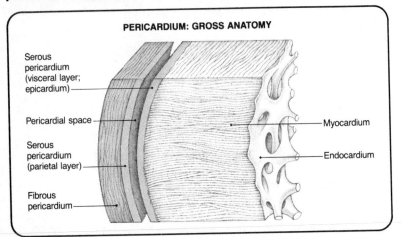

Serous pericardium (visceral layer; epicardium)

Pericardial space

Serous pericardium (parietal layer)

Fibrous pericardium

Myocardium

Endocardium

pericardial tamponade See **cardiac tamponade.**

pericardiocentesis, pericardicentesis A procedure for drawing fluid in the pericardial space between the serous membranes by surgical puncture and aspiration of the pericardial sac.

pericarditis An inflammation of the pericardium owing to trauma, malignant neoplastic disease, infection, uremia, myocardial infarction, collagen disease, or idiopathic causes. Two stages are observed if treatment in the first stage does not halt progress of the condition to the extremely grave second stage. The first stage is characterized by fever, substernal chest pain that radiates to the shoulder or neck, dyspnea, and a dry, nonproductive cough. On examination, a rapid and forcible pulse, a pericardial friction rub, and a muffled heartbeat over the apex are noted. The patient becomes increasingly anxious, tired, and orthopneic. During the second stage, a serofibrinous effusion develops within the pericardium, restricting cardiac activity; the heart sounds become muffled, weak, and distant on auscultation. A bulge is visible on the chest over the precordial area. If the effusion is purulent, owing to bacterial infection, a high fever, sweats, chills, and prostration also occur. Hypothermia treatment may be necessary to reduce the temperature. Antibiotic or antifungal, analgesic, and anti-inflammatory drugs may be ordered. The patient is kept in bed, and the head of the bed is elevated 45° to decrease dyspnea. Oxygen and parenteral fluids are usually given, vital signs are evaluated, and the chest is auscultated frequently. Pericardiocentesis or pericardiotomy may be performed to remove accumulated fluid or to make a diagnosis.

pericardium, *pl.* **pericardia** A fibroserous sac that surrounds the heart and the roots of the great vessels. It consists of the serous pericardium and the fibrous pericardium. The serous pericardium consists of the parietal layer, which lines the inside of the fibrous pericardium, and the visceral layer, which adheres to the surface of the heart. Between the two layers is the pericardial space containing a few drops of pericardial fluid, which lubricates opposing surfaces of the space and allows the heart to move easily during contraction. Injury or disease may cause fluid to exude into the space, causing a wide separation between the heart and the outer pericardium. The fibrous pericardium, which constitutes the outermost sac and is composed of tough, white fibrous tissue lined by the parietal layer of the serous pericardium, fits loosely around the heart and attaches to large blood vessels emerging from the top of the heart but not to the heart itself. It is relatively inelastic and protects the heart and the serous membranes. **—pericardial,** *adj.*

pericholangitis An inflammatory condition of the tissues surrounding the bile ducts in the liver. Pericholangitis is a complication of ulcerative colitis and is characterized by a recurrent fever, chills, jaundice, and, possibly, portal hypertension. Treatment of the ulcerative colitis has little effect on the liver disease. See also **ulcerative colitis.**

peridural anesthesia See **epidural anesthesia.**

perifolliculitis Inflammation of the tissue surrounding a hair follicle. Compare **folliculitis.**

perikaryon The cytoplasm of a cell body exclusive of the nucleus and any processes, specifically the cell body of a neuron. **—perikaryontic,** *adj.*

perilymph The clear fluid separating the osseous labyrinth from the membranous labyrinth in the internal ear. Compare **endolymph.**

perinatal Of or pertaining to the time and process of giving birth or being born.

perinatal death **1.** The death of a fetus weighing more than 1,000 g (2¼ lb) at 28 or more weeks of gestation. **2.** The death of an infant between birth and the end of the neonatal period.

perinatal mortality The statistical rate of fetal and infant death, including stillbirths, from 28 weeks of gestation to the end of the neonatal period of 4 weeks after birth. Perinatal mortality is usually expressed as the number of deaths per 1,000 live births in a specific geographical area or program in a given period of time.

perinatal physiology The physiology of the process of giving birth or being born.

perinatologist A physician who specializes in the practice of perinatology.

perinatology A branch of medicine concerned with the study of the anatomy and physiology of the mother and her unborn and newborn infant and with the diagnosis and treatment of disorders occurring in them during pregnancy, childbirth, and the puerperium. —**perinatologic, perinatological,** *adj.*

perineal care A cleansing procedure prescribed for cleansing the perineum after various obstetric and gynecologic procedures. Sterile or clean perineal care may be prescribed.

perineorrhaphy A surgical procedure in which a tear or defect in the perineum is repaired by suturing.

perineotomy A surgical incision into the perineum. See also **episiotomy.**

perineum The part of the body situated dorsal to the pubic arch and the arcuate ligaments, ventral to the tip of the coccyx, and lateral to the inferior rami of the pubis and the ischium and the sacrotuberus ligaments. The perineum supports and surrounds the distal portions of the urogenital and gastrointestinal tracts of the body. In the female, the central fibrous perineal body between the vagina and the anus is larger than in the male, and the bulbospongiosus, which is a sphincter around the orifice of the vagina and a cover over the clitoris, does not exist in the male perineum. —**perineal,** *adj.*

period *Nontechnical.* Menses.

periodic Of an event or phenomenon: recurring at regular or irregular intervals. —**periodicity,** *n.*

periodical mania A mood disorder in which successive attacks of mania of varied duration occur at regular intervals. See also **mania.**

periodic apnea of the newborn A normal condition in the full-term newborn that is characterized by an irregular pattern of rapid breathing followed by a brief period of apnea, usually associated with rapid-eye-movement (REM) sleep. Apnea in the newborn not associated with REM sleep or with periodic breathing is symptomatic of intracranial bleeding, seizure activity, infection, pneumonia, hypoglycemia, drug depression, or various cardiac defects. See also **sudden infant death syndrome.**

periodic deep inspiration In respiratory therapy: periodic deep, forced inspiration of compressed gas or air in controlled ventilation. Many ventilators can be set to provide a selected number of deep respirations each hour. The process helps to prevent atelectasis. Also called sigh.

periodontal Of or pertaining to the area around a tooth, as the peridontium.

periodontal disease Disease of the tissues around a tooth, as an inflammation of the periodontal membrane.

periodontics, periodontia A branch of dentistry concerned with the diagnosis, treatment, and prevention of diseases of the periodontium. —**periodontic, periodontal,** *adj.*

periodontist A dentist who specializes in periodontics.

periodontitis Inflammation of the periodontium, which includes the periodontal ligament, the gingiva, and the alveolar bone. See also **periodontal, periodontal disease, periodontics.**

periorbita The periosteum of the orbit of the eye. It is continuous with the dura mater and the sheath of the optic nerve and extends a process at the margin of the orbit to form the orbital septum. The periorbita is loosely connected to the bones of the orbit, from which it can be easily detached.

periosteum A fibrous vascular membrane covering the bones, except at their extremities. It consists of an outer layer of collagenous tissue containing a few fat cells and an inner layer of fine elastic fibers. Periosteum is permeated with the nerves and blood vessels that innervate and nourish underlying bone.

peripheral Of or pertaining to the outside, surface, or surrounding area of an organ or other structure.

peripheral acrocyanosis of the newborn A normal, transient condition of the newborn, characterized by pale cyanotic discoloration of the hands and feet, especially the fingers and toes. The blueness fades as the infant begins to breathe easily but returns if the infant is allowed to get chilled.

peripheral glioma See **schwannoma.**

peripheral nervous system The motor and sensory nerves and ganglia outside the brain and spinal cord. The system consists of 12 pairs of cranial nerves, 31 pairs of spinal nerves, and the various branches of the 43 pairs in body organs. Sensory, or afferent, peripheral nerves transmitting information to the central nervous system and motor, or efferent, peripheral nerves carrying impulses from the brain usually travel together but separate at the cord level into a posterior sensory root and an anterior motor root. Fibers innervating the body wall are designated somatic, and those supplying internal organs are termed visceral. The autonomic system includes the peripheral nerves involved in regulating cardiovascular, respiratory, endocrine, and other automatic body functions. Nerves in the sympathetic or thoracolumbar division of the autonomic system secrete norepinephrine and cause peripheral vasoconstriction, cardiac acceleration, coronary artery dilation, bronchodilation, and inhibition of peristalsis. Parasympathetic nerves constitute the craniosacral division of the autonomic system, secrete acetylcholine, and cause peripheral vasodilation, cardiac inhibition, bronchoconstriction, and

---

PERITONEAL DIALYSIS: COMPARISON WITH HEMODIALYSIS

PERITONEAL DIALYSIS

Advantages
- Can be performed immediately

- Requires less complex equipment and less specialized personnel than hemodialysis

- Requires small amounts of heparin or none at all

- No blood loss, minimal cardiovascular stress

- Can be performed by patient anywhere (continuous ambulatory peritoneal dialysis), without assistance and with minimal patient teaching

- Allows patient independence without long interruptions in daily activities

- Lower cost

Disadvantages
- Contraindicated within 72 hours of abdominal surgery

- Requires 48 to 72 hours for significant response to treatment

- Severe protein loss necessitates high-protein diet (up to 100 g/day).

- High risk of peritonitis; repeated bouts may cause adhesions, preventing further treatments with peritoneal dialysis.

- Urea clearance less than with hemodialysis (60%)

HEMODIALYSIS

Advantages
- Takes only 3 to 8 hours per treatment

- Faster results in an acute situation

- Total number of hours of maintenance treatment is only half that of peritoneal dialysis.

- In an acute situation, can use an I.V. route without a surgical access route

Disadvantages
- Requires surgical creation of a vascular access between circulation and dialysis machine

- Requires complex water treatment, dialysis equipment, and highly trained personnel

- Requires administration of larger amounts of heparin

- Confines patient to special treatment unit

---

stimulate peristalsis. Injury to a peripheral nerve results in loss of movement and sensation in the area innervated distal to the lesion.

peripheral plasma cell myeloma   See **plasmacytoma.**

peripheral polyneuritis   See **multiple peripheral neuritis.**

peripheral vascular disease   Any abnormal condition which affects the blood vessels outside the heart and the lymphatic vessels. Signs and symptoms include numbness, pain, pallor, elevated blood pressure, and impaired arterial pulsations. Causes include obesity, cigarette smoking, stress, sedentary occupations, and numerous metabolic disorders. Peripheral vascular disease in association with bacterial endocarditis may involve emboli in terminal arterioles and produce gangrenous infarctions of distal parts of the body. Large emboli may occlude peripheral vessels and cause atherosclerotic occlusive disease. Treatment of severe cases may require amputation of gangrenous body parts. Less severe cases may be treated by eliminating causative factors, especially cigarette smoking, and by the administration of various drugs, such as vasodilators. Some kinds of peripheral vascular disease are **arteriosclerosis, atherosclerosis.**

peripheral vision   A capacity to see objects that reflect light to areas of the retina distant from the macula.

peristalsis   The coordinated, rhythmic, serial contraction of smooth muscle that forces food through the digestive tract, bile through the bile duct, and urine through the ureters.

peritoneal cavity   The potential space between the parietal and the visceral layers of the peritoneum. Normally, the two layers are in contact. The peritoneal cavity is divided by a narrow constriction into a greater sac—the peritoneal cavity—and a lesser sac —the omental bursa. The omental bursa is associated with the dorsal surface of the stomach and the surrounding structures. See also **epiploic foramen.**

peritoneal dialysis   A procedure performed to correct an imbalance of fluid or of electrolytes in the blood or to remove toxins, drugs, or other wastes normally excreted by the kidney. The peritoneum is used as a diffusible membrane. Peritoneal dialysis may be performed nightly for chronically ill children while they sleep and may also be carried out regularly at home. It is contraindicated in patients with extensive intra-abdominal adhesions, localized peritoneal infection, and gangrenous or perforated bowels, although peritonitis may itself sometimes be treated by peritoneal lavage and antibiotics, using peritoneal dialysis. Under local anesthesia, a many-eyed catheter is sutured in place, and a sterile dressing is applied. The catheter is connected to the inflow and outflow tubing with a Y-connector, and the air in the tubing is displaced by the dialysate to avoid introducing air into the peritoneal cavity. The amount and the kind of dialysate and the length of time for each exchange cycle vary with the age, size, and condition of the patient. There are three phases in each cycle. During inflow, the dialysate is introduced into the peritoneal cavity. During equilibration, the dialysate remains in the peritoneal cavity; by means of osmosis, diffusion, and filtration, the needed electrolytes pass to the bloodstream via the vascular peritoneum to the blood vessels of the abdominal cavity, and the waste products pass from the blood vessels through the vascular peritoneum into the dialysate. During the third phase, called outflow, the dialysate is allowed to drain from the peritoneal cavity by gravity. The fluid is warmed to body temperature before instillation, and heparin antibiotics or other additives may be added to the dialysate. The patient's fluid balance, respirations, pulse, blood pressure, temperature, and mental state are frequently evaluated, and blood glucose and electrolytes are tested regularly. The amount of fluid instilled and the amount and character of the fluid drained are noted. Bacteriologic cultures of the drainage are performed regularly, and a low-sodium, high-carbohydrate, high-fat, 20- to 40-g protein diet is usually given. Medication for pain may be necessary. The need for dialysis and the techniques, dangers, and advantages of peritoneal dialysis are explained to the patient and the patient's family. Peritoneal dialysis may result in several complications, including perforation of the bowel, peritonitis, atelectasis, pneumonia, pulmonary edema, hyperglycemia, hypovolemia, hypervolemia, and adhesions. Peritonitis, the most common problem, is usually caused by failure to use aseptic technique and is characterized by fever, cloudy dialysate, leukocytosis, and abdominal discomfort. Dialysis may usually be continued while the infection is treated with antibiotics, which are given systemically or intraperitoneally. Atelectasis and pneumonia may result from compression of the thoracic cavity, with decreased respiratory excursion and blood flow to the bases of the lungs caused by an excessive volume of dialysate in the peritoneal cavity. Dyspnea, tachypnea, rales, and tachycardia require reevaluation of the amount of dialysate, the raising of the head of the bed, and respiratory therapy to prevent atelectasis and pneumonia. As diabetics are at risk of developing hyperglycemia, serum and urine glucose levels are monitored, and, if necessary, sorbitol may be substituted for glucose in the dialysate. If dialysate fluid is retained in the peritoneal cavity, hypervolemia may occur, predisposing the patient to pulmonary edema and congestive failure. If the dialysate is removed too rapidly or if the dialysate used is a hypotonic glucose solution, hypovolemia may result. Adhesions often develop because of local irritation to the surrounding tissues caused by the intraperitoneal catheter.

peritoneal dialysis solution A solution of electrolytes and other substances introduced into the peritoneum to remove toxic substances from the body and to correct electrolyte and acid-base imbalances. Also called **dialysate.**

peritoneoscope See **laparoscope.**

peritoneum An extensive serous membrane that covers the entire abdominal wall of the body and is reflected over the contained viscera. It is divided into the parietal peritoneum and the visceral peritoneum. In men, it is a closed membranous sac. In women, it is perforated by the free ends of the uterine tubes. The free surface of the peritoneum is smooth mesothelium lubricated by serous fluid, which permits the viscera to glide easily against the abdominal wall and against one another. The mesentery of the peritoneum fans out from the main membrane to suspend the small intestine. Other parts of the peritoneum are the transverse mesocolon, the greater omentum, and the lesser omentum. —**peritoneal,** *adj.*

peritonitis An inflammation of the peritoneum produced by bacteria or irritating substances introduced into the abdominal cavity by a penetrating wound or perforation of an organ in the gastrointestinal tract or the reproductive tract. Peritonitis is caused most commonly by rupture of the vermiform appendix but also occurs following perforations of intestinal diverticuli, peptic ulcers, gangrenous gallbladder, gangrenous obstructions of the small bowel, or incarcerated hernias, as well as ruptures of the spleen, liver, ovarian cyst, or fallopian tube, especially in ectopic pregnancy. In some cases, peritonitis is secondary to the release of pancreatic enzyme, bile, or digestive juices of the upper gastrointestinal tract, and there are reports of postoperative peritonitis caused by cornstarch used to powder surgical gloves. The genera most frequently identified as causative agents in peritonitis are *Escherichia coli, Bacteroides, Fusobacterium,* anaerobic and aerobic streptococci, *Klebsiella* and *Proteus* are uncommon and *Clostridium, Staphylococcus aureus,* and gonococci are rare. Pneumococci occasionally found in peritonitis in young females are thought to enter the abdominal cavity via the vagina and fallopian tubes. Characteristic signs and symptoms of peritonitis include abdominal distention, rigidity and pain, rebound tenderness, decreased or absent bowel sounds, nausea, vomiting, and tachycardia. The patient has chills and fever, breathes rapidly and shallowly, is anxious, dehydrated, unable to defecate, and may vomit fecal material. Leukocytosis, an electrolyte imbalance, and hypovolemia are usually present, and shock and heart failure may ensue. Paracentesis may be performed to withdraw ascitic fluid that is turbid or purulent in pyogenic peritonitis. Repair of the perforation or rupture responsible for the infection may be indicated, but surgery is usually delayed until the patient is stabilized.

NURSING CONSIDERATIONS: The patient is placed in bed in a semi-Fowler's position with the knees flexed to facilitate breathing and localize pus in the lower abdomen. Parenteral fluids with electrolytes, large doses of antibiotics, and emetics are administered as ordered. A nasogastric or nasointestinal tube is passed, an indwelling catheter is inserted, and a rectal tube may be

PERMANENT DENTITION

Maxillary
1. Central incisor: age 7 to 8
2. Lateral incisor: age 8 to 9
3. Canine: age 11 to 12
4. First premolar: age 9 to 11
5. Second premolar: age 10 to 12
6. First molar: age 6 to 7
7. Second molar: age 12 to 13
8. Third molar: age 17 to 25

Mandibular
9. Central incisor: age 6 to 7
10. Lateral incisor: age 7 to 8
11. Canine: age 11 to 12
12. First premolar: age 9 to 12
13. Second premolar: age 11 to 12
14. First molar: age 6 to 7
15. Second molar: age 12 to 13
16. Third molar: age 17 to 25

used. Measurements are made of the intake and output of fluids, and the character, color, odor, and amount of drainage are noted. The patient is observed for changes in blood pressure, apical pulse, respiration, rectal temperature, bowel sounds, and abdominal distention. Pain is controlled with analgesia. The patient acutely ill with peritonitis is usually very apprehensive and needs constant care.

peritonsillar abscess   An infection of tissue between the tonsil and pharynx, usually following acute follicular tonsillitis. The symptoms include dysphagia, pain radiating to the ear, and fever. Redness and swelling of the tonsil and adjacent soft palate are present. Treatment includes penicillin, warm saline irrigation, incision and drainage with suction if there is no spontaneous rupture of the abscess, and, sometimes, tonsillectomy. Also called **quinsy.** Compare **parapharyngeal abscess, retropharyngeal abscess.** See also **tonsillitis.**

periungual   Of or pertaining to the area around the fingernails or the toenails.

perivascular goiter   An enlargement of the thyroid gland surrounding a large blood vessel.

perivitelline   Surrounding the vitellus or yolk mass.

perivitelline space   The space between the ovum and the zona pellucida of mammals into which the polar bodies are released at the time of maturation. In some animals it is a fluid-filled space that separates the fertilization membrane from the vitelline membrane surrounding the ovum after the penetration of the spermatozoon.

perlèche   See **cheilosis.**

permanent dentition   The eruption of the 32 permanent teeth, beginning with the appearance of the first permanent molars at about 6 years of age. The process is completed by age 12 or 13 except for the 4 wisdom teeth, which do not erupt until 18 to 25 years of age, or later. Also called **secondary dentition.** Compare **deciduous dentition.** See also **tooth.**

permanent tooth   One of the set of 32 teeth that appear during and after childhood and last until old age. In each jaw they include 4 incisors, 2 canines, 4 premolars, and 6 molars. They are divided into the permanent teeth, which replace the 20 deciduous teeth of infancy, and the superadded teeth, which include 12 molars, 3 on each side of the upper and lower jaws. The permanent teeth start to develop in the 9th week of fetal life with the thickening of the epithelium along the line of the future jaw. The permanent teeth start to calcify soon after birth; the teeth in the lower jaw proceeding somewhat faster than those in the upper jaw. The permanent teeth erupt first in the lower jaw; the first molars in about the 6th year; the two central incisors, about the 7th year; the two lateral incisors, about the 8th year; the first premolars, about the 9th year; the second premolars, about the 10th year;

the canines, between the 11th and the 12th years; the second molars, between the 12th and the 13th years; the third molars, between the 17th and the 25th years. The third molars ('wisdom teeth') in many people are underdeveloped, badly oriented, or so deeply buried in bone that they must be surgically removed. Compare **deciduous tooth**. See also **tooth**.

permissible dose In radiotherapy: the amount of radiation that may be received by an individual in a specified period of time with the expectation of no significantly harmful results.

pernicious anemia A progressive, megaloblastic, macrocytic anemia, affecting mainly older people, that results from a lack of intrinsic factor essential for the absorption of vitamin B_{12}. The maturation of red blood cells in bone marrow becomes disordered, the posterior and lateral columns of the spinal cord deteriorate, the white blood cell count is reduced, and the polymorphonuclear leukocytes become multilobed. Extreme weakness, numbness and tingling in the extremities, fever, pallor, anorexia, and loss of weight may occur. The condition is usually treated with vitamin B_{12} injection and with folic acid and iron therapy.

pernio See **chilblain**.

pero- A combining form meaning 'maimed or deformed': *perobrachius, perodactylus.*

perobrachius A fetus or individual with deformed arms.

perochirus A fetus or individual with malformed hands.

perocormus See **perosomus**.

perodactylus A fetus or an individual with a deformity of the fingers or the toes, especially the absence of one or more digits.

perodactyly, perodactylia A congenital anomaly characterized by a deformity of the digits, primarily the complete or partial absence of one or more fingers or toes.

peromelia, peromely A congenital anomaly characterized by the malformation of one or more of the limbs. —**peromelus**, *n*.

peroneal Of or pertaining to the outer part of the leg, over the fibula and the peroneal nerve.

peroneal muscular atrophy An abnormal condition characterized by the symmetrical weakening or atrophy of the foot and the ankle muscles and by hammertoes. This disease is a dominantly inherited condition and occurs in a neuronal form or as a hypertrophic neuropathy. The hypertrophic neuropathy results in demyelination of nerve fibers and characteristic onion-bulb formations. Affected individuals usually have high plantar arches and an awkward gait, caused by weak ankle muscles. In the neuronal form, this condition usually starts in the second decade of life and causes muscle weaknesses similar to those associated with the hypertrophic neuropathy. Both forms of the disease may also involve mild sensory loss in the lower limbs. Corrective surgery and leg braces may stabilize weak ankle joints.

peroneus brevis The smaller of the two lateral muscles of the leg, lying under the per-

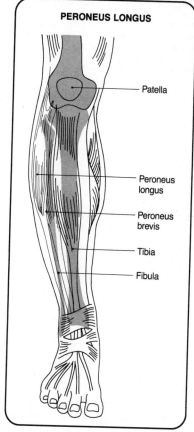

PERONEUS LONGUS

Patella

Peroneus longus

Peroneus brevis

Tibia

Fibula

oneus longus. The peroneus brevis arises from the fibula and inserts into the fifth metatarsal bone. It contains fibers from the fourth and the fifth lumbar and the first sacral nerves. It pronates and plantar flexes the foot. Compare **peroneus longus**.

peroneus longus The more superficial of the two lateral muscles of the leg. It arises from the head and the body of the fibula, converges to a long tendon that crosses the sole of the foot, and inserts into the first metatarsal bone and the medial cuneiform bone. The muscle pronates and plantar flexes the foot. Compare **peroneus brevis**.

peronia A congenital malformation or developmental anomaly.

peropus A fetus or individual with malformed feet, often associated with some defect of the legs.

perosomus A fetus or individual whose body, especially the trunk, is severely malformed. Also called **perocormus**.

perosplanchia A congenital anomaly characterized by the malformation of the viscera.

peroxide See **hydrogen peroxide**.

perphenazine A phenothiazine antipsychotic agent.

PERRLA Acronym for *p*upils *e*qual, *r*ound, *r*eact to *l*ight, *a*ccommodation. In the process of performing an assessment of the eyes, the size and shape of the pupils, their reaction to light, and their ability to accommodate are evaluated.

persistent cloaca A congenital anomaly in which the intestinal, urinary, and reproductive ducts open into a common cavity resulting from the failure of the urorectal septum to form during prenatal development. Also called **congenital cloaca.**

persona, *pl.* **personae** In analytic psychology: the personality or role that a person presents to the outer world in order to satisfy the demands of society or as an expression of some intrapsychic conflict. The persona masks the person's inner being or unconscious self. Compare **anima.** See also **archetype.**

personal and social history In a health history: an account of the personal and social details that serve to identify a person. This includes place of birth, religion, race, marital status, number of children, military status, occupational history, and place of residence, but it may often include education, current living situation, and smoking, alcohol, and drug habits. The personal and social history is obtained at the initial interview and becomes a part of the permanent record.

personality 1. The composite of the behavioral traits and attitudinal characteristics by which one is recognized as an individual. **2.** The pattern of behavior each person evolves, both consciously and unconsciously, as a means of adapting to a particular environment.

personality disorder Any of a large group of mental disorders characterized by rigid, inflexible, and maladaptive behavior patterns that impair a person's ability to function in society by severely limiting adaptive potential. Such a disorder, which is generally recognized during childhood or adolescence, tends to continue through adulthood. Some kinds of personality disorders are **antisocial personality disorder, histrionic personality disorder, paranoid personality disorder, passive-aggressive personality disorder, schizoid personality disorder.** Also called **character disorder.**

personality test Any of a variety of standardized tests used to evaluate or assess facets of personality structure, emotional status, and behavioral traits. Compare **achievement test, aptitude test, intelligence test, psychological test.**

personal orientation 1. A continually evolving process in which a person determines and evaluates the relationships that exist between the person and other people. **2.** The assessment derived by a person regarding those relationships.

personal unconscious In analytic psychology: the thoughts, ideas, emotions, and other mental phenomena that are acquired and repressed during one's lifetime. Compare **collective unconscious.**

perspiration 1. The act or process of perspiring; the excretion of fluid by the sweat glands through pores in the skin. **2.** The fluid excreted by the sweat glands. It consists of water containing sodium chloride, phosphate, urea, ammonia, and other waste products. Perspiration serves as a mechanism for excretion and for regulating body temperature. Kinds of perspiration are **insensible perspiration, sensible perspiration.** See also **diaphoresis.**

Perthes' disease Osteochondrosis of the head of the femur in children, characterized initially by epiphyseal necrosis or degeneration followed by regeneration or recalcification. Also called **coxa plana, Legg-Calvé-Perthes' disease, pseudocoxalgia, Waldenström's disease.**

pertussis An acute, highly contagious respiratory disease characterized by paroxysmal coughing that ends in a loud whooping inspiration. It occurs primarily in children less than 4 years of age who have not been immunized. The causative organism, *Bordetella pertussis,* is a small, nonmotile, gram-negative coccobacillus. A similar organism, *B. parapertussis,* causes a less severe form of the disease called parapertussis. Transmission occurs directly by contact or by inhalation of infectious particles, usually spread by coughing and sneezing, and indirectly through freshly contaminated articles. Diagnosis consists of positive identification of the organism in nasopharyngeal secretions. The incubation period averages 7 to 14 days, followed by 6 to 8 weeks of illness divided into three distinct stages: catarrhal, paroxysmal, and convalescent. Onset of the catarrhal stage is gradual, usually beginning with coryza, sneezing, a dry cough, a slight fever, listlessness, irritability, and anorexia. The cough becomes paroxysmal after 10 to 14 days and occurs as a series of short rapid bursts during expiration followed by the characteristic whoop, a hurried, deep inhalation that has a high-pitched crowing sound. There is usually no fever, and the respiratory rate between paroxysms is normal. During the paroxysm there is marked facial redness or cyanosis and vein distention; the eyes may bulge, the tongue may protrude, and the facial expression usually indicates severe anxiety and distress. Large amounts of a viscid mucus may be expelled during or following paroxysms, which occur from 4 to 5 times a day in mild cases to as many as 40 to 50 times a day in severe cases. Vomiting frequently occurs after the paroxysms because of gagging or choking on the mucus. In infants, choking may be more common than the characteristic whoop. This stage lasts from 4 to 6 weeks. Attacks are most frequent and severe during the first 1 to 2 weeks; then they gradually decline and disappear. During the convalescent stage, a simple, persistent cough is usual. For a period of up to 2 years after the initial attack, paroxysmal coughing may accompany respiratory infections. Routine treatment consists of bed rest, a good diet, and adequate amounts of fluid. Antibiotics may be prescribed to reduce contagiousness or to control secondary infection. Hospitalization may be necessary for infants and children and for those with dehydration or other complications. Oxygen may be needed to relieve dyspnea and cyanosis; intravenous therapy may be necessary when prolonged vomiting interferes with adequate nutrition. Endotracheal intubation is rarely necessary but may be lifesaving in infants if the thick mucus cannot easily be suctioned from the air passages. Pertussis immune globulin is available, but its efficacy has not been established and its use is not recommended. Active immunization is recommended with pertussis vaccine, usually in combination with diphtheria and tetanus toxoids in a series of three injections. One attack of the disease usually confers immunity. Also called **whooping cough.**

pertussis immune globulin A passive immunizing agent against pertussis.

pertussis vaccine An active immunizing agent against pertussis.

perversion **1.** Any deviation from what is considered normal or natural. **2.** The act of causing a change from what is normal or natural. **3.** *Informal.* In psychiatry: any of a number of sexual practices that deviate from what is considered normal adult behavior. See also **paraphilia.**

pervert **1.** *Informal.* A person whose sexual pleasure is derived from stimuli almost universally regarded as unnatural, as a fetishist or sadomasochist; a paraphiliac. **2.** One whose sexual behavior deviates from a social or statistical norm but is not necessarily pathological.

pes cavus A deformity of the foot characterized by an excessively high arch with hyperextension of the toes at the metatarsophalangeal joints, flexion at the interphalangeal joints, and shortening of the Achilles tendon. The condition may be present at birth or appear later owing to contractures or an imbalance of the muscles of the foot, as in neuromuscular diseases. Surgical treatment is indicated in severe cases, especially in childhood, although in milder forms the pain from the excessive pressure under the metatarsal heads can be relieved by spongerubber or leather insoles fitted into the shoes. Also called **clawfoot, gampsodactyly, griffe des orteils, talipes cavus.**

pes planus See **flatfoot.**

pessary A device inserted in the vagina to treat uterine prolapse, uterine retroversion, or cervical incompetence. It is employed in the treatment of women whose advanced age or poor general condition precludes surgical repair. A vaginal cream containing estrogen is usually prescribed to cause the vaginal epithelium to thicken and become more resistant to irritation from the pessary. Pessaries are also used in younger women in evaluating symptomatic uterine retroversion; if pelvic pain is relieved by anteversion of the uterus with the pessary in place and returns when retroversion recurs after the pessary is removed, retroversion is demonstrated to be the cause of pain, and surgical

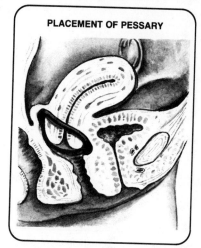

PLACEMENT OF PESSARY

uterine suspension can be expected to provide long-term relief. The pessary is also used in the management of cervical incompetence in pregnancy. It holds the uterus in a forward position in which intra-abdominal and intrauterine pressure cause less stress on the neck of the womb. A pessary must be removed, usually daily, for cleaning. Left in place, the pessary is likely to cause severe irritation, leading to vaginal infection. A **Smith-Hodge pessary** is a rubber or vinyl covered wire rectangle that fits between the pubic bone and the posterior vaginal fornix, supporting the uterus and holding the cervix in a posterior position. A **Gelhorn pessary** is an inflexible device made of lucite in the form of a large collar button. It has a canal through the stem that allows drainage of vaginal secretions. The large end of the pessary is placed deep in the vagina, the small end of the stem protruding at the introitus. A doughnut pessary is a permanently inflated flexible rubber doughnut that is inserted to support the uterus by blocking the canal of the vagina. An inflatable pessary is a collapsible rubber doughnut to which is attached a flexible stem containing a rubber valve. The pessary is inserted collapsed, inflated with a bulb similar to that of a sphygmomanometer, and deflated for removal. A **Bee-cell pessary** is a soft rubber cube wherein each face of the cube is a conical depression that acts as a suction cup when the pessary is in the vagina. A **diaphragm pessary** is a contraceptive diaphragm used for uterovaginal support. A stem pessary is a slim curved rod that is fitted into the cervical canal for uterine positioning. It is rarely used today.

pessimism The inclination to anticipate the worst possible results from any action or situation or to emphasize unfavorable conditions. —**pessimist,** *n.*

pesticide poisoning A toxic condition caused by the ingestion or inhalation of a substance used for eradicating pests. Kinds of pes-

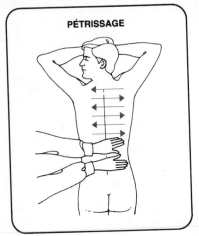

PÉTRISSAGE

ticide poisoning include **malathion poisoning, parathion poisoning.** See also **herbicide poisoning, rodenticide poisoning.**

pestis See **bubonic plague.**

PET *abbr* **positron emission tomography.**

petalo- A combining form meaning 'of or related to a leaf': *petalobacteria, petalococcus.*

petechiae, *sing.* **petechia** Tiny purple or red spots that appear on the skin as a result of minute hemorrhages within the dermal or submucosal layers. Petechiae range from pinpoint to pinhead size and are flush with the surface. Compare **ecchymosis. —petechial,** *adj.*

petechial fever Any febrile illness accompanied by small petechiae on the skin, as seen in the late stage of typhoid fever.

petit mal See **absence seizure.**

petr- A combining form meaning 'of or pertaining to stone': *petrifaction, petroleum.*

pétrissage A technique in massage in which the muscles are alternately kneaded and stroked. Pétrissage promotes circulation and relaxes the muscles. Compare **effleurage, friction, rolling effleurage.**

petrolatum A semisolid mixture of hydrocarbons used as a topical protectant and emollient.

petrolatum gauze Absorbent gauze permeated with white petrolatum.

petroleum distillate poisoning A toxic condition caused by the ingestion or inhalation of a petroleum distillate, as fuel oil, lubricating oil, glue, and various solvents. Nausea, vomiting, chest pain, dizziness, and severe depression of the central nervous system characterize the condition. Severe or fatal pneumonitis may occur if the substance is aspirated; therefore, induced emesis is contraindicated. Gastric lavage with water, a saline cathartic, and oxygen administration, if required, are recommended. See also **gasoline poisoning, kerosene poisoning.**

petrosphenoidal fissure A fissure on the floor of the cranial fossa between the posterior edge of the wing of the sphenoid bone and the

petrous part of the temporal bone.

Peutz-Jeghers syndrome An inherited disorder, transmitted as an autosomal dominant trait, characterized by multiple intestinal polyps and abnormal mucocutaneous pigmentation, usually over the lips and buccal mucosa. If obstruction or bleeding occurs, surgical removal of the polyps may be indicated.

-pexia See **-pexis.**

-pexis A combining form meaning 'a fixation of' something specified: *glycopexis, hemopexis.* Also **-pexia, -pexy.**

-pexy See **-pexis.**

Peyer's patches Groups of lymph nodes in the terminal ileum near its junction with the colon opposite to the juncture of the mesentery. In certain infectious diseases, as typhoid fever, they become ulcerated and enlarged.

peyote 1. A cactus, *Lophophora,* from which a hallucinogenic drug, mescaline, is derived. 2. Mescaline.

Peyronie's disease A disease of unknown cause characterized by fibrous induration of the corpora cavernosa of the penis. An association with Dupuytren's contracture of the palm has been recognized. The chief symptom of Peyronie's disease is painful erection. Palliative treatment includes radiation therapy and intralesional corticosteroid injections. There is no known cure.

PFT *abbr* **pulmonary function test.**

PG *abbr* **prostaglandin.**

PGY *abbr* postgraduate year.

pH A scale representing the relative acidity (or alkalinity) of a solution, in which a value of 7 is neutral, below 7 is acid, and above 7 is alkaline. The numerical pH value indicates the relative concentration of hydrogen ions in the solution compared to that of a standard solution. See also **acid, acid-base balance.**

phaco- A combining form meaning 'of or related to a lens': *phacocele, phacocyst.* Also **phako-.**

phacomalacia An abnormal condition of the eye in which the lens of the eye becomes soft because of a soft cataract.

phacomatosis See **phakomatosis.**

phage See **bacteriophage.**

-phage A combining form meaning 'something that eats' the matter specified: *mycophage, osteophage.* Also **-phag.**

-phagia A combining form meaning: 1. An 'eating of a substance': *autophagia, chthonophagia.* 2. 'Desire for food': *amylophagia, monophagia.*

phago- A combining form meaning 'of or pertaining to eating or ingestion': *phagokaryosis, phagology.*

phagocyte A cell that is able to surround, engulf, and digest microorganisms and cellular debris. **Fixed phagocytes,** which do not circulate, include the fixed macrophages and the cells of the reticuloendothelial system. **Free phagocytes,** which circulate in the bloodstream, include the leukocytes and the free macrophages. **—phagocytic,** *adj.*

PHAGOCYTOSIS: FOUR STAGES

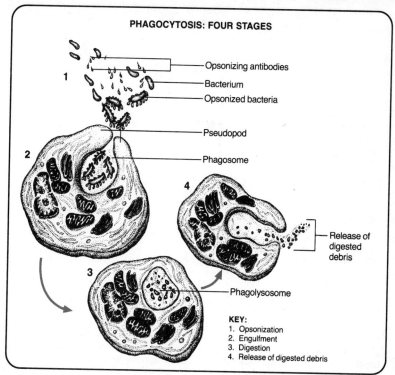

1 — Opsonizing antibodies
— Bacterium
— Opsonized bacteria

— Pseudopod

2 — Phagosome

4

— Release of digested debris

3 — Phagolysosome

KEY:
1. Opsonization
2. Engulfment
3. Digestion
4. Release of digested debris

phagocytosis The process by which certain cells engulf and dispose of microorganisms and cell debris.

-phagy A combining form meaning the 'practice of eating' something specified: *biophagy, coprophagy.* Also **-phagia.**

-phakia A combining form meaning a 'lens': *aphakia.*

phako- See **phaco-.**

phakomatosis, phacomatosis, *pl.* **phakomatoses** In opthalmology: a hereditary syndrome characterized by benign tumorlike nodules of the eye, skin, and brain. The four disorders designated phakomatoses are neurofibromatosis (Recklinghausen's disease), tuberous sclerosis (Bourneville's disease), encephalotrigeminal angiomatosis (Sturge-Weber syndrome), and cerebroretinal angiomatosis (von Hippel-Lindau disease).

-phalangia A combining form meaning a 'condition of the bones of the fingers or toes': *bradyphalangia, symphalangia.*

phalanx, *pl.* **phalanges** Any one of the 14 tapering bones comprising the fingers of each hand and the toes of each foot. They are arranged in 3 rows at the distal end of the metacarpus and the metatarsus. The fingers each have 3 phalanges; the thumb has 2. The toes each have 3 phalanges; the great toe has 2. The phalanges of the foot are smaller and less flexible than those of the hand.

phall- See **phallo-.**

phallic stage In Freudian psychoanalysis: the period in psychosexual development occurring between the ages of 3 and 6 years when emerging awareness and self-manipulation of the genitals are the predominant source of pleasurable experience. Fixation at this stage may lead to extreme aggressiveness in adulthood, or it may be a precipitating factor in the development of psychosexual disorders. See also **psychosexual development.**

phallo-, phall- A combining form meaning 'of or related to the penis': *phallocampsis, phallodynia.*

phalloidine, phalloidin A poison present in the mushroom *Amanita phalloides*. Ingestion of phalloidine results in bloody diarrhea, vomiting, severe abdominal pain, kidney failure, and liver damage. Approximately 50% of phalloidine poisonings are fatal.

phallus See **penis.**

-phane A combining form meaning a 'thing with a (specified) appearance': *diaphane, xanthophane.* Also **-phan.**

phanero- A combining form meaning 'visible or apparent': *phanerogenetic, phaneromania.*

phantom limb syndrome A phenomenon common after amputation of a limb in which sensation or discomfort is experienced in the missing limb. In some people severe pain per-

PHARYNGEAL TONSIL

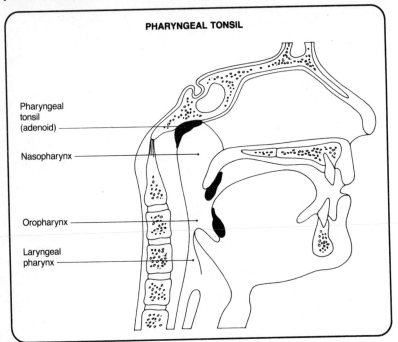

Pharyngeal tonsil (adenoid)

Nasopharynx

Oropharynx

Laryngeal pharynx

sists. See also **pseudesthesia.**

phantom tumor A swelling resembling a tumor, usually caused by muscle contraction or gaseous distention of the intestines.

phao- See **pheo-.**

pharmaceutical 1. Of or pertaining to pharmacy or drugs. **2.** A drug.

pharmaceutical chemistry The science dealing with the composition and preparation of chemical compounds used in medical diagnoses and therapies.

pharmacist A specialist in formulating and dispensing medications. Pharmacists are licensed by the various states to practice pharmacy.

pharmaco- A combining form meaning 'of or related to drugs or medicine': *pharmacochemistry, pharmacomania.*

pharmacogenetics The study of the effect that the genetic factors belonging to a group or to an individual have on the response of the group or the individual to certain drugs.

pharmacokinetics In pharmacology: the study of the action of drugs within the body, including the routes and mechanisms of absorption and excretion, the rate at which a drug's action begins and the duration of the effect, the biotransformation of the substance in the body, and the effects and routes of excretion of the metabolites of the drug.

pharmacological treatment See **treatment.**

pharmacologist A specialist in pharmacology.

pharmacology The study of the preparation, properties, uses, and actions of drugs.

pharmacopoeia, pharmacopeia 1. A compendium containing descriptions, recipes, strengths, standards of purity, and dosage forms for selected drugs. **2.** The available stock of drugs in a pharmacy. **3.** The total of all authorized drugs available within the jurisdiction of a given geographical or political area.

pharmacy 1. The study of preparing and dispensing drugs. **2.** A place for preparing and dispensing drugs.

PharmD *abbr* Doctor of Pharmacy. One trained to practice in a clinical setting, rather than dispensing medication.

-pharmic A combining form meaning 're-lated to drugs and medicinal remedies': *alexipharmic, antipharmic.*

pharyng- See **pharyngo-.**

pharyngeal aponeurosis A sheet of connective tissue just beneath the mucosa of the pharynx.

pharyngeal bursa A blind sac at the base of the pharyngeal tonsil.

pharyngeal reflex See **gag reflex.**

pharyngeal tonsil One of two masses of lymphatic tissue situated on the posterior wall of the nasopharynx behind the posterior nares. During childhood these masses often swell and block the passage of air from the nasal cavity into the pharynx, preventing the child from breathing through the nose.

pharyngitis Inflammation or infection of the pharynx, usually causing symptoms of a sore throat. Some causes of pharyngitis are diphtheria, herpes simplex virus, infectious mononucleosis, and streptococcal infection. Specific treatment depends upon the cause. Symptoms may be relieved by analgesic medication, drinking warm or cold liquids, or saline irrigation of the throat. See also **strep throat.**

pharyngo-, pharyng- A combining form meaning 'of or related to the pharynx': *pharyngocele, pharyngoglossus.*

pharyngoconjunctival fever An adenovirus infection characterized by fever, sore throat, and conjunctivitis. It is an epidemic illness, particularly prevalent in summer, that is spread by droplet infection and direct contact. Contaminated water in lakes and swimming pools is a common source of infection. Also called **swimming pool conjunctivitis.** See also **adenovirus.**

pharynx A tubular structure about 13 cm (5 inches) long that extends from the base of the skull to the esophagus and is situated just in front of the cervical vertebrae. The pharynx serves as a passageway for the respiratory and digestive tracts and changes shape to allow the formation of various vowel sounds. The pharynx is composed of muscle, is lined with mucous membrane, and is divided into the nasopharynx, the oropharynx, and the laryngopharynx. It contains the openings of the right and the left auditory tubes, those of the two posterior nares, the fauces, and those into the larynx and the esophagus. It also contains the pharyngeal tonsils, the palatine tonsils, and the lingual tonsils. Also called **throat.** See also **larynx.**

phase microscope A microscope with a special condenser and objective containing a phase-shifting ring that allows the viewer to see small differences in refraction indexes as differences in image intensity or contrast. Used especially for examining transparent specimens, as living or unstained cells and tissues.

phase of maximum slope The time of rapid cervical dilatation and rapid fetal descent in the active phase of labor. See **Friedman curve.**

-phasia A combining form meaning a 'speech disorder': *agitophasia, logaphasia.*

phasic Referring to a process proceeding in stages or phases.

-phasic A combining form meaning 'relating to a speech disorder': *endophasic, paraphasic.*

-phasis A combining form meaning 'speech, utterance': *allophasis, heterophasis.* Also **-phasia, -phasy.**

-phasy See **-phasis.**

PhD *abbr* Doctor of Philosophy.

-phemia A combining form meaning a '(specified) disorder of speech': *dysphemia, paraphemia.*

phen- A combining form indicating derivation from benzene: *phenacitin, phenicate.*

phenacemide A hydantoin anticonvulsant.

phenacetin A nonnarcotic analgesic and antipyretic agent.

phenazopyridine hydrochloride A urinary tract analgesic.

phencyclidine hydrochloride (PCP) A piperidine derivative administered parenterally to achieve neurolept anesthesia. Because of its marked hallucinogenic properties, it is illegal in the United States for human use.

phendimetrazine tartrate An amphetaminelike central nervous system stimulant used for appetite suppression.

-phene A combining form denoting members of the phenol group: *camphene, phlobaphene.* Also **-phen.**

phenelzine sulfate An MAO (monoamine oxidase) inhibitor antidepressant.

phenic acid See **carbolic acid.**

phenindione An oral anticoagulant of the indandione type.

phenmetrazine hydrochloride An amphetaminelike central nervous system stimulant.

phenobarbital, p. sodium Barbiturate sedative and hypnotic agents.

phenocopy A phenotypic trait or condition that is induced by nongenetic factors but closely resembles a phenotype usually produced by a specific genotype. The trait is neither inherited nor transmitted to offspring. Such conditions as deafness, cretinism, mental retardation, and congenital cataracts are caused by mutant genes but can also result from a number of different agents, as the rubella virus in congenital cataracts. Phenocopies may present problems in genetic screening and counseling so that all exogenous factors must be ruled out before any congenital trait or defect is labeled hereditary.

phenol A coal-tar derivative used as a topical antipruritic agent.

phenol camphor An oily mixture of camphor and phenol, used as an antiseptic and toothache remedy.

phenolphthalein A stimulant laxative.

phenol poisoning Corrosive poisoning caused by the ingestion of compounds containing phenol, as carbolic acid, creosote, and naphthol. Characteristics are burns of the mucous membranes, weakness, pallor, pulmonary edema, convulsion, and respiratory, circulatory, cardiac, and renal failure. In treatment, the skin around the mouth and nose is washed, as are any external burns; the mouth, throat, esophagus, and stomach are lavaged with water and charcoal. Oxygen, intravenous fluids, electrolytes, and pain medication may be necessary. Rarely, esophageal stricture may develop.

phenomenon A sign that is often associated with a specific illness or condition and is, therefore, diagnostically important.

phenothiazine Any of a group of drugs which have a three-ring structure in which two benzene rings are linked by a nitrogen and a sulfur. The most widely used are the two prototypes, chlorpromazine and prochlorperazine; closely related are trimeprazine and triflupromazine. The phenothiazines exert significant influence on many organ systems of the body at once; for example, they exert antiadrenergic, anticholinergic, and antihistaminic activity. All phenothiazines are withheld from patients with

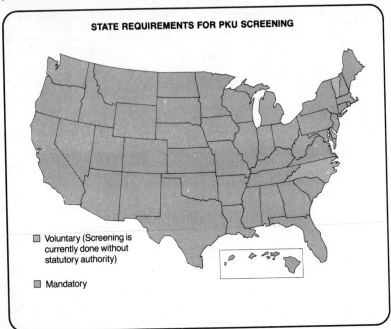

STATE REQUIREMENTS FOR PKU SCREENING

☐ Voluntary (Screening is
   currently done without
   statutory authority)

▨ Mandatory

severe central nervous system depression or epilepsy and are given with caution to those with
liver disease. These drugs are not recommended
for use in pregnancy. See also specific drugs.

phenotype **1.** The complete observable
characteristics of an organism or group, including anatomical, physiological, biochemical,
and behavioral traits, as determined by the interaction of both genetic makeup and environmental factors. **2.** A group of organisms that
resemble each other in appearance. Compare
genotype. —phenotypic, *adj.*

phenoxy- A combining form indicating the
presence of a chemical group composed of phenyl
and an atom of oxygen: *phenoxycaffeine.*

phenoxybenzamine hydrochloride A
sympatholytic antihypertensive that is an alpha-
adrenergic blocking agent.

phenoxymethyl penicillin See **penicillin
V.**

phenprocoumon An oral anticoagulant of
the coumarin type.

phensuximide A succinimide anticonvulsant agent.

phentermine hydrochloride An amphetaminelike central nervous system stimulant.

**phentolamine hydrochloride, p. me-
sylate, p. methanesulfonate** Sympath-
olytics that act as alpha-adrenergic blocking
agents.

phenylacetic acid A metabolite of phenylalanine excreted in urine in conjugation with
glutamine.

phenylalanine An essential amino acid
necessary for the normal growth and develop-

ment of infants and children and for normal
protein metabolism throughout life. It is abundant in milk, eggs, and other common foods.
See also **phenylketonuria.**

phenylalaninemia The presence of phenylalanine in the blood. See also **hyperphenylalaninemia.**

phenylbutazone A nonsteroidal anti-inflammatory agent.

phenyl carbinol See **benzyl alcohol.**

phenylephrine hydrochloride A sympathomimetic adrenergic mydriatic and nasal
decongestant.

phenylethyl alcohol A colorless, fragrant
liquid with a burning taste, used as a bacteriostatic agent and preservative in medicinal solutions. Also called **benzyl carbonol.**

phenylic acid See **carbolic acid.**

phenylic alcohol See **carbolic acid.**

phenylketonuria (PKU) Abnormal presence of phenylketone and other metabolites of
phenylalanine in the urine, characteristic of an
inborn metabolic disorder caused by the absence or a deficiency of phenylalanine hydroxylase, the enzyme responsible for the conversion
of the amino acid phenylalanine into tyrosine.
Accumulation of phenylalanine is toxic to brain
tissue. Untreated individuals have very fair hair,
eczema, a musty (mousy) odor of the urine and
skin, and progressive mental retardation. Treatment consists of a diet free of phenylalanine.
Phenylketonuria occurs approximately once in
16,000 births in the United States. Most states
require a screening test for all newborns. See
also **Guthrie test. —phenylketonuric,** *adj.*

phenylmercuric nitrate   A disinfectant.

phenyl methanol   See **benzyl alcohol.**

phenylpropanolamine hydrochloride
A sympathomimetic agent commonly used to relieve nasal congestion. This drug is also an over-the-counter appetite suppressant.

phenylpyruvic acid   A product of the metabolism of phenylalanine. Phenylpyruvic acid in the urine is indicative of phenylketonuria.

phenylpyruvic amentia   See **phenylketonuria.**

phenyltoloxamine citrate   An antihistamine usually used in a fixed-combination drug with an analgesic.

phenytoin, p. sodium   Group II antiarrhythmic and anticonvulsant agents used mainly to control epilepsy.

pheo-   A combining form meaning 'dusky': *pheochrome, pheochromoblast.* Also **phao-.**

pheochromocytoma, *pl.* **pheochromocytomas, pheochromocytomata**   A vascular tumor of chromaffin tissue of the adrenal medulla or sympathetic paraganglia, characterized by hypersecretion of epinephrine and norepinephrine, causing persistent or intermittent hypertension. Typical signs include headache, palpitation, sweating, nervousness, hyperglycemia, nausea, vomiting, and syncope. There may be weight loss, myocarditis, cardiac arrhythmia, and heart failure. The tumor occurs most frequently in young people, and only a small percentage of the lesions are malignant. Surgical excision is the usual treatment; patients with nonresectable tumors may be treated with adrenergic blocking agents or with metyrosine, a drug that reduces norepinephrine production.

pheromone   A hormonal substance secreted by an individual that elicits a response from another individual of the same species.

phil-   A combining form meaning 'having an affinity for': *philanthropist, philocatalase.*

-phil   A combining form meaning 'of that which combines with or is stained by': *hydrophil, liopophil.* Also **-philic, -philous.**

Philadelphia chromosome   A translocation of the long arm of chromosome 22, often seen in the abnormal myeloblasts, erythroblasts, and megakaryoblasts of patients who have chronic myelocytic leukemia.

-philia   A combining form meaning: **1.** A 'tendency towards an action': *calciphelia, spasmophilia.* **2.** 'Abnormal appetite for a thing': *lygophilia, necrophilia.* Also **-phily.**

-philous   A combining form meaning 'having an affinity for': *calciphilous, cyanophilous.*

-phily   A combining form meaning: **1.** A 'fondness for something': *necrophily.* **2.** An 'affinity for something': *hydrophily, xerophily.*

phimosis   Tightness of the prepuce of the penis that prevents its retraction over the glans. The condition is usually congenital but may be the result of infection. Circumcision is the usual treatment. An analogous condition of the clitoris occurs rarely. Compare **paraphimosis.** See also **phimosis vaginalis.**

phimosis vaginalis   Congenital narrow-

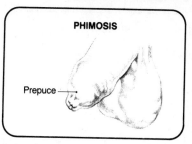

PHIMOSIS

Prepuce

ness or closure of the vaginal opening.

phleb-   See **phlebo-.**

phlebitis   See **thrombophlebitis.**

phlebo-, phleb-   A combining form meaning 'of or related to a vein or veins': *phlebocarcinoma, phlebograph.*

phlebogram   **1.** An X-ray film obtained by phlebography. **2.** A graphic representation of the venous pulse, obtained by phlebograph. Also called **venogram.**

phlebograph   A device for producing a graphic record of the venous pulse.

phlebography   **1.** The technique of preparing an X-ray image of veins injected with a radiopaque contrast medium. **2.** The technique of preparing a graphic record of the venous pulse by means of a phlebograph. Also called **venography.**

phlebothrombosis   An abnormal venous condition in which a clot forms within a vein, usually owing to hemostasis, hypercoagulability, or occlusion. In contrast to thrombophlebitis, the wall of the vein is not inflamed.

phlebotomus fever   An acute, mild infection, caused by one of five distinct arboviruses transmitted to man by the bite of an infected sandfly, (genus *Phlebotomus*), characterized by rapidly developing fever, headache, eye pain, conjunctivitis, myalgia, and, occasionally, a macular or urticarial rash. Aseptic meningitis may also occur. Phlebotomus fever is self-limiting, no fatalities have been recorded, and no specific therapy is available. Bed rest, fluids, and aspirin are recommended. A second attack may occur a few weeks after the first. Also called **pappataci, sandfly fever.**

phlebotomy   The incision of a vein for the letting of blood, as in collecting blood from a donor. Phlebotomy is the chief treatment for polycythemia vera and may be performed every 6 months, or more frequently if required. The procedure is sometimes used to decrease the amount of circulating blood and pulmonary engorgement in acute pulmonary edema. Also called **venesection.**

phleg-   See **phlogo-.**

phlegm   Thick mucus secreted by the tissues lining the respiratory passages.

phlegmasia   An inflammation.

phlegmasia alba dolens   Thrombophlebitis of the femoral vein, resulting in leg pain and edema. It may occur after childbirth or after a severe febrile illness.

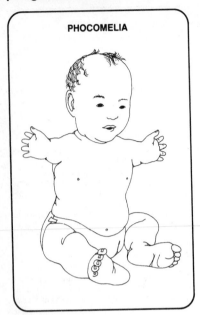

PHOCOMELIA

phlegmasia cerulea dolens   A severe form of thrombosis of a deep vein, usually the femoral vein. The condition is acute and fulminating and is usually accompanied by vast edema and cyanosis of the limb distal to the occluding thrombosis.

phlegmonous gastritis   A rare but severe form of gastritis, involving the connective tissue layer of the stomach wall. It occurs as a complication of systemic infection, peptic ulcer, cancer, surgery, or other severe stress and represents an acute abdominal emergency. Treatment includes surgery, antibiotics, and nonaspirin analgesics.

phlogo-, phleg-   A combining form meaning 'of or related to inflammation': *phlogocyte, phlogogen.*

phlyctenular keratoconjunctivitis   An inflammatory condition of the cornea and conjunctiva, characterized by tiny, ulcerating vesicles. The condition is believed to be a hypersensitivity reaction to a bacterial protein. It is seen most often in children as a response to allergens found in tuberculin, gonococci, monilia, or various parasites. Vitamin deficiency may be a factor. The condition responds to topical corticosteroids, but corneal scars may remain, possibly obscuring vision. Also called **phlyctenulosis, scrofulous keratitis.** See also **eczematous conjunctivitis.**

phlyctenulosis   See **phyctenular keratoconjunctivitis.**

phob-   A combining form meaning 'of or pertaining to fear or morbid dread': *phobia, phobophobia.*

-phobe   A combining form meaning 'one who fears' something specified: *dermatophobe, he-*

liophobe. Also **-phobiac, -phobist.**

phobia   An anxiety disorder characterized by an obsessive, irrational, and intense fear of a specific object, as an animal or dirt, of an activity, as meeting strangers or leaving the familiar setting of the home, or of a physical situation, as heights and open or closed spaces. Typical manifestations of phobia include faintness, fatigue, palpitations, perspiration, nausea, tremor, and panic. The fear, which is out of proportion to reality, usually results from some early painful or unpleasant experience involving the particular object or situation, or it may arise from displacing an unconscious conflict to an external object or situation to which it is symbolically related. Treatment includes psychotherapy and behavior therapy. Some kinds of phobias are **agoraphobia, claustrophobia, gynephobia, laliophobia, photophobia, simple phobia, social phobia, zoophobia.** Also called **phobic disorder, phobic neurosis, phobic reaction.** Compare **compulsion.** —**phobiac,** *n.,* **phobic,** *adj.*

-phobia   A combining form meaning 'abnormal fear' of the object, experience, or place specified: *agoraphobia.*

phobiac   A person who exhibits or is afflicted with a phobia.

-phobiac   See **-phobe.**

-phobic   A combining form meaning: **1.** 'Exhibiting or possessing an aversion for or fear of (something)': *Anglophobic, zoophobic.* **2.** The 'absence of a strong affinity': *chromophobic, osmiophobic.* Also **-phobous.**

phobic disorder   See **phobia.**

phobic neurosis   See **phobia.**

phobic reaction   See **phobia.**

phobic state   A condition characterized by extreme anxiety resulting from the excessive, irrational fear of a particular object, situation, or activity. See also **phobia.**

-phobist   See **-phobe.**

-phobous   See **-phobic.**

phocomelia   A developmental anomaly characterized by the absence of the upper portion of one or more of the limbs so that the feet or hands or both are attached to the trunk of the body by short, irregularly shaped stumps, resembling the fins of a seal. The condition, caused by interference with the embryonic development of the long bones, is rare and is seen primarily as a side effect of the drug thalidomide taken during early pregnancy. Also called **seal limbs.** Compare **amelia.** —**phocomelic,** *adj.*

phocomelic dwarf   A dwarf in whom the long bones of any or all of the extremities are abnormally short.

phocomelus   An individual who has phocomelia.

phon-   See **phono-.**

-phone   A combining form meaning: **1.** A 'device for transmitting sound': *auriphone, ossiphone.* **2.** A 'device for monitoring body sounds': *miophone, sphygmophone.*

phonic   Of or pertaining to voice, sounds, or speech.

PHONOCARDIOGRAM WAVEFORMS IN RELATION TO ELECTROCARDIOGRAM

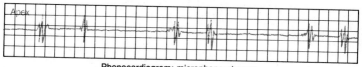

Phonocardiogram: microphone at apex

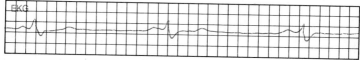

Electrocardiogram

-phonic A combining form meaning 'sounds made in a (specified) part of the body': *bronchiophonic, leptophonic.*

phono-, phon- A combining form meaning 'of or related to sound, often specifically the sound of the voice': *phonocardiograph, phonopathy.*

phonocardiogram A graphic recording obtained from a phonocardiograph.

phonocardiograph An electroacoustical device that produces graphic heart sound recordings, used in the diagnosis and monitoring of heart disorders. This instrument produces phonocardiograms by using a system of microphones and associated recording equipment. The microphone placed over the base of the heart records the timing of the aortic and the pulmonary components of the second heart sound and the loudest murmurs. The microphone placed over the apex is connected to special filters that allow the recording of low-frequency sounds, as those associated with atrial and ventricular gallops, as well as high-frequency sounds, such as those associated with mitral regurgitation and ventricular septal defect. To assure an accurate recording, the examiner also uses audiophones to monitor the sounds and an oscilloscope to monitor cardiac impulses. —**phonocardiographic,** *adj.*

-phony A combining form meaning: **1.** 'Sound': *echophony, laryngophony.* **2.** A 'speech disorder' of a (specified) type: *autophony, gutturophony.* Also **-phonia.**

phor- A combining form meaning 'bearing, carrying': *phoresis, phoroblast.*

-phore A combining form meaning a 'bearer or possessor': *physaliphore, trochophore.* Also **-phor.**

-phoresis A combining form meaning a 'movement in a (specified) manner or medium': *aphoresis, cataphoresis.*

-phoria A combining form meaning: **1.** A '(condition of) visual axes of the eye': *anophoria, esophoria.* **2.** An 'emotional state': *adiaphoria, euphoria.*

phosphatase An enzyme that acts as a cat-

alyst in chemical reactions involving phosphorus. See also **catalyst, enzyme.**

phosphate A compound of phosphoric acid. Phosphates are important in the storage and utilization of energy and the transmission of genetic information within a cell and from one cell to another. See also **adenosine diphosphate, adenosine triphosphate, phosphorus.**

phosphoglycerate kinase An enzyme that catalyzes the reversible transfer of a phosphate group from adenosine triphosphate to D-3-phosphoglycerate, forming D-1,3-diphosphoglycerate. The reaction is one of the steps in glycolysis.

phospholipid One of a class of compounds, widely distributed in living cells, containing phosphoric acid, fatty acids, and a nitrogenous base. Two kinds of phospholipids are **lecithin, sphingomyelin.**

phosphomevalonate kinase An enzyme that catalyzes the transfer of a phosphate group from adenosine triphosphate to produce adenosine diphosphate and 5-pyrophosphomevalonate.

phosphoric acid A clear, colorless, odorless liquid that is irritating to the skin and eyes and moderately toxic if ingested. It is used in the production of fertilizers, soaps, detergents, animal feeds, and certain drugs.

phosphorus (P) A nonmetallic chemical element occurring in nature as a component of phosphate rock. Its atomic number is 15; its atomic weight is 30.975. Phosphorus forms a series of sulfides used in the manufacture of matches. It can be prepared in yellow or white, red, and black allotropic forms. Essential for the metabolism of protein, calcium, and glucose, phosphorus is used by the body in its combined forms, which are obtained from milk, cheese, meat, legumes, and nuts. A deficiency of phosphorus can cause weight loss, anemia, and abnormal growth. Phosphorus is essential to the body for the production of adenosine triphosphate. It is also needed for the process of glycolysis. Chronic poisoning from phosphorus is characterized by anemia, cachexia, bronchitis,

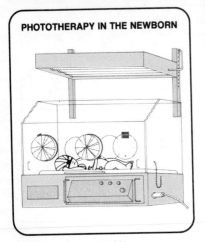

PHOTOTHERAPY IN THE NEWBORN

and necrosis of the mandible.

phosphorus poisoning A toxic condition caused by the ingestion of white or yellow phosphorus, sometimes found in rat poisons, certain fertilizers, and fireworks. Intoxication is characterized initially by nausea, throat and stomach pain, vomiting, diarrhea, and an odor of garlic on the breath. Following a few days of apparent recovery, nausea, vomiting, and diarrhea recur with renal and hepatic dysfunction. Treatment includes gastric lavage and administration of mineral oil, vitamin K, intravenous fluids, and medication to counteract shock. Physical contact with the patient's vomitus and feces is avoided.

phot- See **photo-**.

-photic A combining form meaning 'pertaining to the ability to see at a (specified) light level': *euryphotic, sthenophotic*.

photo-, phot- A combining form meaning 'of or pertaining to light': *photoelectric, photoreceptor*.

photoallergic Exhibiting a delayed hypersensitivity reaction after exposure to light. Compare **phototoxic**. See also **photoallergic contact dermatitis**.

photoallergic contact dermatitis A papulovesicular, eczematous, or exudative skin reaction occurring 24 to 48 hours after exposure to light in a previously sensitized person. The sensitizing substance concentrates in the skin and requires chemical alteration by light to become an active antigen. Among common photosensitizers are phenothiazines, hexachlorophene, and oral hypoglycemic agents. Prevention requires avoidance of the photosensitizer and sunlight. Treatment is the same as that for any other inflammatory dermatitis.

photochemotherapy A kind of chemotherapy in which the effect of the administered drug is enhanced by exposing the patient to light, as the treatment of psoriasis with oral methoxsalen followed by exposure to ultraviolet light. See also **chemotherapy**.

photophobia 1. Abnormal sensitivity to light, especially by the eyes. It is prevalent in albinism and diseases of the conjunctiva and cornea and may be a symptom of measles, psittacosis, encephalitis, Rocky Mountain spotted fever, and Reiter's syndrome. 2. In psychiatry: a morbid fear of light with an irrational need to avoid light places. The anxiety disorder is seen more often in women than in men and is usually caused by a repressed intrapsychic conflict symbolically related to light. Treatment consists of psychotherapy followed by behavior therapy. —**photophobic**, *adj*.

photosensitive Increased reactivity of skin to sunlight caused by a disorder, as albinism or porphyria, or more frequently resulting from the use of certain drugs. Relatively brief exposure to sunlight or to an ultraviolet lamp may cause edema, papules, urticaria, or acute burns in individuals with endogenous or acquired photosensitivity. Drugs inducing photosensitivity include phenothiazines, tetracyclines, griseofulvin, nalidixic acid, oral hypoglycemic agents, and halogenated salicylanides used in antifungal soaps. Treatment involves avoidance of exposure to sunlight or the photosensitizing agent. Methoxsalen and trioxsalen are potent photosensitizers sometimes used to enhance pigmentation or increase tolerance to sunlight, but overexposure or overdosage can cause severe reactions. —**photosensitivity**, *n*.

photosynthesis A process by which green plants containing chlorophyll synthesize chemical substances, chiefly carbohydrates, from atmospheric carbon dioxide and water, using light for energy and liberating oxygen in the process.

phototherapy A treatment by the use of light, especially ultraviolet light, which may be employed in the therapy of acne, decubiti and other indolent ulcers, psoriasis, and hyperbilirubinemia. —**phototherapeutic**, *adj*.

phototherapy in the newborn A treatment for hyperbilirubinemia and jaundice in the newborn that involves the exposure of an infant's skin to intense fluorescent light. The blue range of light accelerates the excretion of bilirubin in the skin, decomposing it by photo-oxidation. Bilirubin levels usually decrease by 3 to 4 mg/100 ml in the first 8 to 12 hours of therapy; thus, simple jaundice clears rapidly. Excess bilirubin and jaundice that are the result of hemolytic disease or infection may be controlled with phototherapy, but the underlying cause is treated separately. Recovery is usually complete. The long-term safety of phototherapy has not been established; short-term efficacy is certain. NURSING CONSIDERATIONS: The nurse performs phototherapy and may be responsible for collecting specimens for serial tests for serum bilirubin. The infant's eyes should be covered.

phototoxic Characterized by a rapidly developing, nonimmunologic reaction of the skin when it is exposed to a photosensitizing substance and light. Compare **photoallergic**. See also **phototoxic contact dermatitis**.

phototoxic contact dermatitis A rap-

PHRENIC PACEMAKER

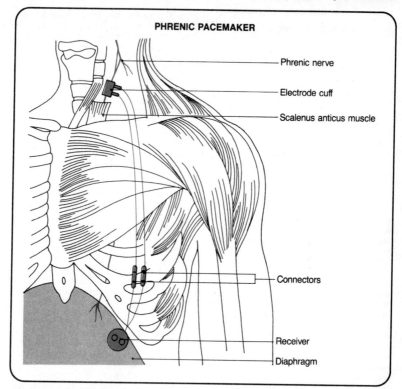

- Phrenic nerve
- Electrode cuff
- Scalenus anticus muscle
- Connectors
- Receiver
- Diaphragm

idly appearing, sunburnlike response of areas of skin that have been exposed to the sun after contact with a photosensitizing substance. Hyperpigmentation may follow the acute reaction. Known photosensitizing materials are coaltar derivatives, oil of bergamot (often used in cosmetics), and plants containing furocoumarin (cowslip, buttercup, carrot, parsnip, mustard, yarrow, etc.). Treatment includes Burow's solution, acid mantle cream, and topical corticosteroids.

-phragma A combining form meaning a 'septum or musculomembranous barrier between cavities': *inophragma, telophragma.* Also **-phragm.**

-phrasia A combining form meaning an 'abnormal condition of speech': *aphrasia, echophrasia.*

phren- A combining form meaning: **1.** 'Of or related to the mind': *phrenoblabia, phrenology.* **2.** 'Of or related to the diaphragm': *phrenodynia, phrenohepatic.*

-phrenia A combining form meaning a 'disordered condition of mental activity': *hebephrenia, ideophrenia.*

phrenic **1.** Of or pertaining to the diaphragm. **2.** Of or pertaining to the mind.

-phrenic A combining form meaning: **1.** The 'diaphragm or adjacent regions of the body': *costophrenic, postphrenic.* **2.** 'Characteristic of a

disorder of the mind': *hebephrenic, ideophrenic.*

phrenic nerve One of a pair of muscular branches of the cervical plexus, arising from the fourth cervical nerve. It contains about half as many sensory as motor fibers and is generally known as the motor nerve to the diaphragm, although the lower thoracic nerves also help to innervate the diaphragm. The phrenic nerve lies on the ventral surface of the scalenus anterior, crossing from its lateral to its medial border. It continues with the scalenus anterior between the subclavian vein and the subclavian artery, enters the thorax, passes over the cupula of the pleura, along the lateral aspect of the pericardium, and reaches the diaphragm, where it divides into terminal branches. The right phrenic nerve is deeper and shorter than the left. The pleural branches of the phrenic nerve are very fine filaments supplying the mediastinal pleura. The pericardial branches are delicate filaments passing to the upper pericardium. The terminal branches diverge after passing separately through the diaphragm and are distributed on the abdominal surface of the diaphragm. Also called **internal respiratory nerve of Bell.** Compare **accessory phrenic nerve.**

phrenic pacemaker A surgically implanted device that regularly stimulates the phrenic nerve, causing the diaphragm to descend and draw air into the lungs. An external

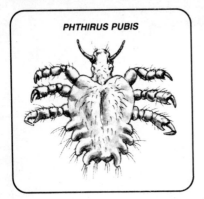

PHTHIRUS PUBIS

transmitter and antenna activate this device, which is used to treat patients with chronic dysfunction of the respiratory control center or with muscle paralysis caused by spinal cord trauma or by innervational or synaptic malfunction.

phthi- A combining form meaning 'decay, wasting away': *phthisiogenesis, phthisis.*

Phthirus A genus of bloodsucking lice that includes the species *Phthirus pubis*, the pubic louse, or crab.

-phthongia A combining form meaning a 'condition of speech': *diphthongia, heterophthongia.*

phyco- A combining form meaning 'of or pertaining to seaweed': *phycochrome, phycocyan.*

phycomycosis A fungal infection caused by a species of the order Phycomycetes. These organisms are common in the soil and are not usually pathogenic. Severe nosocomial pulmonary phycomycosis sometimes occurs with advanced diabetes mellitus that is untreated or out of control and complicated by ketoacidosis. See also **zygomycosis.**

phyl- A combining form meaning 'guarding or preservation': *phylacagogic, phylaxis.*

-phyll A combining form meaning a 'coloring matter in plants': *chlorophyll, leukophyll.* Also **-phyl.**

phyllo- A combining form meaning 'of or pertaining to leaves': *phyllochlorin, phyllode.*

phylloquinone See **vitamin K₁.**

phylo- A combining form meaning 'type, kind': *phylobiology, phylogenesis.*

phylogenesis See **phylogeny.**

phylogenetic, phylogenic 1. Relating to or acquired during phylogeny. 2. Based on a natural evolutionary relationship, as a system of classification.

phylogeny The development of the structure of a particular race or species as it evolved from simpler forms of life. Compare **ontogeny.**

-phyma A combining form meaning a 'swelling tumor': *adenophyma, onychophyma.*

physi- See **physio-.**

-physical A combining form meaning 'natural': *iatrophysical, medicophysical.*

physical allergy An allergic response to physical factors, as cold, heat, light, or trauma. Usually, specific antibodies are found in people having physical allergies. Common characteristics include pruritis, urticaria, and angioedema. Prophylaxis usually includes an attempt to remove the stimulus, and treatment involves the use of antihistamines or steroids. Compare **contact dermatitis.** See also **atopic.**

physical assessment The part of the health assessment representing a synthesis of the information obtained in a physical examination by using four basic techniques: inspection, palpation, percussion, and auscultation (IPPA).

physical chemistry The natural science dealing with the relationship between chemical and physical properties of matter.

physical diagnosis The process accomplished by the study of the physical manifestations of health and illness revealed in the physical examination, the patient's complete history, and laboratory tests. Physical diagnosis is to medicine what the health assessment is to nursing.

physical examination An investigation of the body to determine its state of health, using any or all of the techniques of inspection, palpation, percussion, auscultation, and smell. The physical examination, medical history, and initial laboratory tests constitute the data base from which a diagnosis is made and treatment is developed.

physical science The study of the laws and properties of nonliving matter. Some kinds of physical science are **chemistry, physics.** Compare **life science.**

physical therapist A person who is licensed to assist in the examination, testing, and treatment of physically disabled or handicapped people through the use of special exercise, application of heat or cold, use of sonar waves, and other techniques.

physical therapy The treatment of disorders with physical agents and methods, as massage, manipulation, therapeutic exercises, cold, heat (including shortwave, microwave, and ultrasonic diathermy), hydrotherapy, electrical stimulation, and light, to assist in rehabilitating patients and in restoring normal function following an illness or injury. Also called **physiotherapy.**

physician 1. A health professional who has earned a degree of Doctor of Medicine (MD) after completion of an approved course of study at an approved medical school and satisfactory completion of National Board Examinations. 2. A health professional who has earned a degree of Doctor of Osteopathy (DO) by satisfactorily completing a course of education in an approved college of osteopathy.

physician's assistant (PA) A person trained in certain aspects of the practice of medicine to provide assistance to a physician. A physician's assistant is trained by physicians and practices under the direction and supervision and within the legal license of a physician. Training programs vary in length from a few months to 2 years. Health-care experience or academic preparation may be a prerequisite to admission to some programs. Most physician's assistants are prepared for the practice of primary care, but some practice subspecialities, including surgical assisting, dialysis, or radiology. National certification is available to qualified graduates of approved training programs. The national organization is the American Association of Physician's Assistants (AAPA). Also called **physician's associate.**

physician's associate   See **physician's assistant.**

Physician's Desk Reference (PDR)   A compendium compiled annually, containing information about drugs, primarily prescription drugs and products used in diagnostic procedures, supplied by their manufacturers.

physics   The study of the laws and properties of matter and energy, particularly as related to motion and force.

-physics   A combining form meaning the 'science of the nature of' something specified: *cytophysics, medicophysics.*

physio-, physi-   A combining form meaning 'related to nature or to physiology': *physiochemical, physiognosis.*

physiological chemistry   See **biochemistry.**

physiological dead space   An area in the respiratory system that includes the anatomical dead space together with the space in the alveoli occupied by air that does not contribute to the oxygen-carbon dioxide exchange. Compare **anatomical dead space.**

physiological motivation   A bodily need, as food or water, that initiates behavior directed toward satisfying the particular need. Also called **organic motivation.** Compare **achievement motivation, social motivation.**

physiologic contracture   A temporary condition in which muscles may contract and shorten for a considerable period of time. Drugs, extremes of temperature, and local accumulation of lactic acid are causes. Compare **hypertonic contracture.**

physiologic dwarf   See **primordial dwarf.**

physiologic psychology   The study of the interrelationship of physiologic and psychologic processes, especially the effects of a change from normal to abnormal.

physiologic retraction ring   A ridge around the inside of the uterus that forms during the second stage of normal labor at the junction of the thinned lower uterine segment and thickened upper segment as a result of progressive lengthening of the muscle fibers of the lower segment and concomitant shortening of the muscle fibers of the upper segment. Compare **constriction ring, pathologic retraction ring.**

physiologic third heart sound   A low-pitched extra heart sound heard early in diastole in a healthy child or young adult. It is of no clinical significance and usually disappears with age. The same sound, heard in an older person who has heart disease, is an abnormal finding called a ventricular gallop. See also **gallop.**

physiotherapy   See **physical therapy. — physiotherapeutic,** *adj.* **physiotherapist,** *n.*

-physis   A combining form meaning a 'growth or growing': *metaphysis, zygapophysis.*

physo-   A combining form meaning 'of or pertaining to air or gas': *physocele, physocephaly.*

physostigmine salicylate   A cholinergic (parasympathomimetic) used as a miotic.

phytanic acid storage disease   A rare genetic disorder of lipid metabolism in which phytanic acid accumulates in the plasma and tissues. The condition is characterized by ataxia, peripheral neuropathy, retinitis pigmentosa, and abnormalities of the bone and skin. Also called **Refsum's syndrome.**

-phyte   A combining form meaning a 'plant which grows in or on or produces': *epiphyte, paraphyte.*

phyto-   A combining form meaning 'of or pertaining to a plant or plants': *phytobezoar, phytoncide.*

phytonadione   See **vitamin K$_1$.**

PI   In the patient record: *abbr* present illness.

pia mater   The innermost of the three meninges covering the brain and the spinal cord. It is closely applied to both structures and carries a rich supply of blood vessels, which nourish the nervous tissue. The cranial pia mater covers the surface of the brain and dips deeply into the fissures and the sulci of the cerebral hemispheres. Extending into the transverse cerebral fissure, the cranial pia mater forms the tela choroidea of the third ventricle, combines with the ependyma to form the choroid plexuses of the third and the lateral ventricles, and passes over the roof of the fourth ventricle to form its tela choroidea and its choroid plexus. The spinal pia mater is thicker, firmer, and less vascular than the cranial pia mater and consists of two layers. The outer layer is composed of longitudinal collagenous fibers which are concentrated along the anterior median fissure as the linea splendens. The inner layer closely wraps the entire spinal cord and, at the end of the cord, is prolonged into the filum terminale. The pia mater also forms the denticulate ligament, which extends the entire length of the spinal cord on both sides between the dorsal and the ventral spinal nerve roots. Compare **arachnoid, dura mater.**

pian   See **yaws.**

pica   A craving to eat substances that are not foods, as dirt, clay, chalk, glue, starch, or hair. The appetite disorder may occur with some nutritional deficiency states, pregnancy, and in some forms of mental illness.

Pick's disease   A form of presenile dementia occurring in middle age. It affects mainly the frontal and temporal lobes of the brain and produces neurotic behavior; slow disintegration of intellect, personality, and emotions; and degeneration of cognitive abilities. See also **dementia.**

Pickwickian syndrome   An abnormal condition characterized by obesity, decreased pulmonary function, somnolence, and polycythemia.

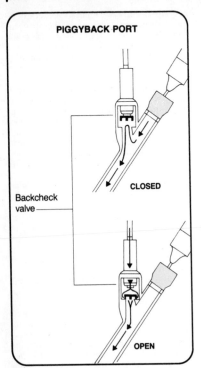

PIGGYBACK PORT

Backcheck valve

CLOSED

OPEN

pico- A combining form meaning 'one trillionth' (10^{-12}) of the unit designated: *picogram*, *picoliter*.

picornavirus A member of a group of small RNA viruses that includes the enteroviruses, rhinoviruses, and causative organisms of encephalomyocarditis and foot-and-mouth disease.

picro- A combining form meaning 'bitter': *picroadonidin*, *picropyrine*.

picrotoxin A central nervous system stimulant obtained from the seeds of *Anamirta cocculus*. It was formerly used as an antidote for acute barbiturate poisoning.

PID *abbr* pelvic inflammatory disease.

piebald Having patches of white hair or skin owing to an absence of melanocytes in those nonpigmented areas. It is a hereditary condition. Compare **albinism.** See also **vitiligo.**

Piedmont fracture An oblique fracture of the distal radius, with fragments of bone pulled into the ulna.

Pierre Robin syndrome A complex of congenital anomalies including a small mandible, cleft lip, cleft palate, other craniofacial abnormalities, and defects of the eyes and ears. Intelligence is usually normal. Treatment includes plastic surgery, speech therapy, orthodontia, and psychological counseling and support.

piez- A combining form meaning 'of or related to pressure': *piezesthesia, piezotherapy*.

pigeon breast A congenital structural defect characterized by a prominent anterior projection of the xiphoid and the lower part of the sternum and by a lengthening of the costal cartilages. It may cause cardiorespiratory complications but rarely warrants surgical correction. Also called **pectus carinatum.** —**pigeonbreasted,** *adj.*

pigeon breeder's lung A respiratory disorder caused by acquired hypersensitivity to antigens in bird droppings. Also called **bird breeder's lung.**

piggyback port A special coupling for the primary I.V. tubing which allows a supplementary, or piggyback, solution to run into the I.V. system. The piggyback port includes a backcheck valve which automatically prevents the primary I.V. solution from flowing while the piggyback solution is flowing. When the piggyback solution stops flowing, the backcheck valve starts the flow of the primary I.V. solution. Piggyback ports are part of piggyback I.V. sets, which are used solely for intermittent drug administration.

pigment 1. Any organic coloring material produced in the body, as melanin. 2. Any colored, paintlike, medicinal preparation applied to the skin surface. —**pigmentary, pigmented,** *adj.,* **pigmentation,** *n.*

pigmy See **pygmy.**

pilar cyst An epidermoid cyst of the scalp. Its keratinized contents are firmer and less cheesy than the material in epidermoid cysts found elsewhere. The cyst originates from the middle portion of the epithelium of a hair follicle. Treatment is surgical excision. Also called **sebaceous cyst.** Compare **epidermoid cyst.**

piles See **hemorrhoid.**

pill See **tablet.**

pillion fracture A T-shaped fracture of the distal femur with displacement of the condyles posterior to the femoral shaft, caused by a severe blow to the knee.

pilo- A combining form meaning 'resembling or composed of hair': *pilocystic, pilomotor*.

pilocarpine hydrochloride, p. nitrate Miotic agents.

pilomotor reflex Erection of the hairs of the skin in response to a chilly environment, emotional stimulus, or irritation of the skin. This normal reaction is abolished below the level of a transverse spinal cord lesion and may be exaggerated on the affected side in a patient with hemiplegia. Also called **gooseflesh, horripilation.**

pilonidal cyst A cyst in the midline of the upper portion of the gluteal fold, formed during embryologic development by the inclusion of a small amount of endothelial tissue in a space beneath the skin. It may sometimes be recognized at birth by a depression, sometimes a hairy dimple, in the midline of the back, sacrococcygeal area. Usually these cysts do not cause any problems, but occasionally a sinus or fistula develops in early adulthood that communicates with the skin, resulting in infection. A fistula may also develop to the spinal tract from a pilonidal

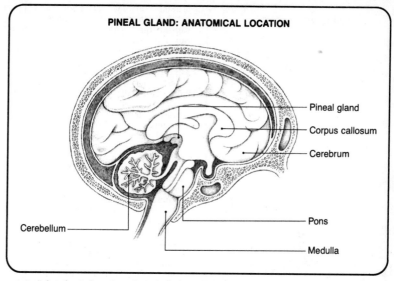

PINEAL GLAND: ANATOMICAL LOCATION

Pineal gland

Corpus callosum

Cerebrum

Pons

Medulla

Cerebellum

cyst. An infected or inflamed cyst is excised, the infection or inflammation is treated, and the space is surgically closed.

pilonidal fistula An abnormal channel containing a tuft of hair, situated most frequently over or close to the tip of the coccyx but also occurring in other regions of the body. Also called **pilonidal sinus.**

pilonidal sinus See **pilonidal fistula.**

pilosebaceous Of or pertaining to a hair follicle and its oil gland.

pimaricin See **natamycin.**

pimelo- A combining form meaning 'of or related to fat': *pimeloma, pimelopterygium.*

pimozide An investigational antipsychotic agent.

pimple A small papule, pustule, or furuncle.

pin 1. In orthopedics: to secure and immobilize fragments of bone with a nail. 2. See **nail,** definition 2. 3. In dentistry: a small metal rod or peg, used as a support in rebuilding a tooth.

pineal body See **pineal gland.**

pineal gland A small, somewhat flattened, cone-shaped structure about 8 mm (¼ inch) long, suspended by a stalk in the epithalamus, situated between the superior colliculi, the pulvinar, and the splenium of the corpus callosum. It consists of glial cells and pineglocytes, and it may secrete the hormone melatonin, which appears to inhibit the secretion of luteinizing hormone. Its precise function has not been established. Also called epiphysis cerebri, pineal body.

pinealocytoma See **pinealoma.**

pinealoma, *pl.* **pinealomas, pinealomata** A rare neoplasm of the pineal body in the brain. It is characterized by hydrocephalus, papillary changes, gait disturbances, headache, nausea, and vomiting. Precocious puberty occurs in some patients with pinealomas, probably owing to extension of the tumor into the hypothalamus. Also called pinealocytoma.

pineal tumor A neoplasm of the pineal body. See also **pinealoma.**

pine tar A topical antieczematic and a rubefacient. It is a common ingredient in creams, soaps, and lotions used to treat chronic skin conditions, as eczema.

ping-ponging *Slang.* A fraudulent practice involving passing a patient from one physician to another so that a health program or facility can charge a third party for several cursory examinations.

pinhole test A test performed in examining a person who has diminished visual acuity to distinguish a refractive error from organic disease. A refractive error may be corrected with glasses and is not medically dangerous. Loss of visual acuity owing to organic disease is serious as it may indicate a systemic, particularly a neurologic, disease and may signal the development of avoidable blindness. The pinhole effect results from blocking peripheral light waves, those most distorted by refractive error.

pinkeye See **conjunctivitis.**

Pinkus' disease See **lichen nitidus.**

pinna, *pl.* **pinnas, pinnae** See **auricule.** —**pinnal,** *adj.*

pinocytosis The process by which extracellular fluid is taken into a cell. The cell membrane develops a saccular indentation filled with extracellular fluid, then closes around it, forming a vaccule of fluid within the cell.

pinta An infection of the skin caused by *Treponema carateum,* an organism common in South and Central America. The bacterium enters the body through a break in the skin. Prolonged exposure and close contact appear to be needed for transmission. The primary lesion is a slowly enlarging papule with regional lymph node enlargement, followed in 1 to 12 months

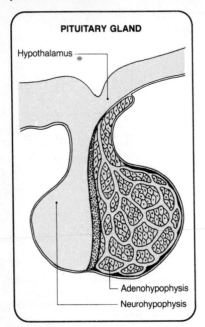

PITUITARY GLAND

Hypothalamus

Adenohypophysis

Neurohypophysis

by a generalized red to slate-blue macular rash. Eventually these lesions become depigmented. Diagnosis is based on serologic tests and dark-field microscopic examination of scrapings from skin lesions. Treatment with penicillin G is effective. The major complication of the disease is social ostracism resulting from the permanent skin disfiguration. Also called **azul, carate, mal del pinto.** Compare **yaws.**

pin track infection An abnormal condition associated with skeletal traction and characterized by infection of superficial, deep, or soft tissues or by osteomyelitis. These infections may develop at skeletal traction pin sites. Signs include erythema at the pin sites, drainage and odor, pin slippage, elevated temperature, and pain. Superficial infection at the pin site is treated with antibiotics administered topically or orally. Deeper infection at the pin sites usually requires removal of the pins and antibiotic therapy.

pinworm See *Enterobius vermicularis.*

pio- A combining form meaning 'of or pertaining to fat': *pionemia, piorthopnea.*

pion See **negative pi meson.**

piperacetazine A phenothiazine antipsychotic agent.

piperacillin sodium A penicillin antibiotic.

piperazine adipate, p. citrate, p. phosphate, p. tartrate Anthelmintic agents.

Piper forceps See **obstetric forceps.**

piperocaine hydrochloride An ester local anesthetic for topical application to oral mucous membranes.

pipette 1. A calibrated, transparent open-ended tube of glass or plastic used for measuring

or transferring small quantities of a liquid or gas. 2. Using a pipette to dispense liquid.

pipobroman An alkylating agent used in cancer chemotherapy.

piriform aperture The anterior nasal opening in the skull.

piriformis A flat, pyramidal muscle lying almost parallel with the posterior margin of the gluteus medius. It is partly within the pelvis and partly at the back of the hip joint. It arises from the sacrum, the greater sciatic foramen, and the sacrotuberous ligament, and it inserts, by a rounded tendon, into the greater trochanter of the femur. It functions to rotate the thigh laterally and to abduct and to help extend it. Compare **obturator externus, obturator internus.**

piroxicam A nonsteroidal anti-inflammatory agent.

Pirquet test A tuberculin skin test that consists of scratching the tuberculin material onto the skin. Also called **von Pirquet test.** See also **tuberculin test.**

pisiform bone A small, spheroidal carpal bone in the proximal row of carpal bones. It is attached to the flexor retinaculum, the flexor carpi ulnaris, and the abductor digiti minimi.

pitch The quality of a tone or sound dependent on the relative rapidity of the vibrations by which it is produced.

pitting 1. Small, punctate indentations in fingernails or toenails, often a result of psoriasis. 2. An indentation that remains for a short time after pressing edematous skin with a finger. 3. Small, depressed scars in the skin or other organ of the body. 4. The removal by the spleen of material from within erythrocytes without damage to the cells.

pituit- A combining form meaning 'of or related to phlegm': *pituitary, pituitous.*

pituitary adamantinoma See **craniopharyngioma.**

pituitary cachexia See **panhypopituitarism.**

pituitary dwarf A dwarf whose retarded development is owing to a deficiency of growth hormone resulting from hypofunction of the anterior lobe of the pituitary. In most cases the cause is unknown, and the defect is limited to a lack of somatotropin, although in some instances gonadotropins, adrenocorticotropic hormone, and thyroid-stimulating hormone may also be deficient. The body is properly proportioned, with no facial or skeletal deformities, and there is normal mental and sexual development. The condition is usually diagnosed in childhood by radiographic examination of the bones and radioimmunoassay of levels of plasma growth hormone. Also called **hypophyseal dwarf, Lévi-Lorain dwarf, Paltauf's dwarf.**

pituitary gland The small gland attached to the hypothalamus and couched in the sphenoid bone. It is divided into an anterior adenohypophysis and a smaller posterior neurohypophysis. The adenohypophysis secretes growth hormone (somatotropin), thyrotropic hormone, adrenocorticotropic hormone (ACTH), two gonadotropic hormones—follicle-stimulating hormone (FSH) and luteinizing hormone (LH)—and prolactin, the hormone that promotes milk secretion. The neurohypophysis stores two hormones, oxytocin and vasopressin. Oxytocin stimulates the contraction of smooth muscle, especially in the uterus. Vasopressin inhibits diuresis and raises blood pressure. The pituitary gland is larger in females than in males and becomes further enlarged during pregnancy. Also called **hypophysis cerebri.** See also **adenohypophysis, neurohypophysis.**

pituitary nanism A type of dwarfism associated with hypophyseal infantilism. See also **pituitary dwarf.**

pituitary-snuff lung A type of hypersensitivity pneumonitis that sometimes occurs among takers of pituitary snuff. The antigens to which the hypersensitivity reaction occurs are found in serum proteins of cows and pigs and in pituitary tissue. Symptoms of the acute form of the disease include chills, cough, fever, dyspnea, anorexia, nausea, and vomiting. The chronic form of the disease is characterized by fatigue, chronic cough, weight loss, and dyspnea on exercise.

pit viper Any one of a family of venomous snakes found in the Western Hemisphere and Asia, characterized by a heat-sensitive pit between the eye and nostril and hollow, perforated fangs. With the exception of coral snakes, all indigenous poisonous snakes in the United States are pit vipers. See also **copperhead, cottonmouth, rattlesnake.**

pityriasis alba A common idiopathic dermatosis characterized by round or oval, finely scaling patches of hypopigmentation. The lesions are sharply demarcated, occasionally pruritic, and occur primarily in children and adolescents. The condition may recur, but spontaneous clearing is the usual prognosis. Treatment includes lubricating creams, topical corticosteroids, and, less commonly, coal-tar creams. Compare **pityriasis rosea.**

pityriasis rosea A self-limiting skin disease in which a slightly scaling, pink, macular rash spreads over the trunk and other unexposed areas of the body. A characteristic feature is the **herald patch,** a larger, more scaly lesion which precedes the diffuse rash by several days. Mild itching is the only symptom. The disease lasts 4 to 8 weeks and rarely recurs. It is unusual, apparently not contagious, and its cause is unknown.

pivot joint A synovial joint in which movement is limited to rotation. The joint is formed by a pivotlike process that may turn within a ring composed partly of bone and partly of ligament. The proximal radioulnar articulation is a pivot joint in which the head of the radius rotates within the ring formed by the radial notch of the ulna and the annular ligament. Also called **trochoid joint.** Compare **gliding joint, hinge joint.** See also **condyloid joint.**

PK *abbr* **psychokinesis.**

PKD *abbr* **polycystic kidney disease.**

PK test *abbr* **Prausnitz-Küstner test.**

PKU *abbr* **phenylketonuria.**

placebo An inactive substance, as saline, distilled water, or sugar, or a less than effective dose of a harmless substance, as a vitamin, prescribed as if it were an effective dose of a needed medication. Placebos are used in experimental drug studies to compare the effects of the placebo with those of the experimental drug. They are also prescribed for patients who cannot be given the medication they request or who, in the judgment of the health-care provider, do not need that medication. Placebo therapy is effective in some cases, and side effects often occur as they would from the actual medication. The benefit to the patient of a placebo should clearly outweigh the ethical, moral, and legal problems posed by its administration.

placebo effect A physical or emotional change occurring after a substance is taken or administered that is not the result of any special property of the substance. The change is usually beneficial and reflects the expectations of the patient and, often, the expectations of the person giving the substance.

placent- A combining form meaning 'a cakelike mass': *placenta, placentapepton.*

placenta A highly vascular fetal organ through which the fetus absorbs oxygen, nutrients, and other substances and excretes carbon dioxide and other wastes. It begins to form on approximately the 8th day of gestation when the blastocyst touches the wall of the uterus and adheres to it. The blastocyst becomes surrounded by an outer layer of syncytiotrophoblast and an inner layer of cytotrophoblast. The trophoblast is able to digest cells of the endometrium, causing a small erosion on the uterine wall in which an embryo nidates. Under the influence of increasing amounts of progesterone, secreted by the corpus luteum of the ovary, the embryo and the placenta continue to develop. A hormone, chorionic gonadotropin, is secreted by the developing placenta and is present in the maternal blood and urine. The trophoblastic layer continues to infiltrate the maternal tissues with fingerlike projections, called chorionic villi. Separating the villi are lakes of blood in the eroded tissue. The maternal blood flows into the lakes surrounding the villi, allowing nutrients, gases, and other substances to pass into the fetal circulation by diffusion, hydrostatic pressure, and osmosis. The placenta is able to secrete large amounts of progesterone by the 3rd month of pregnancy, enough to relieve the corpus luteum of that function. At term the normal placenta weighs ½ to ⅓ of the weight of the infant. The maternal surface is lobulated and divided into cotyledons. It has a dark red, rough, liverlike appearance. The fetal surface is smooth and shiny, covered with the fetal membranes, marked by the large white blood vessels beneath the membranes that fan out from the centrally inserted umbilical cord. The time between the delivery of the infant and the expulsion of the placenta is the third and last stage of labor.

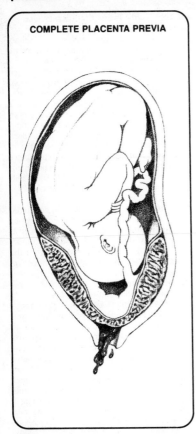

COMPLETE PLACENTA PREVIA

-placenta   A combining form meaning an 'organ shaped like a flat cake': *ectoplacenta*, *subplacenta*.

placental hormone   One of the several hormones produced by the placenta, including human placental lactogen, chorionic gonadotropin, estrogen, progesterone, and a thyrotropinlike hormone.

placental insufficiency   An abnormal condition of pregnancy that retards fetal and uterine growth. One or more placental abnormalities cause dysfunction of maternal-placental or fetal-placental circulation sufficient to compromise fetal nutrition and oxygenation. Some of these abnormalities are abnormal implantation of the placenta, multiple pregnancy, abnormal attachments of the umbilical cord or anomalies of the cord itself, and abnormalities of the placental membranes. Histopathologic abnormalities that can cause placental insufficiency include intravillous thrombi, and breaks in the placental membrane that result in fetal bleeding into the maternal circulation. Placental insufficiency may also result from placental senescence in postmaturity, from systemic diseases, as erythroblastosis fetalis and diabetes

mellitus, or from infections. See also **intrauterine growth retardation.**

placenta previa   A condition of pregnancy in which the placenta is implanted abnormally in the uterus so that it impinges upon or covers the internal os of the uterine cervix. It is the most common cause of painless bleeding in the third trimester of pregnancy. Its etiology is unknown. The incidence of the condition increases with increased parity from approximately 1 in 1,500 primiparas to approximately 1 in 20 grand multiparas. Even slight dilatation of the internal os can cause enough local separation of an abnormally implanted placenta to result in bleeding. If severe hemorrhage occurs, immediate cesarean section is usually required to stop the bleeding and to save the mother's life; it is performed regardless of the stage of fetal maturity. Prior to hemorrhage, placenta previa may be diagnosed by ultrasonography and treated with complete bed rest under close observation. Even at rest, sudden massive hemorrhage can occur without warning. Vaginal examination is usually contraindicated if placenta previa is present or suspected because palpation can cause local placental separation and precipitate hemorrhage. Cautious and very gentle intracervical palpation may be performed to determine the existence and exact extent of previa. Before this examination, an intravenous infusion is begun, the woman's blood is typed and cross-matched, and preparations for immediate cesarean section are made. If the placenta is next to or near rather than touching or covering the cervical os, labor and vaginal delivery may be attempted. Types of placenta previa are **complete** or **total placenta previa, marginal placenta previa, partial placenta previa.** Compare **abruptio placentae.**

Plafon fracture   A fracture that involves the buttress portion of the malleolus of a bone.

plagiocephaly, plagiocephalism   A congenital malformation of the skull in which premature or irregular closure of the coronal or lambdoidal sutures results in asymmetrical growth of the head, giving it a twisted, lopsided appearance so that the maximum length is not along the midline but on a diagonal. See also **craniostenosis. —plagiocephalic, plagiocephalous,** *adj.*

plague   An infectious disease caused by the bite of a flea infected by a rat infected with the bacillus *Yersinia pestis.* Plague is primarily an infectious disease of rats: the rat fleas feed on humans only when their preferred hosts have been killed by the plague in a rat epizootic; therefore, epidemics occur after rat epizootics. Kinds of plague include **bubonic plague, pneumonic plague, septicemic plague.** See also *Yersinia pestis.*

plague vaccine   An active immunizing agent prepared with killed plague bacilli.

plaintiff   In law: a person who files a civil lawsuit initiating a legal action. In criminal actions, the prosecution is the plaintiff, acting in behalf of the people of the jurisdiction.

-plakia A combining form meaning 'patches on mucous membrane': *leukoplakia, malocoplakia.*

planar xanthoma A yellow or orange flat macule or slightly raised papule containing foam cells and occurring in clusters in localized areas, as the eyelids, or widely distributed over the body, as in generalized planar xanthoma or xanthelasmatosis. Also called **plane xanthoma, xanthoma planum.** See also **xanthelasmatosis.**

plane **1.** A flat surface determined by three points in space. **2.** An extension of a longitudinal section through an axis, as the coronal, the horizontal, and the sagittal planes used to identify the position of various parts of the body in the study of anatomy. **3.** The act of paring or of rubbing away. **4.** A superficial incision in the wall of a cavity or between tissue layers, especially in plastic surgery. **—planar,** *adj.*

planes of anesthesia See **Guedel's signs.**

-plania A combining form meaning 'deviation from its normal location': *choloplania, spiloplania.*

planned parenthood A philosophical framework central to the development of contraceptive methods, contraceptive counseling, and family-planning programs and clinics. Advocates hold that it is the right of each woman to decide when to conceive and bear children, and that contraceptive and gynecologic care and information should be available to help her become or avoid becoming pregnant.

planning In five-step nursing process: a category of nursing behavior in which a strategy is designed for the achievement of care goals for a patient, as established in assessing and analyzing. Planning includes developing and modifying a care plan for the patient, cooperating with other personnel, and recording relevant information. To develop the plan, the nurse anticipates the patient's needs; involves the patient and the patient's family in designing the plan; uses all information necessary for managing care of the patient, including recorded information from other health professionals and the patient's age, sex, culture, ethnicity, and religion; plans for the patient's comfort, activity, and function; and chooses appropriate nursing measures. With the cooperation of other health personnel, the nurse coordinates patient care and identifies resources in the hospital or community for social or health assistance. Planning follows analyzing and precedes implementing in the five-step nursing process. See also **assessing, evaluating.**

plano- A combining form meaning 'wandering': *planocyte, planotopokinesia.*

plantago seed A bulk-forming laxative.

plantar Of or pertaining to the sole of the foot. Also called **volar.**

plantar aponeurosis The tough fascia surrounding the muscles of the soles of the feet. Also called **plantar fascia.**

plantar fascia See **plantar aponeurosis.**

plantaris One of three superficial muscles at

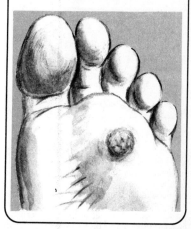

PLANTAR WART

the back of the leg, between the soleus and the gastrocnemius. The plantaris is a small muscle that arises from the distal part of the linea aspera of the femur and from the oblique popliteal ligament of the knee joint. It has a small, fusiform belly, ending in a long, slender tendon that inserts into the calcaneus. It flexes the foot and the leg. Compare **gastrocnemius, soleus.**

plantar neuroma A neuroma of the sole of the foot.

plantar reflex The normal response elicited by stroking the outer surface of the sole from heel to toes, characterized by flexion of the toes. Compare **Babinski's reflex.**

plantar wart A painful verrucous lesion on the sole of the foot, primarily at points of pressure, as over the metatarsal heads and the heel. Caused by the common wart virus, it appears as a soft, central core and is surrounded by a firm, hyperkeratotic ring resembling a callus. Multiple tiny black spots on the surface represent bits of coagulated blood in the wart. Treatment methods include electrodesiccation, cryotherapy, topical acids, cantharadin, and even mental suggestion. See also **mosaic wart, verruca.**

plantigrade **1.** Of, pertaining to, or characterizing the human gait. **2.** Walking on the sole of the foot with the heel touching the ground.

plaque **1.** A flat, often raised, patch on the skin or any other organ of the body. **2.** A patch of atherosclerosis. **3.** A thin film on the teeth made up of mucin and colloidal material found in saliva and often secondarily invaded by bacteria. Also called **dental plaque.**

-plasia A combining form meaning '(condition of) formation or development': *alloplasia, anosteoplasia.*

-plasm A combining form meaning 'cell or tissue substance': *deutoplasm, phytoplasm.* Also **-plasma.**

plasma The watery, colorless, fluid portion

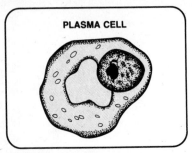

PLASMA CELL

of the lymph and the blood in which the leukocytes, erythrocytes, and platelets are suspended. It contains no cells and is made up of water, electrolytes, proteins, glucose, fats, bilirubin, and gases. It is essential for carrying the cellular elements of the blood through the circulation, transporting nutrients, maintaining the acid-base balance of the body, and transporting wastes from the tissues. Plasma and interstitial fluid correspond closely in content and protein concentration; therefore, plasma is important in maintaining the osmotic pressure and exchange of fluids and electrolytes between capillaries and tissues. Compare **serum**.

plasma-   A combining form meaning 'the liquid portion of the blood': *plasmablast, plasmacyte.*

-plasma   A combining form meaning 'fluid part of cytoplasm or protoplasm': *ectoplasma, hydroplasma.*

plasma cell   A lymphoid or lymphocyte-like cell found in the bone marrow, connective tissue, and, sometimes, in the blood. It contains an eccentric nucleus with deeply staining chromatin material arranged in a pattern resembling the spokes of a wheel. Plasma cells are involved in the immunologic mechanism and are formed in large numbers in multiple myeloma. Also called **plasmacyte**.

plasma cell leukemia   An unusual neoplasm of blood-forming tissues in which the predominant cells in peripheral blood are plasmacytes. The disease may develop in the course of multiple myeloma or arise independently. Bence Jones proteinuria, abnormal serum globulins, hepatomegaly, and splenomegaly are usual in plasma cell leukemia. In most cases, plasma cell leukemia is rapidly fatal, but some patients respond to treatment with alkylating agents and glucocorticoids.

plasma cell myeloma   See **multiple myeloma**.

plasma cell tumor   See **plasmacytoma**.

plasmacyte   See **plasma cell**.

plasmacytoma, *pl.* **plasmacytomas, plasmacytomata**   A focal neoplasm containing plasma cells. It may develop in the bone marrow, as in multiple myeloma, or outside the bone marrow, as in certain tumors of the viscera and the mucosa of the nasal, oral, and pharyngeal areas. Also called **peripheral plasma cell myeloma, plasma cell tumor**.

plasma membrane   See **cell membrane**.

plasmapheresis   See **therapeutic plasma exchange**.

plasmaphoresis   A laboratory procedure in which the plasma proteins are separated by electrophoresis for identification and evaluation of the proportion of the various proteins.

plasma protein   Any one of the various proteins, including albumin, fibrinogen, and the gamma globulins, which constitute about 6% to 7% of the blood plasma in the body. These substances aid in the maintenance of water balance affecting osmotic pressure, increase blood viscosity, and help maintain blood pressure. Fibrinogen and prothrombin are essential to blood coagulation, and the gamma globulins are important in immunoregulation. All the plasma proteins except the gamma globulins are synthesized in the liver. See also **serum**.

plasma thromboplastin antecedent (PTA)   A blood factor essential in the coagulation process. Thromboplastin cannot be formed in its absence. Also called **antihemophilic C factor, factor IX complex**.

plasma thromboplastin component deficiency   See **hemophilia**.

plasmid   In bacteriology: any type of intracellular inclusion considered to have a genetic function, especially a molecule of DNA separate from the bacterial chromosome that determines traits not essential for the viability of the organism but that in some way changes the organism's ability to adapt. R (resistance) factor is an example: a bacterium containing the factor is able to resist many antibacterial drugs that act in many different ways. Plasmid may be passed from one bacterium to another, and it is replicated in later generations of any bacterium carrying it.

plasmidotrophoblast   See **syncytiotrophoblast**.

plasmin   See **fibrinolysin**.

plasminogen   See **fibrinogen**.

plasmo-   A combining form meaning 'of or related to plasma or to the substance of a cell': *plasmocyte.*

Plasmodium   A genus of protozoa, several species of which cause malaria, transmitted to humans by the bite of an infected *Anopheles* mosquito. *Plasmodium falciparum* causes falciparum malaria, the most severe form of the disease; *P. malariae* causes quartan malaria; *P. ovale* causes mild tertian malaria with oval red blood cells; and *P. vivax* causes common tertian malaria. See also *Anopheles*, **blackwater fever, malaria**.

plasmosome, plasmasome   The true nucleolus of a cell as distinguished from the karyosomes in the nucleus.

plast-   A combining form meaning 'formed': *plastidogenetic, plastodynamia.*

-plast   A combining form meaning a 'primitive cell': *chondroplast, gymnoplast.*

plaster   **1.** Any composition of a liquid and a powder that hardens when it dries, used in shaping a cast to support a fractured bone as it heals, as plaster of paris. **2.** A home remedy consisting of a semisolid mixture applied to a part of the body as a counterirritant or for other therapeutic reasons, as a mustard plaster.

-plastia A combining form meaning '(condition of) cell or tissue formation or development': *macroplastia, mastplastia.* Also **-plasia.**

-plastic A combining form meaning 'pertaining to the development of' (something specified): *entoplastic, hemoplastic.*

plastic surgery The alteration, replacement, or restoration of visible portions of the body, performed to correct a structural or cosmetic defect. In performing corrective plastic surgery, the surgeon may use tissue from the patient, from another person, or from an inert material that is nonirritating, has an appropriate consistency, and can hold its shape and form indefinitely. Implants are commonly used in mammoplasty for breast augmentation. Skin grafting is the most common procedure in plastic surgery. Z-plasty and Y-plasty are simpler techniques often performed instead of a graft in areas of the body covered by skin that is loose and elastic, as the neck, axilla, throat, and inner aspect of the elbow. Dermabrasion is used to remove pockmarks, scars from acne, or signs of traumatic skin damage. Chemical peeling is used primarily for removing fine facial wrinkles. Tattooing, in which a pigment is tattooed into the skin of a graft, changes the color of the graft to resemble the surrounding skin. Reconstructive plastic surgery corrects birth defects, repairs structures destroyed by trauma, and replaces tissue removed in other surgical procedures. Cleft lip and cleft palate repair and other maxillofacial surgical procedures, including rhinoplasty, otoplasty, and rhytidoplasty, are among these reconstructive procedures. Since the patient may be exceedingly uncomfortable about the real or perceived appearance of the defect, all staff members should exhibit an accepting, nonjudgmental attitude. Optimal nutritional status helps a graft to 'take' and speeds healing. Each procedure and technique involves particular kinds of care in the preoperative and postoperative periods. Instructions and assistance in self-care activities are also specific to these procedures. See also specific procedures.

-plasty A combining form meaning 'plastic surgery on a (specified) body part or by (specified) means': *bronchoplasty, cervicoplasty.*

plate A flat structure or layer, as a thin layer of bone or the frontal plate between the sides of the ethmoid cartilage and the sphenoid bone in the fetus.

platelet The smallest of the cells in the blood. Platelets are disk-shaped and contain no hemoglobin. They are essential for the coagulation of blood. Normally, between 200,000 and 300,000 platelets are found in 1 cubic mm of blood. See also **thrombocytopenia, thrombocytosis.**

platinum (Pt) A silvery-white, soft metallic element. Its atomic number is 78; its atomic weight is 195.09. Platinum is used in jewelry and in the manufacture of chemical apparatus that must

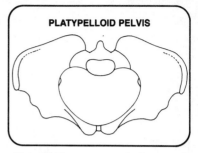

PLATYPELLOID PELVIS

withstand high temperatures. It also occurs as a spongy substance and a black powder.

platy- A combining form meaning 'broad or flat': *platybasia, platyenemic.*

platypelloid pelvis A rare type of pelvis (present in 3% of women) in which the inlet is round like the gynecoid type in the anterior section, but the posterior section is foreshortened by its flat and heavy border. The sacrum is hollow and inclines posteriorly, and the sidewalls are convergent. In the midplane, the transverse diameter is much wider than the narrowed anteroposterior diameter. Vaginal delivery is not usually possible in a woman who has a platypelloid pelvis.

platysma One of a pair of wide muscles at the side of the neck. It arises from the fascia covering the superior parts of the pectoralis major and the deltoideus, crosses the clavicle, and rises obliquely and medially along the side of the neck. The anterior fibers of the platysma interlace, inferior and posterior to the symphysis menti, with the fibers of the muscle of the opposite side. The posterior fibers of the platysma cross the mandible, some inserting into the bone below the oblique line, others into the skin and the subcutaneous tissue of the lower part of the face. The platysma covers the external jugular vein as the vein descends from the angle of the mandible to the clavicle. It serves to draw down the lower lip and the corner of the mouth. When the platysma fully contracts, the skin over the clavicle is drawn toward the mandible, increasing the diameter of the neck.

play Any spontaneous or organized activity that provides enjoyment, entertainment, or diversion. It is essential in childhood for the development of a normal personality. Play provides an outlet for releasing tension and stress as well as a means for testing and experimenting with new or fearful roles or situations. An indispensable part of the nursing care of children, especially in the hospital, play offers the nurse one of the most effective methods of communicating with and gaining the trust of the child and helping the child to understand treatments and procedures. Kinds of play include **active play, associative play, cooperative play, dramatic play, parallel play, passive play, skill play, solitary play.** See also **play therapy.**

play therapy A form of psychotherapy in which a child plays in a protected and struc-

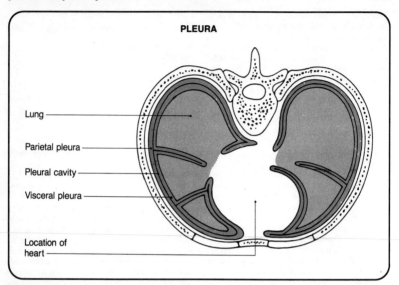

PLEURA

Lung

Parietal pleura

Pleural cavity

Visceral pleura

Location of heart

tured environment with games and toys provided by a therapist, who observes the child in order to gain insight into the child's thoughts, feelings, and fantasies. As conflicts are discovered, the therapist often helps the child to understand and work through them.

pleasure principle In psychoanalysis: the need for immediate gratification of instinctual drives. Compare **reality principle.**

pledget A small, flat compress made of cotton gauze, or a tuft of cotton wool, lint, or a similar synthetic material, used to wipe the skin, absorb drainage, or clean a small surface.

-plegia A combining form meaning 'a (specified) paralysis': *colicoplegia, esophagoplegia.*

-plegic A combining form meaning: **1.** 'Of or pertaining to a specific paralysis': *cycloplegic, ganglionoplegic.* **2.** A 'sufferer from a specific paralysis': *diplegic, ophthalmoplegic.*

pleiades A mass of enlarged lymph nodes.

pleio- See **pleo-.**

pleiotropy In genetics: a variable factor, such as a gene, that modifies basic patterns of inheritance. It is the multiple, different, and apparently unrelated manifestation of a particular disorder, as the cluster of symptoms in Marfan's syndrome: aortic aneurysm, dislocation of the optic lens, skeletal deformities, and arachnodactyly, any or all of which may be present.

pleo-, pleio- A combining form meaning 'more': *pleochromatic, pleomastia.*

plessimeter See **pleximeter.**

plethysmogram A tracing produced by a plethysmograph.

plethysmograph An instrument which measures and records changes in the sizes and volumes of extremities and organs by measuring changes in their blood volumes. —**plethysmographic,** *adj.,* **plethysmography,** *n.*

pleur- See **pleuro-.**

pleura, *pl.* **pleurae** A delicate serous membrane enclosing the lung, composed of a single layer of flattened mesothelial cells resting on a delicate membrane of connective tissue. Beneath the membrane is a stroma of collagenous tissue containing yellow elastic fibers. The pleura divides into the visceral pleura, which covers the lung, dipping into the fissures between the lobes, and the parietal pleura, which lines the chest wall, covers the diaphragm, and reflects over the structures in the mediastinum. The parietal and visceral pleurae are separated from each other by a small amount of fluid that acts as a lubricant as the lungs expand and contract during respiration. See also **pleural cavity, pleural space.** —**pleural,** *adj.*

pleural cavity The cavity within the thorax that contains the lungs. Between the ribs and the lungs is a serous membrane which divides into the visceral and parietal pleurae.

pleural effusion An abnormal accumulation of fluid in the interstitial and air spaces of the lungs, characterized by fever, chest pain, dyspnea, and nonproductive cough. The fluid involved is an exudate or a transudate from inflamed pleural surfaces. A transudate which accumulates in pulmonary edema is commonly aspirated. An exudate may result from pulmonary infarction, trauma, tumor, or infection, as tuberculosis. The specific cause of the exudate is treated, and the exudate may be aspirated or surgically drained. Other treatment may include the administration of corticosteroids, diuretics, vasodilators, and oxygen therapy.

pleural space The potential space between the visceral and parietal layers of the pleurae. The space contains a small amount of fluid that acts as a lubricant, allowing the pleurae to slide smoothly over each other as the lungs expand and contract with respiration.

pleurisy Inflammation of the parietal pleura of the lungs, characterized by dyspnea and stabbing pain, leading to restriction of ordinary breathing with spasm of the chest on the affected side. A friction rub may be heard on auscultation. Simple pleurisy with undetectable exudate is called fibrinous or dry; pleural effusion indicates extensive inflammation with considerable amounts of exudate in the pleural spaces. Common causes of pleurisy include bronchial carcinoma, lung or chest wall abscess, pneumonia, pulmonary infarction, and tuberculosis. The condition may result in permanent adhesions between the pleura and adjacent surfaces. Treatment consists of relief of pain and therapy for the primary disease. See also **pleural effusion, pleurodynia, pulmonary edema.**

pleuro-, pleur- A combining form meaning 'of or pertaining to the pleura, to a side, or to a rib': *pleurocentrum, pleurography.*

pleurodynia **1.** Acute inflammation of the intercostal muscles and the muscular attachment of the diaphragm to the chest wall. It is characterized by sudden severe pain and tenderness, fever, headache, and anorexia. These symptoms are aggravated by movement and respiration. The lungs are not affected and characteristically there is no cough or pleural effusion. **2.** See **epidemic pleurodynia.**

pleuropericardial rub An abnormal coarse friction sound heard on auscultation of the lungs during late inspiration and early expiration. It is caused by the visceral and parietal pleural surfaces rubbing against each other. The sound is not affected by coughing. A pleural rub indicates primary inflammatory, neoplastic, or traumatic pleural disease or inflammation secondary to infection or neoplasm. See also **breath sound, Kussmaul respirations, rale, rhonchi, wheeze.**

pleuroperitoneal cavity See **splanchnocoele.**

pleuropneumonia **1.** A combination of pleurisy and pneumonia. **2.** An infection of cattle resulting in inflammation of both the pleura and lungs, caused by microorganisms of the *Mycoplasma* group. See also *Mycoplasma,* **pleuropneumonia-like organism.**

pleuropneumonia-like organism (PPLO) A group of filterable organisms of the genus *Mycoplasma* similar to *M. mycoides,* the cause of pleuropneumonia in cattle.

pleurothotonos An involuntary, severe, prolonged contraction of the muscles of one side of the body, resulting in an acute arch to that side. Pleurothotonos is usually associated with tetanus infection or strychnine poisoning. Compare **emprosthotonos, opisthotonos, orthotonos. —pleurothotonic,** *adj.*

plex- A combining form meaning 'a stroke or to strike': *plexalgia, pleximeter.*

-plex A combining form meaning a 'network': *brachiplex, cerviplex.* Also **-plexus.**

-plexia, -plexy A combining form meaning '(condition resulting from a) stroke': *apoplexia, pagoplexia.*

plexiform neuroma A neoplasm composed of twisted bundles of nerves. Also called **Verneuil's neuroma.**

pleximeter A mediating device, as a percussor or finger, used to receive light taps in percussion. Also called **plessimeter.** See also **percussion.**

plexor See **percussor.**

plexus, *pl.* **plexuses** A network of intersecting nerves and blood vessels or of lymphatic vessels. The body contains many plexuses, as the brachial plexus, the cardiac plexus, the cervical plexus, and the solar plexus.

plic- A combining form meaning a 'fold or ridge': *plicadentin, plication.*

plica, *pl.* **plicae** A fold of tissue within the body, as the plicae transversales of the rectum and the plicae circulares of the small intestine. **—plical,** *adj.*

plica circularis, *pl.* **plicae circulares** See **circular fold.**

plicae transversales recti Semilunar, transverse folds in the rectum that support the weight of feces. Also called **Houston's valves.** See also **rectum.**

plica semilunaris The semilunar fold of the conjunctiva that extends laterally from the lacrimal caruncle. It has a concave free border directed toward the cornea. In some individuals it contains smooth muscular fibers.

plica umbilicalis lateralis See **lateral umbilical fold.**

plica umbilicalis mediana See **middle umbilical fold.**

Plimmer's bodies Small, round, encapsulated bodies found in cancers and once thought to be the causative parasites. Also called **Behla's bodies, cancer bodies.**

-ploid A combining form meaning 'having a (specified) number of chromosome sets': *heptaploid, octaploid.*

ploidy The status of a cell nucleus in regard to the number of complete chromosome sets it contains.

-ploidy A combining form meaning the 'condition of having a (specified) number of chromosome sets': *alloploidy, haploidy.*

plug A mass of tissue cells, mucus, or other matter that blocks a normal opening or passage of the body.

Plummer's disease Goiter characterized by a hyperfunctioning nodule or adenoma and thyrotoxicosis. Also called **toxic nodular goiter.**

Plummer-Vinson syndrome A rare disorder associated with severe and chronic iron-deficiency anemia, characterized by dysphagia owing to esophageal webs at the level of the cricoid cartilage. Also called **sideropenic dysphagia.** Compare **Paterson-Kelly syndrome.**

plunging goiter See **diving goiter.**

pluri- A combining form meaning 'more': *pluriceptor.*

pluripolar mitosis See **multipolar mitosis.**

plutonium (Pu) A man-made, metallic, radioactive element formed by adding neutrons to uranium. Its atomic number is 94; its atomic weight is 242. A highly toxic waste product of nuclear power plants, plutonium was used in the assembly of early nuclear weapons.

Pm Symbol for **promethium.**

PMD *abbr* private medical doctor. Also called **LMD.**

PMI *abbr* **point of maximum impulse.**

PMT *abbr* **premenstrual tension.**

PND *abbr* **1. postnasal drip. 2. paroxysmal nocturnal dyspnea.**

-pnea A combining form meaning 'breath or breathing': *brachypnea, dyspnea.* Also **-pnoea.**

pneo- A combining form meaning 'of or pertaining to the breath, or to breathing': *pneodynamics, pneograph.*

pneumato-, pneuma- A combining form meaning 'of or related to air or gas, or to respiration': *pneumatology.*

pneumo-, pneumono- A combining form meaning 'of or related to the lungs, to air, or to the breath': *pneumobacillin, pneumocele.*

pneumococcal Of or pertaining to bacteria of the genus *Pneumococcus.*

pneumococcal vaccine An active immunizing agent containing antigens of the 14 types of *Pneumococcus* associated with 80% of the cases of pneumococcal pneumonia.

pneumococcus, *pl.* **pneumococci** A gram-positive diplococcal bacterium of the species *Diplococcus pneumoniae,* the most common cause of bacterial pneumonia. More than 85 subtypes of this organism are known. See also **lobar pneumonia, pneumonia.**

pneumoconiosis Any disease of the lung caused by chronic inhalation of dust, usually mineral dusts of occupational or environmental origin. Some kinds of pneumoconioses are **anthracosis, asbestosis, silicosis.**

pneumocystosis Infection with the parasite *Pneumocystis carinii,* usually seen in infants or debilitated or immunosuppressed people and characterized by fever, cough, tachypnea, and, frequently, cyanosis. The diagnosis is difficult to make and usually requires lung biopsy and special staining techniques. Mortality nears 100% in untreated patients. Treatment with pentamidine isethionate or a combination of trimethoprim and sulfamethoxazole is effective. Also called **interstitial plasma cell pneumonia.**

pneumoencephalogram A radiograph of the brain made during pneumoencephalography.

pneumoencephalography A procedure for the radiographic visualization of the ventricular space, basal cisterns, and subarachnoid space overlying the cerebral hemispheres of the brain. Air, helium, or oxygen is injected into the lumbar subarachnoid space after intermittent removal of cerebrospinal fluid by lumbar puncture. See also **encephalography, ventriculography. —pneumoencephalographic,** *adj.*

pneumogastric nerve See **vagus nerve.**

pneumomediastinum The presence of air or gas in the mediastinal tissues, which in infants may lead to pneumothorax or pneumopericardium, especially in those with respiratory distress syndrome or aspiration pneumonitis. In older children, the condition may result from bronchitis, acute asthma, pertussis, cystic fibrosis, or bronchial rupture from cough or trauma.

pneumonia An acute inflammation of the lungs, usually owing to inhaled pneumococci of the species *Diplococcus pneumoniae,* causing the alveoli and bronchioles of the lungs to become plugged with a fibrous exudate. Pneumonia may be caused by other bacteria, as well as by viruses, rickettsiae, and fungi, but in 85% of the cases, pneumococcus infection is the cause. Characteristic of pneumonia are severe chills, a high fever (which may reach 40.6°C, or 105°F), headache, cough, and chest pain. Inflammation of the lower lobe of the right lung may produce a pain suggesting appendicitis. An effusion of red blood cells into the alveolar spaces, resulting from histolytic damage by the microorganism, produces rust-colored sputum that may signal pneumococcal infection. As the disease progresses, sputum may become thicker and more purulent, and the person may experience painful attacks of coughing. Respiration usually becomes more difficult, painful, shallow, and rapid. The pulse increases, often measuring 120 or more beats per minute. Other signs may include profuse sweating and cyanosis. In children, pneumonia may be accompanied by febrile convulsion. As the alveoli become filled with exudate, the affected area of a lobe becomes increasingly firm and consolidated. A distinctive kind of rale is heard on auscultation. X-ray films are taken to evaluate consolidation; sputum analysis and blood cultures help in identifying the causative organism. The treatment of pneumonia includes bed rest, fluids, antibiotics, analgesics, antipyretics, and, if necessary, oxygen. The antibiotic prescribed is specific for the bacterium identified in the laboratory analysis of sputum or blood. Expectorants, postural drainage, and aspiration of the bronchi are often prescribed. Chest X-rays are advised during the acute phase, after therapy has been completed, and at a follow-up examination 4 to 6 weeks later.

NURSING CONSIDERATIONS: Fluid and electrolytes are often lost during prolonged high fever; intravenous replacement is often required. Ice packs or cold, wet compresses may be needed to reduce the fever. Fever, loss of fluids, and breathing through the mouth result in a need for care of the mouth and the nares, where herpes lesions frequently develop. The nurse collects samples of sputum for laboratory analysis, administers antibiotics and other medications, and notes temperature, pulse, and respiration as often as necessary.

-pneumonia A combining form meaning an 'inflammation of the lungs': *necropneumonia, splenopneumonia.*

-pneumonic A combining form meaning: **1.** 'Related to pneumonia': *peripneumonic, pleu-*

ropneumonic. **2.** 'Related to the lungs': *hepatopneumonic.*

pneumonic plague A highly virulent and rapidly fatal form of plague characterized by bronchopneumonia. There are two forms: primary pneumonic plague results from involvement of the lungs in the course of bubonic plague; secondary pneumonic plague results from the inhalation of infected particles of sputum from a person having pneumonic plague. Compare **bubonic plague, septicemic plague.** See also **plague, Yersinia pestis.**

pneumonitis, *pl.* **pneumonitides** Inflammation of the lung. Pneumonitis may be caused by a virus, or it may be an allergic reaction to chemicals or organic dusts, as bacteria, bird droppings, or molds. It is usually an interstitial granulomatous fibrosing inflammation of the lung, especially of the bronchioles and alveoli. Dry cough is a common sign. Treatment depends on the cause but includes removal of any offending agents and the administration of corticosteroids to reduce inflammation. See also **hypersensitivity pneumonitis.** Compare **pneumonia.**

pneumono- See **pneumo-.**

pneumothorax A collection of air in the pleural space causing the lung to collapse. It may be the result of an open chest wound that permits the entrance of air into the pleural space or of the rupture of a vesicle on the surface of the lung, possibly without apparent cause. A tension pneumothorax results when air enters the pleural space with each inspiration and becomes trapped, causing pressure buildup. This increased pressure may cause a mediastinal shift. The onset of pneumothorax is accompanied by a sudden, sharp chest pain, followed by difficult, rapid breathing, cessation of normal chest movements on the affected side, tachycardia, a weak pulse, hypotension, diaphoresis, an elevated temperature, pallor, dizziness, and anxiety. The patient is urged to remain quiet and is placed in bed in Fowler's position. Oxygen is administered through a nasal cannula, unless contraindicated. The air is aspirated from the pleural space by a chest tube inserted and attached to a water seal drainage system; the tube is not removed until air no longer is expelled through the underwater drainage system and an X-ray shows that the lung is completely expanded. Pain may be controlled by administering appropriate analgesics; respiratory depressants are avoided. The patient is taught how to turn, cough, and breathe deeply.

PNH *abbr* **paroxysmal nocturnal hemoglobinuria.**

-pnoea See **-pnea.**

PNP *abbr* **pediatric nurse practitioner.**

Po Symbol for **polonium.**

PO₂ Symbol for partial pressure of oxygen. See **partial pressure.**

pod- See **podo-.**

podiatrist A health professional trained to diagnose and treat diseases and other disorders of the feet. A podiatrist receives a degree of DPM

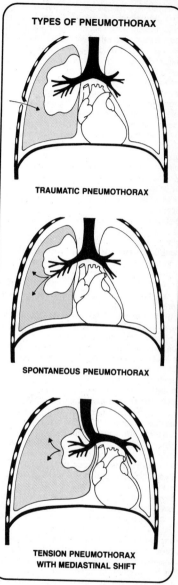

TYPES OF PNEUMOTHORAX

TRAUMATIC PNEUMOTHORAX

SPONTANEOUS PNEUMOTHORAX

TENSION PNEUMOTHORAX WITH MEDIASTINAL SHIFT

(doctor of podiatric medicine) and is licensed by state and national boards of podiatry.

podiatry The diagnosis and treatment of diseases and other disorders of the feet.

-podium A combining form meaning 'something footlike': *axiopodium, phyllopodium.*

podo-, pod- A combining form meaning 'of or related to the foot': *podogram, podology.*

podophyllotoxin Any one of a group of substances derived from the roots of *Podophyllum peltatum,* a common plant species known as mayapple or mandrake. Podyphillin, a resinous preparation of podophyllotoxin, is prescribed in the topical treatment of condyloma acuminatum. Several semisynthetic podophyllotoxins are being studied for their antineoplastic effects. They are not recommended for use in early pregnancy.

podophyllum resin A caustic topical agent.

-poetic A combining form meaning 'referring to production of something specified': *cholepoetic, oenopoetic*. Also **-poietic.**

-poiesis, -poesis A combining form meaning 'production of': *cholanopoiesis, hemopoiesis*.

-poietic A combining form meaning 'producing something specified': *cholepoietic, gonepoietic*. Also **-poetic.**

poikilo- A combining form meaning 'varied or irregular': *poikiloderma, poikilothymia*. Also **pecilo-.**

poikilocytosis An abnormal degree of variation in the shape of the erythrocytes in the blood. Compare **macrocytosis, microcytosis.**

poikiloderma atrophicans vasculare An abnormal skin condition characterized by hyperpigmentation or hypopigmentation, telangiectasia, and atrophy of the epidermis. It may be symmetrical or patchy, localized or widespread. It tends to be permanent.

poikiloderma of Civatte A common benign, progressive dermatitis characterized by dry and scaly erythmatous patches on the face and neck. As the condition progresses, pigment is deposited around the hair follicles extending down the lateral aspects of the neck. Photosensitivity is possible.

poikilothermic See **cold-blooded.**

point of maximum impulse (PMI) The place in the fifth intercostal space of the thorax, just medial to the left midclavicular line.

poison Any substance that impairs health or destroys life when ingested, inhaled, or absorbed by the body in relatively small amounts. Some toxicologists suggest that, depending on dosages, all substances are poisons. The real concern is the risk or hazard associated with the use of any substance, as the high risk that may be associated with a life-saving drug that would not be acceptable as a food additive. Clinically, all poisons are divided into those which respond to specific treatments or antidotes and those for which there is no specific treatment. Research continues to develop effective antitoxins for poisons, but there are relatively few effective antidotes. Treatment is based mainly on eliminating the toxic agent from the body before it can be absorbed, while maintaining respiration and circulation. Some substances that may be poisonous are the saps of certain plants, bacterial toxins, animal venoms, corrosives, heavy-metal compounds, certain gases, various volatile and nonvolatile substances, industrial chemicals, and numerous drugs. The toxic effects of poisons may be reversible or irreversible. The capacity of body tissue to recover from poison determines the reversibility of the effect. Poisons

that injure the central nervous system (CNS) create irreversible effects because CNS neurons of the brain cannot regenerate. Toxic effects of drugs or chemicals may be divided into local effects and systemic effects. Local effects, as those caused by the ingestion of caustic substances and the inhalation of irritants, involve the site of the first contact between the biological system and the toxicant. Systemic effects depend on the absorption and the distribution of the toxicant. Systemic toxicity most often affects the CNS but may also affect the circulatory system, the blood and hematopoietic system, the skin, and the visceral organs, as the liver, kidneys, and lungs. The muscles and the bones are less often affected by systemic toxicity. The precise incidence of poisoning in the United States is not known, but about 150,000 cases are voluntarily reported to the National Clearinghouse for Poison Control Centers each year. Authorities, however, estimate that the real incidence is at least 10 times the number of reported cases. The total number of poisoning cases increases each year, but the incidence of poisoning in children under 5 years has significantly decreased, probably because of safer packaging of household drugs and products. About 60% of all poisoning involves children 1 to 2 years old and the ingestion of chemicals other than drugs. Approximately 75% of the cases of poisoning in individuals over 15 years of age are drug-related. About 4,000 persons die each year in the United States from poisoning by toxic liquid and solid substances. Another 7,000 persons are bitten by poisonous snakes, as the pit viper and coral snake. Such bites may cause severe pain and swelling, numbness, respiratory distress, paralysis, impaired coagulation, coma, and death. Snake bites may be treated with antivenin, tetanus toxoid, and broad spectrum antibiotics. Systemic antihistamines and topical antipyretics are commonly used to treat toxic skin reactions from poisonous plants, as poison ivy, poison sumac, and poison oak. Common treatments for acute poisoning from toxic chemicals and liquids involve emesis and gastric lavage. Most toxic effects of drugs occur shortly after administration, but carcinogenic effects of chemicals may take 15 to 45 years to develop fully. Chemical carcinogenesis is a complex process involving the conversion of secondary carcinogens into primary carcinogens and the possible development of tumors through reactions of the toxicant with deoxyribonucleic acid. **—poisonous,** *adj.*

poison control center One of a nearly worldwide network of facilities that provide information regarding all aspects of poisoning or intoxication, maintain records of their occurrence, and refer patients to treatment centers.

poisoning **1.** The act of administering a toxic substance. **2.** The condition or physical state produced by the ingestion, injection, or inhalation of or exposure to a poisonous substance. Identification of the poison and the presentation of a container label are critical to expeditious diagnosis and treatment. Kinds of poisoning include **food poisoning, heavy metal poisoning, petroleum distillate poisoning, salicylate poisoning.** See also **alcohol poisoning, carbon monoxide poisoning, cyanide poisoning, nicotine poisoning, pesticide poisoning, poison ivy, poison oak, poison sumac.**

poison ivy Any of several species of climbing vine of the genus *Rhus*, characterized by shiny, three-pointed leaves. Skin contact results in localized vesicular eruption with itching and burning, which may be treated with antipruritic lotions, cold compresses, or topical corticosteroid ointment or cream. Severe cases may require corticosteroids given intramuscularly or orally. In people who are hypersensitive, prophylactic treatment with *Rhus* antigen may be given after contact, before symptoms develop. Careful washing of the exposed skin after suspected contact may prevent the reaction. See also **rhus dermatitis, urushiol.**

poison oak Any of several species of shrub of the genus *Rhus*, common in North America. Skin contact results in allergic dermatitis in many people. The characteristics and treatment are similar to those of poison ivy. See also **rhus dermatitis, urushiol.**

poison sumac A shrub of the genus *Rhus*, common in North America. Skin contact results in allergic dermatitis in many people. The characteristics and treatment are similar to those of poison ivy. See also **rhus dermatitis, urushiol.**

poker spine See **bamboo spine.**

polar body One of the small cells produced during the two meiotic divisions in the maturation process of female gametes, or ova. It is nonfunctional and incapable of being fertilized. See also **oogenesis.**

polarity **1.** The existence or manifestation of opposing qualities, tendencies, or emotions, as pleasure and pain, love and hate, strength and weakness, dependence and independence, masculinity and femininity. The concept is central to various psychotherapeutic approaches, as client-centered therapy, in which the key to self-actualization lies in accepting polarity within oneself. **2.** In physics: the distinction between a negative and a positive electrical charge.

poloxamer iodine A disinfectant.

pole **1.** In biology: an end of an imaginary axis drawn through the symmetrically arranged parts of a cell, organ, ovum, or nucleus. **2.** In anatomy: the point on a nerve cell at which a dendrite originates. —**polar,** *adj.*

polio *Informal.* **Poliomyelitis.**

polio- A combining form meaning 'of or related to gray matter in the nervous system': *polioclastic, poliomyelitis.*

polioencephalitis An inflammation of the gray matter of the brain caused by infection by a poliovirus.

polioencephalomyelitis Inflammation of the gray matter of the brain and the spinal cord, caused by infection by a poliovirus.

poliomyelitis An infectious disease caused by one of the three polioviruses. Asymptomatic,

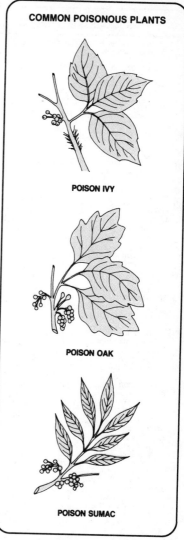

COMMON POISONOUS PLANTS

POISON IVY

POISON OAK

POISON SUMAC

mild, and paralytic forms of the disease occur. Several factors influence susceptibility to the virus and the course of the disease: more boys than girls are severely affected, stress increases susceptibility, more pregnant than nonpregnant women acquire the paralytic form of the disease, and the severity of the infection increases with age. It is transmitted from person to person through fecal contamination or oropharyngeal secretions. Asymptomatic infection has no clinical features, but it confers immunity. Abortive poliomyelitis lasts only a few hours and is characterized by minor illness with fever, malaise, headache, nausea, vomiting, and slight abdominal discomfort. Nonparalytic poliomyelitis is

SUGGESTED GENERAL TREATMENT FOR POISONING

1. No treatment necessary after ingestion of small amounts. Fluids may be given.

2. Induce vomiting. Give syrup of ipecac in the following doses:
Under 1 year of age:
2 teaspoons followed by at least 2 or 3 glasses of fluid (except milk).
1 year or older:
1 tablespoon followed by at least 2 or 3 glasses of fluid (except milk).
Vomiting may be induced up to a minimum of 4 hours after ingestion.
Do not induce vomiting if the patient is semi-comatose, comatose, or convulsing.
Administer an adsorbant. Give activated charcoal in the following doses:

Under 2 years of age: 25 g
2 years or older: 50 g

Note: Mix with water. Most effective if given within 30 minutes after ingestion; however, it may be used up to 3 hours after ingestion.

To be administered after vomiting has been induced.
Do not give before the use of syrup of ipecac.

3. Dilute or neutralize with water or milk. *Do not induce vomiting.* Gastric lavage is indicated. Call Poison Center for specific instructions.

4. Treat symptomatically unless botulism is suspected. Call Poison Center for specific information regarding botulism.

Acetaminophen	2, 8
Acetone	2
Acids	
Ingestion	5
Eye contamination	7
Topical	6
Inhalation if mixed with bleach	9
Aerosols	
Eye contamination	7
Inhalation	9
After-shave	
lotions	*See Cologne*
Airplane glue	10
Alcohol	
Ingestion	2
Eye contamination	7
Alkali	
Ingestion	5
Eye contamination	7
Topical	6
Inhalation	9
Ammonia	
Ingestion	5
Eye contamination	7
Inhalation	9
Amphetamines	2, 8
Analgesics	10
Aniline dyes	
Ingestion	2, 8
Inhalation	8, 9
Topical	6, 8
Antacids	1
Antibiotics	
Less than 2 to 3 times total daily dose	1
More than 3 times total daily dose	2
Antidepressants	
Tricyclic	2, 8
Others	2
Antifreeze (ethylene glycol)	
Ingestion	2
Eye contamination	7
Antihistamines	2, 8
Antiseptics	2
Ant trap	
Kepone type	1
Others	2
Aquarium products	1
Arsenic	2, 8
Aspirin	2
Baby oil	1
Ball-point ink	1
Barbiturates	

Short-acting	10
Long-acting	2
Bathroom bowl cleaner	
Ingestion	5
Eye contamination	7
Inhalation if mixed with bleach	9
Topical	6
Batteries	
Dry cell (flashlight)	1
Mercury (hearing aid)	2
Wet cell (automobile)	5
Benzene	
Ingestion	10
Inhalation	9
Topical	6
Birth control pills	1
Bleaches	
Liquid ingestion	1
Solid ingestion	5
Eye contamination	7
Inhalation when mixed with acids or alkalies	9
Boric acid	2
Bromides	2
Bubble bath	1
Caffeine	2
Camphor	2
Candles	1
Caps for cap pistols	
Less than one roll	1
More than one roll	2
Carbon monoxide	9
Carbon tetrachloride	
Ingestion	2
Inhalation	9
Topical	6
Chalk	1
Chlorine	
bleach	*See Bleaches*
Cigarettes	
Less than one	1
One or more	2
Clay	1
Cleaning fluids	10
Cleanser (household)	1
Clinitest tablets	5
Cocaine	10
Codeine	2, 8
Cold remedies	10
Cologne	
Less than 15 ml	1
More than 15 ml	2
Contraceptive pills	1
Corn/wart removers	5

Cosmetics	*See specific type*
Cough medicines	10
Crayons	
Children's	1
Others	2
Cyanide	8
Dandruff shampoo	2
Darvon	*See Propoxaphene*
Dehumidifying packets	1
Denture adhesives	1
Denture cleansers	5
Deodorants	1
Deodorizer cakes	2
Deodorizers, room	10
Desiccants	1
Detergents	
Liquid/powder (general)	1
Electric dishwasher and phosphate-free	5
Dextromethorphan hydrobromide	2, 8
Diaper rash ointment	1
Digitalis glycosides	10
Dishwasher detergents	*See Detergents*
Disinfectants	3
Drain cleaners	*See Lye*
Dyes	
Aniline	*See Aniline dyes*
Others	2
Electric dishwasher detergent	*See Detergents*
Epoxy glue	
Catalyst	5
Resin or when mixed	10
Epsom salts	2
Ethyl	
alcohol	*See Alcohol*
Ethylene	
glycol	*See Antifreeze*
Eye makeup	1
Fabric softeners	2
Fertilizers	10
Fishbowl additives	1
Food poisoning	4
Furniture polish	10
Gas (natural)	9
Gasoline	10

SUGGESTED GENERAL TREATMENT FOR POISONING (cont.)

5. Dilute or neutralize with water or milk. *Do not induce vomiting.* Gastric lavage should be avoided. This substance may cause burns of the mucous membranes. Consult ear, nose, and throat specialist following emergency treatment. Call Poison Center for specific information.

6. Immediately wash skin thoroughly under running water. Call Poison Center for further information.

7. Immediately wash eyes with a gentle stream of running water. Continue for 15 minutes. Call Poison Center for further information.

8. Specific antagonist may be indicated. Call Poison Center.

9. Remove to fresh air. Support respirations. Call Poison Center for further information.

10. Call Poison Center for specific instructions.

11. Symptomatic and supportive treatment. *Do not induce vomiting for ingestion.* I.V. naloxone hydrochloride to be given as indicated for respiratory depression. *Dosage:*
Adult: 0.4 to 2.0 mg I.V.
May be repeated at 2- to 3-minute intervals.
Child: 0.01 to 0.1 mg/kg I.V.
May be repeated at 2- to 3-minute intervals.

Glue	10
Gun products	10
Hair dyes	
Ingestion	3
Eye contamination	7
Topical	6
Hallucinogens	5, 8
Hand cream	1
Hand lotions	1
Herbicides	10
Heroin	8, 11
Hormones	1
Hydrochloric acid	*See Acids*
Inks	
Ball-point pen	1
Indelible	2
Laundry marking	2
Printer's	2
Insecticides	
Ingestion	8
Topical	6, 8
Iodine	5, 8
Iron	10
Isopropyl alcohol	*See Alcohol*
Kerosene	10
Laundry marking ink	2
Laxatives	2
Lighter fluid	10
Liniments	2
Lipstick	1
Lye	
Ingestion	5
Eye contamination	7
Inhalation when mixed with bleach	9
Topical	6
Magic Markers	1
Makeup	1
Marijuana	10
Markers	
Indelible	2
Water-soluble	1
Matches	
Less than 12 wood or 20 paper	1
More than the above	2
Mercurochrome	
Less than 15 ml	1
More than 15 ml	2
Mercury	

Metallic (thermometer)	1
Salts	2
Merthiolate	
Less than 15 ml	1
More than 15 ml	2
Metal cleaners	10
Methadone	8, 11
Methyl alcohol	2, 8
Methyl salicylate	2
Mineral oil	1
Model cement	10
Modeling clay	1
Morphine	8, 11
Mothballs	2
Mushrooms	2, 8
Nail polish	1
Nail polish remover	
Less than 15 ml	1
More than 15 ml	2
Narcotics	8, 11
Natural gas	9
Nicotine	*See Cigarettes*
Oil of wintergreen	2
Opium	8, 11
Oven cleaner	*See Lye*
Paint	
Acrylic	10
Latex	10
Lead base	10
Oil base	10
Paint chips	10
Paint thinner	10
PCP	*See Phencyclidine hydrochloride*
Pencils	1
Perfume	*See Cologne*
Permanent wave solution	
Ingestion	5
Eye contamination	7
Peroxide (hydrogen)	1
Pesticides	
Ingestion	8
Topical	6, 8
Petroleum distillates	10
Phencyclidine hydrochloride	10
Phosphate-free detergents	5
Pine oil	10
Plants	10
Polishes	10
Printer's ink	10
Propoxyphene	2, 8
Putty	1

Rodenticides	10
Rubbing alcohol	*See Alcohol*
Saccharin	1
Sachet	1
Sedatives	10
Shampoo	
Ingestion	1
(See also Dandruff shampoo)	
Shaving cream	1
Shaving lotion	*See Cologne*
Shoe dyes	2
Shoe polish	2
Sleep aids	10
Soaps	1
Soldering flux	5
Starch, washing	1
Strychnine	10
Sulfuric acid	*See Acids*
Suntan preparations	10
Swimming pool chemicals	5
Talc	
Ingestion	1
Inhalation	10
Tear gas	9
Teething rings	1
Thermometers	1
Toilet bowl cleaner	*See Bathroom bowl cleaner*
Toilet water	*See Cologne*
Toothpaste	1
Toys, fluid-filled	1
Tranquilizers	2, 10
Tricyclic antidepressants	2, 8
Turpentine	10
Typewriter cleaners	10
Varnish	10
Vitamins	
Water-soluble	1
Fat-soluble	2
With iron	10
Wart removers	5
Weed killers	10
Window cleaner	10
Windshield washer fluid	2, 8
Wood preservatives	5

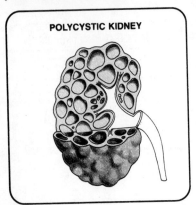

POLYCYSTIC KIDNEY

longer lasting and is marked by meningeal ir-ritation with pain and stiffness in the back and by all the signs of abortive poliomyelitis. Paralytic poliomyelitis begins as abortive poliomyelitis. The symptoms abate, and for several days the person seems well. Malaise, headache, and fever recur; pain, weakness, and paralysis develop. The peak of paralysis is reached within the 1st week. Treatment of the abortive and nonparalytic forms of the disease is symptomatic, consisting of bed rest, good nutrition, and avoidance, for at least 2 weeks, of overexertion, stress, and fatigue. Treatment of the paralytic form includes hospitalization, application of hot packs and the giving of baths, range-of-motion exercise, and assisted ventilation when necessary. As soon as the acute febrile stage is over, active, comprehensive rehabilitation is promptly begun. Poliomyelitis, which has not been eradicated, may be prevented by immunization. Also called **polio** (*informal*). See also **poliovirus**.

poliomyelitis vaccine See **poliovirus vaccine.**

poliosis Depigmentation of the hair on the scalp, eyebrows, eyelashes, mustache, beard, or body. The condition may be inherited and generalized or acquired and localized in patches. Acquired localized poliosis often occurs in alopecia areata.

poliovirus The causative organism of poliomyelitis. There are three serologically distinct types of this very small RNA virus. Infection with or immunization against one type does not protect against the others.

poliovirus vaccine A vaccine prepared from poliovirus to confer immunity to it. TOPV, the trivalent live oral form of the vaccine, is recommended for all children under 18 years who have no specific contraindications. The inactivated poliovirus vaccine (IPV) is recommended for infants and children who are immunodeficient and for unvaccinated adults. TOPV is called Sabin vaccine; IPV is called Salk vaccine. IPV is given subcutaneously. Rarely, vaccine-associated paralysis occurs following administration of TOPV; this reaction has not occurred with IPV.

pollakiuria An abnormal condition characterized by unduly frequent voiding of urine.

pollen coryza Acute seasonal rhinitis caused by exposure to an allergenic. Also called **hay fever.** See also **coryza.**

pollinosis See **hay fever.**

pollution **1.** The act of defiling or rendering impure. **2.** Voluntary or involuntary discharge of semen without sexual intercourse.

polonium (Po) A radioactive element which is one of the disintegration products of uranium; its atomic number is 84; its atomic weight is approximately 210.

polus, *pl.* **poli** Either of the opposite ends of any axis; the official anatomical designation for the extremity of an organ. See also **pole.** —**polar,** *adj.*

poly- A combining form meaning 'many or much': *polyacid, polycholia, polydactylia.*

polyarteritis An abnormal inflammatory condition of several arteries.

polyarteritis nodosa A severe and poorly understood collagen vascular disease in which there is widespread inflammation and necrosis of small- and medium-sized arteries and ischemia of the tissues they serve. Any organ or organ system may be affected. The disease attacks men and women between the ages of 20 to 50. Its cause is unknown, although immunologic factors are suspected. Polyarteritis nodosa may be acute and rapidly fatal, or chronic and wasting. It is characterized by fever, abdominal pain, weight loss, neuropathy, and, if the kidneys are affected, hypertension, edema, and uremia. Some symptoms may mimic gastrointestinal or cardiac disorders. Diagnosis is based upon the clinical signs, laboratory tests, and biopsy of affected sites. Mortality in polyarteritis nodosa is high, especially if there is kidney involvement. Aggressive treatment includes massive doses of corticosteroids. Immunosuppressive drugs have been used experimentally with some success. Physical therapy helps maintain muscle tone and prevents or slows disability.

polychromasia See **polychromatophilia.**

polychromatophile Any cell that may be stained by several different dyes.

polychromatophilia An abnormal tendency of a cell, particularly an erythrocyte, to be dyed by a variety of laboratory stains. Also called **polychromasia.**

polyclonal **1.** Of, pertaining to, or designating a group of identical cells or organisms derived from several identical cells. **2.** Of, pertaining to, or designating several groups of identical cells or organisms (clones) derived from a single cell.

polyclonal gammopathy See **gammopathy.**

polycystic kidney disease (PKD) An abnormal condition in which the kidneys are enlarged and contain many cysts. **Adult polycystic disease (APD)** may be unilateral, bilateral, acquired, or congenital. The condition is characterized by flank pain and high blood pressure. Kidney failure eventually develops, progressing to uremia and death. **Childhood polycystic disease (CPD)** is uncommon and may be differentiated from adult or congenital polycystic disease by genetic, morphologic, and clinical facets. Death usually occurs within a few years as the result of portal hypertension and liver and kidney failure. A portocaval shunt may prolong life into the twenties. **Congenital polycystic disease (CPD)** is a rare congenital aplasia of the kidney involving all or only a small segment of one or both kidneys. Severe bilateral aplasia results in death shortly after birth. Minor aplasia may cause no dysfunction and may never be diagnosed.

polycystic ovary An abnormal condition characterized by anovulation, amenorrhea, hirsutism, and infertility. It is caused by an endocrine imbalance with increased levels of testosterone, estrogen, and luteinizing hormone (LH) and decreased secretion of follicle-stimulating hormone (FSH). The increased level of LH may be the result of an increased sensitivity of the pituitary to stimulation by releasing hormone or of excessive stimulation by the adrenal gland. Polycystic ovary may also be associated with problems in the hypothalamic-pituitary-ovarian axis, with extragonadal sources of androgens, or with androgen-producing tumors. This condition is transmitted as an X-linked dominant or autosomal dominant trait. The depressed but continuous production of FSH associated with this disorder causes continuous partial development of ovarian follicles. Numerous follicular cysts, 2 to 6 mm (about $\frac{1}{12}$ to $\frac{1}{4}$ inch) in diameter, may develop. The affected ovary commonly doubles in size and is invested by a smooth, pearly white capsule. The increased level of estrogen associated with this abnormality raises the risk of cancers of the breast and the endometrium. Depending on the severity of symptoms and whether or not the patient wants to become pregnant, treatment involves suppression of hormonal stimulation of the ovary, usually using female hormones or resection of part of one or both ovaries.

polycythemia An abnormal increase in the number of erythrocytes in the blood. It may be secondary to pulmonary or heart disease or to prolonged exposure to high altitudes. In the absence of a demonstrable cause, it is considered idiopathic. Compare **leukemia.** See also **erythrocytosis.**

polydactyly, polydactylia, polydactylism A congenital anomaly characterized by the presence of more than the normal number of fingers or toes. The condition is usually inherited as an autosomal dominant characteristic and can usually be corrected by surgery shortly after birth. Also called **hyperdactyly.**

polydipsia 1. Excessive thirst characteristic of several conditions, including diabetes mellitus in which an excessive concentration of glucose in the blood osmotically increases the excretion of fluid via increased urination, leading to hypovolemia and thirst. In diabetes insipidus,

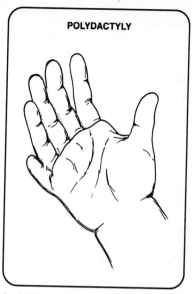

POLYDACTYLY

the deficiency of the pituitary antidiuretic hormone results in excretion of copious amounts of dilute urine, reduced fluid volume in the body, and polydipsia. In nephrogenic diabetes insipidus, there is also copious excretion of urine and consequent polydipsia. Polyuria resulting from other forms of renal dysfunction also leads to polydipsia. The condition may also be psychogenic in origin. 2. *Informal.* Alcoholism.

polygene Any of a group of nonallelic genes that individually exert a small effect but together interact in a cumulative manner to produce a particular characteristic within an individual, usually of a quantitative nature, as size, weight, skin pigmentation, or degree of intelligence. Also called **cumulative gene, multiple factor, multiple gene.** See also **multifactorial inheritance. —polygenic,** *adj.*

polygenic inheritance See **multifactorial inheritance.**

polyhybrid In genetics: pertaining to or describing an individual, organism, or strain that is heterozygous for more than three specific traits, that is the offspring of parents differing in more than three specific gene pairs, or that is heterozygous for more than three particular characteristics or gene loci being followed.

polyhybrid cross In genetics: the mating of two individuals, organisms, or strains that have different gene pairs that determine more than three specific traits or in which more than three particular characteristics or gene loci are being followed.

polyhydramnios See **hydramnios.**

polyleptic Describing a disease or condition marked by numerous remissions and exacerbations.

polyleptic fever A fever occurring paroxysmally, as smallpox and relapsing fever.

polymicrogyria See **microgyria**.

polymorphism **1.** The state or quality of existing or occurring in several different forms. **2.** The state or quality of appearing in different forms at different stages of development. Kinds of polymorphism are **balanced polymorphism, genetic polymorphism.** —**polymorphic,** *adj.*

polymorphocytic leukemia A neoplasm of blood-forming tissues in which mature, segmented granulocytes are predominant. Also called **mature cell leukemia, neutrophilic leukemia.**

polymorphonuclear Having a nucleus with a number of lobules or segments connected by a fine thread.

polymorphonuclear leukocyte A white blood cell containing a segmented lobular nucleus; an eosinophil, basophil, or neutrophil. See also **granulocyte.**

polymorphous Occurring in many forms, possibly changing in structure or appearance at different stages.

polymorphous light eruption A common, recurrent, superficial vascular reaction to sunlight or ultraviolet light in susceptible individuals. Within 1 to 4 days after exposure to the light, small, erythematous papules and vesicles appear on otherwise normal skin, then disappear within 2 weeks. A delayed allergic response is a possible cause. Tanning reduces the severity of the reaction.

polymyalgia rheumatica A chronic, episodic, inflammatory disease of the large arteries that usually develops in people over the age of 60 years. Polymyalgia rheumatica and cranial arteritis may represent the same disease process with slightly different symptoms. Polymyalgia rheumatica primarily affects the muscles. It is characterized by pain and stiffness of the back, shoulder, or neck, usually more severe on rising in the morning; and a cranial headache, as in cranial arteritis, which affects the temporal and occipital arteries, causing a severe, throbbing headache. Serious complications include arterial insufficiency, coronary occlusion, stroke, or blindness. Usually, patients with polymyalgia rheumatica or cranial arteritis have marked elevations of the erythrocyte sedimentation rate. Both forms of the disease may follow a self-limiting course; however, adrenocorticosteroids effectively reduce inflammation and speed recovery. Both forms are probably autoimmune conditions. Also called **temporal arteritis.**

polymyositis Inflammation of many muscles, usually accompanied by deformity, edema, insomnia, pain, sweating, and tension. Some forms of polymyositis are associated with malignancy. See also **dermatomyositis.**

polymyxin An antibiotic used topically and systemically in the treatment of gram-negative bacterial infections.

polymyxin B sulfate An otic and ophthalmic antibiotic anti-infective.

polyneuritic psychosis See **Korsakoff's psychosis.**

polypeptide A chain of amino acids joined by peptide bonds. A polypeptide has a larger molecular weight than a peptide but a smaller molecular weight than a protein. Polypeptides are formed by partial hydrolysis of proteins or by synthesis of amino acids into chains.

polyphagia Eating to the point of gluttony. See also **bulimia.**

polyploid, polyploidic **1.** Of or pertaining to an individual, organism, strain, or cell that has more than the two complete sets of chromosomes normal for the somatic cell. The multiple of the haploid number characteristic of the species is denoted by the appropriate prefix, as in triploid, tetraploid, pentaploid, hexaploid, heptaploid, octaploid, and so on. Polyploidy is rare in animals, producing organisms that are abnormal in appearance and usually infertile, but it is common in plants, which are generally larger, have larger cells, and are more hardy than those with the normal diploid number. **2.** Such an individual, organism, strain, or cell. Compare **aneuploid.** —**polyploidy,** *n.*

polypoid adenocarcinoma See **papillary adenocarcinoma.**

polyradiculitis Inflammation of many nerve roots, as found in Guillain-Barré syndrome.

polyribosome See **polysome.**

polysome In genetics: a group of ribosomes joined together by a molecule of messenger RNA containing the genetic code. The structure is found in the cytoplasm during protein synthesis. Also called **ergosome, polyribosome.** See also **translation.**

polysomy The presence of a chromosome in at least triplicate in an otherwise diploid somatic cell as the result of chromosomal nondisjunction during meiotic division in the maturation of gametes. The chromosome may be replicated three (trisomy), four (tetrasomy), or more times. In males with Klinefelter's syndrome the genotype may be XXXY or XXXXY instead of the usual XXY associated with the syndrome. Among polysomic females with three, four, or five X chromosomes there is a higher frequency of mental retardation.

polytene chromosome An excessively large type of chromosome consisting of bundles of unseparated chromonemata filaments. It is found primarily in the saliva of certain insects. See also **giant chromosome.**

polythiazide A thiazide diuretic.

polyunsaturated fatty acid See **unsaturated fatty acid.**

polyuria The excretion of an abnormally large quantity of urine. Some causes of polyuria are diabetes insipidus, diabetes mellitus, and diuretics.

polyvalent antiserum See **antiserum.**

polyvinyl chloride (PVC) A common synthetic thermoplastic material.

POMP Acronym for a combination drug regimen used in the treatment of cancer, containing three antineoplastics: Purinethol (mercaptopurine), Oncovin (vincristine sulfate), methotrexate, and prednisone (a glucocorticoid).

Pompe's disease   A form of muscle glycogen storage disease in which there is a generalized accumulation of glycogen, resulting from a deficiency of acid maltase (alpha-1,4-glucosidase). It is usually fatal in infants, owing to cardiac or respiratory failure. Children with Pompe's disease appear imbecilic and hypotonic, seldom living beyond 20 years. In adults muscle weakness is progressive, but the disease is not fatal. There is no effective treatment. Also call **glycogen storage disease, type II.** See also **glycogen storage disease.**

pompholyx   See **dyshidrosis.**

POMR   *abbr* **problem-oriented medical record.**

pono-   A combining form meaning 'of or related to pain': *ponograph, ponopalmosis.*

ponos   See **kala-azar.**

pons, *pl.* **pontes**   **1.** Any slip of tissue connecting two parts of a structure or an organ of the body. **2.** A prominence on the ventral surface of the brain stem, between the medulla oblongata and the cerebral peduncles of the midbrain. The pons consists of white matter and a few nuclei and is divided into a ventral portion and a dorsal portion. The ventral portion consists of transverse fibers separated by longitudinal bundles and small nuclei. The dorsal portion comprises the tegmentum, which is a continuation of the reticular formation of the medulla. Also called **bridge of Varolius.**

pont-   A combining form meaning 'bridge': *pontic, ponticulus.*

Pontiac fever   See **Legionnaires' disease.**

pooled plasma   A liquid component of whole blood, collected and pooled from multiple donors to prepare various plasma products or to use directly as a plasma expander when whole blood is unavailable or is contraindicated. It is useful in surgery and in the treatment of hypovolemia because of its stability and availability in freeze-dried form. It is collected from blood banks or prepared directly from donors by plasmapheresis. It is thin and colorless or slightly yellow. Of the total volume of normal blood, 55% to 65% is plasma.

poorly differentiated lymphocytic malignant lymphoma   A lymphoid neoplasm containing many cells resembling lymphoblasts that have a fine nuclear structure and one or more nucleoli. Also called **lymphoblastic lymphoma, lymphoblastic lymphosarcoma, lymphoblastoma.**

popliteal artery   A continuation of the femoral artery, extending from the opening in the abductor magnus, passing through the popliteal fossa at the knee, dividing into eight branches, and supplying various muscles of the thigh, leg, and foot.

popliteal node   A node in one of the groups of lymph glands in the leg. Approximately seven small popliteal nodes are imbedded in the fat of the popliteal fossa at the back of the knee. One node is near the terminal section of the saphenous vein and drains the area around the vein. Another node lying between the popliteal artery

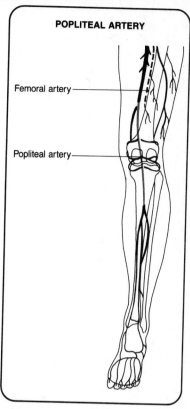

POPLITEAL ARTERY

Femoral artery

Popliteal artery

and the posterior surface of the knee joint drains that region. The other popliteal nodes lie along the popliteal vessels and receive the afferent trunks accompanying the anterior and posterior tibial vessels. Compare **anterior tibial node, inguinal node.**

popliteal pulse   The pulse of the popliteal artery, palpated behind the knee of a person lying prone with the knee flexed.

population   **1.** In genetics: an interbreeding group of individuals, organisms, or plants characterized by genetic continuity through several generations. **2.** A group of individuals collectively occupying a particular geographical locale. **3.** Any group that is distinguished by a particular trait or situation. **4.** Any group measured for some variable characteristic from which samples may be taken for statistical purposes.

population at risk   A group of people who share a characteristic that causes each member to be vulnerable to a particular event, as nonimmunized children who are exposed to poliovirus.

population genetics   A branch of genetics that applies Mendelian inheritance to groups and studies the frequency of alleles and genotypes in breeding populations. See also **Hardy-Weinberg equilibrium principle.**

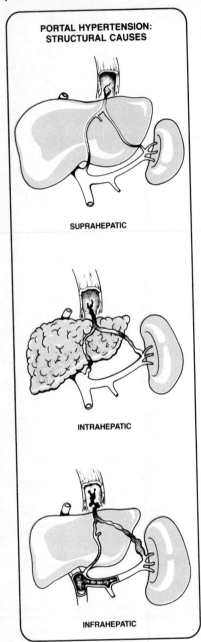

PORTAL HYPERTENSION: STRUCTURAL CAUSES

SUPRAHEPATIC

INTRAHEPATIC

INFRAHEPATIC

por- A combining form meaning 'passage or pore': *porencephalia, porion.*

-pore A combining form meaning 'passageway': *metapore, myelopore.*

poriomania A tendency to leave home impulsively or to be a vagabond.

pork tapeworm See *Taenia solium.*

pork tapeworm infection An infection of the intestine or the tissues, caused by the adult and larval forms of the tapeworm *Taenia solium.* The pork tapeworm can use humans as both intermediate hosts for larvae and definitive hosts for the adult worm. Humans are usually infected with the adult worm after eating contaminated, undercooked pork. The infection is rare in the United States but relatively common in South America, Asia, and Russia. See also **cysticercosis, tapeworm infection.**

poro- A combining form meaning 'callus': *porokeratosis.*

porphobilinogen A substance that appears in the urine of persons with porphyria, representing an error of metabolism. See also **porphyria.**

porphyria A group of inherited disorders in which there is abnormally increased production of substances called porphyrins. Two major classifications of porphyria are **erythropoietic porphyria,** characterized by the production of large quantities of porphyrins in the blood-forming tissue of the bone marrow, and **hepatic porphyria,** in which large amounts of porphyrins are produced in the liver. Common to both classifications are photosensitivity, abdominal pain, and neuropathy.

porphyrin Any iron- or magnesium-free pyrrole derivative occurring in many plant and animal tissues.

portacaval shunt A shunt created surgically to increase the flow of blood from the portal circulation by carrying it into the vena cava.

portal fissure A fissure on the visceral surface of the liver along which the portal vein, the hepatic artery, and the hepatic ducts pass. Also called porta hepatis.

portal hypertension An increased venous pressure in the portal circulation caused by compression or by occlusion in the portal or hepatic vascular system. It results in splenomegaly, large collateral veins, ascites, and, in severe cases, systemic hypertension and esophageal varices. Portal hypertension is frequently associated with alcoholic cirrhosis, but also results from tricuspid valve incompetence, hepatic or portal vein thrombosis, and constrictive pericarditis. Also called **renovascular hypertension.**

portal system The network of veins that drains the blood from the abdominal portion of the digestive tube, the spleen, the pancreas, and the gallbladder and conveys blood from these viscera to the liver.

portal-systemic encephalopathy See **hepatic coma.**

portal vein A vein that ramifies like an artery in the liver and ends in capillarylike sinusoids that convey the blood to the inferior vena cava through the hepatic veins. In the adult, the portal vein has no valves; but in the fetus and during a brief postnatal period the tributaries of the portal vein contain valves that soon atrophy and disappear. In some individuals, the valves persist as degenerate structures. About 8 cm (3½ inches) long, the portal vein is formed at the level of the second lumbar vertebra by the junction of the superior mesenteric and the splenic veins. The portal vein passes behind the duodenum and ascends through the lesser omentum to the porta hepatis, where it divides into the right and the left branches. The right branch of the portal vein enters the right lobe of the liver and the left branch enters the left lobe.

Porter-Silber reaction A reaction, visible as a change in color to yellow, that indicates the amount of adrenal steroids (the 17-hydroxycorticosteroids) excreted per day in the urine. It is used to evaluate adrenocortical function.

port-wine stain See **nevus flammeus.**

position Any one of many postures of the body, as the anatomical position, lateral recumbent position, or semi-Fowler's position. See specific positions.

-position A combining form meaning 'to put, set in place': *juxtaposition, reposition.*

positive 1. Of a laboratory test: indicating that a substance or a reaction is present. 2. Of a sign: indicating on physical examination that a finding is present, often meaning a pathologic change. 3. Of a substance: tending to carry or carrying a positive chemical charge.

positive end-expiratory pressure (PEEP) In respiratory therapy: ventilation controlled by a flow of air delivered in cycles of constant pressure through the respiratory cycle. The patient is intubated and a respirator cycles the air through an endotracheal or tracheostomy tube. PEEP is used for the relief of respiratory distress secondary to shock, pulmonary edema, trauma, surgery, or other conditions in which arterial levels of oxygen are deficient. During PEEP therapy close observation and monitoring of blood gases and vital signs are necessary. Compare **continuous positive airway pressure.**

positive euthanasia See **active euthanasia.**

positive feedback 1. In physiology: an increase in function in response to a stimulus, as micturition increases once the flow of urine has started or as the uterus contracts more frequently and with greater strength once it has begun to contract in labor. 2. *Informal.* An encouraging, favorable, or otherwise positive response from one person to what another person has communicated.

positive identification The unconscious modeling of one's personality on that of another who is admired and esteemed. See also **identification.**

positive pressure 1. A greater-than-ambient atmospheric pressure. 2. In respiratory therapy: any technique in which compressed air or gas is delivered to the respiratory passages at greater-than-ambient pressure. Positive-pressure techniques in respiratory therapy require a flow-regulating device and a delivery system, as a cannula, mouthpiece, endotracheal tube, or tracheostomy tube.

positive-pressure breathing unit See **IPPB unit.**

positive relationship In research: a direct relationship between two variables; as one increases the other can be expected to increase. Also called **direct relationship.** Compare **negative relationship.**

positive signs of pregnancy Three unmistakable signs of pregnancy: fetal heart tones, heard on auscultation; fetal skeleton, seen on X-ray film or ultrasonogram; and fetal parts, felt on palpation.

positron emission tomography (PET) A computerized radiographic technique that employs radioactive substances to examine the metabolic activity of body structures. The patient either inhales or is injected with a biochemical, as glucose, carrying a radioactive substance that emits positively charged particles called positrons. When the positrons combine with negatively charged electrons normally found in body cells, gamma rays are emitted. The electronic circuitry and computers of the PET device detect the gamma rays and convert them into color-coded images that indicate the intensity of the metabolic activity of the organ involved. The radioactive substances used in the PET technique are very short-lived to minimize the patient's exposure to radiation. Researchers use PET to study blood flow and the metabolism of the heart and the blood vessels. There is also a growing application of the technique in the study and diagnosis of cancer and in studies of the biochemical activity of the brain.

post- A combining form meaning 'after or behind': *postarbortal, postcerebellar.*

postcommissurotomy syndrome A condition of unknown etiology occurring within the first few weeks following cardiac valvular surgery. Intermittent episodes of pain and fever may last weeks or months and then resolve spontaneously.

postconcussional syndrome A condition following head trauma, characterized by dizziness, poor concentration, headache, hypersensitivity, and anxiety. It usually resolves itself without treatment.

posterior 1. Of or pertaining to or situated in the back part of a structure, as of the dorsal surface of the human body. 2. The back part of something. 3. Toward the back.

posterior atlantoaxial ligament One of five ligaments connecting the atlas to the axis. It is broad and thin and fixed to the inferior border of the anterior arch of the atlas and to the ventral surface of the body of the axis. Compare **anterior atlantoaxial ligament.**

posterior atlanto-occipital membrane One of a pair of thin, broad, fibrous sheets that forms part of the atlanto-occipital joint between the arch of the atlas and the occipital bone at the posterior margin of the foramen magnum and contains an opening for the vertebral artery and the suboccipital nerve. Also called posterior atlanto-occipital ligament. Compare **anterior atlanto-occipital membrane.**

posterior auricular artery One of a pair of small branches from the external carotid arteries, dividing into auricular and occipital branches and supplying parts of the ear, scalp, and other structures in the head.

posterior costotransverse ligament One of the five ligaments of each costotransverse joint, comprised of a fibrous band passing from the neck of each rib to the base of the vertebra above. Compare **superior costotransverse ligament.**

posterior fossa A depression on the posterior surface of the humerus, above the trochlea, that lodges the olecranon of the ulna when the elbow is extended.

posterior longitudinal ligament A thick, strong ligament attached to the dorsal surfaces of the vertebral bodies, extending from the occipital bone to the coccyx. Also called posterior common ligament.

posterior mediastinal node A node in one of three groups of thoracic visceral nodes, connected to the part of the lymphatic system that serves the esophagus, pericardium, diaphragm, and convex surface of the liver. Compare **anterior mediastinal node.**

posterior mediastinum The irregularly shaped caudal portion of the mediastinum, parallel with the vertebral column. It is bounded ventrally by the pericardium, caudally by the diaphragm, dorsally by the vertebral column from the 4th to the 12th thoracic vertebra, and laterally by the mediastinal pleurae. It contains the bifurcation of the trachea, two primary bronchi, esophagus, thoracic duct, many large lymph nodes, and various vessels, as the thoracic portion of the aortic arch. Compare **anterior mediastinum, middle mediastinum, superior mediastinum.**

posterior nares A pair of posterior openings in the nasal cavity that connect the nasal cavity with the nasopharynx and allow the inhalation and the exhalation of air. Each is an oval aperture that measures about 2.5 cm (1 inch) vertically and is about 1.5 cm (⅗ inch) in diameter. Also called **choana.** Compare **anterior nares.**

posterior neuropore The opening at the caudal end of the embryonic neural tube. It closes at about the 25 somite stage, which indicates the end of horizon XII in the numerical anatomical charting of human embryonic development. Compare **anterior neuropore.** See also **horizon.**

posterior pituitary gland See **neurohypophysis.**

posterior tibial artery One of the divisions of the popliteal artery, starting at the distal border of the popliteus muscle, passing behind the tibia, dividing into eight branches, and supplying various muscles of the lower leg, foot, and toes. Its eight branches are the peroneal, nutrient (tibial), muscular, posterior medial malleolar, communicating, medial calcaneal, medial plantar, and lateral plantar. Compare **anterior tibial artery.**

posterior tibialis pulse The pulse of the posterior tibialis artery palpated on the medial aspect of the ankle, just posterior to the prominence of the ankle bone.

posterior vein of the left ventricle One of the five tributaries of the coronary sinus that drains blood from the capillary bed of the myocardium. It courses along the diaphragmatic surface of the left ventricle, accompanying the circumflex branch of the left coronary artery. In some individuals, it ends in the great cardiac vein. Compare **great cardiac vein, middle cardiac vein, small cardiac vein.**

postero- A combining form meaning 'of or related to the posterior part': *posteroanterior, posteromedian.*

posthepatic cirrhosis See **cirrhosis.**

postictal Of or pertaining to the period following a convulsion. —**postictus,** *n.*

postinfectious Occurring after an infection.

postinfectious encephalitis See **encephalitis.**

postinfectious glomerulonephritis The acute form of glomerulonephritis, which may follow 1 to 6 weeks after a streptococcal infection. Characteristics are hematuria, oliguria, and proteinuria, especially in the form of granular casts. There is slight impairment of renal function, but most patients recover in 1 to 3 months. There is no specific treatment; the dietary restriction of protein and the prescription of diuretics may be necessary until kidney function returns to normal. See also **glomerulonephritis.**

postmastectomy exercises Exercises essential to the prevention of shortening of the muscles and contracture of the joints following mastectomy.

postmature 1. Overly developed or matured. 2. Of or pertaining to a postmature infant. See also **dysmaturity.** —**postmaturity,** *n.*

postmature infant An infant, born after the end of the 42nd week of gestation, bearing the physical signs of placental insufficiency. Characteristically, the infant has dry, peeling skin, long fingernails and toenails, and folds of skin on the thighs and, sometimes, on the arms and buttocks. Hypoglycemia and hypokalemia are common. Postmature infants often look as if they have lost weight in utero. The newborn is fed early and the calcium and potassium levels in the blood are monitored and corrected, if necessary, to avoid seizures and neurologic damage. To avoid the syndrome, labor may be induced as gestation approaches 42 weeks. To anticipate the problems associated with the syndrome, the fetus and the mother may be electronically monitored through labor.

postmenopausal 1. Of or pertaining to the period of life following the menopause. 2. Being postmenopausal.

postmortem 1. After death. 2. *Informal.* Postmortem examination. Also called **autopsy, necropsy.**

postmyocardial infarction syndrome

A condition that may occur days or weeks after an acute myocardial infarction. It is characterized by fever, pericarditis with a friction rub, pleurisy, pleural effusion, and joint pain. It tends to recur and often provokes severe anxiety, depression, and fear that it is another heart attack. Treatment includes aspirin and a short course of corticosteroids. Nursing care includes close observation, emotional support, and reassurance, especially when debilitating anxiety and depression are present.

postnasal drip (PND) A drop-by-drop discharge of nasal mucus into the posterior pharynx, often accompanied by a feeling of obstruction, an unpleasant taste, and fetid breath, caused by rhinitis, chronic sinusitis, or hypersecretion by the nasopharyngeal mucosa. Treatment include the application of drops or sprays of phenylephrine or ephedrine sulfate to constrict blood vessels and reduce hyperemia, sinus irrigation to improve drainage, and the use of appropriate antibiotics. Therapy for allergies may be indicated in some cases, and surgery may be required if the nasal passages are obstructed by polyps or a deviated septum.

postnecrotic cirrhosis A nodular form of cirrhosis that may follow hepatitis or other inflammation of the liver. Also called **posthepatic cirrhosis.** See also **cirrhosis.**

postoperative Of or pertaining to the period of time following surgery. It begins with the patient's emergence from anesthesia and continues through the time required for the acute effects of the anesthetic to abate.

postoperative atelectasis A form of atelectasis in which collapse of lung tissue is caused by the depressant effects of anesthetic drugs. Deep breathing and coughing are encouraged at frequent intervals postoperatively to prevent this condition.

postoperative bed A bed prepared for a patient who is weak or unconscious, as when recovering from anesthesia. The bed is in the flat position. The top linen is fan-folded to the far side of the bed and not tucked in. The bed is made in this way to simplify transferring a patient from a stretcher into the bed.

postoperative care The management of a patient following surgery.

NURSING CONSIDERATIONS: The recovery room nurse performs the immediate postoperative procedures, and the clinical-unit nurse provides ongoing care, emotional support, and instructions for the patient and family. Special attention is given to preventing trauma postoperatively, as may occur when confused or elderly patients fall getting out of bed. The airway patency, rate, depth, and character of respirations, pulse, blood pressure, temperature, skin color, level of consciousness, and condition of dressings and drainage tubes are assessed. If respirations are noisy, the patient is assisted in coughing. A rapid, weak, thready pulse may indicate increased bleeding and is reported, especially if other signs of impending shock, as hypotension or decreased consciousness, are evident. The dressing

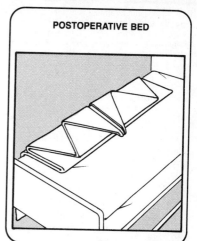

POSTOPERATIVE BED

is examined at frequent intervals and excessive drainage is reported immediately. The patient is positioned for comfort and good ventilation with the side rails of the bed raised for safety and the head slightly elevated, except after spinal anesthesia, neurosurgery, and certain kinds of ocular surgery. A cardiac monitor may be connected. Parenteral fluids and medication for pain are administered as ordered. Fluid intake and output are measured and ambulation, when ordered, is assisted. See also **preoperative care.**

postoperative cholangiography In diagnostic radiology: a procedure for outlining the major bile ducts. A radiopaque contrast material is injected into the common bile duct via a T-tube inserted during surgery. It is usually performed after a cholecystectomy to discover any residual calculi. See also **cholangiography.**

postpartal care Care of the mother and her newborn infant during the first few days of the puerperium. See also **newborn intrapartal care.**

postpartum After giving birth.

postpartum depression An abnormal psychiatric condition that occurs following childbirth, typically, from 3 days to 6 weeks postpartum. Symptoms range from mild 'postpartum blues' to an intense, suicidal, depressive psychosis. The etiology is not proven; neurochemical and psychologic influences have been implicated. Approximately one third of patients have had some degree of psychiatric abnormality predating the pregnancy. The disorder recurs in subsequent pregnancies in 25% of cases. Depending on the severity of the disorder, psychoactive medication or psychiatric hospitalization may be necessary.

postperfusion syndrome A cytomegalovirus (CMV) infection, occurring between 2 to 4 weeks after the transfusion of fresh blood containing CMV. Postperfusion syndrome is characterized by prolonged fever, hepatitis, rash, atypical lymphocytosis, and, occasionally, jaundice. No specific treatment is available.

postpericardiotomy syndrome A condition that sometimes occurs days or weeks after pericardiotomy, characterized by symptoms of pericarditis, often without any fever. It appears to be an autoimmune response to damaged muscle cells of the myocardium and pericardium. See also **pericarditis.**

postpill amenorrhea Failure of normal menstrual cycles to resume within 3 months following discontinuation of oral contraception. The pathophysiology of this uncommon, rarely permanent condition is poorly understood. See also **amenorrhea, oral contraceptive.**

postpolycythemic myeloid metaplasia A common late development in polycythemia vera, characterized by anemia owing to sclerosis of the bone marrow. The production of red blood cells then occurs only in extramedullary tissue, as the liver and spleen. This condition is frequently complicated by leukemia. See also **myeloid metaplasia, polycythemia.**

postprandial (pp) After a meal.

postpubertal panhypopituitarism See **panhypopituitarism.**

postpuberty, postpubescence A period of approximately 1 to 2 years following puberty during which skeletal growth slows and the physiologic functions of the reproductive years are established. —**postpuberal, postpubertal, postpubescent,** *adj.*

postsynaptic 1. Situated after a synapse. 2. Occurring after a synapse has been crossed.

postsynaptic element Any neurological structure, as a neuron, situated distal to a synapse.

postterm infant See **postmature infant.**

posttraumatic stress disorder An anxiety disorder characterized by an acute emotional response to a traumatic event or situation involving severe environmental stress, as a natural disaster or serious automobile accident. Symptoms include recurrent, intrusive recollections or nightmares, diminished responsiveness to the external world, hyperalertness or an exaggerated startle response, sleep disturbances, irritability, memory impairment, difficulty in concentrating, depression, anxiety, headaches, and vertigo. Treatment usually consists of sedation in extreme cases followed by supportive psychotherapy. Also called **stress reaction, stress response syndrome. See also combat fatigue, shell shock.**

postural albuminuria See **orthostatic proteinuria.**

postural drainage The use of positioning to drain secretions from specific segments of the bronchi and the lungs into the trachea. Coughing normally expels secretions from the trachea. Positions are selected that promote drainage from the affected parts of the lungs. Pillows and raised sections of the hospital bed support or elevate parts of the body. Effectiveness of the procedure depends on positioning that allows drainage by gravity and on liquefaction, ciliary action, and effective breathing.

NURSING CONSIDERATIONS: A patient with dyspnea, hemoptysis, signs of cerebral hemorrhage, increased intracerebral pressure, or lung abscess is placed in a head-down position with caution and only with a specific medical order. Suction is kept available for the patient who might not be able to expel the secretions that have drained into the trachea. The patient's tolerance for the procedure and the position is carefully observed; fatigue is avoided. See also **cupping and vibrating.**

postural hypotension See **orthostatic hypotension.**

postural proteinuria See **orthostatic proteinuria.**

postural vertigo See **cupulolithiasis.**

posture The position of the body with respect to the surrounding space. A posture is determined and maintained by coordination of the various muscles that move the limbs, by proprioception, and by the sense of balance.

pot *Slang.* See **cannabis.**

pot- A combining form meaning 'of or related to drinking': *potable, potocytosis.*

potassium (K) An alkali-metal element, the seventh most abundant element in the earth's crust. Its atomic number is 19; its atomic weight is 39.102. Potassium occurs in a wide variety of silicate rocks; in its elemental form it is easily oxidized and extremely reactive. Potassium salts are necessary to the life of all plants and animals. Potassium in the body constitutes the predominant intracellular cation, helping to regulate neuromuscular excitability and muscle contraction. Sources of potassium in the diet are whole grains, meat, legumes, fruit, and vegetables. The average adequate daily intake for most adults is 2 to 4 g. Potassium is important in glycogen formation, protein synthesis, and in the correction of imbalances of acid-base metabolism, especially in association with the action of sodium and hydrogen ions. Most of the dietary potassium in the body is absorbed from the gastrointestinal tract and, in homeostasis, the amount of potassium excreted in the urine is essentially equal to the amount of potassium in the diet. Potassium salts are very important as therapeutic agents but are extremely dangerous if used improperly. The kidneys play an important role in controlling potassium secretion and absorption. Aldosterone stimulates sodium reabsorption and potassium secretion by the kidneys; the major extrarenal adaptation to this process involves the absorption of potassium by the body tissues, especially the tissues of the muscles and the liver. The intracellular concentrations of potassium and hydrogen are higher than those of the extracellular fluid of the body, and when the extracellular hydrogen ion concentration increases, as in acidosis, potassium ions move from the cells into the extracellular fluid. When the extracellular hydrogen ion decreases, as in alkalosis, potassium ions move from the extracellular fluid into the cells. Extracellular acidosis produces hyperkalemia. Extracellular alkalosis produces hypokalemia. Increased gas-

POSITIONS FOR POSTURAL DRAINAGE

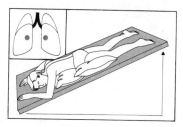

THE POSTERIOR BASAL SEGMENTS

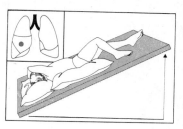

THE MEDIAL AND LATERAL SEGMENTS

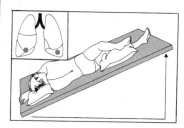

THE LATERAL BASAL SEGMENTS

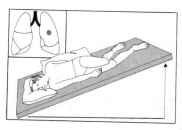

THE SUPERIOR AND INFERIOR SEGMENTS
OF THE LINGULAR PORTION

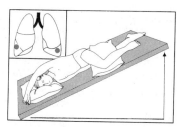

THE ANTERIOR BASAL SEGMENTS

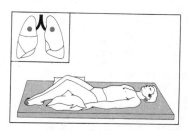

THE ANTERIOR SEGMENTS

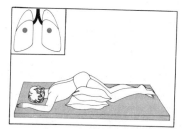

THE SUPERIOR SEGMENTS

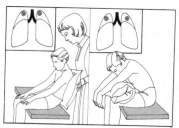

APICAL
SEGMENT

POSTERIOR
SEGMENT

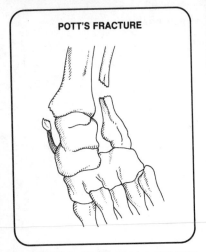

POTT'S FRACTURE

trointestinal secretion of potassium may occur with the loss of gastrointestinal fluid through vomiting, diarrhea, surgical drainage, or the chronic use of laxatives.

potassium acetate, p. bicarbonate, p. chloride, p. gluconate, p. phosphate Sources of potassium in electrolyte replacement solutions.

potassium hydroxide (KOH) A white, soluble, highly caustic compound. Occasionally used in solution as an escharotic for bites of rabid animals, KOH has many laboratory uses as an alkalinizing agent, including the preparation of clinical specimens for examination of fungi under a microscope.

potassium iodide (SSKI) An expectorant.

potassium penicillin V See **penicillin V.**

potassium permanganate An antiseptic.

potassium-sparing diuretic See **diuretic.**

potency In embryology: the range of developmental possibilities of which an embryonic cell or part is capable, regardless of whether the stimulus for growth or differentiation is natural, artificial, or experimental. See also **competence.**

-potent A combining form meaning 'able to do' something specified: *pluripotent, viripotent.*

potential trauma In dentistry: a change in tissue that may occur because of existing malocclusion or dental disharmony.

potentiation An action in which the effect of two drugs given simultaneously is greater than the effect of the drugs given separately.

Pott's disease See **tuberculous spondylitis.**

Pott's fracture A fracture of the fibula near the ankle, often accompanied by a break of the malleolus of the tibia or rupture of the internal lateral ligament. Also called **Dupuytren's fracture.**

pouch of Douglas See **rectouterine pouch.**

poultice A soft, moist, pulp spread between layers of gauze or cloth and applied hot to an area to provide heat or counterirritation.

povidone-iodine A disinfectant commonly applied to the skin before surgery and to the urinary meatus after catheterization.

Powassan virus infection An uncommon form of encephalitis caused by a tick-borne arbovirus found in eastern Canada and the northern United States.

pox 1. Any of several vesicular or pustular exanthematous diseases. 2. The pitlike scars of smallpox. 3. Syphilis.

poxvirus A member of a family of viruses that includes the organisms that cause molluscum contagiosum, smallpox, and vaccinia.

PPD *abbr* **Purified protein derivative,** the material used in testing for tuberculin sensitivity. Also called PPD of Seibert, PPD-S. See also **Mantoux test, tine test, tuberculin test, tuberculosis.**

PPLO *abbr* **pleuropneumonia-like organism.** See *Mycoplasma.*

PPO *abbr* Diphengloxazole, a scintillator used in radiology.

PPV *abbr* positive pressure ventilation. See **positive pressure,** definition 2.

Pr Symbol for **praseodymium.**

practice theory In nursing research: a theory that describes, explains, and prescribes nursing practice. It serves as the basis for specific items in the curriculum of nursing education and for the development of theories in the administration of nursing.

practicing medicine without a license In law: practicing activities defined under state law in the medical practice act without physician supervision, direction, or control.

practitioner A person qualified to practice in a special professional field, as a nurse practitioner.

Prader-Willi syndrome A metabolic condition characterized by congenital hypotonia, hyperphagia, obesity, mental retardation, and the development of diabetes mellitus in later life. Associated with a less-than-normal secretion of gonadotropic hormones by the pituitary gland.

prae- See **pre-.**

-pragia A combining form meaning 'quality of action': *bradypragia, dyspragia.*

pralidoxime chloride An antidote for organophosphate poisoning.

pramoxine hydrochloride A topical anesthetic and antipruritic agent.

prandial Pertaining to a meal, used in relation to timing, as postprandial. **—prandiality,** *n.*

praseodymium (Pr) A rare-earth metallic element. Its atomic number is 59; its atomic weight is 140.91.

Prausnitz-Küstner (PK) test A skin test in which an allergic response is transferred to a nonallergic person who acts as a surrogate to permit identification of the allergen. After screening the allergic patient for hepatitis and other serum-borne diseases, a small amount of the patient's serum is injected intradermally into several sites on a nonallergic person (usually a relative). After 24 to 48 hours, suspected antigens are applied to these sites on the nonallergic person. A sensitive skin response (wheal-flare reaction), indicates that the suspect antigen is indeed causing hypersensitivity in the allergic patient. The test is only performed when skin sensitivity testing cannot be performed directly on the allergic person. Also called **passive transfer test, PK test.** Compare **patch test, radioallergosorbent test.** See also **anaphylaxis.**

-praxia A combining form meaning a 'condition concerning the performance of movements': *dyspraxia.*

-praxis A combining form meaning a 'therapeutic treatment involving a (specified) method': *actinopraxis.*

prazepam A benzodiazepine antianxiety agent.

prazosin hydrochloride A vasodilator antihypertensive.

pre- A combining form meaning 'before': *preataxic, precritical, pregenital, preconscious.* Also **prae-.**

preagonal ascites A rapid accumulation of fluid within the peritoneal cavity, representing the transudation of serum from the circulatory system. Preagonal ascites immediately precedes death in some cases. See also **ascites.**

preanesthetic medication **1.** Any sedative, tranquilizer, hypnotic, or anticholinergic medication administered prior to anesthesia. Pentobarbital, secobarbital, phenobarbital, morphine, scopolamine, and atropine are commonly used. The choice of drug depends on such variables as the patient's age and physical condition and the specific operative procedure. **2.** The administration of such medications.

preaortic node A node in one of the three sets of lumbar lymph nodes that serve various abdominal viscera supplied by the celiac, superior mesenteric, and inferior mesenteric arteries. The preaortic nodes lie ventral to the aorta and are divided into the celiac nodes, superior mesenteric nodes, and inferior mesenteric nodes. Most of the efferents from the preaortic nodes unite to form the lymphatic intestinal trunk, which enters the cisterna chyli. Compare **lateral aortic node, retroaortic node.**

precancerous dermatitis See **intraepidermal carcinoma.**

precipitate **1.** To cause a substance to separate or to settle out of solution. **2.** A substance that has separated from or settled out of a solution. **3.** Occurring hastily or unexpectedly.

precipitate delivery Childbirth that occurs with such speed or in such a situation that the usual preparations cannot be made. See also **emergency childbirth.**

precipitin An antibody that causes formation of an insoluble complex when combined with a specific soluble antigen.

precocious Pertaining to the early, often

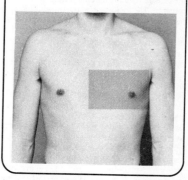

PRECORDIAL AREA

premature, development of physical or mental qualities.

precocious dentition The abnormal acceleration of the eruption of the deciduous or permanent teeth, usually associated with an endocrine imbalance, as hyperthyroidism. Compare **retarded dentition.**

preconscious **1.** Prior to the development of self-consciousness and self-awareness. **2.** In psychiatry: the mental function in which thoughts, ideas, emotions, or memories not in immediate awareness can be brought into the consciousness, usually through associations, without encountering any intrapsychic resistance or repression. **3.** The mental phenomena capable of being recalled, although not present in the conscious mind.

precordial Of or pertaining to the precordium, which forms the region over the heart and the lower part of the thorax.

precordial movement Any motion of the anterior wall of the thorax localized in the area over the heart. Kinds of precordial movements include apical impulse, left ventricular thrust, right ventricular thrust.

predeciduous dentition The epithelial structures found in the mouth of the infant preceding the eruption of the deciduous teeth. See also **deciduous dentition, teething.**

predictive hypothesis In research: a hypothesis that predicts the nature of a relationship among the variables to be studied.

predictive validity Validity of a test or a measurement tool that is established by demonstrating its ability to predict the results of an analysis of the same data using another test instrument or measurement tool. See also **validity.**

predictor variable See **independent variable.**

prednisolone, p. acetate, p. sodium phosphate, p. tebutate Topical glucocorticoid ophthalmic anti-inflammatory agents.

prednisone A glucocorticoid.

preeclampsia An abnormal condition of pregnancy characterized by the onset of acute hypertension after the 24th week of gestation.

The classic triad of preeclampsia is hypertension, proteinuria, and edema. The etiology of the disease remains unknown despite extensive research. The incidence increases with increasing gestational age, and it is more common with multiple gestation, hydatidiform mole, or hydramnios. A typical lesion in the kidneys, glomeruloendotheliosis, is pathognomonic. Termination of the pregnancy results in resolution of the signs and symptoms of the disease and in healing of the renal lesion. Mild preeclampsia is diagnosed if one or more of the following signs develop after the 24th week of gestation: systolic blood pressure of 140 mmHg or more or a rise of 30 mmHg or more above the woman's usual systolic blood pressure; diastolic blood pressure of 90 mmHg or more or a rise of 15 mmHg or more above the woman's usual diastolic blood pressure; proteinuria; edema. Severe preeclampsia is diagnosed if one or more of the following is present: systolic blood pressure of 160 mmHg or more or a diastolic blood pressure of 110 mmHg or more on two occasions 6 hours apart with the woman at bed rest; proteinuria of 5 g or more in 24 hours; oliguria of less than 400 ml (13½ oz) in 24 hours; ocular or cerebral vascular disorders; cyanosis or pulmonary edema. Preeclampsia commonly causes abnormal metabolic function, including negative nitrogen balance, increased central nervous system irritability, hyperactive reflexes, compromised renal function, hemoconcentration, and alterations of fluid and electrolyte balance. Complications include premature separation of the placenta, hypofibrinogenemia, hemolysis, cerebral hemorrhage, ophthalmologic damage, pulmonary edema, hepatocellular changes, fetal malnutrition, and lowered birth weight. The most serious complication is eclampsia, which can result in mternal and fetal death. Healthy living conditions, including a diet high in protein, calories, and essential nutritional elements, and rest and exercise are associated with a decreased incidence of preeclampsia. Treatment includes rest, sedation, magnesium sulfate, and antihypertensives. Ultimately, if eclampsia threatens, delivery by induction of labor or cesarean section may be necessary. See also **eclampsia.**

preferential anosmia   The inability to smell certain odors. The condition is often caused by psychological factors concerning either a particular smell or the situation in which the smell occurs.

prefix   A portion of a word, usually derived from Latin or Greek, occurring at the beginning of a compound word. In this dictionary, prefixes are called combining forms. In the words *antiseptic, epidermis, hypoglycemia, periosteum,* and *semipermeable, anti-, epi-, hypo-, peri-,* and *semi-* are prefixes.

preformation   An early theory in embryology in which the organism is contained in minute and complete form within the germ cell and after fertilization grows from microscopic to normal size. Compare **epigenesis.**

pregnancy   The gestational process, comprising the growth and development within a woman of a new individual from conception through the embryonic and fetal periods to birth. Pregnancy lasts approximately 266 days (38 weeks) from the day of fertilization, but it is clinically considered to last 40 weeks from the 1st day of the last menstrual period. The expected date of confinement is calculated on the latter basis even if a woman's periods are irregular. Pregnancy begins following coitus at or near the time of ovulation (usually about 14 days prior to a woman's next expected menstrual period). Of the millions of ejaculated sperm cells, thousands reach the female ovum in the outer end of the fallopian tube, but usually only one penetrates the egg for union of the male and female pronuclei and conception. The zygote, genetically a unique entity, begins cell division as it is transported to the uterine cavity where it implants in the uterine wall. Maternal and embryologic elements together form the beginnings of the placenta, which grows into the substance of the uterus. The placenta functions in maternal-fetal exchange of nutrients and waste products, though the maternal and fetal bloods do not normally mix. See **expected date of confinement.**

pregnancy rate   In statistics: the ratio of pregnancies per 100 woman-years, calculated as the product of the number of pregnancies in the women observed, multiplied by 1,200 (months), divided by the product of the number of women observed, multiplied by the number of months observed. If 50 women used one contraceptive method for 12 months, and 5 of them became pregnant, the pregnancy rate would be 10 per 100 woman-years.

pregnanediol   A crystalline, biologically inactive compound found in the urine of women during pregnancy or the secretory phase of the menstrual cycle. A dihydroxy derivative of the saturated steroid pregnane, pregnanediol is formed by the reduction of progesterone.

preinvasive carcinoma   See **carcinoma in situ.**

Preisner model   See **nurse-therapist model.**

premalignant fibroepithelioma   An elevated flesh-colored sessile neoplasm formed of interlacing ribbons of epithelial cells on a hyperplastic mesodermal stroma. The tumor occurs most often on the lower trunk of older people and may be found in association with a superficial basal cell carcinoma or may develop into a basal cell carcinoma.

premature   **1.** Not fully developed or mature. **2.** Occurring before the appropriate or usual time. **3.** Of or pertaining to an infant born before 37 weeks of gestation.

premature atrial contraction (PAC)   A cardiac arrhythmia characterized by an atrial beat occurring before the expected excitation, indicated electrocardiographically as an early P wave followed by a normal QRS complex. Premature atrial beats may occur occasionally, in a regular pattern, or several may occur in se-

STAGES OF PREGNANCY

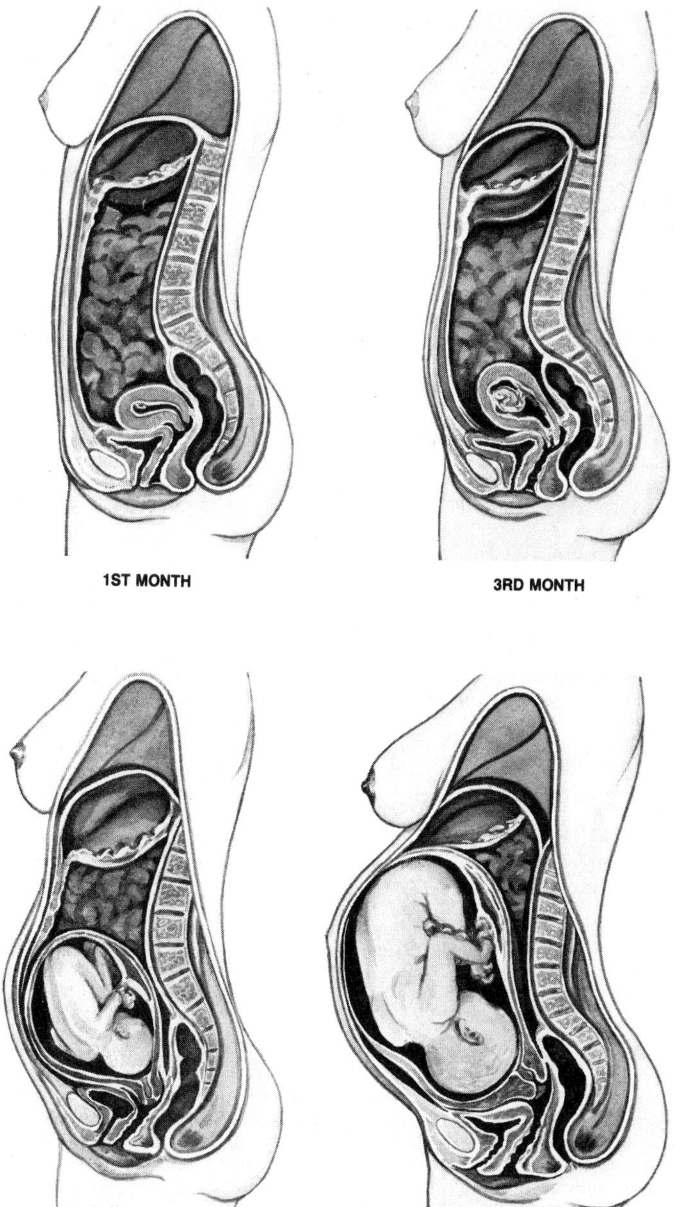

1ST MONTH

3RD MONTH

6TH MONTH

9TH MONTH

THE PREMATURE AND THE TERM INFANT COMPARED

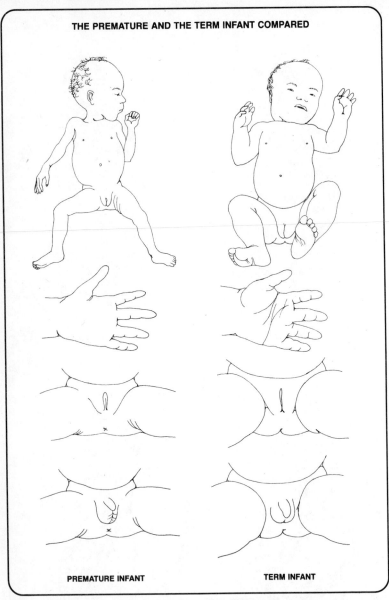

PREMATURE INFANT   TERM INFANT

quence. The arrhythmia may be the result of atrial enlargement or ischemia or may be caused by stress, caffeine, or nicotine.

premature ejaculation Uncontrollable, untimely ejaculation of semen, often owing to anxiety during sexual intercourse. Behavioral techniques can be learned by the man and his partner to extend the length of time between erection and ejaculation. See also **ejaculation, erection.**

premature infant Any neonate, regardless of birth weight, born prior to 37 weeks of gestation. Since exact gestational age is often difficult to determine, low birth weight is a significant criterion for identifying the high-risk infant with incomplete organ system development. Predisposing factors associated with prematurity include multiple pregnancy, toxemia, chronic disease, acute infection, sensitization to blood incompatibility, and any severe trauma that may interfere with normal fetal development. In most instances the etiology is unknown. The premature infant usually appears small and scrawny, has a large head in relation to body size, and weighs less than 2,500 g (5½ lb). The skin is bright pink, smooth, shiny, and translucent with the underlying vessels clearly visible. The arms and legs are extended, not flexed, as in the full-term infant. There is little subcutaneous fat, sparse hair, few creases on the soles and palms, and poorly developed ear cartilage. In boys, the scrotum has few rugae, and the testes may be undescended; in girls, the labia gape, and the clitoris is prominent. Common problems are variations of body temperature, apnea, respiratory distress, poor sucking and swallowing reflexes, small stomach capacity, lowered tolerance of the alimentary tract that may lead to necrotizing enterocolitis, immature renal function, hepatic dysfunction often associated with hyperbilirubinemia, incomplete enzyme systems, and susceptibility to various metabolic upsets, as hypoglycemia, hyperglycemia, and hypocalcemia. The degree of complications and the rate of survival of premature infants are directly related to the state of physiological and anatomical maturity of the various organ systems at the time of birth, the condition of the infant other than prematurity, and the quality of postnatal care. With treatment in a neonatal intensive care unit, survival rates improve yearly. Increasing numbers of very small infants develop normally, and those who do not have seizures or apneic spells in the first few days will not suffer neurologic or physical sequelae. Of primary concern for the nurse is the stabilization of body temperature by maintaining a neutral thermal environment, the maintenance of respiration, the prevention of infection, the provision of adequate nutrition and hydration, and the conservation of energy. Also called **preterm infant.** Compare **postmature infant.**

premature labor Labor that occurs earlier in pregnancy than normal, either before the fetus has reached a weight of 2,000 to 2,500 g (4½ to 5½ lb) or before the 37th or 38th week of gestation. No single measure of fetal weight or gestational age is used universally to designate premature birth. Prematurity is a concomitant of 75% of births that result in neonatal mortality. It may occur spontaneously or iatrogenically. The incidence of premature labor increases in inverse proportion to maternal age, weight, and socioeconomic status. Incidence is higher for black women, for women who have not had adequate prenatal care or whose obstetric history is abnormal, and for women who smoke or whose diets are deficient in protein or calories. Predisposing conditions include maternal infection, low weight gain, uterine bleeding, multiple gestation, polyhydramnios, uterine abnormalities, incompetent cervix, premature rupture of membranes, and intrauterine fetal growth retardation. The etiology of premature labor is poorly understood; in some cases, there may be several contributing causes. In some pregnancies, premature labor may be homeostatic, resulting in the best possible outcome under the particular, abnormal conditions. If premature labor itself constitutes a threat to the fetus, the outcome of pregnancy may be improved if labor can be inhibited. Determining accurately which pregnancies are likely to benefit from the inhibition of labor and which are not is difficult. Medications used to stop labor are not always effective. Misdiagnosis of gestational age and fetal condition may lead to induction of labor that is inadvertently premature; premature infants whose births have been brought about inappropriately early account for 15% of admissions to newborn intensive care nurseries. Also called **preterm labor.** See also **premature infant, small-for-gestational-age infant.**

premature ventricular contraction (PVC) A cardiac arrhythmia characterized by a ventricular beat preceding the expected electrical impulse, shown on the electrocardiogram as an early, wide QRS complex without a preceding P wave. Premature ventricular contractions may occur occasionally, in a regular pattern, or as several in sequence. They may be caused by stress, acidosis, electrolyte imbalance, hypoxemia, hypercapnia, ventricular enlargement, or a toxic reaction to drugs, especially to digitalis or quinidine. Isolated PVCs are not clinically significant, but they may produce tachycardia, and frequent occurrence of the arrhythmia indicates myocardial irritability and may be a precursor of ventricular tachycardia or fibrillation and lead to inadequate cardiac output. Agents used in treating PVCs include procainamide, lidocaine, oxygen, sodium bicarbonate, and potassium. Also called **premature venticular beat.**

premenopausal **1.** Of or pertaining to the time of life preceding the menopause. **2.** Being premenopausal.

premenstrual tension (PMT) A syndrome of nervous tension, irritability, weight gain, edema, headache, mastalgia, dysphoria, and lack of coordination occurring during the last few days of the menstrual cycle preceding the onset of menstruation. There are several theories that attempt to explain the etiology of the syndrome, including nutritional deficiency, stress, hormonal imbalance, and various emotional disorders. None has proved valid.

premolar One of eight teeth, four in each dental arch, located lateral to and posterior to the canine teeth. The premolars appear during childhood and remain until old age. They are smaller and shorter than the canine teeth. The crown of each premolar is compressed anteroposteriorly and surmounted by two cusps. The neck of the premolar is oval; the root is usually single and compressed, with an anterior and a posterior groove. The upper premolars are larger than the lower premolars. Also called **bicuspid.** Compare **canine tooth, incisor, molar.**

premolar tooth See **bicuspid.**

prenatal Prior to birth; occurring or existing before birth, referring both to the care of the woman during pregnancy and the growth and development of the fetus. Also called **antenatal.**

prenatal development The entire process of growth, maturation, differentiation, and development that occurs between conception and birth. On approximately the 14th day before the next expected menstrual period, ovulation usually occurs. If fertilization occurs, the ovum undergoes cell division several times during the first 2 weeks, becoming a morula and then a blastocyst that is able to implant in the uterine wall. From the beginning of the 3rd to the end of the 7th week of embryonic development, implantation deepens and completes. Primitive uteroplacental circulation originates between the enlarging trophoblast and the maternal endometrial tissue of the uterus. The amniotic cavity appears as an opening between the inner cell mass and the invading trophoblast. A thin lining in the cavity becomes the amnion. At this point, the embryo is a two-layered embryonic disk composed of an ectoderm and an endoderm. As the disk thickens in the middle, giving rise to the third cell layer, or mesoderm, the basic structural systems of the body begin to form. The neural tube develops as a precursor of the central nervous system in the midline of the cranial portion of the ectoderm. Primitive blood vessels and blood cells, a heart tube, and umbilical vessels are formed and begin to function. Arm and leg buds may be seen, and rudimentary gut, lungs, and kidneys form. By the 5th week, the brain has begun to grow rapidly, the heart tube is divided into chambers, the palate and the upper lip are forming, and the urogenital system is developing. By the end of the 7th week, all essential systems are present. The period of time from the 8th week to birth is called the fetal stage. From the 8th to the 10th week, the fetus continues to grow and develop rapidly. The head is almost one half of its total length, and arms, legs, and face are clearly recognizable. The fetus floats in the amniotic fluid of the amniotic sac within the uterus; the umbilical vessels in the cord extend to a rapidly growing placenta. By the 12th week, the features of the face are formed, and the eyelids are present but not yet closed, as they have not divided into upper and lower eyelids. The palate is fusing, there is a neck between the large head and the body, and tooth buds and nail beds have begun to form. Identification of the external genitalia is possible for the first time. From the 13th to the 16th weeks, the arms, legs, and trunk grow rapidly, and the fetus is active. Scalp hair develops, and the skeleton of the fetus is calcified. Between the 17th and the 20th weeks of pregnancy, movement begins. At the 24th week, the external ears are smooth and soft, and the skin is wrinkled and translucent. The body is covered with lanugo and vernix and weighs a little more than 454 g (1 lb). At 28 weeks, subcutaneous fat begins to develop; fingernails and toenails are present; the eyelids are separate, and the eyes may open; scalp hair is well developed; and, in males, the testes are at or below the internal

inguinal ring. By the 32nd week, the fetus weighs between 1,361 to 1,814 g (3 to 4 lb). The hair is fine and woolly, the fingernails and toenails have grown to the tips of the fingers and toes, and there are one or two creases on the anterior part of the soles of the feet. The areolae of the breasts are visible but flat. In females, the clitoris is prominent, and the labia majora are small and separated. At 36 weeks, the body and the limbs are fuller and more rounded, creases involve the anterior two thirds of the soles, and the skin is thicker and less translucent. As the fetus reaches term, between 38 and 42 weeks, the vernix decreases, and the ear cartilage is developed. In males, the testes are in the scrotum; in females, the labia majora meet in the midline and cover the labia minora and the clitoris. At 40 weeks, the average fetus weighs 3,289 g (7¼ lb) and is between 48 and 56 cm (19 and 22 inches) long. Prenatal development may be adversely affected by several factors. Between 2 and 14 weeks of gestation, ionizing radiation, drugs, various viruses, malnutrition, trauma, or maternal disese may have profound effects on morphologic and functional development. During the first 10 days of development, any damage usually kills the conceptus. After 14 weeks when all the organs, systems, and parts of the body have formed, any adverse effects are largely functional; major morphologic damage does not occur.

prenatal diagnosis Any of various diagnostic techniques to determine if a developing fetus in the uterus is affected with a genetic disorder or other abnormality. X-ray examination and ultrasound scanning can be used to follow fetal growth and detect structural abnormalities; amniocentesis enables fetal cells to be obtained from the amniotic fluid for culture and biochemical assay to detect metabolic disorders and for chromosomal analysis; fetoscopy enables fetal blood to be withdrawn from a blood vessel on the placenta and examined for disorders, as thalassemia, sickle-cell anemia, and Duchenne's muscular dystrophy. If any of the tests are positive, and the child is likely or certain to be born with a severe defect or disease, the parents need support and advice from genetic counselors on whether to terminate the pregnancy. Also called **antenatal diagnosis.** See also **genetic counseling, genetic screening.**

preoperative Of or pertaining to the period of time preceding a surgical procedure. Commonly, the preoperative period begins with the first preparation of the patient for surgery. It ends with the induction of surgical anesthesia in the operating suite.

preoperative care The preparation and management of a patient prior to surgery. NURSING CONSIDERATIONS: The nurse performs and explains the preoperative procedures, reinforces the doctor's explanation of the operation, provides instruction and emotional support, answers the patient's questions as honestly as possible, and reassures the patient that medication

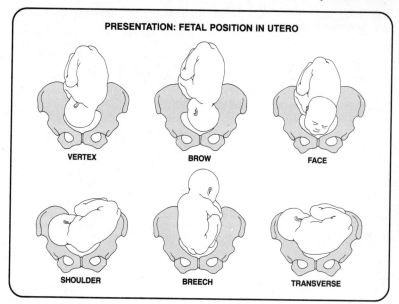

PRESENTATION: FETAL POSITION IN UTERO

VERTEX   BROW   FACE

SHOULDER   BREECH   TRANSVERSE

will be available to relieve postoperative pain. Depending on the surgical procedure, the nurse shows the patient how to turn, cough, deep breathe, and support the incision during coughing. The nurse informs the patient and the patient's family about the postoperative period in the recovery room or the intensive care unit, if indicated.

prepatellar bursa A bursa between the tendon of the quadriceps and the lower part of the femur continuous with the cavity of the knee joint.

preprandial Before a meal.

prepubertal panhypopituitarism See panhypopituitarism.

prepuberty The period immediately preceding puberty, lasting approximately 2 years and characterized by preliminary physical changes, as accelerated growth and appearance of secondary sex characteristics, that lead to sexual maturity. —**prepuberal, prepubertal,** *adj.*

prepubescence The state of being prepubertal. —**prepubescent,** *adj.*

prepuce A fold of skin that forms a retractable cover, as the foreskin of the penis or the fold around the clitoris. —**prepucial, preputial,** *adj.*

presbycardia An abnormal cardiac condition, especially affecting elderly individuals and associated with heart failure in the presence of other complications, as heart disease, fever, anemia, mild hyperthyroidism, and excess fluid administration. Presbycardia may be associated with decreased elasticity of the musculature of the heart and with mild fibrotic changes of the heart valves, but the basis for these changes and the associated pigmentation of the heart is not known.

presbyopia Farsightedness resulting from a loss of elasticity of the lens of the eye. It commonly develops with advancing age. —**presbyopic,** *adj.*

prescreen **1.** To evaluate a patient or a group of patients to identify those who are at greater risk of developing a particular condition in order to select those who are in particular need of special diagnostic procedures or health care. **2.** *Informal.* A rapid, superficial examination of a person who does not appear to be acutely ill. It may include taking a medical history.

prescription An order for medication, therapy, or a therapeutic device given by a properly authorized person to a person properly authorized to dispense or perform the order. A prescription is usually in written form and includes the name and address of the patient, the date, the b symbol (superscription), the medication prescribed (inscription), directions to the pharmacist or other dispenser (subscription), directions to the patient that must appear on the label, the prescriber's signature, and, in some instances, an identifying number.

prescription drug A drug that can be dispensed to the public only with a prescription. The designation of a drug as a prescription drug is made by the Food and Drug Administration. See also **ethical drug.**

prescriptive theory A theory that is comprised of a description of a specific activity, a statement of the goal of the activity, and an analysis of the elements of the activity that, together, constitute a prescription for reaching the goal.

presenile dementia See **Alzheimer's disease.**

presentation The position of an infant in utero with reference to the part of the infant that

ARTERIAL PRESSURE POINTS

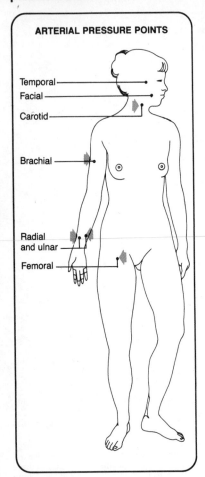

Temporal

Facial

Carotid

Brachial

Radial
and ulnar

Femoral

is directed toward or into the birth canal. Kinds of presentations are breech presentation, brow presentation, face presentation, shoulder presentation, transverse presentation, vertex presentation. Also called **fetal lie.** —**present,** *v.*

present health In a health history: a chronologic, succinct account of any recent changes in the health of the patient and of the circumstances or symptoms that prompted the person to seek health care.

presenting symptom See **symptom.**

presomite embryo An embryo in any stage of development prior to the appearance of the first pair of somites, which, in humans, usually occurs around 19 to 21 days following fertilization of the ovum.

pressor Describing a substance that tends to cause a rise in blood pressure.

pressure A force, or stress, applied to a surface by a fluid or an object. Pressure is usually measured in units of mass per unit of area, as

pounds per square inch (psi).

pressure acupuncture A system of acupuncture involving the application of pressure, as by the tip of a finger, to certain specified points of the body. See also **acupuncture.**

pressure bandage A bandage applied to stop bleeding, prevent edema, or provide support for varicose veins.

pressure dressing A dressing firmly applied to exert pressure, usually on a wound for hemostasis.

pressure point 1. A point over an artery where the pulse may be felt. Pressure on the point may be helpful in stopping the flow of blood from a wound distal to the point. 2. A site that is extremely sensitive to pressure, as the phrenic pressure point along the phrenic nerve between the sternocleidomastoid and the scalenus anticus on the right side; such pressure may indicate gallbladder dysfunction.

pressure sore See **decubitus ulcer.**

preswing stance stage One of the five stages in the stance phase of walking or gait, involving a brief transitional period of double limb support during which one leg of the body is rapidly relieved of body-bearing weight and prepared for the swing forward. The type of preswing used by an individual is a factor in the diagnoses of many abnormal orthopedic conditions. Compare **initial contact stance stage, loading response stance stage, midstance, terminal stance.** See also **swing phase of gait.**

presynaptic 1. Situated near or before a synapse. 2. Occurring before a synapse is crossed.

presynaptic element Any neurological structure, as a neuron, situated proximal to a synapse.

presystolic Pertaining to the period preceding systole.

preterm infant See **premature infant.**

preterm labor See **premature labor.**

pretibial Of or pertaining to the area of the leg in front of the tibia.

pretibial fever An acute infection caused by *Leptospira autumnalis*, characterized by headache, chills, fever, enlarged spleen, myalgia, low white blood cell count, and a rash on the anterior surface of the legs. Also called **Fort Bragg fever.**

pretrial discovery See **discovery.**

prevalence In epidemiology: the number of all new and old cases of a disease or occurrences of an event during a particular time period, expressed as a ratio in which the number of events is the numerator and the population at risk is the denominator. See also **rate.**

prevention In nursing care: any action directed toward preventing illness and promoting health to avoid the need for primary, secondary, or tertiary health care. Prevention includes assessment and promotion of health potential; application of prescribed measures, as immunization; health teaching; early diagnosis and treatment; and recognition of disability limitations and rehabilitation potential. In acute-care nursing, many interventions are simultaneously therapeutic and preventive.

preventive   Tending to slow, stop, or interrupt the course of an illness or to decrease the incidence of a disease.

preventive care   A pattern of nursing and medical care that focuses on the prevention of disease and on health maintenance and includes early diagnosis of disease, discovery and identification of people at risk of developing specific problems, counseling, and other intervention to avert a health problem. Examples are screening tests, health education, and immunization programs.

preventive treatment   A procedure, measure, substance, or program designed to prevent a disease from occurring or a mild disorder from becoming more severe. Various diseases are prevented by immunizations with vaccines, antiseptic measures, the avoidance of smoking, regular exercise, a prudent diet, adequate rest, the correction of congenital anomalies, and screening programs. Also called **prophylactic treatment.**

previa, praevia   *Informal.* Placenta previa.

previllous embryo   An embryo of a placental mammal at any stage prior to the development of the chorionic villi, which, in humans, begin to form between the 1st and 2nd months following fertilization of the ovum.

previtamin   See **provitamin.**

priapism   An abnormal condition of prolonged or constant penile erection, often painful and seldom associated with sexual arousal. It may result from a lesion within the penis or the central nervous system and sometimes occurs in men who have acute leukemia.

priapitis   Inflammation of the penis.

priapus   See **penis.**

prickle cell layer   See **stratum spinosum.**

prickly heat   See **miliaria.**

prilocaine hydrochloride   An amide local anesthetic agent.

prim-   A combining form meaning 'first': *primerite, primigravida.*

primaquine phosphate   An antimalarial agent.

primary   **1.** First in order of time, place, development, or importance. **2.** Not derived from any other source or cause; specifically, the original condition or set of symptoms in disease processes, as a primary infection or a primary tumor. **3.** In chemistry: noting the first and most simple compound in a related series, formed by the substitution of one of two or more atoms or of a group in a molecule, as in amine or carboxyl radicals. Compare **secondary, tertiary.**

primary afferent fiber   A sensory nerve fiber that transmits impulses from the intrafusal fibers of the muscle spindle to the central nervous system during muscle contraction. See also **gamma efferent fiber.**

primary amputation   Amputation that is performed after severe trauma occurs, after the patient has recovered from shock and before infection has set in. Compare **secondary am-**

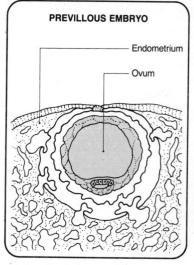

PREVILLOUS EMBRYO

— Endometrium

— Ovum

putation. See also **amputation.**

primary apnea   A self-limited condition characterized by an absence of respiration. It may follow a blow to the head and is common immediately after birth in the newborn, who breathes spontaneously when the carbon dioxide in the circulation reaches a certain level. Reflexes are present and the heart is beating, but the skin may appear pale or cyanotic and muscle tone is diminished. No treatment is necessary, but careful observation, maintenance of body temperature, and oral pharyngeal aspiration are usually performed. Within seconds, the newborn usually begins breathing, becomes pinker, moves the arms and legs, and cries. Compare **periodic apnea of the newborn, secondary apnea.**

primary atelectasis   Failure of the lungs to expand fully at birth. Commonly seen in premature infants or those narcotized by maternal anesthesia. The infant is usually cared for in an incubator in which the temperature and humidity may be closely monitored. Nursing care includes frequent changes of position of the infant to assist respiration, suctioning to remove bronchial secretions, and very slow feedings to avoid abdominal distention.

primary atypical pneumonia   See **mycoplasma pneumonia.**

primary biliary cirrhosis   A chronic inflammatory condition of the liver. It is characterized by generalized pruritus, enlargement and hardening of the liver, weight loss, and diarrhea with pale, bulky stools. Petechiae, epistaxis, or hemorrhage resulting from hypoprothrombinemia may also be evident. Pathological fractures and collapsed vertebrae may develop as the result of the associated malabsorption of vitamin D and calcium. Xanthomas commonly develop when the serum cholesterol level exceeds 450 mg/100 ml. The etiology of primary biliary cir-

PRIMARY BRONCHI

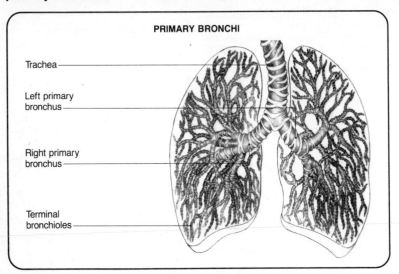

Trachea

Left primary bronchus

Right primary bronchus

Terminal bronchioles

rhosis is unknown; it most often affects women aged 40 to 60. The diagnosis is confirmed by liver biopsy and cholangiography. Jaundice, dark urine, pale stools, and cutaneous xanthosis may occur in the later stages of this disease. Treatment commonly includes the administration of fat-soluble vitamins A, D, E, and K to prevent and correct deficiencies caused by malabsorption. Drugs, including cholestyramine, may relieve associated pruritus. D-penicillamine may help correct this disorder over the long term. When treatment is begun in the early, asymptomatic stages of the condition, the prognosis is excellent. The life expectancy is about 5 years for symptomatic patients after the onset of jaundice. Compare **secondary biliary cirrhosis.**

primary bronchus One of the two main air passages that branch from the trachea and convey air to the lungs as part of the respiratory system. The right primary bronchus is about 2.5 cm (1 inch) long, is wider and shorter than the left primary bronchus, and enters the right lung nearly opposite the fifth thoracic vertebra. The left primary bronchus is about 5 cm (2 inches) long, passes under the aortic arch, and courses ventral to the esophagus, the thoracic duct, and the descending aorta before dividing into bronchi for the superior and the anterior lobes of the lung. The bronchi, like the trachea, are composed of rings of hyaline cartilage, fibrous tissue, mucous membrane, and glands. The carina at the bottom of the trachea separates the two primary bronchi and is situated to the left of the middle line so that the right primary bronchus is a more direct extension of the trachea than the left. Hence, foreign objects entering the trachea usually drop into the right bronchus rather than the left.

primary carcinoma A neoplasm at its site of origin.

primary constriction See **centromere.**

primary cutaneous melanoma A primary melanoma on the skin.

primary degenerative dementia See **senile psychosis.**

primary dental caries Dental caries developing in the enamel of a tooth that was previously unaffected.

primary dentition See **deciduous dentition.**

primary fissure A fissure that marks the division of the anterior and posterior lobes of the cerebellum.

primary gain A benefit, primarily relief from emotional conflict and freedom from anxiety, attained through the use of a defense mechanism or other psychological process. Compare **secondary gain.**

primary health care A basic level of health care that includes programs directed at the promotion of health, early diagnosis of disease or disability, and prevention of disease. Primary health care is provided in an ambulatory facility to limited numbers of people, often those living in a particular geographic area. In any episode of illness, it is the first patient contact with the health-care system.

primary histoplasmosis See **histoplasmosis.**

primary host See **definitive host.**

primary nurse A nurse who is responsible for the planning, implementation, and evaluation of the nursing care of one or more clients 24 hours a day for the duration of the hospital stay. In primary nursing, nursing care usually includes the development and implementation of a care plan; participation in conferences on the care of a client; collaboration with the client, the health-care team members, and the client's family; referral to community resources; and evaluation of care.

primary nursing A system for the distri-

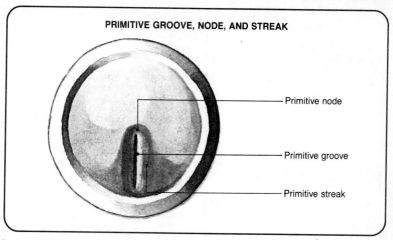

PRIMITIVE GROOVE, NODE, AND STREAK

- Primitive node
- Primitive groove
- Primitive streak

bution of nursing care in which one nurse directs and coordinates nurses and other personnel; schedules all tests, procedures, and daily activities for one patient; and cares for that patient personally when on duty. In an acute-care situation, the primary-care nurse might be responsible for only one patient; in an intermediate-care situation, she might be responsible for three or more patients. Advantages include continuity of patient care; accountability of the nurse for that care; patient-centered care that is comprehensive, individualized, and coordinated; and the professional satisfaction of the nurse. Compare **team nursing.**

primary organizer   The part of the dorsal lip of the blastopore that is self-differentiating and induces the formation of the neural plate that gives rise to the main axis of the embryo.

primary physician   1. The physician who usually takes care of a person; the physician who first sees a patient for the care of a given health problem. **2.** A family practice physician or general practitioner. See also **family medicine.**

primary sequestrum   A piece of dead bone that completely separates from sound bone during the process of necrosis. Compare **secondary sequestrum.**

primary shock   A state of physical collapse comparable to fainting. It may be the result of slight pain, as that produced by venipuncture, or may be caused by fright. Primary shock is usually mild, self-limited, and of short duration. Severe injury may prolong and merge primary shock with secondary shock. Compare **hemorrhagic shock.**

primary tooth   See **deciduous tooth.**

primary tuberculosis   The childhood form of tuberculosis, most commonly occurring in the lungs, the posterior pharynx, or, rarely, the skin. Infants lack resistance to the disease and are easily infected and especially vulnerable to rapid and extensive spread of the infection through their bodies. In childhood, the disease is usually brief and benign, characterized by regional lymphadenopathy, calcification of the tubercles, and residual immunity. The tuberculin test will be positive for life. See also **tuberculosis.**

prime mover   A muscle that acts directly to produce a desired movement amid other muscles acting to indirectly produce the same movement. Most movements of the body require the combined actions of numerous muscles. Compare **antagonist, fixation muscle, synergist.**

primidone   A barbiturate anticonvulsant.

primigravida   A woman who is pregnant for the first time. Also called **gravida I. —primigravid,** *adj.*

primitive   1. Undeveloped; undifferentiated; rudimentary; showing little or no evolution. **2.** Embryonic; formed early in the course of development; existing in an early or simple form. Compare **definitive. 3.** First or early in terms of time; original; primary.

primitive fold   See **primitive ridge.**

primitive groove   A furrow in the posterior region of the embryonic disk that indicates the cephalocaudal axis resulting from the active involution of cells forming the primitive streak.

primitive gut   See **archenteron.**

primitive line   See **primitive streak.**

primitive node   A knoblike gathering of cells at the cephalic end of the primitive streak in the early stages of embryonic development in humans and higher animals. It consists of mesoderm cells that give rise to the notochord and corresponds to the dorsal lip of the blastopore in lower animals.

primitive pit   A minute indentation at the anterior end of the primitive groove in the early developing embryo. It lies posterior to the primitive node and probably functions as an opening into the notochordal canal in man and the higher animals and into the neurenteric canal in the lower animals.

primitive reflex   Any reflex not normally found in an adult but normal in an infant or fetus. In an adult, the presence of such a reflex usually indicates serious neurological disease.

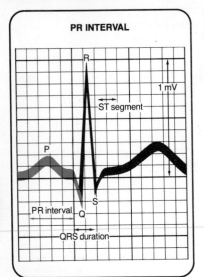

PR INTERVAL

1 mV

ST segment

P

PR interval — Q

S

QRS duration

Some kinds are **grasp reflex, Moro reflex, sucking reflex.**

primitive ridge A ridge that bounds the primitive groove in the early stages of embryonic development. Also called **primitive fold.** See also **primitive streak.**

primitive streak A dense area on the central posterior region of the embryonic disk, formed by the morphogenetic movement of a rapidly proliferating mass of cells that spreads between the ectoderm and endoderm, giving rise to the mesoderm layer. This seamlike elongation indicates the cephalocaudal axis along which the embryo develops and corresponds to the blastopore of lower animal groups. Also called **primitive line.**

primordial 1. Characteristic of the most undeveloped or primitive state, specifically those cells or tissues that are formed in the early stages of embryonic development. **2.** First or original; primitive.

primordial dwarf A person of extremely short stature who is otherwise perfectly formed, with the usual proportions of body parts and normal mental and sexual development. The condition may be genetically related, involving a defect in the ability to utilize growth hormone, or it may occur sporadically within a particular population. Also called **hypoplastic dwarf, normal dwarf, physiologic dwarf, pure dwarf, true dwarf.** See also **pituitary dwarf, pygmy.**

primordial germ cell Any of the large spherical diploid cells that are formed in the early stages of embryonic development and are precursors of the oogonia and spermatogonia. Primordial germ cells are formed outside of the gonads and migrate to the embryonic ovaries and testes for maturation. See also **oogenesis, spermatogenesis.**

primordial image In analytic psychology: the archetype or original parent, representing the source of all life. It occurs in the memory as a stage preceding the differentiation of the actual mother and father. See also **collective unconscious.**

primordium, *pl.* **primordia** The first recognizable stage in the embryonic development and differentiation of a particular organ, tissue, or structure; anlage; rudiment.

principal cell See **chief cell.**

PR interval The component of the cardiac cycle shown on an electrocardiogram as an inverted U-shaped curve from the beginning of the P wave that tails off in an abrupt, flat downward direction (Q wave) until it angles sharply upward to a peak (R wave). It represents the interval of time required for atrial depolarization and for the impulse from the sinoatrial node to reach the ventricles, preparing them for contraction.

Prinzmetal's angina A form of angina pectoris. Attacks occur during rest and are associated with an elevation of the ST segment on the electrocardiogram.

-privia A combining form meaning a '(specified) condition of loss or deprivation': *calciprivia, hormonoprivia.*

PRL *abbr* **prolactin.**

p.r.n. In prescriptions: *abbr pro re nata,* a Latin phrase meaning 'as needed.' The times of administration are determined by the needs of the patient.

pro- A combining form meaning 'first or in front of': *procallus, procheilon.*

proaccelerin See **factor V.**

probability The likelihood that a given event will occur, stated as a ratio with the number of times it is expected to occur over the number of possible occurrences.

proband See **propositus.**

probenecid A uricosuric agent.

problem-oriented medical record (POMR) A method of recording data about the health status of a patient in a problem-solving system. The POMR method, developed by Dr. Lawrence Weed, preserves the data in an easily accessible way that encourages ongoing assessment and revision of the health-care plan by health-care team members. The format varies from setting to setting, but the components of the method are similar. A data base is collected prior to identifying the patient's problems. The data base consists of information collected from an interview with the patient and family or others, a health assessment or physical examination of the patient, and laboratory tests. Weed recommends that the data base be as complete as possible, limited only by potential hazard of pain or discomfort to the patient or by excessive expense of the diagnostic procedure. The interview, augmented by prior records, provides the patient's history, including the reason for contact; a descriptive profile of the person; a history of family illness, the current illness, and past illness; an account of the patient's current health practices; and a review of systems. The physical examination or health assessment comprises the second major part of the data base. The next section of the POMR is the master problem list, whose formulation is similar to the assessment phase of the nursing process. Each problem represents a conclusion or a decision resulting from examination, investigation, and analysis of the data base. A problem is defined as anything that causes concern to the patient or to the care-giver, including physical abnormalities, psychologic disturbance, and socioeconomic problems. The master problem list usually includes active, inactive, temporary, and potential problems. The list serves as an index to the rest of the record and is arranged in five columns: a chronological list of problems; the date of onset; the action taken; the outcome of the problem (often its resolution); and its date. Problems may be added, and intervention or plans for intervention may be changed; thus, the status of each problem is available for all health-care professionals involved in caring for the client. The third major section of the POMR is the initial plan. Each problem is named and described, usually written on the progress note in a SOAP format: S stands for the subjective data from the patient's point of view; O for the objective data acquired by inspection, percussion, auscultation, and palpation and from laboratory tests; A is an assessment of the problem, or an analysis of the subjective and objective data; and P is the plan, including further diagnostic work, therapy, and education or counseling. After an initial plan for each problem is formulated and recorded, the problems are followed in the progress notes by narrative notes in the SOAP format or by flow sheets showing data in a tabular manner. A discharge summary is formulated and written, relating the overall assessment of progress during treatment and the plans for follow-up or referral. The summary allows a review of all the problems initially identified and encourages continuity of care for the patient.

problem-solving approach to patient-centered care In nursing: a conceptual framework that incorporates the patient's overt physical needs with covert psychological, emotional, and social needs. It provides a model for caring for the whole person as an individual, not as an example of a disease or a medical diagnosis. Nursing is defined as a problem-solving process. The patient is viewed as a person in an impaired state, less than usually able to perform self-care activities. Nursing problems are conditions experienced by the patient or the patient's family in which the nurse may provide professional service. The nurse makes a nursing diagnosis that identifies the impaired state and determines the care needed to augment the patient's ability to perform self-care. The requirements for care are classified in four levels: care given to sustain life is sustenal care; care given to assist the patient in self-care is remedial care; care that helps the patient to develop new skills and goals in self-care is restorative care; and

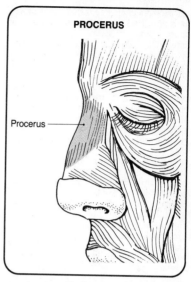

PROCERUS

Procerus

care given to guide the patient to a level of self-help beyond the normal level is preventive care. Twenty-one nursing problems are identified and sorted into four groups: problems relating to comfort, hygiene, and safety; physiological balance; psychological and social factors; and sociologic and community factors.

probucol An antilipemic agent.

procainamide hydrochloride A group I antiarrhythmic, also used as a local anesthetic.

procaine hydrochloride An ester local anesthetic.

procarbazine hydrochloride An antineoplastic agent.

procaryon See **prokaryon.**

procaryosis See **prokaryosis.**

Procaryotae In bacteriology: a kingdom of plants that includes all microorganisms in which the nucleoplasm has no basic protein and is not surrounded by a nuclear membrane. The kingdom has two divisions, Cyanobacteria and Bacteria.

procaryote See **prokaryote.** —**procaryotic,** *adj.*

procerus One of three muscles of the nose. Arising from the fascia of the nasal bone and the lateral nasal cartilage and inserting into the skin over the lower part of the forehead between the eyebrows, it is a small pyramidal muscle, innervated by buccal branches of the facial nerve. The procerus draws down the eyebrows and wrinkles the nose. Compare **depressor septi, nasalis.**

process 1. A series of related events that follow in sequence from a particular state or condition to a conclusion or resolution. 2. A natural growth that projects from a bone or other part.

process recording In nursing education: a system used for teaching nursing students to understand and analyze verbal and nonverbal interaction. The conversation between nurse and patient is written on special forms or in a special format. The student nurse records observations, perceptions, thoughts, feelings, and the words exchanged. The process recording helps the student nurse identify patterns of difficulty in communicating with the patient.

process schizophrenia A form of schizophrenia caused by organic changes in the brain. The onset of the disease is usually gradual, but it progresses to irreversible psychosis. Compare **reactive schizophrenia.** See also **schizophrenia.**

prochlorperazine, p. maleate Phenothiazine antipsychotic agents.

prochromosome See **karyosome.**

proconvertin See **factor VII.**

proct- See **procto-.**

-proctia A combining form meaning '(condition of the) anus': *ankyloproctia, cacoproctia.*

proctitis Inflammation of the rectum and anus caused by infection, trauma, drugs, allergy, or radiation injury. Acute or chronic, it is accompanied by rectal discomfort and the repeated urge to pass feces with the inability to do so. Pus, blood, or mucus may be present in the stools, and tenesmus may be present. Also called **rectitis.**

procto-, proct- A combining form meaning 'of or pertaining to the rectum': *proctocele, proctorrhea.*

proctodeum, proctodaeum, *pl.* **proctodea, proctodaea** An invagination of the ectoderm, located behind the urorectal septum of the developing embryo, and which forms the anus and the anal canal when the cloacal membrane ruptures. —**proctodaeal, proctodeal,** *adj.*

proctologist A physician who specializes in proctology.

proctology The branch of medicine that treats disorders of the colon, rectum, and anus.

proctoscope An instrument used to examine the rectum and the distal portion of the colon. It consists of a light and a magnifying lens mounted on a tube or speculum. Compare **sigmoidoscope.**

procyclidine hydrochloride A cholinergic (parasympatholytic) blocking agent.

prodromal labor The early period in parturition before uterine contractions become forceful and frequent enough to result in progressive dilatation of the uterine cervix.

prodrome 1. An early sign of a developing condition or disease. 2. The earliest phase of a developing condition or disease. —**prodromal,** *adj.*

productive cough A sudden, noisy expulsion of air from the lungs that effectively removes sputum from the respiratory tract and helps to clear the air passages, permitting oxygen to reach the alveoli. Coughing is stimulated by irritation or by inflammation of the respiratory tract, caused most frequently by infection. Deep breathing, with contraction of the diaphragm and intercostal muscles and forceful exhalation, promotes productive coughing in patients with respiratory infections. Mucolytic agents liquefy mucus in the respiratory tract so that it can be raised and expectorated more easily. Anticholinergic drugs, as atropine, decrease respiratory secretions. See also **nonproductive cough.**

professional corporation (PC) A corporation formed according to the law of a particular state for the purpose of delivering a professional service.

professional liability A legal concept describing the obligation of a professional person to pay a patient or client for damages caused by the professional's act of omission, commission, or negligence. Professional liability better describes the responsibility of all professionals to their clients than does the concept of malpractice, but the idea of professional liability is central to malpractice.

professional network In psychiatric nursing: the network of professional resources available to support the psychiatric outpatient in the community. The network may include a therapist, a hospital day-treatment program, social work agency, and other agencies.

professional organization An organization created to deal with issues of concern to its members, who share a professional status.

Professional Standards Review Organization (PSRO) An organization formed under Social Security Act Amendments of 1972 to review the services provided under Medicare, Medicaid, and Maternal Child Health programs.

profibrinolysin See **fibrinogen.**

progenitive Capable of producing offspring; reproductive.

progenitor 1. A parent or ancestor. 2. One who, or anything that, originates or precedes; precursor.

progeny 1. Offspring; an individual or organism resulting from a particular mating. 2. The descendants of a known or common ancestor.

progeria An abnormal congenital condition characterized by premature aging and the appearance in childhood of gray hair and wrinkled skin and by small stature, absence of pubic and facial hair, and the posture and habitus of an aged person. Death usually occurs before the age of 20. Compare **infantilism.**

progestagen See **progestogen.**

progestational Of or pertaining to a drug with effects similar to those of progesterone, the hormone produced by the corpus luteum and adrenal cortex during the luteal phase of the menstrual cycle that prepares the uterus for reception of the fertilized ovum. Natural and synthetic preparations of progesterone and its derivative, medroxyprogesterone acetate, are used in the treatment of secondary amenorrhea and abnormal uterine bleeding. Progestational compounds, as norethindrone and norgestrel, are constituents of oral contraceptives. The use of progestogens to prevent habitual or threatened abortion is no longer recommended.

progesterone A progestational hormone.

progestogen, progestagen Any natural or synthetic progestational hormone. Also called progestin.

proglottid An egg-bearing segment of a tapeworm, containing both male and female reproductive organs.

prognosis A prediction of the probable outcome of a disease based on the person's condition and the usual course of the disease as noted in similar situations.

progressive Describing the course of a disease or condition in which the signs and symptoms become more prominent and severe, as progressive muscular atrophy.

progressive histoplasmosis See **histoplasmosis.**

progressive patient care A system of care in which patients are placed in units on the basis of their needs for care as determined by the degree of illness, as intensive care, intermediate care, and minimal care, rather than in units based on a medical specialty.

progressive resistance exercise A method of increasing the strength of a weak or injured muscle by gradually increasing the resistance against which the muscle works, as by using graduated weights over a period of time. Also called **graduated resistance exercise.** See also **active resistance exercise.**

progressive spinal muscular atrophy of infants See **Werdnig-Hoffmann disease.**

progressive systemic sclerosis (PSS) The most common form of scleroderma.

progress notes In the patient record: notes made by a nurse and physician that describe the patient's condition and the treatments given or planned. Progress notes may follow the problem-oriented medical record (POMR) format. The physician's progress notes usually focus on the medical or therapeutic aspects of the patient's condition and care; the nurse's progress notes, while noting the medical conditions of the patient, usually focus on the objectives stated in the nursing-care plan, as the person's ability to perform activities of daily living or acceptance or understanding of a particular condition or treatment. Progress notes in an in-hospital setting are recorded daily; progress notes in a clinic or office setting are usually preceded by an episodic or an interval history and are written as an account of each visit.

projection 1. A protuberance; anything that thrusts or juts outward. 2. The act of perceiving an idea or thought as an objective reality. 3. In psychology: an unconscious defense mechanism by which individuals attribute their own unacceptable traits, ideas, or impulses to others.

projective test A kind of diagnostic, psychological, or personality test that uses unstructured or ambiguous stimuli (such as inkblots, a series of pictures, abstract patterns, or incomplete sentences) to illicit responses that reflect a projection of various aspects of the subject's per-

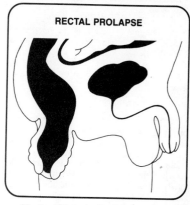

RECTAL PROLAPSE

sonality. See also **Rorschach test.**

prokaryocyte, procaryocyte A cell without a true nucleus and with nuclear material scattered throughout the cytoplasm. These include bacteria, viruses, rickettsiae, chlamydiae, mycoplasmas, actinomycetes, and certain algae. Compare **eukaryocyte.**

prokaryon, procaryon 1. Nuclear elements that are not bound by a membrane but are spread throughout the cytoplasm, as in bacteria, viruses, and other unicellular organisms. 2. An organism containing such unbound nuclear elements. Compare **eukaryon.**

prokaryosis, procaryosis The condition of not containing a true nucleus surrounded by a nuclear membrane, as in bacteria and viruses. Compare **eukaryosis.**

prokaryote, procaryote An organism that does not contain a true nucleus surrounded by a nuclear membrane, characteristic of lower forms, as bacteria, viruses, and blue-green algae. The nuclear elements are spread throughout the cytoplasm, and division occurs through simple fission. Compare **eukaryote. —prokaryotic,** *adj.*

prolactin (PRL) A hormone produced and secreted into the bloodstream by the anterior pituitary. Prolactin, acting with estrogen, progesterone, thyroxine, insulin, growth hormone, glucocorticoids, and human placental lactogen, stimulates the development and growth of the mammary glands. After parturition, prolactin, together with glucocorticoids, is essential for the initiation and maintenance of milk production. Prolactin synthesis and release from the pituitary is mediated by the central nervous system in response to suckling by the infant. When suckling or its mechanical equivalent ceases, prolactin secretion slows and milk production ceases. Prolactin is similar to growth hormone in its chemical structure. It is unknown in males. Also called **lactogen, lactogenic hormone, luteotropin.**

prolapse The falling, sinking, or sliding of an organ from its normal position or location in the body, as uterine prolaspe, rectal prolapse, or anal prolapse.

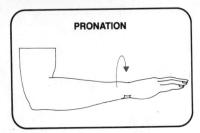

PRONATION

prolonged release Designed to deliver a dose of a drug over an extended period. The most common device for this purpose is a soft, soluble capsule containing minute pellets of the drug for release at different rates in the gastrointestinal tract, depending on the thickness and nature of the oil, fat, wax, or resin coating on the pellets. Another system consists of a porous plastic carrier impregnated with the drug and a surfactant that facilitates the entry of gastrointestinal fluids that slowly leach out the drug. Ion exchange resins that bind to drugs and liquids containing suspensions of slow-release drug granules are also used to provide medication over an extended period. Various mechanisms and vehicles have also been developed to prolong the release of drugs after injection intramuscularly or subcutaneously.

promazine hydrochloride A phenothiazine antipsychotic agent.

promethazine hydrochloride A phenothiazine antihistamine.

promethium (Pm) A radioactive, rare-earth, metallic element. Its atomic number is 61; its atomic weight is 147.

promoter In molecular genetics: a DNA sequence that initiates RNA transcription of the genetic code.

prompt insulin zinc suspension A fast-acting noncrystalline semilente insulin prescribed in the treatment of diabetes mellitus when a prompt, intense, and short-acting response is desired. This type of insulin is only slightly slower to act than insulin injection. See also **fast-acting insulin.**

promyelocyte A large mononuclear blood cell abnormally present in the circulating blood. It contains a single, regular, symmetric nucleus and a few undifferentiated cytoplasmic granules. It is intermediate in development between a myeloblast and a myelocyte and is indicative of leukemia. See also **leukemia, metamyelocyte, myeloblast.**

pronation **1.** Assumption of a prone position, one in which the ventral surface of the body faces downward. **2.** The rotation of the forearm so the palm of the hand faces downward and backward. **3.** The lowering of the medial edge of the foot while turning it outward. —**pronate,** *v.,* **prone,** *adj.*

pronator reflex A reflex elicited by holding the patient's hand vertically and tapping the distal end of the radius or ulna, resulting in pronation of the forearm. Hyperactivity of the reflex

may be seen with lesions of the pyramidal system above the level of the sixth cervical nerve root.

pronator teres A superficial muscle of the forearm, arising from a humeral and an ulnar head. The humeral head is the larger and more superficial, originating near the medial epicondyle, from the tendon common to the superficial muscles of the forearm, from certain intermuscular septa, and from the antebrachial fascia. The ulnar head originates in the coronoid process of the ulna. Fibers from both portions of the muscle pass obliquely across the forearm, ending in a flat tendon that inserts into the radius. The pronator functions to pronate the hand. Compare **flexor carpi radialis, flexor carpi ulnaris, flexor digitorum superficialis, palmaris longus.**

prone **1.** Lying with the face downward. **2.** Referring to the hand with the palm facing downward. Compare **supine.**

proneness profile A screening process that evaluates the probability of developmental problems occurring early in life, ideally beginning in the course of prenatal care and continuing after delivery. Significant variables in selecting the infants who are at risk are the perinatal health status of the mother and infant, especially complications of pregnancy, delivery, the neonatal period, and the puerperium; characteristics of the mother, especially her temperament, educational level, perception of the life situation, and perception of the infant; characteristics of the infant, including alertness, activity pattern, and responsiveness; and the behaviors of the infant and care-giver as they interact. The proneness profile is followed by a developmental profile that assesses the current status of the infant and care-giver. Three areas to be considered are: characteristics of the infant, including adaptation and response to the environment, the ability to give interpretable cues, and the developmental progress as compared with established norms; characteristics of the care-giver, including adaptation to the new infant, sensitivity to cues from the infant, and techniques for relieving distress; and the healthful quality of the environment.

pronephric duct One of the paired ducts that connects the tubules of each of the pronephros with the cloaca in the early developing vertebrate embryo. They later become the functional mesonephric ducts. Also called **archinephric canal, archinephric duct.**

pronephric tubule Any of the segmentally arranged excretory units of the pronephros in the early developing vertebrate embryo. The tubules open into the pronephric duct and communicate with the coelom through a nephrostoma. In humans and the higher vertebrates, the tubules are present only in vestigial form; in lower animals, they are functional.

pronephros, pronephron, *pl.* **pronephroi, pronephra** The primordial excretory organ in the developing vertebrate embryo. It consists of a series of pronephric tubules that arise along the anterior portion of the nephrotome and empty into the cloaca by way of the pronephric duct. In humans and other mammals, the structure is nonfunctional, representing the first of three excretory systems formed one after the other in an anterior to posterior sequence, which disappear with the formation of the mesonephros. The organ is functional in primitive fishes, as lampreys, and serves as a provisional kidney in some fishes and amphibians. Also called **archinephron, head kidney.** See also **mesonephros, metanephros. —pronephric,** *adj.*

pronucleus, *pl.* **pronuclei** The nucleus of the ovum or the spermatozoon after fertilization but prior to the fusion of the chromosomes to form the nucleus of the zygote. Each contains the haploid number of chromosomes, is larger than the normal nucleus, and is diffuse in appearance. The female pronucleus of the mature ovum is formed only after penetration by the sperm and the completion of the second mitotic division and polar body formation. The nucleus then loses its nuclear envelope to release the chromosomes so that synapsis can occur with the chromosomes of the male pronucleus, which is contained in the head of the spermatozoon. Also called **germinal nucleus.** See also **oogenesis, spermatogenesis.**

propantheline bromide A gastrointestinal anticholinergic agent.

proparacaine hydrochloride A topical ophthalmic anesthetic.

prophase The first of four stages of nuclear division in mitosis and in each of the two divisions of meiosis. In mitosis, the chromosomes progressively shorten and thicken to form individually recognizable elongated double structures composed of two chromatids held together by a centromere; the nucleolus and nuclear membrane disappear, the spindle and polar bodies are formed, and the chromosomes begin to migrate toward the midplane of the developing spindle. In the first meiotic division, prophase is complex and subdivided into five stages: leptotene, zygotene, pachytene, diplotene, and diakinesis. In the second meiotic division, the same processes occur as in mitotic prophase. See also **anaphase, interphase, meiosis, metaphase, mitosis, telophase.**

prophylactic 1. Preventing the spread of disease. 2. An agent that prevents the spread of disease. **—prophylactically,** *adv.*

prophylactic forceps See **low forceps.**

prophylactic treatment See **preventive treatment.**

prophylaxis Prevention of or protection against disease, often involving the use of a biological, chemical, or mechanical agent to destroy or prevent the entry of infectious organisms.

propiomazine hydrochloride A phenothiazine used as a preanesthetic sedative.

propionicacidemia A rare, inherited metabolic defect caused by the body's failure to metabolize the amino acids threonine, isoleucine, and methionone, characterized by lethargy and mental and physical retardation. Acidosis occurs as a result of the accumulation of propionic acid in the body. A diet low in these amino acids is difficult to achieve but is the only treatment. **—propionicacidemic,** *adj.*

propionic fermentation The production of propionic acid by the action of bacteria on sugars or lactic acid.

propositus A person from whom a genealogical lineage is traced, as is done to discover the pattern of inheritance of a familial disease or a physical trait.

propoxyphene A mild, centrally acting narcotic analgesic prescribed to relieve mild to moderate pain.

propoxyphene hydrochloride, p. napsylate Synthetic analgesics structurally related to opioids.

propranolol hydrochloride A sympatholytic beta-adrenergic blocking agent used as an antihypertensive and group III antiarrhythmic.

proprietary 1. Of or pertaining to an institution or other organization that is operated for profit. 2. Of a product, as a drug or device, made for profit.

proprietary hospital A hospital operated as a profit-making organization. Many are owned and operated by physicians primarily for their own patients, but they also accept patients from other physicians. Others are owned by investor groups or large corporations.

proprietary medicine Any pharmaceutical preparation or medicinal substance protected from commercial competition because its ingredients or method of manufacture are kept secret or protected by trademark or copyright.

proprioception Sensation pertaining to stimuli originating from within the body regarding spatial position and muscular activity or to the sensory receptors that they activate. Compare **exteroceptive, interoceptive.**

proprioceptive reflex Any reflex initiated by stimulation of proprioceptive receptors, as the increase in respiratory rate and volume induced by impulses arising from muscles and joints during exercise.

proprioceptor Any sensory nerve ending, as those located in muscles, tendons, joints, and the vestibular apparatus, that responds to stimuli originating from within the body regarding movement and spatial position. Compare **exteroceptor, interoceptor.** See also **mechanoreceptor.**

proptosis Bulging, protrusion, or forward displacement of a body organ or area.

propylformic acid See **butyric acid.**

propylthiouracil (PTU) A thyroid hormone antagonist.

proscribe To forbid, as forbidding of certain acts or services by the members of an organization by its bylaws. **—proscriptive,** *adj.*

prosencephalon The part of the brain that includes the diencephalon and the telencephalon. It develops from the anterior of the three primary vesicles of the embryonic neural tube and contains structures, as the thalamus and

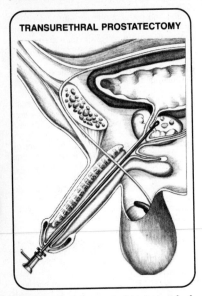

TRANSURETHRAL PROSTATECTOMY

hypothalamus, that control important body functions and affect the consciousness, the appetite, and the emotions. Also called **forebrain.** Compare **mesencephalon.** —**prosencephalic,** *adj.*

proso-, pros- A combining form meaning 'forward or anterior': *prosocoele, prosodemic.*

prosopalgia See **trigeminal neuralgia.**

-prosopia A combining form meaning '(condition of the) face': *lipoprosopia, schizoprosopia.*

prosopo- A combining form meaning 'of or related to the face': *prosopoanoschisis, prosopodiplegia.*

prosoposternodidymus A fetal monster consisting of conjoined twins united laterally from the head through the sternum.

prosopothoracopagus Conjoined symmetrical twins who are united laterally in the frontal plane from the thorax through most of the head.

prospective study A study designed to determine the relationship between a condition and a characteristic shared by some members of a group. Initially, the population selected is healthy. Some of the group members share a characteristic, as cigarette smoking. Over a period of time, the rate at which a condition, as lung cancer, occurs in the smokers and in the nonsmokers is noted. A study may involve many variables or only two; it may seek to demonstrate a relationship that is an association or one that is causal. The kinds of data collected, the number of people studied, and other details of the study affect the kind of analysis and the interpretation of the data.

prostaglandin (PG) One of several potent hormonelike unsaturated fatty acids that act in very low concentrations on local target organs.

They are produced in small amounts and have significant effects. Prostaglandins given by nebulizer, in tablets, or in solutions for oral or intravenous use, effect changes in vasomotor tone, capillary permeability, smooth-muscle tone, aggregation of platelets, endocrine and exocrine functions, and in the autonomic and central nervous systems. Uses include termination of pregnancy and treatment of asthma and gastric hyperacidity.

prostate A gland in males that surrounds the neck of the bladder and the urethra and elaborates a secretion that liquefies coagulated semen. It is a firm structure about the size of a chestnut, composed of muscular and glandular tissue. It is located in the pelvic cavity, below the caudal part of the symphysis pubis and ventral to the rectum, through which it can be felt, especially when enlarged. A depression on its cranial border accommodates the entry of the two ejaculatory ducts and divides the posterior surface of the gland into the middle lobe above and a larger portion below. A sinus about 6 mm (¼ inch) long runs upward and backward in the gland behind the middle lobe and is part of the urethra. The prominent lateral surfaces of the prostate are covered by a plexus of veins and by the ventral portions of the levator ani. The portion of the gland in front of the urethra is comprised of dense muscular tissue. In most men the urethra lies along the junction of the anterior portion and the middle third of the prostate. Ejaculatory ducts pass obliquely through the gland's posterior part. Prostatic secretion consists of alkaline phosphatase, citric acid, and various proteolytic enzymes. —**prostatic,** *adj.*

prostatectomy Surgical removal of a portion of the prostate gland, performed for benign prostatic hypertrophy or the total excision of the gland in malignancy. An indwelling urinary catheter is inserted, and a type and cross-match of blood is done to prepare for possible transfusion. Either a general or a spinal anesthetic is used. Kinds of approaches include transurethral, the most common, in which a resectoscope is inserted and through it shavings of prostatic tissue are cut off at the bladder opening with a loop; suprapubic; and retropubic. The perineal approach is used for biopsy when early cancer is suspected or for the removal of calculi. In a suprapubic approach, the patient returns with a large catheter positioned into the bladder through the abdomen. Wound drains are left in place in both the perineal and the suprapubic types. After surgery, hematuria is expected for several days. On the first day the bleeding is frank, usually venous, and may be controlled by increasing the pressure in the balloon end of the urethral catheter. If arterial in nature, the bleeding will be bright red with numerous clots and increased viscosity and may lead to hemorrhagic shock, requiring transfusion and surgical intervention. Bladder spasm may occur if a catheter becomes blocked or from the irritation of the balloon of the catheter in the bladder. Antispasmodic drugs may prevent spasm but are

PROSTATIC UTRICLE

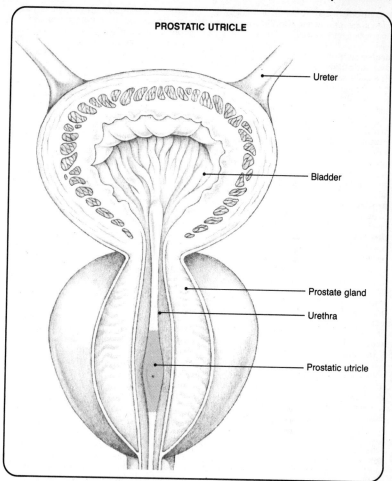

- Ureter
- Bladder
- Prostate gland
- Urethra
- Prostatic utricle

not given in severe cardiac disease or glaucoma. The nurse assesses the patient's ability to void in adequate amounts when the urethral catheter is removed. Complications of prostatectomy include urethral stricture (especially with the transurethral approach), urinary incontinence, and impotence.

prostatic Pertaining to the prostate gland.

prostatic catheter A catheter about 40 cm (16 inches) long with an angled tip used in male catheterization to pass an enlarged prostate gland obstructing the urethra.

prostatic ductule Any one of 12 to 20 tiny excretory tubes that convey the alkaline secretion of the prostate gland and open into the floor of the prostatic portion of the urethra. The ductules are joined together by areolar tissue, supported by extensions of the fibrous capsule of the prostate and its muscular stroma, and wrapped in a delicate network of capillaries.

prostatic utricle The part of the urethra in males that forms a cul-de-sac about 6 mm (¼ inch) long behind the middle lobe of the prostate. It is composed of fibrous tissue, muscular fibers, and mucous membrane; numerous small glands open on its inner surface. Derived from the atrophied paramesonephric ducts, the prostatic utricle is homologous with the uterus in females. Also called **uterus masculinis**. See **prostate.**

prostatitis Acute or chronic inflammation of the prostate gland, usually the result of infection. The patient complains of burning, frequency, and urgency of urination. Treatment consists of administration of antibiotics, sitz baths, bed rest, and fluids. Compare **benign prostatic hypertrophy.**

prosthesis, *pl.* **prostheses** **1.** An artificial replacement for a missing body part. **2.** A device designed and applied to improve function, as a hearing aid. See also **maxillofacial prosthesis, Starr-Edwards prothesis.**

prosthodontics A branch of dentistry devoted to the construction of artificial appliances that replace missing teeth or restore parts of the face.

prot- See **proto-**.

protactinium (Pa) A radioactive element. Its atomic number is 91; its atomic weight is 231. The longest-lived isotope of protactinium is ^{231}Pa, which has a half life of 34,000 years and is produced as an intermediate in the radioactive decay of uranium 235.

protamine sulfate A heparin antagonist.

protamine zinc insulin suspension A long-acting insulin that is absorbed slowly at a steady rate. Some patients can be treated with only one injection daily, but combination therapy with regular insulin may be necessary for adequate control.

protanopia See **daltonism**.

protease An enzyme that is a catalyst in the breakdown of protein. See also **proteolytic**.

protein Any of a large group of naturally occurring, complex, organic nitrogenous compounds. Each is composed of large combinations of amino acids containing the elements carbon, hydrogen, nitrogen, oxygen, usually sulfur, and, occasionally, phosphorus, iron, iodine, or other essential constituents of living cells. Twenty-two amino acids have been identified as vital for proper growth, development, and maintenance of health. The body can synthesize 14 of these amino acids (nonessential), while the remaining 8 (essential) must be obtained from dietary sources. Protein is the major source of building material for muscles, blood, skin, hair, nails, and the internal organs. It is necessary for the formation of hormones, enzymes, and antibodies; as a source of heat and energy; and it functions as an essential element in proper elimination of waste materials. Rich dietary sources are meat, poultry, fish, eggs, milk, and cheese, which are classified as complete proteins since they contain the eight essential amino acids. Nuts and legumes, including navy beans, chick-peas, soybeans, and split peas, are also good sources but are incomplete proteins, since they do not contain all the essential amino acids. Protein deficiency causes abnormal growth and tissue development in children, leading to kwashiorkor and marasmus, while in adults it results in lack of vigor and stamina, weakness, mental depression, poor resistance to infection, impaired healing of wounds, and slow recovery from disease. Excessive intake of protein may in some conditions result in fluid imbalance.

protein-bound iodine (PBI) Iodine that is firmly bound to protein in serum, the measurement of which indirectly indicates the concentration of circulating thyroxine (T_4). PBI less than the normal range of 4 to 8 microns/ml of serum is indicative of hypothyroidism, and a PBI of more than the normal values indicates hyperthyroidism. The test is currently used less frequently because of the availability of more sensitive measurements of T_4.

protein kinase A protein that catalyzes the transfer of a phosphate group from adenosine triphosphate to produce a phosphoprotein.

protein metabolism The processes whereby protein foodstuffs are used by the body to make tissue proteins, together with the processes of breakdown of tissue proteins in the production of energy. Food proteins are first broken down into amino acids, then absorbed into the bloodstream, and finally used in body cells to form new proteins. Amino acids in excess of the body's needs may be converted by liver enzymes into keto acids and urea. Growth hormones and androgens stimulate protein formation, and adrenal cortical hormones tend to cause breakdown of body proteins. Diseases affecting protein metabolism include homocystinuria, liver disease, maple sugar urine disease, and phenylketonuria.

proteinuria The presence in the urine of abnormally large quantities of protein, usually albumin. Healthy adults excrete less than 250 mg of protein per day. Persistent proteinuria is usually a sign of renal disease or renal complications of another disease, as hypertension or heart failure. However, proteinuria can result from heavy exercise or fever. Also called **albuminuria**.

proteo- A combining form meaning 'of or pertaining to protein': *proteocrasis*, *proteolysis*.

proteolipid A type of lipoprotein in which lipid material forms more than one half of the molecule. It is insoluble in water and occurs primarily in the brain.

proteolysis A process in which water added to the peptide bonds of proteins breaks the protein molecule. Numerous enzymes may catalyze this process. The action of mineral acids and heat may also induce proteolysis. —**proteolytic**, *adj.*

Proteus A genus of motile, gram-negative bacilli often associated with nosocomial infections, normally found in feces, water, and soil. *Proteus* may cause urinary tract infections, pyelonephritis, wound infections, diarrhea, bacteremia, and endotoxic shock. Some species are sensitive to penicillin; most respond to aminoglycoside antibiotics.

prothrombin A plasma protein that is the precursor of thrombin. It forms thrombin, the first step in blood clotting, when exposed to thromboplastin and calcium. It is synthesized in the liver if adequate vitamin K is present. Also called **factor II**. See also **blood clotting**.

prothrombin time (PT) A one-stage test for detecting certain plasma coagulation defects owing to a deficiency of factors V, VII or X. Thromboplastin and calcium are added to a sample of the patient's plasma and, simultaneously, to a sample from a normal control. The length of time required for clot formation in both samples is observed. Thrombin is formed from prothrombin in the presence of adequate calcium, thromboplastin, and the essential tissue coagulation factors. A prolonged PT therefore indicates deficiency in one of the factors, as in liver disease, vitamin K deficiency, or anticoagulation therapy with the coumarin derivatives. Compare **partial thromboplastin time.** See also **blood clotting.**

proto-, prot- A combining form meaning 'first': *protoblast, prototoxin.*

protocol A written plan specifying procedures for giving a particular examination, in conducting research, or in providing care for a particular condition. See also **standing orders.**

proton A positively charged particle that is a fundamental component of the nucleus of all atoms. The number of protons in the nucleus of an atom equals the atomic number of the element. Compare **electron, neutron.** See also **atomic weight.**

protoplast 1. In biology: the protoplasm of a cell without its containing membrane. 2. A first entity or an original. —**protoplastic,** *adj.*

protoporphyria Increased excretion of protoporphyrin in the feces.

protoporphyrin A kind of porphyrin that combines with iron and protein to form important organic molecules including catalase, hemoglobin, and myoglobin.

protostoma See **blastopore.**

protozoa, *sing.* **protozoön** Single-celled microorganisms of the class Protozoa, the lowest form of animal life. Protozoa are more complex than bacteria, forming a self-contained unit with organelles that carry on such functions as locomotion, nutrition, excretion, respiration, and attachment to other objects or organisms. Approximately 30 protozoa are pathogenic to humans. —**protozoal, protozoan,** *adj.*

protozoal infection Any disease caused by single-celled organisms of the class Protozoa. Some kinds are **amebic dysentery, kala-azar, malaria, trichomonas vaginalis.**

protracted dose In radiotherapy: a low amount of radiation delivered continuously over a relatively long period of time. See also **blood clotting.**

protriptyline hydrochloride A tricyclic antidepressant.

protrusio bulbi See **exophthalmia.**

proud flesh Excessive granulation tissue. See also **pyogenic granuloma.**

Provincial Territorial Nurses' Association (PTNA) An association of nurses organized at the provincial or territorial level. The Canadian Nurses' Association is a federation of the 11 PTNAs.

provitamin A precursor of a vitamin; a substance found in certain foods that in the body may be converted into a vitamin. Also called **previtamin.**

provocative diagnosis A diagnosis in which the identity and etiology of an illness are discovered by inducing an episode of the condition, as in immunology where an allergen causing an allergic response is shown to be an etiologic factor in the allergic condition.

proximal Nearer to a point of reference, frequently the trunk of the body, than other parts of the body. Proximal interphalangeal joints are those closest to the hand.

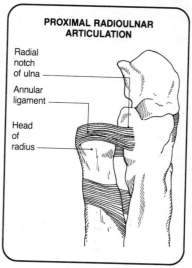

PROXIMAL RADIOULNAR ARTICULATION

Radial notch of ulna

Annular ligament

Head of radius

proximal radioulnar articulation The pivot joint between the circumference of the head of the radius and the ring formed by the radial notch of the ulna and the annular ligament. The joint allows the rotary movements of the head of the radius in pronation and supination. Also called **superior radioulnar joint.** Compare **distal radioulnar articulation.**

proximal renal tubular acidosis (proximal RTA) An abnormal condition characterized by excessive acid accumulation and bicarbonate excretion. It is caused by the defective reabsorption of bicarbonate in the proximal tubules of the kidney and the resulting flow of excessive bicarbonate into the distal tubules which normally secrete hydrogen ions. This disruption impedes the formation of titratable acids and ammonium for excretion and leads to metabolic acidosis. Treatment is as for renal tubular acidosis. In **primary proximal RTA,** the defective reabsorption of bicarbonate is the sole causative factor. In **secondary proximal RTA,** the reabsorptive defect is one of several causative factors and may result from tubular cell damage produced by various disorders, as Fanconi's syndrome. Compare **distal renal tubular acidosis.**

proxymetacaine See **proparacaine hydrochloride.**

prudent person In law: one who exercises sound judgment in adapting a means to an end, conducts oneself in a sensible manner, and carefully weighs the consequences of his or her actions.

prurigo Any of a group of chronic inflammatory conditions of the skin characterized by severe itching and multiple, dome-shaped, small papules capped by tiny vesicles. As a result of repeated scratching, crusting and lichenification may occur. Causes are allergies, drugs, endocrine abnormalities, malignancies, and parasites. Treatment depends on the cause. Symptomatic therapy is the same as for pruritus. A mild form is called **prurigo mitis** and a more severe form, **prurigo agria** or **prurigo ferox.** See also **pruritus.** —**pruriginous,** *adj.*

pruritus The symptom of itching, an uncomfortable sensation leading to the urge to scratch, which often results in secondary infection. Causes are allergy, infection, jaundice, lymphoma, and skin irritation. Treatment depends on the cause; symptomatic relief may be obtained by antihistamines, starch baths, topical corticosteroids, cool water, or alcohol applications. —**pruritic,** *adj.*

pruritus ani A common chronic condition of itching of the skin around the anus. Some causes are candida infection, contact dermatitis, external hemorrhoids, pinworms, psoriasis, and psychogenic illness. Treatment depends on the cause; symptomatic relief may be obtained by careful cleansing, soothing creams or lotions, topical corticosteroids, antihistamines, and tranquilizers.

pruritus vulvae Itching of the external genitalia of a female that may become chronic and result in lichenification, atrophy, and occasionally malignancy. Some causes are contact dermatitis, lichen sclerosus et atrophicus, psychogenic pruritus, trichomoniasis, and vaginal candidiasis. Treatment depends on its cause.

psammo- A combining form meaning 'of or related to sand or to sandlike material': *psammocarcinoma.*

psammoma, *pl.* **psammomas, psammomata** A neoplasm containing small calcified granules (psammoma bodies) that occurs in the meninges, choroid plexus, pineal body, and ovaries. Also called **sand tumor.**

psammoma body A round, layered mass of calcareous material occurring in benign and malignant epithelial and connective tissue neoplasms and in some chronically inflamed tissue.

-pselaphesia, -pselaphesis A combining form meaning '(condition of the) tactile sense': *apselaphesia.*

psuedesthesia A sensation without an external stimulus or a sensation that does not correspond to the causative stimulus, as phantom limb pain.

pseudo-, pseud- A combining form meaning 'false': *pseudoangina, pseudocyst.*

pseudoallele In genetics: one of two or more closely linked genes on a chromosome that appear to function as a single member of an allelic pair but occupy distinct, nearly corresponding loci on homologous chromosomes. Such gene pairs produce a mutant effect in the diploid state when located on homologous chromosomes but are capable of being separated by crossing over during meiosis to produce a wild-type effect when recombined on either of the homologues. —**pseudoallelic,** *adj.,* **pseudoallelism,** *n.*

pseudoanorexia A condition in which an individual eats secretly while claiming a lack of appetite and inability to eat. Also called **false anorexia.**

pseudochylous ascites Abnormal accumulation in the peritoneal cavity of a milky fluid that resembles chyle. The turbidity of the fluid is caused by cellular debris. It is indicative of an abdominal tumor or infection. Compare **chylous ascites.** See also **ascites.**

pseudocoxalgia See **Perthes' disease.**

pseudocyst A space or cavity containing gas or liquid but without a lining membrane. It commonly occurs after pancreatitis when digestive juices break through the normal pancreas ducts and collect in spaces lined by fibroblasts and surfaces of adjacent organs. Symptoms are due to displacement of abdominal structures or fluid or to atelectasis at the base of the left lung. Ultrasound and computerized tomography are useful in diagnosis; surgical drainage is the best therapy. See also **pancreatitis.**

pseudoephedrine hydrochloride, p. sulfate Sympathomimetic vasoconstrictors used as decongestants.

pseudogene In molecular genetics: a sequence of nucleotides that resembles a gene and may be derived from one but lacks a genetic function.

pseudogout See **chondrocalcinosis.**

pseudohermaphroditism A condition in which the gonads are of one sex, but one or more contradictions exist in the morphologic criteria of the sex.

pseudojaundice A yellow discoloration of the skin that is not caused by hyperbilirubinemia. Excessive ingestion of carotene results in a form of pseudojaundice.

pseudomembranous enterocolitis See **necrotizing enterocolitis.**

pseudomembranous stomatitis A severe inflammation of the mouth that produces a membranelike exudate. The condition may be caused by a variety of bacteria or by chemical irritants. It may produce dysphagia, pain, fever, and swelling of the lymph glands, or it may remain localized and mild.

pseudomonad A bacterium of the genus *Pseudomonas.*

Pseudomonas A genus of gram-negative bacteria that includes several free-living species found in soil and water and some opportunistic pathogens, as *Pseudomonas aeruginosa,* isolated from wounds, burns, and infections of the urinary tract. Pseudomonads are notable for their fluorescent pigments and their resistance to disinfectants and antibiotics.

pseudoneurotic schizophrenia, pseudopsychopathic schizophrenia See **latent schizophrenia.**

pseudorubella See **roseola infantum.**

pseudosclerema See **adiponecrosis subcutanea neonatorum.**

pseudotumor A false tumor. Kinds of pseudotumors are **orbital pseudotumor, pseudotumor cerebri.**

pseudotumor cerebri A condition characterized by increased intracranial pressure, headache, vomiting, and papilledema without neurological signs, except, occasionally, palsy of the sixth cranial nerve. Also called **benign intracranial hypertension, meningeal hydrops.**

pseudoxanthoma elasticum See **Grönblad-Strandberg syndrome.**

psi *abbr* pounds per square inch.

psilocybin A psychedelic drug and an active ingredient of various Mexican hallucinogenic mushrooms of the genus *Psilocybe mexicana.* It can produce altered states of mood and consciousness and has no acceptable medical use in the United States. Psilocybin is controlled under Schedule I of the Comprehensive Drug Abuse Prevention and Control Act of 1970, which bans the prescription of psilocybin and numerous other drugs and allows their procurement and use only for special research projects authorized by the Drug Enforcement Administration of the United States Department of Justice.

psittacosis An infectious illness caused by the bacterium *Chlamydia psittaci,* characterized by respiratory, pneumonialike symptoms and transmitted to humans by infected birds, especially parrots. Variable clinical manifestations resemble many infectious diseases, but fever, cough, anorexia, and severe headache are almost always present. A history of exposure to birds is highly suggestive, because all chlamydiae are difficult to isolate and culture. A demonstrated rise in antibody titer confirms a diagnosis. Tetracycline is usually used to treat psittacosis and is continued for 10 to 14 days after the fever subsides. Isolation is advised. Also called **ornithosis, parrot fever.** See also *Chlamydia.*

psoas major A long abdominal muscle originating from the transverse processes of the lumbar vertebrae and the fibrocartilages and sides of the vertebral bodies of the lower thoracic vertebrae and the lumbar vertebrae. It joins the iliacus to form the iliopsoas deep in the pelvis as it passes under the inguinal ligament and inserts in the lesser trochanter. It acts to flex and laterally rotate the thigh and to flex and laterally bend the spine.

psoas minor A long, slender muscle of the pelvis, ventral to the psoas major. Many individuals do not have this muscle. It arises from the bodies of the 12th thoracic and the 1st lumbar vertebrae and from the disk between them and ends in a long, flat tendon that inserts into the pectineal line of the pelvis and into the iliac fascia. It functions to flex the spine. Compare **iliacus, psoas major.**

psor- A combining form meaning 'of or related to itching': *psora, psorocomium.*

psoralen-type photosynthesizer Any one of the chemical compounds that contain photosensitizing psoralen and that react on exposure to ultraviolet light to increase the melanin in the skin. Naturally occurring psoralen photosynthesizers, as 5- and 8-methoxypsoralen, are found in carrot greens, celery, dill, figs, limes, parsley, and other plants. Some psoralen-type photosynthesizers produced as pharmaceuticals are methoxsalen and trioxalen; both are used to

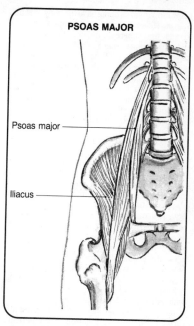

PSOAS MAJOR

Psoas major

Iliacus

enhance skin pigmentation or tanning in the treatment of skin diseases, as psoriasis and vitiligo.

psoriasis A common, chronic, heritable skin disorder, characterized by circumscribed red patches covered by thick, dry, silvery, adherent scales that are the result of excessive development of epithelial cells. Exacerbations and remissions are typical. Lesions may be anywhere on the body but are more common on extensor surfaces, bony prominences, scalp, ears, genitalia, and the perianal area. An arthritis, particularly of distal small joints, may accompany the skin disease. Treatment includes topical and intralesional corticosteroids, ultraviolet light, tar solution baths, creams and shampoos, methotrexate, and photochemotherapy. Subcategories of psoriasis include **guttate psoriasis** and **pustular psoriasis.** See also **photochemotherapy, psoriatic arthritis. —psoriatic,** *adj.*

psoriatic arthritis A form of rheumatoid arthritis associated with psoriatic lesions of the skin and nails, particularly at the distal interphalangeal joints of the fingers and toes, resulting in a characteristic 'pencil in cup' deformity seen on X-ray examination.

PSRO *abbr* **Professional Standards Review Organization.**

PSS *abbr* **progressive systemic sclerosis.**

PSSO *abbr* peer specialist second opinion.

psych- See **psycho-.**

psychasthenia See **obsessive-compulsive neurosis.**

psyche 1. The aspect of one's mental faculty that encompasses the conscious and unconscious processes. 2. The vital mental or spiritual entity of the individual as opposed to the body or soma. **3.** In psychoanalysis: the total components of the id, ego, and superego, including all conscious and unconscious aspects. Compare **soma.**

psychedelic **1.** Of or describing a mental state characterized by altered sensory perception and hallucination, accompanied by euphoria or fear, usually caused by the deliberate ingestion of drugs or other substances known to produce this effect. **2.** Of or describing any drug or substance that causes this state, as mescaline or psilocybin.

psychiatric disorder See **mental disorder.**

psychiatric nurse practitioner A nurse practitioner who, by advanced study and clinical practice, has gained expert knowledge in the care and prevention of mental disorders. See also **psychiatric nursing.**

psychiatric nursing The branch of nursing concerned with the prevention and cure of mental disorders and their sequelae. It employs theories of human behavior as its scientific framework and requires the use of the self as its art or expression in nursing practice. Some of the activities of the psychiatric nurse include the provision of a safe therapeutic milieu; working with patients, or clients, concerning the real day-to-day problems that they face; identifying and caring for the physical aspects of the patient's problems, including drug reactions; assuming the role of social agent or parent for the patient in various recreational, occupational, and social situations; conducting psychotherapy; and providing leadership and clinical assistance for other nurses and health care workers. Psychiatric nurses work in many settings; their responsibilities vary with the setting and with the level of expertise, experience, and training of the individual nurse. Also called **mental health nursing.**

psychiatry The branch of medical science that deals with the causes, treatment, and prevention of mental, emotional, and behavioral disorders. Some kinds of psychiatry are **community psychiatry, descriptive psychiatry, dynamic psychiatry, existential psychiatry, forensic psychiatry, orthopsychiatry. —psychiatric,** *adj.*

-psychic A combining form meaning 'relating to the relation between mind and body': *allopsychic, biopsychic.*

psychic infection The spread of neurotic or psychic effects on a small scale, as in folie à deux, or on a large scale, as in the dance and witch manias of the Middle Ages or the spread of hysterical or panic reactions in a crowd. Also called psychic contagion. See also **sympathy.**

psychic suicide The termination of one's own life without the use of physical means or agents, as an older person widowed after many years of marriage who becomes sufficiently depressed to lose 'the will to live.'

psychic trauma An emotional shock or injury or a distressful situation that produces a lasting impression, especially on the subconscious mind. Common causes are abuse or neglect in childhood, rape, and loss of a loved one. Psychotherapeutic sessions in which the injured person can express feelings can alleviate psychic trauma.

psycho-, psych- A combining form meaning 'of or related to the mind': *psychoauditory, psychodynamics.*

psychoanalysis A branch of psychiatry founded by Sigmund Freud devoted to the study of the psychology of human development and behavior. It is a system of psychotherapy based on the concepts of a dynamic unconscious, utilizing free association, dream interpretation, and the analysis of defense mechanisms, especially resistance and transference. Through these devices, emotions and behavior are traced to repressed instinctual drives in the unconscious. Treatment consists of helping the patient recognize repressed emotional conflicts, analyzing their origin, and bringing them into the consciousness so that irrational and maladaptive behavior can be altered. See also **psychosexual development.**

psychoanalyst A psychotherapist, usually a psychiatrist, who has had special training in psychoanalysis and who applies the techniques of psychoanalytic theory.

psychoanalytic **1.** Of or pertaining to psychoanalysis. **2.** Using the techniques or principles of psychoanalysis.

psychobiology **1.** The study of personality development and functioning in terms of the interaction of the body and the mind. **2.** A school of psychiatric thought introduced by Adolf Meyer that stresses total life experience, including biological, emotional, and sociocultural factors, in assessing the psychological makeup or mental status of an individual. Mental disorders are interpreted as dynamic adaptive reactions to stress or conflict, with little or no emphasis on unconscious factors. Also called **biopsychology.** See also **distributive analysis and synthesis.**

psychocatharsis See **catharsis.**

psychodrama A form of group therapy, originated by J. L. Moreno, in which people act out their emotional problems through dramatization and role playing. Also called **role-playing therapy.**

psychogenesis **1.** The development of the mind or of a mental function or process. **2.** The development or production of a physical symptom or disease from mental or psychic origins rather than organic factors. **3.** The development of emotional states, either normal or abnormal, from the interaction of conscious and unconscious psychological forces. Compare **somatogenesis.**

psychogenic, psychogenetic **1.** Originating within the mind. **2.** Any physical symptom, disease process, or emotional state of psychological rather than physical origin. See also **psychosomatic.**

psychogenic pain disorder A disorder characterized by persistent and severe pain with no apparent organic cause. The condition is often accompanied by other sensory or motor dysfunction, as paresthesia or muscle spasm. The cause may be one or many unresolved needs or conflicts. Treatment consists of immediate alleviation of the symptoms followed by long-term psychotherapy to uncover the unconscious emotional conflicts that influenced the development and maintenance of the pain. See also **psychogenesis.**

psychokinesia 1. Impulsive, maniacal behavior resulting from deficient or defective inhibitions. 2. In parapsychology: psychokinesis.

psychokinesis (PK) The direct influence of the mind or will upon matter usually resulting in the production of motion in objects without the intervention of the physical senses or a physical force.

psychokinetics The study of psychokinesis.

psychological test Any of a group of standardized tests designed to measure or ascertain such characteristics as intellectual capacity, motivation, perception, role behavior, values, level of anxiety or depression, coping mechanisms, and general personality integration. Compare **achievement test, aptitude test, intelligence test, personality test.**

psychologist A specialist in the study of psychology.

psychology 1. The study of behavior and of the functions and processes of the mind, especially as related to environment. 2. A profession that involves practical applications of knowledge, skills, and techniques in the understanding of, prevention of, or solution to individual or social problems, especially to the interaction between the individual and the physical and social environment. 3. The mental, motivational, and behavioral characteristics and attitudes of an individual or group. Kinds of psychology include **analytic psychology, behaviorism, clinical psychology, cognitive psychology, experimental psychology, humanistic psychology, social psychology.** —**psychologic, psychological,** *adj.,* **psychologically,** *adv.*

psychometrics, psychometry The development, administration, or interpretation of psychological and intelligence tests.

psychomotor development The progressive attainment by the child of skills that involve both mental and muscular activity, as the ability of the infant to turn over, sit, or crawl at will and of the toddler to walk, talk, control bladder and bowel functions, and begin solving cognitive problems.

psychomotor seizure A temporary impairment of consciousness, often associated with temporal lobe disease and characterized by psychic symptoms, loss of judgment, automatic behavior, and abnormal acts. No apparent convulsions occur, but there may be loss of consciousness or amnesia for the episode. During the seizure the individual may appear drowsy, intoxicated, or violent; asocial acts or crimes may be committed but normal activities, as driv-

ing a car, typing, or eating, may continue at an automatic level. Psychic symptoms include visual and auditory hallucinations, a sense of unreality, and déjà vu. Visceral symptoms may include chest pain, transient respiratory arrest, tachycardia, gastrointestinal discomfort, and abnormal sensations of smell and taste.

psychoneurosis See **neurosis.**

psychoneurotic See **neurotic.**

psychoneurotic disorder See **neurotic disorder.**

psychopath A person who has an antisocial personality disorder. Also called **sociopath.**

psychopathia See **psychopathy.**

psychopathia sexualis A mental disease characterized by sexual perversion.

psychopathic Of or pertaining to antisocial behavior. Also called **sociopathic.** See also **antisocial personality, antisocial personality disorder.**

psychopathic personality See **antisocial personality.**

psychopathologist One who specializes in the study and treatment of mental disorders. —**psychopathology,** *n.*

psychopathology 1. The study of the causes, processes, and manifestations of mental disorders. 2. The behavioral manifestation of any mental disorder.

psychopathy Any disease of the mind, congenital or acquired, not necessarily associated with subnormal intelligence. Also called **psychopathia.**

psychopharmacology The scientific study of the effects of drugs in the treatment of mental disorders.

psychophylaxis See **mental hygiene.**

psychophysical preparation for childbirth A program that prepares women for giving birth by teaching them the physiology of the process, exercises to improve muscle tone and physical stamina, and techniques of breathing and relaxation to promote control and comfort during labor and delivery. Goals of all of the methods are a decrease in the mother's fear and pain, a decrease in or elimination of the use of analgesia and anesthesia in childbirth, and an increase in the mother's participation and cooperation, thus requiring less obstetric intervention. Methods include **Bradley method, Lamaze method, Read method.**

psychophysics The branch of psychology concerned with the relationships between physical stimuli and sensory responses.

psychophysiologic 1. Of or pertaining to psychophysiology. 2. Having physical symptoms resulting from psychogenic origins; psychosomatic.

psychophysiological disorder Any of a group of mental disorders characterized by the dysfunction of an organ or organ system controlled by the autonomic nervous system, as a peptic ulcer, which may be caused or aggravated by emotional factors, as stress or anxiety. Also called **psychosomatic illness, psychosomatic reaction.**

psychophysiology **1.** The study of physiology as related to aspects of psychological or behavioral function. See also **psychophysiological disorder. 2.** The study of mental activity by physical examination and observation.

psychoprophylactic preparation for childbirth A system of prenatal education for giving birth using the Lamaze method of natural childbirth.

psychosexual Of or pertaining to the psychological and emotional aspects of sex. See also **psychosexual development, psychosexual disorder.** —**psychosexuality,** *n.*

psychosexual development In psychoanalysis: the emergence of the personality through a series of stages from infancy to adulthood, each relatively fixed in time and characterized by a dominant mode of achieving libidinal pleasure through the interaction of biological drives and environmental restraints. Resolution of the conflicts encountered at each stage theoretically leads to a balanced, heterosexual adjustment and normal development, while a lack of resolution results in personality disturbances, fixated at the stage during which the unresolved conflicts occurred. Disturbances may be latent or may result in behavioral or personality disorders. The stages of development are the oral stage, anal stage, phallic stage, latency stage, and genital stage. Also called **libidinal development.** See also **psychomotor development.**

psychosexual disorder A condition characterized by abnormal sexual attitudes, desires, or activities resulting from psychological rather than organic causes. See also **gender identity disorder, paraphilia, psychosexual dysfunction.**

psychosexual dysfunction Any of a large group of sexual maladjustments or disorders caused by an emotional or psychological problem.

psychosis, *pl.* **psychoses** Any major mental disorder of organic or emotional origin characterized by extreme personality derangement or disorganization, often with severe depression, agitation, regressive behavior, illusions, delusions, and hallucinations that so greatly impair perception, thinking, emotional response, and personal orientation that the individual loses touch with reality, is incapable of functioning normally, and usually requires hospitalization. Kinds of psychoses include **alcoholic psychosis, bipolar disorder, Korsakoff's psychosis, paranoia, schizophrenia, senile psychosis.** See also **major affective disorder, organic mental disorder.**

-psychosis A combining form meaning a 'serious mental disorder': *autopsychosis, encephalopsychosis.*

psychosocial assessment An assessment of a person's mental and social status and function. The person's self-image and self-esteem, goals, values, beliefs, and relationships are observed and evaluated.

psychosocial development In child development: a description devised by Erik Erik-son of the normal serial development of trust, autonomy, identity, and intimacy that begins in infancy and progresses as the infantile ego interacts with the environment. To reach a new stage, the preceding one must be fully realized. The sequence and chronology of the stages coincide with the psychosexual stages of development as described by Freud.

psychosomatic **1.** Of or pertaining to psychosomatic medicine. **2.** Relating to, characterized by, or resulting from the interaction of the mind or psyche and the body. **3.** The expression of an emotional conflict through physical symptoms. See also **psychogenic, psychophysiological disorder.**

psychosomatic approach The interdisciplinary or holistic study of physical and mental disease from a biological, psychosocial, and sociocultural point of view.

psychosomatic illness See **psychophysiological disorder.**

psychosomatic medicine The branch of medicine concerned with the interrelationships between mental and emotional reactions and somatic processes; in particular, the manner in which intrapsychic conflicts influence physical symptoms. It maintains that the body and mind are one inseparable entity and that both physiological and psychological techniques should be applied in the study and treatment of illness. Also called **psychosomatics.**

psychosomatic reaction See **psychophysiological disorder.**

psychosurgery Surgical interruption of certain nerve pathways in the brain, performed to treat chronic, unremitting anxiety, agitation, or obsessional neuroses when the condition is severe and alternative treatments, as psychotherapy, drugs, and electroshock, have proven ineffective. The procedure may be a limited prefrontal lobotomy (in which connecting fibers in the frontal region are cut) or a modified bifrontal tractotomy (in which nerve tracts of the brain stem are severed). Light general anesthesia is given. Postoperative nursing care includes observation for signs of leakage of cerebrospinal fluid. A marked alteration of personality is unavoidable. Various cognitive and affective functions are also affected, depending on the location of the induced lesion, the extent of destruction of nerve tissue, and the age, sex, and condition of the patient. Modern psychotherapeutic drugs have replaced psychosurgery in most cases.

psychotherapeutics The treatment of personality disorders by means of psychotherapy.

psychotherapist One who practices psychotherapy, including psychiatrists, licensed psychologists, psychiatric nurses, psychiatric social workers, and persons trained in counseling. Compare **psychoanalyst.**

psychotherapy Any of a large number of related methods of treating mental and emotional disorders by psychological techniques rather than by physical means. Included are reinforcement, persuasion, suggestion, reassur-

PSYCHOSEXUAL AND PSYCHOSOCIAL DEVELOPMENT

FREUD'S THEORY	ERIKSON'S THEORY
Oral stage (ages 0 to 18 months) • Uses mouth as source of satisfaction • **Passive phase:** Is helpless, narcissistic, and egocentric. Operates on pleasure principle, feels omnipotent, wants to satisfy hunger, sucking, and security needs • **Active phase:** Bites as a mode of pleasure, experiments and associates continuously, exhibits sensory discrimination, differentiates between mental images and reality, differentiates between others, discovers self	**Orosensory stage (ages 0 to 12 months)** • Develops basic attitudes of trust vs. mistrust (through mother's reaction to infant needs) • Uses mouth as source of satisfaction and means of dealing with anxiety-producing situations
Anal stage (ages 1½ to 3) • Learns muscular control of urination and defecation *(toilet-training period)* • Exhibits increasing self-control (walks, talks, dresses, and undresses) • Asserts independence by learning to say *no (negativism)* • Delays gratification until proper time *(reality principle)* • Begins ego and superego development • Engages in parallel play	**Anal-muscular stage (ages 1 to 3)** • Focuses on development of basic attitudes of autonomy vs. shame and doubt • Learns limits of ability to affect the environment by direct manipulation • Exerts self-control and willpower
Phallic stage (ages 3 to 6) • Focuses libidinal energy on genitalia • Learns sexual identity • Experiences internalization of superego • Engages in sibling rivalry • Manipulates parents • Experiences refinement of intellectual and motor activities • Increases socialization and associative play	**Genitolocomotor stage (ages 3 to 6)** • Experiences development of basic attitudes of initiative vs. guilt • Learns limits of ability to affect the environment through assertiveness • Explores the world through senses, thoughts, and imagination • Demonstrates direction and purpose through activities • Engages in first real social contacts through cooperative play • Develops conscience
Latency stage (ages 6 to 12) • Enters quiet stage: sexual development lies dormant; emotional tension eases • Experiences normal homosexual phase: boys join gangs and girls form cliques • Increases intellectual capacity • Starts school • Identifies with teachers and peers • Weakens home ties • Recognizes authority figures outside home *(hero worship)*	**Latency stage (ages 6 to 12)** • Experiences development of basic attitudes of industry vs. inferiority • Creates, develops, and manipulates • Initiates and completes tasks • Understands rules and regulations • Displays competence and productivity
Genital stage (ages 12 to young adult) • Develops secondary sex characteristics and experiences reawakened sex drives • Exhibits increased concern over physical appearance • Strives toward independence • Exhibits sexual maturity • Identifies member of opposite sex as love object • Matures intellectually • Plans future • Experiences identity crisis	**Puberty and adolescent stage (ages 12 to 18)** • Experiences development of basic attitudes of identity vs. role diffusion • Integrates life experiences • Seeks partner of opposite sex • Begins to establish identity and place in society

Adapted from Kreigh and Perko, *Psychiatric and Mental Health Nursing,* 1979, pp. 126-133. Reprinted with permission of Reston Publishing Co., a Prentice-Hall Co., 11480 Sunset Hills Rd., Reston, Va. 22090

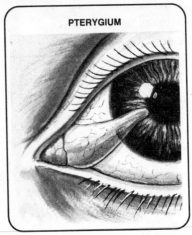

PTERYGIUM

ance, support, and abreaction. Some of the aims are to change maladaptive behavioral patterns, improve interpersonal relationships, resolve inner conflicts, modify inaccurate assumptions about the self and the environment, and foster a sense of self-identity to promote individual growth leading to a more meaningful and fulfilling existence. Kinds of psychotherapy are **behavior therapy, group therapy, humanistic-existential therapy, interpersonal therapy, psychoanalysis.**

psychotic 1. Of or pertaining to psychosis. 2. A person exhibiting the characteristics of a psychosis.

psychotic disorder See **psychosis.**

psychotic reaction See **psychosis.**

psychro- A combining form meaning 'of or pertaining to cold': *psychrophilic, psychrophore.*

psyllium A bulk-forming laxative.

psyllium seed See **plantago seed.**

Pt Symbol for **platinum.**

PT *abbr* **prothrombin time.**

PTA *abbr* **plasma thromboplastin antecedent.**

PTCA *abbr* **percutaneous transluminal coronary angioplasty.**

pteroylglutamic acid See **folic acid.**

pterygium A thick, triangular bit of pale tissue that extends medially from the nasal border of the cornea to the inner canthus of the eye.

-pterygium A combining form meaning a '(specified) abnormality of the conjunctiva': *loxopterygium, pimelopterygium.*

pterygoideus lateralis One of the four muscles of mastication. Extending almost horizontally from the infratemporal fossa and the condyle of the mandible, it is a short, thick, somewhat conical muscle, arising by two heads from the great wing of the sphenoid, the infratemporal crest, and the lateral pterygoid plate. It inserts into the condyle of the mandible and into the articular disk of the temporomandibular articulation. The pterygoideus lateralis func-

tions to open the jaws, protrude the mandible, and move it from side to side. Also called **external pterygoid muscle.** Compare **masseter, pterygoideus medialis, temporalis.**

pterygoideus medialis One of the four muscles of mastication. Arising from the pyramidal process of the palatine bone and from the tuberosity of the maxilla and inserting into the medial surface of the ramus of the mandible, it acts to close the jaws. Also called **internal pterygoid muscle.** Compare **masseter, pterygoideus lateralis, temporalis.**

pterygoid plexus One of a pair of extensive networks of veins between the temporalis and the pterygoideus lateralis, extending between surrounding structures in the infratemporal fossa. The plexus receives deoxygenated blood from various tributaries that correspond with branches of the maxillary artery; it communicates with the cavernous sinus through the foramen of Vesalius and with the facial vein through the deep facial and with the angular veins. Compare **maxillary vein.**

PTH *abbr* **parathyroid hormone.**

PTNA *abbr* **Provincial Territorial Nurses' Association.**

ptoma- A combining form meaning 'of or related to a corpse': *ptomaine, ptomatopsia.*

ptosis An abnormal condition of one or both upper eyelids. The eyelid droops because of congenital or acquired weakness of the levator muscle or paralysis of the third cranial nerve. Partial ptosis and a small pupil may be caused by a hemologic disorder of the sympathetic portion of the autonomic nervous system. May be treated surgically by shortening the levator muscle.

-ptosis A combining form meaning a 'prolapse of an organ': *hepaptosis, uvulaptosis.*

ptotic kidney A kidney that is abnormally situated in the pelvis, usually over the sacral promontory behind the peritoneum. The condition may be either congenital or secondary to trauma and is usually asymptomatic, but obstruction of the flow of urine from the kidney may result from pregnancy.

PTT *abbr* **partial thromboplastin time.**

ptyalin A starch-digesting enzyme present in saliva. Also called **amylase.**

ptyalism Excessive salivation. Sometimes occurs in early pregnancy. Also called **hyperptyalism.**

ptyalo- A combining form meaning 'of or related to the saliva': *ptyalocele, ptyalogenic.*

-ptysis A combining form meaning a 'spitting of matter': *albuminoptysis, hemoptysis.*

Pu Symbol for **plutonium.**

pub- A combining form meaning 'adult': *puberal, pubescence.*

pubarche The onset of puberty, marked by initial development of secondary sexual characteristics.

-pubic A combining form meaning 'of, referring, or relating to the frontal part of the pelvis': *iliopubic, retropubic.*

pubic bone See **pubis.**

pubic symphysis The slightly movable interpubic joint of the pelvis, consisting of two pubic bones separated by a disk of fibrocartilage and connected by two ligaments. Also called **symphysis pubis.**

pubis, *pl.* **pubes** One of a pair of pubic bones that, with the ischium and the ilium, form the hip bone and join the pubic bone from the opposite side at the symphysis pubis. The pubis forms one fifth of the acetabulum and is divisible into the body, the superior ramus, and the inferior ramus. The external surface of the pubis is rough and serves as the origin of the adductor longus, the obturator externus, the adductor brevis, and the proximal part of the gracilis. The internal surface of the pubis is smooth; it forms part of the anterior wall of the pelvis, giving origin to the levator ani and the obturator internus, and attachment to the puboprostatic ligaments and a few muscular fibers from the bladder. The pubic crest affords attachment to the rectus abdominus, the pyramidalis, and the inguinal falx. The lateral portion of the superior ramus of the pubis presents the superior, the inferior, and the dorsal surfaces. The superior surface presents the iliopectineal line, and the inferior ramus gives origin to the gracilis, a portion of the obturator externus, the adductor brevis, the adductor magnus, the obturator internus, and the constrictor urethrae. Compare **ilium, ischium.**

publish or perish *Informal.* A practice followed in many academic institutions in which a contract for employment is renewed at the same or higher rank only if a candidate has demonstrated scholarship and professional status by having published work in a book or in a national professional journal.

pubococcygeus exercises A regimen of isometric exercises involving a series of voluntary contractions of the muscles of the pelvic diaphragm and perineum to increase the contractility of the vaginal introitus or to improve retention of urine. Also called **Kegel exercises.**

pudendal block A form of regional anesthetic block administered to relieve the discomfort of the expulsive second stage of labor. The pudendal nerves are anesthetized by the injection of a local anesthetic in the trunk of each nerve as it passes over the sacrospinous ligament, just below the ischial spine. Pudendal block anesthetizes the perineum, vulva, clitoris, labia majora, and the perirectal area without affecting the muscular contractions of the uterus. When properly administered, the risk is minimal.

pudendal canal See **Alcock's canal.**

pudendal nerve One of the branches of the pudendal plexus that arises from the second, third, and fourth sacral nerves, passes between the piriformis and coccygeus, and leaves the pelvis through the greater sciatic foramen. It crosses the spine of the ischium and reenters the pelvis through the lesser sciatic foramen. It accompanies the internal pudendal vessels through a fascial tunnel along the lateral wall of the ischiorectal fossa and divides into two terminal branches near the urogenital diaphragm. The

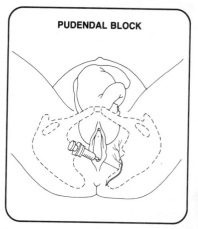

PUDENDAL BLOCK

branches of the pudendal nerve form the inferior rectal nerve and then divide to form the perineal nerve and dorsal nerve of the penis or clitoris. See also **pudendal plexus.**

pudendal plexus A network of motor and sensory nerves formed by the anterior branches of the second, third and all of the fourth sacral nerves. It is often considered part of the sacral plexus. The pudendal plexus lies in the posterior hollow of the pelvis, on the ventral surface of the piriformis. The branches of the plexus are the visceral branches, the muscular branches, and the pudendal nerve. The visceral branches arise from the second, third, and fourth sacral nerves and supply the bladder, prostate, seminal vesicles, uterus, external genitalia, and some of the intestinal tract. The muscular branches arise from the fourth, and, sometimes, the third and fifth sacral nerves and supply the levator ani, sphincter ani, and coccygeus. The pudendal nerve arises from the second, third, and fourth sacral nerves and divides into five branches supplying the genital structures and the pelvic region. Compare **lumbar plexus, sacral plexus.**

pudendum, *pl.* **pudenda** The external genitalia, especially of women. In a woman it comprises the mons veneris, the labia majora, the labia minora, the vestibule of the vagina, the urinary meatus, and the vestibular glands. In a man it comprises the penis, scrotum, and testes. **—pudendal,** *adj.*

puer- A combining form meaning 'child': *puericulture, puerilism, puerperium.*

puericulture The specialty of rearing and training children. **—puericulturist,** *n.*

puerile Of or pertaining to children or childhood; juvenile. **—puerility,** *n.*

puerperal **1.** Of or pertaining to the period immediately after childbirth. **2.** Of or pertaining to a woman (puerpera) who has just given birth to an infant.

puerperal endometritis See **puerperal fever.**

puerperal fever A syndrome associated with systemic bacterial infection and septicemia that

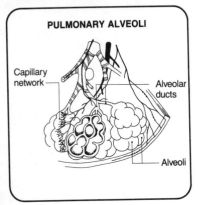

PULMONARY ALVEOLI

Capillary network

Alveolar ducts

Alveoli

occurs following childbirth, usually as a result of unsterile obstetric technique. Puerperal fever is characterized by endometritis, fever, tachycardia, uterine tenderness, and foul-smelling lochia; if untreated, prostration, renal failure, bacteremic shock, and death may occur. The causative organism is most often one of the hemolytic streptococci. Puerperal fever was little known before hospital childbirth became common, early in the 19th century; but then it became an endemic and frequently epidemic scourge that resulted in the deaths of many thousands of mothers and infants. Maternal mortality rates of 20% and higher were not uncommon in parts of the world where childbirth occurred in hospitals. Ignaz Philipp Semmelweis, in Vienna, noted that women attended by midwives were much less likely to contract the disease than those attended by physicians and medical students. Midwives did not perform frequent vaginal examinations during labor and did not participate in autopsies. Though the germ theory of disease had not yet been elaborated, Semmelweis deduced that the causative agent of the disease was being transmitted by doctors and students from the infected cadavers in the autopsy room to women in labor on the maternity wards. By instituting a policy requiring that the hands and instruments of obstetric attendants be disinfected, maternal mortality in his clinic dropped dramatically. His work was widely ignored or discredited for almost half a century because physicians were unwilling to believe that they were the agents of transmission. Late in the 19th century, following Pasteur's discovery of microbes, Semmelweis was posthumously vindicated. Sterile techniques were gradually instituted, but not until the 4th decade of the 20th century did puerperal fever cease to be the leading cause of maternal death. Postpartum uterine infection still is not uncommon, but it is effectively treated with massive parenteral doses of antibiotics before it becomes a systemic illness. Also called **puerperal metritis.**

puerperal mania   A rare, acute mood disorder that sometimes occurs in women following childbirth, characterized by a severe manic re-

action. See also **mania, postpartum depression.**

puerperal metritis   See **puerperal fever.**

puerperium   The time following childbirth, lasting approximately 6 weeks, during which the anatomic and physiologic changes brought about by pregnancy resolve, and a woman adjusts to the new or expanded responsibilities of motherhood and nonpregnant life.

Pulex   A genus of fleas. Some species transmit arthropod-borne infections, as plague and epidemic typhus.

PULHES   A system for recording the physical and mental status of recruits in the U.S. military. The term represents physical capacity (P), upper limbs (U), lower limbs (L), hearing (H), eyesight (E), and emotional stability (S).

pulmo-, pulmon-   A combining form meaning 'of or pertaining to the lungs': *pulmogram.*

pulmonary, pulmonic   Of or pertaining to the lungs or the respiratory system.

pulmonary alveolus   One of the lung's terminal air sacs in which oxygen and carbon dioxide are exchanged.

pulmonary anthrax   See **woolsorter's disease.**

pulmonary arteriolar resistance (PAR) Pressure loss per unit of blood flow from the pulmonary artery to a pulmonary vein.

pulmonary atrium   Any of the spaces at the end of an alveolar duct into which alveoli open.

pulmonary capillary wedge pressure (PCWP)   The pressure in the capillary end of the pulmonary artery, which reflects mean left atrial pressure and left ventricular end-diastolic pressure. It is measured by threading a catheter into a branch of the pulmonary artery and inflating a balloon at its tip. Also called **pulmonary wedge pressure.**

pulmonary carcinosis   See **alveolar cell carcinoma.**

pulmonary edema   The accumulation of extravascular fluid in lung tissues and alveoli, caused most commonly by congestive heart failure and also occurring in barbiturate and opiate poisoning, diffuse infections, hemorrhagic pancreatitis, and renal failure, and following neardrowning, the inhalation of irritating gases, and the rapid administration of whole blood, plasma, serum albumin, or intravenous fluids. In congestive heart failure, serous fluid is pushed back through the pulmonary capillaries into alveoli and quickly enters bronchioles and bronchi. The patient breathes rapidly and shallowly with difficulty, is usually restless, apprehensive, pale or cyanotic, and may cough up frothy, pink sputum. The peripheral and neck veins are usually engorged; the blood pressure and heart rate are increased, and the pulse may be full and bounding or weak and thready. There may be edema of the extremities, diffuse rales in the lungs, respiratory acidosis, and profuse diaphoresis. Acute pulmonary edema is an emergency requiring prompt treatment. The patient is placed in bed in a high Fowler's position and the immediate administration of intravenous mor-

827

---

phine sulfate is usually ordered to relieve pain, quiet breathing, and allay apprehension. A cardiotonic, often digitalis; a fast-acting diuretic, often furosemide or ethacrynic acid; and a bronchodilator, often aminophylline, may be given. Oxygen is administered, usually by mask or nonrebreather mask. While the patient is acutely ill the blood pressure, respiration, apical pulse, and breath sounds are continually monitored. Parenteral fluids, if indicated, are infused slowly in limited quantities; the patient's intake and output of fluids are measured. The patient is weighed daily and any sudden gain is noted and reported.

pulmonary embolism (PE) The blockage of a pulmonary artery by foreign matter, as fat, air, tumor tissue, or a thrombus that usually arises from a peripheral vein. Predisposing factors include an alteration of blood constituents with increased coagulation, damage to blood vessel walls, and stagnation or immobilization, especially when associated with prolonged bed rest, childbirth, congestive heart failure, or surgery. Pulmonary embolism is difficult to distinguish from myocardial infarction and pneumonia. It is characterized by dyspnea, sudden chest pain, shock, and cyanosis. Pulmonary infarction, which often occurs within 6 to 24 hours after the formation of a pulmonary embolus, is further characterized by pleural effusion, hemoptysis, leukocytosis, fever, tachycardia and atrial arrhythmias, and a striking distention of the neck veins. Analysis of blood gases reveals decreased PO_2. Pulmonary embolism is detected by chest X-rays, pulmonary angiography, and radioscanning of the lung fields. Two thirds of patients with a massive pulmonary embolus and resultant infarction die within 2 hours. Initial resuscitative measures include external cardiac massage, oxygen, vasopressor drugs, embolectomy, and correction of acidosis. The formation of further emboli is prevented by the use of anticoagulants, and, sometimes, streptokinase or urokinase.

pulmonary function test (PFT) A series of tests for determining the capacity of the lungs to exchange oxygen and carbon dioxide efficiently. There are two general kinds of pulmonary function tests. One measures ventilation or the ability of the bellows action of the chest and lungs to move gas in and out of alveoli; the other kind measures the diffusion of gas across the alveolar capillary membrane and the perfusion of the lungs by blood. Efficient gas exchange in the lungs requires a balanced ventilation/perfusion ratio, with areas receiving ventilation well perfused and areas receiving blood flow capable of ventilation. Basic ventilation studies are performed with a spirometer and recording device as the patient breathes through a mouthpiece and connecting tube; a nose clip prevents nasal breathing. Measurements or calculations are made of the tidal volume (V_T), or gas inspired and expired in a normal breath; the inspiratory reserve volume (IRV), or the maximal volume that can be inspired after a normal respiration;

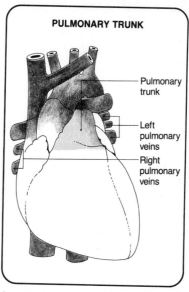

PULMONARY TRUNK

- Pulmonary trunk
- Left pulmonary veins
- Right pulmonary veins

the expiratory reserve volume (ERV), or the maximal volume that can be expired forcefully after a normal expiration; the residual volume (RV), or the gas remaining in the lungs following maximal expiration; and the minute volume, or the gas inspired and expired in a minute of normal breathing. The vital capacity of the lungs is equal to V_T + IRV + ERV and the total lung capacity to V_T + IRV + ERV + RV. The forced expiratory volume (FEV), or the amount of air forcefully expelled in the 1st second after a maximal inspiration, and the maximal breathing capacity (MBC), or the amount of gas exchanged per minute with maximal rate and depth of respiration, each have special clinical significance. Bronchospirometric measurements of the ventilation and oxygen consumption of each lung separately are performed using a specially constructed double-lumen catheter with two balloons. Arterial blood gas studies, including determinations of the acidity, partial pressure of carbon dioxide and of oxygen, and the oxyhemoglobin saturation, provide information on the diffusion of gas across the alveolar capillary membrane and the adequacy of oxygenation.

pulmonary sulcus tumor A destructive, invasive neoplasm that develops at the apex of the lung and infiltrates the ribs, vertebrae, and the brachial plexus. Also called **Pancoast's tumor.**

pulmonary surfactant A surfactant agent found in the lungs that functions to reduce the surface tension of the fluid on the surface of the cells of the lower respiratory system, enhancing the elasticity of the alveoli and bronchioles and, thus, the exchange of gases in the lungs.

pulmonary trunk The short, wide vessel that conveys venous blood from the right ventricle of the heart to the lungs. It is about 5 cm

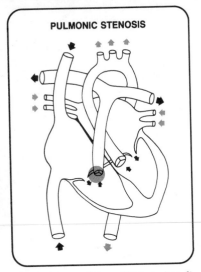

PULMONIC STENOSIS

(2 inches) long and 3 cm (1¼ inches) in diameter; it ascends obliquely, dividing into right and left branches.

pulmonary vascular resistance (PVR) Pressure loss per unit of blood flow from the pulmonary artery to the left ventricle.

pulmonary vein One of a pair of large vessels that return oxygenated blood from each lung to the left atrium of the heart. The right pulmonary veins pass dorsal to the right atrium and the superior vena cava. The left pulmonary veins pass ventral to the descending thoracic aorta. Compare **pulmonary trunk.**

pulmonary wedge pressure See **pulmonary capillary wedge pressure.**

pulmonary Wegener's granulomatosis A rare, fatal disease of young or middle-aged men, characterized by granulomatous lesions of the respiratory tract, focal necrotizing arteritis, and, finally, widespread inflammation of body organs. Pulmonary infarction and glomerulonephritis may occur.

pulmonic See **pulmonary.**

-pulmonic A combining form meaning 'relating to the lungs': apulmonic, gastropulmonic.

pulmonic stenosis An abnormal cardiac condition, characterized by concentric hypertrophy of the right ventricle with relatively little increase in diastolic volume. When the ventricular septum is intact this condition may be caused by valvular stenosis, infundibular stenosis, or both. It produces a pressure difference during systole between the right ventricular cavity and the pulmonary artery. It is most often congenital but may also be produced after birth by any of a number of types of lesions. Severe pulmonic stenosis may result in heart failure and death, but mild to moderate forms are relatively well tolerated by some patients. See also **valvular heart disease.**

pulmonic valve A cardiac structure composed of three semilunar cusps that close during each heartbeat to prevent blood from flowing back into the right ventricle from the pulmonary artery. The cusps are separated by sinuses which resemble tiny buckets when they are closed and filled with blood. These flaps grow from the lining of the pulmonary artery and, when they collapse from the inflow of ventricular blood, open the valve and allow deoxygenated blood to flow through the pulmonary artery to the lungs. Also called **semilunar valve.** Compare **aortic valve, mitral valve, tricuspid valve.**

pulp Any soft, spongy tissue, as that contained within the spleen, the pulp chamber of the tooth, or the distal phalanges of the fingers and the toes. —**pulpy,** adj.

pulpitis Infection or inflammation of the dental pulp. See also **caries.**

pulse **1.** A rhythmical beating or vibrating movement. **2.** A brief electromagnetic wave. **3.** The regular, recurrent expansion and contraction of an artery produced by waves of pressure caused by the ejection of blood from the left ventricle of the heart as it contracts. The phenomenon is easily detected on superficial arteries, as the radial and carotid arteries, and corresponds to each beat of the heart. The normal number of pulse beats per minute in the average adult varies from 50 to 100; fluctuations occur with exercise, injury, illness, and emotional reactions.

pulse deficit The discrepancy between the ventricular rate auscultated at the apex of the heart and the arterial rate of the radial pulse.

pulseless disease See **Takayasu's arteritis.**

pulse point Any one of the sites on the surface of the body where arterial pulsations can be easily palpated. The most commonly used pulse point is over the radial artery at the wrist. Other pulse points are over the temporal artery in front of the ear, over the common carotid artery at the lower level of the thyroid cartilage, over the brachial artery in the antecubital fossa, over the femoral artery in the inguinal area, over the popliteal artery behind the knee, over the dorsalis pedis artery on the top of the foot, and over the posterior tibialis artery behind the medial malleolus.

pulse pressure The difference between the systolic and diastolic pressures, normally 30 to 40 mmHg.

-pulsion A combining form meaning the 'action or condition of pushing': lateropulsion, retropulsion.

pulsus alternans A pulse with regular alternation of weak and strong beats without changes in the length of the cycle.

pulsus paradoxus An abnormal decrease in systolic pressure and pulse-wave amplitude during inspiration. The normal fall in pressure is less than 10 mmHg, and an excessive decline may be a sign of cardiac tamponade in acute pericarditis.

pump **1.** An apparatus used to move fluids or gases by suction or by positive pressure, as an infusion pump, or stomach pump. **2.** A physiologic mechanism by which a substance is moved, usually by active transport across a cell membrane, as a sodium pump. **3.** To move a liquid or gas by suction or positive pressure.

pump lung See **congestive atelectasis.**

punch biopsy The removal of living tissue for microscopic examination, usually bone marrow from the sternum, by means of a punch.

punch forceps A surgical instrument used to cut out a disk of dense or resistant tissue, as bone and cartilage. The ends of the blades are perforated to grip the involved tissue.

punct- A combining form meaning 'a point, or like a point': *punctate, punctiform.*

punctum lacrimale, *pl.* **puncta lacrimalia** A tiny aperture in the margin of each eyelid that opens into the lacrimal duct. The puncta release the tears that travel from the lacrimal glands through the lacrimal ducts to the conjunctiva. Puncta clogged with mucus or dirt cause irritation.

puncture wound A traumatic injury caused by the penetration of the skin by a narrow object, as a knife or slender fragment of glass. In such an injury to the eye, a lung, or a visceral organ, the object or implement is not removed until the person has been transported to a medical facility. Minor puncture wounds are treated with thorough cleansing. If a puncture wound closes at the skin before deeper healing has occurred, suppuration often results. A tetanus booster inoculation is usually given for such wounds, if inoculation has not been given within the last 10 years.

punitive damages See **damages.**

Punnett square A checkerboard, graphlike diagram, used in charting genetic ratios, that shows all of the possible combinations of male and female gametes when one or more pairs of independent alleles are crossed. See also **pedigree.**

pupil A circular opening in the iris of the eye, located slightly to the nasal side of the center of the iris. The pupil lies behind the anterior chamber of the eye and the cornea and in front of the lens. Its diameter changes with contraction and relaxation of the muscular fibers of the iris as the eye responds to changes in light, emotional states, and other kinds of stimulation. The pupil is the 'window' of the eye through which light passes to the lens and the retina. See also **dilatator pupillae, sphincter pupillae. —pupillary,** *adj.*

pupill- See **pupillo-.**

pupillary reflex **1.** See **light reflex. 2.** See **accommodation reflex.**

pupillary-skin reflex See **ciliospinal reflex.**

pupillo-, pupill- A combining form meaning 'of or pertaining to the pupil': *pupillometer, pupilloplegia.*

pur- A combining form meaning 'of or related to pus': *puric, puriform.*

pure dwarf See **primordial dwarf.**

pure tone audiometry See **audiometry.**

pure vegetarian See **strict vegetarian.**

purgation See **catharsis.**

purge **1.** To evacuate the bowels, as with a cathartic. **2.** A cathartic. **—purgation,** *n.,* **purgative,** *n., adj.*

purified protein derivative (PPD) A dried form of tuberculin used in testing for past or present infection with tubercle bacilli. This product is usually introduced into the skin during such tests and may produce a tuberculin-positive reaction within 48 to 72 hours.

purine Any one of a large group of nitrogenous compounds. Purines are produced as end products in the digestion of certain proteins in the diet, but some are synthesized in the body. Purines are also present in many medications and other substances, including caffeine, various diuretics, muscle relaxants, and myocardial stimulants. Hyperuricemia may develop in some people as a result of an inability to metabolize and excrete purines. Foods that are high in purines include anchovies and sardines, sweetbreads, liver, kidneys, and other organ meats, legumes, and poultry.

Purkinje network A complex network of muscle fibers that spread through the right and the left ventricles of the heart and carry the impulses that contract those chambers almost simultaneously. The Purkinje fibers ramify from cardiac muscle fibers spreading into the right ventricle and are continuous with the muscle of the right ventricle. The fibers that connect with the Purkinje fibers start in the atrioventricular (AV) node in the right atrium of the heart, along the lower part of the interatrial septum. Impulses generated in the sinoatrial (SA) node travel swiftly through the muscle fibers of both atria of the heart, starting atrial contraction. As the impulse enters the AV node from the right atrium it slows and allows both atria to contract completely before traveling into the ventricles. The velocity of the impulse increases after the impulse leaves the AV node and spreads to the Purkinje fibers. The Purkinje fibers, which can be identified only with the aid of a microscope, are larger in diameter than ordinary cardiac muscle and contain relatively few peripheral myofibrillae.

purpur- A combining form meaning 'purple': *purpuriferous, purpuriparous.*

purpura Any of several bleeding disorders characterized by hemorrhage into the tissues, particularly beneath the skin or mucous membranes, producing ecchymoses or petechiae. **—purpuric,** *adj.*

purulent Producing or containing pus.

pus A creamy, viscous, pale yellow or yellow green fluid exudate that is the result of liquefaction necrosis. Its main constituent is an abundance of polymorphonuclear leukocytes. Bacterial infection is its most common cause.

pustular psoriasis A severe form of psoriasis consisting of bright red patches and sterile pustules all over the body. Crops of lesions lasting 4 to 7 days occur every few days in cycles over weeks or months. Recurrences are inevitable. Fever, leukocytosis, and hypoalbuminemia are associated. In rare cases, hypovolemia and kidney failure occur. Hospitalization may be necessary for fluid replacement, steroid therapy, and sedation. Compare **guttate psoriasis.** See also **psoriasis.**

pustule   A small, circumscribed elevation of the skin containing fluid that is usually purulent. —**pustular,** *adj.*

P value   In research: the statistical probability attached to the occurrence of a given finding by chance alone in comparison with the known distribution of possible findings, considering the kinds of data, the technique of analysis, and the number of observations. The P value may be noted as a decimal: p $<$ .01 means that the likelihood of the phenomena tested occurring by chance alone is less than 1%.

PVC   *abbr* **1.** polyvinyl chloride. **2.** premature ventricular contraction.

PVR   *abbr* **pulmonary vascular resistance.**

P wave   The cardiac cycle component shown on an electrocardiogram as an inverted U-shaped curve that follows the end of the T wave and precedes the spike of the QRS complex. It represents atrial depolarization, during which the atria contract, pumping blood into the ventricles from the superior vena cava and the pulmonary vein.

PWP   *abbr* **pulmonary wedge pressure.**

pyel-   See **pyelo-.**

pyelitis   An inflammation of the pelvis of the kidney. See **pyelonephritis.**

pyelo-, pyel-   A combining form meaning 'of or pertaining to the pelvis of the kidney': *pyelocaliectasis.*

pyelogram   An X-ray of the kidneys and ureters. An intravenous pyelogram (I.V.P), taken following the injection of a radiopaque dye, shows the size and location of the kidneys, the outline of the ureters and bladder, the filling of the renal pelvises, the patency of the urinary tract, and any cysts or tumors within the kidneys. Preparation for an I.V.P includes bowel cleansing, withholding of fluids for 8 hours, and testing for sensitivity to the iodine in the radiopaque dye; persons with known sensitivity are not tested lest anaphylaxis occur. Patients able to tolerate the dye may feel warm and experience a salty taste when the material is injected. Retrograde pyelograms, which demonstrate filling of the renal collecting structures, are taken after the contrast medium is injected into the ureters by means of catheters in a cystoscope introduced through the urethra into the bladder.

pyelography   See **intravenous pyelography.**

pyelonephritis   A diffuse pyogenic infection of the pelvis and parenchyma of the kidney. Acute pyelonephritis is usually the result of an infection that ascends from the lower urinary tract to the kidney. *Escherischia coli* contamination of the urethral meatus is a common cause in females. Infection may spread to the kidney from other locations in the body. The onset of acute pyelonephritis is rapid, characterized by

fever, chills, flank pain, nausea, and urinary frequency. A urinalysis reveals the presence of bacteria and white blood cells. Antimicrobial treatment is continued for 10 days to 2 weeks. Relapse or reinfection is common. Chronic pyelonephritis develops slowly following bacterial infection of the kidney and may progress to renal failure. Most cases are associated with some form of obstruction. Treatment includes removal of the cause of obstruction and long-term antimicrobial therapy.

pygmalianism   A psychosexual abnormality in which the individual directs erotic fantasies toward a self-made object.

pygmy, pigmy   An extremely small person whose bodily parts are proportioned accordingly; a primordial dwarf.

pygo-   A combining form meaning 'of or pertaining to the buttocks': *pygoamorphus, pygodidymus.*

pygoamorphus   Asymmetrical, conjoined twins in which the parasitic member is represented by an undifferentiated amorphous mass attached to the autosite in the sacral region.

pygodidymus   **1.** A malformed fetus that has a double pelvis and hips. **2.** Conjoined twins that are fused in the cephalothoracic region but separated at the pelvis.

pygomelus   A malformed fetus that has an extra limb or limbs attached to the buttock. Also called **epipygus.**

pygopagus   Conjoined twins consisting of two fully formed or nearly formed fetuses that are united in the sacral region so that they are back to back.

pyknic   Describing a body structure characterized by short, round limbs, a full face, a short neck, stockiness and a tendency toward obesity. Compare **asthenic habitus, athletic habitus.** See also **endomorph.**

pykno-   A combining form meaning 'thick, compact, or frequent': *pyknocardia, pyknomorphous.*

pyle-   A combining form meaning 'of or related to the portal vein': *pylemphraxis, pylephlebitis.*

pyloric orifice   The opening of the stomach into the duodenum lying to the right of the middle line at the level of the cranial border of the first lumbar vertebra. The orifice is usually indicated on the surface of the stomach by the circular, duodenopyloric constriction.

pyloric sphincter   A thickened muscular ring in the stomach, separating the pylorus from the duodenum. Also called **pyloric valve.**

pyloric stenosis   A narrowing of the pyloric sphincter at the outlet of the stomach, causing an obstruction that blocks the flow of food into the small intestine. The condition occurs as a congenital defect in 1 of 200 newborns and, occasionally, in older adults secondary to an ulcer or fibrosis at the outlet. Diagnosis is made in infants by the presence of forceful projectile vomiting and palpation of a hard, prominent pylorus, and in adults by X-ray following barium ingestion. After surgery, a stomach tube re

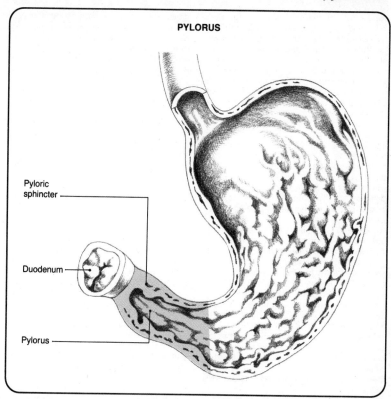

PYLORUS

Pyloric
sphincter

Duodenum

Pylorus

mains in place and observation is maintained
for signs of hemorrhage or of blockage of the
tube.

pyloric ulcer See **peptic ulcer.**

pyloric valve See **pyloric sphincter.**

pyloro- A combining form meaning 'of or
related to the pylorus': *pylorodilator, pyloroplasty.*

pyloroplasty A surgical procedure performed to relieve pyloric stenosis resulting from
chronic gastric ulcer. Before surgery, any electrolyte imbalances or fluid deficiencies are corrected; sodium chloride and potassium chloride
solutions may be given to correct ion losses from
vomiting, which is characteristic of the condition. The passageway is dilated. The operation
allows the alkaline secretions of the duodenum
to flow back into the stomach. Branches of the
vagus nerve that supply the acid-secreting portion of the stomach may be cut, reducing the
acidity of the stomach contents. Diarrhea is a
common postoperative complication.

pylorospasm A spasm of the pyloric
sphincter of the stomach, as occurs in pyloric
stenosis.

pylorus, *pl.* **pylori, pyloruses** A tubular
portion of the stomach that angles to the right
from the body of the stomach toward the duodenum. The most common position of the py-

lorus is about 3 cm (1¼ inch) to the right of the
sagittal axis. It is marked by the thickening of
the pyloric sphincter and its lining is composed
of an intestinal kind of epithelium rather than
the gastric kind common to the body of the stomach. **—pyloric,** *adj.*

pyo- A combining form meaning 'of or related
to pus': *pyocalyx, pyocele.*

pyoderma Any purulent skin disease, as impetigo.

pyogenic Pus-producing.

pyogenic granuloma A small, nonmalignant mass of excessive granulation tissue, usually found at the site of an injury. Most often a
dull red color, it contains numerous capillaries,
bleeds easily, and is very tender. Treatment is
with electric cautery or topical silver nitrate.
Also called **telangiectatic granuloma.**

pyorrhea **1.** A discharge of pus. **2.** A purulent inflammation of the tissues surrounding
the teeth. **—pyorrheal,** *adj.*

pyosalpinx An accumulation of pus in a
fallopian tube. See also **salpingitis.**

pyramidal Of or pertaining to the shape of
a pyramid.

pyramidalis One of a pair of anterolateral
muscles of the abdomen, contained in the lower
end of the sheath of the rectus abdominis. It is
a small, triangular muscle that arises from the

pubis and inserts into the linea alba. It functions to tense the linea alba. Compare **obliquus externus abdominis, obliquus internus abdominis, rectus abdominis, transversus abdominis.**

pyramidal tract   A pathway comprised of groups of nerve fibers in the white matter of the spinal cord through which motor impulses are conducted to the anterior horn cells from the opposite side of the brain. These descending fibers, the nerve cells of which are found in the precentral cortex, regulate the voluntary and reflex activity of the muscles through the anterior horn cells.

pyrantel pamoate   An anthelmintic agent.

pyrazinamide   An antitubercular agent.

pyrethrins   A pediculicide.

pyreto-   A combining form meaning 'of or pertaining to fever': *pyretogen, pyretography.*

pyrexia   See **fever.**

-pyrexia   A combining form meaning a 'febrile condition': *apyrexia, electropyrexia.*

pyridostigmine bromide   A cholinergic (parasympathomimetic) agent.

pyridoxal phosphate   A body enzyme that acts with pyridoxamine phosphate and transaminase to catalyze the reversible transfer of an amino group from an alpha-amino acid to an alpha-keto acid, especially alpha-ketoglutaric acid, a process essential to metabolism.

pyridoxamine phosphate   An enzyme that acts with pyridoxal phosphate and transaminase in the reversible transfer of an amino group from an alpha-amino acid to an alpha-keto acid, especially alpha-ketoglutaric acid, a process essential in body metabolism.

pyridoxine   A water-soluble, white, crystalline vitamin that is part of the B complex group, derived from pyridine, and converted in the body to pyridoxal and pyridamin for synthesis. It functions as a coenzyme essential for the synthesis and breakdown of amino acids, the conversion of tryptophan to niacin, the breakdown of glycogen to glucose-1-phosphate, the production of antibodies, the formation of heme in hemoglobin, the formation of hormones important in brain function, the proper absorption of vitamin B_{12}, the production of hydrochloric acid and magnesium, and the maintenance of the balance of sodium and potassium, which regulates body fluids and the functioning of the nervous and musculoskeletal systems. Rich dietary sources are meats, especially organ meats, whole-grain cereals, soybeans, peanuts, wheat germ, and brewer's yeast; milk and green vegetables supply smaller amounts. The most common symptoms of deficiency are seborrheic dermatitis about the eyes, nose, mouth, and behind the ears, cheilosis, glossitis and stomatitis, nervousness, depression, peripheral neuropathy, and lymphopenia, leading to convulsions in infants and anemia in adults. Several drugs interfere with the use of pyridoxine, notably isoniazid and penicillamine, and supplements of the vitamin are recommended with their use. The need for increased amounts of pyridoxine occurs during pregnancy, lactation, exposure to radiation, cardiac failure, aging, and use of oral contraceptives. The vitamin is considered nontoxic. Also called **vitamin B_6.**

pyridoxine hydrochloride   See **vitamin B_6.**

pyrilamine maleate   An ethylenediamine antihistamine.

pyrimethamine   An antimalarial agent.

pyrimidine   An organic compound of heterocyclic nitrogen found in nucleic acids and in many drugs, including the antiviral drugs, acyclovir and ribavirin.

pyro-   A combining form meaning 'of or related to fire or heat, or produced by heating': *pyrocatechin, pyrodextrin.*

pyrogen   Any substance or agent that tends to cause a rise in body temperature, as some bacterial toxins. See also **fever. —pyrogenic,** *adj.*

pyrolagnia   Sexual stimulation or gratification from watching or setting fires.

pyromania   An impulse neurosis characterized by an uncontrollable urge to set fires. The condition is found predominantly in men and is usually associated with alcohol intoxication, chronic personal frustrations, resentment of authority figures, or some other psychological or psychosexual dysfunction. Treatment consists of psychotherapy to uncover the causative emotional problems and often institutionalization for the protection of the person and of society.

pyromaniac   **1.** A person with or displaying characteristics of pyromania. **2.** Of, pertaining to, or exhibiting pyromania. **—pyromaniacal,** *adj.*

pyrosis   A precordial, substernal, or epigastric burning sensation, often associated with the eructation of acid contents of the stomach. It may be a symptom of esophagitis. Also called **heartburn.**

pyrrole   Any of several organic compounds whose derivatives may be added to whole blood or to plasma as a preservative.

pyruvate kinase   An enzyme in all body tissues that catalyzes the transfer of a phosphate group from adenosine triphosphate to produce adenosine diphosphate and phosphoenolpyruvate.

pyruvate kinase deficiency   A congenital hemolytic disorder transmitted as an autosomal recessive trait. The homozygous condition is characterized by severe chronic hemolysis. The heterozygous form may occur with a mild to severe anemia but is usually asymptomatic and of no clinical significance.

pyruvic acid   A compound formed as an end product of glycolysis, the anaerobic stage of glucose metabolism. Exposed to oxygen and acetylcoenzyme A at the entrance to the Krebs' citric acid cycle, the compound is changed to citric acid.

pyrvinium pamoate   An anthelmintic agent.

pyuria   The presence of white blood cells in urine, usually a sign of urinary tract infection. See also **bacteriuria.**

q.d. In prescriptions: *abbr quaque die,* a Latin phrase meaning 'everyday.' Also called **quotid.**

Q fever An acute febrile illness, usually respiratory, caused by the rickettsia *Coxiella burnetii.* It is spread through tick bite or contact with infected animals, especially sheep, goats, and cattle, by inhalation or by drinking their contaminated milk. Abrupt onset and prolonged high fever are characteristic. The disease responds to tetracycline. A vaccine is available. Also called **Australian Q fever.**

q.h. In prescriptions: *abbr quaque hora,* a Latin phrase meaning 'every hour.'

q.2h. In prescriptions: *abbr quaque secunda hora,* a Latin phrase meaning 'every 2 hours.'

q.i.d. In prescriptions: *abbr quater in die,* a Latin phrase meaning 'four times a day.'

QRS complex The component of the cardiac cycle shown on an electrocardiogram as a sharp positive or negative deflection following the less acute curve of the P wave and preceding the ST segment. It represents ventricular depolarization, in which the electrical impulse is conducted over the bundle of His and the Purkinje fibers, causing ventricular contraction.

q.s. In prescriptions: *abbr quantum sufficiat,* a Latin phrase meaning 'quantity required.'

Q's test See **Queckenstedt's test.**

quadr- A combining form meaning 'four': *quadrangular, quadribasic, quadrivalent.*

quadratus labii superioris See **zygomaticus minor.**

quadriceps femoris The great extensor muscle of the anterior thigh, comprised of the rectus femoris, the vastus lateralis, the vastus medialis, and the vastus intermedius, and forming a large dense mass covering the front and sides of the femur. Tendons of the four parts of the muscle unite at the distal part of the thigh, forming a large strong tendon that inserts into the patella. The quadriceps is innervated by branches of the femoral nerve, which contain fibers from the second, third, and fourth lumbar nerves, and it functions to extend the leg.

quadriceps reflex See **patellar reflex.**

quadrigeminal 1. In four parts. 2. A fourfold increase in size or frequency.

quadrigeminal pulse A pulse in which a pause occurs after every fourth beat.

quadriplegia A condition characterized by paralysis of the arms, the legs, and the trunk of the body below the level of an associated injury to the spinal cord. It may be caused by spinal cord injury, especially in the area of the fifth to the seventh vertebrae. Automobile accidents and sporting mishaps are common causes. Signs and symptoms commonly include flaccidity of the arms and the legs and the loss of power and sensation below the level of the injury. Cardiovascular complications may also develop from any injury that damages the spinal cord above the fifth cervical vertebra because of an associated block of the sympathetic nervous system. A major cause of death from such injury is respiratory failure. Other symptoms may include low body temperature, bradycardia, impaired peristalsis, and autonomic dysreflexia. Diagnosis is based on a complete physical and neurological examination, X-rays, and myelography. Treatment includes immobilization, catheterization, aggressive respiratory therapy, the use of diuretics to decrease spinal cord edema, and surgery to fuse unstable spinal sections and remove bone fragments. Complications, as hypothermia, bradycardia, catheter obstruction, and fecal impaction may occur. A quadriplegic patient who suffers hypothermia is wrapped in blankets instead of being warmed with hot water bottles or electromechanical devices because such devices can burn the skin of the patient experiencing severe sensory loss. Abdominal binders and antiembolism hose are used when placing the patient in an upright position. Patients who develop bradycardia are commonly connected to a cardiac monitor and intravenously administered an antimuscarinic drug, as atropine. Fecal impaction may cause hypertension and is always a possible complication. Manipulation of the rectum to free such impaction may aggravate the associated hypertension. A common precaution in removing an obstructive fecal mass is first to apply a topical anesthetic ointment, as tetracaine. NURSING CONSIDERATIONS: Maintaining adequate respiration and the integrity of the gastrointestinal system is very important. Compare **hemiplegia, paraplegia.**

quadruplet Any one of four offspring born of the same gestation period during a single pregnancy. See also **Hellin's law.**

quale, *pl.* **qualia** 1. The quality of a particular thing. 2. A quality considered as an independent entity. 3. In psychology: a feeling, sensation, or other conscious process that has its own unique, particular quality regardless of its external meaning or frame of reference.

qualitative Of or pertaining to the quality, value, or nature of something.

quality assurance In health care: any evaluation of services provided and the results achieved as compared to accepted standards. In one form of quality assurance, various attributes of health care, as cost, place, accessibility, treatment, and benefits, are scored in a two-part

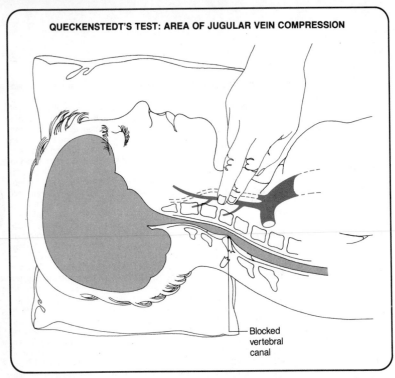

QUECKENSTEDT'S TEST: AREA OF JUGULAR VEIN COMPRESSION

Blocked
vertebral
canal

process. First, the actual results are compared with standard results; then, any deficiencies noted or identified serve to prompt recommendations for improvement.

quantitative inheritance See **multifactorial inheritance.**

quantum mechanics See **quantum theory.**

quantum theory In physics: a theory dealing with the interaction of matter and electromagnetic radiation, particularly at the atomic and subatomic levels, according to which radiation consists of small units of energy called quanta. Radiation can be absorbed only in whole quanta, and the energy content of a quantum is inversely proportional to its wavelength. Also called **quantum mechanics.**

quarantine **1.** Isolation of people with communicable disease or of those exposed to communicable disease during the contagious period in an attempt to prevent spread of the illness. **2.** The practice of detaining travelers or vessels coming from places of epidemic disease, originally for 40 days, for the purpose of inspection or disinfection.

quartan Recurring on the 4th day or at about 72-hour intervals. See also **quartan malaria.**

quartan malaria A form of malaria that is caused by the protozoan *Plasmodium malariae* and characterized by febrile paroxysms that occur every 72 hours. Compare **falciparum ma-**laria, tertian malaria. See also **malaria.**

quarti- A combining form meaning 'fourth': *quartipara, quartisect, quartisternal.*

Queckenstedt's test A test for an obstruction in the spinal canal in which the jugular vein on each side of the neck is compressed alternately. The pressure of the spinal fluid is measured by a manometer connected to a lumbar puncture needle or catheter. Normally, occlusion of the veins of the neck causes an immediate rise in spinal fluid pressure; if the vertebral canal is blocked, no rise occurs. If increased intracranial pressure is suspected, this test should not be performed.

Queensland tick typhus An infection caused by *Rickettsia australis,* occurring in Australia, transmitted by ticks, and resembling mild Rocky Mountain spotted fever. Treatment includes the administration of chloramphenicol or tetracycline. Prevention depends on avoiding tick bites and on the prompt removal of attached ticks. See also **rickettsiosis.**

quellung reaction The swelling of the capsule of a bacterium, seen in the laboratory when the organism is exposed to specific antisera. This phenomenon is used to identify the genera, species, or subspecies of the bacteria causing a disease, including *Haemophilus influenzae, Neisseria meningitides,* and many kinds of streptococci. Also called **capsular swelling test.**

Quengle cast A two-section, hinged ortho-

Q WAVE

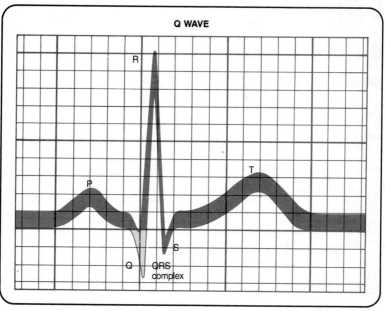

pedic cast for immobilizing the lower extremities from the foot or ankle to below the knee and the upper thigh to a level just above the knee. The two parts of the cast are connected by special hinges at knee level, medially and laterally. The Quengle cast is used for the gradual correction of knee contractures.

quercetin A yellow, crystalline, flavonoid pigment found in oak bark and the juice of lemons, asparagus, and other plants. It is used to reduce abnormal capillary fragility.

querulous paranoia A form of paranoia characterized by extreme discontent and habitual complaining, usually about imagined slights by others. Also called **paranoia quaerula.**

quickening The first fetal movement in utero, usually felt at 16 to 20 weeks of gestation.

quin- A combining form meaning 'of or related to quinine': *quiniretin, quinometry, quinotoxin.*

-quin, -quine A combining form naming medicinal compounds from quinine: *aminoquin, floraquin.*

quinacrine hydrochloride An antihelmintic agent.

Quincke's pulse An abnormal alternate blanching and reddening of the skin that may be observed in several ways, as by pressing the front edge of the fingernail and watching the blood in the nail bed recede and return. This pulsation is characteristic of aortic insufficiency and other abnormal conditions but may also occur in otherwise normal individuals. For-

merly, it was thought to be caused by pulsation of the capillaries, but study has shown it occurs because of pulsation of subpapillary arteriolar and venous plexuses.

quinestrol A synthetic estrogen.

quinethazone A thiazidelike diuretic agent.

quinidine bisulfate, q. gluconate, q. polygalacturonate, q. sulfate Group I antiarrhythmic agents.

quinine A white, bitter crystalline alkaloid, made from cinchona bark, used in antimalarial medications.

quinine dihydrochloride See **quinine sulfate.**

quinine sulfate An antimalarial with antipyretic, analgesic, and muscle relaxant activity.

quinque- A combining form meaning 'five': *quinquecuspid, quinquetubercular, quinquevalent.*

quinsy See **peritonsillar abscess.**

quint- A combining form meaning 'fifth or fivefold': *quintessence, quintipara, quintuplet.*

quintan Recurring on the 5th day or at about 96-hour intervals.

quintana fever See **trench fever.**

quotid See **q.d.**

Q wave The component of the cardiac cycle shown on an electrocardiogram as a short abrupt downward line from the end of the tail of the P wave. It represents the first part of the QRS complex. It is usually not prominent, and its absence may be without clinical significance.

R *abbr* **1. metabolic respiratory quotient. 2. respiratory exchange ratio.**

Ra Symbol for **radium.**

rabbit fever See **tularemia.**

rabies An acute, usually fatal, viral disease of the central nervous system transmitted from animals to people by infected blood, tissue, or, most commonly, saliva. The reservoirs of the virus are chiefly animals, including skunks, bats, foxes, dogs, raccoons, and cats, but almost never rodents. After introduction into the human body, often by a bite of an infected animal, the virus travels along nerve pathways to the brain and, later, to other organs. An incubation period ranges from 10 days to 1 year and is followed by a prodromal period characterized by fever, malaise, headache, paresthesia, and myalgia. After several days, severe encephalitis, delirium, agonizingly painful muscular spasms, seizures, paralysis, coma, and death ensue. Few nonfatal cases have been documented in humans; survival has been the result of intensive supportive nursing and medical care. There is no treatment once the virus has reached the tissue of the nervous system. A series of intramuscular injections with a vaccine is begun. NURSING CONSIDERATIONS: Rabies virus infection may be eradicated from most communities by prophylactic immunization of and stringent measures for the control of domestic animals and the elimination of any wild animals acting as reservoirs of infection. The nurse may teach the necessity of avoiding wild animals and the importance of immediate medical treatment for any animal bite. Also called **hydrophobia.** —**rabid,** *adj.*

rabies immune globulin (RIG) A solution of antirabies immune globulin.

rabies vaccine A sterile suspension of killed rabies virus prepared from human diploid cells. Also called **HDCV.**

race A group of genetically related people who share certain physical characteristics.

racemose Resembling a bunch of grapes, used in describing a structure in which many branches terminate in nodular, cystlike forms.

racemose aneurysm A marked dilatation of lengthened, tortuous blood vessels, some of which may be distended to 20 times their normal size. Also called **cirsoid aneurysm.**

rachi- See **rachio-.**

rachio- A combining form meaning 'of or related to the spine': *rachiotome, rachiotomy.* Also **rachi-, rhachi.**

rachiopagus, rachipagus Conjoined symmetrical twins that are united back to back along the spinal column.

rachischisis See **spina bifida.**

rachischisis totalis See **complete rachischisis.**

rachitic **1.** Of or pertaining to rickets. **2.** Resembling the condition of one afflicted with rickets.

rachitic dwarf A person whose retarded growth is owing to rickets. See also **Fanconi's syndrome.**

rachitis **1.** Rickets. **2.** An inflammatory disease of the vertebral column.

racial immunity A form of natural immunity shared by most of the members of a race. Compare **individual immunity, species immunity.**

racial unconscious See **collective unconscious.**

rad *abbr* radiation absorbed dose; basic unit of absorbed dose of ionizing radiation. One rad is equal to the absorption of 100 ergs of radiation energy per gram of matter. See also **rem.**

radi- A combining form meaning 'root': *radiciform, radicotomy.*

radial artery An artery in the forearm, starting at the bifurcation of the brachial artery, passing in 12 branches to the forearm, wrist, and hand. In the forearm, it extends from the neck of the radius to the forepart of the styloid process; in the wrist, from the styloid process to the carpus; in the hand, from the carpus, across the palm, to the little finger. In the forearm, the branches of the radial artery are the radial recurrent, muscular, palmar carpal, and superficial palmar; in the wrist, the branches are the dorsal carpal and the first dorsal metacarpal. In the hand, the branches are the princeps pollicis, radialis indicis, deep palmar arch, palmar metacarpal, perforating, and recurrent.

radial keratotomy A surgical procedure in which a series of tiny shallow incisions are made on the cornea, causing it to bulge slightly. The operation, which is performed under local anesthesia, requires only 30 minutes. Hospitalization is not necessary. Radial keratotomy corrects myopia.

radial nerve The largest branch of the brachial plexus, arising on each side as a continuation of the posterior cord. It supplies the skin of the arm and forearm and their extensor muscles. It crosses the tendon of the latissimus dorsi beneath the axillary artery, passes the inferior border of the teres major, and winds around the medial side of the humerus to enter the triceps between the medial and the long heads of that muscle. It spirals down the arm close to the humerus in the groove separating the origins of the medial and the long heads of the triceps, accompanied by the deep brachial artery. On the lateral side of the arm, it pierces the lateral intermuscular septum, runs between the brachialis and the brachioradialis, and divides into the superficial and the deep branches. The branches of the radial nerve are the medial muscular branches, the posterior brachial cutaneous nerve, the posterior muscular branches, the posterior antebrachial cutaneous nerve, the lateral muscular branches, the superficial branch, and the deep branch. Also called **musculospiral nerve.** Compare **median nerve, musculocutaneous nerve, ulnar nerve.**

radial notch of ulna The narrow, lateral depression in the coronoid process of the ulna that receives the head of the radius.

radial pulse The pulse of the radial artery palpated at the wrist over the radius. The radial pulse is the one most often taken, owing to the ease with which it is palpated.

radial recurrent artery A branch of the radial artery, arising just distal to the elbow, ascending between the branches of the radial nerve, and supplying several muscles of the arm and the elbow.

radial reflex A normal reflex elicited by tapping over the distal radius, with the response being flexion of the forearm. Flexion of the fingers may also occur if the reflex is hyperactive.

radiant energy The energy emitted by electromagnetic radiation, as radio waves, light, X-rays, and gamma rays.

radiate To diverge or spread from a common point. —**radiation**, *n.*

radiate ligament A ligament that connects the head of a rib with a vertebra and an associated intervertebral disk. Each of the 24 radiate ligaments consists of 3 flat fasciculi attached to the head of a rib. The superior fasciculus connects with the vertebra above, the inferior fasciculus connects with the vertebra below, and the middle fasciculus connects to the disk between the two vertebrae. Radiate ligaments to the 10th, 11th, and 12th ribs have only 2 fasciculi.

radiation 1. The emission of energy, rays, or waves. 2. In medicine: the use of a radioactive substance in the diagnosis or treatment of disease. —**radiate**, *adj., v.*

radiation caries Tooth decay caused by ionizing radiation of the oral and maxillary structure. Radiation caries is often a side effect of treatment for oral malignancies. See also **dental caries.**

radiation detector A device for converting radiant energy to an observable form, used for detecting the presence and, sometimes, the amount of radiation. A Geiger-Müller detector counts and registers the number of particles or photons reaching it from a radioactive source and can be designed with sufficient sensitivity to detect cosmic radiation. An ionization chamber detects exposure to radiation by collecting the ion pairs formed by the passage of radiation through the device.

radiation exposure A measure of the ion-

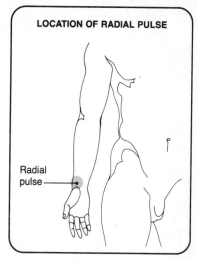

LOCATION OF RADIAL PULSE

Radial pulse

ization produced in air by X-rays or gamma rays. It is the sum of the electrical charges on all ions of one sign that are produced when all electrons liberated by photons in a volume of air are completely stopped, divided by the mass of air in the volume element. The unit of exposure is the roentgen.

radiation sickness A condition resulting from exposure to ionizing radiation. The severity of the condition is determined by the volume of radiation, the length of time of exposure, and the area of the body affected. Moderate exposure may cause headache, nausea, vomiting, anorexia, and diarrhea; long-term exposure may result in sterility, damage to the fetus in pregnant women, leukemia or other forms of cancer, alopecia, and cataracts.

radiation syndrome See **radiation sickness.**

radiation therapy See **radiotherapy.**

radical 1. A group of atoms that acts together and forms a component of a compound. The group tends to remain bound together when a chemical reaction removes it from a compound and attaches it to another. A radical does not exist freely in nature. 2. Drastic therapy, as the surgical removal of an organ, limb, or other part of the body.

radical dissection The surgical removal of tissue in an extensive area surrounding the operative site. Most often it is performed to identify and excise all tissue that may be malignant to decrease the chance of recurrence.

radical mastectomy Surgical removal of an entire breast, pectoral muscles, axillary lymph nodes, and all fat, fascia, and adjacent tissues. It is performed in the treatment of cancer of the breast. Preoperatively, the staff encourages verbalization of the patient's fears about the potential loss of her breast, if diagnosis is not known preoperatively. Her self-image is usually severely threatened, and she characteristically grieves in

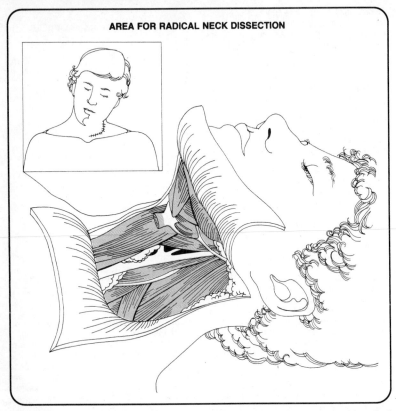

AREA FOR RADICAL NECK DISSECTION

anticipation of a loss of a body part and feared loss of femininity. The postoperative period is physically and emotionally painful; the woman is best warned by supportive but realistic explanations prior to surgery. Edema of the arm on the affected side is the rule, as the axillary lymphatic structures that drain the lymph from the arm are removed during surgery. A pressure dressing is usually applied and left in place until bleeding and drainage have decreased. A drain is usually left in the wound for several days. The woman may be anxious, depressed, angry, withdrawn, or reflect hopelessness. In addition to the usual postoperative measures, the nurse elevates the affected arm above the level of the right atrium; checks the color, sensation, and motion of the fingers; checks the donor site if a graft was performed; and applies reinforcement to the pressure dressing as necessary. Later, the patient is assisted in range-of-motion exercises for all extremities and is taught to perform gradually increasing arm and shoulder exercises. In discussion and in providing physical care, the loss of the breast is dealt with frankly; to avoid the fact is not helpful to the patient. On discharge, the patient is encouraged to shower daily, to apply an emollient, like cocoa butter, to the incision, and to examine the remaining breast

monthly. **Reach to Recovery** may be involved in counseling and support before and after a mastectomy. Chemotherapy and radiation therapy may continue after surgery. The woman is told never to allow blood to be drawn from the affected arm; intravenous injection is also to be avoided in that arm. Blood pressure measurement, vaccination, and other injections are best performed on the other arm. Compare **modified radical mastectomy, simple mastectomy.**

radical neck dissection Dissection and removal of all lymph nodes and removable tissues under the skin of the neck, performed to prevent the spread of malignant tumors of the head and neck that have a reasonable chance of being controlled. Before surgery, thorough mouth hygiene is given and antibiotics are begun. Under general anesthesia, a tracheostomy is done; the tumor, surrounding tissues, and lymph nodes on the affected side are then removed in one mass from the angle of the jaw to the clavicle, forward to the midline, and back to the angle of the jaw. A total laryngectomy may be done as part of the surgery. After surgery, the nurse suctions the tracheostomy as necessary and observes vital signs for indications of hemorrhage or difficulty in breathing. A humidifier or vaporizer will ease coughing and production of mucus. I.V. fluids are continued in the nondominant arm. Extensive work with a speech pathologist may be necessary to learn esophageal speech. Radiation of the tumor site may be begun and chemotherapy may continue. Compare **neck dissection.**

radical therapy **1.** A treatment intended to cure, not palliate. **2.** A definitive, extreme treatment; not conservative, as radical rather than partial mastectomy.

radical vulvectomy See **vulvectomy.**

radio- A combining form meaning 'of or related to radiation, sometimes specifically to emission of radiant energy, to radium, or to the radius': *radioactive, radiobiology.*

radioactive Giving off radiation as the result of the disintegration of the nucleus of an atom.

radioactive contamination The undesirable addition of radioactive material to the skin or part of the environment. Beta radiation contamination of the bodies of health-care personnel is only possible through the ingestion, inhalation, or absorption of the source, as when the skin is contaminated with a beta emitter contained in an absorbable chemical form. Instruments, drapes, surgical gloves, and clothing that come in contact with serous fluids, blood, and urine of patients containing beta or gamma radiation emitters may be contaminated. The severity of the contamination is directly related to the elapsed time between the administration of the isotope and surgery; on completion of the procedure, possibly contaminated material is isolated and checked. If found to be contaminated, it is disposed of according to institutional or federal standards.

radioactive contrast media A solution or colloid containing materials of high atomic number, used for visualizing soft tissue structures in diagnostic radiology. Diagnostic radiopharmaceuticals indicate their positions in the body by their gamma ray emissions.

radioactive decay The disintegration of the nucleus of an unstable nuclide by the spontaneous emission of charged particles or photons, or both.

radioactive element An element subject to spontaneous degeneration of its nucleus, accompanied by the emission of alpha particles, beta particles, or gamma rays. All elements with atomic numbers greater than 83 are radioactive. Some kinds of radioactive elements are radium, thorium, uranium. Compare **stable element.** See also **radioactivity.**

radioactive iodine (sodium iodide) (^{131}I) A thyroid hormone antagonist.

radioactive iodine excretion The elimination by the body of radioactive iodine (RAI) administered in a test of thyroid function and in the treatment of hyperthyroidism. Most RAI is excreted in urine, but small amounts may be found in sputum, perspiration, feces, and vomitus.

radioactive iodine excretion test A method of evaluating thyroid function by measuring the amount of radioactive iodine (RAI)

**RADIOALLERGOSORBENT
TEST VALUES
(Measurement of allergen-specific
IgE antibody)**

Negative	< 150% of control
Borderline	150% to 400% of control
Positive	> 400% of control

in urine after the patient is given an oral tracer dose of the radioisotope ^{131}I. Normally, 5% to 35% of the dose is absorbed by the thyroid, but absorption is increased in hyperthyroidism and decreased in hypothyroidism, and the amount excreted in urine is inversely proportional to the uptake of RAI. Following administration of the tracer, a scintillation detector is placed over the patient's neck at 2, 6, and 24 hours to measure the RAI accumulated by the thyroid, and the amount excreted is assayed in urine collected for 24 hours after the oral dose. Diarrhea can result in low values of RAI in urine; renal failure, by decreasing excretion, can cause high readings. See also **radioactive iodine uptake.**

radioactive iodine uptake (RAIU) The absorption and incorporation by the thyroid of radioactive iodine (RAI), administered orally as a tracer dose in a test of thyroid function and as larger doses for the treatment of hyperthyroidism. The radioisotope ^{131}I is rapidly absorbed in the stomach and is concentrated in the thyroid. A normal thyroid absorbs 5% to 35% of a tracer dose, while the uptake is increased in hyperthyroidism. Patients receiving a large therapeutic dose of RAI may require hospitalization for several days. See also **radioactive iodine excretion test.**

radioactivity The emission of corpuscular or electromagnetic radiations as a consequence of nuclear disintegration. Natural radioactivity is a property exhibited by all chemical elements with an atomic number greater than 83; artificial radioactivity is man-made through the bombardment of naturally occurring isotopes with subatomic particles or high levels of gamma or X-radiation.

radioallergosorbent test (RAST) A test in which a technique of radioimmunoassay is used to identify and quantify IgE in serum that has been mixed with any of 45 known allergens. If an atopic allergy to a substance exists, an antigen-antibody reaction occurs with conjugation and clumping. The test is an in vitro method of demonstrating allergic reactions. Compare **patch test, Prausnitz-Küstner test.**

radiobiology The branch of the natural sciences dealing with the effects of radiation on

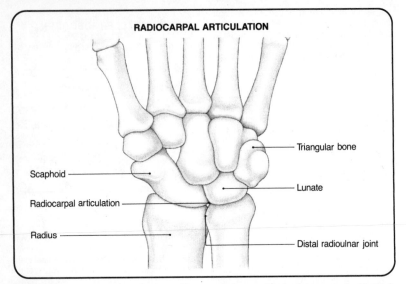

RADIOCARPAL ARTICULATION

Scaphoid

Radiocarpal articulation

Radius

Triangular bone

Lunate

Distal radioulnar joint

biological systems. —**radiobiologic, radiobiological,** *adj.*

radiocarpal articulation The condyloid joint at the wrist that connects the radius and distal surface of an articular disk with the scaphoid, the lunate, and the triangular bones. The joint involves four ligaments and allows all movements but rotation. Also called **wrist joint.**

radiochemistry The branch of chemistry that deals with the properties and behavior of radioactive materials and the use of radionuclides in the study of chemical and biological problems.

radiographic magnification Visualization of small areas through magnification achieved with a small X-ray tube, a common diagnostic tool in orthopedics.

radiography The production of shadow images on photographic emulsion through the action of ionizing radiation. The image is the result of the differential attenuation of the radiation in its passage through the object being radiographed. —**radiographic,** *adj.*

radioimmunoassay (RIA) A technique in radiology used to determine the concentration of an antigen, antibody, or other protein in the serum. A radioactively labeled substance known to react in a certain way with the suspected protein is injected, and any reaction is monitored.

radioiodine A radioactive isotope of iodine used in radiotherapy in the treatment of some thyroid conditions and in diagnostic radiology in various scanning techniques. A common form of radioiodine is ^{131}I.

radioisotope A radioactive isotope of an element, used for therapeutic and diagnostic purposes.

radioisotope scan A two-dimensional representation of the gamma rays emitted by a radioisotope, showing its concentration in a body site, as the thyroid gland, brain, or kidney. Radioisotopes used in diagnostic scanning may be administered intravenously or orally.

radiologist A physician who specializes in radiology.

radiology The branch of medicine concerned with radioactive substances and, using various techniques of visualization, with the diagnosis and treatment of disease using any of the various sources of radiant energy. —**radiologic, radiological,** *adj.*

radiopaque Not permitting the passage of X-rays or other radiant energy. Bones are relatively radiopaque and therefore show as white areas on an exposed X-ray film. Lead is markedly radiopaque and therefore is widely used to shield X-ray equipment and atomic power sources. See also **radioactive element, radioactivity, radiopaque dye.** —**radiopacity,** *n.*

radiopaque dye A chemical substance that does not permit the passage of X-rays. Various radiopaque iodine compounds are used to outline the interior of such hollow organs as heart chambers and blood vessels.

radiopharmaceutical A drug that exhibits spontaneous disintegration of unstable nuclei with the emission of nuclear particles or photons. Kinds of radiopharmaceuticals are **diagnostic radiopharmaceutical, research radiopharmaceutical, therapeutic radiopharmaceutical.**

radiopharmacist A trained professional responsible for the formulation and dispensing of prescribed radioactive tracers and for the clinical aspects of radiopharmacy. Radiopharmacists must receive training in radioactive tracer techniques, in the safe handling of radioactive materials, in the preparation and quality control of drugs for administration to humans, and in the basic principles of nuclear medicine. Some states require that radioactive drugs be dispensed by licensed pharmacists, while others recognize radiopharmaceutical specialists who are not necessarily graduates of a school of pharmacy.

radiopharmacy A facility for the preparation and dispensing of radioactive drugs and for the storage of radioactive materials, inventory records, and prescriptions of radioactive substances. The radiopharmacy is usually the correlation point for radioactive wastes, the unit responsible for waste disposal or storage, and a center for clinical investigations employing radioactive tracers. It may also be a center for research and for the training of students and residents in radiology and nuclear medicine.

radioresistance The relative resistance of cells, tissues, organs, organisms, chemical compounds, or any substances to the effects of radiation. Compare **radiosensitivity. —radioresistant,** adj.

radioresistant Unchanged by or protected against damage by such radioactive emissions as X-rays, alpha particles, or gamma rays. Compare **radiosensitive.** See also **radioactivity.**

radiosensitive Capable of being changed by or reacting to such radioactive emissions as X-rays, alpha particles, or gamma rays. Compare **radioresistant.** See also **radioactivity.**

radiosensitivity The relative susceptibility of cells, tissues, organs, organisms, or any living substances to the effects of radiation. Cells of self-renewing systems, as those in the crypts of the intestine, are the most radiosensitive. Cells that divide regularly but mature between divisions, as spermatogonia and spermatocytes, are next in radiosusceptibility. Long-lived cells that usually do not undergo mitosis unless there is a suitable stimulus include the less radiosensitive liver, kidney, and thyroid cells. Least sensitive are fixed postmitotic cells that have lost the ability to divide, as neurons. Connective tissue and blood vessels are intermediate in radiosensitivity; parenchymal cells are affected by moderate doses of radiation that do not damage connective tissue.

radiotherapy The treatment of neoplastic disease by using X-rays or gamma rays, usually from a cobalt source, to deter the proliferation of malignant cells by decreasing the rate of mitosis or impairing DNA synthesis. Prior to radiotherapy, the procedure, its purpose, duration, painlessness, and the need to remain completely still during irradiation are explained to the patient. Potential sequelae, as erythema, edema, desquamation, hyperpigmentation, atrophy, pruritus or skin pain, altered taste, anorexia, nausea, vomiting, headache, hair loss, malaise, tachycardia, and increased susceptibility to infection, may be discussed in response to specific questions raised by the patient. A preliminary visit to the radiology department may be arranged so that the equipment and the room in which the patient will be positioned on a table can be seen. From this position, the patient is able to communicate with the radiotherapist in an adjoining booth. Daily hygiene measures are completed before treatment; on returning from irradiation, the patient is placed in a noninfectious environment or, if necessary, in protective isolation; friends, family, other patients, and staff members with infections, especially upper respiratory infections, are not permitted to visit. Skin care is administered following irradiation and every 4 hours thereafter, but the ink markings placed by the radiologist on the skin to mark the focus of treatment are not removed between treatments, and the treated area is not washed with water; sterile mineral oil, lanolin, or petroleum jelly may be applied if the radiologist approves. The patient wears loose garments, rests on an air mattress, foam or gel pad, or sheepskin, and a footboard or bed cradle is used to elevate the top sheet and blanket. Cosmetics are avoided and underarm deodorants or antiperspirants are contraindicated if the axillary area is irradiated. If hair loss occurs, the patient may wear a wig, scarf, cap, or toupee. High-protein supplements, soothing gelatins, and ice cream are provided, and other food is served when desired by the patient; six small, bland feedings may be tolerated more easily than regular meals. Quiet periods are maintained before and after meals. Antiemetics and vitamins are administered as ordered, and tube feedings or total parenteral nutrition may be indicated if the patient's food intake is severely decreased. Oral hygiene, using a soft-bristled brush and dilute mouthwash or, if needed, foam or sponge swabs and a saline rinse, is administered whenever required, and a fluid intake of 2,000 to 3,000 ml (68 to 101 oz) daily is maintained, unless contraindicated. In preparation for discharge, the patient is instructed to follow the hospital practices for skin care, oral hygiene, fluid intake, and a high-protein, nutritious diet but to avoid eating immediately before and after irradiation. The patient is told to avoid, until ordered, tight clothing; extremes of temperature; exposure to sunlight, tub baths or showers, and persons with infections and to report to the physician any symptom of infection, inability to eat, severe diarrhea, increasing headache, fatigue, or increasing redness, swelling, itching, or pain at the site of therapy. The nurse offers thorough explanation of the radiotherapy, provides care after treatment, and prepares the patient for discharge and, if indicated, continued therapy on an outpatient basis. Radiotherapy can control or arrest the development of a number of forms of cancer and provide palliation in some inoperable tumors; the maintenance of adequate nutrition and meticulous care of the skin may allow the person to avoid the most serious and unpleasant side effects of radiotherapy.

radioulnar articulation The articulation of the radius and the ulna, consisting of a proximal articulation, a distal articulation, and three sets of ligaments.

radium (Ra) A radioactive metallic element of the alkaline-earth group. Its atomic number

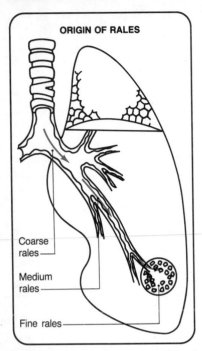

ORIGIN OF RALES

Coarse rales

Medium rales

Fine rales

is 88. Four radium isotopes occur naturally and have different atomic weights: 223, 224, 226, and 228. The isotope with atomic weight 226 is the most abundant. The element occurs in the uranium minerals carnotite and pitchblende. Radium salts have been used extensively as radiation sources in the treatment of cancer but are gradually being replaced in such therapy by cobalt and cesium.

radius, *pl.* radii   One of the bones of the forearm, lying parallel to the ulna. Its proximal end is small and forms a part of the elbow joint. The distal end is large and forms a part of the wrist joint. The radius articulates with the humerus, ulna, scaphoid, and lunate bones.

radix, *pl.* radices   See **root. —radical,** *adj.*

radon (Rn)   A radioactive, inert, gaseous, nonmetallic element. Its atomic number is 86; its atomic weight is 222. Radon is used in radiation cancer therapy.

RAI   *abbr* **radioactive iodine.**

RAIU   *abbr* **radioactive iodine uptake.**

RA latex test   *abbr* **rheumatoid arthritis latex test.** See **latex fixation test.**

rale   A common abnormal respiratory sound heard on auscultation of the chest during inspiration, characterized by discontinuous bubbling noises. Fine rales have a crackling sound produced by air entering distal bronchioles or alveoli that contain serous secretions, as in congestive heart failure. Medium rales are medium-pitched bubbling or gurgling sounds caused by air passing through secretions in the bronchioles or by separation of bronchiolar walls previously adhered by exudate. Coarse rales originate in the larger bronchi or trachea and have a lower pitch. Kinds of rales are **sibilant rale, sonorous rale.** Compare **rhonchi, wheeze.**

rami-   A combining form meaning 'branch': *ramicotomy, ramification.*

Ramsay Hunt's syndrome   A neurologic condition resulting from invasion of the seventh nerve ganglia and the geniculate ganglion by varicella-zoster virus, characterized by severe ear pain, facial nerve paralysis, vertigo, hearing loss, and, often, mild, generalized encephalitis. The vertigo may last days or weeks, but usually resolves itself. The facial paralysis may be permanent, and the hearing loss, which is rarely permanent, may be partial or total. Treatment usually includes the prescription of corticosteroid drugs. Also called **herpes zoster oticus.**

ramus, *pl.* rami   A small, branchlike structure extending from a larger one or dividing into two or more parts, as a branch of a nerve or artery or one of the rami of the pubis. —**ramification,** *n.* **ramify,** *v.*

random genetic drift   See **genetic drift.**

random sample   A representative part of a larger whole selected without specific method or pattern so that each member has equal chance of being chosen.

range of motion (ROM) exercise   Any body action involving the muscles, the joints, and natural directional movements, as abduction, extension, flexion, pronation, and rotation. Such exercises are usually applied in the treatment of orthopedic deformities, in the assessment of injuries and deformities, and in athletic conditioning.

ranula   A cyst beneath the tongue owing to obstruction of a salivary duct or mucous gland.

rape   A sexual assault, homosexual or heterosexual, the legal definitions for which vary from state to state. Rape is a crime of violence or one committed under the threat of violence, and its victims are treated for medical and psychological trauma.

NURSING CONSIDERATIONS: Characteristically, the victim is frightened, humiliated, and personally violated. General physical examination may reveal cuts, bruises, and other injuries. Pelvic or genital examination may show traumatic injury to the genitalia or anus. Careful physical examination is performed, and a detailed history and specimens are obtained. Ideally, counseling is offered immediately to all rape victims. In the case of a woman raped by a man, a pregnancy test is performed and specific injuries are treated. If the test is positive, prophylaxis against conception may be administered. Usually, antibiotics are given to prevent the development of venereal disease. Arrangements for ongoing emotional support are made. A trained, sympathetic nurse of the same sex is assigned to stay with the victim. Privacy for the history, examination, and police interview is assured. The victim may or may not choose to talk to the police, but the police must be informed in every case. The victim must sign a special form to allow specimens to be released to a law enforcement agency. In general, it is the role of the nurse and other medical workers to examine, to treat, and to collect specimens as necessary, not to decide whether rape has occurred. See also **statutory rape.**

rape counseling Counseling by a trained person provided to a victim of rape. Rape counseling ideally begins at the time the crime is first reported, as in an emergency room. Initially, the counselor offers sensitive support for the victim by accepting the person in a nonprejudicial, noncritical way. The victim's response to the trauma of the assault is empathetically elicited, and three basic statements are made: the counselor is sorry that the rape happened, is glad that the injuries are not worse, and does not think that the victim was wrong or did anything wrong. Counseling personnel may provide supportive services and advocacy and liaison between the victim and medical, legal, and law-enforcement authorities. This involves staying with the victim during medical examination, police or district attorney's questioning, and throughout the criminal justice process.

rape-trauma syndrome A nursing diagnosis accepted by the Fifth National Conference on the Classification of Nursing Diagnoses. The syndrome results from the experience of being raped and includes an acute phase of disorganization and a longer phase of reorganization in the victim's life. The etiology of the syndrome is the trauma of the rape. The defining characteristics are divided into three subcomponents: rape-trauma, compound reaction, and silent reaction. The defining characteristics of rape-trauma in the acute phase are emotional reactions of anger, guilt, embarrassment, and humiliation; fear of physical violence and death; wish for revenge; and multiple physical complaints, including gastrointestinal distress, genitourinary discomfort, tension, and disturbance of the normal sleep pattern. The long-term phase of rape-trauma is characterized by changes in the usual patterns of daily life (even a change in residence), nightmares and phobias, and a need for support from friends and family. The compound reaction is characterized by all of the defining characteristics of rape-trauma, reliance on alcohol or drugs, or the reoccurrence of the symptoms of previous conditions, including psychiatric illness. The silent reaction sometimes occurs in place of the rape-trauma or compound reaction. The defining characteristics are an abrupt change in the person's usual sexual relationships, an increase in nightmares, an increasing anxiety during the interview about the rape incident, a marked change in sexual behavior, denial of the rape or refusal to discuss it, and the sudden development of phobic reactions. See also **nursing diagnosis.**

raphe, rhaphe A line of union of the halves of various symmetrical parts, as the abdominal raphe of the linea alba or the raphe penis.

rapid-acting insulin See **short-acting insulin.**

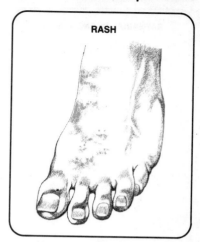

RASH

rapid eye movement (REM) See **sleep.**

rapport A sense of mutuality and understanding; harmony, accord, confidence, and respect underlying a relationship between two persons. It is an essential bond between a therapist and patient in psychotherapy.

raptus 1. A state of intense emotional or mental excitement, often characterized by uncontrollable activity or behavior resulting from an irresistible impulse; ecstasy; rapture. 2. Any sudden or violent seizure or attack. Kinds of raptus include **raptus haemorrhagicus, raptus maniacus, raptus melancholicus, raptus nervorum.**

raptus haemorrhagicus A sudden, massive hemorrhage.

raptus maniacus A sudden, violent attack of mania. See also **mania.**

raptus melancholicus An attack of extreme agitation or frenzy that occurs during depression.

raptus nervorum A sudden, violent attack of nervousness.

rare-earth element A metallic element having an atomic number between 57 and 71 inclusive. These closely related substances are classified in three groups: the cerium metals are lanthanum, cerium, praesodynium, neodynium, promethium, and samarium; the terbium metals are europium, gadolinium, and terbium; the yttrium metals are dysprosium, holmium, erbium, thulium, yttrium, ytterbium, and lutetium. Also called rare-earth metal.

RAS *abbr* **reticular activating system.**

rash A skin eruption. Kinds of rashes include **butterfly rash, diaper rash, heat rash.**

Rashkind procedure The enlargement of an opening in the cardiac septum between the right and left atria, performed to relieve congestive heart failure in newborns with certain congenital heart defects by improving the oxygenation of the blood. The procedure allows more mixing between oxygenated blood from the lungs and systemic blood, without the risk of surgery,

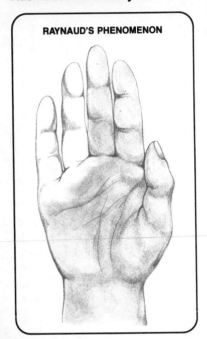

RAYNAUD'S PHENOMENON

sustaining life until the infant is 2 to 3 years old, when a shunt can be created to carry systemic blood to the lungs. Preoperatively, a cardiac catheterization is done to pinpoint the defect. Under light general anesthesia, a deflated balloon is passed through the foramen ovale into the left atrium. The balloon is inflated and pulled across the septum to enlarge the opening. Postoperatively, the infant is observed for respiratory difficulty and signs of hypoxia or decreasing cardiac output. Humidified oxygen is administered. Also called **balloon septostomy.**

Rasmussen's aneurysm A localized dilatation of a blood vessel in a tuberculous cavity that causes hemorrhage when it ruptures.

rat-bite fever Either of two distinct infections transmitted to humans by the bite of a rat or mouse, characterized by fever, headache, malaise, nausea, vomiting, and rash. In the United States, the disease is more commonly caused by *Streptobacillus moniliformis,* and its unique features are rash on palms and soles, painful joints, prompt healing of the wound, and a duration of 2 weeks. In the Far East, rat-bite fever is usually caused by *Spirillum minus* and is associated with an asymmetric rash on the extremities, no joint symptoms, a relapsing fever, swelling at the site of the wound, regional lymphadenopathy, and a duration of from 4 to 8 weeks. Relapse is common. Penicillin is effective in treating either form of the disease. Rat-bite fever resulting from infection caused by *Streptobacillus moniliformis* is also called **Haverhill fever;** infection caused by *Spirillum minus* is also called **sodoku.**

rate A numerical ratio, often used in the compilation of data concerning the prevalence and incidence of events, in which the number of actual occurrences appears as the numerator, and the number of possible occurrences appears as the denominator, as when 1 person in 15 fails an examination, the failure rate is said to be 1/15 (or 1 in 15). Standard rates are stated in conventional units of population, as neonatal mortality per 1,000.

Rathke's pouch tumor See **craniopharyngioma.**

ratio The relationship of one quantity to one or more other quantities, expressed as a proportion of one to the others and written either as a fraction (8/3) or linearly (8:3).

rational **1.** Of or pertaining to a measure, method, or procedure based on reason. **2.** Of or pertaining to a therapeutic method based on an understanding of the cause and mechanisms of a disease and the potential effects of the drugs or procedures used in treating the disorder. **3.** Sane; capable of normal reasoning or behavior.

rationale A system of reasoning or a statement of the reasons to explain data or phenomena.

rational emotive therapy (RET) A form of psychotherapy, originated by Albert Ellis, that emphasizes a reorganization of one's cognitive and emotional functions, a redefinition of one's problems, and a change in one's attitudes to develop more effective patterns of behavior. RET is conducted with individuals or with groups.

rational treatment See **treatment.**

rattle An abnormal sound heard by lung auscultation in some forms of pulmonary disease. It consists of a coarse vibration caused by the movement of moisture and the separation of the walls of small air passages in respiration.

rat typhus See **murine typhus.**

rauwolfia The dried roots of *Rauwolfia serpentina,* which provide the extracts for such hypotensive agents as reserpine.

rauwolfia alkaloid Any one of more than 20 alkaloids derived from the root of a climbing shrub, *Rauwolfia serpentina,* indigenous to India. Formerly used as an antipsychotic agent, its use today is confined to the treatment of hypertension. Numerous trade name formulations of the principal alkaloid, reserpine, are available.

rauwolfia serpentina A sympatholytic antihypertensive that acts peripherally.

ray A beam of radiation, as heat or light, moving away from a source.

Raynaud's phenomenon Intermittent bilateral attacks of ischemia of the fingers or toes and, sometimes, the ears or nose, marked by severe pallor and often accompanied by paresthesia and pain. It is brought on characteristically by cold or emotional stimuli and relieved by heat and is due to an underlying disease or anatomical abnormality.

Raynaud's sign See **acrocyanosis.**

Rb Symbol for **rubidium.**

RBC *abbr* red blood cell. See **erythrocyte.**

RBE *abbr* **relative biological effectiveness.**

RCP *abbr* **Royal College of Physicians.**

RCPSC *abbr* **Royal College of Physicians and Surgeons of Canada.**

RCS *abbr* **Royal College of Surgeons.**

RDA *abbr* recommended daily allowance; dietary needs as outlined by the Food and Nutritional Board, National Academy of Sciences Research Council.

RDS *abbr* respiratory distress syndrome. See **respiratory distress syndrome of the newborn.**

re- A combining form meaning 'back, again, contrary, etc.': *reaction, recombination.*

Re Symbol for **rhenium.**

Reach to Recovery A national volunteer organization that offers counseling and support to women who have breast cancer and to their families. Many of the members have had mastectomies themselves.

reaction A response in opposition to a substance, treatment, or other stimulus, as an antigen-antibody reaction in immunology. —**react,** *v.,* **reactive,** *adj.*

reaction formation A defense mechanism in which a person avoids anxiety through behavior and attitudes that are the opposite of his repressed impulses and drives and that serve to conceal those unacceptable feelings.

reactive depression An emotional disorder characterized by an acute feeling of despondency, sadness, and depressive dysphoria, which varies in intensity and duration. The condition is caused by an unrealistic and inappropriate reaction to some identifiable external situation or intrapsychic conflict and is relieved when the circumstance is altered or the conflict understood and resolved. Also called **exogenous depression, situational depression.** Compare **endogenous depression.** See also **depression.**

reactive schizophrenia A form of schizophrenia caused by environmental factors rather than by organic changes in the brain. The onset of the disease is usually rapid; symptoms are of brief duration, and the affected individual appears well both immediately before and following the schizophrenic episode. Compare **process schizophrenia.** See also **schizophrenia, schizophreniform disorder.**

reading In molecular genetics: the linear process in which the genetic information contained in a nucleotide sequence is decoded, as in the translation of the messenger RNA directives for the sequence of the amino acids in a polypeptide.

Read method A method of psychophysical preparation for childbirth designed by Dr. Grantly Dick-Read. It was the first 'natural childbirth' program, a term coined by Dick-Read, who held that childbirth is a normal, physiologic procedure and that the pain of labor and delivery is of psychologic origin: the fear-tension-pain syndrome. He countered women's fears with education about the physiologic process, encouraged a positive, welcoming attitude, corrected false information, and led tours of the hospital before birth. To decrease tension, he developed a series of breathing exercises for use during the various stages of labor. To foster relaxation and optimal physical function in labor and in recovery after delivery, he incorporated a series of physical exercises to be performed regularly in classes and in practice at home during pregnancy. Throughout labor, the woman is helped to understand what is occurring and to participate and accept the experience. Currently, many authorities who advocate use of other aspects of the Read method recommend that a woman in labor not lie on her back. Supine hypotension is frequently the result of this position, as the uterus can fall back, occluding the vena cava and decreasing the volume of blood returned to the heart, thus reducing the volume of the cardiac output. Maternal hypotension follows, resulting in decreased placental perfusion and an inadequate supply of oxygen to the fetus. Today, the woman using the Read method spends most of labor lying on her side or in a semisitting position with her knees, back, and head well supported. Compare **Bradley method, Lamaze method.**

readthrough In molecular genetics: transcription of RNA beyond the normal termination sequence in the DNA template, caused by the occasional failure of RNA polymerase to respond to the end point signal.

reagent A chemical substance known to react in a specific way. A reagent is used to detect or synthesize another substance in a chemical reaction.

reagin **1.** An antibody associated with human atopy, as asthma and hay fever. It attaches to mast cells and basophils and sensitizes the skin and other tissues. It is associated with gamma-E-globulin and, when involved in antigen-antibody reactions, triggers the release of histamine and other mediators that cause atopic symptoms. **2.** A nonspecific, nontreponemal antibodylike substance found in the serum of individuals with syphilis. It can combine with an antigen prepared as a lipid extract of normal tissue, a phenomenon that constitutes the basis of the serologic tests for syphilis. —**reaginic,** *adj.*

reagin-mediated disorder A hypersensitivity reaction, as hay fever or an allergic response to an insect sting, produced by reaginic antibodies (IgE immunoglobulins) that bind exogenous antigen to the surface of mast cells and basophils, causing degranulation and the release of histamine, bradykinin, serotonin, and other vasoactive amines. An initial sensitizing dose of the antigen induces the formation of specific IgE antibodies, and their attachment to mast cells and basophils results in hypersensitivity to a subsequent challenging dose of the antigen. Reactions range from a simple wheal and flare on the skin to life-threatening anaphylactic shock, depending on the amount and route of entrance of the sensitizing dose and challenging dose, the amount and distribution of IgE antibodies, the responsiveness of the host, the timing of expo-

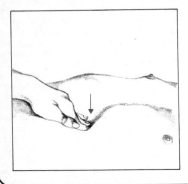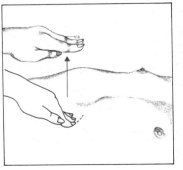

TESTING FOR REBOUND TENDERNESS

sure to the allergen, and the tissues in which the antigen-antibody reaction occurs. Allergens that commonly cause these reactions include plant spores, pollens, animal danders, stings, serum proteins, foods, and certain drugs. See also **allergy, generalized anaphylaxis, hay fever.**

reality principle   An awareness of the demands of the environment and the need for an adjustment of behavior to meet those demands, expressed primarily by the renunciation of immediate gratification of instinctual pleasures in order to obtain long-term and future goals. In psychoanalysis, this function is held to be performed by the ego. Compare **pleasure principle.**

reality testing   A process of evaluating the physical and social aspects of one's environment so as to differentiate between external reality and any inner imaginative world and to behave in a manner that exhibits an awareness of accepted norms and customs.

reality therapy   A form of psychotherapy in which the aims are to help define and assess basic values within the framework of a current situation and to evaluate the person's present behavior and future plans in relation to those values. The emphasis in treatment is on the present rather than the past.

reapproximate   To rejoin tissues separated by surgery or trauma so that their anatomic relationship is restored. **—reapproximation,** *n.*

reasonable person   In law: a hypothetical person who possesses the qualities that are used as an objective standard upon which to judge a defendant's action in a negligence suit. In such suits, it must be decided whether or not a reasonable person, under the same circumstances, would have acted in the same way as the defendant.

rebound   1. Recovery from illness. 2. A sudden contraction of muscle following a period of relaxation, often seen in conditions in which inhibitory reflexes are lost.

rebound tenderness   A sign of inflammation of the peritoneum in which pain is elic-

ited by the sudden release of a hand pressing on the abdomen. See also **appendicitis, peritonitis.**

rebreathing bag   In anesthesia: a flexible bag attached to a mask. The rebreathing bag may function as a reservoir for anesthetic gases during surgery or for oxygen during resuscitation. It may be squeezed to pump the gas or air into the lungs.

recapitulation theory   The theory, formulated by German naturalist Ernst Heinrich Haeckel, that an organism during the course of embryonic development passes through stages that resemble the structural form of several ancestral types of the species as it evolved from a lower to a higher form of life. It is summarized by the statement "Ontogeny recapitulates phylogeny." Also called **biogenetic law, Haeckel's law.**

receiver   In communication theory: the person or persons to whom a message is sent.

recess   A small hollow cavity, as the epitympanic recess in the tympanic cavity of the inner ear.

recessive gene   1. Of, pertaining to, or describing a gene, the effect of which is masked or hidden if there is a dominant gene at the same locus. If both genes are recessive and produce the same trait, the trait is expressed in the individual. 2. The member of a pair of genes that lacks the ability to express itself in the presence of its more dominant allele; it is expressed only in the homozygous state. Compare **dominant gene.**

reciprocal gene   See **complementary gene.**

reciprocal inhibition   A theory in behavior therapy that if an anxiety-producing stimulus occurs simultaneously with a response that diminishes anxiety, the stimulus may cause less anxiety, as deep chest breathing and relaxation of the deep muscles appear to diminish anxiety and pain in childbirth. See also **systemic desensitization.**

reciprocal translocation   The mutual exchange of genetic material between two non-

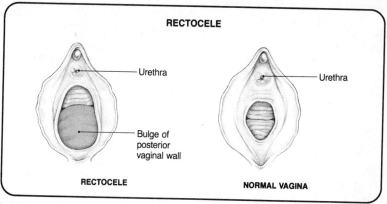

RECTOCELE

Urethra

Bulge of posterior vaginal wall

Urethra

RECTOCELE   NORMAL VAGINA

homologous chromosomes. Also called **interchange.**

Recklinghausen's canal The small lymph space in the connective tissues of the body.

Recklinghausen's disease See **neurofibromatosis.**

Recklinghausen's tumor A benign tumor, derived from smooth muscle containing connective tissue and epithelial elements, that occurs in the wall of the oviduct or posterior uterine wall.

reclining Leaning backward. —**recline,** *v.*

recluse spider See **brown spider.**

recombinant The cell or organism that results from the recombination of genes within the DNA molecule, regardless of whether naturally or artificially induced. See also **recombinant DNA.**

recombinant DNA A DNA molecule in which rearrangement of the genes has been artificially induced. Enzymes are used to break isolated DNA molecules into fragments that are then rearranged in the desired sequence. Portions of DNA material from another organism of the same or a different species may also be introduced into the molecule, which is then replicated, resulting in both genotypic and phenotypic alterations in the organism. See also **genetic engineering, recombination.**

recombination In genetics: the formation of new combinations and arrangements of genes within the chromosome as a result of independent assortment of unlinked genes, crossing over of linked genes, or intracistronic crossing over of nucleotides.

recon In molecular genetics: the smallest genetic unit that is capable of recombination, thought to be a triplet of nucleotides.

recovery room (RR, R.R.) An area adjoining the operating room to which surgical patients are taken while still under anesthesia, before being returned to their rooms. Vital signs and adequacy of ventilation are carefully observed as the patient recovers conciousness. It has a specially trained nursing staff with a nurse anesthetist or anesthesiologist available. See also **postoperative care.**

recreational therapy A form of adjunctive psychotherapy in which games or other group activities are used as a means of modifying maladaptive behavior, awakening social interests, or improving the ability to communicate in depressed, withdrawn people.

recrudescent hepatitis A form of acute viral hepatitis marked by a relapse during the period of recovery. A minority of patients experience it, and the prognosis for ultimate recovery is rarely affected.

recrudescent typhus See **Brill-Zinsser disease.**

rectal anesthesia General anesthesia achieved by the insertion, injection, or infusion of an anesthetic agent into the rectum; this procedure is rarely performed because of the unpredictability of absorption of the drug into the blood.

rectal cancer See **colorectal cancer.**

rectal reflex The normal response (defecation) to the presence of an accumulation of feces in the rectum. Also called **defecation reflex.**

rectitis See **proctitis.**

rectocele A protrusion of the rectum and the posterior wall of the vagina into the vagina. The condition, which occurs after the muscles of the vagina and pelvic floor have been weakened by childbearing, old age, or surgery, may reflect a congenital weakness in the wall and may, if severe, result in dyspareunia and difficulty in evacuating the bowel. Reconstructive surgery is often helpful. Also called proctocele.

rectosigmoid A portion of the anatomy that includes the lower portion of the sigmoid and the upper portion of the rectum.

rectouterine excavation See **rectouterine pouch.**

rectouterine pouch A deep pouch between the uterus and the rectum at the top of the posterior wall of the vagina, formed by the posterior ligament extending from the posterior surface of the uterus to the rectum. Also called **cul-de-sac of Douglas, rectouterine excavation.**

rectum, *pl.* **rectums, recta** The portion

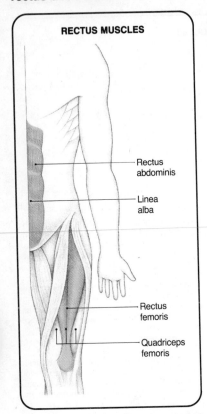

RECTUS MUSCLES

- Rectus abdominis
- Linea alba
- Rectus femoris
- Quadriceps femoris

of the large intestine, about 12 cm (4¾ inches) long, continuous with the descending sigmoid colon, just proximal to the anal canal. It follows the sacrococcygeal curve, ends in the anal canal, and usually contains three transverse semilunar folds. Each fold is about 12 mm (½ inch) wide. The folds overlap when the intestine is empty. —**rectal,** *adj.*

rectus abdominis   One of a pair of an-terolateral muscles of the abdomen, extending the whole length of the ventral aspect of the abdomen and separated by the linea alba. Each rectus arises in a lateral tendon from the crest of the pubis and is interlaced by a medial tendon with that of the opposite side. The rectus ab-dominis inserts into the 5th, 6th, and 7th ribs. It is innervated by branches of the 7th through the 12th intercostal nerves and functions to flex the vertebral column, tense the anterior abdom-inal wall, and assist in compressing the abdom-inal contents. Compare **obliquus externus ab-dominis, obliquus internus abdominis, pyramidalis, transversus abdominis.**

rectus femoris   A fusiform muscle of the anterior thigh, one of the four parts of the quad-riceps femoris. It arises in an anterior tendon originating in the iliac spine and in a posterior tendon originating in the brim of the acetabu-

lum. The two tendons unite and spread into a broad, thick aponeurosis, which extends down-ward over the thigh in the center of the quad-riceps femoris. The rectus femoris is innervated by branches of the femoral nerve, which contain fibers from the second, third, and fourth lumbar nerves, and it functions to flex the leg. Compare **vastus intermedius, vastus lateralis, vastus medialis.** See also **quadriceps femoris.**

rectus muscle   A muscle of the body that has a relatively straight form. Some kinds of rectus muscles are **rectus abdominis, rectus femoris.**

recumbent   Lying down or leaning back-ward. See also **reclining.** —**recumbency,** *n.*

recurrent bandage   A bandage that is wrapped several times around itself, as on a finger.

recurrent fever   See **relapsing fever.**

recurvatum   Backward thrust of the knee caused by weakness of the quadriceps.

red blood cell (RBC)   See **erythrocyte.**

Red Book of the American Academy of Pediatrics   A book that serves as the stan-dard reference source of immunization proce-dures for children and adults. It is available from the American Academy of Pediatrics Inc., Ev-anston, Ill.

red bug   See **chigger.**

red cell   See **erythrocyte.**

red cell indices   A series of relationships that characterize the red cell population in terms of size, hemoglobin content, and hemoglobin concentration. Derived mathematically from the red cell count and the hemoglobin and hemat-ocrit values, the indices are useful in making differential diagnoses of several kinds of anemia. The values reported are the mean corpuscular hemoglobin, the mean corpuscular hemoglobin concentration, and the mean corpuscular vol-ume.

red corpuscle   See **erythrocyte.**

Red Cross   1. See **International Red Cross Society.** 2. See **American Red Cross.**

red fever   See **dengue.**

red marrow   The red vascular substance consisting of connective tissue and blood vessels containing primitive blood cells, macrophages, megakaryocytes, and fat cells. It is found in the cavities of many bones, including the flat and the short bones, the bodies of the vertebrae, the sternum, the ribs, and the articulating ends of the long bones. Red marrow manufactures and releases leukocytes and erythrocytes into the bloodstream. See also **bone marrow.**

redon   The smallest unit of the DNA molecule capable of recombination; it may be as small as one deoxyribonucleotide pair. Compare **cis-tron, muton.**

reduce   In surgery: the restoration of a part to its original position after displacement, as in the reduction of a fractured bone by bringing ends or fragments back into alignment or of a hernia by returning the bowel to its normal po-sition. A fracture may be reduced under local or general anesthesia. If performed by outside

REFERRED PAIN FROM VISCERAL ORGANS

ORGAN	REFERRED PAIN AREA
Gallbladder	• Right upper quadrant • Right posterior infrascapular area
Diaphragm	• Posterior neck • Posterior shoulder area
Duodenum	• *Most commonly:* midline of the abdominal wall, just above the umbilicus
Appendix	• Umbilicus • Parietal peritoneal involvement, right lower quadrant
Ureter	• Inguinal region • Loin

manipulation alone, the reduction is said to be closed; if surgery is necessary, it is said to be open. See also **fracture, hernia, invagination, traction. —reduce,** *v.*

reducing diet A diet that is low in calories, used for reduction of body weight. The diet must supply fewer calories than the individual expends each day, while supplying all the essential nutrients for maintaining health. A usual diet of this type provides 1,200 calories per day from the basic food groups. Meats are usually broiled, roasted, stewed, or sauteed; vegetables are steamed or eaten raw; starches and fats are limited; and fresh fruits replace desserts. Foods to be avoided are sweetened carbonated beverages, fried foods, pastries, and most snack foods. Vitamin and mineral deficiencies may result if such a diet is not carefully planned. Also called **lowcaloric diet.**

reduction 1. The addition of hydrogen to a substance. Also called **hydrogenation. 2.** The removal of oxygen from a substance. **3.** The decrease in the valence of the electronegative part of a compound. **4.** The addition of one or more electrons to a molecule or atom of a substance. **5.** The correction of a fracture, hernia, or luxation. **6.** The reduction of data, as in converting interval data to an ordinal or nominal scale of measurement.

reduction division See **meiosis.**

Reed-Sternberg cell One of a number of large, abnormal, multinucleated reticuloendothelial cells in the lymphatic system in Hodgkin's disease. The number and proportion of these cells identified form the basis for the histopathologic classification of Hodgkin's disease.

reefer *Slang.* See **cannabis.**

refereed journal A professional or literary journal in which articles or papers are selected for publication by a panel of referees who are experts in the field. The important national professional journals in medicine and nursing are refereed.

referential idea See **idea of reference.**

referred pain Pain felt at a site different from that of an injured or diseased organ or part of the body. Angina, the pain of coronary artery insufficiency, may be felt in the left shoulder, arm, or jaw.

refined birth rate The ratio of total births to the total female population, considered during a period of 1 year. Compare **birth rate, crude birth rate, true birth rate.**

reflection of content The return of a verbal message, using the same words in which it was sent.

reflection of feelings The disclosure of feelings sensed during conversation but not yet spoken.

reflex action The involuntary functioning or movement of any organ or part of the body in response to a particular stimulus. The function or action occurs immediately, without the involvement of the will or consciousness.

reflex apnea Involuntary cessation of respiration owing to irritating, noxious vapors or gases.

reflex bladder See **spastic bladder.**

reflex dyspepsia An abnormal condition characterized by impaired digestion associated with the disease of an organ not directly involved with digestion. See also **dyspepsia.**

reflux An abnormal backward or return flow of a fluid. Kinds of reflux include **gastroesophageal reflux, hepatojugular reflux, vesicoureteral reflux.**

refracting medium See **medium.**

refraction 1. The change of direction of energy as it passes from one medium to another of different density. **2.** An examination to determine and to correct refractive errors of the eye.

refractory period The interval following the excitation of a neuron or the contraction of a muscle during which repolarization of the cell membrane occurs. The period is divided into two phases. During the absolute stage, the cell is incapable of responding to any stimulus, regardless of its strength, because of total depolarization. During the relative phase, as repolarization is underway, a stimulus intensity above the threshold may elicit a response even though the normal resting potential of the cell has not been reached.

Refsum's syndrome A rare, hereditary disorder of lipid metabolism in which phytanic acid cannot be broken down. The syndrome is characterized by ataxia, abnormalities of the bones and skin, peripheral neuropathy, and retinitis pigmentosa. Foods containing phytanic acid must be avoided to prevent progressive deterioration. Also called **phytanic acid storage disease.**

regional Of or pertaining to a geographical area, as a regional medical facility, or to a part of the body, as regional anesthesia.

regional anatomy The study of the structural relationships within the organs and the parts of the body. Kinds of regional anatomy are **surface anatomy** and **cross-sectional anatomy.**

regional anesthesia Anesthesia of an area of the body by injecting a local anesthetic to block a group of sensory nerve fibers. Kinds of regional anesthesia include **brachial plexus anesthesia, epidural anesthesia, paracervical block, pudendal block, spinal.**

regional enteritis See **Crohn's disease.**

regionalization In health-care planning: the organization of a system for the delivery of health care within a region to avoid costly duplication of services and to ensure availability of essential services. Hospitals are classified as primary, secondary, and tertiary health centers, depending on the facilities and personnel available, the population served, the number of beds in the institution, and other criteria.

registered nurse (RN) 1. *U.S.* A professional nurse who has completed a course of study at a school of nursing accredited by the National League for Nursing and who has taken and passed the State Board Test Pool Examination. A registered nurse may use the initials RN following the signature. RNs are licensed to practice by individual states. 2. *Canada* A professional nurse who has completed a course of study at an approved school of nursing and who has taken and passed an examination administered by the Canadian Nurses' Association Testing Service. See also **nurse, nursing.**

Registered Therapist (RT) A title awarded by the American Registry of Radiologic Technicians as certification of qualification to act as an X-ray technician.

registrar An administrative officer whose responsibility is to maintain the records of an institution.

registry 1. An office or agency in which lists of nurses and records pertaining to nurses seeking employment are maintained. 2. In epidemiology: a listing service for incidence data pertaining to the occurrence of specific diseases or disorders, as a tumor registry.

regression 1. A retreat or backward movement in conditions, signs, or symptoms. 2. A return to an earlier, more primitive form of behavior. 3. A tendency in physical development to become more typical of the population than of the parents. —**regress,** *v.*

regular diet A full, well-balanced diet containing all of the essential nutrients needed for optimal growth, repair of the tissues, and normal functioning of the organs. Also called **full diet.**

Regular Iletin A trade name for insulin injection (crystalline zinc insulin).

Regular Insulin A trade name for insulin injection (crystalline zinc insulin).

regulative cleavage See **indeterminate cleavage.**

regulative development A type of embryonic development in which the fertilized ovum undergoes indeterminate cleavage, producing blastomeres that have similar developmental potencies and are each capable of giving rise to a single embryo. Determination of the particular organs and parts of the embryo occurs during later stages of development and is influenced by inductors and intercellular interaction. Damage or destruction of various cells during the early stages of development results in readjustments and substitutions so that a normal organism is formed. Compare **mosaic development.**

regulatory gene In molecular genetics: a genetic unit that regulates or suppresses the activity of one or more structural genes.

regulatory sequence In molecular genetics: a series of DNA nucleotides that regulate the expression of a gene.

regurgitation 1. The return of swallowed food into the mouth. 2. The backward flow of blood through a defective heart valve, named for the affected valve, as in **aortic regurgitation.**

rehabilitation The restoration of an individual or a part to normal or near-normal function following a disabling disease, injury, addiction, or incarceration. —**rehabilitate,** *v.*

rehabilitation center A facility providing therapy and training for rehabilitation. The center may offer occupational therapy, physical therapy, vocational training, and such special training as speech therapy.

Rehfuss stomach tube A specially designed gastric tube with a graduated syringe, used for withdrawing specimens of the contents of the stomach for study following a test meal.

Reifenstein's syndrome Male hypogonadism of unknown etiology, marked by azoospermia, undescended testes, gynecomastia, testosterone deficiency, and elevated gonadotropin titers. The condition appears to be inherited as an X-linked recessive trait, but no chromosomal abnormality has been identified.

reinforcement In psychology: a process in which a response is strengthened by the fear of punishment or the anticipation of reward.

Reiter's syndrome An arthritic disorder of adult males, believed to result from a myxovirus or *Mycoplasma* infection. The syndrome most often affects the ankles, feet, and sacroiliac joints and is usually associated with conjunctivitis and urethritis. The onset may be marked by unexplained diarrhea and low-grade fever, followed in 2 to 4 weeks by conjunctivitis. Lesions that become superficial ulcers may form on the palms and the soles. Arthritis usually persists after the conjunctivitis and urethritis subside, but it may become episodic. Treatment includes a short course of tetracycline to treat the infection and phenylbutazone to relieve pain and inflammation in the joint.

rejection **1.** In medicine: an immunological response to organisms or substances that the system recognizes as foreign, including grafts or transplants. **2.** In psychiatry: the act of excluding or denying affection.

relapse **1.** To exhibit again the symptoms of a disease from which a patient appears to have recovered. **2.** The recurrence of a disease after apparent recovery. —**relapsing,** *adj.*

relapsing fever Any one of several acute infectious diseases, marked by recurrent febrile episodes, caused by various strains of the spirochete *Borrelia*. The disease is transmitted by both lice and ticks and is often seen during wars and famines. It has occurred in several western states of the United States but is more commonly found in South America, Asia, and Africa. The first episode usually starts with a sudden high fever, 40° to 40.6°C, (104° to 105°F), accompanied by chills, headache, neuromuscular pain, and nausea. A rash may appear over the trunk and extremities; and jaundice is common during the later stages. Each attack lasts 2 or 3 days and culminates in a crisis of high fever, profuse sweating, and a rise in heart and respiratory rate. This is followed by an abrupt drop in temperature and a return to normal blood pressure. People typically relapse after 7 to 10 days of normal temperature and eventually recover completely. In louse-borne disease, there is usually only a single relapse; in tick-borne disease, several successively milder relapses may occur. To make a diagnosis, the spirochete must be seen on a blood smear obtained during an attack. Treatment is with a long-acting penicillin, tetracycline, or chloramphenicol. Antimicrobial therapy may induce a Herxheimer reaction, so treatment is withheld during a febrile crisis. Disinfection of clothing and bedding is necessary to destroy any lice or ticks. Also called **African tick fever, famine fever, recurrent fever, spirillum fever, tick fever.**

relapsing polychondritis A rare disease of unknown cause resulting in inflammation and destruction of cartilage with replacement by fibrous tissue. Autoimmunity may be involved in this condition. Most commonly, the ears and noses of middle-aged people are affected with episodes of tender swelling, often accompanied by fever, arthralgias, and episcleritis. Consequences include floppy ears, collapsed nose, hearing loss, or hoarseness and airway obstruction owing to laryngeal and tracheal cartilage involvement. Corticosteroids suppress the activity of the disease.

relation searching In nursing research: a study design used to discover and describe relationships between and among variables. It may be used to describe various nursing situations in order to examine the efficacy of certain aspects of nursing care.

relative biological effectiveness (RBE) In radiotherapy: the ratio of the effect of an absorbed dose of a form of radiation under study to the effect of a standard, reference form of radiation.

relative cephalopelvic disproportion See **cephalopelvic disproportion.**

relative growth The comparison of the various increases in size of similar organisms, tissues, or structures at different time intervals.

relative refractory period See **refractory period.**

relative risk An assessment of the degree or incidence of adverse effects that may be expected in the presence of a particular factor or event as compared with the expected adverse effects in the absence of the factor or event.

relaxation **1.** A reducing of tension, as when a muscle relaxes between contractions. **2.** A lessening of pain.

relaxation therapy Treatment in which patients are taught to perform breathing and relaxation exercises and to concentrate on pleasant situations when a noxious stimulus is applied. An integral part of the Lamaze method of childbirth, relaxation therapy is also used to relieve various kinds of pain and physical manifestations of stress. Some patients learn through relaxation therapy to relax taut muscles at will, to abort migraine attacks, or to reduce their blood pressure. See also **Lamaze method.**

releasing hormone (RH) One of several peptides produced by the hypothalamus and secreted directly into the anterior pituitary via a portal system. Each of the releasing hormones stimulates the pituitary to secrete a specific tropic hormone, such as corticotropic-releasing hormone, which stimulates the pituitary to secrete adrenocorticotropic hormone. These tropic hormones travel to receptive target organs or glands. The target organ or gland then releases its hormones into the blood. Compare **inhibiting hormone.**

relevant verbal mesage A spoken idea that fits the context of the immediate situation.

reliability In research: the extent to which a test measurement or a device produces the same results with different investigators, observers, or administration of the test over time.

rem Acronym for roentgen equivalent man. A dose of ionizing radiation that produces in humans the same effect as one roentgen of x-radiation or gamma radiation.

REM *abbr* **rapid eye movement.** See **sleep.**

remission The partial or complete disappearance of the clinical and subjective characteristics of a chronic or malignant disease. Remission may be spontaneous or the result of therapy. In some cases, remission is permanent, and the disease is cured. Compare **cure.**

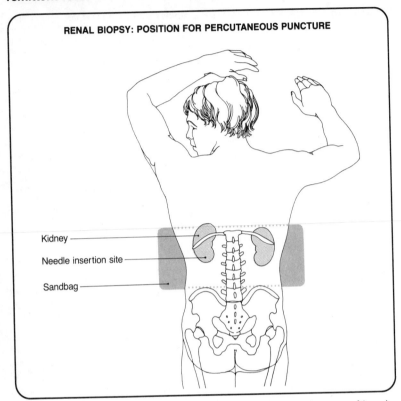

RENAL BIOPSY: POSITION FOR PERCUTANEOUS PUNCTURE

Kidney

Needle insertion site

Sandbag

remittent fever Diurnal variations of an elevated temperature with exacerbations and remissions but never a return to normal.

remote afterloading In radiotherapy: a technique in which an applicator, as an acrylic mold of an area to be irradiated, is placed in or on the patient and then loaded from a safe source with a high-activity radioisotope. The mold or applicator contains grooves for the insertion of nylon tubes into which the radioactive material can be introduced. Remote afterloading is used in the treatment of head, neck, vaginal, and cervical tumors.

ren- A combining form meaning 'of or pertaining to the kidneys': *renicardiac, reniform.*

renal Of or pertaining to the kidney.

renal adenocarcinoma See **renal cell carcinoma.**

renal artery One of a pair of large, visceral branches of the abdominal aorta, arising caudally to the superior mesenteric artery at the level of the disk between the first and second lumbar vertebrae. The left renal artery is somewhat more cranial than the right. The renal arteries supply the kidney, suprarenal glands, and the ureters.

renal biopsy The removal of kidney tissue for microscopic examination to establish the diagnosis of a renal disorder and to aid in determining the stage of the disease, the appropriate therapy, and the prognosis. An open biopsy involves an incision, permits better visualization of the kidney, and carries a lower risk of hemorrhage; a closed or percutaneous biopsy performed by aspirating a specimen of tissue with a needle requires a shorter period of recovery and is less likely to cause infection. Prior to biopsy, the procedure is explained and the patient is medically evaluated and tested for bleeding or coagulation time. The patient's blood is usually typed and crossmatched with two units of donor blood that are held for a possible transfusion until there is no threat of bleeding after the procedure. An open biopsy is generally carried out in the operating room, but the percutaneous procedure may be performed in the radiology department or in the patient's room. The location of the kidney, determined by a plain X-ray film, dye contrast study, or fluoroscopic examination, is marked on the patient's skin in ink for a needle biopsy. A local anesthetic is injected and the physician inserts the biopsy needle in the lower pole of the kidney, since this area contains the smallest number of large renal vessels. The needle is quickly withdrawn and, after pressure is applied to the site for 20 minutes, a pressure bandage is applied; the patient is turned and kept supine and motionless for the next 4 hours. The dressing, blood pressure,

RENAL CORTEX

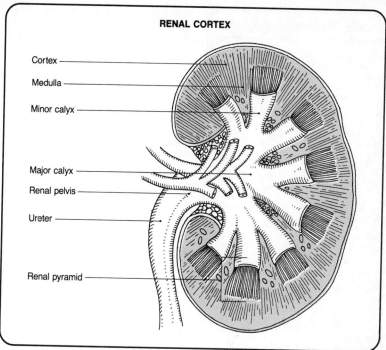

Cortex
Medulla
Minor calyx
Major calyx
Renal pelvis
Ureter
Renal pyramid

and pulse are checked every 15 to 60 minutes for 2 hours, the temperature every 4 hours for 24 hours; excessive drainage, decreased blood pressure, tachycardia, or elevated temperature are reported to the physician. Fluids are forced to the maximum allotted for the patient's condition; the amount and character of urinary output are noted and the physician is informed if hematuria occurs. The patient is kept in bed for at least 24 hours and is cautioned not to lift any heavy objects for 10 days.

NURSING CONSIDERATIONS: The nurse offers an explanation of the procedure, prepares and positions the patient for the percutaneous procedure, and, on its completion, provides care and emotional support.

renal calculus   A calculus formed in the pelvis of the kidney.

renal calyx   The first unit in the system of ducts in the kidney carrying urine from the renal pyramid of the cortex to the renal pelvis for excretion through the ureters. There are two divisions: the **minor calyx,** with several others, drains into a larger major calyx, which in turn joins other major calyces to form the renal pelvis.

renal cell carcinoma   A malignant neoplasm of the kidney, composed predominantly of large cells with clear cytoplasm that originate in tubular epithelium. The tumor may develop in any part of the kidney, becoming a large mass that may grow into the tributaries of the renal vein. Hematuria and pain are usually present.

Metastasis, especially to the lungs and bones, may occur early in the course of development. Treatment includes surgery and radiotherapy. Also called **adenocarcinoma of the kidney, clear cell carcinoma of the kidney.** See also **Wilms' tumor.**

renal colic   Sharp, severe pain in the lower back over the kidney, radiating forward into the groin. Renal colic usually accompanies forcible dilation of a ureter followed by spasm as a stone is lodged or passed through it. See also **urinary calculus.**

renal corpuscle   See **Malpighian corpuscle.**

renal cortex   The soft, granular, outer layer of the kidney, containing approximately 1.25 million renal tubules, which remove body wastes in the form of urine.

renal diet   A diet prescribed in chronic renal failure and designed to control the intake of protein, potassium, sodium, phosphorus, and fluids, depending on individual conditions. Carbohydrates and fats are the principal sources of energy. Protein is limited; the amount is determined by the patient's condition and is usually supplied from milk, eggs, and meat. Cereals, bread, rice, and pasta are the primary sources of calories. Some vegetables and fruits are included, depending on the degree of restriction of potassium and phosphorus. The low potassium level of the diet also makes it useful in hyperkalemia. The diet is nutritionally inadequate and should be supplemented with vita-

STAGES OF RENAL FAILURE

Acute
● During the first *(oliguric)* phase, urine output suddenly decreases to less than 400 ml/day, with elevated blood urea nitrogen (BUN), serum creatinine, and potassium levels. This phase may last from a few days to more than a month.
● During the second *(diuretic)* phase, the urine output increases to more than 400 ml/day. It may be as high as 8 liters/day. BUN, serum creatinine, and potassium stabilize at elevated levels, then decrease, and eventually reach normal levels. This phase also may last from a few days to a month. If not reversed, the patient's condition deteriorates to chronic renal failure.

Chronic
● In the first *(diminished renal reserve)* stage, renal tissue is destroyed, but the patient remains asymptomatic.
● In the second *(renal insufficiency)* stage, the patient may exhibit elevated BUN and creatinine levels but show only vague signs and symptoms, such as increased blood pressure, lassitude, and decreased mental acuity. However, the patient may also have more severe signs and symptoms, such as muscular hyperactivity, gastrointestinal disturbances, or congestive heart failure.
● In the third stage, called *end stage renal disease (ESRD)*, the patient shows elevated BUN and serum creatinine levels; fluid and electrolyte level imbalances; and worsening of all previously mentioned signs and symptoms.

mins and electrolytes. See also **Giordano-Giovannetti diet.**

renal dwarf A dwarf whose retarded growth is caused by renal failure.

renal failure Inability of the kidneys to excrete wastes, concentrate urine, and conserve electrolytes. The condition may be acute or chronic. Acute renal failure is characterized by oliguria and by the rapid accumulation of nitrogenous wastes in the blood. It is caused by hemorrhage, trauma, burn, toxic injury to the kidney, acute pyelonephritis or glomerulonephritis, or lower urinary tract obstruction. Treatment includes restricted intake of fluids and of all substances that require excretion by the kidney. Antibiotics and diuretics are also used. Chronic renal failure may result from many other diseases. The early signs include sluggishness, fatigue, and mental dullness. Later, anuria, convulsions, gastrointestinal bleeding, malnutrition and various neuropathies may occur. Congestive heart failure and hypertension are frequent complications, the results of hypervolemia. Urinalysis reveals greater than normal amounts of urea and creatinine, waxy casts, and a constant volume of urine regardless of variations in water intake. Anemia frequently occurs.

Treatment usually includes restricted water and protein intake and the use of diuretics. When medical measures have been exhausted, long-term hemodialysis is often begun, and kidney transplantation is considered.

renal hypertension Hypertension resulting from kidney disease, including chronic glomerulonephritis, chronic pyelonephritis, renal carcinoma, and renal calculi. Analgesic abuse and certain drug reactions may also result in renal hypertension. Therapy depends on the cause and may include administration of antibiotics or diuretics or surgery. Untreated renal hypertension is likely to result in kidney damage and cardiovascular disease.

renal nanism Dwarfism associated with infantile renal osteodystrophy.

renal papilla See **papilla.**

renal rickets A condition characterized by rachitic changes in the skeleton and caused by chronic nephritis.

renal tubular acidosis (RTA) An abnormal condition associated with persistent dehydration, metabolic acidosis, hypokalemia, hyperchloremia, and nephrocalcinosis. It is caused by the inability of the kidneys to conserve bicarbonate and to adequately acidify the urine. Prolonged RTA can cause hypercalciuria and the formation of kidney stones. Depending on treatment and the extent of renal damage, prognosis is usually good. Some common signs and symptoms of RTA, especially in children, may include anorexia, vomiting, constipation, retarded growth, polyuria, nephrocalcinosis, and rickets. RTA can also cause urinary tract infections and pyelonephritis. Confirming diagnosis of distal RTA is based on laboratory tests that show impaired urine acidification in association with systemic metabolic acidosis. Confirming diagnosis of proximal RTA is based on tests that show bicarbonate wasting owing to impaired reabsorption. Other significant laboratory findings may show decreased sodium bicarbonate, pH, potassium, and phosphorus; increased serum chloride, alkaline phosphatase, urinary bicarbonate, and potassium; and urine with low specific gravity. Treatment seeks to replace excessively secreted substances, especially bicarbonate, and may include the administration of sodium bicarbonate tablets, potassium to counter low potassium levels, vitamin D to preserve calcium metabolism, and antibiotics to counter pyelonephritis. Surgery may be required to excise renal calculi.

NURSING CONSIDERATIONS: The urine of the patient is strained to capture any kidney stones for analysis, and the nurse is alert to any signs of hematuria. Patients with low potassium levels are usually advised to eat potassium-rich foods, as bananas, oranges, and baked potatoes. The patient and family also benefit from advice and encouragement in seeking genetic counseling and RTA screening. Compare **distal renal tubular acidosis, proximal renal tubular acidosis, metabolic acidosis, respiratory acidosis.**

Rendu-Osler-Weber syndrome See **Os-**

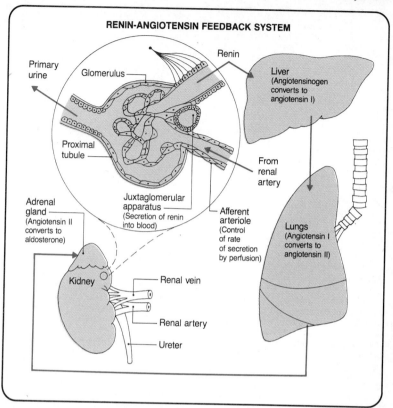

RENIN-ANGIOTENSIN FEEDBACK SYSTEM

Primary urine

Glomerulus

Renin

Liver (Angiotensinogen converts to angiotensin I)

Proximal tubule

From renal artery

Adrenal gland (Angiotensin II converts to aldosterone)

Juxtaglomerular apparatus (Secretion of renin into blood)

Afferent arteriole (Control of rate of secretion by perfusion)

Lungs (Angiotensin I converts to angiotensin II)

Kidney

Renal vein

Renal artery

Ureter

ler-Weber-Rendu syndrome.

renin A proteolytic enzyme, produced by and stored in the juxtaglomerular apparatus that surrounds each arteriole. The enzyme affects the blood pressure by catalyzing the change of angiotensinogen to angiotensin, a strong pressor. Compare **rennin**.

rennin A milk-curdling enzyme that occurs in the gastric juices of infants and is also contained in the rennet produced in the stomach of calves and other ruminants. It is an endopeptidase that converts casein to paracasein and was formerly used extensively as a curdling agent by the cheese industry. An artificially produced microbial rennet, rather than the enzyme extracted from rennet in calves, is used in one half of the cheese produced in the United States today. Compare **renin**.

renovascular hypertension See **portal hypertension**.

reovirus Any one of three ubiquitous, double-stranded RNA viruses found in the respiratory and alimentary tracts in healthy and in sick people. Reoviruses have been implicated in some cases of upper respiratory disease and infantile gastroenteritis.

repetition compulsion An unconscious need to revert to and repeat earlier situations, patterns of behavior, and acts in order to experience previously felt emotions or relationships. See also **compulsion**.

replacement The substitution of a missing part or substance with a similar structure or substance, as the replacement of an amputated limb with a prosthesis.

replication 1. A process of duplicating, reproducing, or copying; literally, a folding back of a part to form a duplicate. 2. In research: the exact repetition of an experiment, performed to confirm the initial findings. 3. In genetics: the duplication of the polynucleotide strands of DNA, or the synthesis of DNA. The process involves the unwinding of the double helix molecule to form two single strands, each of which acts as a template for the synthesis of a complementary strand. The two resulting molecules of DNA each contain one new and one parental strand which coil to form the double helix. Also called semiconservative replication. —**replicate**, v.

replicator In genetics: the segment of the DNA molecule that initiates and controls the replication of the polynucleotide strands.

replicon In genetics: a replication unit; the segment of the DNA molecule that is undergoing replication. The unit is regulated by a section of the molecule, called the regulator, which con-

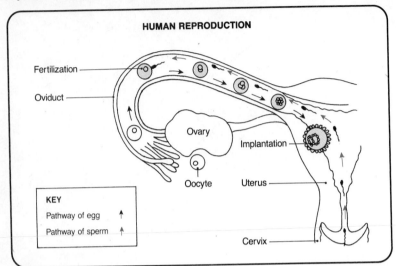

HUMAN REPRODUCTION

Fertilization

Oviduct

Ovary

Implantation

Oocyte

Uterus

KEY

Pathway of egg ↑

Pathway of sperm ↑

Cervix

---

trols replication and coordinates it with cell division.

report In nursing: the transfer of information from the nurses on one shift to the nurses on the following shift. Report is given at the time of change of shift. The head nurse, team leader, or primary nurse conducts the report, summarizing the progress and status of each patient for the nurses who will next assume responsibility. The provider of the information is said to 'give report' and the oncoming staff to 'take report.' Report may be given to the assembled oncoming staff, or it may be tape-recorded so that staff members can listen to it individually or in a group on their own schedule. The Kardex and medcard of each patient are updated before report, and staff members are informed of the changes during report.

repression 1. The act of restraining, inhibiting, or suppressing. **2.** In psychoanalysis: an unconscious defense mechanism whereby unacceptable thoughts, feelings, ideas, impulses, or memories, especially those concerning some traumatic past event, are pushed from the consciousness because of their painful guilt association or disagreeable content and are submerged in the unconscious, where they remain dormant but operant and dynamic. Such repressed emotional conflicts are the source of anxiety, which may lead to any of the anxiety disorders. Compare **suppression.—repress,** *v,* **repressive,** *adj.*

repressor In molecular genetics: a protein that binds to a sequence of nucleotides regulating an adjacent gene. The repressor, when bound, blocks the transcription of the gene.

repressor gene In molecular genetics: a unit of genetic information that represses the activity of another gene.

reproduction 1. The process by which animals and plants give rise to offspring; procrea-

tion; the total of the cellular and genetic phenomena involved in the transmission of organic life from one organism to successive generations similar to the parents, so that the perpetuation and continuity of the species is maintained. In humans, the spermatozoa in the male and the ova in the female, which are produced by the testes and ovaries, unite during fertilization to form the new individual. **2.** The creation of a similar structure, situation, or phenomenon; duplication; replication. **3.** In psychology: the recalling of a former idea, impression, or something previously learned. See also **fertilization, oogenesis, pregnancy, spermatogenesis. —reproductive,** *adj.*

repulsion 1. The act of repelling, disjoining; a force that separates two bodies or things. **2.** In genetics: the situation in linked inheritance in which the alleles of two or more mutant genes are located on homologous chromosomes so that each chromosome of the pair carries one or more mutant and wild-type genes, which are located close enough to be inherited together. Compare **coupling.** See also **trans configuration.**

request for proposal (RFP) A solicitation by a funding agency for proposals to accomplish a particular goal. The RFP lists the requirements a project must meet to receive funding.

RES *abbr* **reticuloendothelial system.**

rescinnamine A sympatholytic antihypertensive that is peripherally acting.

research instrument A testing device for measuring a given phenomenon, as a paper-and-pencil test, a questionnaire, an interview, or a set of guidelines for observation.

research measurement An evaluation of the quantity or incidence of a given variable as obtained by using a research instrument.

research radiopharmaceutical A drug that is labeled with a small quantity of a ra-

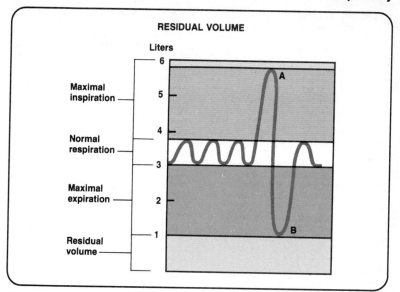

RESIDUAL VOLUME

Liters

Maximal inspiration

Normal respiration

Maximal expiration

Residual volume

dioactive tracer in order to study its biodistribution; it may later be used in a nonradioactive form.

resect To remove tissue from the body by surgery. Resection of an organ may be partial or complete.

resection The cutting out of a significant portion of an organ or structure. A kind of resection is a **wedge resection.**

reserpine A sympatholytic antihypertensive that acts peripherally.

reserve A potential capacity to maintain the vital functions of the body in homeostasis by adjusting to increased need, as cardiac reserve, pulmonary reserve, and alkali reserve. See also **homeostasis.**

reserve cell carcinoma See **oat cell carcinoma.**

reservoir bag A component of an anesthesia machine in which gas accumulates, forming a reserve supply of gas for use when the flow is inadequate. This component also permits bagging, or manual control of ventilation, and serves as a visible monitor of machine function.

reservoir host A nonhuman host that serves to sustain an infectious organism as a potential source of human infection. Wild monkeys are reservoir hosts for the yellow fever virus.

reservoir of infection A continuous source of infectious disease. People, animals, and plants may be reservoirs of infection.

resident A physician in one of the postgraduate years of clinical training following the 1st, or internship, year. The length of residency varies according to the specialty. See also **PGY.** Compare **intern, extern.**

residual volume The volume of gas in the lungs at the end of a maximum expiration.

residue schizophrenia A form of schizo-

phrenia in which there is a history of at least one psychotic schizophrenic episode and objective signs of the illness, in which social withdrawal, eccentric behavior, illogical thinking, and inappropriate emotional reactions persist. The symptoms are less severe than those manifested by persons classified as psychotic. See also **schizophrenia.**

res ipsa loquitur Latin for 'the thing speaks for itself.' A legal concept that is important in many malpractice suits. It describes a situation in which an injury occurred when the defendant was solely and exclusively in control and in which the injury would not have occurred had due care been exercised. Classic examples are a sponge left in the abdomen after abdominal surgery and the amputation of the wrong extremity.

resistance transfer factor See **R factor.**

resonance An echo or other sound produced by percussion of an organ or cavity of the body during a physical examination. **—resonant,** *adj.*

resorcinated camphor A mixture of camphor and resorcinol, used for the treatment of pediculosis and itching.

resorcinol A topical keratolytic agent.

resorcinol test See **Boas' test.**

respiration 1. External respiration is the act of inhaling and exhaling. Some kinds of external respiration are **Biot's respiration, Cheyne-Stokes respiration, Kussmaul respiration.** 2. Internal respiration is the process of the molecular exchange of oxygen and carbon dioxide within the pulmonary system. The rate varies with the age and condition of the person.

respirator An apparatus used to modify air for inspiration or to improve pulmonary ventilation. See also **nebulizer.**

respiratory Of or pertaining to respiration.

respiratory acidosis   A condition characterized by increased arterial PCO_2, excess carbonic acid, and increased plasma hydrogen-ion concentration. It is caused by reduced alveolar ventilation. The hypoventilation associated with this condition inhibits the excretion of carbon dioxide, which consequently combines with water in the body to produce excessive carbonic acid and thus reduces blood pH. Some common signs and symptoms of respiratory acidosis are headache, lethargy, shallow and irregular respirations, fine tremors, tachycardia, hypertension, and vasodilation. Confirming diagnosis is usually based on arterial blood gas values for PCO_2 over the normal 45 mmHg and on pH values below the normal range of 7.35 to 7.45. Ineffective treatment of acute respiratory acidosis can lead to coma and death. Treatment of this condition seeks to remove or to inhibit the underlying causes of associated hypoventilation. Any airway obstructions are immediately removed. Treatment may include oxygen therapy and the intravenous administration of bronchodilators and sodium bicarbonate. NURSING CONSIDERATIONS: The patient with respiratory acidosis is carefully monitored for any changes in respiratory, cardiovascular, and CNS functions, arterial blood gas pressures, and electrolyte concentrations. In patients requiring mechanical ventilation, clear airways are maintained, and tracheal tubes are regularly suctioned. Also called primary carbon dioxide excess. Compare **metabolic acidosis.** See also **metabolic alkalosis, respiratory alkalosis.**

respiratory alkalosis   A condition characterized by decreased PCO_2, decreased hydrogen-ion concentration, and increased blood pH. It is caused by pulmonary and nonpulmonary problems. The hyperventilation associated with respiratory alkalosis most commonly stems from extreme anxiety. Respiratory alkalosis may also be iatrogenically induced by excessive mechanical ventilation. Deep and rapid breathing at rates as high as 40 respirations per minute is a major sign of respiratory alkalosis. Other symptoms are light-headedness, dizziness, peripheral paresthesia, spasms of the hands and the feet, muscle weakness, tetany, and cardiac arrhythmia. Confirming diagnosis is often based on PCO_2 levels below 35 mmHg, but the measurement of blood pH is critical in differentiating between metabolic acidosis and respiratory alkalosis. In the acute stage, blood pH rises in proportion to the fall in PCO_2, but in the chronic stage remains within the normal range of 7.35 to 7.45. The carbonic acid concentration is normal in the acute stage of this condition but below normal in the chronic stage. Treatment of respiratory alkalosis concentrates on removing the underlying causes. Severe cases, especially those caused by extreme anxiety, may be treated by having the patient breathe into a paper bag and inhale exhaled carbon dioxide to compensate for the deficit being created by hyperventilation. Sedatives may also be administered to decrease the respiration rate. Also called primary CO_2 deficit. Compare **metabolic alkalosis.** See also **metabolic acidosis, respiratory acidosis.** NURSING CONSIDERATIONS: The nurse monitors neurologic, neuromuscular, and cardiovascular functions, arterial blood gases, and serum electrolytes.

respiratory assessment   An evaluation of the condition and function of a person's respiratory system. The nurse asks if the person coughs, wheezes, is short of breath, tires easily, or experiences chest or abdominal pain, chills, fever, excessive sweating, dizziness, or swelling of feet and hands. Noted if present are signs of confusion, anxiety, or restlessness; flaring nostrils; cyanotic lips, gums, earlobes, or nails; clubbing of extremities; fever; anorexia; and a tendency to sit upright. The person's breathing is closely observed for evidence of slow, rapid, irregular, shallow, or Cheyne-Stokes respiration, hyperventilation, a long expiratory phase or periods of apnea, and for retractions in the suprasternal, supraclavicular, substernal, or intercostal areas during breathing. The presence of tachycardia, bradycardia, or sinus arrhythmia or evidence of congestive heart failure, as rales, rhonchi, edema, hepatosplenomegaly, abdominal distention, and pain, is recorded. The thorax is examined for scoliosis, kyphosis, funnel or barrel chest, or unequal shoulder height and is palpated for indications of thoracic expansion, tracheal deviation, crepitations, and fremitus. Percussion is performed to evaluate resonance, hyperresonance, tympany, dull or flat sounds; rales, rhonchi, wheezing, friction rubs, the transmission of spoken words through the chest wall, and decreased or absent breath sounds are detected by auscultation. Background information pertinent to the evaluation includes allergies, recent exposure to infection, immunizations, exposure to environmental irritants, previous respiratory disorders and operations, preexisting chronic conditions, medication currently taken, the persons's smoking habits, and the family history. Valuable diagnostic aids are a chest X-ray, complete blood count, electrocardiogram, pulmonary function tests, bronchoscopy, determinations of blood gases and electrolytes, studies of sputum, throat, or nasopharyngeal cultures, and gastric washings, lung scans, and biopsies. The nurse collects the background information and the results of diagnostic tests and may perform the examination. In a respiratory-care unit, a nurse clinician or practitioner may have greatly expanded responsibilities, as interpreting data from electrocardiographic tracings, setting up and adjusting a respirator, titrating medications, and obtaining specimens for blood gas determination. An accurate and thorough assessment of respiratory function is an essential component of the physical examination and is vital to the diagnosis or ongoing care of a respiratory illness.

respiratory burn   Tissue damage occurring in the respiratory system, resulting from the inhalation of a hot gas or burning particles, as may occur during a fire or explosion. Compare smoke inhalation. See also **burn**.

respiratory center A group of nerve cells in the pons and medulla of the brain that control the rhythm of breathing in response to changes in levels of oxygen and carbon dioxide in the blood and cerebrospinal fluid. Change in the concentration of oxygen and carbon dioxide or hydrogen ion levels in the arterial circulation and in cerebrospinal fluid activate central and peripheral chemoreceptors; these send impulses to the respiratory center, increasing or decreasing the breathing rate. This response is essential for normal breathing. The respiratory center is inhibited by barbiturates, anesthetics, tranquilizing agents, and morphine. See also **hyperventilation, hypoventilation**.

respiratory distress syndrome of the newborn (RDS) An acute lung disease of the newborn, characterized by airless alveoli, inelastic lungs, more than 60 respirations a minute, nasal flaring, intercostal and subcostal retractions, grunting on expiration, and peripheral edema. The condition occurs most often in premature infants and in infants of diabetic mothers. It is caused by a deficiency of pulmonary surfactant, resulting in overdistended alveoli and, at times, hyaline membrane formation, alveolar hemorrhage, severe right-to-left shunting of blood, increased pulmonary resistance, decreased cardiac output, and severe hypoxemia. The disease is self-limiting; the infant dies in 3 to 5 days or completely recovers with no aftereffects. Treatment includes measures to correct shock, acidosis, and hypoxemia and use of continuous positive airway pressure especially developed for infants to prevent alveolar collapse. Also called **hyaline membrane disease**. Compare **adult respiratory distress syndrome**.

respiratory exchange ratio (R) The ratio of the net expiration of carbon dioxide to the concurrent net inspiration of oxygen, expressed by the formula Vco_2/Vo_2.

respiratory failure The inability of the cardiac and pulmonary systems to maintain an adequate exchange of oxygen and carbon dioxide in the lungs. Respiratory failure may be hypoxemic or ventilatory. Hypoxemic failure is characterized by hyperventilation and occurs in diseases that affect the alveoli or interstitial tissues of the lobes of the lungs, as alveolar edema, emphysema, fungal infections, leukemia, lobar pneumonia, lung carcinoma, various pneumoconioses, pulmonary eosinophilia, sarcoidosis, or tuberculosis. Ventilatory failure, characterized by increased arterial tension of carbon dioxide, occurs in acute conditions in which retained pulmonary secretions cause increased airway resistance and decreased lung compliance, as in bronchitis and emphysema. Ventilation may also be reduced by depression of the respiratory center by barbiturates or opiates, hypoxia, hypercarbia, intracranial diseases, trauma, or by lesions of the neuromuscular system or thoracic cage. Treatment includes maintaining patency of airways by suction, broncho-

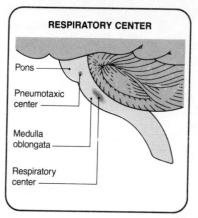

RESPIRATORY CENTER

Pons

Pneumotaxic center

Medulla oblongata

Respiratory center

dilators, or tracheostomy; antibiotics for infections; anticoagulants for pulmonary thromboemboli; and electrolyte replacement in fluid imbalance. Oxygen may be administered in some cases; in others it may further decrease the respiratory reflex by removing the stimulus of an elevated level of carbon dioxide. Respiratory failure may result in cor pulmonale with congestive heart failure and respiratory acidosis. See also **airway obstruction, carbon dioxide, hypercapnia, hyperventilation, hypoxemia, hypoxia, respiratory acidosis**.

respiratory rate The rate of breathing at rest, about 14 breaths per minute in an adult. The hydrogen ion concentration in the cerebrospinal fluid controls the rate of respiration. The rate may be more rapid in febrile states, severe systemic infection, diffuse pulmonary fibrosis, left ventricular failure, thyrotoxicosis, and in states of tension. Slower breathing rates may result from head injury, coma, or narcotic overdose.

respiratory rhythm A regular cycle of inspiration and expiration, controlled by neuronal impulses transmitted between the muscles of inspiration in the chest and the respiratory centers in the brain. The normal breathing pattern may be altered by a prolonged expiratory phase in obstructive diseases of the airway, as asthma, chronic bronchitis, and emphysema, or by Cheyne-Stokes respiration in patients with increased intracranial pressure or heart failure. See also **apnea, Biot's respiration, Hering-Breuer reflex, hyperventilation, hypoventilation, tachypnea**.

respiratory syncytial virus (RSV) A member of a subgroup of myxoviruses that causes formation of giant cells or syncytia in tissue culture. It is a common cause of epidemics of acute bronchiolitis, bronchopneumonia, and the common cold in young children and sporadic acute bronchitis and mild upper respiratory infections in adults. Symptoms of infection with this virus include fever, cough, and severe malaise. Treatment includes rest and the administration of aspirin and nasal decongestants. See also **bron-**

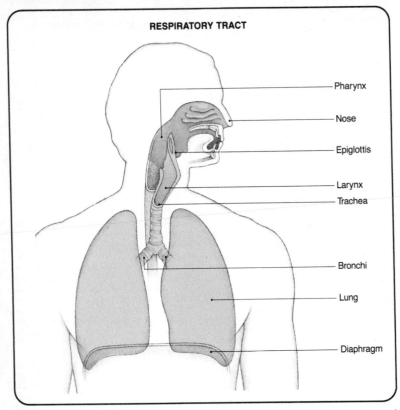

RESPIRATORY TRACT

Pharynx

Nose

Epiglottis

Larynx

Trachea

Bronchi

Lung

Diaphragm

chiolitis, bronchitis, bronchopneumonia, rhinovirus.

respiratory system See **respiratory tract.**

respiratory therapy (RT) **1.** Any treatment that maintains or improves the ventilatory function of the respiratory tract. **2.** *Informal.* The department in a health-care facility that provides respiratory therapy for the clients of the facility.

respiratory tract The complex of organs and structures that performs the pulmonary ventilation of the body and the exchange of oxygen and carbon dioxide between the ambient air and the blood circulating through the lungs. It also warms the air passing into the body and assists in the speech function by providing air for the vocal cords. Every 24 hours about 500 cubic feet of air passes through the respiratory tract of the average adult, who breathes in and out between 12 and 18 times a minute. The respiratory tract is divided into the upper respiratory tract and the lower respiratory tract. Also called **respiratory system.**

respiratory tract infection Any infectious disease of the upper or lower respiratory tract. **Upper respiratory infections** include the common cold, pharyngitis, rhinitis, sinusitis and tonsillitis. **Lower respiratory infections** in-

clude bronchitis, bronchiolitis, pneumonia, and tracheitis.

respondeat superior Latin for 'let the master answer.' A doctrine stating that an employer may be held liable for torts committed by employees acting within the scope of their employment.

respondent conditioning See **classical conditioning.**

restatement A paraphrase or rewording of another's idea without altering its original meaning.

resting cell A cell that is not undergoing division. See also **interphase.**

resting tremor See **passive tremor.**

restless legs syndrome A benign condition of unknown etiology characterized by an irritating sensation of uneasiness, tiredness, and itching deep within the muscles of the leg, especially the lower part of the limb, accompanied by twitching and, sometimes, by pain. The only relief is walking or moving the legs. The condition may be associated with various psychiatric disorders, probably as a form of extrapyramidal hyperkinesis. Also called **anxietas tibiarum, Ekbom syndrome, Wittmaack-Ekbom syndrome.**

restraint Any one of numerous devices used

in aiding the immobilization of patients, especially children, in traction. Some kinds of restraints are specially designed slings, jackets, or diapers. Restraints often involve a certain amount of emotional trauma for the patient involved and must be carefully employed.

restriction endonuclease In molecular genetics: an enzyme that cleaves DNA at a specific site. Each of the many different endonucleases isolated from various bacteria acts at a species-specific cleavage site, making it possible for researchers to divide DNA into discrete segments.

resuscitation The process of sustaining the vital functions of a person in respiratory or cardiac failure while reviving him, using techniques of artificial respiration and cardiac massage, correcting acid-base imbalance, and treating the cause of failure. See also **cardiopulmonary resuscitation. —resuscitate,** *v.*

resuscitator An apparatus for pumping air into the lungs. It consists of a mask snugly applied over the mouth and nose, a reservoir for air, and a manually or electrically powered pump. Often oxygen may be added to the air in the reservoir.

RET *abbr* **rational emotive therapy.**

retarded Of physical, intellectual, social, or emotional development: abnormally slow. **—retard,** *v.*, **retardation,** *n.*

retarded dentition The abnormal delay of the eruption of the deciduous or permanent teeth resulting from malnutrition, malposition of the teeth, a hereditary factor, or a metabolic imbalance, as hypothyroidism. Also called **delayed dentition.** Compare **precocious dentition.**

retarded depression The depressive phase of bipolar disorder.

retch A strong attempt to vomit without bringing up anything. Compare **eructation, vomit.**

rete A network, especially of arteries or veins. **—retial,** *adj.*

retention 1. A resistance to movement or displacement. 2. The ability of the digestive system to hold food and fluid. 3. The inability to urinate or defecate. 4. The ability of the mind to remember information acquired from reading, observation, or other processes. **—retain,** *v.*

retention of urine An abnormal, involuntary accumulation of urine in the bladder as a result of a loss of muscle tone in the bladder, neurologic dysfunction or damage to the bladder, obstruction of the urethra, or the administration of a narcotic analgesic, especially morphine.

reticul- A combining form meaning 'netlike': *recticulation, reticulocyte, reticulopod.*

reticular Of a tissue or surface: having a netlike pattern or structure of veins.

reticular activating system (RAS) A functional (rather than a morphologic) system in the brain essential for wakefulness, attention, concentration, and introspection. A network of

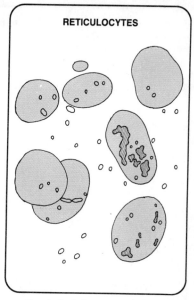

RETICULOCYTES

nerve fibers in the thalamus, hypothalamus, brain stem, and cerebral cortex contribute to the system.

reticular formation A small, thick, cluster of neurons, nestled within the brain stem, that controls breathing, heartbeat, blood pressure, level of consciousness, and other vital functions of the body. The reticular formation constantly monitors the state of the body through connections with the sensory and the motor tracts. Certain nerve cells in the formation regulate the flow of hydrochloric acid in the stomach; other cells regulate swallowing and tongue, eye, and facial movements.

reticulocyte An immature erythrocyte characterized by a meshlike pattern of threads and particles at the former site of the nucleus. Reticulocytes normally make up less than 1% of the circulating erythrocytes; a greater proportion reflects an increased rate of erythropoiesis.

reticuloendothelial system (RES) A functional, rather than anatomical, system of the body involved primarily in defense against infection and in disposal of the products of the breakdown of cells. It is made up of macrophages, the Kupffer's cells of the liver, and the reticulum cells of the lungs, bone marrow, spleen, and lymph nodes. Disorders of this system include **eosinophilic granuloma, Gaucher's disease, Hand-Schüller-Christian syndrome, Niemann-Pick disease.**

reticuloendotheliosis An abnormal condition characterized by increased growth and proliferation of the cells of the reticuloendothelial system. See **reticuloendothelial system.**

reticulosarcoma See **undifferentiated malignant lymphoma.**

reticulum cell sarcoma See **histiocytic**

RETINA

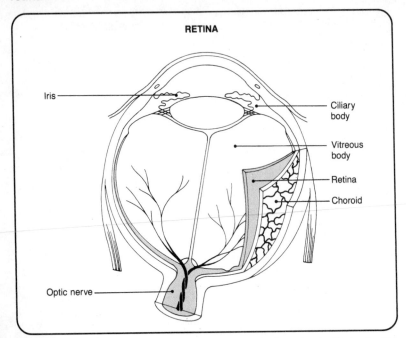

Iris

Ciliary body

Vitreous body

Retina

Choroid

Optic nerve

malignant lymphoma.

retina A 10-layered, delicate, nervous tissue membrane of the eye, continuous with the optic nerve, that receives images of external objects and transmits visual impulses through the optic nerve to the brain. The retina is soft, semitransparent, and contains rhodopsin, which gives it a purple tint. The retina becomes clouded and opaque if exposed to direct sunlight. It consists of an outer pigmented layer and a 9-layered retina proper. The outer surface of the retina is in contact with the choroid; the inner surface with the vitreous body. The retina is thinner anteriorly where it extends nearly as far as the ciliary body and thicker posteriorly, except for a thin spot in the exact center of the posterior surface where focus is best. The nervous fibers end anteriorly in the jagged ora serrata at the ciliary body, but the membrane of the retina extends over the back of the ciliary processes and the iris. See also **Jacob's membrane, macula, optic disk.**

retinaculum, *pl.* **retinacula** 1. A structure that retains an organ or tissue. 2. An instrument for retracting tissues during surgery.

retinaculum extensorum manus The thick band of antebrachial fascia that wraps tendons of the extensor muscles of the forearm at the distal ends of the radius and the ulna. Also called **dorsal carpal ligament, extensor retinaculum of the hand.** Compare **retinaculum flexorum manus.**

retinaculum flexorum manus The thick, fibrous band of antebrachial fascia that wraps the carpal canal surrounding the tendons of flexor

muscles of the forearm at the distal ends of the radius and the ulna. Also called **flexor retinaculum of the hand, volar ligament.**

retinal An aldehyde preform of vitamin A produced by the enzymatic dehydration of retinol. It is the active form of the vitamin necessary for night, day, and color vision. See also **retinene, vitamin A.**

retinal detachment A separation of the retina from the choroid in the back of the eye, usually resulting from a hole in the retina that allows the vitreous humor to leak between the choroid and the retina. Severe trauma to the eye, as a contusion or penetrating wound, may be the proximate cause, but in most cases it is the result of internal changes in the vitreous chamber associated with aging, or, less frequently, owing to inflammation of the interior of the eye. NURSING CONSIDERATIONS: Usually, retinal detachment develops slowly. The first symptom is often the sudden appearance of a large number of spots floating loosely suspended in front of the affected eye. The person may not seek help, as the number of spots tends to decrease during days and weeks following the detachment. The person may also notice a curious sensation of flashing lights as the eye is moved. Because the retina does not contain sensory nerves that relay sensations of pain, the condition is painless. Detachment usually begins at the thin peripheral edge of the retina and extends gradually beneath the thicker, more central areas. The person perceives a shadow that begins laterally and grows in size slowly encroaching on central vision. As long as the center of the retina is unaffected, the vision, when looking straight ahead, is normal; when the center becomes affected, the eyesight is distorted, wavy, and indistinct. If the process of detachment is not halted, total blindness results. Surgery is usually required. If the condition is discovered early, when the hole is small and the volume of vitreous humor lost is not large, the retinal hole may be closed by causing a scar to form on the choroid and to adhere to the retina around the hole. The scar may be produced by heat, lasers, electrical current, or cold. The scar is held against the retina by local pressure achieved by a variety of surgical techniques. The degree of sight restoration depends on the extent and duration of separation.

retinene Either of the two carotenoid pigments found in the rods of the retina that are preforms of vitamin A and are activated by light. See also **retinal, retinol.**

retinoblastoma, *pl.* **retinoblastomas, retinoblastomata** A congenital, hereditary neoplasm developing from retinal germ cells. It is the most common malignancy of the eye in childhood. Characteristic signs are diminished vision, strabismus, retinal detachment, and an abnormal pupillary reflex. The rapidly growing tumor may invade the brain and metastasize to distant sites. Treatment includes removal of the eye and as much of the optic nerve as possible, followed by radiation and chemotherapy.

retinocerebral angiomatosis See **cerebroretinal angiomatosis.**

retinol The cis-trans form of vitamin A. It is found in the retinas of mammals. Also called **vitamin A$_1$.**

retraction of the chest The visible sinking-in of the soft tissues of the chest between and around the firmer tissue of the cartilagenous and bony ribs, as occurs with increased inspiratory effort. Retraction begins in the intercostal spaces. If increased effort is needed to fill the lungs, supraclavicular and infraclavicular retraction may be seen. In infants, sternal retraction occurs with only slight increase in respiratory effort, owing to the pliability of their chests. Compare **intercostal bulging.**

retractor An instrument for holding back the edges of tissues and organs to maintain exposure of the underlying anatomy, particularly during surgery, as an army retractor or a double-ended Richardson retractor.

retro- A combining form meaning 'backward, or located behind': *retronasal, retroperitoneal.*

retroaortic node A node in one of three sets of lumbar lymph nodes that serve various structures in the abdomen and the pelvis. They lie below the cisterna chyli on the bodies of the third and the fourth lumbar vertebrae and receive the lymphatic trunks from the lateral aortic nodes and preaortic nodes. Compare **lateral aortic node, preaortic node.**

retroflexion The bending or flexing backward of an organ, as the bending backward of the body of the uterus at an angle with the cervix.

retrograde 1. Moving backward; moving in

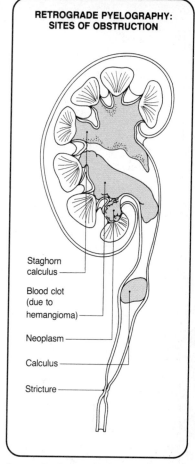

RETROGRADE PYELOGRAPHY: SITES OF OBSTRUCTION

Staghorn calculus

Blood clot (due to hemangioma)

Neoplasm

Calculus

Stricture

the opposite direction to that which is considered normal. **2.** Degenerating; reverting to an earlier state or worse condition. **3.** Catabolic.

retrograde amnesia The loss of memory for events occurring before a particular time in a person's life. The condition may result from disease, brain injury or damage, or a traumatic emotional incident. Compare **anterograde amnesia.** See also **amnesia.**

retrograde cystoscopy A technique in radiology for examining the bladder in which a catheter is inserted through the urethra into the bladder, allowing the urine present in the bladder to pass through the catheter. See also **cystogram, retrograde pyelography.**

retrograde infantilism See **acromegalic eunuchoidism.**

retrograde pyelography A technique in radiology for examining the structures of the kidney's collecting system that is especially useful in locating an obstruction in the urinary tract. A radiopaque contrast medium is injected

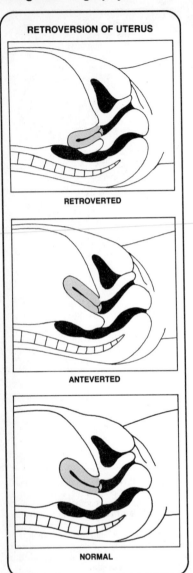

RETROVERSION OF UTERUS

RETROVERTED

ANTEVERTED

NORMAL

through a urinary catheter into the ureters and the calyces of the pelves of the kidneys. Rarely, severe anaphylactoid reaction to the medium may occur, owing to a patient's hypersensitivity to the iodine in the medium.

retrograde urography   See **retrograde pyelography.**

retrogression   A return to a less complex state, condition, or behavioral adaptation; degeneration; deterioration. See also **regression.**

retroperitoneal   Of or pertaining to organs closely attached to the abdominal wall and partly covered by peritoneum, rather than suspended by that membrane.

retroperitoneal fibrosis   A chronic inflammatory process, usually of unknown cause, in which fibrous tissue surrounds the large blood vessels in the lower lumbar area. It frequently causes constriction of the midportion of the ureters, which may lead to hydronephrosis and azotemia. Occasionally the fibrosis spreads upward to involve the duodenum, bile ducts, and superior vena cava. Symptoms include low-back and abdominal pain, weakness, weight loss, fever, and, with urinary tract involvement, frequency of urination, hematuria, polyuria, or anuria. Methysergide, taken to prevent migraine headaches, is one known cause of this condition. Treatment includes stopping methysergide and surgical release of the ureters from the fibrosis with transplantation.

retroperitoneal lymph node dissection   Surgical removal of lymph nodes behind the peritoneum, usually performed in an attempt to eliminate sites of lymphoma or metastases from malignancies originating in pelvic organs or genitalia.

retropharyngeal abscess   A collection of pus in the tissues behind the pharynx accompanied by difficulty in swallowing, fever, and pain. Occasionally, the airway becomes obstructed. Treatment includes appropriate parenteral antibiotics and surgical drainage. Tracheostomy may be necessary. Compare **parapharyngeal abscess, peritonsillar abscess.**

retroplacental   Behind the placenta.

retrospective chart audit   A format for an audit developed by the Joint Commission on the Accreditation of Hospitals. The audit involves several steps that outline a procedure for evaluating the effectiveness of the care given at a particular institution and for correcting any deficiencies found by reviewing the patient's records after discharge and comparing the data with standards held to be adequate by the Commission.

retrospective study   A study in which a search is made for a relationship between one (usually current) phenomenon or condition and another that occurred in the past.

retrouterine   Behind the uterus.

retroversion   A common condition in which an organ is tipped backward, usually without flexion or other distortion. The uterus may be retroverted in as many as one fourth of normal women. No treatment is necessary. Compare **anteversion.** See also **anteflexion, retroflexion.** —**retrovert,** *v.*

retrovirus   A member of a family of viruses that includes the oncoviruses.

Reverdin's needle   A surgical needle with an eye that can be opened and closed with a slide.

reverse anaphylaxis   See **inverse anaphylaxis.**

reverse Barton's fracture   A fracture of the volar articular surface of the radius with associated displacement of the carpal bones and radius.

reversed bandage   A roller bandage that is reversed on itself with a half twist so that it lies smoothly, conforming to the contour of the extremity. See also **roller bandage**.

reversed coarctation   See **Takayasu's arteritis.**

reverse isolation   Isolation procedures designed to protect a patient from infectious organisms that might be carried by the staff, other patients, or visitors, or on droplets in the air or on equipment or materials. Absolute reverse isolation is rarely necessary and requires elaborate specialized equipment. Protective modified reverse isolation is less restrictive but is not prolonged needlessly as the patient usually feels lonely and sensorily deprived. Handwashing, gowning, gloving, sterilization or disinfection of materials brought into the area, and other details of housekeeping vary with the reason for the isolation and the usual practices of the hospital.

review committee   A group of individuals delegated to inspect and report on the quality of health care in a given institution.

review of systems (ROS)   In a health history: a system-by-system review of the functions of the body. The ROS is begun during the initial interview with the patient and completed during the physical examination, as physical findings prompt further questions. One outline of the systems and some of the signs and symptoms that might be noted or reported are as follows:

SKIN: bruising, discoloration, pruritus, birthmarks, moles, ulcers, decubiti, changes in the hair or nails.

HEMATOPOIETIC: spontaneous or excessive bleeding, fatigue, enlarged or tender lymph nodes, pallor, history of anemia.

HEAD AND FACE: pain, traumatic injury, ptosis.

EARS: ringing in the ears, change in hearing, running or discharge from the ears, deafness, dizziness.

EYES: change in vision, pain, inflammation, infections, double vision, scotomata, blurring, tearing.

MOUTH AND THROAT: dental problems, hoarseness, dysphagia, bleeding gums, sore throat, ulcers or sores in the mouth.

NOSE AND SINUSES: discharge, epistaxis, sinus pain, obstruction.

BREASTS: pain, change in contour or skin color, lumps, discharge from the nipple.

RESPIRATORY TRACT: cough, sputum, change in sputum, night sweats, nocturnal dyspnea, wheezing.

CARDIOVASCULAR SYSTEM: chest pain, dyspnea, palpitations, weakness, intolerance of exercise, varicosities, swelling of extremities, known murmur, high blood pressure, asystole.

GASTROINTESTINAL SYSTEM: nausea, vomiting, diarrhea, constipation, quality of appetite, change in appetite, dysphagia, gas, heartburn, melena, change in bowel habits, use of laxatives or other drugs to alter the function of the GI tract.

REYE'S SYNDROME: CLINICAL STAGES

Stage I: vomiting, lethargy, hepatic dysfunction

Stage II: hyperventilation, delirium, hepatic dysfunction, hyperactive reflexes

Stage III: coma, hyperventilation, decorticate rigidity, hepatic dysfunction

Stage IV: deepening coma; decerebrate rigidity; large, fixed pupils; minimal hepatic dysfunction

Stage V: seizures, loss of deep tendon reflexes, flacidity, respiratory arrest, ammonia above 300 mg/100 ml

---

URINARY TRACT: dysuria, change in color of urine, change in frequency of urination, pain with urgency, incontinence, edema, retention.

GENITAL TRACT, MALE: penile discharge, pain or discomfort, pruritus, skin lesions, hematuria, history of venereal disease.

GENITAL TRACT, FEMALE: menstrual history, obstetric history, contraceptive use, discharge, pain or discomfort, pruritus, history of venereal disease.

SKELETAL SYSTEM: heat, redness, swelling, limitation of function, deformity, crepitation, pain in a joint or an extremity, the neck, or back, especially with movement.

NERVOUS SYSTEM: dizziness, tremor, ataxia, difficulty in speaking, change in speech, paresthesia, loss of sensation, seizures, syncope.

ENDOCRINE SYSTEM: tremor, palpitations, intolerance of heat or cold, polyuria, polydipsia, polyphagia, diaphoresis, exophthalmos, goiter.

PSYCHOLOGIC STATUS: nervousness, instability, despression, phobia, sexual disturbances, criminal behavior, insomnia, night terrors, mania, memory loss, perseveration, disorientation.

Reye's syndrome   A combination of acute encephalopathy and fatty infiltration of the internal organs that may follow acute viral infections. This syndrome has been associated with influenza B, chicken pox (varicella), the enteroviruses, and the Epstein-Barr virus. It has also been epidemiologically associated, in children, with administration of aspirin and other salicylates. The syndrome usually affects people under 18 years old, characteristically causing an exanthematous rash, vomiting, and confusion about 1 week after the onset of a viral illness. Mortality varies between 20% and 80%, depending on the severity of symptoms. The cause of Reye's syndrome is unknown and there is no specific treatment available.

R factor   An episome in bacteria that is responsible for drug resistance and is transmissible to progeny and to other bacterial cells by conjugation. The portion of the episome involved in replication and transmission is called resistance transfer factor.

RFP *abbr* **request for proposal.**

RF (rheumatoid factor) test See **latex fixation test.**

Rh Symbol for **rhodium.**

-rh- For combining forms containing -rh-, see **-(r)rhachia, -(r)rhage,** etc.

rhabdo-, rhabdi- A combining form meaning 'rod-shaped, or of or pertaining to a rod': *rhabdocyte, rhabdomyoma.*

rhabdomyoma, *pl.* **rhabdomyomas, rhabdomyomata** A tumor of striated muscle that may occur in the uterus, vagina, pharynx, and tongue, and in the heart as congenital neoplastic nodules. Also called **myoma striocellulare.**

rhabdomyosarcoma, *pl.* **rhabdomyosarcomas, rhabdomyosarcomata** A highly malignant tumor, derived from primitive striated muscle cells, that occurs most frequently in the head and neck and is also found in the genitourinary tract, extremities, body wall, and retroperitoneum. In some cases, the onset is associated with trauma. The initial symptoms depend on the site of tumor development and indicate local tissue or organ destruction, as dysphagia, vaginal bleeding, hematuria, or the obstruction of the flow of urine. Diagnostic measures may include barium X-ray studies, angiography, or tomography. Embryonal rhabdomyosarcoma occurs in the head, neck, or trunk of young children; alveolar rhabdomyosarcoma is usually seen in the extremities of adolescents, and the pleomorphic form is most common in the legs of adults. Surgical excision is rarely possible, because the tumor is poorly encapsulated and tends to spread. Amputation of an affected limb or extremity may be curative. Radiotherapy and chemotherapy with combinations of actinomycin D, adriamycin, cyclophosphamide, and vincristine may greatly increase the length of survival.

rhabdovirus A member of a family of viruses that includes the organism causing rabies.

rhachi- See **rachio-.**

rhagades Cracks or fissures in skin that has lost its elasticity, especially common around the mouth. See also **cheilosis.**

rhaphe See **raphe.**

Rh₀(D) immune globulin A passive immunizing agent given after abortion, miscarriage, ectopic pregnancy, or delivery. It is prescribed to prevent Rh sensitization. It is not given to an $Rh_0(D)$ positive patient or to the infant. The most serious adverse reaction is anaphylaxis.

rhenium (Re) A hard, brittle, metallic element. Its atomic number is 75; its atomic weight is 186.2. Rhenium has a high melting point and is used in thermometers for measuring high temperatures.

rheo- A combining form meaning 'of or pertaining to electric current, or to a flow': *rheobase, rheoscope, rheotaxis.*

Rhesus factor See **Rh factor.**

-rheumatic A combining form meaning 'relating to or exhibiting traits of rheumatism': *postrheumatic, prerheumatic.*

rheumatic Of or pertaining to rheumatism.

rheumatic aortitis Inflammation of the aorta, occurring in rheumatic fever and characterized by disseminated focal lesions that may progressively form fibrosis.

rheumatic arteritis A complication of rheumatic fever characterized by generalized inflammation of arteries and arterioles. Fibrin, mixed with cellular debris, may invade, thicken, and stiffen the vessel wall, and the vessel may be surrounded by hemorrhage and exudate.

rheumatic chorea See **Sydenham's chorea.**

rheumatic fever An inflammatory disease that may develop as a delayed reaction to inadequately treated Group A beta-hemolytic streptococcal infection of the upper respiratory tract. This disorder usually occurs in young school-age children and may affect the brain, heart, joints, skin, or subcutaneous tissues. The onset is usually sudden, often occurring in from 1 to 5 symptom-free weeks following recovery from a sore throat or from scarlet fever. Early symptoms usually include fever, joint pain, nose bleeds, abdominal pain, and vomiting. The major manifestations of this disease include migratory polyarthritis affecting numerous joints and carditis, which causes palpitations, chest pain, and, in severe cases, symptoms of cardiac failure. Sydenham's chorea, which may develop, is usually the sole, late sign of rheumatic fever and may initially be manifested as an increased awkwardness and an associated tendency to drop objects. As the chorea progresses, irregular body movements may become extensive, occasionally involving the tongue and the facial muscles. Other developments may include transient erythema marginatum with circular lesions and subcutaneous rheumatic nodules on various joints and tendons, the spine, and the back of the head. There is no specific diagnostic test for rheumatic fever. The development of serum antibodies to streptococcal antigens is a positive diagnostic sign. Affected individuals may also develop leukocytosis, moderate anemia, and proteinuria. C-reactive protein, evaluated in a specimen of blood, is abnormally high. Recurrences of rheumatic fever are common. Except for carditis, all the manifestations of this disease usually subside without any permanent effects. Mild cases may last 3 to 4 weeks. Severe cases with associated arthritis and carditis may last 2 to 3 months. Management of this disease includes bed rest and severe restriction of normal activity. Penicillin is often administered, even if throat cultures are negative, and steroids or salicylates may be used, depending on the severity of any associated carditis and arthritis.

NURSING CONSIDERATIONS: Symptoms largely determine the type of nursing care. Large volumes of fluids are usually administered. The nurse also provides emotional support and helps minimize joint pain by properly positioning the patient.

rheumatic heart disease　Damage to heart muscle and heart valves caused by episodes of rheumatic fever. When a susceptible person acquires a group A beta-hemolytic streptococcal infection, an autoimmune reaction may occur in heart tissue, resulting in permanent deformities of heart valves or chordae tendineae. Involvement of the heart may be evident during acute rheumatic fever, or it may be discovered long after the acute disease has subsided. It is characterized by heart murmurs owing to stenosis or insufficiency of the valves and by compensatory alterations in the size of the chambers of the heart and the thickness of their walls. Abnormalities of pulse rate and rhythm, heart block, and congestive heart failure are also common. Deaths are usually due to heart failure or bacterial endocarditis. Episodes of acute rheumatic fever must be vigorously treated and supportive therapy given for heart failure. Chronic rheumatic heart disease may require no immediate treatment except for close observation. If signs of inefficient or decompensating heart action occur, digitalis, diuretics, and a low-sodium diet are often prescribed. In some patients, surgical commissurotomy or valve replacement is necessary. Patients with a history of rheumatic fever or evidence of rheumatic heart disease, in order to prevent streptococcal infection, should receive daily prophylactic penicillin by mouth or monthly intramuscular injections of benzathene penicillin, at least during childhood and adolescence. Patients with evidence of deformed heart valves should be given prophylactic antibiotics before surgical and dental procedures to prevent bacterial endocarditis. See also **aortic stenosis, mitral stenosis, rheumatic fever.** NURSING CONSIDERATIONS: Nurses have a responsibility to help educate patients about the disease and how to recognize the early symptoms and signs of its complications. It is especially important to stress the regular use of prophylactic penicillin to prevent streptococcal infections and the need to take special prophylactic antibiotics before surgery and all dental procedures.

rheumatism　*Nontechnical.* **1.** Any of a large number of inflammatory conditions of the bursae, joints, ligaments, or muscles characterized by pain, limitation of movement, and structural degeneration of single or multiple parts of the musculoskeletal system. **2.** The syndrome of pain, limitation of movement, and structural degeneration of elements in the musculoskeletal system as may occur in gout, rheumatoid arthritis, systemic lupus erythematosus, ankylosing spondylitis, and many other diseases. —**rheumatic,** *adj.,* **rheumatoid,** *adj.*

rheumatoid arthritis　A chronic, destructive, sometimes deforming, collagen disease that has an autoimmune component. It is characterized by symmetrical inflammation of the synovium and increased synovial exudate, leading to thickening of the synovium and swelling of

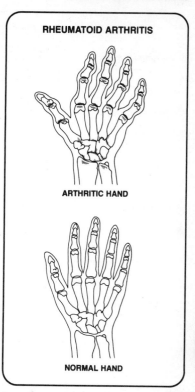

RHEUMATOID ARTHRITIS

ARTHRITIC HAND

NORMAL HAND

the joint. It usually first appears in early middle age, between 36 and 50 years of age, and most commonly in women. The course of the disease is variable but is most frequently marked by remission and exacerbation. A kind of rheumatoid arthritis that occurs in younger people is **Still's disease.** Rheumatoid arthritis may first present itself with constitutional symptoms, including fatigue, weakness, and poor appetite. Other early signs include low-grade fever, anemia, and an increased erythrocyte sedimentation rate. The symptoms listed by the American Rheumatism Association include morning stiffness, joint pain or tenderness, swelling of at least two joints, subcutaneous nodules (called arthritic nodules and usually found at pressure points, as the elbows), structural changes in the joint seen on X-ray film, a positive rheumatoid factor agglutination test, decreased precipitation of mucin from synovial fluid, and characteristic histologic changes on pathologic examination of the fluid. Immune complexes are characteristically present in both the blood serum and the synovial fluid. Rheumatoid factor (RF) is present in serum and joint fluid of most persons with rheumatoid arthritis, and higher titers of RF are correlated with more severe forms of the disease, in particular those forms with extra-articular manifestations. Antinuclear antibodies and special rheumatoid precipitins are

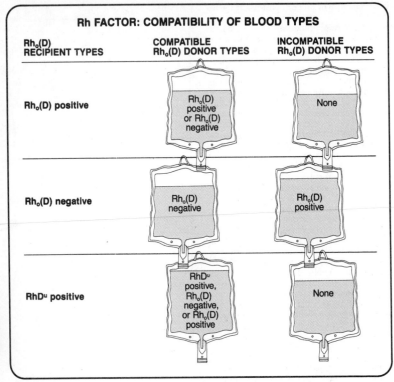

Rh FACTOR: COMPATIBILITY OF BLOOD TYPES

$Rh_o(D)$ RECIPIENT TYPES	COMPATIBLE $Rh_o(D)$ DONOR TYPES	INCOMPATIBLE $Rh_o(D)$ DONOR TYPES
$Rh_o(D)$ positive	$Rh_o(D)$ positive or $Rh_o(D)$ negative	None
$Rh_o(D)$ negative	$Rh_o(D)$ negative	$Rh_o(D)$ positive
RhD^u positive	RhD^u positive, $Rh_o(D)$ negative, or $Rh_o(D)$ positive	None

also occasionally present. Extra-articular manifestations may include cardiac involvement, vasculitis, pulmonary disease, and proteinuria. There may also be a thickening of the synovium, called pannus formation. In long-term, severe, chronic rheumatoid arthritis, Felty's syndrome may be present, characterized by splenomegaly, leukopenia, and frequent infections. The basic treatment includes sufficient rest, exercise to maintain joint function, medication for the relief of pain and the reduction of inflammation, orthopedic intervention to prevent or correct deformities, and excellent nutrition, with weight loss, if necessary. Salicylates are usually given to alleviate inflammation. If improvement is not achieved other anti-inflammatories, as indomethacin, phenylbutazone, penicillamine, antimalarials, gold salts, or some antineoplastic drugs may be used. Corticosteroids are prescribed with caution because of side effects. Other treatments, including diathermy, ultrasonography, warm paraffin applications, hydrotherapy with exercise, and applications of heat are occasionally used. Also called **arthritis deformans, atrophic arthritis.**

NURSING CONSIDERATIONS: As rheumatoid arthritis is not always progressive, deforming, or debilitating and as early treatment may help the person to recover and perhaps to avoid future attacks, most people who have rheumatoid arthritis may continue in their jobs. As stress often precedes exacerbation of the condition, the person is counseled to avoid situations known to cause anxiety, fatigue, infection, and other stressors.

rheumatoid coronary arteritis An abnormal condition, characterized by a thickening of the tunica intima of the coronary arteries, which may produce coronary insufficiency. This collagen disease causes inflammation and fibrinoid degeneration of connective tissue and is commonly treated with glucocorticoids.

rheumatoid factor (RF) Antiglobulin antibodies often found in the serum of patients with rheumatoid arthritis. Rheumatoid factors are present in about 70% of such cases, but they may also be found in such widely divergent diseases as tuberculosis, parasitic infections, and leukemia. See also **latex fixation test.**

rheumatologist A specialist in rheumatology.

rheumatology The study of disorders characterized by inflammation, degeneration, or metabolic derangement of connective tissue. These disorders are sometimes referred to collectively as rheumatism.

Rh factor, $Rh_o(D)$ antigen An antigenic substance present in the erythrocytes of most people. A person having the factor is Rh+ (Rh positive); a person lacking the factor is Rh−

(Rh negative). Transfusion, blood typing, and cross matching depend on Rh+ and ABO classification. If an Rh− person receives Rh+ blood, hemolysis and anemia occur. Rh+ infants may be exposed to antibodies to the factor produced in the Rh− mother's blood, resulting in red blood cell destruction and erythroblastosis fetalis. If a person has the D^u variant of the Rh factor, he is considered an Rh+ donor, but an Rh− recipient to avoid a possible mild hemolytic reaction. The Rh factor was first isolated and identified in the blood of a species of the rhesus monkey. It is present in the red blood cells of 85% of the population.

rhigo-   A combining form meaning 'cold': *rhigolene*, *rhigosis*.

rhin-   See **rhino-**.

Rh incompatibility   In hematology: a lack of compatibility between two groups of blood cells that are antigenically different owing to the presence of the Rh factor in one group and its absence in the other. See also **Rh factor**.

rhinencephalon, *pl.* **rhinencephala**   A portion of each cerebral hemisphere that contains the limbic system, which is associated with the emotions. See also **limbic system**. —**rhinencephalic**, *adj.*

rhinitis   Inflammation of the nasal mucous membranes, usually accompanied by mucosal swelling and nasal discharge. It may be complicated by sinusitis. Also called **coryza**.

rhino-, rhin-   A combining form meaning 'of or pertaining to the nose or to a noselike structure': *rhinocephalia*, *rhinolalia*.

rhinopathy   Any disease or malformation of the nose.

rhinophyma   A form of rosacea in which there is sebaceous hyperplasia, redness, prominent vascularity, swelling, and distortion of the skin of the nose. Treatment includes dermabrasion, electrosurgery, and plastic surgery. See also **rosacea**.

rhinoplasty   A procedure in plastic surgery in which the structure of the nose is changed. Bone or cartilage may be removed, tissue grafted from another part of the body, or synthetic material implanted to alter the shape. Under local anesthesia, intranasal incisions are made, and the nose is reshaped. Postoperatively, any respiratory difficulty is reported immediately and the patient is kept in mid-Fowler's position. Frequent oral care is given and ice compresses are applied to decrease the pain and edema that usually occur. Edema and discoloration around the eyes last for several days. The procedure is often performed for cosmetic reasons.

rhinoscope   An instrument for examining the nasal passages through the anterior nares or through the nasopharynx.

rhinoscopy   An examination of the nasal passages to inspect the mucosa and detect inflammation, deformities, or asymmetry, as in deviation of the septum. The nasal passages may be examined anteriorly, by introducing a speculum into the anterior nares, or posteriorly, by introducing a rhinoscope through the naso-

pharynx. —**rhinoscopic**, *adj.*

rhinosporidiosis   An infection caused by the fungus *Rhinosporidium seeberi*, characterized by fleshy red polyps on mucous membranes of the nose, conjunctiva, nasopharynx, and soft palate. The disease may be acquired by swimming or bathing in infected water. The most effective treatment is electrocautery.

rhinotomy   A surgical procedure in which an incision is made along one side of the nose, performed to drain accumulated pus from an abcess or a sinus infection.

rhinovirus   Any of about 100 serologically distinct, small RNA viruses that cause about 40% of acute respiratory illnesses. Infection is characterized by dry, scratchy throat, nasal congestion, malaise, and headache. Fever is minimal. Nasal discharge lasts 2 or 3 days. Children may also develop a cough. Treatment is nonspecific and may include rest, analgesics, antihistamines, and nasal decongestants. Complete recovery is usual. Compare **adenovirus, parainfluenza virus, respiratory syncytial virus**.

rhitid-   See **rhytid-**.

rhitidosis, rhytidosis   A wrinkling, especially of the cornea.

rhizo-   A combining form meaning 'of or related to a root': *rhizodontropy*, *rhizome*.

Rh negative   See **Rh factor**.

Rhodesian trypanosomiasis   An acute form of African trypanosomiasis, caused by the parasite *Trypanosoma brucei rhodesiense*. The disease may progress rapidly, causing encephalitis, coma, and death in only a few weeks. Also called **kaodzera**. Compare **Gambian trypanosomiasis**. See also **African trypanosomiasis**.

rhodium (Rh)   A gray-white metallic element. Its atomic number is 45; its atomic weight is 102.91. It is used to provide a hard lustrous coating on other metals and to make mirrors.

rhodo-   A combining form meaning 'red': *rhodocyte*, *rhodoplast*.

rhodopsin   The purple pigmented compound in the rods of the retina, formed by a protein, opsin, and a derivative of vitamin A, retinal. Rhodopsin adapts the eye to low-density light. The compound breaks down when struck by light, and this chemical change triggers the conduction of nerve impulses. Brief periods of darkness allow the opsin and the retinal to reconstitute the rhodopsin, which accounts for the short delay a person experiences in adapting to sudden or drastic changes in lighting, as when moving out of bright sunlight into a darkened room or from darkness into bright light. Closing the eyes is a natural reflex that allows reconstitution of rhodopsin. Compare **iodopsin**.

rhomboideus major   A muscle of the upper back below and parallel to the rhomboideus minor. Arising from the spinous processes of the third, fourth, and fifth thoracic vertebrae and inserting into the lower half of the medial border of the scapula, it is innervated by the dorsal scapular nerve from the brachial plexus and, with the rhomboideus minor, functions to draw

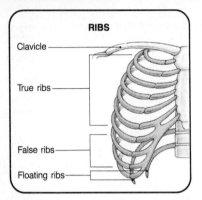

RIBS

Clavicle

True ribs

False ribs

Floating ribs

the scapula toward the vertebral column while supporting it and drawing it slightly upward. Compare **latissimus dorsi, levator scapulae, rhomboideus minor, trapezius.**

rhomboideus minor   A muscle of the upper back, above and parallel to the rhomboideus major. It arises from the ligamentum nuchae and from the spinous processes of the seventh cervical and first thoracic vertebrae. It inserts into the upper part of the medial border at the root of the spine of the scapula. It is innervated by the dorsal scapular nerve from the brachial plexus, which contains fibers from the fifth cervical nerve, and, with the rhomboideus major, acts to draw the scapula toward the vertebral column, while supporting the scapula and drawing it slightly upward. Compare **latissimus dorsi, levator scapulae, rhomboideus major, trapezius.**

rhomboid glossitis   See **median rhomboid glossitis.**

rhonchi, *sing.* **rhonchus**   Abnormal sounds heard on auscultation of a respiratory airway obstructed by thick secretions, muscular spasm, neoplasm, or external pressure. The continuous rumbling sounds are more pronounced during expiration, and they characteristically clear on coughing. Rhonchi may be sibilant or sonorous. Sibilant rhonchi are high pitched and are heard in the small bronchi, as in asthma. Sonorous rhonchi are lower pitched and are heard in the large bronchi, as in tracheobronchitis. Compare **rale, wheeze.**

rhotacism   A speech disorder characterized by a defective pronunciation of words with the sound 'r,' by the excessive use of the sound 'r,' or by the substitution of another sound for 'r.' Compare **lallation, lambdacism.**

Rh positive   See **Rh factor.**

rhus dermatitis   A skin rash resulting from contact with a plant of the genus *Rhus*, as poison ivy, poison oak, or poison sumac. See also **contact dermatitis.**

rhyp-   A combining form meaning 'of or pertaining to filth': *rhyparia, rhypophagy.*

rhythm method   See **natural family-planning method.**

rhytid-, rhitid-   A combining form meaning

'wrinkle or wrinkled': *rhytidectomy.*

rhytidoplasty, rhitidoplasty   A procedure in reconstructive plastic surgery in which the skin of the face is tightened, wrinkles are removed, and the skin is made to appear firm and smooth. A pressure dressing is applied and left in place for 24 to 48 hours. Postoperative medication for pain is often necessary. The sutures are removed several days after discharge in an outpatient facility or in the surgeon's office.

rhytidosis   See **rhitidosis.**

RIA   See **radioimmunoassay.**

rib   One of the 12 pairs of elastic arches of bone forming a large part of the thoracic skeleton. The first 7 ribs on each side are called the **true ribs,** because they articulate directly with the sternum and the vertebrae. The remaining 5 ribs are called the **false ribs.** The first 3 attach ventrally to the ribs above them; the last 2 are free at their ventral extremities and are called **floating ribs.**

riboflavin   A yellow, crystalline, water-soluble pigment, one of the heat-stable components of the B vitamin complex. It combines with specific flavoproteins and functions as a coenzyme in the oxidative processes of carbohydrates, fats, and proteins. It is also important in the prevention of some visual disorders, especially cataracts. It is not stored to any great degree in the body and must be supplied regularly in the diet. Common sources are organ meats, milk, cheese, eggs, green leafy vegetables, meat, whole grains, and legumes. Deficiency of riboflavin produces cheilosis, local inflammation, desquamation, encrustation, glossitis, photophobia, corneal opacities, proliferation of corneal vessels, seborrheic dermatitis about the nose, mouth, forehead, ears, and scrotum, trembling, sluggishness, dizziness, edema, inability to urinate, and vaginal itching. Also called **vitamin B$_2$.** See also **ariboflavinosis.**

ribonucleic acid (RNA)   A nucleic acid, found in both the nucleus and cytoplasm of cells, that transmits genetic instructions from the nucleus to the cytoplasm. In the cytoplasm, RNA functions in the assembly of proteins. See also **deoxyribonucleic acid.**

ribosome   A cytoplasmic organelle composed of ribonucleic acid and protein that functions in the synthesis of cellular protein. Ribosomes interact with messenger RNA and transfer RNA to join together amino acid units into a polypeptide chain according to the sequence determined by the genetic code. The structures appear singly or in clusters as polysomes, or they may be attached to endoplasmic reticulum. See also **translation.**

rice diet   A diet consisting only of rice, fruit, fruit juices, and sugar, supplemented with vitamins and iron. Salt is strictly forbidden. It is prescribed for the treatment of hypertension, chronic renal disease, and obesity. The diet is somewhat modified after blood pressure is lowered and other symptoms are alleviated. It should not be followed for any length of time, since the severe dietary restrictions may lead to nutri-

right bundle branch block

tional deficiencies or imbalance. Also called **Duke diet, Kempner rice-fruit diet.**

rickets A condition caused by the deficiency of vitamin D, calcium, and, usually, phosphorus, seen primarily in infancy and childhood, and characterized by abnormal bone formation. Symptoms include soft, pliable bones, causing deformities as bowlegs and knock-knees, nodular enlargements on the ends and sides of the bones, muscle pain, enlarged skull, chest deformities, spinal curvature, enlargement of the liver and spleen, profuse sweating, and general tenderness of the body when touched. Prophylaxis and treatment include a diet rich in calcium, phosphorus, and vitamin D and adequate exposure to sunlight. Kinds of rickets include **acute rickets, adult rickets, celiac rickets, renal rickets, vitamin D resistant rickets.** See also **osteodystrophy, osteomalacia, vitamin D.**

rickettsia, *pl.* **rickettsiae** Any organism of the genus *Rickettsia.* Rickettsiae are small, round, or rod-shaped bacteria that live as intracellular parasites in lice, fleas, ticks, and mites. They are transmitted to humans by bites from these insects. Rickettsial diseases have been responsible for many of history's worst epidemics. The various species are distinguished on the basis of similarities in the diseases they cause: the spotted fever group includes Rocky Mountain spotted fever, rickettsialpox, and others; the typhus group includes endemic and epidemic typhus; the tsutsugamushi group includes scrub typhus; a miscellaneous group includes Q fever and trench fever. Tetracycline or chloramphenicol is usually prescribed. —**rickettsial,** *adj.*

rickettsialpox A mild, acute infectious disease caused by *Rickettsia akari* and transmitted from mice to humans by mites. It is characterized by an asymptomatic, crusted primary lesion, chills, fever, headache, malaise, myalgia, and a rash resembling chicken pox. About 1 week after onset of symptoms, small, discrete, maculopapular lesions appear on any part of the body, but rarely on palms or soles. These lesions become vesicular and dry and form scabs. Eventually the scabs fall off, leaving no scars. Chloramphenicol or tetracycline will hasten recovery. Also called **Kew Gardens spotted fever.** Compare **chickenpox, smallpox.** See also **rickettsia.**

rickettsiosis, *pl.* **rickettsioses** Any of a group of infectious diseases caused by microorganisms of the genus *Rickettsia.* Kinds of rickettsioses include a spotted fever group (**boutonneuse fever, North Asian tick-borne rickettsiosis, Queensland tick typhus, rickettsialpox, Rocky Mountain spotted fever**), a typhus group (**epidemic typhus, murine typhus, scrub typhus**), and a miscellaneous group (**Q fever, trench fever**). See also **rickettsia.**

rider's bone A bony deposit that sometimes develops in horseback riders on the lower end of the tendon of the adductor muscle of the thigh. Also called **cavalry bone.**

ridge A projection or projecting structure,

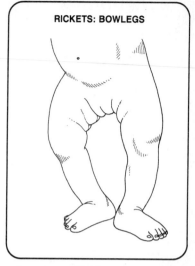

RICKETS: BOWLEGS

as the gastrocnemial ridge on the posterior surface of the femur, giving attachment to the gastrocnemius muscle.

Riedel's thyroiditis See **fibrous thyroiditis.**

Rieder cell leukemia A malignant neoplasm of blood-forming tissues, characterized by the presence in blood of large numbers of atypical myeloblasts with immature cytoplasm and relatively mature lobulated, indented nuclei.

rifampin An antibacterial antitubercular agent.

Rift Valley fever An arbovirus infection of east and south Africa spread by mosquitoes or by handling infected sheep and cattle. It is characterized by abrupt fever, chills, headache, and generalized aching, followed by epigastric pain, anorexia, loss of taste, and photophobia. The disease is of short duration, and recovery is usually complete. There is no specific treatment.

RIG *abbr* rabies immune globulin.

right atrioventricular valve See **tricuspid valve.**

right brachiocephalic vein A vessel, about 2.5 cm (1 inch) long, that starts in the root of the neck at the junction of the internal jugular and the subclavian veins on the right side and descends vertically from behind the sternal end of the clavicle to join the left brachiocephalic vein and form the superior vena cava. Compare **left brachiocephalic vein.**

right bundle branch block An abnormal cardiac condition, characterized by an impaired electrical signal associated with the bundle of fibers that transmits impulses from the atrioventricular (AV) bundle to the right ventricle. This dysfunction may be a complete or an incomplete block of action impulses for ventricular contraction and may be caused by a small focal lesion in the AV bundle. A right bundle branch

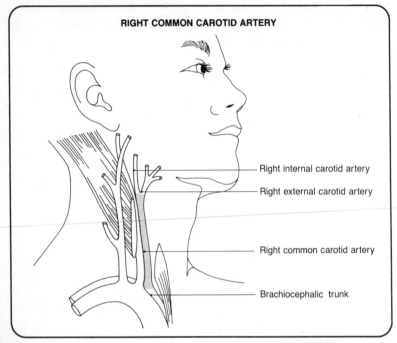

RIGHT COMMON CAROTID ARTERY

Right internal carotid artery

Right external carotid artery

Right common carotid artery

Brachiocephalic trunk

block is often associated with right ventricular hypertrophy, especially in individuals under 40 years of age. In older individuals, a right bundle branch block is commonly caused by coronary artery disease. A complete right bundle branch block commonly occurs following surgical closure of a ventricular defect.

right common carotid artery The shorter of the two common carotid arteries, springing from the brachiocephalic trunk, passing obliquely from the level of the sternoclavicular articulation to the cranial border of the thyroid cartilage, and dividing into the right internal and the right external carotid arteries. Compare **left common carotid artery.**

right coronary artery One of a pair of branches of the ascending aorta, arising in the right posterior aortic sinus, passing along the right side of the coronary sulcus, dividing into the right interventricular artery and a large marginal branch, supplying both ventricles, the right atrium, and the sinoatrial node. Compare **left coronary artery.**

right coronary vein See **small cardiac vein.**

right-handedness A natural tendency to favor the use of the right hand. Also called **dextrality.** See also **cerebral dominance, handedness.**

right-heart failure An abnormal cardiac condition characterized by the impairment of the right side of the heart and congestion and elevated pressure in the systemic veins and capillaries. Right-heart failure is usually related to left-heart failure, because both sides of the heart are part of a circuit, and what affects one side will eventually affect the other. The most common cause of right-heart failure is left-heart failure. Also called **right-sided failure.** Compare **left-heart failure.**

right hepatic duct The duct that drains bile from the right lobe of the liver into the common bile duct.

righting reflex Any reflex that tends to return an animal to its normal body position in space when it has been moved from the normal position. These reflexes involve a number of sensory receptors including the eyes, labyrinth, and muscles.

right interventricular artery See **dorsal interventricular artery.**

right lymphatic duct A vessel that conveys lymph from the right upper quadrant of the body into the bloodstream in the neck at the junction of the right internal jugular and the right subclavian veins. About 1.25 cm (½ inch) long, it courses over the medial border of the scalenus anterior. At its orifice are two semilunar valves that prevent venous blood from flowing backward into the duct. Lymph drains into the right lymphatic duct from numerous capillaries and vessels and from three lymphatic trunks in the right quadrant. Compare **thoracic duct.** See also **lymphatic system.**

right pulmonary artery The longer and slightly larger of the two arteries conveying blood from the heart to the lungs, rising from the pulmonary trunk, bending to the right behind the

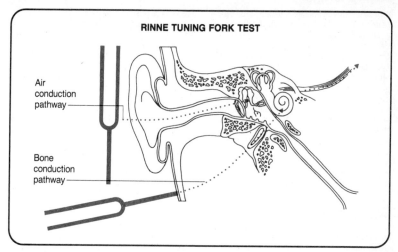

RINNE TUNING FORK TEST

Air conduction pathway

Bone conduction pathway

aorta, and dividing into two branches at the root of the right lung. Compare **left pulmonary artery.**

right-sided failure See **right-heart failure.**

right subclavian artery A large artery that arises from the brachiocephalic artery. It has several important branches: the axillary, vertebral thoracic, and internal thoracic arteries and the cervical and costocervical trunks, perfusing the right side of the upper body.

rigidity A condition of hardness, stiffness, or inflexibility. **—rigid,** *adj.*

rigidus A deformity characterized by limited motion, especially dorsiflexion of the great toe. This condition causes pain and may ultimately produce degenerative changes of involved joints.

rigor **1.** A rigid condition of the tissues of the body, as in rigor mortis. **2.** A violent attack of shivering that may be associated with chills and fever.

rigor mortis The rigid stiffening of skeletal and cardiac muscle shortly after death.

rim- A combining form meaning 'crack, fissure': *rimal, rimose.*

ring chromosome A circular chromosome formed by the fusion of the two ends. It is the primary type of chromosome found in bacteria.

Ringer's injection A fluid and electrolyte replacement solution.

Ringer's injection, lactated A fluid and electrolyte replacement solution closely approximating the electrolyte concentration in blood plasma.

ringworm See **tinea.**

Rinne tuning fork test A method of assessing auditory acuity, useful in distinguishing conductive from sensorineural hearing loss. The test is performed with tuning forks of 256, 512, and 1,024 cycles, and while each ear is tested, the other is masked. The stem of a vibrating fork is alternately placed 1.25 cm (½ inch) from the external auditory meatus of the

ear and on the adjacent mastoid bone until the sound is no longer heard at each of these positions. The person with normal hearing perceives the sound for a longer period when conduction is by air than by bone. If the patient has a conductive loss, the sound is heard for a longer period when conducted by bone than by air. In sensorineural loss, the sound is heard longer when conducted by air, but perception by both air and bone conduction is diminished.

Rio Grande fever See **abortus fever.**

risk factor A factor that causes a person or a group of people to be particularly vulnerable to an unwanted, unpleasant, or unhealthful event, as immunosuppression, which increases the incidence and severity of infection.

risorius One of the 12 muscles of the mouth. Arising in the fascia over the masseter and inserting into the skin at the corner of the mouth, it is innervated by mandibular and buccal branches of the facial nerve and acts to retract the angle of the mouth, as in a smile.

Risser cast An orthopedic device for encasing the entire trunk of the body, extending over the cervical area to the chin. In rare cases, it extends over the hips to the knees. The Risser cast is of plaster of paris or fiberglass and is used to immobilize the trunk of the body in the treatment of scoliosis and in the preoperative or the postoperative correction or the maintenance of correction of scoliosis. It often has a hole cut in front to allow room for abdominal expansion. Compare **body jacket, turnbuckle cast.**

risus sardonicus A wry, masklike grin caused by spasm of the facial muscles, as seen in tetanus.

ritodrine hydrochloride Used in the management of preterm labor.

Ritter's disease A rare, staphylococcal infection of newborns that begins with red spots about the mouth and chin, gradually spreading over the entire body and followed by generalized exfoliation. Vesicles and yellow crusts may also be present. Ritter's disease is usually fatal unless treated with antibiotics, which should be selected on the basis of bacterial sensitivity tests. Also called **dermatitis exfoliativa neonatorum.** Compare **toxic epidermal necrolysis.**

river blindness See **onchocerciasis.**

r-loop In molecular genetics: a distinctive loop formation seen under an electron microscope. It is composed of a single helical strand of DNA, wound with a hybrid strand containing another single strand of DNA with a strand of RNA.

RMSF *abbr* **Rocky Mountain spotted fever.**

Rn Symbol for **radon.**

RN *abbr* **registered nurse.**

RNA *abbr* **ribonucleic acid.**

RNA nucleotidyltransferase See **RNA polymerase.**

RNA polymerase In molecular genetics: an enzyme that catalyzes the assembly of ribonucleoside triphosphates into RNA, with single-stranded DNA serving as the template. Also called **RNA nucleotidyltransferase.**

RNA splicing In molecular genetics: the process by which base pairs that interrupt the continuity of genetic information in DNA are removed from the precursors of messenger RNA.

RN,C *abbr* **registered nurse, certified.**

Robertsonian translocation The exchange of entire chromosome arms, with the break occurring at the centromere, usually between two nonhomologous acrocentric chromosomes, to form one large metacentric chromosome and one small chromosome that carries little genetic material and may be lost through successive cell divisions, leading to a reduction in total chromosome number.

rock fever See **brucellosis.**

Rocky Mountain spotted fever (RMSF) A serious tick-borne infectious disease occurring throughout the temperate zones of North and South America, caused by *Rickettsia rickettsii* and characterized by chills, fever, severe headache, myalgia, mental confusion, and rash. Erythematous macules first appear on wrists and ankles, spreading rapidly over the extremities, trunk, face, and, usually, the palms and soles. Hemorrhagic lesions, constipation, and abdominal distention are also common. Early treatment with chloramphenicol or tetracycline is important, as more than 20% of untreated patients die from shock and renal failure. A diet high in protein is important to avoid hypoproteinemia. Nursing care is especially important to avoid decubitus ulcers and hypostatic or aspiration pneumonia. Immunity follows recovery. Also called **mountain fever, mountain tick fever, spotted fever.** Compare **measles, meningococcemia, rickettsialpox, scrub typhus, typhus.**

rod 1. A straight cylindrical structure. 2. One of the tiny cylindrical elements arranged perpendicular to the surface of the retina. Rods contain the chemical rhodopsin, which adapts the eye to detect low-intensity light and gives the rods a purple color. Each rod is 40 to 60 microns in length and about 2 microns thick and consists of a slender, reactive outer segment and an inner granular segment. When bright light strikes a rod, rhodopsin rapidly breaks down; it reforms gradually in low-intensity light. Compare **cone.** See also **iodopsin, Jacob's membrane.**

rodenticide poisoning A toxic condition caused by the ingestion of a substance intended for the control of rodent populations. See also **phosphorus poisoning, thallium poisoning, warfarin poisoning.**

rodent ulcer A slowly developing serpiginous ulceration of a basal cell carcinoma of the skin. See also **basal cell carcinoma.**

roentgen The quantity of X- or gamma radiation that creates 1 electrostatic unit of ions in 1 cc of air (0.001293 g) at 0°C (32° F) and 760 mmHg of pressure. In radiotherapy or radiodiagnosis, the roentgen is the unit of the emitted dose. See also **rad, rem.**

roentgen fetometry The use of radiographic techniques to measure the fetus in utero.

roentgenology The study of the diagnostic and therapeutic uses of X-rays. See also **radiology, roentgen, X-ray.**

roentgen ray See **X-ray.**

Rokitansky's disease See **Budd-Chiari syndrome.**

Rolando's fracture A fracture of the base of the first metacarpal.

role playing A psychotherapeutic technique in which a person acts out a real or simulated situation as a means of understanding intrapsychic conflicts.

role-playing therapy See **psychodrama.**

Rolfing See **structural integration.**

roller bandage A long, tightly wound strip of material, which may vary in width. It is generally applied as a circular bandage.

roller clamp A device, usually made of plastic, equipped with a small roller that may be rolled counterclockwise to close off primary intravenous tubing or clockwise to open it. The roller clamp may also be manipulated to increase and decrease the flow of the intravenous solution and is easily moved with the thumb, making it a one-handed convenience in the administration of intravenous therapy. Compare **screw clamp, slide clamp.**

rolling effleurage A circular, rubbing stroke used in massage to promote circulation and muscle relaxation, especially on the shoulders and buttocks. Compare **effleurage, pétrissage.**

Romberg sign An indication of loss of the sense of position in which the patient loses balance when standing erect, feet together, and eyes closed. Also called Romberg test.

rongeur forceps A strong, heavy-biting forceps used for cutting bone. Also called rongeur.

rooming-in In a hospital: a recent practice that allows mothers and newborn infants to share accommodations, remaining together in the hospital as they would at home.

root The lowest part of an organ or a structure

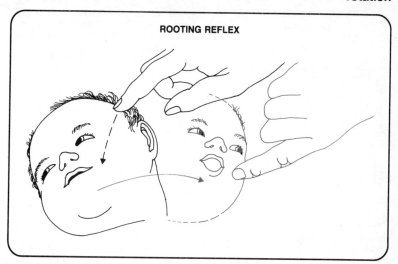

ROOTING REFLEX

by which something is firmly attached, as the anatomical root of the tooth. Also called **radix.**

rooting reflex   A normal response in newborns when the cheek is touched or stroked along the side of the mouth to turn the head toward the stimulated side and to begin to suck. The reflex usually disappears by 3 to 4 months of age but may persist until 12 months of age.

Rorschach test   A projective personality assessment test developed by the Swiss psychiatrist Hermann Rorschach. It consists of 10 pictures of inkblots—5 in black and white, 3 in black and red, and 2 multicolored—to which the subject responds by telling, in as many interpretations as are desired, what images and emotions each design evokes. Replies are evaluated according to whether the response is to the entire image or only part of it; whether color, shading, shape, or location of individual elements is significant; whether movement is seen; and the degree of complexity of each interpretation. The test assesses the degree to which intellectual and emotional factors are integrated in the subject's perception of the environment. See also **Holtzman inkblot technique.**

ROS   *abbr* **review of systems.**

rosacea   A chronic form of acne seen in adults of all ages and associated with telangiectasia, especially of the nose, forehead, and cheeks. Also called **acne rosacea.** See also **rhinophyma.**

rose fever   A common misnomer for seasonal allergic rhinitis caused by pollen, most frequently of grasses, that is airborne at the time roses are in bloom. Roses are not the cause of common spring and summer allergic reactions; their pollen is not dispersed by the wind but is carried from flower to flower by insects.

Rosenmüller's organ   See **epoophoron.**

Rosenthal's syndrome   See **hemophilia C.**

roseola   1. Any rose-colored rash. 2. See **roseola infantum.**

roseola infantum   A benign, presumably viral, endemic illness of infants and young children, characterized by abrupt, high, sustained or spiking fever, mild pharyngitis, and lymph node enlargement. Febrile convulsions may occur. After 4 or 5 days, the fever suddenly drops to normal, and a faint, pink, maculopapular rash appears on the neck, trunk, and thighs. The rash may last a few hours to 2 days. Sequelae may occur as a result of the convulsions. There is no specific therapy or vaccine. Aspirin or acetaminophen is often used to try to control fever. Also called **exanthem subitum, sixth disease, Zahorsky's disease.**

rose spots   Small erythematous macules occurring on the upper abdomen and anterior thorax and lasting 2 or 3 days, characteristic of typhoid and paratyphoid fevers.

rost-   A combining form meaning 'of or pertaining to a beak': *rostellum, rostrad, rostriform.*

rostral   Beak-shaped. **—rostrum,** *n.*

rot-   A combining form meaning 'turned or to turn': *rotate, rotatory, rotexion.*

rotameter   A device that is operated by a needle valve in an anesthetic gas machine that measures gases by speed of flow, according to their viscosity and density. Also called **flowmeter.**

rotating tourniquet   One of four constricting devices used in a rotating order to pool blood in the extremities in order to relieve congestion in the lungs in acute pulmonary edema. The procedure is no longer recommended for the treatment of this condition.

rotation   1. A turning around an axis. 2. One of the four basic kinds of motion allowed by various joints; the rotation of a bone around its central axis, which may lie in a separate bone, as in the pivot formed by the dens of the axis around which the atlas turns. A bone, as the humerus, may also rotate around its own lon-

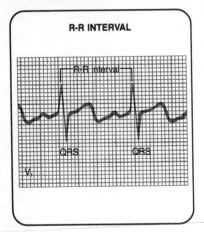

R-R INTERVAL

gitudinal axis, or the axis of rotation may not be quite parallel to the long axis of the rotating bone, as in movement of the radius on the ulna during pronation. Compare **circumduction.** See also **angular movement, gliding.**

Rotor syndrome A rare condition of the liver inherited as an autosomal recessive trait. It is similar to Dubin-Johnson syndrome but can be distinguished by the normal functioning of the gallbladder and normal pigmentation of the liver. See also **Dubin-Johnson syndrome.**

rotula See **troche.**

roughage See **dietary fiber.**

rouleaux, *sing.* **rouleau** An aggregation of red cells in what looks like a stack of coins or checkers. The formation may sometimes be caused by abnormal proteins, as in multiple myeloma or macroglobulinemia, but it is most often a microscopic artifact. Compare **hemagglutination.** See also **erythrocyte sedimentation rate.**

rounds *Informal.* A teaching conference or a meeting in which the clinical problems encountered in the practice of nursing, medicine, or other service are discussed. Kinds of rounds include **grand rounds, nursing rounds, teaching rounds, walking rounds.**

roundworm Any worm of the class Nematoda, including *Ancylostoma duodenale, Ascaris lumbricoides, Enterobius vermicularis,* and *Strongyloides stercoralis.*

route of administration Of a drug: any one of the ways in which a drug may be administered, as intramuscularly, intranasally, intravenously, intra-arterially, intrathecally, orally, rectally, subcutaneously, sublingually, topically, or vaginally.

Rovsing's sign An indication of acute appendicitis in which pressure on the left lower quadrant of the abdomen causes pain in the right lower quadrant. See also **appendicitis.**

Royal College of Physicians (RCP) A professional organization of physicians in the United Kingdom.

Royal College of Physicians and Sur-

geons of Canada (RCPSC) A national Canadian organization that recognizes and confers membership on certain qualified physicians and surgeons.

Royal College of Surgeons (RCS) A professional organization of surgeons in the United Kingdom.

RPF *abbr* renal plasma flow.

RR *abbr* recovery room.

-(r)rachia A combining form meaning a '(specified) foreign chemical substance': *calciorrhachia, glycorrhachia.*

-(r)rhage A combining form meaning a 'rupture; an excessive fluid discharge': *hemorrhage, lymphorrhage.*

-(r)rhagia A combining form meaning a 'fluid discharge of excessive quantity': *lymphorrhagia, meningorrhagia.*

-(r)rhagic A combining form meaning 'of, pertaining to, or referring to a kind or condition of excessive fluid discharge': *haemorrhagic, lymphorrhagic.*

-(r)rhaphy, -(r)rhaphia A combining form meaning a 'suturing in place': *cysticorrhaphy, meningeorrhaphy.*

-(r)rhea A combining form meaning: 'fluid discharge, flow': *anarrhea, cystirrhea.* Also **-(r)rhoeica.**

-(r)rheal See **-(r)rheic.**

-(r)rheic A combining form meaning 'pertaining to a fluid discharge': *cryptorrheic, diarrheic.* Also **-(r)rheal, -(r)rhetic.**

-(r)rhetic See **-(r)rheic.**

-(r)rhexis A combining form meaning a 'rupture of a (specified) body part': *arteriorrhexis, cardiorrhexis.*

-(r)rhine A combining form meaning 'having a (specified type of) nose': *leptorrhine, mesorrhine.*

-(r)rhinia A combining form meaning '(condition of the) nose': *arrhinia, birhinia.*

-(r)rhoeica A combining form meaning 'fluid discharge': *seborrhoeica, gonorrhoeica.* Also **-(r)rhea.**

-(r)rhythmia A combining form meaning '(condition of the) heartbeat or the pulse': *bradyrhythmia, dysrhythmia.*

R-R interval The interval from the peak of one QRS complex to the peak of the next as shown on an electrocardiogram. See also **cardiac cycle.**

RRT *abbr* registered respiratory therapist.

RSV *abbr* respiratory syncytial virus. See **bronchiolitis.**

RT *abbr* respiratory therapy.

RTA *abbr* renal tubular acidosis.

rtc *abbr* return to clinic. It is noted on the chart, usually followed by a date on which a subsequent appointment has been made for the patient.

Ru Symbol for **ruthenium.**

rub- A combining form meaning 'red': *rubedo, ruber, rubor.*

rubbing alcohol A disinfectant for skin and instruments. It contains 70% ethyl or isopropyl alcohol by volume, the remainder consisting of water and denaturants. It may cause dryness of the skin. Rubbing alcohol is for external use only and is flammable.

rubefacient **1.** A substance or agent that increases the reddish coloration of the skin. **2.** Increasing the reddish coloration of the skin.

rubella A contagious viral disease characterized by fever, symptoms of a mild upper respiratory infection, lymph node enlargement, arthralgia, and a diffuse, fine, red, maculopapular rash. The virus is spread by droplet infection, and the incubation time is from 12 to 23 days. The symptoms usually last only 2 or 3 days, except for arthralgia, which may persist longer or recur. One attack confers lifelong immunity. If a woman acquires rubella in the 1st trimester of pregnancy, fetal anomalies may result, including heart defects, cataracts, deafness, and mental retardation. An infant exposed to the virus in utero at any time during gestation may shed the virus for up to 30 months after birth. The illness itself is mild and needs no special treatment. Live attenuated rubella vaccine is advised for all children to reduce chances of an epidemic and thus to protect pregnant women. The vaccine is not given to women already pregnant, and it is recommended that pregnancy be avoided for 3 months after the administration of rubella vaccine. Immune serum globulin containing rubella antibodies may help prevent fetal infection in exposed susceptible pregnant women, but ordinary gamma globulin will not protect the fetus.

NURSING CONSIDERATIONS: Temporary arthralgia is common after vaccination. Women of childbearing age working with children may be tested for immunity to rubella and vaccinated if not immune. The only proof of immunity is the laboratory demonstration of antibodies to the rubella virus. The rash and malaise of rubella resemble those of scarlet fever, some cases of mononucleosis, and allergic drug reactions, leading some people to think they have had rubella when they have not. Also called **German measles**, **three-day measles.** Compare **measles, scarlet fever.**

rubella and mumps virus vaccine A suspension containing live attenuated mumps and rubella viruses.

rubella embryopathy Any congenital abnormality in an infant caused by maternal rubella in the early stages of pregnancy.

rubella virus vaccine A suspension containing live attenuated rubella virus.

rubeola See **measles.**

rubescent Reddening.

rubidium (Rb) A soft metallic element of the alkali metals group. Its atomic number is 37; its atomic weight is 85.47. Slightly radioactive, it is used in radioisotope scanning.

Rubin's test A test performed in the process of evaluating the cause of infertility by assessing the patency of the fallopian tubes. Carbon dioxide gas (CO_2) is introduced into the tubes under pressure through a cannula inserted into the cervix. The CO_2 is passed through it from a syringe connected to a manometer at pressures of up to 200 mmHg. If the tubes are open, the gas enters the abdominal cavity and the recorded pressure falls below 180 mmHg. A high-pitched bubbling can be heard through the abdominal wall with the stethoscope as the gas escapes from the tubes. The patient may complain of shoulder pain from diaphragmatic irritation; an X-ray will show free gas under the diaphragm. If the tubes are blocked, gas cannot escape from the tubes into the abdominal cavity, and the pressure recorded on the manometer remains at 200 mmHg. A tracing may be made to show tubal peristalsis, any leakage in the system, tubal spasm, or partial obstruction. After the test, the patient rests for a 3-hour period. Crampy pain, dizziness, nausea, and vomiting may occur; positioning with the pelvis higher than the head, in knee-chest position, or in Trendelenberg's position, allows the gas to stay in the pelvis and gives some relief by avoiding diaphragmatic irritation.

rubivirus A member of the togavirus family, which includes the rubella virus.

rubor Redness, especially when accompanying inflammation.

ructus See **eructation.**

rudiment An organ or tissue that is incompletely developed or nonfunctional. —**rudimentary,** *adj.*

Ruffini's corpuscles A variety of oval-shaped nerve endings in the subcutaneous tissue of the human finger, located principally at the junction of the corium and the subcutaneous tissue. Ruffini's corpuscles consist of strong connective-tissue sheaths enclosing nerve fibers with many branches that end in small knobs. Compare **Golgi-Mazzoni corpuscles, Pacini's corpuscles.**

ruga, *pl.* **rugae** A ridge or fold, as the rugae of the stomach, which present large folds in the mucous membrane of that organ.

rule of nines A formula for estimating the amount of body surface covered by burns by assigning 9% to the head and each arm, twice 9% to each leg and to the anterior and posterior trunk, and 1% to the perineum. This system is used for emergency assessment only, because it does not take into account age-related variations in body build.

rumination Habitual regurgitation of small amounts of undigested food with little force after every feeding, a condition commonly seen in infants. It may be a symptom of overfeeding, of eating too fast, or of swallowing air. It has little or no clinical significance. More copious and forceful regurgitation may indicate a more serious condition, as an allergic intestinal reaction or a metabolic disorder. See also **vomit.**

rupture **1.** A tear or break in the continuity or configuration of an organ or body tissue, including those instances when other tissue protrudes through the opening. See also **hernia. 2.** To cause a break or tear.

ruptured intervertebral disk See **herniated disk.**

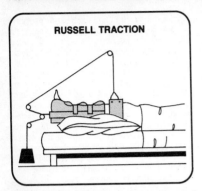

RUSSELL TRACTION

Rural Clinics Assistance Act An act of Congress that permitted the establishment of clinics in certain areas designated rural and underserved and in some inner cities. The clinics are designed to provide primary care through teams of physicians and nurse practitioners. The act is significant to nursing by being the first federal legislation which allows third-party reimbursement directly to nurses practicing in expanded roles.

Russell dwarf A person affected with Russell's syndrome, a congenital disorder in which short stature is associated with various anomalies of the head, face, and skeleton and with varying degrees of mental retardation.

Russell's bodies The mucoprotein inclusions that are found in globular plasma cells in cancer. The bodies contain surface gamma globulins, probably derived from the condensation of internal cellular secretions. Also called **cancer bodies, fuchsin bodies.**

Russell traction A unilateral or bilateral orthopedic mechanism that combines suspension and traction to immobilize, position, and align the lower extremities in the treatment of fractured femurs and hip and knee contractures and in the treatment of disease processes of the hip and the knee. Russell traction is applied as adhesive or nonadhesive skin traction and employs a sling to relieve the weight of the lower extremities subjected to traction pull. Compare **split Russell traction.**

Russian bath A hot steam bath followed by a cold plunge. Also called **Finnish bath.**

ruthenium (Ru) A hard, brittle, metallic element. Its atomic number is 44; its atomic weight is 101.07.

rutin A bioflavonoid obtained from buckwheat and used in the treatment of capillary fragility.

RV *abbr* **residual volume.**

RVC *abbr* responds to verbal commands.

R wave The component of the cardiac cycle shown on an electrocardiogram as a steep, straight, upward line to the beginning of the sharp downward slant of the S wave. It represents the middle part of the QRS complex.

S

S Symbol for: **1. sulfur. 2.** saturation of hemoglobin.

S₁ The first heart sound in the cardiac cycle, occurring with ventricular systole. It is associated with closure of the mitral and tricuspid valves. Auscultated at the apex, it is louder, longer, and lower than the second sound (S₂), which follows it.

S₂ The second heart sound in the cardiac cycle. It is associated with closure of the aortic and pulmonary valves just before ventricular diastole. Auscultated at the base of the heart, the second sound is louder than the first.

S₃ The third heart sound in the cardiac cycle, occurring early in diastole. Normally, it is audible only in children and physically active young adults. It is an abnormal finding in older people and usually indicates myocardial failure.

S₄ The fourth heart sound in the cardiac cycle. It occurs late in diastole upon contraction of the atria. Rarely heard in normal subjects, it indicates an abnormally increased resistance to ventricular filling, as in hypertensive cardiovascular disease, coronary artery disease, myocardiopathy, and aortic stenosis.

SA *abbr* **1. surgeon's assistant. 2.** sinoatrial. **3.** surface area.

Sabin-Feldman dye test A diagnostic test for toxoplasmosis that depends on the presence of specific antibodies that block the uptake of methylene blue dye by the cytoplasm of the *Toxoplasma* organisms.

Sabin vaccine See **poliovirus vaccine.**

sac A pouch or a baglike organ, as the abdominal sac of the embryo that develops into the abdominal cavity.

saccharide Any of a large group of carbohydrates including all sugars and starches. Almost all carbohydrates are saccharides. See also **carbohydrate, sugar.**

saccharin, saccharine **1.** A white, crystalline substance sweeter than table sugar (sucrose). Saccharin is often used as a sugar substitute. **2.** Having a cloyingly sweet taste.

saccharo-, sacchari- A combining form meaning 'of or pertaining to sugar': *saccharobiose, saccharorrhea.*

Saccharomyces A genus of yeast fungi, including brewer's and baker's yeast as well as some pathogenic fungi that cause such diseases as bronchitis and pharyngitis.

saccharomycosis **1.** Infection with yeast fungi, as the genera *Candida* or *Cryptococcus.* **2.** Cryptococcosis or European blastomycosis.

saccule A small bag or sac, as the air saccules of the lungs. See also **sacculus. —saccular,** *adj.*

sacculus, *pl.* **sacculi** A little sac or bag, especially the smaller of the two divisions of the membranous labyrinth of the vestibule, which communicates with the cochlear duct through the ductus reuniens in the inner ear. See also **saccule.**

Sachs' disease See **Tay-Sachs disease.**

sacral Of or pertaining to the sacrum.

sacral foramen One of several openings between the fused segments of the sacral vertebrae in the sacrum through which the sacral nerves pass.

sacral node A node in one of the seven groups of parietal lymph nodes of the abdomen and pelvis, situated within the sacrum. The sacral nodes receive lymphatics from the rectum and the posterior wall of the pelvis. Compare **lumbar node.** See also **lymph, lymphatic system, lymph node.**

sacral plexus A network of motor and sensory nerves formed by the lumbosacral trunk from the fourth and fifth lumbar and the first, second, and third sacral nerves. These nerves converge toward the caudal portion of the greater sciatic foramen and unite to become a large, flattened band, most of which continues into the thigh as the sciatic nerve. Compare **lumbar plexus.**

sacral vertebra One of the five segments of the vertebral column that fuse in the adult to form the sacrum. The ventral border of the first sacral vertebra projects into the pelvis. The bodies of the other sacral vertebrae are smaller than that of the first and are flattened and curved ventrally, forming the convex, anterior surface of the sacrum. Compare **cervical vertebra, coccygeal vertebra, lumbar vertebra, thoracic vertebra.** See also **sacrum, vertebra.**

sacro- A combining form meaning 'of or pertaining to the sacrum': *sacrococcyx, sacroiliac, sacrolumbalis.*

sacroiliac articulation An immovable joint in the pelvis formed by the articulation of each side of the sacrum with an iliac bone.

sacrospinalis A large, fleshy muscle of the back that divides into a lateral iliocostalis column, an intermediate longissimus column, and a medial spinalis column. Also called **erector spinae.**

sacrum The large, triangular bone at the dorsal part of the pelvis, inserted like a wedge between the two hip bones. The base of the sacrum articulates with the last lumbar vertebra, and its apex articulates with the coccyx; various muscles attach to its spinal crest. The sacrum is shorter and wider in women than in men. **—sacral,** *adj.*

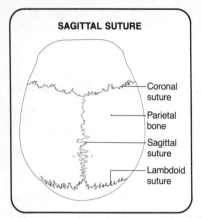

SAGITTAL SUTURE

- Coronal suture
- Parietal bone
- Sagittal suture
- Lambdoid suture

saddle block anesthesia A form of regional nerve block affecting the parts of the body that would touch a saddle, were the patient sitting in one. It is performed by injecting a local anesthetic into the spinal cavity. Saddle block anesthesia is common in some centers for anesthesia during childbirth. See also **obstetric anesthesia.**

saddle joint A synovial joint in which surfaces of contiguous bones are reciprocally concavo-convex. A saddle joint permits no axial rotation but allows flexion, extension, adduction, and abduction, as in the carpometacarpal joint of the thumb. Also called **articulatio sellaris.** Compare **condyloid joint, pivot joint.**

sadism **1.** Abnormal pleasure derived from inflicting physical or psychological pain on others; cruelty. **2.** In psychiatry: a psychosexual disorder characterized by the infliction of physical or psychological pain or humiliation on another person, either a consenting or nonconsenting partner, to achieve sexual excitement or gratification. The condition is usually chronic and seen predominantly in men. Kinds of sadism are **anal sadism, oral sadism.** Also called **active algolagnia.** Compare **masochism.** See also **algolagnia, sadomasochism.** —**sadist,** *n.,* **sadistic,** *adj.*

sadist A person who practices sadism.

sadomasochism See **algolagnia.**

safe period See **natural family-planning method.**

sagittal In anatomy: of or pertaining to a suture or an imaginary line extending from the front to the back in the midline of the body or a part of the body.

sagittal plane The anteriorposterior plane or the section parallel to the median plane of the body. Compare **frontal plane, median plane, transverse plane.**

sagittal suture The serrated connection between the two parietal bones of the skull, coursing down the midline from the coronal suture to the upper part of the lambdoidal suture.

SaH, SAH *abbr* subarachnoid hemorrhage.

SAIN *abbr* **Society for Advancement in Nursing.**

salicylamide A salicylate nonnarcotic analgesic and antipyretic agent.

salicylate Any of several widely prescribed drugs derived from salicylic acid. Salicylates exert analgesic, antipyretic, and anti-inflammatory actions. The most important is acetylsalicylic acid, or aspirin.

salicylate poisoning A toxic condition caused by the ingestion of salicylate, most often in aspirin or oil of wintergreen. Intoxication is characterized by rapid breathing, vomiting, headache, irritability, ketosis, hypoglycemia, and, in severe cases, by convulsions and respiratory failure.

salicylazosulfapyridine See **sulfasalazine.**

salicylic acid A keratolytic agent that is applied topically.

saline cathartic One of a large group of cathartics administered to achieve prompt, complete evacuation of the bowel. The most common indication is preparation of the bowel for diagnostic examination. Various preparations may be used to achieve catharsis.

saline infusion The therapeutic introduction of a physiologic salt solution into a vein or under the skin.

saline irrigation The washing out of a body cavity or wound with a stream of salt solution, usually an isotonic aqueous solution of sodium chloride.

saline solution A solution containing sodium chloride. Depending on the use, it may be hypotonic, isotonic, or hypertonic with body fluids.

saliva The clear, viscous fluid secreted by the salivary and mucous glands in the mouth. Saliva contains water, mucin, organic salts, and the digestive enzyme ptyalin. It moistens the oral cavity to initiate the digestion of starches and to aid in chewing and swallowing.

salivary Of or pertaining to saliva or its formation.

salivary duct Any one of the ducts through which saliva passes. Kinds of salivary ducts are **Bartholin's duct, duct of Rivinus, parotid duct, submandibular duct.**

salivary fistula An abnormal communication from a salivary gland or duct to an opening in the mouth or on the skin of the face or neck.

salivary gland One of the three pairs of glands that pour their secretions into the mouth, thus aiding the digestive process. The salivary glands are the parotid, the submandibular, and the sublingual glands. They are racemose structures consisting of numerous lobes subdivided into smaller lobules connected by dense areolar tissue, vessels, and ducts. The ducts ramify inside each lobule, ending in alveoli. One kind of alveolus secretes a viscid fluid containing mucin. The other kind secretes serous fluid. The sublingual gland secretes mucus; the parotid gland, serous fluid; and the submandibular gland se-

CLINICAL VARIANTS OF SALMONELLOSIS

	CAUSE	CLINICAL FEATURES
Entero-colitis	Any species of nontyphoidal *Salmonella*, but usually *S. enteritidis*. Incubation period: 6 to 48 hours.	Mild to severe abdominal pain, diarrhea, sudden fever to 38.8°C (102°F), nausea, vomiting; usually self-limiting, but may progress to enteric fever (resembling typhoid), local abscesses (usually abdominal), dehydration, septicemia
Paratyphoid	*S. paratyphi* and *S. schottmülleri* (formerly *S. paratyphi B*). Incubation period: 3 weeks or more.	Fever and transient diarrhea; generally resembles typhoid but less severe
Bacteremia	Any *Salmonella* species, but most commonly *S. choleraesuis*. Incubation period varies.	Fever, chills, anorexia, weight loss (without gastrointestinal symptoms), joint pains
Localized infections	Usually follows bacteremia caused by *S. choleraesuis*.	Site of localization determines symptoms; localized abscesses may cause osteomyelitis, endocarditis, bronchopneumonia, pyelonephritis, and arthritis.
Typhoid fever	*S. typhi* enters GI tract and invades the bloodstream via the lymphatics, setting up intracellular sites. During this phase, infection of biliary tract leads to intestinal seeding with millions of bacilli. Involved lymphoid tissues (especially Peyer's patches in ileum) enlarge, ulcerate, and necrose, resulting in hemorrhage. Incubation period: usually 1 to 2 weeks.	Symptoms of enterocolitis may develop within hours of ingestion of *S. typhi*; usually subside before onset of typhoid fever symptoms. **First week:** Gradually increasing fever, anorexia, myalgia, malaise, headache **Second week:** Remittent fever up to 40°C (104°F) usually in the evening; chills, diaphoresis, weakness, delirium, increasing abdominal pain and distention, diarrhea or constipation, cough, moist rales, tender abdomen with enlarged spleen, maculopapular rash (especially on abdomen) **Third week:** Persistent fever, increasing fatigue and weakness; usually subsides end of third week, although relapses may occur **Complications:** Intestinal perforation or hemorrhage, abscesses, thrombophlebitis, cerebral thrombosis, pneumonia, osteomyelitis, myocarditis, acute circulatory failure, chronic carrier state

cretes both mucus and serous fluid.

salivary gland cancer A malignant neoplastic disease of a salivary gland, occurring most frequently in a parotid gland. Malignant tumors are rapid-growing, hard, lumpy, fixed, and frequently tender. Pain, trismus, and facial palsy may occur. Diagnostic tests include X-rays, with sialographic studies and mandibular and chest films, and cytologic studies. The most common malignant neoplasms are mucoepidermoid, adenoid cystic, solid, and squamous cell carcinomas. Treatment usually consists of the surgical removal of a lobe with a benign tumor and total parotidectomy with a radical neck dissection if the lesion is advanced. Radiotherapy is administered for residual, recurrent, or inoperable cancers, and chemotherapy may be palliative.

Salk vaccine See **poliovirus vaccine.**

salmon calcitonin See **calcitonin.**

Salmonella A genus of motile, gram-negative, rod-shaped bacteria that includes species causing typhoid fever, paratyphoid fever, and some forms of gastroenteritis.

salmonellosis A form of gastroenteritis caused by ingestion of food contaminated with *Salmonella*, characterized by an incubation period of 6 to 48 hours followed by sudden, colicky abdominal pain; fever; and bloody, watery diarrhea. Nausea and vomiting are common and abdominal signs may resemble acute appendicitis or cholecystitis. Symptoms usually last from

2 to 5 days, but diarrhea and fever may persist for 2 weeks. There is no specific treatment. See also **food poisoning.**

salol camphor A clear, oily mixture of two parts of camphor and three parts of phenyl salicylate, used as a local antiseptic.

Salonica fever See **trench fever.**

salpingectomy Surgical removal of one or both fallopian tubes, to remove a cyst, a tumor, or an abscess. Often the operation is done at the same time as a hysterectomy or an oophorectomy.

salpingitis An inflammation or infection of the fallopian tube. See also **pelvic inflammatory disease.**

salpingo- A combining form meaning 'of or pertaining to a tube, especially a fallopian tube': *salpingocele, salpingolysis, salpingoplasty.*

salpingostomy Formation of an artificial opening in a fallopian tube, in order to restore patency in a tube whose fimbriated opening has been closed by infection or chronic inflammation or to drain an abcess or an accumulation of fluid. A prosthesis may be inserted to maintain the patency of the fallopian tube and to direct the route of the ova to assist fertilization.

salpinx, *pl.* **salpinges** A tube, as the salpinx auditiva and the salpinx uterina. **—salpingian,** *adj.*

salsalate A salicylate nonnarcotic analgesic and antipyretic.

salt **1.** A compound formed by the chemical reaction of an acid and a base. Salts are usually composed of a metal and a nonmetal. Some salts contain groups of atoms that behave chemically as metals or nonmetals. **2.** Sodium chloride (common table salt). **3.** A substance, as magnesium sulfate (Epsom salt), used as a purgative.

saltation In genetics: a mutation causing a significant difference in appearance between parent and offspring or an abrupt variation in the characteristics of the species. **—saltatorial, saltatoric, saltatory,** *adj.*

saltatory evolution The appearance of a sudden, abrupt change within a species, caused by mutation; the progression of a species by sudden major changes. The phenomenon occurs predominantly in plants as a result of polyploidy. See also **emergent evolution.**

salt depletion The loss of salt from the body through excessive elimination of body fluids by perspiration, diarrhea, vomiting, or urination, without corresponding replacement. See also **electrolyte balance, heat exhaustion.**

Salter fracture See **epiphyseal fracture.**

salt-free diet See **low-sodium diet.**

salve See **ointment.**

samarium (Sm) A rare-earth, metallic element. Its atomic number is 62; its atomic weight is 150.35.

sand bath The application of warm, dry sand or of damp sand to the body.

sandfly fever See **phlebotomus fever.**

Sandhoff's disease A variant of Tay-Sachs disease that includes defects in the enzymes hexosaminidase A and B. It has a progressively more rapid course and is found in the general population. Also called **gangliosidosis type II.** See also **Tay-Sachs disease.**

sand tumor See **psammoma.**

sangui- A combining form meaning 'of or pertaining to blood': *sanguicolous, sanguiferous, sanguinolent.*

sanguineous Pertaining to blood.

sanita- A combining form meaning 'of or pertaining to health': *sanitarium, sanitas, sanitation.*

San Joaquin fever Primary stage of coccidioidomycosis.

SA node See **sinoatrial node.**

saphenous nerve The largest and longest branch of the femoral nerve, supplying the skin of the medial side of the leg. It accompanies the great saphenous vein along the medial side of the leg, and at the medial border of the tibia in the distal third of the leg it divides into two terminal branches. One branch joins the medial cutaneous and the obturator nerves to form the subsartorial plexus. A large infrapatellar branch passes to the skin over the patella and on the lateral side of the knee joins with branches of the lateral femoral cutaneous nerve to form the patellar plexus. One branch of the saphenous nerve below the knee supplies the ankle. Another branch below the knee supplies the medial side of the foot. See also **femoral nerve.**

saphenous vein See **great saphenous vein.**

sapo- A combining form meaning 'of or pertaining to soap': *sapogenin, saponaceous, sapotoxin.*

saponin A soapy material found in some plants, especially bouncing bet (soapwort) and certain lilies. It is used in demulcent medications to provide a sudsy quality.

-sarc A combining form meaning '(specified type of) flesh': *ectosarc, endosarc, perisarc.*

sarco- A combining form meaning 'of or related to the flesh': *sarcoadenoma, sarcode, sarcolyte.*

Sarcodina A class of one-celled organisms, belonging to the phyllum Protozoa and subphyllum Plasmodroma. The class includes four species of amebae parasitic in humans: *Entamoeba coli* and *E. hartmanni,* which inhabit the colon; *E. gingivalis,* found in tartar and on the gums; and *E. histolytica,* which causes amebic dysentery and hepatic amebiasis. See also **ameba, amebiasis, amebic abscess, amebic dysentery,** *Entamoeba, Entamoeba histolytica,* **hepatic amebiasis.**

sarcoidosis A chronic disorder of unknown etiology characterized by the formation of tubercles of nonnecrotizing epithelioid tissue. Common sites are the lungs, spleen, liver, skin, mucous membranes, and lacrimal and salivary glands, usually with involvement of the lymph glands. The lesions usually disappear over a period of months or years but progress to widespread granulomatous inflammation and fibrosis. Also called **Boeck's sarcoid.**

sarcoidosis cordis A form of sarcoidosis in which granulomatous lesions develop in the myocardium. Mild cases with few infiltrates are asymptomatic. In severe cases, the myocardium may be infiltrated with many tumors and cardiac failure may follow. See also **sarcoidosis.**

sarcoma, *pl.* **sarcomas, sarcomata** An uncommon, malignant neoplasm of the soft tissues arising in fibrous, fatty, muscular, synovial, vascular, or neural tissue. About 40% of sarcomas occur in the lower extremities, 20% in the upper extremities, 20% in the trunk, and the rest in the head, neck, or retroperineum. The tumor, composed of closely packed cells in a fibrillar or homogeneous matrix, tends to be vascular and is usually highly invasive. Sarcomas may arise in burn or radiation scars. Small tumors may be managed by local excision and postoperative radiotherapy. Bulky sarcomas of the extremities may require amputation followed by irradiation and combination chemotherapy. See specific sarcomas.

-sarcoma A combining form meaning a 'malignant neoplasm': *angiosarcoma, hemangiosarcoma, myelosarcoma.*

sarcoma botryoides A tumor derived from primitive striated muscle cells, occurring most frequently in young children and characterized by a painful, edematous, polypoid, grapelike mass in the upper vagina or on the uterine cervix or the neck of the urinary bladder. See also **rhabdomyosarcoma.**

sarcomagenesis The process of initiating and promoting the development of a sarcoma. Compare **oncogenesis, tumorigenesis. —sarcomagenetic,** *adj.*

sarcoplasmic reticulum A network of tubules and sacs in skeletal muscles that aids muscle contraction and relaxation by releasing and storing calcium ions.

Sarcoptes scabiei The genus of itch mite that causes scabies.

sartorius The longest muscle in the body, extending from the pelvis to the calf of the leg. It is a narrow muscle that arises from the anterior superior iliac spine, passes obliquely across the proximal anterior part of the thigh from the lateral to the medial side, and inserts, by a tendon and an aponeurosis, into the tibia. It is innervated by branches of the femoral nerve. It acts to flex the thigh and rotate it laterally and to flex the leg and rotate it medially. Compare **quadriceps femoris.**

saturated In chemistry: **1.** Unable to absorb, dissolve, or accept any more of a given substance. **2.** Term applied to a hydrocarbon having all carbon bonds filled, without any double or triple bonds, and unable to unite directly with another compound. See also **saturated solution.**

saturated fatty acid Any of a number of glyceryl esters of certain organic acids in which all the atoms are joined by single valence bonds. These fats are chiefly of animal origin, though ordinary oleomargarine and hydrogenated shortenings also contain them. A diet high in

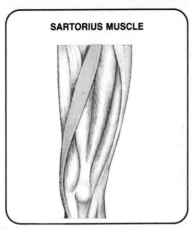

SARTORIUS MUSCLE

saturated fatty acids may contribute to a high serum cholesterol level, which seems to be associated with an increased incidence of coronary heart disease. Compare **unsaturated fatty acid.**

saturated solution A solution in which the solvent contains the maximum amount of solute it can take up. See also **solute, solvent.**

saturn- A combining form meaning 'lead': *saturnine, saturnism, saturnotherapy.*

satyriasis Excessive, uncontrollable sexual desire in males, of organic or psychological origin. Also called satyromania. Compare **nymphomania.**

sauna bath A bath in which hot vapor induces sweating, followed by rubbing of the body, and ending with a cold shower. Also called **Finnish bath, Russian bath.**

Sayre's jacket A cast applied for support and immobilization to treat certain spinal column abnormalities.

Sb Symbol for **antimony.**

SBE *abbr* **1. self-breast examination. 2. sub-acute bacterial endocarditis.**

Sc Symbol for **scandium.**

scab See eschar.

scabicide Any one of a large group of topical drugs that destroy the itch mite, *Sarcoptes scabiei.* All are potentially toxic and irritating to the skin. Kinds of scabicides include **crotamiton, gamma benzene hexachloride, lindane.**

scabies An age-old disease caused by *Sarcoptes scabiei,* the itch mite, characterized by intense itching of the skin and excoriation from scratching. The mite, transmitted by close contact, as in institutions, burrows into outer layers of the skin where the female lays eggs. Within 2 to 4 months after the first infection, sensitization to the mites and their products begins, resulting in a pruritic, papular rash most common on the webs of fingers, flexor surfaces of wrists, and thighs. Secondary bacterial infection may occur. Diagnosis may be made by microscopic identification of adult mites, larvae, or eggs in scrapings of the burrows.

SCAPHOID BONES OF THE HAND AND FOOT

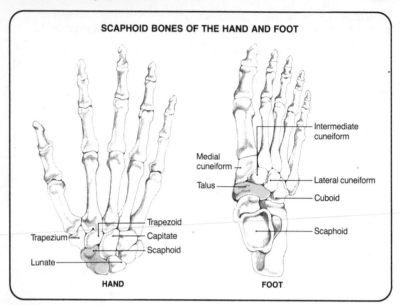

Intermediate cuneiform

Medial cuneiform

Lateral cuneiform

Talus

Cuboid

Trapezoid

Trapezium

Capitate

Scaphoid

Scaphoid

Lunate

HAND   **FOOT**

scalded skin syndrome See **toxic epidermal necrolysis.**

scale **1.** A small, thin flake of keratinized epithelium. **2.** A thin layer of tartar on the teeth. **3.** A weighing device. **4.** The scoring on an instrument that measures or registers, as on a ruler. **5.** To form a scale on. **6.** To remove encrusted material from a surface, as from a tooth.

scalp Skin covering the head, excluding the face and ears.

scalp-vein needle A thin-gauge needle designed for use on small veins, as in children.

scamping speech Abnormal speech in which consonants or whole syllables are left out of words owing to the person's inability to shape the sounds.

scandium (Sc) A gray metallic element. Its atomic number is 21; its atomic weight is 44.956.

scanning Carefully studying an area, organ, or system of the body by recording and displaying an image of the concentration of an injected radioactive substance that has an affinity for that specific tissue. The liver, brain, and thyroid can be examined by various scanning techniques. See specific scanning techniques. —**scan,** *n., v.*

scanning electron microscope (SEM) An instrument similar to an electron microscope in that a beam of electrons rather than visible light is used to scan the surface of a specimen. An SEM differs from an electron microscope in that the sample may be of any convenient size or shape, and the image, produced on a television screen, appears three-dimensional. Compare **electron microscope, transmission scanning electron microscope.**

scanning electron microscopy The technique using a scanning electron microscope

in which a beam of electrons is accelerated and focused on an electrically conducting sample. The beam is moved in a point-to-point manner over the surface of the specimen. The number of electrons emerging from the sample is proportionate to the shape, density, and other properties of the sample. Compare **electron microscopy, transmission scanning electron microscope.**

scanning speech Abnormal speech in which words are broken because of pauses between syllables.

Scanzoni rotation An obstetric operation in which forceps having a curved shank are applied to the fetal head while it is high in the pelvis. The head is displaced upward and rotated to the occiput anterior position. The forceps are removed and repositioned, and the delivery is accomplished by axis traction. The operation has been largely replaced by cesarean section. See also **forceps delivery, obstetric forceps.**

scapho- A combining form meaning 'boatshaped': *scaphocephaly, scaphohydrocephaly, scaphoid.*

scaphocephaly, scaphocephalis, scaphocephalism A congenital malformation of the skull in which premature closure of the sagittal suture results in restricted lateral head growth. The head is abnormally long and narrow with a cephalic index of 75 or less. The condition is often associated with mental retardation. Also called **dolichocephaly, mecocephaly.** See also **craniostenosis. —scaphocephalic, scaphocephalous,** *adj.*

scaphoid bone Either of two similar bones of the hand and the foot. The scaphoid bone of the hand is slanted at the radial side of the carpus and articulates with the radius, trapezium, trapezoid, capitate, and lunate bones. Also called **navicular bone.**

scapula One of the pair of large, flat, triangular bones that form the dorsal part of the shoulder girdle. It has two surfaces, three borders, three angles, and a prominent dorsal spine. Also called **shoulder blade.**

-scapula A combining form meaning a 'shoulderblade or a part of it': *mesoscapula, prescapula, proscapula.*

scapulohumeral Of or pertaining to the structures of muscles and the area around the scapula and humerus.

scapulohumeral muscular dystrophy A form of limb-girdle muscular dystrophy that begins in the shoulder girdle. Also called **Erb's muscular dystrophy.**

scapulohumeral reflex A normal response to tapping the vertebral border of the scapula, resulting in arm adduction. Absence of the reflex may indicate a lesion in the region of the fifth cervical segment of the spinal cord.

scar See **cicatrix.**

scarification Multiple superficial scratches or incisions in the skin, as are made for the introduction of a vaccine. Erroneously used to mean 'producing a scar.'

scarify To make multiple superficial incisions into the skin; to scratch. Vaccination against smallpox is achieved by scarifying the skin under a drop of vaccine.

scarlatina See **scarlet fever.**

scarlatiniform Resembling the rash of **scarlet fever.**

scarlet fever An acute contagious disease of childhood caused by an erythrotoxin-producing strain of group A hemolytic *Streptococcus*, characterized by sore throat, fever, enlarged lymph nodes in the neck, prostration, and a diffuse bright red rash. Also called **scarlatina.**

scarlet red **1.** An azo dye used in pharmaceutical preparations. **2.** A dermatomucosal agent used to treat decubitus ulcers.

scato-, skato A combining form meaning 'of or related to dung, or to fecal matter': *scatophagy, scatophilia.*

scattergram A graph representing the distribution of two variables in a sample population. One variable is plotted on the vertical axis; the second on the horizontal axis. The scores or values of each sample unit are usually represented by dots.

scattering In radiology: a change in direction path of subatomic particles caused by collision or interaction.

scavenging system See **gas scavenging system.**

scel- A combining form meaning 'leg': *scelalgia, scelotyrbe.*

-scelia A combining form meaning '(condition of the) legs': *macroscelia, polyscelia, rhaeboscelia.*

Schedule I A category of drugs not considered legitimate for medical use by the Drug En-

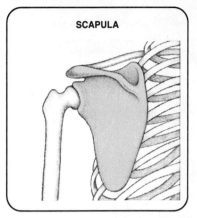

SCAPULA

forcement Agency. The category includes cannabis, heroin, LSD, and mescaline. Special licensing procedures are required to use Schedule I substances.

Schedule II A category of drugs considered to have a strong potential for abuse or addiction, but which have legitimate medical use. The category includes cocaine, methadone, methaqualone, morphine, and pentobarbital.

Schedule III A category of drugs that have less potential for abuse or addiction than Schedule I or II drugs. The category includes glutethimide and various analgesic compounds containing codeine.

Schedule IV A category of drugs that have less potential for abuse or addiction than those of Schedules I to III. The category includes chloral hydrate, chlordiazepoxide, and oxazepam.

Schedule V A category of drugs that have a small potential for abuse or addiction. The category includes many commonly prescribed medications that contain small amounts of codeine or diphenoxylate.

Schedule of Drugs A classification system that categorizes drugs by their potential for abuse. The schedule is divided into five groups: Schedules I to V. The assignment of drugs to the categories varies from state to state. All substances in Schedules II to V require a written prescription signed by a physician. See also specific schedules.

Scheuermann's disease An abnormal skeletal condition characterized by a fixed kyphosis that develops at puberty and is caused by wedge-shaped deformities of one or several vertebrae. The cause of the disease is unknown. The most striking pathologic feature is the presence of wedge-shaped vertebral bodies, seen on radiographic examination, that create an excessive curvature. Scheuermann's disease occurs most frequently in children between the ages of 12 and 16, with onset at puberty, and the incidence is greater in girls than in boys. The onset is insidious and often associated with a history of unusual physical activity or participation in sports. The most frequent symptom

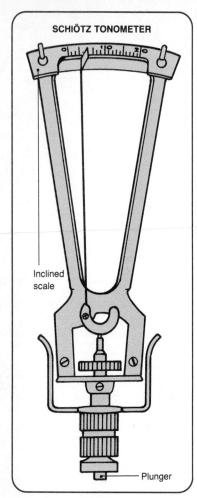

SCHIÖTZ TONOMETER

Inclined scale

Plunger

is poor posture with accompanying symptoms of fatigue and pain in the involved area. In most affected individuals the kyphosis is within the thoracic vertebrae. If the disease is diagnosed at the onset, the associated posture may be corrected actively and passively. Otherwise, the associated posture becomes fixed within a period of 6 to 9 months. The most effective treatment of Scheuermann's disease is immobilization with a plaster cast or with a Milwaukee brace. In adults, persistent pain in the thoracic area may indicate a degenerative alteration secondary to this disease process, and spinal arthrodesis may be required to relieve the symptoms. Also called **adolescent vertebral epiphysitis, juvenile kyphosis.**

Schick test A skin test to determine immunity to diphtheria in which diphtheria toxin is injected intradermally. A positive reaction is marked by redness and swelling at the site of injection; a negative reaction is marked by absence of redness or swelling.

Schilder's disease Eponym for a group of progressive, severe, neurologic diseases beginning in childhood and characterized by demyelination of the white matter of the brain with muscle spasticity, optic neuritis, aphasia, deafness, adrenal insufficiency, and dementia. Many of the signs resemble those of multiple sclerosis. There is no known treatment. The cause may be viral or genetic.

Schiller's test A procedure for indicating areas of abnormal epithelium in the vagina or on the cervix of the uterus as a guide in selecting biopsy sites for cancer detection. A potassium iodide or aqueous iodine solution is painted on the vaginal walls and cervix under direct visualization. Normal epithelium contains glycogen and stains a deep brown color; abnormal epithelium, containing no glycogen, will not stain, and nonstaining sites may then be included in tissue biopsies. The test is not specific for malignancy, since inflammation, ulceration, and keratotic lesions also may not accept the iodine stain.

Schilling's leukemia See **monocytic leukemia.**

Schilling test A diagnostic test for pernicious anemia in which vitamin B_{12} tagged with radioactive cobalt is administered orally, and gastrointestinal absorption is measured by determining the radioactivity of urine samples collected over a 24-hour period. In persons with pernicious anemia, the ability to absorb vitamin B_{12} is reduced, so that excretion of radioactive material is reduced.

Schiötz tonometer A tonometer that measures intraocular pressure by gauging the depth of corneal indentation made by the weighted plunger on the device.

schisto- A combining form meaning 'split, or cleft': *schistocelia, schistocephalus, schistomelia.*

Schistosoma A genus of blood flukes that may cause urinary, gastrointestinal, or liver disease and that requires fresh water snails as intermediate hosts. *S. hematobium,* found chiefly in Africa and the Middle East, affects the bladder and pelvic organs, causing painful, frequent urination and hematuria. *S. japonicum,* found in Japan, the Philippines, and Eastern Asia, causes gastrointestinal ulcerations and fibrosis of the liver. *S. mansoni,* found in Africa, the Middle East, the Caribbean, and South America, causes symptoms similar to those caused by *S. japonicum.* See also **schistosomiasis.**

schistosomiasis A parasitic infection caused by a species of fluke of the genus *Schistosoma,* transmitted to man, the definitive host, by contact with fresh water contaminated by human feces. A single fluke may live in one part of the body, depositing eggs frequently, for up to 20 years. The eggs are irritating to mucous membrane, causing it to thicken and become papillomatous. Pain, obstruction, dysfunction of the affected organ, and anemia may result. Diagnosis requires morphologic identification of the ova or the parasite. Treatment is difficult; oxyamniquine is the current drug of choice. Second only to malaria in the number of people affected, schistosomiasis is particularly prevalent in the tropics and in the Orient. Also called **bilharziasis.** See also **blood fluke, *Schistosoma.***

schistosomicide   A drug destructive to schistosomes. Niridazole, metrifonate, oxamniquine hycanthone hydrochloride, and various salts of antimony, including stibophen, are potent antischistosomal agents. —**schistosomicidal,** *adj.*

schizo-   A combining form meaning 'divided, or related to division': *schizocephalia, schizogenesis, schizophrenia.*

schizoaffective disorder   A condition that includes characteristics of schizophrenia and bipolar disorder or of other major affective disorders.

schizogenesis   Reproduction by fission. —**schizogenetic, schizogenic, schizogenous,** *adj.*

schizogony   **1.** Reproduction by multiple fission. **2.** The asexual reproductive stage of sporozoans, specifically the portion of the life cycle of the malarial parasite that occurs in the erythrocytes or liver cells. See also *Plasmodium.* —**schizogonic, schizogonous.** *adj.*

schizoid   **1.** Characteristic of or resembling schizophrenia; schizophrenic. **2.** A person, not necessarily a schizophrenic, who exhibits the traits of a schizoid personality.

schizoid personality   A functioning but maladjusted person whose behavior is characterized by extreme shyness, oversensitivity, introversion, seclusiveness, and avoidance of close interpersonal relationships.

schizoid personality disorder   A condition characterized by a defect in the ability to form social relationships. The condition may precede schizophrenia.

schizont   The multinucleated cell stage during the sexual reproductive phase in the life cycle of a sporozoan, specifically the malarial parasite *Plasmodium.* Also called **agamont.** Compare **sporont.** See also **schizogony.**

schizonticide   A substance that destroys schizonts. —**schizonticidal,** *adj.*

schizophasia   Incomprehensible speech characteristic of some forms of schizophrenia. See also **word salad.**

schizophrene   A person afflicted with schizophrenia.

schizophrenia   Any one of a large group of psychotic disorders characterized by gross distortion of reality, disturbances of language and communication, withdrawal from social interaction, and the disorganization and fragmentation of thought, perception, and emotional reaction. Apathy and confusion; delusions and hallucinations; rambling or stylized patterns of speech, as evasiveness, incoherence, and echolalia; withdrawn, regressive, and bizarre behavior; and emotional lability often occur. No

single cause of the disease is known. Treatment often requires the use of antipsychotics, and antidepressant and antianxiety drugs. Kinds of schizophrenia include **acute schizophrenia, catatonic schizophrenia, childhood schizophrenia, disorganized schizophrenia, latent schizophrenia, paranoid schizophrenia, process schizophrenia, reactive schizophrenia, residual schizophrenia.** Also called schizophrenic disorder, schizophrenic reaction.

schizophrenic   **1.** Of or pertaining to schizophrenia. **2.** A person afflicted with schizophrenia.

schizophreniform disorder   A condition exhibiting the same symptoms as schizophrenia but characterized by an acute onset with resolution in 2 weeks to 6 months.

schizophrenogenic   Tending to cause or produce schizophrenia.

Schizotrypanum cruzi   See **Chagas' disease.**

schizotypal personality disorder   A condition characterized by oddities of thought, perception, speech, and behavior that are not severe enough to meet the clinical criteria for schizophrenia. Symptoms include magical thinking, ideas of reference, recurrent illusions, social isolation, peculiar speech patterns, and exaggerated anxiety or hypersensitivity to real or imagined criticism. See also **schizoid personality disorder, schizophrenia.**

Schlatter-Osgood disease, Schlatter's disease   See **Osgood-Schlatter disease.**

Schlemm's canal   See **canal of Schlemm.**

Schneiderian carcinoma   An epithelial malignancy of the nasal mucosa and paranasal sinuses.

Schönlein Henoch purpura   See **Henoch-Schönlein purpura.**

School Nurse Practitioner (SNP)   A registered nurse qualified by postgraduate study to act as a nurse practitioner in a school.

school phobia   An extreme separation anxiety disorder of children, usually in the elementary grades, characterized by a persistent, irrational fear of going to school.

Schultz-Chariton phenomenon   A cutaneous reaction to the intradermal injection of scarlatina antiserum in a person who has a scarletiniform rash. The rash blanches.

Schwabach test   A hearing test, using a 256-, 512-, 1024-, or 2048-cycle tuning fork, in which tester and patient occlude one ear and the tester then alternates the vibrating fork between the mastoid process of the patient's open ear and his own until one of them ceases to hear the tone. The result is 'Schwabach normal' if both hear the sound the same length of time. 'Schwabach shortened,' when the patient hears the sound a shorter time, indicates a sensorineural hearing loss. 'Schwabach prolonged,' when the patient hears it longer, means conductive hearing loss.

schwannoma, *pl.* **schwannomas, schwannomata**   A benign, solitary, encapsulated tumor arising in the neurilemma

SCLERA

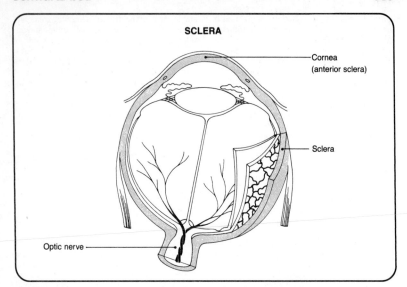

Cornea
(anterior sclera)

Sclera

Optic nerve

(Schwann's sheath) of peripheral, cranial, or autonomic nerves. Also called Schwann-cell tumor, neurilemoma.

Schwartz bed   See **hyperextension bed.**

Schwartzman-Sanarelli phenomenon A phenomenon induced experimentally. Animals injected twice with a bacterial endotoxin develop massive disseminated intravascular coagulation with thrombosis of the blood vessels in the kidneys. Also called Schwartzman phenomenon.

scia-   See **skia-.**

sciatic   Near the ischium, as the sciatic nerve.

sciatica   Condition stemming from irritation or swelling of the sciatic nerve and involving severe pain that courses down the sciatic nerve from the hip and along the posterior or lateral aspect of the leg or appears at any point on this path. See also **meralgia, neuralgia, neuritis.**

SCID   *abbr* **severe combined immunodeficiency disease.**

science   A systematic attempt to establish theories to explain observed phenomena. Pure science is concerned with the gathering of information solely for the sake of obtaining new knowledge. **Applied science** is the practical application of scientific theory and laws. See also **hypothesis, law, scientific method, theory.**

scientific method   A systematic, ordered approach to gathering data and solving problems. The basic approach is the statement of the problem followed by the statement of a hypothesis. An experimental method is established to help prove or disprove the hypothesis. The results of the experiment are observed, and conclusions are drawn from the observed results.

scintillascope   A device with a fluorescent screen and a magnifying lens for viewing alpha emissions, used in diagnostic tests to locate radioactive isotope concentrations in the body. Also

called a spinthariscope.

scintillation   **1.** An emission of sparks or flashes. **2.** A subjective sensation as of seeing sparks. **3.** The spontaneous emissions of alpha, beta, and sometimes gamma particles produced by the disintegration of radioactive substances.

scintiphotography   Use of a camera to photograph the scintillations of radioactive substances introduced into the body for diagnostic purposes. The process depicts the contours and functions of organs or tissues that concentrate or metabolize the radioisotope.

scintiscan   The pattern, plotted on paper, made by scintillations of radioactive substances introduced into the body for diagnostic purposes, showing graphically the concentration or metabolism of the substances in organs or tissues.

scirrho-   A combining form meaning 'hard, or related to a hard cancer or scirrhus': *scirrhoid, scirrhoma.*

scirrhous carcinoma   A hard, fibrous, particularly invasive tumor in which the malignant cells occur singly or in small clusters or strands in dense connective tissue. It is the most common form of breast cancer. Also called **carcinoma fibrosum.** See also **breast cancer.**

scissors   A sharp instrument composed of two opposing cutting blades, held together by a central pin. The most common dissecting scissors are the straight Mayo, for cutting sutures; the long, curved Mayo, for deep, heavy, or tough tissue; the short, curved Metzenbaum, for superficial, delicate tissue; the long, blunt, curved Metzenbaum, for deep, delicate tissue; and the Snowden-Pencer, for deep, delicate tissue.

scler-, sclero-   A combining form meaning 'hard,' often used to show relationship to the sclera: *scleroadipose, sclerocorneal.*

sclera   The tough, inelastic, opaque membrane covering the posterior five sixths of the eye bulb. It maintains the size and form of the bulb and attaches to muscles that move the bulb. Posteriorly, it is pierced by the optic nerve and, with the transparent cornea, comprises the outermost of three tunics covering the eye bulb.

scleredema An idiopathic skin disease characterized by nonpitting induration beginning on the face or neck and spreading downward over the body, sparing the hands and feet. Symptoms may include swelling of the tongue; restricted eye movement; and pericardial, pleural, and peritoneal effusions. Resolution occurs after several months, but recurrences are common. The condition often follows a streptococcal infection or an exanthem of childhood. There is no specific treatment. Compare **scleroderma.**

sclerema neonatorum A progressive, generalized hardening of the skin and subcutaneous tissue of the newborn. It is usually a fatal condition that occurs as a result of severe cold stress in severely ill, premature infants subject to such life-threatening conditions as metabolic acidosis, hypoglycemia, gastrointestinal or respiratory infection, or gross malformation. Also called scleredema neonatorum, sclerema adiposum.

sclerodactyly A musculoskeletal deformity affecting the hands of patients with scleroderma. The fingers are fixed in a semiflexed position with the fingertips pointed and ulcerated.

scleroderma A relatively rare autoimmune disease affecting the blood vessels and connective tissue, characterized by fibrous degeneration of the connective tissue of the skin, lungs, and internal organs. Scleroderma is most common in middle-aged women. Signs include skin changes, joint deformity, and pain on movement. Scleroderma may occur in a mild form with the person living 30 to 50 years, or there may be early death owing to cardiac, renal, pulmonary, or intestinal involvement. Localized forms of scleroderma may occur; these cases are benign and occur only as small circumscribed patches on the skin. A biopsy of the lesion may be done to diagnose the condition. X-ray examination of the lungs and gastrointestinal tract may be diagnostic in the systemic form of the disease. Blood tests may reveal antinuclear antibodies. Corticosteroids may help treat the symptoms, and salicylates and mild analgesics may ease joint pain.

-scleroma A combining form meaning an 'induration, a hardening of the tissues': *laryngoscleroma, pharyngoscleroma, rhinoscleroma.*

scleromalacia perforans A condition of the eyes in which devitalization and sloughing of the sclera occur as a complication of rheumatoid arthritis. The pigmented uvea becomes exposed, and glaucoma, cataract formation, and detachment of the retina may result.

sclerose To harden or to cause hardening. **—sclerotic,** *adj.*

sclerosing hemangioma A solid, cellu-

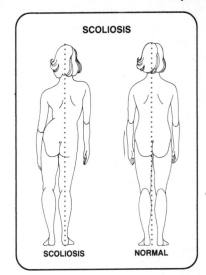

SCOLIOSIS

SCOLIOSIS   NORMAL

lar, tumorlike nodule of the skin or a mass of histiocytes, thought to arise from a hemangioma by the proliferation of endothelial and connective tissue cells.

sclerosis A condition characterized by hardening of tissue resulting from any of several causes, including inflammation. **—sclerotic,** *adj.*

sclerotome In embryology: the part of the segmented mesoderm layer in the developing embryo that originates from somites and gives rise to the skeletal body tissue, specifically, the paired segmented masses of mesodermal tissue that lie on each side of the notochord and develop into the vertebrae and ribs. See also **somite.**

scoleco- A combining form meaning 'of or pertaining to a worm': *scolecoid, scolecoidectomy, scolecology.*

scolex, *pl.* **scoleces** The headlike segment or organ of an adult tapeworm that has hooks, grooves, or suckers by which it attaches itself to the wall of the intestine.

scolio- A combining form meaning 'twisted or crooked': *scoliodontic, scoliokyphosis, scoliosiometry.*

scoliosis Lateral curvature of the spine, a common abnormality of childhood. Causes include congenital malformations of the spine, poliomyelitis, skeletal dysplasias, spastic paralysis, and unequal leg length. Early recognition and orthopedic treatment may prevent progression. Treatment includes braces, casts, exercises, and corrective surgery. See also **kyphoscoliosis, kyphosis, lordosis, spinal curvature.**

scop- A combining form meaning 'to examine, observe': *scopograph, scopometer, scopophilia.*

-scope A combining form meaning an 'instrument for observation': *ciliariscope, episcope, pelviscope.*

-scopia A combining form meaning 'observation': *aknephascopia, mixoscopia.*

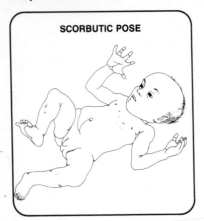

SCORBUTIC POSE

scopolamine, s. hydrobromide Antiemetic, mydriatic, and cholinergic (parasympatholytic) blocking agents.

scopophilia, scoptophilia 1. Sexual pleasure derived from looking at sexually stimulating scenes or at another person's genitals; voyeurism. 2. A morbid desire to be seen; exhibitionism. —**scopophiliac, scopophilic, scoptophiliac, scoptophilic;** *adj., n.*

scopophobia An anxiety disorder characterized by a morbid fear of being seen or stared at by others. The condition is common in schizophrenia. See also **phobia.**

-scopy A combining form meaning 'observation': *bioscopy, stomachoscopy, thoracoscopy.*

-scorbic A combining form meaning 'of or referring to the prevention or treatment of scurvy': *antiscorbic, ascorbic, glucoascorbic.*

-scorbutic, -scorbic, -scorbutical A combining form meaning 'pertaining to scurvy': *antiscorbutic, postscorbutic, scorbutic.*

scorbutic pose The characteristic posture of a child with scurvy—thighs and legs semiflexed and hips rotated outward. See also **scurvy.**

scorbutus See **scurvy.**

scorpion sting A painful wound produced by a scorpion, an arachnid with a hollow stinger in its tail. The stings of many species are only slightly toxic, but some, including *Centruroides sculpturatus* of the southwestern United States, may inflict fatal injury, especially in small children. Initial pain is followed within several hours by numbness, nausea, muscle spasm, dyspnea, and convulsion. Treatment includes ice applied to the wound and intravenous calcium gluconate to control muscle spasm, if necessary. Severe cases may require oxygen and respiratory assistance. An antivenin is available in some areas.

scoto- A combining form meaning 'of or related to darkness': *scotodinia, scotogram, scotographic.*

scratch test A skin test for identifying an allergen, performed by placing a small quantity of a solution containing a suspected allergen on a lightly scratched skin area. Wheal formation in 15 minutes is a positive reaction.

screamer's nodule See **vocal cord nodule.**

screening 1. A preliminary procedure, as a test or examination, to detect the most characteristic sign or signs of a disorder that may require further investigation. 2. The examination of a large sample of a population to detect a specific disease or disorder.

screen memory A consciously tolerable memory that replaces one that is emotionally painful to recall.

screw clamp A device, usually plastic, equipped with a screw that can be manipulated to close and open the primary I.V. tubing for regulating flow. Compare **roller clamp, slide clamp.**

scrib-, script- A combining form meaning 'write': *scribble, scribomania, prescription.*

Scribner shunt A type of arteriovenous bypass, used in hemodialysis, consisting of a special tube connection outside the body.

scrofula Primary tuberculosis with abscess formation, usually of the cervical lymph nodes.

scrofulous keratitis See **phlyctenular keratoconjunctivitis.**

scrotal cancer An epidermoid malignancy of the scrotum, characterized initially by a small sore that may ulcerate. The lesion occurs most frequently in elderly men who have been exposed to soot, pitch, crude oil, mineral oils, polycyclic hydrocarbons, or arsenical fumes from copper smelting. Treatment involves wide surgical excision of the tumor and resection of inguinal nodes. Also called **chimney-sweeps' cancer, soot wart.**

scrotum The pouch of skin containing the testes and parts of the spermatic cords. It is divided on the surface into two lateral portions by a ridge that continues ventrally to the undersurface of the penis and dorsally along the middle line of the perineum to the anus. In young, robust individuals the scrotum is short, corrugated, and closely wraps the testes. In older persons, in debilitated individuals, and in warm environments, the scrotum becomes elongated and flaccid. The lateral left portion of the scrotum hangs lower than the right, corresponding with the longer length of the left spermatic cord. The scrotum is highly vascular and contains no fat. See also **testis.** —**scrotal,** *adj.*

scrub See **surgical scrub.**

scrub room A special hospital area where surgeons and surgical teams use disposable sterile brushes and bactericidal soaps to wash and scrub their fingernails, hands, and forearms before performing or assisting in surgical operations.

scrub typhus An acute, febrile disease of Asia, India, northern Australia, and the western Pacific islands, caused by several strains of the genus *Rickettsia tsutsugamushi* and transmitted from infected rodents to humans by mites. It is characterized by a necrotic papule or black eschar at the bite site. Tender, enlarged regional lymph nodes, fever, severe headache, eye pain, muscle aches, and a generalized rash usually occur. In severe cases, the myocardium and the central nervous system may be involved. The Weil-Felix reaction and indirect fluorescent antibody tests are useful in diagnosis. Treatment with broad-spectrum antibiotics, as chloramphenicol, doxycycline, or tetracycline, has reduced mortality to nearly zero. Person-to-person transmission is not known to occur. Also called **Japanese river fever, mite typhus, tsutsugamushi disease.** Compare **Q-fever, Rocky Mountain spotted fever, typhus.**

scruple   A measure of weight in the apothecaries' system, equal to 20 grains or 1.296 gm. See also **apothecaries' weight, metric system.**

scultetus binder   A many-tailed binder with an attached central piece. The tails are overlapped; the last two tied or pinned act to secure the others. A scultetus bandage may be opened or removed without moving the bandaged part of the body.

scurvy   A condition resulting from lack of ascorbic acid in the diet. It is characterized by weakness; anemia; edema; spongy gums, often with ulceration and loosening of the teeth; a tendency to mucocutaneous hemorrhages; and induration of the muscles of the legs. Treatment and prophylaxis of the disease consist of administration of ascorbic acid and the inclusion of fresh vegetables and fruits in the diet. Also called scorbutus. See also **ascorbic acid, citric acid, infantile scurvy.**

scyt-   A combining form meaning 'skin': *scytitis, scytoblastema.*

Se   Symbol for **selenium.**

sealed source   In radiotherapy: a source of radiant energy in which the radioactive material is permanently encased in a container or bonding material in a manner to prevent leakage. Sealed sources, as seeds, needles, and specially designed applicators, are used in the implantation of cesium 137, iodine 125, iridium 192, radium 226, and other radionuclides for the treatment of various malignant tumors.

seal limbs   See **phocomelia.**

seatworm   See *Enterobius vermicularis.*

sea urchin sting   An injury inflicted by any of a variety of sea urchins, in which the skin is punctured and in some species, venom released. A venomous sting is characterized by pain, muscular weakness, numbness around the mouth, and dyspnea. See also **stingray.**

seawater bath   A bath taken in warm seawater or in a saline solution.

sebaceous   Fatty, oily, or greasy, usually referring to the oil-secreting glands of the skin or to their secretions.

sebaceous cyst   A misnomer for epidermoid cyst or pilar cyst.

sebaceous gland   One of the many small sacculated organs in the dermis. They are located throughout the body in close association with all types of body hair. Each gland consists of a single duct which emerges from a cluster of oval alveoli. Each alveolus is composed of a transparent basement membrane enclosing epithelial cells. The ducts from most sebaceous

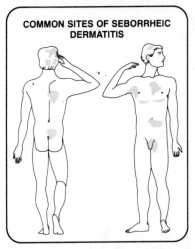

COMMON SITES OF SEBORRHEIC DERMATITIS

glands open into the hair follicles but some open on the general surface of the skin. The sebum secreted by the glands oils the hair and the surrounding skin, helps to prevent evaporation of sweat, and aids in the retention of body heat. Compare **sudoriferous gland.**

seborrhea   Any of several common skin conditions in which an overproduction of sebum causes excessive oiliness or dry scales. See also **seborrheic blepharitis, seborrheic dermatitis. —seborrheic,** *adj.*

seborrheic blepharitis   A form of seborrheic dermatitis in which the eyelids are erythematous and the margins are covered with a granular crust.

seborrheic dermatitis   A common, chronic, inflammatory skin disease characterized by dry or moist greasy scales and yellowish crusts. Common sites are the scalp, eyelids, face, external surfaces of the ears, axillae, breasts, groin, and gluteal folds. In acute stages there may be exudate and infection resulting in secondary furunculosis. Occasionally, generalized exfoliation results. Kinds of seborrheic dermatitis include **cradle cap, dandruff, seborrheic blepharitis.**

seborrheic keratosis   A benign, well-circumscribed, raised, tan-to-black, warty skin lesion on the face, neck, chest, or upper back. The macules are loosely covered with a greasy crust that leaves a raw pulpy base when removed. Itching is common. Also called basal cell acanthoma, basal cell papilloma, seborrheic wart.

seborrheic wart   See **seborrheic keratosis.**

sebum   The normal secretion of the sebaceous glands of the skin, composed of keratin, fat, and cellular debris. Combined with sweat, sebum forms a moist, oily, acidic film that is mildly antibacterial and antifungal and protects the skin against drying.

Seckel's syndrome   See **bird-headed dwarf.**

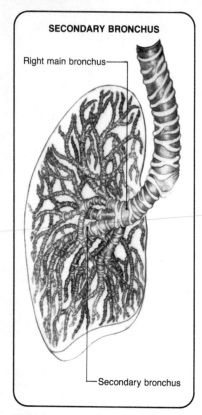

SECONDARY BRONCHUS

Right main bronchus

Secondary bronchus

seclusion In psychiatric nursing: the isolation of a patient in a special room in order to decrease stimuli which might be causing or exacerbating the patient's emotional distress.

secobarbital, s. sodium Barbiturate sedative-hypnotic agents.

secondary amputation Amputation performed after suppuration has begun following severe trauma. An area is left open for drainage, and antibiotics are given. Compare **primary amputation.** See also **amputation.**

secondary areola A second ring appearing around the areola of the breast during pregnancy that is more pigmented than the areola before pregnancy.

secondary biliary cirrhosis An abnormal hepatic condition characterized by bile duct obstruction with or without infection. It involves periportal inflammation with progressive fibrosis, destruction of parenchymal cells, and nodular degneration. Compare **primary biliary cirrhosis.**

secondary bronchus A lobar or segmental bronchus. See also **bronchus, primary bronchus.**

secondary dementia Dementia resulting from another, concurrent form of psychosis. See also **dementia.**

secondary dental caries Dental caries developing in a tooth already affected by the condition; often a new cavity forms adjacent to or beneath the restorative filling of an old cavity.

secondary dentition See **permanent dentition.**

secondary fissure A fissure between the uvula and the pyramid of the cerebellum.

secondary fracture See **neoplastic fracture.**

secondary gain An indirect benefit, usually obtained through an illness or debility. Such gains may include monetary and disability benefits, personal attentions, or escape from unpleasant situations and responsibilities. Compare **primary gain.**

secondary health care An intermediate level of health care that includes diagnosis and treatment, performed in a hospital having specialized equipment and laboratory facilities.

secondary host Any animal in which the larval or intermediate stages of a parasite develop. Certain snails are secondary hosts for liver flukes and schistosomes. Humans are secondary hosts for malaria parasites. Also called intermediate host. Compare **dead-end host, definitive host, reservoir host.** See also **host,** definition 1.

secondary hypertrophic osteoarthropathy See **clubbing.**

secondary nutrient A substance that acts as a stimulant to activate the flora of the gastrointestinal tract to synthesize other nutrients.

secondary port A device for regulating the flow of a primary and a secondary I.V. solution. It consists of a Y-shaped plastic apparatus that attaches to the primary I.V. tubing and allows the two solutions to flow separately or simultaneously. Compare **piggyback port.**

secondary sequestrum A piece of dead bone that partially separates from sound bone during the process of necrosis but may be pushed back into position. Compare **primary sequestrum.**

secondary sex characteristic Any of the physical characteristics of sexual maturity secondary to hormonal stimulation that develops in the maturing individual.

secondary shock A state of physical collapse and prostration caused by numerous traumatic and pathological conditions. It develops over a period of time following severe tissue damage and may merge with primary shock, accompanied by various signs, as weakness, restlessness, low body temperature, low blood pressure, cold sweat, and reduced urinary output. Death may occur within a relatively short time, unless appropriate treatment intervenes. Secondary shock is often associated with heat stroke, crushing injuries, myocardial infarction, poisoning, fulminating infections, burns, and other life-threatening conditions. The pathology of this state reflects changes in the capillaries, which become dilated and engorged with blood. Petechial hemorrhages develop in the serous membranes, edema swells the soft tissues, and

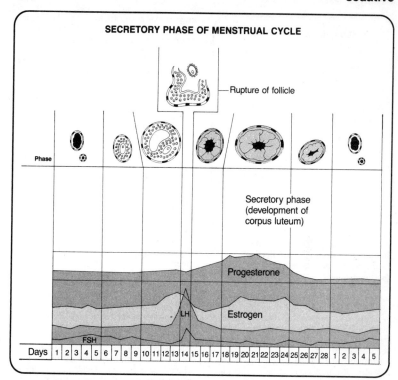

SECRETORY PHASE OF MENSTRUAL CYCLE

Rupture of follicle

Phase

Secretory phase
(development of
corpus luteum)

Progesterone

LH

Estrogen

FSH

Days 1 2 3 4 5 6 7 8 9 10 11 12 13 14 15 16 17 18 19 20 21 22 23 24 25 26 27 28 1 2 3 4 5

the vital organs undergo degenerative changes. Compare **hemorrhagic shock, primary shock.**

second cuneiform bone See **intermediate cuneiform bone.**

second filial generation See **F₂.**

second nerve See **optic nerve.**

second sight An improvement in the near vision of the aged owing to the myopia associated with increasing lenticular nuclear sclerosis. This type of sclerosis commonly leads to the development of nuclear cataracts.

secrete To discharge a substance into a cavity, a vessel, or an organ or onto the skin surface. —**secretion,** *n.*

secretin A digestive hormone produced by certain cells lining the duodenum and jejunum when acidic, partially digested food enters the intestine from the stomach. It stimulates the pancreas to produce a fluid high in salts but low in enzymes. Secretin has a limited stimulating effect on the production of bile. See also **pancreas.**

secretin test A test of pancreatic function after stimulation with secretin. The test measures the volume and bicarbonate concentration of pancreatic secretions. A lower than normal volume suggests an obstructing malignancy. Reduced bicarbonate and amylase concentration may indicate chronic pancreatitis.

secretory duct Of a gland: a small duct that has a secretory function and joins with an excretory duct.

secretory phase The phase of the menstrual cycle following the release of an ovum from a mature ovarian follicle. The corpus luteum, stimulated by luteinizing hormone (LH), develops from the ruptured follicle. It secretes progesterone, which stimulates the development of the glands and arteries of the endometrium, causing it to become thick and spongy. In a negative-feedback response to the increased progesterone level in the blood, LH secretion decreases. If an embryo does not implant on the endometrium, chorionic gonadotropin is not secreted, and the secretory phase ends. The corpus luteum involutes, progesterone levels plummet, and menstruation occurs. Also called **luteal phase.**

sect- A combining form meaning 'to cut': *sectio, section.*

-sect A combining form meaning 'to cut': *dissect, medisect, quadrisect.*

secund- A combining form meaning 'second, or following': *secundigravida, secundina, secundine.*

secundigravida A woman pregnant for the second time. Also called **gravida II.** —**secundigravid,** *adj.*

sedation An induced state of quiet, calmness, or sleep, as by means of a sedative or hypnotic medication.

sedative **1.** Of or pertaining to a substance, procedure, or measure that has a calming effect.

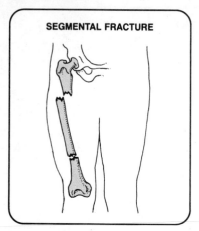

SEGMENTAL FRACTURE

2. An agent that decreases functional activity, diminishes irritability, and allays excitement. Some sedatives have a general effect on all organs; others affect principally the activities of the heart, stomach, intestines, nerve trunks, respiratory system, or vasomotor system. Barbiturates and nonbarbiturate sedatives are used to induce sleep, reduce pain, help induce anesthesia, and treat convulsive conditions, anxiety states, and irritable bowel syndrome. See also **sedative-hypnotic.**

sedative bath The immersion of the body in water for a prolonged period of time, used especially as a calming procedure for agitated patients.

sedative-hypnotic A drug that reversibly depresses the central nervous system activity, used chiefly to induce sleep and to allay anxiety. Barbiturates and many nonbarbiturate sedative-hypnotics depress the activity of all excitable tissue and affect the arousal center in the brainstem. Various sedative-hypnotics and minor tranquilizers with similar effects are used to treat insomnia, acute convulsive conditions, anxiety states, and to help induce anesthesia. Although sedative-hypnotics have a soporific effect, they may interfere with rapid eye movement (REM) sleep associated with dreaming and, when administered to patients with fever, may cause excitement rather than relaxation. Sedative-hypnotics may interfere with temperature regulation, depress oxygen consumption in various tissues, produce nausea and skin rashes, and, in elderly patients, may cause dizziness, confusion, and ataxia. Acute reactions to an overdose of a sedative-hypnotic may be treated with an emetic, activated charcoal, gastric lavage, and measures to maintain airway patency. See also **barbiturate.**

sedimentation rate See **erythrocyte sedimentation rate.**

sed. rate Erythrocyte sedimentation rate.

segment A section or portion of a body, organ, or object, occurring naturally or having its borders artificially established.

segmental bronchus A bronchus branching from a lobar bronchus to a bronchiole.

segmental fracture A bone break which produces several large bone fragments. The fragments may pierce the skin, as in an open fracture, or may be contained within the skin, as in a closed fracture.

segmental resection A surgical procedure in which a part of an organ, gland, or other body part is excised, as a segmental resection of an ovary to diminish the hormonal secretion.

segmentation **1.** The repetition of structured parts or the process of dividing into segments or similar parts, as the formation of somites or metameres. **2.** The division of the zygote into blastomeres; cleavage.

segmentation cavity See **blastocoele.**

segmentation cell See **blastomere.**

segmentation nucleus The nucleus of the zygote resulting from the fusion of the male and female pronuclei in the fertilized ovum. It is the final stage in fertilization and initiates the first cleavage of the zygote. Also called **cleavage nucleus.**

segmented hyalinizing vasculitis A chronic, relapsing inflammatory condition of the blood vessels of the lower legs associated with nodular or purpuric skin lesions that may become ulcerated and leave scars. Also called **livedo vasculitis.**

segregation In genetics: a principle stating that the chromosome pairs bearing genes from both parents are separated during meiosis. Chance alone determines which gene, maternal or paternal, travels to which gamete. See also **dominance, independent assortment.**

seizure See **convulsion.**

seizure threshold The amount of stimulus needed to cause a convulsive seizure. Any person can have seizures if the stimulus is sufficient. Those who have spontaneous convulsions are said to have a 'low seizure threshold.'

selection In genetics: the process by which various factors or mechanisms determine and modify the reproductive ability of a genotype within a specific population, thus influencing evolutionary change. Kinds of selection are **artificial selection, natural selection, sexual selection.**

selective angiography A graphic procedure that allows selective visualization of the aorta, the major arterial systems, or a particular vessel.

selenium (Se) A metalloid element of the sulfur group. Its atomic number is 34; its atomic weight is 78.96. Selenium also occurs as a trace element in foods. It is used externally to control seborrheic dermatitis, dandruff, and other forms of dermatosis.

selenium sulfide A dermatomucosal agent used to treat psoriasis and other skin conditions.

self *pl.* **selves. 1.** The total essence or being of a person; the individual. **2.** Those affective, cognitive, and spiritual qualities that distinguish one person from another; individuality. **3.** A person's awareness of his own being or identity; consciousness; ego. See also **personality**.

self-actualization In humanistic psychology: the fundamental tendency toward the maximum realization and fulfillment of one's human potential.

self-alien See **ego-dystonic**.

self-alienation See **depersonalization**.

self-anesthesia Self-administered inhalational anesthesia using a hand-held breathing device. It is most common in England; trilene is the usual gas.

self-breast examination (SBE) A procedure in which a woman examines her breasts and their accessory structures for evidence of a malignant process. The SBE is usually performed 1 week to 10 days after the first day of the menstrual cycle, when the breasts are smallest and cyclic nodularity is least apparent. Also called **breast self-examination.** See also **breast examination.**

self-care **1.** The personal and medical care performed by the patient, usually in collaboration with and after instruction by a professional medical person. **2.** The medical care by laypersons of their families, friends, and themselves, including identification and evaluation of symptoms, medication, and treatment. Self-care is self-limited, voluntary, and wholly outside professional health-care systems but may include consultation with a physician or other health-care professional as a resource. **3.** Personal care accomplished without technical assistance, as eating, washing, and dressing. The goal of rehabilitation medicine is maximal personal self-care.

self-care deficit: feeding, bathing/hygiene, dressing/grooming, toileting A nursing diagnosis accepted by the Fifth National Conference on the Classification of Nursing Diagnoses. The etiology of the condition may be an intolerance for activity owing to decreased strength or endurance, pain or discomfort, impairment of cognitive or perceptual function, depression or marked anxiety, or impairment of mobility or of neuromuscular or musculoskeletal function. The kinds of deficit are separated into functional categories and are graded from I to IV. Level I requires use of equipment or devices. Level II requires help from another person. Level III requires help from another person and the use of equipment or devices. Level IV requires complete dependence. See also **nursing diagnosis.**

self-care theory A model used to provide a conceptual framework for nursing care to achieve the greatest possible degree of patient self-care. The need for care includes biophysical and psychosocial needs and the specific needs that are the result of the illness.

self-catheterization A procedure performed by a patient to empty the bladder, using sterile technique. The patient who cannot empty the bladder completely but can retain urine for 2 to 4 hours at a time can be taught self-catheterization if he has some manual dexterity and the ability to palpate the bladder.

self-concept The composite of ideas, feelings, and attitudes that a person has about his own identity, worth, capabilities, and limitations. Such factors as the values and opinions of others, especially in the formative years of early childhood, play an important part in the development of the self-concept.

self-concept, disturbance in: body image, self-esteem, role performance, personal identity A nursing diagnosis accepted by the Fifth National Conference on the Classification of Nursing Diagnoses. The disturbance represents a disruption in the way one sees oneself. There are four subcomponents, each with its own etiology and defining characteristics. The etiology of a disturbance in body image may be a biophysical, cognitive, perceptual, psychosocial, cultural, or spiritual factor. The defining characteristics of the deficit include verbal or nonverbal responses to a real or perceived change in structure or function, a missing body part, personalization of the missing part by giving it a name, refusal by the client to look at a part of the body, negative feelings about the body, trauma to a nonfunctioning part, a change in general social involvement or life-style, and a fear of rejection by others. The etiology of a disturbance in self-esteem is to be developed at a later conference. The defining characteristics of a disturbance in self-esteem are an inability to accept praise or encouragement, a lack of participation in treatment and therapy, observed self-neglect, self-destructive behavior, or a lack of eye contact with others. The etiology of a disturbance in role performance is to be developed at a later conference. The defining characteristics of a disturbance in role performance include a change in the person's perception of the role or a denial of the role, a change in the physical capacity to perform the actions of the role, and a lack of knowledge of the functions of the role. The etiology and the defining characteristics of a disturbance in personal identity are to be developed at a later conference. See also **nursing diagnosis.**

self-conscious **1.** The state of being aware of oneself as an individual entity that experiences, desires, and acts. **2.** A heightened awareness of oneself and one's actions as reflected by the observations and reactions of others; socially ill-at-ease. —**self-consciousness,** *n.*

self-differentiation Specialization and diversification of a tissue or part resulting solely from intrinsic factors.

self-disclosure The process by which one's inner being, thoughts, and emotions are revealed to another. It is important for psychological growth in individual and group psychotherapy.

self-fulfilling prophecy A principle that states that a belief in or the expectation of a particular resolution is a factor that contributes to its fulfillment.

self-help group A group of people who meet to improve their health through discussion

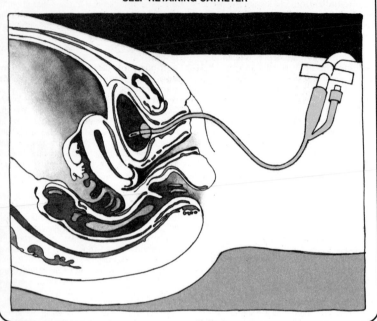

SELF-RETAINING CATHETER

and special activities. Characteristically, self-help groups are not led by a professional. A women's self-help group may be primarily supportive or it may be concerned with learning to perform basic tests, like a Pap test. Compare **group therapy.**

self-image The total concept, idea, or mental image one has of oneself and of one's role in society.

self-limited Of a disease or condition: tending to end without treatment.

self-radiolysis A process in which a compound is damaged by radioactive decay products originating in an atom within the compound.

self-retaining catheter An indwelling urinary catheter that has a double lumen. One channel allows urine to drain from the bladder into a collecting bag; the other channel has a balloon at the bladder end, and a diaphragm at the other end.

self-theory A personality theory that utilizes one's self-concept in integrating the function and organization of the personality. See also **humanistic psychology.**

sella turcica A transverse depression crossing the midline on the superior surface of the body of the sphenoid bone and containing the pituitary gland.

SEM See **scanning electron microscope.**

-seme A combining form meaning '(one) having an orbital index of less than 84, more than 89, or in between' as specified by the prefix:

megaseme, mesoseme, microseme.

semeio- A combining form meaning 'sign, or symptom': *semeiography, semeiology, semeiotic.*

semen The thick, whitish secretion of the male reproductive organs discharged from the urethra upon ejaculation. It contains various constituents, including spermatozoa in their nutrient plasma. Also called **seminal fluid, sperm.** —**seminal,** *adj.*

semi- A combining form meaning 'one-half or partly': *semicoma, semisupination.*

semicircular canal Any of three bony, fluid-filled loops in the osseous labyrinth of the internal ear, associated with the sense of balance. The posterior, superior, and lateral canals open into the cochlea.

semicircular duct One of three ducts that make up the membranous labyrinth of the inner ear. See also **membranous labyrinth.**

semicoma See **coma.** —**semicomatose,** *adj.*

semi-Fowler's position Placement of the patient in an inclined position, with the upper half of the body raised by elevating the head of the bed.

semilente insulin See **short-acting insulin.**

semilunar bone See **lunate bone.**

semilunar valve 1. A valve with half-moon-shaped cusps, as the aortic valve and the pulmonic valve. 2. Any one of the cusps constituting such a valve. Also called **tricuspid valve.** See also **heart valve.**

semimembranosus One of three posterior femoral muscles situated at the back and medial side of the thigh. It originates in a thick tendon attached to the ischial tuberosity and inserts into the horizontal groove on the medial condyle of the tibia. The muscle is innervated by several branches of the tibial portion of the sciatic nerve, and functions to flex the leg, rotate it medially after flexion, and extend the thigh. Compare **biceps femoris, hamstring muscle, semitendinosus.**

seminal duct Any duct through which semen passes, as the deferent duct or the ejaculatory duct.

seminal fluid See **semen.**

seminal vesiculitis Inflammation of a seminal vesicle.

seminarcosis See **twilight sleep.**

seminiferous Producing, containing, or transmitting semen.

semitendinosus One of three posterior femoral muscles of the thigh, remarkable for the great length of its tendon of insertion. The muscle is innervated by branches of the tibial portion of the sciatic nerve. It functions to flex the leg, rotate it medially after flexion, and extend the thigh. Compare **biceps femoris, hamstring muscle, semimembranosus.**

sender In communication theory: the person by whom a message is encoded and sent.

senescent Aging. See also **senile.** —**senescence,** *n.*

Sengstaken-Blakemore tube A thick catheter having a triple lumen and two balloons, used to produce pressure by balloon tamponade to arrest hemorrhaging from esophageal varices. Attached to a tube, one balloon is blown up in the stomach and exerts pressure against the upper orifice. Similarly attached, another longer and narrower balloon exerts pressure on the walls of the esophagus. The third tube is used for withdrawing gastric contents. See also **tube.**

senile Of, pertaining to, or characteristic of the aging process, especially the physical or mental deterioration accompanying aging. —**senescent,** *adj.,* **senility,** *n.*

senile angioma See **cherry angioma.**

senile cataract A kind of cataract, associated with aging, in which a hard opacity forms in the nucleus of the lens of the eye.

senile delirium Disorientation and mental feebleness associated with extreme age and characterized by restlessness, insomnia, aimless wandering, and, less commonly, by hallucination. See also **delirium, senile psychosis.**

senile dementia See **senile psychosis.**

senile dental caries Tooth decay occurring at an advanced age. Senile dental caries is usually characterized by cavity formation in or around the cementum layer of the tooth. See also **dental caries.**

senile endometritis Endometritis in a postmenopausal woman.

senile involution A pattern of retrograde changes occurring with advancing age and resulting in the progressive shrinking and degen-

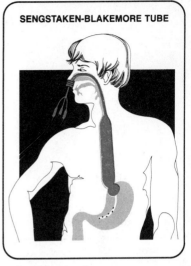

SENGSTAKEN-BLAKEMORE TUBE

eration of tissues and organs.

senile keratosis See **actinic keratosis.**

senile memory See **anterograde memory.**

senile nanism Dwarfism associated with progeria.

senile psychosis An organic mental disorder of the aged, resulting from the generalized atrophy of the brain with no evidence of cerebrovascular disease. Symptoms include loss of memory, impaired judgment, confusion, confabulation, and irritability. The condition, which is irreversible, is more common in women than in men, runs a gradual and progressive course, and may be a late form of Alzheimer's disease. Also called **primary degenerative dementia, senile dementia.** See also **multi-infarct dementia.**

senile wart See **actinic keratosis.**

senna The dried leaflets or pods of *Cassia acutifolia* or *Cassia augustifolia*, used as a cathartic.

sens- A combining form meaning 'perception or feeling': *sensation, sensimeter, sensitinogen.*

sensible perspiration Fluid loss from the body through the sweat glands in an observable quantity. Compare **insensible perspiration.**

sensitivity 1. Capacity to feel, transmit, or react to a stimulus. 2. Susceptibility to a substance, as a drug or an antigen. See also **allergy, hypersensitivity.** —**sensitive,** *adj.*

sensitivity-training group A group that offers members a supportive atmosphere in which to experiment with and alter behavioral patterns and interpersonal reactions. The purpose is to learn what occurs during group interactions, test and refine new behavioral responses, and apply those responses to situations outside the group. Also called **T-group.** See also **psychotherapy.**

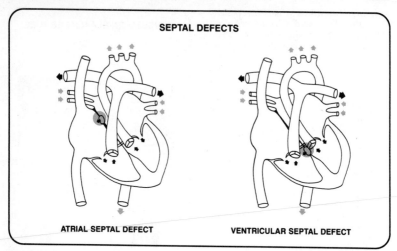

SEPTAL DEFECTS

ATRIAL SEPTAL DEFECT   VENTRICULAR SEPTAL DEFECT

sensitization   1. An acquired reaction in which specific antibodies develop in response to an antigen. This is deliberately caused in immunization by injecting a disease-causing organism that has been altered so it can no longer cause disease yet remains able to cause antibody production. Allergic reactions are hypersensitivity reactions that result from excess sensitization to a foreign protein. **2.** A photodynamic method of destroying microorganisms. **3.** *Nontechnical.* Anaphylaxis. **—sensitize,** *v.*

sensorimotor   Both sensory and motor.

sensorineural hearing loss   A form of hearing loss in which sound is conducted through the external and middle ear in a normal way, but a defect in the inner ear results in its distortion, making discrimination difficult. Amplification of the sound with a hearing aid helps some people with sensorineural hearing loss, but many have an intolerance to loud noises and will not be helped. Compare **conductive hearing loss.**

sensorium   1. The center in the brain that controls sensation. **2.** The entire sensory apparatus of the body.

sensory   1. Pertaining to the senses or sensation. **2.** Referring to a structure for receiving and transmitting impulses from the sense organs to the reflex and higher centers of the brain, as a nerve.

sensory apraxia   See **ideational apraxia.**

sensory deprivation   An involuntary loss of physical awareness caused by detachment from external sensory stimuli. Such deprivation often results in psychological disorders. Sensory deprivation may be associated with various handicaps and conditions, as blindness, heavy sedation, and prolonged isolation.

sensory nerve   A nerve consisting of afferent fibers that conduct sensory impulses from the periphery of the body to the brain or spinal cord via the dorsal spinal roots. Compare **motor nerve.**

sensory-perceptual alterations: visual, auditory, kinesthetic, gustatory, tactile, olfactory perception   A nursing diagnosis accepted by the Fifth National Conference on the Classification of Nursing Diagnoses. The etiology of the alteration may be excessive or insufficient environmental stimulation; changes in the reception, transmission, or integration of stimuli; endogenous or exogenous chemical alteration in the perception of stimuli; or psychological stress or disturbance. The defining characteristics of the disturbance include disorientation; change in the ability to abstract, conceptualize, or solve problems; change in behavior and in sensory acuity; restlessness; irritability; inappropriate response to stimuli; and hallucination. See also **nursing diagnosis.**

sensory process   The first step in communication or action, involving the constant and mostly unconscious reception of environmental stimuli by the sense organs and their transmission to the brain. See also **perception, transmission.**

SEP   *abbr* **somatosensory evoked potential.**

separation anxiety   Fear and apprehension caused by separation from familiar surroundings and significant persons. It occurs commonly in an infant when separated from its mother or when it is approached by a stranger. See also **anxiety, anxiety neurosis.**

seps-   A combining form meaning 'of or pertaining to decay': *sepsin, sepsis, sepsometer.*

sepsis   Infection, contamination. Compare **asepsis. —septic,** *adj.*

-sepsis   A combining form meaning 'decay due to a (specified) cause or of a (specified) sort': *colisepsis, endosepsis, typhosepsis.*

sept-   A combining form meaning: **1.** 'Of or pertaining to the nasal septum': *septectomy, septometer.* **2.** 'Seven': *septigravida, septipara.*

septal defect   An abnormal, usually congenital defect in the wall separating two cham-

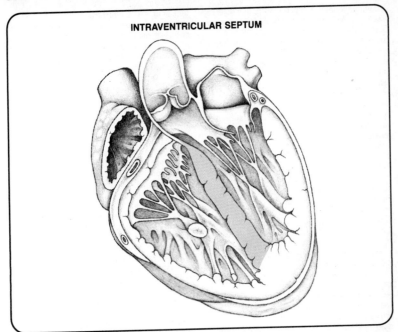

INTRAVENTRICULAR SEPTUM

bers of the heart. Depending on the size and the site of the defect, various amounts of oxygenated and deoxygenated blood mix, resulting in decreased oxygen in the blood. Kinds of septal defects are **atrial septal defect, ventricular septal defect.**

-septic A combining form meaning 'referring to decay of a sort or due to a (specified) cause': *aseptic, colyseptic.*

septic abortion Spontaneous or induced termination of a pregnancy in which the life of the mother may be threatened because of the invasion of pathogens into the endometrium, myometrium, and other tissues, requiring immediate and intensive care, massive antibiotic therapy, evacuation of the uterus, and, often, emergency hysterectomy to prevent death. Compare **infected abortion.** See also **criminal abortion, induced abortion.**

septic arthritis An acute form of arthritis, characterized by bacterial inflammation of a joint caused by bacteria carried in the bloodstream from another infection or by joint contamination during trauma or surgery. The joint is stiff, painful, tender, warm, and swollen. The diagnosis is confirmed by bacteriologic identification of an organism in a specimen obtained by joint aspiration. Parenteral antibiotics are given to prevent joint destruction. Repeated aspiration of the joint or surgical incision and drainage may be performed to relieve pressure. Also called **acute bacterial arthritis.**

septicemia Systemic infection of the bloodstream. It is diagnosed by blood culture and vigorously treated with antibiotics. Characteristi-

cally, septicemia causes fever, chills, prostration, pain, headache, nausea, or diarrhea. Also called **blood poisoning.** Compare **bacteremia.** See also **septic shock. —septicemic,** *adj.*

-septicemia A combining form meaning '(condition of the) blood caused by virulent microorganisms': *pneumosepticemia, pyosepticemia.* Also **-septicaemia.**

septicemic plague A rapidly fatal form of bubonic plague in which septicemia with meningitis precedes formation of buboes. Compare **bubonic plague, pneumonic plague.** See also **plague,** *Yersinia pestis.*

septic fever An elevation of body temperature associated with infection by pathogenic microorganisms or in response to a toxin secreted by a microorganism.

septic shock A form of shock that occurs in septicemia when endotoxins are released from certain bacteria in the bloodstream. The endotoxins cause decreased vascular resistance, resulting in a drastic fall in blood pressure. Fever, tachycardia, increased respirations, confusion, or coma may also occur. Septic shock is usually preceded by signs of severe infection, often of the genitourinary or gastrointestinal system. The causative organism is most frequently gramnegative. Antibiotics, vasopressors, and intravenous fluids and volume expanders are usually given. Also called **bacteremic shock.** A kind of septic shock is **toxic shock syndrome.**

septum, *pl.* **septa** A partition, as the interauricular septum that separates the atria of the heart.

sequela, *pl.* **sequelae** Any abnormal condition that follows and is the result of a disease, treatment, or injury, as paralysis following poliomyelitis.

sequential imaging In nuclear medicine: a diagnostic procedure in which a series of closely timed images of the rapidly changing distribution of an administered radioactive tracer is used to determine a physiologic process or processes within the body.

sequester To detach, separate, or isolate, as a patient sequestered to prevent the spread of an infection.

sequestered antigens theory A theory of autoimmunity, maintaining that immunologic tolerance depends on a certain degree of contact between immunologic cells and body cells and on a certain degree of antigen exposure. The theory holds that certain sequestered antigens in the brain, the lenses of the eye, and spermatozoa are isolated from the circulations of the blood and the lymph and do not contact the immune system. When body tissues are damaged, the sequestered antigens suddenly are exposed to the immune system but are not recognized as such by the body, and an autoimmune reaction results. Compare **forbidden clone theory.**

sequestered edema Edema localized in the tissues surrounding a newly created surgical wound.

sequestrum, *pl.* **sequestra** A fragment of dead bone partially or entirely detached from the surrounding or adjacent healthy bone.

sequestrum forceps A forceps with small, powerful teeth used for extracting necrotic or sharp fragments of bone from surrounding tissue.

sequoiasis A type of hypersensitivity pneumonitis common among workers in sawmills where redwood is processed. The antigens are the fungus *Pullularia pullulans* and species of the genus *Graphium*, found in moldy redwood sawdust.

sero- A combining form meaning 'of or pertaining to blood serum': *seroculture, serogenesis, serolin.*

serological diagnosis A diagnosis made through laboratory examination of antigen-antibody reactions in the serum. Also called **immunodiagnosis, serum diagnosis.**

serology The branch of laboratory medicine that studies blood serum for evidence of infection by evaluating antigen-antibody reactions in vitro. **—serologic, serological,** *adj.*

serosa Any serous membrane, as the tunica serosa, that lines the walls of body cavities and secretes a watery exudate.

serosanguineous Of a discharge: thin and red; composed of serum and blood.

serotonin A naturally occurring derivative of tryptophan found in platelets and in cells of the brain and the intestine. Serotonin is released from platelets upon damage to the blood vessel walls. It acts as a potent vasoconstrictor. Serotonin in intestinal tissue stimulates the smooth muscle to contract. In the central nervous system, it acts as a neurotransmitter.

serous membrane One of the many thin sheets of tissue that line closed cavities of the body, as the pleura lining the thoracic cavity. Between the visceral layer of serous membrane covering various organs and the parietal layer lining the cavity containing such organs is a potential space moistened by serous fluid. The fluid reduces the friction of the structures covered by the serous membrane, as the lungs, which move against the thoracic walls in respiration. Compare **mucous membrane, skin, synovial membrane.**

serpent ulcer A skin ulceration that heals in one area but extends to another. Also called **serpiginous ulcer.**

Serratia A genus of motile, gram-negative bacilli capable of causing infection in humans. *Serratia* organisms are frequently acquired in hospitals. See also **nosocomial infection.**

serratus anterior A thin muscle of the chest wall extending from the ribs under the arm to the scapula. Arising from the outer surface and upper border of the first eight or nine ribs, it inserts into the medial angle, the vertebral border, and the inferior angle of the scapula. It is innervated by the long thoracic nerve of the brachial plexus. It acts to rotate the scapula and to raise the shoulder, as in full flexion and abduction of the arm. Compare **pectoralis major, pectoralis minor, subclavius.**

Sertoli-Leydig cell tumor See **arrhenoblastoma.**

serum 1. The clear, thin, sticky fluid portion of the blood. Like plasma, it contains no blood cells or platelets; unlike plasma, it contains no fibrinogen. See also **blood clotting. 2.** A vaccine or toxoid prepared from the serum of a hyperimmune donor for prophylaxis against an infection or poison.

serum albumin A major protein in blood plasma that helps maintain blood's oncotic pressure.

serum C-reactive protein See **C-reactive protein.**

serum diagnosis See **serological diagnosis.**

serum glutamic oxaloacetic transaminase (SGOT) A catalytic enzyme found in various parts of the body, especially the heart, liver, and muscle tissue. Increased amounts of the enzyme occur in the serum as a result of myocardial infarction, acute liver disease, the actions of certain drugs, and any disease or condition in which cells are seriously damaged. See also **transaminase.**

serum glutamic pyruvic transaminase (SGPT) A catalytic enzyme normally found in high concentration in the liver. Increased SGPT levels in serum indicates liver damage. See also **transaminase.**

serum hepatitis See **hepatitis B.**

serum sickness An immunologic disorder occurring 2 to 3 weeks after antiserum administration. It is caused by an antibody reaction to an antigen in the donor serum and is characterized by fever, splenomegaly, swollen lymph glands, skin rash, and joint pain. Treatment is symptomatic and supportive and may include corticosteroids. See also **antigen-antibody reaction, Arthus reaction.**

service of process In law: the delivery of a writ, summons, or complaint to a defendant. The original of the document is shown; a copy is served. Service of process gives reasonable notice to allow the person to appear, testify, and be heard in court.

sesamoid bone Any one of numerous small, round, bony masses embedded in certain tendons that may be subjected to compression as well as tension. The largest sesamoid bone is the patella, which is embedded in the tendon of the quadriceps femoris at the knee.

sesqui- A combining form meaning 'one and a half': *sesquibasic, sesquibo, sesquihora.*

sessile **1.** In biology: attached by a base rather than by a stalk or a peduncle, as a leaf that is attached directly to its stem. **2.** Permanently connected.

set- A combining form meaning 'of or related to a bristle': *setaceous, setiferous, seton.*

settlement In law: an agreement made between parties to a suit before a judgment is rendered by a court.

seventh nerve See **facial nerve.**

severe combined immunodeficiency disease (SCID) An abnormal condition characterized by the absence or marked deficiency of B cells and T cells with the consequent lack of humoral immunity and cell-mediated immunity. This disease occurs as an X-linked recessive disorder only in males and as an autosomal recessive disorder affecting both males and females. It results in a pronounced susceptibility to infection. The precise cause of SCID is not known, but research indicates it may be caused by a cytogenic dysfunction of the embryonic stem cells in differentiating B cells and T cells. The affected individual consequently has a very small thymus and little or no protection against infection. Pronounced susceptibility to infection usually becomes obvious in affected individuals 3 to 6 months after birth, when maternal immunoglobulin reserves diminish. Infants with SCID commonly fail to thrive and develop a variety of complications, as sepsis, watery diarrhea, persistent pulmonary infections, and common viral infections that are often fatal. Some of the more obvious symptoms after the infant has used most of the maternal immunoglobulin stores are cyanosis, rapid respirations, and normal chest sounds with an abnormal chest X-ray. Most infants with SCID die of severe infection within 1 year after birth. The only satisfactory treatment available is a histocompatible bone marrow transplant, but such a procedure may cause a graft-versus-host reaction. Placing the infant with SCID in a completely sterile environment for a long time may prolong life if the infant has not had recurring infections. Supportive treatment is the primary approach in managing SCID.

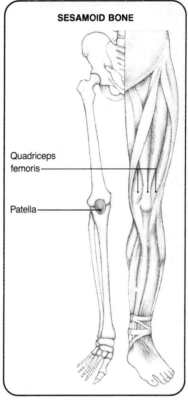

SESAMOID BONE

Quadriceps femoris

Patella

sex **1.** A classification of male or female based on many criteria, among them anatomic and chromosomal characteristics. **2.** Coitus. Compare **gender.**

sex- A combining form meaning 'six': *sexdigitate, sexivalent, sextan.*

sex chromatin A densely staining mass within the nucleus of all nondividing cells of normal mammalian females. It represents the facultative heterochromatin of the inactivated X chromosome. Examination of cells obtained by amniocentesis for the presence or absence of sex chromatin is a technique used for determining the sex of a fetus. Sex chromatin is also found as a drumsticklike mass attached to one of the nuclear lobes in polymorphonuclear leukocytes in normal females. Also called **Barr body.** See also **Lyon hypothesis.**

sex chromosome A chromosome responsible for the sex determination of offspring; it carries genes that transmit sex-linked traits and conditions. Two distinct sex chromosomes, the X and the Y, are unequally paired and appear in females in the XX combination and in males as XY. Compare **autosome.**

sex chromosome mosaic An individual or organism whose cells contain variant chromosomal numbers involving the X or Y chromosomes. Such variations are found in most of the syndromes associated with sex chromosome aberrations, primarily Turner's syndrome, and may be caused by nondisjunction of the chromosomes during the second meiotic division of gametogenesis or by some error in chromosome distribution during cell division of the fertilized ovum. Sex chromosome mosaics often have sexual abnormalities, but because of sex hormones, the overall phenotype is uniform and not mosaic in external characteristics. See also **intersexuality.**

sex factor See **F factor.**

sex-influenced Of or pertaining to an autosomal genetic trait or condition, as patterned baldness, that in one sex is expressed phenotypically in both homozygotes and heterozygotes, while in the other sex a phenotypic effect is produced in homozygotes only. Also called sex-controlled.

sexism A belief that one sex is superior to the other and consequently has endowments, rights, and status greater than those of the inferior sex. **—sexist,** n.

sex-limited Of or pertaining to an autosomal genetic trait or condition that is expressed phenotypically in only one sex, although the genes for them may be carried by both sexes. Such traits or conditions are typically influenced by hormonal or environmental conditions.

sex-linked Pertaining to genes or to the normal or abnormal characteristics or conditions they transmit. See also **sex-linked disorder, X-linked, Y-linked. —sex linkage,** n.

sex-linked disorder Any disease or abnormal condition that is determined by the sex chromosomes. These may involve a deviation in the number of either the X or Y chromosomes, as occurs in Turner's syndrome. Such aberrations in the number of sex chromosomes do not produce the severe clinical effects that are associated with autosomal aberrations, although some degree of mental deficiency is usually apparent. Other sex-linked disorders are transmitted by single gene defects carried on the X chromosome. X-linked dominant mutations, as hypophosphatemic vitamin D–resistant rickets, are rare, and males are more seriously affected than females. In inheritance patterns, X-linked dominant conditions are transmitted by affected males to all of their daughters but none of their sons, by affected heterozygous females to one half of their children regardless of sex, and by affected homozygous females to all of their children. X-linked recessive mutations are more common and are responsible for such traits and disorders as color blindness, hemophilia, the Duchenne type of muscular dystrophy, and inborn errors of metabolism. Such conditions are always transmitted by females so that those predominantly affected are males, since they have only one X chromosome, and all genes, whether recessive or dominant, are expressed. Affected males never transmit the condition to their sons, but all of their daughters will be carriers; they, in turn, will transmit the trait to half of their sons. Occasionally, heterozygous females for X-linked recessive disorders show varying degrees of expression but never as severe as those of the affected male. There are no known clinically significant traits or conditions associated with the genes on the Y chromosome; its only known function is triggering the development of male characteristics.

sex-linked ichthyosis A congenital skin disorder characterized by large, thick, dry scales that are dark and that cover the neck, scalp, ears, face, trunk, and flexor surfaces of the body. It is transmitted by females as an X-linked recessive trait and appears only in males. The condition is managed by topical applications of emollients and the use of keratolytic agents to facilitate removal of the scales. Also called **X-linked ichthyosis.** See also **ichthyosis.**

sex mosaic See **sex chromosome mosaic.**

sexual Of or pertaining to sex.

sexual dwarf An adult dwarf whose genital organs are normally developed.

sexual dysfunction A nursing diagnosis accepted by the Fifth National Conference on the Classification of Nursing Diagnoses. The etiology of the condition may be a biological, psychological, or social alteration in sexuality caused by an ineffectual or absent role model; physical abuse; psychosocial abuse, as in a harmful relationship; misinformation or lack of information; a conflict in values; a lack of privacy; or an alteration in body structure or function, as may result from surgery, congenital anomalies, or trauma. The defining characteristics of the condition include a statement by the client of the perceived dysfunction, a physical alteration or limitation imposed by disease or treatment, a reported inability to achieve sexual satisfaction, an alteration in the sexual relationship with the partner, and a change in interest in the self or in others. See also **nursing diagnosis.**

sexual generation Reproduction by the union of male and female gametes.

sexual harassment An aggressive, sexually motivated act of physical or verbal violation of a person over whom the aggressor has power. Sexual harassment in the workplace is against the law, since it abridges the victim's right to equal opportunity, privacy, and freedom from assault.

sexual history In a patient record: the portion of the patient's personal history concerned with sexual function and dysfunction. A sexual history is particularly important in gathering data from a patient who has a disease of the reproductive tract, who experiences sexual dysfunction, or who requests contraception, abortion, or sterilization. It may include age at onset of sexual intercourse, the kind and frequency of sexual activity, and the satisfaction derived from it.

sexual intercourse See **coitus.**

sexuality 1. The sum of the physical, functional, and psychologic attributes that are expressed by one's gender identity and sexual behavior, whether or not related to the sex organs or to procreation. **2.** The genital characteristics that distinguish male from female.

sexually transmitted disease See venereal disease.

sexual melancholia A state of depression in a man resulting from the belief that he is impotent. See also **bipolar disorder, depression.**

sexual psychopath An individual whose sexual behavior is openly perverted, antisocial, and criminal. See also **antisocial personality disorder.**

sexual reassignment A change in the gender identity of a person by legal, surgical, hormonal, or social means.

sexual reflex In males: a reflex in which tactile or cerebral stimulation results in penile erection, in priapism, or in ejaculation. Also called **genital reflex.**

sexual selection The theory that mates are chosen according to the attraction of or preference for certain characteristics, as coloration or behavior patterns, so that eventually only those particular traits appear in succeeding generations. The theory explains the wide variety of sexual characteristics among the various species.

SFD *abbr* small for dates. See **small-for-gestational-age infant.**

SGA *abbr* small for gestational age. See **small-for-gestational-age infant.**

SGOT *abbr* **serum glutamic oxaloacetic transaminase.**

SGPT *abbr* **serum glutamic pyruvic transaminase.**

shadow chart A copy of the data from a permanent patient record, made for use when retrieval from the record room may be difficult or time-consuming.

shaping A behavioral therapy procedure for conditioning a person to develop new behavioral responses. Initially, any act remotely resembling the desired behavior is reinforced; gradually, the criterion is made more stringent until the desired response is attained.

shared paranoid disorder See **folie à deux.**

SHCC *abbr* **Statewide Health Coordinating Committee.**

sheath A tubular structure that surrounds an organ or any other body part, as the sheath of the rectus abdominis muscle.

sheep cell test A method that mixes human blood cells with the red blood cells of sheep to determine the absence or the deficiency of human T-lymphocytes. The sheep cell test is used to diagnose several diseases, as DiGeorge's syndrome.

sheet bath The application of wet sheets to the body, used primarily as an antipyretic procedure.

shellfish poisoning A toxic, neurologic condition that results from eating clams or mussels that have ingested the poisonous protozoa commonly called the red tide. Treatment includes I.V. injection of a weak prostigmin meth-

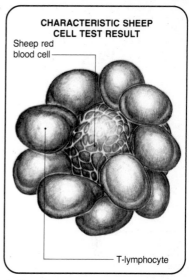

CHARACTERISTIC SHEEP CELL TEST RESULT

Sheep red blood cell

T-lymphocyte

ylsulfate solution, oxygen administration, and artificial respiration.

shell shock Any of a number of mental disorders believed to be caused by the noise and concussion of exploding shells or bombs but actually owing to a traumatic reaction to combat stress. See also **combat fatigue, posttraumatic stress disorder.**

shield In radiation technology: a material for preventing or reducing the passage of charged particles or radiation. A shield may be designated by the radiation it is intended to absorb, as a gamma-ray shield, or according to the kind of protection it is intended to give, as a background, biological, or thermal shield. Lucite and aluminum can be used for beta-radiation shields, but lead is required for gamma-ray shields.

shift to the left In hematology: a predominance of immature lymphocytes, noted in a differential white blood cell count. It is usually indicative of an infection or inflammation. The term derives from a graph of blood components in which immature cell frequencies appear on the left side of the graph.

shift to the right In hematology: a preponderance of polymorphonuclear neutrophils having three or more lobes, indicating cell maturity. The phenomenon is common in severe liver disease and advanced pernicious anemia. It indicates a relative lack of blood-forming activity.

Shigella A genus of gram-negative pathogenic bacteria that cause gastroenteritis and bacterial dysentery, as *Shigella dysenteriae*. See also **shigellosis.**

shigellosis An acute bacterial infection of the bowel, characterized by diarrhea, abdominal pain, and fever, that is transmitted by hand-to-mouth contact with the feces of individuals infected with bacteria of a pathogenic species

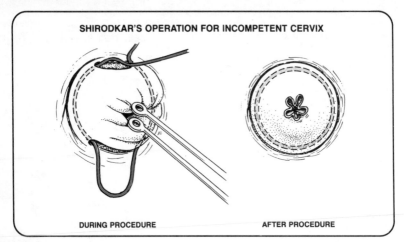

SHIRODKAR'S OPERATION FOR INCOMPETENT CERVIX

DURING PROCEDURE   AFTER PROCEDURE

of the genus *Shigella*. The disease occurs in isolated outbreaks in the United States but is endemic in underdeveloped areas of the world. It is especially common and usually most severe in children. Diagnosis is made by isolating and identifying *Shigella* in a stool specimen. The preferred treatment is supportive, and the major goal is to prevent dehydration. Antimicrobials are given if the disease is severe or the likelihood of further transmission great. Isolation and strict handwashing precautions are instituted. Shigellosis infections must be reported to the public health department. Also called **bacillary dysentery.**

shin bone   See **tibia.**

shindylesis   An articulation of certain bones of the skull in which a thin plate of one bone enters a cleft formed by the separation of two layers of another bone, as the insertion of the vomer bone into the fissure between the maxillae and the palatine bones.

shingles   See **herpes zoster.**

shin splints   A painful condition of the lower leg caused by strain of the long flexor muscle of the toes following strenuous athletic activity. Treatment usually involves rest and exercise therapy. Surgery is sometimes necessary.

Shirodkar's operation   A surgical procedure called a cerclage in which the cervical canal is closed by a purse-string suture embedded in the uterine cervix encircling the canal. It is performed to correct an incompetent cervix that has failed to retain previous pregnancies. Under spinal block or general anesthesia, a band of nonabsorbable material is buried beneath the mucosa of the cervix and pulled in a purse-string manner to close the cervix. The band may be left in place permanently, in which case subsequent deliveries are by cesarean section. Occasionally, a temporary cerclage is done. The band is then removed prior to labor and vaginal delivery. Postoperatively, infection or vaginal fistula may occur.

shock   An abnormal physiological state, the first phase of the body's alarm reaction to trauma. The common clinical signs of shock include reduced cardiac output, circulatory insufficiency, tachycardia, hypotension, restlessness, pallor, and diminished urinary output. Shock often results from severe tissue damage and may be primary, secondary, or hemorrhagic. See also **cardiogenic shock, electric shock, hypovolemic shock.**

shock lung   A form of pulmonary edema that causes acute respiratory failure, resulting from increased permeability of the alveolar capillary membrane. Fluid accumulates in the lung interstitium, alveolar spaces, and small airways, causing lungs to stiffen. Effective ventilation is impaired causing inadequate oxygenation of blood. Also called adult respiratory distress syndrome.

shock trousers   Pneumatic trousers designed to counteract hypotension, associated with internal or external bleeding, and hypovolemia. Shock trousers may be contraindicated in patients with pulmonary edema, cardiogenic shock, increased intracranial pressure, or eviscerations. Also called MAST (Medical Anti-Shock Trousers) suit.

short-acting   Pertaining to or characterizing a therapeutic agent, usually a drug, with a brief period of effectiveness, usually beginning soon after administration.

short-acting insulin   An aqueous preparation of the antidiabetic principle of beef pancreas or pork pancreas that begins to act within an hour of injection and reaches a peak of action in 2 to 4 hours. The duration of action of regular insulin is 4 to 6 hours and of crystalline zinc insulin 5 to 8 hours. Also called **rapid-acting insulin.** See also **insulin.** Compare **intermediate-acting insulin, long-acting insulin.**

shortage area   A geographic area designated by the federal government as undersupplied with certain kinds of health-care services, hence, possibly eligible for aid under certain federal programs, including the National Health

Service Corps or the Rural Clinics Assistance Act.

short arm cast An orthopedic cast applied to immobilize the hand or the wrist. It is used in treating fractures, for postoperative positioning, and for correction or maintenance of correction of deformities. Compare **long arm cast.**

shorting The fraudulent practice of dispensing a quantity of drug less than that called for in the prescription and of charging for the quantity specified in the prescription. See also **kiting.**

short leg cast An orthopedic cast used for immobilizing fractures in the lower extremities from the toes to the knee. The short leg cast is also used in severe sprains and torn soft tissue of the ankle, for postoperative positioning and immobilization, and for correction or maintenance of correction of a deformity. Compare **long leg cast.**

short leg cast with walker An orthopedic cast applied to immobilize the lower extremities from the toes to the knee while allowing the patient to walk by using a rubber walker on the bottom of the cast. The short leg cast with walker is used when weight-bearing ambulation is desired.

short sight See **myopia.**

short-term memory Memory of recent events.

shotgun therapy *Informal.* Any treatment that has a wide range of effect and which, therefore, can be expected to correct the abnormal condition even though the particular cause is unknown. Shotgun therapy may cause more than an acceptable rate of side effects and is rarely desirable or necessary.

shoulder blade See **scapula.**

shoulder joint The ball-and-socket articulation of the humerus with the scapula. The joint includes eight bursae and five ligaments, including the glenoidal labrum, which deepens the articular cavity and protects the edges of articulating bones. Also called **humeral articulation.**

shoulder spica cast An orthopedic cast applied to immobilize the trunk of the body to the hips, the wrist, and the hand. It incorporates a diagonal shoulder support between the hip and arm portions. The shoulder spica cast is used to treat shoulder dislocations and injuries and to position and immobilize the shoulder after surgery.

show See **vaginal bleeding.**

shreds Glossy mucous filaments in the urine, indicating urinary tract inflammation. Also called **mucous shreds.**

shunt **1.** To redirect the flow of a body fluid from one cavity or vessel to another. **2.** A tube or device implanted in the body to redirect fluid from one cavity or vessel to another.

Shy-Drager syndrome A rare, progressive neurologic disorder of young and middle-aged adults. It is characterized by orthostatic hypotension, bladder and bowel incontinence, atrophy of the iris, anhidrosis, tremor, rigidity,

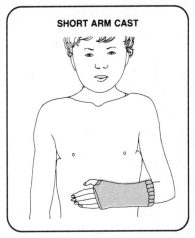

SHORT ARM CAST

incoordination, ataxia, and muscle wasting. Treatment includes drug therapy to control motor symptoms and to maintain an adequate blood pressure. Antigravity stockings may prevent pooling of blood in the lower extremities. See also **orthostatic hypotension.**

Si Symbol for **silicon.**

SIADH *abbr* **syndrome of inappropriate antidiuretic hormone secretion.**

sial-, sialo- A combining form meaning 'of or related to saliva or to the salivary glands': *sialoaerophagy, sialoangitis, sialostenosis.*

-sialia A combining form meaning '(condition of the) saliva': *asialia, oligosialia, polsialia.*

sialogogue Anything that stimulates saliva secretion.

sialography A technique in radiology in which a salivary gland is filmed after an opaque substance is injected into its duct. —**sialogram,** *n.,* **sialographic,** *adj.*

sialolith A calculus formed in a salivary gland or duct.

Siamese twins Conjoined, equally developed twin fetuses produced from the same ovum. The severity of the condition ranges from superficial fusion, as of the umbilical vessels, to that in which the heads or complete torsos are united and several internal organs are shared. With modern surgical techniques, most Siamese twins can be successfully separated. See also **conjoined twins.**

Siberian tick typhus A mild, acute febrile illness seen in north, central, and east Asia, caused by *Rickettsia siberica,* transmitted by ticks, and characterized by a diffuse maculopapular rash, headache, conjunctival inflammation, and a small ulcer or eschar at the site of the tick bite. Treatment with chloramphenicol or tetracycline is associated with an excellent prognosis. Also called **North Asian tick typhus.** See also **rickettsia, typhus.**

sibilant rale An abnormal whistling sound produced by the lungs in respiratory disorders or diseases. It is caused by the passage of air

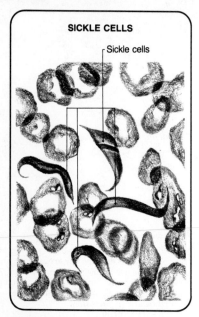

SICKLE CELLS

Sickle cells

through a lumen narrowed by the accumulation of mucus or other viscid fluid.

sibling **1.** One of two or more children who have both parents in common; a brother or sister. Also called sib *(informal)*. **2.** Of or pertaining to a brother or sister.

sibship **1.** The state of being related by blood. **2.** A group of people descended from a common ancestor who are used as a basis for genetic studies. **3.** Brothers and sisters considered as a group.

sicc- A combining form meaning 'dry': *siccative, siccolabile.*

sickle cell An abnormal, crescent-shaped red blood cell containing hemoglobin S, an abnormal form of hemoglobin characteristic of sickle cell anemia.

sickle cell anemia A severe, chronic, incurable, anemic condition that occurs in people homozygous for hemoglobin S (Hb S). The abnormal hemoglobin results in distortion and fragility of the erythrocytes. Sickle cell anemia is characterized by crises of joint pain, thrombosis, and fever and by chronic anemia, with splenomegaly, lethargy, and weakness.

sickle cell crisis An acute, episodic condition that occurs in children with sickle cell anemia. It may be vaso-occlusive, resulting from the aggregation of misshapen erythrocytes, or anemic, resulting from bone marrow aplasia, increased hemolysis, folate deficiency, or splenic sequestration of erythrocytes. Painful vaso-occlusive crisis is the most common type. It is usually preceded by an upper respiratory or gastrointestinal infection without an exacerbation of anemia. The clumps of sickled erythrocytes obstruct blood vessels, resulting in occlusion,

ischemia, and infarction of adjacent tissue. Characteristic of this kind of crisis are leukocytosis; acute abdominal pain from visceral hypoxia; painful swelling of the soft tissue of the hands and feet (hand-foot syndrome); and migratory, recurrent, or constant joint pain, often so severe that movement of the joint is limited. Anemic crisis is characterized by a dramatic, rapid drop in hemoglobin levels resulting from various causes. Aplastic crisis resulting in severe anemia occurs as red blood cell production is diminished by acute viral, bacterial, or fungal infection. Megaloblastic anemia (another form of anemic crisis) results from folic acid deficiency during periods of accelerated erythropoiesis. Hyperhemolytic crisis, characterized by anemia, jaundice, and reticulocytosis, results from glucose-6-phosphate dehydrogenase deficiency or in reaction to multiple transfusions. Acute sequestration crisis, which occurs in children aged 6 months to 5 years, results when large quantities of blood suddenly accumulate in the spleen, causing massive splenic enlargement, severe anemia, shock, and, ultimately, death. Therapy consists of immediate transfusion of packed red blood cells in the acute anemic crisis and alleviation of severe abdominal and joint pain with analgesics or narcotics as needed in vaso-occlusive crisis. Short-term oxygen therapy, hydration by oral or by intravenous means, electrolyte replacement to counteract metabolic acidosis resulting from hypoxia, and antibiotics to treat any existing infection may be necessary. Pneumococcal and meningococcal vaccination is recommended for all children between the ages of 2 and 5 years because they are highly susceptible to infection. Partial exchange transfusions are often mandatory in life-threatening crises, as when sickling occurs in the vessels of the brain or of the lungs, and may be used as a preventive technique, although multiple transfusions increase the risk of hepatitis, hemosiderosis, and transfusion reactions. Oral anticoagulants have been used to relieve the pain of vaso-occlusion, but these drugs increase the risk of bleeding. In children with recurrent splenic sequestration, a splenectomy may be a lifesaving procedure.

NURSING CONSIDERATIONS: The primary concern during a crisis is to initiate procedures that reduce sickling. Foremost is prevention of tissue deoxygenation and resulting hypoxia. This is done by maintaining bed rest to minimize energy expenditure and oxygen utilization, although some exercise is necessary to promote circulation. Hydration and electrolyte balance are essential. Serum sodium is monitored closely to avoid hyponatremia. The nurse constantly monitors the child's condition for splenomegaly, infection, evidence of shock or cerebrovascular accident, hypervolemia, transfusion reaction, or increasing anemia.

sickle cell thalassemia A heterozygous blood disorder in which the genes for sickle cell and for thalassemia are both inherited. A mild form and a severe form may be identified, depending on the degree of suppression of beta-chain synthesis by the thalassemia gene. In the mild form, synthesis is only partially suppressed, and the red blood cell may contain from 25% to 35% normal hemoglobin A along with a somewhat greater concentration of hemoglobin S. The clinical course is relatively mild. When beta-chain synthesis is completely suppressed, as in the severe form, only hemoglobin S appears in the red blood cells, and the clinical course is generally severe, as in homozygous sickle cell anemia. See also **hemoglobinopathy, hemoglobin variant.**

sickle cell trait The heterozygous form of sickle cell anemia, characterized by the presence of both hemoglobin S and hemoglobin A in the red blood cells. It is of little clinical significance. Anemia and the other signs of sickle cell anemia do not occur. People who have the trait are informed and counseled regarding the possibility of having an infant with sickle cell disease if both parents have the trait. See **hemoglobin S.**

sick role A pattern of behavior in which a person adopts the symptoms of a physical or mental disorder in order to be cared for, sympathized with, and protected from the demands and stresses of life.

sidero- A combining form meaning 'of or pertaining to iron': *siderocyte, siderofibrous, sideropenic.*

sideroblastic anemia Any one of a heterogenous group of chronic hematologic disorders characterized by normocytic or slightly macrocytic anemia, hypochromic and normochromic red blood cells, and decreased erythropoiesis and hemoglobin synthesis. The red blood cells contain a perinuclear ring of iron-stained granules. The condition may be acquired or hereditary, primary or secondary to another condition or situation. The etiology of the disease is not understood. Treatment may include extract of liver, pyridoxine, folic acid, and blood transfusion. Compare **iron-deficiency anemia, siderosis.**

sideropenic dysphagia See **Plummer-Vinson syndrome.**

siderosis 1. A variety of pneumoconiosis caused by the inhalation of iron dust or particles. 2. The introduction of color in any tissue owing to the presence of excess iron. 3. An increase in the amounts of iron in the blood. See also **hemochromatosis, hemosiderosis.**

SIDS *abbr* **sudden infant death syndrome.**

sigh See **periodic deep inspiration.**

Sigma Theta Tau A national honor society for nurses.

sigmoid 1. Of or pertaining to an S shape. 2. The sigmoid colon.

sigmoid colon The portion of the colon that extends from the end of the descending colon in the pelvis to the juncture of the rectum.

sigmoidectomy Excision of the sigmoid flexure of the colon, most commonly performed to remove a malignant tumor.

sigmoid mesocolon A fold of peritoneum that connects the sigmoid colon with the pelvic

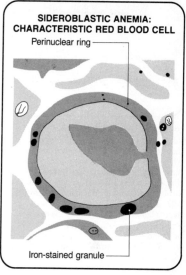

SIDEROBLASTIC ANEMIA: CHARACTERISTIC RED BLOOD CELL
Perinuclear ring
Iron-stained granule

wall, forming a curved line of attachment. The apex of the curve is located at the division of the left common iliac artery. Compare **mesentery proper, transverse mesocolon.**

sigmoidoscope An endoscope used to examine the lumen of the sigmoid colon. It allows direct visualization of the mucous membrane lining the colon. Compare **proctoscope.**

sign An objective finding as perceived by an examiner, as a fever or a rash. Many signs accompany symptoms, as erythema and a maculopapular rash are often seen when a patient complains of pruritus. Compare **symptom.**

signal symptom See **symptom.**

significance 1. In research: the statistical probability that a given finding is very unlikely to have occurred by chance alone. The conventional standard for attributing significance is a finding that occurs fewer than 5 times in 100 by chance alone ($p < 0.05$). 2. The importance of a study in developing a practice or theory, as in nursing practice.

silent mutation In molecular genetics: an alteration in a sequence of nucleotides that does not result in an amino acid change.

silicon (Si) A nonmetallic element, second to oxygen as the most abundant of the elements. Its atomic number is 14; its atomic weight is 28.086. Protracted inhalation of silica dusts can cause silicosis, which increases susceptibility to other pulmonary diseases.

silicone 1. Any organic silicon polymer compound used in medicine as a lubricant or a rubber substitute. 2. A topical protectant used to promote healing by reducing irritation and friction.

silicosis A lung disorder caused by continued, long-term inhalation of silicon dioxide dust, which is found in sands, quartzes, flints, and in many other stones. Silicosis is characterized

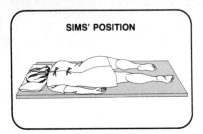

SIMS' POSITION

by the development of nodular fibrosis in the lungs. The incidence of silicosis is highest among industrial workers exposed to silica powder; those who work with ceramics, sand, or stone, and those who mine silica. Also called **grinder's disease, quartz silicosis.** See also **chronic obstructive pulmonary disease, inorganic dust.**

silk suture   A braided, fine, black suture material, usually used to close incisions, wounds, and cuts in the skin. It is not absorbed by the body and is removed after approximately 7 days.

silo filler's disease   A rare, acute respiratory condition seen in agricultural workers who have inhaled nitrogen oxide as they work with fermented fodder in closed, poorly ventilated spaces like silos. Characteristically, symptoms of respiratory distress and pulmonary edema occur several hours after exposure.

silver (Ag)   A whitish, precious metal occurring mainly as a sulfide. Its atomic number is 47; its atomic weight is 107.88. It is used extensively as a component of amalgams of dental fillings and many medications, especially antiseptics and astringents.

Silver dwarf   A person who has Silver's syndrome, a congenital disorder in which short stature is associated with lateral asymmetry; various anomalies of the head, face, and skeleton; and precocious puberty.

silver-fork fracture   See **Colles' fracture.**

silver nitrate   A topical caustic agent.

silver nitrate 1%   An ophthalmic anti-infective.

silver protein, mild   A disinfectant.

silver salts poisoning   A toxic condition caused by the ingestion of silver nitrate, characterized by discoloration of the lips, vomiting, abdominal pain, dizziness, and convulsions. Treatment includes gastric lavage with salt water. Anticonvulsant and antihypotensive therapy may be necessary.

silver sulfadiazine   A local anti-infective.

simethicone   An antiflatulent.

simian crease   A single crease across the palm from the fusion of the proximal and distal palmar creases; seen in congenital disorders, as Down's syndrome. Also called simian line.

simian virus 40   A vacuolating virus isolated from the kidney tissue of rhesus monkeys.

simil-   A combining form meaning 'like': *similimum.*

Simmonds' disease   See **panhypopituitarism.**

simple angioma   A tumor consisting of a

network of small vessels or distended capillaries surrounded by connective tissue.

simple fission   See **binary fission.**

simple fracture   An uncomplicated, closed fracture in which the bone does not break the skin. Compare **compound fracture.**

simple mastectomy   A surgical procedure in which a breast is completely removed and the underlying muscles and adjacent lymph nodes are left intact. The procedure may be performed to remove small malignant neoplasms of the breast, or it may be done as a palliative measure to remove an ulcerated carcinoma in advanced breast cancer. Compare **modified radical mastectomy, radical mastectomy.**

simple phobia   An anxiety disorder characterized by a persistent, irrational fear of specific things, such as animals, dirt, light, or darkness. Some kinds of simple phobias are **algophobia, mysophobia, nyctophobia.** Compare **social phobia.** See also **phobia.**

simple protein   A protein yielding amino acids as its only or chief product upon hydrolysis. The class includes albumins, globulins, glutelins, alcohol-soluble proteins, albuminoids, histones, and protamines. See **complex protein.**

simple schizophrenia   A slow, insidiously progressive form of schizophrenia characterized by apathy, withdrawal, lack of initiative, gradual depletion of emotional reactions, and an impoverishment in human relationships. See also **schizotypal personality disorder.**

simple tubular gland   One of the many multicellular glands with only one tube-shaped duct, as various glands within the epithelium of the intestine.

Simpson forceps   See **obstetric forceps.**

Sims' position   A position in which the patient lies on the left side with the right knee and thigh drawn upward toward the chest.

sin-   A combining form meaning 'hollow, cavity': *sinography, sinus.*

sinap-   A combining form meaning 'of or related to mustard': *sinapine, sinapiscopy.*

sinew   A tendon, as the thick, flattened tendon attached to the short head of the biceps brachii. See also **tendon.**

singer's nodule   See **vocal cord nodule.**

single-blind study   An experiment in which either the subject or the person collecting data does not know whether the subject is in the control group or the experimental group. See also **double-blind study.**

single monster   A fetus with a single body and head but severely malformed or duplicated parts or organs.

singultus   See **hiccup.**

sinistrality   See **left-handedness.**

sinistro-   A combining form meaning 'left, or related to the left side': *sinistrocardia, sinistrophobia, sinistrotorsion.*

sinoatrial (SA) block   A conduction disturbance in the heart during which an impulse formed within the SA node is blocked from depolarizing the atrial myocardium. Causes in-

SINOATRIAL NODE

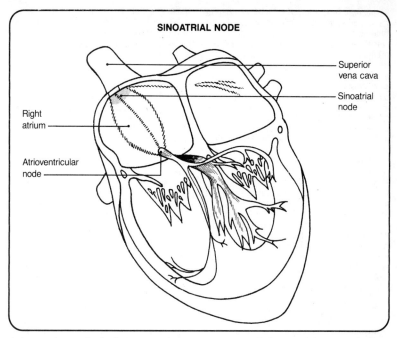

Superior vena cava

Sinoatrial node

Right atrium

Atrioventricular node

---

clude excessive vagal stimulation, acute infections, and atherosclerosis. Treatment for symptomatic SA block includes the use of atropine, isoproterenol, and, if these are not effective, stimulation and regulation of the heart with an electronic impulse generated by a pacemaker.

sinoatrial (SA) node A cluster of hundreds of cells located in the right atrial wall of the heart near the opening of the superior vena cava. It comprises a knot of modified heart muscle that generates impulses that cause the muscle fibers of both atria to contract. Specialized pacemaker cells in the node have an intrinsic rhythm that is independent of stimulation by nerve impulses from the brain and the spinal cord. The sinoatrial node will normally 'fire' at a rhythmic rate of 70 to 75 beats per minute. If the node fails to generate an impulse, pacemaker function will shift to another excitable component of the cardiac conduction system, as the atrioventricular node or the Purkinje fibers. Also called Keith-Flack node. Compare **atrioventricular node, Purkinje network.** See also **pacemaker.**

sinus bradycardia See **bradycardia.**

sinus headache See **headache.**

sinusitis An inflammation of one or more paranasal sinuses. It may be a complication of an upper respiratory infection, dental infection, allergy, a change in atmosphere, or a structural defect of the nose. With swelling of nasal mucous membranes the openings from sinuses to the nose may be obstructed, resulting in an accumulation of sinus secretions, causing pressure, pain, headache, fever, and local tenderness.

Treatment includes steam inhalations, nasal decongestants, analgesics, and, if infection is present, antibiotics.

sinus tachycardia See **tachycardia.**

sinus venosus defect See **atrial septal defect.**

sippy diet A severely restricted dietary regimen for peptic ulcer patients. It consists of hourly servings of milk and cream for several days, with the gradual addition of eggs, refined cereals, pureed vegetables, crackers, and other simple foods as tolerated until the regular bland diet is reached. Supplementary iron and vitamins are indicated to prevent deficiency states. See also **bland diet.**

sireniform fetus See **sirenomelus.**

sirenomelia A congenital anomaly in which there is complete fusion of the lower extremities and no feet. Also called **apodial symmelia.**

sirenomelus An infant who has sirenomelia. Also called **sympus apus.**

siriasis Sunstroke. See also **heat hyperpyrexia.**

-sis A combining form meaning an 'action, process, or result of': *centesis, genesis.*

Sister Kenny's treatment Poliomyelitis therapy in which the patient's limbs and back are wrapped in warm, moist woolen cloths and, after the pain subsides, the patient exercises affected muscles, especially by swimming.

-site A combining form meaning an 'organism living inside another form from which it derives sustenance': *celiosite, hemosite.*

site visit A visit made by designated officials to evaluate or to gather information about a department or institution. A site visit is a step in the accreditation of an institution and in the funding of many major projects.

-sitia A combining form meaning '(condition of) appetite for food': *apositia, asitia.*

sito- A combining form meaning 'of or pertaining to food': *sitomania, sitophobia.*

sitosterol A mixture of sterols derived from plants, used for treating hyperbetalipoproteinemia and hypercholesterolemia that are unresponsive to dietary measures. Its use is controversial, since it causes loose bowel movements and may lead to diarrhea or interfere with the absorption of other medications. Use in pregnancy is not recommended.

situational anxiety A state of apprehension, discomfort, and anxiety precipitated by the experience of new situations or events. It is not abnormal, requires no treatment, and usually disappears as the person adjusts to the new experiences. See also **anxiety, anxiety neurosis.**

situational crisis In psychiatry: a crisis that arises suddenly in response to an external event or a conflict concerning a specific circumstance. The symptoms are transient and the episode is usually brief.

situational depression In psychiatry: an episode of emotional and psychological depression that occurs in response to a specific set of external circumstances.

situational psychosis In psychiatry: a psychotic episode that results from a specific set of external circumstances.

situational therapy In psychiatry: a kind of psychotherapy in which the milieu is part of the treatment program. See also **milieu therapy.**

situation therapy See **milieu therapy.**

situs The normal position or location of a body organ or part.

sitz bath A bath in which only the hips and buttocks are immersed in water or saline solution. The procedure is used for patients who have had rectal or perineal surgery. Also called **hip bath.**

sixth disease See **roseola infantum.**

sixth nerve See **abducent nerve.**

Sjögren-Larsson syndrome A congenital condition, inherited as an autosomal recessive trait, characterized by ichthyosis, mental deficiency, and spastic paralysis.

skato- See **scato-.**

skeletal enchondromatosis See **enchondromatosis.**

skeletal fixation Any method of holding together the fragments of a fractured bone by attaching wires, screws, plates, or nails. See also **external pin fixation.**

skeletal muscle See **striated muscle.**

skeletal traction One of the two basic kinds of orthopedic traction used to treat fractured bones and correct orthopedic abnormalities. Skeletal traction is applied to the affected structure by a metal pin or wire inserted in the tissue of the structure and attached to traction ropes. Skeletal traction is often used when continuous traction is desired to properly immobilize, position, and align a fractured bone during the healing process. Infection of the pin tract may develop. Compare **skin traction.**

skeleton The supporting framework for the body, comprising 206 bones that protect delicate structures, provide attachments for muscles, allow body movement, serve as major reservoirs of blood, and produce red blood cells. The skeleton is divided into the axial skeleton, which has 74 bones, the appendicular skeleton, with 126 bones, and the 6 auditory ossicles. The skeleton changes throughout life as bone formation and bone destruction proceed concurrently. During childhood and adolescence, bone formation proceeds faster than bone destruction. Between the ages of 35 and 40 bone destruction proceeds faster than bone formation. In advanced age bone destruction increases, bones become thin and brittle, the length of vertebrae diminishes due to reduction in thickness of the disks and to exaggeration of the curvatures, particularly in the thoracic region, and height decreases. See also **bone. —skeletal,** *adj.*

Skene's duct See **paraurethral duct.**

Skene's glands The largest of the glands that open into the urethra of women. They contain ducts that open just within the urethral orifice.

skew A deviation from a line or symmetrical pattern, as data in a research study that do not follow the expected statistical curve.

skia-, scia- A combining form meaning 'of or related to shadows, especially of internal structures as produced by roentgen rays': *skiabaryt, skiagenol, skiagraph.*

skilled nursing facility (SNF) An institution or part of an institution that meets criteria for accreditation established by the sections of the Social Security Act that determine the basis for Medicaid and Medicare reimbursement for skilled nursing care, including rehabilitation and various medical and nursing procedures.

Skillern's fracture An open fracture of the distal radius associated with a greenstick fracture of the distal ulna.

skill play A form of play in which a child persistently repeats an action or activity until it has been mastered.

skim milk Milk from which the fat has been removed. Most of the vitamin A is removed with the cream, although all other nutrients remain. Also called **nonfat milk, skimmed milk.**

skin The tough, supple cutaneous membrane that covers the entire surface of the body. It is the largest organ of the body and serves as a waterproof covering that also protects the body against parasites, bacteria, and viruses. This versatile membrane also serves as the outer sensory network of the body, lubricates the exterior of the body with secretions, and helps to control body temperature. The main layers of the skin are the epidermis and the thicker underlying dermis. A tough, scaly layer of dead cells on the surface of the skin constantly flakes away and is replaced by new epidermal cells, which fill with keratin as they migrate to the surface. The dermis is elastic and durable and contains a complex network of nerve endings, sweat glands, hair follicles, lymphatic vessels, and blood vessels. Just below the dermis are fat cells that store energy and help provide the substance and the shape of the human form. All the hairs of the body grow from the dermis; the only parts of the body without hair are the palms of the hands and the soles of the feet. Also called **integument**.

skin cancer A cutaneous neoplasm caused by ionizing radiation, certain genetic defects, chemical carcinogens, or by overexposure to the sun. Skin cancers, the most common and most curable malignancies, are also the most frequent secondary lesions in patients with cancer in other sites. Risk factors are a fair complexion, xeroderma pigmentosa, vitiligo, senile and seborrheic keratitis, Bowen's disease, radiation dermatitis, and hereditary basal cell nevus syndrome. The most common skin cancers are basal cell carcinomas and squamous cell carcinomas. A definitive diagnosis may be established by biopsy, which may be the only treatment required for small lesions. Depending on the type of skin cancer, topical medications, radiotherapy, or surgery may be indicated. Despite the curability of skin cancer it causes many deaths because of failure to seek treatment at early stages.

skinfold calipers An instrument used to measure the breadth of a fold of skin, usually on the posterior aspect of the upper arm or over the lower ribs of the chest.

skinfold thickness The thickness of a fold of skin gripped by calipers. The measurement approximates the amount of subcutaneous fat for use in determining nutritional needs. The most common test sites are the triceps and the subscapular area.

skin graft A portion of skin implanted to cover areas where skin has been lost through burns, injury, or by surgical removal of diseased tissue. To prevent tissue rejection, the graft is taken from the patient's own body or from the body of an identical twin. Skin from another person can be used as a temporary cover for large burned areas to decrease fluid loss. The area from which the graft is taken is called the donor site, and that on which it is placed is called the recipient site. Various techniques are used to graft skin. A successful new graft of any type is well established in about 72 hours and can be expected to survive unless a severe infection or trauma occurs. Preoperatively, both the donor and the recipient site must be free of infection and the recipient site must have a good blood supply. Postoperatively, stretching or motion of the recipient site is prevented. Strict sterile technique is used for handling dressings, and antibiotics may be given prophylactically to prevent infection. Good nutrition with a high-protein, high-calorie diet is essential.

skin integrity, impairment of: actual A nursing diagnosis accepted by the Fifth National Conference on the Classification of Nursing Diagnoses. The etiology of the condition may be

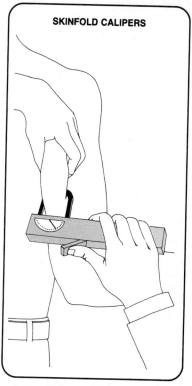

SKINFOLD CALIPERS

environmental (external) or somatic (internal). Environmental factors that may affect the development of impaired skin integrity include heat or cold; chemical substances; mechanical factors, as a shearing force or pressure, restraint, or laceration; radiation; physical immobilization; and humidity. Somatic factors that may result in impairment of integrity of the skin include drugs, obesity or emaciation, malnutrition, metabolic disturbance, circulatory disturbance, altered sensation or pigmentation, developmental factors, immunologic deficit, or change in the turgor of the skin. The defining characteristics of the problem are disruption of the surface of the skin, destruction of cell layers of the skin, and invasion of structures of the body through the skin. See also **nursing diagnosis**.

skin integrity, impairment of: potential A nursing diagnosis accepted by the Fifth National Conference on the Classification of Nursing Diagnoses. The defining characteristics of the problem are the environmental (external) or somatic (internal) risk factors that may contribute to the etiology of the breakdown of the integument. Among the environmental factors are hypothermia or hyperthermia; presence of an injurious chemical substance; shearing force or pressure, restraint, or laceration; radiation; physical immobilization; presence on the skin

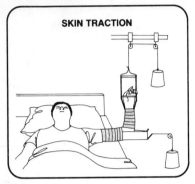

SKIN TRACTION

of excretions or secretions; and an abnormally high humidity. Somatic factors include reaction to some medications; obesity or emaciation; an abnormal metabolic state; alteration in circulation, sensory function, or pigmentation; bony prominences; adverse developmental factors; decrease in normal skin turgor; and psychogenic or immunologic abnormalities. See also **nursing diagnosis.**

Skinner box A boxlike laboratory apparatus used in operant conditioning in animals, usually containing a lever or other device that, when pressed, produces reinforcement by either giving a reward, as food or an escape outlet, or avoiding a punishment, as an electric shock. Also called **standard environmental chamber.** See also **operant conditioning.**

skin prep A procedure for cleansing the skin with an antiseptic before surgery or venipuncture. Skin preps are performed to kill bacteria and pathologic organisms and to reduce the risk of infection.

skin tag See **cutaneous papilloma.**

skin test A test to determine the reaction of the body to a substance by observing the results of injecting the substance intradermally or applying it topically to the skin. Skin tests are used to detect allergens, to determine immunity, and to diagnose disease. Kinds of skin tests include **patch test, Schick test, tuberculin test.**

skin traction One of the two basic types of traction used in orthopedics for the treatment of fractured bones and the correction of orthopedic abnormalities. Skin traction applies pull to an affected body structure by straps attached to the skin surrounding the structure. Kinds of skin traction include **adhesive skin traction, nonadhesive skin traction.** Compare **skeletal traction.**

sklero- See **sclero-.**

skull The bony structure of the head, consisting of the cranium and the skeleton of the face. The cranium, which contains and protects the brain, consists of 8 bones. The skeleton of the face is composed of 14 bones.

SL *abbr* **1. soda lime. 2. sublingual.**

SLE *abbr* **systemic lupus erythematosus.**

sleep A state marked by reduced consciousness, diminished activity of the skeletal muscles, and depressed metabolism. People normally experience sleep in patterns that follow four observable, progressive stages: during Stage 1, the brain waves are of the theta type, followed in Stage 2 by the appearance of distinctive sleep spindles; during Stages 3 and 4, the theta waves are replaced by delta waves. These four stages represent 75% of a period of typical sleep and are called collectively, **nonrapid eye movement (NREM)** sleep. The remaining time is usually occupied with **rapid eye movement (REM)** sleep. The REM sleep periods, lasting from a few minutes to half an hour, alternate with the NREM periods. Dreaming occurs during REM time. Individual sleep patterns normally change throughout life as daily requirements for sleep gradually diminish from as much as 20 hours a day in infancy to as little as 6 hours a day in old age. Infants tend to begin a sleep period with REM sleep, whereas REM activity usually follows the four stages of NREM sleep in adults.

sleeping pill *Informal.* **1.** A sedative taken for insomnia or for postoperative sedation. **2.** A nonprescription drug that is classified pharmaceutically as an aid to sleeping. Antihistamines, as pyrilamine maleate and doxylamine succinate, depend on their side effects for sedative action, which may disappear with continued use of such agents.

sleeping sickness See **African trypanosomiasis.**

sleep pattern disturbance A nursing diagnosis accepted by the Fifth National Conference on the Classification of Nursing Diagnoses. The condition is a disruption of the hours of sleep, causing discomfort or interference with normal daily activities. The etiology of the problem may be change in bodily sensation, illness, psychological disturbance, stress, or various environmental changes. Characteristics of a sleep pattern disturbance include changes in behavior and performance, as increased irritability; restlessness; disorientation; lack of energy; and fatigue. The critical defining characteristics, at least one of which must be present in order to make the diagnosis, are difficulty in falling asleep, wakening earlier than usual, interruption of the night's sleep by periods of wakefulness, or not feeling rested after sleep. See also **nursing diagnosis.**

sleep terror disorder A condition occurring during stages 3 or 4 of nonrapid eye movement sleep, characterized by repeated episodes of abrupt awakening, usually with a panicky scream, accompanied by intense anxiety, confusion, agitation, disorientation, unresponsiveness, marked motor movements, and total amnesia concerning the event. The disorder is seen usually in children, is more common in boys than in girls, and is extremely variable in frequency but is more likely to occur if the individual is fatigued, under stress, or has been given a tricyclic antidepressant or neuroleptic at bedtime. Compare **nightmare.** See also **pavor nocturnus.**

sleepwalking See **somnambulism.**

slide clamp A device, usually constructed of plastic, employed to regulate the flow of I.V. solution. It has a graduated opening through which the intravenous tubing passes. Compare **roller clamp, screw clamp.**

sling A bandage or device used to support an injured part of the body.

sling restraint A therapeutic device, usually constructed of felt, used to assist in the immobilization of patients, especially orthopedic patients in traction. The sling is placed over the pelvis to reduce pelvic motion with lower extremity traction or over the abdominal area as countertraction with Dunlop traction. Compare **diaper restraint, jacket restraint.**

slip-on blood pump A plastic mesh device with an attached squeeze bulb, rubber tubing, and pressure gauge, used to help administer large amounts of blood quickly. The plastic mesh slips over the blood bag and applies pressure to the bag when the bulb is squeezed.

slipped disk *Informal.* See **herniated intervertebral disk.**

slit lamp An instrument used in ophthalmology for examining the conjunctiva, lens, vitreous humor, iris, and cornea. A high-intensity beam of light is projected through a slit, and a cross section of the illuminated part of the eye is examined through a magnifying lens.

slit lamp microscope A microscope for ophthalmic examination. It permits the viewer to examine the endothelium of the posterior surface of the cornea in a projected band of light that is shaped like a slit.

slough **1.** To shed or cast off dead tissue cells of the endometrium, which are shed during menstruation. **2.** The tissue that has been shed.

slow-acting insulin See **long-acting insulin.**

slow virus A virus that remains dormant in the body after initial infection. Years may elapse before symptoms occur. Several degenerative diseases of the central nervous system are believed to be caused by slow viruses, including subacute sclerosing panencephalitis and kuru.

Sm Symbol for **samarium.**

SMA 12, SMA 24 A trade name for a system that uses a small computer to perform 12 or 24 different blood chemistry tests from a single blood sample.

small cardiac vein One of the five tributaries of the coronary sinus that drains blood from the myocardium. It runs through the coronary sulcus between the right atrium and the right ventricle and opens into the right side of the coronary sinus. It conveys blood from the back of the right atrium and the right ventricle and, in some individuals, is joined by the right marginal vein. Also called **right coronary vein.** Compare **great cardiac vein, middle cardiac vein, posterior vein of the left ventricle.**

small cell carcinoma See **oat cell carcinoma.**

smallest cardiac vein One of the tiny vessels that drain deoxygenated blood from the

SLIDE CLAMPS ON I.V. SETUP

myocardium into the atria. A few of these vessels end in the ventricles. Also called **vein of Thebesius.** Compare **anterior cardiac vein.** See also **coronary vein.**

small-for-gestational-age (SGA) infant An infant whose weight and size at birth falls below the 10th percentile of appropriate-for-gestational-age infants. Factors associated with smallness or retardation of intrauterine growth other than genetic influences include any disorder causing short stature, as dwarfism; malnutrition owing to placental insufficiency; and certain infectious agents. Other factors associated with an SGA infant include cigarette smoking by the mother during pregnancy and maternal addiction to alcohol or heroin. Asphyxia may be a significant risk for the SGA infant during labor and delivery if the condition is the result of placental insufficiency. Such an infant has a low Apgar score, becomes acidotic in labor and at birth, and is likely to develop hypoglycemia within the first hours or days of life. Given

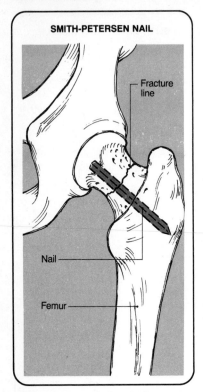

SMITH-PETERSEN NAIL

Fracture line

Nail

Femur

adequate nutrition and caloric intake, some SGA infants show phenomenal catch-up growth. Also called small-for-dates infant. Compare **large-for-gestational-age infant**. See also **dysmaturity**.

small intestine   The longest portion of the digestive tract, extending for about 7 m (23 feet) from the pylorus of the stomach to the iliocecal junction. It is divided into the duodenum, jejunum, and ileum. Decreasing in diameter from beginning to end, it is situated in the central and caudal part of the abdominal cavity, surrounded by large intestine. Compare **large intestine**.

small omentum   See **lesser omentum**.

smallpox   A highly contagious viral disease characterized by fever, prostation, and a vesicular, pustular rash. Smallpox is caused by one of two species of poxvirus: variola minor (alastrim) or variola major. Worldwide vaccination with vaccinia, a related poxvirus, has eradicated smallpox. For several years, no natural case of the disease has been reported. Also called **variola**.

smallpox vaccine   A vaccine prepared from dried smallpox virus.

smear   A laboratory specimen for microscopic examination prepared by spreading a thin film of tissue on a glass slide. To make the specimen diagnostically useful, dye, stain, reagent, diluent, or lysing agent may be applied to it.

smegma   A secretion of sebaceous glands, especially the cheesy, foul-smelling secretion found under the foreskin of the penis and at the base of the labia minora near the glans clitoris.

Smith fracture   A reverse Colles' fracture of the wrist, involving volar displacement and angulation of a distal bone fragment.

Smith-Hodge pessary   See **pessary**.

Smith-Petersen nail   A three-flanged stainless steel nail used in orthopedic surgery to anchor the fractured neck of the femur to its head. It is introduced below the prominence of the greater trochanter and passed through the fractured part into the head of the femur. See also **nail, pin**.

smoke inhalation   The inhalation of noxious fumes or irritating particulate matter that may cause severe pulmonary damage. Chemical pneumonitis, asphyxiation, and physical trauma to the respiratory passages may occur. Characteristics include irritation of the upper respiratory tract, singed nasal hairs, dyspnea, hypoxia, dusty gray sputum, rhonchi, rales, restlessness, anxiety, cough, hoarseness, and pulmonary edema. The characteristics of smoke inhalation and its treatment vary with the nature of the fumes or matter inhaled and the extent of exposure.

smooth muscle   One of two kinds of muscle, composed of elongated, spindle-shaped cells in muscles not under voluntary control, as the smooth muscle of the intestines. The heart muscle is an exception because it is a striated involuntary muscle. The nucleated cells of smooth muscle are arranged parallel to one another and to the long axis of the muscle they form. Also called **involuntary muscle, unstriated muscle**. Compare **cardiac muscle, striated muscle**.

Sn   Symbol for tin.

SN   *abbr* student nurse.

SNA   *abbr* **1**. State Nurses' Association. **2**. Student Nurses' Association.

snail   An invertebrate of the order Gastropoda, several species of which are intermediate hosts of the blood flukes that cause schistosomiasis in humans. See also *Schistosoma*.

snakebite   A wound resulting from penetration of the flesh by the fangs of a snake. Bites by snakes known to be nonvenomous are treated as puncture wounds; those produced by an unidentified or poisonous snake require immediate intervention, which consists of retarding venom absorption and then removing the toxin. Pit vipers are responsible for 98% of the poisonous snakebites in the United States.

snare   A device for holding a wire noose, used to remove small pedunculated growths. The operator tightens the wire around the peduncle to remove the growth.

sneeze   A sudden, forceful, involuntary expulsion of air through the nose and mouth resulting from irritation to mucous membranes of the upper respiratory tract, as by dust, pollen, or viral inflammation. Also called **sternutation**.

Snellen chart One of several charts used in testing visual acuity. Letters, numbers, or symbols are arranged on the chart in decreasing size from top to bottom.

Snellen test A test of visual acuity using a Snellen chart. The person being tested stands 20 feet (about 6 m) from the chart and reads as many of the symbols as possible, reading each line and proceeding downward from the top. A score is assigned in the form of a ratio, comparing the subject's performance with that of a statistically normal subject's performance. A person who can read what the average person can read at 20 feet has 20/20 vision.

SNF *abbr* **skilled nursing facility.**

snout reflex An abnormal sign elicited by tapping the nose, resulting in a marked facial grimace. It usually indicates bilateral corticopontine lesions.

Snowden-Pencer scissors See **scissors.**

SNP *abbr* **School Nurse Practitioner.**

snuffles A nasal discharge in infancy characteristic of congenital syphilis. See **syphilis.**

soap 1. A compound of fatty acids and an alkali. Soap cleanses because fat molecules are attracted to soap molecules in a water solution and are pulled off the dirty surface into the water. 2. A metallic salt of any salt produced from an acid. Compare **detergent.**

SOAP method A method of taking and charting a patient history and physical examination in which information is classified as subjective (S), objective (O), with assessment (A), and plan (P). This SOAP statement is made for each syndrome, problem, symptom, or diagnosis. Patient histories charted by this method are said to be SOAPed and charts produced using it are called SOAP charts. The method is used widely in the United States, but not in Canada. See also **problem-oriented medical record (POMR).**

socialization 1. The process by which an individual learns to live in accordance with the expectations and standards of a group or society, acquiring its beliefs, habits, values, and behavior primarily through imitation, family interaction, and educational systems; the procedure by which society integrates the individual. 2. In psychoanalysis: the process of adjustment that begins in early childhood by which the individual becomes aware of the need to accommodate inner drives to the demands of external reality. See also **internalization.**

socialized medicine A system for the delivery of health care in which the expense of care is borne by the government.

social medicine An approach to disease prevention and treatment based on the study of human heredity, environment, social structures, and cultural values.

social motivation An incentive or drive resulting from a sociocultural influence that initiates behavior toward a particular goal. Compare **achievement motivation, physiological motivation.**

social phobia An anxiety disorder char-

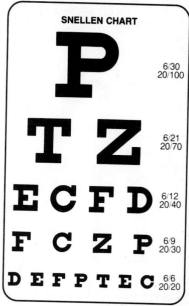

SNELLEN CHART

P	6/30 20/100
T Z	6/21 20/70
E C F D	6/12 20/40
F C Z P	6/9 20/30
D E F P T E C	6/6 20/20

acterized by a persistent, irrational fear of situations in which the individual may be exposed to scrutiny by others and a compelling desire to avoid those situations. Some kinds of social phobia are **erythrophobia, laliophobia, xenophobia.** Compare **simple phobia.** See also **phobia.**

social psychiatry A branch of psychiatry based on the study of social influences on the development and course of mental diseases. In treatment, social psychiatry favors the use of milieu or other situational approaches.

social psychology In psychology: the study of the effects of group membership on the behavior, attitudes, and beliefs of the individual.

Social Security Act A federal statute that provides for a national system of old-age assistance, survivors' and old-age insurance benefits, unemployment insurance and compensation, and other public welfare programs, including Medicare and Medicaid.

Society for Advancement in Nursing (SAIN) A group established to advance the nursing profession through higher education.

sociopath See **psychopath.**

sociopathic See **psychopathic.**

sociopathic personality See **antisocial personality.**

socket A hollow in a bone that fits around a correspondingly shaped bone or organ, as a hip socket or eye socket.

soda A compound of sodium, particularly sodium bicarbonate, sodium carbonate, or sodium hydroxide.

soda lime (SL) A chemical compound used to absorb exhaled carbon dioxide in an anesthesia rebreathing system.

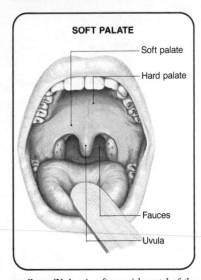

SOFT PALATE

— Soft palate

— Hard palate

— Fauces

— Uvula

sodium (Na) A soft, grayish metal of the alkaline metals group. Its atomic number is 11; its atomic weight is 22.99. Sodium is one of the most important elements in the body. Sodium ions are involved in acid-base balance, water balance, the transmission of nerve impulses, and the contraction of muscles. It is an important component of secretions, including saliva, gastric and intestinal secretions, bile, and pancreatic fluid. It is also the chief electrolyte in interstitial fluid. A decrease in the sodium concentration of the interstitial fluid immediately decreases osmotic pressure, making it hypotonic to intracellular fluid osmotic pressure. Sodium is also important in the transport of sodium and potassium ions through the cytoplasmic membrane. The kidney is the chief regulator of sodium levels in body fluids. Sodium salts, as sodium bicarbonate, are widely used in medications.

sodium acid glutamate See **sodium glutamate.**

sodium aminosalicylate An antitubercular agent.

sodium arsenite poisoning A toxic condition caused by the ingestion of sodium arsenite, an insecticide and weed killer. The symptoms of and treatment for arsenite poisoning are similar to those for arsenic poisoning.

sodium bicarbonate A systemic alkalinizer and an antacid.

sodium biphosphate A stimulant laxative.

sodium chloride Common table salt (NaCl), which is used as a fluid and electrolyte replenisher, isotonic vehicle, irrigating solution, and enema.

sodium chloride 20% solution An oxytocic agent.

sodium chloride and dextrose See **dextrose and sodium chloride injection.**

sodium chloride, hypertonic A solution used in ophthalmology to reduce edema.

sodium etidronate See **etidronate disodium.**

sodium glutamate A salt of glutamic acid used for the treatment of hepatic coma and the enhancement of the flavor of foods. Also called **monosodium glutamate, sodium acid glutamate.**

sodium hypochlorite solution A disinfectant.

sodium iodide See **radioactive iodine.**

sodium lactate A systemic alkalinizer.

sodium lactate injection An electrolyte replenisher that is prescribed for metabolic acidosis.

sodium morrhuate See **morrhuate sodium injection.**

sodium nitroprusside (SNP) See **nitroprusside sodium.**

sodium phosphate A hyperosmolar laxative.

sodium phosphate P32 An antineoplastic, antipolycythemic, radioactive agent.

sodium polystyrene sulfonate A potassium-removing resin.

sodium pump A theoretical mechanism for transporting sodium ions across cell membranes against an opposing concentration gradient. Sodium is normally moved from a region of low concentration within a cell to the extracellular fluid, which contains a much higher concentration. Energy for this transport system is obtained from the hydrolysis of adenosine triphosphate by special enzymes. See also **calcium pump, electrolyte balance.**

sodium-restricted diet See **low-sodium diet.**

sodium salicylate A salicylate nonnarcotic analgesic and antipyretic.

sodium stibocaptate An investigational parasiticide for certain schistosomal infections. It is available from the Centers for Disease Control. Also called **stibocaptate.**

sodium thiosalicylate A salicylate nonnarcotic analgesic and antipyretic.

sodoku See **rat-bite fever.**

sodomy 1. Unnatural sexual intercourse. 2. Intercourse with an animal. 3. Oral or anal intercourse or copulation. —**sodomite,** *n.,* **sodomize,** *v.*

soft diet A diet that is soft in texture, low in residue, easily digested, and well tolerated. It provides the essential nutrients in the form of liquids and semisolid foods. Omitted are raw fruits and vegetables, coarse breads and cereals, rich desserts, strong spices, all fried foods, veal, pork, nuts, and raisins. It is commonly recommended for people who have gastrointestinal disturbances, acute infections, or for anyone unable to tolerate a normal diet.

soft fibroma A fibroma that contains many cells. Also called **fibroma molle.**

soft palate The structure composed of mucous membrane, muscular fibers, and mucous glands that is suspended from the posterior border of the hard palate, forming the roof of the mouth. Suspended from the posterior border is the conical, pendulous, palatine uvula. Arching laterally from the base of the uvula are the two curved, musculomembranous pillars of the fauces. Compare **hard palate.**

soft radiation   Radiation of low energy and low penetrating power.

software   The programs and procedures for operating a system, especially a computer system. See also **hardware.**

-sol   A combining form meaning a 'colloidal solution': *electrosol, nitromersol.*

solar-   A combining form meaning 'of or pertaining to the sun': *solarium, solarization.*

solar fever   **1.** See **dengue. 2.** See **sunstroke.**

solarium   A large, sunny room serving as a lounge for ambulatory patients in a hospital.

solar plexus   A dense network of nerve fibers and ganglia that surrounds the roots of the celiac and the superior mesenteric arteries at the level of the first lumbar vertebra. It is one of the great autonomic plexuses of the body in which the nerve fibers of the sympathetic system and the parasympathetic system combine. Also called **celiac plexus.**

solar radiation   The emission and diffusion of rays from the sun. Overexposure may result in sunburn, keratosis, skin cancer, or lesions associated with photosensitivity.

soleus   One of three superficial posterior muscles of the leg. It is a broad, flat muscle lying just under the gastrocnemius and arising by tendinous fibers from the head of the fibula, from the popliteal line, and from the medial border of the tibia. Compare **gastrocnemius, plantaris.**

solid   **1.** A body, figure, structure, or substance that has length, breadth, and thickness; contains no cavity or hollowness; is not a liquid or a gas; and has no breaks or openings on its surface. **2.** Describing such a body, figure, structure, or substance.

solitary play   A form of play among a group of children within the same room or area in which each child engages in an independent activity using toys that are different from the others', concentrating solely on the particular activity, and showing no interest in joining in or interfering with the play of others. Compare **cooperative play.** See also **associative play, parallel play.**

-soluble   A combining form meaning 'able to be dissolved': *acetosoluble, hydrosoluble, liposoluble.*

solute   A substance dissolved in a solution.

solution   A mixture of two or more substances dissolved in another substance. The molecules of each of the substances disperse homogeneously and do not change chemically. A solution may be a gas, a liquid, or a solid. Compare **colloid, suspension.** See also **solute, solvent.**

-solve   A combining form meaning 'to loosen': *dissolve, resolve.*

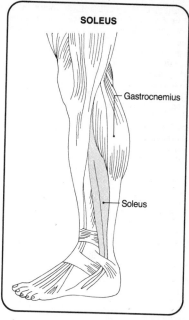

SOLEUS

— Gastrocnemius

— Soleus

solvent   Any liquid in which another substance can be dissolved. The term is used informally to refer to organic liquids like benzene, carbon tetrachloride, and other volatile petroleum distillates that, when inhaled, can cause intoxication as well as damage to mucous membranes of the nose and throat and the tissues of the kidney, liver, and brain. Repeated, prolonged exposure can result in addiction, brain damage, blindness, and other serious consequences, some of them fatal. See also **benzene poisoning, carbon tetrachloride, glue sniffing, petroleum distillate poisoning.**

soma, *pl.* **somata, somas**   **1.** The body as distinguished from the mind or psyche. **2.** The body, excluding germ cells. **3.** The body of a cell. **—somatic, somal,** *adj.*

soma-   See **somato-.**

-soma   A combining form meaning a 'body or portion of a body': *hystersoma, microsoma, prosoma.*

-somatia   A combining form meaning '(condition of the) body, especially concerning size': *diplosomatia, macrosomatia, microsomatia.*

somatic   Pertaining to the body. Compare **psychic.** See also **psychosomatic. —soma,** *n.*

-somatic   A combining form meaning: **1.** The 'cause of effects on the body': *exsomatic, neurosomatic, psychosomatic.* **2.** 'Concerning a type of human body': *eurysomatic, leptosomatic.*

somatic cavity   See **coelom.**

somatic cell   Any of the body tissue cells with the diploid number of chromosomes, as distinguished from those with the haploid number. Compare **germ cell.**

somatic chromosome   Any chromosome

in a diploid or somatic cell, as contrasted to those in a haploid or gametic cell; an autosome.

somatic delusion A false notion or belief concerning body image or body function. See also **delusion.**

somatist A psychotherapist or psychiatrist who believes every neurosis and psychosis has an organic cause.

somatization disorder A disorder characterized by recurrent, multiple, physical complaints and symptoms for which there is no organic cause. The condition typically occurs in adolescence or in the early adult years and in women. The symptoms vary according to the individual and the underlying emotional conflict. Some common symptoms are gastrointestinal dysfunction, paralysis, temporary blindness, cardiopulmonary distress, painful or irregular menstruation, sexual indifference, and pain during intercourse. Hypochondriasis may develop if the condition is untreated. Also called **Briquet's syndrome.**

somato-, soma- A combining form meaning 'of or pertaining to the body': *somatoceptor, somatogenic.*

somatoform disorder Any of a group of neurotic disorders, characterized by symptoms suggesting physical illness or disease, for which there are no demonstrable organic causes or physiological dysfunctions. The symptoms are usually the physical manifestations of some unresolved intrapsychic factor or conflict. Kinds of somatoform disorders are **conversion disorder, hypochondriasis, psychogenic pain disorder, somatization disorder.**

somatogenesis **1.** In embryology: the development of the body from the germ plasm. **2.** The development of a physical disease or of symptoms from an organic pathophysiologic cause. Compare **psychogenesis.** —**somatogenic, somatogenetic,** *adj.*

somatoliberin See **growth hormone–releasing factor.**

somatomegaly A condition in which the body is abnormally large owing to an excessive secretion of somatotropin or an inadequate secretion of somatostatin.

somatoplasm The nonreproductive protoplasmic material of the body cells, as distinguished from the reproductive material of the germ cells. Compare **germ plasm.**

somatopleure The tissue layer that forms the body wall of the early developing embryo. Consisting of an outer layer of ectoderm lined with somatic mesoderm, it continues as the amnion and chorion external to the embryo. Compare **splanchnopleure.** —**somatopleural,** *adj.*

somatosensory evoked potential (SEP) Evoked potential elicited by repeated stimulation of the pain and touch systems. It is the least reliable of the evoked potentials currently being studied as monitors of neurologic function during surgery.

somatosplanchnic Of or pertaining to the trunk of the body and the visceral organs.

somatostatin A hormone produced in the

hypothalamus that inhibits the factor that stimulates release of somatotropin from the anterior pituitary gland. It also inhibits the release of certain hormones and enzymes. Also called **growth hormone–release-inhibiting hormone.**

somatotropic hormone Also called **somatotropin.** See **growth hormone.**

-some A combining form meaning 'a body' of a specified sort: *chromosome, microsome.*

-somia A combining form meaning '(condition of) possessing a body': *agenosomia, diplosomia.*

somite Any of the paired, segmented masses of mesodermal tissue that form along the length of the neural tube during the early stage of embryonic development in vertebrates. These structures give rise to the vertebrae and differentiate into various tissues of the body, including the voluntary muscle, bone, connective tissue, and the dermal layers of the skin.

somite embryo An embryo in any stage of development between the formation of the first and the last pairs of somites, which in humans occurs in the 3rd and 4th weeks following fertilization of the ovum.

somn-, somni- A combining form meaning 'of or pertaining to sleep': *somnifacient, somniferous.*

somnambulism **1.** A condition occurring during Stages 3 or 4 of nonrapid-eye-movement sleep that is characterized by complex motor activity, usually culminating in walking about, with no recall of the episode on awakening. The episodes, which usually last from several minutes to half an hour or longer, occur primarily in children, are more common in boys than in girls, and are more likely to occur if the individual is fatigued, under stress, or has taken a sedative or hypnotic medication. Seizure disorders, central nervous system infections, and trauma may be predisposing factors, but the condition is more commonly related to anxiety. In adults, the condition is less common and is classified as a dissociative reaction. Also called **noctambulation, sleepwalking. 2.** A hypnotic state in which one has full possession of the senses but no recollection of the episode.

-somnia A combining form meaning '(condition of or like) sleep': *asomnia, hyposomnia.*

somnolent **1.** The condition of being sleepy or drowsy. **2.** Tending to cause sleepiness. —**somnolence,** *n.*

-somus A combining form meaning a 'fetal monster with a body': *disomus, hemisomus.*

son- A combining form meaning 'of or pertaining to sound': *sonitus, sonometer.*

sonogram See **ultrasonography.**

sonography See **ultrasonography.**

sonorous rale A snoring sound that may be produced by the vibration of thick secretions lodged in a bronchus.

soot wart See **scrotal cancer.**

soporific **1.** Of or pertaining to a substance, condition, or procedure that causes sleep. **2.** A soporific drug. See also **hypnotic, sedative.**

sorbic acid A compound occurring naturally in berries of the mountain ash. Commercial sorbic acid derived from acetaldehyde is used in fungicides, food preservatives, lubricants, and plasticizers.

sordes, *pl.* **sordes** Dirt or debris, especially the crusts consisting of food, microorganisms, and epithelial cells that accumulate on teeth and lips during a febrile illness or one in which the patient takes nothing by mouth. Sordes gastricae is undigested food and mucus in the stomach.

sore **1.** A wound, ulcer, or lesion. **2.** Tender or painful.

souffle A soft murmur heard through a stethoscope, usually over the uterus in a pregnant woman. It is coincident with the maternal pulse and is caused by blood circulating in the large uterine arteries.

sound **1.** A form of mechanical radiant energy that travels in longitudinal waves through air, liquid, or solids and produces auditory sensations in the ear. See also **cochlea, ear. 2.** Auditory sensations produced in the ear by vibrations of 20 to 20,000 cycles per second, measured in decibels; noise. See also **decibel. 3.** A normal or abnormal noise that originates inside the body. See also **bruit, fremitus, murmur, rale, souffle. 4.** An instrument used to locate an opening, test for patency or create patency, ascertain depth, or reveal contents in a cavity or canal. A sound is used to determine the depth of the uterus, to detect calculi in the bladder, and, less commonly, to assist in correctly inserting a urinary catheter in the urethra through the urinary meatus. **5.** Free of disease or injury; healthy.

South African genetic porphyria See **variegate porphyria.**

South American blastomycosis See **paracoccidioidomycosis.**

South American trypanosomiasis See **Chagas' disease.**

Southey's tube A small, very thin cannula introduced into edematous tissue to withdraw fluid, especially from the legs or feet, to relieve the edema of congestive heart failure. Also called Southey-Leech tube. See also **cannula, tube.**

sp, *pl.* **sp, spp** *abbr* **species.**

space An actual or a potential cavity of the body, as the complemental spaces in the pleural cavity that are not occupied by lung tissue.

Spanish fly See **cantharis.**

spano- A combining form meaning 'scanty or scarce': *spanogyny, spanomenorrhea, spanopnea.*

sparganosis An infection with the fish tapeworm larvae, characterized by painful subcutaneous or eye swellings. It is acquired by ingesting larvae in contaminated water or in inadequately cooked, infected frog flesh. Treatment includes surgery and local injection of ethyl alcohol.

spasm **1.** An involuntary muscle contraction of sudden onset, as habit spasms, hiccups, stuttering, or a tic. **2.** A convulsion or seizure. **3.**

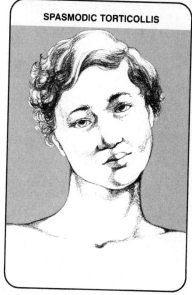

SPASMODIC TORTICOLLIS

A sudden, transient constriction of a blood vessel, bronchus, esophagus, pylorus, ureter, or other hollow organ. Compare **stricture.** See also **bronchospasm, pylorospasm.**

-spasm A combining form meaning a 'convulsion' of a specified sort: *gastrospasm, neurospasm.*

spasmo- A combining form meaning 'of or pertaining to spasm(s)': *spasmodermia, spasmophemia.*

-spasmodic, -spasmodical A combining form meaning 'of or pertaining to a convulsion': *angiospasmodic, antispasmodic.*

spasmodic torticollis A form of torticollis characterized by episodes of neck muscle spasms. The condition is often transient, and examination seldom reveals a physical cause.

spastic Of or pertaining to spasms or other uncontrolled contractions of the skeletal muscles. See also **cerebral palsy. —spasticity,** *n.*

spastic aphonia A condition in which a person is unable to speak because of spasmodic contraction of the abductor muscles of the throat.

spastic bladder A form of neurogenic bladder caused by a lesion of the spinal cord above the voiding reflex center. It is marked by loss of bladder control and bladder sensation, incontinence, and automatic, interrupted, incomplete voiding. It is often caused by trauma but may be a result of tumor or multiple sclerosis. Also called **automatic bladder, reflex bladder.** Compare **flaccid bladder.**

spastic colon See **irritable bowel syndrome.**

spastic paralysis An abnormal condition characterized by the involuntary contraction of one or more muscles with associated loss of muscular function. Compare **flaccid paralysis.**

spastic pseudoparalysis   See **Creutz-feldt-Jakob disease.**

spatial summation   See **summation,** definition 2.

SPE   *abbr* **sucrose polyester.**

Spearman's rho   In statistics: a statistical test for correlation between two rank-ordered scales.

special gene system   A plasmid, transposon, or other genetic fragment that is able to transfer genetic information from one cell to another.

specialing   *Informal.* **1.** In psychiatric nursing: the constant attendance of a professional staff member upon a disturbed patient to prevent self-inflicted harm and also to observe the patient's behavior. The patient so 'specialed' is accompanied in all activities by the staff member. **2.** In nursing: the giving of nursing care to only one person, as a private-duty nurse.

specialist   A health-care professional who practices a specialty. A specialist usually has advanced clinical training and may have a postgraduate academic degree.

special sense   The sense of sight, smell, taste, or hearing.

specialty   A branch of medicine or nursing.

species (Sp)   The category of living things below genus in rank. A species includes individuals of the same genus who are similar in structure and chemical composition and who can interbreed. See also **genus.**

species immunity   A form of natural immunity shared by all members of a species. Compare **individual immunity, racial immunity.**

specific activity   In nuclear medicine: **1.** The radioactivity of a radioisotope per unit mass of the element or compound, expressed in microcuries per millimol or disintegrations per second per milligram. **2.** The relative activity per unit mass, expressed as counts per minute per milligram. The specific activity of potassium in the human body is the same as that of the environment or diet, and, since potassium is associated chiefly with muscle tissue, a whole body count of ^{40}K, following administration of the radioisotope, can be used to distinguish lean-body mass from total-body mass.

specific gravity   The ratio of the density of a substance to the density of another substance accepted as a standard. The usual standard for liquids and solids is water. Hydrogen is the usual standard for gases. See also **density, mass.**

specificity theory   A theory of pain, proposing that pain messages travel distinct physical paths from receptors in skin and viscera via the spinal cord to the brain's pain center for interpretation and response. It explains the efficacy of regional nerve blocks and surgical severing of nerves, but does not explain phantom limb syndrome.

specimen   A small sample of something, intended to show the nature of the whole, as a urine specimen.

spectinomycin dihydrochloride   An antibiotic.

spectr-   A combining form meaning 'image': *spectrograph, spectrophobia.*

spectrometer   An instrument for measuring wavelengths of rays of the spectrum, the deviation of refracted rays, and the angles between faces of a prism. Kinds of spectrometers are **mass spectrometer, Mossbauer spectrometer.**

spectrometry   The procedure of measuring wavelengths of light and other electromagnetic waves. See also **spectrometer.** —**spectrometric,** *adj.*

spectrophotometry   The measurement of color in a solution by determining the amount of light absorbed in the ultraviolet, infrared, or visible spectrum, widely used in clinical chemistry to calculate the concentration of substances in solution. —**spectrophotometric,** *adj.*

spectrum, *pl.* **spectra**   **1.** A range of phenomena or properties occurring in increasing or decreasing magnitude. Radiant or electromagnetic energy is arranged on the basis of wavelength and frequency. Electromagnetic radiation includes spectra of radio waves, infrared, visible light, ultraviolet, X-rays, and gamma rays. See also **electromagnetic radiation, wave. 2.** The range of effectiveness of an antibiotic. A broad-spectrum antibiotic is effective against a wide range of microorganisms. See also **antibiotic.**

speculum   A retractor to separate the walls of a cavity for examination.

speech   **1.** The expression of thoughts in verbal sounds. **2.** The act of communicating verbally, requiring the coordination of larynx, mouth, lips, tongue, lungs, throat, and abdomen.

speech audiometry   See **audiometry.**

speech dysfunction   Any defect or abnormality of speech, including aphasia, alexia, stammering, stuttering, aphonia, and slurring. Speech problems may develop from any of a variety of causes.

speech pathology   **1.** The study of abnormalities of speech or of the organs of speech. **2.** The diagnosis and treatment of abnormalities of speech as practiced by a speech pathologist or a speech therapist.

speech therapist   A person trained in speech pathology who treats people with disorders affecting normal oral communication. Also called speech pathologist.

speed   The rate of change of position with time. Compare **velocity.**

sperm   **1.** See **semen. 2.** See **spermatozoon.**

-sperm   A combining form meaning a 'seed': *gymnosperm, oosperm.*

spermatic cord   A structure extending from the deep inguinal ring in the abdomen to the testis, descending nearly vertically into the scrotum. The left spermatic cord is usually longer than the right; consequently, the left testis usually hangs lower than the right. Each cord consists of arteries, veins, lymphatics, nerves, and the excretory duct of the testis.

spermatic duct   See **deferent duct.**

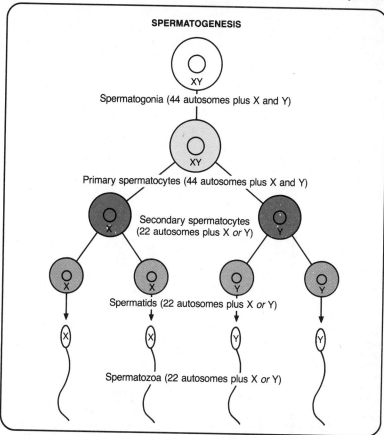

SPERMATOGENESIS

Spermatogonia (44 autosomes plus X and Y)

Primary spermatocytes (44 autosomes plus X and Y)

Secondary spermatocytes (22 autosomes plus X *or* Y)

Spermatids (22 autosomes plus X *or* Y)

Spermatozoa (22 autosomes plus X *or* Y)

spermatic fistula An abnormal passage communicating with a testis or a seminal duct.

spermatid A male germ cell that arises from a spermatocyte and that becomes a mature spermatozoon in the last phase of the continual process of spermatogenesis.

spermato-, spermo- A combining form meaning 'of or pertaining to seed, specifically to the male generative element': *spermatoblast, spermatocyst.*

spermatocele A cystic swelling, either of the epididymis or of the rete testis, that contains spermatozoa. It lies above, behind, and separate from the testis; it is usually painless and requires no therapy.

spermatocide A chemical substance that kills spermatozoa by reducing their surface tension, causing the cell wall to break down by a bactericidal effect or by creating a highly acidic environment. Various spermatocidal agents are used in contraceptive creams. Also called **spermicide.**

spermatocyte A male germ cell that arises from a spermatogonium. Each spermatocyte gives rise to two haploid secondary spermatocytes that redivide to become spermatids.

spermatocytogenesis See **spermatogenesis.**

spermatogenesis The process of development of spermatozoa, including the first stage, called **spermatocytogenesis,** in which spermatogonia become spermatocytes that develop into spermatids, and the second stage, called **spermiogenesis,** in which the spermatids become spermatozoa.

spermatogonium, *pl.* **spermatogonia** A male germ cell that gives rise to a spermatocyte early in spermatogenesis.

spermatozoon, *pl.* **spermatozoa** A mature male germ cell that develops in the seminiferous tubules of the testes. Resembling a tadpole, it is about 50 micrometers ($\frac{1}{500}$ inch) long, and has a head with a nucleus, a neck, and a tail that provides propulsion. It is the generative component of the semen, impregnating the ovum and resulting in fertilization. See **spermatogenesis.**

-spermia, -spermy A combining form meaning '(condition of) possessing or producing seed': *aspermia, asthenospermia.*

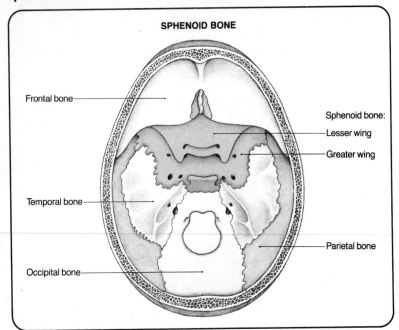

SPHENOID BONE

Frontal bone

Temporal bone

Occipital bone

Sphenoid bone:
Lesser wing
Greater wing

Parietal bone

spermicidal Destructive to spermatozoa.

spermicide See **spermatocide.**

spermiogenesis See **spermatogenesis.**

sphacel- A combining form meaning 'of or pertaining to gangrene': *sphaceloderma, sphacelotoxin.*

sphaero- See **sphero-.**

spheno- A combining form meaning 'of or pertaining to the sphenoid bone or to a wedge': *sphenocephaly, sphenoidotomy.*

sphenoidal fissure A cleft between the great and small wings of the sphenoid bone.

sphenoidal sinus One of a pair of cavities in the sphenoid bone of the skull, lined with mucous membrane that is continuous with that of the nasal cavity. Each sinus is approximately spheroidal, with a diameter of about 2 cm (¾ inch), but its shape and size vary from person to person. A large sphenoidal sinus may extend into the roots of the pterygoid processes, into the great wings, or into the occipital bone. Compare **ethmoidal air cells, frontal sinus, maxillary sinus.**

sphenoid bone The bone at the base of the skull, anterior to the temporal bones and the basilar part of the occipital bone. It resembles a bat with its wings extended.

sphenomandibular ligament One of a pair of flat, thin ligaments comprising part of the temporomandibular joint between the mandible and the temporal bone. It is attached to the spine of the sphenoid bone and becomes broader as it descends to the lingula of the mandibular foramen.

-sphere, -sphaera, -sphaere A combining form meaning: **1.** A 'spherical body': *chondriosphere, onconosphere.* **2.** A 'realm that supports life': *biosphere, vivosphere.*

sphero-, sphaero- A combining form meaning 'round or pertaining to a sphere': *spherocyte, spherolith.*

spherocyte An abnormal spherical red cell that contains more than the normal amount of hemoglobin. It can be seen and identified under the microscope on the stained blood specimen. Its presence in large numbers causes increased osmotic fragility of red blood cells. —**spherocytic,** *adj.*

spherocytic anemia A hematologic disorder characterized by hemolytic anemia owing to the presence of spherocytes. The cells are fragile and tend to hemolyze in the oxygen-poor peripheral circulatory system. Episodic crises of abdominal pain, fever, jaundice, and splenomegaly occur. As repeated transfusions are often needed to treat the anemia, siderosis may develop. Splenectomy may then be necessary. The condition is inherited as an autosomal dominant trait.

spherocytosis The abnormal presence of spherocytes in the blood. Compare **elliptocytosis.**

spheroidea See **ball-and-socket joint.**

sphincter A circular band of muscle fibers that constricts a passage or closes a natural opening in the body, as the hepatic sphincter in the muscular coat of the hepatic veins near their union with the superior vena cava.

sphincter pupillae A muscle that expands the iris, narrowing the diameter of the pupil of the eye. It is composed of circular fibers arranged in a narrow band about 1 mm wide, surrounding the margin of the pupil toward the posterior surface of the iris. The circular fibers near the free margin of the iris are closely packed; those that are near the periphery of the band are more separated and form incomplete circles. Compare **dilatator pupillae.**

sphingomyelin A group of phospholipids that, on hydrolysis, yields phosphoric acid, choline, sphingosine, and a fatty acid. Sphingomyelins occur primarily in nervous tissue and generally in membranes.

sphingomyelin lipidosis Any of a group of diseases characterized by an abnormality in the ability of the body to store sphingolipids. Kinds of sphingomyelin lipidosis include **Gaucher's disease, Niemann-Pick disease, Tay-Sachs disease.** See also **angiokeratoma corporis diffusum.**

sphygm-, sphygmo- A combining form meaning 'pulse': *sphygmoid, sphygmomanometer.*

-sphygmia A combining form meaning '(condition of the) pulse': *anisosphygmia, hemisphygmia.*

sphygmo- A combining form meaning 'of or related to the pulse': *sphygmobologram, sphygmoscope.*

sphygmogram A tracing produced by a sphygmograph. A curve occurs on the tracing with each atrial pulsation. An upward, primary elevation is followed by a sudden drop to a point slightly above the baseline. The curve then gradually descends to the baseline in small decrements of amplitude. Sphygmographic abnormalities of rate, rhythm, and form may aid in cardiovascular assessment.

sphygmograph An instrument that records the force of the atrial pulse. —**sphyamographic,** *adj.*

sphygmomanometer A device for measuring the arterial blood pressure, consisting of a cuff with an air bladder connected to a tube with a bulb for pumping air into the bladder and a gauge for indicating the air pressure being exerted over the artery. See also **manometer.**

spica bandage A figure-eight bandage in which each turn generally overlaps the next to form a succession of V-like designs. It may be used to give support, to apply pressure, or to hold a dressing in place on the chest, limbs, thighs, or pelvis.

spica cast An orthopedic cast applied to immobilize part or all of the trunk of the body and part or all of one or more extremities. It is used to treat various fractures, as of the hip and the femur, and in correcting or maintaining the correction of hip deformities. Kinds of spica casts are **bilateral long leg spica cast, one-and-a-half spica cast, shoulder spica cast, unilateral long leg spica cast.**

spicule A sharp body with a needlelike point.

spider angioma A form of telangiectasis characterized by a central, elevated, red dot the size of a pinhead from which small blood vessels

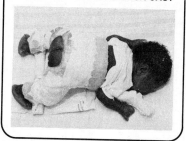

BILATERAL LONG LEG SPICA CAST

radiate. Spider angiomas are often associated with elevated estrogen levels. Also called **spider nevus.** See also **telangiectasia.**

spider antivenin See **black widow spider antivenin.**

spider bite A puncture wound produced by the bite of a spider, an arachnid related to ticks and mites. Fewer than 100 of some 30,000 species of spiders are known to bite. Two of them, the black widow spider and the brown spider, found in the United States, are poisonous.

spider nevus See **spider angioma.**

spina, *pl.* **spinae** A spine or a thornlike projection, as the bony projection on the anterior border of the ilium, forming the anterior end of the iliac crest.

spina bifida A relatively common congenital neural tube defect characterized by a developmental anomaly in the posterior vertebral arch. It may occur with only a small deformed lamina separated by a midline gap, or it may be associated with the complete absence of laminae surrounding a large area. In cases where the separation is wide enough, contents of the spinal canal protrude posteriorly, and a myelomeningocele is evident. This more serious deformity is associated with gross deficits not normally manifested in spina bifida. Also called **spinal dysrhaphia.**

spina bifida anterior Incomplete closure along the anterior surface of the vertebral column. The defect is often associated with developmental anomalies of the abdominal and thoracic viscera.

spina bifida cystica A developmental defect of the central nervous system in which a hernial cyst containing meninges (meningocele), spinal cord (myelocele), or both (myelomeningocele) protrudes through a congenital cleft in the vertebral column. The protruding sac is encased in a layer of skin or a fine membrane that can easily rupture, causing the leakage of cerebrospinal fluid and an increased risk of meningeal infection. The severity of neurological dysfunction and associated defects depends directly on the degree of nerve involvement. The most severe type is lumbosacral myelomeningocele, which is frequently associated with hydrocephalus and the Arnold-Chiari malformation. Compare **spina bifida occulta.** See also

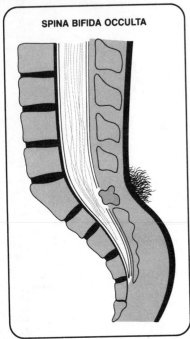

SPINA BIFIDA OCCULTA

myelomeningocele, neural tube defect.

spina bifida occulta Defective closure of the laminae of the vertebral column in the lumbosacral region without hernial protrusion of the spinal cord or meninges. The defect occurs in about 5% of the population and is identified externally by a skin depression or dimple, dark tufts of hair, telangiectasis, or soft, subcutaneous lipomas at the site. Since the neural tube has closed, no neurological impairments are usually associated with the defect. However, any abnormal adhesion of the spinal cord to the area of the malformation may lead to neuromuscular disturbances, usually problems with gait and foot weakness and with the bowel and bladder sphincters. Compare **spina bifida cystica.**

spinal 1. Of or pertaining to the spine, especially the spinal column. 2. *Informal.* Spinal anesthesia, as saddle block or caudal anesthesia.

spinal accessory nerve See **accessory nerve.**

spinal aperture A large opening formed by the body of a vertebra and its arch.

spinal canal The cavity within the vertebral column.

spinal caries See **tuberculous spondylitis.**

spinal column See **vertebral column.**

spinal cord A long, nearly cylindrical structure lodged in the vertebral canal and extending from the foramen magnum at the skull base to the upper lumbar region. A major component of the central nervous system, the spinal cord of the adult is about 1 cm (⅜ inch) in diameter with an average length of 42 to 45 cm (16½ to 18 inches). The cord conducts sensory and motor impulses to and from the brain and controls many reflexes. There are 31 spinal nerves originating from the cord: 8 cervical, 12 thoracic, 5 lumbar, 5 sacral, and 1 coccygeal. The cord has an inner core of gray material consisting mainly of nerve cells and is enclosed by 3 protective membranes (meninges): the dura mater, arachnoid, and pia mater. It is an extension of the medulla oblongata of the brain and ends caudally between the 12th thoracic and 3rd lumbar vertebrae, often at or adjacent to the disk between the 1st and 2nd lumbar vertebrae. Also called **chorda spinalis, medulla spinalis.**

spinal cord compression An abnormal and often serious condition resulting from pressure on the spinal cord. The symptoms range from temporary numbness of an extremity to permanent quadriplegia, depending on the cause, severity, and location of the pressure. Causes include spinal fracture, vertebral dislocation, tumor, hemorrhage, and edema associated with contusion. See also **herniated disc, spondylolisthesis.**

spinal cord injury Any one of the traumatic disruptions of the spinal cord, often associated with extensive musculoskeletal involvement. Common spinal cord injuries are spinal fractures and dislocations. Such trauma may cause varying degrees of paraplegia and quadriplegia. Injuries to spinal structures below the first thoracic vertebra may produce paraplegia. Injuries to the spine above the first thoracic vertebra may cause quadriplegia. Injuries that completely transect the spinal cord cause permanent loss of motor and sensory functions activated by neurons below the level of the lesions involved. Spinal cord injuries produce a state of spinal shock, characterized by placid paralysis, and complete loss of skin sensation at the time of the injury. Within a few weeks the muscles affected may become spastic, and the skin sensation may return to a slight degree. The motor and the sensory losses that prevail a few weeks after the injury are usually permanent. Treatment of spinal cord injuries varies considerably and involves numerous approaches, as orthopedic exercises, ambulatory techniques, and special physical and psychological therapy.

spinal cord tumor A neoplasm of the spinal cord of which more than 50% are extramedullary, about 25% are intramedullary, and the rest are extradural. Symptoms usually develop slowly and may progress from unilateral paresthesia and a dull ache to lancinating pain, weakness in one or both legs, abnormal deep tendon reflexes, and, in advanced cases, monoplegia, hemiplegia, or paraplegia. Function of the autonomic nervous system is sometimes disturbed, causing areas of dry, cold, blue-pink skin or profuse sweating of the lower extremities. The diagnosis is made by X-ray and myelographic examination. Most extramedullary and nonmetastatic extradural tumors are surgically removed; intramedullary lesions are enucleated, whenever possible; and inoperable tumors are treated with radiotherapy and chemotherapy.

spinal curvature Any persistent, abnormal deviation of the vertebral column from its normal position. Kinds of spinal curvature are **kyphoscoliosis, kyphosis, lordosis, scoliosis.**

spinal dysrhaphia See **spina bifida.**

spinal fasciculi See **spinal tract.**

spinal fluid See **cerebrospinal fluid.**

spinal fusion The fixation of an unstable segment of the spine, accomplished by skeletal traction or immobilization of the patient in a body cast but most frequently by a surgical procedure. Also called **spondylosyndesis.**

spinal headache A headache occurring after spinal anesthesia or lumbar puncture, caused by a loss of cerebrospinal spinal fluid (CSF) from the subarachnoid space, resulting in traction of the meninges on the pressure-sensitive intracranial structures. Severe spinal headache may be accompanied by diminished aural and visual acuity. Treatment usually includes keeping the patient flat in bed to relieve the meningeal irritation, encouraging increased fluid intake to increase CSF production and volume, and administering analgesics to reduce pain. If severe headache persists, an anesthesiologist may perform an autologous blood patch procedure in which a clot of the patient's blood is formed and planted over the leaking puncture site in the dura to prevent further CSF loss.

spinal manipulation The forced passive flexion, extension, and rotation of vertebral segments, carrying the elements of articulation beyond the usual range of movement to the limit of anatomic range. It may be used effectively in physiotherapy to treat vertebral and sacroiliac dislocations, sprains, and adhesions.

spinal muscular atrophy See **Duchenne's disease.**

spinal nerves The 31 pairs of nerves without special names that are connected to the spinal cord and numbered according to the level of the cord at which they emerge. There are 8 cervical, 12 thoracic, 5 lumbar, and 5 sacral pairs, and 1 coccygeal pair. Emerging from the cord, each spinal nerve divides into the anterior, the posterior, and the white rami, with the anterior and posterior rami serving the voluntary nervous system and the white rami serving the autonomic nervous system. See also **spinal cord.**

spinal puncture See **lumbar puncture.**

spinal tract Any one of the ascending and descending pathways for motor or sensory nerve impulses that is found in the white matter of the spinal cord. Twenty-one different tracts are found in the dorsal, the ventral, and the lateral funiculi of the white substance. Ascending tracts conduct impulses up the spinal cord to the brain; descending tracts conduct impulses down the cord from the brain. The four major ascending tracts are the lateral spinothalmic, the ventral spinothalmic, the fasciculi gracilis and cuneatus, and the spinocerebellar. The four major descending tracts are the lateral corticospinal, the ventral corticospinal, the lateral reticulospinal,

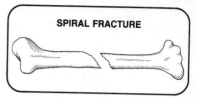

SPIRAL FRACTURE

and the medial reticulospinal.

spindle **1.** The fusiform figure of achromatin in the cell nucleus during the late prophase and the metaphase of mitosis. It consists of tiny fibers radiating out from the centrosomes and connecting them with one another. **2.** A type of brain wave, consisting of a short series of changes in electrical potential with a frequency of 14/second. **3.** Any one of the special receptor organs comprising the neurotendinous and the neuromuscular spindles distributed throughout the body. These kinds of spindles serve as special receptor organs that detect the degree of stretch in a muscle or at the junction of a muscle with its tendon and are essential in maintaining muscle tone.

spindle cell carcinoma A rapidly growing neoplasm composed of fusiform squamous cells. It may be difficult to distinguish from a sarcoma.

spindle cell nevus See **benign juvenile melanoma.**

spinnbarkheit The clear, slippery, elastic consistency characteristic of cervical mucus during ovulation. It has the consistency of an uncooked egg white, and it is a valuable sign of the peak fertile period in a woman's menstrual cycle. Observation of spinnbarkheit is useful in natural methods of family planning, in infertility studies, and for artificial insemination. See also **ovulation method of family planning.**

spino- A combining form meaning 'of or pertaining to the spine': *spinocain, spinoglenoid.*

spinocerebellar Of or pertaining to the spinal cord and the cerebellum.

spinocerebellar disorder An inherited disorder characterized by a progressive degeneration of the spinal cord and cerebellum, often involving other parts of the nervous system as well. These disorders tend to occur within families and can be inherited as dominant or recessive traits. Onset is usually early, during childhood or adolescence. No effective treatment is known. Some kinds of spinocerebellar degeneration are **Charcot-Marie-Tooth atrophy, Dejerine-Sottas disease, Friedreich's ataxia, Refsum's syndrome.**

spinofallopian tube shunt See **ventriculofallopian tube shunt.**

spinth- A combining form meaning 'spark': *spinthariscope, spintherometer.*

spir- A combining form meaning: **1.** 'A coil, or coiled': *spiradenitus, spireme.* **2.** 'Of or pertaining to the breath, or to breathing': *spiracle, spirogram.*

spiral fracture A bone break in which the disruption of bone tissue is spiral, oblique, or

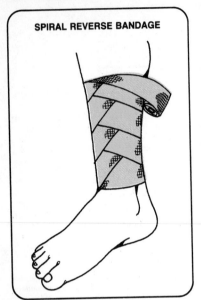

SPIRAL REVERSE BANDAGE

transverse to the long axis of the fractured bone.

spiral organ of Corti　See **Corti's organ.**

spiral reverse bandage　A spiral bandage that is turned and folded back on itself as necessary to make it fit the contour of the body more securely.

spirillary rat-bite fever　See **rat-bite fever.**

spirillum fever　See **rat-bite fever.**

spirit　1. Any volatile liquid, particularly one that has been distilled. 2. A volatile substance dissolved in alcohol. See also **volatile.**

spiritual distress (distress of the human spirit)　A nursing diagnosis accepted by the Fifth National Conference on the Classification of Nursing Diagnoses. The etiology of the condition may be separation from religious or cultural ties or a change in beliefs or value system, intense suffering, severe stress, or prolonged treatment. The defining characteristics include stated anger against a deity or questions about the meaning of the suffering being experienced. The client may joke in a macabre fashion, have nightmares, cry, act in a hostile or apathetic manner, express anger or resentment against religious figures, and cease participation in religious practices. See also **nursing diagnosis.**

spirochete　Any bacterium that is motile and spiral-shaped. Compare **bacillus, coccus, vibrio.** —**spirochetal,** *adj.*

spirogram　A visual record of respiratory movements made by a spirometer.

spirograph　A device for recording respiratory movements. See also **spirometer.** —**spirographic,** *adj.*

spirometer　An instrument that measures and records the volume of inhaled and exhaled air,

used to assess pulmonary function. Volumetric information is recorded on a chart, called a spirogram. —**spirometric,** *adj.*

spirometry　Laboratory evaluation of the air capacity of the lungs by means of a spirometer. Compare **blood gas determination.** —**spirometric,** *adj.*

spironolactone　A potassium-sparing diuretic.

Spitz nevus　See **benign juvenile melanoma.**

splanchn-, splanchno-　A combining form meaning 'of or pertaining to a viscus, or to the splanchnic nerve': *splanchnocele, splanchnography.*

splanchnic　Of or pertaining to the internal organs; visceral.

-splanchnic　A combining form meaning 'viscera, entrails': *somaticosplanchnic, trisplanchnic.*

splanchnocele　1. See **splanchnocoele. 2.** Hernial protrusion of any abdominal viscera.

splanchnocoele, splanchnocele　A part of the embryonic body cavity, or coelom, that gives rise to the abdominal, pericardial, and pleural cavities. Also called **pleuroperitoneal cavity.**

splanchnopleure　A layer of tissue in the early developing embryo, formed by the union of endoderm and splanchnic mesoderm. It gives rise to the embryonic gut and the visceral organs and continues external to the embryo as the yolk sac and allantois. Compare **somatopleure.** —**splanchnopleural,** *adj.*

S-plasty　A plastic surgery technique in which an S-shaped incision is made to reduce tension and improve healing in areas of loose skin.

spleen　A soft, highly vascular, roughly ovoid organ situated between the stomach and the diaphragm in the left hypochondriac region. The spleen is considered part of the lymphatic system, because it contains lymphatic nodules. It is dark purple and varies in shape in different individuals and within the same individual at different times. The precise function of the spleen has baffled physiologists for more than 100 years, but the most recent research indicates it performs various tasks, as defense, homopoiesis, blood storage, and the destruction of red blood cells and platelets. Macrophages lining the sinuses of the spleen destroy microorganisms by phagocytosis. The spleen also produces leukocytes, monocytes, lymphocytes, and plasma cells. It produces red blood cells before birth and is believed to produce red blood cells after birth only in extreme and hemolytic anemia. If the body suffers severe hemorrhage, the spleen can increase the blood volume from 350 to 550 ml in less than 60 seconds. Compare **thymus.** —**splenic,** *adj.*

splen- See **spleno-.**

splenectomy　The surgical excision of the spleen.

-splenia　A combining form meaning '(condition of the spleen': *asplenia, eusplenia, microsplenia.*

splenic flexure syndrome   A recurrent pain and abdominal distention in the left upper quadrant of the abdomen owing to a pocket of gas trapped in the large intestine below the spleen, at the flexure of the transverse and descending colon. The symptoms are relieved by defecation or passing flatus.

splenic gland   See **pancreaticolienal node.**

splenic vein   See **lienal vein.**

splenius capitis   One of a pair of deep muscles of the back. Arising from the ligamentum nuchae, the seventh cervical vertebra, and the first three or four thoracic vertebrae, it inserts in the occipital bone and the mastoid process of the temporal bone.

splenius cervicis   One of a pair of deep muscles of the back. Arising from a narrow tendinous band from the spinous processes of the third through the sixth thoracic vertebrae, it inserts into the transverse processes of the upper two or three cervical vertebrae. Also called splenius colli.

spleno-, splen-   A combining form meaning 'of or pertaining to the spleen': *splenocele, splenodiagnosis, splenomalacia.*

splenomedullary leukemia   See **acute myelocytic leukemia, chronic myelocytic leukemia.**

splenomegaly   An abnormal enlargement of the spleen, as associated with portal hypertension, hemolytic anemia, Niemann-Pick disease, or malaria.

splenomyelogenous leukemia   See **acute myelocytic leukemia, chronic myelocytic leukemia.**

splint   1. An orthopedic device for immobilization, restraint, or support of any part of the body. It may be rigid or flexible. 2. In dentistry: a device for anchoring the teeth or modifying the bite. Compare **brace, cast.**

splinter fracture   A comminuted fracture with thin, sharp, bone fragments.

splinter hemorrhage   Linear bleeding under a finger- or toenail, resembling a splinter. It is seen after trauma and in patients with bacterial endocarditis.

split gene   In molecular genetics: a genetic unit whose continuity is interrupted.

split personality   See **multiple personality.**

split Russell traction   An orthopedic mechanism that combines suspension and traction to immobilize, position, and align the lower extremities in the treatment of congenital hip dislocation, hip and knee contractures, and in the correction of orthopedic deformities. Split Russell traction, usually applied as adhesive or nonadhesive skin traction, employs a sling to relieve the weight of the lower extremities. The traction weights are suspended from pulley and rope systems at the foot and the head of the bed; a jacket restraint is often incorporated to aid immobilization. Split Russell traction may be used as a unilateral or as a bilateral mechanism. Compare **Russell traction.**

spodo-   A combining form meaning 'of or

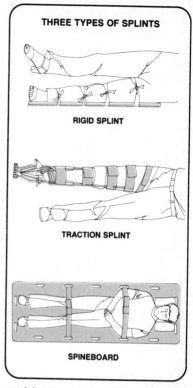

THREE TYPES OF SPLINTS

RIGID SPLINT

TRACTION SPLINT

SPINEBOARD

pertaining to waste materials': *spodogenous, spodophagous.*

-spondylic   A combining form meaning 'referring to the vertebrae': *cyclospondylic, monospondylic.*

spondylitis   An inflammation of any of the spinal vertebrae, usually characterized by stiffness and pain. The condition may result from trauma, infection, or rheumatoid disease. See also **ankylosing spondylitis.**

spondylo-   A combining form meaning 'of or pertaining to a vertebra, or to the spinal column': *spondylocace, spondylodidymia.*

spondylolisthesis   The partial forward dislocation of one vertebra over the one below it, most commonly the fifth lumbar vertebra over the first sacral vertebra. See also **spinal cord compression.**

spondylosis   A spinal condition characterized by fixation or stiffness of a vertebral joint. See also **Marie-Strümpell disease, spondylitis.**

spondylosyndesis   See **spinal fusion.**

sponge   1. A resilient, absorbent mass used to absorb fluids, apply medication, or cleanse. The sponge may be the internal skeleton of a marine animal, or it may be manufactured from cellulose, rubber, or synthetic material. 2. *Informal.* A folded gauze square used in surgery.

sponge bath   The procedure of washing the

patient with a damp washcloth or sponge, used when a full bath is not necessary or as a method of reducing body temperature.

spongio- A combining form meaning 'like a sponge, or related to a sponge': *spongioblast*, *spongiopilin*.

spongioblastoma, *pl.* **spongioblastomas, spongioblastomata** A neoplasm composed of spongioblasts, embryonic epithelial cells that develop around the neural tube and transform into cells of the supporting connective tissue of nerve cells or cells of lining membranes of the ventricles and the spinal cord canal. A kind of spongioblastoma is **spongioblastoma unipolare.** Also called **glioblastoma, gliosarcoma, spongiocytoma.**

spongioblastoma multiforme See **glioblastoma multiforme.**

spongioblastoma unipolare A rare neoplasm composed of approximately parallel spongioblasts. It may occur near the third ventricle, in the pons and brain stem, in basal ganglia, or in the spinal cord's terminal filament.

spongiocytoma See **spongioblastoma.**

spontaneous Occurring naturally and without apparent cause, as spontaneous remission.

spontaneous abortion A termination of pregnancy before the 20th week of gestation caused by abnormalities of the conceptus or maternal environment. More than 10% of pregnancies end as spontaneous abortions, almost all owing to blighted ova that have congenital defects incompatible with life. Compare **induced abortion.**

spontaneous delivery A vaginal birth occurring without the mechanical assistance of obstetric forceps or a vacuum aspirator.

spontaneous evolution The unassisted delivery of a fetus in the transverse position. See also **Denman's spontaneous evolution.**

spontaneous fracture See **pathologic fracture.**

spontaneous generation The theoretical origin of living organisms from inanimate matter; abiogenesis.

spontaneous labor A labor beginning and progressing without mechanical or pharmacologic stimulation.

spor-, sporo- A combining form meaing 'of or pertaining to a spore': *sporocyst, sporogenesis.*

sporadic Of a number of events: occurring at scattered, intermittent, and apparently random intervals.

-sporangium A combining form meaning an 'encasement of spores': *haplosporangium, oosporangium.*

spore **1.** A reproductive unit of some genera of fungi or protozoa. **2.** A form, assumed by some bacteria, that is resistant to heat, drying, and chemicals. Under proper environmental conditions the spore may revert to the actively multiplying form of the bacterium. Diseases caused by spore-forming bacteria include anthrax, botulism, gas gangrene, and tetanus.

-spore A combining form meaning a 'reproductive element': *archespore, chlamydospore.*

sporicide Any agent effective in destroying spores, as compounds of chlorine and formaldehyde.

sporiferous Producing or bearing spores.

sporoblast Any cell that gives rise to a sporozoite or spore during the sexual reproductive phase of the life cycle of a sporozoan, specifically the cells resulting from the multiple fission of the encysted zygote of the malarial parasite *Plasmodium* from which the sporozoites develop.

sporocyst **1.** Any structure containing spores or reproductive cells. **2.** A saclike structure, or oocyst, secreted by the zygote of certain protozoa before sporozoite formation. **3.** The second larval stage in the life cycle of parasitic flukes. The saclike organism develops from the miracidium, or first larval stage, in the body of a freshwater snail host and contains germinal cells that give rise either to daughter sporocysts that develop into cercariae or to rediae. See also **fluke.**

sporogenesis **1.** The formation of spores; sporogeny. **2.** Reproduction by means of spores. **—sporogenic,** *adj.*

sporogenous Describing an animal or plant that reproduces by spores.

sporogeny The formation of spores.

sporogony Reproduction by means of spores, specifically the formation of sporozoites during the sexual stage of the life cycle of a sporozoan, primarily the malarial parasite *Plasmodium.* Compare **schizogony.**

sporont A mature protozoan parasite in the sexual reproductive stage of its life cycle. It undergoes conjugation to form a zygote, which produces sporozoites by multiple fission. Compare **schizont.** See also **sporogony.**

sporonticide Any substance that destroys sporonts, as chloroquine and other antimalarial drugs. **—sporonticidal,** *adj.*

sporophore That part of an organism or plant that produces spores.

sporophyte The asexual, spore-bearing stage in plants that reproduce by alternation of generations.

sporotrichosis A common, chronic fungal infection caused by the species *Sporothrix schenckii*, usually characterized by skin ulcers and subcutaneous nodules along lymphatic channels. It rarely spreads to bones, lungs, joints, or muscles. The fungus is found in soil and decaying vegetation and usually enters the skin by accidental injury. Treatment may include amphotericin B.

Sporotrichum A genus of soil-inhabiting fungi formerly thought to cause sporotrichosis.

Sporozoa A class of parasite in the phylum Protozoa that is characterized by the absence of any external organs of locomotion. Included in this class are the genera *Toxoplasma* and *Plasmodium.*

sporozoite Any of the cells resulting from the sexual union of spores during the life cycle of a sporozoan. It refers specifically to the elongated nucleated cells produced by the multiple fission of the zygote contained in the oocyst in the female *Anopheles* mosquito during the sexual reproductive stage of the life cycle of the malarial parasite *Plasmodium*. Upon release from the oocyst, the sporozoites migrate to the salivary glands of the mosquito, from which they are transmitted to humans and develop within the parenchymal cells of the liver as merozoites. Also called **falciform body.** See also **malaria, Plasmodium.**

sport In genetics: **1.** An individual or organism that differs drastically from its parents or others of its type because of genetic mutation; a mutant. **2.** A genetic mutation. **3.** See **lusus naturae.**

sporulation **1.** A type of reproduction that occurs in lower plants and animals, as fungi, algae, and protozoa, and involves the formation of spores by the spontaneous division of the cell into four or more daughter cells, each of which contains a portion of the original nucleus. **2.** The formation of a refractile body, or resting spore, within certain bacteria that makes the cell resistant to unfavorable environmental conditions. The cell regains its viability when the conditions become favorable. See also **spore.**

spotted fever See **Rocky Mountain spotted fever.**

sprain A traumatic injury to the tendons, muscles, or ligaments around a joint, characterized by pain, swelling, and skin discoloration over the joint. The duration and severity of the symptoms vary with the extent of damage to the supporting tissues. Treatment requires support, rest, and alternating cold and heat. Ultrasound therapy may speed recovery. X-rays are often indicated to rule out a fracture.

sprain fracture A fracture that results from a tendon or ligament separation at the point of insertion, associated with the bone separation at the same site.

spring forceps A kind of forceps that includes a spring mechanism, used for grasping an artery to arrest or prevent hemorrhage. Also called **bulldog forceps.**

spring lancet A lancet with a spring-triggered blade. It may be used for collecting small specimens of blood for laboratory tests. See also **lancet.**

sprinter's fracture A fracture of the anterior superior or the anterior inferior spine of the ilium, caused by a bone fragment being forcibly pulled by a violent muscle spasm.

sprue A chronic disorder resulting from malabsorption of nutrients from the small intestine. Symptoms include diarrhea, weakness, weight loss, poor appetite, pallor, muscle cramps, bone pain, and a smooth, shiny tongue. It occurs in both tropical and nontropical forms and affects both children and adults. Also called **catarrhal dysentery.** See also **malabsorption syndrome, nontropical sprue, tropical sprue.**

SPSS In statistics: *abbr* **Statistical Package for the Social Sciences,** a computer program used in clinical nursing research to analyze complex data from large samples.

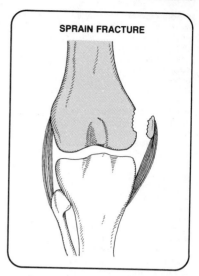

SPRAIN FRACTURE

spurious aperture of facial canal An opening in the petrous part of the temporal bone for the greater petrosal nerve and a branch of the middle meningeal artery.

sputum Material coughed up from the lungs and expectorated through the mouth. It contains mucus, cellular debris, microorganisms, and possibly blood or pus. The amount, color, and constituents of the sputum are important in the diagnosis of many illnesses, including tuberculosis, pneumonia, and lung cancer.

squam- A combining form meaning 'of or pertaining to scales': *squamatization, squamocellular, squamopetrosal.*

squamous cell carcinoma A slow-growing, malignant tumor of squamous epithelium, often found in the lungs and skin but also in the anus, cervix, larynx, nose, bladder, and other sites. The typical skin lesion—a firm, red, horny, painless nodule, ranging from less than one to several centimeters in size—often results from overexposure to the sun. The neoplastic cells characteristically resemble prickle cells and form keratin pearls on the lesion surface. Also called **epidermoid carcinoma.**

squeeze dynamometer A dynamometer for measuring the muscular strength of the grip of the hand.

squint See **strabismus.**

squinting eye The abnormal eye of strabismus that cannot be focused with the fixated eye. See also **strabismus.**

Sr Symbol for **strontium.**

ss *abbr* **steady state.**

SSSS *abbr* **staphylococcal scalded skin syndrome.**

S's test See **Sulkowitch's test.**

stab form See **band.**

-stabile A combining form meaning 'stable, resistant to change': *coctostabile, hydrostabile, tempostabile.*

stable element A nonradioactive element, one not subject to spontaneous nuclear degeneration. Some kinds of stable elements are calcium, iron, lead, potassium, and sodium. Compare **radioactive element.** See also **element.**

staccato speech Abnormal speech in which pauses between words break phrase or sentence rhythm. The condition is sometimes associated with multiple sclerosis.

stadium, *pl.* **stadia** A stage in a fever or illness, as the prodromal stage of a viral infection.

staff **1.** The people who work toward a common goal and are employed or supervised by someone of higher rank, as the nurses in a hospital. **2.** A designation by which a staff nurse is distinguished from a head nurse or other nurse. **3.** In nursing education: the nonprofessional employees of the institution, as librarians, technicians, secretaries, and clerks. **4.** In nursing service administration: the units of the organization that provide service to the 'line,' or administratively defined hierarchy, as the personnel office is 'staff' to the director of nursing and the nursing service administration.

staff development In nursing: a process that assists individual nurses in attaining new skills and knowledge, gaining increasing levels of competence, and growing professionally. Various resources outside the agency employing the nurse may be used. The process may include such programs as orientation, in-service education, and continuing education.

staffing pattern In hospital or nursing administration: the number and kinds of staff assigned to the particular units and departments of a hospital. Staffing patterns vary with the unit, department, and shift.

staff of Æsculapius A staff carried by Æsculapius, the Greek god of medicine. It is used as the traditional symbol of the physician. A single serpent entwines the staff, which is often confused with the caduceus, a staff with two serpents, symbolizing the U.S. Army Medical Corps.

staff position In management theory: a position outside an institution's hierarchy of authority, such as clinical specialist or consultant, counselor, or in-service training or patient education director, as opposed to a line position. A staff person provides a specific service or product and usually reports directly to the administrator or a line supervisor.

-stage A combining form meaning a '(specified) phase': *aecidiostage, multistage, uredostage.*

stages of anesthesia See **Guedel's signs.**

stages of dying The five emotional and behavioral stages that often occur after a person first learns of approaching death. The stages, identified and described by Elisabeth Kübler-Ross, are denial and isolation, anger, bargaining, depression, and acceptance. The stages may occur in sequence or they may recur, as the person moves forward and backward; especially between denial, anger, and bargaining. See ac-

ceptance, anger, bargaining, denial and isolation, depression. See also **hospice.**

staging **1.** The classification of a disease, organism, or biological process into distinct developmental periods or phases. **2.** The classification of neoplasms according to tumor size, nodal involvement, and metastatic progress. See also **TNM.** **3.** The determination of the current developmental phase of a progressive disease or malignant tumor. See also **cancer staging.**

stain **1.** A pigment, dye, or substance used to impart color to microscopic objects or tissues to facilitate examination and identification. Kinds of stains include **acid-fast stain, Gram's stain, Wright's stain.** **2.** To apply pigment to a substance or tissue to examine it under a microscope. **3.** An area of discoloration.

-stalsis A combining form meaning a 'contraction in the alimentary canal': *antistalsis, catastalsis, retrostalsis.*

stance phase of gait The first phase of the normal gait cycle that begins with the strike of the heel on the ground and ends with the lift of the toe at the beginning of the swing phase of gait; the brief period in which both feet are on the ground.

standard **1.** An evaluation that serves as a basis for comparison for evaluating similar phenomena or substances, as a standard for the practice of a profession. **2.** A pharmaceutical preparation or a chemical substance of known quantity, ingredients, and strength that is used to determine the constituents or the strength of another preparation. **3.** Of known value, strength, quality, or ingredients. —**standardize,** *v.,* **standardization,** *n.*

standard death certificate A form for a death certificate commonly used throughout the United States. It is the preferred form of the United States Census Bureau.

standard deviation In statistics: a mathematical statement of the dispersion of a set of values or scores from the mean. Each sample value is subtracted from the sample mean and squared, and the squares are summed. The square root of the summed squares gives a mathematically standardized value so that sample deviations can be compared.

standard environmental chamber See **Skinner box.**

standard error In statistics: the variability in scores that can be expected if measurements are made on random samples of the same size from the same universe of population, phenomena, or observations. The standard error provides a framework within which a determination of the difference between groups may be made. It is an element used in determining statistical significance by means of a wide variety of formulas and methods.

standardized death rate The number of deaths per 1,000 people of a specified population during 1 year. This rate is adjusted, using a standard population, to avoid distortion by the age composition of the specified group. Also called **adjusted death rate.**

STAPES

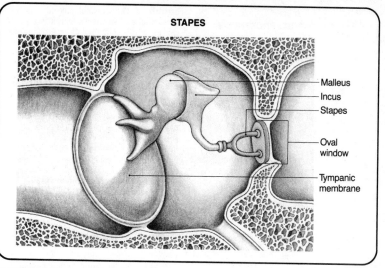

- Malleus
- Incus
- Stapes
- Oval window
- Tympanic membrane

standing orders A written document containing rules, policies, procedures, regulations, and orders for the conduct of patient care in various stipulated clinical situations. The standing orders are usually formulated collectively by the professional members of a department in a hospital or other health-care facility.

stann- A combining form meaning 'of or pertaining to tin': *stanniferous, stanniform.*

stanozolol An anabolic steroid.

stapedectomy Removal of the stapes of the middle ear and insertion of a graft and prosthesis, performed to restore hearing in the treatment of otosclerosis. The stapes, which has become fixed, is replaced so vibrations transmit sound waves through the oval window to the fluid of the inner ear. Under local anesthesia, the stapes is removed and the opening into the inner ear is covered with a graft of body tissue. Headache and dizziness are expected early in the postoperative period. Possible complications include infection of the outer, middle, or inner ear; displacement or rejection of the graft or the prosthesis; and leaking of perilymph around the prosthesis into the middle ear, with ringing in the ear and dizziness. Compare **incudectomy.**

stapes One of the three ossicles in the middle ear, resembling a tiny stirrup. It transmits sound vibrations from the incus to the internal ear. Compare **incus, malleus.** See also **middle ear.**

staphylo-, staphyl- A combining form meaning 'resembling a bunch of grapes,' used especially to show relationship to the uvula: *staphyloangina, staphylococcide.*

staphylococcal infection An infection caused by a pathogenic species of *Staphylococcus,* commonly characterized by the formation of abscesses of the skin or other organs. Staphylococcal infections of the skin include carbuncles, folliculitis, furuncles, and hidradenitis suppurativa. Bacteremia is common and may

result in endocarditis, meningitis, or osteomyelitis. Staphylococcal pneumonia often follows influenza or other viral disease and may be associated with chronic or debilitating illness. Acute gastroenteritis may result from an enterotoxin produced by certain species of staphylococci in contaminated food. Treatment usually includes bed rest, analgesics, and an antimicrobial drug that is resistant to penicillinase, an enzyme secreted by many species of *Staphylococcus.* Surgical drainage, especially of deep abscesses, is often necessary.

staphylococcal scalded skin syndrome (SSSS) An abnormal skin condition, characterized by epidermal erythema, peeling, and necrosis, that gives the skin a scalded appearance. This disorder primarily affects infants 1 to 3 months old and children, but it may also affect adults. It is caused by strains of *Staphylococcus aureus,* especially phage type 71. Deficient immune functions and renal insufficiency may be predisposing factors. SSSS is more common in the neonate because of undeveloped immunity and renal systems. A prodromal upper respiratory tract infection with concomitant purulent conjunctivitis is commonly associated with SSSS. Epidermal complications develop in the erythemal stage, the exfoliation stage, and the desquamation stage. Erythema often spreads around the mouth and other orifices and may extend over the entire body in wide circles as the skin becomes tender and the superficial layer of the skin sloughs from friction. The exfoliation stage follows the erythema stage by 24 to 48 hours and is commonly manifested by slight crusting and erosion, which may spread from around the orifices to wider skin areas. The desquamation stage of SSSS, following the exfoliation stage, is characterized by the drying up of affected areas and the formation of powdery scales. Normal skin replaces the scales within

STARR-EDWARDS PROSTHESIS

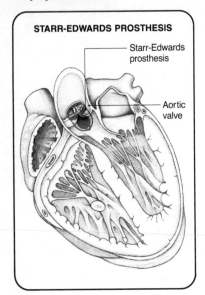

Starr-Edwards prosthesis

Aortic valve

5 to 7 days. Diagnosis is based on close observation of the development of SSSS through its three characteristic stages. Confirming diagnosis is usually made by isolating Group 2 *Staphylococcus aureus* in cultures of skin lesions. The mortality in SSSS is 2% to 3%, death usually being caused by complications of fluid and electrolyte loss, sepsis, and involvement of other body systems.

NURSING CONSIDERATIONS: Treatment of SSSS commonly includes the administration of systemic antibiotics to prevent secondary infections and the replacement of body fluids to maintain fluid and electrolyte balance. Nursing care includes monitoring vital signs to check for sepsis, maintaining skin integrity using strict aseptic technique, and giving warm baths and soaks to aid healing. Special care for the neonate may include maintaining body temperature by using an incubator.

Staphylococcus A genus of nonmotile, spherical, gram-positive bacteria. Some species are normally found on the skin and in the throat; certain species cause severe, purulent infections or produce an enterotoxin, which may cause nausea, vomiting, and diarrhea. Life-threatening staphylococcal infections may arise in hospitals. *Staphylococcus aureus* is a species frequently responsible for abscesses, endocarditis, impetigo, osteomyelitis, pneumonia, and septicemia. *S. epidermidis,* formerly called *S. albus,* occasionally causes endocarditis in the presence of intracardiac prostheses. See also **staphylococcal infection. —staphylococcal,** *adj.*

staphylokinase An enzyme, produced by certain strains of staphylococci, that catalyzes the conversion of plasminogen to plasmin in various animal hosts of the microorganism.

starch 1. The principal molecule used for the storage of food in plants. Starch is a polysaccharide and is composed of long chains of glucose subunits. In animals, excess glucose is stored as glycogen. The molecular structure of glycogen is similar to that of starch. **2.** A demulcent. See also **carbohydrate, glucose, glycogen.**

Starr-Edwards prosthesis An artificial cardiac valve. A caged-ball form of device, it obstructs the valve opening, preventing the backward flow of blood. See also **prosthesis.**

start codon See **initiation codon.**

startle reflex See **Moro reflex.**

start point In molecular genetics: the initial nucleotide transcribed from the DNA template in the formation of messenger RNA.

starvation 1. A condition resulting from prolonged deficiency of essential nutrients and characterized by multiple physiologic and metabolic dysfunctions. **2.** The act or state of starving or being starved. See also **malnutrition.**

stas- A combining form meaning 'stopped, or related to standing or walking': *stasibasiphobia, stasidynic, stasis.*

-stasia A combining form meaning: **1.** A '(specified) condition involving the ability to stand': *astasia, dysstasia.* **2.** A '(condition of) stoppage or inhibition': *hemostasia, menostasia.* Also **-stasis.**

stasis 1. A disorder in which the normal flow of a fluid through a vessel of the body is slowed or halted. **2.** Stillness.

-stasis A combining form meaning a 'stoppage': *enterostasis, mecystasis, proctostasis.*

stasis dermatitis A common result of venous insufficiency of the legs beginning with ankle edema and progressing to tan pigmentation, patchy erythema, petechiae, and induration. Ultimately, there may be atrophy and fibrosis of the skin and subcutaneous tissue, with ulcerations that are slow to heal. The tan pigment is hemosiderin from blood leaking through capillary walls under elevated venous pressure. The involved skin is easily irritated or sensitized to topical medications. The dermatitis is often treated by bed rest, Burow's solution for oozing lesions, antibiotics for infection, and corticosteroids to reduce inflammation. Also called venous stasis dermatitis. See also **stasis ulcer.**

stasis ulcer A necrotic, craterlike skin lesion of the lower leg owing to chronic venous congestion. The ulcer is often associated with stasis dermatitis and varicose veins. Healing is slow. Bed rest, elevation, and pressure bandages are usually ordered and appropriate antibiotics, Burow's solution compresses, Unna's paste boot, pinch grafts, and surgery to improve venous flow are useful in treatment. Also called **varicose ulcer.** See also **stasis dermatitis.**

-stat A combining form meaning: **1.** A 'device for keeping stationary': *catheterostat, ophthalmostat.* **2.** An 'instrument for the regulation of' something specified: *hemostat, rheostat.* **3.** An 'apparatus for the reflection of in one direction of' something specified: *siderostat.* **4.** A 'device for studying in a state of rest': *hydrostat, mi-*

crostat. **5.** An 'agent for stopping the growth of': *bacteriostat, fungistat.*

-state A combining form meaning the 'result of a (specified) process': *anastate, catastate, mesostate.*

State Board Test Pool Examination An examination prepared by the National Council of State Boards of Nursing for testing the competency of a person to perform as a newly licensed registered nurse. Each jurisdiction within the United States and its territories regulates entry into the nursing practice; each requires the candidate to pass the examination. The content is planned to test the candidates' knowledge of the nursing process as applied to the broad areas of nursing practice, including maternal and child health, medical and surgical nursing, and psychiatric nursing. The process includes five steps: assessing, analyzing, planning, implementing, and evaluating. Knowledge, comprehension, application, and analysis of the nursing process are tested as they apply to decision-making situations.

state medicine *Informal.* See **socialized medicine.**

State Nurses' Association (SNA) An association of nurses at the state level. The various State Nurses' Associations are constituent units of the American Nurses' Association.

Statewide Health Coordinating Committee (SHCC) A component of the national network of Health Systems Agencies.

static Without motion, at rest, in equilibrium. Compare **dynamic.**

static imaging In nuclear medicine: a diagnostic procedure in which a radioactive substance is administered to a patient to visualize an internal organ or body compartment. An image or set of images is made of the fixed or slowly changing distribution of the radioactivity.

Statistical Package for the Social Sciences See **SPSS.**

station The level of the biparietal plane of the fetal head relative to the level of the ischial spines of the maternal pelvis. An imaginary plane at the level of the spines is designated 'zero station.' Higher and lower stations are numbered at intervals of 1 cm; minus above, plus below. In breech presentation, the bitrochanteric diameter of the breech is used to determine station. See also **dilatation, effacement, labor.**

statotonic reflex See **attitudinal reflex.**

status **1.** A specified state or condition, as emotional status. **2.** An unremitting state or condition, as status asthmaticus.

status asthmaticus An acute, severe, and prolonged asthma attack in which bronchospasm does not respond to oral medication. Hypoxia, cyanosis, and unconsciousness may follow. Treatment includes aminophylline given intravenously, controlled positive pressure ventilation, heavy sedation, frequent bronchial hygiene therapy, and emotional support. A bronchodilator may be given by aerosol inhalation from a ventilator.

status dysraphicus See **dysraphia.**

status epilepticus A medical emergency characterized by continual attacks of convulsive seizures occurring without intervals of consciousness. Unless convulsions are arrested, irreversible brain damage results. Status epilepticus can be precipitated by the sudden withdrawal of anticonvulsant drugs, inadequate body levels of glucose, a brain tumor, a head injury, a high fever, or by poisoning. Therapy includes intravenous administration of anticonvulsant drugs, nutrients, and electrolytes, preferably given in an intensive care unit. An adequate airway is usually maintained with an oral pharyngeal or endotracheal tube.

statute of limitations In law: a statute that sets a limit of time during which a suit may be brought or criminal charges may be made. In a malpractice suit, dispute may arise as to whether the time set by the particular statute of limitations begins to run at the time of the injury or at the time of the discovery of the injury.

statutory rape In law: sexual intercourse with a female below the age of consent, which varies from state to state. See also **rape.**

steady state (SS) A basic physiologic concept implying that the various forces and processes of life are in a state of homeostasis. Living organisms are in constant flux, working to balance the internal and external environments in an effort to avoid a deficiency or an excess that might cause illness. Steady state is a complete state of well-being involving total adaptation.

-stearic A combining form meaning '(specified) fat or fat derivatives': *aleostearic, ketostearic.*

Stearns' alcoholic amentia A form of insanity caused by alcohol and characterized by an emotional disturbance less severe than that of delirium tremens but of longer duration and with greater mental clouding and amnesia.

stearo-, steap-, stear-, steato- A combining form meaning 'of or pertaining to fat': *stearoconotum, stearodermia.*

stearyl alcohol A solid substance, prepared by the catalytic hydrogenation of stearic acid, used in various ointments.

steatorrhea Greater than normal amounts of fat in the feces, characterized by frothy, foul-smelling fecal matter that floats, as in celiac disease, some malabsorption syndromes, and any condition in which fats are poorly absorbed by the small intestine.

Steele-Richardson-Olszewski syndrome A rare, progressive, neurologic disorder of unknown etiology, occurring in middle age, more often in men. It is characterized by paralysis of eye muscles, ataxia, neck and trunk rigidity, pseudobulbar palsy, and parkinsonian facies. Dementia and inappropriate emotional responses are also common. Treatment usually includes the antiparkinsonian drug levodopa for control of extrapyramidal symptoms. See also **Parkinson's disease.**

steeple head See **oxycephaly.**

Steimart's disease See **myotonic muscular dystrophy.**

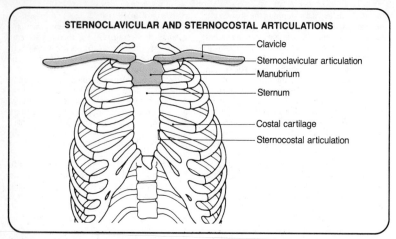

STERNOCLAVICULAR AND STERNOCOSTAL ARTICULATIONS

Clavicle
Sternoclavicular articulation
Manubrium
Sternum
Costal cartilage
Sternocostal articulation

stell- A combining form meaning 'of or pertaining to a star': *stellate, stellectomy.*

stellate Star-shaped or arranged in the pattern of a star.

stellate fracture A fracture that involves the central point of impact or injury and radiates numerous fissures throughout surrounding bone tissue.

stem cell leukemia A malignant neoplasm of blood-forming organs in which the predominant neoplastic cell is too immature to classify. The disease is extremely acute and has a rapid, relentless course. Also called **embryonal leukemia, hemoblastic leukemia, hemocytoblastic leukemia, lymphoidocytic leukemia, undifferentiated cell leukemia.**

stem cell lymphoma See **undifferentiated malignant lymphoma.**

steno- A combining form meaning 'contracted or narrow': *stenobregmate, stenocephaly.*

stenosis An abnormal condition characterized by the constriction of an opening or passageway. Kinds of stenosis include **aortic stenosis, pyloric stenosis.** —**stenotic,** *adj.*

Stensen's duct See **parotid duct.**

stent 1. A compound used in making dental impressions and medical molds. 2. A mold or device made of stent, used in anchoring skin grafts and for supporting body openings and cavities during grafting, or vessels and tubes of the body during surgical anastomosis.

step reflex See **dance reflex.**

sterco- A combining form meaning 'of or pertaining to feces': *stercobilin, stercolith.*

stereo- A combining form meaning 'solid, three-dimensional, or firmly established': *stereoblastula, stereograph.*

stereognostic perception The ability to recognize objects by the sense of touch.

stereoscopic microscope A microscope that produces an object with a three-dimensional appearance through the use of a double optical system with independent light paths. Also

called **Greenough microscope.**

stereoscopic parallax See **binocular parallax.**

stereotypy The persistent, inappropriate, mechanical repetition of actions, body postures, or speech patterns, usually occurring without variation in thought processes or ideas. It is often seen in schizophrenia. —**stereotypical,** *adj.*

sterile 1. Barren; unable to produce children owing to a physical abnormality, often the absence of spermatogenesis in a man or blockage of the fallopian tubes in a woman. Compare **impotence.** 2. Free from living microorganisms. —**sterility,** *n.*

sterilization 1. A process or act that renders a person unable to produce children. See also **hysterectomy, tubal ligation, vasectomy.** 2. A technique for destroying microorganisms using heat, water, chemicals, radiation, or gases. —**sterilize,** *v.*

-sternal A combining form meaning 'pertaining to the sternum': *adsternal, presternal.*

sternal node A node in one of the three groups of thoracic parietal lymph nodes. They are situated at the anterior ends of the intercostal spaces, adjacent to the internal thoracic artery. Also called **internal mammary node.** Compare **diaphragmatic node, intercostal node.** See also **lymphatic system, lymph node.**

-sternia A combining form meaning '(condition of the) sternum': *asternia, koilosternia.*

sterno- A combining form meaning 'of or pertaining to the sternum': *sternocleidal, sternocostal.*

sternoclavicular articulation The double gliding joint between the sternum and the clavicle. It involves the sternal end of the clavicle, the superior and lateral part of the manubrium, the cartilage of the first rib, and six ligaments.

sternocostal articulation The gliding articulation of the cartilage of each true rib and the sternum, except for the articulation of the first rib in which the cartilage is directly united with the sternum to form a synchondrosis. Each sternocostal articulation also involves five ligaments.

sternohyoideus One of the four infrahyoid muscles. Arising from the medial end of the clavicle, the posterior sternoclavicular ligament, and the manubrium sterni and inserting into the inferior border of the hyoid bone, it is a thin, narrow muscle innervated by fibers from the first, second, and third cervical nerves. It acts to depress the hyoid bone. Also called sternohyoid muscle. Compare **sternothyroideus.**

sternothyroideus One of the four infrahyoid muscles. Arising from the dorsal surface of the manubrium sterni and inserting into the thyroid cartilage, it is innervated by fibers from the first, second, and third cervical nerves and it acts to depress the thyroid cartilage. Also called **sternothyroid muscle.** Compare **sternohyoideus.**

sternothyroid muscle See **sternothyroideus.**

sternum The elongated, flattened bone forming the middle portion of the thorax. It supports the clavicles, articulates with the first seven pairs of ribs, and comprises the manubrium, the gladiolus, and the xiphoid process. It is composed of highly vascular tissue covered by a thin layer of bone. The sternum is longer in men than in women.

sternutation See **sneeze.**

sterognosis 1. The faculty of perceiving and understanding the form and nature of objects by touch. 2. Perception by the senses of the solidity of objects. —**sterognostic,** *adj.*

stertorous Having a snoring sound.

stetho-, steth- A combining form meaning 'of or pertaining to the chest': *stethometer, stethomyitis, stethospasm.*

stethoscope An instrument, used in mediate auscultation, consisting of two earpieces connected by means of flexible tubing to a diaphragm, which is placed against the skin of the patient's chest or back.

Stevens-Johnson syndrome A serious, sometimes fatal inflammatory disease affecting children and young adults. It is characterized by the acute onset of fever, bullae on the skin, and ulcers on the mucous membranes of the lips, eyes, mouth, nasal passage, and genitalia. Pneumonia, pain in the joints, and prostration are common. It may be an allergic reaction to some drugs, or it may follow pregnancy, herpesvirus I, or other infection. Treatment includes bed rest, antibiotics for pneumonia, glucocorticoids, analgesics, mouthwashes, and sedatives.

-sthenia A combining form meaning 'power or strength': *angiosthenia, eusthenia.*

sthenic fever High body temperature associated with thirst, dry skin, and, often, delirium.

stheno-, sthen- A combining form meaning 'of or pertaining to strength': *sthenometer, sthenoplastic.*

-sthenuria A combining form meaning '(condition of) urination or of the specific gravity of urine': *hypersthenuria, isosthenuria.*

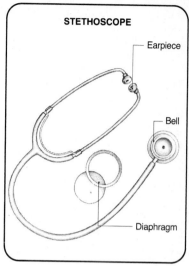

STETHOSCOPE

Earpiece

Bell

Diaphragm

stib- A combining form meaning 'of or pertaining to antimony': *stibamine, stibophen.*

-stichia A combining form meaning a 'condition involving rows of eyelashes': *distichia, tristichia.*

sticky ends See **cohesive termini.**

Stieda's fracture A fracture of the internal condyle of the femur.

stiff lung See **adult respiratory distress syndrome.**

stigma, *pl.* **stigmata** 1. A moral or physical blemish. 2. A physical characteristic that identifies a disease or a condition.

stilet, stilette See **stylet.**

stilbestrol See **diethylstilbestrol.**

stillbirth 1. The birth of a fetus that died before or during delivery. 2. A fetus, born dead, that weighs more than 1,000 gm (2 lb, 3 oz) and would usually have been expected to live.

stillborn 1. An infant that was born dead. 2. Of or pertaining to an infant that was born dead.

Still's disease A form of rheumatoid arthritis, usually affecting the larger joints of children under age 16. As bone growth in children depends on the epiphyseal plates of the distal epiphyses, skeletal development may be impaired. Treatment includes analgesia, anti-inflammatory medication, and rest. The recovery rate in this juvenile form is better than in the adult forms of rheumatoid arthritis. Also called **juvenile rheumatoid arthritis.**

stimulant cathartic A cathartic that promotes bowel motility, especially the longitudinal peristalsis of the colon. Kinds of stimulant cathartics are **cascara sagrada, senna.**

stimulating bath A bath taken in water that contains an aromatic substance, an astringent, or a tonic.

stimulus, *pl.* **stimuli** Anything that excites or incites an organism or part to function, be-

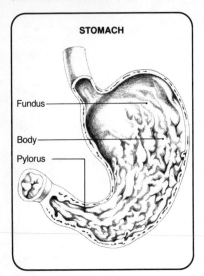

STOMACH

Fundus

Body

Pylorus

come active, or respond. **—stimulate,** *v.*

stimulus duration The length of time a stimulus must be applied for the resulting nerve impulse to produce excitation in the receptor tissue. In general, more intense stimuli require shorter excitation times to effect cellular response.

sting An injury caused by a sharp, painful penetration of the skin, often accompanied by exposure to an irritating chemical or animal venom. In cases of hypersensitivity, a highly venomous sting, or multiple stings, anaphylactic shock may occur. Kinds of stings include **bee sting, jellyfish sting, scorpion sting, sea urchin sting.** See also **stingray, wasp.**

stingray A flat, long-tailed fish bearing barbed spines connected to sacs of venom. Spasm of the skeletal muscles, severe local pain, seizures, and dyspnea may occur if the skin is broken by the spines. See also **sea urchin sting.**

St. Louis encephalitis An arbovirus brain infection transmitted from birds to man by the bite of an infected mosquito. Most common in the central and southern United States, it is characterized by headache, malaise, fever, stiff neck, delirium, and convulsions. Sequelae may include visual and speech disturbances, difficulty in walking, and personality changes. Convalescence may be prolonged, and death may result. Compare **California encephalitis, equine encephalitis.** See also **encephalitis.**

stoker's cramp See **heat cramp.**

Stokes-Adams syndrome See **Adams-Stokes syndrome.**

-stole A combining form the meaning 'contraction, retraction, or dilatation of various organs': *anastole, diastole.*

stoma, *pl.* **stomas, stomata 1.** A pore, orifice, or opening on a surface. **2.** An artificial opening of an internal organ on the surface of the body, created surgically, as for a colostomy

or tracheostomy. **3.** A new opening created surgically between two body structures, as for a gastroenterostomy or pancreaticogastrostomy.

-stoma A combining form meaning a 'mouth': *hypostoma, metastoma, tetrastoma.*

stomach The major organ of digestion, located in the right upper quadrant of the abdomen and divided into the fundus, the body, and the pylorus. It receives and partially processes food and drink funneled from the mouth and esophagus and moves nutritional bulk into the intestines. The stomach lies in the epigastric and left hypogastric regions bounded by the anterior abdominal wall and the diaphragm between the liver and the spleen. The shape of the stomach is modified by the amount of contents, stage of digestion, development of gastric musculature, and condition of the intestines. It is lined with a mucous coat, a submucous coat, a muscular coat, and a serous coat, all richly supplied with blood vessels and nerves, and contains fundic, cardiac, and pyloric gastric glands. Also called **gaster.**

stomach pump A pump for withdrawing stomach contents through a tube passed through the mouth or nose into the stomach.

stomadeum See **stomodeum.**

stomal peptic ulcer A marginal peptic ulcer. See also **peptic ulcer.**

stomatitis Any inflammatory condition of the mouth. It may result from infection by bacteria, viruses, or fungi; from exposure to certain chemicals or drugs; from vitamin deficiency; or from a systemic inflammatory disease. Kinds of stomatitis include **aphthous stomatitis, pseudomembranous stomatitis, thrush, Vincent's infection.**

stomato-, stomo- A combining form meaning 'of or pertaining to the mouth': *stomatodysodia, stomatogastric.*

-stomia A combining form meaning '(condition of the) mouth': *atelostomia, atretostomia.*

stomodeum, stomodaeum, *pl.* **stomodeums, stomodea, stomodaeums, stomodaea, stomadeums, stomadea** An invagination in the ectoderm located in the foregut of the developing embryo that forms the mouth. Compare **proctodeum. —stomodeal, stomodaeal, stomadeal,** *adj.*

-stomy A combining form meaning 'surgical opening': *gastrostomy, lobostomy.*

stone See **calculus.**

-stone A combining form meaning a 'calculus in a human organ or duct': *bilestone, gallstone.*

stool See **feces.**

stool softener See **fecal softener.**

stop needle A needle with a shoulder flange that stops it from penetrating beyond a certain distance.

storing fermentation The rapid, gaseous clotting of milk caused by *Clostridium perfringens.*

stork bite See **telangiectatic nevus.**

STPD *abbr* standard temperature, standard pressure, dry.

strab- A combining form meaning 'squinting': *strabismometer, strabometry.*

strabismus An abnormal ocular condition in which each eye's optic axis is misaligned. In convergent strabismus, one eye turns toward the bridge of the nose; in divergent strabismus, one eye is turned away. These conditions may be sporadic or permanent. Paralytic convergent strabismus results from inability of the ocular muscles to move the eye owing to neurologic deficit or muscular dysfunction, which may be caused by tumor, infection, or injury to the brain or eye. Nonparalytic convergent strabismus is an inherited defect in the position of the two eyes in relation to each other. The person cannot use the two eyes together but has to fix with one or the other. The eye that looks straight at a given time is the fixing eye. Some people have alternating strabismus, using one eye and then the other; some have monocular strabismus affecting only one eye. Nonparalytic strabismus is treated most successfully in early childhood. Treatment consists mainly of covering the fixing eye, forcing the child to use the deviating eye. Other kinds of strabismus may be correctd by surgery or the use of prisms, or both. Also called **squint. —strabismal, strabismic, strabismical,** *adj.*

straight-line blood set A common device used for delivering blood infusions. It includes the plastic tubing, the clamp, the drip chamber, and the filter. Straight-line blood sets contain filters within the drip chamber. Compare **component drip set, component syringe set, microaggregate recipient set, Y-set.**

straight sinus One of the six posterior superior venous channels of the dura mater, which helps to drain blood from the brain into the internal jugular vein. It has no valves and is located at the junction of the falx cerebri with the tentorium cerebelli. Compare **inferior sagittal sinus, superior sagittal sinus, transverse sinus.**

strain **1.** To exert excessive physical force that may result in injury, usually muscular. **2.** To separate solids or particles from liquid with a filter or sieve. **3.** The damage, usually muscular, that results from excessive physical effort. **4.** A taxon that is a subgroup of a species. **5.** An emotional state reflecting mental pressure or fatigue.

straitjacket A coatlike garment of canvas with long sleeves that can be tied behind the wearer's back to prevent movement of the arms. It is used for restraining violent or uncontrollable people who might be a danger to themselves or to others.

strangulation The constriction of a tubular structure of the body, as the trachea, that impedes circulation or prevents function. See also **intestinal strangulation. —strangulate,** *v.,* **strangulated,** *adj.*

strapping The application of overlapping strips of adhesive tape to an extremity or body area to exert pressure and hold a structure in place, performed in the treatment of strains,

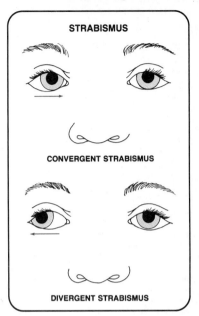

STRABISMUS

CONVERGENT STRABISMUS

DIVERGENT STRABISMUS

sprains, dislocations, and certain fractures.

strati- A combining form meaning 'layer': *stratification, stratiform.*

stratiform cartilage See **fibrocartilage.**

stratiform fibrocartilage A structure made of fibrocartilage that forms a thin coating of osseous grooves through which tendons of certain muscles glide. Small masses of stratified fibrocartilage also develop in the tendons of some muscles that glide over bones, as in the tendons of the peroneus longus and the tibialis posterior. Compare **circumferential fibrocartilage, connecting fibrocartilage, interarticular fibrocartilage.**

stratum, *pl.* **strata** A uniformly thick sheet or layer, usually associated with other layers, as the stratum basale and the stratum spinosum of the epidermis.

stratum basale One of the five layers of the epidermis, situated beneath the stratum spinosum. It consists of a single layer of columnar cells. In the stratum basale and the stratum spinosum, new cells are formed to replace the ones being worn away from the surface.

stratum corneum The horny, outermost layer of the skin, composed of dead cells converted to keratin that continually flakes away. The thickness of the layer is correlated with the normal wear of the area it covers. The stratum corneum is thick on the palms of the hands and the soles of the feet but thin over more protected areas. Also called **horny layer.** See also **skin.**

stratum germinativum See **stratum basale.**

stratum granulosum One of the five layers of the epidermis, situated just below the stratum corneum except in the palms and the soles, where

STRATA OF THE SKIN

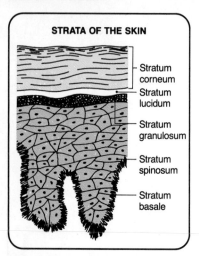

- Stratum corneum
- Stratum lucidum
- Stratum granulosum
- Stratum spinosum
- Stratum basale

it lies just under the stratum lucidum. The stratum granulosum contains visible granules in the cytoplasm of its cells, which die, become keratinized, move to the surface, and flake away. See also **skin.**

stratum lucidum One of the five layers of the epidermis, situated just beneath the stratum corneum and present only in the thick skin of the palms and the soles. It contains translucent eleidin which forms keratin. See also **skin.**

stratum spinosum One of the five layers of the epidermis, composed of several layers of polygonal cells. It lies on top of the stratum basale and beneath the stratum granulosum and contains tiny fibrils within its cellular cytoplasm. When the cells of the stratum spinosum are pulled apart, they present minute spines at their surfaces. Also called **prickle cell layer.** See also **skin.**

stratum spongiosum One of the three layers of the endometrium of the uterus, containing tortuous, dilated uterine glands and a small amount of interglandular tissue. With the stratum compactum, it forms the functional part of the endometrium during pregnancy. Compare **stratum basale.** See also **decidua, placenta.**

strawberry gallbladder A tiny, yellow gallbladder spotted with deposits on the red mucous membrane, typical of cholesterolosis.

strawberry hemangioma See **capillary hemangioma.** Also called **hemangioma simplex.**

strawberry mark See **capillary hemangioma.**

streak A line or a stripe, as the primitive streak at the caudal end of the embryonic disk.

strepho-, streph- A combining form meaning 'twisted': *strephopodia, strephosymbolia.*

strep throat *Informal.* An infection of the oral pharynx and tonsils caused by a hemolytic species of *Streptococcus,* usually belonging to group A. The infection is characterized by sore throat, chills, fever, swollen lymph nodes in the

neck, and, sometimes, by nausea and vomiting. The symptoms usually begin abruptly a few days after exposure to the organism in airborne droplets or after direct contact with an infected person. The throat is diffusely red and tonsils often are covered with a yellow or white exudate. Diagnosis is confirmed by bacteriologic culture and identification of the streptococcal bacteria in a specimen taken from the throat. Complications of strep throat are otitis media, scarlet fever, and sinusitis; other complications include acute glomerulonephritis and acute rheumatic fever. Treatment usually includes intramuscular injection of benzathine penicillin G or the administration of penicillin for 10 days. Erythromycin may be given to people allergic to penicillin. For recurrent infections, tonsillectomy may be recommended. Analgesics and throat irrigation with warm saline solution may give relief from pain. Also called **streptococcal sore throat.**

strepto- A combining form meaning 'twisted': *streptobacilli, streptococcal.*

streptobacillary rat-bite fever See **Haverhill fever.**

Streptobacillus A genus of necklace-shaped bacteria that can cause rat-bite fever in humans.

streptococcal infection An infection caused by pathogenic bacteria of one of several species of the genus *Streptococcus* or their toxins. Almost any organ of the body may be involved. The infections occur in many forms including cellulitis, endocarditis, erysipelas, impetigo, meningitis, pneumonia, scarlet fever, tonsillitis, and urinary tract infection. See also **strep throat.**

Streptococcus A genus of nonmotile, gram-positive cocci classified by serologic types (Lancefield groups A through T), by hemolytic action (alpha, beta, gamma) when grown on blood agar, and by reaction to bacterial viruses (phage types 1 to 86). Many species cause disease in humans. *Streptococcus fecalis,* a penicillin-resistant, Group D enterococcus and normal inhabitant of the gastrointestinal tract, may cause infection of the urinary tract or endocardium. *S. pneumoniae* (formerly, *Diplococcus pneumoniae*) causes 90% of the cases of bacterial pneumonia in the United States. *S. pyogenes* belongs to group A and may cause tonsillitis or respiratory, urinary, or skin infections. Some beta-hemolytic strains may lead to rheumatic fever or to glomerulonephritis. *S. viridans,* a member of the normal flora of the mouth, is the most common cause of bacterial endocarditis, especially when introduced into the bloodstream during dental procedures.

streptokinase An enzyme, produced by streptococci, that catalyzes the conversion of plasminogen to plasmin in various animal hosts of the microorganism.

streptolysin A filterable substance, produced by various streptococci, that liberates hemoglobin from red blood cells.

streptomycin sulfate An aminoglycoside antibiotic and antitubercular agent.

streptozocin An alkylating agent and chemotherapy drug.

stress Any emotional, physical, social, economic, or other factor that requires a response or change, as dehydration, which can cause an increase in body temperature, or a separation from parents, which can cause a young child to cry. Stress may also be applied therapeutically to promote change, as implosion therapy for phobic patients, in which the patient is given support while being exposed to the situation that produces anxiety and is thereby gradually desensitized. The nature and degree of stress are frequently evaluated by the nurse as part of her ongoing holistic nursing assessment.

stress fracture A fracture, especially of one or more of the metatarsal bones, caused by repeated, prolonged, or abnormal stress.

stress reaction 1. See **general adaptation syndrome.** 2. See **post-traumatic stress disorder.**

stress response syndrome See **post-traumatic stress disorder.**

stress test A test that measures the function of a body system when subjected to carefully controlled amounts of stress. The data produced allow evaluation of the condition of the body system. Cardiopulmonary function, respiratory function, and intrauterine fetal-placental function are tested with stress tests. See also **exercise electrocardiogram, oxytocin challenge test.**

stress ulcer A gastric or duodenal ulcer that develops in previously unaffected individuals subjected to severe stress, as when severely burned. See also **Curling's ulcer.**

stri- A combining form meaning 'line or streak': *striation, striocellular, striomuscular.*

stria, *pl.* **striae** A streak or a linear scar, often resulting from rapidly developing skin tension, as seen on the abdomen after pregnancy. Purplish striae are one of the classical findings in hyperadrenocorticism. Also called **stretch mark.**

striated muscle One of two kinds of muscle, including all the skeletal muscles. Striated muscles are composed of bundles of parallel, striated fibers under voluntary control; the heart, a striated involuntary muscle, is an exception. Each striated muscle is covered by a thin connective epimysium and divided into bundles of sheathed fibers containing smaller myofibrils. Also called **skeletal muscle, voluntary muscle.** Compare **cardiac muscle, smooth muscle.**

stricture An abnormal narrowing of the lumen of a hollow organ, as the esophagus, ureter, or urethra, owing to inflammation, external pressure, or scarring. Treatment varies depending on the cause. Compare **spasm.**

strict vegetarian A vegetarian whose diet excludes the use of all foods of animal origin. Such diets, unless adequately planned, may be deficient in many essential nutrients. Also called **pure vegetarian, vegan.**

stridor An abnormal, high-pitched, musical respiratory sound, caused by an obstruction in

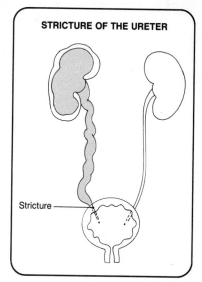

STRICTURE OF THE URETER

Stricture

the trachea or larynx. It is usually heard during inspiration. Stridor may indicate several neoplastic or inflammatory conditions. Compare **pleuropericardial rub, rale, rhonchi, wheeze.**

string carcinoma A malignancy of the large intestine, usually of the ascending or transverse colon that, on radiologic visualization, causes the intestine to appear to be tied in segments like a string of large beads.

strip membranes In obstetrics: a procedure in which an examiner digitally frees the membranes of the amniotic sac from the wall of the lower segment of the uterus in the small area around the cervical os. It is done to stimulate labor, but, as infection or hemorrhage may result, it is not recommended.

stripping *Nontechnical.* A surgical procedure for the removal of the long and the short saphenous veins of the legs. See also **milking, varicose vein.**

stroke See **cerebrovascular accident.**

-stroke A combining form meaning a 'condition caused by or resembling an apoplectic stroke': *bloodstroke, lightstroke.*

stroke prone profile A predictive index using a complex of risk factors that indicate susceptibility of a person to cerebrovascular accident (CVA). The factors include age, hypertension, a history of transient ischemic attacks, cigarette smoking, heart disorders, associated embolism, family hisory of CVA, use of oral contraceptives, diabetes mellitus, physical inactivity, obesity, hypercholesteremia, and hyperlipidemia.

stroma- A combining form meaning 'a covering': *stromatin, stromatogenous.*

stroma, *pl.* **stromata** An organ's supporting tissue or the matrix as distinguished from its parenchyma, as the vitreous stroma, which encloses the vitreous humor of the eye, and Rol-

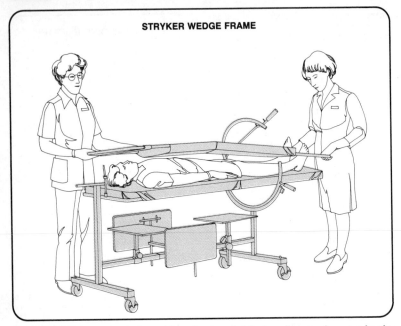

STRYKER WEDGE FRAME

let's stroma, which contains the hemoglobin of a red blood cell. **—stromatic,** *adj.*

-stroma A combining form meaning the 'supporting tissue of an organ': *blastostroma, mesostroma.*

Strongyloides A genus of parasitic intestinal nematode.

strongyloidiasis Infection of the small intestine by the roundworm *Strongyloides stercoralis,* acquired when larvae from the soil penetrate intact skin, incidentally causing a pruritic rash. The larvae pass to the lungs via the bloodstream, sometimes causing pneumonia. Larvae then migrate up the air passages to the pharynx, are swallowed, and develop into adult worms in the small intestine. Bloody diarrhea and intestinal malabsorption may result. Rarely, fatal disseminated strongyloidiasis occurs. Diagnosis depends on finding larvae in freshly passed feces. Treatment often includes administration of thiabendazole.

strontium (Sr) A metallic element. Its atomic number is 38; its atomic weight is 87.62. Chemically similar to calcium, it is found in bone tissue. Isotopes of strontium are used in radioisotope scanning procedures of bone. Strontium-85 (^{85}Sr) and strontium-87 (^{87}Sr) mimic calcium metabolism and are used in studies of bone physiology and disorders. Strontium-90, the longest lived, is the most dangerous constituent of nuclear fallout. It can replace some of the calcium in food, become concentrated in teeth and bones, and continue to emit electrons that can cause death in the host. Cows concentrate strontium-90 in their milk.

-strophe A combining form meaning 'turn-

ing or twisting': *cardianastrophe, enstrophe.* Also **-strophy.**

stropho- A combining form meaning 'twisted': *strophocephalus.*

-strophy A combining form meaning a 'twisting or turning': *dystrophy, exstrophy.* Also **-strophe.**

structural chemistry The science dealing with the molecular structure of chemical substances.

structural gene In molecular genetics: a unit of genetic information that specifies the amino acid sequence of a polypeptide.

structural integration A technique of deep massage intended to help in body realignment by altering the length and tone of myofascial tissues. The basis of the practice is the belief that misalignment of myofascial tissues, caused by improper posture and emotional and physical traumas, may have an overall detrimental effect on a person's energy level, self-image, muscular efficiency, perceptions, and general health. Also called **Rolfing.**

structure A part of the body, such as the heart, a bone, a gland, a cell, or a limb.

strum- A combining form meaning 'of or pertaining to a goiter, or to scrofula': *strumectomy.*

struma lymphomatosa See **Hashimoto's disease.**

Stryker wedge frame An orthopedic bed that allows the patient to be rotated as required to either the supine or prone position. Like the Foster bed, the Stryker wedge frame is used to immobilize patients with unstable spines, for postoperative management of multilevel spinal fusions, and to manage patients with severe burns.

Use of the Stryker wedge frame is not recommended if hyperextension of the spine is required or if lower extremity traction is needed. Most hospitals provide the nursing staff with charts to determine the elevation needed for countertraction according to the weight of the patient and the pull forces of traction weights. Compare **Foster bed, hyperextension bed.**

ST segment The component of the cardiac cycle shown on an electrocardiogram as a short, gradual upward curve following the spiked QRS complex, preceding the ascent of the T wave. It represents the interval between complete depolarization at the end of ventricular contraction and the beginning of repolarization.

Stuart-Power factor See **factor X.**

stump The part of a limb following amputation that is proximal to the portion amputated.

stump hallucination The sensation of the continued presence of an amputated limb. See also **hallucination, phantom limb syndrome.**

stupor A state of lethargy and unresponsiveness in which a person seems unaware of his surroundings. The condition occurs in neurologic as well as psychiatric disorders. Kinds of stupor are **anergic stupor, benign stupor, delusion stupor, epileptic stupor. —stuporous,** adj.

Sturge-Weber syndrome A congenital neurocutaneous disease marked by a port winecolored capillary hemangioma over a sensory dermatome of a branch of the trigeminal nerve of the face. X-ray of the skull reveals intracranial calcification. The cerebral cortex may atrophy, and generalized or focal seizures, angioma of the choroid, secondary glaucoma, optic atrophy, and new cutaneous hemangiomas may develop. There is no known cure. Treatment is supportive.

sty, stye A purulent infection of a Meibomian or sebaceous gland of the eyelid, often caused by a staphylococcal organism. Also called **hordeolum.**

-style A combining form meaning a 'bone attached to an internal structure': *cephalostyle, sarcostyle.*

stylet, stilet, stilette A thin, metal probe for inserting into or passing through a needle, tube, or catheter to clean the hollow bore, or for inserting in a soft, flexible catheter to make it shift as the catheter is placed in a vein or passed through an orifice of the body.

stylo- A combining form meaning 'like a stake or pole,' used especially to show relationship to the styloid process of the temporal bone: *stylomastoid, stylomyloid, stylostixis.*

stylohyoid bone See **stylohyoideus.**

stylohyoideus One of four suprahyoid muscles, lying anterior and superior to the posterior belly of the digastricus. It is a slender muscle that arises from the styloid process and inserts into the hyoid bone. It is pierced near its insertion by the tendon of the digastricus. It is innervated by fibers of the mandibular branch of the facial nerve, and it serves to draw the hyoid bone up and back. Also called **stylohyoid**

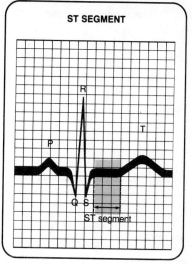

ST SEGMENT

bone. Compare **digastricus, geniohyoideus, mylohyoideus.**

stylohyoid ligament The ligament attached to the tip of the styloid process of the temporal bone and to the lesser cornu of the hyoid bone. It frequently contains a small cartilage in its center and is often partially ossified.

stylomandibular ligament One of a pair of specialized bands of cervical fascia, forming an accessory part of the temporomandibular joint. It extends from the styloid process of the temporal bone to the ramus of the mandible between the masseter and pterygoideus muscles and separates the parotid gland from the submandibular gland. Compare **sphenomandibular ligament.**

styptic 1. A substance used as an astringent, often to control bleeding. A chemical styptic induces blood coagulation. A cotton pledget used as a compress to control bleeding is a mechanical styptic. 2. Acting as an astringent or agent to control bleeding.

sub- A combining form meaning 'under, near, almost, or moderately': *subacid, subcapsular.* Also **suf-, sup-.**

subacromial bursa The bursa separating the acromion and deltoid muscle from the insertion of the supraspinatus muscle and the greater tubercle of the humerus.

subacute 1. Less than acute. 2. Of or pertaining to a disease or other abnormal condition present in a person who appears to be clinically well. The condition may be discovered by a laboratory test or X-ray.

subacute bacterial endocarditis (SBE) A chronic bacterial infection of the heart valves, characterized by a slow, quiet onset with fever, heart murmur, splenomegaly, and the development of clumps of abnormal tissue, called vegetations, around an intracardiac prosthesis or on the flaps of a valve. Various species of *Strep-*

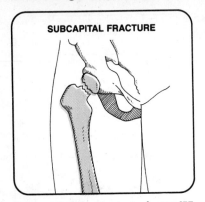

SUBCAPITAL FRACTURE

tococcus or *Staphylococcus* commonly cause SBE. Dental procedures are associated with infection by *Streptococcus viridans*, surgical procedures with *Streptococcus fecalis*, and self-infection (especially by drug abusers) with *Staphylococcus aureus*. The infected vegetations may separate from the valve or prosthesis and form emboli. Oster's nodes, petechiae, Roth's spots, and splinter hemorrhages under the fingernails are common manifestations of blood-borne metastases of these emboli. Bacteriologic examination of blood cultures may allow specific diagnosis and treatment. Treatment requires prolonged and regular administration of an effective antibiotic. During the acute phase of illness, the fever is treated with antipyretic medication and bed rest; adequate high-protein diet and fluids are encouraged. Sometimes bed rest and hospitalization may be necessary for several weeks. See also **endocarditis.**

subacute glomerulonephritis   An uncommon noninfectious disease of the renal glomerulus, characterized by proteinuria, hematuria, decreased urine production, and edema. Of unknown cause, the disease may progress rapidly, and renal failure may occur. Kidney transplantation and dialysis are the only treatments. See also **acute glomerulonephritis, chronic glomerulonephritis, uremia.**

subacute sclerosing panencephalitis An uncommon, slow-virus infection caused by the measles virus and characterized by diffuse inflammation of brain tissue, personality change, seizures, blindness, dementia, fever, and death. The condition occurs in children and in adolescents who have had measles at a very early age. No effective therapy is known. See also **slow virus.**

subacute thyroiditis   See **de Quervain's thyroiditis.**

subarachnoid   Situated under the arachnoid membrane and above the pia mater.

subarachnoid block anesthesia   A form of spinal anesthesia involving the injection of an anesthetic into the space between the arachnoidea and pia mater. This procedure is an especially effective form of rapid spinal anesthesia but one requiring great skill to avoid contamination or neurologic trauma. See also **obstetric anesthesia.**

subarachnoid hemorrhage (SaH, SAH) An intracranial hemorrhage into the cerebrospinal fluid-filled space between the arachnoid and pial membranes on the surface of the brain. The hemorrhage may extend into the brain if the force of the bleeding from the broken vessel is sudden and severe. The cause may be trauma, or rupture of a berry aneurysm or an arteriovenous anomaly. The first symptom of a subarachnoid hemorrhage is a sudden extremely severe headache that begins in one localized area and then spreads, becoming dull and throbbing. Other characteristics of subarachnoid hemorrhage include dizziness, rigidity of the neck, pupillary inequality, vomiting, drowsiness, sweating and chills, stupor, and loss of consciousness. A brief period of unconsciousness immediately following the rupture is common; severe hemorrhage may result in continued unconsciousness, coma, and death. Delirium and confusion often persist through the first weeks of recovery and permanent brain damage is not uncommon. Treatment has three basic goals: preservation of life, limitation of disability, and prevention of recurrence. Bed rest is recommended for as long as 4 to 6 weeks. Care for the person who is unconscious owing to a subarachnoid hemorrhage is the same as for the person who is unconscious from other neurologic causes: an airway is maintained, the bladder is emptied, and fluid and electrolyte balance is maintained. The patient who is conscious needs relief from pain, especially in the first days after hemorrhage. Surgical repair of a vessel or excision of an aneurysm may be performed if the patient is conscious, relatively young, healthy, and normotensive.

subcapital fracture   A fracture of tissue just distal to the head of a bone that pivots in a ball-and-socket joint, as the head of the femur.

subclavian   Situated under the clavicle.

subclavian artery   One of a pair of arteries that vary in origin, course, and the height to which they rise in the neck, having six similar main branches supplying the vertebral column, spinal cord, ear, and brain. See also **left subclavian artery, right subclavian artery.**

subclavian steal syndrome   A vascular syndrome caused by an occlusion in the subclavian artery proximal to the origin of the vertebral artery. The block results in a reversal of the normal blood pressure gradient in the vertebral artery and decreased blood flow distal to the occlusion. This condition is characterized by episodes of flaccid paralysis of the arm, pain in the mastoid and occipital areas, and a diminished or absent radial pulse on the involved side.

subclavian vein   The continuation of the axillary vein in the upper body, extending from the lateral border of the first rib to the sternal end of the clavicle, where it joins the internal jugular to form the brachiocephalic vein. It usually contains a pair of valves near its junction

SUBCUTANEOUS INJECTION SITES

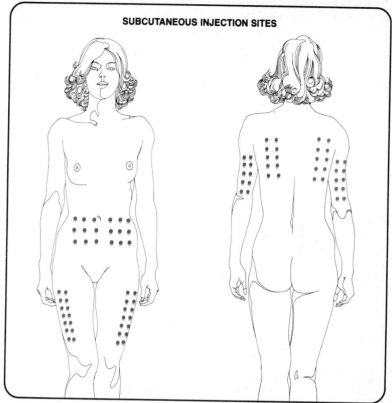

with the internal jugular vein. The subclavian vein receives deoxygenated blood from the external jugular vein and, on the left side, at the junction with the internal jugular vein, receives lymph from the thoracic duct. On the right side, at the corresponding junction, it receives lymph from the right lymphatic duct.

subclavius A short muscle of the chest wall. It is a small, cylindrical muscle between the clavicle and the first rib and arises in a short, thick tendon from the junction of the first rib and its cartilage. The subclavius is innervated by a special nerve from the lateral trunk of the brachial plexus, which contains fibers from the fifth and sixth cervical nerves, and it acts to draw the shoulder down and forward. Compare **pectoralis major, pectoralis minor, serratus anterior.**

subclinical Of or pertaining to a disease or abnormal condition that is so mild it produces no symptoms.

subconscious **1.** Imperfectly or partially conscious. **2.** In psychiatry: the preconscious and the unconscious. —**subconsciousness,** *n.*

subconscious memory A thought, sensation, or feeling that is not immediately available for recall to the conscious mind.

subcutaneous Beneath the skin.

subcutaneous fascia A continuous layer of connective tissue over the entire body between the skin and the deep fascial investment of the body's specialized structures. It consists of an outer, normally fatty layer and an inner, thin, elastic layer. Between the two layers lie superficial blood vessels, nerves, lymphatics, the mammary glands, most of the facial muscles, and the platysma. Compare **deep fascia, subserous fascia.**

subcutaneous fat necrosis See **adiponecrosis subcutanea neonatorum.**

subcutaneous infusion See **hypodermoclysis.**

subcutaneous injection An injection into the subcutaneous tissue beneath the skin, usually on the upper arm, thigh, or abdomen. A 24- or 25-gauge, ⅝-inch-long needle is used. If subcutaneous injections are repeated, each is performed at least 5 cm (2 inches) from the previous site. A diagram of a plan for the rotation of injection sites helps to avoid overuse of one area of skin.

subcutaneous mastectomy A surgical procedure in which all the breast tissue of one or both breasts is removed, leaving the skin, areola, and nipple intact. The adjacent lymph nodes and the pectoralis major and pectoralis

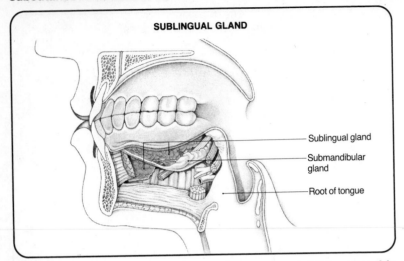

SUBLINGUAL GLAND

Sublingual gland

Submandibular gland

Root of tongue

minor are not removed. It may be performed on women who are at great risk of developing breast cancer. Reconstruction of the breasts is performed, with the assistance of a plastic surgeon, through the insertion of prostheses to restore the breasts' normal contour.

subcutaneous nodule   A small, solid boss, or node, beneath the skin that can be detected by touch. Subcutaneous nodules consisting chiefly of Aschoff bodies are found in patients with rheumatic fever. Minute subcutaneous nodules formed by the perivascular infiltration of mononuclear cells occur in typhus fever.

subdural   Situated under the dura mater and above the arachnoid membrane.

suberosis   See **cork worker's lung.**

subgerminal cavity   See **blastocoele.**

subinvolution   Delayed or absent involution of the uterus during the postpartum period. The causes of subinvolution include retained fragments of placenta, uterine fibromyomas, and infection. The condition is characterized by longer and heavier bleeding after childbirth and, on pelvic examination, a larger and softer uterus than would be expected at that time. Treatment includes ergonovine given by mouth for 2 or 3 days, and, if an infection is present, an antibiotic. The hemoglobin or hematocrit is also evaluated and iron is given if necessary.

subjective   **1.** Pertaining to the essential nature of an object as perceived in the mind rather than to the entity itself. **2.** Existing only in the mind. **3.** That which arises within or is perceived by the individual, such as pain, as contrasted with something that is modified by external circumstances or something that may be evaluated by objective standards. **4.** A person who places excessive importance on his own moods, attitudes, or opinions; egocentric.

subjective data collection   The process in which the patient describes his problem and the interviewer records the description. The in-

terviewer encourages a full description of the onset, the course, and the character of the problem and any factors that aggravate or ameliorate it. Compare **objective data collection.**

sublethal gene   A gene whose presence causes abnormalities or impairs the functioning of an organism but does not cause its death. Compare **lethal gene.**

subleukemic leukemia   A malignant neoplasm characterized by anemia, thrombocytopenia, and abnormally functioning leukocytes that infiltrate tissues but are not present in circulating blood in abnormal numbers. Also called **aleukemic leukemia, aleukocythemic leukemia, hypocytic leukemia, leukopenic leukemia.**

sublimate   To refine or divert instinctual impulses and energy from their immediate goal to one that can be expressed in a social, moral, or aesthetic manner acceptable to the person and to society.

sublimation   **1.** A defense mechanism by which an unacceptable instinctive drive is unconsciously diverted to and expressed through a personally approved, socially accepted means. **2.** In psychoanalysis: the process of diverting certain components of the sex drive to a socially acceptable, nonsexual goal. Compare **displacement.**

subliminal   Taking place below the threshold of sensory perception or outside the range of conscious awareness.

sublingual   Beneath the tongue.

sublingual administration of medication   The administration of a drug, usually in tablet form, by placing it beneath the tongue until the tablet dissolves.

sublingual duct   **1.** See **Bartholin's duct. 2.** See **duct of Rivinus.**

sublingual gland   One of a pair of small salivary glands situated under the mucous membrane of the floor of the mouth, beneath the tongue.

It is a narrow, almond-shaped structure. It is in relation, inferiorly, with the mylohyoideus; posteriorly, with the submandibular gland; laterally, with the mandible; and, medially, with the genioglossus, from which it is separated by the lingual nerve and the submandibular duct. It has from 8 to 20 ducts, some of which join to form the sublingual duct. The sublingual gland secretes mucus produced by its alveoli. Compare **parotid gland, submandibular gland.**

subluxation A partial dislocation.

submandibular duct A duct through which a submandibular gland secretes saliva. Also called **submaxillary duct.**

submandibular gland One of a pair of round, walnut-sized salivary glands in the submandibular triangle, reaching anteriorly to the anterior belly of the diagastricus and posteriorly to the stylomandibular ligament. The ligament lies between the submandibular gland and the parotid gland. The submandibular gland extends superiorly under the inferior border of the mandible and extends a deep process anteriorly above the mylohyoideus muscle. The gland secretes both mucus and a thinner serous fluid, which aid the digestive process. Compare **parotid gland, sublingual gland.** See also **salivary gland.**

submaxillary duct See **submandibular duct.**

submetacentric Pertaining to a chromosome in which the centromere is located approximately equidistant between the center and one end so that the arms of the chromatids are not equal in length. Compare **acrocentric, metacentric, telocentric.**

submucous Beneath a mucous membrane.

subperiosteal fracture A fracture in a bone beneath the periosteum that does not disrupt the periosteal covering.

subpoena In law: a document from a court commanding that a person appear at a certain time and place to testify on a specific matter.

subpoena duces tecum In law: a subpoena commanding a person to bring books, papers, records, or other items to the court.

subserous fascia One of three kinds of fascia, lying between the internal layer of deep fascia and the serous membranes lining the body cavities in much the same manner as the subcutaneous fascia lies between the skin and the deep fascia. Compare **deep fascia, subcutaneous fascia.**

subspecialty A professional and highly specialized field of practice, as nursing in dialysis, or neurology. Compare **specialty.**

substance P A neurotransmitting substance that is synthesized by the body and acts to stimulate vasodilation and contraction of intestinal and other smooth muscles. It also plays a part in salivary secretion, diuresis, and natriuresis, and it affects the function of the peripheral and central nervous systems.

substernal goiter An enlargement of the thyroid gland, a portion of which is beneath the sternum.

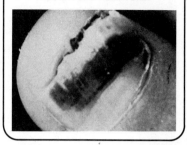

SUBUNGUAL HEMATOMA

subthalamus A portion of the diencephalon that serves as a correlations center for optic and vestibular impulses relayed to the globus pallidus. It is a transition zone between the thalamus and the tegmentum mesencephali, squeezed between the cerebral peduncle and the mammillary area. It accommodates prolongations of the red nucleus and the substantia nigra and contains fibrous masses of the fields of Forel. Compare **epithalamus, hypothalamus, metathalamus, thalamus.** —**subthalamic,** *adj.*

subtle Having a low intensity; not severe and having no serious sequelae, as a mild infection or inflammation.

subungual Under a fingernail or toenail.

subungual hematoma A collection of blood beneath a nail, usually resulting from trauma. The pain accompanying this condition may be quickly alleviated by burning or drilling a small hole through the nail to release the blood.

succ- A combining form meaning 'of or pertaining to a juice': *succagogue, succorrhea, succus.*

succinic acid A compound found in certain hydatid cysts and in lichens, amber, and fossils. Commercial succinic acid is used in lacquer and dyes. Succinic acid was formerly used to treat diabetic ketoacidosis.

succinylcholine chloride A depolarizing neuromuscular blocking agent.

succus, *pl.* **succi** A juice or fluid, usually one secreted by an organ of the gastrointestinal system.

succussion splash The sound elicited by shaking the body of an individual who has free fluid and air or gas in a hollow organ or body cavity. It may be present over a normal stomach and in hydropneumothorax, large hiatal hernia, or intestinal or pyloric obstruction.

suck **1.** To draw a liquid or semiliquid into the mouth by creating a partial vacuum through motions of the lips and tongue. **2.** To hold on the tongue and dissolve by the movements of the mouth and action of the saliva. **3.** To draw fluid into the mouth, specifically to draw milk from the breast or nursing bottle.

sucking blisters The pale, soft pads on an infant's upper and lower lips that look like blisters but are not. They form as soon as the infant begins to suck well. They seem to augment the

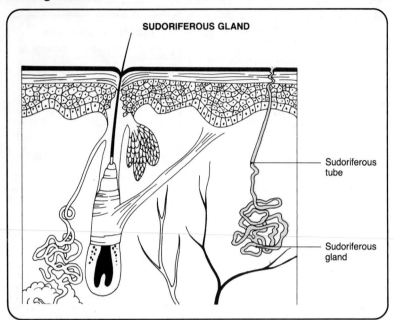

SUDORIFEROUS GLAND

Sudoriferous
tube

Sudoriferous
gland

seal of the lips around the nipple or breast. Some infants are born with them, having sucked on their own fingers, hand, or arm before birth.

sucking reflex Involuntary sucking movements of the circumoral area in newborns in response to stimulation. The reflex continues throughout infancy and often occurs without stimulation. Compare **rooting reflex.**

suckle **1.** To provide nourishment, specifically to breast-feed. **2.** To take in as nourishment, especially by breast-feeding.

suckling An infant who has not been weaned.

sucralfate A drug used to treat a duodenal ulcer by forming a local ulcer-adherent complex.

sucrose Sugar derived from sugar cane, sugar beets, and sorghum.

sucrose polyester (SPE) A synthetic, nonabsorbable fat that, when added to the diet, reduces plasma cholesterol levels by increasing the excretion of cholesterol in the feces. It is formulated to have the characteristic texture, taste, and consistency of regular margarine or vegetable oil and adds no calories to the diet.

suction curettage A method of curettage in which a specimen of the endometrium or the products of conception are removed by aspiration. Under local or light general anesthesia the cervix is dilated, a catheter is introduced into the uterus, and suction is applied. Also called **vacuum aspiration.** Compare **dilatation and curettage.**

suction drainage See **drainage.**

sudden infant death syndrome (SIDS) The unexpected and sudden death of an apparently normal and healthy infant that occurs during sleep and with no physical or autopsic ev-

idence of disease. It is the most common cause of death in infants between the ages of 2 weeks and 1 year, with an incidence rate of 1 in every 300 to 350 live births. The etiology is unknown but multiple causes have been proposed, including lack of biotin in the diet, abnormality of the endogenous-opioid system, mechanical suffocation, a defect in respiratory mucosal defense, prolonged apnea, an unknown virus, anatomical abnormality of the larynx, and immunoglobulin abnormalities. It is known that the condition occurs more often during the winter months in infants 10 to 14 weeks old, especially those born prematurely, and in males more often than in females. Also, it is seen more often among infants who have recently had a minor illness such as upper respiratory infection, or in infants born to women less than 20 years of age who have had at least one previous child, who begin prenatal care in the third trimester, or who smoke or are anemic or drug dependent. The syndrome is neither contagious nor hereditary, although there is a greater than average risk of its occurrence within the same family, which may indicate the influence of polygenic factors. Also called **cot death, crib death.** See also **parental grief.**

sudo- A combining form meaning 'of or pertaining to sweat': *sudogram, sudokeratosis, sudorrhea.*

sudoriferous duct A duct leading from a sudoriferous gland to the surface of the skin. Also called **sweat duct.**

sudoriferous gland One of about three million tiny structures within the dermis that produces sweat. The average quantity of sweat secreted in 24 hours varies from 700 to 900 ml (about 23 to 30 fluid ounces). Most of these glands are eccrine glands, producing sweat, which carries away sodium chloride, the waste products urea and lactic acid, and the breakdown products from garlic, spices, and other substances. (Apocrine sweat glands associated with the coarse hair of the armpits and the pubic region are larger and secrete fluid which is much thicker than that secreted by the eccrine glands.) Each sudoriferous gland consists of a single tube with a deeply coiled body and a superficial duct. In the superficial layers of the dermis the duct is straight; in the deeper layers it is convoluted. In the thick dermis of the palms of the hands and the soles of the feet the duct is spirally coiled. The number of glands per square centimeter of skin varies in different parts of the body. Compare **sebaceous gland.**

sudorific 1. Of or pertaining to a substance or condition, as heat or emotional tension, that promotes sweating. 2. A sudorific agent. Sweat glands are stimulated by cholinergic drugs. The alkaloid pilocarpine is a potent sudorific drug, but it is rarely used for that purpose in modern medicine. Also called **diaphoretic.**

suf- See **sub-.**

suffocative goiter An enlargement of the thyroid gland causing pressure and a sensation of suffocation.

sugar Any of several water-soluble carbohydrates. The two principal categories of sugars are monosaccharides and disaccharides. A monosaccharide is a single sugar, as glucose, fructose, or galactose. A disaccharide is a double sugar, as sucrose (table sugar) or lactose. See also **carbohydrate, fructose, galactose, glucose, saccharide, sucrose.**

sugar alcohol An alcohol produced by the reduction of an aldehyde or ketone of a sugar.

suggestion 1. The process by which one thought or idea leads to another, as in the association of ideas. 2. The use of persuasion, exhortation, or other devices to implant an idea, thought, attitude, or belief in the mind of another as a means of influencing or altering behavior or states of mind. See also **hypnosis.** 3. An idea, belief, or attitude implanted in the mind of another. Compare **autosuggestion.**

suicidal melancholia A state of severe depression in which suicidal tendencies are prominent.

suicide 1. The intentional taking of one's own life. 2. *Informal.* The ruin or destruction of one's own interests. 3. A person who commits or attempts self-destruction. Early signs of suicidal intent include depression; expressions of guilt, tension, and agitation; insomnia; loss of weight and appetite; neglect of personal appearance; and direct or indirect threats to commit suicide. —**suicidal,** *adj.*

suicide gesture In psychiatric nursing: an apparent attempt to cause self-injury without lethal consequences and generally without actual intent to commit suicide. A suicide gesture serves to attract attention to the patient's disturbed emotional status but is not as serious as a suicide attempt.

suicidology The study of the prevention and the causes of suicide. —**suicidologist,** *n.*

sulcus, *pl.* **sulci** A shallow groove, depression, or furrow on the surface of an organ. A sulcus is usually not as deep as a fissure, but, in the terminology of anatomy, 'sulcus' and 'fissure' are often used interchangeably. —**sulcate,** *adj.*

sulcus pulmonalis A depression on each side of the vertebral bodies that accommodates the posterior portion of the lung.

sulfa (6%) in petrolatum A scabicide.

sulfacetamide, s. sodium An ophthalmic anti-infective.

sulfacytine A sulfonamide antibiotic.

sulfadiazine A sulfonamide antibiotic.

sulfamethizole A sulfonamide antibiotic.

sulfamethoxazole A sulfonamide antibiotic.

sulfamethoxazole and trimethoprim See **co-trimoxazole.**

sulfanilic acid A red-tinged, white crystalline compound used in the synthesis of sulfonamides and as a reagent in tests for phenol, fecal matter in water, albumen, aldehydes, and glucose. Also called **anilinparasulfonic acid.**

sulfapyridine A sulfonamide antibiotic.

sulfasalazine A sulfonamide used to treat colitis.

sulfate A salt of sulfuric acid. A sulfate is usually a combination of a metal with sulfuric acid. Natural sulfates, as sodium sulfate, calcium sulfate, and potassium sulfate, are plentiful in the body.

sulfhemoglobin A form of hemoglobin containing an irreversibly bound sulfur molecule that prevents normal oxygen binding. It is present in the blood in trace amounts.

sulfinpyrazone A uricosuric agent.

sulfisoxazole A sulfonamide antibiotic.

sulfo- A combining form naming chemical compounds, showing presence of divalent sulfur or of the group SO_2OH: *sulfoamide, sulfomethane, sulfophenol.*

sulfobromophthalein A substance used in its disodium salt form for evaluating the function of the liver. See also **Bromsulphalein test.**

sulfonamide One of a large group of synthetic, bacteriostatic drugs that are effective in treating infections caused by many gram-negative and gram-positive microorganisms. The drugs act by preventing the normal growth, development, and multiplication of the bacteria but do not kill mature organisms. Some sulfonamides are short-acting, some are intermediate-acting, and some are long-acting, depending on the speed with which they are excreted. They are used in treating many urinary tract infections, as well as systemic infections. Some people are hypersensitive to the drugs. Hemolytic anemia, agranulocytosis, thrombocytopenia, or aplastic anemia, drug fever, and jaundice may occur. Dosage varies with the particular drug and with the age, size, and condition of the

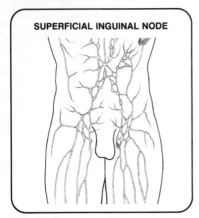

SUPERFICIAL INGUINAL NODE

patient. Most sulfonamides are given orally.

sulfonylurea   An oral antidiabetic agent that stimulates the pancreatic production of insulin. Hypersensitivity to sulfonamides is a contraindication for using such agents, and ethanol consumption is incompatible with all sulfonylureas. Aspirin or other salicylates taken with any sulfonylurea intensifies the hypoglycemic effect.

sulfosalicylic acid   A white or faintly pink crystalline substance that is highly water-soluble, used as a reagent in tests for albumin and as an intermediate compound in the manufacture of dyes and surfactants.

sulfoxone, s. sodium   An antileprotic agent.

sulfur, sulphur (S)   **1.** A nonmetallic, multivalent, tasteless, odorless chemical element that occurs abundantly in yellow crystalline form or in masses, especially in volcanic areas. Its atomic number is 16; its atomic weight is 32.06. **2.** A topical keratolytic agent.

sulfurated lime solution   A topical keratolytic agent.

-sulfuric, -sulphuric   A combining form meaning 'compounds containing sulfur, especially in its highest valences': *hydrosulfuric, persulfuric, thiosulfuric.*

sulfuric acid   A clear, colorless, oily, highly corrosive liquid that generates great heat when mixed with water. An extremely toxic substance, sulfuric acid causes severe skin burns, blindness on contact with the eyes, serious lung damage if the vapors are inhaled, and death if it is ingested. In industry, sulfuric acid is used in the manufacture of fertilizers, dyes, glue, and other acids, in the purifying of petroleum, and in the pickling of metals. Weak solutions of sulfuric acid are used in the treatment of gastric hypoacidity and serous diarrhea. It was formerly called **oil of vitriol.**

sulindac   A nonsteroidal anti-inflammatory agent.

Sulkowitch's test   An examination of the urine for the presence of calcium. A reagent, containing oxalic acid, ammonium oxalate, and glacial acetic acid, mixed with urine, causes calcium to precipitate out of the urine. Also called

S's test. See also **hypercalciuria.**

summary judgment   In law: a judgment requested by any party to a civil action to end the action when it is believed that there is no genuine issue or material fact in dispute.

summation   **1.** An accumulative effect or action; a total aggregate; totality. **2.** In neurology: the accumulation of the concentration of a neurotransmitter at a synapse, either by increasing the frequency of nerve impulses in each fiber (temporal summation) or by increasing the number of fibers stimulated (spatial summation), so that the threshold of the postsynaptic neuron is overcome and an impulse is transmitted. See also **facilitation,** definition 2.

summons   In law: a document issued by a clerk of the court upon the filing of a complaint. A sheriff, marshall, or other appointed person serves the summons, notifying a person that an action has been begun against him. See also **service of process.**

sundowning   A condition in which elderly institutionalized patients tend to become confused or disoriented at the end of the day. Many of them have diminished visual acuity and varying degrees of sensorineural and conduction hearing loss.

sunstroke   A morbid condition caused by overexposure to the sun and characterized by a high fever, convulsions, and coma. See also **heat hyperpyrexia.**

sup-   See **sub-.**

super-   A combining form meaning 'above, or implying excess': *superduct, superfunction.*

superego   In psychoanalysis: that part of the psyche, functioning mostly in the unconscious, that develops as the standards of the parents and of society are incorporated into the ego. The superego has two parts, the conscience and the ego ideal. See also **ego, ego ideal, id.**

superfecundation   The fertilization of two or more ova released during one menstrual cycle by spermatozoa released during separate acts of sexual intercourse.

superfetation   The fertilization of a second ovum after the onset of pregnancy, resulting in the presence of two fetuses of different degrees of maturity developing within the uterus simultaneously. Also called **superimpregnation.**

superficial   **1.** Of or pertaining to the skin or another surface. **2.** Not grave or dangerous.

superficial fading infantile hemangioma   A superficial, transient, salmon-colored patch in the center of the forehead, face, or occiput of many newborns. It fades during the first 2 years of life, but it may temporarily deepen in color if the child becomes flushed or angry.

superficial implantation   In embryology: the partial embedding of the blastocyst within the uterine wall so that it and, later, the chorionic sac protrude into the uterine cavity. Also called **central implantation, circumferential implantation.**

superficial inguinal node   A node in one of the two groups of inguinal lymph glands in

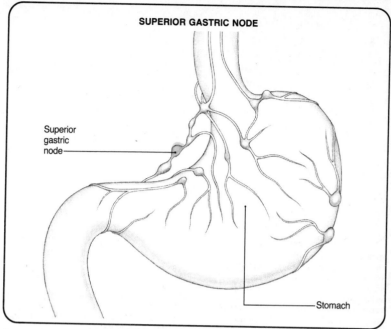

SUPERIOR GASTRIC NODE

Superior gastric node

Stomach

the upper femoral triangle of the thigh. The nodes form a chain distal to the inguinal ligament and receive afferents from the skin of the penis, scrotum, perineum, buttocks, and abdominal wall below the level of the umbilicus. Compare **anterior tibial node, popliteal node.**

superficial reflex   Any neural reflex initiated by stimulation of the skin. Kinds of superficial reflexes are **abdominal reflex, cremasteric reflex.** Compare **deep tendon reflex.**

superficial sensation   The awareness or perception of feelings in the superficial layers of the skin in response to touch, pressure, temperature, and pain. Such sensations are conveyed to the brain via the spinothalamic system. Compare **deep sensation.**

superficial spreading melanoma   A melanoma that grows outward, spreading over the surface of the affected organ or tissue, most commonly on the lower legs of women. Occurring in late middle age, it is raised and palpable, is usually unevenly pigmented, and has an irregular shape and unclear border.

superficial temporal artery   An artery at each side of the head that can be easily felt in front of the ear and is used to take the pulse. It is the smaller of the two terminal branches of the external carotid and arises in the substance of the parotid gland. It crosses the zygomatic process of the temporal bone and about 5 cm (2 inches) above the process divides into the frontal branch and the parietal branch. Compare **deep temporal artery, middle temporal artery.**

superficial vein   One of the many veins that lie between the subcutaneous fascia just under the skin. Compare **deep vein.**

superimpregnation   See **superfetation.**

superinfection   An infection occurring during antimicrobial treatment for another infection. It is usually a result of change in the normal tissue flora favoring replication of some organisms by diminishing the vitality and then the number of competing organisms.

superior   Situated above or oriented toward a higher place as the head is superior to the torso. Compare **inferior.**

superior aperture of the minor pelvis   An opening bounded by the crest and pecten of the pubic bones, the arch-shaped lines of the ilia, and the anterior margin of the base of the sacrum.

superior aperture of the thorax   An elliptical opening at the summit of the thorax bounded by the first thoracic vertebra, the first ribs, and the upper margin of the sternum.

superior costotransverse ligament   One of five ligaments associated with each costotransverse joint, except that of the first rib. It passes from the neck of each rib to the transverse process of the vertebra immediately above and is associated with the intercostal vessels and the intercostal nerves. Compare **posterior costotransverse ligament.**

superior gastric node   A node in one of two sets of gastric lymph glands, accompanying the left gastric artery, and divided into the upper group of nodes on the stem of the artery, the lower group of nodes accompanying branches of the artery along the cardiac half of the lesser curvature of the stomach, and the paracardial

SUPERIOR SAGITTAL SINUS

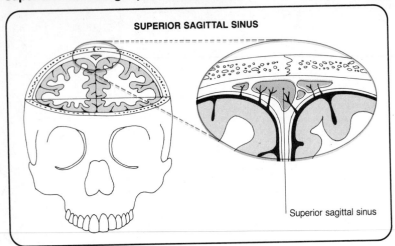

Superior sagittal sinus

group of nodes around the neck of the stomach. The superior gastric nodes receive their afferents from the stomach and pass their efferents to the celiac group of preaortic nodes. Compare **inferior gastric node.**

superior hemorrhagic polioencephalitis See **Wernicke's encephalopathy.**

superior mediastinum The cranial portion of the mediastinum in the middle of the thorax, containing the trachea, the esophagus, the aortic arch, and the origins of the sternohyoidei and the sternothyroidei. It is bounded by the superior aperture of the thorax, the plane of the superior limit of the pericardium, the manubrium, the upper four thoracic vertebrae, and laterally by the mediastinal aspect of the parietal pleurae of the lungs. Compare **anterior mediastinum, middle mediastinum, posterior mediastinum.**

superior mesenteric artery A visceral branch of the abdominal aorta, arising caudal to the celiac artery, dividing into five branches, and supplying most of the small intestine and parts of the colon. The branches are the inferior pancreaticoduodenal, intestinal, ileocolic, right colic, and middle colic.

superior mesenteric node A node in one of the three groups of visceral lymph nodes that serve the viscera of the abdomen and the pelvis. The superior mesenteric nodes are associated with branches of the superior mesenteric artery and are divided into mesenteric nodes, iliocolic nodes, and mesocolic nodes. Compare **gastric node, inferior mesenteric node.**

superior mesenteric vein A tributary of the portal vein that drains the blood from the small intestine, the cecum, and the ascending and transverse colons. It begins in the right iliac fossa, ascends between the two mesenteric layers to the right of the superior mesenteric artery, and joins the lienal vein to form the portal vein, dorsal to the neck of the pancreas. The tributaries of the superior mesenteric vein are the

intestinal vein, the ileocolic vein, the right colic vein, the middle colic vein, the gastroepiploic vein, and the pancreaticoduodenal vein. See also **portal vein.**

superior profunda artery See **deep brachial artery.**

superior radioulnar joint See **proximal radioulnar articulation.**

superior sagittal sinus One of the six venous channels in the posterior of the dura mater, draining blood from the brain into the internal jugular vein. It has no valves and presents a triangular section as the sinus courses posteriorly through a groove in the frontal bone and passes along the convex margin of the falx cerebri to the occipital protuberance, usually continuing as the right transverse sinus. The superior sagittal sinus receives the superior cerebral veins, veins from the diploe, and, near the posterior extremity of the sagittal suture, the anastomosing emissary veins from the pericranium and the veins from the dura mater. It also anastomoses with veins of the nose, the scalp, and the diploe. Compare **inferior sagittal sinus, straight sinus, transverse sinus.**

superior subscapular nerve One of two small nerves on opposite sides of the body that arise from the posterior cord of the brachial plexus. It supplies the superior part of the subscapularis. Compare **inferior subscapular nerve.**

superior thyroid artery One of a pair of arteries in the neck, usually rising from the external carotid artery, that supplies the thyroid gland and several head muscles.

superior ulnar collateral artery A long, slender division of the brachial artery, arising just distal to the middle of the arm, descending to the elbow, and anastomosing with the posterior ulnar recurrent and inferior ulnar collateral arteries.

superior vena cava The second largest vein of the body, returning deoxygenated blood from the upper half of the body to the right atrium. It is about 2 cm (¾ inch) in diameter and 7 cm (2¾ inches) long and is formed by the junction of the two brachiocephalic veins at the level of the first intercostal space behind the sternum on the right side. The section of the superior vena cava closest to the heart is within the pericardial sac, covered by the serous pericardium. It has no valves. Just before it enters the pericardium, it receives the azygous vein and several small pericardial veins. Compare **inferior vena cava.**

supination 1. The position of lying on the back, face up. 2. One of the kinds of rotation allowed by certain skeletal joints, as by the elbow and the wrist joints, which allow the palm of the hand to turn up. Compare **pronation.** —**supinate,** *v.,* **supine,** *adj.*

supinator longus See **brachioradialis.**

supine Lying horizontally on the back. Compare **prone.** See also **body position.**

supplemental inheritance The acquisition or expression of a genetic trait or condition from the presence of two independent pairs of nonallelic genes that interact so that one gene supplements the action of the other.

supplementary gene One of two pairs of nonallelic genes that interact so that one pair needs the presence of the other to be expressed, while the other pair can produce an effect independently.

support 1. To sustain, hold up, or maintain in a desired position or condition. 2. The assistance given to this end, as physical support, emotional support, or life support.

supportive psychotherapy A form of psychotherapy that concentrates on creating an effective means of communication with an emotionally disturbed person rather than on trying to produce psychological insight into his underlying conflicts. Compare **nondirective therapy.**

suppository An easily melted medicated mass for insertion in the rectum, urethra, or vagina. Theobroma oil, glycerinated gelatin, and high–molecular-weight polyethylene glycols are common vehicles for drugs in suppositories that are cone- or spindle-shaped for insertion in the rectum, globular or egg-shaped for use in the vagina, and pencil-shaped for insertion in the urethra. Drugs administered by rectal suppository are absorbed systemically, and this route is especially useful in infants, uncooperative patients, and in patients who are vomiting.

suppressant An agent that suppresses or diminishes a physical or mental activity, as a medication that reduces hyperkinetic behavior.

suppression In psychoanalysis: the conscious inhibition or effort to conceal unacceptable or painful thoughts, desires, impulses, feelings, or acts. Compare **repression.**

suppression amblyopia A partial loss of vision, usually in one eye, owing to cortical suppression of central vision to avoid diplopia. It occurs commonly in strabismus in the eye that deviates and does not fixate. Early recognition

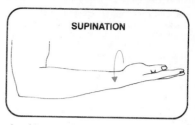

SUPINATION

of strabismus and amblyopia is essential; if begun early, occlusive therapy that forces use of the bad eye may dramatically improve a child's vision.

suppressor gene In molecular genetics: a genetic unit that reverses the effect of a specific gene mutation.

suppressor mutation In molecular genetics: a mutation that partially or completely restores a function lost by a primary mutation occurring in a different genetic site.

suppressor T cell See **T cell.**

suppurate To produce purulent matter. —**suppuration,** *n.,* **suppurative,** *adj.*

supra- A combining form meaning 'above or over': *suprabuccal, supradural.*

supraclavicular nerve One of a pair of cutaneous branches of the cervical plexus, arising from the third and mostly the fourth cervical nerve. It emerges from the posterior border of the sternocleidomastoideus and crosses the posterior triangle of the neck under the deep fascia. Near the clavicle it pierces the fascia and the platysma in the anterior, the middle, and the posterior groups. The anterior group supplies the skin of the infraclavicular region, the middle group supplies the skin over the pectoralis major and the deltoideus, and the posterior group supplies the skin of the cranial and the dorsal parts of the shoulder.

supracondylar fracture A fracture involving the area between the condyles of the humerus or the femur.

suprainfection A secondary infection usually caused by an opportunistic pathogen, as a fungal infection following the antibiotic treatment of another infection.

suprapubic Located above the symphysis pubis.

suprarenal Situated above the kidney.

suprascapular nerve One of a pair of branches from the cords of the brachial plexus. It arises from the superior trunk, passes to the scapular notch, and, in the supraspinatous fossa, branches to the supraspinatus, the shoulder joint, the infraspinatus, and the scapula.

suprasellar cyst See **craniopharyngioma.**

supraspinal ligament The ligament that connects the apices of the spinous processes from the seventh cervical vertebra to the sacrum. Between the spinous processes, it is continuous with the interspinal ligaments; from the seventh cervical vertebrae, it continues upward to the external occipital protuberance and the medial nuchal line as the ligamentum nuchae.

suramin sodium An antitrypanosomal and an antifilarial available from the Centers for Disease Control. It is used primarily for treatment and prophylaxis of African trypanosomiasis.

surface anatomy The study of the structural relationships of the external features of the body to the internal organs and parts. Compare **cross-sectional anatomy.**

surface anesthesia See **topical anesthesia.**

surface area (SA) The total area exposed to the outside environment. The surface area of an object increases with the square of the object's linear dimensions; volume increases as the cube of the object's linear dimensions. Thus, the larger of two objects of the same shape will have less surface area per unit volume than the smaller object.

surface biopsy The removal of living tissue for microscopic examination by scraping the surface of a lesion. The procedure is used primarily to diagnose cancer of the uterine cervix. See also **exfoliative cytology.**

surface tension The tendency of the surface of a liquid to minimize the area of its surface by contracting. This property causes liquids to rise in a capillary tube, affects the exchange of gases in the pulmonary alveoli, and alters the ability of various liquids to wet another surface.

surface therapy A form of radiotherapy administered by placing one or more radioactive sources on or near an area of body surface. The resulting array of sources is called a surface mold, surface applicator, or plaque.

surface thermometer A device that detects and indicates the temperature of the surface of any body part.

surfactant 1. An agent, as soap or detergent, dissolved in water to reduce its surface tension or the tension at the interface between the water and another liquid. 2. Certain lipoproteins that reduce the surface tension of pulmonary fluids, allowing gas exchange in the alveoli and contributing to the elasticity of pulmonary tissue. See also **alveolus, atelectasis, surface tension.**

surfer's nodules Nodules on the skin of the knees, ankles, feet, or toes of a surfer, caused by repeated contact of the skin with an abrasive, sandy surfboard. The nodules will slowly disappear if surfing is discontinued.

surgeon's assistant (SA) A medical professional trained to assist in surgery and in the preoperative and postoperative periods under the supervision of a licensed medical doctor. An SA is required to attend 2 years of college studying anatomy, physiology, pharmacology, and other subjects, followed by 2 years of special clinical training and clinical experience.

surgery A branch of medicine concerned with diseases and trauma requiring operative procedures. —**surgical,** *adj.*

-surgery A combining form meaning the 'treatment of illness or deformity': *cardiosurgery, chemosurgery, radiosurgery.* Also **-chirurgia.**

surgical anatomy In applied anatomy: the study of the structure and morphology of the tissues and organs of the body as they relate to surgery.

surgical anesthesia The third stage of general anesthesia. See also **general anesthesia, Guedel's signs.**

surgical diathermy See **electrocoagulation.**

surgical microscope See **operating microscope.**

surgical pathology The study of disease through examination of tissue specimens obtained during surgery. The surgical pathologist often examines specimens during surgery to determine how the operation should be modified or completed.

surgical scrub 1. A bactericidal soap or solution used by surgeons and surgical nurses before performing or assisting in surgery. 2. The act of washing the fingernails, hands, and forearms with a bactericidal soap or solution.

surrogate 1. A substitute; a person or thing that replaces another. 2. In psychoanalysis: a substitute parental figure; a symbolic image or representation of another, as may occur in a dream. The identity of the person represented often remains unconscious.

sursum- A combining form meaning 'upward': *sursumduction, sursumvergence, sursumversion.*

susceptibility The condition of being more than normally vulnerable to a disease or disorder. —**susceptible,** *adj.*

suspension 1. A liquid in which small particles of a solid are dispersed but not dissolved and in which the dispersal is maintained by stirring or shaking the mixture. 2. A treatment, used primarily in spinal disorders, consisting of suspending the patient by the chin and shoulders. 3. A temporary cessation of pain or of a vital process.

suspensory ligament of the lens See **zonula ciliaris.**

sustained release See **prolonged release.**

sustenance 1. The act or process of supporting or maintaining life or health. 2. The food or nutrients essential for maintaining life.

sutilains A proteolytic enzyme used as a cleansing and debriding agent.

sutura, *pl.* **suturae** An immovable fibrous joint in which certain bones of the skull are connected by a thin layer of fibrous tissue. Compare **gomphosis, syndesmosis.**

sutura dentata An immovable fibrous joint that is one kind of true suture in which toothlike processes interlock along the margins of connecting bones of the skull. Compare **sutura limbosa, sutura serrata.**

sutura limbosa An immovable fibrous joint that is one kind of true suture in which beveled and serrated edges of certain connecting bones of the skull, as the parietal and temporal bones, overlap and interlock. Compare **sutura dentata, sutura serrata.**

sutura plana A fibrous joint that is one kind

FOUR-LUMEN SWAN-GANZ CATHETER

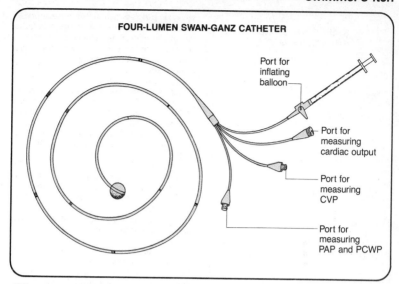

Port for inflating balloon

Port for measuring cardiac output

Port for measuring CVP

Port for measuring PAP and PCWP

of false suture in which rough, contiguous edges of certain bones of the skull, as the maxillae, form a connection. Compare **sutura squamosa.**

sutura serrata An immovable fibrous joint that is one kind of true suture in which connecting bones interlock along serrated edges that resemble fine-toothed saws. Compare **sutura dentata, sutura limbosa.**

sutura squamosa An immovable fibrous joint that is one kind of false suture in which overlapping, beveled edges unite certain bones of the skull, as the temporal and the parietal bones. Compare **sutura plana.**

suture **1.** A border or a joint, as between the bones of the cranium. **2.** To stitch together cut or torn edges of tissue with suture material. **3.** A surgical stitch taken to repair an incision, tear, or wound. **4.** Material used for surgical stitches, as absorbable or nonabsorbable silk, catgut, wire, or synthetic material.

SV40 *abbr* **simian virus 40.**

swab A stick or clamp for holding absorbent gauze or cotton, used for washing, cleansing, or drying a body surface, for collecting a specimen for laboratory examination, or for applying a topical medication.

swamp fever **1.** See **leptospirosis. 2.** See **malaria.**

Swan-Ganz catheter A long, thin cardiac catheter with a tiny balloon at the tip. It is used to determine left ventricular function by measuring pulmonary capillary wedge pressure and pulmonary arterial pressure. It may also have a thermistor at the end, which allows for measurement of cardiac output.

swan-neck deformity A structural abnormality of the kidney tubules associated with rickets. The kidney tubule connecting the glomerulus with the convoluted portion of the tu-

bule is narrowed into a configuration referred to as 'swan neck.' There is also a thinning and atrophy of the distal tubule and a shortening of the convoluted portion.

S wave The component of the cardiac cycle shown on an electrocardiogram as a line slanting downward sharply from the peak of the R wave to the beginning of the upward curve of the T wave. It represents the final phase of the QRS complex.

sweat See **perspiration.**

sweat bath A bath given to induce sweating.

sweat duct Any one of the tiny tubules conveying sweat to the skin surface from about 3 million sweat glands in the body. Each sweat duct is the most superficial part of a coiled tube that forms the body of each sweat gland and opens onto the surface through a funnel-shaped opening. Each duct is composed of a basement membrane with two or three layers of polyhedral cells and is lined with a thin cuticle.

sweat gland See **sudoriferous gland.**

sweat test A method for evaluating sodium and chloride excretion from the sweat glands, often the first test performed in the diagnosis of cystic fibrosis. The sweat glands are stimulated with a drug, as pilocarpine, and the perspiration produced is analyzed. The exocrine glands of patients with cystic fibrosis produce sodium and chloride concentrations that are three to six times that of the normal. The test is very reliable. See also **cystic fibrosis.**

swimmer's ear *Informal.* Otitis externa resulting from infection transmitted in the water of a swimming pool.

swimmer's itch An allergic dermatitis caused by sensitivity to schistosome cercarias, which die under the skin, leading to erythema, urticaria, and a papular rash lasting 1 or 2 days. Treatment usually includes oral antihistamines

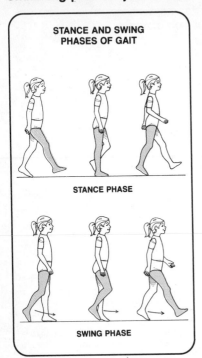

**STANCE AND SWING
PHASES OF GAIT**

STANCE PHASE

SWING PHASE

and antipruritic lotions. See also **schistosomiasis.**

swimming pool conjunctivitis See
pharyngoconjunctival fever.

swing phase of gait One of the two phases
in the rhythmic process of walking. The swing
phase of gait follows the stance phase and is
divided into the initial swing stage, the mid-
swing stage, and the terminal swing stage. The
analyses of pathological gaits and the diagnoses
of many abnormal orthopedic conditions focus
on walking as a specialized function of the musculoskeletal system and the swing phase of gait
as the kinetic conclusion of one complete gait
cycle. Compare **stance phase of gait.**

sy- See **syn-.**

sycosis barbae An inflammation of hair
follicles of shaved skin. Treatment includes light,
infrequent shaving; topical and systemic antibiotics; and daily plucking of infected hairs. Also
called **barber's itch, sycosis vulgaris.**

sycosis vulgaris See **sycosis barbae.**

Sydenham's chorea A form of chorea associated with rheumatic fever, usually occurring during childhood. The cause is a streptococcal infection of the vascular and perivascular
brain tissues. The choreic movements increase
over the first 2 weeks, reach a plateau, and then
diminish. The child is usually well within 10
weeks. With undue exertion or emotional strain,
the condition may recur. Also called **chorea
minor, rheumatic chorea.**

syl- See **syn-.**

sylvatic plague An endemic disease of wild
rodents caused by *Yersinia pestis* and transmissible to humans by the bite of an infected
flea. It is found on every continent except Australia. See also **bubonic plague.**

sym- See **syn-.**

symbiosis **1.** In biology: a mode of living
characterized by close association between organisms of different species, usually in a mutually beneficial relationship. **2.** In psychiatry:
a. A state in which two mentally disturbed people are emotionally interdependent. **b.** Pathologic inability of a child to separate from its
mother emotionally and, sometimes, physically.
—**symbiotic,** *adj.*

**symbiotic infantile psychotic syn-
drome** A condition in which children, usually between ages 2 and 4, have an abnormal
relationship with their mother, characterized by
severe regression, intense separation anxiety,
cessation of useful speech, and autism.

symbol **1.** An image, object, action, or other
stimulus that represents something else by reason of conscious association, convention, or other
relationship. **2.** An object, mode of behavior, or
feeling that disguises a repressed emotional conflict through an unconscious association rather
than through an objective relationship, as in
dreams and neuroses.

-symbolia A combining form meaning
'(condition involving) the ability to interpret
symbols': *asymbolia, dyssymbolia, strephosymbolia.*

symbolism In psychiatry: an unconscious
mental mechanism characteristic of all human
thinking in which a mental image stands for,
but disguises, some other object, person, or
thought, especially one associated with emotional conflict. The mechanism is a principal
factor in the formation of dreams and in various
symptoms resulting from such neurotic and psychotic conditions as conversion reactions, ob-
sessions, and compulsions. Also called **symbolization.**

symbolization See **symbolism.**

symelus See **symmelus.**

symmelia A fetal anomaly characterized by
the fusion of the lower limbs, with or without
feet. Kinds of symmelia are apodial symmelia,
monopodial symmelia, tripodial symmelia.

symmelus, symelus A malformed fetus
characterized by symmelia.

Symmer's disease See **giant follicular
lymphoma.**

symmetrical, symmetric Of the body or
parts of the body: equal in size or shape; different in placement or arrangement about an
axis. Compare **asymmetrical.** —**symmetry,** *n.*

symmetrical lipomatosis See **nodular
circumscribed lipomatosis.**

symmetric tonic neck reflex A normal
response in infants to assume the crawl position
by extending the arms and bending the knees
when the head and neck are extended. The reflex
disappears when neurological and muscular development enables independent limb movement

for actual crawling. Also called **crawling reflex.** See also **tonic neck reflex.**

sympathectomy A surgical interruption of part of the sympathetic nerve pathways, performed for the relief of chronic pain in vascular diseases, as arteriosclerosis. The sheath around an artery carries the sympathetic nerve fibers that control constriction of the vessel. Removal of the sheath causes the vessel to relax and expand and allows more blood to pass through it. The operation may also be done with a vascular graft to increase the blood flow through the graft area. Postoperatively, the adequacy of circulation in the affected extremity is monitored. An arteriogram shows a widened pathway.

sympathetic nervous system See **autonomic nervous system.**

sympathetic ophthalmia A granulomatous inflammation of the uveal tract of both eyes occurring after an injury to the uveal tract of one eye. Corticosteroids may be helpful in treatment, but surgical enucleation of the originally injured eye may be necessary to preserve vision in the uninjured eye. Also called **metastatic ophthalmia, migratory ophthalmia.**

sympathetic trunk One of a pair of chains of ganglia extending along the side of the vertebral column from the base of the skull to the coccyx. Each trunk is part of the sympathetic nervous system and consists of a series of ganglia connected by cords containing various types of fibers. The cranial end of the trunk is formed by the superior cervical ganglion from the internal carotid nerve of the head. In some individuals, the caudal ends of both trunks merge into a single ganglion at the coccyx. Interconnection of the trunks is common but rarely occurs above the fifth lumbar nerve. The central ganglia of each trunk are irregularly shaped structures with diameters ranging from 1 to 10 mm. Each sympathetic trunk distributes branches with postganglionic fibers to the autonomic plexuses, the cranial nerves, the individual organs, the nerves accompanying arteries, and the spinal nerves.

sympathizing eye In sympathetic ophthalmia: the uninfected eye that becomes infected by lymphatic or blood-born metastasis of the microorganism.

sympatholytic See **antiadrenergic.**

sympatholytic agent See **antiadrenergic.**

sympathomimetic Noting a pharmacologic agent that mimics the effects of stimulation of organs and structures by the sympathetic nervous system by occupying adrenergic receptor sites and acting as an agonist or by increasing the release of the neurotransmitter norepinephrine at postganglionic nerve endings. Various sympathomimetic agents are used as decongestants of nasal and ocular mucosa. They are also used for maintaining normal blood pressure during operations under spinal anesthesia. Adverse effects of sympathomimetic drugs may be nervousness, severe headache, anxiety, vertigo, nausea, vomiting, dilated pupils, glycosuria, and

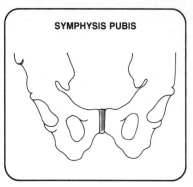

SYMPHYSIS PUBIS

dysuria. Also called **adrenergic.**

sympathomimetic amine See **adrenergic.**

sympathy 1. An expressed interest or concern regarding the problems, emotions, or states of mind of another. Compare **empathy.** 2. The relation that exists between the mind and body causing the one to be affected by the other. 3. Mental contagion or the influence exerted by one individual or group on another and the effects produced, as the spread of panic. 4. The physiologic or pathologic relationship between two organs, systems, or parts of the body. —**sympathetic,** *adj.,* **sympathize,** *v.*

symphalangia 1. A condition, usually inherited, characterized by ankylosis of the fingers or toes. 2. A congenital anomaly in which webbing of the fingers or toes occurs in varying degrees, often in conjunction with other defects of the hands or feet. Also called symphalangism. See also **syndactyly.**

symphocephalus Twin fetuses joined at the head. It is often used as a general designation for fetuses with varying degrees of the anomaly. See also **cephalothoracopagus, craniopagus, syncephalus.**

symphysic teratism A congenital anomaly in which there is a fusion of normally separated parts or organs, as a horseshoe kidney, or in which parts close prematurely, as the skull bones in craniostenosis.

symphysis, *pl.* **symphyses** 1. A line of union, especially a cartilaginous joint in which adjacent bony surfaces are firmly united by fibrocartilage. Also called **fibrocartilaginous joint.** 2. *Informal.* Symphysis pubis. —**symphysic,** *adj.*

symphysis pubis See **pubic symphysis.**

sympodia A congenital developmental anomaly characterized by fusion of the lower extremities. See also **sirenomelus, sympus.**

symptom A subjective indication of a disease or a change in condition as perceived by the patient. Many symptoms are accompanied by objective signs, as pruritus, which is often reported with erythema and a maculopapular eruption on the skin. Some symptoms may be objectively confirmed, as numbness of a body part, which may be confirmed by absence of

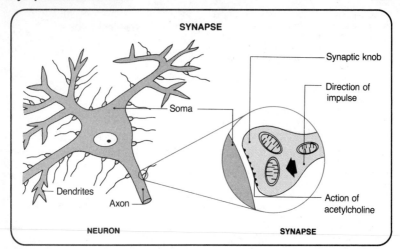

SYNAPSE

Synaptic knob

Direction of impulse

Soma

Dendrites

Axon

Action of acetylcholine

NEURON   SYNAPSE

response to a pinprick. Compare **sign.**

symptomatic nanism   Dwarfism associated with defects in bone growth, tooth formation, and sexual development.

symptothermal method of family planning   A natural method of family planning that incorporates the ovulation and basal body temperature methods of family planning. It is more effective than either method used alone and requires fewer days of abstinence.

sympus   A malformed fetus in which the lower extremities are completely fused or rotated, and the pelvis and genitalia are defective. Kinds of sympuses are **sirenomelus, sympus dipus, sympus monopus.** See also **symmelus.**

sympus apus   See **sirenomelus.**

sympus dipus   A malformed fetus in which the lower extremities are fused, and both feet are formed.

sympus monopus   A malformed fetus in which the lower extremities are fused, and one foot is formed. Also called **monopodial symmelia, uromelus.**

syn-, sy-, syl-, sym-   A combining form meaning 'union or association': *synalgia, syncephalus.*

synadelphus, syndelphus, *pl.* **synadelphi**   A conjoined twin fetal monster with a single head and trunk and eight limbs. Also called **cephalothoracoiliopagus.**

synapse   **1.** The region surrounding the point of contact between two neurons or between a neuron and an effector organ, across which nerve impulses are transmitted through the action of a neurotransmitter, as acetylcholine or norepinephrine. When an impulse reaches the terminal point of one neuron, it causes the release of the neurotransmitter, which diffuses across the gap between the two cells to bind with receptors in the other neuron, muscle, or gland, triggering electrical changes that either inhibit or continue the transmission of the impulse. Synapses are polarized so that nerve impulses travel in only

one direction. **2.** To form a synapse or connection between neurons. **3.** In genetics: to form a synaptic fusion between homologous chromosomes during meiosis. Kinds of synapses include **axoaxonic synapse, axodendritic synapse, axodendrosomatic synapse, axosomatic synapse, dendrodendritic synapse.** Compare **ephapse. —synaptic,** *adj.*

synapsis, *pl.* **synapses**   The pairing of homologous chromosomes during the early meiotic prophase stage in gametogenesis to form double or bivalent chromosomes. **—synaptic,** *adj.*

synaptic cleft   The microscopic, extracellular space at the synapse that separates the membrane of the terminal nerve endings of a presynaptic neuron and the membrane of a postsynaptic cell. Nerve impulses are transmitted across this cleft by means of a neurotransmitter. See also **neuromuscular junction.** Also called synaptic gap.

synaptic junction   The membranes of both the presynaptic neuron and the postsynaptic receptor cell, together with the synaptic cleft. See also **synapse.**

synaptic transmission   The passage of a neural impulse across a synapse from one nerve fiber to another by a neurotransmitter. Compare **ephaptic transmission.**

synarthrosis, *pl.* **synarthroses**   See **fibrous jo′nt.**

syncephalus   A conjoined twin monster having a single head and two bodies. Also called **monocephalus.**

synchilia, syncheilia   A congenital anomaly in which the lips are completely or partially fused; atresia of the mouth.

synchondrosis, *pl.* **synchondroses**   A cartilaginous joint between two immovable bones, as the synchondroses of the cranium.

synchorial   Pertaining to multiple fetuses that share a common placenta, as in monozygosity.

synclitism   **1.** In obstetrics: a condition in which the sagittal suture of the fetal head is in line with the transverse diameter of the inlet, equidistant from the maternal symphysis pubis and sacrum. This position is usually found on examination either late in pregnancy or early in labor, as the fetal head descends into the pelvic inlet. As labor progresses, posterior asynclitism develops and, as the head descends further, anterior asynclitism is evident owing to the shape of the true pelvis below the inlet. **2.** In hematology: the normal condition in which the nucleus and the cytoplasm of the blood cells mature simultaneously and at the same rate.

syncopal attack Any episode of unconsciousness or fainting, especially one associated with fear or pain.

syncope A brief lapse in consciousness caused by transient cerebral hypoxia. It is usually preceded by a sensation of light-headedness and may often be prevented by lying down or by sitting with the head between the knees.

syncretic thinking A stage in the development of the cognitive thought processes of the child. During this phase, thought is based purely on what is perceived and experienced. The child is incapable of reasoning beyond the observable or of making deductions or generalizations. In Piaget's classification, this stage occurs between 2 and 7 years of age. Compare **abstract thinking, concrete thinking.** —**syncresis,** *n.*

syncytial trophoblast See **syncytiotrophoblast.**

syncytiotrophoblast The outer syncytial layer of the trophoblast of the early mammalian embryo that erodes the uterine wall during implantation and gives rise to the villi of the placenta. Also called **plasmidotrophoblast, syncytial trophoblast, syntrophoblast.** Compare **cytotrophoblast.** —**syncytiotrophoblastic,** *adj.*

syndactylus A person with webbed fingers or toes.

syndactyly, syndactylia, syndactylism A congenital anomaly characterized by the fusion of the fingers or toes. It varies in severity from incomplete webbing of the skin of two digits to complete union of digits and fusion of the bones and nails. —**syndactyl, syndactylous,** *adj.*

syndelphus, *pl.* **syndelphi** See **synadelphus.**

syndesmo- A combining form meaning 'of or pertaining to the connective tissue or, particularly, the ligaments': *syndesmochorial, syndesmography.*

syndesmosis, *pl.* **syndesmoses** A fibrous articulation in which two bones are connected by interosseous ligaments, as the anterior and the posterior ligaments in the tibiofibular articulation. Compare **gomphosis, sutura.**

syndrome A complex of signs and symptoms resulting from a common cause or appearing, in combination, to present a clinical picture of a disease or inherited abnormality. See also specific syndromes.

syndrome of inappropriate antidiuretic hormone secretion (SIADH) An

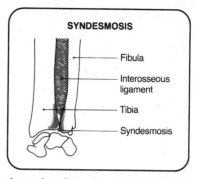

SYNDESMOSIS

- Fibula
- Interosseous ligament
- Tibia
- Syndesmosis

abnormal condition characterized by the excessive release of antidiuretic hormone (ADH), which upsets the fluid and electrolytic balances of the body. It results from various malfunctions, as water retention, increased extracellular fluid volume, the inability of the body to produce and secrete dilute urine, and hyponatremia. SIADH develops in association with diseases that affect the osmoreceptors of the hypothalamus. Oat cell carcinoma of the lung is the most common cause, affecting about 80% of involved patients. Prognosis depends on the underlying disease and the response of the patient to treatment. Common signs and symptoms of SIADH are weight gain despite anorexia, vomiting, nausea, muscle weakness, and irritability. In some patients, SIADH may produce coma and convulsions. Confirming diagnosis is based on urine osmolality that exceeds 150 milliosmols/kg of water and serum osmolality of less than 280 milliosmols/kg of water. Normal urine osmolality is 1.5 times serum osmolality. Other significant results include less than normal concentrations of blood urea nitrogen, serum creatinine, and albumin and a higher than normal concentration of sodium in the urine. Treatment of SIADH commonly includes restriction of water intake and may require administration of normal saline to raise the serum sodium level if water intoxication is severe. Furosemide may be administered to block circulatory overload, and drugs, as demeclocycline hydrochloride and lithium, may be administered to block renal response to ADH. Nursing care includes monitoring for signs of hyponatremia, weight change, and fluid imbalance.

synechia, *pl.* **synechiae** An adhesion, especially of the iris to the cornea or lens of the eye. It may develop from glaucoma, cataracts, uveitis, keratitis, or as a complication of surgery or trauma to the eye. Synechiae prevent or impede flow of aqueous fluid between the anterior and posterior chambers of the eye and may lead rapidly to blindness. Immediate treatment consists of dilating the pupils with a mydriatic agent.

synergist An organ, agent, or a substance that augments the activity of another organ, agent, or substance. —**synergistic, synergetic,** *adj.*

synergy The process in which two organs, substances, or agents work simultaneously to enhance the function and effect of one another. Also called synergism. **—synergistic,** *adj.*

synophthalmia See **cyclopia.**

synotia A congenital malformation characterized by the union or approximation of the ears in front of the neck, often accompanied by the absence or defective development of the lower jaw. Compare **agnathia.** See also **otocephaly.**

synotus A fetus with synotia.

synovia A transparent, viscous fluid, resembling the white of an egg, secreted by synovial membranes and acting as a lubricant for many joints, bursae, and tendons. Also called **synovial fluid. —synovial,** *adj.*

synovial bursa One of the many closed sacs filled with synovial fluid in the connective tissue between the muscles, the tendons, the ligaments, and the bones. The synovial bursae facilitate the gliding of muscles and tendons over bony and ligamentous prominences. Compare **synovial membrane, synovial tendon sheath.**

synovial chondroma A rare cartilaginous growth developing in the connective tissue below the synovial membrane of the joints, tendon sheaths, or bursa. Foci on the surface may develop stalks and then detach, resulting in loose bodies within the joint. Also called **synovial chondromatosis.**

synovial chondromatosis A rare condition in which masses of cartilage develop in the synovial membranes of bursae, joints, and tendon sheaths. Metaplastic foci on the membrane surface may become sessile, pedunculate, and may then separate, forming loose masses.

synovial crypt A pouch in the synovial membrane of a joint.

synovial fluid The clear, viscid fluid secreted in the bursae and tendon sheaths of the joints. It contains mucin, albumin, fat, and mineral salts and serves to lubricate the joints.

synovial joint A freely movable joint in which contiguous bony surfaces are covered by articular cartilage and connected by ligaments lined with synovial membrane. Kinds of synovial joints are **ball-and-socket joint, condyloid joint, gliding joint, hinge joint, pivot joint, saddle joint.** Also called abarthrosis, diarthrosis. Compare **cartilaginous joint, fibrous joint.**

synovial membrane The inner layer of an articular capsule surrounding a freely movable joint. The synovial membrane is loosely attached to the external fibrous capsule. It secretes into the joint a thick fluid that normally lubricates the joint. Compare **synovial bursa, synovial tendon sheath.**

synovial sarcoma A malignant tumor, composed of synovioblasts, that begins as a soft swelling and often metastasizes through the bloodstream to the lung before it is discovered.

synovial sheath Any one of the membranous sacs that enclose a tendon of a muscle and facilitate the gliding of a tendon through a fibrous or a bony tunnel, as that under the flexor retinaculum of the wrist.

synovial tendon sheath One of the many membranous sacs enclosing various tendons that glide through fibrous and bony tunnels in the body, as those under the flexor retinaculum of the wrist. One layer of the synovial sheath lines the tunnel; the other covers the tendon. The sheath secretes synovial fluid, which lubricates the tendon. Compare **synovial bursa, synovial membrane.**

synovitis An inflammatory condition of the synovial membrane of a joint as the result of an aseptic wound or a traumatic injury. The knee is most commonly affected. Fluid accumulates around the capsule; the joint is swollen, tender, and painful; and motion is restricted. In most cases, the inflammation subsides, and the fluid is resorbed without medical or surgical intervention.

synteny In genetics: the presence on the same chromosome of two or more genes that may or may not be transmitted as a linkage group but that appear to be able to undergo independent assortment during meiosis. The term is used primarily in human genetics where linked inheritance patterns are more difficult to determine. See also **linkage.**

-synthesis A combining form meaning 'putting together or formation of': narcosynthesis, psychosynthesis.

synthetic Of or pertaining to a substance produced by an artificial process or material.

synthetic chemistry The science dealing with the formation of chemical compounds from simpler substances.

synthetic oleovitamin D See **viosterol.**

syntrophoblast See **syncytiotrophoblast.**

syphilis A venereal infection caused by the spirochete *Treponema pallidum*, usually transmitted by sexual contact and characterized by distinct stages of effects over a period of years. Any organ system may become involved. The spirochete is able to pass through human placenta, producing congenital syphilis. The first stage (**primary syphilis**) is marked by the appearance of a small, painless, red pustule on the skin or mucous membrane between 10 and 90 days after exposure. The lesion may appear anywhere on the body where contact with a lesion on an infected person has occurred, but it is seen most often in the anogenital region. It quickly erodes, forming a painless, bloodless ulcer, called a chancre, exuding a fluid that swarms with spirochetes. It heals spontaneously within 10 to 40 days, often creating the mistaken impression that the sore was not a serious event. The second stage (**secondary syphilis**) occurs about 2 months later, after the spirochetes have increased in number and spread throughout the body. This stage is characterized by general malaise, anorexia, nausea, fever, headache, alopecia, bone and joint pain, or the appearance of a morbiliform rash that does not itch, flat white sores in the mouth and throat, or condylomata lata papules on the moist areas of the skin. The disease remains highly contagious at this stage and can be spread by kissing. The symptoms usually continue for 3 weeks to 3 months but may be recurrent over a period of 2 years. The

959

third stage (**tertiary syphilis**) may not develop for 3 to 15 or more years. It is characterized by the appearance of soft, rubbery tumors, called gummas, that ulcerate and heal by scarring. Gummas may develop anywhere on the body surface and in the eyes, liver, lungs, stomach, or reproductive organs. Tertiary syphilis may be painless or accompanied by deep, burrowing pain. The ulceration of the gummas may result in punched-out areas of the palate, nasal septum, or larynx. Various tissues and structures of the body may be damaged or destroyed, leading to mental or physical disability and premature death. **Congenital syphilis** resulting from prenatal infection may result in the birth of a deformed or blind infant. In some cases, the infant appears to be well until, at several weeks of age, snuffles, sometimes with a blood-stained or mucopurulent discharge, and skin lesions are observed, particularly on the palms and soles or in the genital region. Such children may also have visual or hearing defects and progeria, and poor health may develop. Diagnosis of syphilis is made by darkfield microscopy of fluid from primary or secondary stage lesions, by bacteriologic study of blood samples, and by an examination of cerebrospinal fluid. Patients with primary or secondary syphilis are usually given benzathine penicillin or an equivalent in a single dose of 2.4 million units or in two doses of 1.2 million units intramuscularly. Treatment of an infected mother with penicillin during the first 4 months of pregnancy usually prevents the development of congenital syphilis. Treating the mother with antibiotics later in the pregnancy usually eliminates the infection but may not protect the fetus. See also **chancre, Hutchinson's teeth, snuffles.**

syphilitic aortitis An inflammatory condition of the aorta, occurring in tertiary syphilis and characterized by diffuse dilatation with gray, wheallike plaques containing calcium on the inner coat and scars and wrinkles on the outer coat. The middle layer of the vascular wall is usually infiltrated with plasma cells and contains fragments of damaged elastic tissue and many newly formed blood vessels. There may be damage to the aortic valves, narrowing of the mouths of the coronary arteries, and the formation of thrombi. Cerebral embolism may result. Signs of syphilitic aortitis are substernal pain, dyspnea, bounding pulse, and high systolic blood pressure. Penicillin may slow the course of the disease, but it cannot reverse the structural damage to the vessels and the heart. Also called **Döhle-Heller disease, luetic aortitis.**

syphilitic meningoencephalitis See **general paresis.**

syphilitic periarteritis An inflammatory condition of the outer coat of one or more arteries occurring in tertiary syphilis and characterized by soft, gummatous, perivascular lesions infiltrated with lymphocytes and plasma cells. Also called **periarteritis gummosa.** See also **syphilitic aortitis.**

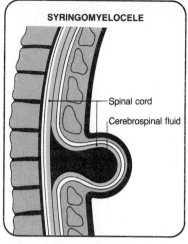

SYRINGOMYELOCELE

— Spinal cord
Cerebrospinal fluid

syring-, syringo- A combining form meaning 'of or pertaining to a tube or a fistula': *syringobulbia, syringocystoma.*

syringe A device for withdrawing, injecting, or instilling fluids. A syringe for the injection of medication usually consists of a calibrated glass or plastic cylindrical barrel having a close-fitting plunger at one end and a small opening at the other to which the head of a hollow-bore needle is fitted.

syringomyelocele A hernial protrusion of the spinal cord through a congenital defect in the vertebral column in which the cerebrospinal fluid within the central cavities of the cord is greatly increased so that the cord tissue forms a thin-walled sac that lies close to the membrane of the cavity. See also **myelomeningocele, neural tube defect, spina bifida.**

system A collection or assemblage of parts that, unified, make a whole. Physiologic systems, as the cardiovascular system, are made up of structures specifically able to engage in processes that are essential for a vital function.

systematic tabulation In research: mechanical or manual techniques for recording and classifying data for statistical analysis.

systemic Of or pertaining to the whole body rather than to a localized area or regional portion of the body.

systemic desensitization A technique used in behavior therapy for eliminating maladaptive anxiety associated with phobias. The procedure involves the construction by the person of a hierarchy of anxiety-producing stimuli and the general presentation of these stimuli until they no longer elicit the initial response of fear. Also called **desensitization.** Compare **flooding.** See also **reciprocal inhibition.**

systemic lupus erythematosus (SLE) A chronic inflammatory disease affecting many body systems. The pathophysiology of the disease includes severe vasculitis, renal involvement, and lesions of the skin and nervous system.

The primary cause of the disease has not been determined; viral infection or dysfunction of the immune system has been suggested. Four times more women than men have SLE. The initial manifestation is often arthritis. An erythematous rash over the nose and malar eminences, weakness, fatigue, and weight loss are also frequently seen early in the disease. Photosensitivity, fever, skin lesions on the neck, and alopecia where the skin lesions extend beyond the hairline may occur. The skin lesions may spread to the mucous membranes and other tissues of the body. Depending on the organs involved, the patient may also have glomerulonephritis, pleuritis, pericarditis, peritonitis, neuritis, or anemia. Renal failure and severe neurologic abnormalities are among the most serious manifestations of the disease. Diagnosis of SLE is based on physical examination and laboratory findings, including antinuclear antibodies in the cerebrospinal fluid and a positive lupus erythematosus cell reaction in a lupus erythematosus preparation. In many cases, SLE may be controlled with corticosteroid medication administered systemically. Also called **disseminated lupus erythematosus, lupus erythematosus.**

systemic remedy A medicinal substance that is given orally, parenterally, or rectally to be absorbed into the circulation for treatment of a health problem. Many remedies or medications administered locally or regionally are, to some degree, absorbed systemically.

systemic vein One of a number of veins that drain deoxygenated blood from most of the body. Systemic veins arise in tiny plexuses that receive blood from the billions of capillaries lacing the body tissues and converge into trunks, which increase in size as they pass toward the heart. They are larger and more numerous than the arteries, have thinner walls, and collapse when they are empty. Kinds of systemic veins are identified according to location, as deep veins, superficial veins, and venous sinuses.

system of care A framework within which health care is delivered, comprised of actors or agents; recipients, consumers, or patients; energy resources or dynamics; organizational and political contexts or frameworks; and processes or procedures. Current theory recognizes that an analysis of the delivery of health care requires knowledge of the systems of care.

systole The normal contraction of the heart, especially of the ventricles, driving blood into the aorta and pulmonary artery. The occurrence of systole is indicated by the first heart sound heard on auscultation, by the palpable apex beat, and by the peripheral pulse. Systole is sometimes described as occurring in three phases: pre-ejection, ejection, and relaxation periods.

-systole A combining form referring to 'types and locations of the higher blood pressure measurement': *dyssystole, hysterosystole.*

systolic click An extra heart sound that occurs in midsystole or in late systole. It is usually of no significance but may be associated with abnormal function of the mitral valve. Compare **ejection click.**

systolic gradient The difference in pressure in the left atrium and left ventricle during systole.

systolic murmur Cardiac murmur occurring during systole. Systolic murmurs are generally less significant than diastolic murmurs and occur in many people with no evidence of heart disease. Systolic murmurs include ejection murmurs often heard in pregnancy or in people with anemia, thyrotoxicosis, or aortic or pulmonary stenosis; pansystolic murmurs heard in people with incompetence of the mitral or tricuspid valve; and late systolic murmurs, also caused by mitral valve incompetence.

T

T 1. *abbr* **tumor** in the TNM system for staging malignant neoplastic disease. See **cancer staging.** 2. Symbol for **temperature.**

T₃ Symbol for **triiodothyronine.**

T₄ Symbol for **thyroxine.**

Ta Symbol for **tantalum.**

TA *abbr* **transactional analysis.**

ta- See **tono-.**

tabe- A combining form meaning 'of or pertaining to wasting (away)': *tabefaction, tabescent.*

tabes dorsalis An abnormal condition characterized by the slow degeneration of all or part of the body and the progressive loss of peripheral reflexes. This disease involves the posterior columns and the posterior roots of the spinal cord and destroys the large joints of affected limbs in some individuals. It is often accompanied by incontinence and impotence and severe flashing pains in the abdomen and the extremities. The cause of tabes dorsalis is unclear and it is believed to be an uncommon disorder.

tablet A small, solid dosage form of a medication. It may be compressed or molded in its manufacture. Most tablets are intended to be swallowed whole, but some may be dissolved in the mouth, chewed, or dissolved in liquid before swallowing; some may be placed in a body cavity.

tacho- A combining form meaning 'of or pertaining to speed': *tachogram, tachography.*

tachy- A combining form meaning 'swift or rapid': *tachycardia, tachypnea.*

tachycardia A circulatory condition in which the myocardium contracts regularly but at an accelerated rate of 100 to 150 beats per minute. Pathologic tachycardia accompanies anoxia, as caused by anemia, congestive heart failure, hemorrhage, or shock.

tachyphylaxis 1. In pharmacology: a phenomenon in which the repeated administration of some drugs results in a marked decrease in effectiveness. 2. In immunology: rapidly developing immunity to a toxin owing to previous exposure, as from previous injection of small amounts of the toxin. Also called **mithridatism.**

tachypnea An abnormally rapid rate of breathing, as seen with hyperpyrexia. See also **respiratory rate.**

tact- A combining form meaning 'of or pertaining to touch': *tactile, tactilogical.*

-tactic 1. A combining form meaning 'exhibiting agent-controlled orientation or movement': *chemotactic, eosinotactic, thermotactic.* 2. A combining form meaning 'having an arrangement of something': *cytotactic, leukotactic.* Also **-tactical, -taxic.**

tactile Of or pertaining to the sense of touch.

tactile anesthesia The absence or lack of the sense of touch in the fingers, possibly resulting from injury or disease. This condition can be congenital or psychosomatic and may cause the patient to incur severe burns, serious cuts, contusions, or abrasions. See also **traumatic anesthesia.**

tactile corpuscle One of many small, oval end organs associated with the sense of touch, widely distributed throughout the body in peripheral areas, as the papillae of the coria of the hands and feet, front of the forehead, skin of the lips, and skin of the mammary papillae. Each corpuscle consists of a tiny, round structure surrounded by a capsule penetrated by a nerve fiber that spirals through the interior of the capsule and ends in globular enlargements. Also called **Meissner's corpuscle.**

tactile corpuscle of Meissner See **Wagner-Meissner corpuscle.**

tactile fremitus A tremulous vibration of the chest wall during respiration that is palpable. It may indicate inflammation, infection, congestion, or, most commonly, consolidation of a lung or a part of a lung.

tactile image A mental concept of an object as perceived through the sense of touch. See also **image.**

Taenia A genus of large, parasitic, intestinal flatworms of the family Taeniidae, class Cestoda, having an armed scolex and a series of segments in a chain. Taeniae are among the most common parasites infecting humans and include *Taenia saginata* and *T. solium.*

taenia- See **tenia-.**

Taenia saginata A species of tapeworm that inhabits the tissues of cattle during its larval stage and infects the intestine of humans in its adult form. *Taenia saginata* may grow to a length of between 3.6 and 7.6 m (12 and 25 feet) and is the tapeworm species that most often infects humans. Also called **beef tapeworm.** See also **tapeworm, tapeworm infection.**

taeniasis An infection with a tapeworm of the genus *Taenia.* See also **tapeworm infection.**

Taenia solium A species of tapeworm that most commonly inhabits the tissues of pigs during its larval stage and infects the intestine of humans in its adult form. Humans may serve as the intermediate hosts and larval infestation of the muscle and brain tissue may occur. Also called **pork tapeworm.** See also **cysticercosis, tapeworm, tapeworm infection.**

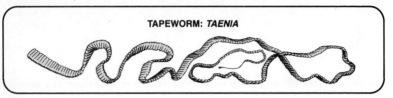

TAPEWORM: *TAENIA*

tail bud See **end bud.**

tail fold A curved ridge formed at the caudal end of the early developing embryo. It consists of the tail bud, which in lower animals gives rise to the caudal appendage and in man forms the hindgut.

tailor's bottom See **weaver's bottom.**

Takayasu's arteritis A disorder characterized by progressive occlusion of the brachiocephalic trunk and the left subclavian and left common carotid arteries above their origin in the aortic arch. Signs of the disorder are the absence of a pulse in both arms and in the carotid arteries, transient paraplegia, transient blindness, and atrophy of the facial muscles. Also called **brachiocephalic arteritis, Martorell's syndrome, pulseless disease, reversed coarctation.**

Takayasu's disease See **aortic arch syndrome.**

talbutal A barbiturate sedative-hypnotic.

talc (magnesium silicate) A protectant and absorbent dusting powder used to treat skin irritations.

talip- A combining form meaning 'clubfooted': *taliped, talipes, talipomanus.*

talipes A deformity, usually congenital, in which the foot is twisted and relatively fixed in an abnormal position. See also **flatfoot, pes cavus.**

talipes cavus See **pes cavus.**

talo- A combining form meaning 'of or pertaining to the ankle': *talocalcaneal, talocrural, talofibular.*

talus, pl. **tali** The second largest tarsal bone. It supports the tibia, rests on the calcaneus, and articulates with the malleoli and with the navicular bones. The talus consists of a body, a neck, and a head. Also called ankle bone, astragalus.

tamoxifen citrate An antineoplastic agent that alters hormone balance.

tampon A pack of cotton, a sponge, or other material used for checking bleeding, absorbing secretions in cavities or canals, or holding displaced organs in position.

tamponade Stoppage of the blood flow to an organ or body part by pressure, as by a tampon or a pressure dressing applied to stop a hemorrhage or by the compression of a blood vessel by an accumulation of fluid, as in cardiac tamponade.

Tangier disease A rare familial deficiency of high-density lipoproteins, characterized by low blood cholesterol and an abnormal orange or yellow discoloration of the tonsils and pharynx. There may also be enlarged lymph nodes, liver, and spleen; muscle atrophy; and peripheral neuropathy. No specific treatment is known.

tannic acid An astringent.

tannin Any of a group of astringent substances obtained from plants, used for the tanning of leather. Tannic acid, a mixture of tannins, is used in the treatment of burns.

tanning A process in which the pigmentation of the skin deepens as a result of exposure to ultraviolet light. Skin cells containing melanin darken immediately. New melanin is formed within 2 to 3 days and moves upward rapidly, allowing the darkening process to continue.

tantalum (Ta) A silvery metallic element. Its atomic number is 73; its atomic weight is 180.95. Relatively inert chemically, tantalum is used in prosthetic devices, such as skull plates and wire sutures.

tantrum A sudden outburst or violent display of rage, frustration, and bad temper, usually occurring in maladjusted children and certain emotionally disturbed persons. The activity is usually not directed at anyone or anything specific but toward the environment in general and is used primarily as a device for attempting to control others and the surroundings. Also called **temper tantrum.**

tapeworm A parasitic, intestinal worm belonging to the class Cestoda and having a scolex and a ribbon-shaped body composed of segments in a chain. Humans usually acquire tapeworms by eating the undercooked meat of intermediate hosts contaminated by the larval form of the tapeworm. In the human alimentary canal, the worm develops into an adult with a scolex and numerous proglottids, each of which is capable of producing eggs. Kinds of tapeworm include *Diphyllobothrium, Taenia.* Also called **cestode.**

tapeworm infection An intestinal infection by one of several species of parasitic worms, caused by eating raw or undercooked meat infested with a tapeworm or its larvae. Symptoms of intestinal infection with adult worms are usually mild or absent, but diarrhea, epigastric pain, and weight loss may occur. Diagnosis is made when eggs or portions of the adult worm are passed in the stool. The drugs niclosamide and quinacrine are used to loosen and dissolve the worm, so it may be excreted. Sanitary disposal of fecal material from affected patients is necessary to prevent the passage of larvae or eggs to humans or other hosts. Certain species of tapeworm can infect humans during the larval stage, causing a serious, often cystic, condition of larval infestation. Also called **cestodiasis.** See also **cysticercosis, tapeworm.**

tapho- A combining form meaning 'of or pertaining to the grave': *taphophilia, taphophobia.*

tapotement A massage in which the body is tapped rhythmically with the fingertips or the sides of the hands, using short, rapid, repetitive movements. The procedure is often used on the chest wall of patients with bronchitis to help loosen the mucus in the air passages. See also **massage.**

tardive dyskinesia An abnormal condition characterized by involuntary, repetitious movements of the muscles of the face, limbs, and trunk. This disorder most commonly affects older people who have been treated for extended periods with phenothiazine drugs to alleviate the symptoms of parkinsonism. The involuntary movements may slacken or disappear after weeks or months and may be significantly reduced by the administration of large doses of choline chloride.

tardy peroneal nerve palsy An abnormal condition and a type of mononeuropathy in which the peroneal nerve is excessively compressed where it crosses the head of the fibula. Such compression may occur when an individual falls asleep with the legs crossed.

tardy ulnar nerve palsy An abnormal condition characterized by atrophy of the first dorsal interosseous muscle and difficulty performing fine manipulations. It may be caused by injury of the ulnar nerve at the elbow and commonly affects individuals with a shallow ulnar groove or those who persistently rest their weight on their elbows. Signs and symptoms of this disorder may include numbness of the small finger, the contiguous half of the proximal and middle phalanges of the ring finger, and the ulnar border of the hand. Treatment concentrates on the prevention of further injury.

target cell 1. An abnormal red blood cell characterized, when stained and examined under a microscope, by a densely stained center surrounded by a pale, unstained ring circled by a dark, irregular band. Target cells occur in the blood after splenectomy, in anemia, in hemoglobin C disease, and in thalassemia. Compare **discocyte, spherocyte. 2.** Any cell having a specific receptor that reacts with a specific hormone, antigen, antibody, antibiotic, sensitized T cell, or other substance.

target organ 1. In radiotherapy: an organ intended to receive a therapeutic dose of irradiation. 2. In nuclear medicine: an organ intended to receive the greatest concentration of a diagnostic radioactive tracer. 3. In endocrinology: an organ most affected by a specific hormone.

tars Antipruritic agents.

tarsal Of or pertaining to the tarsus or ankle bone.

tarsal bone Any one of seven bones comprising the tarsus of the foot, consisting of the talus, calcaneus, cuboid, navicular, and the three cuneiforms.

tarsal gland One of numerous modified sebaceous glands on the inner surfaces of the eye-

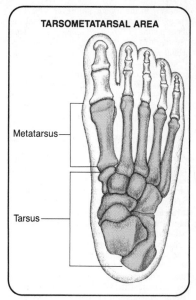

TARSOMETATARSAL AREA

Metatarsus—

Tarsus—

lids. About 30 tarsal glands, resembling tiny, parallel strings of pearls, line each upper eyelid, and somewhat fewer tarsal glands line each lower eyelid. They are embedded in grooves in the inner surfaces of the tarsi, their lengths corresponding to the width of the tarsal plates. The ducts of the tarsal glands open by tiny apertures on the free margins of the eyelids. Each gland consists of a single straight follicle with numerous lateral branches. The follicles are supported by a basement membrane and lined at their mouths by stratified epithelium. Polyhedral cells line the deeper parts of the follicles and their lateral diverticula. Also called **Meibomian gland.** Compare **ciliary gland.**

tarsal tunnel syndrome An abnormal condition and a kind of mononeuropathy, characterized by pain and numbness in the sole of the foot. This disorder may be caused by ankle fractures which compress the posterior tibial nerve and may be corrected by appropriate orthopedic therapy or by surgery.

tarso- A combining form meaning 'of or pertaining to the edge of the foot or to the eyelid': *tarsoclasis, tarsomalacia, tarsometatarsal.*

tarsometatarsal Of or pertaining to the metatarsal bones and the tarsus of the foot, especially the articulations of the metatarsal bones with the cuneiform and cuboid bones at the instep of the foot.

tarsus, *pl.* **tarsi** 1. The area of articulation between the foot and the leg. 2. Any one of the plates of cartilage about 2.5 cm (1 inch) long forming the eyelids. One tarsal plate shapes each eyelid. The superior tarsal plates form the upper eyelids; the inferior tarsal plates, the lower eyelids. The superior tarsal plates are semilunar, about 10 mm wide at the center, and attach anteriorly to the levator palpebrae superioris. The inferior tarsal plates are thin, elliptical, and about 5 mm in vertical diameter. The plates' free margins are thick and straight, with the orbital margins attached to the circumference of the orbit by the orbital septum and the lateral angles attached to the zygomatic bones by the lateral palpebral raphes. The medial angles of the plates end at the lacus lacrimalis and attach to the frontal process of the maxilla by the medial palpebral ligament. —**tarsal,** *adj.*

tartar **1.** A hard, gritty deposit composed of organic matter, phosphates, and carbonates that collects on the teeth and gums. See also **gingivitis. 2.** Any of several compounds containing tartrate, the salt of tartaric acid. See **antimony potassium tartrate.**

tartar emetic See **antimony potassium tartrate.**

tartaric acid A colorless or white powder found in various plants and prepared commercially from maleic anhydride and hydrogen peroxide. It is used in tartar emetic.

-tas A noun-forming combining form: *fragilitas, graviditas, infertilitas.*

taste The sense of perceiving different flavors in soluble substances that contact the tongue and trigger nerve impulses to special taste centers in the cortex and the thalamus of the brain. The four basic traditional tastes are sweet, salty, sour, and bitter. The front of the tongue is most sensitive to salty and sweet substances; the sides of the tongue are most sensitive to sour substances; and the back of the tongue is most sensitive to bitter substances. The middle of the tongue produces virtually no taste sensation. Chemoreceptor cells in the taste buds of the tongue detect different substances. Adults have about 9,000 taste buds, most of them situated on the upper surface of the tongue. The sense of taste is intricately linked with the sense of smell, and taste discrimination is very complex.

taste bud Any one of many peripheral taste organs distributed over the tongue and the roof of the mouth. Each taste bud rests in a spherical pocket, which extends through the epithelium. Gustatory cells and supporting cells form each bud, which has a surface opening and an opening in the basement membrane. Also called **gustatory organ.**

TAT *abbr* **tetanus antitoxin.**

tauto- A combining form meaning 'same': *tautomenial, tautomeral, tautomerism.*

tax- A combining form meaning 'order or arrangement': *taxis, taxology, taxonomy.*

-taxia A combining form meaning: **1.** A '(condition of) impaired mental or physical control': *acroataxia, cardiataxia, hypotaxia.* **2.** A '(condition of) internal ordering or arrangement': *cataxia, heterotaxia, prostaxia.* Also **-taxis, -taxy.**

-taxic See **-tactic.**

-taxis A combining form meaning: **1.** A '(specified) arrangement': *biotaxis, heterotaxis.* **2.** A 'movement of an organism in response to a stimulus': *aerotaxis, geotaxis.* Also **-taxia, -taxy.**

taxonomy A system for classifying organisms on the basis of natural relationships and assigning them appropriate names. —**taxonomic,** *adj.*

-taxy See **-taxia, -taxis.**

Taylor brace A padded steel brace used to support the spine. Also called Taylor splint.

Tay-Sachs disease An inherited, neurodegenerative disorder of lipid metabolism caused by a deficiency of the enzyme hexosaminidase A, which results in the accumulation of sphingolipids in the brain. The condition, which is transmitted as an autosomal recessive trait, occurs predominantly in families of Eastern European Jewish origin, specifically the Ashkenazic Jews, and is characterized by progressive mental and physical retardation and early death. Symptoms first appear by 6 months of age, after which no new skills are learned and there is progressive loss of those skills already acquired. Convulsions and atrophy of the optic nerve head occur after 1 year, followed by blindness, with a cherry-red spot on each retina, spasticity, dementia, and paralysis. Most children die between the ages of 2 and 4 years. There is no therapy for the condition, and intervention is purely symptomatic and supportive. The disease can be diagnosed in utero through amniocentesis. Also called **amaurotic familial idiocy, gangliosidosis type I, infantile cerebral sphingolipidosis, Sachs' disease.** See also **Sandhoff's disease.**

Tay's spot See **cherry-red spot.**

Tb Symbol for **terbium.**

TB *abbr* **tuberculosis.**

T binder A binder in the shape of the letter T. It is used for the perineum and sometimes for the head. Also called **crucial bandage, Heliodorus' bandage.**

TBP *abbr* **1.** bithionol. **2.** total bypass.

Tc Symbol for **technetium.**

T cell A small circulating lymphocyte produced in the bone marrow that matures in the thymus or as a result of exposure to thymosin secreted by the thymus. T cells have several functions but primarily mediate cellular immune responses, as graft rejection and delayed hypersensitivity. One kind of T cell, the **helper cell,** affects the production of antibodies by B cells; a **suppressor T cell** suppresses B cell activity. Compare **B cell.** See also **immune response.**

TD *abbr* **toxic dose.**

TD50 See **median toxic dose.**

tDNA *abbr* **transfer DNA.**

Te Symbol for **tellurium.**

tea *Slang.* See **cannabis.**

teacher's nodule See **vocal cord nodule.**

teaching rounds The somewhat informal conferences held regularly, often at the beginning of the day. Various members of the department and staff may attend, including nurses, residents, interns, students, attending physicians, and faculty. Specific problems in the care of current patients are discussed. See also **nursing rounds.**

team nursing A decentralized system in

which the care of a patient is distributed among the members of a team. The charge nurse delegates authority to a team leader, who must be a professional nurse. The team leader assigns tasks, schedules care, and instructs team members. A conference is held at the beginning and at the end of each shift to allow team members to exchange information and the team leader to make changes in the nursing-care plan for any patient. Compare **primary nursing.**

team practice Professional practice by a group of professionals that may include physicians, nurses, and others, as a social worker, nutritionist, or physical therapist, who manage the care of a specified number of patients as a team, usually in an outpatient setting.

teardrop fracture An avulsion fracture of one of the short bones, as a vertebra, causing a tear-shaped disruption of bone tissue.

tear duct Any duct that carries tears, including the lacrimal ducts, nasolacrimal ducts, and the excretory ducts of the lacrimal glands.

tearing Watering of the eye, usually caused by excessive tear production, as by emotion, infection, or mechanical irritation by a foreign body. If the normal amount of fluid tears is produced but not drained into the lacrimal punctum at the nasal border of the eye, tearing will occur. If the lacrimal punctum, sac, cuniculi, or nasolacrimal duct becomes blocked, tears will also overflow. Also called **epiphora.**

technetium (Tc) A radioactive, metallic element. Its atomic number is 43; its atomic weight is 99. The first man-made element, technetium also occurs in nature. Isotopes of technetium are used in radioisotope scanning procedures of internal organs.

-technic See **-technique.**

-technics A combining form meaning 'the art or mechanics of': *balneotechnics, mnemotechnics.* Also **-technology, -techny.**

technique, technic The method and details followed in performing a procedure, as those used in conducting a laboratory test, a physical examination, or any process requiring certain skills or an ordered sequence of actions.

-technique A combining form meaning 'the skillful way in which something is done': *iatrotechnique, microtechnique, zymotechnique.* Also **-technic.**

techno- A combining form meaning 'art': *technocausis, technology, technopsychology.*

-technology See **-technics.**

-techny A combining form meaning 'the art or mechanics of a specified area: *odontotechny, zootechny, zymotechny.* Also **-technics, -technology.**

tecto- A combining form meaning 'rooflike': *tectocephalic, tectorial.*

teether An object, as a teething ring, on which an infant can bite or chew during the teething process.

teething The physiological process of the eruption of the deciduous teeth through the gums. It normally begins between the 6th and 8th months of life and occurs periodically until the complete

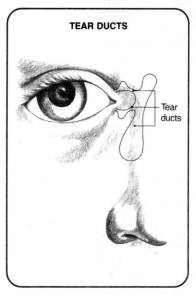

TEAR DUCTS

Tear ducts

set of 20 teeth has appeared at about 30 months. Discomfort and inflammation result from the pressure exerted against the periodontal tissue as the crown of the tooth breaks through the membranes. General signs of teething include excessive drooling, biting on hard objects, irritability, difficulty in sleeping, and refusal of food. Fever or diarrhea often occurs during teething but is indicative of illness rather than of teething. The pain and inflammation may usually be soothed by cold, as with a frozen teething ring, cold metal spoon, or ice wrapped in a washcloth. —**teethe,** *v.*

teething ring A circular device, usually made of plastic or rubber, on which an infant may chew or bite during the teething process.

teg- A combining form meaning 'of or pertaining to a cover': *tegmen, tegmental, tegument.*

TEIB *abbr* triethylene-immuno-benzoquinone.

tela- A combining form meaning 'a web or weblike structure': *telalgia, telangiectasia, telangitis.*

-tela A combining form meaning a 'weblike membrane': *aulatela, epitela, metatela.*

telangiectasia Permanent dilatation of groups of superficial capillaries and venules. Common causes are actinic damage, atrophy-producing dermatoses, rosacea, elevated estrogen levels, and collagen-vascular diseases. See also **Osler-Weber-Rendu syndrome, spider angioma.**

telangiectasis A spot, usually on the skin, produced by dilatation of a capillary or terminal artery.

telangiectatic epulis A benign, red tumor of the gingiva, containing prominent blood vessels. Low-grade or chronic irritation is usually associated, and the lesion is easily traumatized.

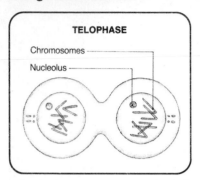

TELOPHASE

Chromosomes

Nucleolus

telangiectatic fibroma See **angiofibroma.**

telangiectatic glioma A tumor composed of glial cells and a network of blood vessels, which give the mass a vivid pink appearance.

telangiectatic granuloma See **pyogenic granuloma.**

telangiectatic lipoma See **angiolipoma.**

telangiectatic nevus A common skin condition of neonates, characterized by flat, deep-pink localized areas of capillary dilatation that occur predominantly on the back of the neck, lower occiput, upper eyelids, upper lip, and bridge of the nose. The dilatated areas disappear by about 2 years of age. Also called **capillary flames, stork bite.**

telangiectatic sarcoma A malignant tumor of mesodermal cells with an unusually rich vascular network.

tele- A combining form meaning: **1.** 'Of or related to the end': *telencephalon, teleneuron, telesystolic.* **2.** 'Operating at a distance or far away': *telecardiogram, teleceptor, telemetry.*

telepathist 1. A person who believes in telepathy. **2.** A person who has or claims to have telepathic powers.

telepathy Thought communication from one person to another by means other than the physical senses. Also called **thought transference.** See also **extrasensory perception, parapsychology.** —**telepathic,** *adj.,* **telepathize,** *v.*

tellurium (Te) An element exhibiting metallic and nonmetallic chemical properties. Its atomic number is 52; its atomic weight is 127.60.

telo- A combining form meaning 'of or pertaining to the end': *telobiosis, telodendron, telosynapsis.*

telocentric Pertaining to a chromosome in which the centromere is located at the end, so that the chromatids appear as straight filaments. Compare **acrocentric, metacentric, submetacentric.**

telogen See **hair.**

telophase The final stage of nuclear division in mitosis and in each of the two divisions in meiosis. The newly produced daughter chromosomes from the preceding anaphase stage assemble at the poles of the division spindle and become long and slender, the nuclear membrane forms around them, the nucleolus reappears,

and the cytoplasm begins to divide. See also **anaphase, interphase, meiosis, metaphase, mitosis, prophase.**

temazepam A benzodiazepine sedative-hypnotic agent.

temperate phage A bacteriophage whose genome is incorporated into the host bacterium. It persists through many cell divisions of the host without destroying it, in contrast to a virulent phage that lyses and kills its host.

temperature 1. A relative measure of sensible heat or cold. **2.** In physiology: a measure of sensible heat associated with the metabolism of the human body, normally maintained at a constant level of 37°C (98.6°F) by the thermotaxic nerve mechanism that balances heat gains and heat losses. **3.** *Informal.* A fever.

temper tantrum See **tantrum.**

template In genetics: the DNA strand that acts as a mold for the synthesis of messenger RNA. This messenger RNA contains the same sequence of nucleic acids as the DNA strand and carries the code to the ribosomes in the cytoplasm for the synthesis of proteins.

tempo- A combining form meaning 'of or pertaining to time': *tempolabile, temporal, tempostabile.*

temporal arteritis A progressive, inflammatory disorder of cranial blood vessels, principally the temporal artery, occurring most in women over the age of 70. Characteristic changes in the involved vessels include granulomatous disruption of the elastic layer and engulfment of fiber fragments by giant cells in the intimal and medial layers. Symptoms are intractable headache, difficulty in chewing, weakness, rheumatic pains, and loss of vision if the central retinal artery becomes occluded. Also called **cranial arteritis, giant cell arteritis, Horton's arteritis.**

temporal artery Any one of three arteries on each side of the head: the superficial temporal artery, the middle temporal artery, and the deep temporal artery.

temporal bone One of a pair of large bones forming part of the lower cranium and containing cavities and recesses associated with the ear, as the tympanic cavity and the auditory tube. Each temporal bone consists of three portions: the squama, the petrous, and the tympanic.

temporal bone fracture A break of the temporal bone of the skull, sometimes characterized by bleeding from the ear. Diminished hearing, facial paralysis, or infection of the tympanic cavity leading to meningitis may occur.

temporalis One of the four muscles of mastication. It is a broad, radiating muscle that arises from the whole of the temporal fossa and from the surface of the temporal fascia. It inserts into the ramus of the mandible near the last molar tooth, and it is innervated by the anterior and the posterior temporal nerves. The temporalis acts to close the jaws and retract the mandible. Also called **temporal muscle.** Compare **masseter, pterygoideus lateralis, pterygoideus medialis.**

temporal lobe The lateral region of the cerebrum, below the lateral fissure. Within the lobe are the center for smell, some association areas for memory and learning, and a region where choice is made of thoughts to express. Compare **frontal lobe, occipital lobe, parietal lobe.**

temporal lobe epilepsy See **psychomotor seizure.**

temporal summation See **summation.**

temporary tooth See **deciduous tooth.**

temporomandibular joint One of two joints connecting the mandible to the temporal bone. It is a combined hinge and gliding joint, formed by the anterior parts of the mandibular fossae of the temporal bone, the articular tubercles, the condyles of the mandible, and five ligaments.

temporomandibular joint pain-dysfunction syndrome An abnormal condition characterized by facial pain and mandibular dysfunction, apparently caused by a defective or dislocated temporomandibular joint. Some common indications of this syndrome are the clicking of the joint when the jaws move, limitation of jaw movement, subluxation, and temporomandibular dislocation. Also called **myofacial pain-dysfunction syndrome.**

temporoparietalis One of a pair of broad, thin scalp muscles, divided into three parts, which fan out over the temporal fascia and insert into the galea aponeurotica. The three parts include an anterior temporal portion, a superior parietal portion, and a triangular portion in between. The temporoparietalis was formerly considered part of the superior and the inferior auricularis. On both sides, it acts with the occipitofrontalis to wrinkle the forehead, widen the eyes, and raise the ears. It is innervated by branches of the facial nerve. Compare **occipitofrontalis.**

TEN *abbr* toxic epidermal necrolysis.

tenaculum, *pl.* **tenacula** A clip or clamp with long handles used to grasp, immobilize, and hold an organ or a piece of tissue. Kinds of tenacula include the abdominal tenaculum, which has long arms and small hooks; the **cervical tenaculum,** which has short hooks or open, eyeshaped clamps used to hold the cervix; and the **forceps tenaculum,** which has long hooks and is used in gynecologic surgery.

tendinitis, tendonitis An inflammatory condition of a tendon, usually resulting from strain. Treatment may include rest, corticosteroid injections, and support.

tendo calcaneus The common tendon of the soleus and gastrocnemius. It is the thickest and strongest tendon in the body and begins near the middle of the posterior part of the leg. In an adult it is about 15 cm (6 inches) long. The tendon becomes contracted about 4 cm (1½ inches) above the heel and flares out again to insert into the calcaneus. Also called **Achilles tendon, calcaneal tendon.**

tendon One of many white, glistening, fibrous bands of tissue that attach muscle to bone. Except at points of attachment, tendons are

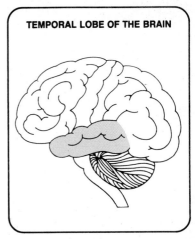

TEMPORAL LOBE OF THE BRAIN

sheathed in delicate fibroelastic connective tissue. Larger tendons contain a thin internal septum, a few blood vessels, and specialized sterognostic nerves. Tendons are extremely strong and flexible, inelastic, and occur in various lengths and thicknesses. Compare **ligament.** **—tendinous,** *adj.*

tendon reflex See **deep tendon reflex.**

tenesmus Persistent, ineffectual spasms of the rectum or bladder, accompanied by the desire to empty the bowel or bladder. Intestinal tenesmus is a common complaint in inflammatory bowel disease and irritable bowel syndrome.

tenia-, taenia- A combining form meaning 'ribbon, band': *taeniasis, teniafuge, taenidium.*

teniposide (VM-26) A podophyllin derivative chemotherapeutic drug.

tennis elbow See **lateral humeral epicondylitis.**

teno-, tenonto- A combining form meaning 'of or pertaining to a tendon': *tenodesis, tenodynia, tenomyotomy.*

Tenon's capsule See **fascia bulbi.**

tenosynovitis Inflammation of a tendon sheath caused by calcium deposits, repeated strain or trauma, high levels of blood cholesterol, rheumatoid arthritis, gout, or gonorrhea. In some instances, movement yields crackling noise over the tendon. Most cases not associated with systemic disease respond to rest.

tenotomy The total or partial severing of a tendon, performed to correct a muscle imbalance, as in the correction of strabismus of the eye or in clubfoot.

TENS *abbr* transcutaneous electrical nerve stimulator.

tension **1.** The act of pulling or straining until taut. **2.** The condition of being taut, tense, or under pressure. **3.** A state or condition resulting from the psychological and physiological reaction to a stressful situation, characterized physically by a general increase in muscle tonus, heart rate, respiration rate, and alertness and

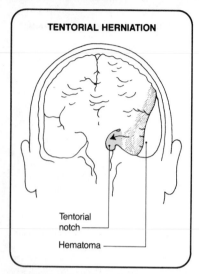

TENTORIAL HERNIATION

Tentorial notch

Hematoma

psychologically by feelings of strain, uneasiness, irritability, and anxiety. See also **stress.**

tension headache A pain that affects the occipital region as the result of overwork or emotional strain, tensing the body and inhibiting rest and relaxation.

tensor Any one of the muscles of the body that tenses a structure. Compare **abductor, adductor, sphincter.**

tensor fasciae latae One of the 10 muscles of the gluteal region, arising from the outer lip of the iliac crest, the iliac spine, and the deep fascia lata. It inserts between the two layers of fascia lata in the proximal third of the thigh. The tensor fasciae latae is innervated by a branch of the superior gluteal nerve, and it functions to flex the thigh and to rotate it slightly medially.

tent 1. A transparent cover, usually of plastic, supported over the upper body by a frame. Used to treat respiratory conditions, it provides a controlled environment into which steam, oxygen, vaporized medication, or droplets of cool water may be sprayed. 2. A cone made of various materials inserted into a cavity or orifice to dilate its opening, as a laminaria tent. 3. A pack placed in a wound to hold it open to ensure that healing progresses from the base of the wound upward.

tenth nerve See **vagus nerve.**

-tention, -tension A combining form meaning: 1. The 'condition of being held': *histortention, retention.* 2. The 'condition of being stretched': *attention, distention, intention.*

tentorial herniation The protrusion of brain tissue into the tentorial notch, caused by increased intracranial pressure from edema, hemorrhage, or a tumor. Characteristic signs are severe headache, fever, flushing, sweating, abnormal pupillary reflex, drowsiness, hypotension, and loss of consciousness. Also called **transtentorial herniation.**

tentorium, *pl.* **tentoria** Any part of the body

that resembles a tent, as the tentorium of the cerebellum.

tentorium cerebelli One of the three extensions of the dura mater that separates the cerebellum from the occipital lobe of the cerebrum. Compare **falx cerebelli, falx cerebri.**

tephr- A combining form meaning 'ash-colored': *tephromalacia, tephromyelitis, tephrylometer.*

tepid Moderately warm to the touch.

teramorphous Of the nature of or characteristic of a monster.

teras, *pl.* **terata** A severely deformed fetus; a monster. —**teratic,** *adj.*

teratism Any congenital or developmental anomaly produced by inherited or environmental factors, or by a combination of the two; any condition in which a severely malformed fetus is produced. Kinds of teratism include **atresic teratism, ceasmic teratism, ectopic teratism, ectrogenic teratism, hypergenetic teratism.** Also called teratosis.

terato- A combining form meaning 'of or related to a monster': *teratoblastoma, teratogenesis, teratoma.*

teratogen Any substance, agent, or process that interferes with normal prenatal development, causing the formation of one or more abnormalities in the fetus. Teratogens act directly on the developing organism or indirectly, affecting such supplemental structures as the placenta or some maternal system. The period of highest vulnerability is from about the 3rd through the 12th week of gestation, when differentiation of the major organs and systems occurs. Susceptibility to teratogenic influence decreases rapidly in the later periods of development. Among the known teratogens are chemical agents, including such drugs as thalidomide, alkylating agents, and alcohol; infectious agents, especially the rubella virus and cytomegalovirus; ionizing radiation, particularly X-rays; and environmental factors, as maternal age and general health. Compare **mutagen.** —**teratogenic,** *adj.*

teratogenesis The development of physical defects in the embryo. —**teratogenetic,** *adj.*

teratogeny See **teratogenesis.** —**teratogenic,** *adj.*

teratoid Of or pertaining to abnormal physical development; resembling a monster.

teratoid tumor See **dermoid cyst.**

teratologist One who specializes in teratology.

teratology The study of the causes and effects of congenital malformations and developmental abnormalities. —**teratologic, teratological,** *adj.*

teratoma, *pl.* **teratomas, teratomata** A tumor composed of different kinds of tissue, none of which normally occur together or at the site of the tumor. Teratomas are most common in the ovaries or testes. Also called **dermoid cyst, organoid cyst, teratoid tumor.**

terbium (Tb) A rare-earth metallic element. Its atomic number is 65; its atomic weight is 158.294.

terbutaline sulfate A sympathomimetic decongestant.

teres, *pl.* **teretes** A long, cylindrical muscle, as the teres minor or the teres major. —**teres,** *adj.*

teres major A thick, flat muscle of the shoulder. Arising from the dorsal surface of the scapula and from the fibrous septa between the teres major, the teres minor, and the infraspinatus, it is innervated by a branch of the lower subscapular nerve from the brachial plexus. It functions to adduct, extend, and rotate the arm medially. Compare **teres minor.**

teres minor A cylindrical, elongated muscle of the shoulder. The teres minor arises from the dorsal surface of the scapula and from two aponeurotic laminae, one of which separates it from the teres major, the other from the infraspinatus. It is inserted into the humerus and is innervated by a branch of the axillary nerve. The teres minor functions to rotate the arm laterally, to weakly adduct the arm, and to draw the humerus toward the glenoid fossa of the scapula, which serves to strengthen the shoulder joint. Compare **teres major.**

terminal Of a structure or process: near or approaching its end, as a terminal bronchiole or a terminal disease. —**terminate,** *v.,* **terminus,** *n.*

terminal nerve A small nerve originating in the cerebral hemisphere in the region of the olfactory trigone, classified by most anatomists as part of the olfactory, or first cranial, nerve. The terminal nerve courses anteriorly along the olfactory tract and passes through the ethmoid bone. Most filaments of the nerve form a single strand, which passes to the membrane near the anterior superior border of the nasal septum and communicates in the nasal cavity with the ophthalmic division of the trigeminal nerve. The central connections of the terminal nerve end in the septal nuclei, the olfactory lobe, and the posterior commissural and supraoptic regions of the brain.

terminal stance One of the five stages in the stance phase of a walking gait, directly associated with the continuation of single limb support or the period during which the body moves forward on the supporting foot. Double limb support is initiated during the latter part of terminal stance, which is often a factor in the analysis of many abnormal orthopedic conditions and the diagnosis of weaknesses that may develop in certain muscles used in walking, as the quadriceps femoris and the gluteus maximus. Compare **initial contact stance stage, loading response stance stage, midstance, preswing stance stage.** See also **swing phase of gait.**

terminal sulcus of the right atrium A shallow channel on the external surface of the right atrium between the superior and inferior venae cavae.

termination codon In molecular genetics: a unit in the genetic code that specifies the end of the sequence of amino acids in a polypeptide.

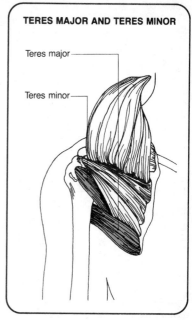

TERES MAJOR AND TERES MINOR

Teres major

Teres minor

termination sequence In molecular genetics: a DNA segment at the end of a unit that is transcribed to messenger RNA from the DNA template.

term infant Any neonate born after the end of the 37th and before the beginning of the 43rd week of gestation. Infants delivered at term usually measure from 48 to 53 cm (19 to 21 inches) dorsally from head to heel and weigh between 2,700 and 4,000 g (6 and 9 lb).

terpin hydrate An expectorant.

territoriality Having proprietary attachment to a domain of nursing, whether geographic or oriented toward a specialty or area of clinical expertise.

terti- A combining form meaning 'third': *tertiary, tertigravida, tertipara.*

tertian Occurring every 3 days, including the first day of occurrence, as **tertian malaria,** in which fever occurs every 3rd day. Compare **quartan.** See also **malaria.**

tertian malaria A form of malaria, caused by the protozoan *Plasmodium vivax* or *P. ovale,* characterized by febrile paroxysms that occur every 48 hours. **Vivax malaria,** caused by *P. vivax,* is the most common form of malaria. Although rarely fatal, it is the most difficult form to cure. Relapses are common. **Ovale malaria,** caused by *P. ovale,* is usually milder and causes only a few, short attacks. Both types of tertian malaria are treated with chloroquine. Compare **falciparum malaria, quartan malaria.** See also **malaria.**

tertiary 1. Third in frequency or in order of use. 2. Belonging to the third level of sophistication of development.

TESTIS

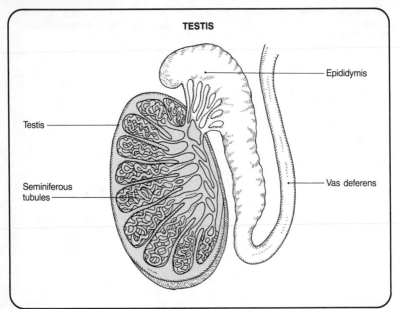

Epididymis

Testis

Vas deferens

Seminiferous
tubules

tertiary health care A specialized, highly technical level of health care that includes diagnosis and treatment of diseases and disabilities. Such care is usually carried on in sophisticated, large research and teaching hospitals. Specialized intensive care units, advanced diagnostic support services, and highly specialized personnel are usually characteristic of tertiary health care. It offers a highly centralized care to the population of a large region and, in some cases, to the world.

test **1.** An examination or trial intended to establish a principle or determine a value. **2.** A chemical reaction or reagent that has clinical significance. **3.** To detect, identify, or conduct a trial. See also **laboratory test.**

test- A combining form meaning 'of or pertaining to the testicles': *testicond, testitoxicosis, testosterone.*

testcross **1.** In genetics: the cross of a dominant phenotype with a recessive phenotype to determine either the degree of genetic linkage or whether the dominant phenotype is homozygous or heterozygous. **2.** The subject undergoing such a test.

testicle See **testis.**

testicular Of or pertaining to the testicle.

testicular artery One of a pair of long, slender branches of the abdominal aorta, arising caudal to the renal arteries and supplying the testis.

testicular cancer A malignant neoplastic disease of the testis occurring most frequently in men between the ages of 20 and 35. An undescended testicle is often affected. In many cases the tumor is detected following an injury, but trauma is not considered an etiologic factor. Pa-

tients with early testicular cancer are often asymptomatic, and metastases may be seeded in lymph nodes, the lungs, and the liver before the primary lesion is palpable. In the later stages there may be pulmonary symptoms, ureteral obstruction, gynecomastia, and an abdominal mass. Diagnostic measures include transillumination of the scrotum, excretory urography, lymphangiography, and a urine or serum test to evaluate circulating levels of luteinizing hormone. Tumors develop more often in the right than in the left testis. Seminomas are the most curable lesions and the most common, representing 40% of all testicular tumors. Embryonal carcinomas are more highly malignant and represent 15% to 20% of these tumors. Teratocarcinomas and choricarcinomas also occur. Radiotherapy and surgical excision are usually recommended to treat seminoma. A combination of drugs, surgery, and radiation is recommended for nonseminomatous tumors.

testicular duct See **deferent duct.**

testicular vein One of a pair of veins that emerge from convoluted venous plexuses, forming the greater mass of the spermatic cords. Veins from each plexus start from small veins at the back of the testes, ascend along the spermatic cords, anterior to the ductus deferens, pass through the deep inguinal ring, and unite to form a single vein. The right testicular vein opens into the inferior vena cava; the left testicular vein into the left renal vein. Both testicular veins contain valves. Compare **ovarian vein.**

testis, *pl.* **testes** One of the pair of male gonads that produce semen. The adult testes are suspended in the scrotum by the spermatic cords; in early fetal life they are contained in the abdominal cavity behind the peritoneum. Before birth they descend into the scrotum and during development are covered with layers of tissue derived from the serous, the muscular, and the fibrous layers of the abdominal parietes. The coverings of the testes are the skin and the dartos tunic of the scrotum, the external spermatic fascia, the cremastic layer, the internal spermatic fascia, and the tunica virginalis. Each testis is a laterally compressed oval body about 4 cm (1½ inch) long, 2.5 cm (1 inch) wide and weighs about 12 g. It lies obliquely in the scrotum, with the cranial extremity directed ventrally and slightly laterally, and the caudal end directed dorsally and slightly medially. The anterior border, the lateral surfaces, and the extremities of the organ are convex, free and smooth, and covered by the tunica virginalis. The convoluted epididymis lying on the posterior border of the testis is about 6 m (20 feet) long and connects with the vas deferens, through which spermatozoa pass during ejaculation. Each testis consists of several hundred conical lobules containing the tiny coiled seminiferous tubules, each about 7.5 cm (3 inches) long, in which spermatozoa develop. The tubules converge to form the rete testis, which is drained by the efferent ducts into the head of the epididymis. The testis, developed in the lumbar region, may be retained in the abdomen, deep inguinal ring, or inguinal canal. The testes are supplied with blood by the two internal spermatic arteries which arise from the aorta, are served by the testicular veins which form the pampiniform plexuses constituting the greater part of the spermatic cords, and are innervated by the spermatic plexuses of nerves from the celiac plexuses of the autonomic nervous system. Compare **ovary.** See also **scrotum.**

testolactone   An antineoplastic agent that alters hormonal balance.

testosterone   An androgenic substance. The primary natural androgen in humans, it is produced by the interstitial cells of the testes under stimulation of luteinizing hormone.

testosterone cypionate, t. enanthate, t. propionate   Androgenic substances.

test tube   A tube made of transparent material having one open end. It is used to grow bacteriologic specimens, for analysis of some chemical functions, and for many other common laboratory functions. See also **tube.**

-tetanic   A combining form meaning 'relating to or producing tetanus or tetany': *antitetanic, posttetanic.*

tetano-   A combining form meaning 'of or pertaining to tetanus': *tetanolysin, tetanometer, tetanophilic.*

tetanus   An acute, potentially fatal infection of the central nervous system caused by an exotoxin, tetanospasmin, elaborated by an anaerobic bacillus, *Clostridium tetani.* More than 50,000 people worldwide die of tetanus infection each year. The toxin is a neurotoxin and is one of the most lethal poisons known. *C. tetani* infects only wounds that contain dead tissue. The bacillus is a common resident of the superficial layers of the soil and a normal inhabitant of the intestinal tracts of cows and horses. The bacillus may enter the body through a puncture wound, laceration, or burn; via the uterus into the bloodstream in septic abortion or postpartum sepsis; or through the stump of the umbilical cord of the newborn. The infection occurs in two clinical forms: one with an abrupt onset, high mortality, and a short incubation period (3 to 21 days); the other with less severe symptoms, a lower mortality, and a longer incubation period (4 to 5 weeks). Wounds of the face, head, and neck are most likely to result in fatal infection, as the bacillus may travel rapidly to the brain. The disease is characterized by irritability, headache, fever, and painful spasms of the muscles resulting in lockjaw, risus sardonicus, opisthotonos, and laryngeal spasm; eventually, every muscle of the body is in tonic spasm. The motor nerves transmit the impulses from the infected central nervous system to the muscles. There is no lesion. Prompt and thorough cleansing and debridement of the wound are essential for prophylaxis. A booster shot of tetanus toxoid is given to previously immunized people; tetanus immune globulin and a series of three injections of tetanus toxoid are given to those not immunized. People who have been immunized within 10 years do not usually require immunization. Treatment includes maintenance of an airway, an antitoxin, sedation, control of the muscle spasms, and assuring a normal fluid balance.

tetanus and diphtheria toxoids   An active immunizing agent containing detoxified tetanus and diphtheria toxoids that slowly produce an antigenic response to the diseases. It is prescribed for immunization against tetanus and diphtheria in children under 7 years of age when pertussis vaccine present in the usual diphtheria, pertussis, and tetanus trivalent vaccine is contraindicated. Immunosuppression, concomitant use of corticosteroids, or acute infection prohibits its use. Among the most serious adverse reactions is anaphylaxis. Stinging at the injection site is common.

tetanus antitoxin (TAT)   A tetanus immune serum that neutralizes exotoxins in tetanus infection. It is prescribed for short-term immunization against tetanus following possible exposure to the organism. It is not given if the more effective tetanus immune globulin is available or if there is a known sensitivity to equine serum. Among the most serious adverse reactions are allergic reactions and pain and inflammation at the injection site.

tetanus immune globulin (TIG)   An injectible solution prepared from the globulin of an immune human. It is effective and much safer than tetanus antitoxin. It is prescribed for short-term immunization against tetanus following possible exposure to the organism. Known hypersensitivity to this drug prohibits its use. The most serious adverse reaction is hypersensitivity. Pain and inflammation at the injection site may occur.

TETRALOGY OF FALLOT

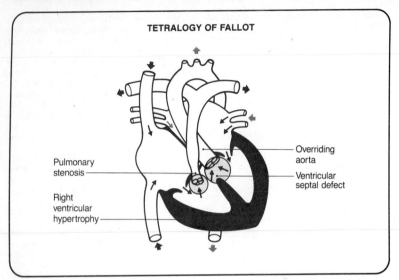

Pulmonary stenosis

Right ventricular hypertrophy

Overriding aorta

Ventricular septal defect

tetanus toxoid An active immunizing agent prepared from detoxified tetanus toxin that produces an antigenic response in the body, conferring permanent immunity to tetanus infection. It is prescribed for active immunization against tetanus. Immunosuppression or acute infection prohibits its use. The most serious adverse reaction to tetanus toxoid is anaphylaxis. Pain and inflammation at the injection site may occur.

tetany A condition characterized by cramps, convulsions, twitching of the muscles, and sharp flexion of the wrist and ankle joints. These symptoms are sometimes accompanied by attacks of stridor. Tetany is a manifestation of an abnormality in calcium metabolism, which can occur in association with vitamin D deficiency, hypoparathyroidism, alkalosis, or the ingestion of alkaline salts. Compare **tetanus.**

tetart- A combining form meaning 'fourth': *tetartanopia, tetartocone.*

tetra- A combining form meaning 'four': *tetracycline, tetrahydric.* Also **tetro-.**

tetracaine, t. hydrochloride Topical antipruritic, ester, and ophthalmic anesthetics.

tetrachlormethane See **carbon tetrachloride.**

tetracycline A broad spectrum antibiotic.

tetracycline hydrochloride, t. phosphate complex Local ophthalmic antibiotics and anti-infectives.

tetrad In genetics: a group of four chromatids of a synapsed pair of homologous chromosomes during the first meiotic prophase stage of gametogenesis. The group is formed to prepare for the two meiotic divisions in the maturation process of gametes. —**tetradic,** *adj.*

tetrahydrocannabinol (THC) The active principle, occurring as two psychomimetic isomers, in the hemp plant *Cannabis sativa,* used in the preparation of marijuana, hashish, bhang, and ganja. THC, a rapidly metabolized beta-adrenergic antagonist, increases pulse rate, causes conjunctival reddening and a feeling of euphoria, and has variable effects on blood pressure, respiratory rate, and pupil size. The drug affects memory, cognition, and the sensorium, decreases motor coordination, and increases appetite. Propranolol blocks the peripheral effects of THC but not the psychic effects. Overdoses of THC may be treated by 'talking down' the patient and administering sedative barbiturates or diazepam parenterally. See also **cannabis.**

tetrahydrozoline hydrochloride An ophthalmic and nasal vasoconstrictor.

tetraiodothyronine See **thyroxine.**

tetralogy of Fallot A congenital cardiac anomaly that consists of four defects: pulmonic stenosis, ventricular septal defect, malposition of the aorta so that it arises from the septal defect or the right ventricle, and right ventricular hypertrophy. The primary symptoms in the infant are cyanosis and hypoxia, usually during crying, difficulty in feeding, failure to gain weight, and poor development. In older children a typical squatting position and clubbing of the fingers and toes are evident. A pansystolic murmur is usually heard and the second heart sound is faint or absent. Diagnosis of the condition is primarily based on the history and physical symptoms, although cardiac catheterization is performed to evaluate the severity of the defects. Treatment consists mainly of supportive measures and palliative surgical procedures, primarily systemic-to-pulmonary anastomoses, to decrease tissue hypoxia and prevent complications until the child is old enough to tolerate total corrective surgery. The optimal age for surgical repair is approximately 4 or 5 years. Also called **blue baby, Fallot's syndrome, Fallot's**

tetralogy. See also **congenital cardiac anomaly, trilogy of Fallot.**

tetraploid, tetraploidic (4n) **1.** Of or pertaining to an individual, organism, strain, or cell that has four complete sets of chromosomes, quadruple the normal haploid number characteristic of the species. In humans, this is extremely rare, found only occasionally in abortuses and stillborn fetuses. **2.** Such an individual, organism, strain, or cell. Compare **diploid, haploid, triploid.** See also **polyploid.**

tetraploidy The state or condition of having four complete sets of chromosomes.

tetro- See **tetra-.**

T fracture An intercondylar fracture in which the fracture lines are T-shaped.

TGF *abbr* **transforming growth factor.**

T-group See **sensitivity-training group.**

Th Symbol for **thorium.**

thalamus, *pl.* **thalami** One of a pair of large, oval organs forming most of the lateral walls of the third ventricle of the brain and part of the diencephalon. It relays sensory impulses to the cerebral cortex, measures about 4 cm (1½ inch) long and 1.5 cm (½ inch) wide, and consists of numerous nuclei arranged in anterior, lateral, intralaminar, medial, and posterior groups. The thalamus extends caudally on each side beyond the third ventricle, with its medial and superior surfaces exposed in the ventricle and its inferior and lateral surfaces buried against other structures. It is composed mainly of gray substance and translates impulses from appropriate receptors into crude sensations of pain, temperature, and touch. It also participates in associating sensory impulses with pleasant and unpleasant feelings, in the arousal mechanisms of the body, and in the mechanisms that produce complex reflex movements. Compare **epithalamus, hypothalamus, subthalamus.** —**thalamic,** *adj.*

thalassemia Hemolytic anemia characterized by microcytic, hypochromic, and short-lived red blood cells caused by deficient hemoglobin synthesis. People of Mediterranean origin are more often affected than others. It is an autosomal recessive, genetically transmitted disease occurring in two forms. **Thalassemia major** (the homozygous form), evident in infancy, is recognized by anemia, fever, failure to thrive, and splenomegaly and confirmed by characteristic changes in the red blood cells on microscopic examination. Frequent transfusions are necessary to maintain the oxygen-carrying capacity of the blood. Red blood cells are rapidly destroyed, freeing large amounts of iron to be deposited in the skin, which becomes bronzed and freckled. The iron is also deposited in the heart, liver, and pancreas, which become fibrotic and dysfunctional. The spleen may become so enlarged that respiratory excursion is impeded, and the abdominal organs are crowded. There is no cure. **Thalassemia minor** (the heterozygous form) is characterized only by a mild anemia and minimal red blood cell changes. Nursing considerations in the care of thalasse-

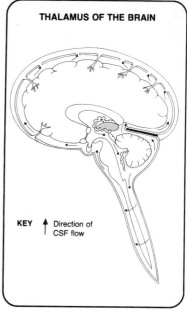

THALAMUS OF THE BRAIN

KEY ↑ Direction of CSF flow

mia patients and their families should include observation for ill effects of transfusion, education and counseling about the disease, and referral for genetic counseling. Also called **Cooley's anemia.** See also **hemochromatosis, hemosiderosis.**

thalasso- A combining form meaning 'of or pertaining to the sea': *thalassophobia, thalassotherapy.*

thalidomide A formerly used sedative-hypnotic, withdrawn because of its potential for teratogenic effects, particularly phocomelia, when taken during pregnancy.

thallium (Tl) A soft, blue-white metallic element that exhibits some nonmetallic chemical properties. Its atomic number is 81; its atomic weight is 204.37.

thallium imaging A diagnostic radiographic procedure in which an isotope of thallium is given intravenously to a patient in a resting state or after a treadmill stress test. The isotope collects in healthy cardiac tissue, but not in areas of poor blood flow and damaged cells, which show up as 'cold spots' on a scanner. The procedure, used to assess myocardial infarction and coronary artery disease, is also known as thallium scintigraphy and cold spot myocardial imaging.

thallium poisoning A toxic condition caused by the ingestion or the absorption through the skin of thallium salts, especially thallium sulfate. Characteristic of the condition are abdominal pain, vomiting, bloody diarrhea, tremor, delirium, and alopecia. Treatment may include gastric lavage, chelation with Prussian blue, and a laxative. Anticonvulsant and antihypotensive

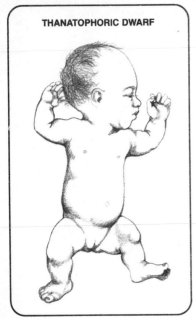

THANATOPHORIC DWARF

medication may be necessary. Thallium has been used in insect and rodent poisons, fireworks, and in some cosmetic hair removers, but this extremely toxic and cumulative poison was banned for use in household products in 1965.

thanato- A combining form meaning 'of or pertaining to death': *thanatobiologic, thanatognomonic, thanatology.*

thanatology The study of death and dying. —**thanatologist,** *n.*

thanatophoric dwarf An infant with severe micromelia, with the limbs usually extending straight out from the trunk, short ribs forming an extremely narrow chest, and flattened vertebral bodies with wide intervertebral spaces. Death usually occurs from respiratory complications shortly after birth.

thanotopsy See **autopsy.**

THC *abbr* tetrahydrocannabinol.

thec- A combining form meaning 'of or pertaining to a sheath, as of a tendon': *thecal, thecitis, thecodont.*

theca, *pl.* **thecae** A sheath or capsule, as the theca cordis.

theca cell tumor An uncommon, benign fibroid tumor of the ovary, composed of theca cells and usually containing granulosa (follicular) cells. These tumors, characteristically solid masses with yellow, fatty streaks, are frequently associated with excessive estrogen production and tend to develop cystic degeneration. Also called fibroma thecocellulare xanthomatodes, thecoma.

-thecium A combining form meaning a 'sack or container': *epithecium, perithecium.*

Theden's bandage A roller bandage applied below the injury and continued upward over a compress, used to stop bleeding. Also called **Genga's bandage.**

thel- A combining form meaning 'of or pertaining to the nipple': *thelalgia, theleplasty, thelitis.*

thelarche The beginning of female pubertal breast development that normally occurs before puberty at the beginning of the rapid growth phase between ages 9 and 13. Premature thelarche is precocious breast development without other evidence of sexual maturation. Compare **menarche.**

-thelia A combining form meaning '(condition of the) nipples': *epithelia, hyperthelia, microthelia.*

-thelioma A combining form meaning a 'tumor in a cellular tissue': *celiothelioma, hemendothelioma, perithelioma.*

-thelium A combining form meaning a 'layer of (a specified kind of) cellular tissue': *desmepithelium, mesothelium.*

thely- A combining form meaning 'female': *thelyblast, thelygenic, thelyplasty.*

thenar **1.** The bulky mass of tissue on the lateral side of the palm of the hand; the ball of the thumb. **2.** Of or pertaining to the palm.

theo- A combining form meaning 'of or pertaining to a god': *theomania, theophobia, theotherapy.*

theophylline, t. sodium glycinate Xanthine derivatives that act as respiratory tract spasmolytics and direct-acting bronchodilators.

theophyllin ethylenediamine See **aminophylline.**

theoretical effectiveness Of a contraceptive method: the effectiveness of a medication, device, or method in preventing pregnancy if used consistently and exactly as intended, without human error. Compare **use effectiveness.**

theory An abstract statement formulated to predict, explain, or describe the relationships among concepts, constructs, or events. Theory is developed and tested by observation and research, using factual data.

theotherapy A therapeutic approach to the prevention, diagnosis, and treatment of disease and dysfunction based on religious or spiritual practices and beliefs.

therapeutic **1.** Beneficial. **2.** Of or pertaining to a treatment.

-therapeutic A combining form meaning 'pertaining to medical treatment by (specified) techniques': *eutherapeutic, kinetotherapeutic, orthotherapeutic.*

therapeutic abortion **1.** A termination of early pregnancy deemed necessary for medical or psychiatric reasons. **2.** *Informal.* Any legal, induced abortion. Compare **elective abortion.** See also **induced abortion.**

therapeutic communication In psychiatric nursing: a process in which the nurse consciously influences a client or helps the client to a better understanding through verbal or nonverbal communication.

therapeutic community (TC) In mental health: a treatment facility in which the entire milieu is part of the treatment. The physical environment, the other clients, the staff, and the policies of the facility influence the individual's activities of daily living in the community. This type of therapy is integral to milieu therapy.

therapeutic equivalent A drug that has essentially the same effect in treating a disease or condition as one or more other drugs. A drug that is a therapeutic equivalent may or may not be chemically equivalent, bioequivalent, or generically equivalent. See also **bioequivalent, chemical equivalence, generic equivalent.**

therapeutic exercise Any exercise planned and performed to attain a specific physical benefit, as maintenance of the range of motion, strengthening of weakened muscles, or increased flexibility of a joint.

therapeutic index The ratio of a drug's toxic dose to its effective dose. The index is used to evaluate the safety of a prescribed dose.

therapeutic plasma exchange (TPE) Removal of plasma from the patient's blood for processing and reinfusion. Blood is withdrawn from the antecubital vein of one arm and passed through a cell separator that removes the formed elements (RBCs, WBCs, platelets) from the plasma. The plasma may be discarded and replaced by substitute protein solutions or filtered through a microporous membrane to remove disease mediators before being reinfused via the antecubital vein of the other arm. TPE is used to treat immune disorders. Also known as plasmapheresis.

therapeutic radiopharmaceutical A radioactive drug administered to a patient to deliver radiation to body tissues internally, as iodine 131, used to ablate thyroid tissue in hyperthyroid patients, or cesium 137, iridium 192, radium 226, or strontium 90, implanted in a sealed source to treat malignant tumors.

-therapeutics A combining form meaning 'medical treatment by (specified) techniques': *hydrotherapeutics, physicotherapeutics, radiotherapeutics.*

-therapia A combining form meaning 'medical care': *balneotherapia, odontotherapia.* Also **-therapy.**

therapy The treatment of any disease or pathological condition. Inhalation therapy, for example, involves administration of various drugs to patients suffering from diseases of the respiratory tract. —**therapeutic,** *adj.*

-therapy A combining form meaning: **1.** 'Medical treatment of disease' by specified means: *chemotherapy, hypnotherapy, kinesitherapy.* **2.** 'Medical treatment of a (specified) disorder or body area': *cardiotherapy, sarcotherapy, urotherapy.* Also **-therapia.**

therio- A combining form meaning 'of or pertaining to beasts': *theriomimicry, theriotherapy, theriotomy.*

-therm A combining form meaning an 'animal with a (specified) body temperature': *allotherm, endotherm.*

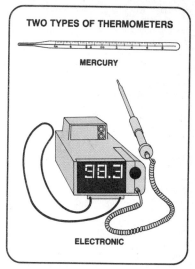

TWO TYPES OF THERMOMETERS

MERCURY

98.3

ELECTRONIC

thermal, thermic Of or pertaining to the production, application, or maintenance of heat.

thermal burn Tissue injury, usually of the skin, caused by exposure to extreme heat. See also **burn.**

-thermia A combining form meaning: **1.** A 'state of body temperature': *monothermia, normothermia, pantothermia.* **2.** 'Generation of body heat': *azothermia, diathermia, transthermia.* Also **-thermy.**

thermic fever See **heat hyperpyrexia.**

thermistor A kind of thermometer for measuring minute changes in temperature. The resistance of a thermistor varies with the ambient temperature, thereby enabling accurate measurements of small temperature changes. See also **temperature, thermometer.**

thermo-, therm- A combining form meaning 'of or pertaining to heat': *thermochemistry, thermogenesis.*

thermocautery The use of a needle or snare that has been heated by direct flame, a heated hydrocarbon vapor, or an electric current, in the destruction of tissue. See also **Paquelin's cautery.**

thermogenesis Production of heat, especially by the cells of the body. —**thermogenetic,** *adj.*

thermography A technique for sensing and recording on film hot and cold areas of the body by means of an infrared detector. It is used to study blood flow to the limbs and to detect breast tumors. —**thermographic,** *adj.*

thermolabile Easily destroyed or altered by heat. Also called **heat labile.** Compare **thermostable.**

thermometer An instrument for measuring temperature. It usually consists of a sealed glass tube, marked in degrees of Celsius or Fahrenheit and containing liquid, usually mercury. The liquid rises or falls as it expands or contracts in response to temperature changes. In electronic thermometers, heat alters the amount of current running through a resistor to provide a digital temperature readout.

thermopenetration The use of diathermic techniques to produce warmth within the body tissues for therapeutic purposes. Also called **transthermia.**

thermoradiotherapy A therapeutic process that applies ionizing radiation to any body part in which the temperature has been raised by artificial means. Thermoradiography seeks to increase the radiosensitivity of the body part being treated.

thermostable Unaffected by or resistant to change by an increase in temperature. Compare **thermolabile.**

thermostat A device for the automatic control of a heating or cooling system. —**thermostatic,** *adj.*

thermotherapy The treatment of disease by the application of heat. Thermotherapy may be administered as dry heat with heat lamps, diathermy machines, electric pads, or hot water bottles or as moist heat with warm compresses or immersion in warm water. —**thermotherapeutic,** *adj.*

-thermy See **-thermia.**

theta rhythm See **theta wave.**

theta wave One of the four types of brain waves, characterized by a relatively low frequency of 4 to 7 hertz and a low amplitude of 10 microvolts. Theta waves are the 'drowsy waves' of the temporal lobes of the brain and are observed in electroencephalograms when the individual is awake but relaxed and sleepy. Also called **theta rhythm.** Compare **alpha wave, beta wave, delta wave.**

-thetic A combining form meaning 'to put, place, set': *metathetic, prosthetic, synthetic.* Also **-thetical.**

-thetical See **-thetic.**

thiabendazole An anthelmintic agent.

thiamine, thiamin A water-soluble, crystalline compound of the B complex vitamin group, essential for normal metabolism and for the health of the cardiovascular and nervous systems. Thiamine combines with pyruvic acid to form a coenzyme necessary for the breakdown of carbohydrates into glucose. Rich sources of thiamine are pork, organ meats, green leafy vegetables, legumes, sweet corn, egg yolk, corn meal, brown rice, yeast, the germ and husks of grains, berries, and nuts. It is not stored in the body and must be supplied daily. A deficiency of thiamine affects chiefly the nervous system, the circulation, and the gastrointestinal tract. Symptoms include irritability, emotional disturbances, loss of appetite, multiple neuritis, increased pulse rate, dyspnea, reduced intestinal motility, and heart irregularities. Severe deficiency causes beriberi. Thiamine is not known to cause any toxic effects. Also called **antiberiberi factor, vitamin B$_1$.**

thiamylal sodium A barbiturate general anesthetic, administered parenterally.

thiethylperazine maleate A phenothiazine antiemetic.

thigh The section of the lower limb between the hip and the knee.

thigh bone See **femur.**

thigm- A combining form meaning 'of or pertaining to touch': *thigmesthesia, thigmocyte, thigmotropic.*

thimerosal A disinfectant.

thinking 1. The cognitive process of forming mental images or concepts. 2. The process of cognitive problem solving through the sorting, organizing, and classification of facts. Kinds of thinking include **abstract thinking, concrete thinking, syncretic thinking.** See also **imagination.**

thio- A combining form designating the presence of sulfur: *thioarsenite, thiocarbamide, thiocyanate.*

thioamide derivative One of a group of antithyroid drugs prescribed in the treatment of hyperthyroidism. Thioamide drugs act by inhibiting the synthesis of thyroid hormone. The principal thioamides are propylthiouricil and methimazole. Adverse reactions include agranulocytosis, hypersensitivity, and a mild, transient pruritus. As agranulocytosis may occur very rapidly, the patient is requested to report immediately instances of sore throat and fever, which often herald the onset of agranulocytosis. Prompt discontinuation of the drug usually results in complete recovery. Use of antithyroid medications in pregnancy may result in fetal hypothyroidism, goiter, and cretinism.

thioctic acid A pyruvate-oxidation factor found in liver and yeast, used in bacterial culture media.

thioguanine An antimetabolite chemotherapeutic drug.

thiopental sodium A barbiturate general anesthetic.

thioridazine hydrochloride A phenothiazine antipsychotic agent.

thiotepa An alkylating agent used in cancer chemotherapy.

thiothixene, t. hydrochloride A thioxanthene antipsychotic agent.

thioxanthene derivative Any one of a group of antipsychotic drugs, each of which is similar to the phenothiazines in indication, action, and adverse effects.

thiphenamil hydrochloride A gastrointestinal anticholinergic agent.

third cuneiform bone See **lateral cuneiform bone.**

third nerve See **oculomotor nerve.**

third-party reimbursement Reimbursement for services rendered to a person in which an entity other than the giver or receiver of the service is responsible for the payment. Third-party reimbursement for the cost of a subscriber's health care is commonly paid by insurance plans.

third ventriculostomy A surgical procedure for draining cerebrospinal fluid into the cisterna chiasmatis of the subarachnoid space in hydrocephalus, usually in the newborn. The procedure is used chiefly when the cisterna magna is not available for the Torkildsen procedure. The third ventriculostomy makes an opening on the anterior wall of the floor of the third ventricle into the interpeduncular cistern and is performed to correct an obstructive type of hydrocephalus.

thirst A perceived desire for water. The sensation of thirst is usually referred to the mouth and throat.

Thiry's fistula An artificial passage from the abdominal surface of an experimental animal to an isolated intestinal segment, created surgically to study internal secretions. The continuity of the animal's gut is restored by anastomosis of the severed sections, and the isolated segment's vascular and nervous connections are maintained. One end of the isolated internal segment is closed, and the other is attached to an opening in the skin of the abdomen.

Thiry-Vella fistula An artificial passage from the abdominal surface of an experimental animal to an isolated intestinal loop, created surgically to study intestinal secretions. The continuity of the animal's gut is restored by anastomosis of the severed sections, and the isolated loop's vascular connections and mesenteric attachment are preserved. The isolated segment ends are attached to two openings in the skin of the abdomen to form a closed internal loop.

thixo- A combining form meaning 'of or pertaining to touch': *thixolabile, thixotropic.*

Thomas splint **1.** A rigid splint made of steel bars curved to fit the involved limb and held in place by a cast or a rigid bandage. It is used to treat chronic joint diseases. **2.** A rigid metal splint that extends from a ring at the hip to beyond the foot. It is used to treat a fractured leg and, in conjunction with traction and suspension devices, to immobilize and position a fractured femur of the preoperative or the postoperative patient. Also called Thomas ring splint.

Thomsen's disease See **myotonia congenita.**

thoracentesis, thoracocentesis The surgical perforation of the chest wall and pleural space with a needle to aspirate fluid for diagnostic or therapeutic purposes or for the removal of a specimen for biopsy. The procedure is usually performed under local anesthesia, with the patient in an upright position. It may be used in the treatment of pleural effusion. Fluid samples may be examined for erythrocyte, leukocyte, and differential white blood cell counts; protein, glucose, and amylase concentrations; and may be cultured for studies of microorganisms that may be present.

thoracic Of or pertaining to the thorax.

-thoracic A combining form meaning 'of, referring, or relating to the chest': *abdominothoracic, extrathoracic.*

thoracic actinomycosis See **actinomycosis.**

thoracic aorta The large, upper portion of the descending aorta, starting at the caudal bor-

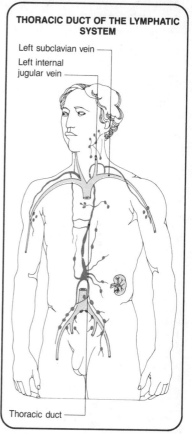

THORACIC DUCT OF THE LYMPHATIC SYSTEM

Left subclavian vein

Left internal jugular vein

Thoracic duct

der of the fourth thoracic vertebra, dividing into seven branches, and supplying many parts of the body, as the heart, ribs, chest muscles, and stomach. Its seven branches are the pericardial, bronchial, esophageal, mediastinal, posterior intercostal, subcostal, and superior phrenic. See also **descending aorta.** Compare **abdominal aorta.**

thoracic duct The common trunk of all the lymphatic vessels, except those on the right side of the head, the neck, and the thorax; the right upper limb; the right lung; the right side of the heart; and the diaphragmatic surface of the liver. It begins high in the abdomen at the cisterna chyli, ventral to the second lumbar vertebra, enters the thorax through the aortic hiatus of the diaphragm, and ascends into the neck through the posterior mediastinum, between the aorta and the azygous vein. In the neck it arches over the clavicle and opens into the junction of the left internal jugular and the left subclavian veins. Compare **right lymphatic duct.** See also **lymphatic system.**

thoracic fistula An abnormal opening in the chest wall that either ends blindly or com-

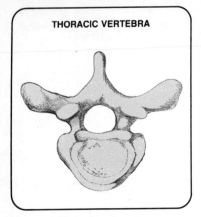

THORACIC VERTEBRA

municates with the thoracic cavity.

thoracic medicine The branch of medicine concerned with the diagnosis and treatment of disorders of the structures and organs of the chest, especially the lungs.

thoracic nerves The 12 spinal nerves on each side of the thorax, including 11 intercostal nerves and 1 subcostal nerve. They are distributed mainly to the walls of the thorax and the abdomen. The thoracic nerves do not enter a plexus but follow independent courses. The first 2 intercostal nerves innervate the upper limb as well as the thorax; the next 4 supply only the thorax; and the lower 5 supply the walls of the thorax and the abdomen. Each subcostal thoracic nerve innervates the abdominal wall and the skin of a buttock. The thoracic portion of the sympathetic trunk contains a series of ganglia often coalesced in a single mass that, when independent, corresponds approximately to the thoracic spinal nerves. The roots of the ganglia are supplied by each thoracic nerve. The 1st thoracic ganglion, larger than the rest, is elongated, lying in the medial end of the first intercostal space, and usually combined with the inferior cervical ganglion into a stellate ganglion. The 2nd to the 10th ganglia lie opposite the intervertebral disk associated with, but slightly lower than, the corresponding thoracic nerve. In most individuals the last thoracic ganglion lies on the body of the 12th thoracic vertebra and, by its connection to both the 11th and the 12th thoracic nerves, serves a dual role as a single ganglion.

thoracic outlet syndrome An abnormal condition and type of mononeuropathy characterized by paresthesia of the fingers. It may be caused by a nerve-root compression by a cervical disk or by carpal tunnel syndrome.

thoracic parietal node One of the lymph glands in the thorax, associated with various lymphatic vessels and divided into sternal nodes, intercostal nodes, and diaphragmatic nodes. See also **lymphatic system, lymph node.**

thoracic vertebra One of the 12 bony segments of the spinal column of the upper back,

designated T1 to T12. T1 is just below the seventh cervical vertebra (C7) and T12 is just above the first lumbar vertebra (L1). The thoracic portion of the spine is flexible and has a concave ventral curvature. Each vertebra has a broad, thick lamina; long, obliquely directed spinous processes; and thick, strong articular facets. The vertebrae become thicker and heavier in descending order from T1 to T12. Compare **cervical vertebra, lumbar vertebra, sacral vertebra.**

thoracic visceral node A node in the three groups of lymph nodes connected to the part of the lymphatic system that serves certain structures within the thorax, as the thymus, pericardium, esophagus, trachea, lungs, and bronchi. The thoracic visceral nodes include the anterior mediastinal nodes, the posterior mediastinal nodes, and the tracheobronchial nodes. Compare **thoracic parietal node.** See also **lymph, lymphatic system, lymph node.**

thoraco- A combining form meaning 'of or pertaining to the chest': *thoracobronchotomy, thoracocentesis.*

thoracocentesis See **thoracentesis.**

thoracodorsal nerve A branch of the brachial plexus, usually arising between the two subscapular nerves. It courses along the posterior wall of the axilla and terminates in branches that supply the latissimus dorsi.

thorax The cage of bone and cartilage containing the principal organs of respiration and circulation and covering part of the abdominal organs. It is formed ventrally by the sternum and costal cartilages and dorsally by the 12 thoracic vertebrae and the dorsal parts of the 12 ribs. Also called **chest.**

thorium (Th) A heavy, gray, radioactive, metallic element. Its atomic number is 90; its atomic weight is 232.04. Thorium is used in radiographic procedures and radiation therapy.

thought processes, alterations in A nursing diagnosis accepted by the Fifth National Conference on the Classification of Nursing Diagnoses. The etiology of the condition is to be developed at a later conference. The defining characteristics of the problem include distraction, egocentrism, abnormal cognitive function, abnormal interpretations of the environment, and attention to environmental cues that is more or less acute than might normally be expected. See also **nursing diagnosis.**

thought transference See **telepathy.**

threadworm See *Enterobius vermicularis.*

thready pulse A pulse that is weak and often fairly rapid. The artery does not feel full, and the rate may be difficult to count. It is characteristic of hypovolemia.

threatened abortion A condition in pregnancy before to the 20th week of gestation characterized by uterine bleeding and cramping sufficient to suggest miscarriage may result. A threatened abortion is generally managed with rest and observation. Compare **incomplete abortion, inevitable abortion.**

three day fever See **phlebotomus fever.**

three-day measles See **rubella.**

threp- A combining form meaning 'of or pertaining to nutrition': *threpsis, threpology.*

threshold The point at which a stimulus is great enough to produce an effect.

thrill A fine vibration, felt by an examiner's hand over the site of an aneurysm or on the precordium, indicating the presence of an organic murmur of grade four or greater intensity. Compare **bruit, murmur.**

throat See **pharynx.**

throb A deep, pulsating discomfort or pain. —**throbbing,** *adj.*

thrombasthenia A rare hemorrhagic disease characterized by a defect in platelet-mediated hemostasis owing to an abnormality in the membrane surface of the platelet. The platelets do not aggregate, a clot does not form, and hemorrhage ensues, often from the mucous membrane. Transfusion with platelets is usually effective in stopping the hemorrhage. The condition is congenital, and is inherited as an autosomal recessive trait.

thrombectomy The removal of a thrombus from a blood vessel, performed as emergency surgery to restore circulation to the affected part. Before surgery, anticoagulant therapy is begun, and an arteriogram is done to locate the thrombus. Under general anesthesia, a longitudinal incision is made into the blood vessel and the clot is removed. Postoperatively, the blood pressure is maintained close to its preoperative level, as a decrease would predispose to further clotting. Compare **embolectomy.**

thrombin **1.** An enzyme formed in plasma during the clotting process from prothrombin, calcium, and thromboplastin. Thrombin causes fibrinogen to change to fibrin, essential in the formation of a clot. **2.** A local hemostatic. See also **blood clot.**

thrombo- A combining form meaning 'of or pertaining to a clot, or thrombosis': *thromboarteritis, thrombocystis.*

thromboangiitis obliterans An occlusive vascular condition, usually of a leg or a foot, in which the small- and medium-sized arteries become inflamed and thrombotic. Early signs of the condition are burning, numbness, and tingling of the foot or leg distal to the lesion. Pulsation in the limb below the damaged blood vessels is often absent. The goal of therapy is to avoid all factors that decrease blood supply to the extremity and to use all means possible to increase the supply. Amputation may be necessary if the condition progresses to gangrene with chronic infection and extensive tissue destruction. Men are affected 75 times more often than women; most of the affected men smoke and are between ages 20 to 40. Also called **Buerger's disease.**

thrombocyte See **platelet.**

thrombocytopathy Any disorder of the blood coagulation mechanism owing to a platelet abnormality or dysfunction. Kinds of thrombocytopathies include **thrombocytopenia,**

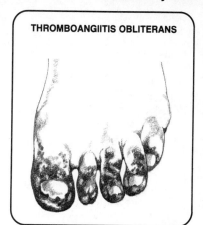

THROMBOANGIITIS OBLITERANS

thrombocytosis. —thrombocytopathic, *adj.*

thrombocytopenia An abnormal hematologic condition in which the number of platelets is reduced, usually by destruction of erythroid tissue in bone marrow because of certain neoplastic diseases or an immune response to a drug. There may be decreased platelet production and survival, increased consumption of platelets, and splenomegaly. Thrombocytopenia is the most common cause of bleeding disorders. Bleeding is usually from many small capillaries. Treatment includes stopping administration of all drugs.

thrombocytopenic purpura A bleeding disorder that is characterized by a marked decrease in the number of platelets, resulting in multiple bruises, petechiae, and hemorrhage into the tissues. It may occur secondary to a number of causes, including infection and drug toxicity. Until recently it was called idiopathic thrombocytopenic purpura (ITP), a diagnosis that was reached only by the exclusion of other causes. Today it is considered to be a manifestation of an autoimmune response. Two distinct entities, acute and chronic thrombocytopenia, can be differentiated from clinical manifestations alone. The acute form usually occurs in children between ages 2 to 6 and is benign, with complete recovery usually apparent within 6 weeks. The chronic form usually occurs in adults between ages 20 to 50. Recovery is rarely spontaneous and often requires adrenocortical steroids or, possibly, splenectomy. Compare **disseminated intravascular coagulation.** See also **hemophilia, hemorrhagic diathesis, thrombasthenia.**

thrombocytosis An abnormal increase in the number of platelets. Benign, or secondary, thrombocytosis is asymptomatic and usually occurs following splenectomy, inflammatory disease, hemolytic anemia, hemorrhage, or iron deficiency; as a response to exercise; or following treatment with vincristine. Thrombocytosis may also occur in advanced carcinoma or Hodgkin's disease or in other lymphomas. Essential

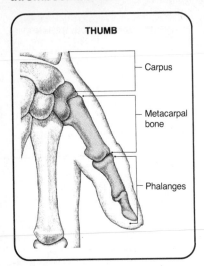

THUMB

Carpus

Metacarpal bone

Phalanges

thrombocythemia is characterized by episodes of spontaneous bleeding alternating with thrombotic episodes. Compare **thrombocytopenia.** See also **polycythemia.**

thromboembolism A condition in which a blood vessel is blocked by an embolus carried in the blood stream from a clot formation site. The area supplied by an obstructed artery may tingle and become cold, numb, and cyanotic. Treatment includes quiet bed rest, warm wet packs, and anticoagulants to prevent the formation of additional thrombi. Embolectomy may be indicated, especially if the aorta or common iliac artery is obstructed. An embolus in the lungs causes a sudden, sharp, thoracic or upper abdominal pain, dyspnea, a violent cough, fever, and hemoptysis. Obstruction of the pulmonary artery or one of its branches may be rapidly fatal. Emboli in smaller pulmonary arteries may be diagnosed by radiologic techniques.

thrombophlebitis Inflammation of a vein, often accompanied by clot formation. It occurs most commonly as the result of trauma to the vessel wall, hypercoagulability of the blood, infection, chemical irritation, postoperative venous stasis, prolonged sitting, standing, or immobilization, or a long period of intravenous catheterization. Thrombophlebitis of a superficial vein is generally evident; the vessel feels hard and thready or cordlike and is extremely sensitive to pressure; the surrounding area may be erythematous and warm to the touch, and the entire limb may be pale, cold, and swollen. Deep vein thrombophlebitis is characterized by aching or cramping pain, especially in the calf when the patient walks or dorsiflexes the foot (Homan's sign). Thrombophlebitis of a vein of the arm or hand caused by an intravenous catheter is usually treated by removing the catheter, elevating the arm, and applying moist heat. When the condition occurs in a vein of the leg, the person is maintained on complete bed rest in a comfortable position that does not restrict venous return. Anticoagulant therapy and streptokinase may be administered and moist heat is applied to the affected area; intense heat, which may burn edematous skin, is avoided. Observation for signs of pulmonary embolism, myocardial infarction, cardiovascular accident, or decreased renal function is constant.

NURSING CONSIDERATIONS: Early postoperative and postpartum ambulation, range of motion exercises for the immobilized patient, good technique in intravenous catheterization, attention to fluid balance, and proper positioning of the patient are common nursing measures to promote good circulation and reduce venous stasis and the development of thrombophlebitis. Also called **phlebitis.**

thrombophlebitis migrans See **migratory thrombophlebitis.**

thrombophlebitis purulenta An inflammation of a vein associated with the formation of a soft, purulent thrombus that infiltrates the wall of the vessel.

thromboplastin A complex substance that initiates the clotting process by converting prothrombin to thrombin in the presence of calcium ions. It is found in most tissue cells and, in somewhat different form, in red blood cells and leukocytes. See also **blood clotting.**

thrombosis, *pl.* **thromboses** An abnormal vascular condition in which a thrombus develops within a blood vessel of the body.

thrombotic phlegmasia See **phlegmasia alba dolens.**

thrombotic thrombocytopenic purpura (TTP) A disorder characterized by thrombocytopenia, hemolytic anemia, and neurological abnormalities. It is accompanied by a generalized purpura with the deposition of microthrombi within the capillaries and smaller arterioles. It is seen in a chronic form and in an acute fulminating form that may be fatal within weeks. Therapy may include corticosteroids and splenectomy. Compare **disseminated intravascular coagulation.** See also **thrombocytopenic purpura.**

thrombus, *pl.* **thrombi** An aggregation of platelets, fibrin, clotting factors, and the cellular elements of the blood attached to the interior wall of a vein or artery, sometimes occluding the lumen of the vessel. Kinds of thrombi include **agonal thrombus, hyaline thrombus, laminated thrombus, marasmic thrombus, parasitic thrombus, white thrombus.** Also called **blood clot.** Compare **embolus.**

thrush See *Candida albicans.*

thulium (Tm) A rare-earth metallic element. Its atomic number is 69; its atomic weight is 168.93. Thulium has been used in portable X-ray devices.

thumb The first and shortest digit of the hand, classified by some anatomists as one of the fingers because its metacarpal bone ossifies in the same manner as those of the phalanges. Other anatomists classify the thumb separately, regarding it as composed of one metacarpal bone and only two phalanges. The metacarpal bone of the thumb articulates with the trapezium of the carpus and is controlled by the thenar muscles and by the abductor pollicis longus, the extensor pollicis brevis, and the extensor pollicis longus. The nerves that innervate the various muscles the thumb include branches of the radial nerve, the deep palmar branch of the ulnar nerve, and a branch of the median nerve.

thumb-sucking The habit of sucking the thumb for oral gratification. It is normal in infants and young children as a pleasure-seeking or comforting device, especially when the child is hungry or tired. The habit reaches its peak when the child is between 18 to 20 months of age. Thumb-sucking beyond ages 4 to 6 may lead to malocclusion of the teeth and deformation of the bony tissue of the thumb. Excessive thumb-sucking, especially in older children, may indicate an emotional problem.

-thymia A combining form meaning '(condition of the) mind or will': amphithymia, barythymia, poikilothymia.

thymic Of or pertaining to the thymus gland.

thymic hypoplasia See **DiGeorge syndrome.**

thymic parathyroid aplasia See **DiGeorge syndrome.**

thymo- A combining form meaning: **1.** 'Of or pertaining to the thymus gland': thymocyte, thymolysis. **2.** 'Of or pertaining to the spirit or mind': thymogenic, thymopathy.

thymol A synthetic or natural thyme oil, used as an antibacterial and antifungal, that is an ingredient in some over-the-counter preparations for the treatment of hemorrhoids, acne, and tinea pedis. It is also used as a stabilizer in various pharmaceutical preparations.

thymoma, pl. **thymomas, thymomata** A usually benign tumor of the thymus gland that may be associated with myasthenia gravis or abnormal or excessive crythropoesis.

thymosin **1.** A naturally occurring immunologic hormone secreted by the thymus gland. It is present in greatest amounts in young children and decreases in amount throughout life. **2.** An investigational drug derived from bovine thymus extracts and prescribed as an immunomodulator in experimental treatments for certain diseases, as systemic lupus erythematosus or rheumatoid arthritis.

thymus, pl. **thymuses, thymi** A single, unpaired gland located in the mediastinum, extending superiorly into the neck to the lower edge of the thyroid gland and inferiorly as far as the fourth costal cartilage. It is the primary central gland of the lymphatic system. The endocrine activity of the thymus is believed to depend on the hormone thymosin, which is composed of biologically active peptides critical to the maturation and the development of the immune system. The T cells of the cell-mediated immune response develop in this gland before migrating to the lymph nodes and the spleen. The gland consists of two lateral lobes closely bound by connective tissue, which also encloses

the entire organ in a capsule. The thymus is about 5 cm (2 inches) long, 4 cm (1½ inches) wide, and 6 mm (¼ inch) thick. The lobes are composed of numerous lobules, which vary from 0.5 to 2 mm in diameter. The lobules are separated by delicate connective tissue. Each lobule is composed of a dense cellular cortex and an inner, less dense medulla. The cortices are composed almost entirely of small lymphocytes secured by reticular tissue with relatively few reticular cells. The medullae contain far fewer lymphocytes than the cortices and are composed of reticular tissue that contains more reticular cells. The gland is supplied by arteries derived from the internal thoracic and from the superior and inferior thyroids.

-thyrea A combining form meaning a 'condition of the thyroid gland': athyrea, hypothyrea. Also **-thyroidism.**

thyro- A combining form meaning 'of or pertaining to the thyroid gland': thyroactive, thyroidectomy.

thyrocalcitonin See **calcitonin.**

thyrocervical trunk One of a pair of short, thick, arterial branches, arising from the first portion of the subclavian arteries, close to the medial border of the scalenus anterior, supplying numerous muscles and bones in the head, neck, and back. Each is divided into three branches: the inferior thyroid, suprascapular, and transverse cervical.

thyroglobulin A thyroid hormone.

thyroid acropathy Swelling of subcutaneous tissue of the extremities and clubbing of the digits. Thyroid acropathy occurs rarely in patients with thyroid disease and is usually associated with pretibial myxedema or with exophthalmos.

thyroid cancer A neoplasm of the thyroid gland, usually characterized by slow growth and a slower and more prolonged clinical course than that of other malignancies. A significant carcinogenic effect of exposure to ionizing radiation is demonstrated by the high rate of thyroid cancer in survivors of atomic bomb explosions and in individuals who have been treated with radiotherapy for an enlarged thymus in infancy. Nontoxic colloid goiters and follicular adenomas may be precursors of malignant thyroid tumors. The first sign of cancer may be an increase in size of the thyroid gland, a palpable nodule, hoarseness, dysphagia, dyspnea, or pain on pressure. Diagnostic measures include X-ray examination, transillumination of the gland, radioisotope scanning, needle biopsy, and ultrasonic examination. More than one half of thyroid malignancies are papillary carcinomas, about one third are follicular carcinomas, and the rest consist of rapidly growing invasive anaplastic carcinomas and medullary carcinomas. Total or subtotal thyroidectomy with excision of involved lymph nodes is usually recommended. Radioactive iodine may be administered postoperatively, and high doses of exogenous thyroid are often used to suppress thyroid-stimulating hormone (TSH), thus aiding the regression of re-

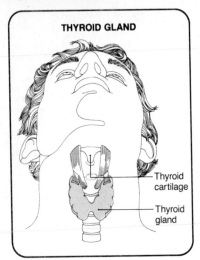

THYROID GLAND

Thyroid
cartilage

Thyroid
gland

sidual tumor. Cancer of the thyroid is twice as common in women as in men; it is diagnosed most frequently in people between ages 30 to 50.

thyroid cartilage   The largest cartilage of the larynx, consisting of two laminae fused at an acute angle in the middle line of the neck to form the Adam's apple. Immediately above this prominence the laminae are separated by the superior thyroid notch. An oblique line runs caudally from the outer surface of each lamina and serves for the attachment of the sternothyroideus, the thyrohyoideus, and the constrictor pharyngis inferior. The cranial border of the thyroid cartilage secures the thyrohyoid membrane; the caudal border holds the cricoid cartilage, and the dorsal border receives insertions of the stylopharyngeus and the pharyngopalatinus. Compare **cricoid.**

thyroid dermoid cyst   A tumor derived from embryonal tissues that is believed to have developed in the thyroid gland or in the thyrolingual duct.

thyroidectomy   The surgical removal of the thyroid gland, performed for colloid goiter, removal of tumors, or hyperthyroidism that does not respond to iodine therapy and antithyroid drugs. All but 5% to 10% of the gland is removed; regrowth usually begins shortly after surgery, and thyroid function may return to normal. For cancer of the thyroid, the entire gland is removed, along with surrounding structures from neck to collarbone, in a radical neck dissection. Postoperatively, the patient is observed for signs of hemorrhage, respiratory difficulty due to edema of the glottis, the muscular twitching of tetany from accidental removal of a parathyroid gland, and thyroid storm.

thyroid function test   Any of several laboratory tests used to evalute thyroid gland function. Often several of the tests are performed simultaneously. Thyroid function tests include protein-bound iodine, butanol-extractable iodine, T-3, T-4, free thyroxine index, thyroxine-binding globulin, thyroid-stimulating hormone, long-acting thyroid stimulator, radioactive iodine uptake, radioactive iodine excretion.

thyroid gland   A highly vascular organ at the front of the neck, usually weighing about 30 g (slightly over 1 ounce), consisting of bilateral lobes connected in the middle by a narrow isthmus. It is slightly heavier in women than in men and enlarges during pregnancy. The thyroid gland secretes the hormone thyroxine directly into the blood and is part of the endocrine system of ductless glands. It is essential to normal body growth in infancy and childhood, and its removal greatly reduces the oxidative processes of the body, producing a lower metabolic rate characteristic of hypothyroidism. The thyroid is activated by the pituitary thyrotrophic hormone and requires iodine to elaborate thyroxine. Compare **parathyroid gland.**

thyroid hormone   An iodine-containing compound secreted by the thyroid gland, predominantly as thyroxine (T_4) and in smaller amounts as triiodothyronine (T_3) which is four times more potent than T_4. These hormones increase the rate of metabolism; affect body temperature; regulate protein, fat, and carbohydrate catabolism in all cells; maintain growth hormone secretion, skeletal maturation, and the cardiac rate, force, and output; promote central nervous system development; stimulate the synthesis of many enzymes; and are necessary for muscle tone and vigor. T_4 accounts for approximately 90% of iodine in circulation and T_3 for 5%. All phases of the production and release of T_4 and T_3 are regulated by the thyroid-stimulating hormone (TSH) secreted by the anterior pituitary gland. The production of thyroid hormones is excessive in Graves' disease and toxic nodular goiter, diminished in myxedema, and absent in cretinism. T_4's normal 6- or 7-day half-life in blood is reduced to 3 or 4 days in hyperthyroidism and extended to 9 or 10 days in myxedema. T_3 has a normal half-life of 2 days or less and, like T_4, is metabolized most actively in the liver. Pharmaceutical preparations of thyroid hormones extracted from animal glands and the synthetic compounds levothyroxine sodium and liothyronine sodium are used as replacement therapy in patients with hypothyroidism.

-thyroidism   See **-thyrea.**

thyroiditis   Inflammation of the thyroid gland. Acute thyroiditis, caused by staphylococcal, streptococcal, or other infections, is characterized by suppuration and abscess formation and may progress to subacute, diffuse disease of the gland. Subacute thyroiditis is marked by fever, weakness, sore throat, and a painfully enlarged gland containing granulomas composed of colloid masses surrounded by giant cells and mononuclear cells. Chronic lymphocytic thyroiditis (Hashimoto's disease), characterized by lymphocyte and plasma cell infiltration of the gland and by diffuse enlargement, seems to be transmitted as a dominant trait and may be associated with various autoimmune disorders. Another chronic form of thyroiditis is Riedel's struma, a rare progressive fibrosis, usually of one lobe of the gland but sometimes involving both lobes, the trachea, and surrounding muscles, nerves, and blood vessels. Radiation thyroiditis occasionally occurs 7 to 10 days following the treatment of hyperthyroidism with radioactive iodine$_{131}$ (^{131}I).

thyroid-stimulating hormone (TSH) A chemical substance, secreted by the anterior lobe of the pituitary gland, that controls the release of thyroid hormone and is needed for thyroid growth and function. The secretion of TSH is regulated by thyrotropin-releasing factor, elaborated in the median eminence of the hypothalamus. Pharmaceutical preparations of bovine thyroid-stimulating hormone are used to increase the uptake of radioactive iodine in the thyroid and the secretion of thyroxine by the thyroid. Also called **thyrotropin**. See also **thyroid hormone**.

thyroid storm A crisis in uncontrolled hyperthyroidism caused by the release into the blood stream of increased amounts of thyroid hormones. The storm may occur spontaneously or be precipitated by infection, stress, or a thyroidectomy performed on a patient who is inadequately prepared with antithyroid drugs. Characteristic signs are fever that may reach 41°C (106°F), a rapid pulse, acute respiratory distress, apprehension, restlessness, irritability, and prostration. The patient may become delirious, lapse into a coma, and die of heart failure.

thyrotoxicosis See **Graves' disease**.

thyrotropin See **thyroid-stimulating hormone**.

thyrotropin-releasing factor (TRF) A chemical substance, secreted by the median eminence of the hypothalamus, that regulates the secretion of thyroid-stimulating hormone by the anterior lobe of the pituitary gland.

thyroxine (T$_4$) A hormone of the thyroid gland, derived from tyrosine, that influences metabolic rate. Also called **tetraiodothyronine**.

thyroxine-binding globulin A plasma protein that binds with and transports thyroxine in the blood.

Ti Symbol for **titanium**.

TI *abbr* therapeutic index.

TIA *abbr* **transient ischemic attack**.

tibia The second longest bone of the skeleton, located at the medial side of the leg. It articulates with the fibula laterally, the talus distally, and the femur proximally, forming part of the knee joint. The tibia attaches to the ligament of the patella and to various muscles. Also called **shin bone**.

tibialis anterior One of the anterior crural muscles of the leg, situated on the lateral side of the tibia. It is a thick, fleshy muscle proximally and tendinous distally, arising from various origins, as the lateral side of the tibia, and inserting into the first cuneiform bone and the first metatarsal bone. It is innervated by a branch of

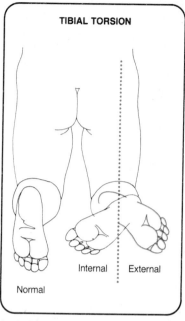

TIBIAL TORSION

Internal : External

Normal

the deep peroneal nerve. The tibialis anterior dorsiflexes and supinates the foot. Also called **tibialis anticus**. Compare **extensor digitorum longus**.

tibialis anticus See **tibialis anterior**.

tibial torsion A lateral or a medial twisting rotation of the tibia on its longitudinal axis, causing an internal or external rotation of the foot. This is a common disorder in toddlers and may correct itself as the child grows. Compare **femoral torsion**.

tic See **mimic spasm**.

ticarcillin disodium A penicillin antibiotic.

tic douloureux See **trigeminal neuralgia**.

tick bite A puncture wound produced by the toothed beak of a blood-sucking tick, a small, tough-skinned arachnid. Ticks transmit several diseases to humans and a few species carry a neurotoxin that may cause ascending paralysis beginning in the legs. Symptoms often disappear when the attached tick is carefully removed with forceps. Placing a drop of alcohol or ether on the tick or coating it with petrolatum or nail polish facilitates removal. See also **Lyme arthritis, Q fever, relapsing fever, Rocky Mountain spotted fever, tularemia**.

tick fever See **relapsing fever**.

tick paralysis A rare, progressive, reversible disorder caused by several species of ticks that release a neurotoxin that causes weakness and paralysis. The tick must feed on the host for several days before symptoms appear; removing the tick leads to rapid recovery.

t.i.d. In prescriptions: *abbr ter in die*, a Latin phrase meaning 'three times a day.'

TINEA: FOUR VARIANTS

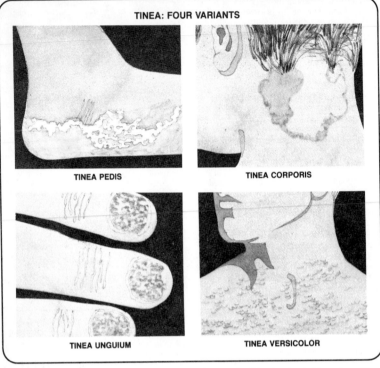

TINEA PEDIS

TINEA CORPORIS

TINEA UNGUIUM

TINEA VERSICOLOR

tidal drainage See **drainage.**

tidal volume (V$_T$) The amount of air inhaled and exhaled during normal ventilation. Inspiratory reserve volume, expiratory reserve volume, and tidal volume make up vital capacity. See also **pulmonary function test.**

tide A variation in the concentration of a particular component of body fluids. —**tidal,** *adj.*

Tietze's syndrome **1.** A disorder characterized by nonsuppurative swellings of one or more costal cartilages causing pain that may radiate to the neck, shoulder, or arm and mimic the pain of coronary artery disease. The syndrome may accompany chronic respiratory infections, and, if the swellings are extremely painful, infiltration with procaine and hydrocortisone may provide relief. **2.** Albinism, except for normal eye pigment, accompanied by deaf mutism and hypoplasia of the eyebrows.

TIG *abbr* **tetanus immune globulin.**

timed release See **prolonged release.**

timolol maleate A sympatholytic antihypertensive, which is a beta-adrenergic blocker, and an ophthalmic agent used to lower intraocular pressure.

tinea A group of fungal skin diseases caused by dermatophytes of several kinds, characterized by itching, scaling, and, sometimes, painful lesions. Diagnosis is made by demonstrating fungus on smear or by culture.

tinea capitis A contagious fungal disease characterized by circular, bald patches of from 1 to 6 cm (½ to 2½ inches) in diameter with slight erythema, scaling, and crusting. Diagnosis is made by bright fluorescence of infected hairs under Wood's light, by microscopic examination of infected hairs, and by culture of the fungus. Also called **ringworm.**

tinea corporis A superficial fungal infection of the nonhairy skin of the body, most prevalent in hot, humid climates and usually caused by species of *Trichophyton* or *Microsporum.*

tinea cruris A superficial fungal infection of the groin, caused by species of *Trichophyton* or *Epidermophyton floccosum.* It is most common in the tropics and among males. Also called **jock itch.**

tinea pedis A chronic, superficial fungal infection of the foot, especially of the skin between the toes and on the soles. It is common worldwide and is usually caused by *Trichophyton mentagrophytes, T. rubrum,* and *Epidermophyton floccosum.* Also called **athlete's foot.**

tinea unguium A superficial fungal infection of the nails caused by various species of *Trichophyton* and, occasionally, by *Candida albicans.* It is more common on the toes than the fingers and can cause complete crumbling and destruction of the nails.

tinea versicolor A fungal infection of the skin characterized by finely desquamating, pale tan patches on the upper trunk and upper arms that may itch and do not tan. In dark-skinned persons the lesions may be depigmented. The fungus fluoresces under Wood's light and may be easily identified in scrapings viewed under a microscope.

Tinel's sign An indication of irritability of a nerve, resulting in a distal tingling sensation upon percussion of a damaged nerve. The sign is often present in carpal tunnel syndrome and is produced by tapping over the median nerve on the volar aspect of the wrist.

Tine test A tuberculin skin test in which a small disk with multiple tines bearing tuberculin antigen is used to puncture the skin. The method is widely used to test for sensitivity to the tuberculin antigen. Induration around the puncture site indicates previous exposure or active disease, requiring further testing. See also **tuberculin test.**

tingling A prickly sensation in the skin or a body part, accompanied by diminished sensitivity to sensory nerve stimulation, felt as the area is numbed by local anesthetic, exposure to the cold, or pressure on a nerve.

tinnitus Tinkling or ringing heard in one or both ears. It may be a sign of acoustic trauma, Ménière's disease, otosclerosis, or presbycusis or of an accumulation of cerumen impinging on the eardrum or occluding the external auditory canal.

tin (Sn) A whitish metallic element. Its atomic number is 50; its atomic weight is 118.69.

tissue activator See **fibrinokinase.**

tissue committee A group that evaluates all surgery performed in a hospital or other health-care facility. See also **tissue review.**

tissue dextrin See **glycogen.**

tissue dose In radiotherapy: the amount of radiation absorbed by tissue in the region of interest, expressed in rads.

tissue fixation A process in which a tissue specimen is placed in a fluid that preserves the cells as nearly as is possible in their natural state.

tissue fixative A fluid that preserves cells in their natural state, so that they may be identified and examined.

tissue kinase See **fibrinokinase.**

tissue perfusion, alteration in: cerebral, cardiopulmonary, renal, gastrointestinal, peripheral A nursing diagnosis accepted by the Fifth National Conference on the Classification of Nursing Diagnoses. The etiology of the diagnosis may be interruption of the venous or arterial circulation to the affected part of the body, hypovolemia or hypervolemia, or a condition that causes abnormal exchange of fluids and nutrients between the cells and the circulation. The defining characteristics of the condition include coldness of the affected extremity, paleness on elevation of the extremity, diminished arterial pulses, and changes in the arterial blood pressure when measured in the affected extremity. Claudication, gangrene, brittle nails, slowly healing ulcers or wounds, shiny skin, and lack of hair are other commonly seen traits. See also **nursing diagnosis.**

tissue response Any reaction or change in living cellular tissue when it is acted upon by disease, toxin, or other external stimulus. Some kinds of tissue responses are **immune response, inflammation, necrosis.**

tissue review A review of the surgery performed in a hospital or other health-care facility. The evaluation is usually made on the basis of the extent of agreement of the preoperative, postoperative, and pathological diagnoses and on the relevance and acceptability of the diagnostic procedures. See also **tissue committee.**

tissue typing A systematized series of tests to evaluate the intraspecies compatibility of tissues of a donor and a recipient prior to transplantation. This is accomplished by identifying and comparing a large series of human leukocyte antigens (HLA) in the cells of the body. See also **immune system, transplant.**

titanium (Ti) A grayish, brittle metallic element. Its atomic number is 22; its atomic weight is 47.90. Titanium dioxide is the active ingredient in a number of topical ointments and lotions.

title A section of the Social Security Act that provides for the establishment, funding, and regulation of a service to a specific segment of the population, as Title XIX, which includes medical coverage under Medicaid.

titubation Posture characterized by a staggering or stumbling gait and a swaying head or trunk while sitting. It may be a manifestation of cerebellar disease. Compare **ataxia.**

Tl Symbol for **thallium.**

TLC *abbr* 1. **total lung capacity.** 2. *Informal.* Tender loving care.

Tm Symbol for **thulium.**

TNM A system for staging malignant neoplastic disease. See also **cancer staging.**

tntc *abbr* too-numerous-to-count. Usually applied to organisms or cells viewed on a slide under a microscope.

toadstool poisoning A toxic condition caused by ingestion of certain varieties of poisonous mushrooms. See **mushroom poisoning.**

tobacco A plant, the leaves of which are dried and used for smoking and chewing, and in snuff. See also **nicotine.**

tobramycin An ophthalmic anti-infective agent.

tobramycin sulfate An aminoglycoside antibiotic.

Tobruk plaster A plaster cast splint with tapes for skin traction coming through openings in the plaster and connected with a Thomas splint. It covers and immobilizes the leg from foot to groin. Also called Tobruk splint.

-tocia A combining form meaning: 1. 'Conditions of labor': *mogitocia, omotocia.* 2. The 'product of parturition': *deuterotocia, odontocia.*

toco-, toko- A combining form meaning 'pertaining to childbirth or labor': *tocodynamometer, tocography.*

TODDLER: NORMAL DEVELOPMENT

Age
1 to 3 years
Physical development
• Anterior fontanel is closed.
• Anal and urinary sphincters can be controlled.
• Height and weight increase at slower rates.
• Birth weight quadruples by age 30 months.
• Arms and legs lengthen from ossification and long-bone growth.
• Primary dentition is complete.
Sensory ability
• Vision is 20/40; accommodation is complete.
• Hearing ability (including ability to localize sounds) fully developed.
Communication skills
• At 15 to 18 months, uses his own jargon—sounds that he understands but that aren't real words
• By 24 months, uses 2- or 3-word phrases and pronounces vowels correctly. Has a 270- to 300-word vocabulary
• By 3 years, has a 900-word vocabulary and uses 4- or 5-word sentences

Motor activity
• Goes up and down stairs alone by placing both feet on a step before climbing to next step
• Jumps down steps without losing balance
• Kicks ball forward without losing balance
• Turns doorknobs
• Rides tricycle
• Holds crayon with fingers; copies crosses and circles
Social skills
• At 15 months, feeds self with little difficulty, tolerates some separation from mother, begins imitating parents
• At 24 months, feeds self well, helps undress himself, becomes possessive of toys. Has daytime elimination control.
• At 36 months, engages in parallel playing (playing in proximity to others but without interaction), puts things away, pulls people to show them something, wants and displays increased independence from mother, begins to recognize sex differences, knows his own sex. May achieve nighttime elimination control.

---

tocodynamometer, tokodynamometer An electronic device for monitoring and recording contractions in labor. It consists of a pressure transducer that is applied to the fundus of the uterus by means of a belt. This is connected to a machine that records the duration of the contractions and the interval between them on graph paper. The tocodynamometer is a component of external monitoring in childbirth. See also **electronic fetal monitor.**

tocopherol Any of a group of pale-yellow, fat-soluble, oily liquid phenolic compounds that possess vitamin E activity in varying degrees. They are stable to heat and acids and acids insoluble to alkalis, ultraviolet light, and oxygen. All are powerful antioxidants and occur naturally in various vegetable oils, oils from seeds, and fish-liver oils. Alpha-tocopherol is the physiologically most active form of the group. See also **vitamin E.**

toddler A child between the ages of 12 to 36 months. During this period, the child acquires a sense of autonomy through the mastery of various specialized tasks, as control of bodily functions, refinement of motor and language skills, and acquisition of socially acceptable behavior, especially toleration of delayed gratification and acceptance of separation from the mother or parents. The period is characterized by exploration of the environment and by rapid cognitive development as the child strives for self-assertion and personal interaction with others while struggling with parental discipline and sibling rivalry. Of primary importance for the nurse is the understanding of the dynamics of the growth and development of the toddler in order to help parents deal effectively with appropriate nutrition, toilet training, temper tantrums, prevention of accidental injury, and childhood fears, especially anxiety as a result of separation from the parents.

toddlerhood The state or condition of being a toddler.

toe Any one of the digits of the feet.

toenail One of the heavy ungual structures covering the terminal phalanges of the toes. Also called **unguis.**

togavirus A family of viruses that includes the organisms causing encephalitis, dengue, yellow fever, and rubella.

toilet training The process of teaching a child to control the functions of the bladder and bowel. Training programs vary, but all emphasize a positive, consistent, nonpunitive, and nonpressured approach, and each program is individualized, depending on the mental and physical age and state of the child, the parent-child relationship, and the readiness of the child to learn. Training often begins between 18 and 24 months of age, when voluntary control of the anal and urethral sphincters is achieved by most children. Bowel training is usually accomplished before bladder training because the urge to evacuate the bowel is stronger than the urge to empty the bladder, and the need is less frequent and more regular. Nighttime bladder control may not be achieved until the child is 4 or 5 years of age or older. Behavior modification, using a system of rewards for each of the various phases of the training, has been successful with both normal and mentally retarded children.

token economy A technique of reinforcement used in behavior therapy to manage a group of people. Individuals are rewarded for specific activities or behavior with tokens they can exchange for desired objects or privileges.

tolazamide An oral sulfonylurea and antidiabetic agent.

tolazoline hydrochloride A peripheral vasodilator.

tolbutamide An oral sulfonylurea and antidiabetic agent.

tolerance The ability to endure hardship, pain, or such ordinarily injurious substances as drugs without apparent physiological or psychological injury.

tolerance dose In radiotherapy: the amount of radiation that can be delivered to a body structure before irreversible damage occurs.

tolmetin sodium A nonsteroidal anti-inflammatory agent.

tolnaftate A local anti-infective.

-tome A combining form meaning: **1.** A 'cutting instrument': *labiotome, neurotome, thyrotome.* **2.** A '(specified) segment or region': *dermomyotome, pleurotome, viscerotome.*

-tomic, -tomical A combining form meaning 'related to incisions or sections of tissue': *dermatomic, phlebotomic.*

tomography An X-ray technique that produces a film representing a detailed cross section of tissue structure at a predetermined depth. Tomography is a valuable diagnostic tool for the discovery and identification of space-occupying lesions.

-tomy A combining form meaning a 'surgical incision': *cystotomy, oncotomy.*

tone See **tonus.**

tongue The principal organ of the sense of taste that also assists in the mastication and the deglutition of food. It is located in the floor of the mouth within the curve of the mandible. Its root is connected to the hyoid bone posteriorly by the hypoglossi and the genioglossi muscles. It is also connected to the epiglottis by three folds of mucous membrane, to the soft palate by the glossopalatine arches, and to the pharynx by the constrictores pharyngis superiores and by the mucous membrane. The apex of the tongue rests anteriorly against the lingual surfaces of the lower incisors. The mucous membrane connecting the tongue to the mandible reflects over the floor of the mouth to the lingual surface of the gum and, in the midline of the floor, is raised into a vertical fold. The dorsum of the tongue is divided into symmetrical halves by a median sulcus, which ends posteriorly in the foramen cecum. A shallow sulcus terminalis runs from this foramen laterally and forward on either side to the margin of the organ. From the sulcus, the

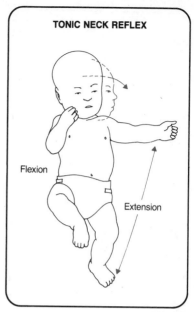

TONIC NECK REFLEX

Flexion

Extension

anterior two thirds of the tongue is covered with papillae. The posterior one third is smoother and contains numerous mucous glands and lymph follicles. The use of the tongue as an organ of speech is not anatomical, but a secondary acquired characteristic. Also called *lingua.*

-tonia A combining form meaning '(condition or degree of) tonus of a sort or in a region of the body': *angiotonia, hemotonia.* Also **-tony.**

-tonic A combining form meaning: **1.** The 'quality of muscle contraction or tonus': *hypertonic, myatonic.* **2.** A 'solution with a comparative concentration': *hypertonic, hypotonic.*

tonicity The quality of possessing tone, or tonus.

tonic neck reflex A normal response of the supine infant to extend the arm and the leg on the side of the body to which the head is quickly turned and to flex the limbs of the opposite side. The reflex, which prevents the infant from rolling over until adequate neurological and motor development occurs, disappears by age 3 to 4 months to be replaced by symmetric positioning of both sides of the body. Absence or persistence of the reflex may indicate central nervous system damage. Also called **asymmetric tonic neck reflex.** See also **symmetric tonic neck reflex.**

tono- A combining form meaning 'pertaining to tone or tension': *tonoclonic, tonoscillograph.*

tonometer An instrument used in measuring tension or pressure, especially intraocular pressure.

tonometry The measuring of intraocular pressure by determining the resistance of the eyeball to indentation by an applied force. Several kinds of tonometers are used. Air-puff tonometers record deflections of the cornea from

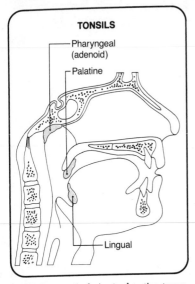

TONSILS

Pharyngeal (adenoid)

Palatine

Lingual

a puff of pressurized air. Applanation tonometers record the pressure needed to flatten the corneal surface.

tonsil A small, rounded mass of tissue, especially lymphoid tissue. Compare **intestinal tonsil, lingual tonsil, palatine tonsil, pharyngeal tonsil.**

tonsillectomy The surgical excision of the palatine tonsils, performed to prevent recurrent streptococcal tonsillitis. Tonsillar tissue is dissected and removed, usually under general anesthesia, and bleeding areas are sutured or cauterized. An airway remains in place until swallowing returns. Tonsillectomy is often combined with adenoidectomy.

tonsillitis An infection or inflammation of a tonsil. Acute tonsillitis, frequently caused by streptococcal infection, is characterized by severe sore throat, fever, headache, malaise, difficulty in swallowing, earache, and enlarged, tender lymph nodes in the neck. Acute tonsillitis may accompany scarlet fever. See also **peritonsillar abscess, scarlet fever, strep throat.**

tonus, tone **1.** The normal state of balanced tension in the body tissues, especially the muscles. Partial contraction or alternate contraction and relaxation of neighboring fibers of a group of muscles hold the organ or the part of the body in a neutral, functional position without fatigue. Tone is essential for many normal body functions, such as holding the spine erect. **2.** The state of the tissues of the body being strong and fit.

-tony A combining form meaning a 'condition of motor control': *arteriotony, neurotony.* Also **-tonia.**

tooth, *pl.* **teeth** One of numerous dental structures that develop in the jaws as part of the digestive system and are used to cut, grind, and process food in the mouth for ingestion. Each

tooth consists of a crown, which projects above the gum; two to four roots, embedded in the alveolus; and a neck, which stretches between the crown and the root. Each tooth also contains a cavity filled with pulp, richly supplied with blood vessels and nerves that enter the cavity through a small aperture at the base of each root. The solid portion of the tooth consists of dentin, enamel, and a thin layer of bone on the root surface. The dentin comprises the bulk of the tooth. The enamel covers the exposed portion of the crown. Two sets of teeth appear at different periods of life: the 20 deciduous teeth appear during infancy, the 32 permanent teeth during childhood and early adulthood. See also **deciduous tooth, permanent tooth.**

tooth germ A primitive cell in the embryo that is the precursor of a tooth.

tophus, *pl.* **tophi** A calculus, containing sodium urate deposits, that develops in periarticular fibrous tissue, typically in patients with gout.

-topia, -topy A combining form meaning '(condition of) placement of organs in the body': *heterotopia, normotopia, skeletopia.*

topical **1.** Of or pertaining to the surface of a body part. **2.** Of or pertaining to a drug or treatment applied topically.

topical anesthesia Surface analgesia produced by application of a topical anesthetic in the form of a solution, gel, or ointment to the skin, mucous membrane, or cornea. The most common ingredients include benzocaine, dibucaine, dimethisoquin, dyclonine, lidocaine, piperocaine, pramoxine, and tetracaine. Also called **surface anesthesia.** Compare **local anesthesia.**

topo- A combining form meaning 'place': *topognosis, toponarcosis.*

TORCH An acronym for *to*xoplasmosis, *o*ther *r*ubella virus, *c*ytomegalovirus, and *h*erpes simplex viruses, a group of agents that can infect the fetus or the newborn causing a constellation of morbid effects.

TORCH syndrome Infection of the fetus or newborn by one of the TORCH agents. The outcome of a pregnancy complicated by a TORCH agent may be abortion or stillbirth, intrauterine growth retardation, or premature delivery. At delivery and during the first days after birth, an infant infected with any one of the organisms may demonstrate various clinical manifestations, as fever, lethargy, poor feeding, petechiae on the skin, purpura, pneumonia, heptosplenomegaly, jaundice, hemolytic and other anemias, encephalitis, microcephaly, hydrocephalus, intracranial calcifications, hearing deficits, chorioretinitis, and micro-ophthalmia. In addition, each of the agents is associated with several other abnormal clinical findings involving abnormal immune response, cataracts, glaucoma, vesicles, ulcers, and congenital cardiac defects. Before pregnancy women may be tested for susceptibility to the rubella virus and inoculated against it if not immune. There are currently no vaccines that confer immunity to the other TORCH agents, but the mother may be serologically tested for antibody levels to them. During pregnancy toxoplasmosis is asymptomatic in about 90% of cases, making diagnosis unlikely. If infection is suspected, serial paired serologic tests are performed. Transplacental infection occurs in 35% of mothers infected during pregnancy. If it is contracted in the first trimester, before the placenta is fully developed, the infant may not become infected; if the infection is contracted, severe congenital manifestations of the syndrome usually occur. If the fetus is infected after the first trimester, the infant is usually born with asymptomatic or mild disease; the infection may be spread from the infant during the newborn period. Primary cytomegalovirus infection during pregnancy is usually asymptomatic. If the infection is suspected, serologic testing may be performed to demonstrate primary infection, as infants born to mothers infected for the first time during pregnancy are much more likely to develop severe congenital anomalies than if the infection were a reactivation of previous cytomegalovirus infection. There is no specific treatment. Transplacental rubella virus infection in pregnancy during the first 8 weeks is likely to cause infection in 50% of fetuses and to result in demonstrable defects in 85% of those infected. The risk becomes less as gestation increases to 24 weeks, after which time infection has not been known to result in defects. Rubella is the only TORCH virus that is usually symptomatic, and, therefore, it is often recognized. There is no treatment for the infection, but screening and immunization before pregnancy could prevent most cases of congenital rubella. Herpesvirus infection (HSV) in pregnancy may rarely be transplacentally transmitted to the fetus. Primary infection during pregnancy may sometimes result in spontaneous abortion or premature delivery. In the newborn the infection is usually systemic and life-threatening. The fetus is most apt to become infected by the virus shed from an active genital lesion during vaginal delivery or as the result of vaginal examination or the placement of an intrauterine catheter or a fetal scalp electrode during labor. There is no treatment: if the mother has active, genital herpesvirus lesions, intrapartal internal monitoring is contraindicated, vaginal examinations are often omitted, regional anesthetic techniques are avoided, and the infant is delivered by cesarean section. The TORCH infections caused by other agents are asymptomatic in pregnancy, revealing themselves by the syndrome evident after birth. The congenital effects are not amenable to change or to amelioration by any known treatment. Newborn infants who are infected with a TORCH agent or who bear the stigmata of TORCH syndrome are considered potential sources of neonatal spread of infection.

Torkildsen procedure See **ventriculocisternostomy.**

torpid idiocy Severe mental retardation associated with dullness and inactivity.

torque A moment of force that tends to pro-

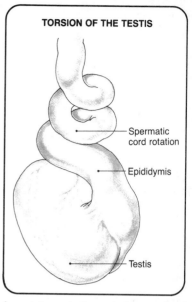

TORSION OF THE TESTIS

Spermatic cord rotation

Epididymis

Testis

duce rotation, or torsion, as the forces produced by contraction of the medial femoral muscles tend to rotate the thigh medially.

torr A unit of pressure, commonly used to mean 1 mm Hg, the amount of pressure required to raise a column of mercury 1 mm.

tors- A combining form meaning 'twisted': *torsiometer, torsive, torsiversion.*

torsion 1. The process of twisting or turning away from the normal position. It may be positive (clockwise) or negative (counterclockwise). 2. The state of being turned.

torsion dystonia See **dystonia musculorum deformans.**

torsion fracture A spiral fracture, usually caused by a torsion injury.

torsion of the testis The axial rotation of the spermatic cord that cuts off the blood supply to the testicle, epididymis, and other structures. Complete ischemia for 6 hours may result in gangrene of the testis. Partial loss of circulation may result in atrophy. Certain testes are anatomically predisposed to torsion because of inadequate connective tissue, but the condition may be caused by trauma with severe swelling. Torsion of the testis is most frequent in the first year of life and during puberty. Surgical correction is required in most cases.

torsion spasm See **dystonia musculorum deformans.**

tort In law: a civil wrong, other than a breach of contract. Torts include negligence, false imprisonment, assault, and battery. The elements of a tort are: a legal duty owed by the defendant to the plaintiff, a breach of duty, and damage from the breach of duty. —**tortious,** *adj.*

tort feasor A person who commits a tort.

torticollis An abnormal condition in which

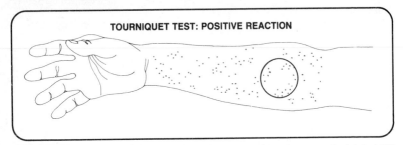

TOURNIQUET TEST: POSITIVE REACTION

the head is inclined to one side as a result of muscle contractions on that side of the neck. It may be congenital or acquired. Treatment may include surgery, heat, support, or immobilization depending on the cause and severity. Also called **wryneck.** See also **spasmodic torticollis.**

Torula histolytica   See *Cryptococcus neoformans.*

torulopsosis   An infection with the yeast *Torulopsis glabrata,* a normal inhabitant of the oropharynx, gastrointestinal tract, and skin, that causes disease in severely debilitated patients, in those with impaired immune function, or, sometimes, in those having prolonged urinary catheterization. Systemic infection is usually treated with amphotericin B or fluorocytosine.

torulosis   See **cryptococcosis.**

torus fracture   See **lead pipe fracture.**

total anomalous venous return   A rare congenital cardiac anomaly in which the pulmonary veins attach directly to the right atrium or to various veins draining into the right atrium rather than directing flow to the left atrium. Clinical manifestations include cyanosis, pulmonary congestion, and heart failure. Other cardiac defects may also be present, as atrial septal defect, which shunts unoxygenated systemic blood to the left side of the heart and helps to decompress the right atrium. Corrective surgery is indicated. See also **congenital cardiac anomaly.**

total cleavage   Mitotic division of the fertilized ovum into blastomeres. Compare **partial cleavage.**

total lung capacity (TLC)   The volume of gas in the lungs at the end of a maximum inspiration.

total parenteral nutrition (TPN)   The administration of a nutritionally adequate hypertonic solution consisting of glucose, protein hydrolysates, minerals, and vitamins through an indwelling catheter into the superior vena cava. The high rate of blood flow results in rapid dilution of the solution and full nutritional requirements can be met indefinitely. The procedure is used when feeding by mouth cannot provide adequate amounts of the essential nutrients. Strict asepsis must be maintained as infection is a grave and present danger. Also called intravenous hyperalimentation. See **hyperalimentation.**

total renal blood flow (TRBF)   The total volume of blood that flows into the renal arteries.

The average TRBF in a normal adult is 1,200 ml/minute.

touch deprivation   A lack of tactile stimulation, especially in early infancy, which if continued may lead to serious developmental and emotional disturbances, as stunted growth, personality disorders, and social regression. In severe cases, a child deprived of adequate physical handling and emotional stimulation may not survive infancy. See also **hospitalism.**

tourniquet   A device used to control hemorrhage, consisting of a wide constricting band applied to the limb proximal to the site of bleeding. Tourniquet use is a drastic measure and is to be employed only if the hemorrhage is life-threatening and if other, safer measures have proved ineffective. See also **hemorrhage.**

tourniquet test   A test of capillary fragility, in which a blood pressure cuff is applied for 5 minutes to a person's arm and is inflated to a pressure halfway between his diastolic and systolic blood pressure. The number of petechiae within a circumscribed area of the skin may be counted, or the results may be reported in a range from negative (no petechiae) to +4 positive (confluent petechiae).

tower head   See **oxycephaly.**

tower skull   See **oxycephaly.**

toxemia   The presence of toxins in the bloodstream. Also called **blood poisoning.** See also **preeclampsia. —toxemic,** *adj.*

-toxemia, -toxaemia   A combining form meaning a '(specified) toxic substance in the blood': *ectotoxemia, gonotoxemia, ophiotoxemia.*

toxemia of pregnancy   See **preeclampsia.**

-toxia   A combining form meaning 'condition resulting from a poison in a (specified) region of the body': *neurotoxia, thyrotoxia.*

toxic   1. Of or pertaining to a poison. 2. Of a disease or condition: severe and progressive.

-toxic, -toxical   A combining form meaning 'pertaining to poison': *cardiotoxic, hematoxic.*

toxic amblyopia   Partial loss of vision owing to retro-optic bulbar neuritis, caused by poisoning with quinine, lead, wood alcohol, arsenic, or certain other poisons.

toxic dementia   Dementia from excessive use of or exposure to a poisonous substance. See also **dementia.**

toxic dose (TD)   In toxicology: the amount of a substance that may be expected to produce a toxic effect. See also **median toxic dose.**

toxic epidermal necrolysis (TEN) A rare skin disease, characterized by epidermal erythema, superficial necrosis, and skin erosions. This condition, which affects mainly adults, makes the skin appear scalded, often leaving scars. The cause of TEN is unknown. It is commonly associated with drug reactions, as those associated with butazones, sulfonamides, penicillins, barbiturates, and hydantoins, and with airborne toxins, as carbon monoxide. TEN may also indicate an immune response, or it may be associated with severe physiologic stress. Early signs of the condition include inflammation of the mucous membranes, fever, malaise, a burning sensation in the conjunctivae, and pervasive tenderness of the skin. As the disease progresses, large, flaccid bullae develop and rupture, exposing wide expanses of denuded skin. Tissue fluids and electrolytes are consequently lost, resulting in extensive systemic complications, as pulmonary edema, bronchopneumonia, gastrointestinal and esophageal hemorrhage, sepsis, shock, renal failure, and disseminated intravascular coagulation. These extreme conditions contribute to the high mortality—about 30%—associated with TEN. Confirming diagnosis is based on symptoms in the third phase of the disease, as skin denuded by even slight friction, affecting the areas of erythema. Treatment of TEN commonly involves the administration of I.V. fluids to replace body fluids and to maintain electrolyte balance.

NURSING CONSIDERATIONS: Nursing care includes meticulous monitoring of vital signs, central venous pressure, and urinary output. Any signs of renal failure, as decreased urinary output, and of bleeding are of immediate concern. It is important to detect and quickly treat any septic infection. Ocular lesions are common with TEN, and frequent eye care is often needed to remove exudate. Protective isolation and prophylactic antibiotic therapy may be required to prevent secondary infection. Nurses also make sure that the TEN patient does not wear tight clothing and is covered loosely to minimize the friction that causes skin sloughing. A Stryker frame or a CircOlectric bed may be helpful. Analgesics are administered as needed, and cool, sterile compresses may be applied to relieve discomfort.

toxic erythema of the newborn See **erythema toxicum neonatorum.**

toxic gastritis See **corrosive gastritis.**

toxic goiter An enlargement of the thyroid gland associated with exophthalmia and systemic disease. See also **Graves' disease.**

toxic hemoglobinuria See **hemoglobinuria.**

toxicity 1. The degree to which something is poisonous. 2. A condition that results from exposure to a toxin or to toxic amounts of a substance that does not cause adverse effects in smaller amounts.

toxic nodular goiter An enlarged thyroid gland characterized by numerous discrete nodules and hypersecretion of thyroid hormones, occurring most frequently in elderly individuals. Typical signs of thyrotoxicosis, as nervousness, tremor, weakness, fatigue, weight loss, and irritability, are usually present, but exophthalmia is rare; anorexia is more common than hyperphagia, and cardiac arrhythmia or congestive heart failure may be a predominant manifestation.

toxico-, toxo- A combining form meaning 'pertaining to poison, poisonous': *toxicomucin, toxicosozin.* Also **toxo-.**

toxicologist A specialist in toxicology.

toxicology The scientific study of poisons, their detection, their effects, and methods of treatment for conditions they produce. —**toxicologic, toxicological,** *adj.*

toxic shock syndrome (TSS) A severe acute disease caused by infection with strains of *Staphylococcus aureus,* phage group I, that produces a unique toxin, enterotoxin F. It is most common in menstruating women using high absorbency tampons but has been seen in newborn infants, children, and men. The onset of the syndrome is characterized by sudden high fever, headache, sore throat with swelling of the mucous membranes, myalgia, diarrhea, nausea, and macular erythematous rash, followed by desquamation 1 to 2 weeks after onset, especially on the fingers and toes. Acute renal failure, abnormal liver function, confusion, and refractory hypotension usually follow, and death may occur. It is probable that mild forms of the syndrome are not reported and, therefore, are not diagnosed. There does not appear to be any seasonal or geographic factor in the etiology of the disease, and there is no evidence of contagion among household or sexual contacts of people who have TSS. *Staphylococcus aureus* may be cultured from many sites, including the pharynx, nares, and cervix, but the drastic effects of infection are the result of the toxin released from the organism rather than from the infection itself. Aggressive volume expansion by the administration of large amounts of intravenous fluid, assisted ventilation, and administration of vasopressors may be necessary in treating severe TSS.

NURSING CONSIDERATIONS: The use of highly absorbent tampons is associated with a greater incidence of the disease than the use of regular tampons. The nurse counsels women to wash their hands before inserting tampons, to avoid the high absorbency tampons, and to report any illness occurring during the menses accompanied by nausea, diarrhea, and fever. Recurrence is likely; a mild, undiagnosed episode during a preceding menstrual period is often reported when severe TSS is diagnosed. Women who have had TSS are usually advised to avoid using any kind of tampons for at least several months and then to use them intermittently with sanitary napkins.

toxin A poison, usually one produced by or occurring in a plant or microorganism. See also **endotoxin, exotoxin.**

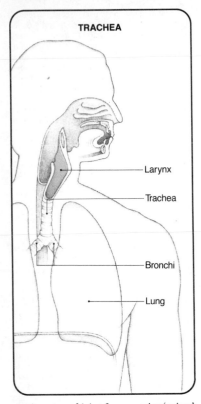

TRACHEA

- Larynx
- Trachea
- Bronchi
- Lung

-toxin A combining form meaning 'poison': *cynotoxin, hypnotoxin, zootoxin.*

toxo- See **toxico-.**

toxocariasis Infection with the larvae of *Toxocara canis,* the common roundworm of dogs and cats. Ingestion of viable eggs, commonly found in soil, leads to the spread of tiny larvae throughout the body, resulting in respiratory symptoms, enlarged liver, skin rashes, eosinophilia, and delayed ocular lesions. Children who eat dirt are particularly subject to this disease. Specific drug therapy is not very useful; the outcome is usually good without therapy. Regular worming of pets helps prevent infection. Also called **visceral larva migrans.**

toxoid A toxin that has been treated with chemicals or with heat to decrease its toxic effect but that retains its antigenic power. It is given to produce immunity by stimulating the creation of antibodies. See also **toxin, vaccine.**

Toxoplasma A genus of protozoa with only one known species, *Toxoplasma gondii,* an intracellular parasite of cats and other hosts that causes toxoplasmosis in man.

toxoplasmosis A common infection with the protozoan intracellular parasite *Toxoplasma gondii,* characterized in the congenital form by liver and brain involvement with cerebral calcification, convulsions, blindness, microcephaly or hydrocephaly, and mental retardation. The acquired form is characterized by rash, lymphadenopathy, fever, malaise, central nervous system disorders, myocarditis, and pneumonitis. Cats acquire the organism by eating infected birds and mice. Cysts of the organism are transmitted from cat feces to humans or by human ingestion of inadequately cooked meat containing the cysts. Transplacental transmission occurs only during acute infection of the mother, but the disease is very serious in the fetus and in those with an impaired immune system. Diagnosis is made by demonstrating rising antibody titers or by immunofluorescent antibody tests. Infection confers immunity. NURSING CONSIDERATIONS: All meat should be heated to at least 60°C (140°F) throughout to kill this parasite. Pregnant women who are not immune are advised not to handle cats, cat feces, or litter boxes.

TPN *abbr* **total parenteral nutrition.**

trabecula carnea, *pl.* **trabeculae carneae** Any one of the irregular bands and bundles of muscle that project from the inner surfaces of the ventricles, except in the arterial cone of the right ventricle. Some of these trabeculae are ridges of muscle along the ventricular walls; others are short projections into the ventricular cavities; still others form the ventricular papillary muscles. See also **heart.**

trabecula septomarginalis See **moderator band.**

trace element An element essential to nutrition or physiological processes, found in such minute quantities that analysis yields a presence of virtually zero amounts.

trace gas A gas or vapor that escapes into the atmosphere during an anesthetic procedure. Because these substances may have adverse effects on the health of personnel exposed to them, scavenging equipment is often installed to clean the air. See also **gas scavenging system.**

tracer **1.** A radioactive isotope used in diagnostic X-ray techniques to allow a biologic process to be seen. The tracer, which is introduced into the body, binds with a specific substance and is followed with a scanner or fluoroscope as it passes through various organs or systems in the body. See also **radioisotope scan.** **2.** A mechanical device that graphically records the outline or movements of an object or part of the body. **3.** A dissecting instrument used to isolate vessels and nerves. **—trace,** *v.*

tracer depot method In nuclear medicine: a technique used to determine local skin or muscle blood flow, based on the rate at which a radioactive tracer deposited in a tissue is removed by diffusion into the capillaries and washed out by the local blood supply. If blood flow is diminished or absent, the deposited tracer does not wash out.

trachea A nearly cylindrical tube in the neck, composed of cartilage and membrane, that extends from the larynx at the level of the sixth cervical vertebra to the fifth thoracic vertebra, where it divides into two bronchi. The trachea conveys air to the lungs; it is about 11 cm (4⅓ inches) long and 2 cm (¾ inch) wide. The ventral surface of the tube is covered in the neck by the thyroid gland isthmus and various other structures. Dorsally, the trachea is in contact with the esophagus. See also **primary bronchus. —tracheal,** *adj.*

tracheal breath sound A normal breath sound heard in trachea auscultation. Inspiration and expiration are equally loud, the expiratory sound being heard during the greater part of expiration, whereas the inspiratory sound stops abruptly at the height of inspiration, with a pause before the expiration sound is heard. Compare **vesicular breath sound.**

tracheitis Any inflammatory condition of the trachea. It may be acute or chronic, resulting from infection, allergy, or physical irritation.

trachelo- A combining form meaning 'pertaining to the neck or a necklike structure': *trachelobregmatic, trachelocystitis.*

trachelodynia See **cervicodynia.**

tracheo- A combining form meaning 'pertaining to the trachea': *tracheobronchial, tracheomalacia, tracheorrhaphy.*

tracheobronchial tree (TBT) An anatomical complex that includes the trachea, the bronchi, and the bronchial tubes. It conveys air to and from the lungs and is a primary structure in respiration. See also **bronchial tree.**

tracheobronchitis Inflammation of the trachea and bronchi, a common form of respiratory infection.

tracheostomy An opening through the neck into the trachea with an indwelling tube inserted. The incision and stoma are created surgically to establish an airway when the pharynx is obstructed by a foreign body, tumor, or edema of the glottis. Local or general anesthesia is usually given. The patient's neck is hyperextended, an incision is made below the Adam's apple, a small opening is made in the fibrous tissues of the trachea, and a tube is slipped in while the hole is held open with a small hemostat, as a mosquito forceps. The tube is suctioned frequently to keep it free from tracheobronchial secretions using a suction catheter attached to a Y-connector. The patient is taught to cough to move secretions up and out of the bronchi. Should the outer tube be expelled, the nurse uses a dilator or hemostat to hold the trachea open until another tube can be inserted. The dressing is changed as necessary, the area is kept dry and clean, and frequent oral care is given. Pen and paper are kept available for communication. Complications of tracheostomy include pneumothorax and mediastinal emphysema. If the procedure was done as an emergency, the tracheostomy is closed once normal breathing is restored. If the tracheostomy is permanent, as with a laryngectomy, the patient is taught self-care. Compare **tracheotomy.**

tracheotomy An incision made into the trachea through the neck below the larynx, performed to gain access to the airway below a blockage with a foreign body, tumor, or edema

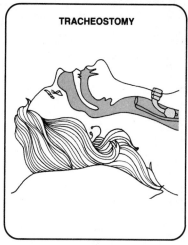

TRACHEOSTOMY

of the glottis. In an emergency any available instrument may be used as a dilator, even the barrel of a ballpoint pen with the inner portion removed, if only that is available. If the blockage persists a tracheostomy tube is inserted; if not, the incision is closed once normal respirations are established. Compare **tracheostomy.**

trachoma A chronic, infectious disease of the eye caused by the bacterium *Chlamydia trachomatis,* characterized initially by inflammation, pain, photophobia, and lacrimation. If untreated, follicles form on the upper eyelids and grow larger until the granulations invade the cornea, eventually causing blindness. Trachoma is a significant cause of blindness and is endemic to hot, dry, poverty-ridden areas. In the United States, it is found on Indian reservations in the Southwest. Also called **Egyptian ophthalmia, granular conjunctivitis.**

tract An elongate group of tissues and structures that function together as a pathway, as the digestive tract.

90-90 traction An orthopedic mechanism, used especially in pediatrics, that combines skeletal traction and suspension with a short leg cast or a splint to immobilize and position the lower extremity in the treatment of a displaced fractured femur. This type of traction is usually unilateral with the opposite leg in Buck's traction or in split Russell traction for immobilization. The pin used in this kind of skeletal traction is inserted into bone in the knee area and attached to a riser running through a pulley on an overhead traction frame to a pulley and weight system fitted over the foot of the bed. The pulley and weight system at the foot of the bed also accommodates additional attachments to the short leg cast or splint of the involved lower limb. Application of 90-90 traction may also incorporate a jacket restraint to help immobilize the patient. A variation of this type of traction is often used with adults in the treatment of low back pain.

TYPES OF TRACTION

Buck's extension

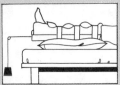

- *Skin traction* usually applied to leg by weight attached to spreader bar below foot, and pulling force is applied with the leg in a straight line.
- Pillow placed under leg keeps pressure off heel.
- *Uses:* dislocated hip after reduction; hip fracture before surgery; after total hip replacement; locked knee; fractured femur before open reduction; irritated hip or knee joint

Dunlop

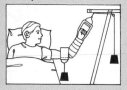

- Applies lateral traction to elbow; temporary; used for children
- Using *skin traction,* shoulder is abducted 90° and elbow extended in 45° position to stretch biceps muscle.
- Uses two pulling forces: one applied laterally to forearm by skin traction, and the other applied downward by sling hanging from distal portion of upper arm. Forces act on elbow from two directions with different magnitudes, causing pull in a third direction.
- *Uses:* transcondylar or supracondylar fracture of humerus; contracture of elbow

Overhead (90°-90°)

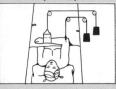

- If applied to arm, upper arm is perpendicular to body, elbow is flexed 90°, and forearm is supported by sling suspended from overhead pulley.
- Usually used with *skeletal traction,* with pin insertion through olecranon
- *Uses:* fracture of humerus or elbow; fracture or injury of shoulder; may also be applied to leg for displaced fractured femur in children and for lower back pain

Russell

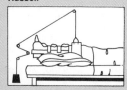

- *Skin traction* to affected leg and sling placed under knee.
- Uses two pulling forces: one applied by double-pulley system at foot and the other applied upward by sling under knee attached to single overhead pulley
- *Uses:* congenital hip dislocation; hip fracture; after total hip replacement; fractured femur; disease of hip or knee

Sidearm

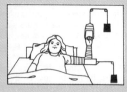

- May be applied by *skin or skeletal traction*
- For lateral-longitudinal traction of humerus, shoulder is abducted 90° and externally rotated, elbow is flexed 90° and kept perpendicular to bed.
- *For skin traction,* separate wraps are used on upper arm and forearm.
- *Skeletal traction* applied by pin through olecranon, with forearm traction by adhesive straps and elastic bandage.
- *Uses:* fractures, dislocations, and other pathologies of upper arm and shoulder; tissue injury around elbow (skin traction)

traction **1.** In orthopedics: the process of putting a limb, bone, or group of muscles under tension using weights and pulleys to align, immobilize, or relieve pressure. **2.** The process of pulling a part of the body along, through, or out of its socket or cavity, as axis traction with obstetric forceps used in delivering an infant.

traction frame An orthopedic apparatus that supports the pulleys, ropes, and weights by which traction is applied to various parts of the body or by which various parts of the body are suspended. Traction frames are used to treat bone fractures and dislocations and disease processes of the musculoskeletal system, to correct various orthopedic deformities, and to immobilize specific areas. The main components of a traction frame are metal uprights, which attach to the bed and support an overhead metal bar. In addition to traction equipment, traction frames are often rigged with trapeze bars that the patient can grasp to help in changing positions and to exercise the muscles of the arms and trunk. Compare **Balkan frame, claw-type traction frame, I.V.-type traction frame.**

trade name The registered trademark assigned to a product by its manufacturer. See also **generic name.**

tragus, *pl.* **tragi** A projection of the cartilage of the auricle at the opening of the external auditory meatus.

trained reflex See **conditioned response.**

traineeship A grant of money allocated to an individual for study in a given field. In nursing, many graduate students have been awarded federal traineeships that provide funds for tuition and living expenses.

training grant A grant of money or other resources to provide training in a particular field. Many schools of nursing receive federal or state grants to provide specific educational programs. Funds may be allocated for faculty salaries, student aid, or other expenses.

trait **1.** A characteristic mode of behavior or a mannerism or physical feature that distinguishes an individual or culture from another. **2.** Any characteristic quality or condition that is genetically determined and inherited as a specific genotype. A trait is expressed in the phenotype as dominant or recessive; it is inherited in the genotype as either homozygous dominant, homozygous recessive, or heterozygous in the ratio of 1:2:1. In medicine, trait is used specifically to denote the heterozygous state of a recessive disorder, as the sickle cell trait. See also **dominance, gene, Mendel's laws, recessive.**

trance **1.** A sleeplike state characterized by the complete or partial suspension of consciousness and loss or diminution of motor activity, as seen in hypnosis, the dissociative form of hysterical neurosis, and various cataleptic and ecstatic states. **2.** A dazed or bewildered condition; stupor. **3.** A state of detachment from one's immediate surroundings, as in deep concentration or daydreaming. Kinds of trances are **alcoholic trance, death trance, hypnotic trance, hysterical trance, induced trance.**

tranquilizer A drug prescribed to calm anxious or agitated people, ideally without decreasing their consciousness. Major tranquilizers (also known as antipsychotic agents), as derivatives of phenothiazine, butyrophenone, and thioxanthene, are used to treat psychoses. Minor tran-

quilizers (also known as antianxiety agents), prescribed for the treatment of anxiety, irritability, tension, or psychoneurosis, include chlordiazepoxide, diazepam, and hydroxyzine. Tranquilizers tend to induce drowsiness and have the potential for causing strong psychological dependence. See also **antipsychotic.**

trans- A combining form meaning 'across, through, over': *transabdominal, transferase.*

transactional analysis (TA) A form of psychotherapy developed by Eric Berne, based on a theory that three different, coherent, organized egos exist throughout life simultaneously in every person, representing the child, the adult, and the parent. Interactions between people are transactions, originating from a person in one of the ego states, received by another person who may be in a complementary or a crossed ego state. Transactions are motivated by a need for recognition and contact called strokes. Transactions occur in six kinds of time structure: withdrawal, rituals, pastimes, games, activities, and intimacy. The goal of transactional analysis is to give the adult ego state decision-making power over the child ego state and the parent ego state.

transaminase An enzyme that catalyzes the transfer of an amino group from an alpha-amino acid to an alpha-keto acid, with pyridoxal phosphate and pyridoxamine phosphate acting as coenzymes. Glutamic-oxaloacetic transaminase (GOT), normally present in serum and various tissues, especially in the heart and liver, is released by damaged cells, and, as a result, a high serum level of GOT may be diagnostic in myocardial infarction or hepatic disease. Glutamic-pyruvic transaminase (GPT), a normal constituent of serum and various tissues, especially in the liver, is released by injured tissue and may be present in high concentrations in the sera of patients with acute liver disease. Also called **aminotransferase.**

transcondylar fracture A fracture that occurs transversally and distal to the epicondyles of any one of the long bones.

trans configuration, trans arrangement, trans position In genetics: **1.** The presence of the dominant allele of one pair of genes and the recessive allele of another pair on the same chromosome. **2.** The presence of at least one mutant gene and one wild-type gene of a pair of pseudoalleles on each chromosome of a homologous pair. Compare **cis configuration.**

transcortical apraxia See **ideomotor apraxia.**

transcription In molecular genetics: the process by which RNA is formed from a DNA template in the manufacture of a protein.

transcultural nursing A field of nursing in which the nurse transcends ethnocentricity and practices nursing in other cultural environments. As current nursing process and theory are not culturally bound and the needs of each person are considered individually, transcultural nursing is potentially a part of all nursing practice.

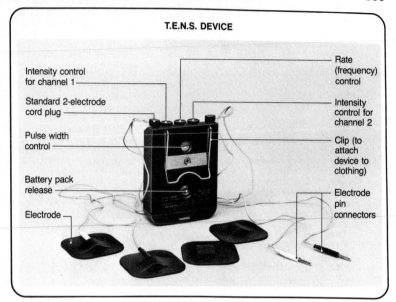

T.E.N.S. DEVICE

Intensity control for channel 1

Standard 2-electrode cord plug

Pulse width control

Battery pack release

Electrode

Rate (frequency) control

Intensity control for channel 2

Clip (to attach device to clothing)

Electrode pin connectors

transcutaneous electrical nerve stimulator (TENS) A portable device that transmits painless electrical impulses to peripheral nerves or directly to a painful area. These impulses block transmission of pain impulses to the brain. TENS, a device used for postoperative patients and those with chronic pain, reduces the need for analgesics and permits resumption of normal activities.

transduction In molecular genetics: a method of genetic recombination by which DNA is transferred from one cell to another by a viral vector.

transfection In molecular genetics: the process by which a cell is infected with DNA or RNA isolated from a virus or a viral vector. Acute transfection is short-term infection.

transfer DNA (tDNA) In molecular genetics: DNA transferred from its original source and present in transformed cells.

transference **1.** The shifting of symptoms from one part of the body to another, as occurs in conversion disorder. **2.** In psychiatry: an unconscious defense mechanism whereby feelings and attitudes originally associated with people and events that were important in one's early life are attributed to others in current situations. **3.** In psychoanalysis and psychotherapy: the feelings of a patient for the analyst to whom the patient has attributed or assigned the qualities, attitudes, and feelings of a person or persons significant in his emotional development, usually a figure from his childhood. See also **countertransference, parataxic distortion.**

transfer factor A leukocyte extract that transfers delayed hypersensitivity from one person to another. Transfer factor is being studied for possible use in treating chronic mucocuta-

neous candidiasis and Wiskott-Aldrich syndrome and as a means of transferring antitumor immunity in patients with various types of cancer.

transferrin A trace protein present in the blood that is essential in iron transport. Its major function is to move iron from the intestine into the bloodstream, making it available to the normoblasts of the bone marrow. It may also take part in a slower exchange with ferritin, hemosiderin, and other iron forms in the tissues. See also **hemosiderin, iron transport.**

transfer RNA (tRNA) In molecular genetics: a kind of RNA that transfers the genetic code from messenger RNA for the production of a specific amino acid. There are at least 20 different kinds of tRNA, each of which is able to combine covalently with a specific amino acid and to bond with at least one messenger RNA nucleotide triplet. Also called **adaptor RNA.**

transformation In molecular genetics: the process in which exogenous genes are integrated into chromosomes in a form that is recognized by the replicative and transcriptive apparatus of the host cell.

transforming growth factor A protein or a group of proteins produced by the cells of a tumor that, when inoculated into a normal cell culture, causes a disorderly and abnormal increase in the number of cells in the culture.

transfusion Introduction into the bloodstream of whole blood or blood components, as plasma, platelets, or packed red blood cells. Whole blood may be infused into the recipient directly from a donor matched for the ABO blood group and antigenic subgroups, but more frequently the donor's blood is collected and stored by a blood bank. See also **blood transfusion.**

transfusion reaction A systemic response to the administration of incompatible blood. The causes include red blood cell incompatibility and allergic sensitivity to the leukocytes, the platelets, or the plasma protein components of the transfused blood, or to the potassium or citrate preservative in banked blood. Fever is the most common transfusion reaction; urticaria is a relatively common allergic response. Asthma, vascular collapse, and renal failure occur less commonly. A hemolytic reaction from red blood cell incompatibility is serious and must be diagnosed and treated promptly. Symptoms emerge shortly after beginning the transfusion, before 50 ml have been given, and include a throbbing headache; sudden, deep, and severe lumbar pain; precordial pain; dyspnea; and restlessness. Objective signs include ruddy facial flushing followed by cyanosis and distended neck veins; rapid, thready pulse; diaphoresis; and cold, clammy skin. Profound shock may occur within 1 hour. When a hemolytic reaction is suspected, the transfusion is promptly terminated and the infusion line kept open with a normal solution of intravenous fluid for therapeutic purposes. The remaining bank blood is saved for a repeat type and cross-match against a fresh sample of blood from the recipient. Direct and indirect Coomb's tests are usually ordered to detect hemolytic antibodies, and a sample of urine is examined for free hemoglobin. In the presence of oliguria, the possibility of acute renal failure is evaluated, and the patient is managed accordingly. Hypovolemia is corrected with saline or plasma expanders but the administration of more whole blood is avoided, if possible. Questioning the patient about previous transfusions may elicit warning indications of possible adverse reactions.

transient ischemic attack (TIA) An episode of cerebrovascular insufficiency, usually owing to a partial occlusion of an artery by an atherosclerotic plaque or an embolism. The symptoms vary with the site and the degree of occlusion. Disturbance of normal vision in one or in both eyes, dizziness, weakness, dysphasia, numbness, or unconsciousness may occur. The attack usually lasts a few minutes; symptoms rarely continue for several hours.

transillumination 1. The passage of light through a solid or liquid substance. **2.** The passage of light through body tissues for the purpose of examining a structure. A diaphanoscope is an instrument introduced into a body cavity to transilluminate tissues.

transitional cell carcinoma A malignant, usually papillary, tumor derived from transitional stratified epithelium, occurring most frequently in the bladder, ureter, urethra, or renal pelvis. The majority of tumors in the collecting system of the kidney are of this kind. They have a better prognosis than squamous cell carcinomas in the same site.

transitional dentition See **mixed dentition.**

transitory mania A mood disorder characterized by the sudden onset of manic reactions, usually lasting from 1 hour to a few days. See also **mania.**

translation In molecular genetics: the process in which the genetic information carried by nucleotides in messenger RNA directs the amino acid sequence in the synthesis of a specific polypeptide.

translocation In genetics: the rearrangement of genetic material within the same chromosome or the transfer of a segment of one chromosome to another nonhomologous one. In simple translocations, one end segment of one chromosome is transferred onto the end of another nonhomologous one, involving a single break in only one of the chromosomes. Translocations in which material from the middle of one chromosome is shifted to the middle of another one are more complex and involve at least three breaks in the participating chromosomes. Such shifting of genetic material can result in serious disorders, as Down's syndrome, which is caused by a 14/21 translocation. Kinds of translocations are **balanced translocation, reciprocal translocation, Robertsonian translocation.**

transmission The transfer or conveyance of a thing or condition, as a neural impulse, infectious or genetic disease, or a hereditary trait, from one person or place to another. —**transmissible,** *adj.*

transmission electron microscopy See **electron microscopy.**

transmission scanning electron microscope An instrument that transmits a highly magnified, well-resolved, three-dimensional image on a television screen. Compare **electron microscope, scanning electron microscope.**

transmission scanning electron microscopy (TSEM) A technique using a transmission scanning electron microscope in which the atomic number of the portion of the sample being scanned is determined and used to modulate a beam of electrons in a cathode-ray tube and in the beam scanning the sample. The image produced is clear, three-dimensional, and highly magnified. Compare **electron microscopy, scanning electron microscopy.**

transmitter substance See **neurotransmitter.**

transneuronal degeneration Degeneration of irreparably damaged nerve cells that may progress proximally or distally to neurons more than one synapse removed.

transovarial transmission The transfer of pathogens to succeeding generations through invasion of the ovary and infection of the egg, as occurs in arthropods, primarily ticks and mites.

transplacental Across or through the placenta, specifically in reference to the exchange of nutrients, waste products, and other material between the fetus and the mother.

transplant 1. To transfer an organ or tissue from one person to another or from one body part to another to replace a diseased structure

TRANSPOSITION OF THE GREAT VESSELS

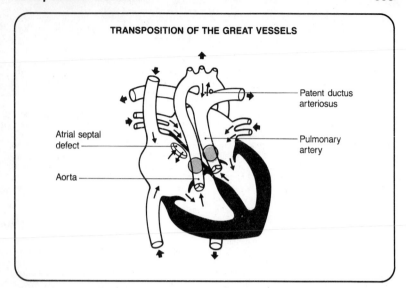

Patent ductus arteriosus

Atrial septal defect

Pulmonary artery

Aorta

or restore function. Skin and kidneys are the most frequently transplanted structures; others include cartilage, bone, corneal tissue, portions of blood vessels and tendons, and, recently but infrequently, hearts and livers. Preferred donors are identical twins or persons having the same blood type and immunologic characteristics. Success of the transplant depends upon overcoming the rejection of the donor tissue by the immune system of the recipient. Under local or general anesthesia, the recipient site is prepared and the donor structure grafted in place; its oxygenation and blood supply are preserved during the procedure until the circulation can be restored at the new site. After surgery, circulation in the area is observed for signs of impairment. Antilymphocytic serum may be given, with steroids, to suppress the production of antibodies to the foreign tissue proteins. Signs of rejection reaction include fever, pain, and loss of function, usually occuring in the first 4 to 10 days following transplantation. The grafted structure may require several weeks to become established. Late rejection may occur several months or even a year later. **2.** Any tissue or organ that is transplanted. **3.** Of or pertaining to a transplanted tissue or organ, to a recipient of a donated tissue or organ, or to a phenomenon associated with the procedure. Also called **graft.** —**transplantation,** *n.*

transposable element In molecular genetics: a DNA fragment or segment that can move or be moved from one site in the genome to another.

transposase In molecular genetics: an enzyme involved in the movement of a DNA fragment or segment from one site in the genome to another.

transposition 1. An abnormality occuring during embryonic development in which a body

part normally on the left is found on the right or vice versa. **2.** The shifting of genetic material from one chromosome to another at some point in the reproductive process, often resulting in a congenital anomaly. —**transpose,** *v.*

transposition of the great vessels A congenital cardiac anomaly in which the pulmonary artery arises from the left ventricle and the aorta from the right ventricle, so that there is no communication between the systemic and pulmonary circulations. Life is impossible without associated cardiac defects, as septal defects or a patent ductus arteriosus, which enable the mixing of oxygenated and unoxygenated blood. The severity of the condition depends on the type and size of the associated defect. The primary symptoms are cyanosis and hypoxia, especially in infants with small septal defects, although cardiomegaly is usually evident a few weeks after birth. Signs of congestive heart failure develop rapidly, especially in those infants with large ventricular septal defects. Definitive diagnosis is based on cardiac catheterization. Surgical correction of the defect is postponed, if possible, until after 6 months of age when the infant can better tolerate the procedure. See also **congenital cardiac anomaly.**

transposon A gene or a group of genes that are mobile and, like plasmids, act to transfer genetic instructions from one place to another. Transposons travel piggyback from virus to virus on bacteriophages. The genetic material is incorporated into the virus when the virus infects a bacterial cell. As the bacteria replicates itself, it also copies the genetic instructions brought by the transposon.

transtentorial herniation A bulge of brain tissue out of the cranium through the tentorial notch, caused by increased intracranial pressure. See also **tentorial herniation.**

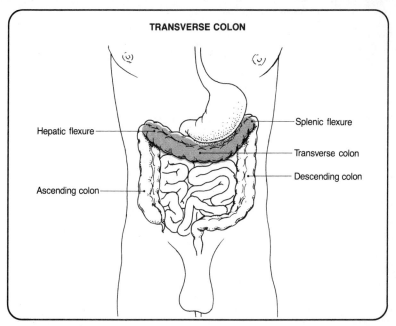

TRANSVERSE COLON

Hepatic flexure

Ascending colon

Splenic flexure

Transverse colon

Descending colon

transthermia   See **thermopenetration.**
transudate   A fluid passed through a membrane or squeezed through a tissue or into the space between the cells of a tissue. It is thin and watery and contains few blood cells or other large proteins. See also **edema.**
transudative ascites   An abnormal accumulation in the peritoneal cavity of a fluid that characteristically contains scant amounts of protein and cells. Ascitic fluids with protein counts of less than 2.5 g/ml are considered to be transudates. Transudative ascites indicates cirrhosis or congestive heart failure.
transurethral   Through the urethra, as in transurethral prostatectomy. Compare **suprapubic.**
transverse   At right angles to the long axis of any common part, as the planes that cut the long axis of the body into upper and lower portions and are at right angles to the sagittal and frontal planes.
transverse colon   The part of the colon extending from the end of the ascending colon at the hepatic flexure on the right side across the midabdomen to the beginning of the descending colon at the splenic flexure on the left side.
transverse fissure   A fissure dividing the dorsal surface of the diencephalon and the ventral surface of the cerebral hemisphere. Also called **fissure of Bichat.**
transverse fracture   A fracture that occurs at right angles to the longitudinal axis of the bone involved.
transverse lie   Abnormal presentation of a fetus in which the long axis of the infant's body

is horizontal to the long axis of the mother's body.
transverse ligament of the atlas   A thick, strong ligament stretched across the ring of the atlas, holding the dens against the anterior arch. As it crosses the dens, it arches cranially and caudally, forming the cruciate ligament of the atlas. The transverse ligament divides the circular opening of the atlas into posterior and anterior parts. The posterior part transmits the spinal cord and its membranes; the anterior part contains the dens.
transverse mesocolon   A broad fold of the peritoneum connecting the transverse colon to the dorsal wall of the abdomen. It is continuous with the greater omentum along the ventral surface of the transverse colon and contains between its layers the vessels that supply the transverse colon. Its two layers diverge along the anterior border of the pancreas. Compare **mesentery proper, sigmoid mesocolon.**
transverse palatine suture   The line of junction between the processes of the maxilla and the horizontal portions of the palatine bones that form the hard palate.
transverse plane   Any one of the planes that cut across the body perpendicular to the sagittal and the frontal planes, dividing the body into caudal and cranial portions. Compare **frontal plane, median plane, sagittal plane.**
transverse sinus   One of a pair of large venous channels in the posterior superior group of sinuses serving the dura mater. Each transverse sinus starts at the internal occipital protuberance, and one, usually the right, is a direct continuation of the superior sagittal sinus, the

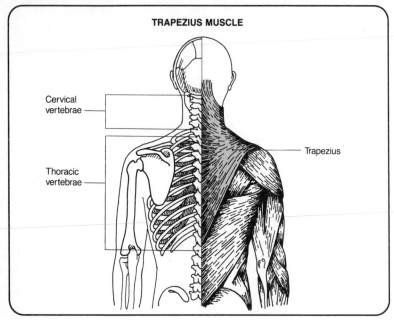

TRAPEZIUS MUSCLE

Cervical vertebrae

Thoracic vertebrae

Trapezius

other a continuation of the straight sinus. Each tranverse sinus curves slightly to the base of the petrous portion of the temporal bone and within the margin of the tentorium. It leaves the tentorium and becomes the sigmoid sinus, which curves inferiorly and medially to the jugular foramen and ends in the internal jugular vein. Compare **confluence of the sinuses, inferior sagittal sinus, occipital sinus, straight sinus, superior sagittal sinus.**

transversus abdominis One of a pair of transverse abdominal muscles that are the anterolateral muscles of the abdomen, lying immediately under the obliquus internus abdominis. Arising from the inguinal ligament, the iliac crest, the thoracolumbar fascia, and the last six ribs, it inserts into the linea alba. It is innervated by branches of the 7th through the 12th intercostal nerves and by the iliohypogastric and the ilioinguinal nerves. It serves to constrict the abdomen and thus assists in micturition, defecation, emesis, parturition, and forced expiration. Compare **obliquus externus abdominis, obliquus internus abdominis, pyramidalis, rectus abdominis.**

tranylcypromine sulfate A monoamine oxidase (MAO) inhibitor antidepressant.

trapezium, *pl.* **trapeziums, trapezia** A carpal bone in the distal row of carpal bones. The trapezium articulates with the scaphoid proximally, the first metacarpal distally, and the trapezoideum and the second metacarpal medially. Also called **greater multangular, os trapezium.**

trapezius A large, flat, triangular muscle of the shoulder and upper back. It arises from the occipital bone, the ligamentum nuchae, and the spinous processes of the seventh cervical and all the thoracic vertebrae. It is innervated by the third and fourth cervical nerves and the spinal accessory nerve. It acts to rotate the scapula, raise the shoulder, and abduct and flex the arm.

trapezoid bone The smallest carpal bone, located in the distal row of carpal bones between the trapezium and the capitate. It resembles a wedge with the broad end at the dorsal surface, the narrow end at the palmar surface. The trapezoid articulates with the scaphoid proximally, the second metacarpal distally, the trapezium laterally, and the capitate medially. Also called **lesser multangular bone, os trapezoideum.**

trauma 1. Physical injury caused by violent or disruptive action or by the introduction into the body of a toxic substance. **2.** Psychic injury resulting from a severe emotional shock. —**traumatic,** *adj.,* **traumatize,** *v.*

-trauma A combining form meaning a 'wound or injury, psychic or physical': *arthrotrauma, barotrauma.*

traumatic anesthesia A total lack of normal sensation in a body part, caused by injury, nerve destruction, or nerve pathway interruptions. See also **tactile anesthesia.**

traumatic delirium Delirium after severe head injury, characterized by alertness and conciousness with disorientation, confabulation, and amnesia. See also **delirium.**

traumatic fever An elevation in body temperature secondary to mechanical trauma, particularly a crushing injury. Such fevers may last 1 or 2 days. The increased body temperature may help provide resistance to subsequent infection, and increased wound temperature may accelerate local healing.

traumatic idiocy Severe mental retardation resulting from injury to the brain received at birth, during infancy, or in early childhood.

traumatic myositis Inflammation of the muscles resulting from a wound or other trauma.

traumatic neuroma A tangled mass of nerve elements and fibrous tissue produced by the proliferation of Schwann cells and fibroblasts following severe nerve injury. A kind of traumatic neuroma is **amputation neuroma.**

traumato- A combining form meaning 'pertaining to trauma, or to an injury or wound': *traumatogenic, traumatopnea, traumatopyra.*

traumatology 1. The study of wounds and injuries. **2.** A surgical specialty dealing with the treatment of wounds, injuries, and resulting disabilities. —**traumatologic, traumatological,** *adj.*

traumatopathy A pathologic condition resulting from a wound or injury. —**traumatopathic,** *adj.*

traumatophilia A psychological state in which a person derives unconscious pleasure from injuries and surgical operations. —**traumatophiliac,** *n.,* **traumatophilic,** *adj.*

traumatopnea Partial asphyxia with collapse of the patient, caused by a penetrating thoracic wound permitting air to enter the pleural space and compress the lungs.

traumatopyra An elevated temperature resulting from a wound or injury.

traumatotherapy The medical, surgical, and psychological treatment of the wounds, injuries, and disabilities that result from trauma. —**traumatotherapeutic,** *adj.*

traumatropism The tendency of damaged tissue to attract microorganisms and promote their growth, frequently causing infections following injuries, especially burns.

travail 1. Physical or mental exertion, especially when distressful. **2.** In obstetrics: the effort of labor and childbirth.

traveler's diarrhea Any of several diarrheal disorders commonly seen in people visiting foreign regions of the world. Some strains of *Escherichia coli* are the common cause. Treatment depends on identification of the cause and includes rehydration with beverages containing electrolytes. Preventive measures include using boiled water for drinking and for brushing the teeth and eating only fruits and vegetables that have a skin or peel. Also called **turista.**

trazodone hydrochloride An antidepressant, chemically unrelated to the cyclic and MAO drugs.

TRBF *abbr* total renal blood flow.

Treacher Collins' syndrome An inherited disorder, characterized by mandibulofacial dysostosis. See also **Pierre Robin syndrome.**

treatment 1. The care and management of a patient to combat, ameliorate, or prevent a disease, disorder, or injury. **2.** A method of combating, ameliorating, or preventing a disease,

disorder, or injury. Active or curative treatment is designed to cure; palliative treatment is directed to relieve pain and distress; prophylactic treatment is for the prevention of a disease or disorder; causal treatment focuses on the etiology of a disorder; conservative treatment avoids radical measures and procedures; empiric treatment employs methods shown to be beneficial by experience; rational treatment is based on a knowledge of a disease process and the action of the measures used. Treatment may be pharmacological, surgical, or supportive. It may be specific for the disorder, or symptomatic to relieve symptoms without effecting a cure.

treatment room A room in a patient-care unit, usually in a hospital, in which various treatments or procedures requiring special equipment are performed.

Trechona A genus of spiders, family Dipluridae, the bite of which is toxic and irritating to humans.

tree In anatomy: an anatomical structure with branches that spread out like those of a tree, as the bronchial tree.

-trema A combining form meaning: **1.** A 'hole, orifice, opening': *gonotrema, helicotrema, peritrema.* **2.** 'Creatures possessing an opening': *Eurytrema, Monotrema, Troglotrema.*

trematode Any species of flatworm of the class Trematoda, some of which are parasitic to humans. Trematodes may infect the liver, the lungs, and the intestines of humans. Kinds of trematodes include the organisms causing **fascioliasis, paragonimiasis, schistosomiasis.** Also called **fluke.**

tremor Rhythmic, purposeless, quivering movements resulting from the involuntary alternating contraction and relaxation of opposing groups of skeletal muscles, occurring in some elderly individuals, certain families, and patients with various neurodegenerative disorders. Senile tremor is characterized by fine, quick movements, especially of the hands, rhythmic head nodding, and increased trembling during purposeful movements. Familial tremor and the tremor occurring in multiple sclerosis also increase during voluntary movement and may be intensified by anxiety, excitement, and self-consciousness. The tremors of Graves' disease, alcoholism, mercury poisoning, and other toxicoses are usually less rhythmic, and the tremor in lead poisoning often affects the lips. Kinds of tremors are **continuous tremor, intention tremor.**

trench fever A rare, self-limited infection caused by *Rochalimaea quintana,* a rickettsial organism transmitted by body lice, and characterized by weakness, fever, rash, and leg pains. Also called **quintana fever.**

trench foot A condition resembling frostbite that results from prolonged exposure of the feet to damp cold. The feet may be pale, edematous, clammy, and numb, and some tissue maceration may occur.

trench mouth An infection of the mouth and gums characterized by ulcerative, destruc-

TREPONEMA PALLIDUM

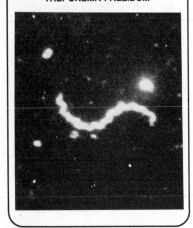

tive lesions of the mucous membrane. It usually occurs in debilitated, malnourished people. The fusiform bacillus and the spirochete found in the ulcers represent secondary infection.

Trendelenburg gait An abnormal gait associated with a weakness of the gluteus medius, characterized by the dropping of the pelvis on the unaffected side of the body at the moment of heel contact on the affected side. The patient with a Trendelenburg gait also shortens the step on the unaffected side and displays a lateral deviation of the entire trunk and affected side during the stance phase of the affected lower limb. Also called **uncompensated gluteal gait.** Compare **compensated gluteal gait.**

Trendelenburg's operation The ligation of varicose veins whose valves are ineffective, performed to remove weakened portions of veins and pockets in which thrombi might lodge. With the patient under general anesthesia, the saphenous vein is ligated at the groin, where it joins the femoral vein. A wire device, called a stripper, is threaded through the lumen of the vein from groin to ankle; the wire and vein are then pulled from the groin incision. Incisions may be made at several sites along the leg. After surgery, a pressure bandage is applied from foot to thigh, and the foot of the bed is elevated. The patient is encouraged to walk but discouraged from standing or sitting. Cyanosis of the toes indicates possible constriction by the dressings. Possible complications include hemorrhage, infection, nerve damage, and thrombosis.

Trendelenburg's position A position in which the head is low and the body and legs are on an inclined plane. It is sometimes used in pelvic surgery to displace the abdominal organs upward, out of the pelvis, or to increase the flow of blood to the brain in hypotension and shock.

Trendelenburg's test A simple test for incompetent valves in a person with varicose veins.

The person lies down and elevates the leg to empty the vein, then stands, and the vein is observed as it fills. If the valves are incompetent, the vein fills from above; if the valves are normal, the vein fills from below.

trephine A circular, sawlike instrument used to remove bone or tissue, usually from the skull. Also called trepan.

Treponema A genus of spirochetes, including some pathogenic to humans.

Treponema pallidum An actively motile, slender spirochetal organism causing syphilis.

treponematosis, *pl.* **treponematoses** Any disease caused by spirochetes of the genus *Treponema.* Kinds of treponematoses are **bejel, pinta, syphilis, yaws.**

-tresia A combining form meaning 'perforation': *atresia, proctotresia, sphenotresia.*

tretinoin (vitamin A acid, retinoic acid) A dermatomucosal agent used to treat acne vulgaris.

TRF *abbr* **thyrotropin releasing factor.**

tri- A combining form meaning 'three or thrice': *triage, tribrachia, tridermoma.*

triacetin An antifungal.

triacetyloleandomycin See **troleandomycin.**

triage 1. In military medicine: a classification of casualties of war and other disasters according to the gravity of injuries, urgency of treatment, and place for treatment. 2. A process in which a group of patients is sorted according to their need for care. The kind of illness or injury, the severity of the problem, and the facilities available govern the process. 3. In disaster medicine: a process in which a large group of patients is sorted in order that care be concentrated on those who are likely to survive.

trial forceps An obstetric operation consisting of an attempt to deliver an infant with obstetric forceps. The forceps are applied to the infant's head, and moderate traction is applied. The delivery is completed only if the trial indicates that delivery can be accomplished safely. Compare **failed forceps.** See also **double setup.**

triamcinolone, t. acetonide, t. diacetate, t. hexacetonide Topical anti-inflammatory agents used on the mucous membranes.

triamterene A potassium-sparing diuretic.

triangular bone The pyramidal carpal bone in the proximal row on the ulnar side of the wrist. It articulates with the lunate bone laterally, the pisiform anteriorly, the hamate distally, and with the triangular articular disk that separates it from the lower end of the ulna. Also called **cuneiform bone, os triquetrum.**

-tribe A combining form meaning a 'surgical instrument used to crush a body part': *cephalotribe, sphenotribe.*

tribromoethyl alcohol See **tribromoethanol.**

TRIC Acronym for *trachoma inclusion conjunctivitis agent,* which refers to *Chlamydia trachomatis.* See also **Chlamydia.**

tricarboxylic acid cycle See **Krebs' citric acid cycle.**

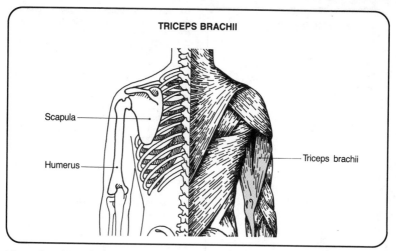

TRICEPS BRACHII

Scapula

Humerus

Triceps brachii

triceps brachii A large muscle that extends the entire length of the dorsal surface of the humerus. Proximally, it has a long head, a lateral head, and a medial head. The long head arises in a flattened tendon originating on the scapula; the lateral head arises from the posterior surface of the humerus, the lateral border of the humerus, and the lateral intermuscular septum; and the medial head arises from the posterior body of the humerus, the medial body of the humerus, and the whole length of the medial intermuscular septum. The three portions of the muscle converge in a long tendon and insert in the posterior aspect of the olecranon. The triceps brachii is innervated by branches of the radial nerve, contains fibers from the seventh and the eighth cervical nerves, and functions to extend the forearm and to adduct the arm. Also called triceps extensor cubiti. Compare **biceps brachii.**

triceps reflex A deep tendon reflex elicited by sharply tapping the triceps tendon proximal to the elbow with the forearm in a relaxed position. The response is a definite, involuntary extension movement of the forearm. The reflex is accentuated by lesions of the pyramidal tract above the level of the seventh or eighth vertebra. Also called triceps jerk. See also **deep tendon reflex.**

triceps surae limp An abnormal action in the walking or gait cycle, associated with a deficiency in the elevating and propulsive factors on the affected side of the body. Such a deficiency prevents the triceps surae from raising the pelvis and carrying it forward. The pelvis consequently sags below its normal level and lags behind in the walking movement.

-trichia A combining form meaning: **1.** A 'pathological condition of the hair': *leukotrichia, melanotrichia, sclerotrichia.* **2.** A '(specified) hairiness': *glossotrichia, polytrichia.* Also **-trichosis.**

trichiasis An abnormal inversion of the eye-

lashes that irritates the eyeball. It usually follows infection or inflammation. Compare **ectropion.**

trichinosis Infestation with the parasitic roundworm *Trichinella spiralis*, transmitted by eating raw or undercooked pork or bear meat. Early symptoms of infection include abdominal pain, nausea, fever, and diarrhea; later, muscle pain, tenderness, fatigue, and eosinophilia are observed. Encysted larvae in improperly cooked pork mature in the intestines of the host, with mature worms depositing their larvae in the intestinal wall. The larvae penetrate the intestinal mucosa and move to other parts of the body through the blood and lymphatic systems, ultimately invading skeletal muscles, especially the diaphragm and the chest muscles, where they encyst. Larval penetration of the brain or the heart may result in death. Serologic tests, skin sensitivity tests, and microscopic examination of specimens of infested muscle obtained by a biopsy often contribute to the diagnosis. Also called **trichinellosis.**

trichlormethiazide A thiazide diuretic.

trichloroethylene A general anesthetic, administered by mask with N_2O, for dentistry, minor surgery, and the first stages of labor. It is too cardiotoxic for deep anesthesia; even in light planes of anesthesia, arrhythmias may occur but may be reversed by administering oxygen and discontinuing the anesthesia.

tricho- A combining form meaning 'pertaining to hair': *trichobezoar, trichomycosis, trichorrhea.*

trichobasalioma hyalinicum See **cylindroma,** definition 2.

trichoepithelioma, *pl.* **trichoepitheliomas, trichoepitheliomata** A benign cutaneous nodule derived from the basal cells of the follicles of the fine body hair of the fetus. Trichoepithelioma is an inherited condition and usually occurs as multiple growths. Also called **acanthoma adenoides cysticum, epithelioma adenoides cysticum.**

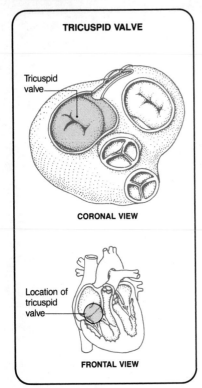

TRICUSPID VALVE

Tricuspid valve

CORONAL VIEW

Location of tricuspid valve

FRONTAL VIEW

trichologia An abnormal condition in which a person pulls out his own hair, usually seen only in delirium.

trichomonacide An agent destructive to *Trichomonas vaginalis*. —**trichomonacidal,** *adj.*

Trichomonas vaginalis A motile protozoan parasite that causes vaginitis with a copious malodorous discharge and pruritus. See also **trichomoniasis.**

trichomoniasis An infection caused by the protozoan *Trichomonas vaginalis*. Vaginal infection is characterized by itching; burning; and frothy, pale yellow-to-green, malodorous vaginal discharge. With chronic infection, all symptoms may disappear, although the organisms are present. In the male, infection is usually asymptomatic but may be evidenced by a persistent or recurrent urethritis. Infection is transmitted by sexual intercourse, rarely by moist washcloths, or, in newborns, by passage through the birth canal. Diagnosis is by microscopic examination of fresh vaginal secretions. Treatment is currently by oral metronidazole.

trichophytic granuloma See **Majocchi's granuloma.**

Trichophyton A genus of fungi that infects skin, hair, and nails. See also **dermatomycosis, dermatophyte.**

-trichosis See **-trichia.**

trichostrongyliasis Infestation with *Trichostrongylus*. Also called **trichostrongylosis.** See also **Nematode.**

Trichostrongylus A genus of roundworm, some species of which are parasitic to man, as *Trichostrongylus orientalis*.

trichotillomania, trichomania A morbid impulse or desire to pull out one's hair, often seen in severe mental retardation and delirium. Also called **hair pulling.** See also **trichologia.** —**trichotillomanic, trichomanic,** *adj.*

trichuriasis, trichiuriasis Infestation with the roundworm *Trichuris trichiura*. The condition is usually asymptomatic, but heavy infestation may cause nausea, abdominal pain, diarrhea, and, occasionally, anemia and rectal prolapse. It is common in tropical areas with poor sanitation. Eggs are passed in feces. Contamination of the hands, food, and water results in ingestion of the eggs, which hatch in the intestines. The adult worms embed two thirds of their length in the submucosa of the colon, where they may live 15 to 20 years. Prevention includes proper disposal of feces and good personal hygiene.

Trichuris A genus of parasitic roundworms of which the species *Trichuris trichiura* infects the intestinal tract. Adult worms, which are 30 to 50 mm (1 to 2 inches) long, resemble a whip, with a threadlike anterior and a thicker posterior. Also called **whipworm.**

triclofos sodium A sedative-hypnotic.

tricrotic pulse An abnormal pulse that has three peaks of elevation on a sphygmogram, representing the pressure wave from the heart in systole followed by two pressure waves in diastole.

tricuspid **1.** Of or pertaining to three points or cusps. **2.** Of or pertaining to the tricuspid valve of the heart.

tricuspid atresia A congenital cardiac anomaly characterized by the absence of the tricuspid valve, so there is no opening between the right atrium and right ventricle. Other cardiac defects, as atrial and ventricular septal defects, are usually present, allowing some shunting of blood into the lungs. Clinical manifestations include severe cyanosis, dyspnea, anoxia, and signs of right-sided heart failure. Definitive diagnosis is made by cardiac catheterization. Immediate palliative treatment includes pulmonary-to-artery anastomoses to increase blood flow to the lungs and atrial septostomy if the atrial septal defect is small. Total corrective surgery has been successful in a limited number of older children. See also **congenital cardiac anomaly.**

tricuspid stenosis See **valvular heart disease.**

tricuspid valve A valve with three main cusps situated between the right atrium and the right ventricle of the heart. The cusps of the tricuspid valve include the anterior, posterior, and medial cusps. The anterior cusp is the largest, the posterior cusp the smallest. The cusps are composed of strong fibrous tissue and are anchored to the papillary muscles of the right ventricle by several tendons. As the right and the left ventricles relax during the diastyle phase of the heartbeat, the tricuspid valve opens, allowing blood to flow into the ventricle. In the systole phase of the heartbeat, both blood-filled ventricles contract, pumping out their contents, while the tricuspid and mitral valves close to prevent any backflow. Also called **right atrioventricular valve.** Compare **mitral valve, semilunar valve.** See also **cuspid valve, heart valve.**

tricyclic antidepressant See **antidepressant.**

tricyclic compound A chemical substance containing three rings in the molecular structure, especially a tricyclic antidepressant drug used to treat reactive or endogenous depression. These drugs also have anticonvulsant, antihistaminic, anticholinergic, hypotensive, and sedative effects. See also **antidepressant.**

tridihexethyl chloride A gastrointestinal anticholinergic agent.

triethanolamine polypeptide oleate-condensate An otic preparation that helps break down cerumen. See also **cerumen.**

trifluoperazine hydrochloride A phenothiazine antipsychotic.

trifluridine An ophthalmic anti-infective agent. Also called **trifluorothymidine.**

trigeminal nerve Either of the largest pair of cranial nerves, essential for the act of chewing, general sensibility of the face, and muscular sensibility of the obliquus superior. The trigeminal nerve divides into three nerves: the ophthalmic, the maxillary, and the mandibular. The trigeminal nerves have sensory, motor, and intermediate roots and connect to three areas in the brain. Also called **fifth nerve, nervus trigeminus, trifacial nerve.**

trigeminal neuralgia A neurologic condition of the trigeminal facial nerve, characterized by paroxysms of flashing, stablike pain radiating along the course of a branch of the nerve from the angle of the jaw. Neuralgia of the first branch results in pain around the eyes and over the forehead; of the second branch, pain in the upper lip, nose, and cheek; of the third branch, pain on the side of the tongue and the lower lip. The momentary bursts of pain recur in clusters lasting many seconds; paroxysmal episodes of the pain may last for hours. Also called **prosopalgia, tic douloureux.**

trigeminal pulse An abnormal pulse in which every third beat is absent. See also **bigeminal pulse, trigeminy.**

trigeminy 1. Grouping in threes. 2. A cardiac arrhythmia that is characterized by the occurrence of three heartbeats in rapid succession. —**trigeminal,** *adj.*

triglyceride A compound consisting of a fatty acid and glycerol. Triglycerides make up most animal and vegetable fats and are the principal lipids in the blood, where they circulate, bound to a protein, forming high- and low-density lipoproteins.

trigone 1. A triangle. 2. The first three dom-

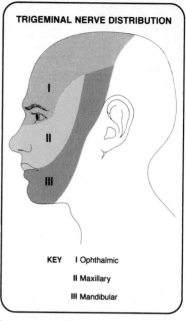

TRIGEMINAL NERVE DISTRIBUTION

I

II

III

KEY I Ophthalmic

II Maxillary

III Mandibular

inant cusps, considered collectively, of an upper molar.

trigonitis Inflammation of the trigone of the bladder, which often accompanies urethritis.

trihexyphenidyl hydrochloride An parasympatholytic anticholinergic blocking agent.

trihybrid In genetics: pertaining to or describing an individual, organism, or strain that is heterozygous for three specific traits, that is the offspring of parents differing in three specific gene pairs, or that is heterozygous for three particular characteristics or gene loci being followed.

trihybrid cross In genetics: the mating of two individuals, organisms, or strains that have different gene pairs that determine three specific traits or in which three particular characteristics or gene loci are being followed.

trihydric alcohol An alcohol with three hydroxyl groups.

triiodothyronine (T$_3$) A hormone which helps regulate growth and development, helps control metabolism and body temperature, and, by a negative feedback system, inhibits thyrotropin secretion by the pituitary. Triiodothyronine is produced mainly from the metabolism of thyroxine in the peripheral tissues but is also synthesized by and stored in the thyroid gland as an amino acid residue of the protein thyroglobulin. Triiodothyronine circulates in the plasma where it is bound mainly to thyroxine-binding globulin and thyroxine-binding prealbumin, proteins that protect the hormone from metabolism and excretion during its half-life of 2 days or less before it is degraded in the liver. The hormone acts principally by complementing thyroxine in the control of protein synthesis. See also **thyroid hormone.**

trilaminar blastoderm   The stage of embryonic development in which all three of the primary germ layers, the ectoderm, mesoderm, and entoderm, have formed. Compare **bilaminar blastoderm.**

trilogy of Fallot   A congenital cardiac anomaly consisting of the combination of pulmonic stenosis, interatrial septal defect, and right ventricular hypertrophy. See also **congenital cardiac anomaly, tetralogy of Fallot.**

trimalleolar fracture   See **Cotton's fracture.**

trimeprazine tartrate   An phenothiazine antihistamine.

trimester   One of the three periods of approximately 3 months into which pregnancy is divided. The 1st trimester includes the time from the 1st day of the last menstrual period to the end of 12 weeks. The 2nd trimester, closer to 4 months in length than 3, extends from the 12th to the 28th week of gestation. The 3rd trimester begins at the 28th week and extends to the time of delivery.

trimethadione   An oxazolidone anticonvulsant agent.

trimethaphan camsylate   A sympatholytic antihypertensive that is a ganglionic blocking agent.

trimethobenzamide hydrochloride   An antiemetic.

trimethoprim   An antibiotic.

trimethoprim and sulfalene   A new, experimental fixed-combination drug for the treatment of chloroquine-resistant falciparum malaria. Its usage is not yet approved by the FDA.

trimethoprim and sulfamethoxazole   See **co-trimoxazole.**

trimethylene   See **cyclopropane.**

trimipramine maleate   A tricyclic antidepressant.

trioxsalen   A melanizing agent.

tripelennamine hydrochloride   An ethylenediamine antihistamine.

triple-dye treatment   The therapy of burns by applying 6% gentian violet, 1% brilliant green, and 0.1% acriflavin base.

triple response   A triad of phenomena that occur in sequence following the intradermal injection of histamine. First, a red spot develops, spreading outward for a few millimeters, reaching its maximal size within 1 minute, and then turning bluish. Next, a brighter red flush of color spreads slowly in an irregular flare around the original red spot. Finally, a wheal, filled with fluid, forms over the original spot. Also called triple response of Lewis.

triple sugar iron reaction   Any one of several reactions in certain bacterial cultures growing on triple sugar iron agar, a culture medium used to aid identification of *Escherichia coli* and other pathogenic enteric bacteria.

triplet   **1.** Any one of three offspring born of the same gestation period during a single pregnancy. See also **Hellin's law. 2.** In genetics: the

unit of three consecutive bases in one polynucleotide chain of DNA or RNA that codes for a specific amino acid. See also **codon, genetic code.**

triploid (3n)   **1.** Of or pertaining to an individual, organism, strain, or cell that has three complete sets of chromosomes, triple the normal haploid number characteristic of the species. In humans, the triploid number is 69, found in rare cases of aborted or stillborn fetuses. Of those triploid fetuses born alive, all have gross and multiple malformations; they live for only a few hours. Also called triploidic. **2.** Such an individual, organism, strain, or cell. Compare **diploid, haploidy, tetraploid.** See also **polyploid.**

triploidy   The state or condition of having three complete sets of chromosomes.

tripodial symmelia   A fetal anomaly characterized by the fusion of the lower extremities and the presence of three feet.

triprolidine hydrochloride   An alkylamine antihistamine.

-tripsis   A combining form meaning a 'chafing or wearing away': *anatripsis, entripsis, syntripsis.*

-tripsy   A combining form meaning a 'crushing of a body part by a surgical instrument': *basiotripsy, lithotripsy.*

trismus   A prolonged tonic spasm of the muscles of the jaw. Also called lockjaw *(informal).* See also **tetanus.**

trisomy, trisomia   A chromosomal aberration that is characterized by the presence of one more than the normal number of chromosomes in a diploid complement; in humans the trisomic cell contains 47 chromosomes and is designated n + 1. The extra member can join any of the normal homologous pairs, although most human trisomies involve the small chromosomes, such as those in the E or the G group, or the sex chromosomes. Partial trisomy occurs when only a portion of a chromosome attaches to another. Trisomies are indicated by the exact chromosome or karyotypic group in which the addition is made, as trisomy 13 or trisomy D. Compare **monosomy.** See also **trisomy syndrome. —trisomic,** *adj.*

trisomy 8   A congenital condition associated with the presence of an extra chromosome 8 within the C group. Those with the condition are slender, of normal height, have a large, asymmetric head, prominent forehead, deep-set eyes, low-set prominent ears, and thick lips. There is mild to severe mental and motor retardation, often with delayed and poorly articulated speech. Skeletal anomalies and joint limitation, especially camptodactyly, may occur, and there are unusually deep palmar and plantar creases, which are diagnostically significant. Most trisomy 8 individuals are mosaic, with no abnormal or only slight clinical manifestations, or they are only partially trisomic and show varying degrees of the clinical symptoms. Trisomy 8 is less severe than other trisomies, especially trisomy 13 and trisomy 18, so that the mortality rate is low. Also called trisomy C syndrome.

trisomy 13   A congenital condition caused by the presence of an extra chromosome in the D group, predominantly chromosome 13 but, in rare instances, chromosome 14 or 15. It is characterized by multiple midline anomalies and central nervous system defects, including holoprosencephaly, microcephaly, myelomeningocele, microphthalmos, and cleft lip and palate. Other characteristics include severe mental retardation, polydactyly, deafness, convulsions, and abnormalities of the heart, viscera, and genitalia. Most infants with the condition are severely affected and do not survive the first 6 months of life. Also called Patau's syndrome, trisomy D syndrome.

trisomy 18   A congenital condition caused by the presence of an extra chromosome 18, characterized by severe mental retardation and multiple deformities. Common defects include scaphocephaly or other skull abnormalities, micrognathia, abnormal facies with low-set malformed ears and prominent occiput, cleft lip and palate, clenched fists with overlapping fingers, especially the index over the third finger, clubfeet, and syndactyly. Ventricular septal defect, patent ductus arteriosus, atrial septal defect, and renal anomalies are also common. The condition occurs predominantly in females, according to a 3:1 sex ratio, and survival beyond a few months is rare. Also called Edward's syndrome, trisomy E syndrome.

trisomy 21   See **Down's syndrome.**

trisomy 22   A congenital condition caused by the presence of an extra chromosome 22 in the G group, characterized by psychomotor retardation and various developmental anomalies. Common defects include microcephaly, micrognathia, hypotonia, hypertelorism, abnormal ears with preauricular tags or fistulas, and congenital heart disease. In partial trisomy 22, the extra chromosome is much smaller than the normal pair and causes coloboma of the iris or anal atresia, or both, as well as various other defects. See also **cat-eye syndrome.**

trisomy D syndrome   See **Patau's syndrome.**

trisomy E syndrome   See **Edward's syndrome.**

trisomy G syndrome   See **Down's syndrome.**

trisomy syndrome   Any condition caused by the addition of an extra member to a normal pair of homologous autosomes or to the sex chromosomes or by the translocation of a portion of one chromosome to another. Most trisomies occur as a result of complete or partial nondisjunction of the chromosomes during cell division. The more severe conditions are related to trisomies of the autosomes rather than the sex chromosomes. The most common trisomy syndromes with clearly established clinical manifestations are trisomy 8, trisomy 13, trisomy 18, trisomy 21, trisomy 22.

trisulfapyrimidines   Three antibacterials in combination (sulfadiazine, sulfamerazine, and sulfamethazine), rarely prescribed today.

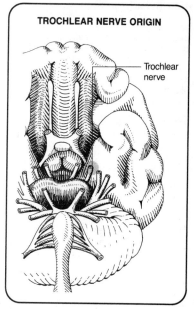

TROCHLEAR NERVE ORIGIN

Trochlear nerve

tRNA   *abbr* **transfer RNA.**

trocar   A sharp, pointed rod that fits inside a tube. It is used to pierce the skin and the wall of a cavity or canal in the body to aspirate fluids, instill a medication or solution, or guide the placement of a soft catheter. See also **cannula.**

trochanter   One of the two bony projections on the proximal end of the femur that serve for the attachment of various muscles. The two protuberances are the greater trochanter and the lesser trochanter.

troche   A small tablet containing a medicinal agent incorporated in a flavored, sweetened mucilage or fruit base that dissolves in the mouth, releasing the drug. Also called **lozenge, rotula, trochiscus.**

trochiscus   See **troche.**

trochlea   A pulley-shaped part or structure. —**trochlear,** *adj.*

trochlear nerve   Either of the smallest pair of cranial nerves, essential for eye movement and eye muscle sensibility. The trochlear nerves branch to the obliquus superior and communicate with the ophthalmic division of the trigeminal nerve, connecting with two areas in the brain. Also called **fourth nerve, nervus trochlearis.**

trochlear notch of ulna   A large depression in the ulna, formed by the olecranon and coronoid processes, that articulates with the trochlea of the humerus.

trochoid joint   See **pivot joint.**

troleandomycin   An antibiotic.

trombiculosis   An infestation with mites of the genus *Trombicula,* some species of which carry scrub typhus.

tromethamine   An systemic alkalinizer.

-tron A combining form meaning a '(specified) type of vacuum tube': *dynatron, magnetron, thyratron.*

trop-, tropo- A combining form meaning 'turn, turning' or 'tendency, affinity': *tropism, tropomyosin.* See also **tropho-**, with which it may be confused.

-tropal See **-tropic.**

-trope A combining form meaning 'influencing or influenced by': *gonadotrope, heliotrope, rheotrope.*

-troph A combining form meaning: **1.** 'That which nourishes an embryo': *embryotroph, hemotroph, histotroph.* **2.** An 'organism that gets nourishment from a (specified) source': *autotroph, metatroph.*

-trophia See **-trophy.**

-trophic A combining form meaning 'referring to a type of nutrition or nutritional requirement': *chondrotrophic, lipotrophic.*

trophic fracture A fracture resulting from the weakening of bone tissue owing to nutritional disturbances.

trophic ulcer A decubitus ulcer caused by external trauma to a part of the body that is in poor condition owing to disease, vascular insufficiency, or loss of afferent nerve fibers. Trophic ulcers may be painless or associated with severe causalgia. See also **decubitus ulcer.**

tropho-, troph- A combining form meaning 'pertaining to food or nourishment': *trophoblast, trophoedema.*

trophoblast The layer of tissue that forms the wall of the blastocyst of placental mammals in the early stages of embryonic development. It functions in the implantation of the blastocyst in the uterine wall and in supplying nutrient to the embryo. At the time of implantation, the cells differentiate into two layers, the inner cytotrophoblast, which forms the chorion, and the syncytiotrophoblast, which develops into the outer layer of the placenta. Also called trophectoderm. —**trophoblastic,** *adj.*

trophoblastic cancer A malignant neoplastic disease of the uterus derived from chorionic epithelium, characterized by the production of high levels of human chorionic gonadotropin (HCG). The tumor may be an invasive hydatid mole (chorioadenoma destruens) formed by grossly enlarged, vesicular chorionic villi or a malignant uterine choriocarcinoma that arises from nonvillous chorionic epithelium. Half the cases of choriocarcinoma follow a molar pregnancy, 25% an abortion, 22.5% a normal pregnancy, and 2.5% an ectopic pregnancy. A hydatid mole invades the myometrium and often forms extrauterine nodules that may spread to distant sites. Choriocarcinoma forms a dark red, hemorrhagic, nodular tumor on or in the uterine wall and metastasizes early in its course to the lungs, brain, liver, bones, vagina, or vulva. Diagnostic measures include serial assays to measure the HCG blood level and histologic examination of specimens obtained by curettage. Hysterectomy is indicated in most cases, but surgery does not eliminate the possibility of a recurrence. Chemotherapy is effective in curing a large percentage of patients with trophoblastic tumors. See also **choriocarcinoma, hydatid mole.**

trophozoite A motile protozoon, as an ameba. Diseases in which trophozoites may be isolated by bacteriologic studies include amebic dysentery and malaria.

-trophy A combining form meaning a 'condition of nutrition or growth': *cyotrophy, lipotrophy.* Also **-trophia.**

-tropia A combining form meaning '(condition of) deviation in the visual axis': *cyclotropia, parectropia.*

-tropic A combining form meaning: **1.** A 'turn or change in the visual axis': *anatropic, hemitropic.* **2.** A 'tendency to have an influence on or be influenced by': *corticotropic.* Also **-tropal.**

tropical medicine The branch of medicine concerned with diagnosis and treatment of diseases common to tropical and subtropical regions.

tropical sore See **oriental sore.**

tropical sprue A malabsorption syndrome of unknown etiology that is endemic in the tropics and subtropics. It is characterized by abnormalities in the small intestinal mucosa, resulting in protein malnutrition and multiple nutritional deficiencies, often complicated by severe infection. Symptoms include diarrhea, anorexia, and weight loss. Megaloblastic anemia may result from folic acid and vitamin B_{12} deficiency. Treatment includes administration of antibiotics, particularly tetracycline; folic acid; iron; calcium; vitamins A, D, K, and the B complex group; and a balanced diet high in protein and normal in fat content. See also **nontropical sprue.**

tropical typhus See **scrub typhus.**

tropicamide A mydriatic agent.

-tropism A combining form meaning a 'condition of having an affinity for something specified': *parasitotropism, phototropism, sitotropism.* Also **-tropy.**

-tropo See **-trop.**

-tropy A combining form meaning 'influenced by or having an affinity for something specified': *allotropy, ergotropy, syntropy.* Also **-tropism.**

Trousseau's sign A test for latent tetany in which carpal spasm is induced by inflating a sphygmomanometer cuff on the upper arm for 3 minutes to a pressure exceeding systolic blood pressure. A positive test may be seen in hypocalcemia and hypomagnesemia.

true birthrate The ratio of total births to the total female population of childbearing age, between ages 15 and 45. Compare **birthrate, crude birthrate, refined birthrate.**

true chondroma See **enchondroma.**

true dwarf See **primordial dwarf.**

true glottis See **glottis.**

true neuroma Any neoplasm composed of nerve tissue.

true rib See **rib.**

true suture An immovable fibrous joint of

the skull in which the edges of bones interlock along a series of processes and indentations. The three kinds of true sutures are the dentata, limbosa, and serrata. Compare **false suture**.

true twins See **monozygotic twins**.

true vocal cord See **vocal cord**.

truncus arteriosus The embryonic arterial trunk that initially opens from both ventricles of the heart and later divides into the aorta and the pulmonary trunk, the two portions separated by the bulbar septum.

trunk incurvation reflex See **Galant reflex**.

truss An apparatus worn to prevent abdominal herniation of the intestines or other organ.

Trypanosoma A genus of parasitic organisms, several species of which cause diseases in humans. Most *Trypanosoma* organisms live part of their life cycle in insects and are transmitted to humans by insect bites. See also **trypanosome, trypanosomiasis.**

Trypanosoma brucei gambiense See **Gambian trypanosomiasis.**

Trypanosoma brucei rhodesiense See **Rhodesian trypanosomiasis.**

Trypanosoma cruzi See **Chagas' disease.**

trypanosome Any one of the organisms of the genus *Trypanosoma*. See also **trypanosomiasis. —trypanosomal,** *adj.*

trypanosomiasis An infection by an organism of the genus *Trypanosoma*. Also called trypanosomal infection.

trypanosomicide A drug destructive to trypanosomes, especially the species of the protozoan parasite transmitted to humans by various insect vectors common in Africa and Central and South America. Various arsenical preparations are used to treat African sleeping sickness and Chagas' disease. **—trypanosomicidal,** *adj.*

trypsin A parenterally administered enzyme. It may also be administered topically or by inhalation.

trypsin crystallized A proteolytic enzyme from the pancreas of the ox, *Bos taurus,* that has been used as a debriding agent for open wounds and ulcers.

tryptophan An amino acid essential for normal growth in infants and for nitrogen balance in adults. Tryptophan is the precursor of several substances, including serotonin and niacin. About 50% of the daily requirement of tryptophan is provided through the metabolism of niacin. The rest is derived from dietary protein. See also **amino acid, protein metabolism.**

TSEM *abbr* **transmission scanning electron microscopy.**

tsetse fly An insect of the genus *Glossina,* found in Africa, which carries the organisms of trypanosomiasis.

TSH *abbr* **thyroid-stimulating hormone.**

TSH releasing factor See **thyrotropin releasing hormone.**

TSS *abbr* **toxic shock syndrome.**

tsutsugamushi disease See **scrub typhus.**

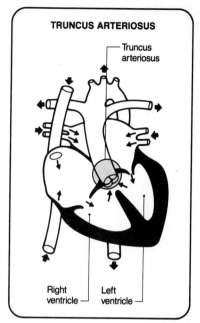

TRUNCUS ARTERIOSUS

Truncus arteriosus

Right ventricle   Left ventricle

TTP *abbr* **thrombotic thrombocytopenic purpura.**

T tube A tubular device in a capital T shape, inserted through the skin into a cavity or a wound, used for drainage.

tubal abortion A condition of pregnancy in which an embryo, ectopically implanted, is expelled from the uterine tube into the peritoneal cavity. It is often accompanied by significant internal bleeding, causing acute abdominal and pelvic pain, but may also be asymptomatic, the products of conception being resorbed. Rarely, the conceptus reimplants on the peritoneum and continues growing to become an abdominal pregnancy. See also **abdominal pregnancy, ectopic pregnancy.**

tubal dermoid cyst A tumor that is derived from embryonal tissues and that develops in an oviduct.

tubal ligation A sterilization procedure in which both fallopian tubes are blocked to prevent conception. Spinal or local anesthesia is used unless the procedure accompanies major surgery. Through a small abdominal incision, the fallopian tubes are ligated in two places with sutures; the intervening segment is burnt, crushed, or excised. The procedure is less commonly performed vaginally. Complications of the procedure, which are rare but serious, include pulmonary embolism, hemorrhage, infection, and tubal pregnancy.

tubal pregnancy An ectopic pregnancy in which the conceptus implants in the fallopian tube. Approximately 2% of all pregnancies are ectopic; of these, approximately 90% are tubal. Tubal pregnancy seldom occurs in primigrav-

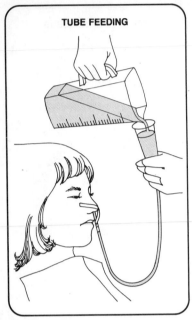

TUBE FEEDING

idas. The most important predisposing factor is prior tubal injury. Most often the tube, which cannot long contain the growing fetus, ruptures, precipitating an intraperitoneal hemorrhage that, if not stopped, can lead rapidly to shock and, often, death. Occasionally, the conceptus does not firmly implant in the tube and is extruded from the fimbriated end of the tube as a tubal abortion. Some conceptuses apparently die and are resorbed in the tube. Diagnosis of tubal pregnancy is often difficult. With rupture of the fallopian tube, women commonly experience sudden sharp pain in one side of the lower abdomen, but the signs and symptoms of tubal pregnancy are insidiously variable, and the classic triad of amenorrhea, pelvic pain, and a tender adnexal mass are present only 50% of the time. Recovery of blood from the cul-de-sac by means of culdocentesis is highly suggestive of a ruptured fallopian tube and tubal pregnancy; it requires immediate surgical exploration of the abdomen. Laparoscopy or laparotomy may be required, particularly if a woman's pregnancy test is positive, the pelvic findings are suggestive, and sonography of the pelvis cannot demonstrate an intrauterine pregnancy. Because of the lethal potential of an undiagnosed tubal pregnancy, women who report any of the characteristic symptoms early in their pregnancies, particularly during the time before the existence of a normal intrauterine pregnancy can be confirmed, must be considered susceptible. Treatment is surgical and involves laparotomy, removal of the entire products of conception and any intraperitoneal blood present, and the removal or repair of the involved tube. A woman

who has had one tubal pregnancy has one chance in five of having another in a subsequent pregnancy. Depending on the location of the developing embryo, the condition is classified as an ampullary, fimbrial, or interstitial tubal pregnancy.

tube   A hollow, cylindrical piece of equipment or structure of the body.

tube feeding   The administration of nutritionally balanced liquefied foods through a tube inserted into the stomach or duodenum. The procedure is used following mouth or gastric surgery, in severe burns, in paralysis or obstruction of the esophagus, in severe cases of anorexia nervosa, and for unconscious patients or those unable to chew or swallow. Also called gavage feeding, nasogastric feeding. See also **parenteral nutrition.**

tubercle   **1.** A nodule or a small eminence, as that on a bone. **2.** A nodule, especially an elevation of the skin that is larger than a papule, as Morgagni's tubercles of the areolae of the breasts. **3.** A small rounded nodule produced by infection with mycobacterium tuberculosis, consisting of a gray translucent mass of small spherical cells surrounded by connective cells.

tuberculin purified protein derivative   A solution containing a purified protein fraction from isolated culture filtrates of strains of *Mycobacterium tuberculosis.* It is used to aid the diagnosis of tuberculosis in the Mantoux test and, for the same purpose in a dried form, in multiple puncture devices. See also **Mantoux test, Tine test.**

tuberculin test   A test to determine past or present tuberculosis infection based on a positive skin reaction, using one of several methods. A purified protein derivative of tubercle bacilli, called tuberculin, is introduced into the skin by scratch, puncture, or intradermal injection. A nonsignificant tuberculin reaction does not rule out a diagnosis of previous or active tuberculosis. Sputum and gastric cultures, acid-fast staining, and X-rays are often needed to establish a diagnosis. Kinds of tuberculin tests include **Heaf test, Mantoux test, Pirquet test, Tine test.**

tuberculoid leprosy   See **leprosy.**

tuberculoma   A rare tumorlike growth of tuberculous tissue in the central nervous system, characterized by symptoms of an expanding cerebral, cerebellar, or spinal mass. Treatment consists of the administration of antimicrobial drugs.

tuberculosis (TB)   A chronic, granulomatous infection caused by an acid-fast bacillus, *Mycobacterium tuberculosis,* generally transmitted by inhalation or ingestion of infected droplets and usually affecting the lungs, although infection of other organ systems by other modes of transmission occurs. Listlessness, vague chest pain, pleurisy, anorexia, fever, and weight loss are early symptoms of pulmonary tuberculosis. Night sweats, pulmonary hemorrhage, expectoration of purulent sputum, and dyspnea develop as the disease progresses. The lung tissues react to the bacillus by producing protective cells that engulf the disease organism, forming tubercles. Untreated, the tubercles enlarge and merge to form larger tubercles that undergo caseation, eventually sloughing off into the cavities of the lungs. Hemoptysis occurs as a result of cavitary spread. Laboratory examination may demonstrate leukocytosis and an increased sedimentation rate, and microscopic study of a sputum specimen stained with carbolfuchsin may be diagnostic. Culture of the tubercle bacillus is slow and requires darkness, carefully controlled temperature, and inoculation on special media. The infecting organism does not produce endotoxins or hemolysins, but tuberculin, a toxic substance, is released as the bacillus disintegrates. Tuberculin has no effect in people who have never been infected but produces a characteristic skin reaction when injected intradermally in people who have or have had tuberculosis. X-ray films of the lungs reveal infiltrates, mediastinal lymphadenopathy, caseation, pleural effusion, and calcification. Tuberculosis may spread from the lungs via the lymphatics and blood vessels; such miliary infection is characterized by tiny, seedlike tubercles in the liver, spleen, and other organs. The bacillus is generally sensitive to isoniazid, para-aminosalicylic acid, streptomycin, rifampin, ultraviolet radiation, and heat. The person is usually hospitalized for several weeks to limit the possible spread of infection, to encourage rest and excellent nutrition, to ensure complete compliance with the prescribed drug regimen, and to observe for adverse drug effects. Care of an outpatient includes continued medication, evaluation for adverse drug effects, sputum analyses, and encouragement to complete the long course of treatment. Before discharge, the patient is taught how to prevent the spread of the disease; the elements of good nutrition; the name, dose, action, and side effects of all medications prescribed; the need to take the drugs regularly; and how and where to get the next supply of drugs. See also **miliary tuberculosis, tuberculin test.**

tuberculosis vaccine   See **BCG vaccine.**
tuberculous spondylitis   A rare, grave form of tuberculosis caused by the invasion of *Mycobacterium tuberculosis* into the spinal vertebrae. The intervertebral disks may be destroyed, resulting in the collapse and wedging of affected vertebrae and the shortening and angulation of the spine. Thoracic vertebrae are more frequently involved than the vertebrae of the lumbar, the cervical, or the sacral segments of the spine. More than one area of the spine may be affected, and normal vertebrae may be evident between affected and unaffected sections. The infection characteristically dissects vertebrae anterolaterally and produces abscesses. The pressure of the abcess may cause ischemic paralysis in the subjacent spinal cord, and abscesses in the cervical area may displace or obstruct the trachea and the esophagus. Also called **Pott's disease, spinal caries.** See also **tuberculosis.**

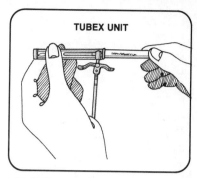

TUBEX UNIT

tuberosity   An elevation or protuberance, especially of a bone.
tuberosity of the tibia   A large, oblong elevation at the proximal end of the tibia that attaches to the ligament of the patella.
tuberous carcinoma   A scirrhous carcinoma of the skin that is characterized by nodular projections. Also called **carcinoma tuberosum.**
tuberous sclerosis   A familial, neurocutaneous disease characterized by epilepsy, mental deterioration, adenoma sebaceum, nodules and sclerotic patches on the cerebral cortex, retinal tumors, depigmented leaf-shaped macules on the skin, tumors of the heart or kidneys, and cerebral calcifications. There is no effective treatment. Also called **epiloia.** See also **adenoma sebaceum.**
tuberous xanthoma   See **xanthoma tuberosum.**
Tubex unit   A trade name for a unit consisting of a cartridge and needle that fits into a holder that has a plunger. The cartridge may be empty or prefilled with a standard dose of a medication. The needle is covered with a rubber protective guard and is permanently attached to the cartridge. The plunger may be unscrewed to allow the cartridge-needle unit to be slipped in place. The holder requires no special care and is reuseable.
tubocurarine chloride   A nondepolarizing neuromuscular blocking agent.
tubule   A small tube, as one of the renal collecting tubules. —**tubular,** *adj.*
tuft fracture   Fracture of one of the distal phalanges.
tularemia   An infectious disease of animals caused by the bacillus *Francisella (Pasteurella) tularensis,* which may be transmitted by insect vectors or direct contact. It is characterized in humans by fever, headache, and an ulcerated skin lesion with localized lymph node enlargement or by eye infection, gastrointestinal ulcerations, or pneumonia, depending on the site of entry and the response of the host. Treatment includes streptomycin, chloramphenicol, and tetracycline. Recovery produces lifelong immunity. A vaccine is available. Also called **deerfly fever, rabbit fever.**
-tumescence   A combining form meaning

TUNING FORK

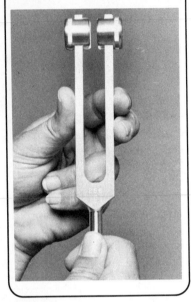

a 'swelling': *detumescence, intumescence.*

tumor 1. A swelling or enlargement occurring in inflammatory conditions. 2. A new growth of tissue characterized by progressive, uncontrolled proliferation of cells. The tumor may be localized or invasive, benign or malignant. Also called **neoplasm.**

tumor albus A white swelling occurring in a tuberculous bone or joint.

tumoricide A substance capable of destroying a tumor. —**tumoricidal,** *adj.*

tumorigenesis The process of imitating and promoting the development of a tumor. Compare **carcinogenesis, oncogenesis, sarcomagenesis.** —**tumorigenic,** *adj.*

Tunga penetrans A small, reddish-brown flea widespread in tropical America and Africa that burrows into the skin, between the toes, and under toenails. Infestation causes pain, itching, and, eventually, a pus-filled ulcer. Secondary septicemia may result from superimposed infection. Also called **chigger, chigoe.**

tungsten (W) A metallic element. Its atomic number is 74; its atomic weight is 183.85.

tunica vasculosa bulbi See **uvea.**

tuning fork A small metal instrument consisting of a stem and two prongs that produces a constant pitch when either prong is struck. It is used in auditory tests of nerve function and of air and bone conduction.

turban tumor A benign neoplasm of multiple pink or maroon nodules that may cover the entire scalp and may also occur on the trunk and extremities. The growth is apparently familial and often recurs after excision.

turbidimetry Measurement of the turbidity (cloudiness) of a solution or suspension in which the amount of transmitted light is quantified with a spectrophotometer or estimated by visual comparison with solutions of known turbidity.

turbinate 1. Of or pertaining to a scroll shape. 2. The concha nasalis.

turgid In a distended, hard, and congested state, usually as a result of an accumulation of fluid. —**turgor,** *n.*

turgor The normal resiliency of the skin caused by the outward pressure of the cells and interstitial fluid. Dehydration results in decreased skin turgor, manifested by lax skin, which, when grasped and raised between two fingers, slowly returns to a position level with the adjacent tissue. Marked edema or ascites results in increased turgor manifested by smooth, taut, shiny skin that cannot be grasped and raised. An evaluation of the turgor of the skin is an essential part of physical assessment.

turista See **traveler's diarrhea.**

turnbuckle cast An orthopedic device used to encase and immobilize the entire trunk, one arm to the elbow, and the opposite leg to the knee. It is constructed of plaster of Paris or fiberglass and incorporates hinges as part of its design in the treatment of scoliosis. The hinges are placed at the level of the apex of the curvature. Employed for pre- and postoperative positioning, it is used less frequently than the Risser cast. An adaptation of the turnbuckle cast is used occasionally as a hyperextension cast for the treatment of kyphosis or kyphoscoliosis.

Turner's sign See **Grey Turner's sign.**

Turner's syndrome A chromosomal anomaly seen in about 1 in 3,000 live female births, characterized by the absence of one X chromosome, congenital ovarian failure, genital hypoplasia, cardiovascular anomalies, dwarfism, short metacarpals, 'shield chest,' extosis of tibia, and underdeveloped breasts, uterus, and vagina. Spatial disorientation and moderate degrees of learning disorders are common. Treatment includes hormone therapy (estrogens, androgens, pituitary growth hormone) and, often, surgical correction of cardiovascular anomalies and the webbing of the neck skin. Also called **Bonnevie-Ullrich syndrome, monosomy X.**

turricephaly See **oxycephaly.**

-tuse A combining form meaning: 1. 'Dull or blunt': *obtuse.* 2. 'To beat or thrust': *contuse.*

T wave The component of the cardiac cycle shown on an electrocardiogram as a short, inverted, U-shaped curve following the ST segment. It represents repolarization, the last phase of the cardiac cycle as the heart recovers from contraction and prepares to begin the cycle again with atrial depolarization during the P wave.

twelfth nerve See **hypoglossal nerve.**

twenty-four-hour-clock system A method of designating time by using the numerical sequence from 00 to 23 for the hours and 00 to 59 for the minutes in a daily cycle beginning with 0000 (midnight) and ending with 2359 (1 minute before the following midnight).

twilight sleep Light anesthesia obtained by parenteral administration of a morphine and scopolamine mixture to reduce pain and obtund recall in childbirth.

twin Either of two offspring born of the same pregnancy and developed from either a single ovum or from two ova released from the ovary simultaneously and fertilized at the same time. The incidence of twin births is about 1 in 80 pregnancies. Kinds of twins include **conjoined twins, dizygotic twins, interlocked twins, monozygotic twins, Siamese twins, unequal twins.** See also **Hellin's law.**

twin monster See **double monster.**

twinning **1.** The development of two or more fetuses during the same pregnancy, either spontaneously or through external intervention for experimental purposes in animals. **2.** The duplication of like structures or parts by division.

two-way catheter A catheter that has a double lumen, one channel for injection of medication or fluids and the other for removal of fluid or specimens.

tybamate An antianxiety agent.

tympanic Of or pertaining to a structure that resonates when struck; drumlike, as a **tympanic abdomen. —tympanum,** *n.* **tympana,** *n., pl.,* **tympani,** *genitive.*

tympanic antrum A relatively large, irregular cavity in the superior anterior portion of the mastoid process of the temporal bone, communicating with the mastoid air cells and lined by the extension of the mucous membrane of the tympanic cavity. The bony tegmen tympani separates the tympanic antrum from the middle fossa of the cranial cavity, and the lateral semicircular part of the internal ear projects into the antrum. See also **mastoid process.**

tympanic cavity See **middle ear.**

tympanic membrane A thin, semitransparent membrane in the middle ear that transmits sound vibrations to the internal ear by means of the auditory ossicles. It is nearly oval in form, with a vertical diameter of about 10 mm, and separates the tympanic cavity from the bottom of the external acoustic meatus. Also called **ear drum, membrana tympani.**

tympanic reflex The reflection of a beam of light shining on the eardrum. In a normal ear, a bright, wedge-shaped reflection is seen; its apex is at the end of the malleus, and its base is at the anterior inferior margin of the eardrum. In disorders of the middle ear or eardrum, this shape may be distorted. Also called **light reflex.**

tympanoplasty Any of the operative procedures on the eardrum or ossicles of the middle ear, used to restore or improve hearing in patients with conductive deafness. These operations may be used to repair a perforated eardrum, for otosclerosis, dislocation of the incus, or necrosis of one of the small bones of the middle ear. See also **myringoplasty.**

-type A combining form meaning a 'representative form or class': *lysotype, serotype, somatotype.*

type A personality A complex of person-

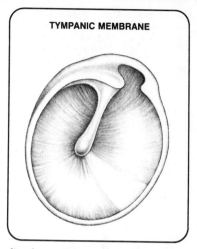

TYMPANIC MEMBRANE

ality characteristics, including chronic impatience, fierce competitiveness, and a compulsion to get things done quickly. Type A personality is a risk factor in myocardial infarction.

type I hyperlipoproteinemia A familial form of primary hyperlipoproteinemia. A relatively rare disease transmitted as an autosomal dominant trait, it is characterized by accumulations of triglycerides and chylomicrons in the blood, resulting in recurrent bouts of severe abdominal pain, usually after ingestion of fats. The symptoms begin in childhood. The disease is caused by a deficiency in the activity of an enzyme, lipoprotein lipase, that normally removes triglycerides from the blood. The accumulation of triglycerides is proportional to the amount of dietary fat. Treatment is primarily dietary; both saturated and unsaturated fats are restricted to amounts that produce less than 500 mg/100 ml of blood, evaluated after an overnight fast. Also called **exogenous hyperlipemia.**

type II hyperlipoproteinemia See **familial hypercholesterolemia.**

type I hypersensitivity See **anaphylactic hypersensitivity.**

type II hypersensitivity See **cytotoxic hypersensitivity.**

type III hypersensitivity See **immune complex hypersensitivity.**

type IV hypersensitivity See **cell-mediated immune response.**

typhlitis See **appendicitis.**

typhlo- A combining form meaning: **1.** 'Pertaining to the cecum': *typhlocolitis, typhlostomy.* **2.** 'Pertaining to blindness': *typhlolexia, typhlology.*

-typhoid A combining form meaning: **1.** A '(specified) form of typus': *bronchotyphoid, meningotyphoid.* **2.** 'Of or resembling typhus': *antityphoid, paratyphoid.* Also **-typhoidal.**

-typhoidal See **-typhoid.**

typhoid fever A bacterial infection that is usually caused by *Salmonella typhi.* Typhoid fever is transmitted by contaminated milk, water, or food and is characterized by headache, delirium, cough, watery diarrhea, rash, and a high fever. The incubation period may be as long as 60 days. Characteristic maculopapular rosy spots are scattered over the skin of the abdomen. Splenomegaly and leukopenia develop first. The diagnosis is made by bacteriologic culture of blood and stool and by a rising titer of agglutinins in the Widal test. The disease may be fatal. Complications include intestinal hemorrhage or perforation and thrombophlebitis. Some people who recover from the disease continue to be carriers and excrete the organism. Prolonged administration of antibiotics or cholecystectomy may eliminate the carrier state. Typhoid vaccine gives some protection but requires annual booster doses. Proper disposal of human wastes is essential to prevent epidemics, and disease carriers should not be permitted to prepare food. Compare **cholera, paratyphoid fever, salmonellosis.**

typhoid pellagra A form of pellagra in which the symptoms also include continued high temperatures.

typhoid vaccine A bacterial vaccine prepared from an inactivated, dried strain of *Salmonella typhi.*

typhus Any of a group of acute infectious diseases caused by various species of *Rickettsia* and usually transmitted from infected rodents to humans by the bites of lice, fleas, mites, or ticks. These diseases are all characterized by headache, chills, fever, malaise, and a maculopapular rash. Kinds of typhus are **epidemic typhus, murine typhus, scrub typhus.** See also **Brill-Zinsser disease.**

-typia A combining form meaning '(condition of) conformity to type': *atypia, ectypia, zelotypia.*

typing The process of ascertaining the classification of a specimen of blood, tissue, or other substance. See also **blood typing, tissue typing.**

tyramine An amino acid synthesized in the body from the essential acid tyrosine. Tyramine stimulates the release of the catecholamines epinephrine and norepinephrine. It is important that people taking monoamine oxidase inhibitors avoid the ingestion of foods and beverages containing tyramine, including beer, wine, broad beans, some cheeses, Chianti wine, chicken livers, caffeine, chocolate, cola drinks, liver, her-

ring, tea, yogurt, and yeast. See also **adrenergic, amine, catecholamine, epinephrine, norepinephrine, vasoconstriction.**

tyro- A combining form meaning 'pertaining to cheese': *tyrogenous, tyroid, tyrometosis.*

tyroma, *pl.* **tyromas, tyromata** A new growth or nodule with a caseous or cheesy consistency.

tyromatosis A process in which necrotic tissue is broken down and degenerates to a granular, amorphous, caseous mass.

tyrosine An amino acid synthesized in the body from the essential amino acid phenylalanine. Tyrosine is found in most proteins and is a precursor of melanin and several hormones, including epinephrine and thyroxin. See also **amino acid, hormone, melanin.**

tyrosinemia **1.** A benign, transient condition of the newborn, especially premature infants, in which an excessive amount of the amino acid tyrosine is found in the blood and urine. The disorder is caused by an anomaly in amino acid metabolism, usually delayed development of the enzymes necessary to metabolize tyrosine, and is controlled by dietary measures and vitamin C therapy. The metabolic defect disappears with treatment, or it may disappear spontaneously. Also called **neonatal tyrosinemia.** **2.** An hereditary disorder involving an inborn error of metabolism of the amino acid tyrosine. The condition, transmitted as an autosomal recessive trait, is caused by an enzyme deficiency and results in liver failure or hepatic cirrhosis, renal tubular defects that can lead to renal rickets and renal glycosuria, generalized aminoaciduria, and mental retardation. Treatment consists of a diet low in tyrosine and phenylalanine and high in doses of vitamin C. Also called **hereditary tyrosinemia.**

tyrosinosis A condition resulting from a defect in amino acid metabolism and characterized by the excretion of an excessive amount of parahydroxyphenylpyruvic acid, an intermediate product of tyrosine, in the urine. See also **tyrosinemia.**

Tzanck test A microscopic examination of cellular material from skin lesions to help diagnose certain vesicular diseases. The tissue is scraped from the base of a vesicle, placed on a slide, and stained with Wright's or Giemsa stain. Multinucleated giant cells are diagnostic of herpesvirus or varicella. Typical pemphigus and other cells can also be identified.

U

u Symbol sometimes used to stand for **micron** (properly μ), as in u/ml, representing μ/ml.

U Symbol for **uranium,** *abbr* unit.

-ular A combining form meaning: **1.** 'Pertaining to' something specified: *appendicular, molecular, pedicular.* **2.** 'Resembling' something specified: *circular, globular, tubular.*

ulcer A circumscribed, craterlike lesion of the skin or mucous membrane resulting from necrosis that accompanies some inflammatory, infectious, and malignant processes. An ulcer may be shallow, involving only the epidermis, as in phemphigus, or deep. Some kinds of ulcer are **decubitus ulcer, peptic ulcer, serpent ulcer.** —**ulcerate,** *v.,* **ulcerative,** *adj.*

ulcerative blepharitis A form of blepharitis in which a staphylococcal infection of the follicles of the eyelashes and glands of the eyelids results in sticky crusts forming on the lid margins. If the crusts are pulled off, the skin beneath bleeds. Tiny pustules develop in the follicles of the eyelashes and break down to form shallow ulcers. Other symptoms include burning, itching, swelling, and redness of the eyelids; a loss of eyelashes; irritation of the conjunctiva with lacrimation; photophobia; and gluing together of the eyelids during sleep by the dried secretions. Compare **nonulcerative blepharitis.**

ulcerative colitis A chronic, episodic, inflammatory disease of the large intestine and rectum, characterized by profuse watery diarrhea containing varying amounts of blood, mucus, and pus, and easily confused with Crohn's disease. The attacks of diarrhea are accompanied by tenesmus, severe abdominal pain, fever, chills, anemia, and weight loss. Children with the disease may suffer retarded physical growth. Diagnosis is aided by X-ray and biopsy. Treatment includes use of corticosteroids or other anti-inflammatory agents, and surgery. NURSING CONSIDERATIONS: Systemic complications of ulcerative colitis include peripheral arthritis, ankylosing spondylitis, kidney and liver disease, and inflammation of the eyes, skin, and mouth. In severe cases, toxic megacolon may develop, which may lead to perforation of the bowel, septicemia, and death. Ulcerative colitis also predisposes the patient to cancer of the colon.

ule- See **ulo-,** definition 2.

-ule See **-ulum.**

-ulent A combining form meaning 'full of, characterized by': *feculent, pulverulent, succulent.*

ulna The bone on the medial or little finger side of the forearm, lying parallel with the radius. Its proximal end bulges into the olecranon and the coronoid processes and dips into the trochlear and the radial notches. The ulna articulates with the humerus and the radius.

ulnar artery A large artery branching from the brachial artery, supplying muscles in the forearm, wrist, and hand; arising near the elbow, it passes obliquely in a distal direction to become the superficial palmar arch. It has nine branches: four in the forearm, two in the wrist, and three in the hand. The forearm branches are the anterior ulnar recurrent, posterior ulnar recurrent, common interosseous, and muscular. The two branches in the wrist are the palmar carpal and dorsal carpal. The branches in the hand are the deep palmar, superficial palmar arch, and common palmar digital.

ulnar nerve One of the terminal branches of the brachial plexus that arises on each side from the medial cord of the plexus and supplies the muscles and the skin on the ulnar side of the forearm and the hand. It can be easily palpated as the 'funny bone' of the elbow as it courses along the groove between the olecranon process and the medial epicondyle of the humerus. It first passes medial to the axillary artery and the brachial artery to the middle of the arm, pierces the medial intermuscular septum, and follows along the medial head of the triceps to the olecranon. It descends into the forearm and in the distal portion on the ulnar side is covered only by the skin and the fascia. Just above the wrist it gives off a large dorsal branch and continues into the hand where it gives off the digital and the muscular branches. The ulnar nerve usually has no branches above the elbow. Below the elbow its branches are the articular branches to the elbow joint, two muscular branches, the palmar cutaneous branch, the dorsal branch, the palmar branch, the superficial branch, and the deep branch. Compare **median nerve, musculocutaneous nerve, radial nerve.**

ulo-, ule- A combining form meaning: **1.** 'Pertaining to a scar or cicatrix': *ulodermatitis, uloid, ulotomy.* **2.** 'Pertaining to the gums or gingivae': *ulectomy, ulocace, ulorrhagia, ulotripsis.*

ulocarcinoma, *pl.* **ulocarcinomas, ulocarcinomata** Any malignant neoplastic disease of the gums that is classified as a carcinoma.

ultra- A combining form meaning 'beyond, farther, beyond a certain limit': *ultragaseous, ultrasound, ultravirus.*

ultracentrifuge A high-speed centrifuge with a rotation rate fast enough to produce sedimentation of viruses, even in blood plasma. It

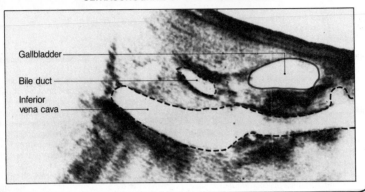

ULTRASONOGRAM OF THE GALLBLADDER

Gallbladder

Bile duct

Inferior
vena cava

---

is used in many kinds of biochemical analyses, including the measurement and separation of some proteins and viruses. Use of an attached microscope may make it possible to see the sediment.

ultrafilter 1. A microporous filter used in laboratory ultrafiltration. 2. A semipermeable membrane.

ultrafiltrate The liquid or very fine particled mass that passes through an ultrafilter.

ultrafiltration Filtration of colloid solutions or fine-particled solids through an ultrafilter, which removes all but the smallest particles. Plasma filtration through the capillary membrane is a natural example. Laboratory ultrafiltration often involves separation of colloid solutions, accelerated by application of pressure.

ultralente insulin See **long-acting insulin.**

ultramicroscopy See **dark-field microscopy.**

ultrasonic cardiography See **echocardiography.**

ultrasonography The process of representing deep structures of the body by measuring and recording the reflection of pulsed or continuous high-frequency sound waves. Also called **sonography.**

ultrasound Very high frequency sound waves, over 20,000 vibrations per second. Medical applications include fetal monitoring, imaging of internal organs, and cleaning dental and surgical instruments.

ultraviolet Light beyond the range of human vision, at the short end of the spectrum. It occurs naturally in sunlight; it burns and tans the skin and converts precursors in the skin to vitamin D. Ultraviolet lamps are used in the control of infectious, airborne bacteria and viruses and in the treatment of psoriasis and other skin conditions. Black light is ultraviolet light used in fluoroscopy. See also **light, radiation, spectrum.**

ultraviolet microscopy See **fluorescent microscopy.**

ultraviolet radiation A range of electromagnetic waves extending from the violet or short-wavelength end of the spectrum to the beginning of the X-ray spectrum. About 5% of the sun's radiation is in the ultraviolet range, but much of it is absorbed by oxygen and ozone in the atmosphere before it reaches earth. Window glass also absorbs this radiation. Artificial sources include the iron arc, carbon arc, and mercury-vapor arc lamps. In medicine, ultraviolet radiation is used in the treatment of rickets and certain skin conditions. Milk and some other foods become activated with vitamin D when exposed to this type of energy. Ultraviolet radiation also causes fluorescence and phosphorescence, useful in such diverse applications as lighting and the identification of minerals.

-ulum, -ulus A combining form meaning 'small one': *ovulum, scutulum, speculum, homunculus, nodulus, ramulus.* Also **-ule.**

umbilical 1. Of or pertaining to the umbilicus. 2. Of or pertaining to the umbilical cord.

umbilical catheterization A procedure in which a radiopaque catheter is passed through an umbilical artery to provide a newborn infant with parenteral fluid, to obtain blood samples, or both, or through the umbilical vein for an exchange transfusion or the emergency administration of drugs, fluids, or volume expanders.

umbilical cord A flexible structure connecting the umbilicus with the placenta in the gravid uterus and giving passage to the umbilical arteries and vein. In the newborn it is about 60 cm (2 feet) long and 1.27 cm (½ inch) in diameter. First formed during the 5th week of pregnancy, it contains the yolk sac and the body stalk with the enclosed allantois. Also called the **chorda umbilicalis, funiculus umbilicalis.**

umbilical duct See **vitelline duct.**

umbilical fissure A groove on the inferior surface of the liver that holds the ligamentum teres and separates the right and left lobes of the liver.

umbilical fistula An abnormal passage from the umbilicus to the intestine or more frequently to the remnant of the canal in the median umbilical ligament that connects the fetal bladder with the allantois.

umbilical hernia A soft, skin-covered protrusion of intestine and omentum through a weakness in the abdominal wall around the umbilicus. It usually closes spontaneously within 1 to 2 years, although large hernias may require surgical closure.

umbilical vein One of a pair of embryonic vessels that return the blood from the placenta and fuse to form a single trunk in the body stalk. They remain separate for a short time in the embryo, opening into the sinus venosus. Development of the fetal liver breaks the connection between the umbilical veins and the sinus venosus, whereupon the right umbilical vein shrivels and disappears. The left umbilical vein remains attached to the placenta, and is contained, with the fetal arteries, in the umbilical cord. After birth, the left umbilical vein and the ductus venosus atrophy and form respectively the ligamentum teres and the ligamentum venosum of the liver.

umbilical vesicle A pear-shaped structure formed from the yolk sac at about the 4th week of prenatal development that protrudes into the cavity of the chorion and connects to the developing embryo by the yolk stalk at the region of the future midgut.

umbilicus The point on the abdomen at which the umbilical cord joined the fetal abdomen, marked in the adult usually by a depression but sometimes by a protrusion.

unciform bone See hamate bone.

uncompensated gluteal gait See Trendelenburg gait.

unconditioned response A normal, instinctive, unlearned reaction to a stimulus; one that occurs naturally and is not acquired by association and training. Also called inborn reflex, instinctive reflex, unconditioned reflex. Compare conditioned response.

unconscious 1. Unaware of the surrounding environment; insensible; incapable of responding to sensory stimuli. 2. In psychiatry: the part of the mental function in which thoughts, ideas, emotions, or memories are outside awareness and not subject to ready recall. It contains data that have never been conscious or that were conscious at one time, usually for a brief period, and later repressed. Compare preconscious. See also collective unconscious.

unconsciousness A state of complete or partial unawareness or lack of response to sensory stimuli as a result of injury, shock, illness, or other bodily disorder, as alcoholic excess, narcotic overdose, poisoning, and sunstroke. Various degrees of unconsciousness can occur during stupor, fugue, catalepsy, and dream states. See also coma.

unction See ointment.

undecylenic acid (zinc undecyclenate) A local anti-infective.

underweight Less than normal in body weight after appropriate adjustments are made

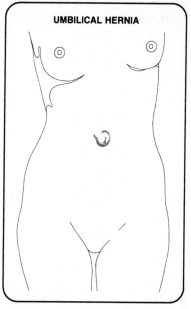

UMBILICAL HERNIA

for height, body build, and age.

undescended testis See cryptorchidism, monorchidism.

undifferentiated cell leukemia See stem cell leukemia.

undifferentiated malignant lymphoma A lymphoid neoplasm containing many large stem cells that have large nuclei, small amounts of pale cytoplasm, and borders that are not well defined. Also called reticulosarcoma, stem cell lymphoma.

undifferentiated schizophrenia See acute schizophrenia.

undisplaced fracture A bone break in which cracks in the osseous tissue may radiate in several directions without the separation or displacement of fragmented sections.

undulant fever See brucellosis.

unengaged head A floating fetal head. See engagement. See also ballottement.

unequal cleavage Mitotic division of the fertilized ovum into blastomeres that are larger near the yolk portion of protoplasm, or vegetal pole, and smaller near the nucleus, or animal pole. Compare equal cleavage.

unequal twins Two nonjoined fetuses born of the same pregnancy in which only one of the pair is fully formed, with the other showing various degrees of developmental defects.

ungual phalanx See distal phalanx.

unguent See ointment.

unguis, *pl.* **ungues** See nail. —**ungual**, *adj.*

uni- A combining form meaning 'one': *unibasal, uniceps.*

UNICEF *abbr* United Nations International Children's Emergency Fund.

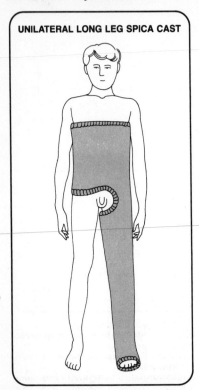

UNILATERAL LONG LEG SPICA CAST

unicellular reproduction The formation of a new organism from a female egg that has not been fertilized; parthenogenesis.

unification model A theoretical framework based on the close relationship of nursing education and clinical nursing service at the University of Rochester, New York. The faculty of the school of nursing hold joint appointments to the school and the hospital, teaching nursing students and providing clinical leadership in nursing service in the hospital. See also **joint appointment.**

unilateral long leg spica cast An orthopedic cast applied to immobilize one leg and the trunk of the body cranially as far as the nipple line. It is used to treat a fractured femur or for the correction or the maintenance of the correction of a hip deformity. Compare **bilateral long leg spica cast, one-and-a-half spica cast.**

unilateral paralysis See **hemiplegia.**

union shop An establishment in which membership in a trade or labor union is required.

uniovular Developing from a single ovum as in monozygotic twins as contrasted with dizygotic twins. Also called **monovular.** Compare **binovular.**

unipolar lead 1. An electrocardiographic conductor in which the exploring electrode is placed on the precordium or a limb while the indifferent electrode is in the central terminal. 2. *Informal.* A tracing produced by such a lead on an electrocardiograph.

unit 1. A single item. 2. A quantity designated as a standard of measurement.

unit dose A method of preparing medications in which individual doses of patient medications are prepared by the pharmacy and delivered in individual labeled packets to the patient's unit to be administered by the nurses on the ordered schedule.

United Nations International Children's Emergency Fund (UNICEF) A fund established by the General Assembly of the United Nations in 1946 to aid children in devastated areas of the world. It is funded by contributions from the member nations and acts to prevent disease, including tuberculosis, whooping cough, and diphtheria, and provides food and clothing to needy children in more than 50 countries.

United States Pharmacopeia (USP) A compendium, recognized officially by the Federal Food, Drug, and Cosmetic Act, that contains descriptions, uses, strengths, and standards of purity for selected drugs and their forms of dosage.

United States Public Health Service (USPHS) An agency of the federal government responsible for the control of the arrival from abroad of any people, goods, or substances that may affect the health of U.S. citizens. The agency sets standards for the domestic handling and processing of food and the manufacture of serums, vaccines, cosmetics, and drugs. It supports and performs research, aids localities in times of disaster and epidemics, and provides medical care for certain groups of Americans.

univalent The capacity of one atom of a chemical element to attract one atom of hydrogen or to displace one atom of hydrogen. See also **valence.**

universal antidote A mixture of 50% activated charcoal, 25% magnesium oxide, and 25% tannic acid, formerly given as an antidote for most acid, heavy metal, alkaloid, and glycoside poisons. It is now believed that the mixture is no more effective than activated charcoal given with water.

universal donor A person with blood of type O, Rh factor negative. Such blood was formerly used for emergency transfusion with minimal risk of incompatibility. However, this practice is seldom used today owing to the widespread availability of plasma expanders and other therapies. See also **blood donor, blood group, transfusion.**

Unna boot A dressing for varicose ulcers formed by applying a layer of a gelatin-glycerin–zinc oxide paste to the leg and then a spiral bandage that is covered with successive coats of paste to produce a rigid boot.

unsaturated alcohol An alcohol derived from an unsaturated hydrocarbon, as an alkene or olefin.

unsaturated fatty acid Any of a number of glyceryl esters of certain organic acids in which some of the atoms are joined by double or triple valence bonds easily split in chemical reactions and joined to other substances. Monounsaturated fatty acids, with one double or triple bond per molecule, are found in such foods as fowl, almonds, pecans, cashew nuts, peanuts, and olive oil. Polyunsaturated fatty acids, with more than one double or triple bond per molecule, occur in fish, corn, walnuts, sunflower seeds, soybeans, cottonseeds, and safflower oil. Diets high in polyunsaturated fatty acids and low in saturated fatty acids have been correlated with low serum cholesterol levels in some study populations. Compare **saturated fatty acid.**

unsocialized aggressive reaction A behavior disorder of childhood characterized by overt and covert hostility, disobedience, physical and verbal aggression, vengefulness, quarrelsome behavior and destructiveness, often manifested in such acts as lying, stealing, temper tantrums, vandalism, and physical violence against others. Most prevalent in boys, the condition results typically from an unstable home environment characterized by harsh and inconsistent application of discipline, general frustration, rejection, marital discord, separation, or divorce. Punitive treatment is ineffective. Recommended treatment reinforces desirable behavioral patterns and attempts to modify unfavorable environmental conditions.

unstriated muscle See **smooth muscle.**

upper extremity suspension An orthopedic procedure used in the treatment of bone fractures and the correction of orthopedic abnormalities of the upper limbs. The procedure uses traction equipment, including metal frames, ropes, and pulleys to relieve the weight of the upper limb involved rather than to exert traction. Upper extremity suspension is usually unilateral but may also be used bilaterally in the postoperative, posttraumatic, or postreduction control of edema. Compare **balanced suspension, hyperextension suspension, lower extremity suspension.**

upper motor neuron paralysis An injury to the lesion in the brain or spinal cord that causes damage to the cell bodies, or axons, or both, of the upper motor neurons, which extend from the cerebral centers to the cells in the spinal column. Clinical manifestations include increased muscle tone and spasticity of the muscles involved with little or no atrophy, hyperactive deep-tendon reflexes, diminished or absent superficial reflexes, the presence of pathological reflexes, as the Babinski's and Hoffmann's reflexes, and no local twitching of muscle groups. Compare **lower motor neuron paralysis.**

upper respiratory infection (URI) See **respiratory tract infection.**

upper respiratory tract One of the two divisions of the respiratory system. The upper respiratory tract consists of the nose, the nasal cavity, the ethmoidal air cells, the frontal sinuses, the sphenoidal sinuses, the maxillary sinus

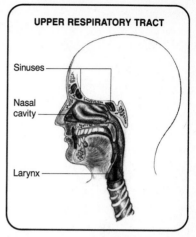

UPPER RESPIRATORY TRACT

Sinuses

Nasal cavity

Larynx

and the larynx. The upper respiratory tract conducts air to and from the lungs and filters, moistens, and warms the air during each inspiration. See also **larynx, nose.** Compare **lower respiratory tract.**

ur- See **uro-.**

uracil mustard An alkylating agent used in chemotherapy.

uranium (U) A heavy, radioactive metallic element. Its atomic number is 92; its atomic weight is 238.03.

urano- A combining form meaning 'pertaining to the palate': *uranoplasty, uranoplegia, uranoschism.*

urate A salt of uric acid, normally present in the urine. See also **gout, uric acid.**

urban typhus See **murine typhus.**

urea 1. An odorless, colorless, crystalline solid, $CO(NH_2)_2$, the diamide of carbonic acid. The natural end product of protein metabolism, urea is formed in the liver from carbon dioxide plus ammonia produced by deamination of amino acids, and found in blood, lymph, and urine. It normally accounts for 80% to 90% of total renal nitrogen, the amount fluctuating in direct proportion to ingestion of protein and rising with fever, diabetes, and increased adrenal activity. Excessive accumulation of urea is a cause of uremia. 2. USP: a drug containing 99% to 100.5% of the amount of urea shown on the label. Given by intravenous infusion as a diuretic to relieve intracranial or intraocular pressure and used in 2% to 25% strengths in topical preparations to hydrate and soften hard, dry skin.

-urea A combining form meaning a 'compound containing urea': *glycolylurea, phenylthiourea, solurea.*

Ureaplasma urealyticum A sexually transmitted microorganism that is a common inhabitant of the urogenital systems of men and women in whom infection is asymptomatic. Neonatal death, prematurity, and perinatal morbidity are statistically associated with colonization of the chorionic surface of the placenta

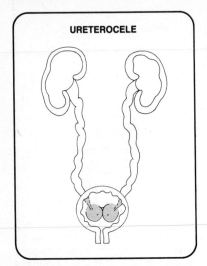

URETEROCELE

branch into calyces, each calyx containing a renal papilla. Urine draining through renal tubules drops into the papillae, passes through the calyces and the pelvis and down each ureter into the bladder. The openings of the ureters in the bladder lie at the lateral angles of the trigone, spaced about 2 cm (¾ inch) apart when the bladder is empty, about 5 cm (2 inches) apart when the bladder is distended. Urine is pumped through the ureters by peristaltic waves that occur an average of three times a minute. Each ureter is composed of a fibrous, a muscular, and a mucous coat and is perfused by arterial branches of the renal, the testicular, the internal iliac, and the inferior vesical arteries. It is innervated by nerves derived from the inferior mesenteric, the testicular, and the pelvic plexi. **—ureteral,** *adj.*

ureteral dysfunction A disturbance of the normal peristaltic flow of urine through a ureter, resulting from dysfunction of ureteral motor nerves. See also **megaloureter.**

ureteritis An inflammatory condition of a ureter caused by infection or by the mechanical irritation of a stone.

ureterocele A prolapse of the terminal portion of the ureter into the bladder. The condition may lead to obstruction of the flow of urine, hydronephrosis, and loss of renal function. Cystoscopy and pyelography reveal the prolapsed ureter. Surgical correction is performed to prevent permanent damage to the kidney.

urethra A small tubular structure that drains urine from the bladder. In women, it is about 3 cm (1 inch) long and lies directly behind the symphysis pubis, anterior to the vagina. In men, it is about 20 cm (8 inches) long and begins at the bladder, passes through the center of the prostate gland, goes between two sheets of tissue connecting the pubic bones, and, finally, passes through the urinary meatus of the penis. In men, the urethra serves as a passageway for semen during ejaculation as well as a canal for urine during voiding. See also **ureter.**

urethral Of or pertaining to the urethra.

urethritis An inflammatory condition of the urethra that is characterized by dysuria, usually the result of an infection in the bladder or kidneys. Medications, as a sulfonamide or other antibacterial, a urinary antiseptic, and an analgesic are usually prescribed once the causative organism is identified by bacteriologic culture of a urine specimen. See also **nongonococcal urethritis.**

urethro- A combining form meaning 'pertaining to the urethra': *urethrocele, urethrocystitis, urethrophraxis.*

urethrocele In women: a herniation of the urethra. It is characterized by a protusion of a segment of the urethra and the connective tissue surrounding it into the anterior wall of the vagina. The herniation may be slight and high in the vagina and only palpable on digital examination when the patient strains downward, or it may be large and low in the anterior wall with visible bulging at the vaginal introitus. A large urethrocele may result in difficulty in voiding,

by the organism. The mechanisms by which the unfavorable effects on pregnancy occur are not understood. There is no characteristic lesion in the fetus or newborn.

uremia 1. The presence of excessive amounts of urea and other nitrogenous waste products in the blood. **2.** The abnormal condition of having an excessive amount of these substances in the blood, as occurs in renal failure. Also called **azotemia.**

uremic frost A pale, frostlike deposit of white crystals on the skin owing to kidney failure and uremia. Urea compounds and other waste products of metabolism that cannot be excreted by the kidneys into the urine are excreted through the small superficial capillaries into the skin, where they collect on the surface.

-uret A combining form designating a binary compound: *bromuret, phosphuret, sulphuret.*

ureter One of a pair of tubes, about 30 cm (12 inches) long, that carry the urine from the kidney into the bladder. They are thick-walled, vary in diameter along their length from 1 mm to 1 cm, and are divided into an abdominal portion and a pelvic portion. The abdominal portion lies behind the peritoneum on the medial side of the psoas major and enters the pelvic cavity by crossing either the termination of the common iliac artery or the commencement of the external iliac artery. In men, the pelvic portion of the ureter runs caudal along the lateral wall of the pelvic cavity and reaches the lateral angle of the bladder just ventral to the upper tip of the seminal vesicle. In women, the pelvic portion of the ureter forms the posterior boundary of the ovarian fossa and runs medially and ventrally along the upper part of the vagina. The ureter enters the bladder through an oblique tunnel that functions as a valve to prevent backflow of urine into the ureter when the bladder contracts. Connecting with the kidneys, the ureters expand into funnel-shaped renal pelves that

URINALYSIS: NORMAL FINDINGS

Macroscopic

ELEMENT	FINDINGS
Color	Straw
Odor	Slightly aromatic
Appearance	Clear
Specific gravity	1.025 to 1.030
pH	4.5 to 8.0
Protein	None
Glucose	None
Ketones	None
Other sugars	None

Microscopic

ELEMENT	FINDINGS
RBCs	0 to 3/high-power field
WBCs	0 to 4/high-power field
Epithelial cells	Few
Casts	None, except occasional hyaline casts
Crystals	Present
Yeast cells	None
Parasites	None

some degree of incontinence, urinary tract infection, and dyspareunia. The condition may be congenital or acquired, secondary to obesity, parturition, and poor muscle tone. Surgical repair is the usual treatment.

URI *abbr* **upper respiratory infection.** See **respiratory tract infection.**

-uria A combining form meaning: **1.** The 'presence of a substance in the urine': *ammoniuria, calciuria, enzymuria.* **2.** '(Condition of) possessing urine': *paruria, polyuria, pyuria.*

uric acid A product of the metabolism of protein present in the blood and excreted in the urine. See also **gout, kidney, liver, purine, urine.**

uricaciduria A greater than normal amount of uric acid in the urine, often associated with urinary calculi or gout.

urico- A combining form meaning 'pertaining to uric acid': *uricocholia, uricosuria, uricotelic.*

urinalysis A physical, microscopic, or chemical examination of urine. The specimen is physically examined for color, turbidity, specific gravity, and pH. Then it is spun in a centrifuge to allow collection of a small amount of sediment that is examined microscopically for blood cells, casts, crystals, pus, and bacteria. Chemical analysis may be performed for the identification and quantification of any of a large

number of substances but most commonly for ketones, sugar, protein, and blood.

urinary Of or pertaining to urine or urine formation.

urinary bladder The muscular membranous sac in the pelvis that stores urine for discharge through the urethra.

urinary calculus A calculus formed in any part of the urinary tract. Calculi may be large enough to cause an obstruction in the flow of urine or small enough to be passed with the urine. See also **calculus.**

urinary elimination, alteration in patterns A nursing diagnosis accepted by the Fifth National Conference on the Classification of Nursing Diagnoses. The etiology of the diagnosis may involve several factors, including anatomical or physical obstruction, impairment of sensory innervation or muscular function of the bladder, or urinary tract infection. Among the characteristics that define the condition are dysuria, urinary frequency, hesitancy, incontinence, nocturia, and urgency of urination. See also **nursing diagnosis.**

urinary frequency A greater than normal frequency of the urge to void without an increase in the total daily volume of urine. The condition is characteristic of inflammation in the bladder or urethra or of diminished bladder capacity or other structural abnormalities. Burning and ur-

URINARY TRACT

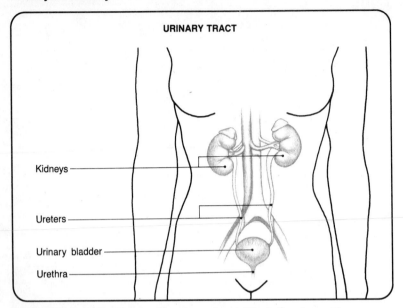

Kidneys

Ureters

Urinary bladder

Urethra

gency with increased frequency herald an infection of the urinary tract. Infection requires precise diagnosis and specific antibacterial medication; structural abnormality may require surgical correction. See also **cystitis, cystocele.**

urinary hesitancy   A decrease in the force of the stream of urine, often with difficulty in beginning the flow. Hesitancy is usually the result of an obstruction or stricture between the bladder and the urethral opening: in men it may indicate an enlargement of the prostate gland; in women, stenosis of the urethral opening. Cold, stress, dehydration, and various neurogenic and psychogenic factors are common causes of this condition.

urinary incontinence   Involuntary passage of urine, with the failure of voluntary control over bladder and urethral sphincters. Among the causes are neurogenic bladder dysfunction resulting from lesions of the brain and spinal cord, a neoplasm of calculus in the bladder, multiple sclerosis, obstruction of the lower urinary tract, trauma, aging, and multiparity in women. In children, incontinence may be psychogenic or the result of allergy. Treatment with medication, surgery, or psychotherapy appropriate to the underlying cause is often effective.

urinary infection   See **urinary tract infection.**

urinary output   The total volume of urine excreted daily, normally between 700 and 2,000 ml (24 and 68 oz). See also **anuria, oliguria, polyuria.**

urinary system assessment   An evaluation of the condition and functioning of the kidneys, bladder, ureters, and urethra and an investigation of concurrent and previous disorders that may be factors in the occurrence of

abnormalities in the urinary system.

urinary tract   All organs and ducts involved in the secretion and elimination of urine from the body.

urinary tract infection (UTI)   An infection of one or more structures in the urinary tract. Most of these infections are caused by gram-negative bacteria, most commonly *Escherichia coli* or species of *Klebsiella, Proteus, Pseudomonas,* or *Enterobacter.* The condition is more common in women than in men and may be asymptomatic. Urinary tract infection is usually characterized by urinary frequency, burning, pain with voiding, and, if the infection is severe, visible blood and pus in the urine. Diagnosis of the cause and the location of the infection is made by microscopic examination of the sediment and supernatant portion of a centrifuged urine specimen, by physical examination of the patient, by bacteriologic culture of a specimen of urine, and, if necessary, by various radiologic techniques, as retrograde pyelography, or by cystoscopy. Treatment includes antibacterial, analgesic, and urinary antiseptic medications. Kinds of urinary tract infections include **cystitis, pyelonephritis, urethritis.**

urination   The act of voiding urine. See also **micturition.**

urine   The fluid secreted by the kidneys, transported by the ureters, stored in the bladder, and voided through the urethra. Normal urine is clear, straw-colored, slightly acid, and has the characteristic odor of urea. The specific gravity of urine is between 1.005 and 1.030. Its constituents include water, urea, sodium chloride and potassium chloride, phosphates, uric acid, organic salts, and the pigment urobilin. Abnormal constituents indicative of disease include ketone bodies, protein, bacteria, blood, glucose, pus, and certain crystals. See also **bacteriuria, glycosuria, hematuria, ketonuria, proteinuria.**

urinoma, *pl.* **urinoma, urinomatas** A urine-filled cyst.

urinometer Any device for determining the specific gravity of urine, including gravitometers and hydrometers.

uro-, ur-, urono- A combining form meaning 'pertaining to urine, the urinary tract, or urination': *urocrisia, uromancy, uropterin.*

urobilin A brown pigment formed by the oxidation of urobilinogen, normally found in feces and, in small amounts, in urine.

urobilinogen A colorless compound formed in the intestine after the breakdown of bilirubin by bacteria. Some of this substance is excreted in feces, and some is resorbed and excreted again in bile or urine. See also **urobilin.**

urogenital Of or pertaining to the urinary and the reproductive systems. Also called **genitourinary.**

urogenital sinus One of the elongated cavities, formed by the division of the cloaca in early embryonic development, into which open the ureter, mesonephric and paramesonephric ducts, and bladder. It also gives rise to the vestibule, urethra, and part of the vagina in the female and part of the urethra in the male.

urogenital system The urinary and genital organs and the associated structures that develop in the fetus to form the kidneys, the ureters, the bladder, the urethra, and the genital structures of the male and female: in women it consists of the ovaries, the uterine tubes, the uterus, the clitoris, and the vagina; in men, the testes, the seminal vesicles, the seminal ducts, the prostate, and the penis. Also called **genitourinary system.**

urogram An X-ray film of the urinary tract, obtained by urography. See also **pyelogram.**

urography Any of a group of X-ray techniques used to examine the urinary system. A radiopaque substance is injected, and X-rays are taken as the substance is passed through or excreted from the part of the system being studied. Some kinds of urography are **cystoscopic urography, intravenous pyelography, retrograde pyelography.**

urokinase An enzyme, produced in the kidney and found in urine, that is a potent activator of the fibrinolytic system. A pharmaceutical preparation of urokinase is administered intravenously in treating pulmonary embolism.

urolith A renal calculus. See also **calculus, renal calculus, urinary calculus.**

urolithiasis See **urinary calculus.**

urologist A licensed physician who has completed an approved residency program and who specializes in the practice of urology.

urology The branch of medicine concerned with the study of the anatomy and physiology, the disorders, and the care of the male and female urinary tracts and the male genital tract.

uromelus See **sympus monopus.**

urono- See **uro-.**

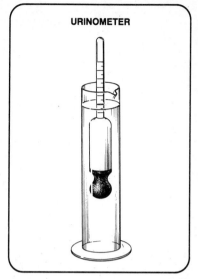

URINOMETER

uropathy Any disease or abnormal condition of any structure located in the urinary tract. **—uropathic,** *adj.*

uroporphyria A rare, genetic disease characterized by excessive secretion of uroporphyrin in the urine, blistering dermatitis, photosensitivity, splenomegaly, and hemolytic anemia. Most patients die from hematologic complications before middle age. See also **porphyria.**

uroporphyrin A porphyrin normally excreted in the urine in small amounts. See also **uroporphyria.**

urorectal septum A ridge of mesoderm covered with endoderm that in the early developing embryo divides the endodermal cloaca into the urogenital sinus and the rectum. Also called **cloacal septum.**

urticaria A pruritic skin eruption characterized by transient wheals with well-defined erythematous margins and pale centers, caused by local release of histamine or other vasoactive substances. Acute urticaria is usually of allergic origin; in chronic cases, causative agents are rarely discovered. Some of the most common causes of urticaria are drugs, foods, insect bites, inhalants, and exposure to the cold or sun. Also called **hives. —urticarial,** *adj.*

urticaria pigmentosa An uncommon form of mastocytosis characterized by pigmented skin lesions that become urticarial upon mechanical or chemical irritation. Although duration of the condition is unpredictable, prognosis is good. Symptomatic treatment usually includes antihistamines. See also **mastocytosis.**

urushiol A toxic resin occurring in the sap of certain plants of the genus *Rhus,* as poison ivy, poison oak, and poison sumac. Urushiol produces allergic contact dermatitis in many people.

USAN Acronym for *United States Adopted*

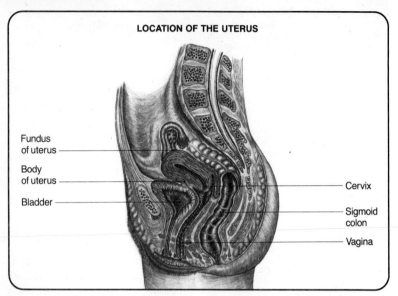

LOCATION OF THE UTERUS

Fundus of uterus

Body of uterus

Bladder

Cervix

Sigmoid colon

Vagina

*N*ames, a list of approved drugs compiled and published by U.S. Pharmacopeial Convention, Inc. (USPC).

use effectiveness Of a contraceptive method: the actual effectiveness of a medication, device, or method in preventing pregnancy. Inconsistent use and human error usually reduce the theoretical effectiveness of any particular method of contraception. Compare **theoretical effectiveness.**

use test A procedure used to identify offending allergens in foods, cosmetics, or fabrics by the systematic elimination and addition of specific items associated with the life-style of the patient involved. Allergic reactions to the use test may be immediate or may be spread over a considerable period of time. See also **allergy testing.**

USP See *United States Pharmacopeia.*

USPHS *abbr* **United States Public Health Service.**

uta A mild cutaneous form of American leishmaniasis, occurring in the Andes of Peru and Argentina, caused by *Leishmania peruana.* See also **American leishmaniasis, leishmaniasis.**

uterine anteflexion An abnormal position of the uterus in which the uterine body is bent forward on itself at the juncture of the isthmus of the uterine cervix and the lower uterine segment.

uterine anteversion A position of the uterus in which the body of the uterus is directed ventrally. Mild degrees of anteversion are of no clinical significance. Slight anteversion is the most common position of the uterus.

uterine cancer Any malignancy of the uterus. It may be cervical cancer affecting the cervix or endometrial cancer affecting the lining of the

body of the uterus. See also **cervical cancer, endometrial cancer.**

uterine retroflexion A position of the uterus in which the body of the uterus is bent backward on itself at the isthmus of the cervix and the lower uterine segment. It has no clinical significance; it does not prevent conception or adversely affect pregnancy.

uterine retroversion A position of the uterus in which the body of the uterus is directed away from the midline, toward the back. Mild degrees of retroversion are common and have no clinical significance. Severe retroversion may be accompanied by vague persistent pelvic discomfort and dyspareunia and may prevent the fitting and use of a contraceptive diaphragm.

uterine tube See **fallopian tube.**

uteritis See **metritis.**

uteroglobulin See **blastokinin.**

utero-ovarian varicocele A swelling of the veins of the pampiniform plexus of the female pelvis. Compare **varicocele, ovarian varicocele.**

uteroplacental apoplexy See **Couvelaire uterus.**

uterovesical See **vesicouterine.**

uterus The hollow, pear-shaped internal female organ of reproduction in which the fertilized ovum is implanted and the fetus develops, and from which the decidua of menses flows. Its anterior surface lies on the superior surface of the bladder separated by a fold of peritoneum, the vesicouterine pouch. Its posterior surface, also covered with peritoneum, is adjacent to the sigmoid colon and some of the coils of the small intestine. The uterus is comprised of three layers: the endometrium, the myometrium, and the parametrium. The endometrium lines the uterus and becomes thicker and more vascular in preg-

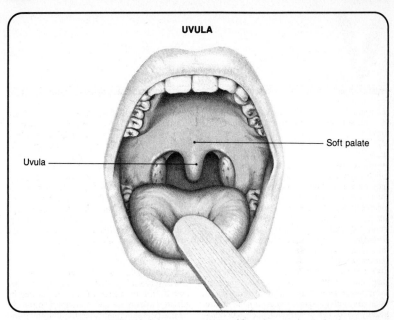

UVULA

Soft palate

Uvula

---

nancy and during the second half of the menstrual cycle under the influence of the hormone progesterone. The myometrium is the muscular layer of the organ. Its muscle fibers wrap around the uterus obliquely, laterally, and longitudinally. After childbirth the meshlike network of fibers contracts, creating a mass of natural ligatures that stop the flow of blood from the large blood vessels supplying the placenta. The parametrium, the outermost layer, is composed of serous connective tissue and extends laterally into the broad ligament. In the adult, the organ measures about 7.5 cm (3 inches) long, 5 cm (2 inches) wide at its fundus, and weighs approximately 40 g (1½ oz). Its growth during pregnancy occurs almost entirely by cellular hypertrophy; few new cells develop. The uterus has two parts: a body and a cervix. The body extends from the fundus to the cervix, just above the isthmus. The cavity within the body is only a potential space, as the walls touch unless the woman is pregnant. The cervix has a vaginal portion, protruding into the vagina, and a supravaginal portion at the juncture of the lower uterine segment. The principal ligaments of the uterus are the broad ligaments, which extend laterally from the sides of the isthmus of the cervix between the folds of the broad ligaments; the cardinal ligaments, crossing the pelvic diaphragm from the top of the cervix to the large muscles of the pelvic outlet; and the uterosacral ligaments, curving back from the cervix to the sacrum around the cul-de-sac of Douglas. The body of the uterus is thus free in the abdominal cavity, fixed only at its base by the series of ligaments from the cervix.

uterus masculinis   See **prostatic utricle.**

UTI   *abbr* **urinary tract infection.**

utilization review   An assessment of the appropriateness and economy of an admission to a health-care facility or a continued hospitalization. The length of the hospital stay is also compared with the average length of stay for similar diagnoses.

utricle   The larger of two membranous pouches in the vestibule of the membranous labyrinth of the ear. It is an oblong structure that communicates with the semicircular ducts by five openings and receives utricular filaments of the acoustic nerve. Compare **saccule.**

utriculosaccular duct   A duct connecting the utricle with an endolymphatic duct of the membranous labyrinth.

uvea   The fibrous tunic beneath the sclera that includes the iris, the ciliary body, and the choroid of the eye. Also called **tunica vasculosa bulbi, uveal tract. —uveal,** *adj.*

uveal tract   See **uvea.**

uveitis   Inflammation of the uveal tract of the eye, including the iris, ciliary body, and choroid. It may be characterized by an irregularly shaped pupil, inflammation around the cornea, pus in the anterior chamber, opaque deposits on the cornea, pain, and lacrimation. Causes include allergy, infection, trauma, diabetes, collagen disease, and skin diseases. A major complication may be glaucoma. See also **chorioretinitis, choroiditis, iritis.**

uvula, *pl.* **uvulae**   The small, cone-shaped process suspended in the mouth above the root of the tongue from the middle of the posterior border of the soft palate. **—uvular,** *adj.*

uvulitis   Inflammation of the uvula. Common causes are allergy and infection.

V

v Symbol for: **1.** venous blood. **2.** vein. **3.** volt.

V Symbol for: **1.** vanadium. **2.** rate of gas flow.

V$_T$ In pulmonary ventilation: *abbr* **tidal volume.**

vaccination Any injection of attenuated or killed microorganisms, as bacteria, to induce immunity or to reduce the effects of associated infectious diseases. Historically, the first vaccinations were administered to immunize against smallpox. Vaccinations are now available to immunize against many diseases.

vaccine A suspension of attenuated or killed microorganisms administered intradermally, intramuscularly, orally, or subcutaneously to induce active immunity to infectious disease. Viruses and rickettsiae used in certain vaccines are grown in avian embryos, rabbit brain tissue, or monkey kidney tissue, and the organisms are usually inactivated by formalin, phenol, or beta-propiolactone. Vaccines may be used as single agents or in combinations.

-vaccine A combining form meaning a 'preparation containing microorganisms for producing immunity to disease': *autovaccine.*

vaccinia An infectious disease of cattle caused by a poxvirus which may be transmitted to humans by direct contact or by deliberate inoculation as a protection against smallpox. A pustule develops at the site of infection, usually followed by malaise and fever which last for several days. After 2 weeks the pustule becomes a crust which eventually drops off, leaving a scar. Individuals with eczema or other preexisting skin disease may develop generalized vaccinia. Rarely, a severe encephalitis may follow vaccinia. Also called **cowpox.** Compare **smallpox.** See also **vaccination.**

vacuole **1.** A clear space or cavity within a cell. **2.** A small space in the body enclosed by a membrane, usually containing fat, secretions, or cellular debris. **—vacuolar, vacuolated,** *adj.*

vacuum aspiration A method of abortion in which the fetus and placenta are removed by suction to terminate an early pregnancy, up to the 14th week. The cervix is dilated and the uterus emptied with suction. Postoperative care includes observation of vital signs for symptoms of blood loss. Also called **suction curettage.** Compare **dilatation and curettage.** See also **therapeutic abortion.**

vagal Of or pertaining to the vagus nerve.

vagina The part of the female genitalia that forms a canal from the orifice through the vestibule to the uterine cervix. It is behind the bladder and in front of the rectum. In the adult woman the anterior wall of the vagina is about 7 cm (2¾ inches) long and the posterior wall is about 9 cm (3½ inches) long. The canal is actually a potential space. The vagina widens from the vestibule upward and narrows toward the top, forming a curved vault around the protruding cervix. The vagina is lined with mucosa covering a layer of erectile tissue and muscle. The mucous membrane of the vagina forms two longitudinal columns from which transverse rugae extend around the canal. The lower end is surrounded by the erectile tissue of the bulb of the vestibule and the bulbocavernosus muscle. The muscular layer is highly vascular.

vagina bulbi See **fascia bulbi.**

vaginal bleeding An abnormal condition in which blood is passed from the vagina, other than during the menses. It may be caused by abnormalities of the uterus or cervix; by an abnormal pregnancy; by endocrine abnormalities; by abnormalities of one or both ovaries or one or both fallopian tubes; or by an abnormality of the vagina. The following terms are commonly used in describing the approximate amount of vaginal bleeding: heavy vaginal bleeding is that which is greater than heaviest normal menstrual flow; moderate vaginal bleeding is that which is equal to heaviest normal menstrual flow; light vaginal bleeding is that which is less than heaviest normal menstrual flow; vaginal staining is a very light flow of blood barely requiring the use of a sanitary napkin or tampon; vaginal spotting is the passage vaginally of a few drops of blood; bloody show is an episode of light vaginal bleeding as often occurs in early labor, during labor, and, particularly, at the time of full dilatation of the cervix at the end of the first stage of labor.

vaginal cancer A malignancy of the vagina occurring rarely as a primary neoplasm and more often as a secondary lesion or extension of vulvar, cervical, endometrial, or ovarian cancer. Clear cell adenocarcinoma occurs in young women exposed in utero to diethylstilbestrol given the mother to prevent abortion, but most primary vaginal cancers arise in white women over 50 years of age. A predisposing factor is cervical carcinoma. Vaginal leukoplakia, erythematosis, erosion, or granulation of the mucosa may prove to be carcinoma in situ. Symptoms of invasive lesions are postmenopausal bleeding, purulent discharge, pain, and dysuria. Diagnostic measures include cervical, endocervical, and vaginal Papanicolaou tests; colposcopy; biopsy; and Schiller's iodine test, in which malignant cells do not stain dark brown. Treatment may be by irradiation or vaginectomy and radical hysterectomy with lymph node dissection. Cryosurgery, topical 5-fluorouracil, and dinitrochlorobenzene (DNCB) may be used, but chemotherapy is not usually effective.

vaginal discharge Any discharge from the vagina. A clear or pearly-white discharge occurs normally. Throughout the reproductive years the amount and character vary in each woman at different times in her menstrual cycle. The discharge is largely composed of secretions of the endocervical glands. Inflammatory conditions of the vagina and cervix often cause an increase in the discharge, which may then have a foul odor and cause pruritus of the perineum and external genitalia.

vaginal instillation of medication The instillation of a medicated cream, a suppository, or a gel into the vagina, usually performed to treat a local infection of the vagina or the uterine cervix.

vaginal jelly A contraceptive containing a spermicide in a jelly medium, usually used with a contraceptive diaphragm or a cervical cap. Some antimicrobial medications are also supplied in the form of a vaginal jelly.

vaginal spotting See **vaginal bleeding.**

vaginal staining See **vaginal bleeding.**

vaginismus A psychophysiologic genital reaction of women, characterized by intense contraction of the perineal and paravaginal musculature, tightly closing the vaginal introitus. It occurs in response to fear of painful intromission prior to coitus or pelvic examination. Vaginismus is considered abnormal if it occurs in the absence of genital lesions and if it conflicts with a woman's desire to participate in coition or to permit examination, but it may be a normal or physiologic response if painful genital conditions exist or if forcible or premature intromission is anticipated. Vaginismus is uncommon. In some cases, the condition is a manifestation of serious mental illness and requires formal psychiatric evaluation and treatment. Gender identity conflict, a history of trauma from rape or incest, or an intense suppression of sexuality in childhood and adolescence are factors often linked with vaginismus.

vagino- A combining form meaning 'pertaining to the vagina': *vaginodynia, vaginolabial.*

vagotomy The cutting of certain branches of the vagus nerve, performed with gastric surgery, to reduce the amount of gastric acid secreted and lessen the chance of recurrence of a gastric ulcer. Since peristalsis will be diminished, a pyloroplasty or an anastomosis of the stomach to the jejunum is done to assure proper emptying of the stomach. See also **anastomosis, gastrectomy, gastric ulcer, pyloroplasty, vagus nerve.**

vagotonus An abnormal increase in the activity and the effects of the stimulation of the vagus nerve, especially bradycardia with decreased cardiac output, faintness, and syncope. Vagotonus may occur in suctioning the oropharynx of a newborn as the syringe, laryngo-

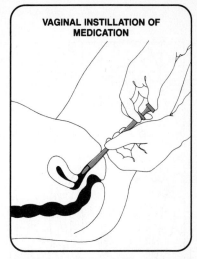

VAGINAL INSTILLATION OF MEDICATION

scope blade, or catheter is inadvertently pressed on the back of the throat, stimulating the nerve. It also occurs in some women following surgical treatment or simple manipulation of the uterine cervix.

vagovagal reflex A stimulation of the vagus nerve by reflex in which irritation of the larynx or the trachea results in slowing of the pulse rate.

vagus nerve Either of the longest pair of cranial nerves essential for speech, swallowing, and the sensibilities and functions of many parts of the body. Also called **nervus vagus, pneumogastric nerve, tenth nerve.**

valence 1. In chemistry: a numerical expression of the capability of an element to combine chemically with atoms of hydrogen or their equivalent. A negative valence indicates the number of hydrogen atoms to which one atom of a chemical element can bond. A positive valence indicates the number of hydrogen atoms that one atom of a chemical element can displace. An element is considered univalent (or monovalent) if each of its atoms can react with only one hydrogen atom or its equivalent; bivalent (or divalent) if each atom can react with two hydrogen or equivalent atoms; tervalent (or trivalent) if each atom can react with three hydrogen atoms; multivalent (or polyvalent) if each atom can react with many hydrogen atoms. 2. In immunology: an expression of the number of antigen-binding sites for one molecule of any given antibody or the number of antibody-binding sites for any given antigen. Most antibody molecules and those belonging to the IgA, IgE, and IgG immunoglobulin classes have two antigen-binding sites.

-valence A combining term meaning the 'combining capacity of an atom compared with that of one hydrogen atom': *quantivalence, trivalence.* Also **-valency.**

-valency See **-valence.**

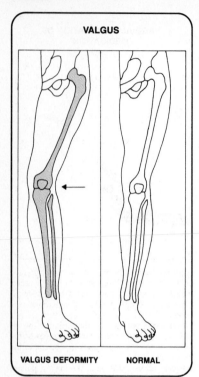

VALGUS

VALGUS DEFORMITY   NORMAL

-valent A combining form meaning 'having a valency of a (specified) magnitude': *octavalent, pentavalent.*

valeric acid An organic acid with a penetrating odor found in the roots of *Valeriana officinalis.* Commercially prepared, it is used in the production of perfumes, flavors, lubricants, and certain drugs.

valgus An abnormal position in which a part of a limb is bent or twisted outward away from the midline, as the heel of the foot in **talipes valgus.** Compare **varus.** See also **hallux valgus.**

validity In research: the extent to which a test or other device measures what it is intended to measure. Kinds of validity include **content validity, current validity, construct validity, face validity, predictive validity.**

valine An essential amino acid produced in the body by the digestion of proteins. It is needed for optimal growth in infants and for nitrogen equilibrium in adults.

vallecula In anatomy: any groove or furrow on the surface of an organ or structure. —**vallecular,** *adj.*

vallecula epiglottica A furrow between the glossoepiglottic folds of each side of the posterior oropharynx.

vallecular dysphagia Difficulty or pain in swallowing as a result of an inflammation of the vallecula epiglottica. Compare **contractile**

ring dysphagia, dysphagia lusoria.

valley fever See **coccidioidomycosis.**

valproic acid, v. sodium Anticonvulsants.

Valsalva maneuver Any forced expiratory effort against a closed airway, as when an individual holds his breath and tightens his muscles in a concerted, strenuous effort to move a heavy object or to change position in bed. Most healthy individuals perform Valsalva maneuvers during normal daily activities without any injurious consequences, but such efforts are dangerous for many patients with cardiovascular diseases, especially if they become dehydrated, increasing the viscosity of their blood and the attendant risk of blood clotting. Constipation increases the risk of cardiovascular trauma in such patients, especially if they perform the Valsalva maneuver in trying to move their bowels. Patients who may be endangered by performing the Valsalva maneuver are commonly instructed to exhale instead of holding their breath when they move. The exhalation decreases the risk of cardiovascular trauma.

Valsalva's test A method for testing the patency of the eustachian tubes. With mouth and nose kept tightly closed, a forced expiratory effort is made; if the eustachian tubes are open, air will enter into the middle ear cavities and the subject will hear a popping sound. See also **Valsalva maneuver.**

values clarification The process of selecting, prizing, and ultimately behaving with regard to a set of beliefs. Values clarification encourages personal growth and facilitates ethical decision-making.

value system The accepted mode of conduct and the set of norms, goals, and values binding any social group.

valve A natural structure or artificial device in a passage or vessel that prevents reflux of the fluid contents passing through it. Valves in veins are membranous folds that prevent backflow of blood. —**valvular,** *adj.*

-valve A combining form meaning 'a thing that regulates the flow of': *bivalve, trivalve.*

valve of Kerkring See **circular fold.**

valve of lymphatics One of the tiny semilunar structures in the vessels and trunks of the lymphatic system that help to regulate the flow of lymph and prevent venous blood from entering the system. There are no valves in the capillaries of the system but there are many in the collecting vessels. The valves are attached by their convex edges to the walls of the vessels, leaving their concave edges free and directed along the course of the lymph's current. Usually, two valves of equal size are found opposite each other. They are more numerous near the lymph nodes. The wall of the vessel just above the attachment of each valve bulges with a small sinus that gives the vessel its beaded appearance. See also **lymphatic system.**

valvotomy The incision into a valve, especially one in the heart, to correct a defect and allow proper opening and closure. Before surgery a cardiac catheterization is performed. The damaged valve is repaired, if possible, or it is removed and a prosthetic valve suture put in its place. Complications peculiar to prosthetic valve surgery are displacement of the valve owing to broken sutures, heart block, leakage and regurgitation from chamber to chamber, infection, and embolus.

valvular heart disease An acquired or congenital disorder of a cardiac valve, characterized by stenosis and obstructed blood flow or by valvular degeneration and regurgitation of blood. Diseases of aortic and mitral valves are most common and may be caused by congenital defects, bacterial endocarditis, syphilis, or, most frequently, by rheumatic fever. Episodes of rheumatic fever often affect cardiac valves, causing them to degenerate and remain open or causing the cusps of the valves to become stiff, calcified, and constricted. Valvular dysfunction results in changes in intracardiac pressure and in pulmonary and peripheral circulation that may lead to cardiac arrhythmia, heart failure, and cardiogenic shock. Malaise, anorexia, embolism, pulmonary edema, and ventricular failure often accompany valvular heart disease. In moderate or severe **aortic stenosis**, pulse pressure is decreased; the carotid pulse is small and slow with a long upstroke, but the apical pulse may be strong and sustained during systole. The patient may experience anginal pain and syncope, and the electrocardiogram may show evidence of left ventricular hypertrophy, conduction defects, or complete heart block. Characteristic signs of aortic regurgitation are dyspnea, profuse sweating, flushed skin, bounding pulsations in neck arteries, and a blowing heart murmur throughout diastole. The electrocardiogram may be normal or reveal left ventricular hypertrophy. The patient with **mitral stenosis** tires easily, is short of breath on exertion, may have paroxysmal nocturnal dyspnea, and may develop hemoptysis and systemic embolism. The first heart sound usually is increased and the second is followed by a decrescendo opening snap. Mitral regurgitation is typified by dyspnea, fatigue, intolerance of exercise, heart palpitation, and a large, laterally placed apical pulse. There may be an apical systolic murmur; a diminished first heart sound; a third heart sound; atrial arrhythmia; or elevated wedge pressure in the left atrium, pulmonary artery, or pulmonary vein. **Tricuspid stenosis** is relatively uncommon, is usually associated with lesions in other valves resulting from rheumatic fever, and, in rare cases, is caused by carcinoid heart disease or endomyocardial fibrosis. Characteristics of tricuspid stenosis are a diastolic pressure gradient between the right atrium and ventricle, jugular vein distention, pulmonary congestion, and, in severe cases, hepatic congestion and splenomegaly. Tricuspid regurgitation, usually secondary to marked dilatation of the right ventricle and the ring of the valve, commonly occurs in late stages of cardiac failure in rheumatic or congenital heart disease with severe pulmonary hypertension. Typical

VALVULAR HEART DISEASE: CAUSES AND INCIDENCE

Mitral stenosis
- Results from rheumatic fever (most common cause)
- Most common in females
- May be associated with other congenital anomalies, such as tetralogy of Fallot

Mitral insufficiency
- Results from rheumatic fever, idiopathic hypertrophic subaortic stenosis (IHSS), mitral valve prolapse, myocardial infarction, severe left ventricular failure, ruptured chordae tendineae
- Associated with other congenital anomalies, such as transposition of the great vessels
- Rare in children without other congenital anomalies

Tricuspid insufficiency
- Results from right ventricular failure, rheumatic fever, and, rarely, trauma and endocarditis
- Associated with congenital disorders

Tricuspid stenosis
- Results from rheumatic fever
- May be congenital
- Associated with mitral or aortic valve disease
- Most common in women

Pulmonic stenosis
- Results from congenital stenosis of valve cusp or rheumatic heart disease (infrequent)
- Associated with other congenital heart defects, such as tetralogy of Fallot

Pulmonic insufficiency
- May be congenital or may result from pulmonary hypertension

Aortic insufficiency
- Results from rheumatic fever, syphilis, hypertension, endocarditis, or may be idiopathic
- Associated with Marfan's syndrome
- Most common in males

Aortic stenosis
- Results from congenital aortic bicuspid valve (associated with coarctation of the aorta), congenital stenosis of valve cusps, rheumatic fever, or atherosclerosis in the aged
- Most common in males

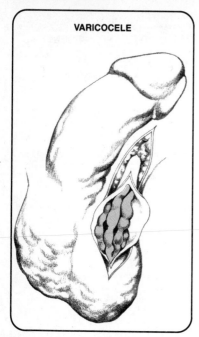

VARICOCELE

signs include engorged neck veins, hepatomegaly, systolic pulsations of the liver, edema, and ascites. The pulmonic valve is affected by rheumatic fever much less frequently than other cardiac valves. **Pulmonic stenosis** may cause the intraventricular septum to bulge into the right ventricular chamber and regurgitation is a consequence of severe pulmonary hypertension, but destruction of the valve does not cause heart failure unless pulmonary hypertension is a serious problem. Cardiotonics, diuretics, analgesics, sodium restriction, and antibiotics, if indicated, are used in the conservative treatment of valvular heart disease, but surgery is usually performed when the symptoms are incapacitating.

valvular stenosis A narrowing or constricture of any of the valves of the heart. The condition may result from a congenital defect, or it may be caused by some disease process. See also **aortic stenosis, congenital cardiac anomaly, mitral stenosis, pulmonic stenosis.**

valvulitis Inflammation of a valve, especially a cardiac valve. Inflammatory changes in the valves of the heart are caused most commonly by rheumatic fever and by bacterial endocarditis and syphilis. Infected valves degenerate or their cusps become stiff and calcified, resulting in stenosis and obstructed blood flow.

vanadium (V) A gray metallic element. Its atomic number is 23; its atomic weight is 50.942. Absorption of vanadium compounds results in a condition called vanadiumism, characterized by anemia, conjunctivitis, pneumonitis, and ir-

ritation of the respiratory tract.

van Bogaert's disease A rare familial disorder of lipid metabolism in which cholestanol is deposited in the nervous system, blood, and connective tissue. Persons with the disease develop progressive ataxia and dementia, premature atherosclerosis, cataracts, and xanthomas of the tendons. No effective treatment is known.

vancomycin hydrochloride An antibiotic.

van den Bergh test A test for the presence of bilirubin in the blood serum. Normal total bilirubin ranges from 0.2 to 1.4 mg per 100 ml of serum, of which about 15% should be what is called direct, or conjugated, bilirubin.

vanillylmandelic acid (VMA) A urinary metabolite of epinephrine and norepinephrine. A greater than normal amount of VMA is characteristic of a pheochromocytoma of the adrenal medulla.

vapor bath The exposure of the body to vapor, as steam.

variable behavior A response, activity, or action that may be modified by individual experience. Compare **invariable behavior.**

variable deceleration An abrupt decrease in the fetal heart rate, unrelated to uterine contraction, that occurs in 50% of all labors. Although usually associated with transitory umbilical cord compression, a severe drop in the fetal heart rate may indicate fetal acidosis or hypoxia.

variance **1.** In statistics: a numerical representation of the dispersion of data around the mean in a given sample. It is represented by the square of the standard deviation and is used principally in performing an analysis of variance. **2.** *Nontechnical.* The general range of a group of findings.

varicella See **chickenpox.**

varicella-zoster virus (VZV) A member of the herpesvirus family, which causes the diseases varicella (chickenpox) and herpes zoster (shingles). The virus has been isolated from vesicle fluid in chickenpox, is highly contagious, and may be spread by direct contact or droplets. Dried crusts of skin lesions do not contain active virus particles. Herpes zoster is produced by reactivation of latent varicella virus, usually several years after the initial infection. There is no simple test for measuring antibodies to this virus; however, zoster immune globulin (ZIG) obtained from convalescing zoster patients, if injected within 3 days of exposure, will prevent varicella in susceptible children. The temporary nature of this protection and the relative scarcity of ZIG warrant reservation of its use to children receiving immunosuppressive therapy or suffering from immune deficiency diseases. Also called herpesvirus varicella-zoster and herpesvirus varicella. See also **chickenpox, herpes zoster.**

varicelliform Resembling chickenpox rash.

varicocele A dilatation of the pampiniform venous complex of the spermatic cord. The varicocele forms a soft, elastic swelling that can cause pain. It is most common in men between the ages of 15 and 25 and affects the left spermatic cord more often than the right. It is usually more pronounced and painful in the standing position. Compare **ovarian varicocele, utero-ovarian varicocele.**

varicose **1.** Of a vein: exhibiting varicosis, or a varicosity. **2.** Abnormally and permanently distended, as the bulging veins in some individuals.

varicose ulcer See **stasis ulcer.**

varicose vein A tortuous, dilated vein with incompetent valves. Causes include congenitally defective valves, thrombophlebitis, pregnancy, and obesity. They are common, especially in women. The saphenous veins of the legs are most often affected. The use of elastic stockings is frequently sufficient therapy for uncomplicated cases. Surgery (ligation and stripping) may be required in severe cases. Injection of sclerosing solutions helps to prevent or to treat postphlebitic syndrome.

varicosis A common condition characterized by one or more tortuous, abnormally dilated, or varicose veins, usually in the legs or the lower trunk, occurring between the ages of 30 and 60. Varicosis may be caused by congenital defects of the valves or walls of the veins or by congestion and increased intraluminal pressure resulting from prolonged standing, poor posture, pregnancy, abdominal tumor, or chronic systemic disease. Symptoms include pain and muscle cramps with a feeling of fullness and heaviness in the legs. Ligation of the vein above the varicosity and removal of the distal portion of the vessel may be indicated for severe cases if deeper vessels can maintain the return of venous blood.

varicosity An abnormal condition, usually of a vein, characterized by swelling and tortuosity.

variegate Having characteristics that vary, especially as to color.

variegate porphyria An uncommon form of hepatic porphyria, characterized by skin lesions and photosensitivity. The condition may be congenital or acquired. The congenital form is more serious, resulting in crises of acute abdominal pain and in certain neurologic complications. See also **porphyria.**

variola See **smallpox.**

variola major See **smallpox.**

variola minor See **alastrim.**

varioloid **1.** Resembling smallpox. **2.** A mild form of smallpox in a vaccinated person or one who has previously had the disease.

varix, *pl.* **varices** **1.** A tortuous, dilated vein. **2.** An enlarged, tortuous artery or a distended, twisting lymphatic.

varus An abnormal position in which a part of a limb is turned inward toward the midline, as the heel and foot in **talipes varus.** Compare **valgus.**

vas, *pl.* **vasa** Any one of the many vessels of the body, especially those that convey blood or lymph.

vascular Of or pertaining to a blood vessel.

vascular hemophilia See **Von Willebrand's disease.**

vascular insufficiency Inadequate peripheral blood flow caused by occlusion of vessels with atherosclerotic plaques, thrombi, or emboli; by damaged, diseased, or intrinsically weak vascular walls; by arteriovenous fistulas; by hematologic hypercoagulability; or by heavy smoking. Signs include pale, cyanotic, or mottled skin over the affected area; swelling of an extremity; absent or reduced tactile sensation; tingling; diminished sense of temperature; muscle pain, as intermittent claudication in the calf; and, in advanced disease, atrophy of muscles of the involved extremity. Diagnosis may be made by checking peripheral pulses in contralateral extremities, or by angiography, plethysmography, ultrasonography, or skin temperature tests. Treatment may include a diet low in saturated fats; moderate exercise; sleeping on a firm mattress; avoidance of smoking, prolonged standing, or prolonged sitting with the knees bent; use of a vasodilating drug; and surgical repair of an arteriovenous fistula or aneurysm. See also **arterial insufficiency.**

vascularization The process by which body tissue becomes vascular and develops proliferating capillaries, naturally or induced by surgery. —**vascularize,** *v.*

vascular leiomyoma A neoplasm composed of a coil of blood vessels surrounded by smooth-muscle fibers.

vascular spider See **spider angioma.**

vasculitis An inflammatory condition of the blood vessels that is characteristic of certain systemic diseases or that is caused by an allergic reaction. Kinds of vasculitis are **allergic vasculitis, necrotizing vasculitis, segmented hyalinizing vasculitis.**

vas deferens, *pl.* **vasa deferentia** The extension of the epididymis of the testis that ascends from the scrotum and joins the seminal vesicle to form the ejaculatory duct. It is enclosed by fibrous connective tissue with blood vessels, nerves, and lymphatics and passes through the inguinal canal as part of the spermatic cord. Extending from the scrotum into the abdominal cavity it passes over the top, then down the posterior surface of the bladder, becomes wider and convoluted, and joins the ampulla of the seminal vesicle. Compare **testis.**

vasectomy A procedure for male sterilization involving the bilateral surgical removal of a portion of the vas deferens. Vasectomy is most commonly performed as an office procedure under local anesthesia. The procedure is also performed routinely prior to removal of the prostate gland in order to prevent inflammation of the testes and epididymides. Potency is not affected.

vaso- A combining form meaning 'pertaining to a vessel or duct': *vasoconstrictor, vasodilatation.*

vasoactive Of a drug: tending to cause vasodilatation or vasoconstriction.

vasoconstriction A narrowing of the lu-

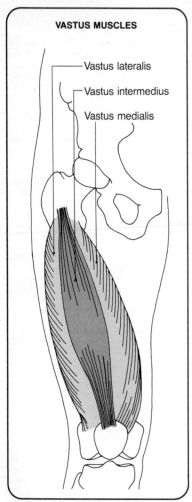

VASTUS MUSCLES

Vastus lateralis

Vastus intermedius

Vastus medialis

tors. Internally secreted epinephrine and nor-epinephrine cause blood vessels to contract by stimulating adrenergic receptors of peripheral sympathetic nerves. Other endogenous vasoconstrictors are angiotensin and antidiuretic hormone. Adrenergic sympathomimetic drugs cause some degree of vasoconstriction, and several are used for this action in maintaining blood pressure during anesthesia and in treating pronounced hypotension. Among these therapeutic agents are metaraminol bitartrate, methoxamine hydrochloride, and norepinephrine (levarterenol).

vasodilatation, vasodilation Widening or distention of blood vessels, particularly arterioles, usually owing to nerve impulses or to certain drugs that cause relaxation of smooth muscle in the walls of the blood vessels. Compare **vasoconstriction.**

vasodilator **1.** A nerve or agent that causes dilatation of blood vessels. **2.** Pertaining to the relaxation of the smooth muscle of the vascular system. **3.** Producing dilatation of blood vessels. Vasodilators are a recent, important addition to the treatment of heart failure. Included are hydralazine, isosorbide dinitrate, nitroglycerin, and nitroprusside.

vasomotor Of or pertaining to the nerves and muscles that control the caliber of the lumen of the blood vessels. Circularly arranged fibers of the muscles of arteries can contract, causing vasoconstriction, or they can relax, causing vasodilatation.

vasomotor rhinitis Chronic rhinitis and nasal obstruction, without allergy or infection, characterized by sneezing, rhinorrhea, nasal obstruction, and vascular engorgement of the mucous membranes of the nose. A vaporizer or humidifier and systemic vasoconstrictive agents are used to alleviate discomfort. Vasomotor rhinitis is common in pregnancy.

vasomotor system That part of the nervous system that controls the constriction and dilatation of the blood vessels. See also **vasoconstriction, vasodilatation.**

vasopressin, v. tannate Antidiuretic hormones.

vasovasostomy A surgical procedure in which the function of the vas deferens on each side of the testes is restored, having been cut and ligated in a preceding vasectomy. The procedure is performed if a man wants to regain his fertility. In most cases, the patency of the canals is achieved, but in many cases fertility does not result, probably owing to circulating autoantibodies that disrupt normal sperm activity. The antibodies apparently develop following vasectomy as the developing sperm cannot be excreted through the urogenital tract.

vastus intermedius One of the four muscles of the quadriceps femoris, situated in the center of the thigh. It arises from the front and lateral surfaces of the femur and from the lateral intermuscular septum. Its fibers end in a superficial aponeurosis which forms the deep part of the quadriceps femoris tendon inserted into

men of any blood vessel, especially the arterioles and the veins in the blood reservoirs of the skin and the abdominal viscera. Vasoconstriction depends on the stimulation of the vasomotor constriction center in the medulla. Impulses from this center travel along the sympathetic nerve fibers and contract the smooth muscle layers of the arteries, the arterioles, the venules, and the veins, causing the constriction of these vessels. Vasoconstriction is also induced by vasomotor pressure reflexes, chemical reflexes, the medullary ischemic reflex, and vasomotor impulses from the cerebral cortex and the hypothalamus. Compare **vasodilatation.**

vasoconstrictor **1.** Of or pertaining to a process, condition, or substance that causes the constriction of blood vessels. **2.** An agent that promotes vasoconstriction. Cold, fear, stress, and nicotine are common exogenous vasoconstric-

the patella. It functions with the other three muscles of the quadriceps to extend the leg. Also called **crureus.** Compare **rectus femoris, vastus lateralis, vastus medialis.**

vastus internus See **vastus medialis.**

vastus lateralis The largest of the four muscles of the quadriceps femoris, situated on the lateral side of the thigh. It is a large, dense mass originating in a broad aponeurosis that is attached to the intertrochanteric line of the femur, the greater trochanter, the lateral lip of the gluteal tuberosity, and the lateral lip of the linea aspera. The fibers of the muscle are gathered to form a strong aponeurosis that converges to become a flat tendon before inserting into the patella. It functions to help extend the leg. Compare **rectus femoris, vastus intermedius, vastus medialis.**

vastus medialis One of the four muscles of the quadriceps femoris, situated in the medial portion of the thigh. It originates from the intertrochanteric line of the femur, the linea aspera, the medial supracondylar line, the tendons of the adductor longus and the adductor magnus, and the medial intermuscular septum. It extends to the lower anterior aspect of the thigh and inserts by an aponeurosis into the patella and the quadriceps femoris tendon. An expansion of the aponeurosis passes to the capsule of the knee joint. It functions in combination with other parts of the quadriceps femoris to extend the leg. Also called **vastus internus.** Compare **rectus femoris, vastus intermedius, vastus lateralis.**

VC *abbr* **vital capacity.**

VD *abbr* **venereal disease.**

VDRL test *abbr* venereal disease research laboratory test, a serological flocculation test for syphilis. It is also positive in other treponemal diseases, as yaws.

Ve Symbol for expired volume.

VE Symbol for volume expired in one minute.

vector **1.** A quantity having direction and magnitude, usually depicted by a straight arrow whose length represents magnitude and whose head represents direction. **2.** A carrier, especially one which transmits disease. A **biological vector** is usually an arthropod in which the infecting organism completes part of its life cycle. A **mechanical vector** transmits the infecting organism from one host to another but is not essential to the life cycle of the parasite. Kinds of vectors include dogs, which carry rabies. —**vector,** *v.,* **vectorial,** *adj.*

VEE *abbr* **Venezuelan equine encephalitis.** See **equine encephalitis.**

vegan See **strict vegetarian.**

veganism The adherence to a strict vegetable diet, with the exclusion of all protein of animal origin.

vegetable albumin Albumin produced in plants.

vegetal pole, vegetative pole The relatively inactive part of the ovum protoplasm where the food yolk is situated. It is usually located opposite the animal pole. Also called **antiger-**

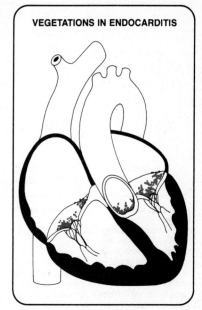

VEGETATIONS IN ENDOCARDITIS

minal pole. Compare **animal pole.**

vegetarian A person whose diet is restricted to foods of vegetable origin, including fruits, grains, and nuts. Many vegetarians eat eggs and milk products but avoid all animal flesh. Kinds of vegetarians are **lacto-ovo-vegetarian, lacto-vegetarian, strict vegetarian.**

vegetarianism The theory or practice of restricting the diet to vegetables, fruits, grains, and nuts.

vegetation An abnormal growth of tissue around a valve, composed of fibrin, platelets, and bacteria.

vegetative **1.** Of or pertaining to nutrition and growth. **2.** Of or pertaining to the plant kingdom. **3.** Denoting involuntary function, as produced by the parasympathetic nervous system. **4.** Resting, not active; denoting the stage of the cell cycle in which the cell is not replicating. **5.** Leading a secluded, dull existence without social or intellectual activity; sluggish; lacking animation. **6.** In psychiatry: emotionally withdrawn and passive, as may occur in schizophrenia. —**vegetate,** *v.*

vegetative nervous system See **autonomic nervous system.**

vehicle **1.** An inert substance with which a medication is mixed to facilitate measurement and administration or application. **2.** Any fluid or structure in the body that passively conveys a stimulus.

Veillonella A genus of gram-negative anaerobic bacteria. The species *Veillonella parvula* is normally present in the alimentary tract, especially in the mouth.

Veillon's tube A transparent tube, the ends of which are closed with removable stoppers,

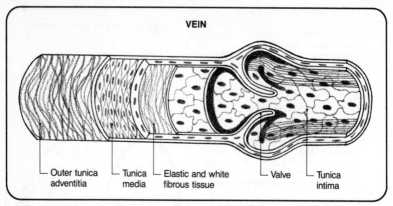

VEIN

Outer tunica adventitia — Tunica media — Elastic and white fibrous tissue — Valve — Tunica intima

used for the laboratory growth of bacteriologic cultures.

vein One of the many vessels that convey blood from the capillaries to the heart as part of the pulmonary venous system, the systemic venous network, or the portal venous complex. Most of the veins of the body are systemic veins that convey blood from the whole body (except the lungs) to the right atrium of the heart. Each vein is a macroscopic structure enclosed in three layers of different kinds of tissue homologous with the layers of the heart. The outer tunica adventitia of each vein is homologous with the epicardium, the tunica media with the myocardium, and the tunica intima with the endocardium. Deep veins course through the more internal parts of the body and superficial veins lie near the surface, where many of them can be seen through the skin. Veins have thinner coatings and are less elastic than arteries and collapse when cut. They also contain semilunar valves at various intervals. Compare **artery.** See also **portal vein, pulmonary vein, systemic vein.**

vein ligation and stripping A surgical procedure consisting of the ligation and removal of the saphenous vein from groin to ankle, performed for the treatment of recurrent thrombophlebitis or severe varicosities or for obtaining a blood vessel to graft in another site.

vein of Thebesius See **smallest cardiac vein.**

veins of the vertebral column The veins that drain the blood from the vertebral column, the adjacent muscles, and the meninges of the spinal cord. Along the entire vertebral column these veins form plexuses that are divided into internal and external groups, according to their locations inside or outside the vertebral canal. The plexuses and the veins of the vertebral network are the external plexus, the internal plexus, the basivertebral veins, the intervertebral veins, and the spinal cord veins.

vellus hair See **lanugo.**

velocity The rate of change in the position of a body moving in a particular direction. Compare **speed.**

velopharyngeal closure The blocking of any escape of air by the raising of the soft palate and the contraction of the posterior pharyngeal wall. Compare **closure, flask closure.**

velopharyngeal insufficiency An abnormal condition resulting from a congenital defect in the velopharyngeal sphincter; closure of the oral cavity beneath the nasal passages is not complete, as seen in cleft palate. Food may be regurgitated through the nose, and speech is impaired. Surgical correction is usually successful.

Velpeau's bandage A roller bandage that immobilizes the elbow and shoulder by holding the brachium against the side and the flexed forearm on the chest. The palm of the hand rests on the clavicle of the opposite side.

vena cava, *pl.* **venae cavae** One of two large veins returning blood from the peripheral circulation to the right atrium of the heart. See also **inferior vena cava, superior vena cava.** —**vena caval,** *adj.*

vena comes, *pl.* **venae comites** One of the deep paired veins that accompany the smaller arteries, one on each side of the artery. The three vessels are wrapped together in one sheath. Some of the arteries accompanied by such venous pairs are the brachial and the tibial.

venereal Pertaining to or caused by sexual intercourse or genital contact.

venereal disease (VD) Any contagious condition acquired by sexual intercourse or genital contact. Kinds of venereal diseases include **chancroid, gonorrhea, granuloma inguinale, herpes genitalis, lymphogranuloma venereum, syphilis.**

venereal sore See **chancre.**

venereal wart See **condylomatum acuminatum.**

venereology The study of venereal diseases. —**venereologic, venereological,** *adj.,* **venereologist,** *n.*

venesection See **phlebotomy.**

Venezuelan equine encephalitis (VEE) See **equine encephalitis.**

venipuncture A technique in which a vein is punctured transcutaneously by a sharp rigid stylet or cannula carrying a flexible plastic catheter or by a steel needle. The purpose is to withdraw a specimen of blood, to perform a phlebotomy, to instill a medication, to start an intravenous infusion, or to inject a radiopaque substance for radiologic examination. See also **intravenous infusion, phlebotomy.**

veno- A combining form meaning 'pertaining to a vein': *venoclysis, venopressor.*

venogram See **phlebogram.**

venography See **phlebography.**

venom A toxic fluid substance secreted by some snakes, arthropods, and other animals and transmitted by their stings or bites.

venom-extract therapy The administration of antivenin as prophylaxis against the toxic effects of the bite of a specific poisonous animal.

venom immunotherapy The reduction of sensitivity to the bite of a venomous insect or animal by the serial administration of gradually increasing amounts of the specific antigenic substance secreted by it.

venous Of or pertaining to a vein.

-venous A combining form meaning 'of or referring to veins': *lymphovenous, perivenous.*

venous blood gas The oxygen and carbon dioxide in venous blood measured by various methods to assess the adequacy of oxygenation and ventilation and to determine the acid-base status. The oxygen tension of venous blood normally averages 40 mmHg; the dissolved oxygen averages 0.1% by volume, the total oxygen content 15.2%, and the oxygen saturation of venous hemoglobin 75%. The carbon dioxide tension normally averages 46 mmHg; the dissolved carbon dioxide 2.9% by volume, and the carbon dioxide content 50%. The normal average pH of venous plasma is 7.37. Venous blood in an extremity when analyzed for gas content provides data chiefly pertaining to that limb. Since a sample from a central venous catheter is usually an incomplete mix of venous blood from various parts of the body, a specimen of completely mixed blood may be obtained from the right ventricle or pulmonary artery for an accurate determination of venous blood gases.

venous insufficiency An abnormal circulatory condition characterized by decreased return of the venous blood from the legs to the trunk of the body. Edema is usually the first sign; pain, varicosities, and ulceration may follow. Treatment consists of elevation of the legs, use of elastic hose, and correction of the underlying condition.

venous pressure The stress exerted by circulating blood on the walls of veins, normally 60 to 120 mm of water in peripheral veins but elevated in congestive heart failure, acute or chronic constrictive pericarditis, and venous obstruction caused by a clot or external pressure against a vein. Indications of increased pressure are continued distention of veins on the back of the hand when it is raised above the sternal notch and distention of the neck veins when the individual is sitting with the head elevated 30° to 45°. Central venous pressure, normally 40 to 100 mm of water, is determined by inserting a catheter into a major vein and threading it through the superior vena cava to the right atrium.

venous pulse The pulse of a vein, usually palpated over the internal or external jugular veins in the neck. The pulse in the jugular vein is taken to evaluate the pressure of the pulse and the form of the pressure wave, especially in a person with a cardiac conduction defect.

venous sinus One of many sinuses that collect blood from the dura mater and drain it into the internal jugular vein. Each sinus is formed by the separation of the two layers of the dura mater, the outer coat of the sinus consisting of fibrous tissue, the inner coat consisting of endothelium continuous with that of the veins.

venous thrombosis A condition characterized by the presence of a clot in a vein in which the wall of the vessel is not inflamed. Pain, swelling, and inflammation may follow if the vein is significantly occluded. Also called **phlebothrombosis.** Compare **thrombophlebitis.**

ventilate 1. To provide with fresh air. 2. To provide the lungs with air from the atmosphere and to oxygenate blood in the pulmonary capillaries. 3. In psychiatry: to open discussion, as to ventilate feelings. —**ventilation,** *n.*

ventilation The process by which gases are moved into and out of the lungs. Compare **respiration.** —**ventilatory,** *adj.*

ventilator Any of several devices used in respiratory therapy to provide assisted respiration and positive pressure breathing.

venting In intravenous therapy: a method for allowing air to enter the vacuum of the intravenous bottle and displace the intravenous solution as it flows out. Venting is not required with a plastic I.V. bag, because the bag collapses as the fluid runs out.

ventral Of or pertaining to a position toward the belly of the body; frontward; anterior. Compare **dorsal.**

-ventral A combining form meaning 'of the stomach or abdominal region': *biventral, dorsoventral.*

ventral hernia See **abdominal hernia.**

ventri- See **ventro-.**

ventricle A small cavity, as one of the cavities filled with cerebrospinal fluid in the brain, or the right and the left ventricles of the heart. —**ventricular,** *adj.*

ventricular Of or pertaining to a ventricle.

ventricular aneurysm A localized dilatation or saccular protrusion in the wall of the left ventricle, occurring most often following a myocardial infarction. Scar tissue is formed in response to the inflammatory changes of the infarction. This tissue weakens the myocardium, allowing its walls to bulge outward when the ventricle contracts. A typical sign of the lesion is a recurrent ventricular arrhythmia that does not respond to treatment with antiarrhythmic drugs. Diagnostic measures are X-ray studies and cardiac catheterization. Treatment may consist of the administration of propranolol, digoxin, or procainamide but usually involves sur-

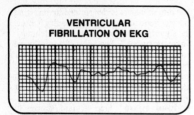

VENTRICULAR FIBRILLATION ON EKG

gical removal of the scar tissue. Also called **cardiac aneurysm.**

ventricular fibrillation A cardiac arrhythmia marked by rapid, disorganized depolarizations of the ventricular myocardium. The condition is characterized by a lack of organized electrical impulse, conduction, and ventricular contraction. Blood pressure falls to zero, resulting in unconsciousness. Death may occur within 4 minutes. Defibrillation and ventilation must be begun immediately.

ventricular gallop An abnormal cardiac rhythm in which a low-pitched extra heart sound is heard early in diastole on auscultation of the heart. When it is heard in an older person with heart disease it indicates myocardial failure. The same sound, heard in a healthy child or young adult, is a physiologic finding (called a physiologic third heart sound) that usually disappears with age. See also **gallop.**

ventricular gradient The algebraic sum of the areas within the QRS complex and within the T wave in the electrocardiogram.

ventricular septal defect (VSD) An abnormal opening in the septum separating the ventricles, permitting blood to flow from the left ventricle to the right ventricle and to recirculate through the pulmonary artery and lungs. It is the most common congenital heart defect, with openings that may be single or multiple and may range in size from 1 to 2 mm to several centimeters (an inch or more). Children who have small defects are usually asymptomatic, while those who have large defects may present with congestive heart failure associated with lower respiratory tract infections, rapid breathing, poor weight gain, restlessness, and irritability. Diagnosis is established by electrocardiography, cardiac catheterization, and angiography. Treatment consists of surgical repair of the defect, preferably in early childhood.

ventricular standstill See **asystole.**

ventriculo- A combining form meaning 'pertaining to a ventricle of the heart or brain': *ventriculocisternostomy, ventriculopuncture.*

ventriculoatrial shunt A surgically created passageway, consisting of plastic tubing and one-way valves, implanted between a cerebral ventricle and the right atrium of the heart in order to drain excess cerebrospinal fluid from the brain in hydrocephalus.

ventriculocisternostomy A surgical procedure performed to treat hydrocephalus. An opening is created that allows cerebrospinal fluid to drain through a shunt from the ventricles of

the brain into the cisterna magna. Also called **Torkildsen procedure.**

ventriculofallopian tube shunt A surgical procedure with limited effectiveness for diverting cerebrospinal fluid into the peritoneal cavity. A polyethylene tube is passed from the lateral ventricle or from the spinal subarachnoid space into a ligated fallopian tube and finally into the peritoneal cavity, where the shunted cerebrospinal fluid is absorbed. This procedure is used to correct both the obstructive and the communicating types of hydrocephalus. Also called **spinofallopian tube shunt.**

ventriculography **1.** An X-ray examination of the head, following injection of air or another contrast medium into the cerebral ventricles. **2.** An X-ray examination of a ventricle of the heart, following injection of a radiopaque contrast medium.

ventriculoperitoneal shunt A surgically created passageway made of plastic tubing and one-way valves between a cerebral ventricle and the peritoneum for draining excess cerebrospinal fluid from the brain in hydrocephalus.

ventriculoperitoneostomy A surgical procedure for temporarily diverting cerebrospinal fluid in hydrocephalus, usually in the newborn. In this procedure, which spares the kidney but is less efficient than a ventriculoureterostomy, a polyethylene tube is passed from the lateral ventricle subcutaneously down the dorsal spine and is reinserted into the peritoneal cavity where the diverted fluid is absorbed. This procedure is used to correct hydrocephalus.

ventriculopleural shunt A surgical procedure for diverting cerebrospinal fluid from engorged ventricles in hydrocephalus, usually in the newborn. Cerebrospinal fluid is diverted from the lateral ventricle into the pleural cavity. It is used to correct both the obstructive and the communicating types of hydrocephalus.

ventriculoureterostomy A surgical procedure for directing cerebrospinal fluid into the general circulation performed in the treatment of hydrocephalus, usually in the newborn. A polyethylene tube is passed from the lateral ventricle down the dorsal spine subcutaneously to the 12th rib; the tube is inserted through the paraspinal muscles into a ureter. Rarely used, the method is an alternative to auriculoventriculostomy. The procedure is performed to correct an obstructive type of hydrocephalus.

ventro-, ventri- A combining form meaning 'pertaining to the belly or to the front of the body': *ventrodorsal, ventrolateral.*

venule Any one of the small blood vessels that gather blood from the capillary plexuses and anastomose to form the veins. **—venular,** *adj.*

VEP *abbr* **visual evoked potential.**

verapamil An antiarrhythmic and antianginal agent.

verbal aphasia See **motor aphasia.**

vermicide An agent that kills worms, particularly those in the intestine. Compare **anthelmintic, vermifuge.**

vermiform appendix   A wormlike, blunt process extending from the cecum. Its length varies from 7.5 to 15 cm (3 to 6 inches) and its diameter is about 0.8 cm (⅓ inch). Also called **appendix vermiformis, cecal appendix.** See also **appendicitis.**

vermifuge   An agent that causes the evacuation of intestinal worms.

vermis, *pl.* **vermes**   **1.** A worm. **2.** A structure resembling a worm, as the median lobe of the cerebellum. —**vermiform,** *adj.*

vernal conjunctivitis   A chronic, bilateral form of conjunctivitis, thought to be allergic in origin, that occurs most frequently in young men under age 20 during the spring and summer months. The most common symptoms include intense itching and crusting discharge. Topical corticosteroids may be applied and desensitization to pollen may be helpful. Compare **allergic conjunctivitis.**

Verneuil's neuroma   See **plexiform neuroma.**

vernix caseosa   A gray-white, cheeselike substance, consisting of sebaceous gland secretions, lanugo, and desquamated epithelial cells, that covers the skin of the fetus and newborn. It acts as a protective agent during intrauterine life and is thought to have an insulating effect against heat loss.

verruca   A fungating, warty skin lesion with a rough, papillomatous surface. Methods of treatment include application of salicylic acid or cantharidin, electrodesiccation, cryosurgery with solid carbon dioxide or liquid nitrogen, and mental suggestion. Also called **wart.** —**verrucose, verrucous,** *adj.*

verruca plana   A small, slightly elevated, smooth, tan or flesh-colored wart, sometimes occuring in large numbers on the face, neck, back of the hands, wrists, and knees, especially in children. Also called **flat wart.**

verruca senillis   See **basal cell papilloma.**

verruca vulgans   See **verruca.** Also called verruca vulgaris.

verrucous carcinoma   A well-differentiated squamous cell neoplasm of the oral cavity, larynx, or genitalia. A slow-growing tumor, it tends to displace rather than invade surrounding tissue; it does not usually metastasize.

verrucous dermatitis   Any skin rash with wartlike lesions.

verruga peruana   See **bartonellosis.**

-verse   A combining form meaning: **1.** 'To turn': *reverse, sacrotransverse.* **2.** 'Turned, changed': *inverse, reverse.*

version and extraction   An obstetric operation in which an infant presenting head first is turned and delivered feet first. It is performed by reaching deeply into the uterus, grasping the infant's feet, and extracting the infant. It is considered outmoded and hazardous and has been replaced by cesarean section, although it may still be done to deliver a second twin. Also called **internal podalic version and total breech extraction.** See also **breech extraction, breech presentation.**

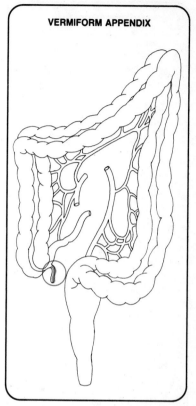

VERMIFORM APPENDIX

-vert   A combining form meaning a 'person who has turned (metaphorically)' in a specified direction: *extrovert.*

vertebra, *pl.* **vertebrae**   Any one of the 33 bones of the spinal column, comprising the 7 cervical, 12 thoracic, 5 lumbar, 5 sacral, and 4 coccygeal vertebrae. The vertebrae, with the exception of the 1st and 2nd cervical vertebrae, are much alike and are composed of a body, an arch, a spinous process for muscle attachment, and pairs of pedicles and processes. The 1st cervical vertebra is called the atlas and has no vertebral body. The 2nd cervical vertebra is called the axis and forms the pivot on which the atlas rotates. The body of the axis also extends into a strong, bony process.

-vertebral   A combining form referring to the spinal column: *pelvivertebral, subvertebral.*

vertebral artery   Each of two arteries branching from the subclavian arteries, arising deep in the neck from the cranial and dorsal subclavian surfaces. Each vertebral artery divides into two cervical and five cranial branches, supplying deep neck muscles, the spinal cord and spinal membranes, and the cerebellum.

vertebral body   The weight-supporting, solid central portion of a vertebra. The pedicles of the arch project from its dorsolateral surfaces.

VERTEBRAL COLUMN

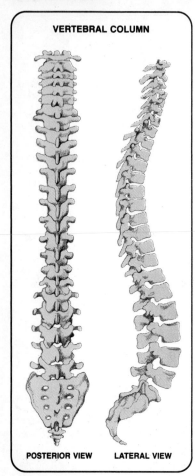

POSTERIOR VIEW   LATERAL VIEW

vertebral column   The flexible structure that forms the longitudinal axis of the skeleton and in the adult includes 26 separate vertebrae arranged in a straight line from the base of the skull to the coccyx. The vertebrae are separated by intervertebral discs. They provide attachment for various muscles, as the iliocostalis thoracis and the longissimus thoracis, which give the column strength and flexibility. The average length of the vertebral column in men is about 71 cm (28 inches). The cervical part measures about 12.5 cm (5 inches), the thoracic part about 28 cm (11 inches), the lumbar part about 18 cm (7 inches), and the sacrum and the coccyx about 12.5 cm (5 inches). The vertebral column in women measures approximately 61 cm (24 inches). The cervical curve is convex ventrally from the apex of the dens to the middle of the 2nd thoracic vertebra and is the least marked of all the curves. The thoracic curve, concave ventrally, starts at the middle of the 2nd and ends at the middle of the 12th thoracic vertebra. The

lumbar curve, more pronounced in women than in men, begins at the middle of the last thoracic vertebra and ends at the sacrovertebral angle. The pelvic curve starts at the sacrovertebral articulation and ends at the point of the coccyx. The thoracic and the sacral curves constitute primary curves, present during fetal life; the cervical and the lumbar curves constitute secondary curves, which develop after birth. The cervical curve develops when the child is able to hold up its head, usually 3 to 4 months after birth; the lumbar curve develops 12 to 18 months after birth, when the child starts to walk. The vertebral column also presents a slight lateral curve, which in most individuals presents a convexity toward the right side. The vertebral canal courses through the vertebral column and contains the spinal cord. The canal is formed by the posterior arches of the vertebrae and is large and triangular in the cervical and the lumbar sections of the column, the most flexible portions. The canal is small and rounded in the thoracic region, where motion is more restricted. Also called **spinal column, spine.** See also **vertebra.**

vertebro-   A combining form meaning 'pertaining to the vertebral column or to a vertebra': *vertebrocostal.*

vertex presentation   In obstetrics: a fetal presentation in which the vertex of the fetus is the part nearest to the cervical os and can be expected to be born first.

vertical plane   See **cardinal frontal plane.**

vertical transmission   The transfer of a disease, condition, or trait from one generation to the next, either genetically or congenitally.

vertigo   A sensation of movement in which the patient feels himself revolving in space (subjective vertigo) or his surroundings revolving about him (objective vertigo). It results from disease of the equilibratory apparatus—the inner ear or the vestibular nerve or its nuclei in the brainstem. Compare **dizziness.**

very low-density lipoprotein (VLDL)   A plasma protein that is composed chiefly of triglycerides with small amounts of cholesterol, phospholipid, and protein. It transports triglycerides primarily from the liver to peripheral sites in the tissues for use or storage. The triglycerides are quickly converted to smaller, more soluble intermediate lipoproteins and eventually to low-density lipoproteins.

vesical fistula   An abnormal passage connecting to the urinary bladder. Vesical fistulae may communicate with the skin, vagina, uterus, or rectum.

vesicle   A tiny blister; a small, thin-walled, raised skin lesion containing clear fluid. —**vesicular,** *adj.*

vesicle reflex   The sensation of a need to urinate when the bladder is moderately distended. See also **micturition reflex.**

vesico-   A combining form meaning 'pertaining to the bladder or to a blister': *vesicocavernous, vesicosigmoid.*

vesicoureteral reflux   An abnormal back-

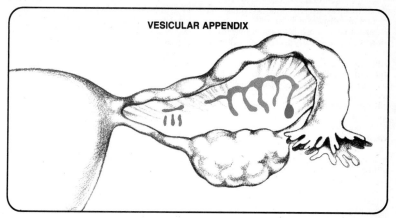

VESICULAR APPENDIX

flow of urine from the bladder to the ureter, resulting from a congenital defect, obstruction of the outlet of the bladder, or infection of the lower urinary tract. Reflux increases the hydrostatic pressure in the ureters and kidneys. The condition is characterized by abdominal or flank pain, enuresis, pyuria, hematuria, proteinuria, and bacteriuria accompanied by persistent or recurrent urinary tract infections. Diagnosis is made by cystoscopy and voiding cystourethrogram. Obstruction or defective implantation of the ureter in the bladder may be surgically corrected. Antibacterial medication, urinary tract antiseptics, and analgesics are usually prescribed for infection.

vesicouterine Of or pertaining to the bladder and uterus. Also called **uterovesical.**

vesicular appendix A cystic structure on the fimbriated end of each of the fallopian tubes.

vesicular breath sound A normal sound of rustling or swishing heard with a stethoscope over the lung periphery, characteristically higher pitched during inspiration and fading rapidly during expiration. Compare **tracheal breath sound.**

vesicular mole See **hydatid mole.**

vesiculitis Inflammation of any vesicle, particularly the seminal vesicles.

vessel Any one of the many tubules throughout the body that convey fluids, as blood and lymph. The main vessels are the arteries, the veins, and the lymphatic vessels.

vestibular Of or pertaining to a vestibule, as the vestibular portion of the mouth, which lies between the cheeks and the teeth.

vestibular gland Any one of four small glands, two on each side of the vaginal orifice. They secrete a lubricating substance. Compare **Cowper's gland.** See also **Bartholin's gland.**

vestibule A space or a cavity that serves as the entrance to a passageway, as the vestibule of the vagina or the vestibule of the ear.

vestibulocochlear nerve See **acoustic nerve.**

vestige An imperfectly developed, relatively useless organ or other structure of the body that had a vital function at an earlier stage of life or in a more primitive form of life, as the vermiform appendix. **—vestigial,** *adj.*

viable Capable of developing, growing, and otherwise sustaining life, as a normal human fetus at 28 weeks of gestation. **—viability,** *n.*

viable infant An infant who at birth weighs 1,000 gm (2¼ lb) or is 28 weeks or more of gestational age.

vibrating See **cupping and vibrating.**

vibration A massage administered by quick tapping with the fingertips, alternating the fingers in a rhythmical manner, or by a mechanical device. See also **massage.**

vibrio Any bacterium that is curved and motile, as those belonging to the genus *Vibrio.* Cholera and several other epidemic forms of gastroenteritis are caused by members of the genus.

Vibrio cholerae The species of comma-shaped, motile bacillus that is the cause of cholera.

vibrio gastroenteritis An infectious disease acquired from contaminated seafood and characterized by nausea, vomiting, abdominal pain, and diarrhea, caused by *Vibrio parahaemolyticus.* Headache, mild fever, and bloody stools may also be present. Spontaneous recovery usually occurs in 2 to 5 days. Compare **salmonellosis, shigellosis.**

Vibrio parahaemolyticus A species of microorganisms of the genus *Vibrio,* the causative agent in food poisoning associated with the ingestion of uncooked or undercooked shellfish, especially crabs and shrimp. This microorganism is a common cause of gastroenteritis in Japan, aboard cruise ships, and in the eastern and southeastern coastal areas of the United States. Thorough cooking of seafood prevents the infection associated with *V. parahaemolyticus,* which causes watery diarrhea, abdominal cramps, vomiting, headache, chills, and fever. The food poisoning from this agent usually subsides spontaneously within 2 days but may be more severe, even fatal, in debilitated and elderly persons. Confirming diagnosis requires bacteriologic examination of the vomitus, stool, and blood. Treatment usually includes bed rest and the oral replacement of fluids.

vidarabine   An ophthalmic anti-infective.

vidarabine monohydrate   An antiviral antibiotic.

villioma   See **villoma.**

villoma, *pl.* **villomas, villomata**   A villous neoplasm or papilloma, occurring chiefly in the rectum. Also called **villioma.**

villous adenoma   A slow-growing, soft, spongy, potentially malignant papillary growth of the mucosa of the large intestine.

villous carcinoma   An epithelial tumor with many long, velvety papillary outgrowths. Also called **carcinoma villosum.**

villous papilloma   A benign tumor with long, slender processes, usually occurring in the bladder, breast, or a cerebral ventricle.

villus, *pl.* **villi**   One of the many tiny projections, barely visible to the naked eye, clustered over the entire mucous surface of the small intestine. The villi diffuse and transport fluids and nutrients. Each villus has a core of delicate areolar and reticular connective tissue supporting the epithelium, various capillaries, and, usually, a single lymphatic lacteal, which fills with milky white chyle during the digestion of a fatty meal. —**villous,** *adj.*

vinblastine sulfate   Alkaloid derivative of the periwinkle plant *(Vinca rosea),* used in cancer chemotherapy.

vincristine sulfate   Alkaloid derivative of the periwinkle plant *(Vinca rosea),* used in cancer chemotherapy.

vindestine sulfate   Alkaloid derivative of the periwinkle plant *(Vinca rosea),* used in cancer chemotherapy.

Vincent's angina   See **acute necrotizing gingivitis.**

Vincent's infection   See **acute necrotizing gingivitis.**

violence, potential for: self-directed or directed at others   A nursing diagnosis accepted by the Fifth National Conference on the Classification of Nursing Diagnoses. The etiology of the condition may be complex and may involve an antisocial personality, mania, organic brain syndrome, panic, rage, suicidal behavior, temporal lobe epilepsy, or a toxic reaction to a medication. Characteristics of clients who are potentially violent include anxiety; fear of the self or other people; lack of verbal ability; complaining or demanding vocalization; provocative, argumentative, or overreactive behavior; poor self-esteem; or psychological depression. Many other factors may also be present, as a history of self-destructive behavior, pacing, excitement, agitation, or the possession of a weapon. See also **nursing diagnosis.**

viomycin sulfate   A tuberculostatic antibiotic.

viosterol   Synthetic vitamin D_2 in an oil base. Also called **synthetic oleovitamin D.** See also **calciferol, ergosterol.**

VIP   *abbr* very important person. A VIP suite in a hospital is one reserved for such persons.

viral disease   See **viral infection.**

viral hepatitis   A viral, inflammatory disease of the liver, caused by one of the hepatitis viruses. Transmission, speed of onset, and probable course of the illness vary with the kind and strain of virus. Characteristics of viral hepatitis are anorexia, malaise, headache, pain over the liver, fever, jaundice, clay-colored stools, dark urine, nausea and vomiting, and diarrhea. Severe infection may be prolonged and result in tissue destruction, cirrhosis, and chronic hepatitis or in hepatic coma and death. Treatment is largely supportive. It includes bed rest; isolation, if necessary; fluids; a low-fat, high-protein, high-calorie diet; special skin care if pruritus is present; emotional support; vitamins B_{12}, K, and C; and monitoring of liver and kidney function. Sedatives, analgesics, antiemetics, and steroids may be ordered. However, the patient is carefully observed for adverse reaction to medication, as the liver may not be able to break down and detoxify the drugs.

NURSING CONSIDERATIONS: The patient with viral hepatitis is taught the importance of washing the hands carefully after urinating or defecating in order to avoid spreading the virus, of eating well, of following written dietary instructions after discharge, and of avoiding alcohol, usually for at least 1 year. The patient is encouraged to have certain blood tests performed periodically, including SGOT and serum bilirubin, to report any symptoms of recurrence immediately, and to avoid contact with people having infections. The patient is told not to donate blood and not to take over-the-counter drugs without medical consultation. See also **hepatitis A; hepatitis B; non-A, non-B hepatitis.**

viral infection   Any of the diseases caused by 1 of approximately 200 viruses pathogenic to humans. Some are the most communicable and dangerous diseases known; some are mild and transient conditions that pass virtually unnoticed. If cells are damaged by the viral attack, disease exists. The signs of the infection reflect the anatomic location of the damaged cells. Viruses are introduced into the body through a break in the skin or through a transfusion into the bloodstream, by droplet infection through the respiratory tract, or by ingestion through the digestive tract into the gastrointestinal system. The pathogenicity of the particular virus depends on the rapidity of action, the enzymes released, the part of the body infected, and the particular action of the virus. The general process of viral infection reflects the life cycle of a virus. The first step in the cycle, after entry into the body, is the attachment of the virus to a susceptible cell and the cell's adsorption of the virus. This is followed by penetration of the viral nucleic acid into the parasitized cell. The dissembled virus at this point causes no symptoms and cannot be recovered from the cells in infectious form. The virus begins to mature within the cell and, carrying its own genetic information, begins to replicate itself, using chemical building blocks and energy available in the parasitized cell. The virus has now taken over the cell. Techniques used in viral identification and immunization are based on the fact that viruses can multiply only inside living cells. Inoculation of susceptible animals, of tissue culture media, and of chick embryos allows cultivation of viruses for study and identification and for the preparation of vaccine. Diagnosis of the cause of viral infection is also possible using various other techniques, including serologic tests, fluorescent antibody microscopic examination, microscopic examination, and skin tests. Exposure to a few viruses results in immunity to that virus and to other closely related viruses. Some vectors are able to spread several viruses, but only one at a time. Other mechanisms of natural resistance to viral infection are poorly understood, but susceptibility to a particular virus is somehow species-specific. See also specific viral infections.

viral pneumonia **1.** Pulmonary infection caused by a virus. **2.** *Informal.* Mycoplasma pneumonia.

viremia The presence of viruses in the blood. Compare **bacteremia, fungemia, parasitemia.**

virile **1.** Of, pertaining to, or characteristic of an adult male; masculine; manly. **2.** Possessing or exhibiting masculine strength, vigor, force, or energy. **3.** Of or pertaining to the male sexual functions; capable of procreation. Compare **virilism.** —**virility,** *n.*

virilism **1.** See **virilization. 2.** Pseudohermaphrodism in a female. **3.** Premature development of masculine characteristics in the male. Kinds of virilism are adrenal virilism, prosopopilary virilism.

virilization A process in which secondary, male sexual characteristics are acquired by a female, usually as the result of adrenal dysfunction or hormonal medication. Also called **masculinization.** See also **adrenal virilism.**

virion A rudimentary virus particle with a central nucleoid surrounded by a protein sheath or capsid. The complete nucleocapsid with a nucleic acid core may constitute a complete virus, as the adenoviruses, or it may be surrounded by an envelope, as in the herpesviruses. Such an envelope is a membrane that contains lipids, proteins, and carbohydrates and projects spikelike structures from its surface. See also **capsid.**

virologist A specialist who studies viruses and diseases caused by viruses.

virology The study of viruses and viral diseases. —**virologic, virological,** *adj.*

virulence The power of a microorganism to produce disease. —**virulent,** *adj.*

virulent Of or pertaining to a highly pathogenic or rapidly progressive condition. —**virulence,** *n.*

virus A minute microorganism much smaller than a bacterium that, having no independent metabolic activity, may only replicate within a cell of a living plant or animal host. A virus consists of a core of nucleic acid (DNA or RNA)

surrounded by a coat of antigenic protein, sometimes surrounded by an envelope of lipoprotein. More than 200 viruses have been identified as capable of causing disease in humans. Some kinds of viruses are **adenovirus, arenavirus, enterovirus, rhinovirus.** See also **viral infection.** —**viral,** *adj.*

visceral Of or pertaining to the viscus.

visceral afferent fibers The nerve fibers of the visceral nervous system that receive stimuli and carry impulses toward the central nervous system and share the sensory ganglia of the cerebrospinal nerves with the somatic sensory fibers. Peripheral distribution of the visceral afferent fibers constitutes the main difference between them and the somatic afferents. The visceral afferents produce sensations different from those of the somatic afferents. The number and extent of the visceral afferents is not clearly established. Their peripheral processes reach the ganglia by various routes. Some of the parts of the body with visceral afferents are the face, scalp, nose, mouth, descending colon, lungs, abdomen, and rectum. See also **autonomic nervous system.**

visceral larva migrans Infestation with parasitic larvae of *Toxocara* or, occasionally, *Ascaris, Strongyloides,* or other nematodes. See **toxocariasis.**

visceral leishmaniasis See **kala-azar.**

visceral lymph node A small oval nodular gland that filters lymph circulating in the lymphatic vessels of the thoracic, abdominal, and pelvic viscera. The visceral lymph nodes of the thorax include the anterior mediastinal nodes, posterior mediastinal nodes, and tracheobronchial nodes. The visceral lymph nodes of the abdomen and pelvis include those that follow the course of the celiac artery, superior mesenteric artery, and inferior mesenteric artery. Compare **parietal lymph node.** See also **lymph, lymphatic system, lymph node.**

visceral nervous system The visceral portion of the peripheral nervous system that comprises the whole complex of nerves, fibers, ganglia, and plexuses by which impulses travel from the central nervous system to the viscera and from the viscera to the central nervous system. It contains the usual afferent fibers that receive stimuli and carry impulses toward the central nervous system and efferent fibers that carry impulses from the appropriate centers to the active effector organs, as the nonstriated muscle, cardiac muscle, and glands of the body. Also called **involuntary nervous system.** See also **autonomic nervous system.**

visceral pain Pain caused by any abnormal condition of the viscera. It is characteristically severe, diffuse, and difficult to localize. Also called visceralgia.

visceral peritoneum One of two portions of the largest serous membrane in the body, which invests the viscera. The free surface of the visceral peritoneum is a smooth layer of mesothelium exuding a serous fluid, which lubricates the viscera and allows them to glide freely against

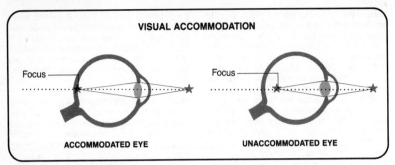

VISUAL ACCOMMODATION

Focus

ACCOMMODATED EYE

Focus

UNACCOMMODATED EYE

the wall of the abdominal cavity or over each other. Compare **parietal peritoneum.** See also **peritoneal cavity.**

visceral pleura The serous membrane that envelops the lungs and lines the fissure between each lobe. See also **parietal pleura.**

viscero- A combining form meaning 'pertaining to the organs of the body': *viscerocranium, visceropleural.*

viscid, viscous Sticky or glutinous.

viscous fermentation The formation of viscous material in milk, urine, and wine by the action of various bacilli.

viscus, *pl.* **viscera** Any one of the large internal organs contained in the abdominal, the thoracic, or the pelvic cavities of the body. **—visceral,** *adj.*

vision The capacity for sight.

visit A meeting between a practitioner and a client or patient.

visual accommodation A process by which the eye adjusts and is able to focus, producing a sharp image at various, changing distances from the object seen. With age, the lens becomes harder and less flexible, resulting in a loss of accommodation and, usually, the ability to focus on nearby objects. Compare **presbyopia.**

visual evoked potential (VEP) An evoked potential elicited by a repeatedly flashing light. The waves produced are too variable to be reliable predictors of injury to nerve tissue. High-risk infants are monitored with VEP to evaluate visual function.

visual field defect One or more spots or defects in the vision that move with the eye, unlike a floater. This fixed defect is usually caused by damage to the retina or visual pathways, as by chorioretinitis, traumatic injury, macular degeneration, glaucoma, or a vascular occlusion of the eye or the brain. Sudden loss of a portion of the visual field warrants ophthalmologic examination.

visual memory The ability to create an eidetic image of visual experiences. Also called **eye memory.**

visual pathway A pathway over which a visual sensation is transmitted from the retina to the brain. A pathway consists of an optic nerve, the fibers of an optic nerve traveling through or along the sides of the optic chiasm

to the lateral geniculate body of the thalamus, and an optic tract terminating in an occipital lobe. The optic tracts, occipital lobe, lateral geniculate bodies of the thalamus, and optic chiasm each contain nerve fibers from both eyes. If the right optic tract were destroyed, a person would lose partial vision in both eyes: the right nasal and the left temporal fields of vision.

visual purple See **rhodopsin.**

vita- A combining form meaning 'pertaining to life': *vitaglass, vital.*

vital capacity (VC) A measurement of the amount of air that can be expelled after a maximum inspiration, representing the greatest possible breathing capacity. Average normal values are 4,000 to 5,000 cc. The vital capacity may be reduced by a decrease in functioning lung tissue, owing to atelectasis, edema, fibrosis, pneumonia, pulmonary resection, or tumors; by limited chest expansion, resulting from ascites, chest deformity, neuromuscular disease, pneumothorax, or pregnancy; or by airway obstruction. Compare **expiratory reserve volume, residual volume, tidal volume.**

vital signs The measurements of pulse rate, respiration rate, and body temperature. Although not strictly a vital sign, blood pressure is also customarily included. Abnormalities of vital signs are often clues to diseases. See also **blood pressure, pulse, respiration, temperature.**

vital statistics Data relating to births or natality, deaths or mortality, marriages, health, and disease or morbidity.

vitamin An organic compound essential in small quantities for normal physiologic and metabolic functioning of the body. With few exceptions, vitamins cannot be synthesized by the body and must be obtained from the diet or dietary supplements. No one food contains all the vitamins. Vitamin-deficiency diseases produce specific symptoms, which are usually alleviated by the administration of the appropriate vitamin. Vitamins are classified according to their fat- or water-solubility, their physiologic effects, or their chemical structures. See specific vitamins. See also **avitaminosis, hypervitaminosis, oleovitamin, provitamin.**

vitamin A A fat-soluble, solid terpene alcohol essential for skeletal growth, maintenance of normal mucosal epithelium, and visual acuity.

It is derived from various carotenoids, mainly carotene, and is present in leafy green vegetables, yellow fruits and vegetables, the liver oils of the cod and other fish, liver, milk, cheese, butter, and egg yolk. Deficiency leads to atrophy of epithelial tissue, resulting in keratomalacia, xerophthalmia, night blindness, and lessened resistance to infection of mucous membranes. Symptoms of hypervitaminosis A are irritability, fatigue, lethargy, abdominal discomfort, painful joints, severe throbbing headache, insomnia and restlessness, night sweats, loss of body hair, brittle nails, and exophthalmos. Also called **antixerophthalmic vitamin.** See also **oleovitamin A.**

vitamin B₁   See **thiamine.**

vitamin B₂   See **riboflavin.**

vitamin B₆   See **pyridoxine.**

vitamin B complex   See **B-complex vitamins.**

vitamin C   See **ascorbic acid.**

vitamin D   See **calciferol.**

vitamin D₂   See **ergocalciferol.**

vitamin D₃   See **cholecalciferol.**

vitamin deficiency   A state or condition resulting from the lack of or inability to utilize one or more vitamins. The symptoms and manifestations of each deficiency vary depending on the specific function of the vitamin in promoting growth and development and maintaining body health.

vitamin D-resistant rickets   A disease clinically similar to rickets but resistant to treatment with large doses of vitamin D. It is caused by a congenital defect in renal tubular reabsorption of phosphate and is usually seen in men. See also **rickets.**

vitamin E   Any or all of the group of fat-soluble vitamins that consist of the tocopherols and are essential for normal reproduction, muscle development, resistance of erythrocytes to hemolysis, and various other biochemical functions. It is an intracellular antioxidant and acts in maintaining the stability of polyunsaturated fatty acids and other fatlike substances, including vitamin A and hormones of the pituitary, adrenal, and sex glands. Deficiency results in muscle degeneration, abnormalities in the vascular system, megaloblastic anemia, hemolytic anemia, infertility, creatinuria, and liver and kidney damage and is associated with the aging process. The richest dietary sources are wheat-germ, soybean, cottonseed, peanut, and corn oils; margarine; whole raw seeds and nuts; soybeans; eggs; butter; liver; sweet potatoes; and the leaves of many vegetables, as turnip greens. It is stored in the body for long periods of time, so severe deficiency is rare. It is considered nontoxic except when taken in megadoses (over 300 units daily). See also **tocopherol.**

vitamin H   See **biotin.**

vitamin K   A group of fat-soluble vitamins known as quinones that are essential for the synthesis of prothrombin in the liver and of several related proteins involved in the clotting of blood. It is also involved with the process of

phosphorylation and electron transport. The vitamin is widely distributed in foods, especially leafy green vegetables, pork liver, yogurt, egg yolk, kelp, alfalfa, fish-liver oils, and blackstrap molasses and is synthesized by the bacterial flora of the gastrointestinal tract. It is also produced synthetically. Deficiency results in hypoprothrombinemia, characterized by poor coagulation of the blood and hemorrhage, and usually occurs from inadequate absorption of the vitamin from the gastrointestinal tract or the inability to utilize it in the liver. It is used to reduce the clotting time in patients with obstructive jaundice and in hemorrhagic states associated with intestinal diseases and diseases of the liver; it is given prophylactically to infants to prevent hemorrhagic disease of the newborn. Natural vitamin K is stored in the body and produces no toxicity. Excessive doses of synthetic vitamin K may cause anemia in newborn infants and hemolysis in persons with glucose-6-phosphate deficiency. See also **vitamin K₁, vitamin K₂, menadione.**

vitamin K₁   A yellow, viscous, oil-soluble vitamin, occurring naturally, especially in alfalfa, and produced synthetically. It is used as a prothrombinogenic agent. Also called **phylloquinone, phytonadione.**

vitamin K₂   A pale-yellow, fat-soluble crystalline vitamin of the vitamin K₂ group that is more unsaturated than vitamin K₁ and slightly less active biologically. It is isolated from putrefied fish meal and synthesized by various bacteria in the gastrointestinal tract. See also **vitamin K.**

vitamin K₃   See **menadione.**

vitaminology   The study of vitamins, including their structures, modes of action, and function in body health.

vitamin P   See **bioflavonoid.**

vitamin P₂   See **calciferol.**

vitamins A and D ointment   An emollient and demulcent.

vitellin   A phosphoprotein containing lecithin, found in the yolk of eggs. Also called **ovovitellin.**

vitelline artery   Any of the embryonic arteries that circulate blood from the primitive aorta of the early developing embryo to the yolk sac. Also called **omphalomesenteric artery.**

vitelline circulation   The circulation of blood and nutrients between the developing embryo and the yolk sac by way of the vitelline arteries and veins. Also called **omphalomesenteric circulation.** See also **fetal circulation.**

vitelline duct   In embryology: the narrow channel connecting the yolk sac with the intestine. Also called **umbilical duct.**

vitelline membrane   The delicate cytoplasmic membrane surrounding the ovum. Also called **yolk membrane.** See also **zona pellucida.**

vitelline sac   See **yolk sac.**

vitelline sphere   See **morula.**

vitelline vein   Any of the embryonic veins that return blood from the yolk sac to the prim-

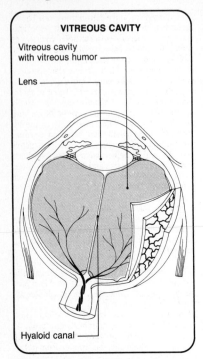

VITREOUS CAVITY

Vitreous cavity with vitreous humor

Lens

Hyaloid canal

itive heart of the early developing embryo. Also called **omphalomesenteric vein.**

vitellogenesis The formation or production of yolk. —**vitellogenetic,** *adj.*

vitellus The yolk of an ovum.

vitiligo A benign, acquired skin disease of unknown cause, consisting of irregular patches of various sizes totally lacking in pigment and often having hyperpigmented borders. Treatment using 8-methoxypsoralen requires extreme care and carefully regulated sun exposure. Waterproof cosmetics are often used to cover the patches. Compare **albinism, piebald, leukoderma.** —**vitiliginous,** *adj.*

vitreous body See **vitreous humor.**

vitreous cavity The cavity posterior to the lens that contains the vitreous body and vitreous membrane and is transected by the vestigial remnants of the hyaloid canal.

vitreous hemorrhage A hemorrhage into the vitreous humor of the eye.

vitreous humor A transparent, semigelatinous substance contained in a thin hyoid membrane filling the cavity behind the crystalline lens of the eye. Some indications of the hyaloid canal may persist in the vitreous humor, but it is not penetrated by any blood vessels and is nourished at its periphery by vessels of the retina and the ciliary processes. Also called **corpus vitreum, vitreous body.**

vitreous membrane A membrane that lines the posterior cavity of the eye and surrounds the vitreous body.

vitriol, oil of See **sulfuric acid.**

vivax malaria See **tertian malaria.**

viviparous Bearing living offspring rather than eggs, as most mammals and some fishes and reptiles. Compare **oviparous, ovoviviparous.**

VMA *abbr* **vanillylmandelic acid.**

Vo$_2$ Symbol for oxygen uptake.

vocal cord Either of two strong bands of yellow elastic tissue in the larynx, enclosed by membranes called vocal folds and attached ventrally to the angle of the thyroid cartilage and dorsally to the arytenoid. Also called true vocal cord, vocal ligament. Compare **false vocal cord.**

vocal cord nodule A small, inflammatory or fibrous growth that develops on the vocal cords of people who constantly strain their voices. Also called **screamer's nodule, singer's nodule, teacher's nodule.** See also **chorditis.**

vocal fremitus The vibration of the chest wall as a person speaks or sings that allows the person's voice to be heard by the examiner during auscultation of the chest with a stethoscope. It is decreased in emphysema, pleural effusion, pulmonary edema, or bronchial obstruction.

voice box See **larynx.**

void To empty or evacuate, as urine from the bladder.

volar Pertaining to the palm of the hand or the sole of the foot.

volar ligament See **retinaculum flexorum manus.**

volatile Of a liquid: the characteristic of boiling at a low temperature and evaporating at room temperature.

volatile solvent An easily evaporated liquid capable of dissolving a substance.

-volemia A combining form meaning '(condition of the) volume of plasma in the body': *hypervolemia, hypovolemia.*

volition 1. The act, power, or state of willing or choosing. 2. The conscious impulse to perform or to abstain from an act. —**volitional,** *adj.*

Volkmann's canal Any one of the small canals connecting Haversian canals in bone tissue. Compare **Haversian canaliculus.** See also **Haversian system.**

Volkmann's contracture A serious, persistent flexion contraction of forearm and hand owing to ischemia. A pressure or crushing injury at the elbow usually precedes this condition, and pressure from a cast or tight bandage about the elbow are common causes. Fibrosis, muscle degeneration, and a clawlike hand may result. Nurses must watch for signs of constriction, such as swelling, pallor, coldness, cyanosis, or pain distal to the injury. Loosening of constriction can restore circulation. Also called **ischemic contracture.**

Volkmann splint A splint that supports and immobilizes the lower leg. It has a footpiece attached to two sides that extends from foot to knee, allowing ambulation.

volsella See **volsella forceps.**

volsella forceps A kind of forceps having

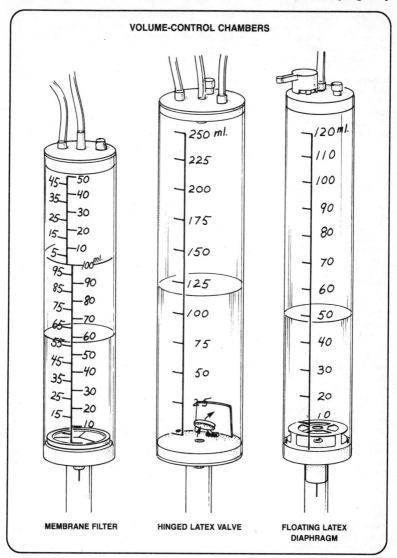

VOLUME-CONTROL CHAMBERS

| MEMBRANE FILTER | HINGED LATEX VALVE | FLOATING LATEX DIAPHRAGM |

a small, sharp-pointed hook at the end of each blade. Also called **volsella, volsellum forceps, vulsella forceps.**

volsellum forceps   See **volsella forceps.**

volt   The unit of electric potential. In an electric circuit, a volt is the force required to send one ampere of current through one ohm of resistance. See also **ampere, circuit, current, ohm, watt.**

volume   The amount of space occupied by a body, expressed in cubic units.

volume-control chamber   Any one of several types of transparent, plastic reservoirs with graduated volumetric markings, used to regu-

late the flow of intravenous solutions. These devices are components of intravenous volume-control sets and accommodate the injection and the mixing of medications by means of special built-in ports. The volume-control fluid chamber contains a valve which prevents air from entering the I.V. tubing. Three types of valves are available: membrane filter, hinged latex valve, and floating latex diaphragm.

volume dose   See **integral dose.**

voluntary   Pertaining to an action or thought originated or accomplished as a result of a person's free will or choice.

voluntary agency   A service agency legally

controlled by volunteers rather than by owners or a paid staff. Most public-health nursing agencies are voluntary; most hospitals are legally controlled by hospital boards, which are composed of lay and professional members who are not paid for their services.

voluntary muscle See **striated muscle.**

-volute A combining form meaning 'to roll, turn around': *cicumvolute, involute.*

volvulus A twisting of the bowel on itself, causing intestinal obstruction. The condition is frequently the result of a prolapsed segment of mesentery and occurs most often in the ileum, the secum, or the sigmoid portions of the bowel. If it is not corrected, the obstructed bowel becomes necrotic; peritonitis and rupture of the bowel occur; and death may ensue. Severe, gripping pain; nausea and vomiting; an absence of bowel sounds; and a tense, distended abdomen suggest the diagnosis, which is confirmed by X-ray examination. Compare **intussusception.**

volvulus neonatorum An intestinal obstruction in a newborn resulting from a twisting of the bowel due to malrotation or nonfixation of the colon. Typical symptoms include abdominal distention; persistent regurgitation, often accompanied by fecal vomiting; and nonpassage of stools. Characteristic barium enema X-rays confirm the diagnosis. The condition requires immediate surgical correction.

vomer The bone forming the posterior and inferior part of the nasal septum and having two surfaces and four borders.

vomit 1. To expel the contents of the stomach through the esophagus and out of the mouth. Also called emesis. 2. The material expelled. Also called vomitus.

von Economo's encephalitis See **epidemic encephalitis.**

von Gierke's disease A form of glycogen storage disease in which abnormally large amounts of glycogen are deposited in the liver and kidneys. The disorder is characterized by hypoglycemia, ketoacidosis, and hyperlipemia. Biopsy of the affected organs reveals the absence of glucose-6-phosphate dehydrogenase, an enzyme necessary for glycogen metabolism. There is no effective treatment for the disorder. Also called **glycogen storage disease, type I.** See also **glycogen storage disease.**

von Hippel-Lindau disease See **cere-**broretinal angiomatosis.

von Pirquet test See **Pirquet test.**

von Recklinghausen's disease See neurofibromatosis.

von Willebrand's disease An inherited disorder characterized by abnormally slow coagulation of the blood and spontaneous epistaxis and gingival bleeding owing to a deficiency of factor VIII. Excessive bleeding is common postpartum, during menstruation, and following injury or surgery. See also **hemophilia, thrombasthenia.**

-vorous A combining form meaning 'of or referring to feeding on' something specified: *leguminivorous.*

vortex, *pl.* **vortexes, vortices** A whirlpool effect produced by the whirling of a more or less cylindrical mass of fluid (liquid or gas). The velocity of the motion increases as the radius of the circle described by the motion decreases; the velocity decreases as the radius increases. Tornadoes and whirlpools are examples of free vortexes.

vox Voice, as vox cholerica.

vox cholerica See **vox.**

voyeur One whose sexual desire is gratified by the practice of voyeurism. Also called **Peeping Tom.**

voyeurism A psychosexual disorder in which a person derives sexual excitement and gratification from looking at the naked bodies and genital organs or observing the sexual acts of others, especially from a secret vantage point.

VSD *abbr* **ventricular septal defect.**

vulsella forceps See **volsella forceps.**

vulva See **pudendum. —vulvar,** *adj.*

vulvar Of or pertaining to the vulva.

vulvectomy The surgical removal of part or all of the tissues of the vulva, performed most frequently in the treatment of malignant or premalignant neoplastic disease. Simple vulvectomy includes the removal of the skin of the labia minora, the labia majora, and the clitoris. **Radical vulvectomy** involves excision of the labia majora, labia minora, clitoris, the surrounding tissues, and the pelvic lymph nodes.

vulvocrural Of or pertaining to the vulva and the thigh.

vulvovaginal Of or pertaining to the vulva and the vagina.

VZV *abbr* **varicella-zoster virus.**

W

W Symbol for **tungsten.**

Wagner-Meissner corpuscle One of a number of small, special sensory end organs with a connective tissue capsule and tiny stacked plates in the corium of the hand and foot, the front of the forearm, the skin of the lips, the mucous membrane of the tongue, the palpebral conjunctiva, and the skin of the mammary papilla. A single nerve fiber penetrates each oval capsule, spirals through the interior, and ends as a globular mass. Also called **tactile corpuscle of Meissner.** Compare **Golgi-Mazzoni corpuscles, Krause's corpuscles.**

Wagstaffe's fracture A fracture characterized by separation of the internal malleolus.

waking imagined analgesia (WIA) The pain relief experienced by a patient who employs the psychological technique, usually with the help of an attending nurse or a hospital aide, of concentrating on previous pleasant personal experiences that produced tranquility, as lying on a summer beach beside cooling ocean water or drifting down a quiet river in a canoe. The patient employing the WIA technique is encouraged to verbalize such experiences, thereby reinforcing recollection with attendant soothing biological responses. This technique is often effective in reducing mild to moderate pain, especially when used with a mild, nonnarcotic analgesic and the compassionate interaction of an attending health-care professional. See also **pain evaluation, pain intervention, pain mechanism.**

Waldenström's disease See **Perthes' disease.**

Waldenström's macroglobulinemia See **macroglobulinemia.**

walker An extremely light, movable apparatus, about waist high, made of metal tubing and used to aid a patient in walking. It has four widely placed, sturdy legs. The patient holds onto the walker and takes a step, then moves the walker forward and takes another step. Compare **crutch.**

walking pneumonia See **mycoplasma pneumonia.**

walking rounds Rounds in which the clinician responsible leads a group of junior clinicians on a tour to visit the patients for whom they are collectively responsible. In some hospitals nurses may participate in walking rounds in lieu of or in addition to report.

wall A limiting structure within the body, as the wall of the abdominal, the thoracic, or the pelvic cavity, or the wall of a cell.

wander **1.** To move about purposelessly. **2.** To cause to move back and forth in an exploratory manner, as, in inserting an intrauterine catheter, the tip of the inserter must usually be wandered around the fetal head in the cervix in order to find a space through which the catheter may be passed upward into the uterus.

wandering goiter See **diving goiter.**

Wangensteen apparatus A nasogastroduodenal catheter and a suction apparatus used for constant, gentle drainage and decompression of the stomach or duodenum. It may be used to relieve abdominal distention that often occurs postoperatively or that may complicate a gastrointestinal disorder, especially an intestinal obstruction. See also **Wangensteen tube.**

Wangensteen tube The catheter portion of a Wangensteen apparatus.

warfarin poisoning A toxic condition caused by the ingestion of warfarin, accidentally in the form of a rodenticide or by overdose of the substance in its pharmacologic anticoagulant form. The poison accumulates in the body and results in nosebleed, bruising, hematuria, melena, and internal hemorrhage. Treatment may include gastric lavage, a cathartic, vitamin K, and blood transfusion. The goal of therapy is to eliminate the poison and to reestablish normal coagulation.

warfarin sodium An anticoagulant.

warm-blooded Having a relatively high and constant body temperature, as the temperatures maintained by humans, other mammals, and birds, despite changes in environmental temperatures. Heat is produced in the warm-blooded human body by the catabolism of foods in proportion to the amount of work performed by the tissues in the body. Heat is lost from the body by evaporation, radiation, conduction, and convection. About 80% of the body heat that is dissipated in humans is lost through the skin; the rest is lost through the mucous membranes of the respiratory, digestive, and urinary systems. The temperature of the average healthy human is 37°C (98.6°F). The human body's tolerance for change in its temperature is very small, and significant changes can have drastic, even fatal consequences. The control mechanism for temperature in the human body consists of thermal receptive neurons in the anterior portion of the hypothalamus, more than two million sweat glands, and the vast network of blood vessels in the skin. Reduced heat loss results from less secretion and slower evaporation of sweat and from vasoconstriction of blood vessels. Increased heat gain results from shivering, which increases the work of body tissues and, hence, increases catabolism. The body's temperature control mechanisms serve to restore normal heat

WX YZ

WASP STING: CLINICAL MANAGEMENT

REACTIONS	DRUG TREATMENT
Localized reaction: painful wound, edema, urticaria, pruritis **Systemic reaction** (anaphylaxis): symptoms of hypersensitivity usually appear within 20 minutes and may include weakness, chest tightness, dizziness, nausea, vomiting, abdominal cramps, and throat constriction. The shorter the interval between the sting and systemic symptoms, the worse the prognosis. Without prompt treatment, symptoms may progress to cyanosis, coma, and death.	• Antihistamines and corticosteroids (in urticaria) • Tetanus prophylaxis *In anaphylaxis:* • Oxygen by nasal cannula or mask • Epinephrine 1:1,000 subcutaneously or I.M. • In bronchospasm, aminophylline and hydrocortisone • In hypotension, metaraminol and isoproterenol

NURSING INTERVENTION

• Cleanse the wound site and apply ice.
• Watch the patient carefully for signs of anaphylaxis. Keep emergency resuscitation equipment available.
• Tell patient who is allergic to bee stings to wear a medical identification bracelet or carry a card, and to carry an anaphylaxis kit. Teach the patient how to use the kit, and refer the patient to an allergist for hyposensitization therapy.
• To prevent stings, tell patient not to wear fragrant cosmetics when outdoors during insect season, to avoid wearing bright colors and going barefoot, to avoid contact with flowers and fruit that attract the insects, and to use insect repellent.

levels during fever. Also called homiothermal, homothermal. Compare **cold-blooded.**

war neurosis See **combat fatigue, shell shock.**

wart See **verruca.**

Warthin's tumor See **papillary adenocystoma lymphomatosum.**

washout The elimination or expulsion of one gas or volatile anesthetic agent by the administration of another.

wasp A slender, narrow-waisted insect with two pairs of membranous wings that are folded lengthwise when at rest like parts of a fan. Many species of wasps may give painful stings that may have severe results in hypersensitive persons. Treatment is as for bee stings.

Wassermann test A diagnostic blood test for syphilis based on the complement-fixation reaction.

wasting A process of deterioration marked by weight loss and decreased physical vigor, appetite, and mental activity.

water (H₂O) A chemical compound, one molecule of which contains one atom of oxygen and two atoms of hydrogen. Almost three quarters of the earth's surface is covered by water. Essential to life as it exists on this planet, water comprises more than 70% of living things. Pure water freezes at 0°C (32°F) and boils at 100°C (212°F) at sea level.

waterborne Carried by water, as a waterborne epidemic of typhoid fever.

Waterhouse-Friderichsen syndrome Overwhelming bacteremia, characterized by the sudden onset of fever, cyanosis, petechiae, and collapse from massive bilateral adrenal hemorrhage. The syndrome requires immediate emergency treatment, hospitalization, and intensive care. Emergency treatment includes vasopressor drugs, intravenous fluids, plasma, and oxygen. No sedatives or narcotics are given. Specific treatment for bacteremia is intensive antibiotic therapy, given parenterally and continued for several days after symptoms subside. Nursing management includes close observation and the maintenance of adequate provision of fluids and nutrients.

water moccasin See **cottonmouth.**

waters *Informal.* See **amniotic fluid.**

watt The unit of electrical power or work in the meter/kilogram/second system of notation. The watt is the product of the voltage and the amperage. One watt of power is dissipated when a current of one ampere flows across a difference in potential of one volt. See also **ampere, current, ohm, volt.**

wave In physics: a disturbance in which energy moves through a medium without permanently altering the constituents of the medium. Electromagnetic waves, as light, X-rays, and radio waves, can travel through a vacuum. Sound waves can be transmitted only through matter. See also **electromagnetic radiation, light, sound, X-ray.**

wavelength The distance between a given point on one wave cycle and the corresponding point on the next successive wave cycle. A pure color is produced by light of a specific wavelength. Electromagnetic waves of different wavelengths account for many of the transmission

WEBER TUNING FORK TEST

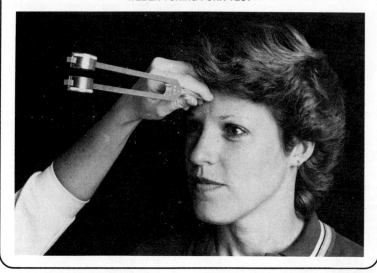

characteristics of radio and television.

wax See **cerumen.**

wax bath See **paraffin bath.**

waxy flexibility See **cerea flexibilitas.**

WBC *abbr* **white blood cell.** See **leukocyte.**

W chromosome, Z chromosome The sex chromosomes of certain insects, birds, and fishes. Females of such species are heterogametic and have one W and one Z chromosome, whereas males are homogametic and have two Z chromosomes. The ZZ-ZW system of nomenclature was chosen to differentiate the chromosomes from the XX-XY type, which occurs in man and various other animals and in which the female is homogametic and the male is heterogametic.

W/D Symbol for well-developed, often used in the initial identifying statement in a patient record. It is used so frequently as to have lost all meaning or use in describing the patient.

wean **1.** To induce a child to give up breast-feeding and to accept other food in place of breast milk. Many children are ready for weaning during the 2nd half of the 1st year; some wean themselves. **2.** To detach or withdraw a person from something on which he is dependent. **—weanling,** *n.*

weanling A child who has recently been weaned.

weaver's bottom A form of bursitis affecting the ischial bursae of the hips of people whose work requires prolonged sitting in one position. Also called **tailor's bottom.**

web A network of fibers forming a tissue or a membrane, as the laryngeal web that spreads between the vocal cords.

Weber tuning fork test A method of assessing auditory acuity, especially useful in determining if defective hearing in an ear is a conductive loss caused by a middle-ear problem or a sensorineural loss, resulting from a disorder in the inner ear or auditory nerve system.

wedge fracture A fracture of vertebral structures with anterior compression.

wedge pressure The capillary pressure in the left atrium, determined by measuring the pressure in a cardiac catheter wedged in the most distal segment of the pulmonary artery.

wedge resection The surgical excision of part of an organ, as a part of an ovary containing a cyst. The segment excised may be wedge-shaped.

WEE *abbr* **western equine encephalitis.** See **equine encephalitis.**

weeping **1.** Crying; lacrimating. **2.** Oozing or exuding fluid, as a sore or rash.

Wegener's granulomatosis An uncommon, chronic inflammatory process leading to the formation of nodules or tumorlike masses in the air passages, necrotizing vasculitis, and glomerulonephritis. Symptoms, depending on the organs involved, may include sinus pain, a bloody, purulent nasal discharge, saddle-nose deformity, chest discomfort and cough, weakness, anorexia, weight loss, and skin lesions. Glomerulonephritis, as a complication, was formerly fatal in a few months, but with the use of cytotoxic drugs, especially cyclophosphamide, a high percentage of patients achieve long-term remissions.

weight The force exerted on a body by the gravity of the earth. On the surface of the earth, mass and weight are the same. As a body moves away from the earth, the weight of the body decreases, but the mass remains constant. In space, a body has mass but no weight. Weight is sometimes measured in units of force, as new-

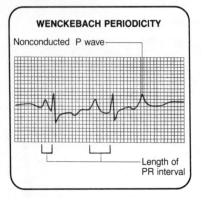

WENCKEBACH PERIODICITY

Nonconducted P wave

Length of PR interval

tons or poundals, but it is usually expressed in pounds or kilograms, as is mass. See also **mass.**

Weil's disease See **leptospirosis.**

Weismannism The basic concepts of heredity and development as proposed by German biologist August Weismann. These state that the vehicle of inheritance is the germ plasm, which is distinct from the somatoplasm and is transmitted from one generation to the next; that during embryonic development the hereditary components are dispersed to the somatoplasm to give rise to inherited characteristics; and that changes in somatoplasm do not affect germ plasm, so that acquired characteristics cannot be inherited. Also called germ plasm theory, Weismann's theory. Compare **pangenesis.** —**Weismannian,** *adj., n.*

Weiss's sign See **Chvostek's sign.**

well-baby care Periodic health supervision for infants and children in order to promote optimal physical, emotional, and intellectual growth and development. Such health-care measures include routine immunizations to prevent disease, screening procedures for early detection and treatment of illness, and parental guidance and instruction in proper nutrition, accident prevention, and specific care and rearing of the child at various stages of development. The recommended preventive health-care schedule for children who are developing normally is monthly for the first 6 months of life, every 2 months until 1 year of age, every 3 months during the 2nd year, and every 6 months during the 3rd year, followed by annual visits. Well-baby care may be provided in a clinic, a convenient local meeting place, a private doctor's office, the public health nurse's office, or a school.

well-differentiated lymphocytic malignant lymphoma A lymphoid neoplasm characterized by the predominance of mature lymphocytes. Also called **lymphocytic lymphoma, lymphocytic lymphosarcoma, lymphocytoma.**

wellness A dynamic state of health.

wen 1. See **pilar cyst.** 2. See **epidermoid cyst.**

Wenckebach heart block See **Mobitz I heart block.**

Wenckebach periodicity A form of second-degree atrioventricular block with a progressive beat-to-beat prolongation of the PR interval, finally resulting in a nonconducted P wave. At this point, the PR interval shortens to normal and the sequence recurs. Also called Wenckebach phenomenon. See also **atrioventricular block.**

Werdnig-Hoffmann disease A genetic disorder beginning in infancy or young childhood, characterized by progressive atrophy of the skeletal muscle resulting from degeneration of the cells in the anterior horn of the spinal cord and the motor nuclei in the brain stem. Onset occurs within the first year of life, with the condition usually apparent at birth. Symptoms include congenital hypotonia; absence of stretch reflexes; flaccid paralysis, especially of the trunk and limbs; lack of sucking ability; fasciculations of the tongue and, sometimes, of other muscles; and, often, dysphagia. Treatment is symptomatic and death generally occurs in early childhood, often from respiratory complications. The condition is transmitted as an autosomal recessive trait and occurs more frequently in siblings than in successive generations. Also called **familial spinal muscular atrophy, Hoffmann's atrophy, infantile spinal muscular atrophy, progressive spinal muscular atrophy of infants, Werdnig-Hoffmann paralysis.** See also **floppy infant syndrome.**

Werdnig-Hoffmann paralysis See **Werdnig-Hoffmann disease.**

Werlhof's disease See **thrombocytopenic purpura.**

Wernicke's encephalopathy An inflammatory, hemorrhagic, degenerative condition of the brain that is characterized by lesions in several parts of the brain including the hypothalamus, mamillary bodies, and tissues surrounding ventricles and aqueducts. Characteristics of the condition include double vision, involuntary and rapid movements of the eyes, lack of muscular coordination, and decreased mental function, which may be mild or severe. Wernicke's encephalopathy is caused by a thiamine deficiency and is seen in association with chronic alcoholism. It also occurs as a complication of gastrointestinal tract disease and hyperemesis gravidarum owing to malabsorption and malnutrition.

West African sleeping sickness See **Gambian trypanosomiasis.**

western equine encephalitis (WEE) See **equine encephalitis.**

West nomogram A nomogram used in estimating the body surface area of children or adults. See also **nomogram.**

wet cough *Nontechnical.* See **productive cough.**

wet dream See **nocturnal emission.**

wet dressing A moist dressing used to relieve symptoms of some skin diseases. As the moisture evaporates, it cools and dries the skin beneath it, softens dried blood and sera, and stimulates drainage. Medication such as povidone-iodine may be added if necessary.

wet lung An abnormal condition of the lungs, characterized by a persistent cough and rales at the lung bases. It occurs in workers exposed to pulmonary irritants, as ammonia, chlorine, sulfur dioxide, volatile organic acids, dusts, and vapors of corrosive chemicals. Treatment consists of removing the person from exposure to the irritant and therapy for possible pulmonary edema. Compare **pulmonary edema.** See also **pleural effusion, pleurisy.**

wet nurse A woman who cares for and breast-feeds another's infant.

W/F Symbol for white female, often used in the initial identifying statement in a patient record.

Wharton's jelly A gelatinous tissue that remains when the embryonic body stalk blends with the yolk sac within the umbilical cord.

wheal A raised, firm lesion with intense localized skin edema, varying in size and shape, and transient in occurrence. It disappears in hours. An example is a hive.

wheat weevil disease A hypersensitivity pneumonitis caused by allergy to weevil particles found in wheat flour.

wheelchair A mobile chair equipped with large wheels and brakes. If long-term use of the chair is expected, a physical therapist may prescribe certain personalized requirements, as size, left- or right-hand propulsion, type of brakes, height of armrests, special seat pads, and various other features.

wheeze 1. A form of rhonchus, characterized by a high-pitched musical quality. It is caused by a high velocity flow of air through a narrowed airway and is heard both during inspiration and expiration. Wheezes are associated with asthma and chronic bronchitis. Unilateral wheezes are characteristic of bronchogenic carcinoma, foreign bodies, and inflammatory stenosing lesions. An asthmatoid wheeze is caused by an obstruction in the trachea or bronchus. 2. To breathe with a wheeze. See also **rale, rhonchi.**

whiplash injury *Informal.* An injury to the cervical vertebrae or their supporting ligaments and muscles causing pain and stiffness, which usually results from sudden acceleration or deceleration of the body, as in a rear-end car collision.

Whipple's disease A rare intestinal disease characterized by severe intestinal malabsorption, steatorrhea, anemia, weight loss, arthritis, and arthralgia. Persons with the disease are severely malnourished and have abdominal pain, chest pain, and a chronic nonproductive cough. The diagnosis is made by jejunal biopsy. Penicillin and tetracycline may alleviate the symptoms. See also **malabsorption syndrome.**

whipworm See *Trichuris.*

whirlpool bath The immersion of the body or a part of the body in a tank of hot water agitated by a jet of equally hot water and air.

white blood cell (WBC) See leukocyte.

white cell *Informal.* White blood cell. See leukocyte.

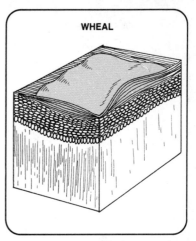

WHEAL

white corpuscle See leukocyte.

white damp See **damp.**

white fibrocartilage A mixture of tough, white fibrous tissue and flexible cartilaginous tissue. It is one of the three kinds of cartilage in the body and is divided into interarticular fibrocartilage, connecting fibrocartilage, circumferential fibrocartilage, and stratiform fibrocartilage. Compare **hyaline cartilage, yellow cartilage.**

whitehead See **milia.**

white leg See **phlegmasia alba dolens.**

white substance The tissue surrounding the gray substance of the spinal cord, consisting of many myelinated nerve fibers and unmyelinated nerve fibers, embedded in a spongy network of neuroglia. It is subdivided in each half of the spinal cord into three funiculi: the anterior, the posterior, and the lateral white column. Each column subdivides into tracts that are closely associated in function. The anterior column divides into two ascending tracts and five descending tracts. The posterior column divides into two large ascending tracts, one small descending tract, and one intersegmental tract. The lateral column divides into six ascending tracts and four descending tracts. Also called **white matter.** Compare **gray substance.** See also **spinal cord, spinal tract.**

white thrombus 1. An aggregation of blood platelets, fibrin, clotting factors, and cellular elements containing few or no erythrocytes. 2. A thrombus comprised chiefly of white blood cells. 3. A thrombus composed primarily of blood platelets and fibrin.

whitlow An inflammation of the end of a finger or toe that results in suppuration. See also **felon.**

WHO *abbr* World Health Organization.

whole blood Blood that is unmodified except for the presence of an anticoagulant. It is used for transfusion. Various components and factors may be separated from whole blood for infusion to replace or to augment a component

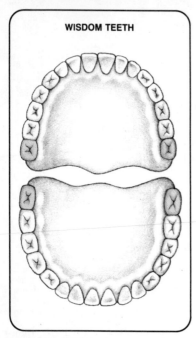

WISDOM TEETH

or factor that is deficient in amount or function owing to a variety of diseases and conditions.

whooping cough   See **pertussis.**

whorl   A spiral turn, as one of the turns of the cochlea or of the dermal ridges that form fingerprints.

WIA   *abbr* **waking imagined analgesia.**

Widal test   An agglutination test used to aid in the diagnosis of salmonella infections, as typhoid fever. A fourfold increase in titer of agglutinins is highly suggestive of active infection. A high titer may persist for years after the disease or after immunization against typhoid fever.

wild-type gene   A normal or standard form of a gene, as contrasted with a mutant form.

will   **1.** The mental faculty that enables one consciously to choose or decide upon a course of action. **2.** The act or process of exercising the power of choice. **3.** A wish, desire, or deliberate intention. **4.** A disposition or attitude toward another or others. **5.** Determination or purpose; willfulness.

Willis's circle   See **circle of Willis.**

Willis's disease   See **diabetes mellitus.**

willow fracture   See **greenstick fracture.**

Wilms' tumor   A malignant neoplasm of the kidney, occurring in children, before the 5th year in 75% of the cases. The most frequent early sign of this large, malignant tumor is hypertension, followed by the appearance of a palpable mass, pain, and hematuria. Diagnosis usually can be established by an excretory urogram with tomography. The tumor, an embryonal adenomyosarcoma, is well encapsulated in the early

stage, but it may later extend into lymph nodes and the renal vein or vena cava and metastasize to the lungs or other sites. Prompt removal of resectable tumors by transperitoneal nephrectomy is recommended. Radiotherapy is used preoperatively or postoperatively; it may be used palliatively in inoperable cases. Cyclic chemotherapy, combined with surgery and irradiation, is proving highly effective.

Wilson's disease   A rare, inherited disorder of copper metabolism, in which copper accumulates slowly in the liver and is then released and taken up in other parts of the body. Hemolysis, then hemolytic anemia occur as the copper accumulates in the red blood cells. Accumulation in the brain destroys certain tissue and may cause tremors, muscle rigidity, dysarthria, and dementia. Kidney function is diminished; the liver becomes cirrhotic. Treatment of Wilson's disease includes a reduction of copper in the diet and the prescription of copper-binding agents and penicillamine. Also called **hepatolenticular degeneration.**

Winckel's disease   See **hemoglobinuria.**

wind chill   The loss of heat from the body when it is exposed to wind of a given speed at a given temperature and humidity. The **wind-chill index** is expressed in kilocalories per hour per square meter of skin surface. The **wind-chill factor** is expressed in degrees Celsius or Fahrenheit as the effective temperature felt by a person exposed to the weather.

winding sheet   A shroud for wrapping a dead body.

window   A surgically created opening in the surface of a structure or an anatomically occurring opening in the surface of or between the chambers of a structure.

windowed   Of an orthopedic cast: having an opening, especially to relieve pressure that may irritate and inflame the skin.

winter cough   *Nontechnical.* A chronic condition characterized by a persistent cough occasioned by cold weather. See also **cough.**

winter itch   Pruritus occurring in cold weather in people who have dry skin, particularly in those who have atopic dermatitis. Warmer temperature, increased humidity, and topical, antipruritic emollients may offer relief.

wiry pulse   An abnormal pulse that is strong but small.

wisdom tooth   Either of the last teeth on each side of the upper and lower jaw. These are third molars and are the last teeth to erupt, usually between the ages of 17 and 21, often causing considerable pain, dental problems, and the need for extraction. Also called **dens serotinus.** See also **molar.**

wish fulfillment   **1.** The gratification of a desire. **2.** In psychology: the satisfaction of a desire or the release of emotional tension through such processes as dreams, daydreams, and neurotic symptoms. **3.** In psychoanalysis: one of the primary motivations for dreams in which an unconscious desire or urge, unacceptable to the ego and superego because of sociocultural restrictions or feelings of personal guilt, is given expression.

wishful thinking   The interpretation of facts or situations according to one's desires or wishes rather than as they exist in reality, usually used as an unconscious device to avoid painful or unpleasant feelings.

Wiskott-Aldrich syndrome   Immunodeficiency inherited as a recessive, X-linked trait, characterized by thrombocytopenia, eczema, inadequate T and B cell function, and an increased susceptibility to viral, bacterial, and fungal infections and to cancer. Treatment includes the prescription of appropriate antibiotics for specific infectious organisms and the administration of transfer factor from activated lymphocytes to increase the resistance to infection and to clear the eczema. See also **transfer factor.**

witch hazel   **1.** A shrub, *Hamamelis virginiana,* indigenous to North America, from which an astringent extract is derived. **2.** A solution comprised of the extract, alcohol, and water, used as an astringent. Also called **hamamelis water.**

witch's milk   A milklike substance secreted from the breast of the newborn, caused by circulating maternal lactating hormone. Also called **hexenmilch.**

withdrawal   **1.** A common response to physical danger or severe stress characterized by a state of apathy, lethargy, depression, retreat into oneself, and, in grave cases, catatonia and stupor. It is pathologic if it interferes with a person's perception of reality and the ability to function in society, as in the various forms of schizophrenia. See also **schizophrenia. 2.** The removal of the penis from the vagina in sexual intercourse prior to ejaculation in an attempt to prevent conception. Withdrawal is not an effective method of contraception. Also called **coitus interruptus.**

withdrawal bleeding   The passage of blood from the uterus, associated with the shedding of endometrium that has been stimulated and maintained by hormonal medication. It occurs when the medication is discontinued. In the endocrine evaluation of a woman with amenorrhea, withdrawal bleeding constitutes evidence that the woman's endometrium is reponsive to hormonal stimulation and that the cause of her amenorrhea is probably not uterine.

withdrawal method   A contraceptive technique in coitus wherein the penis is pulled from the vagina prior to ejaculation. It is not reliable because small amounts of seminal fluid carrying millions of spermatozoa may be emitted without sensation prior to full ejaculation. Also called **coitus interruptus.**

withdrawal symptoms   The unpleasant, sometimes life-threatening physiologic changes that occur when certain drugs are withdrawn after prolonged, regular use. The effects may occur following use of a narcotic, tranquilizer, stimulant, barbiturate, alcohol, or other substance to which the person has become physi-

ologically or psychologically addicted. See symptom.

withdrawn behavior   A condition in which there is a blunting of the emotions and a lack of social responsiveness.

Wittmaack-Ekbom syndrome   See **restless legs syndrome.**

W/M   Symbol for white male, often used in the initial identifying statement in a patient record.

W/N   Symbol for well-nourished, often used in the initial identifying statement in a patient record. It is used so frequently as to have lost all meaning or use in identifying or describing the patient.

Wolffian body   See **mesonephros.**

Wolffian duct   See **mesonephric duct.**

Wolff-Parkinson-White syndrome   A disorder of atrioventricular conduction, characterized by two AV conduction pathways. This syndrome is often identified by a characteristic delta wave seen on an electrocardiogram. See also **Lown-Ganong-Levine syndrome.**

wolfram (W)   See **tungsten.**

woman-year   In statistics: a year in the reproductive life of a sexually active woman; a unit that represents 12 months of exposure to the risk of pregnancy. Woman-years are used in calculating a pregnancy rate in the assessment of the effectiveness of the various methods of family planning and of the adverse effect on the birth rate of various environmental factors.

womb   See **uterus.**

wood alcohol   See **methanol.**

Wood's glass   A nickel-oxide filter that holds back all light except for a few violet rays of the visible spectrum and ultraviolet wavelengths of about 365 nanometers. It is used extensively to help diagnose fungus infections of the scalp and erythrasma and to reveal porphyrins and fluorescent materials.

Wood's light   An ultraviolet light used to diagnose certain scalp and skin diseases. The light causes hairs infected with a fungus, as *tinea capitis,* to become brilliantly fluorescent. Also called Wood's lamp, Wood's rays.

woolsorter's disease   The pulmonary form of anthrax, so named because it is an occupational hazard to those who handle sheep's wool. Early symptoms mimic influenza, but the patient soon develops high fever, respiratory distress, and cyanosis. If the disease is not treated at this stage, it is often fatal. Also called **pulmonary anthrax.** See also **anthrax.**

word association   See **controlled association.**

word association test   See **association test.**

word salad   A jumble of words and phrases that lacks logical coherence and meaning, often characteristic of disoriented individuals and schizophrenics.

work therapy   A therapeutic approach in which the client performs a useful activity or learns an occupation, as in occupational therapy.

work tolerance   The kind and amount of

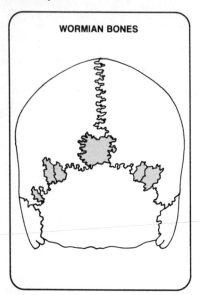

WORMIAN BONES

work that a physically or mentally ill person can or should perform.

work-up   The process of performing a complete evaluation of a patient, including history, physical examination, laboratory tests, and X-ray or other diagnostic procedures in order to acquire an accurate data base upon which a diagnosis and treatment plan may be based.

World Health Organization (WHO)   An agency of the United Nations, affiliated with the Food and Agricultural Organization of the UN, the International Atomic Energy Agency, the International Labor Organization, the Pan American Health Organization, and UNESCO. The WHO is primarily concerned with worldwide or regional health problems, but in emergencies it is authorized to render local assistance on request. Its functions include furnishing technical assistance, stimulating and advancing epidemiologic investigation of diseases, recommending health regulations, promoting cooperation among scientific and professional health groups, and providing information and counsel relating to health matters. Its headquarters are in Geneva, Switzerland. Also called **Organisation Mondiale de la Santé, OMS.**

worm   Any of the soft-bodied, elongated invertebrates of the phyla Annelida, Nemathelminthes, or Platyhelminthes. Some parasitic worms that affect humans are **hookworm, pinworm, tapeworm.** See also **fluke, roundworm.**

wormian bone   Any of several tiny, smooth, segmented bones that are soft, moist, and tepid to the touch, usually found as the serrated borders of the sutures between the cranial bones. Wormian bones were named for the Danish anatomist Claus Worm.

wound   **1.** Any physical injury involving a break in the skin, usually caused by an act or accident rather than by a disease, as a chest wound, gunshot wound, or puncture wound. **2.** To cause an injury, especially one that breaks the skin.

wound irrigation   Rinsing a wound or the cavity formed by a wound using a medicated solution, water, or an antimicrobial liquid preparation.

NURSING CONSIDERATIONS: Wounds are irrigated in order to remove secretions and dried blood and to keep the wound surface open in order to encourage healing from the inside out. When the irrigation solution returns clear, the wound is considered clean. Frequency of irrigation, type of solution, and amount of solution to be used are specifically prescribed. The condition of the wound, amount of irrigating solution used, and the appearance of the returned solution are noted by the nurse.

Wright's stain   A stain containing methylene blue and eosin, used to color blood specimens for microscopic examination, as for complete blood count and for malarial parasites.

wrist   See **carpus.**

wrist joint   See **radiocarpal articulation.**

writer's cramp   A painful involuntary contraction of the muscles of the hand when attempting to write. It often occurs following long periods of writing. Also called **graphospasm.**

wrongful death statute   In law: a statute existing in all states that provides that the death of a person can give rise to a cause of legal action brought by the person's beneficiaries in a civil suit against the person whose willful or negligent acts caused the death. Prior to the existence of these statutes, a suit could be brought only if the injured person survived the injury.

wrongful life action   In law: a civil suit usually brought against a physician or health facility on the basis of negligence that resulted in the wrongful birth or life of an infant. The parents of the unwanted child seek to obtain payment from the defendant for the medical expenses of pregnancy and delivery, for pain and suffering, and for the education and upbringing of the child. Wrongful life actions have been brought and won in several situations, including malpracticed tubal ligations, vasectomies, and abortions. Failure to diagnose pregnancy in time for abortion and incorrect medical advice leading to the birth of a defective child have also led to malpractice suits for a wrongful life.

wryneck   See **torticollis.**

Wuchereria   A genus of filarial worms found in tropical climates. *Wuchereria bancrofti,* transmitted by mosquitoes, is the cause of elephantiasis. See also **filariasis.**

X Symbol for Kienbock's unit of X-ray exposure.

xanthelasma palpebrarum See **xanthoma palpebrarum.**

xanthelasmatosis A disseminated, generalized form of planar xanthoma frequently associated with reticuloendothelial disorders, especially multiple myeloma.

xanthemia See **carotenemia.**

xanthine A nitrogenous by-product of the metabolism of nucleoproteins. It is normally found in the muscles, liver, spleen, pancreas, and urine. —**xanthic,** *adj.*

xanthine derivative Any one of the closely related alkaloids caffeine, theobromine, or theophylline. They are found in plants widely distributed geographically and are variously ingested as components in different beverages, as coffee, tea, cocoa, and cola drinks. The xanthine derivatives or methylxanthines stimulate the central nervous system, produce diuresis, and relax smooth muscles.

xanthinuria 1. The presence of excessive quantities of xanthine in the urine. 2. A rare disorder of purine metabolism, resulting in the excretion of large amounts of xanthine in the urine owing to the absence of an enzyme, xanthine oxidase, that is necessary in xanthine metabolism. This inherited deficiency may cause the development of kidney stones made of xanthine precipitate.

xantho- A combining form meaning 'yellow'.

xanthochromic, xanthochromatic Having a yellow color, as cerebrospinal fluid that contains blood or bile.

xanthogranuloma, *pl.* **xanthogranulomas, xanthogranulomata** A tumor or nodule of granulation tissue containing lipid deposits. A kind of xanthogranuloma is **juvenile xanthogranuloma.**

xanthoma, *pl.* **xanthomas, xanthomata** A benign, fatty, fibrous, yellow plaque, nodule, or tumor that develops in the subcutaneous layer of skin, often around tendons. The lesion is characterized by the intracellular accumulation of cholesterol and cholesterol esters.

xanthoma disseminatum A benign, chronic condition in which small orange or brown papules and nodules develop on many body surfaces, especially on the mucous membrane of the oropharynx, larynx, and bronchi, and in skin folds and fissures. Also called **xanthoma multiplex.**

xanthoma eruptivum See **eruptive xanthoma.**

xanthoma multiplex See **xanthoma disseminatum.**

xanthoma palpebrarum A soft, yellow spot or plaque usually occurring in groups on the eyelids. Also called **xanthelasma palpebrarum.**

xanthoma planum See **planar xanthoma.**

xanthomasarcoma A giant cell sarcoma of the tendon sheaths and aponeuroses which contains xanthoma cells.

xanthoma striatum palmare A yellow or orange, flat plaque or slightly raised nodule occurring in groups on the palms of the hands.

xanthoma tendinosum A yellow or orange, elevated or flat, round papule or nodule that usually occurs in clusters on tendons, especially the extensor tendons of the hands and feet, of individuals with hereditary lipid storage disease.

xanthomatosis An abnormal condition in which there are deposits of yellow fatty material in the skin, internal organs, and reticuloendothelial system. It may be associated with hyperlipoproteinemia, paraproteinemia, lipid storage diseases, and other disorders of adipose tissue. Also called **xanthosis.** See also **hyperlipidemia, xanthoma, xanthoma palpebrarum.**

xanthoma tuberosum A yellow or orange, flat or elevated, round papule occurring in clusters on the skin of joints, especially the elbows and knees, usually in people who have a hereditary lipid storage disease, as hyperlipoproteinemia. The xanthomatous papules may also be associated with biliary cirrhosis and myxedema. Also called **tuberous xanthoma, xanthoma tuberosum multiplex.**

xanthopsia An abnormal visual condition in which everything appears to have a yellow hue. It is sometimes associated with jaundice or digitalis toxicity.

xanthosis 1. A yellow discoloration sometimes seen in degenerating tissues of malignant diseases. 2. See **xanthomatosis.** 3. A reversible yellow discoloration of the skin most commonly caused by the ingestion of large amounts of yellow vegetables containing carotene pigment. The antimalarial drug quinacrine, if taken over a prolonged period, may produce a similar skin color. Xanthosis may be differentiated clinically from jaundice since the sclerae are yellowed in jaundice but not in xanthosis. Also called **carotenosis.** See also **carotenemia.**

xanthureic acid A metabolite of tryptophan that occurs in normal urine and in elevated levels in patients with vitamin B$_6$ deficiency.

X chromosome A sex chromosome that in humans and many other species is present in both sexes, appearing singly in the cells of nor-

XIPHOID PROCESS

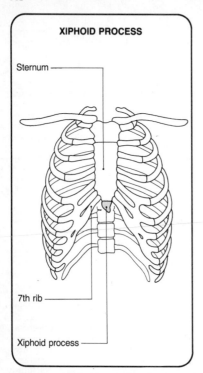

Sternum

7th rib

Xiphoid process

sitivity to ultraviolet light, exposure to which results in freckles, telangiectases, keratoses, papillomas, carcinoma, and, possibly, melanoma. Keratitis and tumors developing on the eyelids and cornea may result in blindness. Exposure to sunlight must be avoided.

xerogram   An X-ray image produced by xeroradiography.

xeroradiography   A diagnostic X-ray technique in which an image is produced electrically rather than chemically, permitting lower exposure times and radiation of lower energy than that of ordinary X-rays. It is used most commonly to discover breast tumors.

X-inactivation theory   See **Lyon hypothesis.**

xerosis   See **dry skin.**

xiphi-   See **xipho.**

xiphisternal articulation   The cartilaginous connection between the xiphoid process and the body of the sternum. This joint usually ossifies at puberty. Compare **manubriosternal articulation.**

xiphisternum   See **xiphoid process.**

xipho-, xiphi-   A combining form meaning 'pertaining to a sword or to the xiphoid process': *xiphodymus, xiphoiditis, xiphopagus.*

xiphoid appendix   See **xiphoid process.**

xiphoid process   The smallest of three parts of the sternum, articulating caudally with the body of the sternum and laterally with the seventh rib. Several muscles of the abdominal wall are attached to the xiphoid process, including the rectus abdominis and the linea alba. Also called **ensiform process, xiphisternum, xiphoid appendix.** Compare **manubrium.**

X-linked   Pertaining to genes or to the characteristics or conditions they transmit that are carried on the X chromosome. Most X-linked traits and conditions, as hemophilia, are recessive and therefore occur predominantly in males, since they have only one X chromosome. Women may inherit the genes but the recessive effects are usually masked by the normal dominant alleles carried on the second X chromosome. Compare **Y-linked.** See also **sex-linked disorder.** —**X linkage,** *n.*

X-linked dominant inheritance   A pattern of inheritance in which the transmission of a dominant gene on the X chromosome causes a characteristic to be manifested. Affected individuals all have an affected parent. All of the daughters of an affected male are affected but none of the sons. Half of the sons and half of the daughters of an affected female are affected. Normal children of an affected parent have normal offspring. The inheritance shows a clear positive family history. Hypophosphatemic vitamin D-resistant rickets is an example of this pattern. X-linked dominant inheritance closely resembles autosomal dominant inheritance. Compare **X-linked recessive inheritance.**

X-linked ichthyosis   See **sex-linked ichthyosis.**

X-linked inheritance   A pattern of inheritance in which the transmission of traits varies

mal males and in duplicate in the cells of normal females. The chromosome is carried as a sex determinant by all of the female gametes and half of all male gametes, is morphologically much larger than the Y chromosome, and has many sex-linked genes associated with clinically significant disorders, as hemophilia, Duchenne's muscular dystrophy, and Hunter's syndrome. Compare **Y chromosome.** See also **X-linked.**

Xe   Symbol for **xenon.**

xeno-   A combining form meaning 'strange or pertaining to foreign matter': *xenodiagnosis, xenogenous, xenology.*

xenogenesis   1. Alternation of generations; heterogenesis. 2. The theoretical production of offspring that are totally different from both of the parents. —**xenogenetic, xenogenic,** *adj.*

xenograft   See **heterograft.**

xenon (Xe)   An inert, gaseous, nonmetallic element. Its atomic number is 54; its atomic weight is 131.30.

xenophobia   An anxiety disorder characterized by a pervasive, irrational fear or uneasiness in the presence of strangers, especially foreigners, or in new surroundings. See also **phobia.**

xero-   A combining form meaning 'pertaining to dryness': *xerocheilia, xeromenia, xerophthalmia.*

xeroderma   A chronic skin condition characterized by dryness and roughness.

xeroderma pigmentosum   A rare, inherited skin disease characterized by extreme sen-

according to the sex of the person, because the genes on the X chromosome have no counterparts on the Y chromosome. The inheritance pattern may be recessive or dominant. The characteristic determined by a gene on the X chromosome is always expressed in males. Transmission from father to son does not occur. Compare **autosomal inheritance.** See also **X-linked dominant inheritance, X-linked recessive inheritance.**

X-linked mucopolysaccharidosis See Hunter's syndrome.

X-linked recessive inheritance A pattern of inheritance in which transmission of an abnormal recessive gene on the X chromosome results in a carrier state in females and characteristics of the condition in males. Affected people have unaffected parents (except for the rare situation in which the father is affected and the mother is a carrier). Half of the female siblings of an affected male carry the trait. Unaffected male siblings do not carry the trait. Sons of affected males are unaffected and daughters of affected males are carriers. Unaffected male children of a carrier female do not carry the trait.

XO In genetics: the designation for the presence of only one sex chromosome; either the X or Y chromosome is missing so that each cell is monosomic and contains a total of 45 chromosomes. See also **Turner's syndrome.**

X-ray **1.** Electromagnetic radiation of shorter wavelength than visible light. X-rays are produced when electrons, traveling at high speed, strike certain materials, particularly heavy metals like tungsten. They can penetrate most substances and are used to investigate the integrity of certain structures, to therapeutically destroy diseased tissue, and to make photographic images for diagnostic purposes, as in radiography and fluoroscopy. Also called **roentgen ray. 2.** A radiograph made by projecting X-rays through organs or structures of the body onto a photographic plate. As some tissue, like bone, is more radiopaque (allowing fewer X-rays to pass through) than other tissue, like skin or fat, a shadow is created on the plate that is the image of a bone or of a cavity filled with a radiopaque substance. **3.** To make a radiograph. See also **contrast medium, electron, fluoroscopy, radiopaque. —X-ray,** *adj.*

X-ray microscope A microscope that produces images by X-rays and records them on fine-grain film or projects them as enlargements. Film images produced by X-ray microscopes may be examined at quite large magnifications with a light microscope.

X-ray pelvimetry A radiographic examination used to determine the dimensions of the female pelvis and, if fetal position permits, the biparietal diameter of the fetal head, performed when there is doubt that the head can pass safely through the pelvis in labor. Because minor degrees of cephalopelvic disproportion are often overcome safely in labor by molding of the fetal skull, and because major disproportions may be detected by clinical pelvimetry or by ultrasonography, the value of X-ray pelvimetry often does not warrant the risk of radiation exposure. Compare **clinical pelvimetry.** See also **cephalopelvic disproportion, contraction, dystocia.**

XX In genetics: the designation for the normal sex chromosome complement in the human female. See also **X chromosome.**

XXY syndrome See **Klinefelter's syndrome.**

XY In genetics: the designation for the normal sex chromosome complement in the human male. See also **X chromosome, Y chromosome.**

xylitol A sweet, crystalline pentahydroxy alcohol obtained by the reduction of xylose and used as an artificial sweetener.

xylo- A combining form meaning 'pertaining to wood': *xyloketosuria, xylose, xylosuria.*

xylometazoline hydrochloride A vasoconstrictor used to relieve nasal congestion.

XYY syndrome The phenotypic manifestation of an extra Y chromosome, which has a positive effect on height and may have a negative effect on mental and psychological development. See also **trisomy.**

Y   Symbol for **yttrium.**

yaws   A nonvenereal infection caused by the spirochete *Treponema pertenue*, transmitted by direct contact and characterized by chronic, ulcerating sores anywhere on the body with eventual tissue and bone destruction, leading to crippling if untreated. It is a disease of unsanitary tropical living conditions and may be effectively treated with penicillin G. All serologic tests for syphilis may be positive in yaws. The infection may afford protection against syphilis. Also called **bouba, buba, frambesia, parangi, patek, pian.** Compare **bejel, pinta, syphilis.**

Yb   Symbol for **ytterbium.**

Y chromosome   A sex chromosome that in humans and many other species is present only in the male, appearing singly in the normal male. It is carried as a sex determinant by half of the male gametes and none of the female gametes, is morphologically much smaller than the X chromosome, and has genes associated with triggering the development and differentiation of male characteristics. There are no known medically significant traits or conditions associated with the genes on the Y chromosome. Compare **X chromosome.**

yeast   Any unicellular, usually oval, nucleated fungus that reproduces by budding. *Candida albicans* is a kind of yeast that can cause fungal infection in humans. See **candidiasis.**

yellow cartilage   The most elastic of the three kinds of cartilage, consisting of elastic fibers in a flexible, fibrous matrix. It is located in various parts of the body, as the external ear, the auditory tube, the epiglottis, and the larynx. Also called **elastic cartilage.** Compare **hyaline cartilage, white fibrocartilage.**

yellow fever   An acute arbovirus infection transmitted by mosquitoes, characterized by headache, fever, jaundice, vomiting, and bleeding. There is no specific treatment and mortality is about 5%. Recovery is followed by lifelong immunity. Immunization for travelers to endemic areas is advised. Nonhuman primates are a reservoir of infection.

yellow fever vaccine   A vaccine produced from live, attenuated yellow fever virus grown in chick embryos and used for immunization against yellow fever. Immunosuppression, pregnancy, or known hypersensitivity to chicken or egg protein prohibits its use. Among the more serious adverse effects are fever, malaise, and hypersensitivity reactions.

yellow marrow   See **bone marrow.**

Yersinia arthritis   A polyarticular inflammation occurring a few days to 1 month after the onset of infection caused by *Yersinia enterocolitica* or *Y. pseudotuberculosis* and usually persisting longer than a month. Knees, ankles, toes, fingers, and wrists are most often affected. Cultures of synovial fluid yield no infectious organism. The clinical presentation may mimic juvenile rheumatoid arthritis, rheumatic fever, or Reiter's syndrome and may be associated with erythema nodosum or erythema multiforme. Treatment is with antibiotics.

Yersinia pestis   A small, gram-negative bacillus that causes plague. The primary host is the rat, but other small rodents also harbor the organism. A person without symptoms may be a carrier, but this happens rarely. *Yersinia pestis* is hardy, living for long periods in infected carcasses, the soil of the host's habitat, or in sputum. Also called ***Pasteurella pestis.*** See also **plague.**

Y fracture   A Y-shaped intercondylar fracture.

-yl   A combining form used in naming radicals: *benzoyl, ethyl, hydroxyl.*

Y-linked   Pertaining to genes or to the characteristics or conditions they transmit that are carried on the Y chromosome. Such traits, as hypertrichosis of the pinna of the ear, can be expressed only in males. Compare **X-linked.** See also **sex-linked disorder. —Y linkage,** *n.*

yogurt   A slightly acid, semisolid, curdled milk preparation made from either whole or skimmed cow's milk and milk solids by fermentation with organisms from the genus *Lactobacillus.* It is rich in vitamins of the B complex group and a good source of protein. It also provides a medium in the gastrointestinal tract that inhibits the growth of harmful bacteria and aids in the absorption of minerals.

yolk   The nutritive material, rich in fats and proteins, contained in the ovum to supply nourishment to the developing embryo. The amount and distribution of the yolk within the egg depend upon the species of animal and type of reproduction and development of offspring. In humans and most mammals the yolk is absent or greatly diffused through the cell, since embryos absorb nutrients directly from the mother through the placenta. See also **deutoplasm.**

yolk membrane   See **vitelline membrane.**

yolk sac   A structure that develops in the inner cell mass of the embryo and expands into a vesicle with a thick part that becomes the primitive gut and a thin part that grows into the cavity of the chorion. The cells of the extraembryonic mesoderm differentiate to develop endothelium, primitive blood plasma, and hemoglobin. After supplying nourishment for the human embryo, the yolk sac usually disappears during the 7th week of pregnancy. See also **allantois, Meckel's diverticulum.**

yolk sphere   See **morula.**

yolk stalk   The narrow duct connecting the yolk sac with the midgut of the embryo during the early stages of prenatal development. It connects at the region of the future ileum and usually undergoes complete obliteration but occasionally may appear as a diverticulum. Also called **omphalomesenteric duct, vitelline duct.** See also **Meckel's diverticulum.**

Young's rule   A method for the calculation of the approximate dose of a drug for a child of 2 years or more using the formula (age in years) ÷ (age + 12) × adult dose. Many clinicians consider this method obsolete.

Y-plasty   A method of surgical revision of a scar, using a Y-shaped incision to reduce scar contractures. See also **S-plasty, Z-plasty.**

Y-set   A device composed of plastic components, used for delivering intravenous fluids through a primary intravenous line connected to a combination drip chamber-filter section from which two separate plastic tubes lead to fluid sources. The Y-set also includes three clamps, one for the primary intravenous line and one for each of the two separate tubes. It is often used to transfuse packed blood cells that must be diluted with saline solution to decrease their viscosity. Compare **component drip set, component syringe set, microaggregate recipient set, straight-line blood set.**

ytterbium (Yb)   A rare-earth metallic element. Its atomic number is 70; its atomic weight is 173.04.

yttrium (Y)   A scaly, gray metallic element. Its atomic number is 39; its atomic weight is 88.905. Radioactive isotopes of yttrium have been used in cancer therapy.

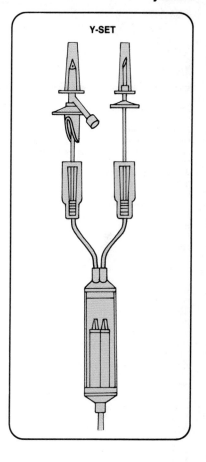

Y-SET

Z

Zahorsky's disease See **roseola infantum.**

Z chromosome A sex chromosome of certain insects, birds, and fishes, appearing singly in normal females of the species and doubly in the males. See also **W chromosome.**

Zenker's diverticulum A circumscribed herniation of the mucous membrane of the pharynx as it joins the esophagus. Food may become trapped in the diverticulum and may be aspirated. Diagnosis is confirmed by X-ray studies. In most cases it is small, causes no dysfunction, is not diagnosed, and requires no treatment.

zero The point on the temperature scale of a thermometer at which the gradations begin. The zero-point of the Celsius (centigrade) and Réamur temperature scales is the freezing point of water; that of the Fahrenheit scale is set at 32 degrees below the freezing point of water.

Ziehl-Neelson stain One of the most widely used methods of acid-fast staining, commonly used in the microscopic examination of a smear of sputum suspected of containing *Mycobacterium tuberculosis.* See also **acid-fast stain.**

ZIG *abbr* **zoster immune globulin.**

zinc (Zn) A blue-white crystalline metal commonly associated with lead ores. Its atomic number is 30; its atomic weight is 65.38. Zinc has many commercial uses, as a protective coating for steel and in printing plates. It is an essential nutrient in the body and is used in numerous pharmaceuticals, as zinc acetate, zinc oxide, zinc permanganate, and zinc stearate.

zinc chill See **metal fume fever.**

zinc deficiency A condition resulting from insufficient amounts of zinc in the diet, characterized by abnormal fatigue, decreased alertness, a decrease in taste and odor sensitivity, poor appetite, retarded growth, delayed sexual maturity, prolonged healing of wounds, and susceptibility to infection and injury. Other conditions that may precipitate the deficiency include alcoholic cirrhosis and other liver diseases, ulcers, myocardial infarction, Hodgkin's disease, mongolism, and cystic fibrosis. Prophylaxis and treatment consist of a diet of foods high in protein and rich in zinc, including meats, eggs, liver, seafood, legumes, nuts, peanut butter, milk, and whole-grain cereals.

zinc gelatin A topical protectant.

zinc oxide A topical astringent, antiseptic, and protectant prescribed for a wide range of minor skin irritations.

zinc salt poisoning A toxic condition caused by the ingestion or inhalation of a zinc salt. Symptoms of ingestion include a burning sensation of the mouth and throat, vomiting, diarrhea, abdominal and chest pain, and, in severe cases, shock and coma. Treatment includes gastric lavage, followed by a demulcent and chelation with calcium edetate, and fluid therapy. Inhalation of zinc salts may cause metal fume fever; skin contact may produce blisters.

zinc sulfate An ophthalmic vasoconstrictor.

ZIP *abbr* zoster immune plasma. See **chickenpox.**

zirconium (Zr) A steel-gray, tetravalent metallic element. Its atomic number is 40; its atomic weight is 91.22. It occurs widely in combined form, especially in zircon and baddeleyite. A component of zirconium dioxide was formerly used in some ointments for the treatment of poison ivy skin rashes, but caused skin granulomas in some individuals. Similar skin conditions developed in individuals using deodorants containing zirconium sodium lactate, and the use of zirconium compounds, except for zirconyl hydroxychloride, has been discontinued in the manufacture of skin ointments. Zirconyl hydroxychloride is still used in antiperspirants.

Zn Symbol for **zinc.**

zoanthropy The delusion that one has assumed the form and characteristics of an animal. —**zoanthropic,** *adj.*

-zoite A combining form meaning a 'simple organism' of a specified sort: *merozoite, saprozoite, sporozoite.*

Zollinger-Ellison syndrome A condition characterized by severe peptic ulceration, gastric hypersecretion, elevated serum gastrin, and gastrinoma of the pancreas or the duodenum. The syndrome is uncommon but not rare; it may occur in early childhood, but is seen more frequently in persons between 20 and 50 years of age. Two thirds of the tumors are malignant. Total gastrectomy may be necessary, but the administration of cimetidine in large doses may control gastric hypersecretion and allow the ulcers to heal. See also **peptic ulcer.**

zomepirac sodium A nonnarcotic analgesic and anti-inflammatory agent.

zona, *pl.* **zonae** A girdlelike, usually striated segment of a rounded or spherical structure. Some kinds of zona are zona arcuata, zona orbicularis, zona pellucida.

zona ciliaris See **ciliary zone.**

zona pellucida The thick, transparent, noncellular membrane that encloses the mammalian ovum. It is secreted by the ovum during its development in the ovary and is retained until near the time of implantation. Also called **oolemma.** See also **vitelline membrane.**

zona radiata A zona pellucida that has a striated appearance caused by radiating canals within the membrane. Also called **zona striata.**

zona striata See **zona radiata.**

Zondek-Ascheim test See **Ascheim-Zondek test.**

zone therapy The treatment of a disorder by mechanical stimulation and counterirritation of a body area in the same longitudinal zone as the affected organ or region.

zooerastia See **bestiality.**

zoogenous Acquired from or originating in animals. See also **zoonosis.**

zoology The study of animal life.

zoomania A psychopathological state characterized by an excessive fondness for and preoccupation with animals. —**zoomaniac,** *n.*

zoonosis A disease of animals that is transmissible to humans from its primary animal host. Kinds of zoonoses are **equine encephalitis, leptospirosis, rabies, yellow fever.**

zooparasite Any parasitic animal organism. Kinds of zooparasites are **arthropod, protozoa, worm.** —**zooparasitic,** *adj.*

zoophilia, zoophilism 1. An abnormal fondness for animals. **2.** In psychiatry: a psychosexual disorder in which sexual excitement and gratification are derived from the fondling of animals or from the fantasy or act of engaging in sexual activity with animals. See also **paraphilia.** —**zoophile,** *n.,* **zoophilic, zoophilous,** *adj.*

zoopsia A visual hallucination of animals or insects, often occurring in delirium tremens.

zootoxin A poisonous substance from an animal, as the venom of snakes, spiders, and scorpions. —**zootoxic,** *adj.*

zoster See **herpes zoster.**

zosteriform Resembling the pocks seen in herpes zoster infection.

zoster immune globulin (ZIG) A passive immunizing agent currently in limited use for preventing or attenuating herpes zoster virus infection in immunosuppressed individuals who are at great risk of severe herpes zoster virus infection.

Z-plasty A method of surgical revision of a scar or closure of a wound using a Z-shaped incision to reduce contractures of the adjacent skin. See also **S-plasty, Y-plasty.**

Z-track An intramuscular injection technique in which the patient's skin is pulled in such a way that the needle track is sealed off after the injection. The technique is done to minimize subcutaneous irritation and discoloration.

Zr Symbol for **zirconium.**

zygogenesis 1. The formation of a zygote. **2.** Reproduction by the union of gametes. —**zygogenetic, zygogenic,** *adj.*

zygoma 1. A long, slender zygomatic process of the temporal bone, arising from the lower part of the squamous portion of the temporal bone, passing forward to join the zygomatic bone, and forming part of the zygomatic arch. **2.** The zygomatic bone that forms the prominence of the cheek.

zygomatic bone One of the pair of bones

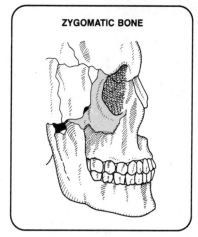

ZYGOMATIC BONE

that forms the prominence of the cheek, the lower part of the orbit of the eye, and parts of the temporal and infratemporal fossae.

zygomatic head See **zygomaticus minor.**

zygomaticus major One of the 12 muscles of the mouth. Arising from the zygomatic bone and inserting into the corner of the mouth, it is innervated by buccal branches of the facial nerve and acts to draw the angle of the mouth up and back to smile or laugh. Also called zygomaticus. Compare **zygomaticus minor.**

zygomaticus minor One of the 12 muscles of the mouth. Arising from the malar surface of the zygomatic bone and inserting into the upper lip, it is innervated by buccal branches of the facial nerve and acts to deepen the nasolabial furrow in a sad facial expression. Also called **quadratus labii superioris, zygomatic head.** Compare **zygomaticus major.**

zygomycosis An acute, often fulminant and sometimes fatal fungous infection caused by a class of water mold, seen primarily in patients with chronic debilitating diseases, especially uncontrolled diabetes mellitus. Characteristically, it begins with fever and with pain and discharge in the nose and paranasal sinuses that progresses to invade the eye and lower respiratory tract. The fungus may enter blood vessels and spread to the brain and other organs. Transmission is usually by inhalation. The diagnosis is confirmed by biopsy and pathologic examination of sputum. Treatment includes improved control of diabetes mellitus, extensive debridement of craniofacial lesions, and amphotericin B administered intravenously. Also called **mucormycosis.** Compare **phycomycosis.**

zygote In embryology: the developing ovum from the time it is fertilized until, as a blastocyst, it is implanted in the uterus.

zygotene The second stage in the first meiotic prophase of gametogenesis in which synapsis of homologous chromosomes occurs. See also **diakinesis, diplotene, leptotene, pachytene.**

zymogenic cell See **chief cell.**

Appendices

Color Atlas of Human Anatomy

Drug Interactions

HEAD, EAR, AND NECK

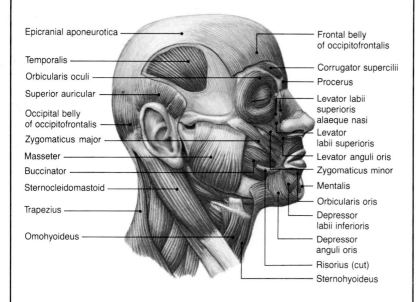

Epicranial aponeurotica

Temporalis

Orbicularis oculi

Superior auricular

Occipital belly
of occipitofrontalis

Zygomaticus major

Masseter

Buccinator

Sternocleidomastoid

Trapezius

Omohyoideus

Frontal belly
of occipitofrontalis

Corrugator supercilii

Procerus

Levator labii
superioris
alaeque nasi

Levator
labii superioris

Levator anguli oris

Zygomaticus minor

Mentalis

Orbicularis oris

Depressor
labii inferioris

Depressor
anguli oris

Risorius (cut)

Sternohyoideus

LATERAL VIEW

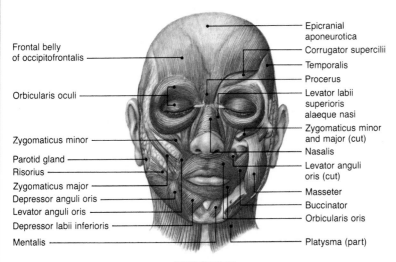

Frontal belly
of occipitofrontalis

Orbicularis oculi

Zygomaticus minor

Parotid gland

Risorius

Zygomaticus major

Depressor anguli oris

Levator anguli oris

Depressor labii inferioris

Mentalis

Epicranial
aponeurotica

Corrugator supercilii

Temporalis

Procerus

Levator labii
superioris
alaeque nasi

Zygomaticus minor
and major (cut)

Nasalis

Levator anguli
oris (cut)

Masseter

Buccinator

Orbicularis oris

Platysma (part)

ANTERIOR VIEW

App

MUSCLES

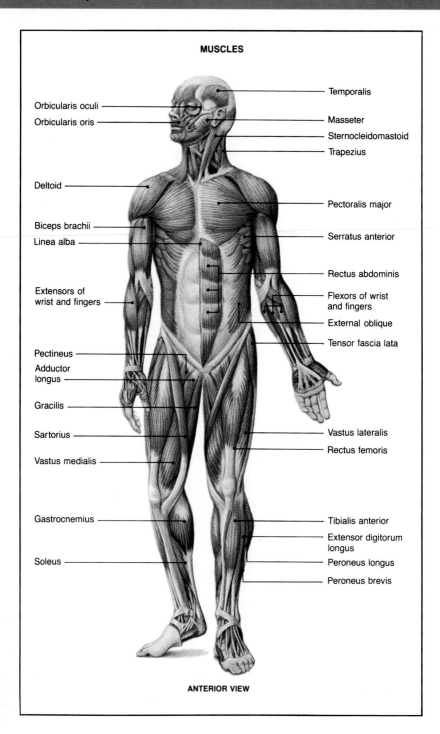

Orbicularis oculi

Orbicularis oris

Deltoid

Biceps brachii

Linea alba

Extensors of
wrist and fingers

Pectineus

Adductor
longus

Gracilis

Sartorius

Vastus medialis

Gastrocnemius

Soleus

Temporalis

Masseter

Sternocleidomastoid

Trapezius

Pectoralis major

Serratus anterior

Rectus abdominis

Flexors of wrist
and fingers

External oblique

Tensor fascia lata

Vastus lateralis

Rectus femoris

Tibialis anterior

Extensor digitorum
longus

Peroneus longus

Peroneus brevis

ANTERIOR VIEW

MUSCLES

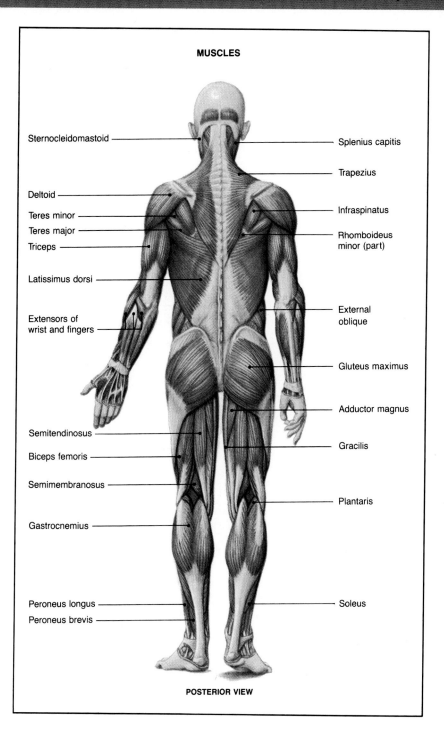

Sternocleidomastoid

Deltoid

Teres minor

Teres major

Triceps

Latissimus dorsi

Extensors of
wrist and fingers

Semitendinosus

Biceps femoris

Semimembranosus

Gastrocnemius

Peroneus longus

Peroneus brevis

Splenius capitis

Trapezius

Infraspinatus

Rhomboideus
minor (part)

External
oblique

Gluteus maximus

Adductor magnus

Gracilis

Plantaris

Soleus

POSTERIOR VIEW

CRANIAL NERVES: ORIGIN AND DISTRIBUTION

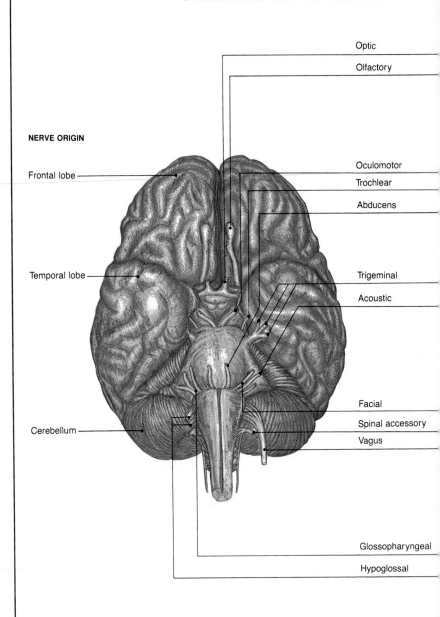

NERVE ORIGIN

Optic

Olfactory

Frontal lobe

Oculomotor

Trochlear

Abducens

Temporal lobe

Trigeminal

Acoustic

Facial

Cerebellum

Spinal accessory

Vagus

Glossopharyngeal

Hypoglossal

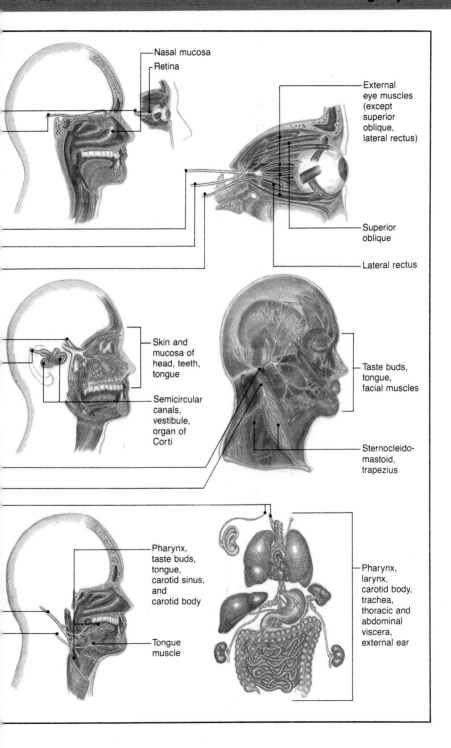

Nasal mucosa

Retina

External
eye muscles
(except
superior
oblique,
lateral rectus)

Superior
oblique

Lateral rectus

Skin and
mucosa of
head, teeth,
tongue

Semicircular
canals,
vestibule,
organ of
Corti

Taste buds,
tongue,
facial muscles

Sternocleido-
mastoid,
trapezius

Pharynx,
taste buds,
tongue,
carotid sinus,
and
carotid body

Tongue
muscle

Pharynx,
larynx,
carotid body,
trachea,
thoracic and
abdominal
viscera,
external ear

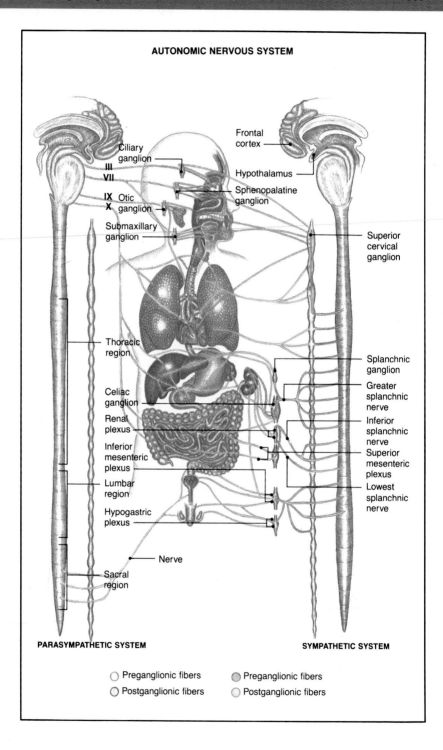

AUTONOMIC NERVOUS SYSTEM

Ciliary ganglion
III
VII
IX Otic
X ganglion
Submaxillary ganglion
Thoracic region
Celiac ganglion
Renal plexus
Inferior mesenteric plexus
Lumbar region
Hypogastric plexus
Nerve
Sacral region

Frontal cortex
Hypothalamus
Sphenopalatine ganglion
Superior cervical ganglion
Splanchnic ganglion
Greater splanchnic nerve
Inferior splanchnic nerve
Superior mesenteric plexus
Lowest splanchnic nerve

PARASYMPATHETIC SYSTEM

SYMPATHETIC SYSTEM

○ Preganglionic fibers
○ Postganglionic fibers

● Preganglionic fibers
○ Postganglionic fibers

EYE

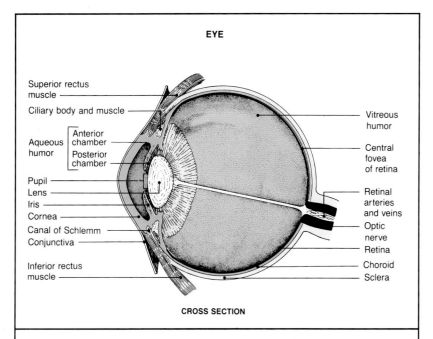

Superior rectus muscle

Ciliary body and muscle

Aqueous humor — Anterior chamber / Posterior chamber

Pupil
Lens
Iris
Cornea
Canal of Schlemm
Conjunctiva

Inferior rectus muscle

Vitreous humor

Central fovea of retina

Retinal arteries and veins

Optic nerve

Retina

Choroid

Sclera

CROSS SECTION

EAR

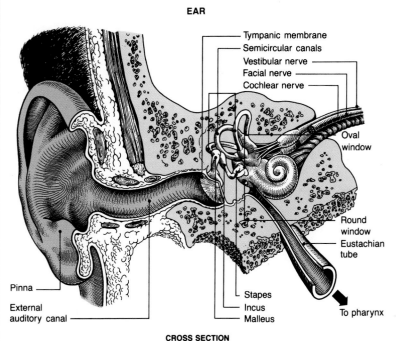

Tympanic membrane
Semicircular canals
Vestibular nerve
Facial nerve
Cochlear nerve

Oval window

Round window
Eustachian tube

To pharynx

Stapes
Incus
Malleus

Pinna

External auditory canal

CROSS SECTION

MAJOR BLOOD VESSELS

ARTERIES

VEINS

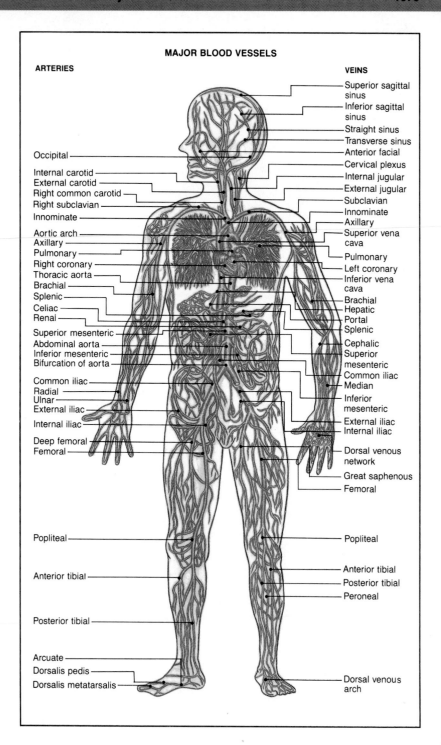

Arteries (left labels):
Occipital
Internal carotid
External carotid
Right common carotid
Right subclavian
Innominate
Aortic arch
Axillary
Pulmonary
Right coronary
Thoracic aorta
Brachial
Splenic
Celiac
Renal
Superior mesenteric
Abdominal aorta
Inferior mesenteric
Bifurcation of aorta
Common iliac
Radial
Ulnar
External iliac
Internal iliac
Deep femoral
Femoral
Popliteal
Anterior tibial
Posterior tibial
Arcuate
Dorsalis pedis
Dorsalis metatarsalis

Veins (right labels):
Superior sagittal sinus
Inferior sagittal sinus
Straight sinus
Transverse sinus
Anterior facial
Cervical plexus
Internal jugular
External jugular
Subclavian
Innominate
Axillary
Superior vena cava
Pulmonary
Left coronary
Inferior vena cava
Brachial
Hepatic
Portal
Splenic
Cephalic
Superior mesenteric
Common iliac
Median
Inferior mesenteric
External iliac
Internal iliac
Dorsal venous network
Great saphenous
Femoral
Popliteal
Anterior tibial
Posterior tibial
Peroneal
Dorsal venous arch

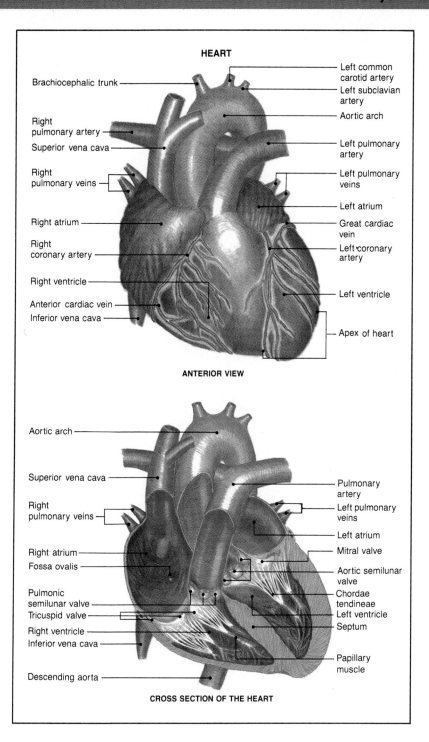

HEART

Brachiocephalic trunk

Right
pulmonary artery

Superior vena cava

Right
pulmonary veins

Right atrium

Right
coronary artery

Right ventricle

Anterior cardiac vein

Inferior vena cava

Left common
carotid artery

Left subclavian
artery

Aortic arch

Left pulmonary
artery

Left pulmonary
veins

Left atrium

Great cardiac
vein

Left coronary
artery

Left ventricle

Apex of heart

ANTERIOR VIEW

Aortic arch

Superior vena cava

Right
pulmonary veins

Right atrium

Fossa ovalis

Pulmonic
semilunar valve

Tricuspid valve

Right ventricle

Inferior vena cava

Descending aorta

Pulmonary
artery

Left pulmonary
veins

Left atrium

Mitral valve

Aortic semilunar
valve

Chordae
tendineae

Left ventricle

Septum

Papillary
muscle

CROSS SECTION OF THE HEART

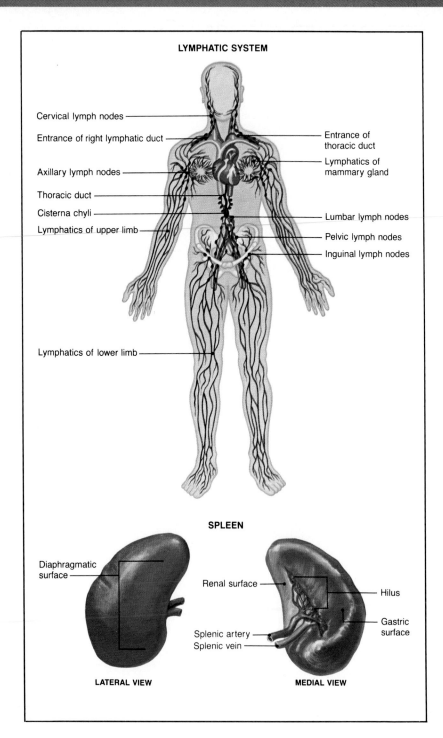

LYMPHATIC SYSTEM

Cervical lymph nodes

Entrance of right lymphatic duct

Entrance of thoracic duct

Lymphatics of mammary gland

Axillary lymph nodes

Thoracic duct

Cisterna chyli

Lymphatics of upper limb

Lumbar lymph nodes

Pelvic lymph nodes

Inguinal lymph nodes

Lymphatics of lower limb

SPLEEN

Diaphragmatic surface

Renal surface

Hilus

Splenic artery

Splenic vein

Gastric surface

LATERAL VIEW

MEDIAL VIEW

NORMAL LUNGS

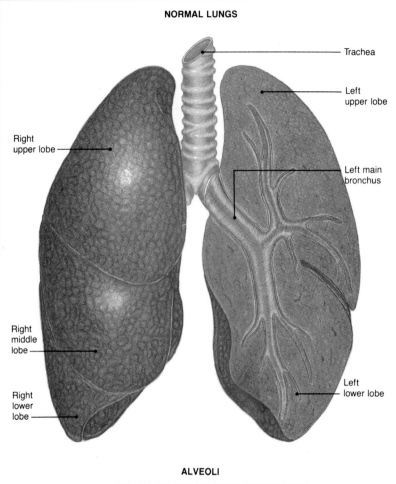

Trachea

Left
upper lobe

Right
upper lobe

Left main
bronchus

Right
middle
lobe

Right
lower
lobe

Left
lower lobe

ALVEOLI

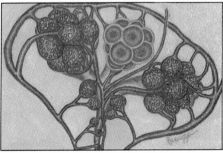

MICROSCOPIC CROSS SECTION

LIVER AND GALLBLADDER

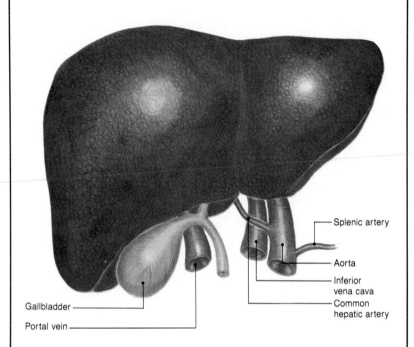

Splenic artery

Aorta

Inferior
vena cava

Common
hepatic artery

Gallbladder

Portal vein

LIVER LOBULE

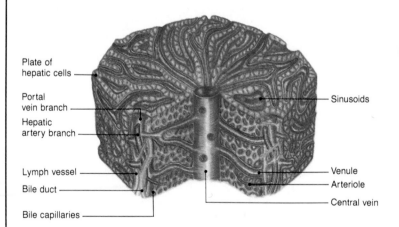

Plate of
hepatic cells

Portal
vein branch

Hepatic
artery branch

Lymph vessel

Bile duct

Bile capillaries

Sinusoids

Venule

Arteriole

Central vein

MICROSCOPIC VIEW

KIDNEY

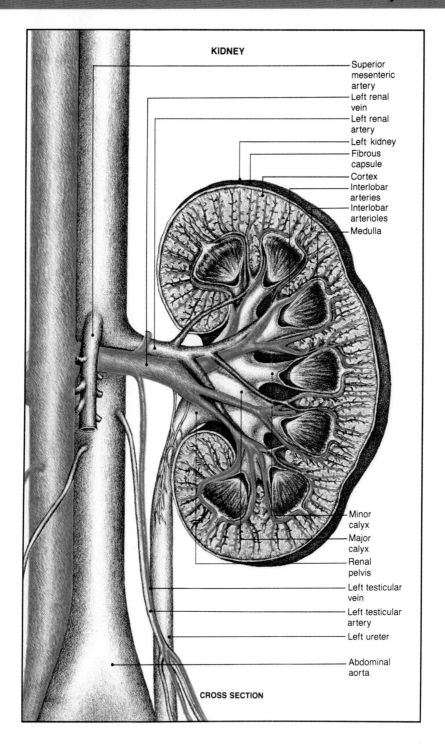

Superior
mesenteric
artery

Left renal
vein

Left renal
artery

Left kidney

Fibrous
capsule

Cortex

Interlobar
arteries

Interlobar
arterioles

Medulla

Minor
calyx

Major
calyx

Renal
pelvis

Left testicular
vein

Left testicular
artery

Left ureter

Abdominal
aorta

CROSS SECTION

FEMALE ORGANS

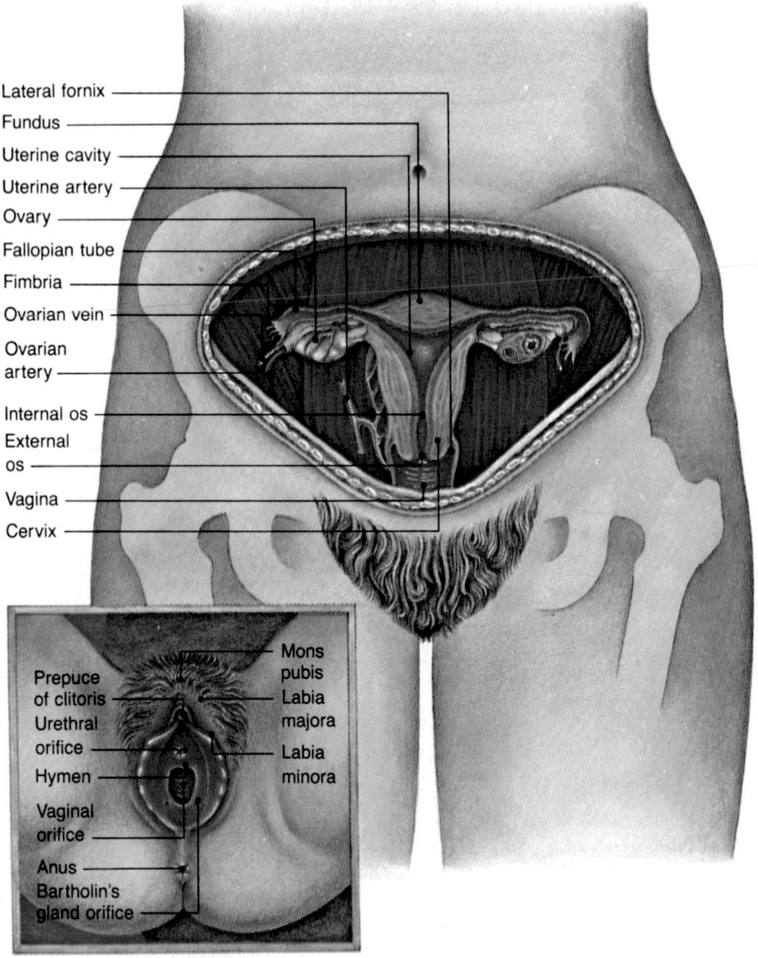

Lateral fornix
Fundus
Uterine cavity
Uterine artery
Ovary
Fallopian tube
Fimbria
Ovarian vein
Ovarian artery
Internal os
External os
Vagina
Cervix

Prepuce of clitoris
Urethral orifice
Hymen
Vaginal orifice
Anus
Bartholin's gland orifice

Mons pubis
Labia majora
Labia minora

FEMALE EXTERNAL GENITALIA

MALE ORGANS

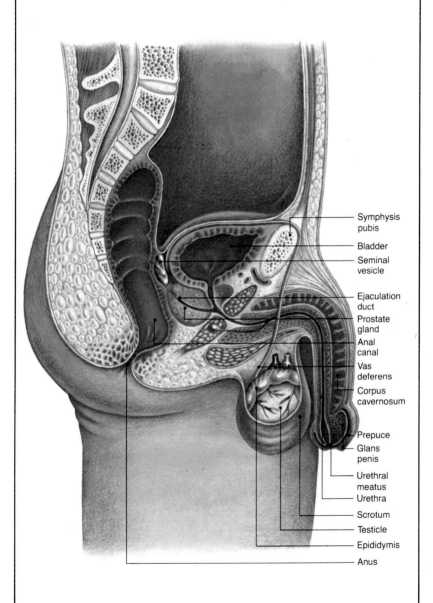

- Symphysis pubis
- Bladder
- Seminal vesicle
- Ejaculation duct
- Prostate gland
- Anal canal
- Vas deferens
- Corpus cavernosum
- Prepuce
- Glans penis
- Urethral meatus
- Urethra
- Scrotum
- Testicle
- Epididymis
- Anus

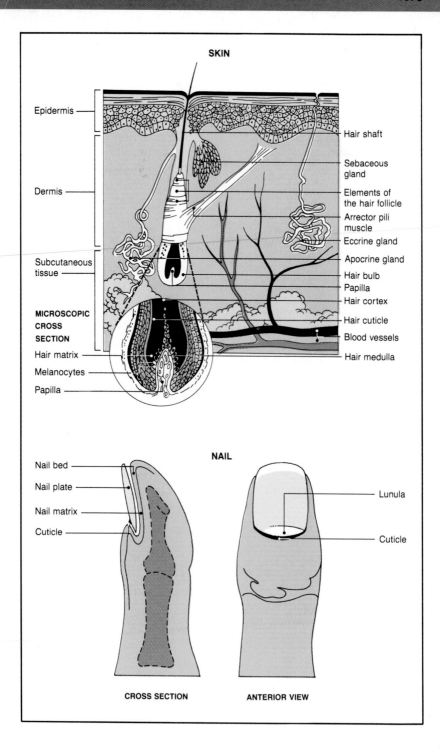

SKIN

Epidermis

Dermis

Subcutaneous tissue

MICROSCOPIC CROSS SECTION

Hair matrix

Melanocytes

Papilla

Hair shaft

Sebaceous gland

Elements of the hair follicle

Arrector pili muscle

Eccrine gland

Apocrine gland

Hair bulb

Papilla

Hair cortex

Hair cuticle

Blood vessels

Hair medulla

NAIL

Nail bed

Nail plate

Nail matrix

Cuticle

Lunula

Cuticle

CROSS SECTION

ANTERIOR VIEW

DRUG INTERACTIONS

A drug interaction takes place when one drug, administered in combination with or within the duration of another drug's effect, changes the effect of one or both drugs. Commonly, the interaction exaggerates or blocks the effect of one or both drugs. Rarely, it produces an effect that cannot be attributed to either drug alone.

Drug interactions may result from alterations of the pharmacokinetics of absorption, distribution, metabolism, or excretion of one drug by another or from a combination of the interacting drugs' actions or effects. One drug may inhibit or stimulate the metabolism or excretion of the other; or it may displace another from plasma-protein–binding sites, freeing it for further action.

Beneficial drug interactions are the basis for combination therapy. One drug, for example, may be given to potentiate, or increase, another drug's effects. Thus, probenecid, which blocks the excretion of penicillin, is sometimes given with penicillin to prolong adequate blood levels of penicillin. Often, two drugs with similar actions are given together for an additive effect. For instance, aspirin and codeine, both analgesics, are given in combination because together they provide greater pain relief than that provided by either drug alone. Drug interactions are also sometimes used to prevent or minimize certain side effects. Hydrochlorothiazide and spironolactone, both diuretics, are administered in combination because the former is potassium-depleting and the latter, potassium-sparing.

Harmful drug interactions may decrease a drug's efficacy or increase its toxicity. For example, in a hypertensive patient well controlled with guanethidine, use of the antidepressant amitriptyline (Elavil) may cause blood pressure to rise to its former high level. Drug combinations that produce such harmful antagonism should be avoided, if possible.

Several other factors commonly contribute to adverse drug interactions, including treatment with multiple drugs, concomitant ingestion of alcohol, self-medication with over-the-counter drugs or another person's prescription, and treatment by more than one doctor for different ailments. Many adverse drug interactions can be prevented by appropriate modifications in dose, time, or route of administration. Patients receiving drugs that may interact must be monitored closely and taught to look for signs and symptoms that may indicate an adverse interaction. The tables that follow summarize the most significant interactions among several major drug groups.

DIGITALIS PREPARATIONS

Digitalis preparations increase the force of myocardial contraction and the refractory period of the atrioventricular (AV) node. These drugs are commonly used to treat congestive heart failure and atrial fibrillation, flutter, and tachycardia. Lowered potassium levels sensitize the myocardium to digitalis, which may make an ordinary dosage potentially toxic. Because many arrhythmias for which digitalis is prescribed cause symptoms that closely resemble those caused by toxic digitalis levels, such toxicity may be difficult to identify and requires careful monitoring of serum digitalis levels.

DIGITALIS PREPARATIONS	INTERACT WITH THESE DRUGS	TO PRODUCE THESE EFFECTS
digitoxin digoxin gitalin	**Diuretics** acetazolamide bendroflumethiazide benzthiazide chlorothiazide chlorthalidone dichlorphenamide ethacrynic acid furosemide hydrochlorothiazide methazolamide methyclothiazide metolazone polythiazide quinethazone trichlormethiazide	• Hypokalemia, predisposing to digitalis toxicity. Monitor serum potassium levels and notify doctor if patient develops leg cramps or any symptoms of digitalis toxicity (nausea and vomiting; loss of appetite; weakness; diarrhea; blurred vision; or appearance of yellow or green halos around objects). • Concomitant use of steroids or ingestion of licorice may also cause potassium loss. • *Note:* Hyperkalemia may also induce arrhythmias. If patient requires potassium supplements (KCl, Kato, K-Lyte, etc.), *monitor potassium levels and EKG frequently.*
	Antihypertensives metoprolol nadolol propranolol	• Excessive bradycardia and increased depressant effect on myocardium. Use together cautiously.
	reserpine reserpine combinations	• Monitor pulse rate regularly. Report any changes in pulse rate or persistent dizziness to doctor.
	Antacids and antacid combinations Aludrox aluminum hydroxide Amphojel Ascriptin Camalox Gelusil Maalox magnesium hydroxide magnesium trisilicate Milk of Magnesia Mylanta	• Decreased absorption and effectiveness of digitalis.
	Over-the-counter asthma preparations Asthmanefrin Bronkaid Mist epinephrine Primatene Mist Vaponefrin Va-Tro-Nol	• May cause or complicate arrhythmias if administered concomitantly with digitalis.

DIURETIC INTERACTIONS

Diuretics increase excretion of water and salt and are commonly used to treat hypertension, edema, cardiac conditions, and renal dysfunction. The carbonic anhydrase inhibitors also decrease ocular secretions of aqueous humor, lowering intraocular pressure, and are sometimes used as an adjunct in glaucoma. Because the thiazide diuretics tend to deplete potassium, close monitoring of potassium levels is necessary, especially in cardiac conditions requiring concomitant digitalis therapy. Lowered potassium levels may cause muscle weakness, leg cramping, and joint or foot pain and may require treatment with supplemental potassium. The potassium-sparing diuretics—spironolactone, amiloride hydrochloride, and triamterene—conserve potassium during diuresis; with these diuretics, potassium supplements may be unnecessary or hazardous.

THESE DIURETICS	INTERACT WITH THESE DRUGS	TO PRODUCE THESE EFFECTS
acetazolamide bendroflumethiazide benzthiazide chlorothiazide chlorthalidone cyclothiazide dichlorphenamide ethacrynic acid furosemide hydrochlorothiazide hydroflumethiazide methazolamide methyclothiazide metolazone polythiazide quinethazone trichlormethiazide	**Digitalis preparations** digitoxin digoxin gitalin	• Potassium loss may lead to hypokalemia, predisposing to digitalis toxicity. Monitor closely for signs of digitalis toxicity. Notify doctor if patient develops any weakness, leg cramps, shortness of breath, abdominal pain, or blurred or yellow vision.
	Cough/cold preparations *(containing antihistamines, decongestants, and possibly alcohol)* Alconefrin Allerest A.R.M. Bayer Decongestant Contac Coricidin Coricidin 'D' Coryban-D Cosanyl-DM Demazin Repetabs and Syrup Dimacol Dristan Tablets, Capsules, and Liquid Epinephrine Fedrazil 4-Way Cold Tablets and Nasal Spray Neo-Synephrine Novahistine Nyquil Ornacol Ornex Orthoxicol phenylephrine Phenylpropranolamine Primatene Privine Romilar CF Sine-Off Tablets Sinutab Cold Tablets and Sinutab II Sudafed SuperAnahist Triaminic Triaminicol Trind Ursinus Vatronol Vicks Inhaler	• Decongestants may negate the diuretic's antihypertensive effect or themselves increase blood pressure. Alcoholic beverages or preparations containing alcohol may increase the potential for severe hypotension and drowsiness.

ORAL ANTICOAGULANT INTERACTIONS

Oral anticoagulants impede clotting by preventing fibrin formation. They are given to the patient at risk of developing clots (thrombosis) and are also used to prevent clot enlargement or fragmentation (thromboembolism). These drugs have no effect on established thrombosis and do not reverse tissue damage; the aim of treatment is to prevent further complications. Since anticoagulants are highly but weakly bound to plasma protein (albumin), they may be easily displaced by other drugs and therefore interact significantly with a great many drugs. Such interactions may be unpredictable and require that the patient be closely monitored. The *in vivo* effect of depressing clotting factors VII, IX, X, II (prothrombin) depends on the dosage. Adverse reactions may include prolonged diarrhea, headaches, fever, loss of appetite, and prolonged or excessive bleeding (from nose, gums, cuts, melena, hematemesis, or unusual menstrual flow).

THESE ORAL ANTICOAGULANTS	INTERACT WITH THESE SUBSTANCES	TO PRODUCE THESE EFFECTS
anisindione bishydroxy- coumarin phenindione phenprocoumon warfarin	allopurinol anabolic steroids clofibrate dextrothyroxine disulfiram glucagon inhalation anesthetics para-aminosalicylic acid sulfonamides thyroid preparations	• Increased prothrombin time. Monitor patient carefully. Consider reduction of anticoagulant dose.
	ethacrynic acid indomethacin mefenamic acid oxyphenbutazone phenylbutazone salicylates	• Increased prothrombin time; ulcerogenic effects. Do not use together.
	Sedatives and hypnotics amobarbital butabarbital ethchlorvynol glutethimide pentobarbital phenobarbital secobarbital Tuinal **Other** carbamazepine rifampin vitamin K	• Decreased anticoagulant activity
	Aspirin and salicylates Alka-Seltzer Alka-2 A.P.C. Ascriptin aspirin Bufferin Coricidin Dristan Tablets Ecotrin Empirin 4-Way Cold Tablets Measurin Midol sodium salicylate SuperAnahist Triaminicin Tablets Vanquish	• Increased anticoagulant activity and risk of excessive bleeding
	Foods Leafy green vegetables, such as cabbage, spinach, kale, cauliflower, alfalfa	• High vitamin K content could reduce anticoagulant effectiveness.

CORTICOSTEROID INTERACTIONS

Corticosteroids are organic or synthetic compounds used in various endocrine, allergic, respiratory, neoplastic, and other disorders to treat adrenal insufficiency, to suppress inflammation, to produce immunosuppression, and to treat shock and anaphylactic reactions. Most are known as glucocorticoids; they produce organic effects regulating carbohydrate, fat, and protein metabolism and have anti-inflammatory activity. The mineralocorticoids desoxycorticosterone and fludrocortisone produce inorganic effects regulating electrolyte and water metabolism. Corticosteroids may mask or exacerbate infection and may cause decreased antibody response after immunization. During glucocorticoid therapy, the patient should carry a card indicating the need for supplemental glucocorticoids during stress.

THESE CORTICOSTEROIDS	INTERACT WITH THESE DRUGS	TO PRODUCE THESE EFFECTS
beclomethasone betamethasone cortisone desoxycortico-sterone dexamethasone fludrocortisone fluprednisolone hydrocortisone methylpredni-solone prednisolone prednisone triamcinolone	**Diuretics** acetazolamide bendroflumethiazide benzthiazide chlorothiazide chlorthalidone diclorphenamide ethacrynic acid furosemide hydrochlorothiazide methazolamide methyclothiazide metolazone polythiazide quinethazone trichlormethiazide	• Increased potassium loss. Possible hypokalemia. Monitor fluid and electrolyte balance carefully.
	Digitalis preparations digitoxin digoxin gitalin	• Hypokalemia predisposing to increased digitalis toxicity. Notify doctor if patient develops shortness of breath, fatigue, prolonged nausea, abdominal pain, cramps, or blurred vision. Monitor serum levels and electrocardiogram.
	Sedatives and hypnotics amobarbital chloral hydrate flurazepam glutethimide pentobarbital secobarbital	• Reduced steroid effectiveness
	Analgesics and cough/cold preparations *(containing antihistamines, salicylates, decongestants, and possibly alcohol)* Alka-Seltzer Allerest A.P.C. Ascriptin aspirin Contac Coricidin Coryban-D Capsules Demazin Ecotrin Empirin Compound Novahistine Nyquil Robitussin A-C Sudafed Plus Triaminicin Vicks Formula 44	• Salicylate- or alcohol-containing preparations and alcoholic beverages can complicate and increase the potential for nausea, ulceration, or decreased steroid effectiveness.

ANTIDEPRESSANT INTERACTIONS

Antidepressants are used to treat psychotic and neurotic endogenous depression and to prevent recurrent depression. Imipramine is used to treat enuresis in children and adolescents. Cyclobenzaprine is primarily a muscle relaxant that interacts like a tricyclic antidepressant.

Tricyclic and tetracyclic antidepressants produce sedative effects within a few hours after oral administration. Anticholinergic side effects (transient drowsiness or dry mouth) occur soon after therapy begins. Antidepressant effects occur 7 to 14 days after onset of therapy due to slow effect on the brain's neurotransmitter mechanism. Onset of antidepressant effect with MAO inhibitors may not occur for several weeks or months and may last up to 2 weeks after therapy ends. Abrupt discontinuation of an antidepressant drug after long-term therapy may cause nausea, headache, and malaise. Sore throat during treatment with cyclic antidepressants may indicate impending agranulocytosis.

THESE ANTI-DEPRESSANTS	INTERACT WITH THESE DRUGS	TO PRODUCE THESE EFFECTS
amitriptyline cyclobenzaprine desipramine doxepin imipramine maprotiline nortriptyline trimipramine antidepressant combinations (Etrafon, Limbitrol, Triavil)	**Antihypertensives** clonidine guanethidine	• Blocked (or reduced) antihypertensive effect; a doctor may adjust required dosage. Use together cautiously.
	MAO inhibitors furazolidone isocarboxazid pargyline phenelzine procarbazine tranylcypromine	• *Severe excitation, increase in blood pressure, fever, convulsions, coma, and possible circulatory collapse* (usually with high dose). Avoid using together. • Increased hypertensive effect. Severe hypertension (hypertensive crisis) possible. Avoid using together.
	Sympathomimetics amphetamine benzphetamine chlorphentermine dextroamphetamine diethylpropion ephedrine epinephrine methamphetamine phendimetrazine phenmetrazine phentermine phenylephrine	• Increased or decreased effect of drugs; possible side effects include increased blood pressure and severe headache. Combinations should be used with caution.
	Cough/cold combinations *(containing antihistamines, decongestants, and possibly alcohol)* Allerest A.R.M. Bayer Decongestant Cheracol Conar Contac Coricidin Coryban-D Cosanyl-DM Demazin Dristan Neo-Synephrine Novahistine Nyquil Pertussin Robitussin A-C and DM Sinutab SuperAnahist Synephricol Triaminicin Triaminicol Vicks Formula 44 Vicks Sinex	• Increased risk of drowsiness or decreased mental alertness. Decongestants may cause increased hypertensive effect.

MAO INHIBITOR INTERACTIONS

Monoamine-oxidase (MAO) inhibitors are used primarily as antidepressants; some are also used to treat anxiety, some infections, or in chemotherapy. These potent drugs have wide-ranging physiologic effects, including a high potential for hazardous interaction with other drugs. Their common side effects include transient drowsiness, dizziness, weakness, or blurred vision. If these symptoms persist or severe headache, rash, dark urine, jaundice, sore throat, or diarrhea occurs, the dosage may need to be adjusted or the drug discontinued. *Because the effects of MAO inhibitors may persist for up to 2 weeks after discontinuing use, no interacting drug should be started within this interval.*

THESE MAO INHIBITORS	INTERACT WITH THESE SUBSTANCES	TO PRODUCE THESE EFFECTS
furazolidone isocarboxazid pargyline phenelzine procarbazine tranylcypromine	**Antihypertensives** guanethidine reserpine-containing drugs	• Severe hypertension (hypertensive crisis) possible. Avoid using together. • *Sudden and severe high blood pressure, hyperpyrexia, fever, excitement and convulsions, and death may result.*
	Sympathomimetics ephedrine epinephrine phenylephrine phenylpropanolamine pseudoephedrine	
	Tricyclic and tetracyclic antidepressants amitriptyline desipramine doxepin imipramine maprotiline nortriptyline protriptyline trimipramine	
	Other levodopa meperidine methylphenidate	• Increased central nervous system excitation or depression can be severe or fatal. Do not use together. • Severe hypertension; possible hypertensive crisis. Do not use together.
	Foods and beverages containing tyramine Most cheeses Caviar Herring Sausage meats Yeast extracts Chocolate Chianti wine and imported beers	• *Severe hypertension, hyperpyrexia, excitement, and convulsions*
	Cough/cold preparations (*containing antihistamines, decongestants, salicylates, and possibly alcohol*) Allerest A.R.M. Bayer Decongestant Bronkaid Cheracol Contac Coricidin 'D' Cosanyl-DM Dristan 4-Way cold products Neo-Synephrine Nyquil Ornacol Ornex Primatene Privine Sudafed Triaminic	

ANTIDIABETIC INTERACTIONS

Antidiabetic drugs supply exogenous insulin or stimulate production of endogenous insulin in patients with diabetes mellitus. Insulin (exogenous or endogenous) lowers blood glucose levels.

Synthetic antidiabetic drugs (sulfonylureas including acetohexamide, chlorpropamide, tolazamide, and tolbutamide) stimulate insulin secretion in diabetic patients who have some beta cell function. Transient side effects may include loss of appetite, nausea, and stomach upset. Prolonged discomfort, sore throat, low fever, diarrhea, or dark urine may require adjustment of dosage or discontinuation of the drug.

THESE ANTI-DIABETICS	INTERACT WITH THESE DRUGS	TO PRODUCE THESE EFFECTS
acetohexamide chlorpropamide insulin tolazamide tolbutamide	**Diuretics** acetazolamide bendroflumethiazide benzthiazide chlorothiazide chlorthalidone dichlorphenamide ethacrynic acid furosemide hydrochlorothiazide methazolamide methyclothiazide metolazone polythiazide quinethazone trichlormethiazide **Steroids**	• Decreased hypoglycemic response. Monitor blood glucose. Notify the doctor if loss of appetite, nausea, vomiting, or excessive thirst and urination occurs.
	Antihypertensives clonidine guanethidine metroprolol nadolol propranolol **MAO inhibitors** furazolidone isocarboxazid pargyline phenelzine tranylcypromine **Anti-inflammatories** oxyphenbutazone pheynlbutazone **Other** clofibrate	• Increased antidiabetic activity (increased hypoglycemic effect) because these drugs may themselves *decrease* blood sugar. Use together cautiously. Monitor blood sugar. Notify the doctor if patient develops excessive hunger, numbness, fatigue, headache, drowsiness, or sweating. Give the patient candy or lump sugar to offset the hypoglycemic reaction. Beta blockers such as metoprolol, nadolol, and propranolol may mask symptoms of hypoglycemia.
	Cough/cold preparations Cheracol and Cheracol D Comtrex Liquid Coryban-D Cosanyl-DM CoTylenol Liquid Demazin Syrup Dristan Cough Formula Neo-Synephrine Elixir Novahistine DH and Novahistine Expectorant Nyquil Pertussin Robitussin, Robitussin A-C, and Robitussin-DM Triaminic Expectorant Valadol Liquid Vicks Formula 44 Cough Mixture	• Altered dosage requirements or increased potential for nausea or stomach upset. • Avoid use with alcoholic beverages or preparations containing alcohol. • Aspirin or other salicylate-containing products may increase hypoglycemic effect. Monitor blood glucose carefully.

ANTIHISTAMINE INTERACTIONS

Antihistamines are thought to block the physiologic action of histamine, the humoral compound that causes symptoms associated with allergic reactions. Antihistamine combinations usually contain a decongestant, such as pseudoephedrine or phenylpropanolamine. Various types of antihistamines are used to treat nasal congestion and drainage, watery eyes, and pruritus resulting from allergic conditions and contact dermatoses. Antihistamines can have a depressant effect on the central nervous system and should be used cautiously with other centrally active drugs and with alcohol.

THESE ANTIHISTAMINES	INTERACT WITH THESE DRUGS	TO PRODUCE THESE EFFECTS
azatadine brompheniramine chlorpheniramine clemastine cyproheptadine dexchlorphenira- mine Dimetapp diphenhydramine Disophrol Drixoral Naldecon Nolamine Novafed A Ornade promethazine tripelennamine triprolidine	**Antianxiety agents** chlordiazepoxide clorazepate diazepam hydroxyzine lorazepam meprobamate oxazepam perphenazine prazepam **Sedatives and sedative combinations** amobarbital chloral hydrate ethchlorvynol Fiorinal flurazepam glutethimide pentobarbital phenobarbital secobarbital Sominex **Antipsychotics** chlorpromazine fluphenazine prochlorperazine promazine thioridazine thiothixene trifluoperazine **Other drugs** clonazepam codeine cyclobenzaprine propoxyphene **Cough/cold preparations** *(containing antihistamines, decongestants, and possibly alcohol)* Allerest A.R.M. Bayer Decongestant Cheracol and Cheracol D Contac Coricidin Coryban-D Cosanyl-DM Dristan Neo-Synephrine Novahistine Nyquil Pertussin Robitussin Sinutab Triaminicin Vicks Formula 44	• Potential central nervous system depression, resulting in drowsiness, dizziness, blurred vision, loss of appetite, and decreased mental alertness. • Warn patient to avoid activities that require mental alertness and good psychomotor coordination (such as driving or operating machinery) until patient's response to combination therapy is established.

GASTROINTESTINAL ANTICHOLINERGIC INTERACTIONS

Anticholinergics inhibit gastrointestinal (GI) smooth-muscle contraction and delay gastric emptying. They are therapeutic adjuncts for pain associated with peptic ulcers. They are also used to treat irritable colon, other functional GI disorders, and neurogenic level disturbances, including splenic flexure syndrome and neurogenic colon. Because these drugs may have central nervous system (CNS) side effects, including drowsiness, dizziness, headache, insomnia, and confusion or excitement (in elderly patients), they should generally be used very cautiously with CNS depressants. The most common side effect of these drugs is dry mouth. If it is severe or if the patient develops skin rash, flushing, or eye pain, the dose may need to be adjusted or discontinued. Because some anticholinergics decrease perspiration, drug-induced fever or heatstroke is possible.

THESE ANTI-CHOLINERGICS	INTERACT WITH THESE DRUGS	TO PRODUCE THESE EFFECTS
atropine belladonna alkaloids dicyclomine l-hyoscyamine sulfate Librax propantheline	**Tricyclic antidepressants** amitriptyline desipramine imipramine nortriptyline	• Constipation, dry mouth, blurred vision, and possible tachycardia. If these drugs must be used together, dose reductions of one or both drugs may be necessary.
	Antipsychotics chlorpromazine haloperidol prochlorperazine **Antiarrhythmics** disopyramide quinidine **Other** cyclobenzaprine meperidine oxybutynin	• Increased anticholinergic activity. Aggravated parkinsonism-like symptoms. Use together with caution. • Increased dry mouth, blurred vision, or drowsiness. These combinations should be avoided if possible.
	Sedatives/hypnotics Compoz Nytol Sleep-Eze Sominex **Cough/cold preparations** (containing antihistamines, decongestants, and possibly alcohol) Allerest A.R.M. Bayer Decongestant chlorpheniramine Chlor-Trimeton Conar Contac Coricidin Coryban-D Demazin Dristan Novahistine Nyquil Nytol Robitussin A-C Sinutab SuperAnahist Triaminic Triaminicin Triaminicol Vicks Formula 44 Cough Mixture Vicks Sinex	• Increased anticholinergic and sedative effect, possibly causing increased drowsiness, dry mouth, or blurred vision.
	Other levodopa	• Possible decreased levodopa effect

ORAL CONTRACEPTIVE INTERACTIONS

Oral contraceptives, usually combinations of estrogen and progestogen, suppress ovulation by increasing the levels of estrogen and progestin, which, through a negative feedback mechanism directed at the hypothalamus, inhibit the follicle-stimulating hormone (FSH) and luteinizing hormone (LH). They are used to prevent pregnancy. High-dose combinations are usually used to treat menstrual cycle disorders, such as endometriosis and hypermenorrhea. This combination of drugs is also used to treat hormone-induced acne but is often ineffective. These drugs should not be used in present or suspected breast cancer or other cancer, hypertension or history of cerebrovascular accident, pregnancy, lactation, or abnormal vaginal bleeding. Cigarette smoking increases the risk of serious cardiovascular side effects and should be avoided during estrogen therapy. These risks also increase with age. Consult individual drug package inserts for additional warnings and precautions.

ESTROGEN WITH ESTROGEN COMBINATIONS	INTERACT WITH THESE SUBSTANCES	TO PRODUCE THESE EFFECTS
Brevicon Demulen Enovid Loestrin Modicon Norinyl Norlestrin Ortho-Novum Ovcon Ovral Ovulen	**Antibiotics** ampicillin rifampin tetracycline **Anticonvulsants** phenytoin	• Increased possibility of breakthrough bleeding or spotting and decreased contraceptive effectiveness. A supplemental form of contraception may be advisable.
	Anticoagulants anisindione bishydroxycoumarin phenindione phenprocoumon warfarin	• Decreased anticoagulant activity. Suggest another form of birth control.
	Vitamins cyanocobalamin (B$_{12}$) folic acid pyridoxine (vitamin B$_6$) vitamin E	• Possible vitamin depletion. Supplemental vitamin therapy advisable.

ANTINEOPLASTIC INTERACTIONS

Antineoplastic drugs destroy cancer cells by interfering with neoplastic cell growth and division. They block the supply or utilization of essential cellular building blocks or interrupt the process of cell division known as the cell cycle. Because of the toxic effects of these drugs on both normal and cancerous cells, chemotherapy is most effective during early stages of tumor growth, when fewer cancer cells are present. Because chemotherapy affects rapidly dividing cells, it is often toxic to actively dividing normal cells and commonly impairs bone marrow, skin, gastrointestinal mucosa, hair follicles, and fetal tissue. However, close monitoring and good patient care (including good hydration and nutrition) can prevent or minimize such effects in many patients. The potential benefits of using chemotherapy in pregnant or lactating women should be weighed against the risks of probable teratogenicity, mutagenicity, and carcinogenicity in fetuses or infants.

THESE ANTINEO-PLASTIC DRUGS	INTERACT WITH THESE SUBSTANCES	TO PRODUCE THESE EFFECTS
azathioprine	allopurinol	• Impaired inactivation of azathioprine. Decrease azathioprine dose to ¼ or ⅓ normal dose.
cyclophosphamide	chloramphenicol corticosteroids	• Reduced activity of cyclophosphamide. Use together cautiously.
	allopurinol	• Possible excessive cyclophosphamide effect. Monitor for enhanced toxicity.
daunorubicin	heparin	• May form a precipitate. Don't mix together.
fluorouracil	acidic foods or beverages (for example, citrus fruit)	• Decreased effectiveness of oral fluorouracil if taken concomitantly with acidic foods or beverages.
mercaptopurine	allopurinol	• Slowed inactivation of mercaptopurine. Decrease mercaptopurine dose to ¼ or ½ normal dose.
methotrexate	alcohol	• Increased hepatotoxicity. Warn patient not to drink alcoholic beverages.
	phenylbutazone probenecid salicylates sulfonamides	• Increased methotrexate toxicity. Avoid using together if possible.
procarbazine	alcohol	• Disulfiram (Antabuse)-like reaction. Warn patient not to drink alcohol while taking this drug.

OVER-THE-COUNTER DRUG INTERACTIONS

This chart deals strictly with drug products that are available without a prescription and points out the potentially hazardous reactions that are possible with careless use. When advising a patient about selecting nonprescription drugs, be sure to evaluate the drugs for possible interactions with others the patient may be taking. *Always read the label.*

THESE ALCOHOL-CONTAINING COMBINATIONS	INTERACT WITH THESE SALICYLATE- AND ANTIHISTAMINE-CONTAINING COMBINATIONS	TO PRODUCE THESE EFFECTS
alcoholic beverages Cheracol, Cheracol D Cosanyl-DM Demazin Syrup Dristan Cough Formula Novahistine-DH and Novahistine Expectorant Nyquil Pertussin Robitussin, Robitussin A-C, Robitussin-DM Triaminic Expectorant Valadol Liquid Vicks Formula 44 Cough Mixture	A.P.C. and A.P.C. Compound A.S.A. and A.S.A. Compound Alka-Seltzer Alka-2 Allerest Anacin Ascriptin Aspergum aspirin Bufferin Cama chlorpheniramine Chlor-Trimeton Compoz Conar Contac Coricidin Coryban-D Demazin Ecotrin Empirin Compound Excedrin 4-Way Cold Tablets Measurin Midol Novahistine Nyquil Nytol P-A-C pyrilamine Robitussin A-C Sinutab Sleep-Eze sodium salicylate Sominex Sudafed Plus Triaminic Triaminicin Triaminicol Vanquish Vicks Formula 44 Cough Mixture	• Increased damage to the stomach lining, possibly causing bleeding. Alcohol-containing combinations taken with antihistamine-containing combinations may cause or increase drowsiness.

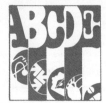

Acknowledgments

p. 68 Adapted with permission from P.B. Lockhart and S.T. Sonis, "Relationship of Oral Complications to Peripheral Blood Leukocyte and Platelet Counts in Patients Receiving Cancer Chemotherapy," *Oral Surgery, Oral Medicine and Oral Pathology* 48:21-28, 1979.

p. 97 Adapted with permission from David T. Purtilo, *Survey of Human Diseases* (Menlo Park, Calif.: Addison-Wesley Publishing Co., 1978), p. 185.

p. 118 Adapted with permission from A. McGehee Harvey et al., eds., *Principles and Practice of Medicine* (New York: Appleton-Century-Crofts, 1980), p. 706.

p. 133 Courtesy of Centers for Disease Control, Atlanta.

p. 172 Courtesy of William C. Nyberg, Scheie Eye Institute, Philadelphia.

p. 197 Adapted with permission from William J. Robbins et al., *Growth* (New Haven, Conn.: Yale University Press, 1928).

p. 200 Courtesy of Marc S. Lapayowker, Department of Radiology, Temple University Hospital, Philadelphia.

p. 211 Courtesy of Marjorie Beyers and Susan Dudas, *Clinical Practice of Medical-Surgical Nursing* (Boston: Little, Brown & Co., 1977), p. 670. Ron Hurst, Photographer.

p. 236 Photography by Paul A. Cohen.

p. 294 Courtesy of National Research Council, Washington, D.C., 1980.

p. 324 Courtesy of Ann Bell, University of Tennessee Center for Health Sciences, Memphis.

p. 345 Courtesy of Centers for Disease Control, Atlanta.

p. 356 Courtesy of Joel I. Hamburger, MD, Northland Radioisotope Lab, Southfield, Mich.

p. 442 Courtesy of Ann Bell, University of Tennessee Center for Health Sciences, Memphis.

p. 457 Courtesy of Maurice Barcos, MD, Roswell Park Memorial Institute, Buffalo.

p. 486 Adapted with permission from Noel R. Rose, "Autoimmune Diseases." Copyright © February 1981 by Scientific American Inc. All rights reserved.

p. 487 Adapted with permission from A.J. Ammann and D.W. Wara, "Evaluation of Infants and Children with Recurrent Infection," in L. Gluck et al., eds., *Current Problems in Pediatrics* 5 (11): entire issue, 1975, by Year Book Medical Publishers, Inc., Chicago.

p. 489 Drawn from X-ray provided courtesy

of Marc S. Lapayowker, Department of Radiology, Temple University Hospital, Philadelphia.

p. 518 Courtesy of Marc S. Lapayowker, Department of Radiology, Temple University Hospital, Philadelphia.

p. 530 Adapted from "Jones Criteria (revised) for Guidance in the Diagnosis of Rheumatic Fever," *Circulation* 32:664, 1965, by permission of the American Heart Association, Inc.

p. 557 Photography by Paul A. Cohen.

p. 605 Adapted with permission from Edmund R. Novak and J. Donald Woodruff, *Novak's Gynecological and Obstetric Pathology* (Philadelphia: W.B. Saunders Co., 1979).

p. 639 Courtesy of Marc S. Lapayowker, Department of Radiology, Temple University Hospital, Philadelphia.

p. 693 Photography by Paul A. Cohen.

p. 699 Courtesy of Samuel L. Moschella et al., *Dermatology* (Philadelphia: W.B. Saunders Co., 1975).

p. 710 Photography by Paul A. Cohen.

p. 762 Information from *State Laws and Regulations on Genetic Disorders*, Office for Maternal and Child Health, Health Services Administration, Public Health Service, U.S. Department of Health and Human Services, July 1980.

p. 784-785 Permission to adapt this chart granted by the National Poison Center Network, Children's Hospital of Pittsburgh.

p. 797 Photography by Paul A. Cohen.

p. 893 Adapted with permission from Griffin T. Ross, "Pituitary and Gonadal Hormones in Women during Spontaneous and Induced Ovulatory Cycles," *Recent Progress in Hormone Research* 26:1, 1970.

p. 923 Photography by Paul A. Cohen.

p. 945 Courtesy of Richard K. Scher and C. Ralph Daniel, *Nail Basics: An Approach to Diagnosis* (Evanston, Ill.: American Academy of Dermatology, 1981).

p. 996 Photography by Thomas Staudenmayer.

p. 1002 Courtesy of Centers for Disease Control, Atlanta.

p. 1010 Courtesy of Marc S. Lapayowker, Department of Radiology, Temple University Hospital, Philadelphia.

p. 1012 Photography by Paul A. Cohen.

p. 1016 Courtesy of Marc S. Lapayowker, Department of Radiology, Temple University Hospital, Philadelphia.

p. 1049 Photography by Paul A. Cohen.

Nursing72
Nursing73
Nursing74
Nursing75
Nursing76
Nursing77
Nursing78
Nursing79
Nursing80
Nursing81
Nursing82
Nursing83
Nursing84
Nursing85

Year after year, one journal delivers more useful clinical information in less time than any other!

Over half a million nurses rely on their subscriptions to keep up with the flood of new drugs, treatments, equipment, and procedures that are changing nursing practice.

Each monthly issue is packed with thoroughly practical, accurate information in concise articles and departments that are clearly written and illustrated in step-by-step detail. You can read an article in minutes and come away with knowledge you can put to work with assurance.

Feature articles focus on demanding problems—ranging from hypertensive crises to cardiogenic shock—that require special skills. You'll quickly learn what to do, how to do it best, when (and when not) to do it.

Drug updates give you critical information quickly—indications, dosages, interactions, contraindications... all you need to administer drugs more confidently.

Assessment aids help you become more proficient in objectively assessing your patients, their conditions, and responses to nursing care.

Self-quizzes bring you the chance to test your knowledge of *current* nursing practices.

Patient-teaching aids help you prepare your patients to follow instructions at home.

Enter your own subscription today with the coupon below. It's a solid, career investment that pays big dividends for you and your patients; (it's even tax-deductible).

MEDICAL PREFIXES AND SUFFIXES *(cont.)*

COLOR

alb-	white. *alb*inism	**flav-**	yellow. ribo*flav*in
chlor-	green. *chlor*ine	**leuko-**	white. *leuko*cyte
chro-	color. poly*chro*matic	**melan(o)-**	black. *melan*in
cyan(o)-	blue. *cyano*sis	**rub-**	red. bili*rub*in
erythro-	red. *erythro*cyte	**xantho-**	yellow. *xantho*ma

DIRECTION

ab-	away from. *ab*ductor	**intra-**	inside. *intra*bronchial
ad-	toward. *ad*duction	**juxta-**	near. *juxta*glomerular
ante-	before, forward. *ante*cubital	**medi-**	middle. *medi*otarsal
circum-	around. *circum*duction	**meta-**	beyond. *meta*carpal
contra-	opposite. *contra*lateral	**par(a)-**	beside. *para*nasal
dextro-	right. *dextro*cardia	**peri-**	around. *peri*cardium
di-	apart, away from. *di*ffraction	**post-**	behind. *post*ocular
ecto-	outside. *ecto*blast	**pre-**	in front of. *pre*maxillary
end(o)-	inward. *endo*derm	**re-**	back, contrary. *re*gurgitation
ep(i)-	on, upon. *epi*canthus	**retro-**	backward. *retro*version
eso-	within. *eso*tropia	**sinistro-**	left. *sinistro*cardia
exo-	outside. *exo*phthalmos	**sub-**	under. *sub*cutaneous
extra-	outside of, beyond. *extra*cellular	**super-**	above, upper. *super*duct
hyper-	above, beyond. *hyper*extension	**supra-**	above, upon. *supra*sternal
hypo-	below, under. *hypo*thermia	**trans-**	across, through. *trans*action
infra-	beneath. *infra*clavicular	**ultra-**	beyond. *ultra*sonic